OXFORD MEDICAL PUBLICATIONS

Mortality from Smoking in Developed Countries 1950-2000

Indirect Estimates from National Vital Statistics

RICHARD PETO
ICRF Cancer Studies Unit
Nuffield Department of Clinical Medicine
Radcliffe Infirmary, Oxford OX2 6HE, UK

ALAN D LOPEZ
Tobacco or Health Programme
World Health Organization
1211 Geneva, Switzerland

JILLIAN BOREHAM
ICRF Cancer Studies Unit
Nuffield Department of Clinical Medicine
Radcliffe Infirmary, Oxford OX2 6HE, UK

MICHAEL THUN
Epidemiology Unit
American Cancer Society
Atlanta, GA 30329, USA

CLARK HEATH Jr
Epidemiology Unit
American Cancer Society
Atlanta, GA 30329, USA

Mortality from Smoking in Developed Countries 1950-2000

Indirect Estimates from National Vital Statistics

Richard Peto Alan D Lopez Jillian Boreham

Michael Thun Clark Heath Jr

Imperial Cancer Research Fund

WORLD HEALTH ORGANIZATION

OXFORD UNIVERSITY PRESS

Oxford New York Tokyo

1994

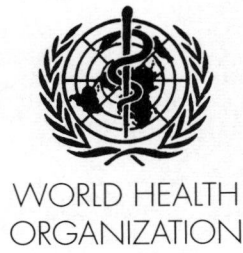

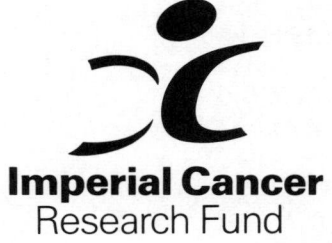

Oxford University Press, Walton Street, Oxford OX2 6DP
Oxford New York
Athens Auckland Bangkok Bombay
Calcutta Cape Town Dar es Salaam Delhi
Florence Hong Kong Istanbul Karachi
Kuala Lumpur Madras Madrid Melbourne
Mexico City Nairobi Paris Singapore
Taipei Tokyo Toronto
and associated companies in
Berlin Ibadan

Published in the United States by
Oxford University Press Inc., New York

A catalogue record for this book is available from the British Library

Library of Congress Cataloging in Publication Data

ISBN 0 19 262619 1

Printed in Great Britain by
The Bath Press, Avon

ACKNOWLEDGEMENTS

The chief acknowledgement is to the millions of doctors, registrars of death, medical statisticians and other supporting staff who, in dozens of countries throughout the past half century, have documented the causes of hundreds of millions of deaths, and rendered publicly available their findings.

The ICRF provided long-term support, and the ICRF/BHF/MRC Clinical Trial Service Unit provided extensive computing facilities, with secretarial assistance from Gale Mead and helpful criticism from Richard Doll. The collaboration of the Division of Epidemiological Surveillance and Health Situation & Trend Assessment at WHO headquarters in providing the basic data for these analyses is gratefully acknowledged. We should also like to acknowledge the support of Dr J Asvall, Regional Director for Europe, and the contribution of the Epidemiology, Statistics & Information Unit and the Action Plan for a Tobacco-free Europe of the WHO Regional Office for Europe in facilitating access to other mortality data. The American Cancer Society Epidemiology Unit provided access to their CPS-II and CPS-I prospective studies of smoking and death among one million Americans in the 1980s and in the 1960s, respectively. The collaboration of the United Nations Population Division (Estimates & Projections Section) in making available supplementary tabulations from their 1992 Global Demographic Assessment is also gratefully acknowledged.

SOURCES OF DATA: PROCEDURES

The aim, where possible, was to get the mortality data for 1955, 1965, 1975, 1985 and 1990, to make projections of the death rates for 1995 that are based on smoothed extrapolation of the age-specific 1985 and 1990 death rates (see text), and to apply these 1995 rates to the UN demographic prediction of the 1995 population. Where (as was sometimes the case) the cause-specific 1955 mortality rates were not available but the all-cause mortality rates were, only the latter were used, and the overall 1955 mortality from smoking was estimated by smoothed extrapolation back to 1955 of the age-specific smoking-attributed mortality rates for 1965 and1975. (The mortality from particular diseases in 1955 was then described as being unknown.)

Where the results from a number of different countries were to be combined (to obtain results for "All Developed", "Former Socialist Economies", "OECD Developed", "European Union" or for "Planned EU") then in a few instances evidence about some particular disease was missing from some of the contributing populations. If it was missing from several then it was treated as missing in the total, but if it was missing for only a few then the rates in the populations for which it was available were applied to the populations for which it was not. (For example, in a few populations Hodgkin's disease was not separated from non-Hodgkin's lymphoma [NHL].) So, where numbers of deaths from some disease are given for a group of populations, that number is intended to apply to the whole group, including the few populations that contributed no data on that disease.

General note: To each of the large totals, 0.2% was added (see foot of page A.48). Here and elsewhere, the "rounding" of certain numbers may cause minor apparent discrepancies in the least significant digits that are displayed.

For a few populations, special methods had to be adopted to deal with missing data (in addition to those described by Peto, Lopez et al, 1992):

Belgium, 1990: The cause-specific 1989 mortality rates were applied to the 1990 population, and the numbers of deaths in each group were then scaled to give known 1990 total mortality.

¶Czech Republic: Mortality data were provided by the Institute of Chest Diseases in Prague. (The 1955 mortality data, which were available only in 10-year age groups, were split into 5-year age groups in the same proportions as the 1955 mortality data for former Czechoslovakia.) Population data for 1995 were estimated by splitting age-specific UN 1995 projections for former Czechoslovakia between the Czech Republic and Slovakia in the same proportions as in 1990.

¶Former German Democratic Republic, 1955 & 1965: Cause-specific, age-specific death rates for the Federal Republic of Germany (within its pre-1990 territories) for 1955 and 1965 were applied to the population of the former GDR for those years and the numbers of deaths in each group were then scaled to give the known 1955 & 1965 total mortality for the former GDR.

¶Germany, 1955, 1965, 1975, 1985 & 1990: By addition of separate estimates for two populations, with projections for 1995 based on 1985 and 1990 rates for the whole of Germany.

Luxembourg, 1955, 1965: Belgian death rates were applied to the Luxembourg population, and scaled to give age-specific Luxembourg totals for all causes.

Romania, 1955: All-cause mortality estimated by applying 1956 rates to 1955 population.

¶Slovakia, 1955, 1965, 1975, 1985, 1990: By subtraction of data for Czech Republic from data for the former Czechoslovakia.

¶Slovenia, 1955 & 1965 not available.

¶Former USSR, 1955: All-cause mortality data were estimated from the 1950-55 & 1955-60 UN population estimates (supplementary tabulations from the UN's "World Population Prospects; the 1992 Revision". For 1985, 1990 & 1995 smoking-attributed deaths were estimated separately for each of the newly independent states of the former USSR, and these results were then added to estimate the numbers for the whole of the former USSR.

SOURCES OF DATA: DISCLAIMER

Most of the national mortality data used in this report have been provided by the World Health Organization, from the official data provided to WHO by its member states. Mortality data for the republics of the ¶former USSR, ¶former Czechoslovakia and ¶former Yugoslavia have, however, been received via a technical collaboration between the WHO European office and the institutions possessing those data, and cannot be regarded as official data provided to WHO by the representative member states: they have not been cleared for all years by the countries concerned, or validated by the WHO.

¶ GENERAL NOTE ON COUNTRY TERMINOLOGY

The designations employed and presentation of material do not imply the expression of any opinion whatsoever on the part of the World Health Organization or other parties involved in the publication concerning the legal status of any country, territory or area, its authorities, its current or former official name or the delimitation of its frontiers or boundaries.

For ease of statistical analysis, various country and regional grouping denominations are used which, although applicable at one particular time in the period of analysis concerned, may not reflect correct terminology at some other point in the current, historical or future context in which they are so used. The use of such terminology is strictly for the purposes of statistical analysis.

In particular, references to the "former Czechoslovakia", the "former USSR" and the "former Yugoslavia" refer to the countries that formerly existed under those names or abbreviations and, when used with respect to data applicable after such countries ceased to exist, to those countries which collectively now cover the same territory as such former countries.

In the case of Armenia, Azerbaijan, Belarus, Estonia, Georgia, Kazakhstan, Kyrgyzstan, Latvia, Lithuania, the Republic of Moldova, the Russian Federation, Tajikistan, Turkmenistan, Ukraine and Uzbekistan, these denominations are used both to refer to these countries as they currently exist and, when used with respect to data relating to before the existence of these countries as independent states, to the republics forming part of the former USSR.

In the case of the Czech Republic, Slovakia and Slovenia, these denominations are used both to refer to these countries as they currently exist and, when used with respect to data relating to before the existence of these countries as independent states, to the republics forming part of the former Czechoslovakia or former Yugoslavia.

In the case of Germany, this denomination is used — unless otherwise indicated — to refer to this country as it currently exists and, when used with respect to data relating to before 3 October 1990, when the German Democratic Republic ("GDR") acceded to the Federal Republic of Germany, to both of these countries collectively.

The terminology "European Union" is used to refer collectively to those countries that currently comprise the European Union, whether or not all the countries concerned were members of the Union at the time the reference is used or whether or not the European Union even existed at the time.

The designation of countries as "developed" is intended for statistical convenience and does not necessarily express a judgement about the stage reached by a particular country in the development process. Following the regional classification used by the United Nations Department of Economic & Social Information & Policy Analysis, the "developed" countries are taken to comprise those of Northern America, all regions of Europe, Japan, Australia, New Zealand and all the countries which were part of the former Union of Soviet Socialist republics (USSR): see United Nations, 1993. World Population Prospects: The 1992 Revision: ST/ESA/SER.A/135, United Nations, New York, p.139.

The terminology "Former Socialist Economies" follows that used by the World Bank in the 1993 World Development Report ("Investing in Health") and comprises Albania (see foot of page A.48), Bulgaria, former Czechoslovakia, Hungary, Poland, Romania, former Yugoslavia, and the republics of the former USSR. It does not include the former German Democratic Republic.

CONTENTS

HAZARDS FOR THE INDIVIDUAL CIGARETTE USER: 1990s US / UK EVIDENCE

BIG risk, especially among those who start smoking cigarettes regularly in their TEENAGE years: if they keep on smoking steadily then about HALF will eventually be killed by tobacco (about one-quarter in old age plus one-quarter in middle age).

— Those killed by tobacco in MIDDLE age (35-69) lose an average of 20-25 YEARS of non-smoker life expectancy.

— Nationwide, tobacco is much the greatest cause of death. (In non-smokers, cancer mortality is decreasing slowly & total mortality is decreasing rapidly.)

— Most of those killed by tobacco were not particularly "heavy" smokers (but, most did start in their teenage years).

STOPPING SMOKING WORKS: Even in middle age, stopping <u>before</u> having cancer or some other serious disease avoids <u>most</u> of the later excess risk of death from tobacco (and, the benefits of stopping at earlier ages are even greater).

Peto, Lopez et al, 1992, 1994

NOTES: Most of those now being killed by tobacco are male, so these numbers are chiefly based on US / UK male hazards in the 1990s. But, the hazards vary from one population to another, from one sex to the other and from one time to another. (Hence, a statement that would be more uniformly correct would be that for young adults who smoke cigarettes regularly, JUST OVER HALF OF THOSE WHO DIE IN MIDDLE AGE will have been killed by tobacco.)

Overall, regular cigarette smokers lose about 8 years of non-smoker life expectancy (or 16 years, for the half who are killed by the habit: 20-25 years for those killed in middle age, plus 5-10 years for those killed at older ages).

1. SUMMARY

PURPOSES AND STRUCTURE OF THE MONOGRAPH

This monograph takes established methods for estimating the mortality from smoking in "developed" populations, and applies them to each of the main developed countries from which appropriate data are available for the 1950s, the 1960s, the 1970s, the 1980s and the 1990s. This provides, in each population, a description of the current level of mortality from smoking, and in many it also provides a description of the trends in smoking-attributed mortality over the past few decades.

At present there are about 2 million deaths per year in developed countries from smoking, so there will be about 20 million deaths from smoking over the decade of the 1990s. But, clear evidence that smoking is a major cause of premature death was first published in 1950, and during the period 1950-1990 about 40 million people were killed by the habit in developed countries alone. Hence, over the whole of the second half of this century (1950-2000) the total number of deaths caused by smoking in developed countries will be about 60 million (40 million at ages 35-69 plus 20 million at older ages).

So far, the large majority of those killed by tobacco have been males in developed countries, but the habit has recently spread to females in developed countries and to much larger numbers of males in the developing countries. (There are, for example, about 300 million smokers in China alone.) If these smoking patterns persist then in the first few decades of the next century there will be much larger numbers killed. It has been plausibly predicted that the current global total of about 3 million deaths per year from tobacco (2 million developed, 1 million not) would, on current smoking patterns, reach about 10 million per year (3 million developed, 7 million not) by the time the children of today reach middle age.

It is the vast size of this epidemic that makes tobacco so uniquely important as a cause of premature death in developed countries, and the chief aim of this book is to facilitate effective communication, first to the reader and then by the reader, of the size of the epidemic.

For that purpose, it makes available in a clear format both detailed and simplified tables and graphs for each of several dozen separate countries (or other developed populations), together with various tables and graphs that bring together and contrast the results for different populations.

Most of the book is taken up with 51 sets of Main Tables and Figures (one set per population) and 54 corresponding sets of detailed Appendix Tabulations (for the same 51 populations, plus 3 others).

After the informative Foreword by Sir Richard Doll, the chapters on Introduction and on Purposes are followed by 3 chapters on Methods, illustrated by a number of results: one explains the format and meaning of the Main Tables and Figures, one explains the format and potential uses of the Appendix Tables, and the third chapter reproduces the Lancet report that originally introduced and discussed the indirect methods that are used to assess the national mortality rates from tobacco. Chapter 8 then extracts, from the Main Tables and Figures and from the Appendices, a range of comparisons between the different developed populations, and the final chapter explores the implications for developing populations.

The emphasis throughout is chiefly on the hazards that entire populations are now suffering, or have suffered over the past few decades, rather than on the hazards that an individual smoker will eventually face. But, some information about individual risks is reviewed in the Introduction, indicating that about half of all regular cigarette smokers will eventually be killed by their habit: about one-quarter in old age and one-quarter in middle age (with those killed by smoking in middle age losing on average about 20-25 years of non-smoker life expectancy: see Box opposite).

These individual hazards, which are directly based on recent epidemiological studies, make plausible the large population hazards that, based on indirect arguments, this monograph describes.

2. FOREWORD

One of the great objectives of medicine is to enable people to live out the span of life to which they are biologically adapted. Extraordinary progress towards this has been made during the past century, even though wars, famines, common infections and acute epidemics have each caused several tens of millions of early deaths, as will the new epidemic of infection with the human immunodeficiency virus. Taking the world as a whole, however, human death rates have decreased substantially over the past few decades, and they are much lower now than they have ever been. This is particularly true in the "developed" countries of the world, which are the chief, but not the only, subject of this monograph. In many of the countries that are now classified as developed, about half the infants born in the 19th century died in childhood or early adult life. But, at current death rates only 4% will do so — indeed, in the "OECD" developed countries, 97% of newborn infants can now expect to survive at least to middle age.

In middle age, however (which this book defines as 35-69 years), progress has been slower, because the control of tuberculosis and of many other infections in developed countries this century has not been accompanied by comparable improvements in control of the chronic diseases of middle age. Indeed, although there have been large decreases in the incidence of some chronic diseases, such as stomach cancer and stroke, there have been large increases in others, such as lung cancer and myocardial infarction. The causes of these chronic diseases are many, but at present one far exceeds all others: namely, the smoking of manufactured cigarettes.

Tobacco contains an addictive drug, and soon after tobacco was introduced to Europe in the 16th century its use in pipes, cigars, snuff or quids spread rapidly around the world. It was not, however, until the beginning of this century that these other forms of tobacco use began to be displaced by cigarettes, the smoke from which is easily inhaled, and it was only after prolonged and widespread use of cigarettes that, during the 1950s, smoking was discovered to be closely associated with some important chronic diseases, and moderately associated with several others. That smoking should be associated with many diseases is not surprising when it is realised that tobacco smoke contains more than 4000 chemicals, over 50 of which are capable of causing cancer in experimental animals, and that inhalation is an effective way of getting noxious chemicals distributed throughout the body. Moreover, it is now clear, as a result of many studies of different types, that the associations that have been observed between smoking and disease are, for the most part, causal in character and that by avoiding smoking the excess risk of disease that occurs in smokers can be largely avoided.

For the past few decades it has been widely known in developed countries that tobacco is dangerous; but it is still insufficiently widely known how large these dangers are. Studies that would directly estimate the proportion of deaths in each country that is attributable to smoking might in principle be straightforward, but would in practice be extremely costly and time-consuming. Peto, Lopez and their colleagues have in this book provided important evidence for those interested in public health, by estimating indirectly the proportion of deaths attributable to smoking in each of the major populations that have been classed by the United Nations as "developed" (including separate estimates for the 15 newly independent countries that constituted the former USSR). For this purpose they have developed an ingenious method. First, they compared national lung cancer mortality rates with the rates that have been observed among US non-smokers, and used the **absolute**

excess mortality from lung cancer in each developed population as an indication of the extent to which that population was being damaged by tobacco (which they were justified in doing because in developed countries lung cancer is so closely related to smoking and so seldom caused by any other factor among non-smokers). Secondly, they used this lung cancer excess as a guide to the fractions of the deaths from other causes that could be attributed to tobacco, calibrating this relationship by epidemiological evidence from the massive cohort study of a million men and women that was carried out by the American Cancer Society in the 1980s.

The number of premature deaths estimated in this way to occur as a result of smoking is enormous. In males it amounted in 1990 to 24 per cent of all the deaths in all developed countries combined (or, at 35-69 years of age, 35% of all male deaths). In females it amounted in 1990 to "only" 7 per cent (or 12%, at ages 35-69), but these proportions are increasing. Indeed, in the few countries where women have smoked cigarettes regularly for several decades, the proportion of female deaths that is attributed to tobacco is now approaching the male figure. In the United States, for example, the proportions of the male and female deaths in 1990 that were attributed to tobacco are respectively 26 and 17 per cent. Elsewhere, the number of female deaths now attributed to smoking is still relatively small, for few of the middle-aged or older women are regular cigarette smokers. But, in many countries (such as France, Spain or Poland) there have in the past few decades been large absolute increases in cigarette use by young women, foreshadowing large increases early next century in female mortality from the habit.

As well as the main analyses that Peto, Lopez et al present, two of their many additional analyses are of special interest. First, they present the trend over the whole of the second half of this century in the proportion of all deaths that is attributed to smoking. Both absolutely and as a proportion of all mortality, when all developed countries are considered together, the mortality they attribute to tobacco is still increasing in both sexes, but it is at last beginning to decline substantially in men in a few countries where the prevalence of male smoking has been substantially reduced, such as Australia and, particularly, the UK.

The second trend that is of particular interest is in the mortality that remains when, for particular diseases, the death rates attributed to smoking are subtracted from the overall death rates, so as to assess what the underlying patterns might have been in the absence of tobacco. This subtraction shows that the mortality rate from cancer that is not attributed to smoking has been approximately constant over the past few decades (indeed, it has if anything been decreasing rather than increasing), and that the mortality rate from non-neoplastic disease that is not attributed to smoking has been falling rapidly nearly everywhere, except in the former socialist economies. Elsewhere (i.e. in the OECD developed countries) non-smoker life expectancy is increasing rapidly. In France, for example, even when neoplastic and other causes are combined, the death rate at ages 35 to 69 that was attributed to factors other than smoking decreased by half in both sexes over the 35-year period from 1955 to 1990.

Interestingly, in developed countries the mortality rate from cancer that is not attributed to smoking is falling slowly not only in middle age (35-69) but also at older ages (70-79). Trends in the mortality from individual types of cancer vary, of course, and some types are clearly becoming more common. But, others are becoming less common, and, reassuringly, the overall mortality rate from cancer that is not attributable to tobacco provides no indication of any general increase in the disease.

In contrast with this reassurance, however, there has been a large increase this century in tobacco-attributable cancer deaths, especially among males. Taking all developed countries together, the cancer death rates have, because of smoking, been increasing rather than decreasing over the past few decades.

Tobacco now accounts for about half of all male cancer deaths in middle age and, when men and women are compared, the men now have much higher cancer death rates than the women. But, the large male excess of cancer is due almost entirely to tobacco. Once the estimated effects of smoking are subtracted out, the cancer death rates in middle age that remain, and that are not attributed to tobacco, are similar in males and in females, in former socialist and in OECD developed countries, and in current and in previous decades.

In addition, however, tobacco kills even more people by other diseases than by cancer, and one great need, both for public and for personal health, is a proper understanding of the numerical importance of such hazards.

It is estimated that the average loss of life for those killed by tobacco was about 16 years — and, since about half of all regular smokers in developed countries are eventually killed by the habit, teenagers or young adults who become regular cigarette smokers must be reducing their life expectancy by the substantial amount of about 8 years. An 8-year loss of life expectancy is also indicated by the most recent evidence from our own 40-year study of smoking and death among British doctors.

Modern medicine and the social conditions that a developed country can provide have not yet reduced mortality in middle age to the same extent as they have done in youth. The figures presented here, however, provide encouraging evidence that, in the absence of smoking, the achievements have been greater than is commonly thought.

Death in old age is inevitable, but death before old age is not. In previous centuries 70 years used to be regarded as humanity's allotted span of life and only about one in five survived to such an age. Nowadays, however, for non-smokers in the "OECD" developed countries, the situation is reversed; in the absence of tobacco, only about one in five will die before 70, and the non-smoker death rates are still decreasing, offering the promise, at least in developed countries, of a world where death before 70 is uncommon.

But, for this promise to be properly realised, ways must be found to limit the vast damage that is now being done by tobacco. Unfortunately, however, as this book shows all too clearly, at present the proportion of premature deaths that is due to smoking is still increasing.

It is the hope of the authors of this book, which I share, that the presentation of their findings in a clear and comprehensible form will help to bring home, not only to the many millions of people in developed countries but also to the far larger populations elsewhere, the great extent to which those who continue to smoke will shorten their expectation of life by so doing.

RICHARD DOLL, FRS
Emeritus Professor of Medicine
University of Oxford, UK

3. INTRODUCTION

THE SCALE OF THE EPIDEMIC

For each major developed country, and for various groups of such countries, tables and graphs are provided that describe the extent to which smoking is now causing death in middle age and in old age. The chief purpose of this book is to facilitate effective communication, first to the reader and then by the reader, of the extraordinary magnitude of the number of deaths that smoking is now causing (Table 1). In developed countries alone, the habit is currently responsible for about two million deaths a year, about half of which are deaths in middle age. There is, however, wide variation between one developed country and another in the current death rates from smoking, and in the trends in those death rates. Hence, for each of the main developed countries (and for a few other developed populations) separate descriptions are provided. Methods to estimate tobacco-attributable mortality have already been introduced and discussed elsewhere (Peto, Lopez et al, 1992), and those methods are used without material change, except for slight improvement in the projections of tobacco-attributed mortality for 1995. What is intended to be new is not the methods, but the clarity of presentation of the results of applying those methods to particular populations.

Table 1

1995 projections

Millions of deaths per year from smoking in developed countries (total: 2 million)

Age at death	Male	Female	Mean years lost per death from smoking
	(M=million)		
35-69	0.9M	0.2M	22 years
70+	0.6M	0.3M	8 years

Peto, Lopez et al, 1992, 1994

Appendix tables: detailed death rates and trends

For convenience of reference, the national death rates in various years that have been used in each population for estimating the effects of tobacco are given in a standard format in a set of Appendices, together with some of the detailed calculations of tobacco-attributed mortality. The Appendices also bring together, in finer detail than is needed for the tobacco calculations, the age-specific 1990 death rates in 54 populations from 44 groups of causes. Although these causes of death include some that are importantly related to smoking, they also include many that are not, the rates of which in these populations are provided in the Appendices for purely descriptive purposes. The 1990 death rates for these populations have not previously been brought together, and comparisons between them are of substantial interest, as are the totals for all developed countries, or for particular groups of developed countries, such as the former socialist economies, the other (i.e. OECD) developed countries or the European Union.

Premature death from smoking: ages 35-69

Throughout this book, "middle age" is defined by convention as 35-69 years of age, and mortality in middle age is analysed separately from that in "old age" (70+). Those killed by tobacco in old age are already, on average, about 80 years old and might soon have died of some other cause. But, those killed by tobacco in middle age would on average, in the absence of tobacco, have been able to look forward to an extra 20 or 25 years of life expectancy, which is substantial. Of course, for the population as a whole tobacco does not reduce life expectancy by 20-25 years of age, but it does do this for the large number of people who are killed by smoking in middle age. Although smoking causes few deaths before middle age, in middle age the habit is now responsible in developed countries for about one-third of all male deaths, plus a growing proportion of all female deaths. Because these risks of premature death are so large, the chief need is to communicate clearly and memorably not just the well-known qualitative fact that tobacco is dangerous, but the less well-known quantitative facts about the sizes of the dangers of tobacco.

Table 2

50-year estimates, 1950-2000
Millions of deaths from smoking in developed countries (total: 60 million)

Age at death	Male (M=million)	Female
35-69	33M	4.8M
70+	19M	5.7M
All	~50M	~10M

Peto, Lopez et al, 1992, 1994

Turning from the projected numbers of deaths in 1995 to the cumulative numbers of deaths throughout the second half of this century, over the 50-year period between the year 1950 and the year 2000 smoking will cause a total of about 60 million deaths in developed countries (Table 2). Of these deaths from smoking in the second half of this century, about 50 million will have been male and 10 million female — or, perhaps more importantly, about 40 million will have been in middle age and 20 million in old age when they are killed.

Sources of evidence: previous under-estimates of the hazards of really prolonged cigarette use

The first major disease to be reliably linked to smoking was cancer of the lung, which in 1950 was shown by Doll & Hill in Britain and by Wynder & Graham in America to be much more common among regular cigarette smokers than among people of the same age and sex who had never smoked regularly. Cancer of the lung is still the disease that is most widely known to be caused by smoking, but in fact the habit causes more deaths by other diseases than it does by lung cancer. This was shown in "prospective" studies, in which large numbers of apparently healthy adults are first asked what they have smoked, and in which their deaths are then monitored over the next several years. This allows the death rates of those who said they were smokers to be compared with the death rates of those of the same age and sex who said they had never smoked regularly (or, more informatively, it allows the death rates from particular diseases to be thus compared).

The first big prospective study of smoking and death was that established by Doll & Hill in 1951, immediately after their 1950 discovery of the relationship between smoking and lung cancer. Within just a few years this study, together with much other evidence, had shown that many different diseases were caused by the habit, and had shown that all-cause mortality was substantially greater in smokers (Doll & Peto, 1976). But, during the 1950s and 1960s the epidemic of death from tobacco was still growing. So, although the results from early prospective studies are still widely cited, in fact they under-estimate the even larger hazards of really prolonged smoking that are now being seen in more recent prospective study results.

At present, the largest such study is the American Cancer Society's Second Cancer Prevention study (CPS-II), a recent prospective study of smoking and death among more than one million US adults. Table 3 shows its main findings during the mid-1980s for middle-aged US males. Because the study was large, and because this was a period when the US epidemic of male death from tobacco was about at its peak, the evidence from that study is particularly reliable about the **ratios** of the death rates of regular smokers to those of men who had never smoked regularly. In Table 3, the death rate from lung cancer is more than twenty times greater among smokers than among non-smokers, while there is only a threefold difference in the death rate from vascular disease (9th ICD 390-459, including heart attacks, strokes and all other diseases of the arteries or veins). But, because vascular disease is so common in America, in absolute terms smoking caused even more deaths from vascular disease than from lung cancer among these men.

Table 3

Smoking and death in middle age, U.S. MALES ACS million-person prospective study, 1984-88

Underlying cause of death	MEAN* ANNUAL MORTALITY RATE per 100,000 males aged 35-69		
	Never smoked regularly	Current cigarette smoker	Excess rate in smokers
Lung cancer	8	196	188
Mouth, larynx, oesoph.	5	28	23
Other cancer	109	188	79
Respiratory	9	62	53
Vascular	176	446	270
Other medical	39	81	42
(Cirrhosis, suicide, homicide, accident)	(37)	(81)	(44)
ALL CAUSES	382	1083	701

* Average of the 7 rates at ages 35-39, 40-44, ..., 65-69 (from Appendix to Peto, Lopez et al, Lancet 339: 1268)

About HALF eventually killed by smoking

The total death rates at the foot of Table 3 are about three times greater among smokers than among non-smokers, and most of the excess is from diseases that can be caused by smoking. This threefold ratio suggests that, of those US male smokers who die in middle age, about two-thirds would not have done so if they had not smoked — or, equivalently, that among US males smoking is now a cause of about two-thirds of all the deaths at ages 35-69 among regular cigarette smokers.

At older ages this same prospective study indicated that smoking is a cause of about half the deaths of US male smokers at 70-79 years of age, and at even older ages the death rates of the smokers still substantially exceeded those of the non-smokers. (Moreover, the smokers who were in their eighties in this study had been born in about 1900, and may not have been regular cigarette smokers throughout their adult lives: if they had been, then the proportion surviving to 80 years of age might have been even smaller, and the excess mortality thereafter even greater.)

Table 4

Smoking and death in middle age, U.S. FEMALES
ACS million-person prospective study, 1984-88

Underlying cause of death	MEAN* ANNUAL MORTALITY RATE per 100,000 females aged 35-69		
	Never smoked regularly	Current cigarette smoker	Excess rate in smokers
Lung cancer	7	111	104
Mouth, larynx, oesoph.	1	10	9
Other cancer	154	177	23
Respiratory	7	39	32
Vascular	65	171	106
Other medical	20	47	27
(Cirrhosis, suicide, homicide, accident)	(16)	(29)	(13)
ALL CAUSES	271	583	312

* Average of the 7 rates at ages 35-39, 40-44, ..., 65-69 (from Appendix to Peto, Lopez et al, Lancet 339: 1268)

If, among a large group of US male cigarette smokers, the habit is a cause of about two-thirds of their deaths at ages 35-69, of about half their deaths at ages 70-79 and of an appreciable fraction of their deaths at older ages, then in the United States about half of all young men who become regular cigarette smokers will eventually be killed by tobacco.

Table 4 shows recent results from the same prospective study for middle-aged US females. But, the lung cancer death rates among US females were still increasing rapidly during the 1980s (Figure 1), suggesting that the eventual hazards for female smokers may be substantially greater in the future than they were during the 1980s.

Figure 1: US lung cancer trends, adjusted for age to US 1970 population. (ACS: non-smoker rates = male 6, female 4)

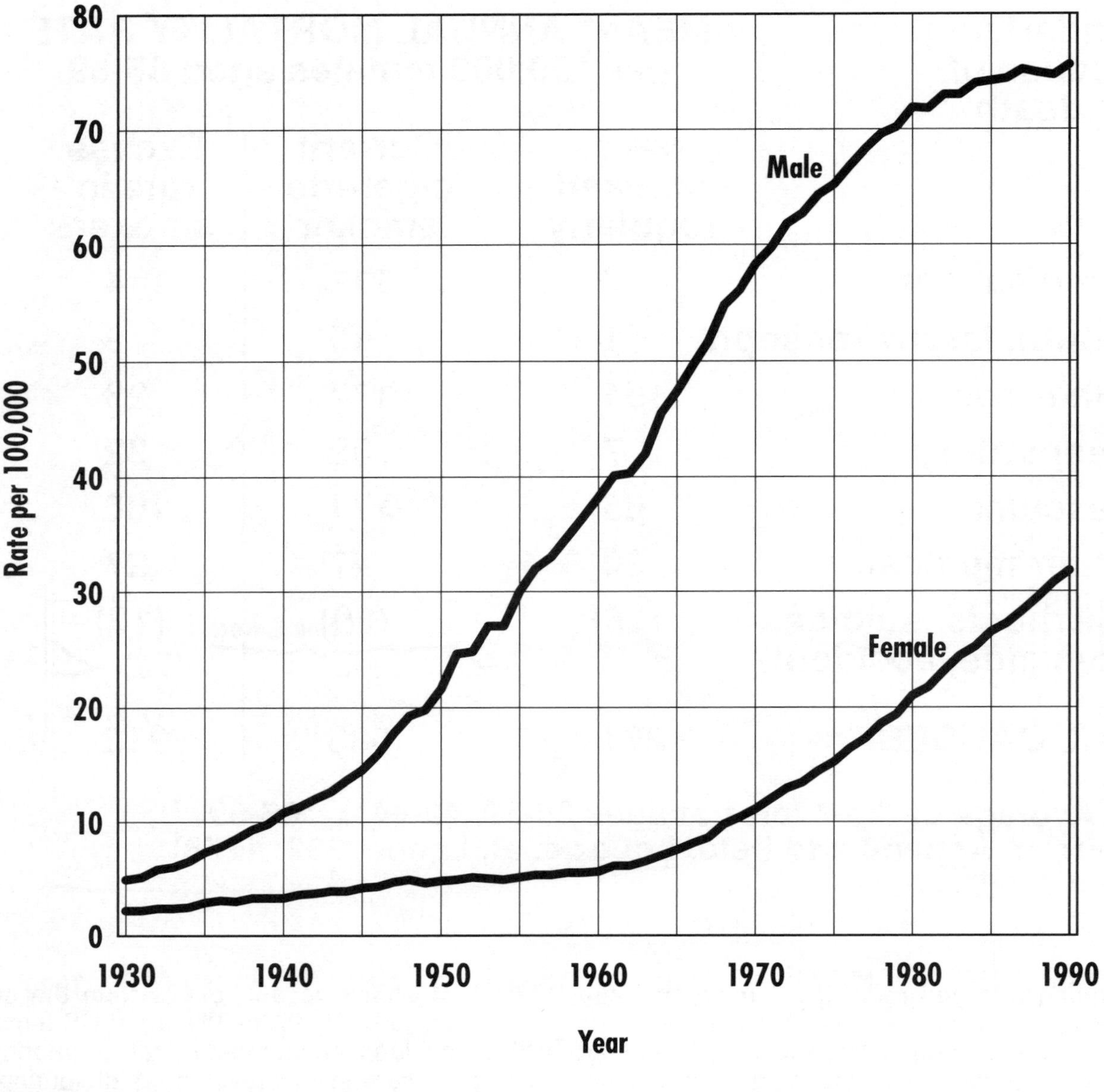

Increasing US mortality from lung cancer, and hence from smoking

Although lung cancer accounts for only a minority of the deaths from tobacco, the closeness of its relationship with cigarette smoking means that any large changes in the lung cancer death rates can provide (at least in developed countries) a useful marker for the evolution of the wider epidemic of death from smoking. Figure 1 describes the increase in the male and female lung cancer death rates that has been seen over the past 60 years in the United States. Figure 2 (males) and Figure 3 (females) compare these lung cancer trends with the trends in the US mortality rates from the other common types of cancer, showing that the increases are specific to lung cancer, and are not part of a generalised increase in the common cancers. The cancer trends in Figures 1, 2 and 3 are not materially affected by changes in the proportions of older people in the

Figure 2: US male cancer trends adjusted for age to US 1970 population. Source: American Cancer Society

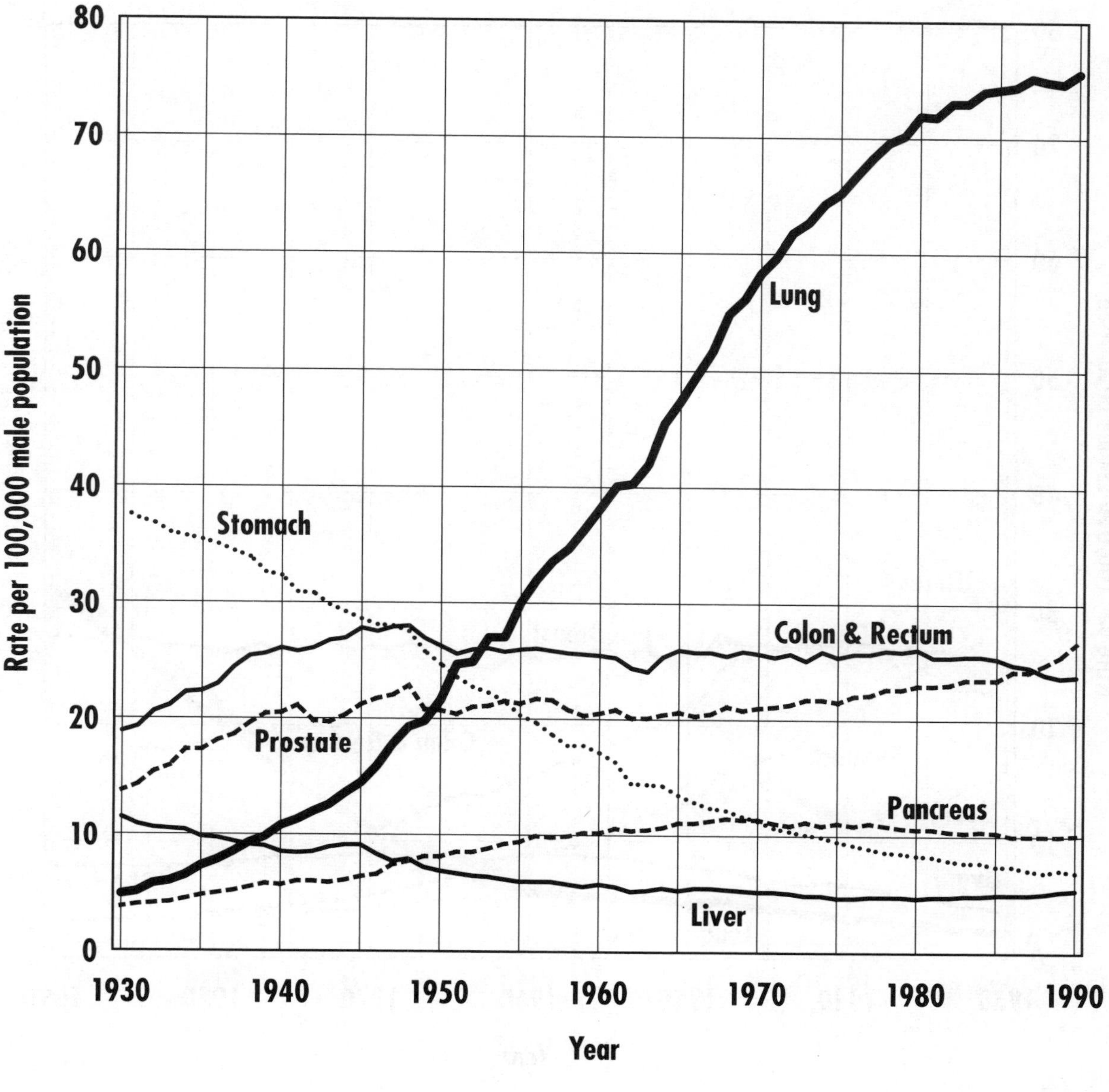

US population, for the rates have been standardised for age (Doll & Peto, 1981, Appendix A). A little of the large absolute increase in the US male lung cancer death rates, especially before 1950, was due to improvements in the reliability with which death certificates were completed and some such artefactual increases may still be in progress, at least in old age (Doll & Peto, 1981, Appendix E). But, in 1950 and from time to time thereafter there have been several large studies of lung cancer in the US that have consistently shown the disease to be rare in non-smokers (see, for example, Table 5).

Hence, the main reason for the large increases in US lung cancer mortality over the past few decades lies in the increasing effects of tobacco, first among males and now among females. It appears that in the 1980s the US male epidemic of lung cancer was about at its peak, while the female epidemic was still rising

Figure 3: US female cancer trends adjusted for age to US 1970 population. Source: American Cancer Society

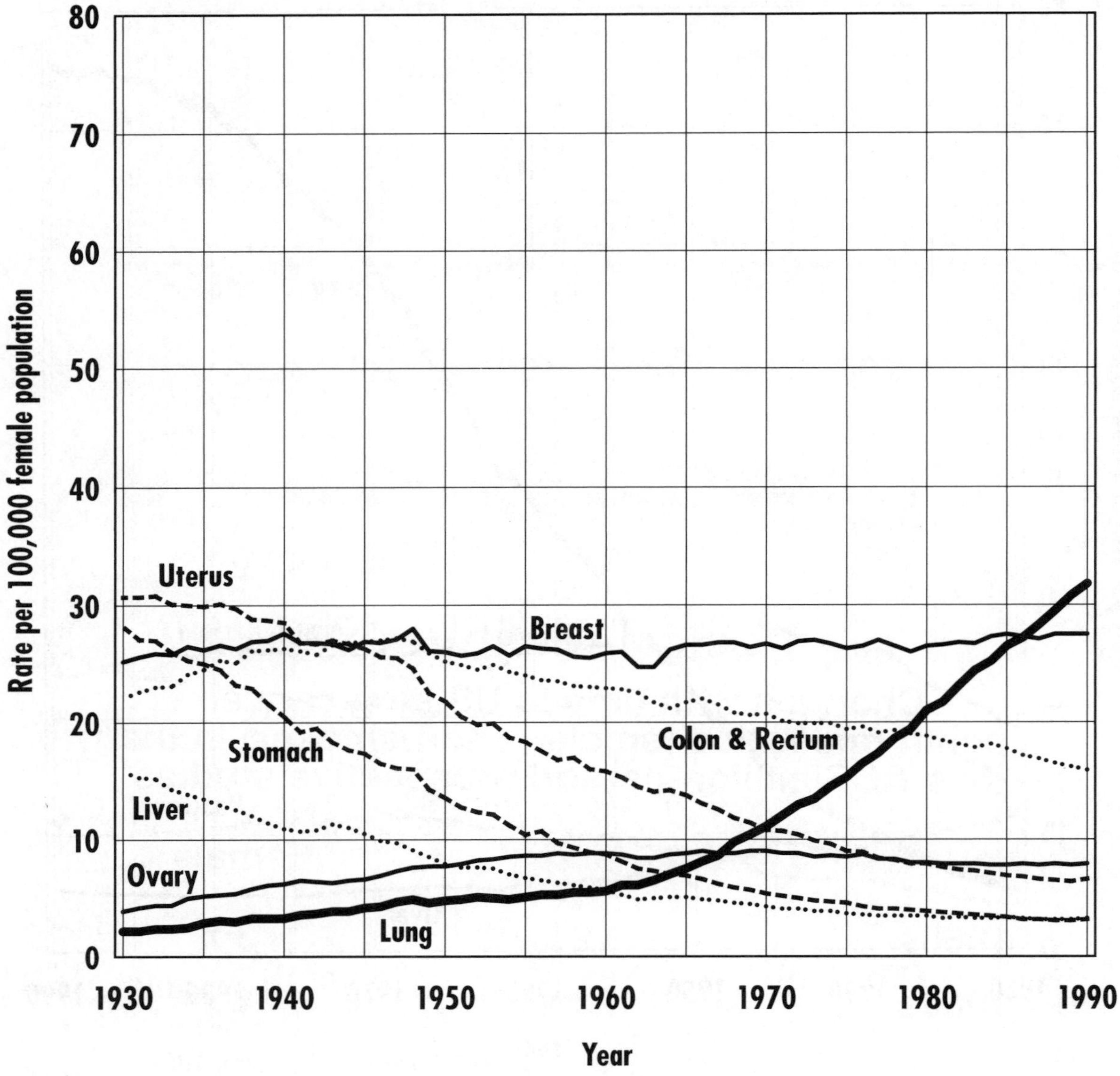

rapidly. If the same is true for some of the other fatal consequences of smoking, then studies of smoking and death among US females in the 1980s may substantially under-estimate the eventual hazards for females of really prolonged cigarette use. Nevertheless, such studies have shown that by the mid-1980s the total female death rates were already about twice as great among smokers as among non-smokers (Table 4). This twofold difference suggests that eventually, among a population of women who smoke cigarettes regularly throughout their adult lives, tobacco will be a cause of at least half, and perhaps substantially more than half, of all their deaths in middle age. The absolute death rates in middle age are smaller in women than in men, but the proportional increase in overall mortality at ages 35-69 that is produced in such populations by really prolonged cigarette smoking will probably eventually be about 2-3 fold in both sexes.

Table 5

Approximate constancy of US non-smoker lung cancer death rates in the two ACS million-person prospective studies

	Male	Female	Both sexes
1960s	6	4	5
1980s	6	5	5
Mean of 2 periods	6	4	5

Annual mortality / 100,000, adjusted (as in Figures 1-3) for age to US 1970 population

Table 6

Changes with time in US lung cancer death rate ratios (smoker : non-smoker) in the two ACS million-person prospective studies

	Male	Female
1960s	12 x	3 x
1980s	22 x	11 x

US Surgeon-General, 1989

The early prospective studies of smoking and death, on which many public warnings about the size of the hazard continue to be based, were done in the 1950s and the 1960s, and Figure 1 shows how greatly studies in those early decades might have under-estimated the eventual hazards of really prolonged tobacco use. The US non-smoker lung cancer death rates were about the same in the 1960s and in the 1980s (Table 5), so there was a substantial change over this 20-year period in the ratio of the lung cancer death rate among smokers to that among non-smokers (Table 6).

Figure 4: Effects of cigarette smoking on survival to age 70 and to age 85, in 40-year prospective study of male British doctors
Source: Doll, Peto et al, 1994

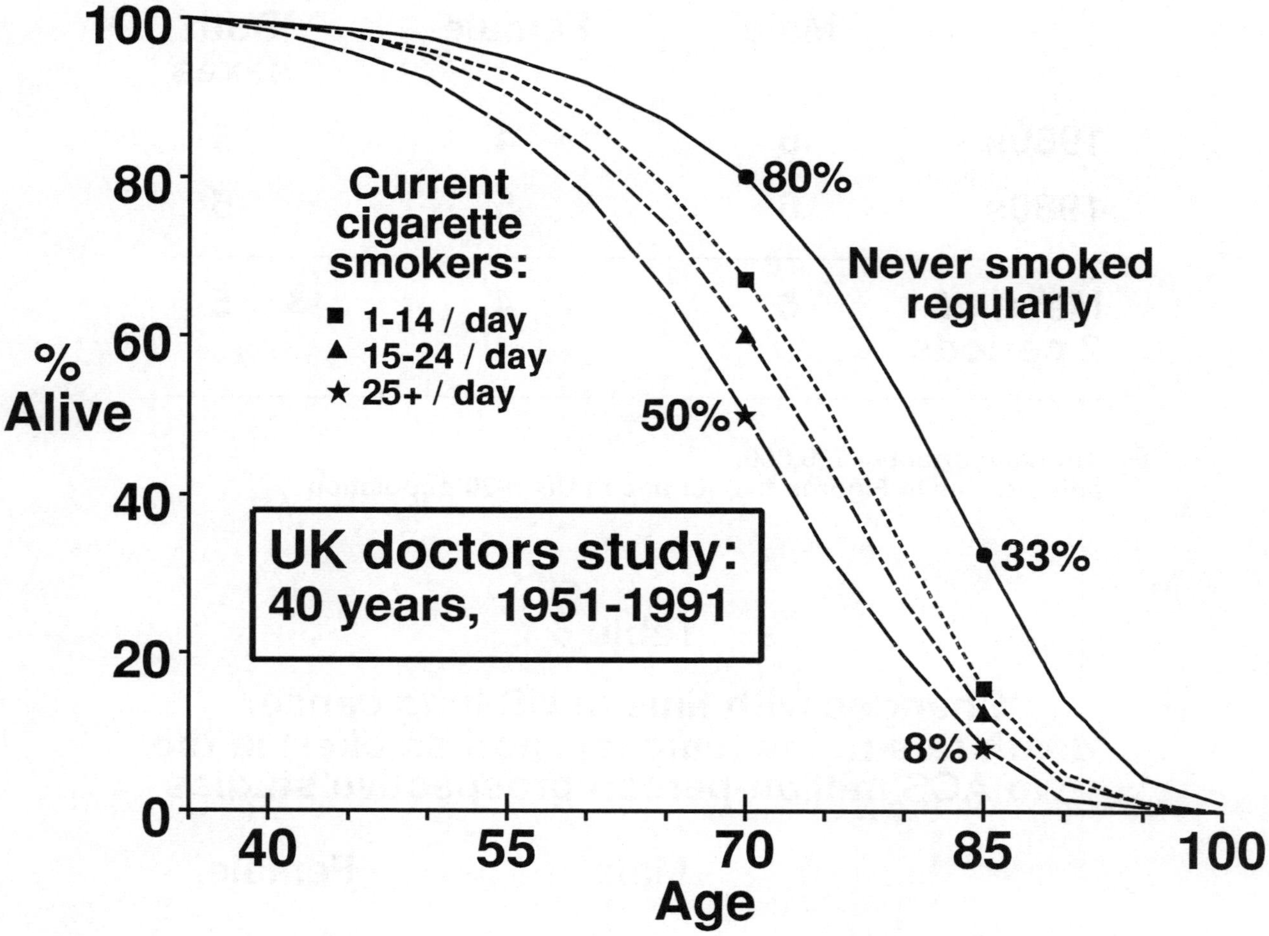

40-year follow-up of British doctors

British data also indicate that the hazards of really prolonged tobacco use are greater than was thought to be the case 20 years ago. The first large prospective study of smoking and death, which was established in Britain in 1951, has now been continued for 40 years, with reliable follow-up even into extreme old age.

Even taking the period 1951-1991 as a whole the hazards of tobacco were substantial, not only among heavy smokers but also among light smokers (Figure 4). But, taking the periods 1951-1971 and 1971-1991 separately, the hazards that are indicated when the current cigarette smokers are compared with men who have never smoked were substantially greater in the more recent period (Figure 5). This recent British evidence indicates almost a three-fold difference in mortality during middle age between the smokers and the non-smokers, which is consistent with the almost three-fold difference in the much larger body of United States evidence in Table 3. In both countries, however, studies in earlier decades had substantially underestimated the male hazards that are now being seen.

Figure 5: Effects of really prolonged cigarette smoking, revealed by the second half of the 40-year prospective study of male British doctors Source: Doll, Peto et al, 1994

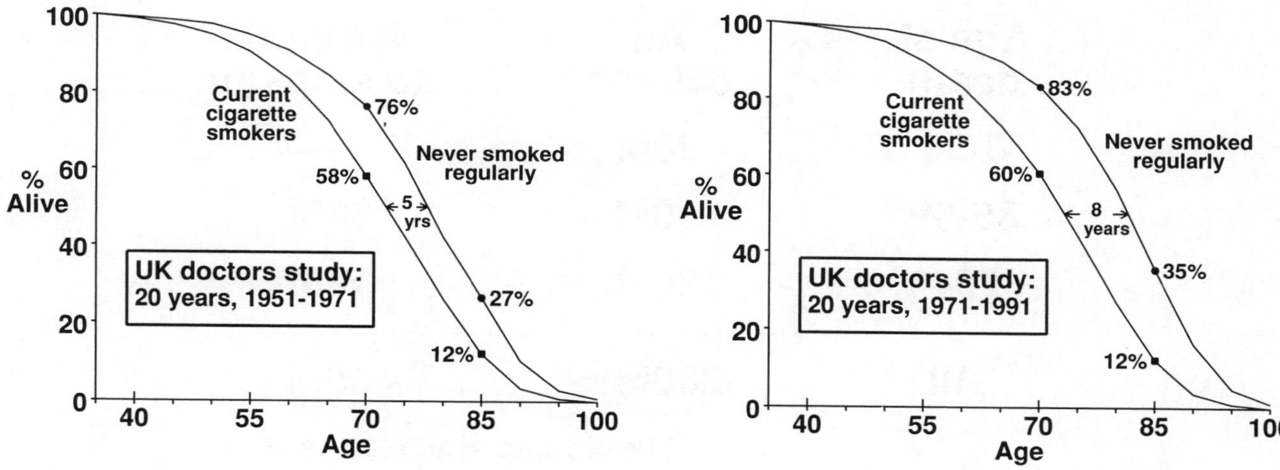

Delay between male and female epidemics

The United Kingdom and the United States are of particular interest not only because they have been well studied epidemiologically but also because the female epidemics are already substantial. This is because, by 1990, substantial proportions of UK and US women had smoked cigarettes regularly for several decades. In many other populations, however, although substantial proportions of women (particularly at younger ages) now smoke cigarettes, their habit was adopted too recently for its main effects to have emerged by 1990. If, therefore, we consider all developed countries, and consider the whole period 1950-2000, then the male epidemic has been substantial (Table 7) but the female epidemic (Table 8) has been much smaller than the UK and US experience suggests it will eventually become.

Table 7

50-year estimates, 1950-2000
Millions (M) of MALE deaths from smoking in developed countries (total: 50 million)

Age at death	All causes	Attributed to smoking
0-34	30M	—
35-69	110M	33M
70+	120M	19M
All	260M	~50M

Peto, Lopez et al, 1992, 1994

Table 8

50-year estimates, 1950-2000
Millions (M) of FEMALE deaths from smoking in developed countries (total: 10 million)

Age at death	All causes	Attributed to smoking
0-34	20M	—
35-69	70M	4.8M
70+	150M	5.7M
All	240M	~10M

Peto, Lopez et al, 1992, 1994

4. PURPOSE OF THIS MONOGRAPH

Quantitative description of hazards

During the present century smoking has become the commonest cause of premature death in developed countries, and over the next few decades it will become a common cause of premature death in many less developed countries as well. Hence, a quantitative description of the situation that now exists in developed countries is of substantial global relevance. The number of deaths now due to smoking is so great that, in terms of public health, what needs to be communicated is not just the qualitative fact that smoking kills, but quantitative facts about how enormously many it kills. This book therefore describes, in several different standard formats, the death rates from smoking in each of the major developed countries and, where possible, the trends in those death rates. The description is not chiefly of the risk of death for the individual who smokes, but of the death rates from tobacco for whole countries (or groups of countries).

[Note that, because the boundaries of many developed countries have changed recently, the populations analysed may have been those of a separate country at one time but not at another. In most places where this might be relevant, the country name is marked with a ¶ sign, and there is an introductory General Note on country terminology.]

The current death rates from smoking vary considerably from one developed population to another and from one period to another. In the 1960s, for example, the UK probably had the worst male death rates in the world from tobacco, but in recent decades the highest male death rates have been in Eastern Europe and the former USSR. For females, the death rates from tobacco were low everywhere in the 1960s, but have now increased substantially in a few countries, such as the UK and US. The current trends in the death rates from tobacco also vary substantially. Among males, the death rates from tobacco are at last decreasing in some developed countries, but are still increasing in others. Among females, large increases in mortality from tobacco are already in progress in some developed countries, but such increases have scarcely begun in other female populations. Despite all this heterogeneity, however, the mortality from tobacco in the aggregate of all developed countries is of some interest (Tables 1 & 2), and this is what will be described to illustrate the standard format of the results for each separate developed population.

Apart from the introductory text, this book has two main sections. The first ("Tables and Figures", pages 1-228) provides, in a format designed for convenient public presentation, the main results for each major developed country, or group of countries. The second section ("Appendix", pages 229-553) then gives finer details.

Indirect estimation of smoking-attributed mortality

The methods used to estimate the effects of tobacco are indirect. They were originally described, and their validity discussed, in a recent report in the Lancet, where space limitations precluded an appropriately full description of the findings for each separate country (Peto, Lopez et al, 1992: reproduced as Chapter 7 of the present monograph). Briefly, in each developed country these indirect methods of estimation depend only on the national mortality statistics (subdivided by sex and age) for lung cancer and for various other diseases, and do not require any knowledge whatever of the past or current smoking patterns in that population.

For lung cancer the method is simply to compare the national lung cancer death rate with the rate that has been seen in the main epidemiological studies of US non-smokers, and to attribute the excess to tobacco. Where, as is often the case, the national lung cancer rates vastly exceed the US non-smoker rates, then uncertainties as to the exact applicability of the US non-smoker rates to other populations have little proportional effect on the lung cancer mortality thus attributed to tobacco.

For other diseases, this absolute excess of lung cancer is then used indirectly, as a guide to the **proportions** of the deaths from other causes that should be ascribed to smoking. (To be conservative, although smoking can cause death from medical causes before middle age, and death from fire, no deaths before age 35 and no deaths at any age from non-medical causes are attributed to the habit.)

These indirect methods may well be reasonably robust (see Chapter 7) despite not taking explicit account of differences between pipes, cigars and various types of cigarettes; differences in the manner and duration of smoking; or, differences in various co-factors. They have the great advantage of providing useful estimates of mortality from tobacco, both for the present decade and for past decades, from each major developed country in any period from which reasonably reliable national mortality statistics are available, even though there will in general be no reliable direct epidemiological evidence about the effects of smoking (or even about the past extent of smoking) in that population.

Materials: 1955, 1965, 1975, 1985 & 1990 national death rates, plus 1995 projections

For most developed countries that, like the UK or US, are members of the Organisation of Economic Cooperation and Development (OECD), the mortality rates for 1955, 1965, 1975, 1985 and 1990 are all available (and those for 1985 and 1990 can be used to estimate those for 1995). For the former socialist economies, some of these rates, particularly in the year 1955, are not reliably available, but the 1955 tobacco-attributed mortality is then estimated by downwards projection of the tobacco-attributed mortality rates in 1965 and in 1975, even though projections for particular medical causes (e.g. cancer) back to 1955 are not attempted. For countries that have only recently gained independence, the 1990 rates are generally provided, but trend analyses are not.

Populations described

The MAIN TABLES AND FIGURES give analyses for 51 developed populations (see box): 44 countries (of which 15 are the newly independent states from the former USSR), 2 former countries (former USSR and former Yugoslavia), and 5 groups of countries: all developed, all former socialist, all others [i.e. all OECD developed] and, for the European Union, the 12 current members of the EU and the 16 planned members of the EU, the four possible extras being Austria, Finland, Norway and Sweden. The APPENDIX TABLES describe these 51 populations plus 3 others: former German Democratic Republic, all Germany except former GDR, and former Czechoslovakia. Where possible, rates are given for 1990, for certain years before 1990 and, by projection, for 1995. Purely for epidemiological convenience (with no political significance intended) this sometimes involves tabulation of death rates for certain "countries" in years after they had ceased to exist, or before they had become independent states.

51 populations in Main Figures and Tables

All 'Developed' Countries
Former Socialist Economies
OECD Developed Countries
European Union (12 countries)
Planned EU (16 countries)

¶Armenia	¶Lithuania
Australia	Luxembourg
Austria	¶Moldova (Rep. of)
¶Azerbaijan	Netherlands
¶Belarus	New Zealand
Belgium	Norway
Bulgaria	Poland
Canada	Portugal
¶Czech Republic	Romania
Denmark	¶Russian Fedn.
¶Estonia	¶Slovakia
Finland	¶Slovenia
France	Spain
¶Georgia	Sweden
¶Germany	Switzerland
Greece	¶Tajikistan
Hungary	¶Turkmenistan
Ireland	¶Ukraine
Italy	United Kingdom
Japan	United States
¶Kazakhstan	¶USSR (Former)
¶Kyrgyzstan	¶Uzbekistan
¶Latvia	¶Yugoslavia (Former)

¶See General Note on country terminology

5. FORMAT OF THE 51 SETS OF MAIN TABLES AND FIGURES

FIRST standard pair of pages: 1990 analyses

For most populations there are three facing pairs of pages, the first pair (here referred to as pages i & ii) describing mortality from tobacco in 1990 and the subsequent two pairs (here referred to as pages iii, iv, v & vi) describing, where possible, projections for 1995 and trends over the past few decades in mortality from smoking and from causes other than smoking.

The first pair of pages (Figure 6) describes in a standard format the mortality from tobacco in 1990. First, the absolute numbers of deaths from smoking in 1990 are given at the top of page i, subdivided by sex and age, showing that most of the loss of life expectancy from smoking is accounted for by the deaths in middle age (Table 9: the loss of life expectancy per death from smoking is calculated at non-smoker death rates).

Figure 6 (pages i & ii of main tables, quarter size) Format of first pair of pages describing mortality from tobacco in 1990

ALL 'DEVELOPED' COUNTRIES: 1990
Relative importance of deaths in MIDDLE age (35–69)

Age range (years)	Deaths attributed to SMOKING / total deaths (millions) Males	Females	Mean years lost PER DEATH FROM SMOKING
0–34	–/0.5	–/0.2	–
35–69	0.9/2.5	0.2/1.4	22 years
70+	0.6/2.9	0.2/4.0	8 years
All ages	1.4/5.8	0.4/5.6	16 years

Peto, Lopez et al, 1992, 1994

ALL 'DEVELOPED' COUNTRIES: 1990 deaths, by cause
Nos. of deaths attributed to smoking / total deaths (thousands)

	Males			Females		
Age:	0–34	35–69	70+	0–34	35–69	70+
Lung Cancer	–/1.2	231/246	141/156	–/0.7	44/64	42/61
All Cancer	–/27	360/736 (49%)	212/600 (35%)	–/23	56/500 (11%)	56/564 (10%)
Vascular	–/27	318/926	163/1467	–/13	57/508	92/2417
Respiratory	–/38	90/140	139/322	–/29	25/66	63/299
All Other	–/413	97/656	40/462	–/179	22/302	25/718
All Causes	–/504	865/2458 (35%)	554/2851 (19%)	–/244	160/1376 (12%)	236/3998 (6%)

ALL 'DEVELOPED' COUNTRIES: 1990
RISKS OF DYING AT AGES 0–34 and 35–69
(Probability that someone entering an age range would die during it, if the death rates in 1990 were to persist unchanged)

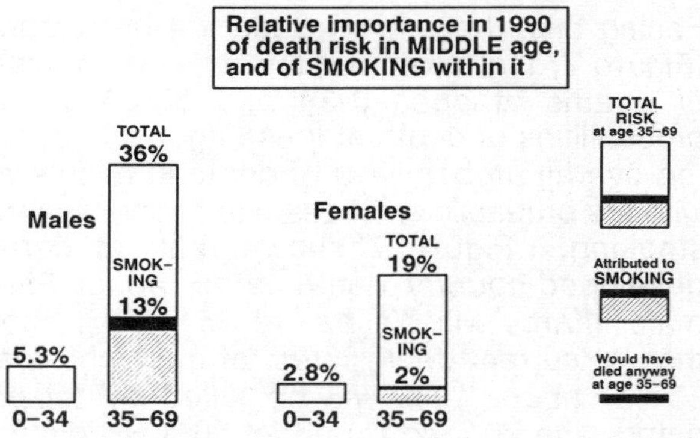

Peto, Lopez et al, 1992, 1994

ALL 'DEVELOPED' COUNTRIES: 1990 deaths, all ages
Nos. of deaths attributed to smoking / total deaths (thousands)

	Males	Females	Males + Females
All Cancer	572/1362 (42%)	112/1087 (10%)	684/2449 (28%)
All Causes	1419/5813 (24%)	396/5618 (7%)	1815/11431 (16%)

Table 9 (from page i of main tables)

ALL "DEVELOPED" COUNTRIES: 1990
Relative importance of deaths in MIDDLE age (35-69)

Age range (years)	Deaths attributed to SMOKING / total deaths (millions) Males	Females	Mean years lost PER DEATH FROM SMOKING
0-34	– / 0.5	– / 0.2	—
35-69	0.9 / 2.5	0.2 / 1.4	22 years
70+	0.6 / 2.9	0.2 / 4.0	8 years
All ages	1.4 / 5.8	0.4 / 5.6	16 years

Peto, Lopez et al, 1992, 1994

Facing this, there is on page ii a bar diagram (Figure 7) that gives not the absolute numbers of deaths at ages 0-34 and 35-69 but the probabilities of death at these ages, contrasting the overall probabilities of death in middle age with the probabilities of death in middle age from smoking. Figure 7 shows that, at current developed-country death rates, about 5% of male infants will die before 35, and it shows that, at current death rates, of men who reach 35 (a) about 13% will be killed by tobacco before age 70, and (b) about 36% will die from any cause before age 70. The last two probabilities cannot be exactly subtracted from each other to find what the probability of death would be in the absence of the deaths attributed to tobacco, because a few of those killed by tobacco would have died before 70 of other causes (solid black shading in Figure 7). This is only a minor correction factor, however: the probability that, in the absence of smoking, a 35-year-old man would die before 70 is not 36% minus 13% (which would be 23%: Figure 7), but instead it is about a quarter. Similar calculations for females are also given, but with few exceptions the female death rates from tobacco are likely to increase sharply over the next few decades, so the real probability that a young woman aged 35 will die from tobacco before age 70 is generally higher than is suggested by the 1990 female mortality from smoking that is illustrated on page ii (Figure 7).

Figure 7 (from page ii of main tables)
ALL "DEVELOPED" COUNTRIES: 1990
Risks of dying at ages 0-34 and 35-69

(Probability that someone entering an age range would die during it, if the death rates in 1990 were to persist unchanged)

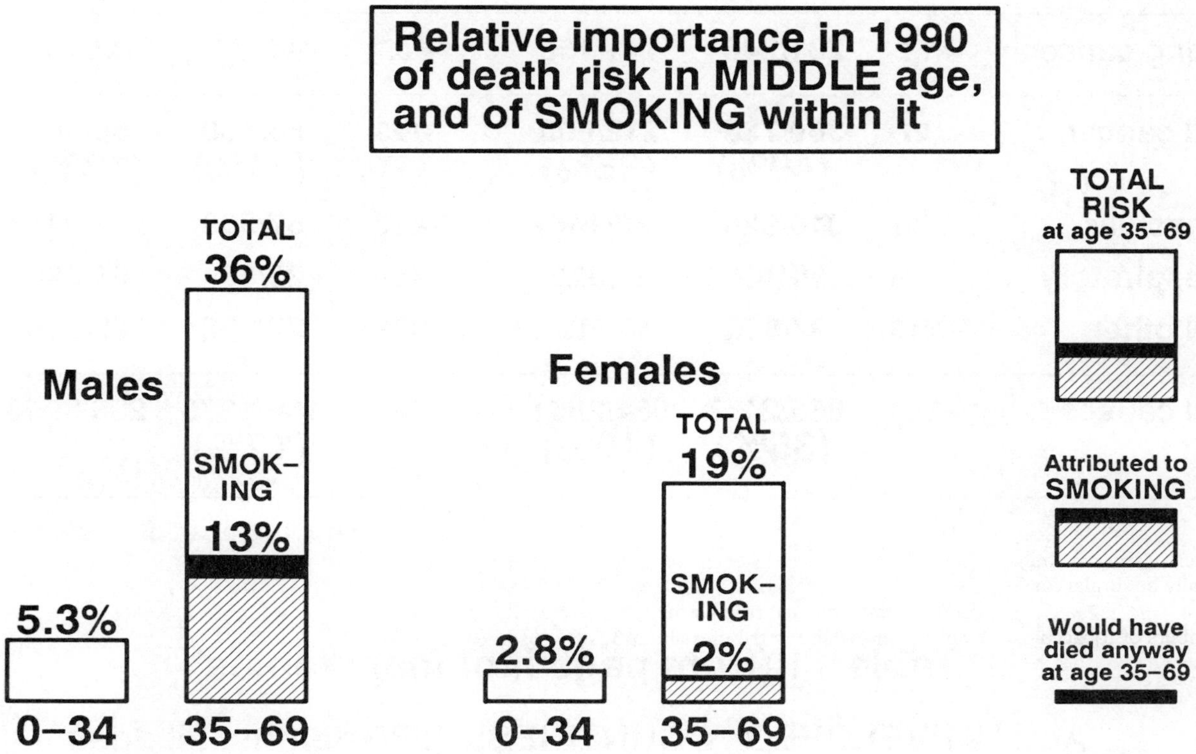

Peto, Lopez et al, 1992, 1994

Returning to page i, at the foot of it are the numbers of tobacco-induced deaths in 1990 from various medical causes (Table 10). For lung cancer, 92% of the male deaths but only 68% of the female deaths in developed countries in 1990 are attributed to smoking (total for both sexes: 87%), but these proportions will vary substantially from one country to another. For cancer as a whole, including lung cancer, tobacco is now responsible, in the aggregate of all developed countries, for about half of all the male cancer deaths in middle age plus about a third of those in old age (Table 10).

Finally, facing this detailed table of age-specific causes, there is a summary of it (Table 11) that combines the numbers of cancer deaths before, during and after middle age. Overall, tobacco was responsible in 1990 for more than a quarter (28%) of all cancer deaths in developed countries, and for about one-sixth (16%) of all deaths in those countries (Table 11). For females, the proportions are smaller (10% of cancer deaths and 7% of all deaths attributed to tobacco), but for males they are larger (42% of cancer deaths and 24% of all deaths in 1990 attributed to tobacco).

Table 10 (from page i of main tables)

ALL "DEVELOPED" COUNTRIES: 1990 deaths, by cause
Nos. of deaths attributed to smoking / total deaths (thousands)

	Males			Females		
Age:	0-34	35-69	70+	0-34	35-69	70+
Lung cancer	–/ 1.2	231/246	141/156	–/ 0.7	44/ 64	42/ 61
All cancer	–/ 27	360/736 (49%)	212/600 (35%)	–/ 23	56/500 (11%)	56/564 (10%)
Vascular	–/ 27	318/926	163/1467	–/ 13	57/508	92/2417
Respiratory	–/ 38	90/140	139/322	–/ 29	25/66	63/299
All other	–/413	97/656	40/462	–/179	22/302	25/718
All causes	–/504	865/2458 (35%)	554/2851 (19%)	–/244	160/1376 (12%)	236/3998 (6%)

Peto, Lopez et al, 1992, 1994

Table 11 (from page ii of main tables)

ALL "DEVELOPED" COUNTRIES: 1990 deaths, all ages
Nos. of deaths attributed to smoking / total deaths (thousands)

	Males	Females	Males + Females
All cancer	572 / 1362 (42%)	112 / 1087 (10%)	684 / 2449 (28%)
All causes	1419 / 5813 (24%)	396 / 5618 (7%)	1815 / 11431 (16%)

Peto, Lopez et al, 1992, 1994

Figure 8 (pages iii & iv of main tables, quarter size) Format of second pair of pages, describing TRENDS IN THE ABSOLUTE NUMBERS of deaths from smoking

ALL 'DEVELOPED' COUNTRIES: 1995 projections
Relative importance of deaths in MIDDLE age (35–69)

Age range (years)	Deaths attributed to SMOKING / total deaths (millions) Males	Females	Mean years lost PER DEATH FROM SMOKING
0–34	–/0.5	–/0.2	–
35–69	0.9/2.4	0.2/1.3	22 years
70+	0.6/2.8	0.3/3.9	8 years
All ages	1.4/5.7	0.5/5.4	16 years

Peto, Lopez et al, 1992, 1994

ALL 'DEVELOPED' COUNTRIES
Smoking–attributed numbers of deaths per year

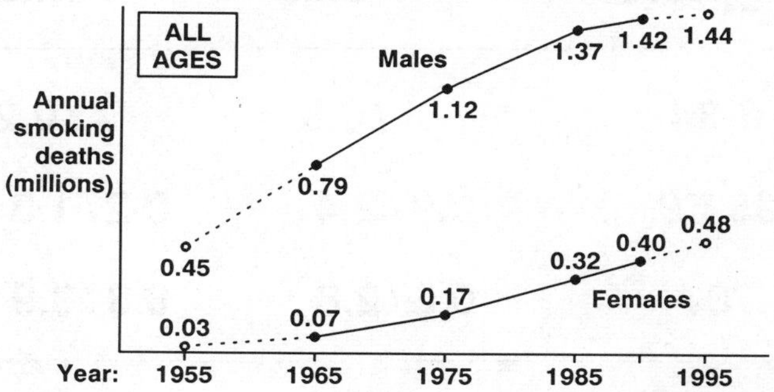

Peto, Lopez et al, 1992, 1994

ALL 'DEVELOPED' COUNTRIES: 1950–2000
Nos. of deaths attributed to smoking / total deaths (thousands)

	Males			Females		
Age:	0–34	35–69	70+	0–34	35–69	70+
1955	–/878	357/1810 (20%)	90/1641 (5%)	–/652	21/1347 (2%)	5.2/2013 (0.3%)
1965	–/664	573/2076 (28%)	220/2019 (11%)	–/426	51/1379 (4%)	19/2496 (0.8%)
1975	–/605	704/2303 (31%)	415/2435 (17%)	–/340	98/1422 (7%)	67/3134 (2%)
1985	–/536	805/2304 (35%)	564/2906 (19%)	–/283	143/1339 (11%)	174/3916 (4%)
1995 (projected)	–/482	870/2435 (36%)	572/2777 (21%)	–/215	171/1312 (13%)	305/3860 (8%)
50–year total* (M=millions), mid–1950 to mid–2000: 62/500M						
1950–2000, by age & sex	–/32M	33/109M (30%)	19/118M (16%)	–/19M	4.8/68M (7%)	5.7/154M (4%)

*Estimated as 10 times the sum of the five annual numbers (for 1955, 1965, 1975, 1985 & 1995)

ALL 'DEVELOPED' COUNTRIES
Smoking–attributed numbers of deaths per year

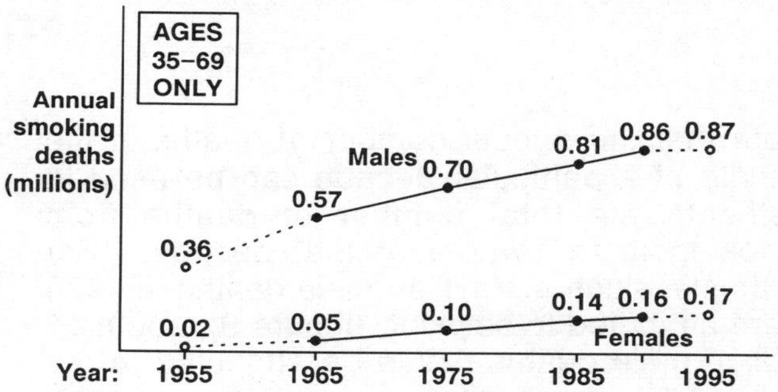

SECOND standard pair of pages: trends in absolute numbers of deaths from smoking, and cumulative 50-year totals

The second and third pairs of pages describe, in a standard format, the trends over the past few decades in the absolute numbers of deaths from tobacco (pages iii & iv) and in the death rates from tobacco (pages v & vi). In populations for which reasonably reliable evidence on trends is not available, the second and third pairs of pages are omitted, and only the first pair remains, describing the 1990 mortality.

Figure 8 illustrates the format of the second pair of pages. The first tabulation is of the projected 1995 numbers (Table 12), which are only very slightly different from the previously tabulated 1990 numbers. On the opposite page there are figures that illustrate, for all ages and then for ages 35-69 only, the numbers of deaths attributed to tobacco in 1955, 1965, 1975, 1985, 1990 and 1995 (Figures 9 & 10).

Table 12 (from page iii of main tables)

ALL "DEVELOPED" COUNTRIES: 1995 projections Relative importance of deaths in MIDDLE age (35-69)

Age range (years)	Deaths attributed to SMOKING / total deaths (millions) Males	Females	Mean years lost PER DEATH FROM SMOKING
0-34	–/0.5	–/0.2	—
35-69	0.9/2.4	0.2/1.3	22 years
70+	0.6/2.8	0.3/3.9	8 years
All ages	1.4/5.7	0.5/5.4	16 years

Peto, Lopez et al, 1992, 1994

Note that the annual number of deaths in the middle of a particular decade can be used to estimate the total number of deaths from smoking in the whole of that decade. For example, since 1.1 million male deaths in 1975 were attributed to smoking (Figure 9), about 11 million male deaths would be attributed to the habit in the decade from mid-1970 to mid-1980. Such arguments yield estimates of numbers of deaths from smoking in these developed countries in each of the past five decades, and hence, by addition, in the whole of the second half of the 20th century.

This total is given, at the foot of page iii, in a tabulation, subdivided by age and sex, of the numbers of deaths from tobacco in each of these five decades (Table 13). In Table 13, the deaths attributed to tobacco are also expressed as a percentage of all deaths, and the changes in these percentages over the past few decades are very different for male and female, and for middle and old age. Among males the proportions of deaths attributed to tobacco have increased moderately in middle age (from 20% in the 1950s to 36% in the 1990s) and substantially in old age (from 5% to 21%), and may well now be about at their maximum. Among females, however, the epidemic continues to increase, with the percentage of deaths attributed to tobacco increasing from a very small number in the 1950s to, by the 1990s, 13% of all deaths in middle age and 8% in old age (Table 13). The 50-year totals at the foot of Table 13 have already been given in Tables 2, 7 and 8. In total, tobacco is estimated to account for about 60 million of the 500 million deaths that will have taken place in developed countries during the second half of the present century. Table 13 suggests that, on present smoking patterns, both the absolute number of deaths and the proportion of all deaths that is attributed to tobacco will be greater next century than this.

Figure 9 (from page iv of main tables)
ALL "DEVELOPED" COUNTRIES, 1955 to 1995
Smoking-attributed numbers of deaths per year at ALL AGES

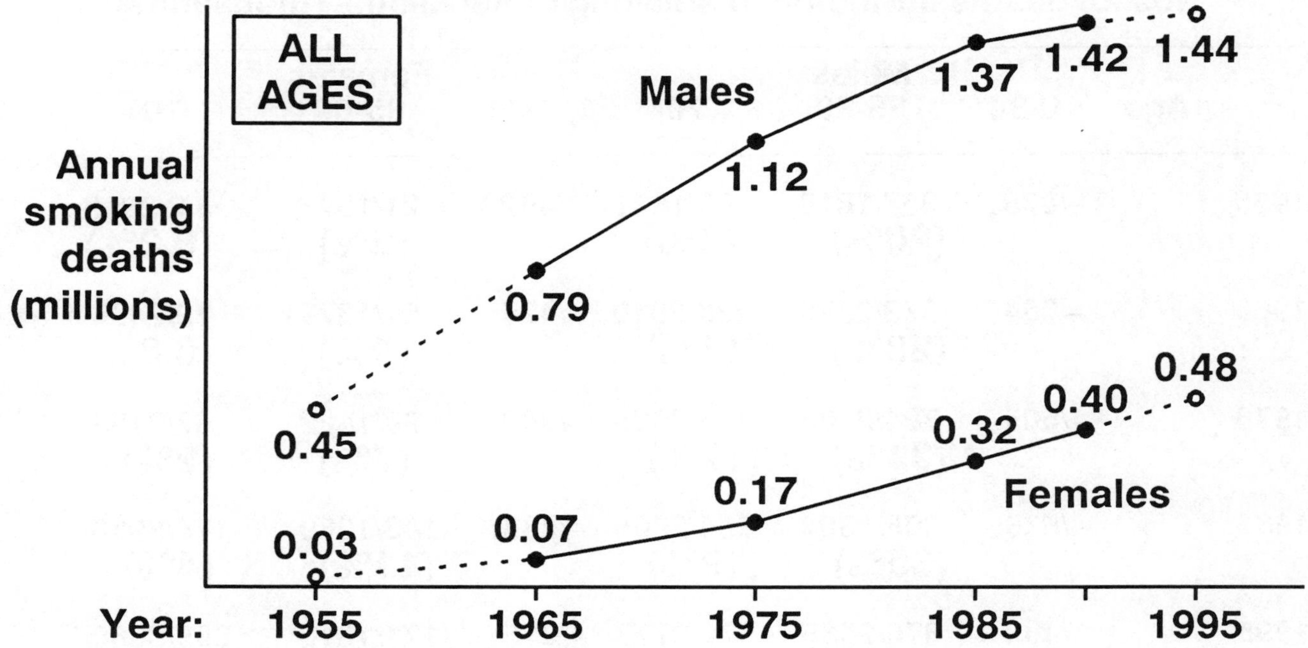

Figure 10 (from page iv of main tables)
ALL "DEVELOPED" COUNTRIES, 1955 to 1995
Smoking-attributed numbers of deaths per year at AGES 35-69 ONLY

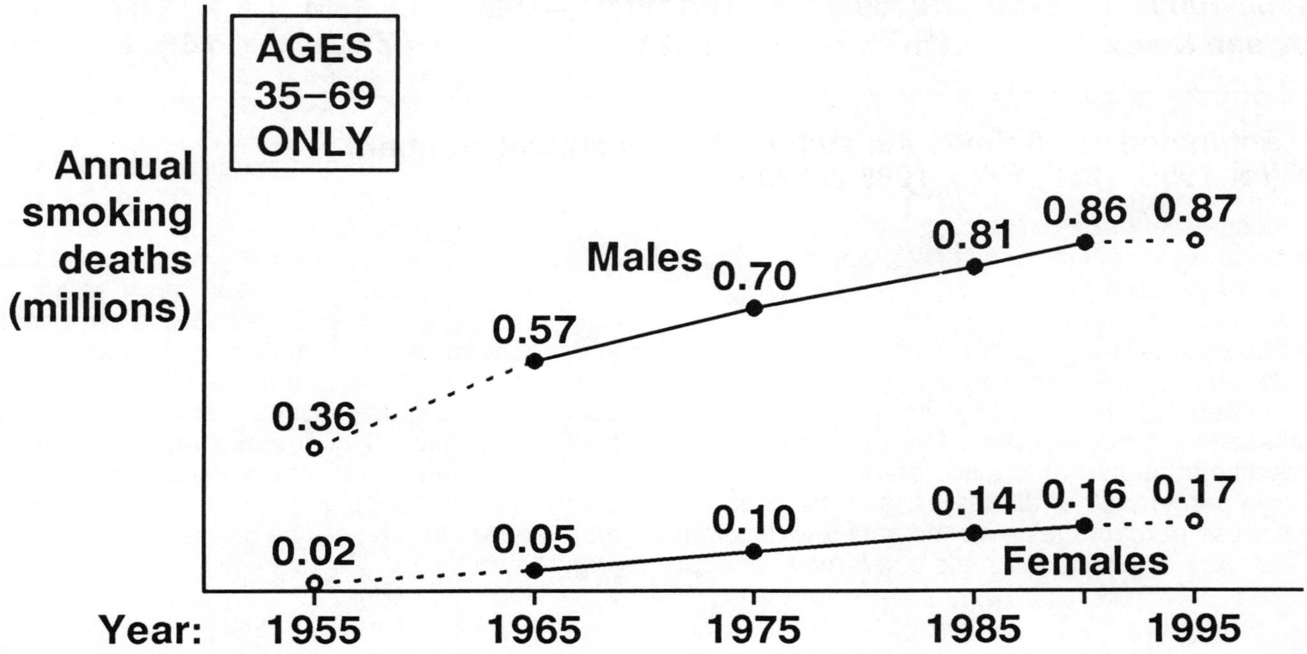

Table 13 (from page iii of main tables)

ALL "DEVELOPED" COUNTRIES: 1950-2000

Nos. of deaths attributed to smoking / total deaths (thousands)

	Males			Females		
Age:	0-34	35-69	70+	0-34	35-69	70+
1955	–/878	357/1810 (20%)	90/1641 (5%)	–/652	21/1347 (2%)	5.2/2013 (0.3%)
1965	–/664	573/2076 (28%)	220/2019 (11%)	–/426	51/1379 (4%)	19/2496 (0.8%)
1975	–/605	704/2303 (31%)	415/2435 (17%)	–/340	98/1422 (7%)	67/3134 (2%)
1985	–/536	805/2304 (35%)	564/2906 (19%)	–/283	143/1339 (11%)	174/3916 (4%)
1995 (projected)	–/482	870/2435 (36%)	572/2777 (21%)	–/215	171/1312 (13%)	305/3860 (8%)
50-year total* (M=millions), mid-1950 to mid-2000:						**62/500M**
1950-2000, by age & sex	–/32M	33/109M (30%)	19/118M (16%)	–/19M	4.8/68M (7%)	5.7/154M (4%)

* Estimated as 10 times the sum of the five annual numbers (for 1955, 1965, 1975, 1985 & 1995)

Figure 11 (pages v & vi of main tables, quarter size)
Format of the final pair of pages, describing TRENDS IN THE DEATH RATES attributed to smoking

ALL 'DEVELOPED' COUNTRIES

ALL DEATHS (annual rates per 1000): Trends in mortality attributed to smoking, and in other mortality

	Males				Females			
	35–69		70–79		35–69		70–79	
Attributed to SMOKING?	Yes	No	Yes	No	Yes	No	Yes	No
1955	3.01	12.7	4.76	71.8	0.14	9.29	0.19	56.0
1965	4.15	11.0	9.33	65.4	0.29	7.68	0.50	49.7
1975	4.50	10.0	13.8	58.9	0.50	6.71	1.17	44.2
1985	4.62	8.70	14.5	52.7	0.71	5.78	2.24	38.3
1990	4.49	8.21	13.6	46.6	0.71	5.35	2.86	33.5

35–69 = mean of 7 age-specific rates; 70–79 = mean of 2 rates (70–74 & 75–79) Peto, Lopez et al, 1992, 1994

ALL 'DEVELOPED' COUNTRIES

ALL CANCER DEATHS (annual rates per 1000): Trends in mortality attributed to smoking, and in other mortality

	Males				Females			
	35–69		70–79		35–69		70–79	
Attributed to SMOKING?	Yes	No	Yes	No	Yes	No	Yes	No
1955	...	...	...	...	...	...	...	...
1965	1.39	2.18	3.16	10.0	0.07	2.29	0.10	7.50
1975	1.61	2.05	4.89	9.62	0.14	2.12	0.26	7.02
1985	1.84	1.99	5.82	9.59	0.23	1.98	0.62	6.83
1990	1.91	2.01	5.96	9.60	0.25	1.94	0.89	6.72

35–69 = mean of 7 age-specific rates; 70–79 = mean of 2 rates (70–74 & 75–79) Peto, Lopez et al, 1992, 1994

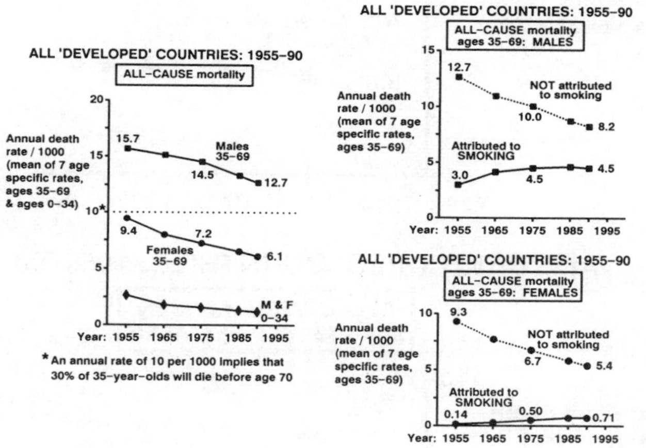

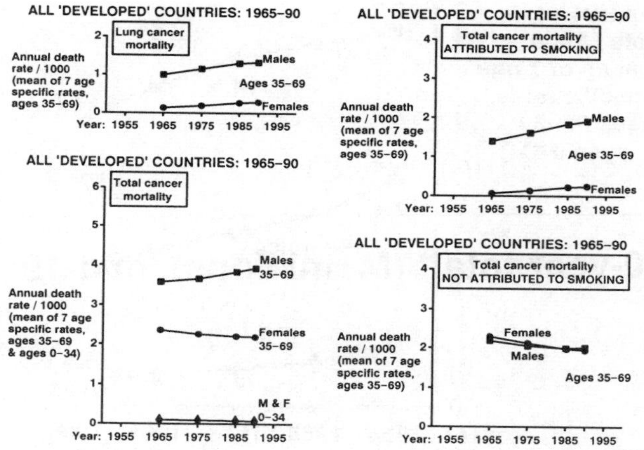

THIRD and final standard pair of pages: trends in death rates from smoking, both for all causes and for neoplastic causes

Figure 11 illustrates the format of the final pair of pages for each population, which describes trends in the death rates that are attributed to tobacco, and trends in the death rates that would remain if the tobacco deaths were subtracted from all deaths. The all-cause death rates are described first (on page v), followed by the cancer death rates (on page vi). "Cancers" comprise all malignant neoplasms (9th ICD 140-208, including leukaemias and lymphomas but excluding solid tumours that are not malignant). On both pages, the trends are given in tabular form at the top of the page, and in graphic form at the bottom.

Figure 12 (from page v of main tables) ALL "DEVELOPED" COUNTRIES Trends from 1955 to 1990 in all-cause mortality rates at ages 0-34 and 35-69, with the overall trends on the left and, on the right, the same male and female trends at ages 35-69 subdivided into the parts attributed to smoking (solid lines) and not attributed to smoking (dotted lines)

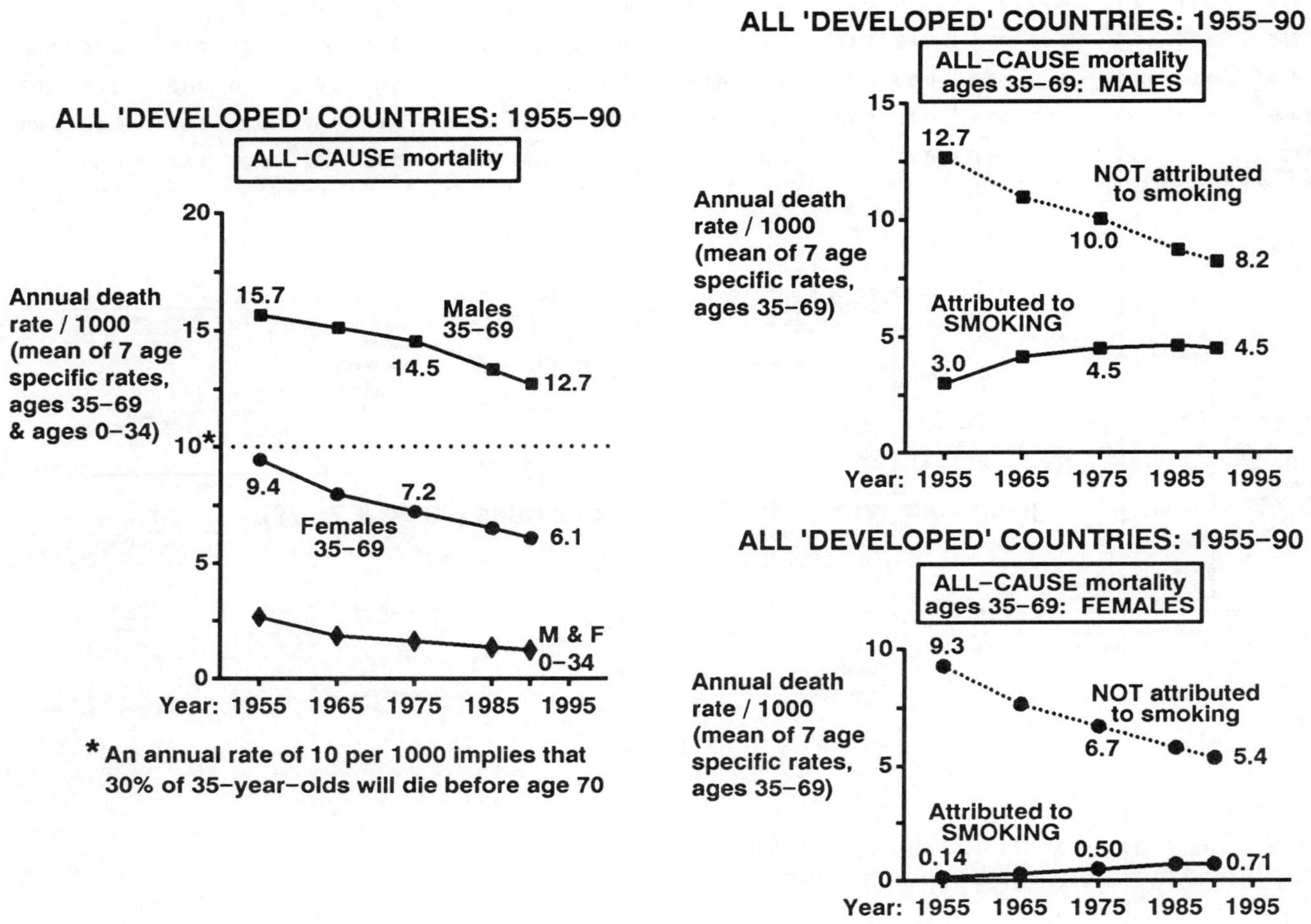

Overall in developed countries the death rates before middle age and in middle age improved substantially over the period 1955 to 1990 (left side of Figure 12), decreasing in middle age from 15.7 down to 12.7 per 1000 in males, and from 9.4 down to 6.1 in females. The horizontal dotted line corresponds to an average annual death rate of 10 per 1000: if this was the average of the death rates from 35 to 69 then it can be shown that the overall probability that a 35-year-old would die before 70 would be 30%.

[Note that the following formula can be used to convert an average death rate of R per 1000 over an age range spanning Y years into P, the probability of surviving: P = exp(-Y * R / 1000). In this case, P = exp(-35 * 10 / 1000) = 0.70.]

Table 14 (from page v of main tables)

ALL "DEVELOPED" COUNTRIES
ALL DEATHS (annual rates per 1000)
Trends in mortality attributed to smoking, and in other mortality

Attributed to SMOKING?	Males 35-69 Yes	Males 35-69 No	Males 70-79 Yes	Males 70-79 No	Females 35-69 Yes	Females 35-69 No	Females 70-79 Yes	Females 70-79 No
1955	3.01	12.7	4.76	71.8	0.14	9.29	0.19	56.0
1965	4.15	11.0	9.33	65.4	0.29	7.68	0.50	49.7
1975	4.50	10.0	13.8	58.9	0.50	6.71	1.17	44.2
1985	4.62	8.70	14.5	52.7	0.71	5.78	2.24	38.3
1990	4.49	8.21	13.6	46.6	0.71	5.35	2.86	33.5

35-69 = mean of 7 age-specific rates; 70-79 = mean of 2 rates (70-74 & 75-79).

Residual mortality trends when smoking-attributed mortality has been subtracted out

The 1990 male and female death rates of 12.7 and 6.1 per 1000 in Figure 12 imply probabilities of 36% and 19% that a 35-year-old would, at these 1990 average death rates, die before age 70, as has already been illustrated (Figure 7). The overall decrease in mortality is, however, composed of an increase in mortality from tobacco, plus an even steeper decrease in the mortality that is not attributed to tobacco (right side of Figure 12), from 12.7 down to 8.2 in males, and from 9.3 down to 5.4 in females. At the top of page v the same data are given in tabular form (Table 14), together with the somewhat less reliable data for males and females at 70-79 years of age, which show similar patterns. The trends at even older ages (80+) would be even less reliable, and are not given. The trends at younger ages are also not given as, to be conservative, none of the deaths before middle age are attributed to tobacco, but there have likewise been substantial decreases between 1955 and 1990 in the average annual death rates at ages 0-34 (from 3.1 down to 1.6 per 1000 for males, and from 2.3 down to 0.8 per 1000 for females: see Appendix tables).

Figure 13 (from page vi of main tables) ALL "DEVELOPED" COUNTRIES Trends from 1965 to 1990 in cancer mortality rates at ages 0-34 and 35-69, with the trends in middle age subdivided into the parts attributed to smoking (upper right) and not attributed to smoking (lower right)

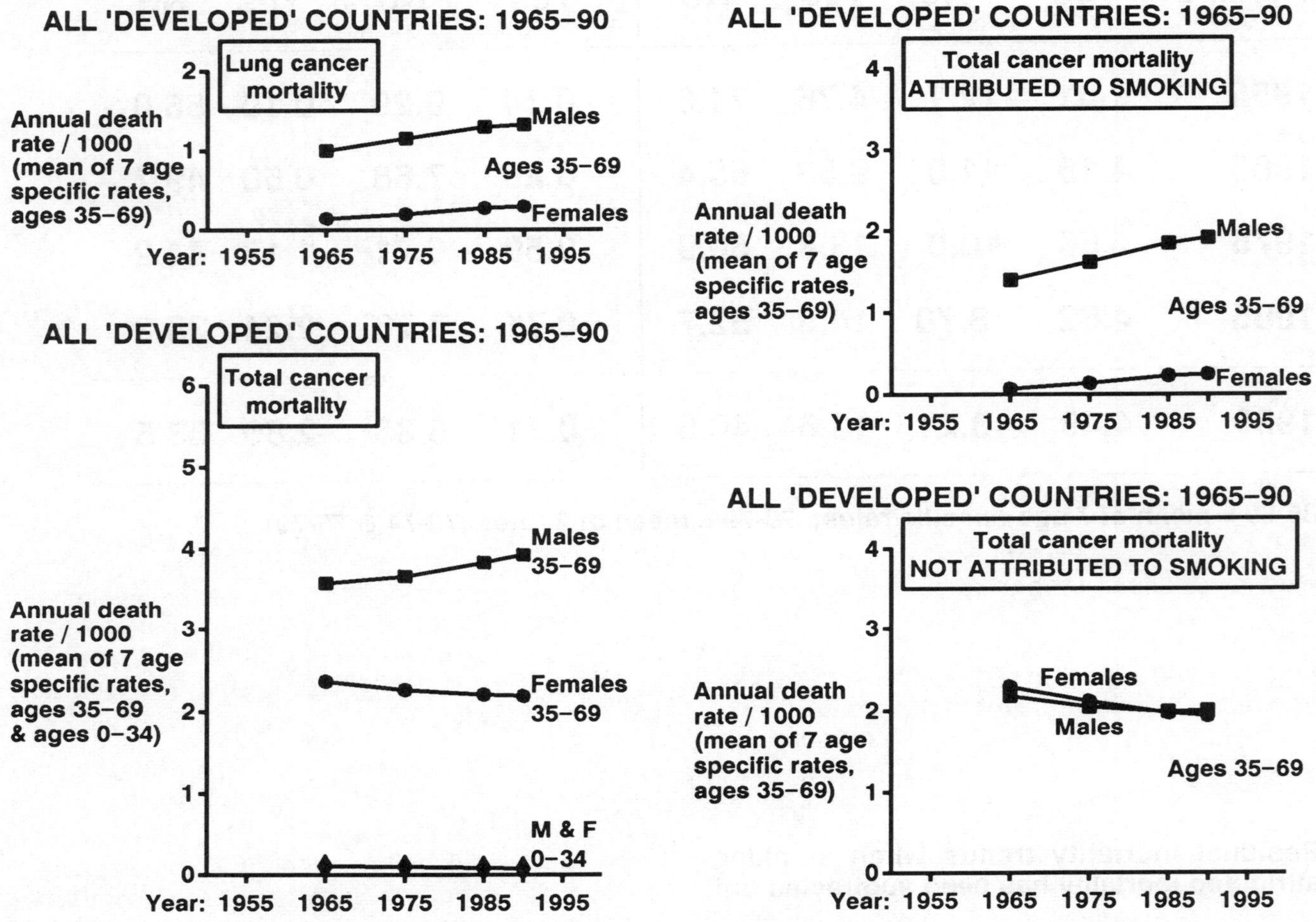

Residual cancer trends: no generalised increase

Death from cancer is, in developed countries, common only in middle and old age. At 0-34 years of age the cancer death rates are already low, and are still decreasing (Figure 13, lower left), because the types of cancer that arise before middle age are uncommon diseases, against which chemotherapy is often effective. In contrast, in middle age cancer remains a substantial cause of death, particularly among males, and in many countries the male cancer death rates at ages 35-69 are not decreasing. But, the commonest neoplastic cause of death in developed countries is lung cancer, and in many developed countries the lung cancer rates are still rising (Figure 13, upper left), as are the overall cancer death rates in middle age that are attributed to tobacco (Figure 13, upper right). These include most of the lung cancer deaths,

Table 15 (from page vi of main tables)

ALL "DEVELOPED" COUNTRIES
ALL CANCER DEATHS (annual rates per 1000)
Trends in mortality attributed to smoking, and in other mortality

	Males				Females			
Attributed to	35-69		70-79		35-69		70-79	
SMOKING?	Yes	No	Yes	No	Yes	No	Yes	No
1955	...	...	...	...	...	...	...	...
1965	1.39	2.18	3.16	10.0	0.07	2.29	0.10	7.50
1975	1.61	2.05	4.89	9.62	0.14	2.12	0.26	7.02
1985	1.84	1.99	5.82	9.59	0.23	1.98	0.62	6.83
1990	1.91	2.01	5.96	9.60	0.25	1.94	0.89	6.72

35-69 = mean of 7 age-specific rates; 70-79 = mean of 2 rates (70-74 & 75-79).

plus a smaller number of tobacco-attributed deaths from other types of cancer. When the tobacco-attributed cancer mortality is subtracted from the overall cancer mortality, to estimate the trends in cancer mortality that might be seen in middle age in the absence of tobacco, the overall rates that remain are similar in males and in females, and are not increasing (Figure 13, lower right).

At the top of page vi the same cancer rates for ages 35-69 are given in tabular form (Table 15), together with the rates for ages 70-79, which exhibit the same pattern of increases in the mortality attributed to smoking and slight decreases in the aggregate of all other cancer mortality. It is noteworthy that there are, if anything, on page vi slight decreases in overall cancer mortality at ages 0-34, and in the cancer mortality at ages 35-69 and 70-79 that is not attributed to smoking. There are, of course, still some uncertainties about exactly how much of the cancer mortality in developed countries should be attributed to tobacco, but still these slight decreases mean that there is in developed countries no good evidence of any generalised increase in overall cancer mortality over and above what might plausibly be ascribed to tobacco.

The fact that there is no generalised increase in cancer among non-smokers does not, of course, mean that there are no new causes to be sought other than smoking, for although some diseases such as stomach cancer are definitely decreasing, others such as melanoma or certain types of non-Hodgkin's lymphoma (NHL) are definitely increasing. It does, however, accurately reflect the overwhelming importance of tobacco as a cause of cancer in developed countries. This is true in OECD developed countries (Figure 14), but it is even more importantly true in the former socialist economies (Figure 15): indeed, once the tobacco-attributed cancer deaths are removed, the trends in the remaining cancer mortality rates in middle age are remarkably similar for male and female and for "East" and "West".

Figure 14 (from page vi of main tables)
OECD DEVELOPED COUNTRIES
Trends from 1955 to 1990 in cancer mortality rates at ages 0-34 and 35-69, with the trends in middle age subdivided into the parts attributed to smoking (upper right) and not attributed to smoking (lower right)

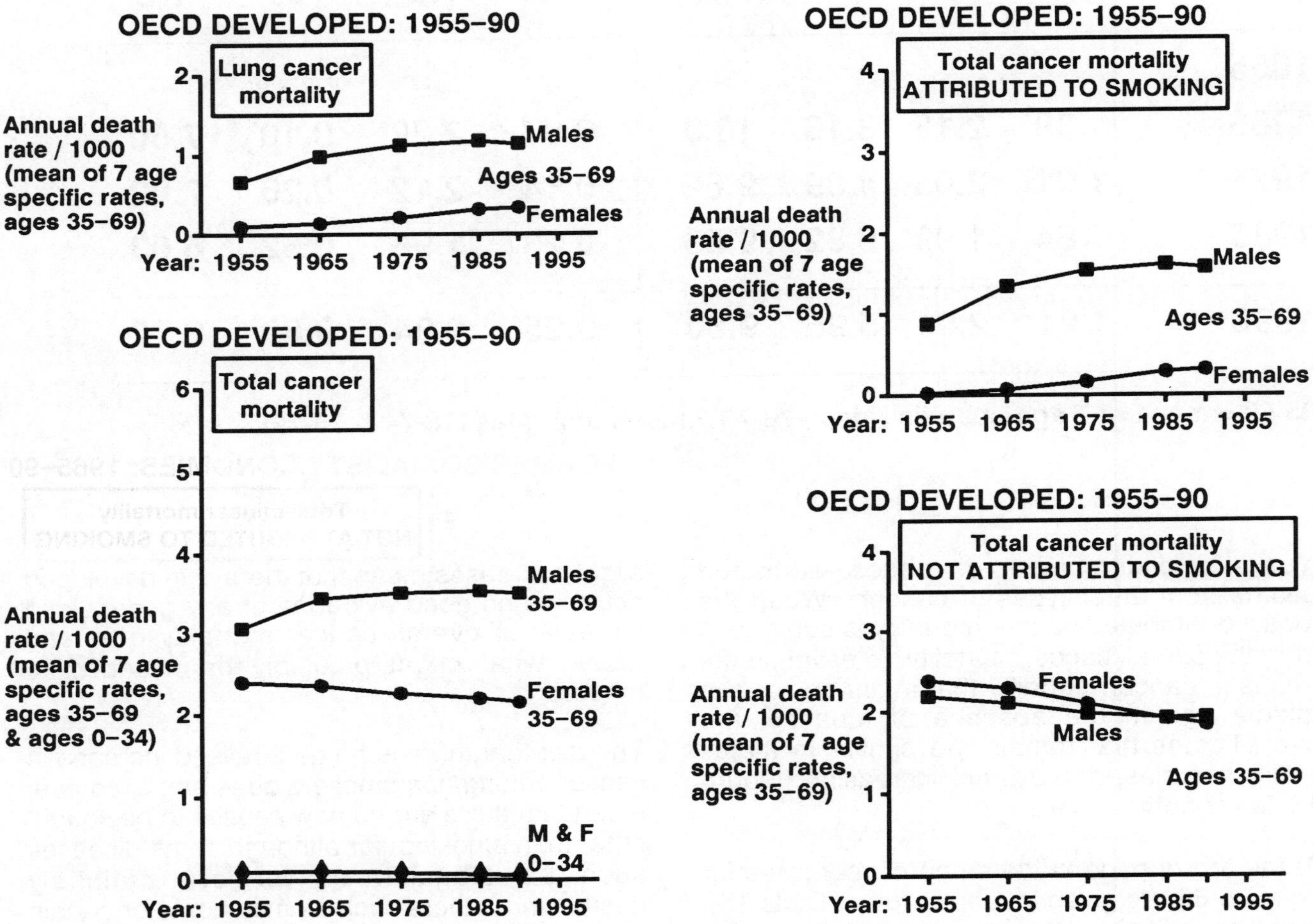

Figure 15 (from page vi of main tables) FORMER SOCIALIST ECONOMIES. Trends from 1965 to 1990 in cancer mortality rates at ages 0-34 and 35-69, with the trends in middle age subdivided into the parts attributed to smoking (upper right) and not attributed to smoking (lower right)

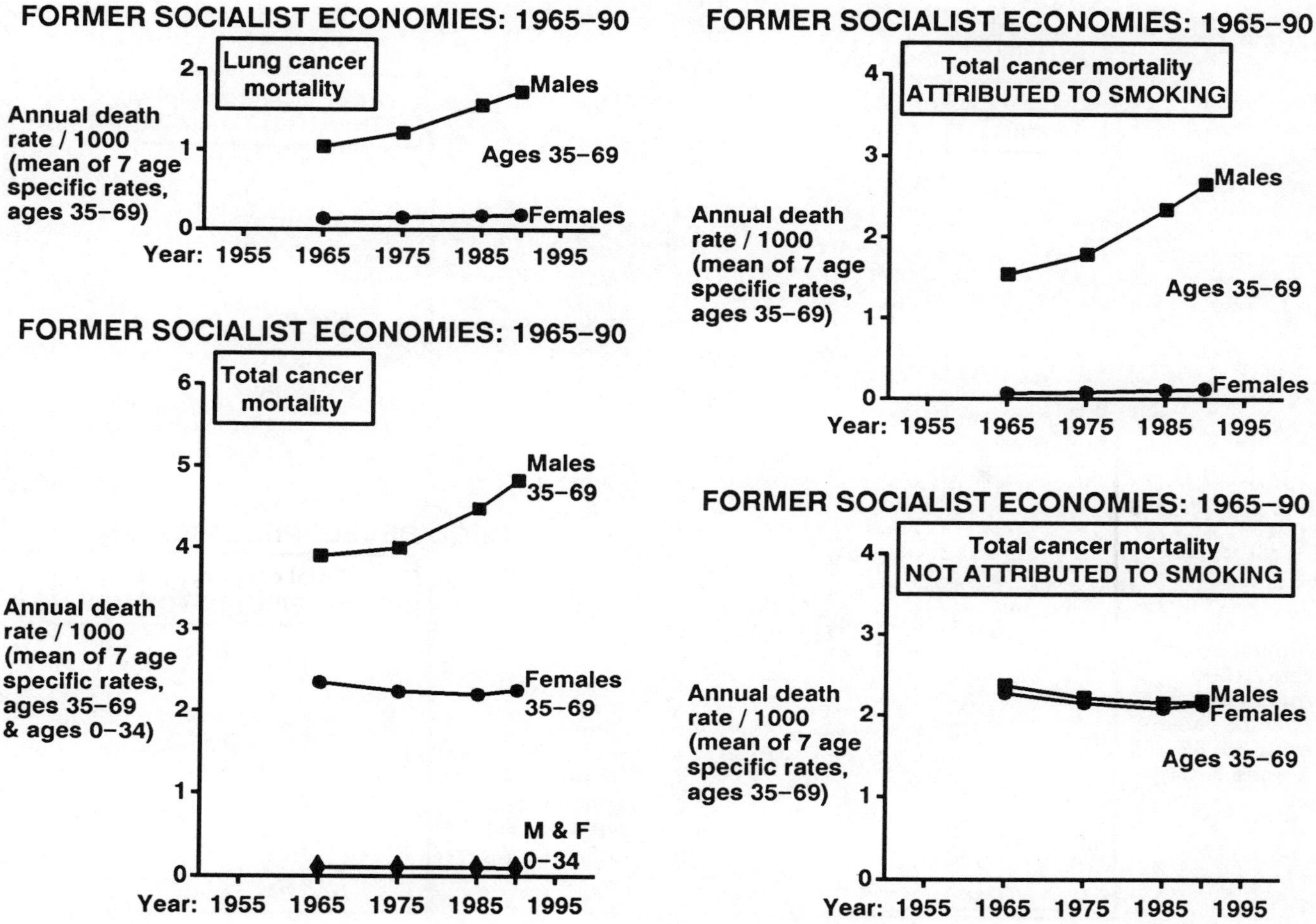

In Figures 14 and 15, the cancer rates for many different populations have been combined, but similar findings will recur when the separate cancer rates in these many different populations are compared with each other in Chapter 8 (Figures 68-76).

Although the cancer mortality that is attributed to smoking is very different in different populations, and is changing rapidly, the residual cancer mortality that is not attributed to smoking is remarkably similar in both sexes and in all these developed populations.

6. FORMAT OF THE 54 SETS OF APPENDIX TABLES

FIRST standard pair of appendix pages for various populations: 1990 ONLY. Age-standardised and age-specific death rates for 44 causes or groups of causes

The death rates on which the main tables and figures were based, together with some of the calculations from them, are given in the 54 sets of Appendix tables, with six standard pages of tables in each set. For each population the death rates are available for 1985 and for 1990, and hence for projected 1995. For the newly independent states of the former USSR no pre-1980 death rates were available, but for other populations the cited data go back to 1975 and 1965 — and, for most of the OECD developed countries, to 1955.

For each population, the FIRST standard pair of Appendix pages always gives the 1990 numbers of deaths, the age-standardised death rates and the age-specific death rates for each of about 44 causes of death, or groups of causes (and, for each, the Appendix table also specifies the 9th ICD categories that it includes, even in populations that did not use the 9th ICD in 1990). These 1990 vital statistics include the numbers used to calculate tobacco-attributed mortality in 1990, and they also provide a useful context for the main tables and figures on death from tobacco. It can be helpful to contrast the mortality from tobacco in a particular country with the mortality in that country from certain other causes or diseases, such as murder, traffic accidents or breast cancer. More generally, those concerned with the public health or with epidemiological research need to be able to refer conveniently to the mortality rates from particular diseases in particular populations, and the tabulations of 1990 data for each country facilitate this. Indeed, for many of the newly independent states of the former USSR such information is not widely known, as it has only recently become available. Also, for the five main groupings of developed countries the overall 1990 death rates provided are themselves of considerable independent interest, and reveal much higher death rates from many conditions in the former socialist economies than in the OECD developed countries.

To illustrate the list of 44 conditions and to show how they can vary between different populations, Tables 16 to 19 bring together some of the numbers from the Appendix tabulations of 1990 mortality for all developed countries (pp.230-1), for the former socialist economies (pp.236-7) and for the OECD developed countries (pp.242-3).

Table 16 describes the cancer mortality patterns. Overall in developed countries, lung cancer now causes twice as many deaths as any other neoplastic disease: indeed, among males it causes three times as many. If cancers of reproductive sites are excluded, then cancer rates as a whole in middle age are substantially higher in males than in females, and in the former socialist economies than in the OECD developed countries (Table 16), but these extreme differences are largely attributable to differences in tobacco-attributed cancer mortality (Figures 14 & 15). Examination of the appendix tables from which Table 16 was abstracted will show only relatively small death rates before middle age from neoplastic disease (the annual male and female cancer death rates per 100,000 in 1990 being 8 and 7 respectively at ages 0-34, as against 392 and 219 at ages 35-69). Stomach cancer rates are still substantial, particularly in the former socialist economies, but experience in many countries suggests that large decreases in this type of cancer over the next few decades can be expected (Figures 2 & 3), even though the disease is somewhat associated with smoking.

Table 16 (from FIRST standard pair of Appendix pages for various populations: pp.230-1, 236-7 & 242-3)

1990 mortality, CANCER

Cause of death (cancer)	Thousands of deaths, ALL DEVELOPED	Rate / 100 000, 35-69* FORMER SOCIALIST		OECD DEVELOPED	
Sex:	M & F	M	F	M	F
Mouth & pharynx	52	21	2	12	2
Oesophagus	62	18	4	14	2
Stomach	244	75	30	28	12
Large intestine	273	36	25	33	22
Liver	55	14	4	13	3
Pancreas	118	18	10	16	10
Larynx	33	20	1	7	1
Lung	530	173	19	114	34
Melanoma	23	4	2	4	2
Breast	177	—	38	—	48
Cervix	33	—	14	—	6
Other uterus	38	—	11	—	6
Ovary	60	—	15	—	14
Prostate	110	12	—	16	—
Bladder	63	10	2	8	2
Other & ill-defined	406	62	37	60	35
Hodgkin's disease	8	2	1	1	1
Myeloma & NHL	89	9	5	14	9
Leukaemia	76	10	6	9	6
ALL CANCER	2449	483	225	351	215

* Mean of the 7 age-specific rates, ages 35-39 to 65-69.

Table 17 (from FIRST standard pair of Appendix pages for various populations: pp.230-1, 236-7 & 242-3)

1990 mortality, VASCULAR

Cause of death (vascular)	Thousands of deaths, ALL DEVELOPED	Rate / 100 000, 35-69 FORMER SOCIALIST		OECD DEVELOPED	
Sex:	M & F	M	F	M	F
Rheumatic	47	14	16	2	3
Hypertensive	167	25	17	10	6
Ischaemic heart*	2309	449	161	197	63
Pulm. embolus, etc**	65	7	5	5	4
Stroke	1470	218	140	57	36
Other vascular*	1300	115	46	83	36
ALL VASCULAR	5358	829	386	354	148

* The distinction between ischaemic heart and other vascular disease is very different in different populations.

** Pulmonary embolism and other venous diseases.

Table 17 describes the main vascular mortality patterns. For rheumatic heart disease the male and female death rates are similar, but for all other vascular causes of death in middle age the rates are far higher for males than for females. Ischaemic heart disease and stroke predominate, and in middle age both are much more common in the former socialist economies than in the OECD developed countries. (Death from ischaemic heart disease is twice as common, and death from stroke is four times as common.) These geographic differences cannot plausibly be accounted for by tobacco. But, vascular disease is the commonest cause of premature death in developed countries, and the high background death rates from vascular disease in the former socialist economies mean that a given level of smoking is likely to produce a much greater absolute risk of vascular death there than it does in the United States (Tables 3 & 4). Moreover, at least among males, the level of smoking is now higher in many former socialist economies than in the USA. Direct evidence of the effects of smoking on vascular diseases in these populations would, however, be of considerable interest.

Table 18 (from FIRST standard pair of Appendix pages for various populations: pp.230-1, 236-7 & 242-3)

1990 mortality, OTHER DISEASES

Cause of death (disease)	Thousands of deaths, ALL DEVELOPED	Rate / 100 000, 35-69 FORMER SOCIALIST		OECD DEVELOPED	
Sex:	M & F	M	F	M	F
Tuberculosis	42	26	4	3	1
Other infective	89	4	2	8	5
Chronic respiratory*	435	96	26	33	16
Other respiratory*	459	22	7	26	12
Peptic ulcer	46	12	3	4	2
Liver cirrhosis	178	50	21	38	14
Renal disease	121	17	14	8	5
Pregnancy, etc	—	—	—	—	—
Congenital/perinatal	146	—	—	—	—
Ill-defined causes	348	28	8	17	7
Other medical causes	892	76	51	84	51
ALL DISEASES except cancer or vascular	**2759**	**332**	**138**	**222**	**113**

* The distinction between chronic respiratory and other respiratory disease is very different in different populations

Table 18 gives the non-neoplastic, non-vascular medical causes of death, and Table 19 gives the non-medical causes. In middle age, all the death rates are higher among males, and most of the death rates are substantially higher in the former socialist economies than in the OECD developed countries. For males, death from respiratory disease is twice as common in the former socialist economies, and the death rate ratio is even more extreme for death from pulmonary tuberculosis, but in absolute terms the greatest difference is in the non-medical causes: homicide, suicide and, particularly, accidents. The death rate of 235 per 100,000 from non-medical causes in the former socialist economies means that, in the absence of other causes of death, about 8% of those aged 35 would die of such causes before 70 (and, further scrutiny of the Appendix tables reveals even higher rates in the Baltic republics and in the Russian Federation).

The totals from Tables 16-19 are brought together in Table 20, displaying again the differences between male and female and between the two groups of countries. Much greater variation, however, can be found when the Appendix tables are used to make comparisons between specific pairs of countries, especially if attention is directed to particular causes of death.

Table 19 (from FIRST standard pair of Appendix pages for various populations: pp.230-1, 236-7 & 242-3)

1990 mortality, NON-MEDICAL

Cause of death (external)	Thousands of deaths, ALL DEVELOPED	Rate / 100 000, 35-69 FORMER SOCIALIST		OECD DEVELOPED	
Sex:	M & F	M	F	M	F
Motor vehicle	213	43	10	19	8
Fire	20	4	2	2	1
Suicide	188	51	13	26	10
Homicide	67	17	6	5	1
ALL NON-MEDICAL	865	235	56	79	28

Table 20 (from FIRST standard pair of Appendix pages for various populations: pp.230-1, 236-7 & 242-3)

1990 mortality, ALL CAUSES

Cause of death	Thousands of deaths, ALL DEVELOPED	Rate / 100 000, 35-69 FORMER SOCIALIST		OECD DEVELOPED	
Sex:	M & F	M	F	M	F
Cancer	2449	483	225	351	215
Vascular disease	5358	829	386	354	148
Other diseases	2759	332	138	222	113
Non-medical	865	235	56	79	28
ALL CAUSES	11431	1879	805	1006	504

SECOND standard pair of appendix pages for various populations: 1990, and also other years. Death rates in middle and in old age from the 11 broad groups of causes that are used for estimating the effects of smoking

Partly so that trends can be seen, and partly to make available the actual numbers from which the tobacco-attributed mortality rates in the main tables and figures were calculated, the SECOND standard pair of appendix pages for each population gives the age-specific death rates in 1990 and in other years from 11 groups of causes in middle and old age. In each such pair of appendix pages, the figures for 1990 are given in a bold typeface, and the projections for 1995 are given in italics. The method of projection from the 1985 and 1990 death rates to the 1995 rates is fairly straightforward: apart from "all causes", or "all cancer" (which are calculated by summation of other categories), there are 9 groups of causes, and the age-specific rates for these in 1995 are estimated by multiplying the 1990 rate by an appropriate extrapolation factor, calculated (with some smoothing) from the 1985-1990 trend.

As well as providing the foundations for the calculations that attribute mortality to tobacco, the trends over the past few decades in all-cause mortality and in particular causes of death are of substantial independent interest, either when large groups of countries are considered or when particular countries are. However, care must be taken when comparing different periods or different countries not to be misled by the effects of changes in traditions of death certification, particularly when considering trends in mortality in old age. In middle age, however, or at earlier ages, the trends may be informative (Table 21), particularly over the period 1975-1990 in which the data from most developed countries should be reasonably reliable.

Over this period, vascular mortality was increasing in the former socialist economies but decreasing rapidly elsewhere, while respiratory mortality was decreasing in parallel in both these groups of countries. More detailed scrutiny of the Appendix tables will, however, show substantial heterogeneity in these and other trends within the former socialist economies, and within the OECD developed countries. (For example, the trends in respiratory mortality are quite different in British and in Canadian women, the former being substantial but decreasing, while the latter is low and constant.)

Extrapolation and smoothing: for any one particular age group (e.g. 0-4, 5-9, 10-14, ..., 70-74, 75-79 or 80+) the extrapolation factor is estimated as follows. Average the (two or three) death rates in that and in any immediately adjacent age groups, do likewise for 1990, and calculate the ratio of the 1990 average to the 1985 average. This is the extrapolation factor that is to be used, except that if it exceeds 1.41 (which would imply a rate of increase more extreme than one doubling per decade) then use 1.41, and if it is less than 0.71 (implying a rate of decrease more extreme than one halving per decade) then use 0.71.

Table 21 (from SECOND standard pair of Appendix pages for various populations: pp.238-9,& 244-5)

(a) Trends in overall & in neoplastic death rates, 35-69*, in FORMER SOCIALIST & in OECD DEVELOPED countries

Year of death	All causes, 35-69*				Neoplastic, 35-69*			
	Former socialist		OECD developed		Former socialist		OECD developed	
Sex:	M	F	M	F	M	F	M	F
1955	1766	1025	1500	908	...	...	307	241
1965	1511	788	1509	800	390	234	345	237
1975	1716	816	1340	672	400	223	352	227
1985	1899	848	1103	553	449	220	354	220
1990	1879	805	1006	504	483	225	351	215
1995 (projected)	*1837*	*762*	*916*	*460*	*512*	*229*	*343*	*208*

* Mean of the 7 age-specific rates per 100,000, ages 35-39 to 65-69.

(b) Trends in vascular & respiratory death rates, 35-69*, in FORMER SOCIALIST & in OECD DEVELOPED countries

Year of death	Vascular, 35-69*				Respiratory, 35-69*			
	Former socialist		OECD developed		Former socialist		OECD developed	
Sex:	M	F	M	F	M	F	M	F
1955	...	...	656	387	...	...	88	36
1965	535	332	675	331	131	46	97	32
1975	697	378	582	255	159	56	89	32
1985	841	420	435	182	149	43	67	29
1990	829	386	354	148	119	33	59	27
1995 (projected)	*793*	*350*	*285*	*119*	*95*	*26*	*54*	*27*

Table 22 (from THIRD standard pair of Appendix pages for all developed countries: pp.234-5*)

Attribution to smoking of 1990 male deaths at ages 35-69 in all developed countries

Cause of death	Thousands attributed to smoking / total	
Lung cancer	231 / 246	(94%)
Mouth / throat cancer	56 / 81	(69%)
Other cancer	73 / 408	(18%)
Chronic respiratory	76 / 93	(82%)
Other respiratory	15 / 48	(31%)
Vascular disease	318 / 926	(34%)
Liver cirrhosis	- / 84	
Other medical cause**	97 / 276	(35%)
Non-medical cause	- / 295	
ALL CAUSES	865 / 2458	(35%)
ALL CANCER	360 / 736	(49%)

* Pages 234-5 give such calculations for 1975, 1985, 1990 and projected 1995 for both sexes and for ages 0-34, 35-69 & 70+

** Includes TB, peptic ulcer and death from ill-defined causes

THIRD standard pair of appendix pages for various populations: smoking-attributed deaths and total deaths for 1990, projected 1995 and earlier periods

Detailed calculations for 1990 and for 1995 are given in the THIRD standard pair of Appendix pages, along with calculations for earlier periods. These provide details of how many of the deaths in recent years were attributed to smoking, and again there is wide variation between one population and another, both in the female numbers and in the male numbers. To illustrate the format, a few of the 1990 numbers are given in Table 22 for males aged 35-69. In this age range, about half of all male cancer deaths plus more than half of all male deaths from respiratory disease are attributed to smoking.

7. METHODS

AS DESCRIBED IN THE ORIGINAL LANCET REPORT (WHICH IS REPRODUCED HERE)

Peto, Lopez et al, 1992

This Lancet paper is provided for convenience of reference to the original scientific description of the materials and methods that are being used to estimate the mortality from smoking, and of the strengths and limitations of the results.

Improved 1995 projections

No material changes have been made in these 1992 methods, or in the 1965, 1975 or 1985 data. But, the 1995 projections (which were based on extrapolation of pre-1985 mortality trends) are now based on extrapolation of post-1985 trends. This should be more reliable, so the 1995 projections in the Lancet report should for most purposes be replaced by the revised projections in this monograph. (The projected 1995 mortality from tobacco is thereby reduced from 1.6 down to 1.4 million among males, but remains 0.5 million among females.)

Mortality from tobacco in developed countries: indirect estimation from national vital statistics

RICHARD PETO ALAN D. LOPEZ JILLIAN BOREHAM
MICHAEL THUN CLARK HEATH, JR

Prolonged cigarette smoking causes even more deaths from other diseases than from lung cancer. In developed countries, the absolute age-sex-specific lung cancer rates can be used to indicate the approximate proportions due to tobacco of deaths not only from lung cancer itself but also, indirectly, from vascular disease and from various other categories of disease. Even in the absence of direct information on smoking histories, therefore, national mortality from tobacco can be estimated approximately just from the disease mortality statistics that are available from all major developed countries for about 1985 (and for 1975 and so, by extrapolation, for 1995). The relation between the absolute excess of lung cancer and the proportional excess of other diseases can only be approximate, and so as not to overestimate the effects of tobacco it has been taken to be only half that suggested by a recent large prospective study of smoking and death among one million Americans.

Application of such methods indicates that, in developed countries alone, annual deaths from smoking number about 0·9 million in 1965, 1·3 million in 1975, 1·7 million in 1985, and 2·1 million in 1995 (and hence about 21 million in the decade 1990–99: 5–6 million European Community, 5–6 million USA, 5 million former USSR, 3 million Eastern and other Europe, and 2 million elsewhere, [ie, Australia, Canada, Japan, and New Zealand]). More than half these deaths will be at 35–69 years of age: during the 1990s tobacco will in developed countries cause about 30% of all deaths at 35–69 (making it the largest single cause of premature death) plus about 14% of all at older ages. Those killed at older ages are on average already almost 80 years old, however, and might have died soon anyway, but those killed by tobacco at 35–69 lose an average of about 23 years of life.

At present just under 20% of all deaths in developed countries are attributed to tobacco, but this percentage is still rising, suggesting that on current smoking patterns just over 20% of those now living in developed countries will eventually be killed by tobacco (ie, about a quarter of a billion, out of a current total population of just under one and a quarter billion).

Lancet 1992; **339**: 1268–78.

Introduction

In countries where cigarette smoking has been common for many decades, tobacco now accounts for a substantial proportion of premature deaths.[1,2] This paper provides estimates for early middle age (35–59), later middle age (60–69), and old age of mortality in developed countries from tobacco during the last few decades of the 20th century. For one particular country in one particular year, its main method is to take the national mortality rates from various categories of disease, and to attribute certain proportions of deaths from those disease categories to tobacco. These attributable proportions vary from one category to another, being largest for lung cancer, upper aerodigestive cancer and chronic obstructive pulmonary disease (COPD),

ADDRESSES: **Imperial Cancer Research Fund Cancer Studies Unit, University of Oxford, Radcliffe Infirmary, Oxford OX2 6HE, UK** (Prof R. Peto, FRS, J. Boreham, PhD); **Tobacco or Health Unit, World Health Organisation, Geneva, Switzerland** (A. D. Lopez, PhD) ; **and Epidemiology Unit, American Cancer Society, Atlanta, Georgia, USA** (M. Thun, MD, C. Heath, MD). Correspondence to Prof Richard Peto.

intermediate for vascular disease, and zero for cirrhosis, accidents, and violence. They also vary with age, sex, and country, being largest in populations where lung cancer is common.

For most developed countries large, nationally representative studies of smoking and mortality are not yet available to provide tobacco-attributable proportions for the main causes of death. Here, these proportions are therefore estimated indirectly, based partly on a large recent prospective study by the American Cancer Society of smoking and mortality among more than a million US adults.[3] That study found that throughout middle age the death rates of current cigarette smokers (most of whom had smoked regularly throughout adult life) were more than twice the rates of non-smokers, who had never smoked regularly. Its results, combined with US smoking patterns, have been used by the US Surgeon-General to estimate that tobacco was responsible for about one-fifth of all US deaths in 1985:[4]

*1985 US deaths attributed to tobacco by US Surgeon-General**

Lung cancer from (active or passive) smoking	110 000
Cancers of other specified sites (eg, mouth, oesophagus, pharynx, larynx, pancreas, cervix, kidney, bladder)	31 000
Cancer of an unspecified site	Not estimated
Coronary artery or cerebral vascular disease	143 000
COPD	57 000
Other vascular or respiratory	45 000
Other medical causes (eg, peptic ulcer)	Not estimated
Fire or neonatal	4000
Total attributed by US Surgeon-General to tobacco (two-thirds male, one-third female)	390 000

*In 1985, there were 2·1 million US deaths.[5]

Only 28% of those tobacco-attributed US deaths involved lung cancer, however (see below).

The hazards of tobacco depend strongly not only on current but also on previous smoking patterns,[6,7] and on several co-factors[8–10] So, the US prospective study cannot be extrapolated directly to other populations, either in the present or, especially, in past decades. Even if the age-specific prevalence of smoking were known, there could be important differences between current smokers in the target population and in the US study. Other methods are therefore needed for other populations, and the chief novelty of the present report is that the *absolute* lung cancer rate in a particular population is used to indicate the *proportions* of the deaths from various other diseases to attribute to smoking. Thus, for example, the high lung cancer rate in the US indicates not only that a large proportion of all US lung cancer deaths are due to smoking (since the US rates are so much higher than would be expected among non-smokers) but also, indirectly, that a moderately large proportion of all other US deaths are due to smoking. Conversely, the low lung cancer rate among Spanish women (which differs hardly at all from what might be expected if none had ever smoked) suggests not only that few of their lung cancer deaths are yet due to smoking but also, indirectly, that few of their other deaths are yet due to the habit.

Such methods do require some form of age-sex-specific "calibration" of the approximate relation between absolute lung cancer rates and the proportions of other diseases attributable to smoking. The ideal might involve nationally representative prospective studies in several very different developed countries. Generally, however, such studies are not yet available so a cruder calibration has been adopted, based on the mortality experience during the 1980s of the current cigarette smokers and never-smokers in the US prospective study.[3] (Actually, the calibration involves attributing to causal effects of smoking none of the deaths from external causes, none of cirrhosis and only half the excesses of diseases other than lung cancer and cirrhosis indicated by that study: see below.)

Once some approximate calibration has been devised, the use of absolute lung cancer rates to estimate the proportions of deaths from other diseases attributable to smoking has the practical advantage that it requires only the national age-sex-specific mortality rates from various causes (which generally are available), and not national details of age-sex-specific past smoking histories (which generally are not). It has also the theoretical advantage that for diseases other than lung cancer it would not be materially biased by differences in other factors that increase by similar percentages the risk among smokers and the risk among non-smokers (for, such an increase will not change the proportion of such deaths that is attributable to smoking). Examples of such "multiplicative confounding" factors might include alcohol[10] for upper aerodigestive cancer or blood lipids[8] or blood pressure[9] for vascular disease.

TABLE I—CIGARETTE SMOKERS VERSUS "NON-SMOKERS" (NEVER SMOKED REGULARLY): SELECTED RISK RATIOS* FROM YEARS 3 TO 6 INCLUSIVE (APPROXIMATELY 1984–88) OF ACS CPS-II PROSPECTIVE STUDY OF ONE MILLION US ADULTS (SEE APPENDIX)

ICD-9	Male	Female
Lung cancer (ICD 162)	24·22	12·50
Upper aerodigestive cancer—mouth, pharynx, larynx or oesophagus (ICD 140–150 and 161)	7·87	6·95
Other cancer (rest of ICD 140–209)	1·69	1·20
Chronic obstructive pulmonary disease (ICD 490–2, 492–6)	13·82	14·21
Cirrhosis, accidents and violence (ICD 571 and 800–999)	—	—
Other medical causes (rest of ICD 000–799)†		
age 35–59	3·05	2·69
" 60–64	2·31	2·68
" 65–69	2·09	2·52
" 70–74	2·00	2·00
" 75 +	1·54	1·44

*Risk ratios are standardised by the method of Mantel and Haenszel for whichever are relevant of the age groups 30–34, 35–39, 40–44, . . ., 75–79, and 80+.
Female risk ratios may rise in future years in the US, at least in the older age groups as women who have smoked for only part of their lives are replaced by lifelong smokers.
†Except in extreme old age, the chief other medical causes were vascular disease, particularly coronary heart disease and stroke. For vascular diseases alone, those age-specific risk ratios were 3·45, 2·33, 2·01, 1·87 and 1·53 for males, and 2·96, 2·89, 2·53, 2·09 and 1·43 for females (and depended similarly on age for stroke and for CHD[4]).

Materials

Prospective study of a million Americans

The American Cancer Society's second Cancer Prevention Study (ACS CPS-II) is a prospective study of smoking and death among more than one million Americans aged 30 or older when they completed a questionnaire in 1982.[3] In 1992, when the current 6-year results were abstracted, mortality follow-up was virtually complete for the first two years, and about 98–99% complete for the next four. Because some conditions that cause death in the first two years might have affected smoking habits at entry, analysis is restricted to years 3–6 inclusive, and relates deaths (subdivided by cause, sex and 5-year age group at the time of death) to person-years (multiplied by 0·985, to allow for the slight incompleteness in 1992 of the mortality follow-up) for those who in 1982 had never smoked regularly, and for those who were then current cigarette smokers (see Appendix). Most of the latter are lifelong cigarette smokers with a mean consumption of about 20 cigarettes per day.[13] In the US,[11] most male smokers under 80 and female smokers under 50 in 1980 had begun smoking in their teenage years, but many older

TABLE II—MORTALITY FROM SELECTED DISEASES IN VARIOUS MIDDLE-AGED POPULATIONS (DEATH CERTIFICATION RATES PER 100 000 AGED 55–64 IN 1985)

Cause of death	Sex	All "developed" countries	EC: 12 countries	Former USSR	USA	USA (ACS prospective study): Current cigarette smoker	Never smoked regularly	67% current +33% never
Lung cancer	M	205	199	265	221	296	12	202
	F	41	33	26	91	164	12	114
Oesophageal cancer	M	23	25	32	19	18	4	13
	F	5	4	8	5	7	0	5
Ischaemic heart disease	M	422	367	609	475	407	160	325
	F	142	95	234	163	117	40	92
Cerebral vascular disease	M	150	100	307	63	52	19	41
	F	106	59	216	47	37	11	28
Respiratory disease	M	112	91	180	102	70	12	51
	F	41	33	47	57	51	9	37
All causes	M	1771	1600	2320	1693	1464	502	1147
	F	866	750	1051	919	815	357	664

Sources: National mortality rates are from the *WHO Statistics Annuals*, and US smoker and non-smoker rates are from years 3–6 of a prospective study of smoking and mortality in a million US adults (American Cancer Society second cancer prevention study: ACS CPS-II).

female smokers had started several years later, so limiting their lung cancer risk.[10] The machine-measured tar levels per US cigarette were about 15 mg in the early 1980s, but had been double this 25 years earlier.[12]

For many diseases, the absolute death rates among the non-smokers and the smokers in the CPS-II study cannot be generalised even to the US, let alone to other populations. For example, the probability that a 35-year-old man will die before 70 is 34% at US 1985 death rates, but only 13% and 32% at the non-smoker and smoker death rates in years 3–6 of CPS-II. This discrepancy is partly because those who agree to join such a study may be of higher socioeconomic status or more interested in health than average (and therefore at lower than average risk of certain diseases). And partly because of the "healthy volunteer" effect: those who already had some evidence of life-threatening disease in 1982 might, as a result of it, have been less likely to join CPS-II, causing much lower death rates during the first year or two (and, unless the disease was something rapidly fatal such as lung cancer, somewhat lower death rates even in years 3–6). Hence, it is only for lung cancer that use will be made of the absolute risks in CPS-II. For all other diseases, it is just the relative risk that will be used (ie, the ratio of the rate among smokers to that among non-smokers), since this ratio may well be more widely generalisable, both to the USA and to some other developed countries, than the absolute risks are.

The relative risks in CPS-II below age 45 are based on only small numbers of deaths among smokers, and are therefore somewhat unreliable (as, for other reasons, are the death rates in extreme old age). The rates from ages 45 onwards are more reliable, and in each 5-year age group from 45 to 74 the death rates of the smokers are more than double those of non-smokers: see Appendix. (Even beyond age 75 they are almost double the non-smoker death rates.) If this approximately twofold difference was largely caused by tobacco, then it would suggest that in each age range about half the deaths of the smokers were caused by tobacco. A persistent twofold difference at each age due to tobacco would mean that about half of all regular cigarette smokers would eventually, either in middle or in old age, be killed by their habit. If, conservatively, it was assumed that "only" two-thirds of the observed more-than-twofold mortality excess is caused by tobacco then the CPS-II study would still suggest that about 40% of all regular cigarette smokers would eventually be killed by their habit.

The main purpose of obtaining the full data (see Appendix) was to match the absolute lung cancer rate in some mixture of CPS-II smokers and CPS-II non-smokers with the absolute lung cancer rate in a particular country, and then to use the proportional excess of various other causes of death in that mixture as a guide to the proportions of those other diseases in that country that might be due to tobacco. For this, the smoker and non-smoker lung cancer rates are needed (Appendix), along with the risk ratios (smoker versus non-smoker) for various groups of diseases (table I).

In table I all upper aerodigestive cancers (ICD-9 140-150, 161) are combined, for statistical stability and because the main such cancers have similarly extreme relative risks with respect to tobacco and with respect to alcohol. Likewise, all vascular diseases are combined because the relative risks for ischaemic heart disease and for stroke depend similarly on age in CPS-II[4] and because the vital statistics may, particularly in old age, interchange some vascular causes of death. Cirrhosis, accidents, and violence are excluded because it is almost impossible to get reliable evidence as to whether smoking can cause them. (Smokers are more likely to commit suicide and to die from cirrhosis, but in the present report no such deaths will be attributed to smoking.)

Routine population and mortality statistics

Age-sex-specific population estimates for each separate developed country are available for five-yearly time periods from 1965 to 2025.[15] For present purposes it is chiefly the populations aged over 35 that will be used, and since people aged over 35 in 2025 were born before 1990, these population estimtes are not affected by uncertainties in future birth rates.

Mortality statistics provided routinely by all major developed countries are published in the WHO's *World Health Statistics Annuals*.[5] Data for 1965, 1975, and 1985 are used here, subdivided by country, by sex, by 5-year age group, and by nine major cause-of-death categories: lung cancer, upper aerodigestive cancer (mouth, pharynx, larynx, oesophagus), other cancer, COPD, other respiratory disease, vascular disease, cirrhosis, other medical causes, and non-medical causes. From these, all-cause death rates for 1995 are estimated by proportional extrapolation of the 1975 and 1985 rates for each country, age, and sex category (subject to the restriction that there should be no more than a twofold difference between a 1985 and a 1995 rate), and the proportion of each such all-cause death rate to attribute to particular causes will be determined by similar extrapolatin of the nine cause-specific rates.

For East Germany, a similar procedure was used to estimate the unavailable 1965 rates by back-extrapolation from the 1975 and 1985 rates. A few other data deficiencies were filled in by applying adjacent rates to the UN population estimates[15] in the relevant years (Belgium, 1986 for 1985; Luxembourg, 1967 for 1965; Romania, 1984 for 1985), and Romanian 1965 cause-specific death numbers in 10-year age ranges (5–14, 15–24, . . ., 65–74, 75+) were subdivided into 5-year numbers (5–9, 10–14, . . ., 80–84, 85+) in the same proportions as Romanian 1969 all-cause mortality. The 1965 Israeli statistics used are those for Jewish deaths only. For secular comparability, subtotals for the twelve European Community (EC) countries in 1965, 1975, or 1985 include all 1992 EC territories. (East and West Germany, although analysed separately, count here as one.) In 1985, 99·8% (10·34 million) of the deaths over age 35 were in the twelve EC and eighteen largest other developed countries. So, in calculating the EC or developed world totals, 0·2% is added to the uncorrected totals and no separate analyses are presented for the 0·02 million deaths in smaller developed populations (0·01M Albania +0·01M others: Andorra,

Channel Is, Faeroes, Gibraltar, Greenland, Iceland, Isle of Man, Lichtenstein, Malta, Monaco, San Marino, Vatican City).

Methods

In estimating the overall scale of the epidemic of death from tobacco in developed countries, there is a range of uncertainty between the lower limits and the upper limits of what is scientifically plausible, and the present report tends to base its calculations chiefly on the lower limits. The uncertainty derives not so much from the million deaths each year from lung cancer, upper aerodigestive cancer, and COPD (the great majority of which can, with only a narrow range of uncertainty, be attributed to tobacco), but from the nine or ten million other deaths each year in developed countries (another million of which may, albeit with a wider range or uncertainty, also be attributed to tobacco). Vascular diseases—chiefly coronary heart disease (CHD) and stroke—account for more than half these other deaths, and the CPS-II study suggests that, at least in North America, tobacco is associated with more deaths from vascular disease than from lung cancer. But, whereas virtually all the excess risk of lung cancer that is associated with smoking in the US (Appendix) is actually caused[10] by the habit, this may not be true for vascular disease: part of the association (table I) may well be due to other differences between US smokers and US non-smokers. Alternatively, if some cardioprotective factor (alcohol use, perhaps) is more common among smokers than among non-smokers then the real cardiotoxicity of tobacco might be underestimated by table I. Hence, even within the CPS-II prospective study itself there is some uncertainty as to what fraction of the vascular mortality among smokers is actually caused by smoking.

Further uncertainties are added when extrapolating from CPS-II to other populations, since even though for lung cancer mortality the absolute rates attributable to smoking in two populations may be equally high, that does not guarantee that for vascular mortality the porportions attributable to smoking in the two populations must be exactly equal to each other. For example (table II), lung cancer mortality just among the middle-aged male smokers in CPS-II is about the same as among all middle-aged males in the USSR, and vascular mortality among the middle-aged male smokers in CPS-II is about 200% higher than in the corresponding non-smokers. Possibly, therefore, vascular mortality among middle-aged USSR males as a whole is also about 200% higher than if none had ever smoked. Perhaps, however, once due allowance has been made for confounding and for the problems of extrapolation from one population to another, this excess percentage in the USSR might be only 100%, not 200% (ie, perhaps only about half, not two-thirds, of the male vascular deaths in middle age are attributable to tobacco).

Conservative underestimation of tobacco hazards

The present report subdivides the diseases that cause death into a few broad categories, and is then conservative in determining what proportions to attribute to tobacco. Conservatively, deaths from external causes (including fires, suicides, and accidents), neonatal deaths (including stillbirths), all other deaths under 35 years, and all deaths from cirrhosis of the liver will not be attributed to tobacco, even though some of these deaths are due to smoking. Lung cancer is dealt with by comparison of the absolute rates in each country with those among US non-smokers. The remaining six disease categories (upper aerodigestive cancer, other cancer, COPD, other pulmonary disease, vascular disease and other medical causes) are dealt with by calculating (on an age-specific basis) the excess percentages suggested indirectly by the national lung cancer rates, and then simply halving each excess percentage, in the hope of obtaining a conservative estimate of the proportions of such deaths to attribute to tobacco (see Discussion).

In populations with high tobacco-attributable mortality from upper aerodigestive cancer or from COPD, halving the large percentage excess makes little difference. For example, whether the excess is 400% or whether it is 800%, the large majority (either 4/5 or 8/9, in this example) of all such deaths will still be attributed to tobacco. But where only a minority of the deaths are attributable to tobacco, halving the percentage excess will almost halve the number attributed to tobacco.

Halving the percentage excess is crude and arbitrary, and although it provides a reasonable degree of protection against overestimation of the epidemic, it does so at the risk of somewhat underestimating the hazards. The degree of underestimation will not be great, however (since the possibility of confounding does have to be allowed for, particularly in diseases where the excess among smokers is only moderate—and the halving has a substantial effect only in these circumstances). Indeed, for the United States itself in 1985 the "conservative" procedures of the present report (by analyses only of national mortality rates) will be found to attribute to tobacco almost exactly the same number of deaths as the US Surgeon-General did by combination of national mortality rates with additional data on the prevalence of smoking in the US. Details of the conservative procedure are summarised below.

Ignore deaths under age 35—Most deaths from tobacco are in middle or old age and, conservatively, attention will be restricted to these. Neonatal deaths, and all other deaths from tobacco before age 35, will therefore be ignored.

Ignore cirrhosis and non-medical causes—Cirrhosis is commoner among smokers than among non-smokers, as is suicide, but it is difficult to assess how much, if any, of these excesses to attribute to smoking. Deaths from cirrhosis (ICD-9 571) will therefore be ignored, along with deaths from suicide, fires and all other external causes (ICD 800-999).

Lung cancer at ages 35–79: compare with US non-smokers—In developed countries, lung cancer is so rare among non-smokers that big studies are needed to describe reliably their age-specific death rates from the disease. The two largest prospective studies of smoking, each of which involved over a million people, both took place in the US, one (CPS-I) in the 1960s and one (CPS-II) in the 1980s. Comparing the lung cancer mortality among the non-smokers (never smoked regularly) in these two studies, there was no significant trend over the 20-year period that separated them[4] (and no significant difference between these studies and the smaller study of British doctors[10]). So, the US non-smoker lung cancer rates in CPS-II (Appendix) may approximately describe non-smokers in other developed countries. Among Spanish women, for example, where smoking cannot yet be causing much lung cancer (since only a few per cent of those in later middle age are smokers) the lung cancer rates are still like those of the US female non-smokers. (Among young Spanish women, however, about half now smoke, and if they continue to do so then when they eventually reach later middle age high death rates must be expected.)

The similarity of non-smoker lung cancer death certification rates in different developed countries is only approximate, for there will be differences not only in the extent to which other diseases are mis-certified as primary lung cancer, or vice versa, but also in the effects on non-smokers of other causative factors such as general air pollution or occupation (or, perhaps, some infective, nutritional or hormonal factors).[10] Among non-smokers, however, the disease is rare even in polluted areas—indeed, even radon and asbestos may cause only a small absolute risk among those who have never smoked. So for each sex the tobacco-attributable lung cancer in each country is estimated by subtracting the smoothed US non-smoker rates in the Appendix from the national rates (with no lung cancer deaths attributed to tobacco in any of the age groups 35–59, 60–64, 65–69, 70–74 or 75–79 in which the national rate was less than the US non-smoker rate or, conservatively, in any subsequent age group): also, because the rates at older ages may be unreliable or unstable, in each population the fraction of lung cancer attributed to smoking was taken to be the same at 80+ as at 75–79.

Other diseases at ages 35–79: conservative halving of apparent excess attributed to tobacco—For the other diseases, a more complicated procedure is needed to estimate the fractions attributable to tobacco, since it cannot be assumed that the absolute rates among non-smokers will be comparable in different populations. First, using the 5-yearly lung cancer rates from the Appendix, a mixture of CPS-II smokers and CPS-II non-smokers aged 35 to 79 is constructed, with the proportions of smokers at ages 35-59, 60–64, 65–69, 70–74 and 75–79 chosen to make the lung cancer rates in each of these age groups in the mixed population equal to those in the country to be analysed. (The ratio of the non-smoker lung cancer rates to the national rates in these five

TABLE III—ALL DEVELOPED COUNTRIES, 1985 MORTALITY: SMOKING-ATTRIBUTED DEATHS/TOTAL DEATHS, IN THOUSANDS

Ages	Sex	Lung cancer	Upper aerodig. cancer	Other cancer	COPD	Other respiratory	Vascular disease	Cirrhosis	Other medical	Non-medical eg, fire, suicide	All fatal conditions
35–69	M	203/217	47/69	64/362	71/87	14/45	297/876	*/90	78/227	*/242	774/2216 (35%)
	F	37/56	4/13	7/399	19/41	3/22	54/496	*/42	18/156	*/84	141/1307 (11%)
70+	M	134/148	19/34	48/383	126/179	15/136	180/1567	*/32	37/321	*/75	561/2876 (20%)
	F	29/48	4/16	6/455	42/120	6/155	72/2462	*/30	16/472	*/91	175/3850 (5%)
All ages†	M	338/367	66/103	112/772	197/270	30/229	477/2470	*/128	115/726	*/536	1335/5601 (24%)
	F	65/104	8/29	13/878	61/163	9/216	126/2972	*/76	34/758	*/236	316/5433 (6%)

*Any relationship of these deaths with smoking is ignored.
†Includes 784 (000) deaths at ages 0–34.

separate age groups determines the proportions not attributed to tobacco.) Second, using for other diseases relative risks from table I (which are taken as if they were independent of age for cancer and for chronic obstructive pulmonary disease), determine the excess in each age group as a percentage of the non-smoker rates. Finally, for a particular disease category in a particular age group, the method of extrapolation from this mixed population to the target country is to assume that the proportion of deaths due to smoking is similar in the target population and in the mixed population. But, it cannot be assumed that all the excess mortality among smokers in the CPS-II study was actually caused by tobacco. Upper aerodigestive cancers, for example, are caused both by tobacco and by alcohol, and smokers may drink more than non-smokers. Likewise, even among non-smokers many diseases are inversely related to social class, and so too is smoking. Hence, in CPS-II part of the excess mortality among smokers may be due to factors other than tobacco. To ensure that the hazards of tobacco are not exaggerated, the excess mortality in the mixed population will be halved before estimating the fraction of deaths attributable to tobacco. For example, if the mixture had 7 times the COPD mortality of non-smokers (ie, a 6-fold excess) then instead of 6/7 of the COPD deaths being attributed to tobacco, only 3/4 would be, a 3-fold excess. In countries where lung cancer is common this does not greatly reduce the fractions of COPD or upper aerodigestive cancer deaths attributed to tobacco, but it does substantially reduce the fractions of other deaths attributed to the habit. This simple halving of the excess risk is obviously not a satisfactory procedure, for it is crude and arbitrary and may seriously under-estimate some of the true hazards of tobacco. Prospective studies in a number of countries of smoking, mortality and various possible confounding factors should eventually clarify the local hazards that are actually caused by tobacco, but in most countries these are not yet available.

Ages 80+: use 75–79 proportions—Because lung cancer rates are particularly unreliable in extreme old age, the proportions of each disease category attributed to smoking will simply be taken to be the same at 80+ as at 75–79.

Results

Does the method produce any obviously anomalous results? Only if its results are generally plausible can their implications be explored. Although brief results will be given for 1965 and 1975, chief emphasis will be on the results for 1985 (the last year for which the results are based on actual mortality rates), on approximate extrapolations to 1995 (the first year for which the results might be directly relevant to current planning of preventive strategies), and on the longer-term trends.

1985 mortality by disease category

Table III gives for 1985 the numbers of tobacco-attributed deaths from various categories of disease. The results are subdivided into middle age (35–69) and old age (70+). Scrutiny of table III does not reveal any obvious implausibilities in particular causes of death, except perhaps for some uncertainty about the large number of "other medical" deaths attributed to smoking. This is such a minor category of death in North America that the excess seen in the CPS-II study cannot reliably be extrapolated to populations where such deaths are common. (Note, however, that some of these "other medical" deaths in national mortality statistics include tobacco-related conditions such as peptic ulcer, tuberculosis, or even some misclassified deaths from a respiratory, neoplastic or vascular cause.)

1985 mortality by age, loss of life expectancy.

Table IV gives, for the same 1985 deaths, a more detailed breakdown by age. The estimates are not reliable below age 45, where the CPS-II study provides only limited data, but the number of deaths attributed to tobacco at these early ages is small. For other reasons,[10] the estimates are also less reliable in old age (particularly above age 80) than in middle age.

From table IV it is possible to estimate the loss of 1985 life expectancy from death at various ages from smoking, since subtraction of the tobacco-attributed deaths leaves the 1985

TABLE IV—AGE DISTRIBUTION OF TOBACCO-ATTRIBUTED DEATHS, ALL DEVELOPED COUNTRIES, 1985, AND YEARS LOSS OF LIFE EXPECTANCY PER DEATH FROM SMOKING (AT THE DEATH RATES REMAINING WITHOUT THE DEATHS ATTRIBUTED TO TOBACCO*)

	Males			Females		
Ages	Deaths (1000) Attrib/Total	Popn. (mill.)	Years lost	Deaths (1000) Attrib/Total	Popn. (mill.)	Years lost
35–39	23/102	42·0	39·1	3/46	42·1	42.4
40–44	34/122	33·6	34·5	4/58	34·3	37·7
45–49	72/215	35·2	30·1	8/101	36·8	33·0
50–54	109/292	31·3	25·7	13/143	33·2	28·5
55–59	184/448	30·5	21·6	24/236	34·6	24·2
60–64	187/512	23·7	17·6	44/335	31·4	20·0
65–69	166/525	16·4	14·0	45/387	23·0	16·1
70–74	210/785	15·2	10·8	59/699	23·8	12·5
75–79	155/836	10·3	8·1	37/914	18·2	9·5
80–84	112/674	5·5	6·0	35/972	11·4	7·1
85+	84/580	2·8	4·0	45/1264	7·4	4·0
0–34	–/509	321·3	**	–/276	311·1	**
35–69	775/2216	212·8	21·5†	141/1306	235·4	22·0†
70+	561/2875	33·8	8·1	176/3849	60·8	8·6
All	1336/5600	567·9	15·9	317/5431	607·3	14·6

Note: Estimates in old age (especially above age 80) may not be reliable.
*Non-smoker life expectancy in a 5-year age range is taken as the mean of that at the start and end of it. At age 85 non-smoker life expectancy is taken as 5 years (male) or 6 years (female), at ages 85+ 4 years (male or female), and at ages 80, 75, . . ., 40, 35 as 2·5 + (2·5 + life expectancy 5 years later) × (probability of surviving 5 more years). If R is the death rate in a particular 5-year period then the probability of surviving that period is exp(−5R), which would, for example, be exp(−5(0·512−0·187)/23·7) for men aged 60 without the deaths attributed to tobacco.
**Since the age distribution from 0 to 34 is fairly uniform, the crude death rates can be used to estimate survival (95% male, 97% female) from birth to 35. But, among those now aged 0–34 most have already escaped the risks of infancy and childhood, so at current death rates larger proportions (98% and 99%) will survive to 35, and so to risk of death at 35–69.
†22·1 and 22·5 at projected 1995 rates (with no change at older ages).

TABLE V—TRENDS IN MORTALITY ATTRIBUTED TO TOBACCO, AND IN ALL MORTALITY, IN DEVELOPED COUNTRIES (NO. = THOUSANDS OF DEATHS, RATE = RATE PER HUNDRED THOUSAND, STANDARDISED FOR AGE*)

		(a) All mortality, irrespective of tobacco							b) Mortality attributed to tobacco					Mortality not attributed to tobacco: (a)–(b)	
		0–34 No.	0–34 Rate	35–69 No.	35–69 Rate	70–79 No.	70–79 Rate	80+ No.	35–69 No.	35–69 Rate	70–79 No.	70–79 Rate	80+ No.	35–69 Rate	70–79 Rate
Male: Lung cancer	1965	1	0	134	100	43	256	8	123	91	36	215	7	(9)	(41)
	1975	1	0	175	115	79	380	18	162	107	70	338	15	(8)	(42)
	1985	1	0	217	130	113	446	36	203	121	102	404	32	(9)	(42)
	1995	**1**	**0**	**292**	**145**	**140**	**535**	**66**	**275**	**137**	**129**	**493**	**61**	**(8)**	**(42)**
Male: Any cancer	1965	31	11	483	357	213	1324	82	189	139	54	323	13	218	1001
	1975	31	10	564	367	297	1472	114	247	161	103	498	28	206	974
	1985	29	9	647	383	386	1548	180	314	184	148	586	54	199	962
	1995	**24**	**8**	**802**	**394**	**419**	**1614**	**259**	**424**	**208**	**181**	**695**	**95**	**186**	**919**
Male: Any fatal condition	1965	665	220	2079	1512	1187	7561	833	573	415	163	969	62	1097	6592
	1975	607	199	2308	1457	1449	7380	991	703	450	294	1412	125	1007	5968
	1985	509	159	2216	1282	1621	6625	1255	774	444	365	1440	196	838	5185
	1995	**392**	**124**	**2429**	**1171**	**1493**	**5864**	**1478**	**941**	**452**	**392**	**1487**	**285**	**719**	**4377**
Female: Lung cancer	1965	1	0	24	14	10	38	3	9	5	2	7	0	(9)	(31)
	1975	1	0	38	19	17	51	7	20	10	7	20	2	(9)	(31)
	1985	1	0	56	27	33	79	15	37	18	20	48	8	(9)	(31)
	1995	**1**	**0**	**84**	**36**	**54**	**126**	**28**	**63**	**27**	**41**	**95**	**19**	**(9)**	**(31)**
Female: Any cancer	1965	27	10	419	235	190	766	95	12	7	3	11	1	228	755
	1975	25	9	452	225	241	738	135	27	14	9	27	4	211	711
	1985	25	8	467	221	310	747	209	47	23	26	63	12	198	684
	1995	**22**	**7**	**505**	**213**	**321**	**751**	**280**	**78**	**34**	**51**	**118**	**28**	**179**	**633**
Female: Any fatal condition	1965	427	141	1382	798	1235	5122	1263	50	28	16	57	6	770	5065
	1975	342	116	1426	718	1457	4596	1682	97	49	43	124	28	669	4472
	1985	276	90	1307	631	1614	3976	2236	141	69	96	224	79	562	3752
	1995	**208**	**70**	**1342**	**571**	**1406**	**3385**	**2690**	**198**	**86**	**150**	**343**	**160**	**485**	**3042**

*Standardised rates are means of seven 5-yearly rates, or of the two rates for 70–74 and 75–79.
Notes: 1995 estimates (in bold type) use national age-specific projections of rates, plus published populations.[15]
The lung cancer death rates (in brackets) that are not attributed to tobacco have been forced to be approximately constant.

death rates that would have been expected in the absence of smoking. Both for males and for females, the average loss of 1985 life expectancy from smoking for those killed by the habit in middle age (35–69) is about 22 years. Indeed, even for those killed in later middle age (60–69) the mean loss is about 16 years, while for those killed by the habit in early middle age (35–59) it is about 27 years. But, many of those killed by the habit in old age (70+) might have have died soon anyway, since their average age at death was about 80. At present, therefore, deaths in early middle age (35–59) account for about half of the loss of life expectancy attributed to smoking, deaths in later middle age (60–69) account for about half of the remainder of it, and deaths in old age (70+) account for under a quarter of the total.

The actual loss of life expectancy of those now being killed by tobacco should, however, be calculated not at 1985 or 1995 non-smoker death rates, but at the progressively lower non-smoker death rates of future years. This will hardly alter the 8-year loss of life expectancy of those killed by tobacco in old age, but will increase the loss of life expectancy of those killed by tobacco in middle age by one or two additional years beyond the 22 years in table IV. Those now being killed by tobacco in middle age are therefore losing about 23 years of non-smoker life expectancy.

Trends in the mortality that is not due to tobacco (table V).

For 1965, 1975, 1985 and (by projection) 1995, table V gives a more detailed breakdown not only of the crude numbers of deaths (which are affected by the size of the population) but also of the standardised death rates (which are not). The analyses are subdivided by age and sex, and are presented separately for lung cancer, for any cancer and for any fatal condition. For each such category of disease, table V gives: *(a)* all mortality, irrespective of tobacco; *(b)* the mortality that is attributed to tobacco; and then, by subtraction, *(c)* the remaining mortality that is not attributed to tobacco. It is the age-standardised rates in table V that are of particular interest, and these are calculated from 0–34, 35–69 and 70–79. Deaths above 80 are not included in these rates, for no sufficiently accurate assessment of the effects of tobacco is possible.

At ages 0–34 the overall mortality is low, the proportion caused by tobacco is small, and the age-standardised death rate is decreasing rapidly. (Both in males and in females it decreased by about one-third over the 20-year period from 1965 to 1985, from an average for both sexes of 181 per 100 000, corresponding to a 6% risk of death by age 35, down to 125, corresponding to a 4% risk.)

At ages 35–69 and at ages 70–79 the male and the female lung cancer mortality rates are both increasing, but the male and female all-cause mortality rates are both decreasing. This suggests that tobacco is responsible for a growing proportion of a decreasing total. In males these opposite effects result in approximately constant overall death rates being attributed to tobacco, but in females the overall death rates attributed to tobacco are beginning to grow rapidly, though they are still far smaller than the male rates.

Cancer—In the present decade, about one-third of all cancer deaths in developed countries are attributed to tobacco (in table V for 1995 the numbers of thousands of cancer deaths attributed to tobacco are: males 700/1504 [47%]; females 157/1128 [14%]; both sexes 857/2632 = 33%). During the 1960s this proportion was much smaller (table V for 1965: 272/1540 = 18%). These changes in the proportions of cancer deaths that are attributed to tobacco are so large that the effects of tobacco have

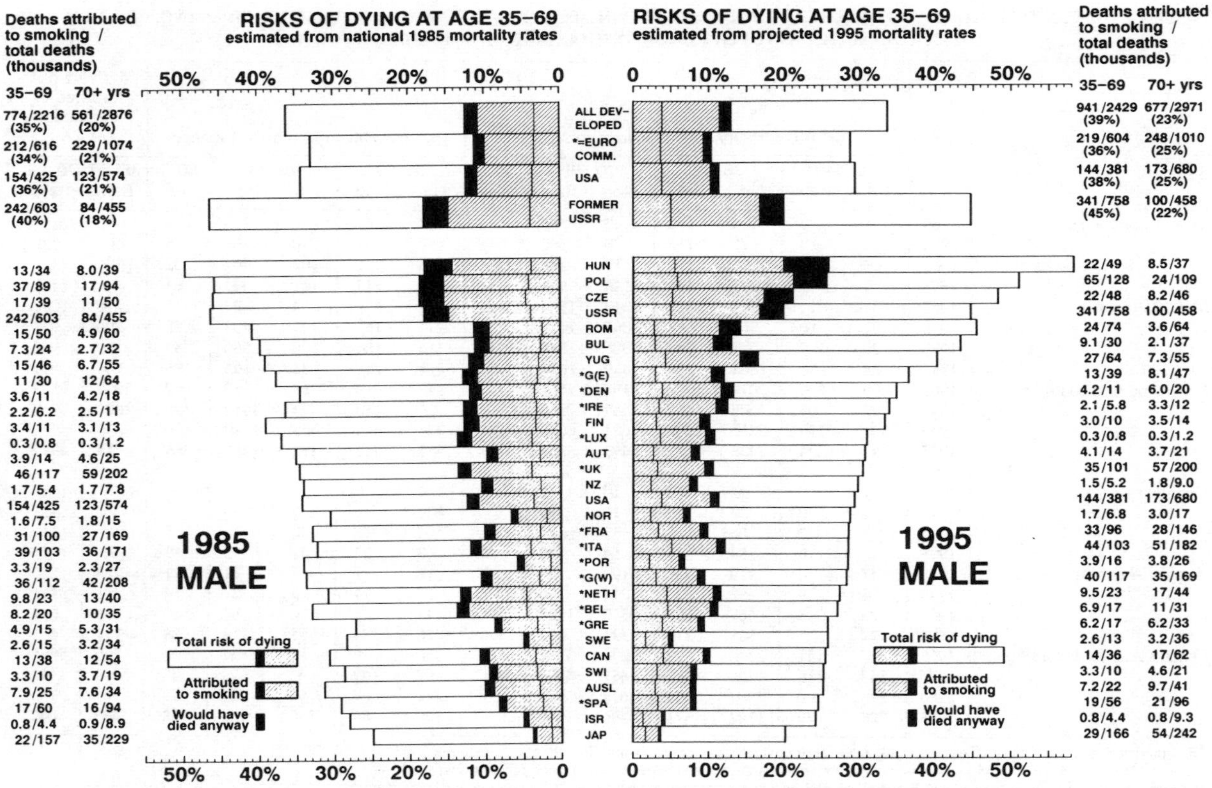

Fig 1—Males, 1985 and 1995: numbers of deaths and risks of death attributed to tobacco and not attributed to tobacco, in various developed populations.

Columns of numbers give deaths (in thousands) attributed to smoking/total deaths, for ages 35–69 and for ages 70+. Bar lengths give risks at age 35 of dying before age 70, at the national death rates of 1985 (left) and at the projected death rates of 1995 (right): total bar length = total risk of dying at 35–69, and solid-plus-shaded bar length = risk of dying from tobacco at 35–69 (solid = would have died before 70 of some other causes; shaded = would have survived to 70 or more; and, within the shaded area, the part between zero and the thin vertical line = probability of dying of lung cancer at age 35–69).

dominated the male trends in overall cancer mortality over the past few decades, causing increases where decreases would otherwise have existed, and are likely to dominate the female trends over the next few decades. Subtraction of the estimated effects of tobacco from the overall trends in cancer mortality (table V, right-hand columns) suggests that, among people who have never smoked, overall cancer death certification rates in developed countries have been decreasing fairly steadily over the past few decades in old age (70–79), in middle age (35–69) and at earlier ages (0–34). The interpretation of such trends has been discussed elsewhere.[10]

All-cause mortality—If, again, the effects of smoking are allowed for by subtraction of the tobacco-attributed deaths, then for the all-cause mortality rates in developed countries that are not attributed to tobacco the decrease is even more striking than for the cancer mortality rates (table V, right-hand columns). Thus, over the past few decades in developed countries non-smokers appear to have experienced decreasing overall cancer mortality rates, together with even more rapidly decreasing mortality from other diseases. (In the particular case of the United States the non-smoker trends can be confirmed directly, since the CPS-I study in the 1960s included many non-smokers, whose experience has been compared[4] with the non-smokers in CPS-II in the 1980s.)

Mortality by country (figs 1 and 2)

Fig 1 (males) and fig 2 (females) describe, for various developed countries or groups of countries, the mortality attributed to tobacco in middle age (35–69) and at older ages. The overall bar lengths (shaded plus white) describe the probabilities of death in middle age, and the shaded parts (hatched plus black) describe the probabilities of death in middle age that are attributed to tobacco. In each figure, the left half describes the analyses of actual 1985 mortality rates, while the right half describes the analyses of projected 1995 mortality rates. Both in 1985 and in 1995, the risks of death in middle age are almost twice as great for males as for females, partly because the male risks currently attributed to smoking (shaded areas) are higher and partly because the other male risks (white areas) are also higher.

Among males (top of fig 1), the lengths of the bars for "all developed countries" indicate that the overall risk of death at ages 35–69 was 36% at the 1985 death rates and 34% at the 1995 rates. In both cases, the risk of death attributed to tobacco was 13%. If this figure of 13% were to continue to be approximately constant for a few decades, it would suggest that about 13% of all men aged 35 in developed countries would be killed by tobacco before 70.

Among females (top of fig 2), the bars for "all developed countries" indicate that the overall risk of death at ages 35–69 was also decreasing (20% at 1985 rates, 18% at 1995 rates). But the risk of death from tobacco at ages 35–69 was increasing (from 2% to 3%) and until, perhaps a few decades hence, it stabilises it cannot be used directly to estimate probabilities of female death in middle age.

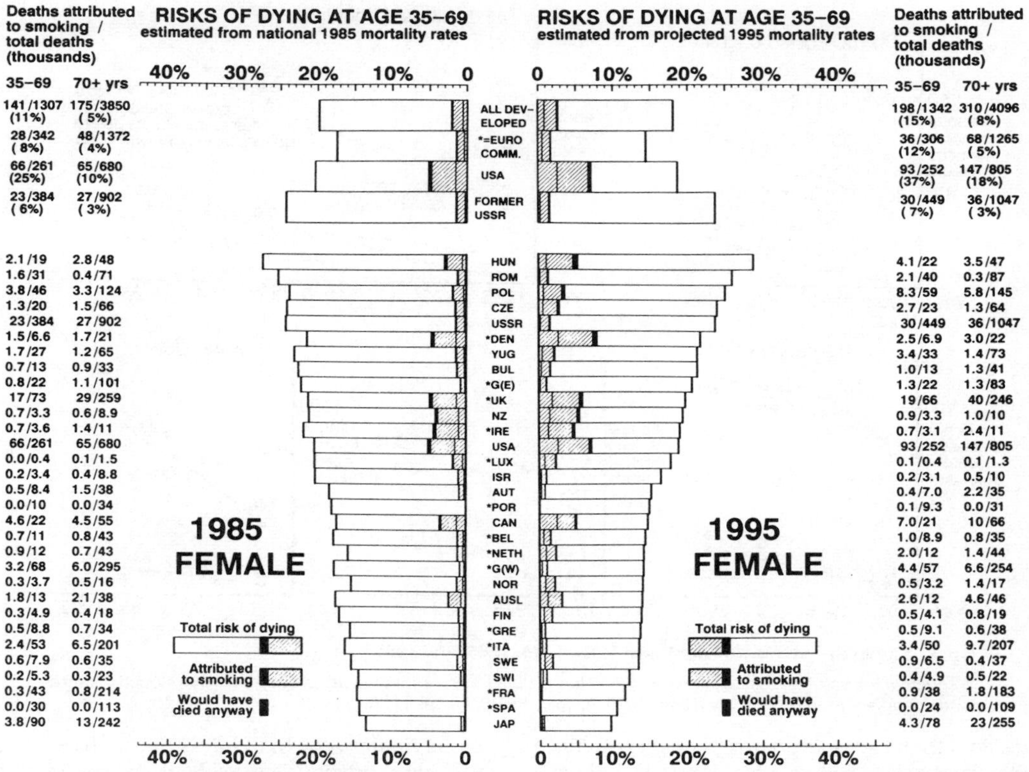

Fig 2—Females, 1985 and 1995: numbers of deaths and risks of death attributed to tobacco and not attributed to tobacco in various developed populations (format as in fig 1).

The overall numbers of deaths (in thousands, male plus female) attributed to tobacco in 1995 were 1139/3771 (30% of all deaths) in middle age and 987/7067 (14% of all deaths) at older ages, the years lost being about 23 each for the former and 8 each for the latter. This predicts a grand total of 2·1 million tobacco-attributed deaths in 1995, of which about 590 000 involve lung cancer. (The vertical lines inside the shaded areas in figs 1 and 2 indicate the lung cancer rates: since the lung cancer prediction is the most reliable, a crude check on the plausibility of this total of about 2 million can be provided by noting that it is 3 or 4 times larger than the lung cancer prediction, this ratio being similar to that in the Surgeon-General's estimate[4] that in 1985 there were about 400 000 tobacco-attributed deaths in the US, of which 110 000 involve lung cancer: see Introduction).

For males (fig 1), the pattern of international differences shows that the epidemic of premature death from tobacco has already become substantial in all developed countries. The all-cause death rates in middle age are especially high in Eastern Europe, one major reason for this being tobacco (shaded areas), and East European death rates are in many cases still increasing. For instance, at the projected 1995 death rates, about half of all Polish males aged 35 could expect to die before 70, with about half these Polish deaths attributed to tobacco. By contrast with this, however, only about a quarter of all Swedish males aged 35 could expect to die before 70, with only about one-fifth of these Swedish deaths attributed to tobacco. However, tobacco is not the only reason for the high male death rates in Eastern Europe because female death rates there are also high.

For females (fig 2), the absolute risks of death in middle age are smaller than for males, and the proportions attributed to tobacco of those deaths are also smaller than for males—indeed, in countries such as France, Spain, and Portugal, the female lung cancer rates are about the same as in US non-smokers, suggesting very small numbers of deaths from tobacco. But, in a few countries the female lung cancer rates are rising rapidly: for example, the proportion of US female deaths attributed to tobacco has risen from 25% at the 1985 death rates to 37% at the 1995 rates, a proportion that is higher in the US than in any other country. At the projected 1995 death rates, about half a million female deaths are atrributed to the habit, including 240 000 in the US and 60 000 in the UK. The low rates in France, Spain, and Portugal are plausible, as are the high rates in the US and UK. What is less plausible in fig 2, however, is that in countries such as the former USSR, a few percent of the female deaths are attributed, perhaps mistakenly, to tobacco. (Even though the female USSR lung cancer death certification rates in 1985 were consistently slightly higher than in US non-smokers, they were, at least in middle age, not yet rising, which suggests that the female epidemic had scarcely begun in the USSR.) But, both in middle and in old age, most of the female deaths attributed to tobacco in fig 2 are from countries such as the Uk or US where the lung cancer epidemic was already well advanced in 1985, so the overall estimates for females remain plausible.

Taking all developed countries together, the European Community (EC), the US and the former USSR each account for about a quarter of the population. Totals for these groupings are shown separately (thick bars) at the top of figs 1 and 2, and longer term trends for the numbers of deaths attributed to tobacco in these groupings are shown in fig 3. For males (or for males and females together), the largest absolute number of tobacco-attributed deaths is in the EC, but for females, the largest number is in the US, and

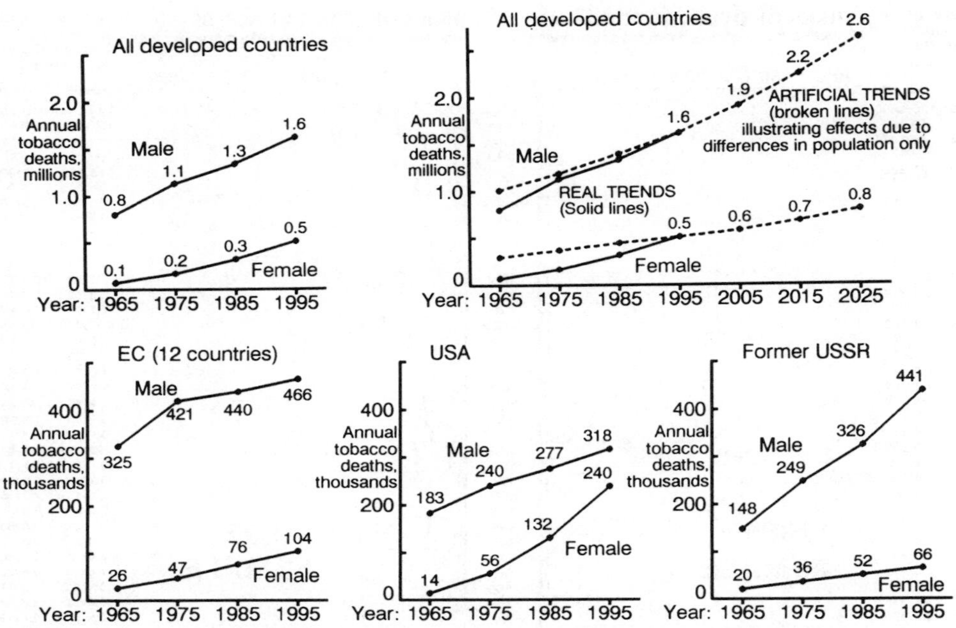

Fig 3—Smoking—attributed deaths in 1965, 1975, 1985, and 1995.

Together with artificial calculations, applying the 1995 tobacco-attributed death rates for all developed countries to the pouplations in other years, 1965–2025, at ages 35–39, 40–44, ..., 80+.

the trends in US tobacco-attributed mortality in fig 3 suggest that the epidemic will, in a decade or two, be killing about as many women as men in the US. (The age-specific rates are lower for women than for men not only for tobacco-attributed deaths but also for other deaths, so the proportion who die of tobacco may eventually be similar for both sexes.)

The trends in fig 3 in the absolute numbers of tobacco-attributed deaths are affected not only by changes in death rates from tobacco but also by changes in the sizes of the populations. For all developed countries together, the effects of population changes alone (broken lines in fig 3) are compared with the real trends. For males, the similarity of the slopes of the broken and the solid lines indicates that the increase in the annual number of deaths is due chiefly to population growth, whereas for females the difference between the slopes shows that the increase is due not just to population growth but, still more, to increasing death rates.

If these constant male death rates from tobacco were to persist for a few more decades, then the annual numbers of male deaths from tobacco would grow from about 1·6 million in 1995 to about 2·6 million by 2025. But the increase in the female rates suggests that the annual numbers of female deaths from tobacco over the next few decades will, on present smoking patterns, become progressively larger than is indicated by the broken line in fig 3. By 2025, therefore, there could well be substantially more than a million female deaths a year in developed countries from tobacco.

Discussion

The strengths and weaknesses of the present method of assessing mortality from tobacco in developed countries were discussed as it was introduced and used. The general conclusion was that in such countries it is likely to be reasonably reliable in middle age but somewhat less reliable at older ages. One simple check on its plausibility is provided by its findings for the United States. Based only on US national mortality data, without the use of any data on smoking habits in the US, it attributes 408 000 US deaths to tobacco in 1985, and 52% fewer in 1965. The US Surgeon-General, by a completely different method that does make use of data on smoking prevalence rates and contemporary relative risks in the US (which might not be available elsewhere) attributes about 390 000 US deaths to tobacco in 1985, and 47% fewer in 1965.[4] This similarity reinforces the plausibility of the present method, at least for populations that are not too different from the US over the past few decades. But, the more different the population or the epoch, the more uncertain the results of the method must be. The plausibility of its overall conclusions will therefore be assessed by discussion not only of the few largest populations that make the largest contributions to the overall total, but also of the populations with the most extreme risks attributed to tobacco.

Populations with low risks, with high risks, or with large absolute numbers of deaths attributed to tobacco

For males, the populations with the lowest and the highest proportions of deaths in middle age now attributed to tobacco are, respectively, Japan (17%) and Poland (50%), and the absolute hazards are even more extremely different than these proportions would suggest (fig 1). A large census-based prospective study of the effects of tobacco already exists in Japan,[16] with results for Japanese males that are reasonably compatible with fig 1. At the projected 1995 Polish death rates about half the males aged 35 would expect to die before 70, with about half of these deaths attributed to tobacco. Direct evidence, preferably from a large, reasonably representative prospective study in a country such as Poland, is needed to test this prediction, to monitor future trends in tobacco-attributable mortality and to seek co-factors that might explain why smoking appears to be even more dangerous in Eastern Europe than elsewhere. Occupational factors and general air pollution must be contributing to differing extents to the lung cancer rates in various countries, and may be particularly important in Eastern Europe. But, they are not likely to be major determinants of the international mortality patterns,[10] and the present approximate methods therefore remain appropriate.

For females, the populations with the lowest and with the highest proportions of deaths in middle age attributed to tobacco are, respectively, Spain (0%) and the USA (37%). In Spain a very low risk is reasonable, as female smoking is rare in middle age and is common only among young women (whose tobacco-attributable death rates will eventually become high if they continue to smoke as they age). In the US a high female death rate from tobacco is well documented for 1985, and a steep trend is well documented from 1965 to 1985.[4] The prediction that there will, during the current decade, be particularly high female death rates from tobacco in the United States is therefore securely based on reliable data from large prospective studies in the same country,[4] and in view of the steep increase in US female mortality from tobacco that is now in progress even larger numbers of deaths from tobacco must be expected among US females during the first few years of the next century.

The validity of the overall estimates for all developed populations in the current decade depends chiefly on the validity of the larger contributions. For females, much the largest contribution involves the reliable estimates from the United States. On average during the 1990s, tobacco is expected to cause about a quarter of a million female deaths a year in the US plus about a quarter of a million female deaths a year in other developed countries. (The second largest contribution is from UK females.) Because the US hazards are well documented, the grand total of half a million female deaths a year (ie, about 5 million female deaths from tobacco in developed countries during the whole decade 1990–1999) can be accepted as reliable.

In each population most of the deaths attributed to tobacco are male, so male mortality is closely correlated with overall (male plus female) mortality from the habit. Either for males alone or for males and females together, the greatest annual number of deaths currently attributed to tobacco in any developed population is in the European Community (fig 3). It is estimated that in the EC there will be about 570 000 deaths per year from tobacco during the current decade, of which about a quarter of a million will still be in middle age (35–69). Within the EC, the countries with the greatest numbers of deaths currently attributed to tobacco are the UK (150 000 per year) and Germany (111 000 per year), although the highest risk of death in middle age from tobacco in the EC (and the most rapid increase in this risk) appears to be in Denmark. A large collaborative European prospective study is currently being organised through the International Agency for Research on Cancer that will monitor the evolution of this epidemic throughout the EC, as well as seeking particularly reliable evidence on possible co-factors for the hazards of tobacco. Within the EC, the UK is the country with much the largest number of deaths attributed to tobacco, and a number of studies of the habit have been conducted there. None, however, has been on a representative sample of the population. All estimates of UK mortality from tobacco have therefore used indirect arguments. A recent estimate of 110 000 deaths a year by the UK Health Education Authority[17] is lower than the present estimate of 150 000 (perhaps because it failed to allow appropriately for the delay between the decrease in male smoking prevalence and the decrease in male death), but is not grossly different.

Extrapolation to future decades

Extrapolation to 1995 is reasonably secure, but the further into the next century the risks are extrapolated (fig 3) the more uncertainty there must be about the age-specific death rates from tobacco. Substantial uncertainty about the age-specific death rates in future decades need not, however, imply similarly large uncertainties about the absolute annual numbers of deaths, for even large changes in death rates (such as, for example, the decreases in causes other than tobacco of vascular mortality) may not have much effect on the proportion of deaths attributable to tobacco. Hence, the age-specific death rates of the future from current smoking patterns cannot be predicted reliably, as they depend on other factors, but the approximate annual number of deaths in the future from tobacco can be.

At the 1995 tobacco-attributed mortality rates among people of a given age there would be about 3·4 million deaths from tobacco in 2025 (2·6 million male plus 0·8 million female: these numbers are larger than the 1·6 million male and 0·5 million female in 1995 only because of population growth). But, although the male tobacco-attributed death rates may, on current smoking patterns, be approximately stable (as they have been for the past few years), the female rates are rising rapidly—indeed, although the age-specific risks are lower for females than for males, if women smoke like men then the US example shows that the absolute number of female deaths from tobacco may eventually be about as great as the male number. The uncertainties in the future predictions are greater than those in the current estimates, but even though the decreasing male death rates from tobacco that have been achieved in a few developed countries may be extended to more developed countries over the next few decades, the female death rates from tobacco are now increasing rapidly and, taking men and women together, of all deaths the proportion attributed to tobacco will for several years continue to increase. Hence, on current smoking patterns in developed countries, at least 3 million deaths a year from tobacco must be expected in 2025, and the actual number could well be considerably higher than this. The UK was the first country to experience high male lung cancer rates, but even in the UK the disease was rare until the second quarter of this century, so worldwide extrapolation of the numbers in fig 3 backwards to low numbers a few decades before 1965 (and taking the number in each decade to be ten times the annual number) indicates that deaths in developed countries from tobacco probably numbered in total "only" a few million from 1930 to 1959, followed by about 9 million in the 1960s, 13 million in the 1970s, 17 million in the 1980s, 21 million in the 1990s and, at the 1995 tobacco-attributed death rates (which will not, of course, really remain constant), 25 million, 29 million and 34 million over the next 3 decades. These numbers total about 150 million from 1930 to 2029, including about 50 million in the 60-year period from 1930 to 1989 and about 100 million in the 40-year period from 1990–2029. Although crude, such estimates suffice to provide a useful guide to the approximate scale of tobacco-related mortality that must be expected in the next century.

An alternative approach to the assessment of these future hazards is to note that in the mid-1990s about one-fifth (2·1 million/10·8 million: figs 1 and 2) of all deaths in developed countries were already attributed to tobacco, and that on current smoking patterns (especially among females) this proportion may well increase a little over the next few decades but is not likely to decrease. This suggests that about one-fifth of the people now living in developed countries (ie, about a quarter of a billion out of one-and-a-quarter billion) will, on current smoking patterns, eventually be killed by tobacco, losing an average of about 15 years of life expectancy per death.

The present methods are obviously crude, and the presentation of a mass of apparently precise figures should not be taken to suggest otherwise. Hence, because the growing worldwide epidemic of premature death from tobacco is so great, its detailed evolution needs to be monitored accurately by large, reliable prospective studies in a number of developed countries (and, particularly importantly,[18] in a number of less developed countries). Such studies could assess not only the effects of tobacco but also some of the factors that importantly modify those effects. The large pattern is, however, now clear: in developed countries tobacco is already causing about two million deaths a year this number is still increasing, and about half those killed by the habit are still only in middle age, making tobacco much the most important cause of premature death. Elsewhere, the epidemic is generally at an earlier stage but recent large increases in cigarette use in countries such as China means that tobacco will, in a few decades, also become one of the most important causes of premature death in less developed countries.[18]

This report originated from the WHO Consultative Group on Statistical Aspects of Tobacco-related Mortality: R. Peto (chairman), A. D. Lopez (scientific secretary), T. Novotny (rapporteur), C. Chollat-Traquet, P. C. Gupta, K. Kuulaasma, M. Parkin, K. D. Stanley. L. Garfinkel first provided CPS-II data, Sir Richard Doll provided helpful criticism, and Gale Mead provided secretarial support (and harrassment).

REFERENCES

1. Zaridze D, Peto R, eds. Tobacco: a major international health hazard. IARC Scientific Publications No. 74, International Agency for Research on Cancer (IARC), Lyon, 1986.
2. IARC Monographs on the Evolution of the Carcinogenic Risk of Chemicals to Humans, Vol 38: tobacco smoking. Lyon: IARC, 1986.
3. Garfinkel L. Selection, follow-up and analysis in the American Cancer Society prospective studies. In: Garfinkel, Ochs O, Mushinksi M, eds. Selection, follow-up and analysis in prospective studies: a workshop. NCI Monograph 67. National Cancer Institute, NIH Publication No. 85–2713, 1985: 49–52.
4. US Department of Health and Human Services. Reducing the health consequences of smoking: 25 years of progress. A report of the Surgeon-General. USDHHS, Public Health Service, Centers for Disease Control Office on Smoking and Health. DHHS Publication No. (CDC) 89-8411, 1989.
5. World Health Organisation (WHO). World health statistics annual. Geneva: WHO, 1987.
6. Peto R. Influence of dose and duration of smoking on lung cancer rates. In: Zaridze D, Peto R, eds. Tobacco: a major international health hazard. IARC Scientific Publications No. 74. Lyon: IARC, 1986: 23–33.
7. Fletcher CM, Peto R. The natural history of chronic airflow obstruction. *Br Med J* 1977; i: 1645–48.
8. Keys A. Seven countries: a multivariate analysis of health and coronary heart disease. Cambridge, Mass: Harvard University Press, 1980.
9. Martin MJ, Hulley SB, Browner WS, Kuller LH, Wentworth D. Serum cholesterol, blood pressure and mortality: implications from a cohort of 361 662 men. *Lancet* 1986; ii: 933–36.
10. Doll R, Peto R. The causes of cancer. *J Natl Cancer Inst* 1981; **66:** 1191–1308.
11. US Department of Health and Human Services. The health consequences of smoking for women. A report of the Surgeon-General. USDHHS, Public Health Service, Centers for Disease Control Office on Smoking and Health, 1980: 86.
12. US Department of Health and Human Services. The health consequences of smoking: cancer. A Report of the Surgeon-General. USDHHS, Public Health Service, Centers for Disease Control Office on Smoking and Health. DHHS Publication No. (CDC) 82-50179, 1982.
13. Garfinkel L, Stellman SD. Smoking and lung cancer in women. *Cancer Res* 1988; **43:** 6951–55.
14. Doll R. The age distribution of cancer: implication for models of carcinogenesis (with discussion). *J Roy Statist Soc A* 1971; **134:** 133–66.
15. UN Department of Economic and Social Affairs. World population prospects 1990 (medium variant). *J Roy Statist Soc A* 1971; **134:** 133–66.
16. Hirayama T. Life-style and mortality: a large-scale census-based cohort study in Japan. *Contrib Epidemiol Biostat* 1990; **6.**
17. Health Education Authority. The smoking epidemic. London: HEA, 1991.
18. World Health Organisation. Tobacco-attributable mortality: global estimates and projections. *Tobacco Alert* 1991; **1:** 4–7.

Appendix: Annual mortality rates per 100,000 in years 3-6 inclusive (approximately 1984-1988) of ACS CPS-II prospective study

Age at death	Current / Never smoker	Lung cancer		Upper aero-dig. cancer		Other cancer		COPD		Other respiratory		Vascular disease		Cirrhosis		Other medical		Non-medical		All causes		Person-years (100,000s)	
		M	F	M	F	M	F	M	F	M	F	M	F	M	F	M	F	M	F	M	F	M	F
35-9	C*	0	7	0	0	0	52	0	0	18	0	55	7	27	7	46	13	64	20	211	104	0.1091	0.1533
	N	7	3	0	0	14	42	0	0	0	0	14	16	0	3	27	0	27	3	89	68	0.1456	0.3081
	(n)	(2)	(2)																				
40-4	C*	23	12	0	4	30	39	0	0	0	4	128	19	0	0	53	16	105	27	338	120	0.1333	0.2580
	N	0	0	7	0	22	70	0	0	0	2	14	15	14	2	7	2	36	17	100	109	0.1393	0.4576
	(n)	(3)	(3)																				
45-9	C	35	49	13	2	45	79	0	3	3	7	209	60	16	2	48	27	61	15	430	243	0.3113	0.5960
	N	9	4	0	0	44	98	0	0	0	5	53	17	0	1	28	5	28	12	162	142	0.3211	1.1687
	(n)	(5)	(4)																				
50-4	C	114	71	29	3	117	139	14	11	4	7	312	93	10	6	46	21	51	14	698	367	0.7625	0.9679
	N	5	5	2	2	71	120	1	1	5	3	86	31	4	2	25	13	27	13	226	188	0.8141	1.9652
	(n)	(7)	(7)																				
55-9	C	227	136	23	11	217	228	27	24	30	20	477	164	19	9	68	52	62	27	1150	669	0.8538	1.0187
	N	3	8	7	1	113	174	3	1	8	6	149	54	1	1	42	29	28	16	355	290	0.8792	2.2411
	(n)	(10)	(10)																				
60-4	C	375	195	54	30	342	300	53	42	32	18	772	298	24	19	118	66	51	12	1821	980	0.7524	0.8987
	N	11	14	6	3	197	239	4	3	9	7	331	103	12	4	60	32	32	17	663	422	0.8057	2.2740
	(n)	(14)	(14)																				
65-9	C	599	310	77	18	567	404	170	101	83	35	1170	553	36	19	188	135	43	24	2934	1600	0.5058	0.6218
	N	24	18	10	4	303	338	7	7	24	12	583	219	7	7	82	57	40	15	1081	676	0.6967	1.9256
	(n)	(20)	(19)																				
70-4	C	899	339	93	48	778	593	324	166	141	67	1977	868	52	11	413	182	96	35	4773	2307	0.2904	0.3746
	N	36	28	12	4	505	449	22	11	57	35	1059	415	8	11	148	107	59	27	1906	1089	0.5053	1.4328
	(n)	(27)	(26)																				
75-9	C*	1168	429	106	36	1380	584	572	250	327	131	3243	1715	82	24	645	292	82	83	7604	3544	0.1224	0.1679
	N	38	42	3	9	821	547	35	19	149	86	1981	961	14	9	391	213	73	46	3504	1932	0.2888	0.9590
	(n)	(35)	(34)																				
80+	C*	1191	400	154	71	1809	872	882	657	684	271	5537	3129	44	14	1103	857	287	57	11691	6330	0.0453	0.0700
	N	88	64	10	19	1264	778	124	54	599	277	4268	3237	0	14	888	573	165	70	7406	5088	0.1938	0.8289
	(n)	(46)	(44)																				

N.B. The absolute risks may be artificially low, but (except for lung cancer) only relative risks are used.
The risks (at age 35) of dying at age 35-69 indicated by these all-causes death rates are: Males: smokers 32%, non-smokers 13%; Females: smokers 18%, non-smokers 9%
* Smoker rates based on less than 20,000 person-years. C=Cigarette smoker in 1982, N=Never smoked regularly, (n)=Smoothed lung cancer rates for these non-smokers.
Smoothing 5-year age-groups with lower limits 35, 40, ..., 70, 75 involved the best-fitting line of slope 4 on a logarithmic graph of non-smoker rates vs these lower limits.[14]

8. SELECTED RESULTS. CONTRASTS BETWEEN DEVELOPED POPULATIONS IN SMOKING-ATTRIBUTED MORTALITY, AND IN OTHER MORTALITY

ABSOLUTE NUMBERS OF DEATHS FROM SMOKING

The reliability of these methods has been discussed in the preceding Lancet report. That discusson remains valid and will not be repeated; here, the chief aim is to use these methods. As well as describing the findings for each separate population, it is of interest to contrast with each other the findings for different populations. Hence, this chapter brings together findings from each separate set (one per population) of the main tables and figures of this monograph. First it contrasts the absolute numbers of deaths in each separate population, then it contrasts the mortality rates, and the trends in those rates.

Maps of Europe (Figs 16 & 17)

The simplest descriptive statistics are the absolute annual numbers of deaths from smoking. These are provided in the detailed tabulations for each country, and in Figures 16 and 17 these annual numbers of deaths are brought together, and are plotted onto maps of Europe. The numbers of deaths for non-European developed populations are given at the foot of each map, together with totals for the European Union and for the former USSR.

The first map (Fig 16, marked ALL AGES) is not subdivided by sex or by age: it combines men and women in middle age (35-69) and in old age (70+), giving the total number of deaths attributed to smoking in each population.

Obviously, the largest numbers of deaths tend to be found in the largest populations. In particular, the numbers of the deaths in 1990 that were attributed to smoking were about half a million in each of three populations: the United States (461,000), the former USSR (457,000) and the planned European Union of 16 countries (shaded areas: EU total 540,000).

These 16 shaded countries of the "Planned EU" include the 12 countries that were already, in 1994, members of the EU, together with the 4 countries that were, in early 1994, planning to become members in the near future (Austria, Finland, Norway and Sweden).

Within the European Union, the countries with the greatest number of deaths in 1990 attributed to smoking are the United Kingdom (138,000) and Germany (112,000).

The mortality attributed to tobacco is, however, known less reliably in old age than in middle age; moreover, those killed by smoking in middle age will, on average, suffer a much greater loss of life expectancy than those killed at older ages by the habit. So, the next map (Fig 17) is restricted to middle age, and gives for 1990 the numbers of deaths at ages 35-69 that were attributed to smoking.

Again, of course, the largest populations predominate, with a few hundred thousand deaths at ages 35-69 from smoking in the United States (223,000), the former USSR (341,000) and the European Union (255,000).

Comparing Figures 16 and 17, it may be seen that the geographic distribution of the deaths from tobacco is very different at different ages. For example, in old age there were far more deaths from smoking in Britain than in Poland, but in middle age this was no longer the case. In these parts of Europe, the largest numbers of deaths in 1990 at ages 35-69 that are attributed to smoking are 54,000 in the United Kingdom, 58,000 in Germany and 50,000 in Poland (Fig 17). These differences reflect, of course, not only the sizes of the individual risks but also the sizes of the populations, and further comparisons between these countries will be deferred until appropriate death rates, and trends in death rates, can be contrasted (see below).

Fig. 16. The geographic distribution of death from smoking

ALL 'DEVELOPED' COUNTRIES, 1990
All ages: 2 million annual deaths from smoking

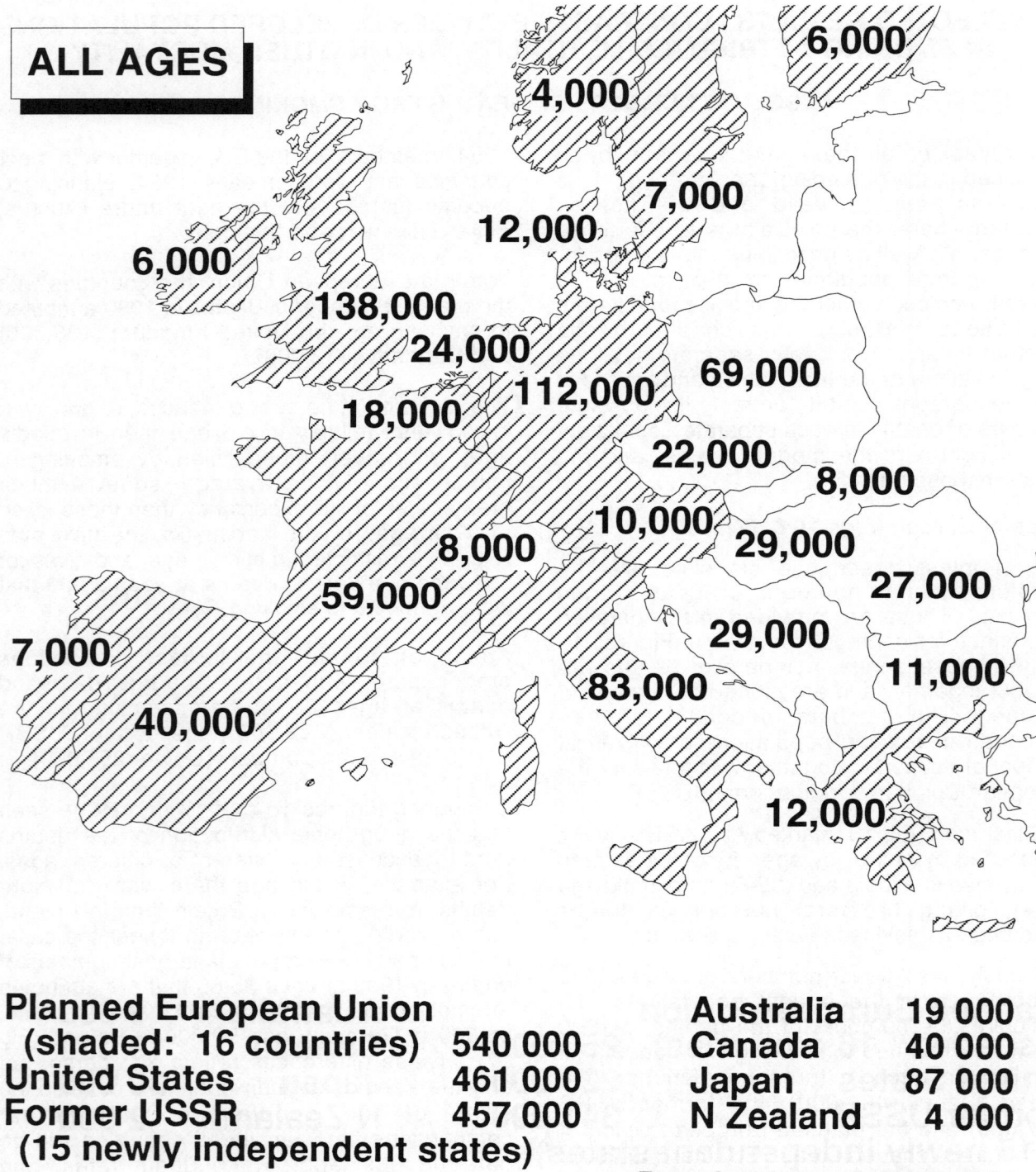

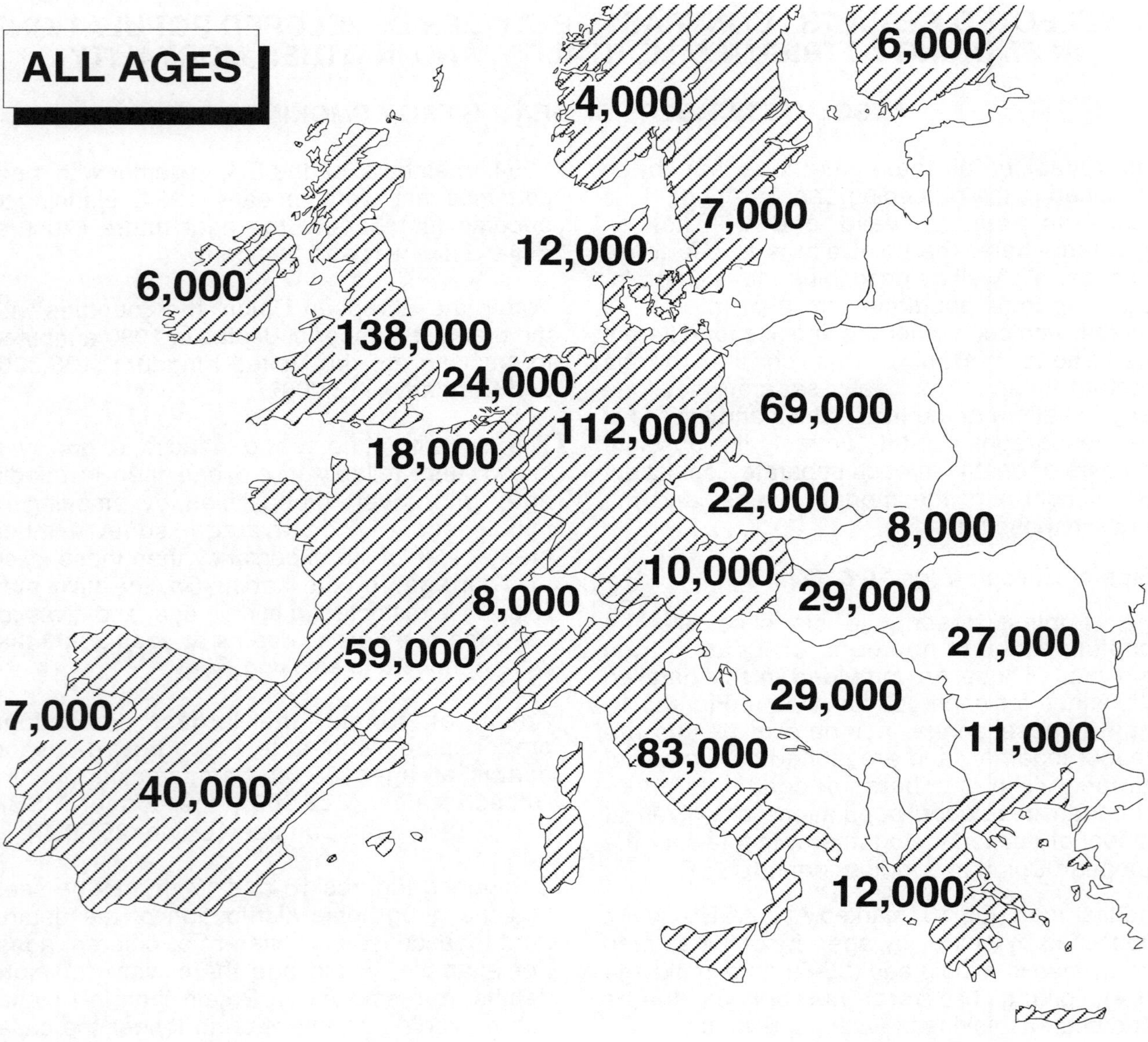

Planned European Union (shaded: 16 countries)	540 000	Australia	19 000
United States	461 000	Canada	40 000
Former USSR (15 newly independent states)	457 000	Japan	87 000
		N Zealand	4 000

Peto, Lopez et al, 1992, 1994

Fig. 17. The geographic distribution of death from smoking in MIDDLE age (35-69 years of age)

ALL 'DEVELOPED' COUNTRIES, 1990
Age 35-69: 1 million annual deaths from smoking

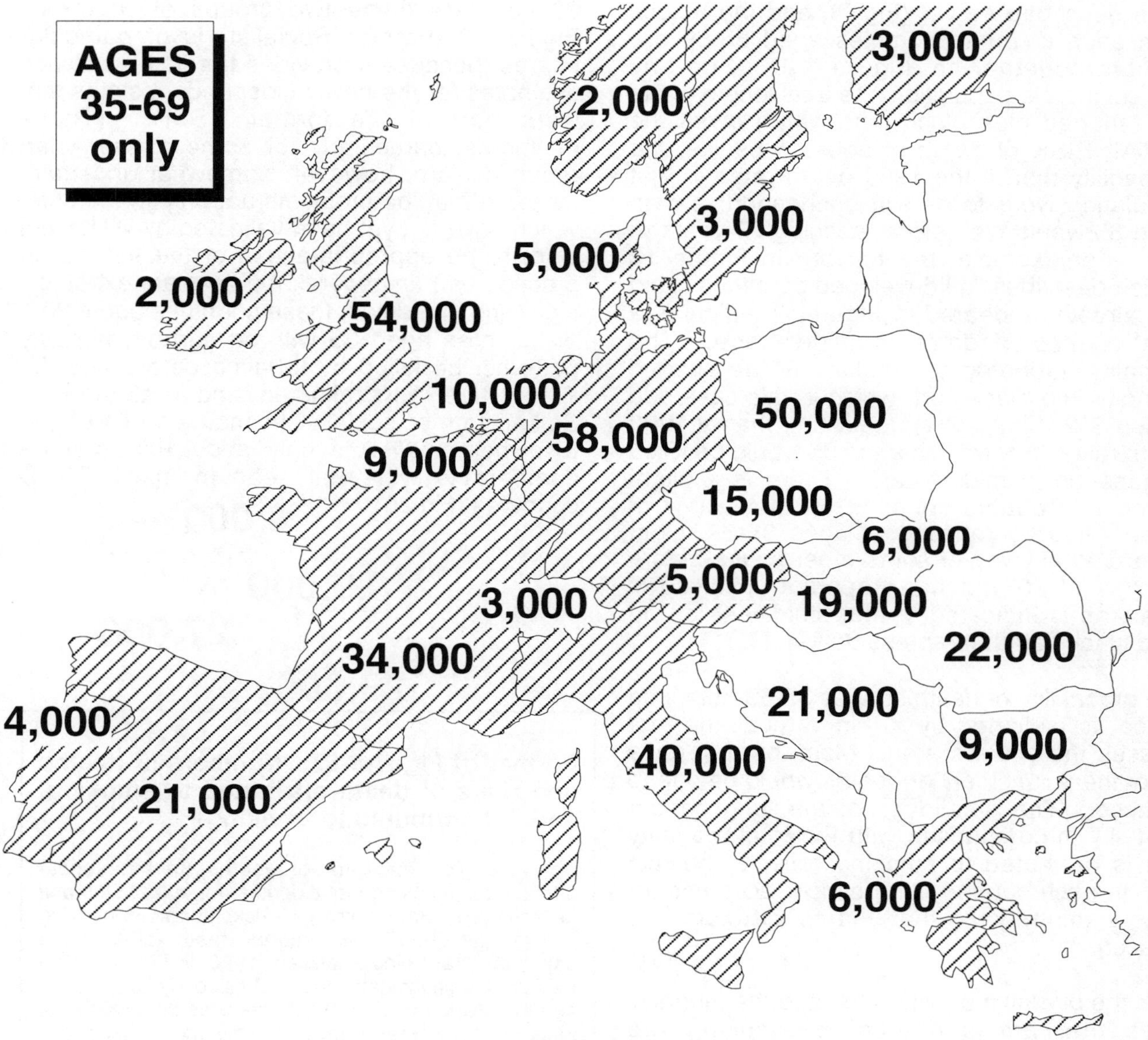

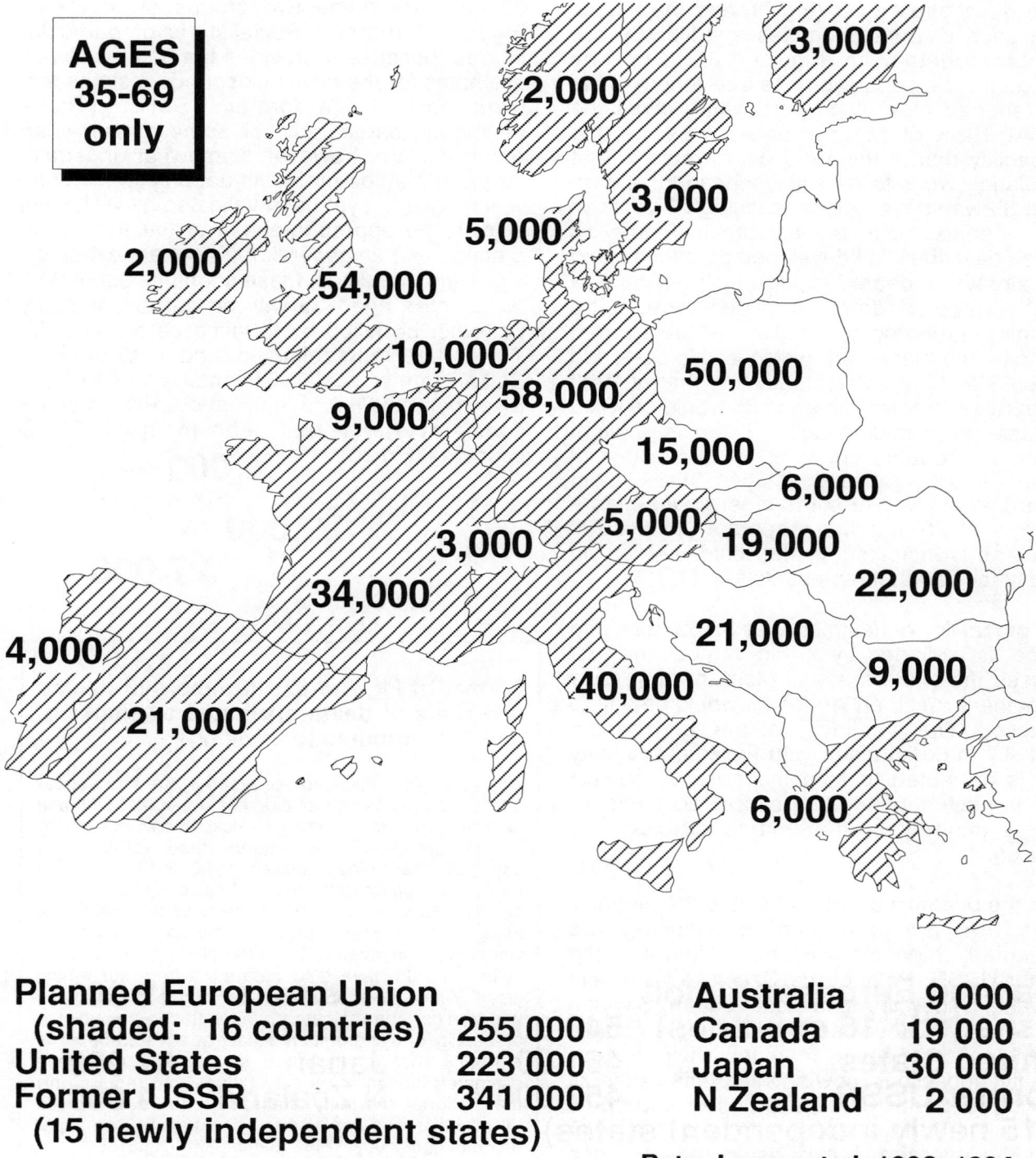

Planned European Union (shaded: 16 countries)	255 000	Australia	9 000
United States	223 000	Canada	19 000
Former USSR (15 newly independent states)	341 000	Japan	30 000
		N Zealand	2 000

Peto, Lopez et al, 1992, 1994

RISKS OF DEATH AT AGES 35-69 FROM SMOKING, OR FROM ANY CAUSE (FIGS 18-57)

Male death risks, and 1955-1995 trends (Figs 18-32)

In the standard set of Main Tables and Figures for each country, a bar diagram is provided that gives the risks of dying at ages 0-34 and at ages 35-69. The format of these bar diagrams has been described earlier (Fig 7), and the results from each country for males aged 35-69 are brought together in Figure 18. For any particular male population, the total length of the bar (shaded plus black plus white) gives the TOTAL RISK of death at ages 35-69, i.e. the probability that, if the 1990 death rates in that population were to persist unchanged, a man aged 35 would die before reaching 70 years of age. For example, the top bar in Figure 18 (which describes "all developed countries", and has already appeared in Figure 7) indicates a 36% chance of death in middle age. The mortality attributed to smoking is the shaded part plus the black part, which in this case add up to 13% (11% + 2%), indicating that at 1990 death rates 13% of men aged 35 would be killed by tobacco in middle age. There is a slight element of double counting, in that a few of those killed by tobacco at ages 35-69 might have died anyway of some other cause before the age of 70, but the proportion involved is small, as is indicated by the smallness of the solid black part that represents it.

The probability of death at ages 35-69 from lung cancer is indicated by a thin vertical line that crosses the shaded area. Most, but not quite all, of these lung cancer deaths would be due to tobacco. The smallness of the lung cancer mortality in comparison with the total mortality that is attributed to smoking reflects the fact that, in each country, lung cancer accounts for only a minority of the deaths attributed to tobacco.

Both the overall mortality rates and the mortality rates that are attributed to smoking are particularly high for men from Hungary, the former USSR, Poland, the Czech republic and Slovakia. They are smallest in Japan, Sweden and Norway. Otherwise, they are more notable for their homogeneity than for their heterogeneity: tobacco is now an important cause of premature death in all developed countries. (The risk in Portugal appears to be a little lower than the average, but is rising rapidly: see below.)

Taken as a whole, however, these male risks of premature death from smoking tend to be greater in former socialist economies than in OECD developed countries, and Figures 19 and 20 separate these two groups of countries. Figure 19 (Former Socialist) is of particular interest because it provides the first-ever such estimates for the newly independent states that were part of the former USSR. (These estimates, particularly for some of the Asian republics, are, however, somewhat uncertain, for there may be problems not only in the data, which have not yet been validated by WHO, but also in the appropriateness of the estimation procedures.) In general, the risks are extremely high, and in many of these countries about 20% of the men aged 35 will, on current mortality patterns, be killed by tobacco before age 70. This is true in Kazakhstan, and in all the non-Balkan former socialist economies of Europe. Elsewhere, the risk is "only" about 10%, which is comparable with that seen in many OECD countries (Fig 20).

Format of Figs 18-57: Numbers of deaths and risks of death attributed to smoking, and not attributed to smoking

Columns give numbers of deaths (in thousands) attributed to smoking / total deaths, for ages 35-69 and for ages 70+. Bar lengths give risks at age 35 of dying before age 70, at the national death rates in the particular year being analysed (1990, in Fig 18). The total bar length indicates the total risk of dying at 35-69, and the shaded-plus-solid part indicates the total risk of being killed at these ages by smoking. (Shaded = would have survived to 70 in the absence of tobacco, solid = would have died before 70 from something else). Within the shaded area, the part to the left of the thin vertical line indicates (where this is known) the probability of dying of lung cancer at ages 35-69. The mortality that is attributed to smoking has been estimated indirectly, by calculations that require only the national mortality statistics: for details, see Introduction, and see also the photoreproduced paper by Peto, Lopez et al, 1992 (Lancet 338: 1268).

Fig. 18. Males, 1990, Developed Populations Smoking–Attributed and Other Mortality

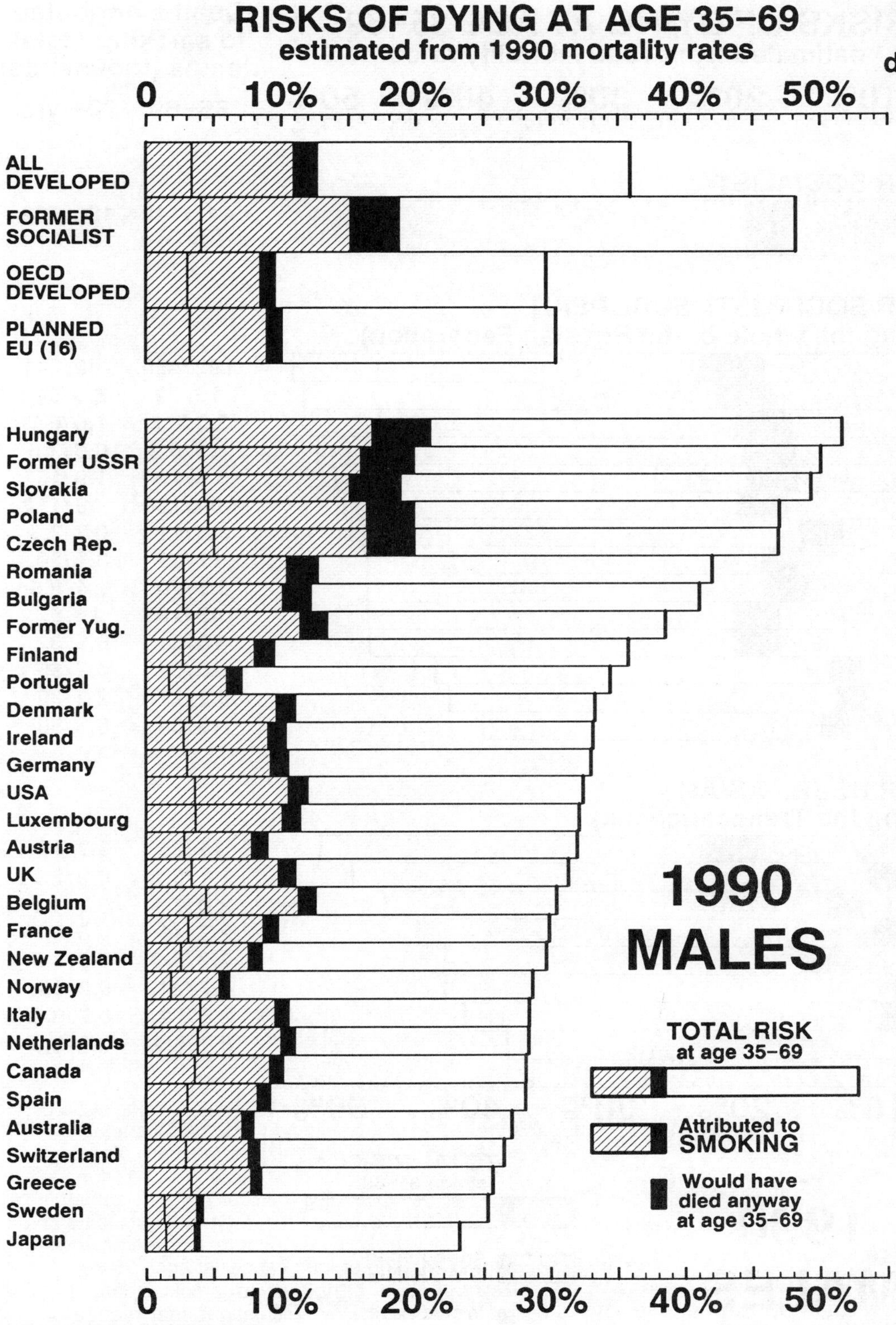

Deaths attributed to smoking / total deaths (thousands)

	35–69	70+ yrs
ALL DEVELOPED	865/2458 (35%)	554/2851 (19%)
FORMER SOCIALIST	441/1124 (39%)	126/763 (17%)
OECD DEVELOPED	424/1334 (32%)	428/2088 (20%)
PLANNED EU (16)	222/673 (33%)	223/1112 (20%)
Hungary	16/39	6.5/34
Former USSR	313/787	84/460
Slovakia	5.8/15	1.9/13
Poland	45/105	15/87
Czech Rep.	13/31	6.1/32
Romania	20/62	4.2/56
Bulgaria	8.2/27	2.2/30
Former Yug.	19/54	6.3/50
Finland	2.6/11	2.7/13
Portugal	4.0/19	2.8/30
Denmark	3.3/10	4.3/20
Ireland	1.7/5.5	2.5/10
Germany	52/162	43/243
USA	150/415	136/595
Luxembourg	0.2/0.7	0.3/1.1
Austria	4.0/14	3.6/22
UK	37/107	52/195
Belgium	7.9/19	8.6/31
France	33/101	25/155
New Zealand	1.4/4.9	1.7/7.7
Norway	1.4/6.9	1.9/16
Italy	38/102	35/166
Netherlands	8.6/22	13/41
Canada	13/38	14/58
Spain	21/63	19/101
Australia	6.7/23	7.3/35
Switzerland	3.1/10	3.7/20
Greece	5.2/16	5.2/32
Sweden	2.1/13	3.2/34
Japan	27/168	42/257

Full legend is on facing page

Peto, Lopez et al, 1992, 1994

Fig. 19. Males, 1990, Former Socialist Countries Smoking–Attributed and Other Mortality

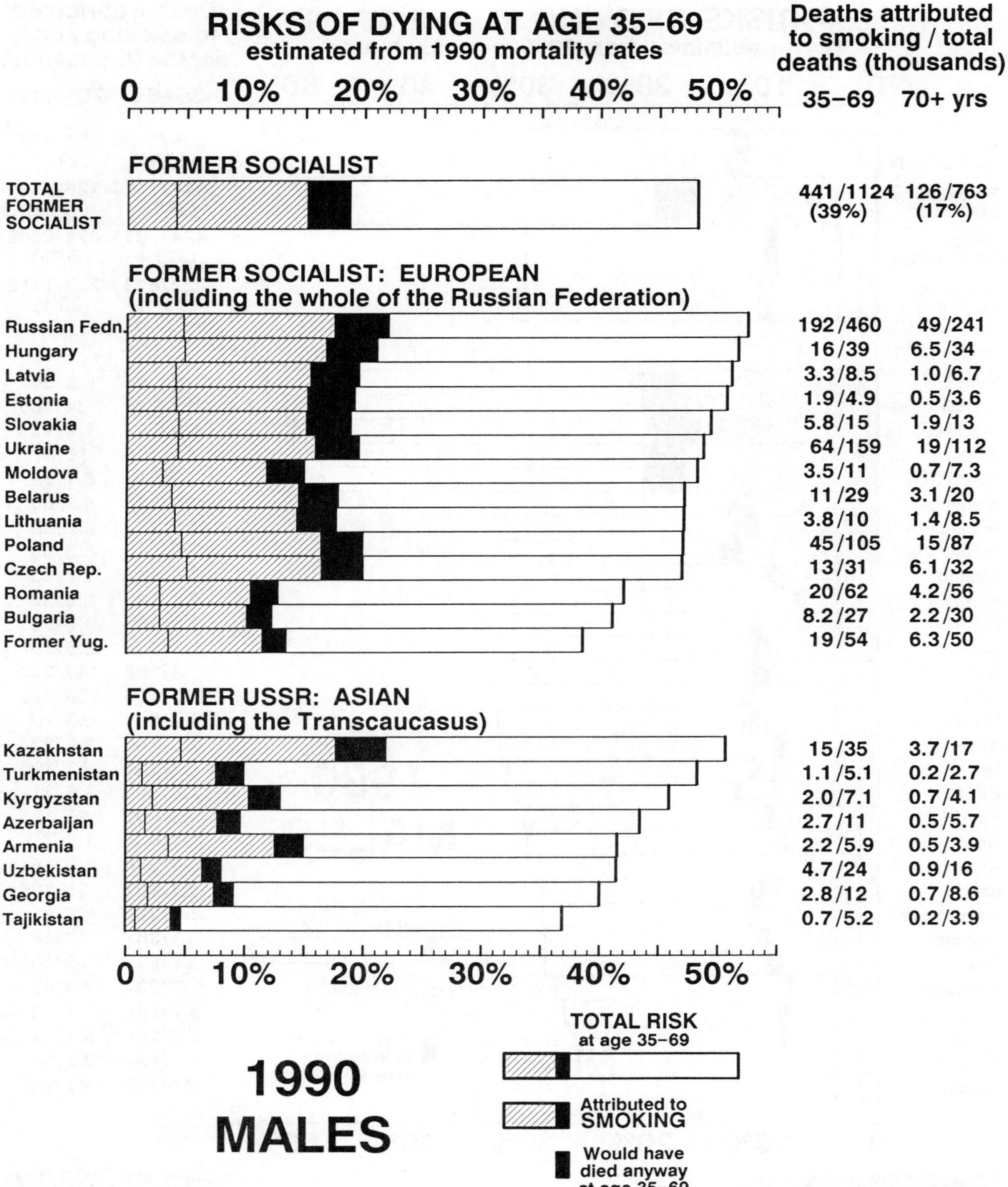

Full legend faces Fig 18

Peto, Lopez et al, 1992, 1994

Fig. 20. Males, 1990, OECD Developed Countries Smoking–Attributed and Other Mortality

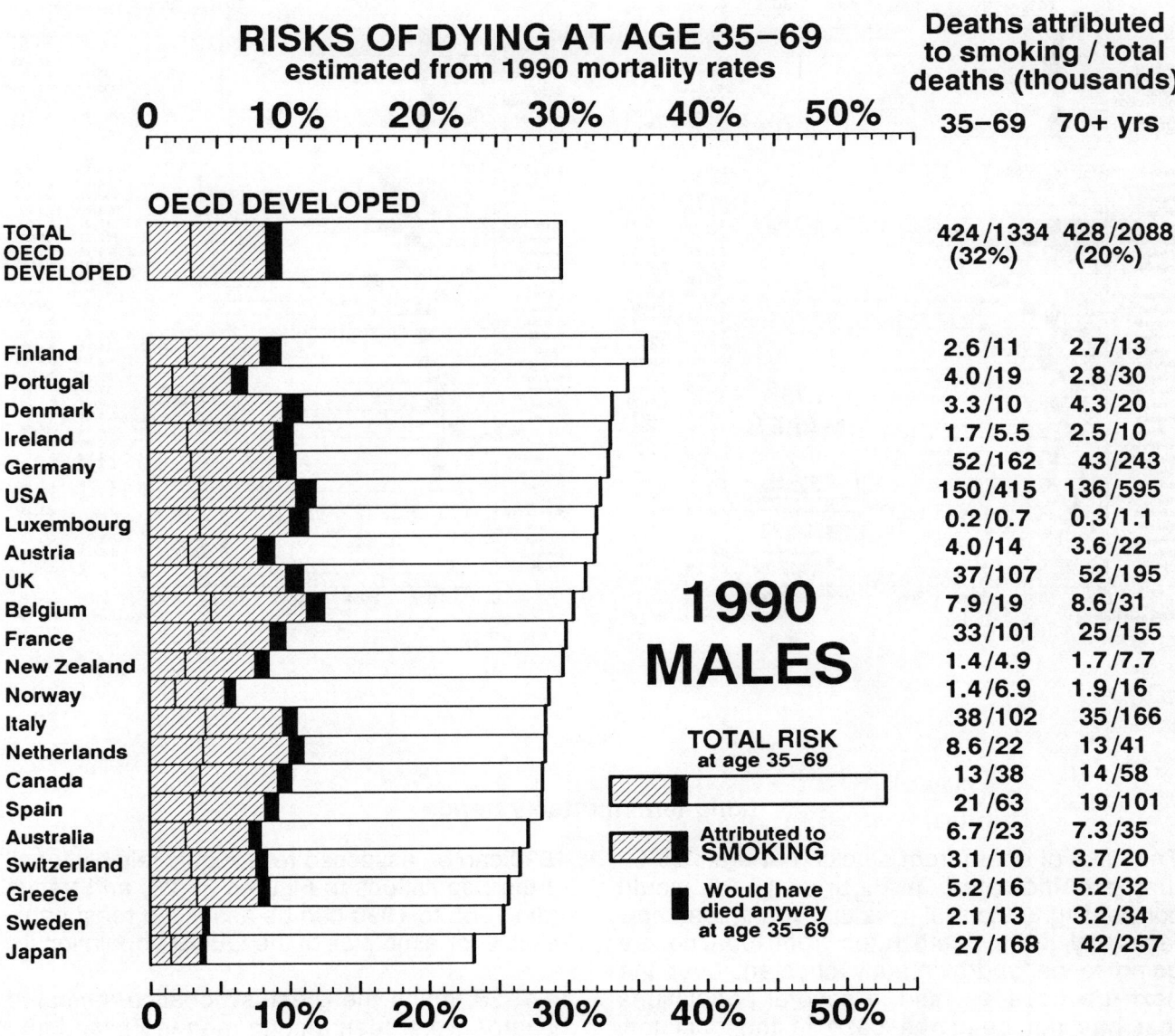

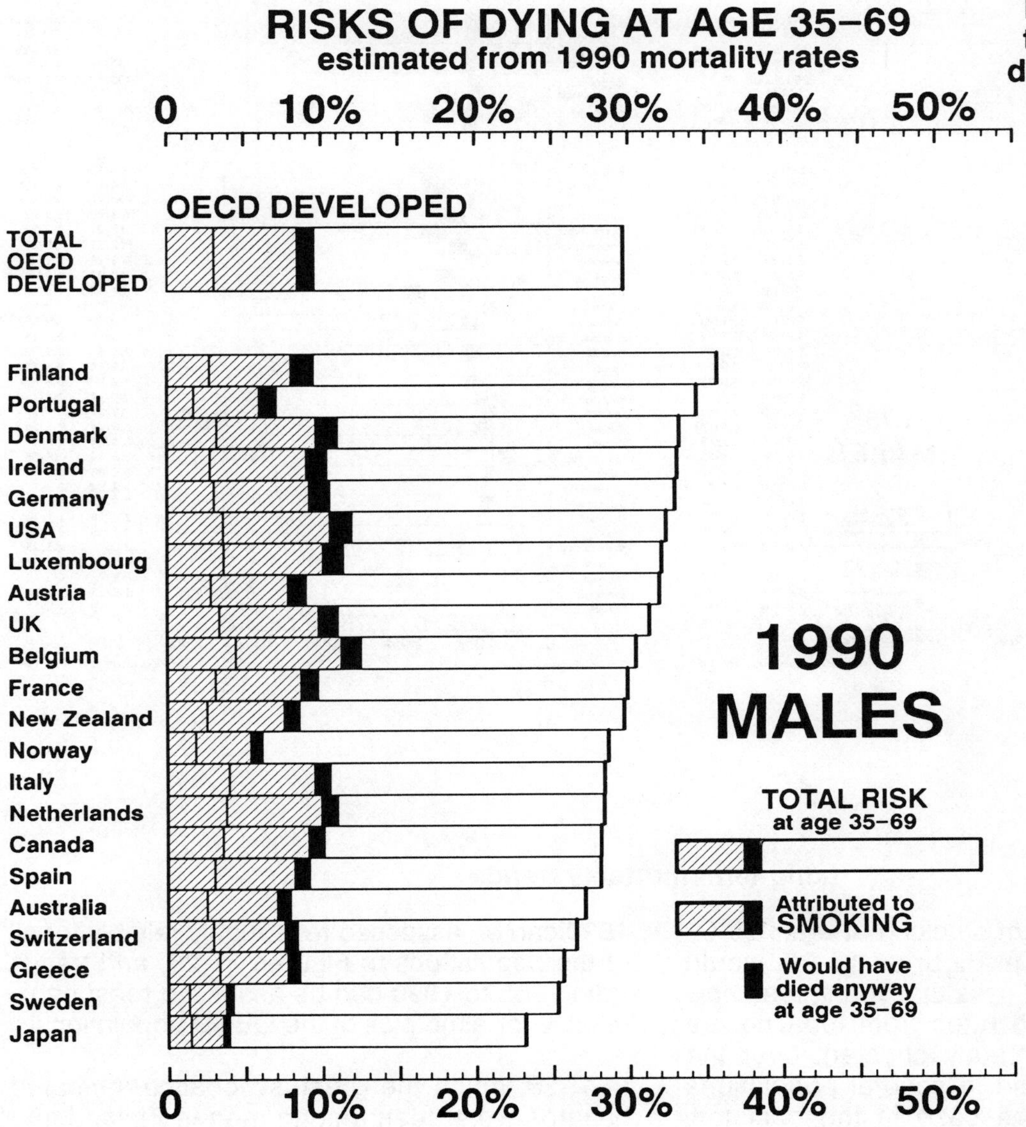

Deaths attributed to smoking / total deaths (thousands)

	35–69	70+ yrs
TOTAL OECD DEVELOPED	424/1334 (32%)	428/2088 (20%)
Finland	2.6/11	2.7/13
Portugal	4.0/19	2.8/30
Denmark	3.3/10	4.3/20
Ireland	1.7/5.5	2.5/10
Germany	52/162	43/243
USA	150/415	136/595
Luxembourg	0.2/0.7	0.3/1.1
Austria	4.0/14	3.6/22
UK	37/107	52/195
Belgium	7.9/19	8.6/31
France	33/101	25/155
New Zealand	1.4/4.9	1.7/7.7
Norway	1.4/6.9	1.9/16
Italy	38/102	35/166
Netherlands	8.6/22	13/41
Canada	13/38	14/58
Spain	21/63	19/101
Australia	6.7/23	7.3/35
Switzerland	3.1/10	3.7/20
Greece	5.2/16	5.2/32
Sweden	2.1/13	3.2/34
Japan	27/168	42/257

Full legend faces Fig 18

Peto, Lopez et al, 1992, 1994

Fig. 21. Males, 1955, Developed Populations
Smoking–Attributed and Other Mortality

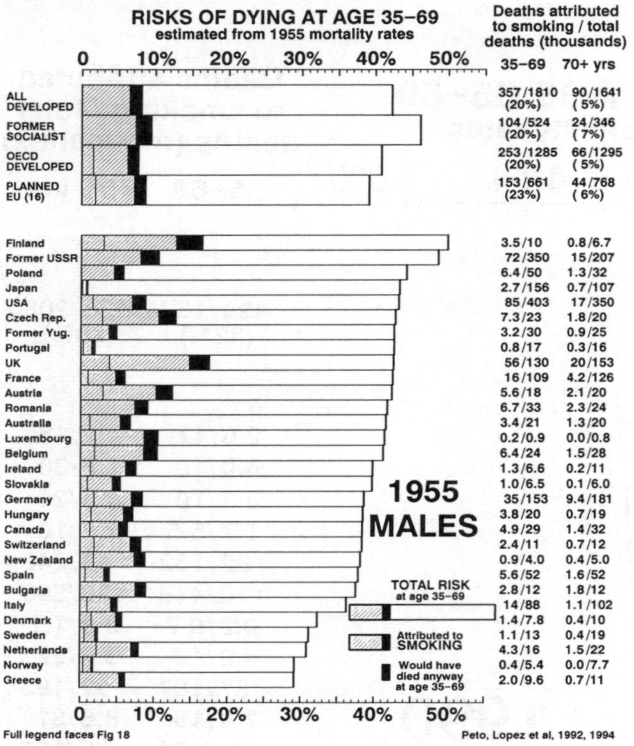

Fig. 22. Males, 1965, Developed Populations
Smoking–Attributed and Other Mortality

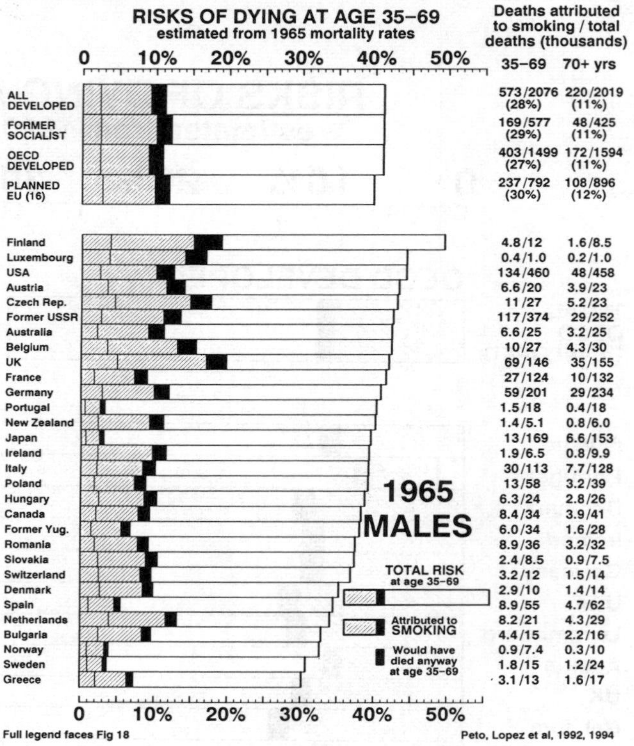

Long-term mortality trends

The risks of death from smoking at ages 35-69 that are indicated in Figures 18-20 would correspond to the real risks that young men now face only if the death rates from tobacco are going to be approximately constant over the next few decades, and in several populations that has not been the case in the past few decades. Figures 21-26 summarise the results of similar calculations for 1955, 1965, 1975, 1985, 1990 and projected 1995 (with the 1995 projections now based on the post-1985 trend from 1985 to 1990, instead of the pre-1985 trend that was used in the original Lancet report of these methods). Some of the earliest rates are rather unreliable. There are, for instance, various uncertainties about the 1965 rates, particularly for some of the former socialist economies, and much larger uncertainties about the 1955 rates for most of the former socialist economies (and for Greece): see the relevant Appendix tables. But, trends from 1975 to 1990 can be assessed reasonably reliably for all of the populations in Figures 21-26, and trends from 1955 to 1990 can be assessed reasonably reliably for almost all of the OECD populations.

In 1955, much the greatest tobacco-attributed hazards were seen among men in Finland and the UK, and these two populations still had the greatest hazards in 1965. By 1975, the UK and Finland still had high rates, but were matched by the Benelux countries, the Czech republic and the former USSR (the republics of which were not then published separately). By 1985 and 1990, however, the pattern had changed substantially. The male rates in the UK had decreased, and had been overtaken by the male rates in several of the former socialist economies. Thes territories are projected to have during the 1990s much the highest risks in the world of male death in middle age from tobacco (Fig 26).

Fig. 23. Males, 1975, Developed Populations Smoking–Attributed and Other Mortality

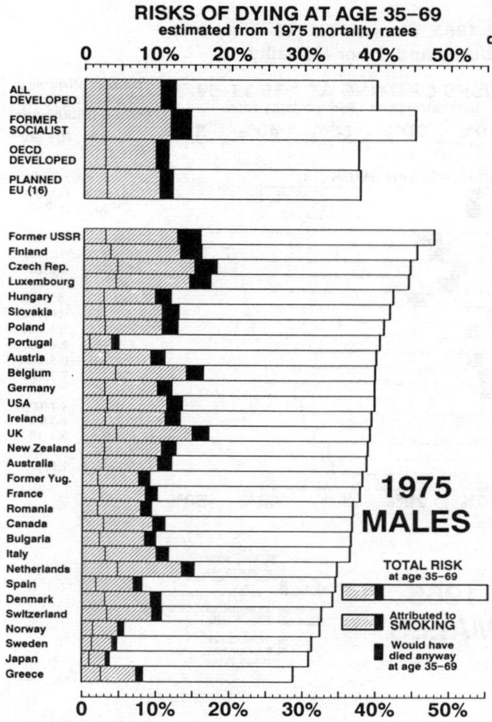

	Deaths attributed to smoking / total deaths (thousands) 35–69	70+ yrs
ALL DEVELOPED	704/2303 (31%)	415/2435 (17%)
FORMER SOCIALIST	256/826 (31%)	94/614 (15%)
OECD DEVELOPED	448/1477 (30%)	321/1821 (18%)
PLANNED EU (16)	246/777 (32%)	201/1056 (19%)
Former USSR	185/583	53/364
Finland	4.2/12	2.2/9.7
Czech Rep.	12/29	8.6/31
Luxembourg	0.4/1.0	0.3/1.1
Hungary	8.0/29	6.3/33
Slovakia	3.3/11	2.1/11
Poland	22/72	10/64
Portugal	2.5/21	1.0/22
Austria	4.7/17	5.2/26
Belgium	9.8/24	8.4/35
Germany	54/180	55/271
USA	157/457	84/485
Ireland	2.3/6.8	1.7/9.8
UK	62/142	52/176
New Zealand	1.9/5.9	1.4/6.3
Australia	8.6/28	5.5/27
Former Yug.	9.4/40	4.9/41
France	31/115	21/155
Romania	11/42	5.1/44
Canada	12/40	8.1/45
Bulgaria	5.5/20	2.9/24
Italy	39/121	23/152
Netherlands	10/24	9.4/36
Spain	14/62	11/78
Denmark	3.3/10	2.7/16
Switzerland	3.8/11	2.7/16
Norway	1.4/7.9	0.9/13
Sweden	2.6/17	2.9/29
Japan	18/156	18/184
Greece	4.2/15	3.9/23

Full legend faces Fig 18 — Peto, Lopez et al, 1992, 1994

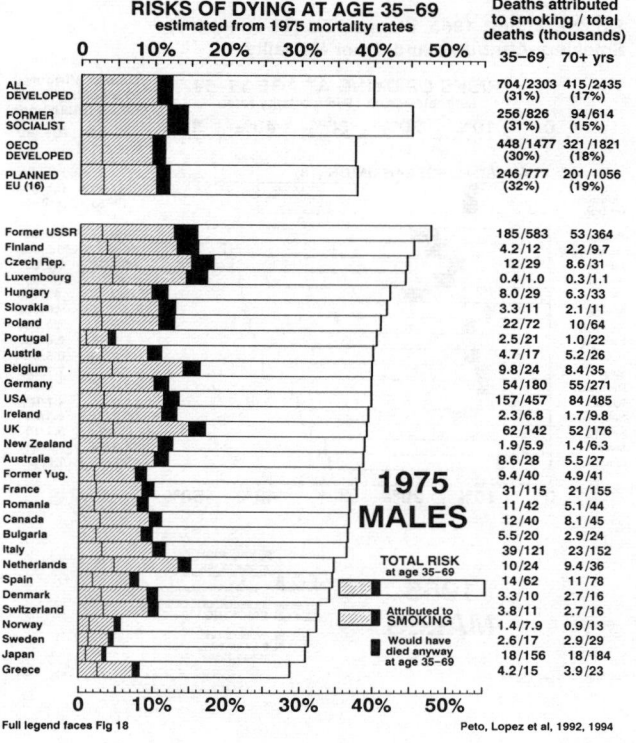

Fig. 24. Males, 1985, Developed Populations Smoking–Attributed and Other Mortality

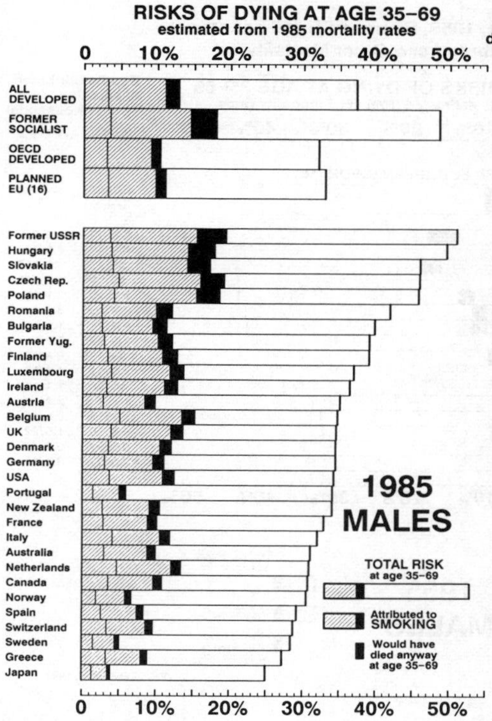

	Deaths attributed to smoking / total deaths (thousands) 35–69	70+ yrs
ALL DEVELOPED	805/2304 (35%)	564/2906 (19%)
FORMER SOCIALIST	379/980 (39%)	138/824 (17%)
OECD DEVELOPED	427/1324 (32%)	426/2082 (20%)
PLANNED EU (16)	224/663 (34%)	242/1161 (21%)
Former USSR	272/693	87/490
Hungary	13/34	8.0/39
Slovakia	4.8/12	2.6/14
Czech Rep.	12/27	8.0/36
Poland	37/89	17/94
Romania	17/53	5.4/63
Bulgaria	7.3/24	2.7/32
Former Yug.	15/46	6.7/55
Finland	3.4/11	3.1/13
Luxembourg	0.3/0.8	0.3/1.2
Ireland	2.2/6.2	2.5/11
Austria	3.9/14	4.6/25
Belgium	8.7/20	10/35
UK	46/117	59/202
Denmark	3.6/11	4.2/18
Germany	46/141	54/272
USA	154/425	123/575
Portugal	3.3/19	2.3/27
New Zealand	1.7/5.4	1.7/7.8
France	31/100	27/169
Italy	39/103	36/171
Australia	7.7/24	7.5/34
Netherlands	9.8/23	13/40
Canada	13/38	12/54
Norway	1.6/7.5	1.8/15
Spain	17/60	16/94
Switzerland	3.3/10	3.7/19
Sweden	2.6/15	3.2/34
Greece	4.9/15	5.3/31
Japan	22/157	35/229

Full legend faces Fig 18 — Peto, Lopez et al, 1992, 1994

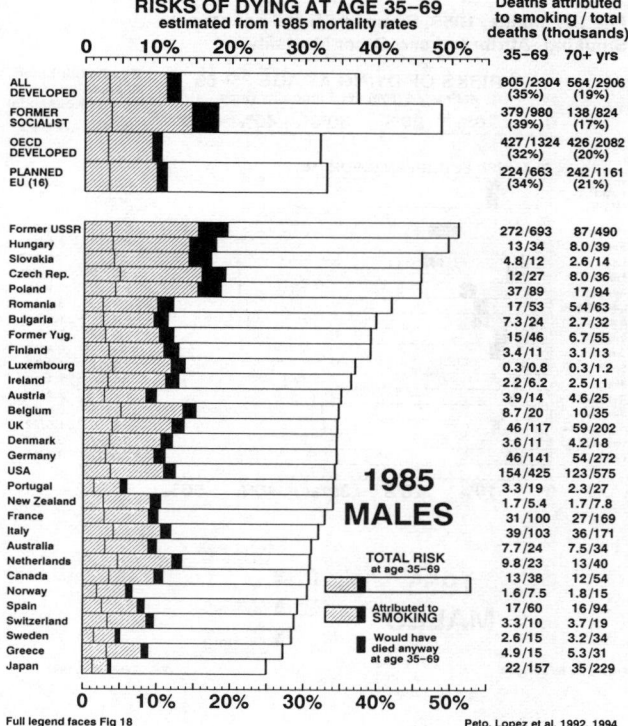

Fig. 25. Males, 1990, Developed Populations Smoking–Attributed and Other Mortality

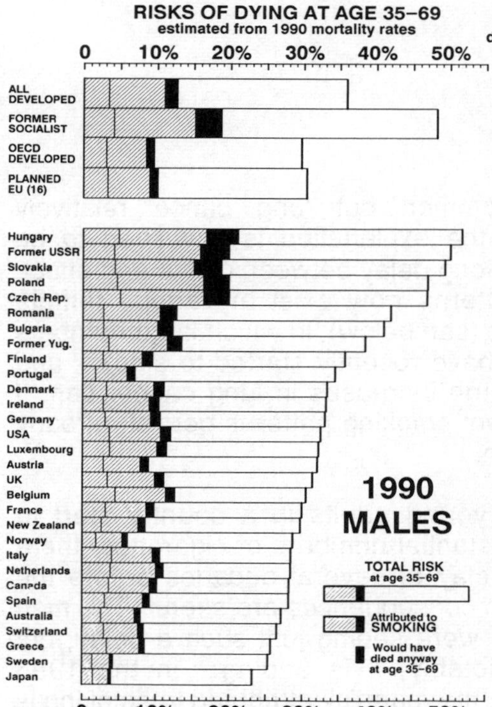

	Deaths attributed to smoking / total deaths (thousands) 35–69	70+ yrs
ALL DEVELOPED	865/2458 (35%)	554/2851 (19%)
FORMER SOCIALIST	441/1124 (39%)	126/763 (17%)
OECD DEVELOPED	424/1334 (32%)	428/2088 (20%)
PLANNED EU (16)	222/673 (33%)	223/1112 (20%)
Hungary	16/39	6.5/34
Former USSR	313/787	84/460
Slovakia	5.8/15	1.9/13
Poland	45/105	15/87
Czech Rep.	13/31	6.1/32
Romania	20/62	4.2/56
Bulgaria	8.2/27	2.2/30
Former Yug.	19/54	6.3/50
Finland	2.6/11	2.7/13
Portugal	4.0/19	2.8/30
Denmark	3.3/10	4.3/20
Ireland	1.7/5.5	2.5/10
Germany	52/162	43/243
USA	150/415	136/595
Luxembourg	0.2/0.7	0.3/1.1
Austria	4.0/14	3.6/22
UK	37/107	52/195
Belgium	7.9/19	8.6/31
France	33/101	25/155
New Zealand	1.4/4.9	1.7/7.7
Norway	1.4/6.9	1.9/16
Italy	38/102	35/166
Netherlands	8.6/22	13/41
Canada	13/38	14/58
Spain	21/63	19/101
Australia	6.7/23	7.3/35
Switzerland	3.1/10	3.7/20
Greece	5.2/16	5.2/32
Sweden	2.1/13	3.2/34
Japan	27/168	42/257

Full legend faces Fig 18 — Peto, Lopez et al, 1992, 1994

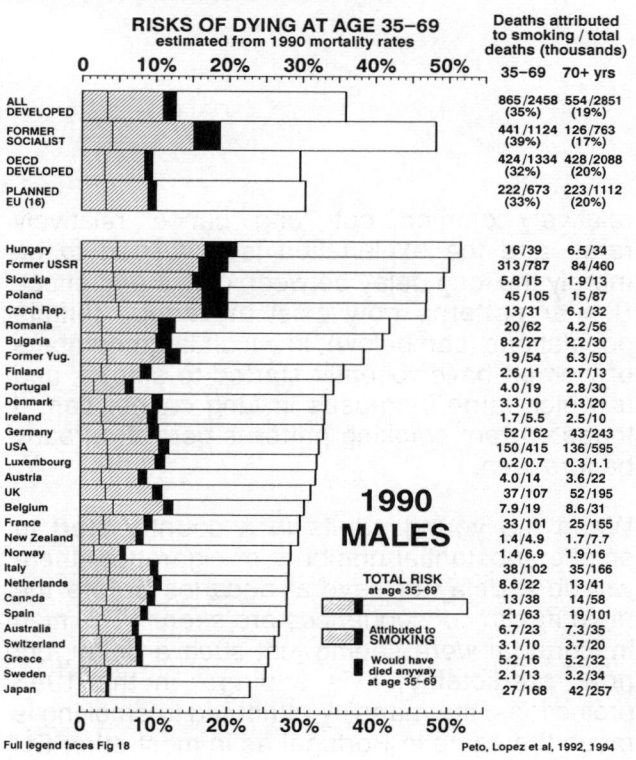

Fig. 26. Males, 1995 (projected), Developed Populations Smoking–Attributed and Other Mortality

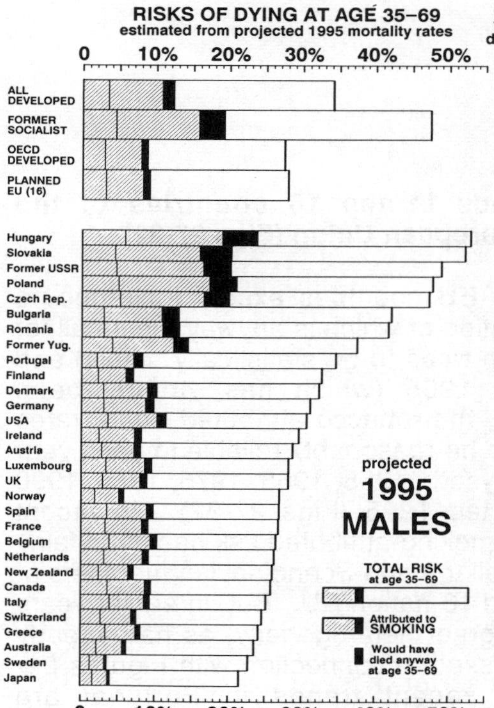

	Deaths attributed to smoking / total deaths (thousands) 35–69	70+ yrs
ALL DEVELOPED	870/2435 (36%)	572/2777 (21%)
FORMER SOCIALIST	463/1143 (41%)	135/741 (18%)
OECD DEVELOPED	407/1292 (31%)	437/2036 (21%)
PLANNED EU (16)	203/629 (32%)	209/1018 (20%)
Hungary	19/42	6.8/33
Slovakia	6.6/17	2.1/13
Former USSR	320/781	89/445
Poland	51/116	17/84
Czech Rep.	14/32	5.8/31
Bulgaria	9.0/29	2.4/31
Romania	21/66	4.4/53
Former Yug.	23/58	7.4/49
Portugal	4.9/21	3.5/33
Finland	2.0/10	2.3/12
Denmark	3.1/10	4.2/20
Germany	51/163	37/212
USA	149/414	154/631
Ireland	1.3/4.9	2.4/9.8
Austria	3.6/13	2.8/18
Luxembourg	0.2/0.7	0.2/0.8
UK	28/92	44/175
Norway	1.3/6.2	2.1/17
Spain	23/63	23/102
France	30/90	22/126
Belgium	6.2/16	8.0/30
Netherlands	7.5/22	14/43
New Zealand	1.2/4.4	1.6/7.4
Canada	13/37	17/63
Italy	33/89	35/154
Switzerland	3.0/9.9	3.8/22
Greece	5.2/16	5.3/31
Australia	5.3/21	6.7/34
Sweden	1.8/11	3.1/34
Japan	31/175	45/258

Full legend faces Fig 18 — Peto, Lopez et al, 1992, 1994

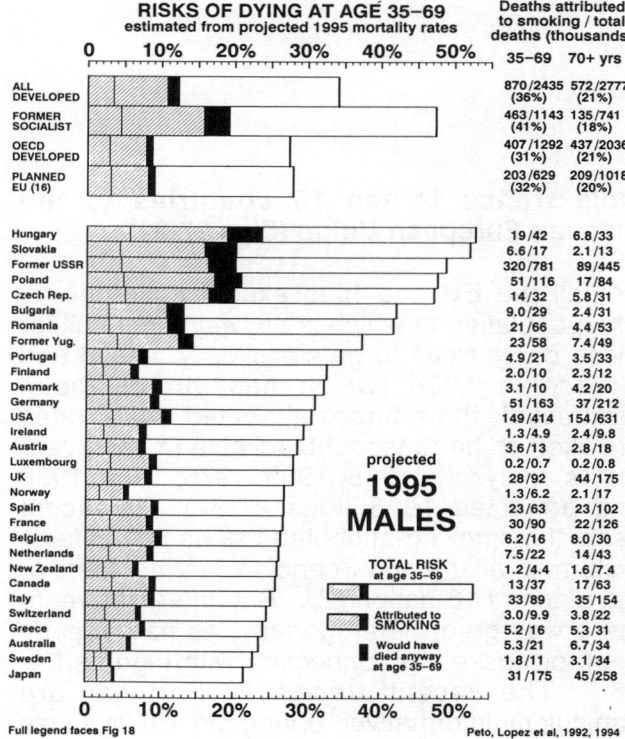

Fig. 27. Males, 1955, Planned EU (16 countries)
Smoking–Attributed and Other Mortality

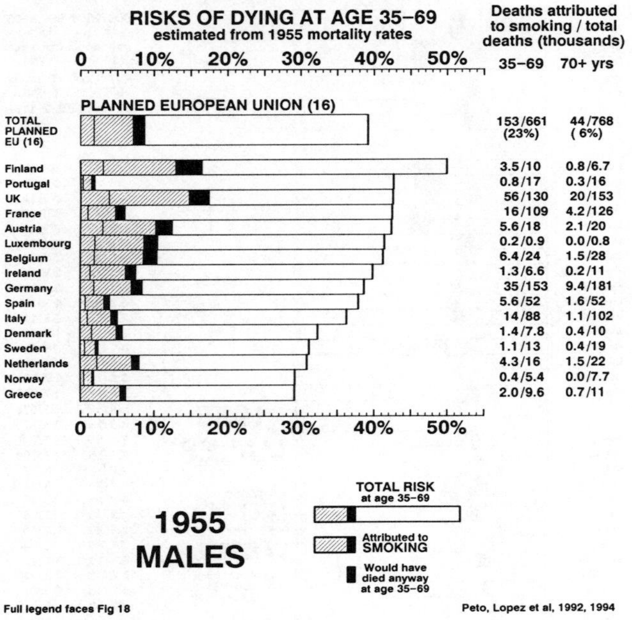

Fig. 28. Males, 1965, Planned EU (16 countries)
Smoking–Attributed and Other Mortality

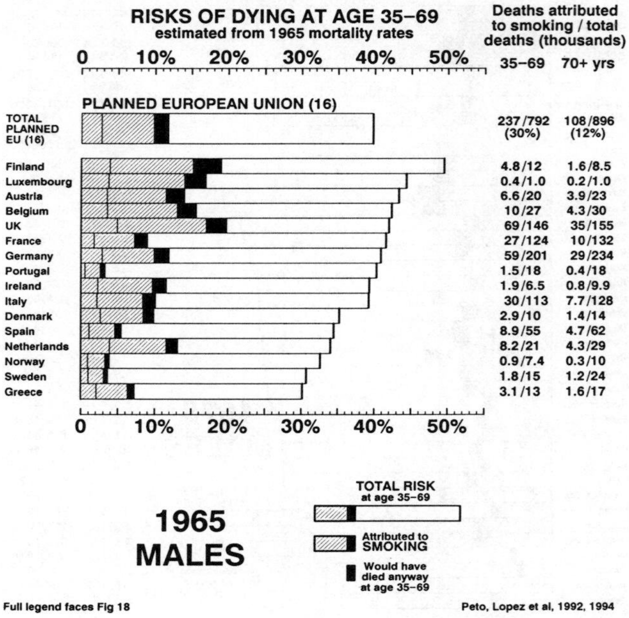

Male trends in the 16 countries of the planned European Union (Figs 27-32)

For all the EU countries except Luxembourg (the population of which is anyway too small for these death rates to be statistically stable) and Greece in 1955 (which has already been discussed), the tobacco-attributed death rates are likely to be reasonably reliable in each year that is analysed: 1955, 1965, 1975, 1985, 1990 and projected 1995 (Figs 27-32). In recent years the smoking-attributed risk has been fairly uniform in all the non-Scandinavian members of the planned 16-nation EU. But, in earlier years there was great heterogeneity, as has already been discussed in connection with Figures 21-26. The recent trends in Portugal are particularly informative: during the 1970s it was noteworthy that in Portugal smoking was relatively common but lung cancer relatively rare, and the explanation is now seen to be merely the long delay between cause and effect. Similar patterns now exist in various female populations (see below), in which large numbers of women have recently started to smoke, and in which large increases in lung cancer can, if these current smoking patterns persist, already be foreseen.

When the young adults in a country start to smoke substantial numbers of cigarettes, there will be a delay of several decades before the main health consequences are seen. The men in Portugal were seeing just such a delay, but now, predictably, it is ending: in the 1995 projections, the mortality attributed to smoking is much the same in Portugal as in most other EU populations.

Fig. 29. Males, 1975, Planned EU (16 countries) Smoking–Attributed and Other Mortality

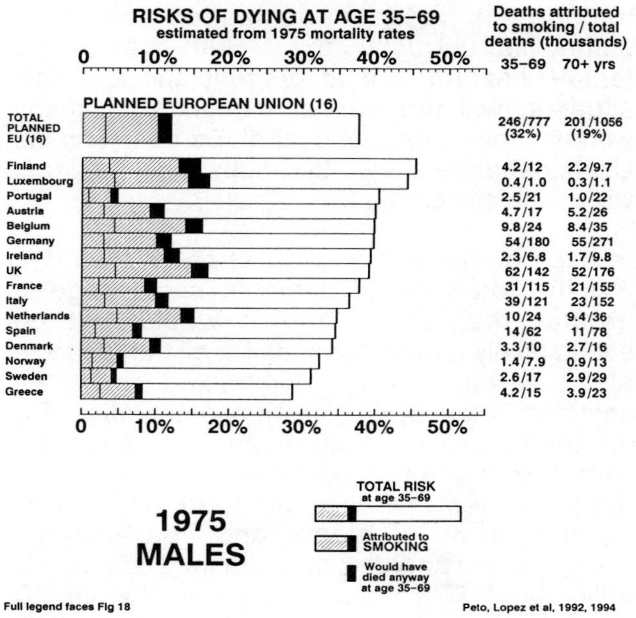

Fig. 30. Males, 1985, Planned EU (16 countries) Smoking–Attributed and Other Mortality

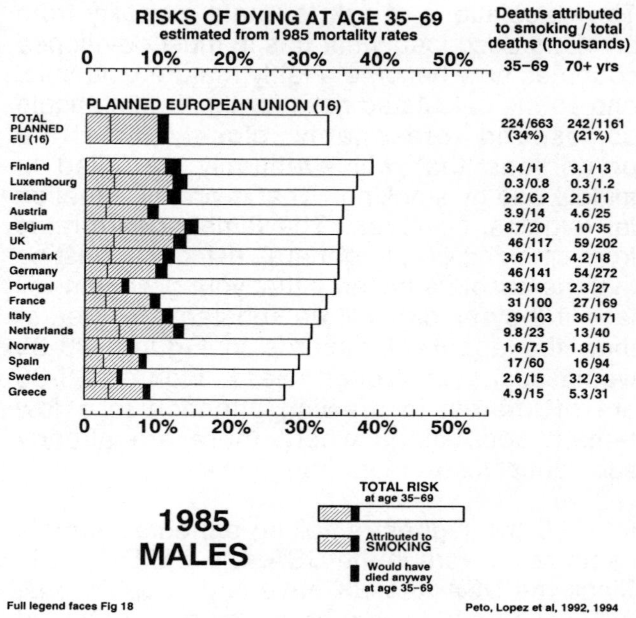

Fig. 31. Males, 1990, Planned EU (16 countries) Smoking–Attributed and Other Mortality

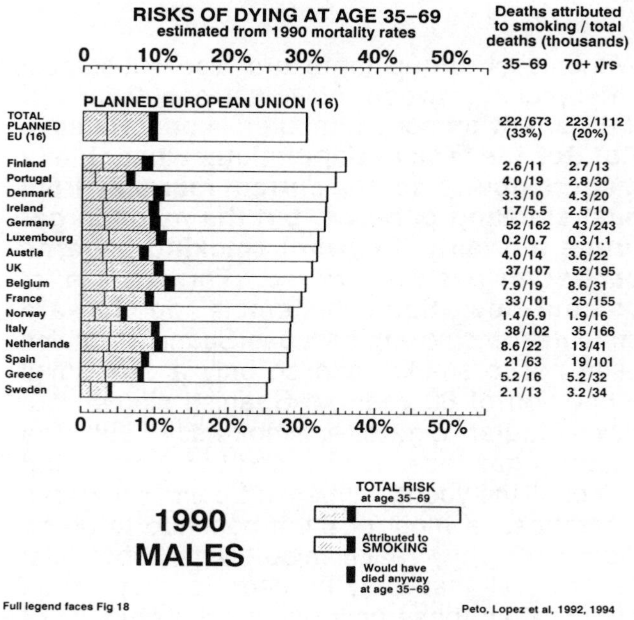

Fig. 32. Males, 1995 (projected), Planned EU (16 countries) Smoking–Attributed and Other Mortality

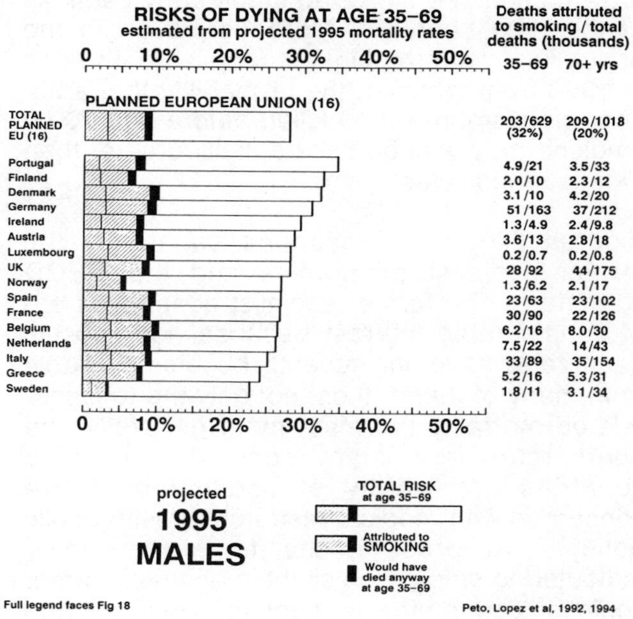

Female death risks, and 1955-1995 trends (Figs 33-47)

The calculations of risk for male mortality from smoking described what has in most developed countries now become a fairly mature epidemic, and so the calculated risks for the 1990s should correspond reasonably closely with the proportions that will eventually be killed in middle age by smoking. That is not the situation for females, however. The female death rates from smoking are, in general, rising, suggesting that the absolute hazards that young women will face if they smoke will be substantially greater than the apparent hazards in Figures 33-35 would suggest. Nevertheless, Figures 33-35 are of interest in drawing attention to a few female populations where there are already substantial death rates from smoking.

In 1990 the highest smoking-attributed female death rates were in the USA, UK and Denmark. Since the USA and UK have large populations, they account between them for well over half of all current female deaths from smoking. But, there have been large increases in cigarette smoking by the young women in many developed populations, so if current smoking patterns persist then much larger female hazards must be expected in the early decades of the next century. Moreover, even in the populations with the highest female death rates in 1990 from tobacco, the probability that a 35-year-old woman will be killed before age 70 by smoking may well be substantially greater than Figure 33 indicates.

Figures 34 and 35 describe separately the former socialist economies and the OECD countries. The former socialist economies are of considerable interest because age-specific death rates have only recently become available from many of them: thus, not only the tobacco-related mortality but also, more generally, the death rates from many conditions in these countries are worthy of scrutiny by those concerned with medical research, or with public policy. At present, the female mortality attributed to smoking is slight in all these former socialist economies (except for Hungary and Kazakhstan), and when this is the case the method of indirect estimation becomes somewhat untrustworthy. But, even if the female hazards are at present still low, this situation will not persist indefinitely: many women now smoke in central Europe, and the US experience shows that substantial hazards will eventually emerge.

In each of the former socialist economies (Fig 34) the total risk of death in middle age is greater than 20%, and it would still be substantially greater than 20% if all the tobacco-attributed mortality was subtracted away. By contrast, in the OECD developed countries (Fig 35) the opposite is true: even in the countries with the highest tobacco-attributed female mortality from tobacco in 1990 (USA, UK, Ireland, New Zealand and, particularly, Denmark) the total risk of death in middle age is only about 20%, and in each of the OECD developed countries the risk of death in middle age would be substantially less than 20% if the tobacco-attributed mortality could be subtracted away (Fig 35). Thus, there are large differences between these two groups of countries in causes other than tobacco of the female deaths in middle age.

Within each group there are also substantial differences between individual populations in the current tobacco-attributed mortality rates. **But, for the female populations what chiefly matters now is not the current mortality from past smoking patterns, but the much larger future mortality if current smoking patterns persist, or even get worse.** For example, at present few Spanish female deaths are attributed to smoking because Spanish females used not to smoke, and so only a very small proportion of 60-year-old Spanish women are now regular cigarette smokers. But, the situation has recently changed completely, and half of all the young women in Spain now smoke cigarettes. If most of them continue to do so then when they reach middle age substantial hazards will inevitably be seen, perhaps even greater than those now being seen among US females.

Fig. 33. Females, 1990, Developed Populations Smoking–Attributed and Other Mortality

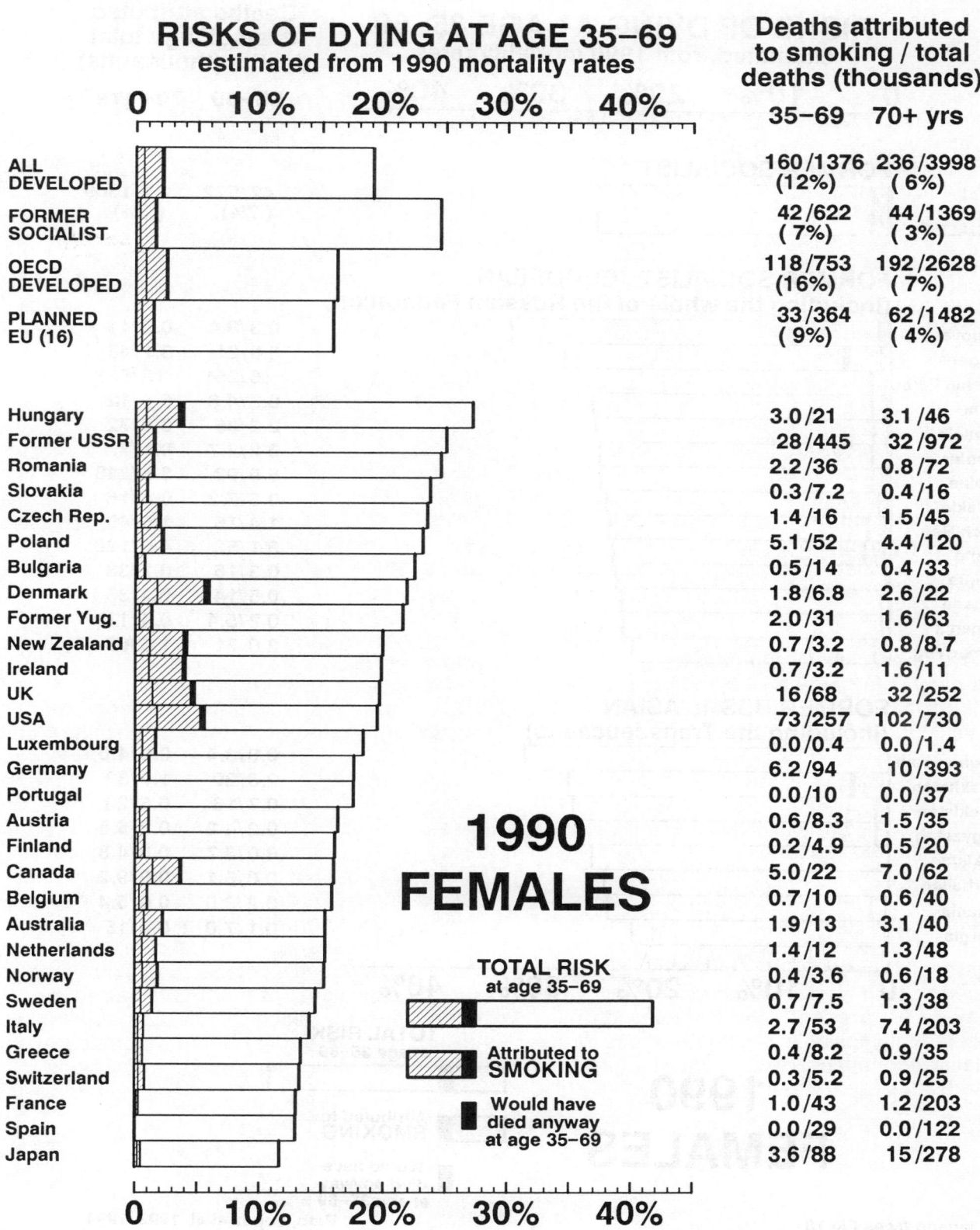

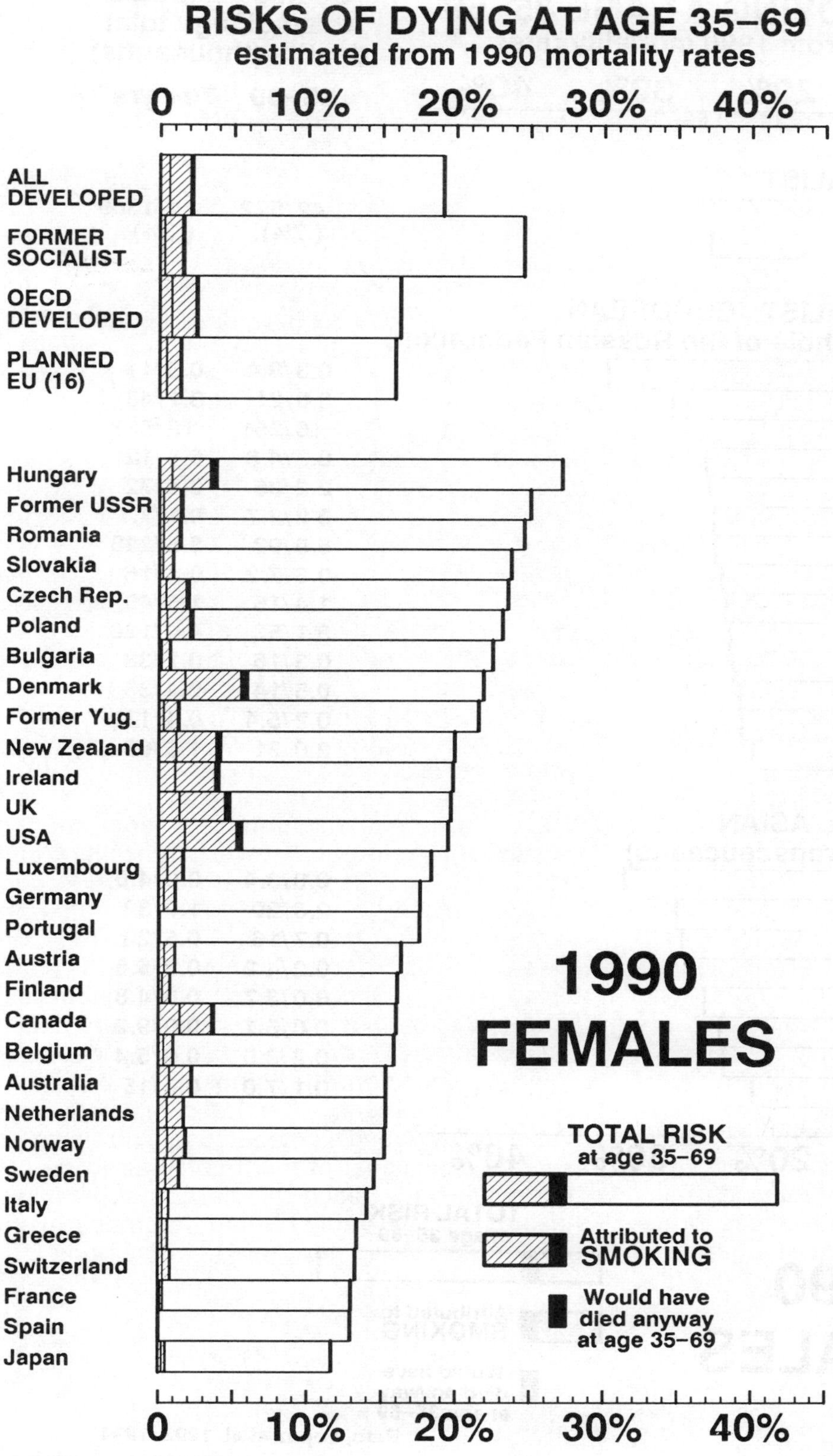

Deaths attributed to smoking / total deaths (thousands)

	35–69	70+ yrs
ALL DEVELOPED	160/1376 (12%)	236/3998 (6%)
FORMER SOCIALIST	42/622 (7%)	44/1369 (3%)
OECD DEVELOPED	118/753 (16%)	192/2628 (7%)
PLANNED EU (16)	33/364 (9%)	62/1482 (4%)
Hungary	3.0/21	3.1/46
Former USSR	28/445	32/972
Romania	2.2/36	0.8/72
Slovakia	0.3/7.2	0.4/16
Czech Rep.	1.4/16	1.5/45
Poland	5.1/52	4.4/120
Bulgaria	0.5/14	0.4/33
Denmark	1.8/6.8	2.6/22
Former Yug.	2.0/31	1.6/63
New Zealand	0.7/3.2	0.8/8.7
Ireland	0.7/3.2	1.6/11
UK	16/68	32/252
USA	73/257	102/730
Luxembourg	0.0/0.4	0.0/1.4
Germany	6.2/94	10/393
Portugal	0.0/10	0.0/37
Austria	0.6/8.3	1.5/35
Finland	0.2/4.9	0.5/20
Canada	5.0/22	7.0/62
Belgium	0.7/10	0.6/40
Australia	1.9/13	3.1/40
Netherlands	1.4/12	1.3/48
Norway	0.4/3.6	0.6/18
Sweden	0.7/7.5	1.3/38
Italy	2.7/53	7.4/203
Greece	0.4/8.2	0.9/35
Switzerland	0.3/5.2	0.9/25
France	1.0/43	1.2/203
Spain	0.0/29	0.0/122
Japan	3.6/88	15/278

Full legend faces Fig 18

Peto, Lopez et al, 1992, 1994

Fig. 34. Females, 1990, Former Socialist Countries Smoking–Attributed and Other Mortality

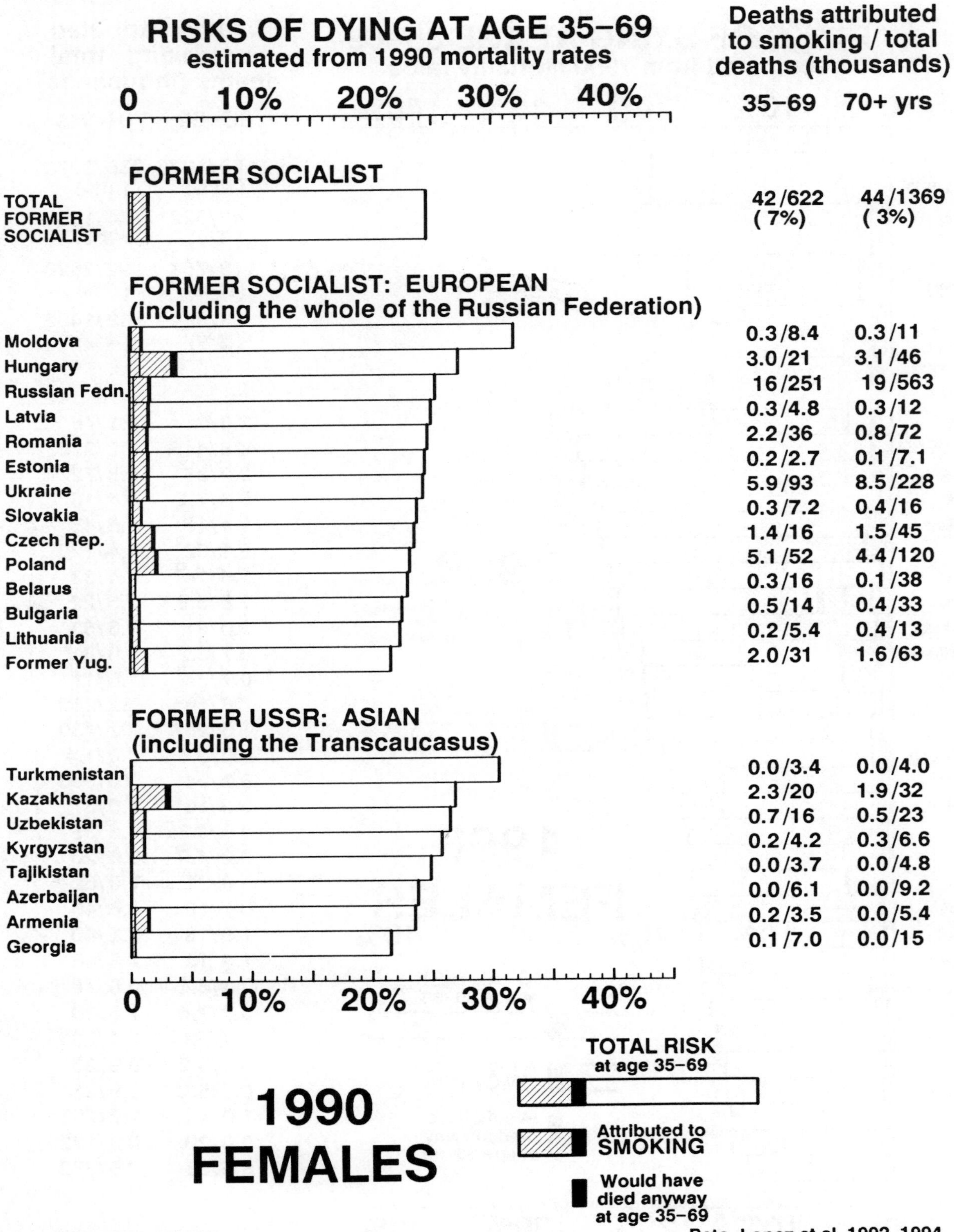

Full legend faces Fig 18

Peto, Lopez et al, 1992, 1994

Fig. 35. Females, 1990, OECD Developed Countries Smoking–Attributed and Other Mortality

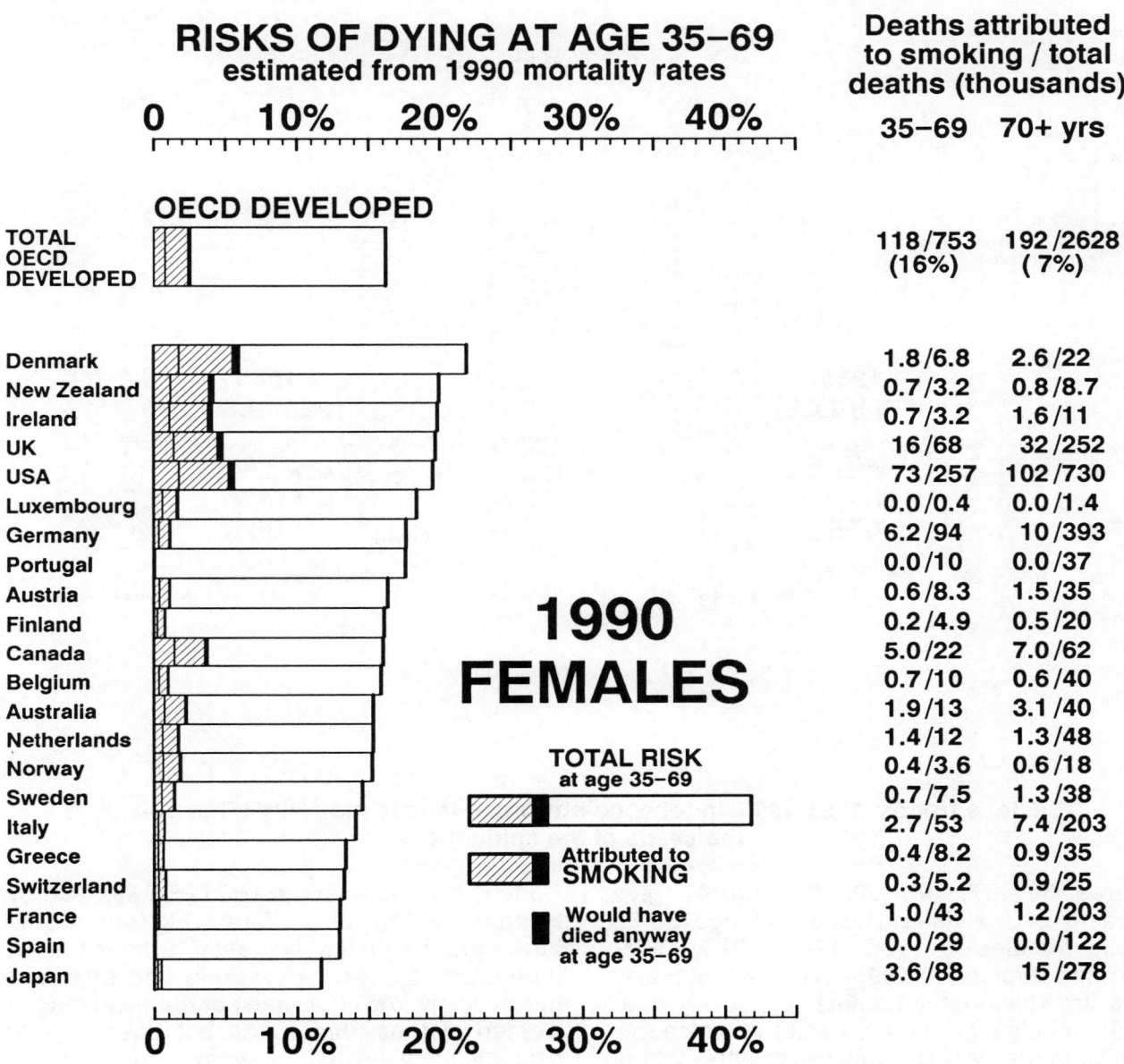

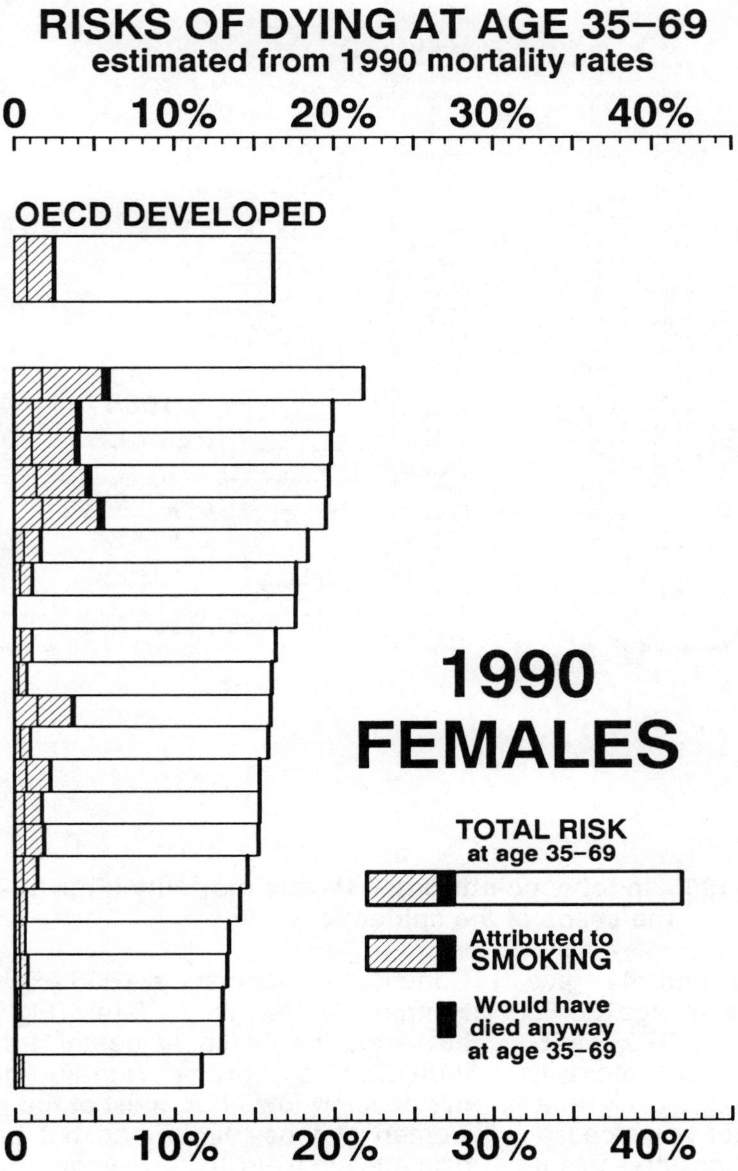

	Deaths attributed to smoking / total deaths (thousands) 35–69	70+ yrs
TOTAL OECD DEVELOPED	118/753 (16%)	192/2628 (7%)
Denmark	1.8/6.8	2.6/22
New Zealand	0.7/3.2	0.8/8.7
Ireland	0.7/3.2	1.6/11
UK	16/68	32/252
USA	73/257	102/730
Luxembourg	0.0/0.4	0.0/1.4
Germany	6.2/94	10/393
Portugal	0.0/10	0.0/37
Austria	0.6/8.3	1.5/35
Finland	0.2/4.9	0.5/20
Canada	5.0/22	7.0/62
Belgium	0.7/10	0.6/40
Australia	1.9/13	3.1/40
Netherlands	1.4/12	1.3/48
Norway	0.4/3.6	0.6/18
Sweden	0.7/7.5	1.3/38
Italy	2.7/53	7.4/203
Greece	0.4/8.2	0.9/35
Switzerland	0.3/5.2	0.9/25
France	1.0/43	1.2/203
Spain	0.0/29	0.0/122
Japan	3.6/88	15/278

Full legend faces Fig 18

Peto, Lopez et al, 1992, 1994

Fig. 36. Females, 1955, Developed Populations
Smoking–Attributed and Other Mortality

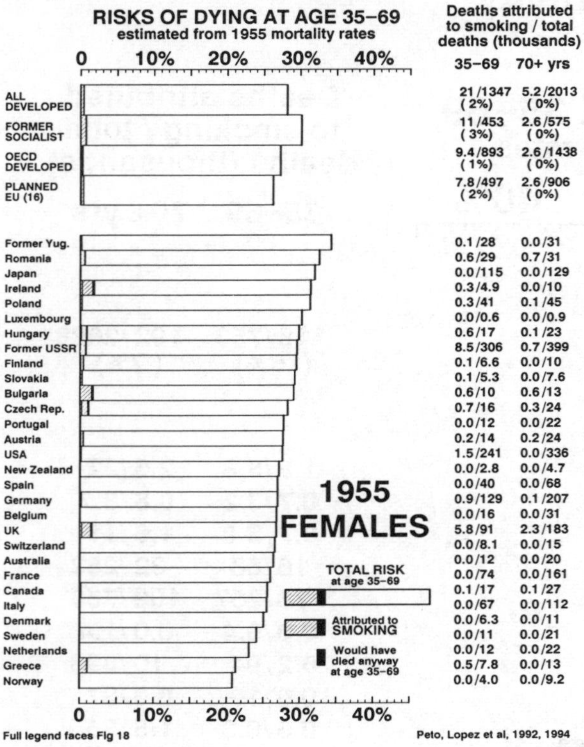

Fig. 37. Females, 1965, Developed Populations
Smoking–Attributed and Other Mortality

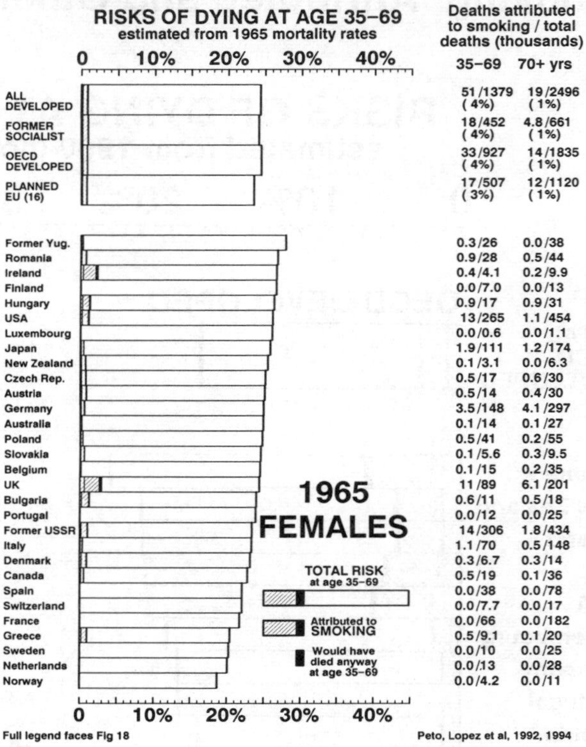

Previous trends, 1955-1995, in tobacco-attributed female mortality (Figs 36-41): the seeds of the epidemic

Figures 36, 37, 38, 39, 40 and 41 give respectively the risks of death at age 35-69 among females in 1955, 1965, 1975, 1985, 1990 and (projected) 1995. The total mortality rates are reasonably reliable, especially after 1965, and although for the earlier years cause-specific mortality is unavailable or unreliable in several countries (particularly Greece and the former socialist economies), the tobacco-attributed hazards in those populations in those years were probably very low, so Figures 36-41 probably provide a trustworthy description not only of the trends in all-cause mortality, but also of the trends in mortality from tobacco.

In 1965 the female mortality from smoking was greatest in the UK and Ireland, and these two countries with high female hazards were joined by the US and New Zealand in 1975 (Fig 38), by Canada and Denmark in 1985 (Fig 39), and by Hungary a few years later (Fig 40). Still, however, the "risks of death" from smoking indicated by these female graphs are misleadingly low. For, most of the middle-aged women at those times had not been regular cigarette smokers in the way that young females are now becoming.

For total mortality the trends in the female rates should be reasonably reliable from 1975 onwards, but in earlier years they may be somewhat unreliable, at least for some of the former socialist countries. (It is, for example, unclear why 1965 should be an exception to the tendency for total female mortality to be greater in the former socialist economies than elsewhere — or, equivalently, how much reliance to put on this apparent exception.)

Fig. 38. Females, 1975, Developed Populations Smoking–Attributed and Other Mortality

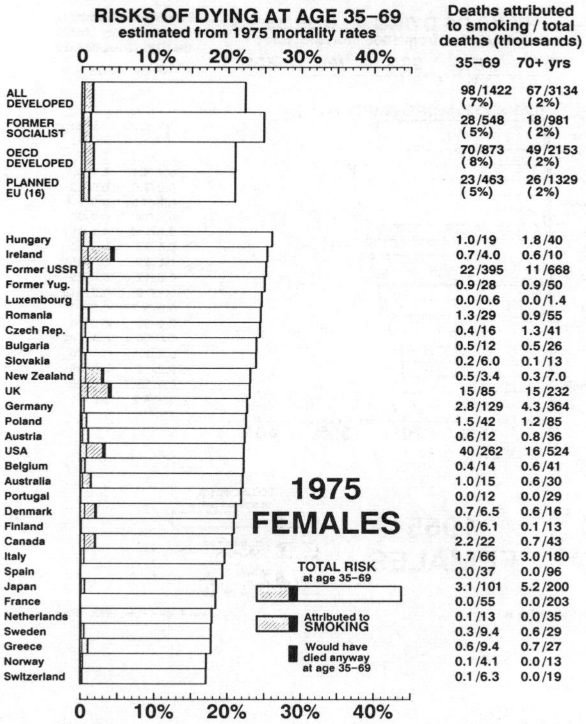

Full legend faces Fig 18 Peto, Lopez et al, 1992, 1994

Fig. 39. Females, 1985, Developed Populations Smoking–Attributed and Other Mortality

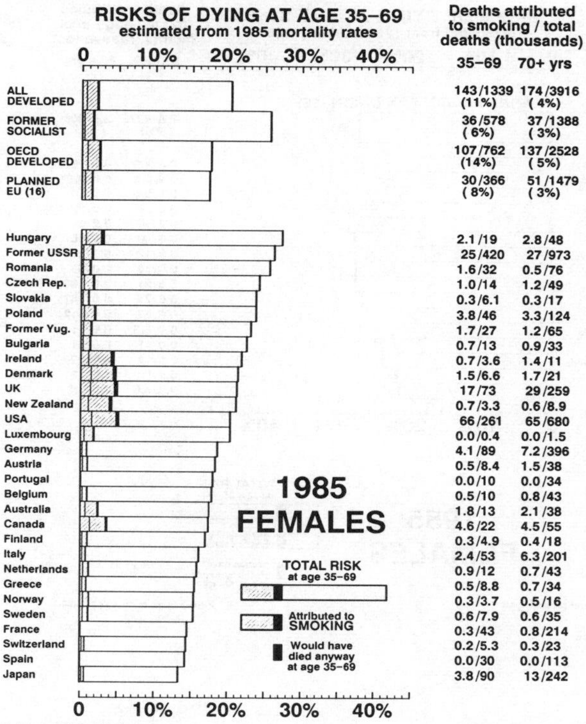

Full legend faces Fig 18 Peto, Lopez et al, 1992, 1994

Fig. 40. Females, 1990, Developed Populations Smoking–Attributed and Other Mortality

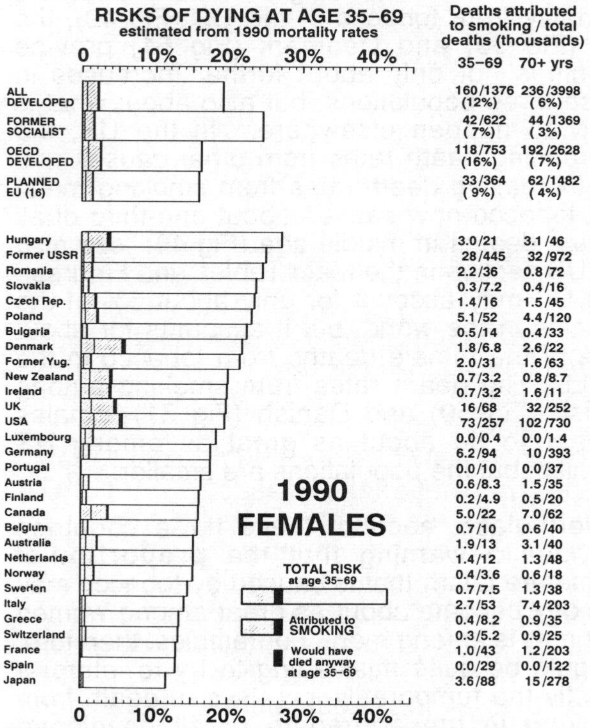

Full legend faces Fig 18 Peto, Lopez et al, 1992, 1994

Fig. 41. Females, 1995 (projected), Developed Populations Smoking–Attributed and Other Mortality

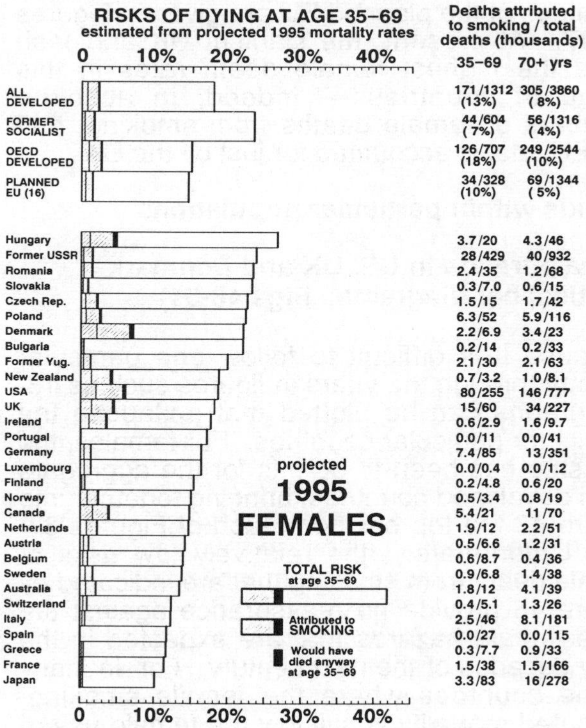

Full legend faces Fig 18 Peto, Lopez et al, 1992, 1994

Fig. 42. Females, 1955, Planned EU (16 countries) Smoking–Attributed and Other Mortality

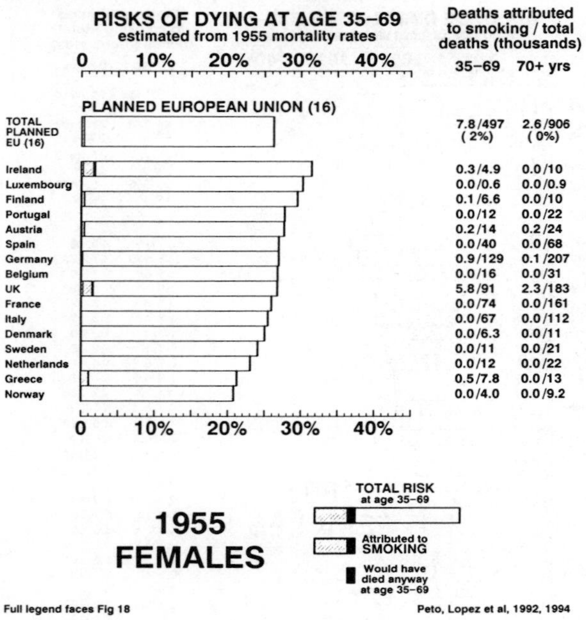

Fig. 43. Females, 1965, Planned EU (16 countries) Smoking–Attributed and Other Mortality

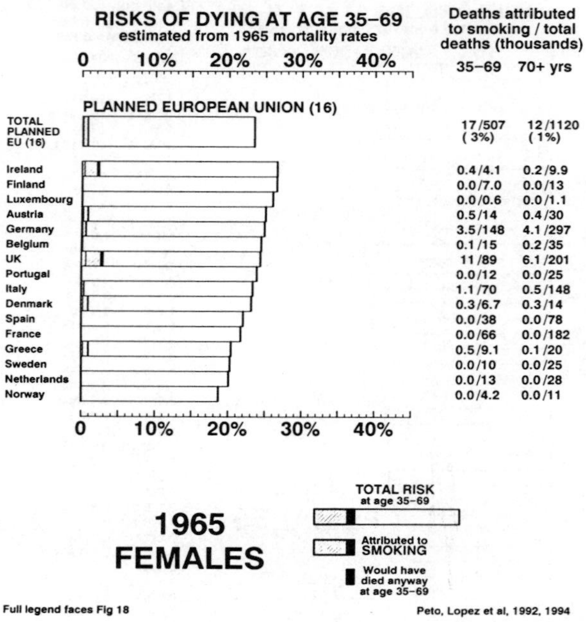

Female trends in the 16 countries of the planned European Union (Figs 42-47)

Trend analyses that are restricted to the 16 countries of the planned EU are given in Figures 42-47. At present, the Danish, UK and Irish have the highest female death rates in this group of countries — indeed, in absolute numbers of female deaths from smoking, half the EU total is accounted for just by the UK.

Trends within particular populations

Female trends in US, UK and Denmark (vertical bar diagrams: Figs 48-51)

Because it is difficult to follow one particular country through the years in figures such as 18-47, graphs can be plotted that juxtapose the results for particular countries. For females, the first step has been to do this for the aggregate of all developed countries, bringing together into Figure 48 the top bar from each of Figures 37-41. Unfortunately, the relatively low risks of female death from smoking that are indicated by Figure 48 provide no reassurance against the large female hazards that are expected in the early decades of the next century. For, in many of the countries where the female smoking-attributed mortality is still low the female use of cigarettes has now increased substantially.

Moreover, the continuing increase in female mortality from tobacco in the US (Fig 49), the UK (Fig 50) and Denmark (Fig 51) provide warnings not only about further increases in those three populations, but also about what is likely to happen elsewhere. In the US, the decreasing death rates from other causes and the increasing death rates from smoking mean that tobacco now causes about one-third of all female deaths in middle age (Fig 49: see also the US section in the Main Tables and Figures). The US may account for only about 5% of the females in the world, but it accounts for about 50% of the female deaths from tobacco in the world. The death rates from smoking among British (Fig 50) and Danish (Fig 51) females appear to be about as great as among US females, but the populations are smaller.

Nevertheless, each of these three countries provides a warning that the **proportion** of premature death that is caused by tobacco may one day become about as great among women as it now is among men. For females, therefore, it would be quite misleading to try to interpret directly the temporarily low risks of death from smoking in the aggregate of all developed countries (Fig 48).

Fig. 44. Females, 1975, Planned EU (16 countries)
Smoking–Attributed and Other Mortality

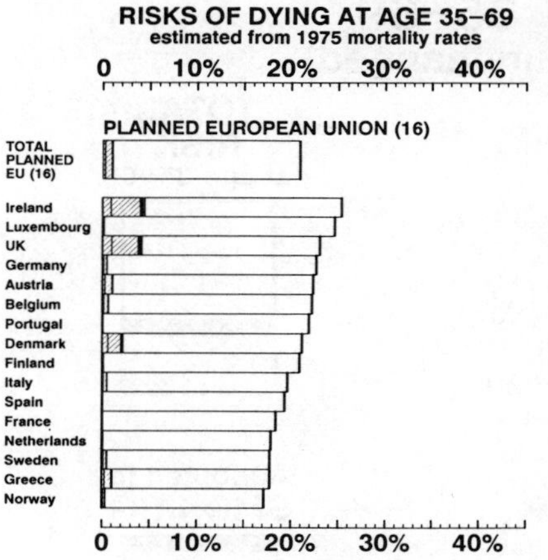

Deaths attributed to smoking / total deaths (thousands)

	35–69	70+ yrs
TOTAL PLANNED EU (16)	23/463 (5%)	26/1329 (2%)
Ireland	0.7/4.0	0.6/10
Luxembourg	0.0/0.6	0.0/1.4
UK	15/85	15/232
Germany	2.8/129	4.3/364
Austria	0.6/12	0.8/36
Belgium	0.4/14	0.6/41
Portugal	0.0/12	0.0/29
Denmark	0.7/6.5	0.6/16
Finland	0.0/6.1	0.1/13
Italy	1.7/66	3.0/180
Spain	0.0/37	0.0/96
France	0.0/55	0.0/203
Netherlands	0.1/13	0.0/35
Sweden	0.3/9.4	0.6/29
Greece	0.6/9.4	0.7/27
Norway	0.1/4.1	0.0/13

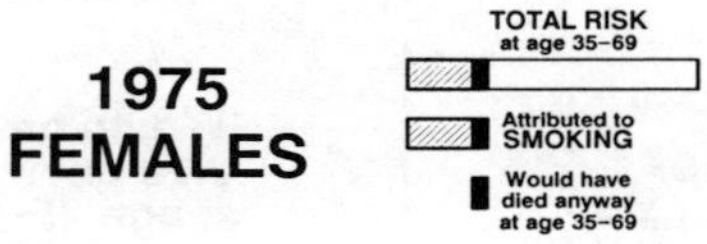

Full legend faces Fig 18

Peto, Lopez et al, 1992, 1994

Fig. 45. Females, 1985, Planned EU (16 countries)
Smoking–Attributed and Other Mortality

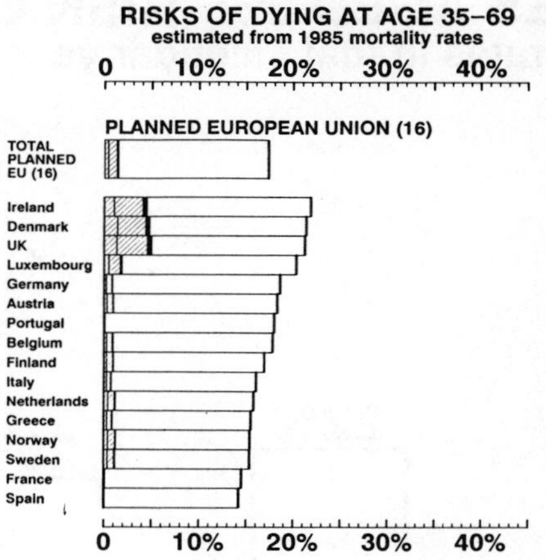

Deaths attributed to smoking / total deaths (thousands)

	35–69	70+ yrs
TOTAL PLANNED EU (16)	30/366 (8%)	51/1479 (3%)
Ireland	0.7/3.6	1.4/11
Denmark	1.5/6.6	1.7/21
UK	17/73	29/259
Luxembourg	0.0/0.4	0.0/1.5
Germany	4.1/89	7.2/396
Austria	0.5/8.4	1.5/38
Portugal	0.0/10	0.0/34
Belgium	0.5/10	0.8/43
Finland	0.3/4.9	0.4/18
Italy	2.4/53	6.3/201
Netherlands	0.9/12	0.7/43
Greece	0.5/8.8	0.7/34
Norway	0.3/3.7	0.5/16
Sweden	0.6/7.9	0.6/35
France	0.3/43	0.8/214
Spain	0.0/30	0.0/113

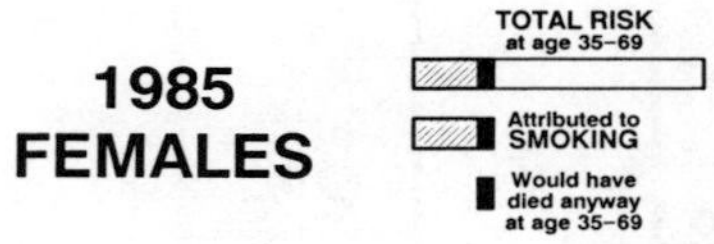

Full legend faces Fig 18

Peto, Lopez et al, 1992, 1994

Fig. 46. Females, 1990, Planned EU (16 countries)
Smoking–Attributed and Other Mortality

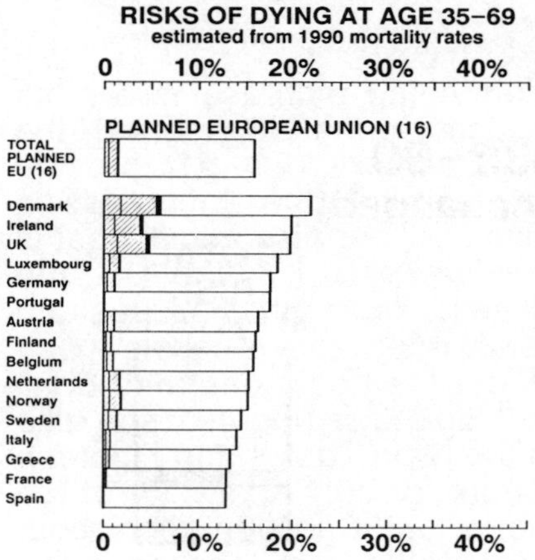

Deaths attributed to smoking / total deaths (thousands)

	35–69	70+ yrs
TOTAL PLANNED EU (16)	33/364 (9%)	62/1482 (4%)
Denmark	1.8/6.8	2.6/22
Ireland	0.7/3.2	1.6/11
UK	16/68	32/252
Luxembourg	0.0/0.4	0.0/1.4
Germany	6.2/94	10/393
Portugal	0.0/10	0.0/37
Austria	0.6/8.3	1.5/35
Finland	0.2/4.9	0.5/20
Belgium	0.7/10	0.6/40
Netherlands	1.4/12	1.3/48
Norway	0.4/3.6	0.6/18
Sweden	0.7/7.5	1.3/38
Italy	2.7/53	7.4/203
Greece	0.4/8.2	0.9/35
France	1.0/43	1.2/203
Spain	0.0/29	0.0/122

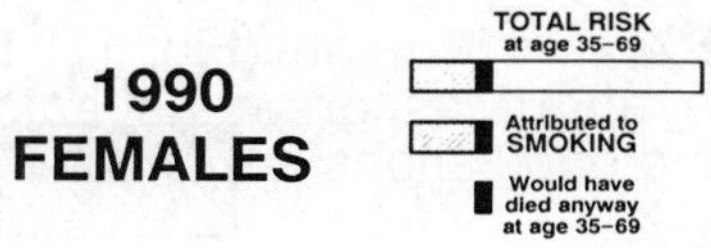

Full legend faces Fig 18

Peto, Lopez et al, 1992, 1994

Fig. 47. Females, 1995 (projected), Planned EU (16 countries)
Smoking–Attributed and Other Mortality

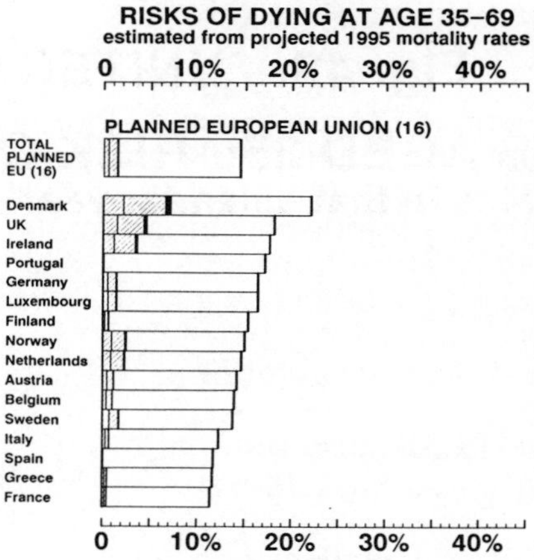

Deaths attributed to smoking / total deaths (thousands)

	35–69	70+ yrs
TOTAL PLANNED EU (16)	34/328 (10%)	69/1344 (5%)
Denmark	2.2/6.9	3.4/23
UK	15/60	34/227
Ireland	0.6/2.9	1.6/9.7
Portugal	0.0/11	0.0/41
Germany	7.4/85	13/351
Luxembourg	0.0/0.4	0.0/1.2
Finland	0.2/4.8	0.6/20
Norway	0.5/3.4	0.8/19
Netherlands	1.9/12	2.2/51
Austria	0.5/6.6	1.2/31
Belgium	0.6/8.7	0.4/36
Sweden	0.9/6.8	1.4/38
Italy	2.5/46	8.1/181
Spain	0.0/27	0.0/115
Greece	0.3/7.7	0.9/33
France	1.5/38	1.5/166

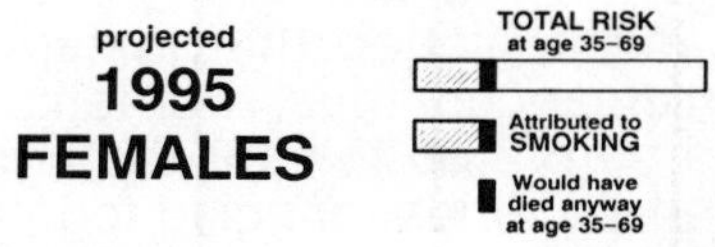

Full legend faces Fig 18

Peto, Lopez et al, 1992, 1994

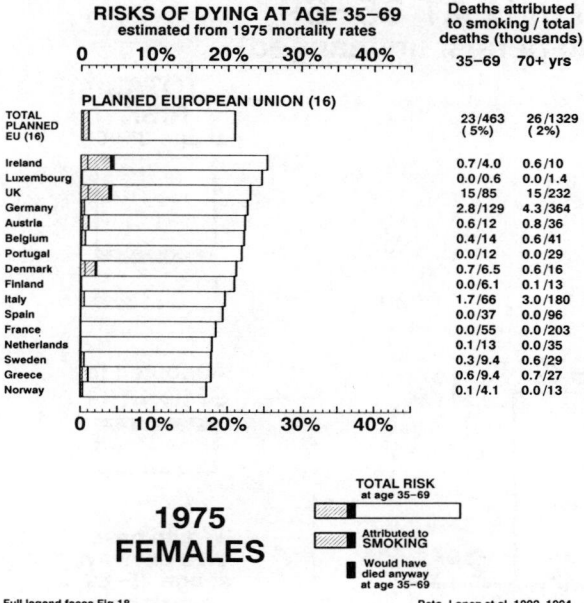

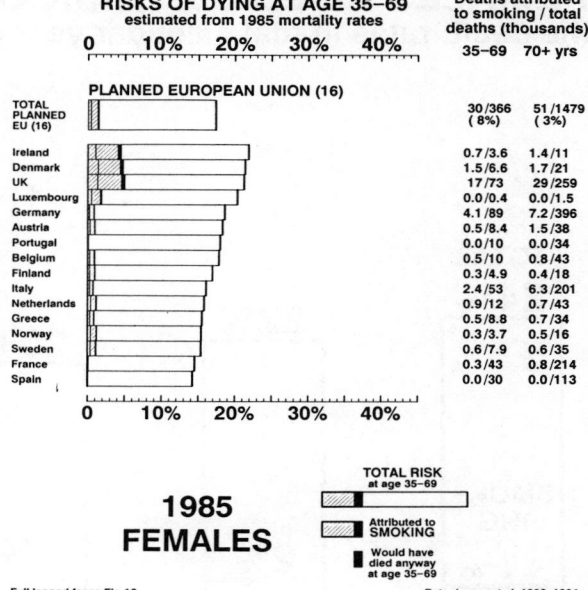

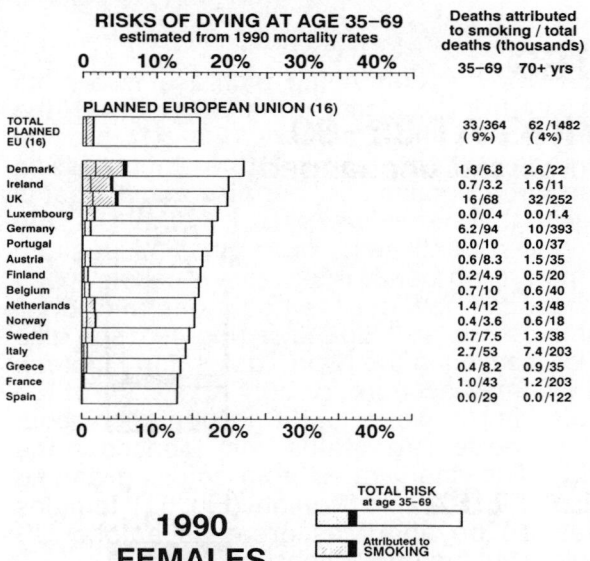

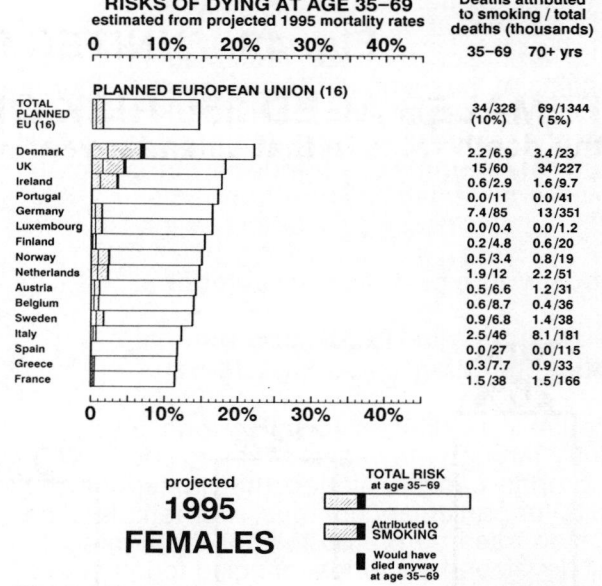

Fig. 48. ALL 'DEVELOPED' COUNTRIES

FEMALES AGED 35: RISK OF DYING AT 35–69

(if the death rates in that calendar year were to persist unchanged)

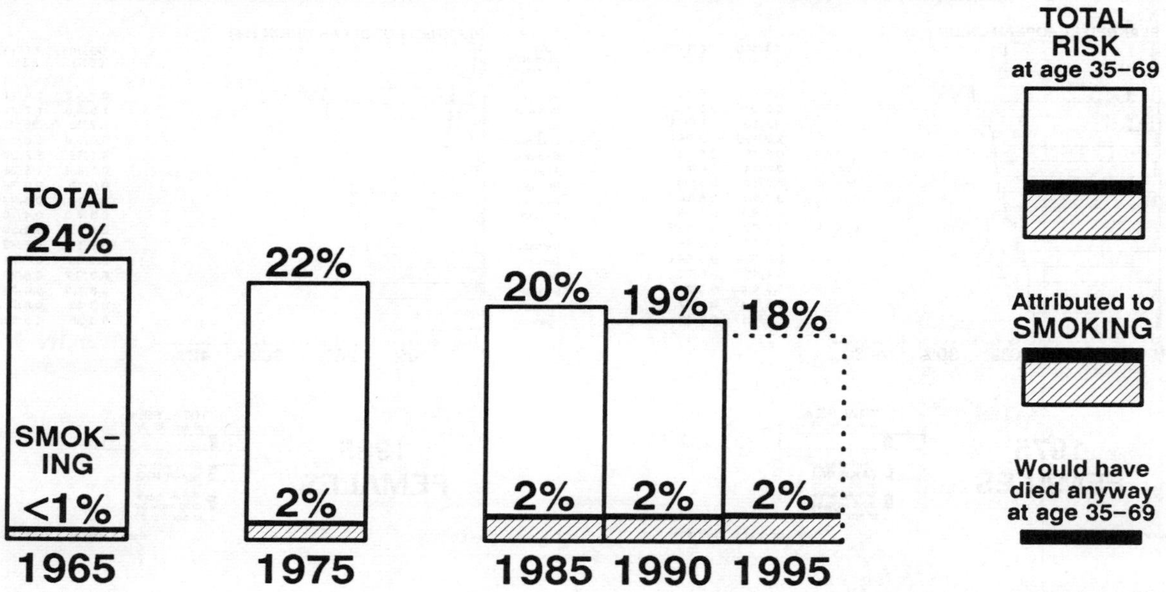

Peto, Lopez et al, 1992, 1994

Fig. 49. UNITED STATES

FEMALES AGED 35: RISK OF DYING AT 35–69

(if the death rates in that calendar year were to persist unchanged)

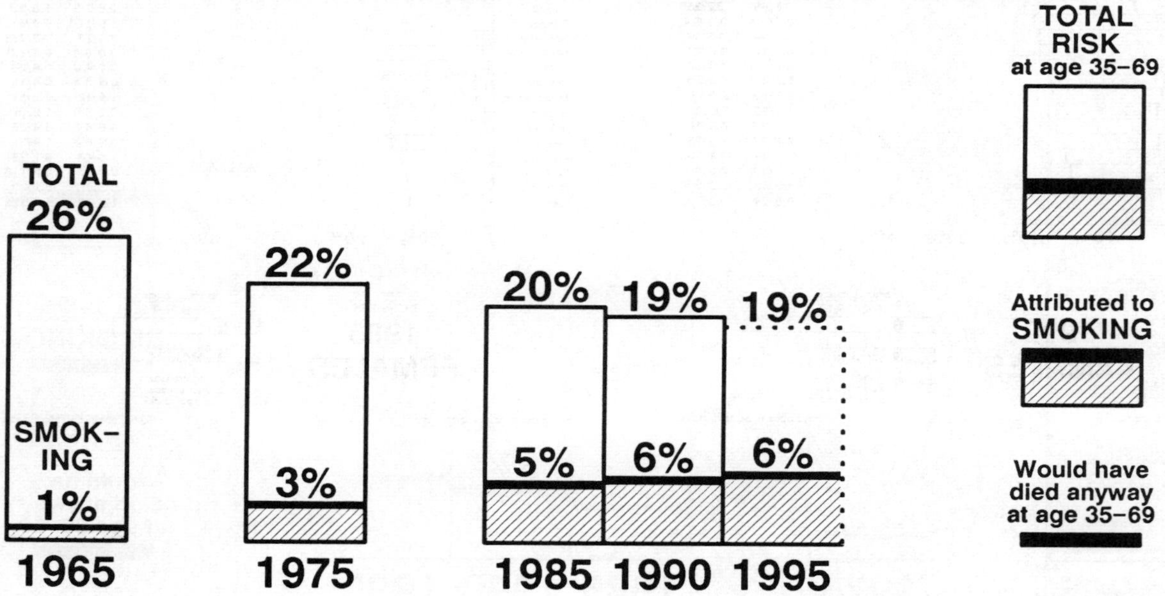

Peto, Lopez et al, 1992, 1994

Fig. 50. UNITED KINGDOM

FEMALES AGED 35: RISK OF DYING AT 35–69
(if the death rates in that calendar year were to persist unchanged)

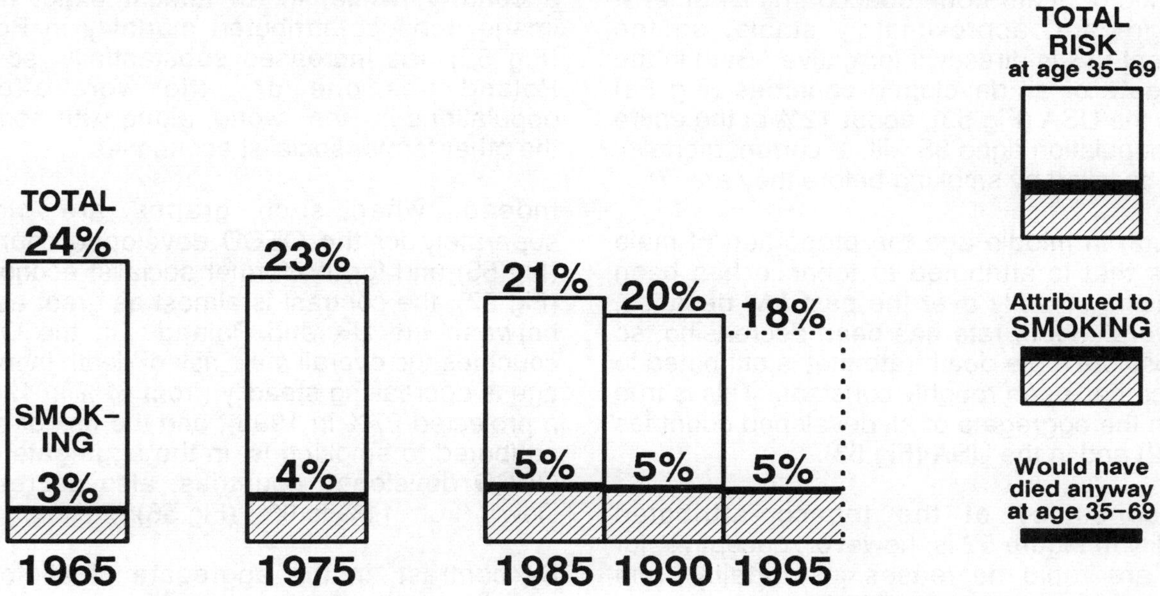

Peto, Lopez et al, 1992, 1994

Fig. 51. DENMARK

FEMALES AGED 35: RISK OF DYING AT 35–69
(if the death rates in that calendar year were to persist unchanged)

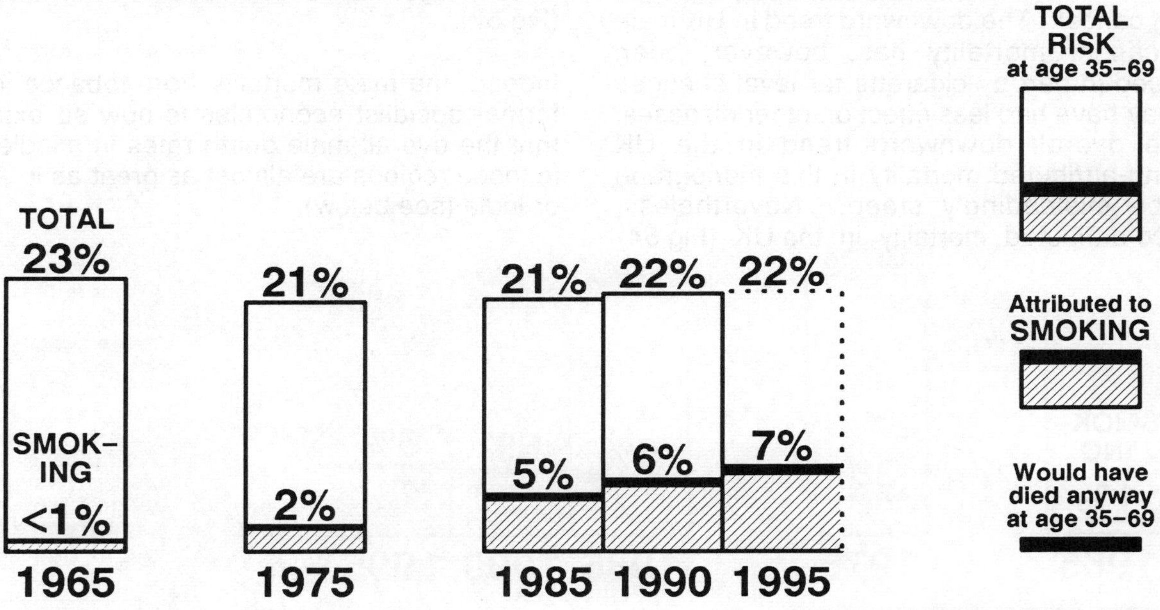

Peto, Lopez et al, 1992, 1994

Male trends in US, UK and Poland (vertical bar diagrams: Figs 52-57)

Similar analyses for males, however, reveal an epidemic of death from tobacco that is, at least in aggregate, approximately stable, so the apparent risk is directly informative. Both in the aggregate of all developed countries (Fig 52) and in the USA (Fig 53), about 12% of the entire male population aged 35 will, at current mortality rates, be killed by smoking before they are 70.

Although in middle age the proportion of male deaths that is attributed to tobacco has been increasing steadily over the past few decades, the overall death rate has been decreasing, so the absolute male death rate that is attributed to tobacco has been roughly constant. This is true both in the aggregate of all developed countries (Fig 52) and in the USA (Fig 53).

The constancy of the tobacco-attributed mortality in Figure 52 is, however, deceptive, for there are rapid decreases in mortality from tobacco in some countries and rapid increases in others. The UK and Poland provide a particularly striking contrast in this respect (see Fig 54: UK, and Fig 55: Poland). In 1965, males in the UK had the worst mortality rates from smoking in the world, while males in Poland had quite low rates. Now, however, the situation is reversed. These downward and upward trends in the UK and Polish smoking-attributed mortality are qualitatively correct, for they parallel large downward and upward trends in lung cancer. The downward trend in UK male lung cancer mortality has, however, been produced in part by cigarette tar level changes that may have had less effect on other diseases, so the overall downward trend in the UK smoking-attributed mortality in this monograph may be misleadingly steep. Nevertheless, tobacco-attributed mortality in the UK (Fig 54) has fallen substantially over the past quarter of a century, while, in an almost exact mirror image, tobacco-attributed mortality in Poland (Fig 55) has increased substantially, so now Poland has one of the worst-affected populations in the world, along with some of the other former socialist economies.

Indeed, when such graphs are plotted separately for the OECD developed countries (Fig 56) and for the former socialist economies (Fig 57), the contrast is almost as great as that between the UK and Poland. In the OECD countries the overall male risk of death in middle age is decreasing steadily (from 41% in 1965 to a projected 27% in 1995), and the risk of death attributed to smoking is, in the aggregate of all OECD developed countries, also decreasing slowly (from 11% to 9%) (Fig 56).

By contrast, in the aggregate of all former socialist economies the overall male death rates are now high (48% in 1990), with no good evidence of any substantial reduction, and the male mortality attributed to tobacco has increased by about half over the past few decades. The 1965 data may be somewhat unreliable, and the 1995 projection is somewhat uncertain, but the 1975-1990 trend should be reasonably reliable, and during that 15-year period the risk attributed to smoking of being killed at ages 35-69 increased from 14% to 19% (Fig 57).

Indeed, the male mortality from tobacco in the former socialist economies is now so extreme that the overall male death rates in middle age in those regions are almost as great as in Africa or India (see below).

Fig. 52. ALL 'DEVELOPED' COUNTRIES

MALES AGED 35: RISK OF DYING AT 35–69

(if the death rates in that calendar year were to persist unchanged)

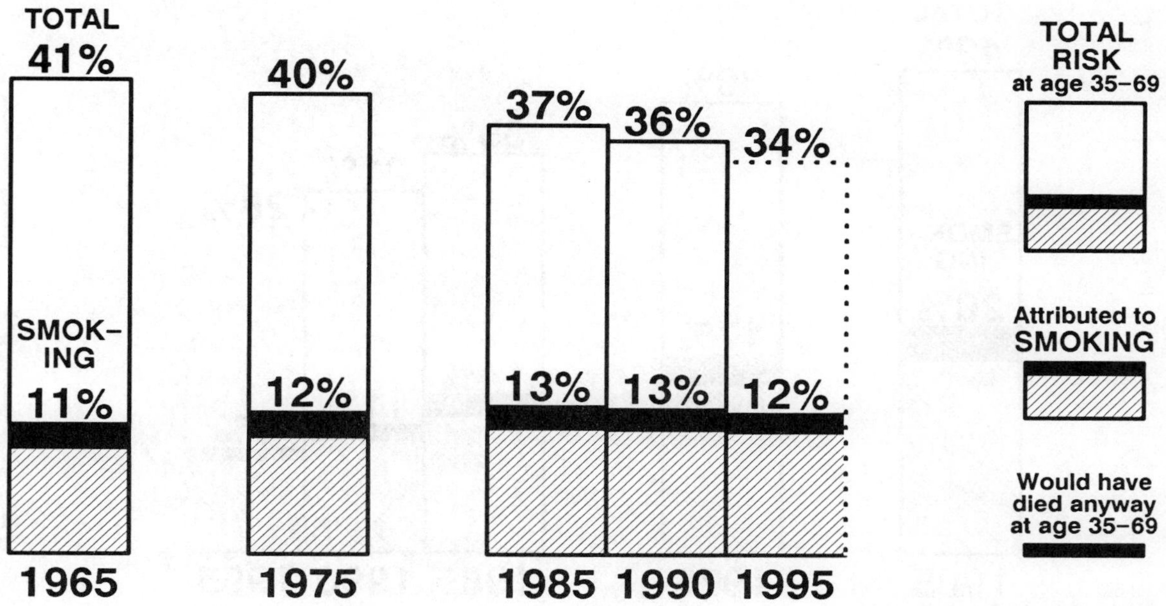

Peto, Lopez et al, 1992, 1994

Fig. 53. UNITED STATES

MALES AGED 35: RISK OF DYING AT 35–69

(if the death rates in that calendar year were to persist unchanged)

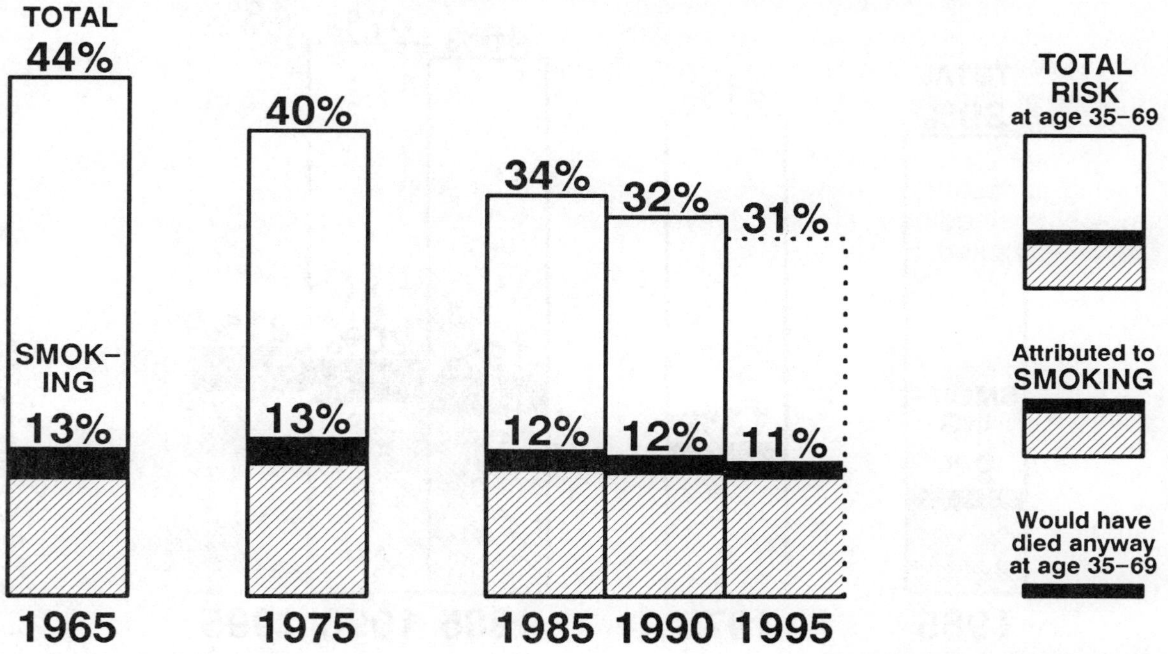

Peto, Lopez et al, 1992, 1994

Fig. 54. UNITED KINGDOM

MALES AGED 35: RISK OF DYING AT 35–69
(if the death rates in that calendar year were to persist unchanged)

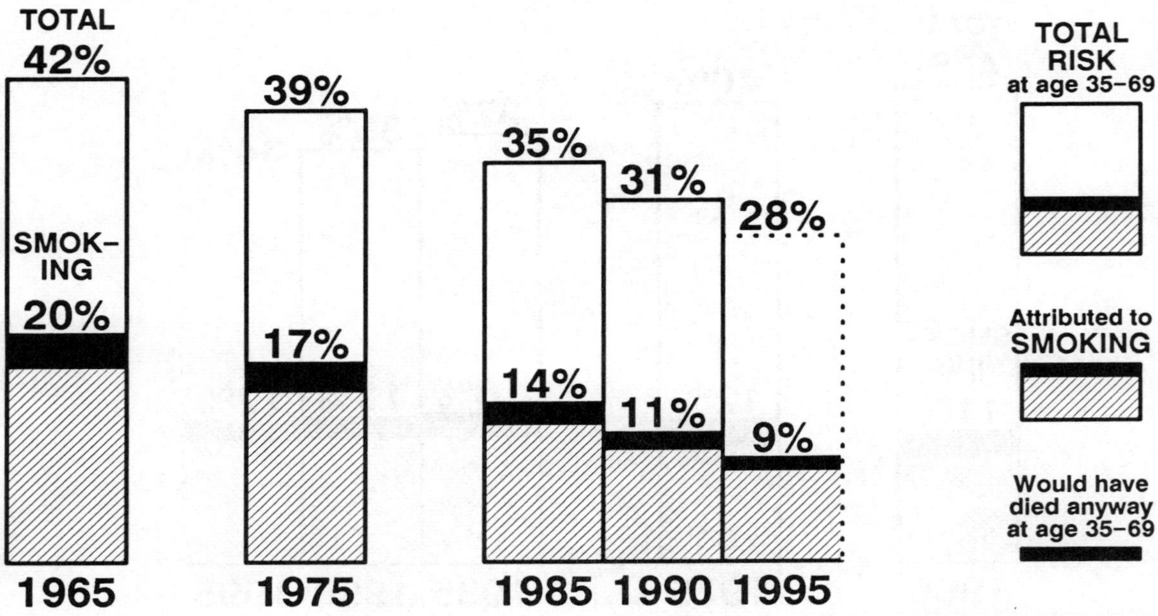

Peto, Lopez et al, 1992, 1994

Fig. 55. POLAND

MALES AGED 35: RISK OF DYING AT 35–69
(if the death rates in that calendar year were to persist unchanged)

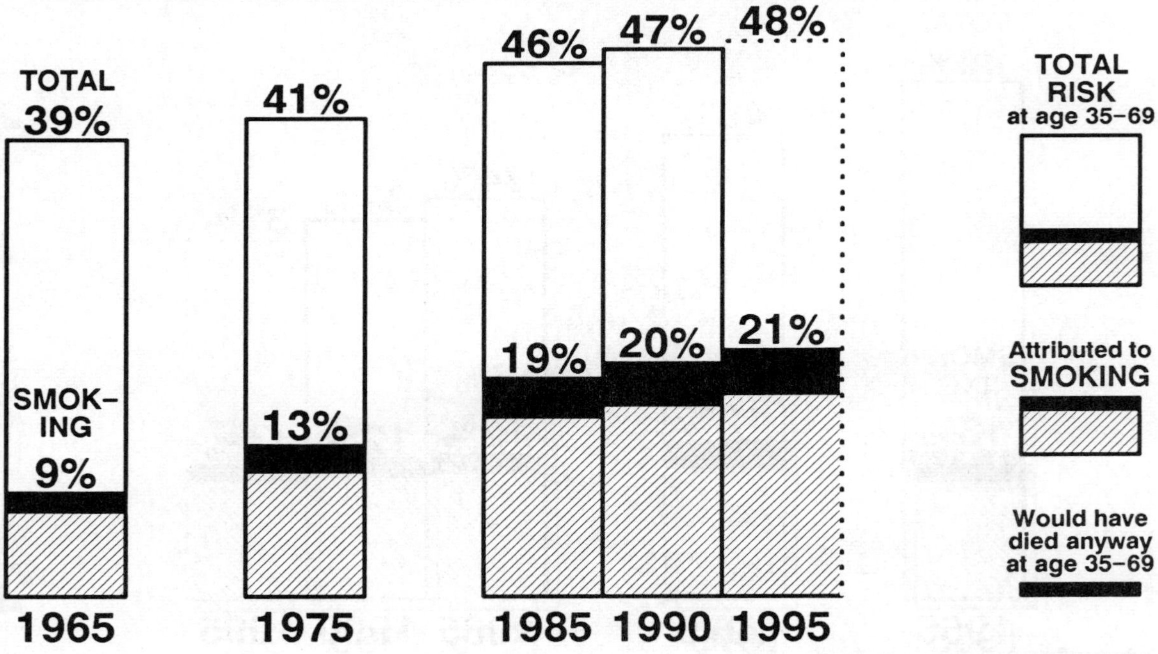

Peto, Lopez et al, 1992, 1994

Fig. 56. OECD DEVELOPED

MALES AGED 35: RISK OF DYING AT 35–69
(if the death rates in that calendar year were to persist unchanged)

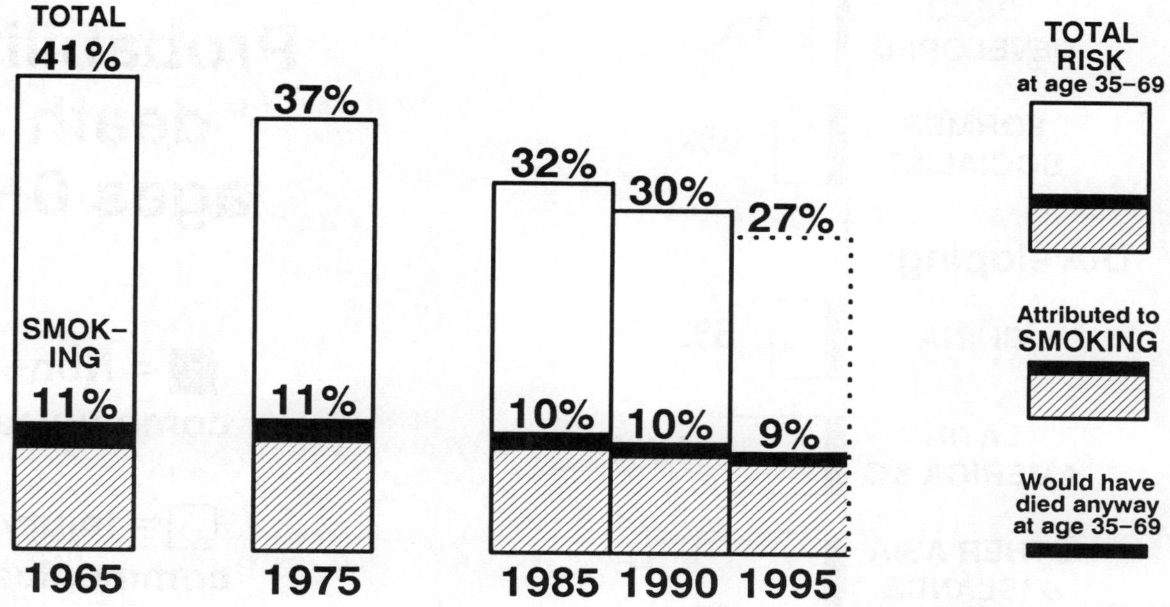

Peto, Lopez et al, 1992, 1994

Fig. 57. FORMER SOCIALIST ECONOMIES

MALES AGED 35: RISK OF DYING AT 35–69
(if the death rates in that calendar year were to persist unchanged)

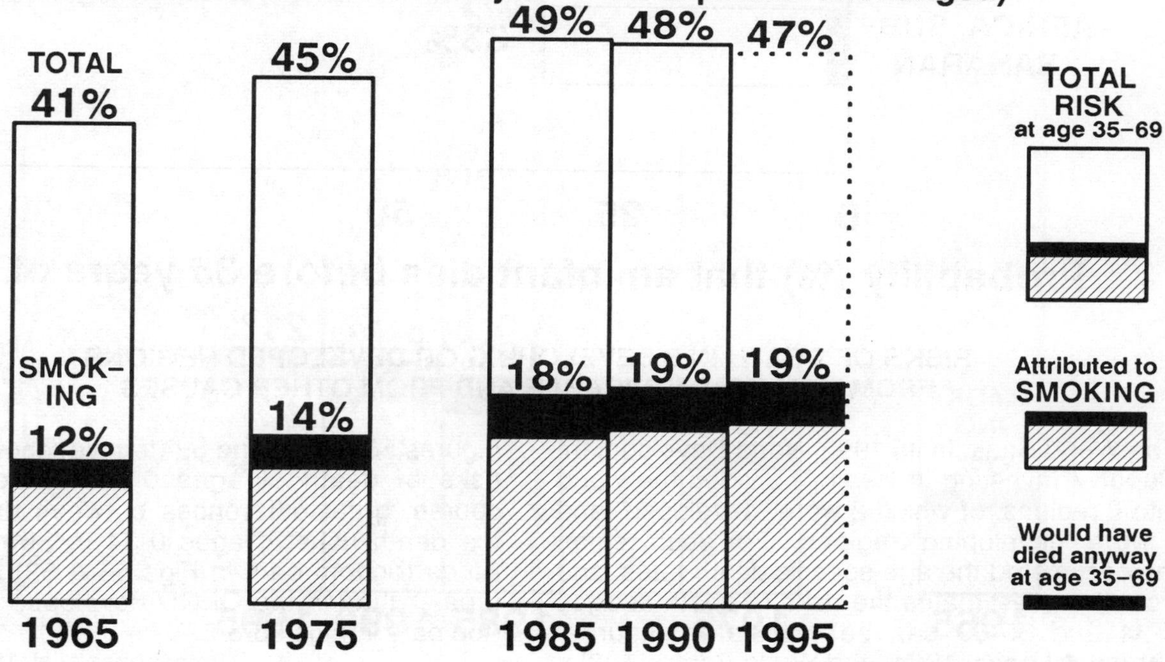

Peto, Lopez et al, 1992, 1994

Fig. 58. Male mortality at ages 0–34 in 8 regions

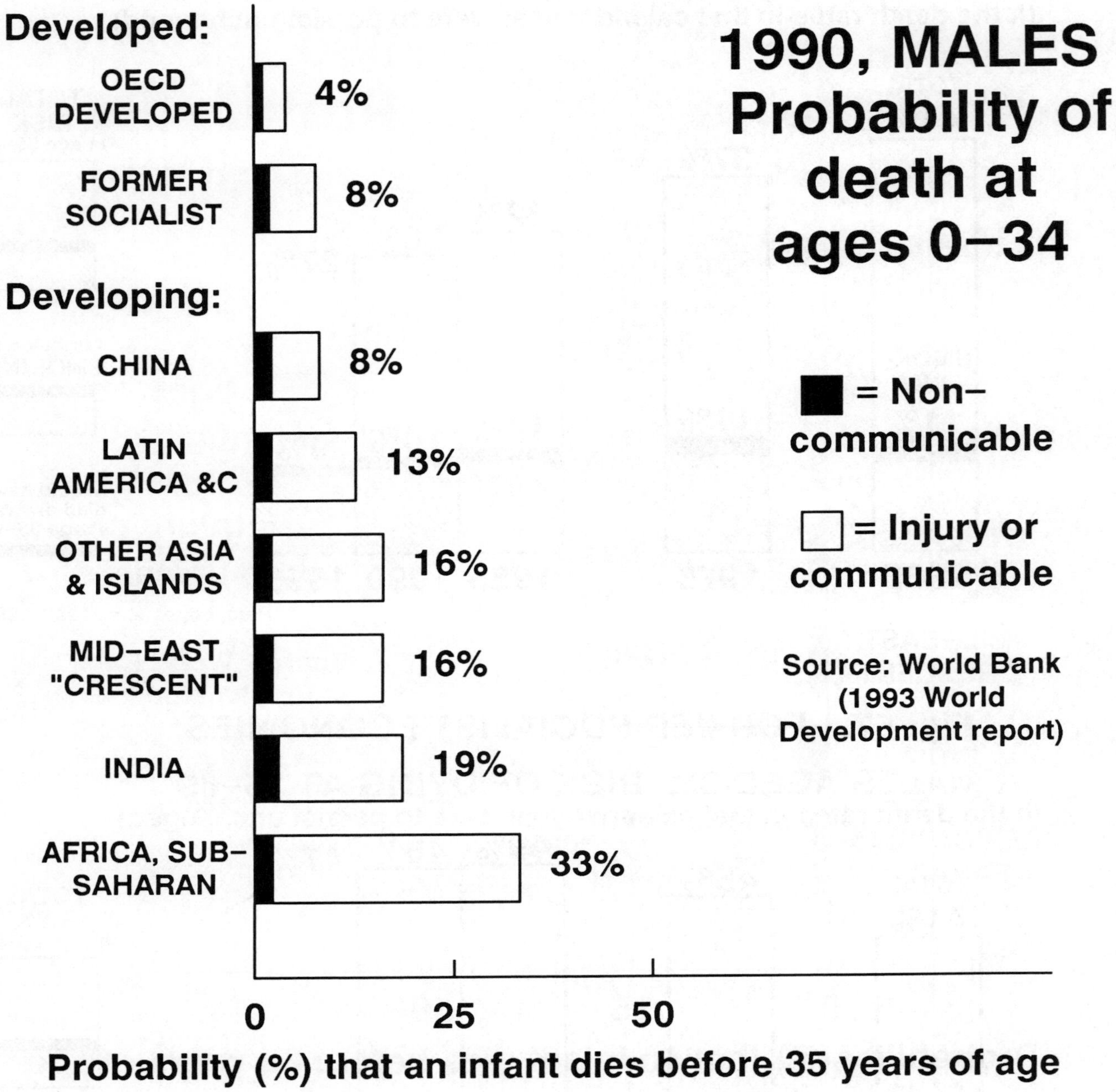

RISKS OF DEATH IN 8 DEVELOPING OR DEVELOPED REGIONS FROM NON-COMMUNICABLE AND FROM OTHER CAUSES

The World Bank, in its 1993 World Development Report ("Investing in Health") divided the world into 8 regions, of which 2 were "developed" and 6 were "developing" regions. For each region they estimated the age-specific death rates, and from these estimates the risks of death at ages 0-34 and 35-69 can be calculated (source: Murray & Lopez, 1994, and World Bank, 1993).

Figures 58 (male) and 59 (female) show these 8 risks of death at ages 0-34. There are, of course, great differences between them, with the death risks at ages 0-34 in Sub-Saharan Africa (bottom bars in Figs 58 & 59) ten times greater than in the OECD developed countries (top bars in Figs 58 & 59).

Fig. 59. Female mortality at ages 0–34 in 8 regions

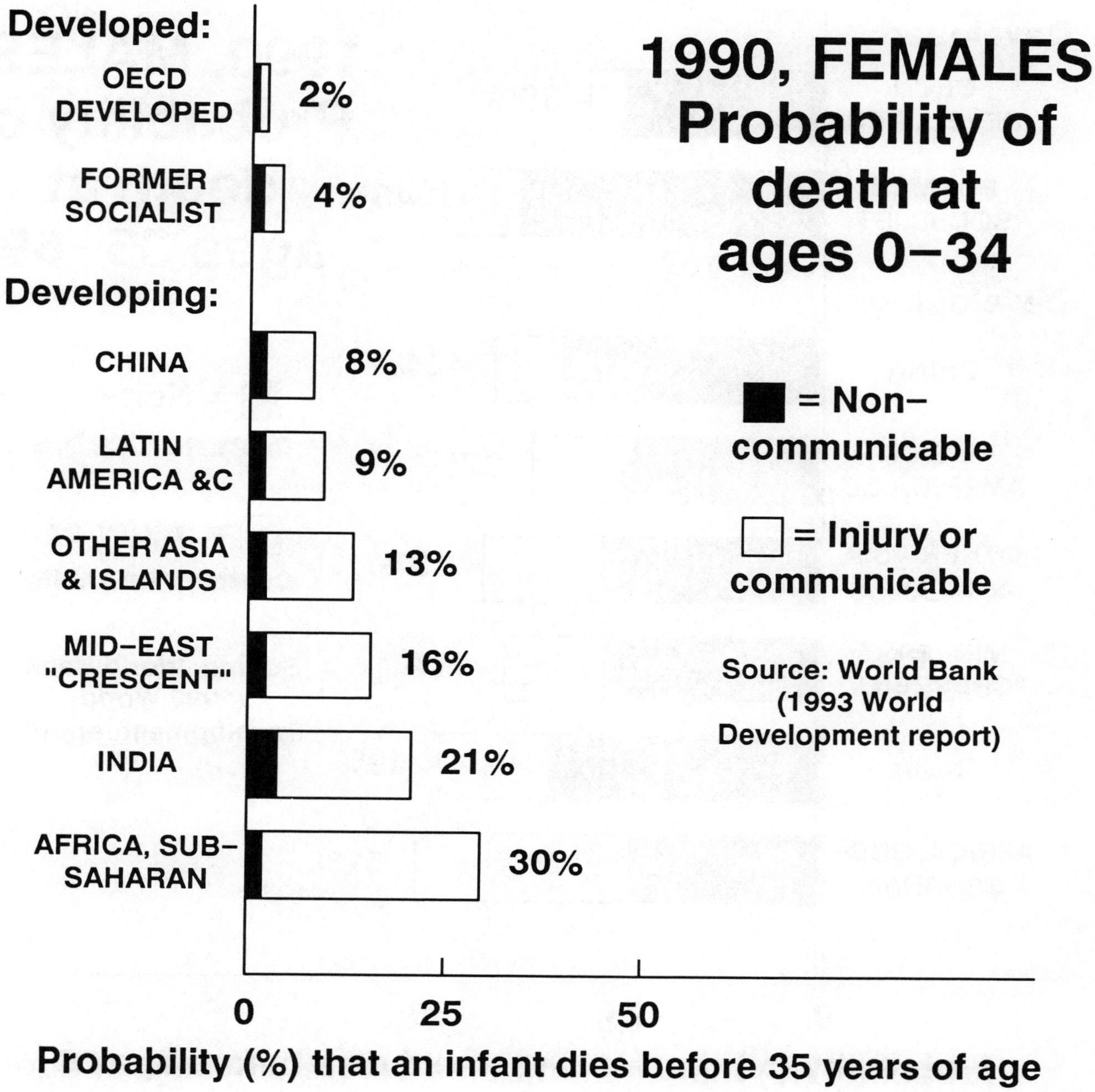

As might be expected, death before age 35 is chiefly caused by infection or by injury (white areas of bars), and the total risk varies greatly from one region of the world to another, being lowest in the developed populations and highest in India and, particularly, in Africa, where about one-third of all newborn infants will die before reaching middle age.

The numbers of deaths from non-communicable diseases at ages 0-34 is relatively small in all 8 regions (solid black areas).

Fig. 60. Male mortality at ages 35–69 in 8 regions

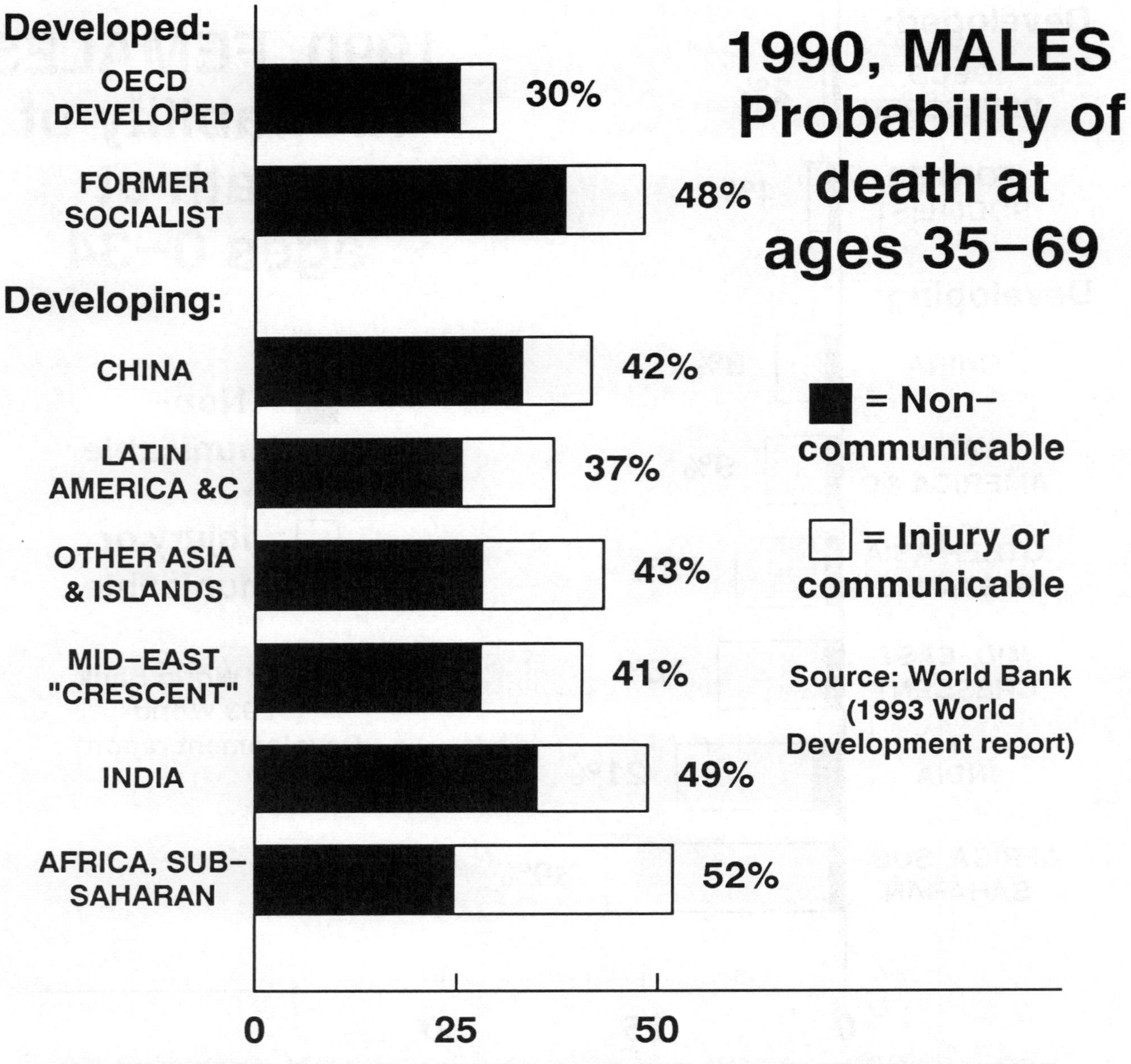

Global patterns at ages 35-69

In contrast, death in middle age is dominated by the non-communicable diseases (solid black areas in Figs 60 & 61), such as stroke, myocardial infarction, emphysema or cancer, each of which can be caused by tobacco. Because the effects of tobacco are so great among males in the former socialist economies, the death rates from non-communicable diseases are higher in that region than in any other. Overall, removal of the effects of tobacco in 1990 from the top two bars in Figure 60 might produce absolute reductions in death from non-communicable disease of 8% and 15% respectively (yielding overall death probabilities of about 22% in OECD and 33% in former socialist: see Figs 19 & 20).

Fig. 61. Female mortality at ages 35–69 in 8 regions

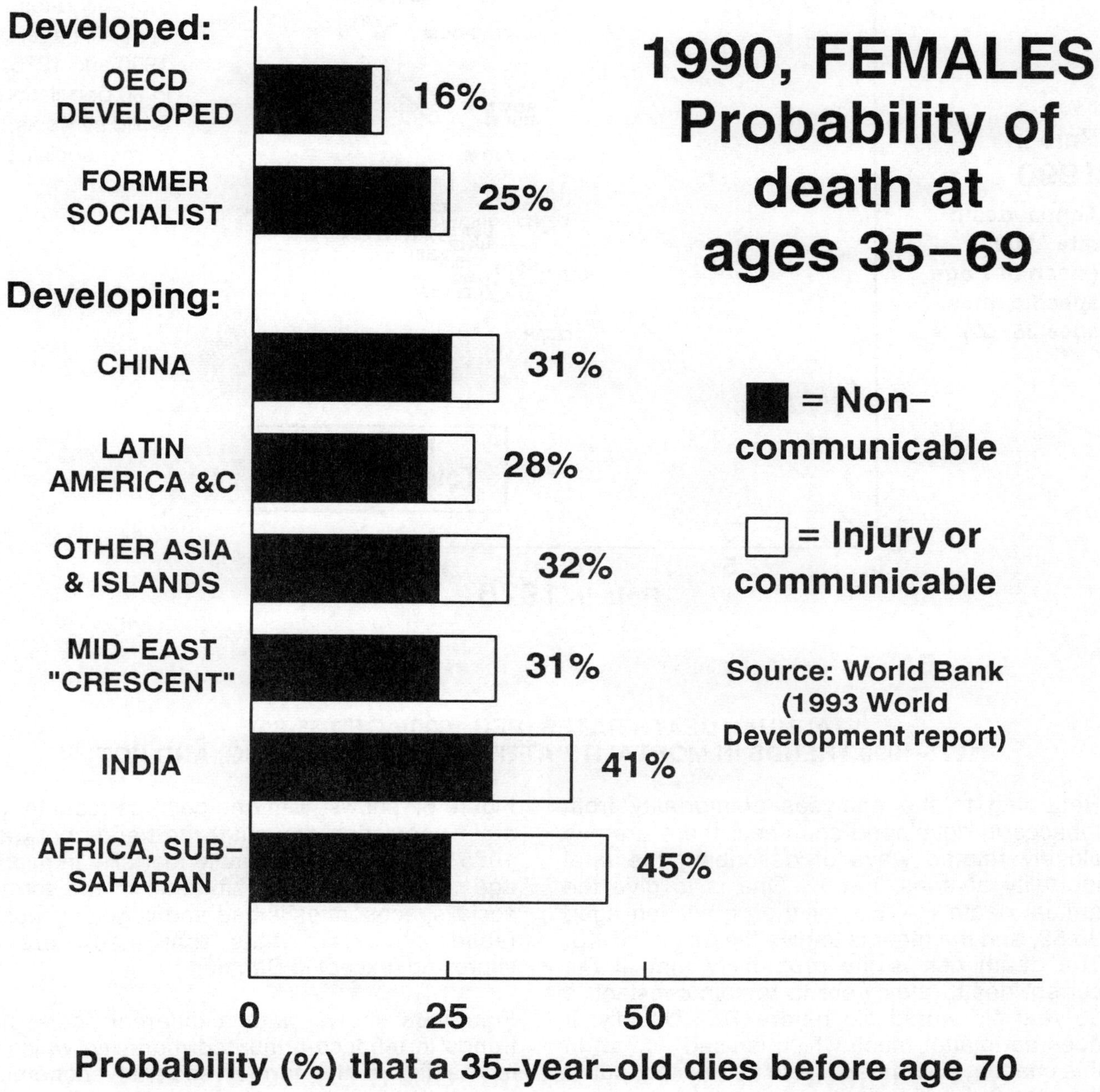

This would remove completely the anomalous excess of male deaths in the former socialist economies (second bar) and would make the male pattern of risk in these 8 regions closely resemble the female pattern at ages 35-69 (Fig 61). Among females, the global mortality patterns are not yet very much influenced by tobacco. In infancy, childhood and early adult life the global female mortality patterns in Figure 59 resemble the male patterns in Figure 58, but in middle age the global female mortality patterns in Figure 61 differ substantially from the male patterns, but do resemble what the male patterns would have been like without the extra burden of tobacco.

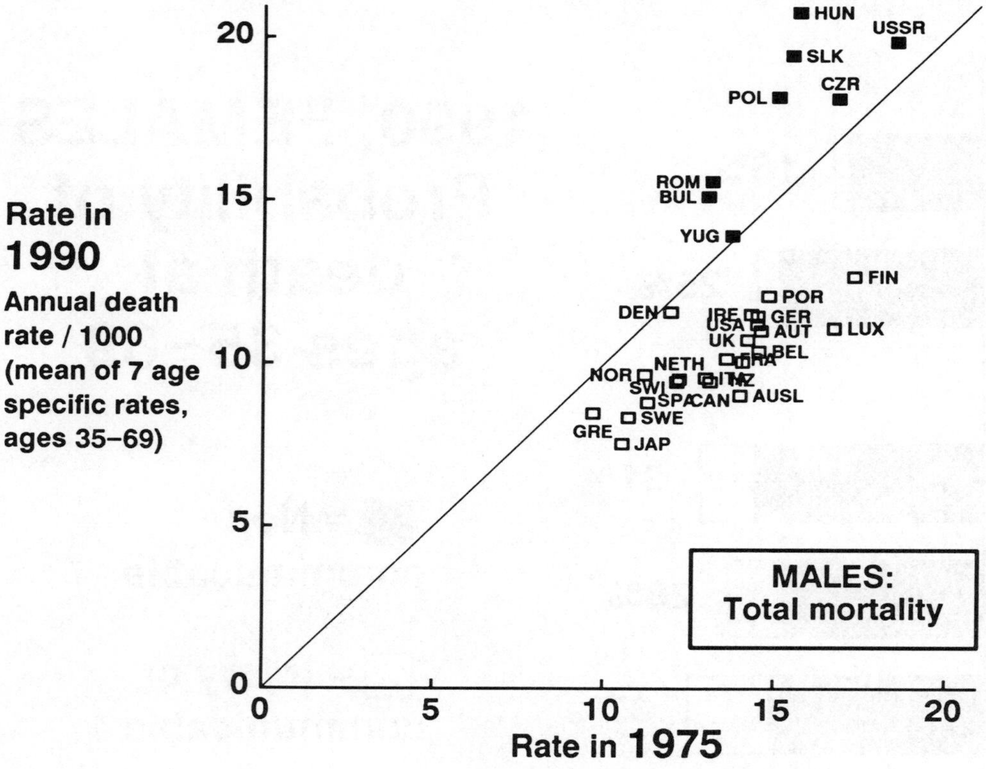

Fig. 62. Males: Total mortality rates in middle age, 1990 and 1975, in 30 populations (solid symbols: former socialist economies)

ANNUAL DEATH RATES (PER 1000 AGED 35-69): 1975-1990 TRENDS IN MORTALITY ATTRIBUTED TO SMOKING, AND NOT

Returning to the analyses of mortality from tobacco in developed countries, there are two closely related ways of describing the total mortality at ages 35-69. One is to give the annual death RATES for the population aged 35-69, and the other is to give the death RISKS. The death risk is the probability that, if the current death rates were to remain constant, a 35-year-old would die before 70. Usually, it does not matter much which is used: so far in this chapter, death risks have been cited, but in the remainder of it death rates will be cited (as they are slightly more convenient for subtracting different causes of death from each other, and for certain analyses of trends).

The period over which trends can best be assessed is 1975-1990. A shorter period might be less reliable, but so too (because of data deficiencies) might a longer period.

Figure 62 shows, with one point per country (or other population grouping) the trends between 1975 and 1990 in total male mortality in middle age. In summary, the situation in the former socialist economies is bad and is getting worse (solid symbols), while that elsewhere is improving (except in Denmark).

Figure 63 shows (with a different scale) the trends in tobacco-attributed mortality, which is increasing in the former socialist economies (and in Portugal) but is constant or decreasing elsewhere.

Figure 64 then shows the remaining trends, in which the mortality attributed to tobacco has been subtracted from the total. This is an indication of what the underlying trends might have been in the absence of tobacco. No large increases remain: the general picture is one of constant hazard in the former socialist economies and decreasing hazard elsewhere.

Fig. 63.
Males: Total mortality rates in middle age ATTRIBUTED TO SMOKING, 1990 and 1975, in 30 populations (solid symbols: former socialist economies)

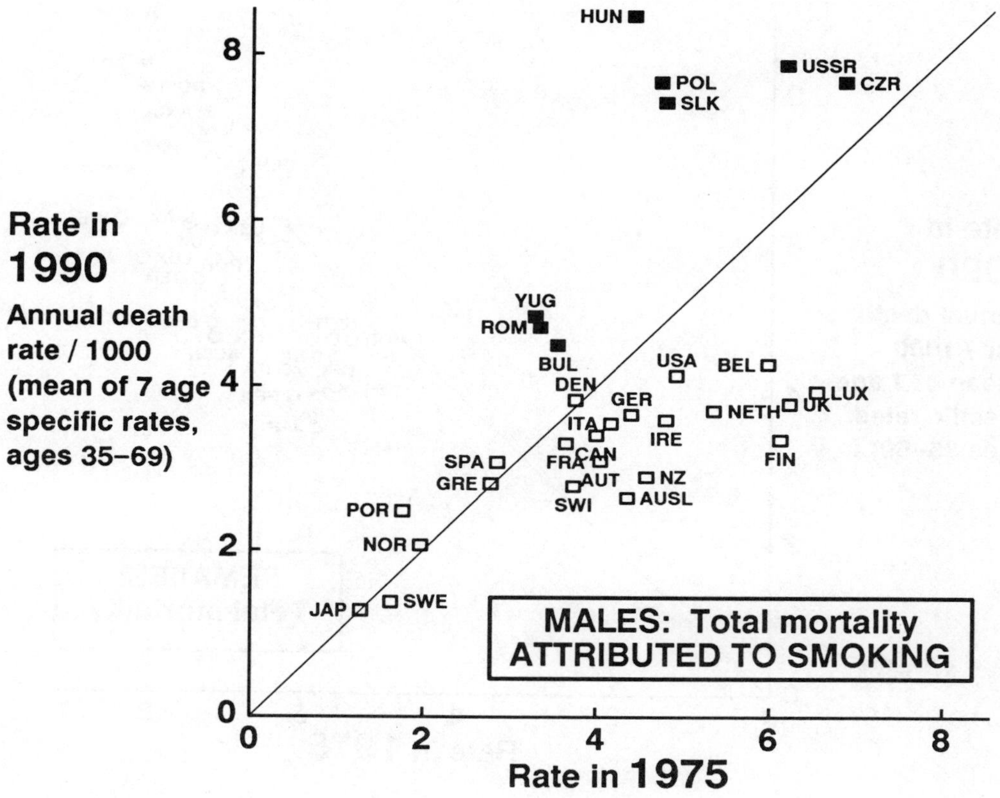

Fig. 64.
Males: Total mortality rates in middle age NOT ATTRIBUTED TO SMOKING, 1990 and 1975, in 30 populations (solid symbols: former socialist economies)

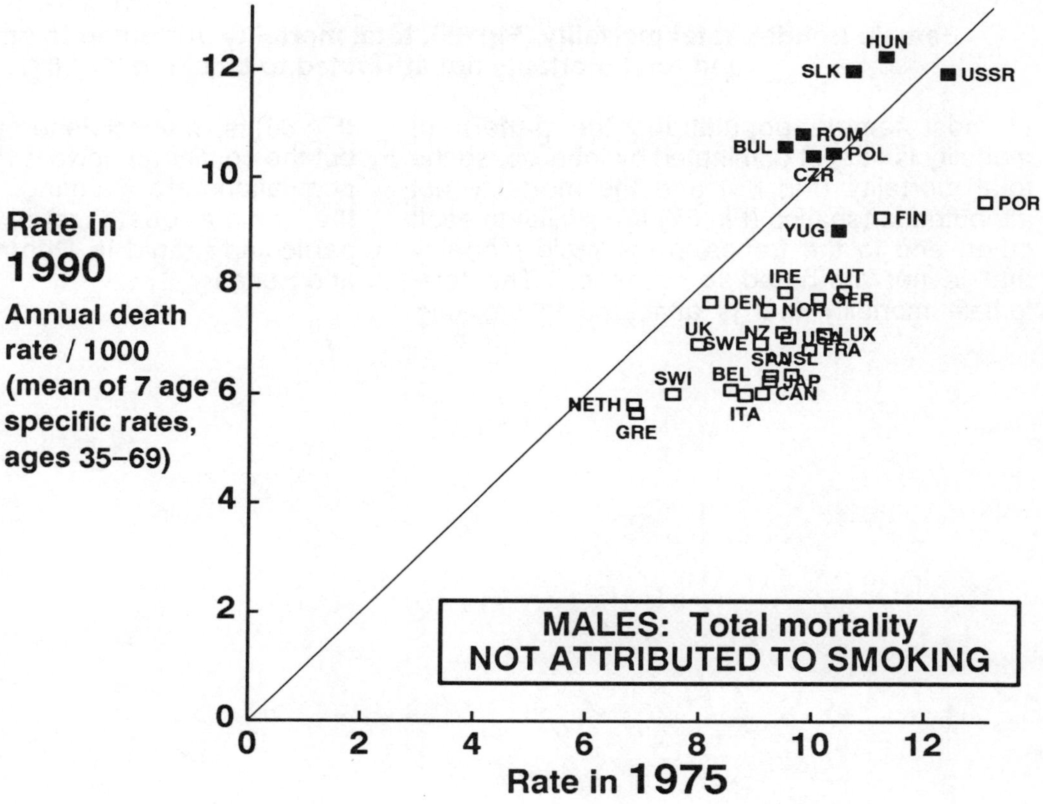

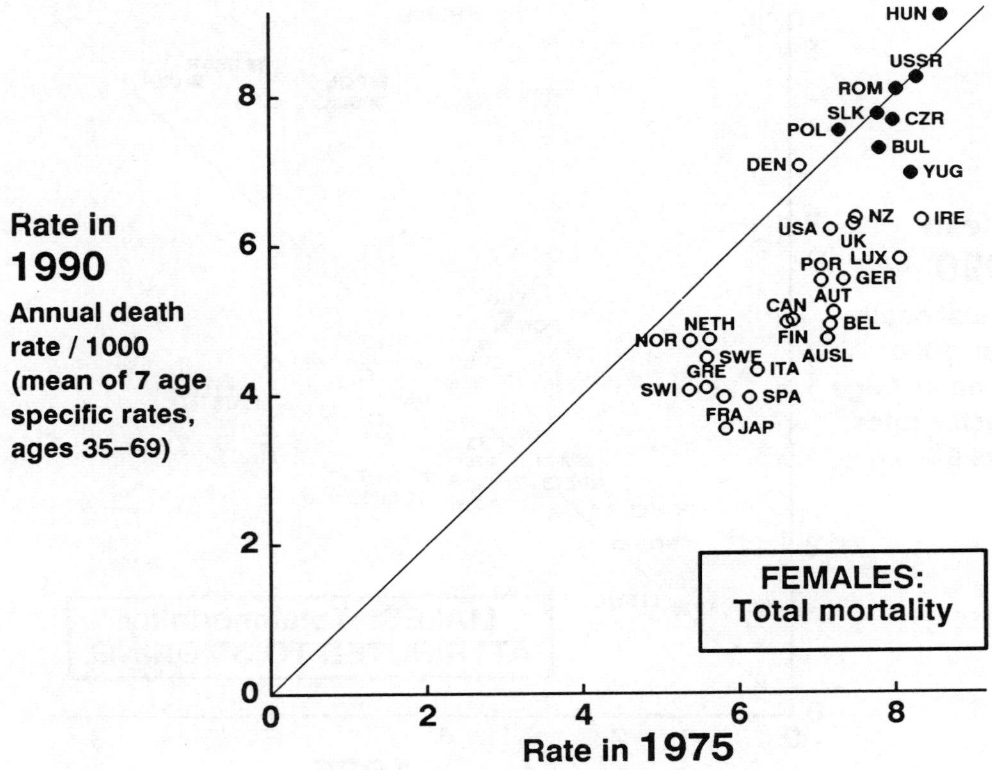

Fig. 65. Females: Total mortality rates in middle age, 1990 and 1975, in 30 populations (solid symbols: former socialist economies)

Female trends: total mortality (Fig 65), total mortality attributed to smoking (Fig 66) and total mortality not attributed to smoking (Fig 67)

In most female populations the pattern of mortality is not yet dominated by tobacco, so the total mortality (Fig 65) and the mortality not attributed to tobacco (Fig 67) are similar to each other, and to the trends in the male mortality that is not attributed to tobacco. The total female mortality that is attributed to smoking (Fig 66) is, in absolute terms, not yet very large, but the continued upward trends in most female populations are alarming. These increases in the female death rates from tobacco are particularly rapid in Denmark, North America and Hungary.

Fig. 66. Females: Total mortality rates in middle age ATTRIBUTED TO SMOKING, 1990 and 1975, in 30 populations (solid symbols: former socialist economies)

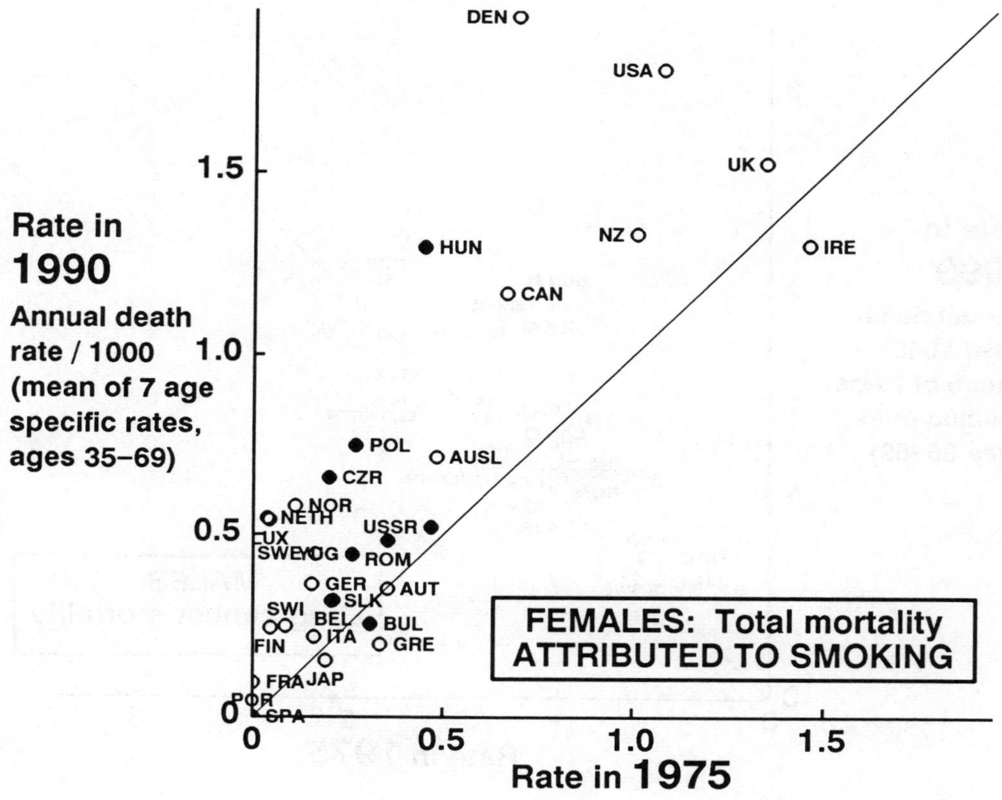

Fig. 67. Females: Total mortality rates in middle age NOT ATTRIBUTED TO SMOKING, 1990 and 1975, in 30 populations (solid symbols: former socialist economies)

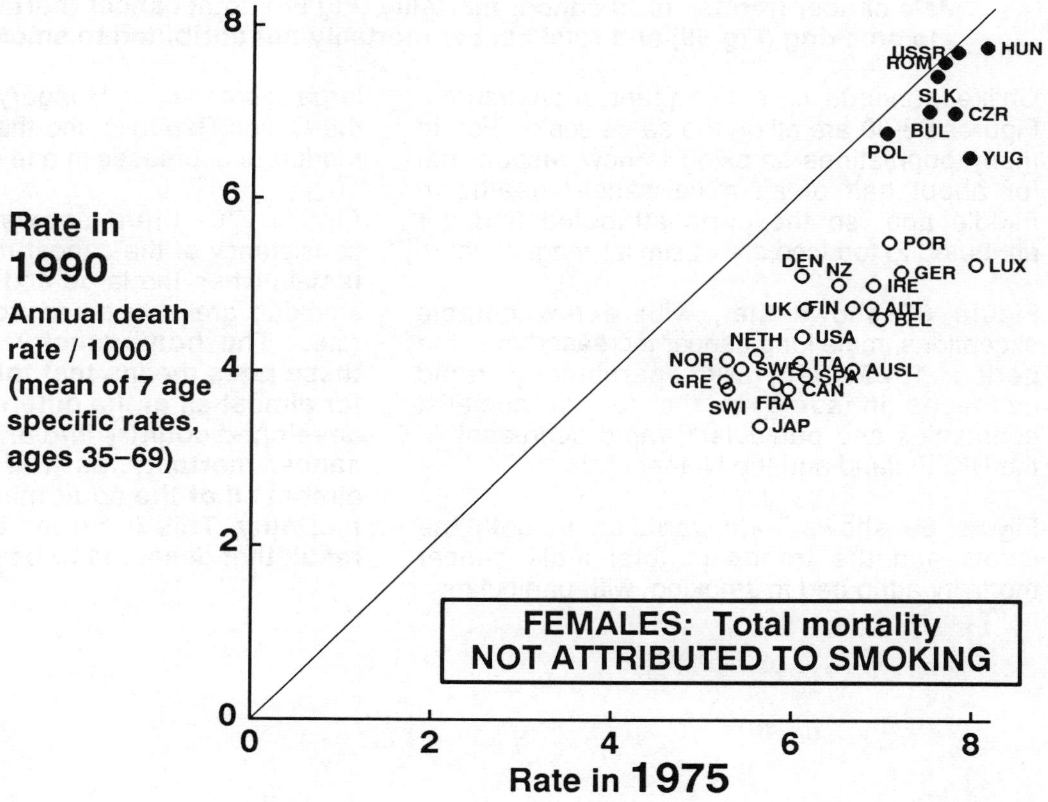

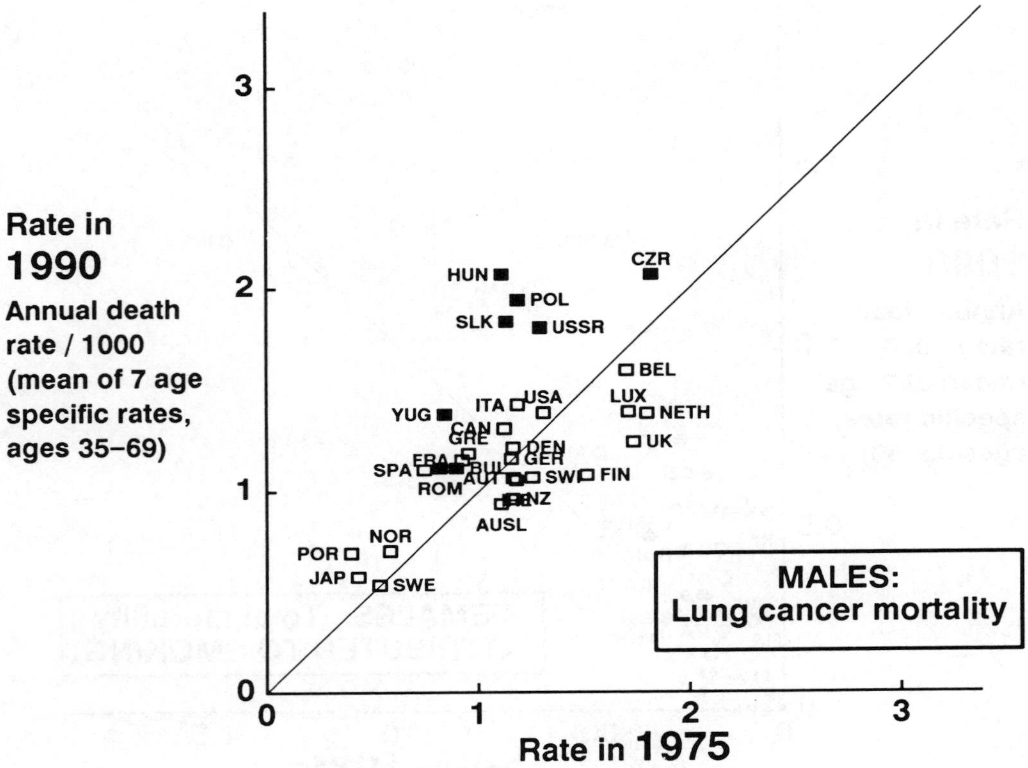

Fig. 68.
Males:
Lung cancer mortality rates in middle age, 1990 and 1975, in 30 populations (solid symbols: former socialist economies)

Male cancer trends: lung cancer mortality (Fig 68), total cancer mortality attributed to smoking (Fig 69) and total cancer mortality not attributed to smoking (Fig 70)

Unlike previous or subsequent such figures, Figures 68-70 are all on the same scale. For, in many populations smoking is now responsible for about half of all male cancer deaths in middle age, so the parts attributed and not attributed to tobacco are of similar magnitude.

Figure 68 shows that, with a few notable exceptions, male lung cancer increased over the period 1975-1990, with particularly rapid increases in some of the former socialist economies and particularly rapid decreases in the UK, Finland and the Netherlands.

Figure 69 shows wide variation in both the levels and the trends in total male cancer mortality attributed to smoking, with particularly large increases in Hungary, Slovakia, Poland, the Czech Republic and the former USSR, and moderate decreases in a few other populations.

Figure 70 then shows the remarkable consistency of the cancer rates and trends that remain when the large and variable hazards of smoking are subtracted from the total cancer rate. **The homogeneity and constancy of these rates means that tobacco can account for almost all of the differences between one developed country and another in adult male cancer mortality, as well as accounting for almost all of the adult male trends in cancer mortality. This is an important and striking result that deserves to be widely recognised.**

Fig. 69.
Males: Cancer mortality rates in middle age ATTRIBUTED TO SMOKING, 1990 and 1975, in 30 populations (solid symbols: former socialist economies)

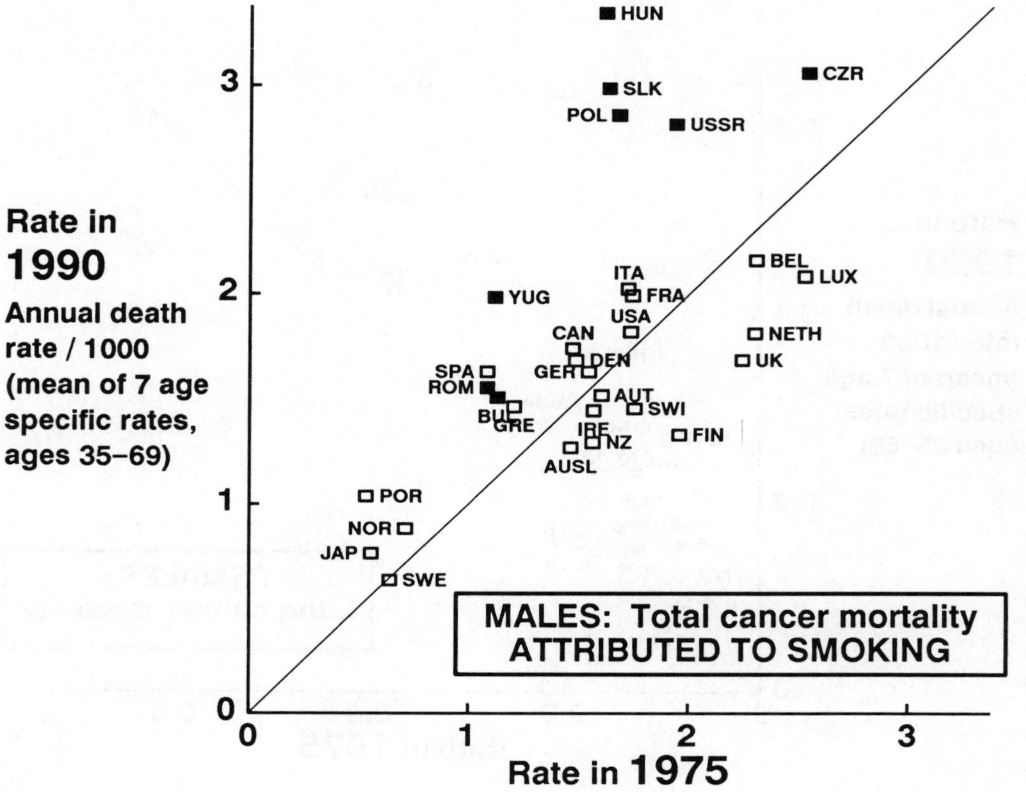

Fig. 70.
Males: Cancer mortality rates in middle age NOT ATTRIBUTED TO SMOKING, 1990 and 1975, in 30 populations (solid symbols: former socialist economies)

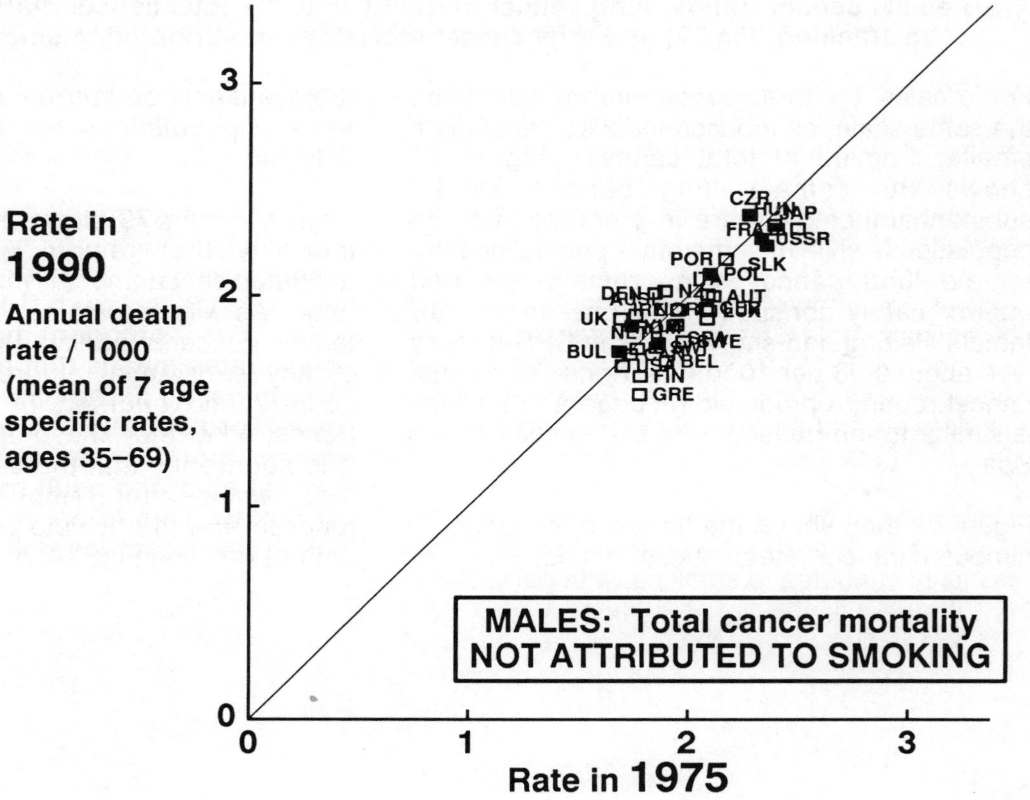

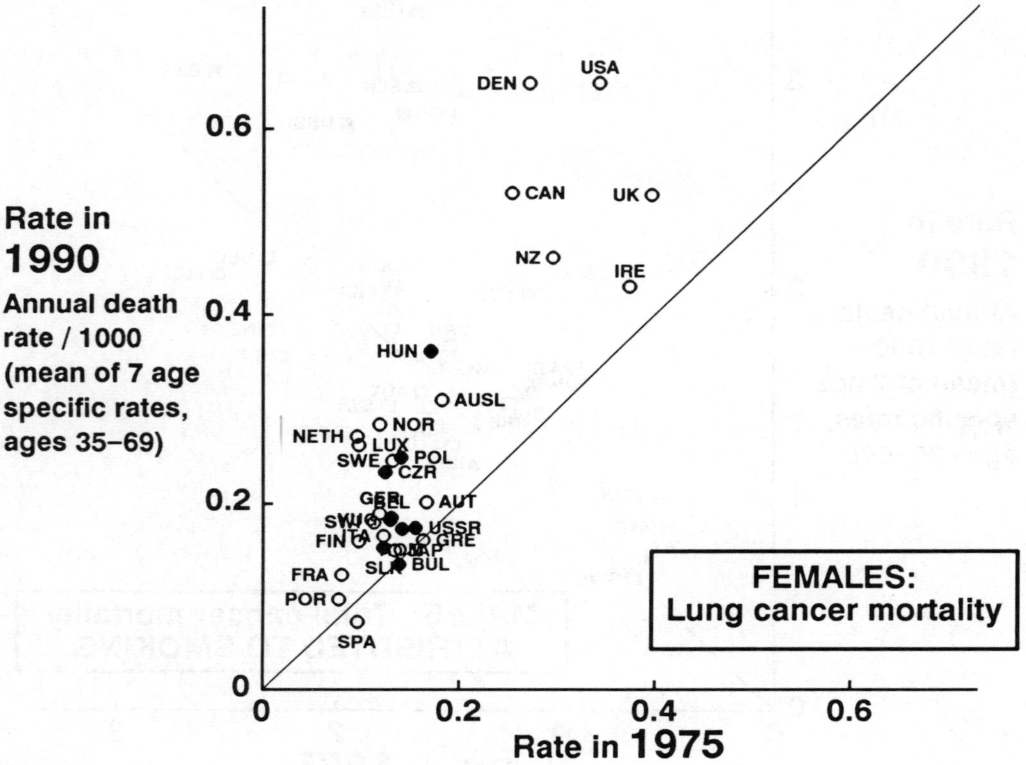

Fig. 71. Females: Lung cancer mortality rates in middle age, 1990 and 1975, in 30 populations (solid symbols: former socialist economies)

Female cancer trends: lung cancer mortality (Fig 71), total cancer mortality attributed to smoking (Fig 72) and total cancer mortality not attributed to smoking (Fig 73)

For females, the three cancer graphs are not on the same scale, as tobacco-induced cancer is a smaller fraction of total cancer. Figure 71 shows the female lung cancer trends: substantial increases are in progress in some populations, while in some other populations the female lung cancer rates remain low and approximately constant. The rate among US female lifelong non-smokers in the CPS-II study was about 0.08 per 1000 (see Annex to original Lancet report, reproduced on page A.56), which is similar to the national rate that is still seen in Spain.

Figure 72 then shows the trends in the tobacco-attributed cancer rates: these do not yet represent a large fraction of all cancer, but in several populations the increases are very definite.

Finally, Figure 73 shows the trends in cancer mortality that remain when the tobacco-attributed cancer mortality is subtracted from the total. As with the males, so too with the adult female cancer mortality: there is a striking lack of any substantial differences between one country and another, or of any substantial trends, other than those attributed to smoking. It is noteworthy that the cancer mortality rates that remain after removal of the effects of tobacco are, in absolute terms, very similar in both sexes (see Figs 74-76 below).

Fig. 72.
Females: Cancer mortality rates in middle age ATTRIBUTED TO SMOKING, 1990 and 1975, in 30 populations (solid symbols: former socialist economies)

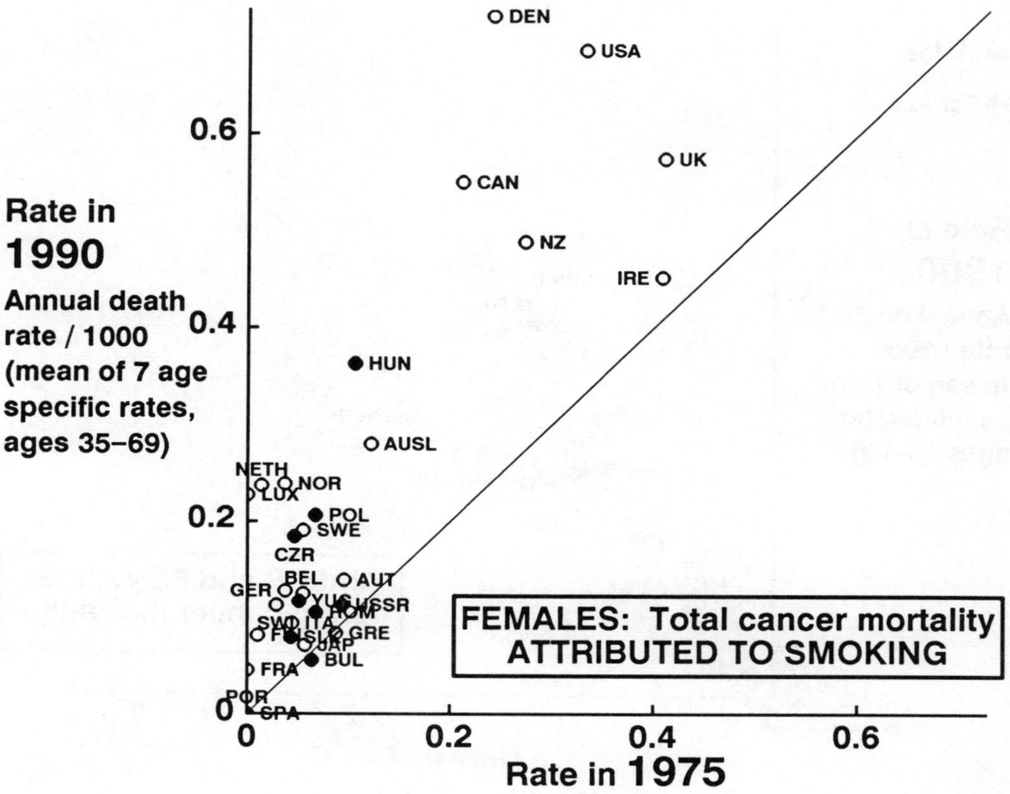

Fig. 73.
Females: Cancer mortality rates in middle age NOT ATTRIBUTED TO SMOKING, 1990 and 1975, in 30 populations (solid symbols: former socialist economies)

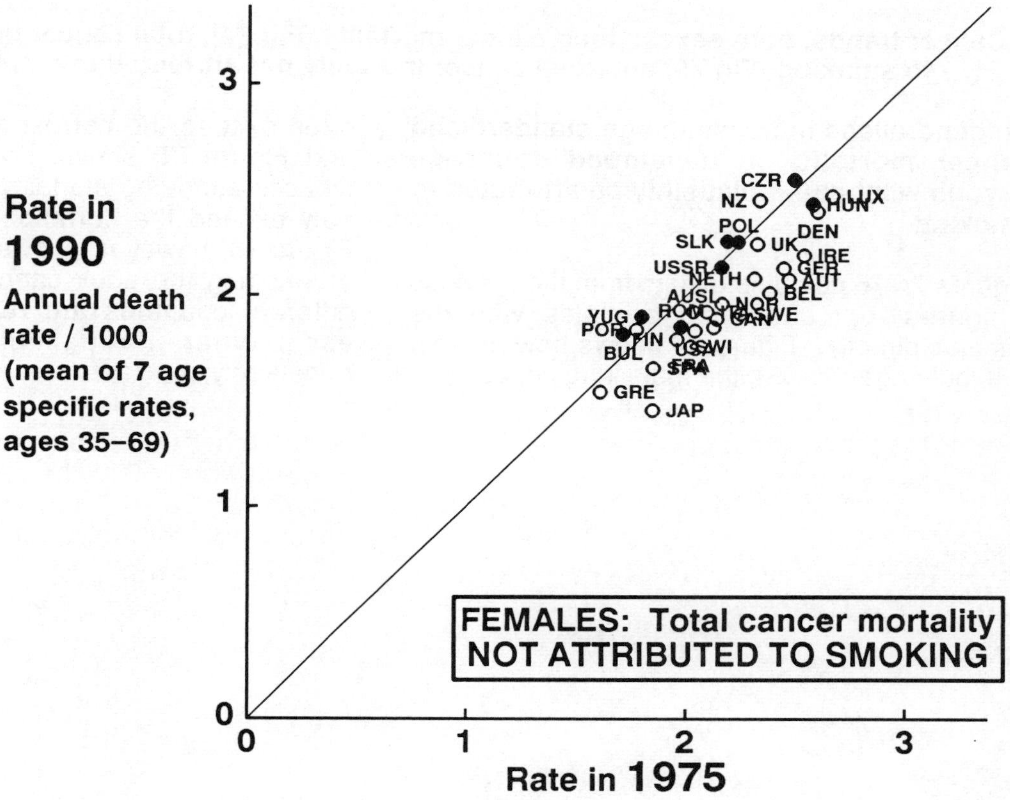

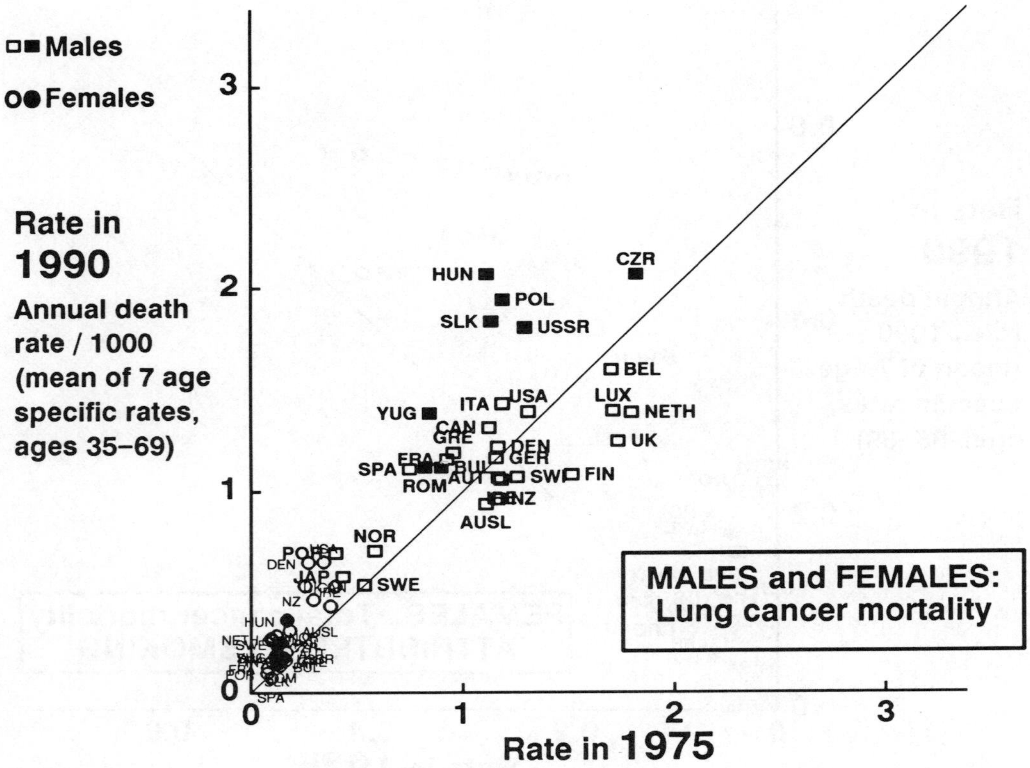

Fig. 74.
Males and females: Lung cancer mortality rates in middle age, 1990 and 1975, in 30 populations (solid symbols: former socialist economies)

Cancer trends, both sexes: lung cancer mortality (Fig 74), total cancer mortality attributed to smoking (Fig 75) and total cancer mortality not attributed to smoking (Fig 76)

No generalised increase in age-standardised cancer mortality in developed countries beyond what could plausibly be attributed to smoking

Figures 74-76 combine results from the previous 6 figures, but contrast the males with the females directly. Figure 74 shows how greatly, in middle age (35-69), the male lung cancer rates exceed the corresponding female rates, and Figure 75 shows how greatly the male tobacco-attributed mortality rates at ages 35-69 now exceed the corresponding female rates. Figure 76, however, shows that in the absence of smoking the adult cancer mortality rates in different countries are remarkably similar to each other throughout the world, and remarkably constant.

Fig. 75.
Males and females: Cancer mortality rates in middle age ATTRIBUTED TO SMOKING, 1990 and 1975, in 30 populations (solid symbols: former socialist economies)

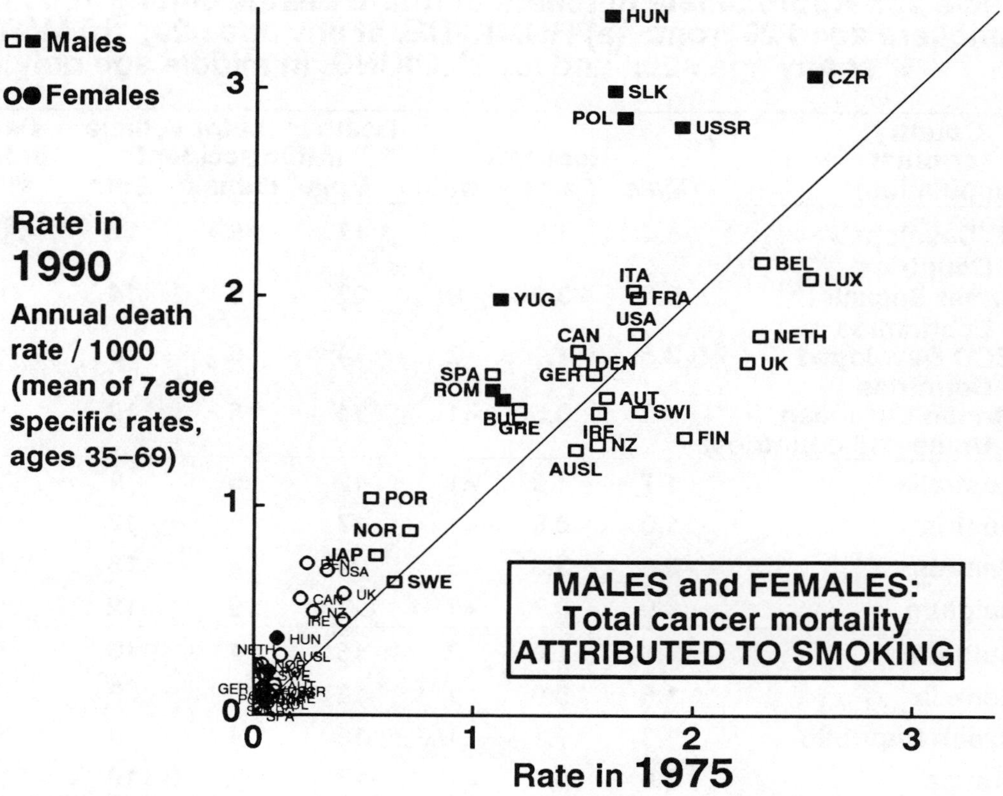

Fig. 76.
Males and females: Cancer mortality rates in middle age NOT ATTRIBUTED TO SMOKING, 1990 and 1975, in 30 populations (solid symbols: former socialist economies)

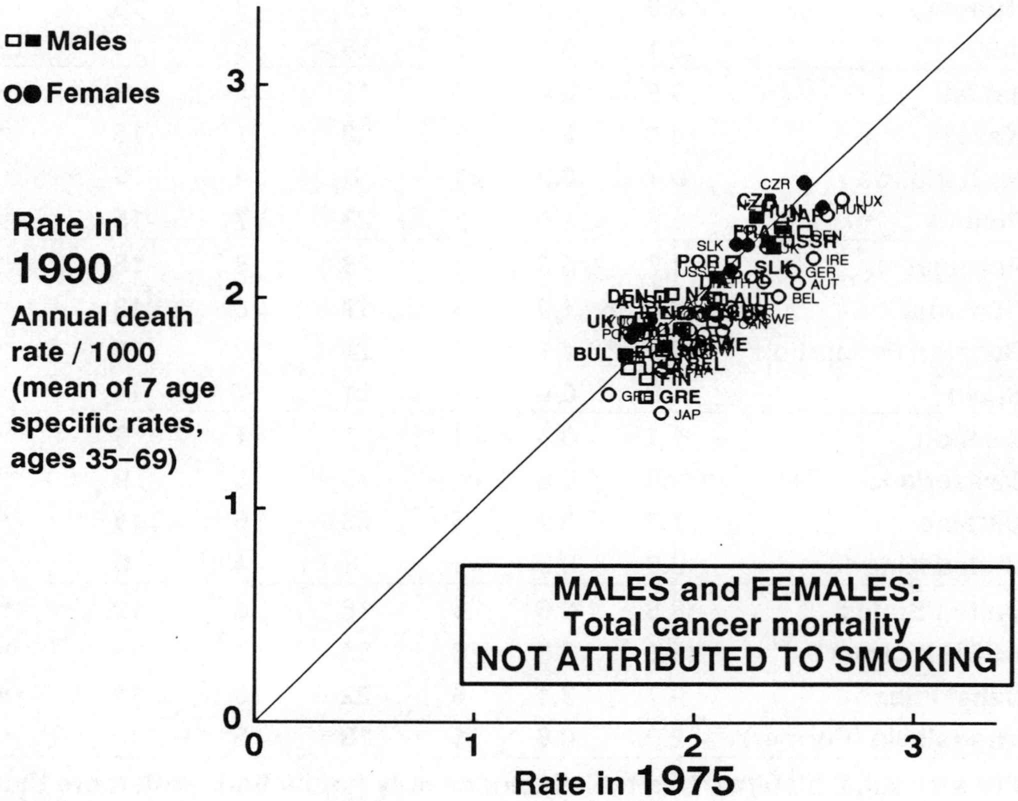

Table 23: Approximate numbers of future deaths among 1000 regular cigarette smokers aged 20 from: (a) HOMICIDE, at any age >20; (b) MOTOR VEHICLES, at any age >20; and (c) SMOKING, in middle age only (35-69)

Country (or other population)*	Homicide			Death in motor vehicle traffic accident			Death from smoking in MIDDLE age ONLY		
	Male	Female	Both	Male	Female	Both	Male	Female	Both
All "Developed" Countries	5.4	1.8	4	17	6	12	~300	~200	~250
Former Socialist Economies	9.0	3.2	6	22	6	14	"	"	"
OECD Developed Countries	3.5	1.1	2	14	6	10	"	"	"
Planned European Union (16 countries)	1.2	0.5	<1	14	5	10	"	"	"
Australia	1.7	1.0	<1	12	6	9	"	"	"
Austria	1.0	0.8	<1	17	6	12	"	"	"
¶Belarus	6.3	3.3	5	24	6	15	"	"	"
Belgium	1.0	0.7	<1	17	6	12	"	"	"
Bulgaria	3.3	1.0	2	15	4	10	"	"	"
Canada	1.6	0.9	1	12	6	9	"	"	"
¶Czech Republic	1.3	1.1	1	12	4	8	"	"	"
France	0.9	0.5	<1	17	7	12	"	"	"
¶Germany	0.7	0.5	<1	11	5	8	"	"	"
Greece	1.0	0.5	<1	22	8	15	"	"	"
Hungary	2.6	1.3	2	23	8	15	"	"	"
Italy	3.1	0.4	2	16	5	11	"	"	"
Japan	0.5	0.4	<1	12	6	9	"	"	"
¶Kazakhstan	13.5	3.7	9	23	7	15	"	"	"
Netherlands	0.7	0.3	<1	8	4	6	"	"	"
Poland	2.8	1.5	2	23	7	15	"	"	"
Portugal	1.7	0.6	1	28	8	18	"	"	"
Romania	5.6	1.9	4	19	6	13	"	"	"
¶Russian Federation	14.1	4.7	9	24	7	15	"	"	"
Spain	1.0	0.4	<1	21	7	14	"	"	"
Sweden	1.1	0.5	<1	7	4	6	"	"	"
Switzerland	1.0	0.8	<1	13	5	9	"	"	"
¶Ukraine	7.7	3.2	5	23	6	15	"	"	"
United Kingdom	0.6	0.3	<1	8	4	6	"	"	"
United States	8.8	2.6	6	16	8	12	"	"	"
¶USSR (Former)	11.6	4.0	8	23	7	15	"	"	"
¶Uzbekistan	9.7	3.1	6	22	6	14	"	"	"
¶Yugoslavia (Former)	2.0	0.8	1	18	5	12	"	"	"

* For statistical stability, this table includes only populations with more than 5 million adults.

9. EXPLANATORY METHODS

Explaining individual hazards

This monograph has been concerned chiefly with the effects of smoking on entire populations, rather than the effects on individuals who smoke. It began, however, with a Box, facing page A.1, that described the hazards for the individual in ways designed to avoid several common misunderstandings (e.g. underestimation of the true hazard; belief that smoking kills only old people; belief that teenage smoking is fairly safe; belief that tobacco is just one among many causes, or that non-smoker mortality patterns are deteriorating; belief that only "heavy" smokers are at serious risk; and underestimation of the substantial benefits of cessation).

More detail may be needed for any of these, but particularly for the comparison of tobacco with other hazards. To help prepare such statements, Table 23 lists the risks of eventual death from homicide or from motor vehicles that a 20-year-old faces in various populations (at 1990 death rates). These could be used as follows for the UK, averaging both sexes:

UNITED KINGDOM: CURRENT RISKS

On average, among 1000 20-year-olds who smoke cigarettes regularly,

— about 1 will die from homicide
— about 6 will die from motor vehicles
— about 250 will be killed by smoking in MIDDLE age alone (+ 250 more in OLD age)

or for the US (where trauma is more common):

UNITED STATES: CURRENT RISKS

On average, among 1000 20-year-olds who smoke cigarettes regularly,

— about 6 will die from homicide
— about 12 will die from motor vehicles
— about 250 will be killed by smoking in MIDDLE age alone (+ 250 more in OLD age)

Explaining population hazards

One useful statistic to cite is the number of children and teenagers (i.e. of those now aged 0-19) who will eventually, on present smoking patterns, be killed by smoking, e.g. for the UK:

- **On present smoking patterns, about 4-5 million of the children and teenagers in the UK today will become regular cigarette smokers in early adult life.**
- **About ONE MILLION of these will be killed by their habit in MIDDLE age alone, losing 20-25 years of non-smoker life expectancy; and, about one million more will be killed in OLD age.**

Such estimates are particularly useful where the epidemic is still at an early stage, for they relate abstract future risks to real individuals. This is relevant in some developed populations (especially for females) and many developing populations (see Chapter 10). The calculation requires just 3 things: (1) the number now aged under 20 (about 15 million in the UK: see Appendix tables, p.524); (2) the proportion of these who will, on present patterns, become regular cigarette smokers, which is roughly the current prevalence of cigarette use in early adult life (about 30%, in the UK); and (3) the proportion of such smokers who will, if they continue, eventually be killed by the habit (which, in developed populations, is about 1/4 in middle age and 1/4 in old age: page A.1).

In developing populations the eventual risks should, conservatively, be estimated to be about 1/3 rather than 1/2, but still the numbers are large. For example, in China there are about 420 million aged under 20, of whom about 40%, or 170 million, will, on present smoking patterns, eventually be smokers by 25 years of age. Even if the risks of being killed are, conservatively, assumed to be "only" 15% in middle age and 15% later, this yields:

On present smoking patterns, about 50 million of the children and teenagers in China today will eventually be killed by the habit. Of these, about half (25 million) will still be only in MIDDLE age when they are killed, losing 20-25 years of non-smoker life expectancy.

Explaining the delay

In talking or lecturing about tobacco, the chief difficulty is often explaining the delay, and the following sequence of material may be useful:

DEATH IN MIDDLE AGE (35-69)

- **Average loss of about 20-25 years of life expectancy for each death from tobacco in MIDDLE age**
- **No effect on population "spiral"**
- **Increasing RELATIVE importance as other causes decrease and the effects of smoking increase**

SEQUENCE OF EVENTS

1. **LARGE INCREASE IN CIGARETTE USE BY YOUNG ADULTS**
2. **MISLEADING DELAY: NO LARGE INCREASE IN LUNG CANCER ETC. FOR SEVERAL DECADES**
3. **EVENTUAL EFFECT: MAYBE ONE-THIRD OF ALL DEATHS IN MIDDLE AGE FROM TOBACCO**

Chief source of misunderstanding: LONG DELAY between increase in smoking and full increase in death risk

Example of long delay: US MALES

Large increase in cigarettes before 1945, but no large increase since

1945:	**male cigarettes high, but male lung cancer still low**
1945-85:	**main lung cancer increase while there was no large increase in male cigarette use**

(then show Fig 1, Table 5 & Figs 2-3)

Smoking kills more people by other diseases than by lung cancer

1985 US deaths attributed to tobacco by the US Surgeon General

Lung cancer	**110,000**
Vascular	**150,000**
Others	**140,000**
Total caused by tobacco	**400,000**
(Tobacco / all deaths	**0.4M / 2M)**

(then show Table 3 from page A.10)

Male mortality ratios (regular cigarette : non-smoker)

3 : 1 at age 35-69 (suggesting about 2/3 of male smoker deaths in middle age caused by tobacco)

All ages: about HALF of all regular cigarette smokers eventually killed by their habit.

DEATH IN MIDDLE AGE (35-69)

By 1990 in the USA, tobacco was causing about 1/3 of all deaths in MIDDLE age (plus "only" about 1/6 of the deaths at older ages)

Those killed by tobacco in MIDDLE age lost on average about 20-25 years of non-smoker life expectancy

Developed countries, 1985-1995: LUNG CANCER deaths in national mortality statistics

0.6M projected on post-1985 trends, with >0.5M attributed to tobacco

DEVELOPED COUNTRIES
~2 million smoking deaths in 1995

	1985 USA	1995, All developed
Lung cancer from smoking	110,000	>500,000
All deaths from smoking (M=million)	~ 0.4M	~ 2.0M

Developed countries, 1995:

More detailed arguments (based on age-specific, cause-specific ratios of other deaths to the excess of lung cancer) yield the same total of about 2M deaths / year.

ADVANTAGE: Can estimate smoking-attributable mortality

(1) in middle and in old age
(2) in earlier times
(3) in each separate country

as long as the lung cancer death rate, and other death rates, are known.

(then show Table 1, Figs 16, 9 & 10, Tables 2, 7, 8 & 13, Figs 12-15 & Table 12)

— Smoking is already causing about one-sixth of all developed-country deaths

— This proportion is still rising. If it stays at or about one-sixth, then at least one-sixth of the population will eventually be killed by tobacco

— 200 million, out of 1.2 billion.

The next chapter deals with developing populations, contrasting the current effects of previous smoking patterns with the much larger future effects if current smoking patterns persist:

Annual deaths attributed to smoking in 1995 and in 2025

	1995	2025
Developed	2M	~ 3M
Developing	~ 1M	~ 7M
World total	3M	~ 10M

M=million deaths / year

Peto, Lopez et al, 1994

CONCLUSIONS, AS REPORTED IN 1990, OF THE WHO CONSULTATIVE GROUP ON STATISTICAL ASPECTS OF TOBACCO-RELATED MORTALITY

The future worldwide health effects of current smoking patterns: 3 million deaths / year in the 1990s, but over 10 million / year eventually

For prevention, what chiefly matters is not current mortality from previous smoking, but future mortality from current smoking patterns. During the 1990s, there will probably be about 3 million deaths per year from tobacco. About 2 million will be in developed countries, but estimates for other countries are not as yet reliable, so the total of 3 million has an uncertainty of about one million either way. Worldwide mortality from tobacco is, however, still rising rapidly (particularly in the less developed countries), partly because of population growth but chiefly because previous large increases in cigarette smoking by young adults will have caused large increases in mortality by the time the young adults of today are middle aged. On the basis of current smoking patterns, the date when worldwide annual mortality from tobacco will exceed 10 million (of which about 3 million will then be in developed countries) probably lies some time in about the 2020s. (Those aged 35-69 in 2025 were aged 0-34 in 1990.) Without large reductions in early smoking uptake or smoking persistence, there will probably be over 10 million deaths per year during the second quarter (2025-2049) of the next century. This would mean that over 200 million of today's children and teenagers will be killed by tobacco, as will a comparable number of today's adults, i.e. that a total of about half a billion of the world's population today will be killed by tobacco. Some will already be over 70 and might have died soon anyway, but about a quarter of a billion will be 35-69, losing on average about 20 years of life. (The world population spiral is not materially affected, however, for few will be of reproductive age.)

These projections are based on the best currently available evidence on mortality patterns, smoking patterns and demographic trends. But, they still need to be reinforced or modified in several different parts of the world (e.g. various parts of China, India, Latin America, Europe) by large prospective studies that record smoking habits once, in the early 1990s, and relate them successively to mortality first 0-4, and then 5-9, 10-14, and 15-19 years afterwards. Such studies will monitor first the current state, and then the evolution, of this great epidemic.

WHO Consultative Group, 1990; R Peto (chair), A D Lopez (secretary) in: Proceedings of the 7th World Conference on Tobacco and Health

10. DEVELOPING POPULATIONS: THE FUTURE HEALTH EFFECTS OF CURRENT SMOKING PATTERNS (Adapted from WHO Collaborative Group, 1990, 1991)

In the present century most of the deaths from smoking have been in developed populations, but next century the opposite will be true. The annual number of deaths from smoking is still increasing in the developed populations, but it will be increasing even faster elsewhere. There has, over the past few decades, been a massive global increase in cigarette consumption, which will have its chief effects on mortality in the next century. Estimates are therefore needed not only (as in much of this book) of the current health effects of past smoking patterns, but of the far larger future health effects of current smoking patterns. These were discussed in 1989 by a WHO collaborative group (Peto & Lopez, 1990; Tobacco Alert, 1991), the conclusions of which are summarised in this chapter: see also the box opposite, which reproduces these conclusions.

Delay between cause and full effect

One of the chief sources of misunderstanding about the real health effects of tobacco is the very long delay, perhaps lasting several decades, between cause and full effect. This is true in developed countries (see preceding chapters), but it is particularly true in developing populations, where there are still many other important causes of death to deal with and where current smoking patterns are having much less effect on current mortality rates than they will on future mortality rates.

The risk of lung cancer depends strongly on the exact duration of smoking, and among regular cigarette smokers in middle or old age those who started in their teenage years will be at much greater risk than those who started later in life. This means that a sudden large persistent increase in cigarette use by a particular generation of teenagers or young adults will have its full effect on mortality in middle age only when, a few decades later, that first persistently exposed generation passes through middle age (and it may have its full effects on mortality in old age only after a delay of several decades (Doll & Peto, 1981; see also IARC Scientific Publication No. 74, 1986). Thus, current lung cancer death rates are strongly affected not only by smoking patterns 25 years ago, but also by the smoking patterns of teenagers and young adults 50 or more years ago. In the United States, for example, the large increase in male cigarette use between 1915 and 1945 resulted in a five-fold increase in age-standardised male lung cancer mortality during the 40-year period 1945 to 1985 (see Figure 1 on page A.12), even though there was no further large increase in cigarette use among American men after 1945 (Doll & Peto, 1981, Appendix E). This pattern of a large increase in cigarette use followed, after a delay of several decades, by a large increase in lung cancer deaths has been seen in many developed countries, and the recent very large increases in cigarette use in China and in many other developing countries are likely to produce comparable increases in male lung cancer during the early decades of the next century.

Other causes of death

Tobacco causes not just lung cancer, but also several other major diseases. In the United States, for example, where a large study of smoking and death has recently been reported, the US Surgeon General (1989) has estimated that in 1985 tobacco caused just over 100,000 of the deaths that were attributed to lung cancer plus just under 300,000 of the other deaths (the total caused by tobacco being about 400,000, or almost 20% of all US deaths that year). Thus, in the United States, tobacco probably caused almost three times as many deaths from other certified causes as from lung cancer.

The extent to which smoking is responsible for deaths from diseases other than lung cancer varies substantially from one population to another. (For example, smoking is particularly cardiotoxic for people who already have other risk factors such as high blood cholesterol, and it causes particularly large risks of cancer of the upper aerodigestive tract for people who already have other risk factors such as regular alcohol use.) But, the range of other diseases that can be caused by smoking is so extensive that the influence of other specific risk factors may effectively average out even in very different populations: for example, in many developing countries, although cholesterol levels are low (limiting the cardiotoxic effects of tobacco), a high prevalence of respiratory diseases may greatly increase pulmonary vulnerability to tobacco. **The general conclusion that smoking causes many more deaths from other diseases than from lung cancer is therefore widely applicable.** Lung cancer is, however, of particular statistical importance because high tobacco-attributable national lung cancer rates can generally be used as an indirect cumulative measure of the effective intensity of past exposure to the hazards of tobacco.

Current effects of smoking in developed countries: 2 million deaths / year

Although more accurate information, particularly about the exact evolution of this epidemic, would still be very desirable, the order of magnitude of the current problem in developed countries has been reasonably reliably established (see earlier chapters): tobacco will cause about 20 million deaths during the last decade of this century. At present most of these deaths from tobacco in developed countries are male, but in many such countries female mortality from tobacco will eventually increase substantially as well, due to the large increases in female smoking over the past few decades. More than half of the deaths from smoking occur at ages 35-69 years, making tobacco much the most important cause of premature death in developed countries.

Current effects in developing countries

For most developing countries the assessment of tobacco-attributable mortality is more difficult. Cigarette sales have increased substantially in recent years (much the largest absolute increase being in China), the male prevalence of smoking now exceeds 50% in many parts of the developing world (although the female prevalence is generally low), and chronic disease mortality rates are already high in many parts of Asia and Latin America. Overall, it was estimated that during the 1990s the annual number of deaths from tobacco in the developing world would be about one million (including several hundreds of thousands in China, plus several hundreds of thousands in India and elsewhere), although this total is necessarily somewhat uncertain.

World total in the 1990s: 3 million / year

Taking both developed and developing countries together, during the 1990s tobacco will be responsible for an average of about 3 million deaths a year worldwide, with a range of uncertainty of perhaps about 2-4 million.

Future deaths from smoking among those now under 20: hundreds of millions

At present there are 2.3 billion children and teenagers in the world, and on current smoking patterns about 30-40 per cent (i.e. about 0.8 billion) will be smokers in early adult life. A large recent prospective study in the United States (Tables 3 & 4 on pages A.10 & A.11: for further details, see p.A.56) indicated that, on average, persistent smokers have more than double the age-standardised death rates of life-long non-smokers. If smoking caused a two-fold excess at all ages it would eventually kill about half of all smokers. Not all the excess mortality associated with smoking is actually caused by smoking, however (though much of it is), the mortality ratio beyond 75 years of age may be less than two-fold, and in developing countries the death rates from some unrelated causes (e.g. infectious diseases) are higher than in the United States. So, in developing countries the proportion of persistent smokers eventually killed by the habit will probably be somewhat less than the proportion of about one-half that is suggested by the North American study. Even if the proportion is "only" about one-third, however, then about 250 million of these 800 million future smokers would be killed by the habit. Neither the accuracy nor the inaccuracy of this estimate of over 200 million deaths should be exaggerated.

If, on current smoking patterns, 200 to 300 million of those born in a 20-year period (e.g. 1970 to 1990) will be killed by tobacco, then at some stage around the middle of the next century (when the majority of these deaths will occur) the average annual number of deaths from tobacco must be about 1/20th of this, or about 10 to 15 million, and at some earlier stage the average annual number of deaths from tobacco will therefore be about 10 million. The uncertainty is not whether, but when, the annual total will, on present smoking patterns, be about 10 million — perhaps in the 2020s, but perhaps not until the 2030s. If the epidemic grows as rapidly in other developing countries as it is likely to do in China (Peto, 1986) then the date might be earlier rather than later: between 1978 and 1992 Chinese annual consumption of manufactured cigarettes increased from 500 billion to 1700 billion (about 30% of the world total), cigarette tar levels are high, case-control studies in China show large effects of prolonged smoking on lung cancer, and the "background" death rates among non-smokers are already unusually high from diseases such as emphysema and cancer of the oesophagus (which suggests that among Chinese smokers the habit will cause particularly large hazards from these diseases). Indeed, the unpublished evidence from the nationwide "spouse-control" study by Liu Boqi et al of several hundred thousand Chinese deaths (plus the same number of controls) suggests that tobacco is already causing about half a million deaths a year in China, of which about half are due to chronic lung disease (a proportion much greater than in developed populations: see Table 3 on page A.10).

Future deaths from smoking among those now aged over 20: hundreds of millions

If annual mortality from tobacco will rise from about 3 million in the 1990s to about 10 million in the 2020s or early 2030s, then the average mortality over this 40-year period will be intermediate between 30 million and 100 million per decade. Since most of those dying from smoking over the next 40 years (plus some of those dying from it more than 40 years hence) are already adults in 1990, about 200 to 300 million of today's 3 billion adults can be expected eventually to die from tobacco.

Eventual world total: half a billion

Combining the estimates for those now under 20 and for those now over 20 years of age, on present smoking patterns about half a billion of the world's population today will eventually be killed by tobacco, and current experience in developed countries suggests that about half of them will be 35-69 years of age when killed. These predictions are summarised below: they will be substantially wrong only if there are substantial changes in global smoking patterns.

FUTURE HEALTH EFFECTS IF CURRENT WORLD-WIDE SMOKING PATTERNS WERE TO PERSIST

3 MILLION DEATHS / YEAR from tobacco in 1990s

10 MILLION DEATHS / YEAR by about the 2020s

ABOUT HALF A BILLION of the world's population today will eventually be killed by tobacco

ABOUT 1/4 OF A BILLION still in middle age (35-69) when killed by tobacco, losing ~20 years of life.

Peto & Lopez, 1990, 1991, for WHO Consultative Group

REFERENCES
AND FURTHER READING

Doll R, Hill AB. Smoking and carcinoma of the lung. Preliminary report. *British Medical Journal* 1950; **2**: 739-748

Doll R, Peto R. Mortality in relation to smoking: 20 years' observations on male British doctors. *British Medical Journal* 1976; **ii**: 1525-1536

Doll R, Gray R, Hafner B, Peto R. Mortality in relation to smoking: 22 years' observations on female British doctors. *British Medical Journal* 1980; **280**: 967-971

Doll R, Peto R. The causes of cancer: quantitative risks of avoidable causes of cancer in the United States today. *Journal of the National Cancer Institute* 1981; **66**: 1191-1308. (Also reprinted as an Oxford University Press paperback, published in 1983)

Doll R, Peto R, Wheatley K, Gray R. Mortality in relation to smoking: 40 years' observations on male British doctors. *British Medical Journal* 1994 (in press)

International Agency for Research on Cancer. *Tobacco: An International Health Hazard.* Zaridze D, Peto R (eds). IARC Scientific Publication No. 74. Lyon, IARC, 1986

International Agency for Research on Cancer. *IARC Monographs on the Evaluation of the Carcinogenic Risk of Chemicals to Humans: Vol. 38, Tobacco Smoking.* Lyon: IARC, 1986

Murray CJL, Lopez AD. Global and regional cause-of-death patterns in 1990. *Bulletin of the World Health Organization* 1994; **72**, No. 3: 447-480

Peto R, Lopez AD. 1990 report to the 7th World Conference on Tobacco or Health, on behalf of the WHO consultative group on statistical aspects of tobacco-related mortality. The future worldwide health effects of current smoking patterns. In: *The Global War: Proceedings of the 7th World Conference on Tobacco or Health.* Durston B, Jamrozik K (eds). Health Dept of Western Australia, Perth, 1990

Peto R, Lopez AD, Boreham J, Thun M, Heath C Jr. Mortality from tobacco in developed countries: indirect estimation from national vital statistics. *Lancet* 1992; **339**: 1268-1278

Peto R. Tobacco: UK and China (letter). *Lancet* 1986; **ii**: 1038

United Nations. *World Population Prospects. The 1992 revision.* ST/ESA/SER.A/135. United Nations, New York, 1993

United States Department of Health & Human Services. *Reducing the health consequences of smoking: 25 years of progress. A report of the US Surgeon-General.* DHHS Publication No. (CDC) 89-8411, Washington, 1989

World Bank. *World Development Report: Investing in Health.* World Bank, Washington, 1993

World Health Organization. *International Classification of Diseases* (ICD), 9th revision. WHO, Geneva, 1977

World Health Organization. Tobacco-attributable mortality: global estimates and projections. *Tobacco Alert* 1991; **1**: 4-7

Wynder EL, Graham EA. Tobacco smoking as a possible etiologic factor in bronchogenic carcinoma. *Journal of the American Medical Association* 1950; **143**: 329-336

MAIN TABLES

AND FIGURES

To facilitate effective communication, the main tables and figures (and all previous ones) are designed for easy reproduction or public projection (and, no copyright over them is claimed)

ALL 'DEVELOPED' COUNTRIES: 1990
Relative importance of deaths in MIDDLE age (35–69)

Age range (years)	Deaths attributed to SMOKING / total deaths (millions) Males	Females	Mean years lost PER DEATH FROM SMOKING
0–34	–/0.5	–/0.2	–
35–69	0.9/2.5	0.2/1.4	22 years
70+	0.6/2.9	0.2/4.0	8 years
All ages	1.4/5.8	0.4/5.6	16 years

Peto, Lopez et al, 1992, 1994

ALL 'DEVELOPED' COUNTRIES: 1990 deaths, by cause
Nos. of deaths attributed to smoking / total deaths (thousands)

	Males			Females		
Age:	0–34	35–69	70+	0–34	35–69	70+
Lung Cancer	–/1.2	231/246	141/156	–/0.7	44/64	42/61
All Cancer	–/27	360/736 (49%)	212/600 (35%)	–/23	56/500 (11%)	56/564 (10%)
Vascular	–/27	318/926	163/1467	–/13	57/508	92/2417
Respiratory	–/38	90/140	139/322	–/29	25/66	63/299
All Other	–/413	97/656	40/462	–/179	22/302	25/718
All Causes	–/504	865/2458 (35%)	554/2851 (19%)	–/244	160/1376 (12%)	236/3998 (6%)

Peto, Lopez et al, 1992, 1994

ALL 'DEVELOPED' COUNTRIES: 1990
RISKS OF DYING AT AGES 0–34 and 35–69

(Probability that someone entering an age range would die during it, if the death rates in 1990 were to persist unchanged)

Relative importance in 1990 of death risk in MIDDLE age, and of SMOKING within it

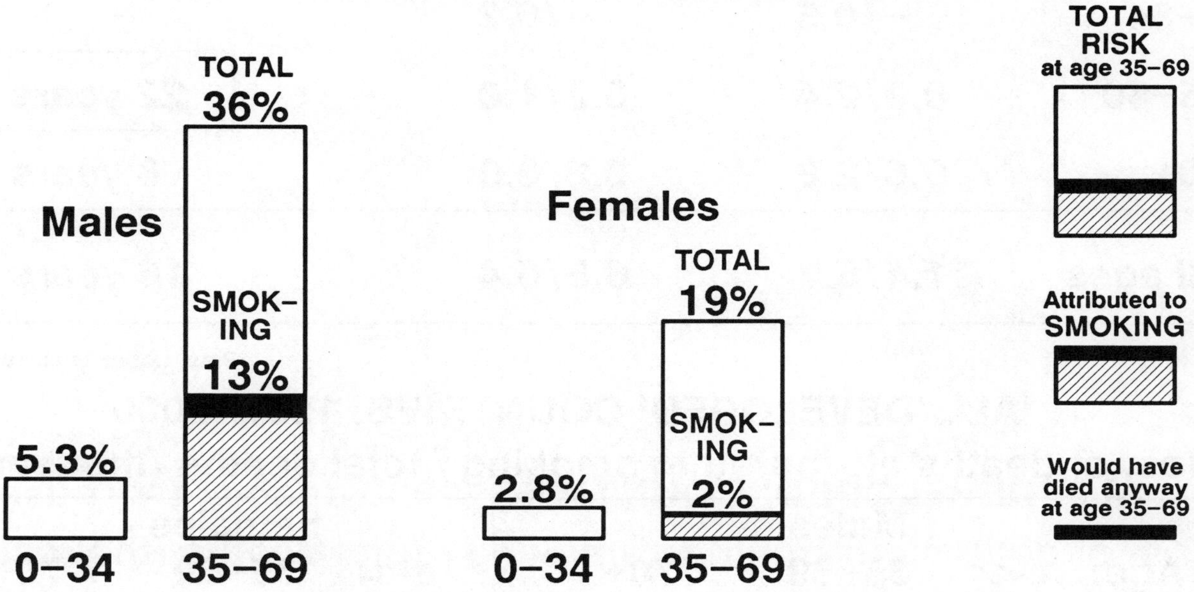

Peto, Lopez et al, 1992, 1994

ALL 'DEVELOPED' COUNTRIES: 1990 deaths, all ages
Nos. of deaths attributed to smoking / total deaths (thousands)

	Males	Females	Males + Females
All Cancer	572/1362 (42%)	112/1087 (10%)	684/2449 (28%)
All Causes	1419/5813 (24%)	396/5618 (7%)	1815/11431 (16%)

Peto, Lopez et al, 1992, 1994

ALL 'DEVELOPED' COUNTRIES: 1995 projections
Relative importance of deaths in MIDDLE age (35–69)

Age range (years)	Deaths attributed to SMOKING / total deaths (millions): Males	Females	Mean years lost PER DEATH FROM SMOKING
0–34	–/0.5	–/0.2	–
35–69	0.9/2.4	0.2/1.3	22 years
70+	0.6/2.8	0.3/3.9	8 years
All ages	1.4/5.7	0.5/5.4	16 years

Peto, Lopez et al, 1992, 1994

ALL 'DEVELOPED' COUNTRIES: 1950–2000
Nos. of deaths attributed to smoking / total deaths (thousands)

	Males			Females		
Age:	0–34	35–69	70+	0–34	35–69	70+
1955	–/878	357 / 1810 (20%)	90 / 1641 (5%)	–/652	21 / 1347 (2%)	5.2 / 2013 (0.3%)
1965	–/664	573 / 2076 (28%)	220 / 2019 (11%)	–/426	51 / 1379 (4%)	19 / 2496 (0.8%)
1975	–/605	704 / 2303 (31%)	415 / 2435 (17%)	–/340	98 / 1422 (7%)	67 / 3134 (2%)
1985	–/536	805 / 2304 (35%)	564 / 2906 (19%)	–/283	143 / 1339 (11%)	174 / 3916 (4%)
1995 (projected)	–/482	870 / 2435 (36%)	572 / 2777 (21%)	–/215	171 / 1312 (13%)	305 / 3860 (8%)
50–year total* (M=millions), mid–1950 to mid–2000:						**62 / 500M**
1950–2000, by age & sex	–/32M	33 / 109M (30%)	19 / 118M (16%)	–/19M	4.8 / 68M (7%)	5.7 / 154M (4%)

*Estimated as 10 times the sum of the five annual numbers (for 1955, 1965, 1975, 1985 & 1995)

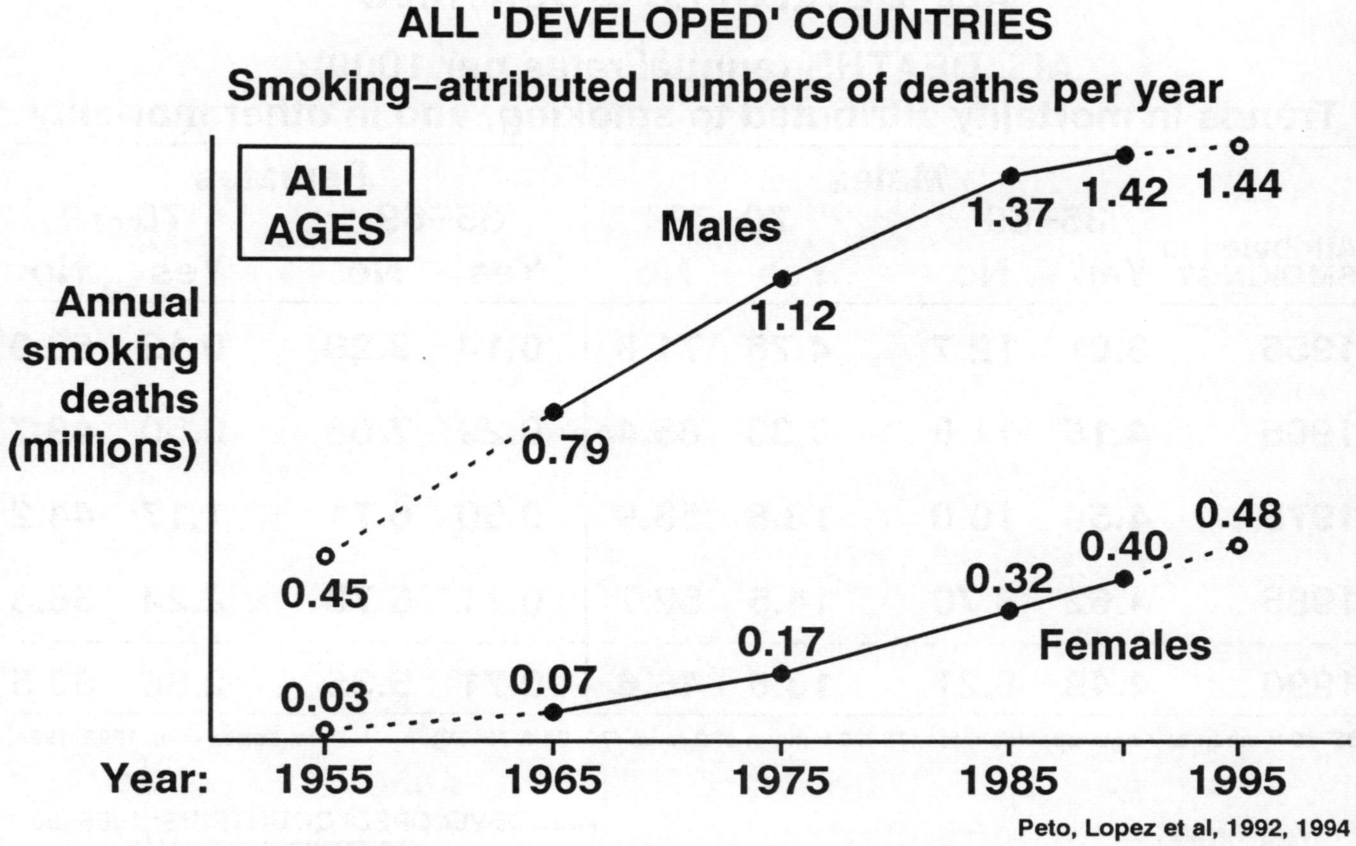
ALL 'DEVELOPED' COUNTRIES
Smoking–attributed numbers of deaths per year
ALL AGES
Annual smoking deaths (millions)
Males
0.45
0.79
1.12
1.37
1.42
1.44
Females
0.03
0.07
0.17
0.32
0.40
0.48
Year: 1955 1965 1975 1985 1995
Peto, Lopez et al, 1992, 1994

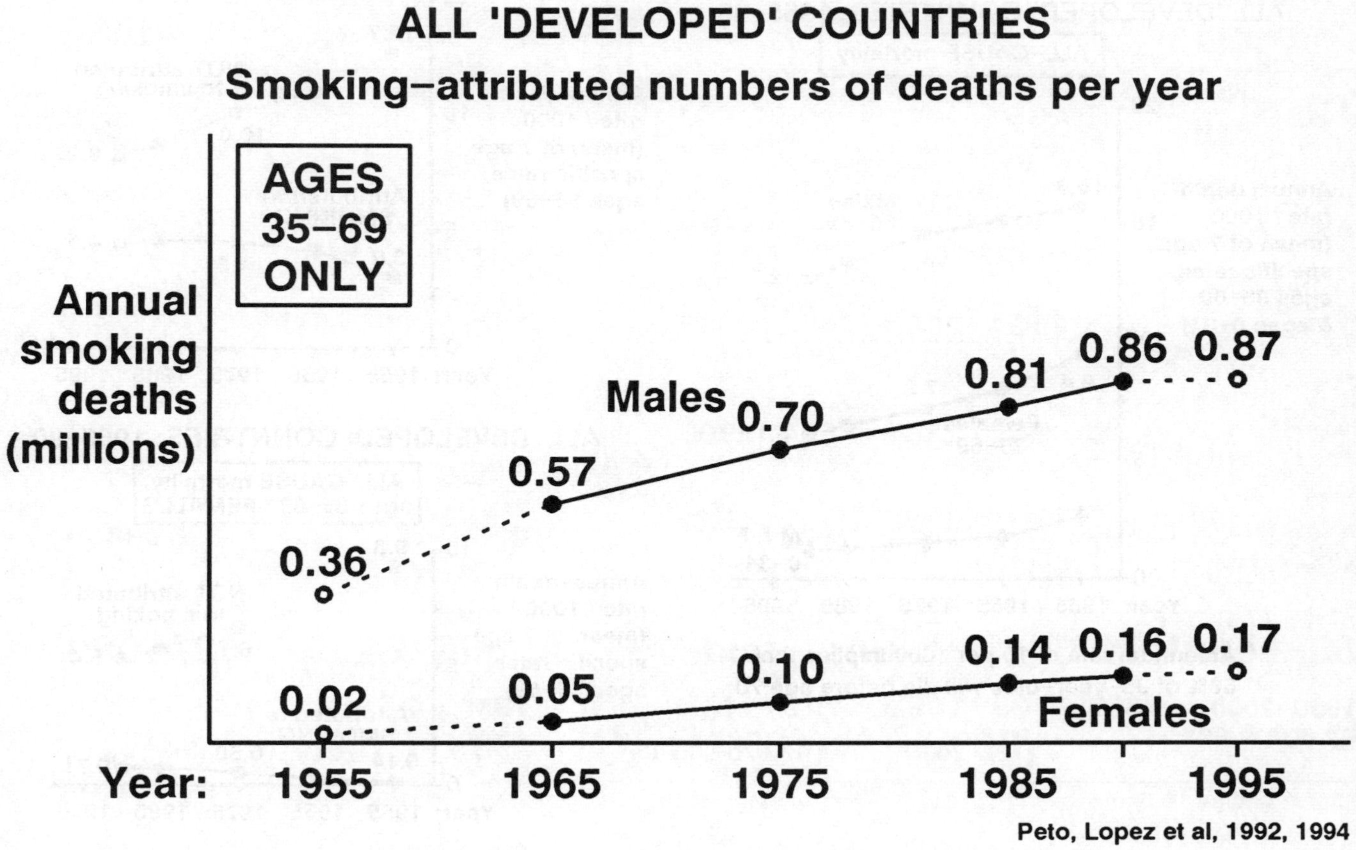
ALL 'DEVELOPED' COUNTRIES
Smoking–attributed numbers of deaths per year
AGES 35–69 ONLY
Annual smoking deaths (millions)
Males
0.36
0.57
0.70
0.81
0.86
0.87
Females
0.02
0.05
0.10
0.14
0.16
0.17
Year: 1955 1965 1975 1985 1995
Peto, Lopez et al, 1992, 1994

ALL 'DEVELOPED' COUNTRIES

ALL DEATHS (annual rates per 1000): Trends in mortality attributed to smoking, and in other mortality

	Males				Females			
	35–69		70–79		35–69		70–79	
Attributed to SMOKING?	Yes	No	Yes	No	Yes	No	Yes	No
1955	3.01	12.7	4.76	71.8	0.14	9.29	0.19	56.0
1965	4.15	11.0	9.33	65.4	0.29	7.68	0.50	49.7
1975	4.50	10.0	13.8	58.9	0.50	6.71	1.17	44.2
1985	4.62	8.70	14.5	52.7	0.71	5.78	2.24	38.3
1990	4.49	8.21	13.6	46.6	0.71	5.35	2.86	33.5

35–69 = mean of 7 age–specific rates; 70–79 = mean of 2 rates (70–74 & 75–79) Peto, Lopez et al, 1992, 1994

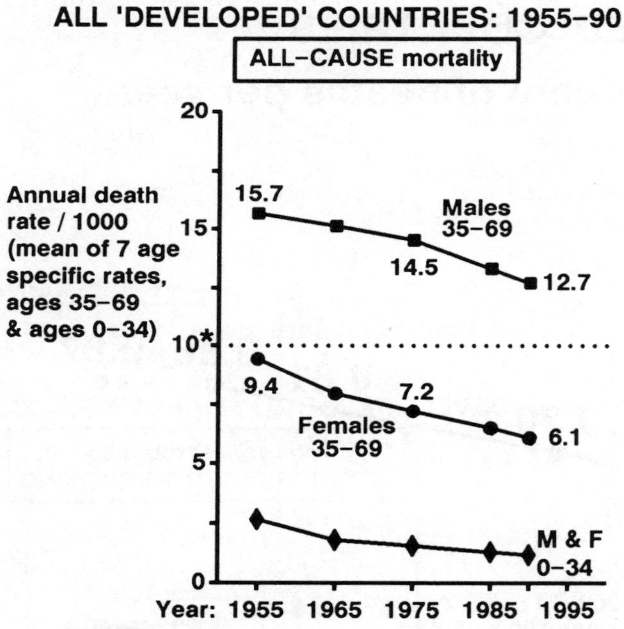

* An annual rate of 10 per 1000 implies that 30% of 35–year–olds will die before age 70

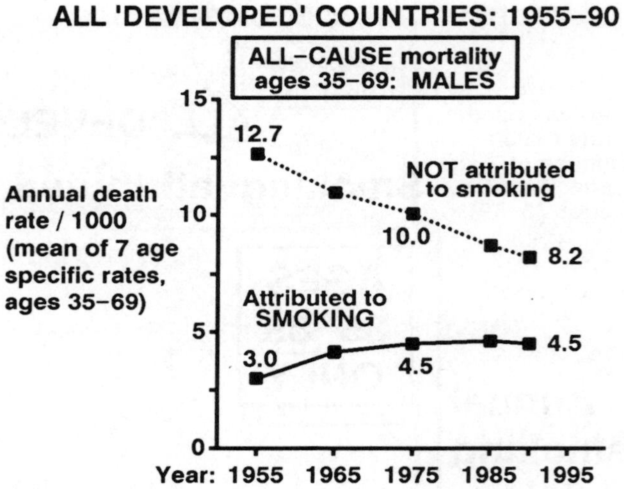

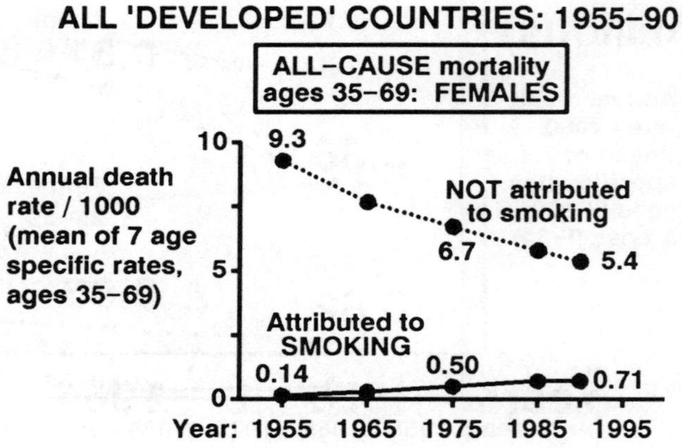

ALL 'DEVELOPED' COUNTRIES

ALL CANCER DEATHS (annual rates per 1000): Trends in mortality attributed to smoking, and in other mortality

	Males				Females			
	35–69		70–79		35–69		70–79	
Attributed to SMOKING?	Yes	No	Yes	No	Yes	No	Yes	No
1955	...	...	...	...	...	...	...	...
1965	1.39	2.18	3.16	10.0	0.07	2.29	0.10	7.50
1975	1.61	2.05	4.89	9.62	0.14	2.12	0.26	7.02
1985	1.84	1.99	5.82	9.59	0.23	1.98	0.62	6.83
1990	1.91	2.01	5.96	9.60	0.25	1.94	0.89	6.72

35–69 = mean of 7 age-specific rates; 70–79 = mean of 2 rates (70–74 & 75–79) Peto, Lopez et al, 1992, 1994

ALL 'DEVELOPED' COUNTRIES: 1965–90

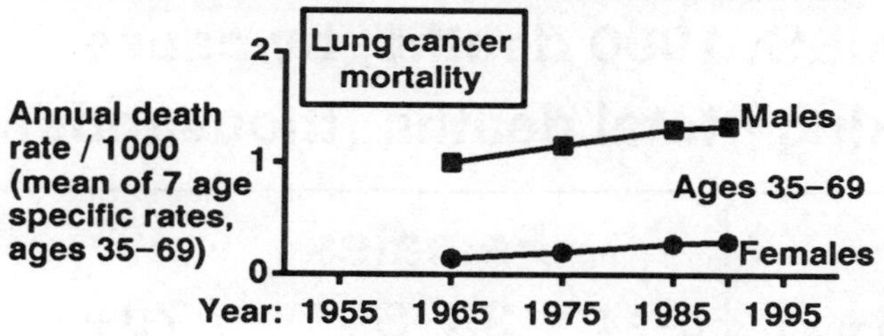

ALL 'DEVELOPED' COUNTRIES: 1965–90

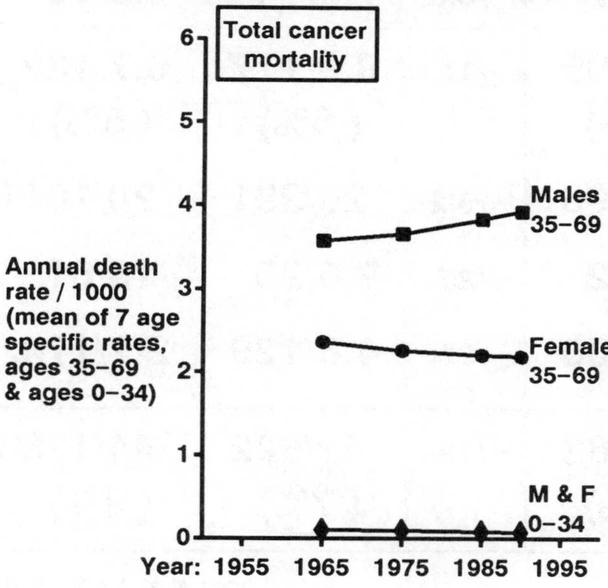

ALL 'DEVELOPED' COUNTRIES: 1965–90

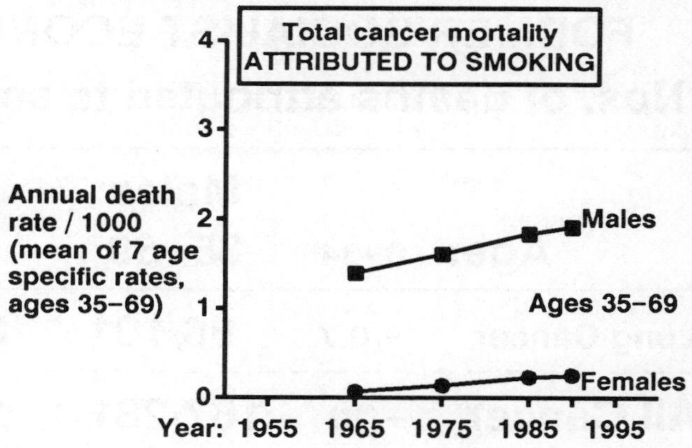

ALL 'DEVELOPED' COUNTRIES: 1965–90

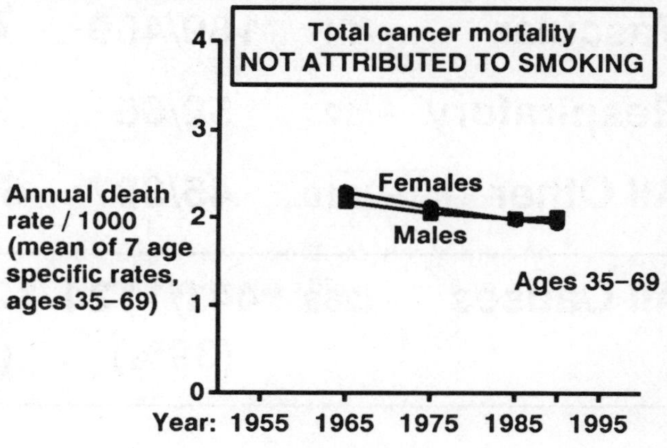

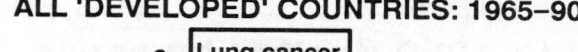

¶FORMER SOCIALIST ECONOMIES: 1990
Relative importance of deaths in MIDDLE age (35–69)

Age range (years)	Deaths attributed to SMOKING / total deaths (thousands) Males	Females	Mean years lost PER DEATH FROM SMOKING
0–34	–/268	–/134	–
35–69	441/1124	42/622	20 years
70+	126/763	44/1369	8 years
All ages	567/2154	87/2125	17 years

Peto, Lopez et al, 1992, 1994

FORMER SOCIALIST ECONOMIES: 1990 deaths, by cause
Nos. of deaths attributed to smoking / total deaths (thousands)

	Males			Females		
Age:	0–34	35–69	70+	0–34	35–69	70+
Lung Cancer	–/0.7	96/101	24/27	–/0.3	7.4/14	4.9/10
All Cancer	–/12	157/281 (56%)	36/105 (35%)	–/11	9.9/177 (6%)	6.7/122 (5%)
Vascular	–/14	189/469	48/496	–/6.2	20/291	20/1011
Respiratory	–/32	50/66	35/62	–/25	7.5/25	15/61
All Other	–/210	45/307	6.7/100	–/91	4.6/129	2.7/174
All Causes	–/268	441/1124 (39%)	126/763 (17%)	–/134	42/622 (7%)	44/1369 (3%)

Peto, Lopez et al, 1992, 1994

FORMER SOCIALIST ECONOMIES: 1990
RISKS OF DYING AT AGES 0–34 and 35–69
(Probability that someone entering an age range would die during it, if the death rates in 1990 were to persist unchanged)

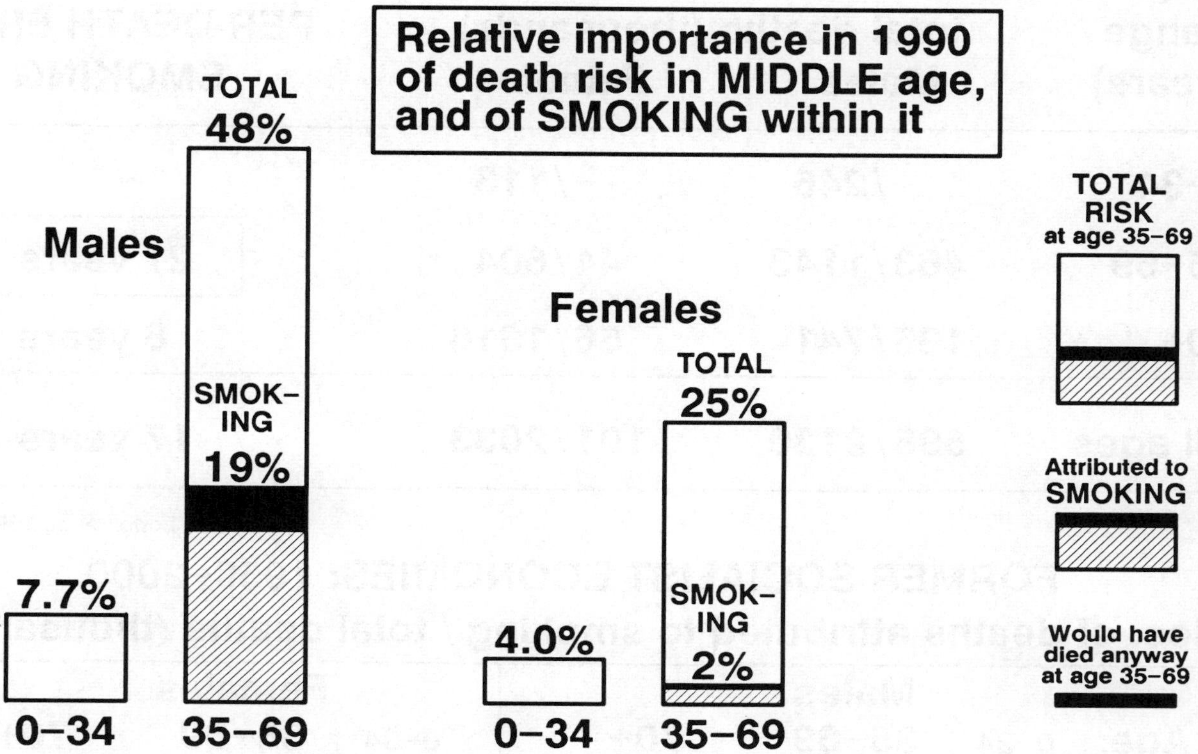

Peto, Lopez et al, 1992, 1994

FORMER SOCIALIST ECONOMIES: 1990 deaths, all ages
Nos. of deaths attributed to smoking / total deaths (thousands)

	Males	Females	Males + Females
All Cancer	193/399 (48%)	17/310 (5%)	210/709 (30%)
All Causes	567/2154 (26%)	87/2125 (4%)	654/4279 (15%)

Peto, Lopez et al, 1992, 1994

FORMER SOCIALIST ECONOMIES: 1995 projections
Relative importance of deaths in MIDDLE age (35–69)

Age range (years)	Deaths attributed to SMOKING / total deaths (thousands) Males	Females	Mean years lost PER DEATH FROM SMOKING
0–34	–/246	–/113	–
35–69	463/1143	44/604	21 years
70+	135/741	56/1316	8 years
All ages	598/2130	101/2033	17 years

Peto, Lopez et al, 1992, 1994

FORMER SOCIALIST ECONOMIES: 1950–2000
Nos. of deaths attributed to smoking / total deaths (thousands)

Age:	Males 0–34	Males 35–69	Males 70+	Females 0–34	Females 35–69	Females 70+
1955	–/395	104/524 (20%)	24/346 (7%)	–/298	11/453 (3%)	2.6/575 (0.5%)
1965	–/282	169/577 (29%)	48/425 (11%)	–/181	18/452 (4%)	4.8/661 (0.7%)
1975	–/300	256/826 (31%)	94/614 (15%)	–/171	28/548 (5%)	18/981 (2%)
1985	–/301	379/980 (39%)	138/824 (17%)	–/164	36/578 (6%)	37/1388 (3%)
1995 (projected)	–/246	463/1143 (41%)	135/741 (18%)	–/113	44/604 (7%)	56/1316 (4%)
50–year total* (M=millions), mid–1950 to mid–2000:						21/170M
1950–2000, by age & sex	–/15M	14/41M (34%)	4.4/30M (15%)	–/9.3M	1.4/26M (5%)	1.2/49M (2%)

*Estimated as 10 times the sum of the five annual numbers (for 1955, 1965, 1975, 1985 & 1995)

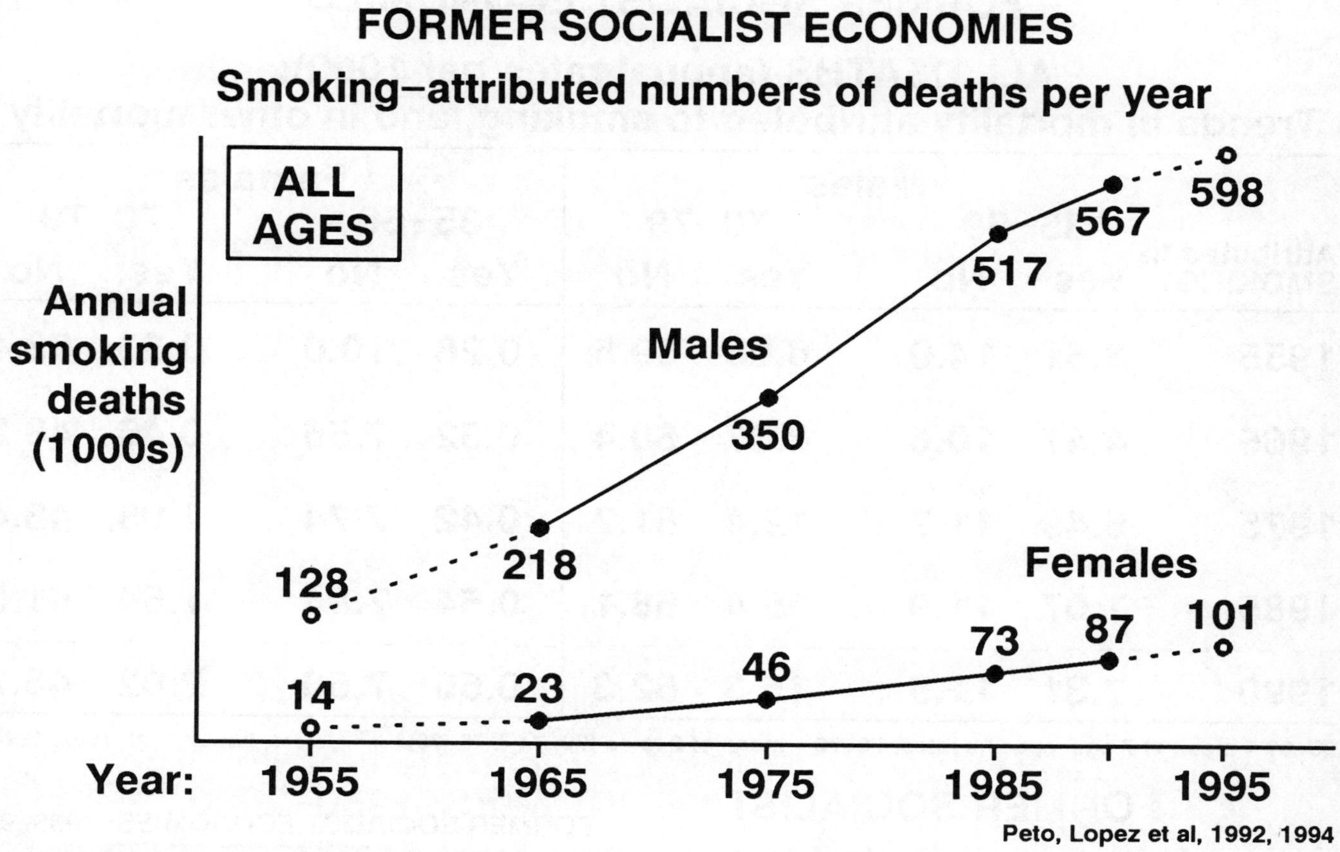
FORMER SOCIALIST ECONOMIES
Smoking–attributed numbers of deaths per year
ALL AGES
Annual smoking deaths (1000s)
Males
128
218
350
517
567
598
Females
14
23
46
73
87
101
Year:
1955
1965
1975
1985
1995
Peto, Lopez et al, 1992, 1994

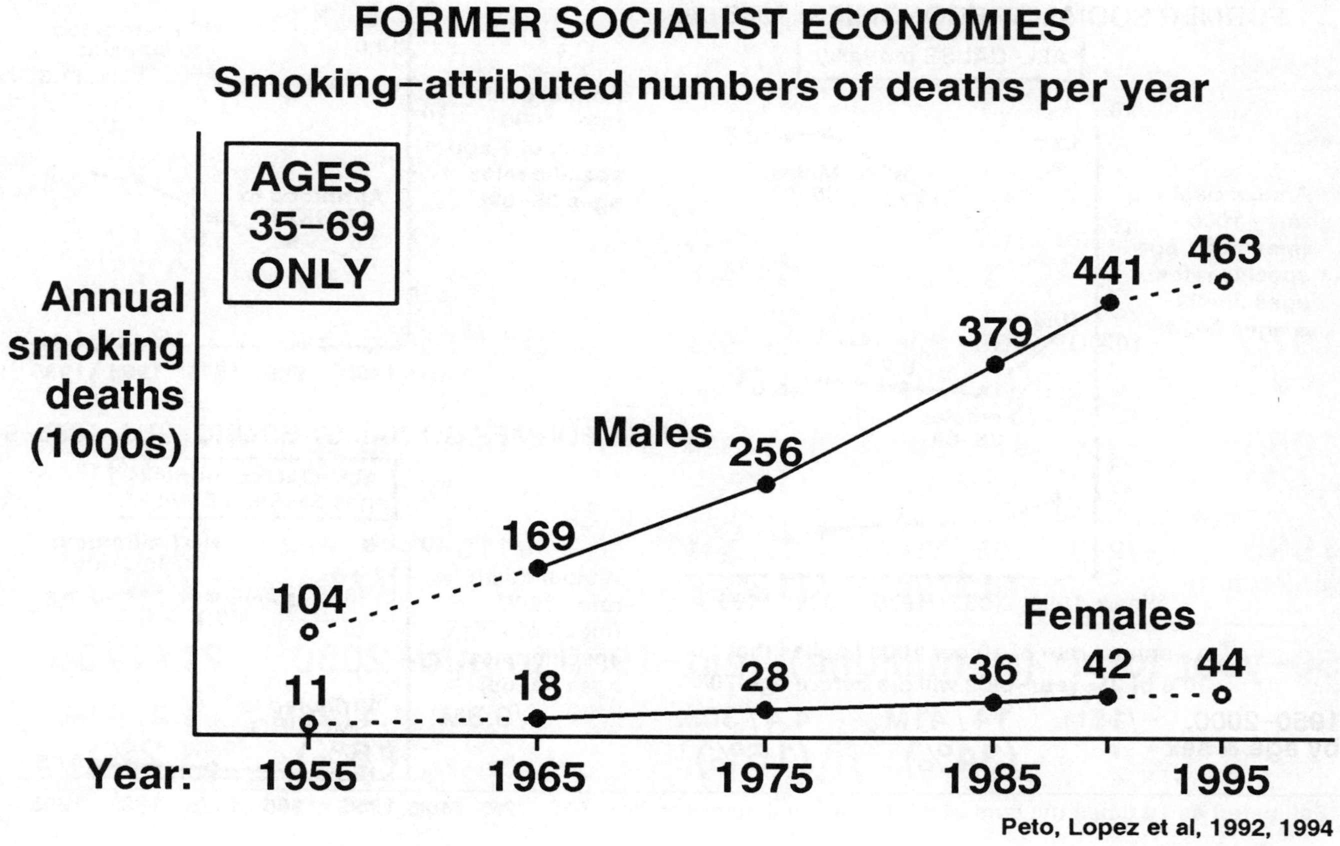
FORMER SOCIALIST ECONOMIES
Smoking–attributed numbers of deaths per year
AGES 35–69 ONLY
Annual smoking deaths (1000s)
Males
104
169
256
379
441
463
Females
11
18
28
36
42
44
Year:
1955
1965
1975
1985
1995
Peto, Lopez et al, 1992, 1994

FORMER SOCIALIST ECONOMIES

ALL DEATHS (annual rates per 1000): Trends in mortality attributed to smoking, and in other mortality

	Males				Females			
	35–69		70–79		35–69		70–79	
Attributed to SMOKING?	Yes	No	Yes	No	Yes	No	Yes	No
1955	3.61	14.0	6.05	69.5	0.26	10.0	0.33	53.4
1965	4.47	10.6	8.87	60.4	0.32	7.56	0.46	48.2
1975	5.49	11.7	12.4	61.7	0.42	7.74	1.05	48.4
1985	7.07	11.9	15.4	68.1	0.54	7.94	1.64	51.3
1990	7.31	11.5	15.3	62.3	0.55	7.50	2.02	46.7

35–69 = mean of 7 age-specific rates; 70–79 = mean of 2 rates (70–74 & 75–79) Peto, Lopez et al, 1992, 1994

FORMER SOCIALIST ECONOMIES: 1955–90

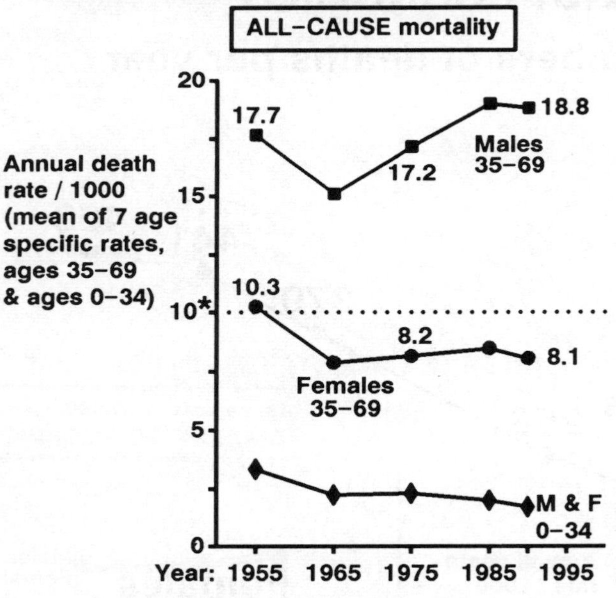

* An annual rate of 10 per 1000 implies that 30% of 35-year-olds will die before age 70

FORMER SOCIALIST ECONOMIES: 1955–90

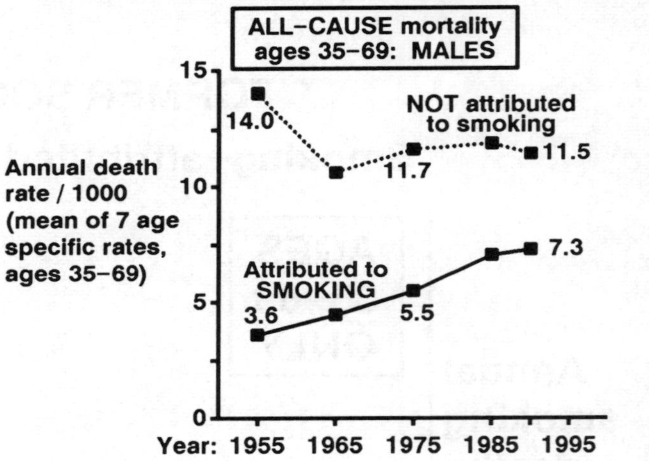

FORMER SOCIALIST ECONOMIES: 1955–90

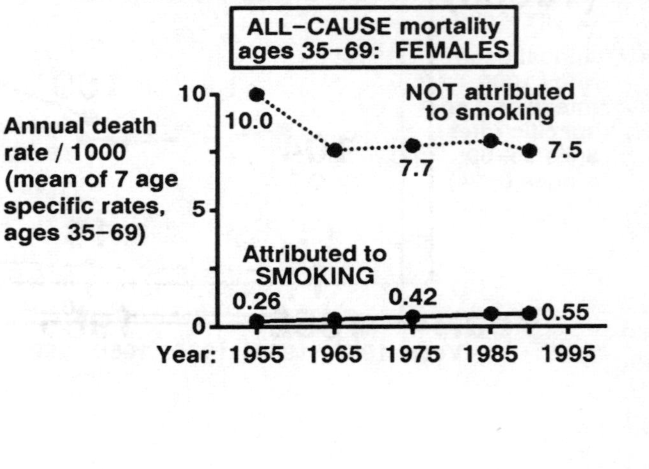

FORMER SOCIALIST ECONOMIES

ALL CANCER DEATHS (annual rates per 1000): Trends in mortality attributed to smoking, and in other mortality

	Males				Females			
	35–69		70–79		35–69		70–79	
Attributed to SMOKING?	Yes	No	Yes	No	Yes	No	Yes	No
1955	...	...	...	...	...	...	...	...
1965	1.54	2.37	2.71	8.82	0.07	2.27	0.07	6.18
1975	1.78	2.22	3.56	8.15	0.09	2.15	0.15	5.83
1985	2.34	2.15	4.61	8.72	0.11	2.08	0.27	6.08
1990	2.65	2.18	5.23	8.99	0.13	2.13	0.40	6.40

35–69 = mean of 7 age–specific rates; 70–79 = mean of 2 rates (70–74 & 75–79) Peto, Lopez et al, 1992, 1994

FORMER SOCIALIST ECONOMIES: 1965–90

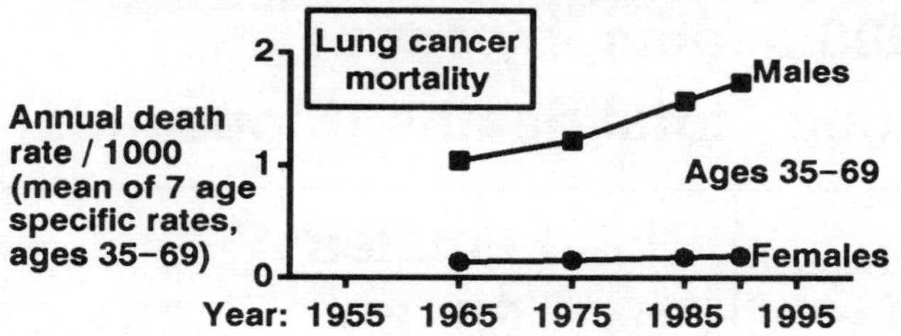

FORMER SOCIALIST ECONOMIES: 1965–90

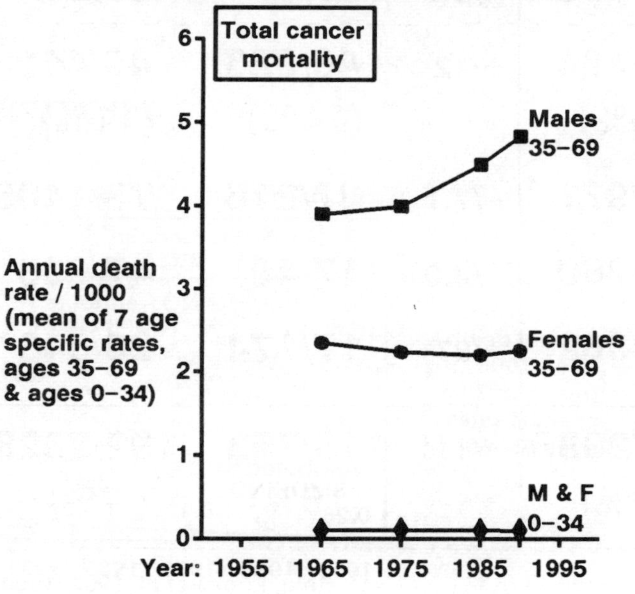

FORMER SOCIALIST ECONOMIES: 1965–90

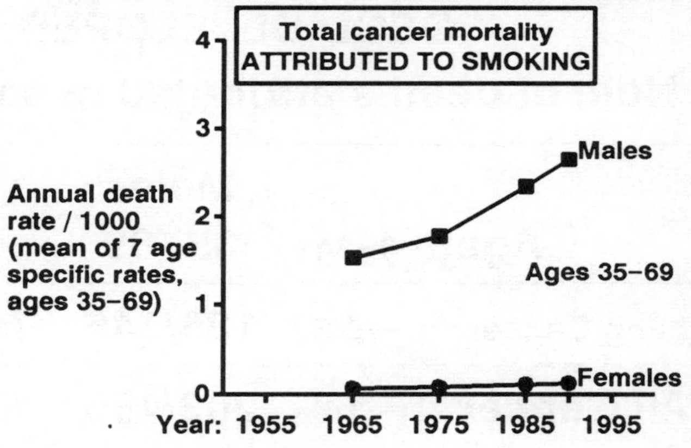

FORMER SOCIALIST ECONOMIES: 1965–90

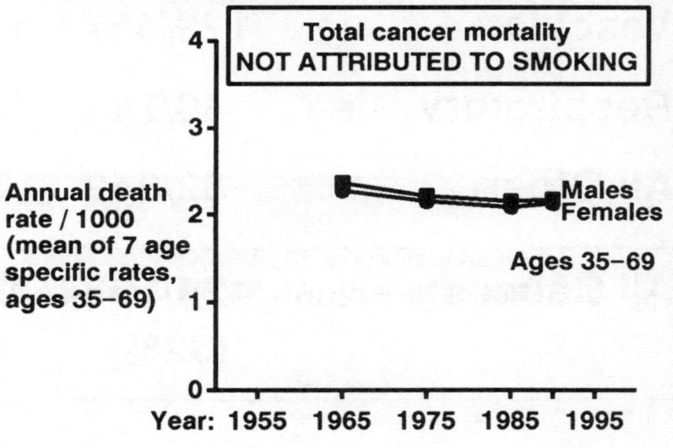

OECD DEVELOPED: 1990
Relative importance of deaths in MIDDLE age (35–69)

Age range (years)	Deaths attributed to SMOKING / total deaths (thousands) Males	Females	Mean years lost PER DEATH FROM SMOKING
0–34	–/236	–/111	–
35–69	424/1334	118/753	22 years
70+	428/2088	192/2628	8 years
All ages	851/3659	309/3493	14 years

Peto, Lopez et al, 1992, 1994

OECD DEVELOPED: 1990 deaths, by cause
Nos. of deaths attributed to smoking / total deaths (thousands)

	Males			Females		
Age:	0–34	35–69	70+	0–34	35–69	70+
Lung Cancer	–/0.6	135/146	117/129	–/0.3	37/50	37/51
All Cancer	–/14	203/455 (45%)	176/494 (36%)	–/12	46/323 (14%)	49/441 (11%)
Vascular	–/12	129/457	116/971	–/7.1	37/216	73/1406
Respiratory	–/5.9	40/74	103/260	–/4.0	17/40	47/238
All Other	–/204	52/349	33/362	–/87	17/174	23/543
All Causes	–/236	424/1334 (32%)	428/2088 (20%)	–/111	118/753 (16%)	192/2628 (7%)

Peto, Lopez et al, 1992, 1994

OECD DEVELOPED: 1990
RISKS OF DYING AT AGES 0–34 and 35–69

(Probability that someone entering an age range would die during it, if the death rates in 1990 were to persist unchanged)

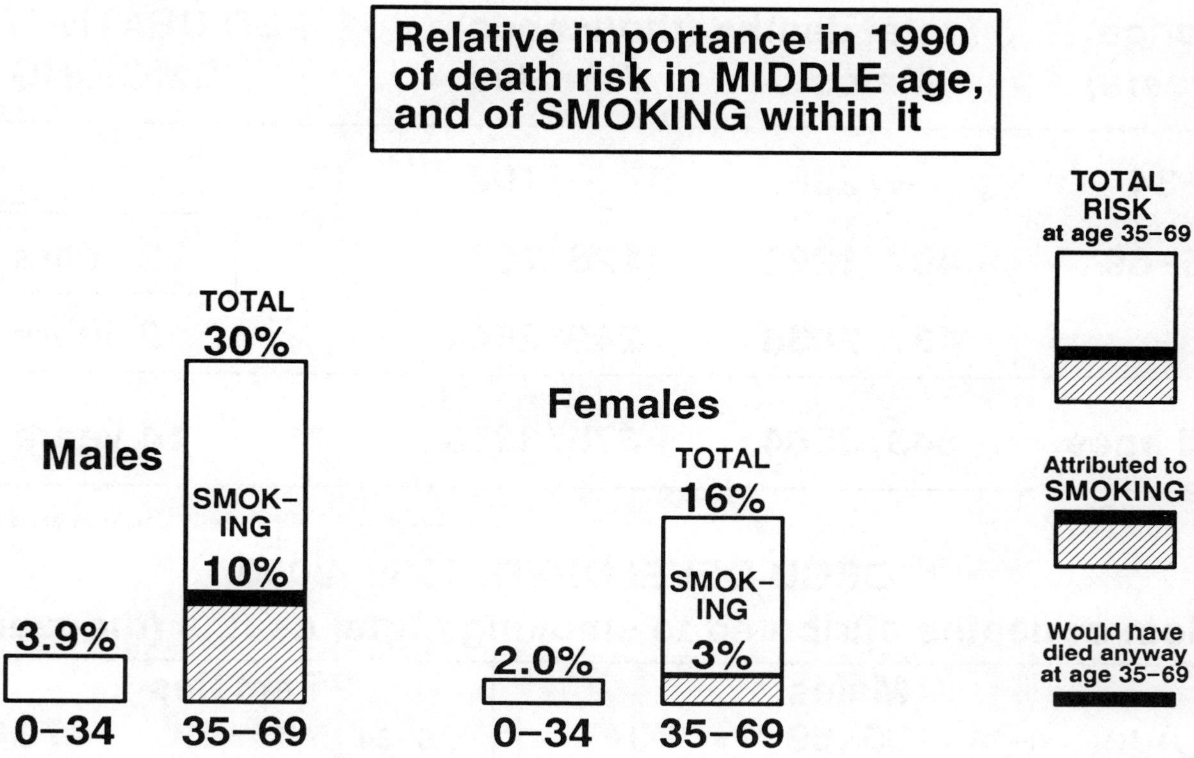

Peto, Lopez et al, 1992, 1994

OECD DEVELOPED: 1990 deaths, all ages
Nos. of deaths attributed to smoking / total deaths (thousands)

	Males	Females	Males + Females
All Cancer	379/963 (39%)	95/777 (12%)	474/1740 (27%)
All Causes	851/3659 (23%)	309/3493 (9%)	1161/7151 (16%)

Peto, Lopez et al, 1992, 1994

OECD DEVELOPED: 1995 projections
Relative importance of deaths in MIDDLE age (35–69)

Age range (years)	Deaths attributed to SMOKING / total deaths (thousands) Males	Females	Mean years lost PER DEATH FROM SMOKING
0–34	–/236	–/102	–
35–69	407/1292	126/707	22 years
70+	437/2036	249/2544	8 years
All ages	843/3564	375/3353	14 years

Peto, Lopez et al, 1992, 1994

OECD DEVELOPED: 1950–2000
Nos. of deaths attributed to smoking / total deaths (thousands)

	Males			Females		
Age:	0–34	35–69	70+	0–34	35–69	70+
1955	–/483	253/1285 (20%)	66/1295 (5%)	–/354	9.4/893 (1%)	2.6/1438 (0.2%)
1965	–/382	403/1499 (27%)	172/1594 (11%)	–/246	33/927 (4%)	14/1835 (0.8%)
1975	–/305	448/1477 (30%)	321/1821 (18%)	–/170	70/873 (8%)	49/2153 (2%)
1985	–/235	427/1324 (32%)	426/2082 (20%)	–/119	107/762 (14%)	137/2528 (5%)
1995 (projected)	–/236	407/1292 (31%)	437/2036 (21%)	–/102	126/707 (18%)	249/2544 (10%)
50–year total* (M=millions), mid–1950 to mid–2000:						42/330M
1950–2000, by age & sex	–/16M	19/69M (28%)	14/88M (16%)	–/9.9M	3.5/42M (8%)	4.5/105M (4%)

*Estimated as 10 times the sum of the five annual numbers (for 1955, 1965, 1975, 1985 & 1995)

OECD DEVELOPED

Smoking–attributed numbers of deaths per year

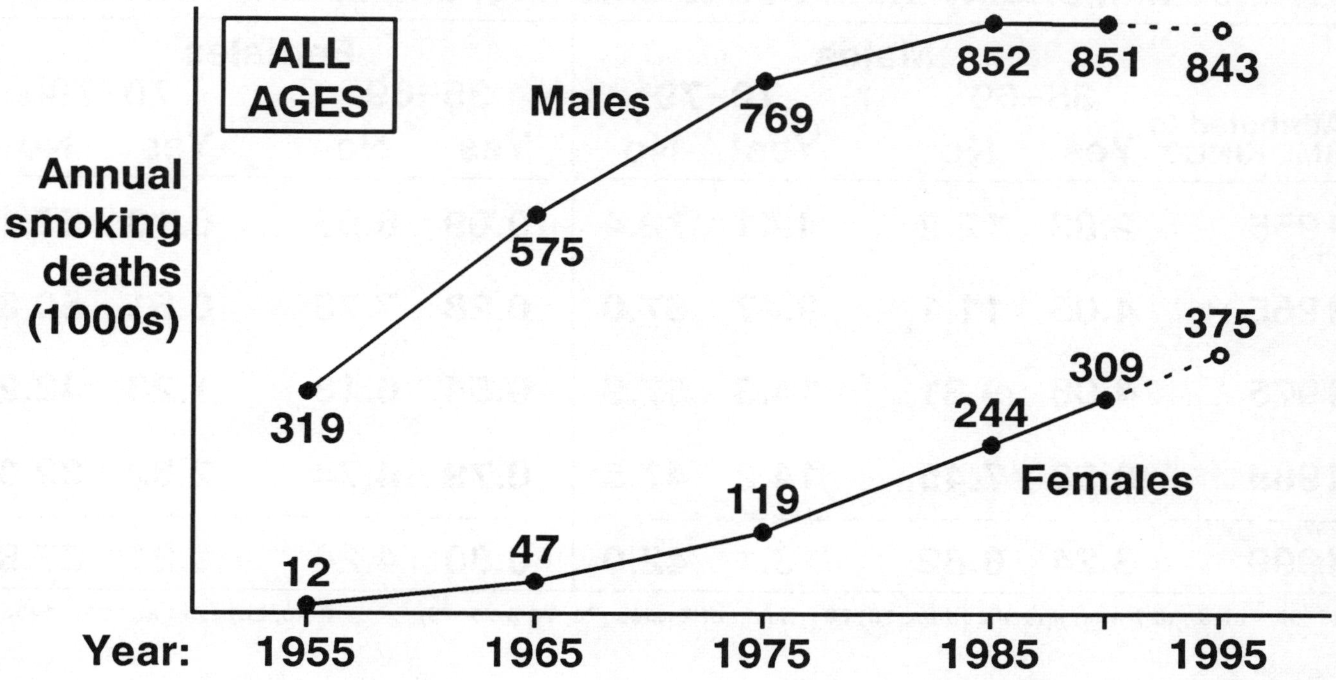

Peto, Lopez et al, 1992, 1994

OECD DEVELOPED

Smoking–attributed numbers of deaths per year

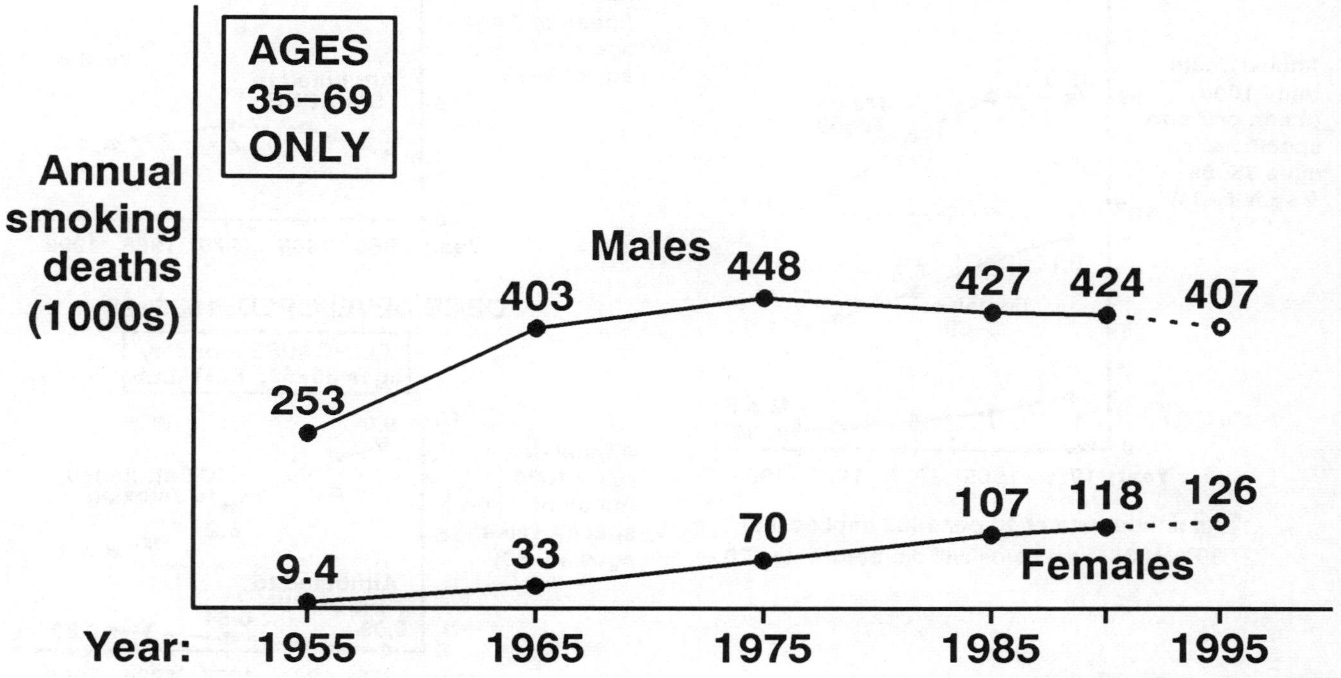

Peto, Lopez et al, 1992, 1994

OECD DEVELOPED

ALL DEATHS (annual rates per 1000): Trends in mortality attributed to smoking, and in other mortality

	Males 35–69		Males 70–79		Females 35–69		Females 70–79	
Attributed to SMOKING?	Yes	No	Yes	No	Yes	No	Yes	No
1955	2.83	12.2	4.41	72.4	0.09	8.98	0.13	57.1
1965	4.03	11.1	9.47	67.0	0.28	7.73	0.51	50.3
1975	4.08	9.31	14.3	57.9	0.54	6.18	1.23	42.2
1985	3.58	7.45	14.2	47.5	0.79	4.74	2.52	32.3
1990	3.24	6.82	13.1	42.0	0.80	4.24	3.21	27.8

35–69 = mean of 7 age-specific rates; 70–79 = mean of 2 rates (70–74 & 75–79)   Peto, Lopez et al, 1992, 1994

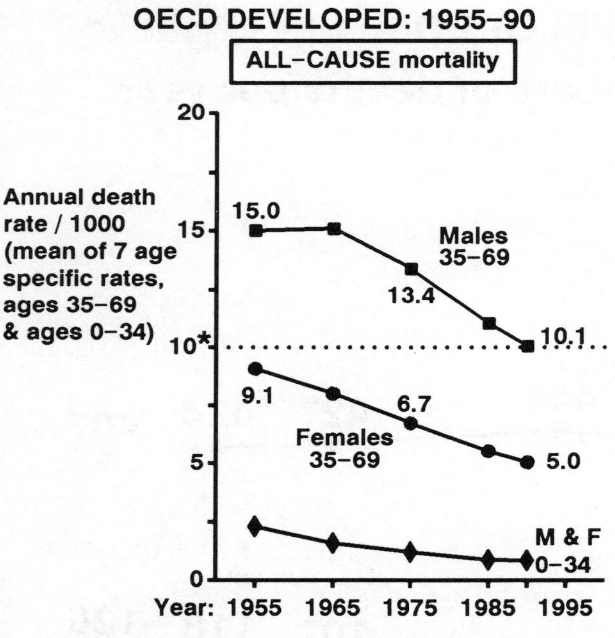

* An annual rate of 10 per 1000 implies that 30% of 35-year-olds will die before age 70

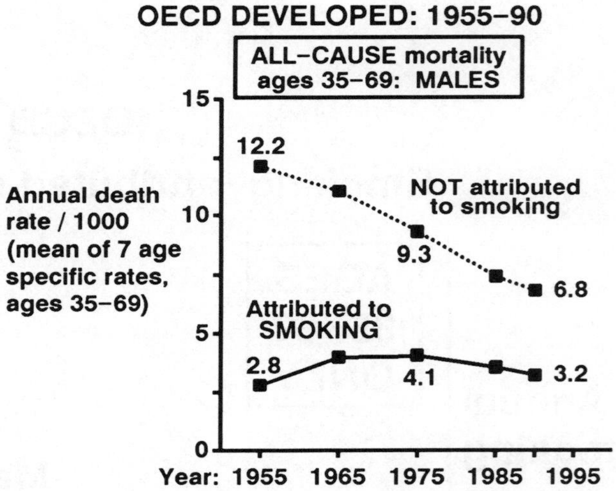

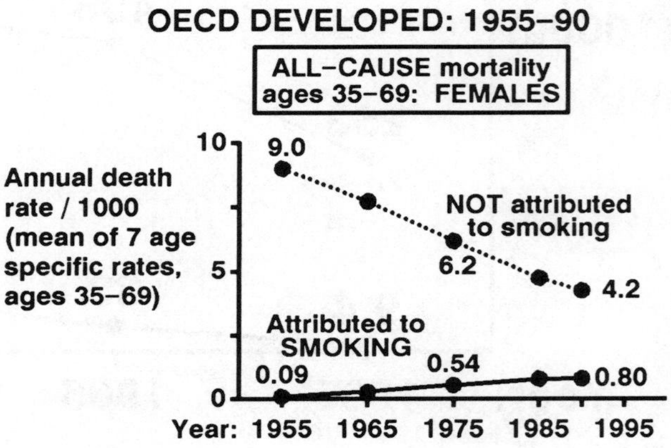

OECD DEVELOPED

ALL CANCER DEATHS (annual rates per 1000): Trends in mortality attributed to smoking, and in other mortality

	Males				Females			
	35–69		70–79		35–69		70–79	
Attributed to SMOKING?	Yes	No	Yes	No	Yes	No	Yes	No
1955	0.87	2.19	1.48	10.5	0.02	2.39	0.02	8.18
1965	1.34	2.11	3.30	10.4	0.07	2.30	0.11	8.05
1975	1.54	1.98	5.35	10.1	0.16	2.10	0.31	7.57
1985	1.62	1.92	6.22	9.88	0.28	1.92	0.78	7.17
1990	1.58	1.94	6.19	9.79	0.31	1.84	1.10	6.87

35–69 = mean of 7 age-specific rates; 70–79 = mean of 2 rates (70–74 & 75–79) Peto, Lopez et al, 1992, 1994

OECD DEVELOPED: 1955–90

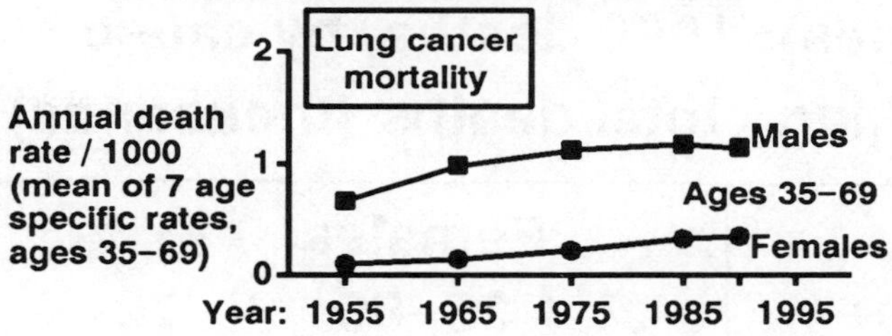

OECD DEVELOPED: 1955–90

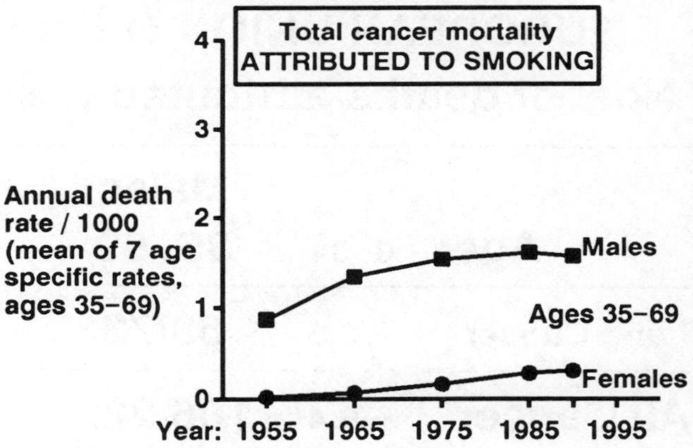

OECD DEVELOPED: 1955–90

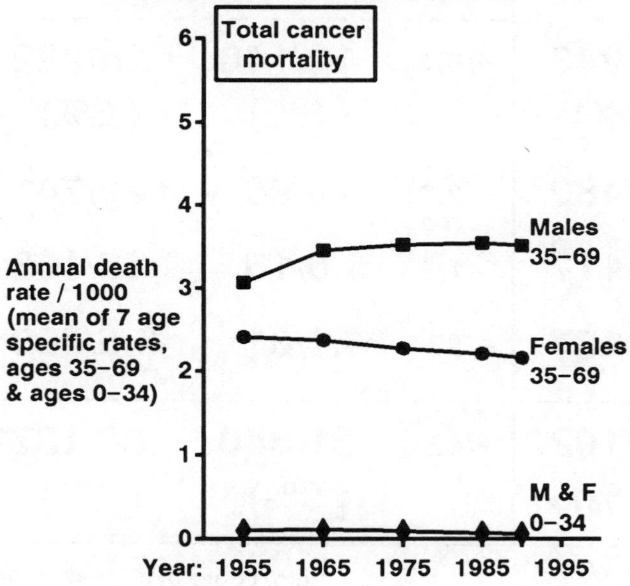

OECD DEVELOPED: 1955–90

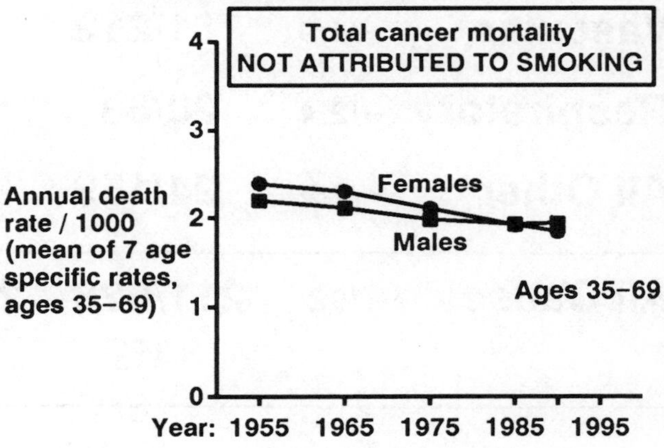

EUROPEAN UNION (12 countries): 1990
Relative importance of deaths in MIDDLE age (35–69)

Age range (years)	Deaths attributed to SMOKING / total deaths (thousands) Males	Females	Mean years lost PER DEATH FROM SMOKING
0–34	–/92	–/42	–
35–69	211/628	31/340	21 years
70+	211/1027	58/1371	8 years
All ages	423/1747	90/1753	14 years

Peto, Lopez et al, 1992, 1994

EUROPEAN UNION (12 countries): 1990 deaths, by cause
Nos. of deaths attributed to smoking / total deaths (thousands)

	Males			Females		
Age:	0–34	35–69	70+	0–34	35–69	70+
Lung Cancer	–/0.3	68/73	54/60	–/0.1	9.2/15	9.8/17
All Cancer	–/6.4	106/225 (47%)	85/243 (35%)	–/5.4	12/148 (8%)	14/222 (6%)
Vascular	–/4.9	61/212	57/480	–/2.7	10/96	22/741
Respiratory	–/2.4	20/33	53/117	–/1.5	5.0/15	15/108
All Other	–/78	24/159	17/187	–/33	4.1/81	6.6/300
All Causes	–/92	211/628 (34%)	211/1027 (21%)	–/42	31/340 (9%)	58/1371 (4%)

Peto, Lopez et al, 1992, 1994

EUROPEAN UNION (12 countries): 1990
RISKS OF DYING AT AGES 0–34 and 35–69

(Probability that someone entering an age range would die during it, if the death rates in 1990 were to persist unchanged)

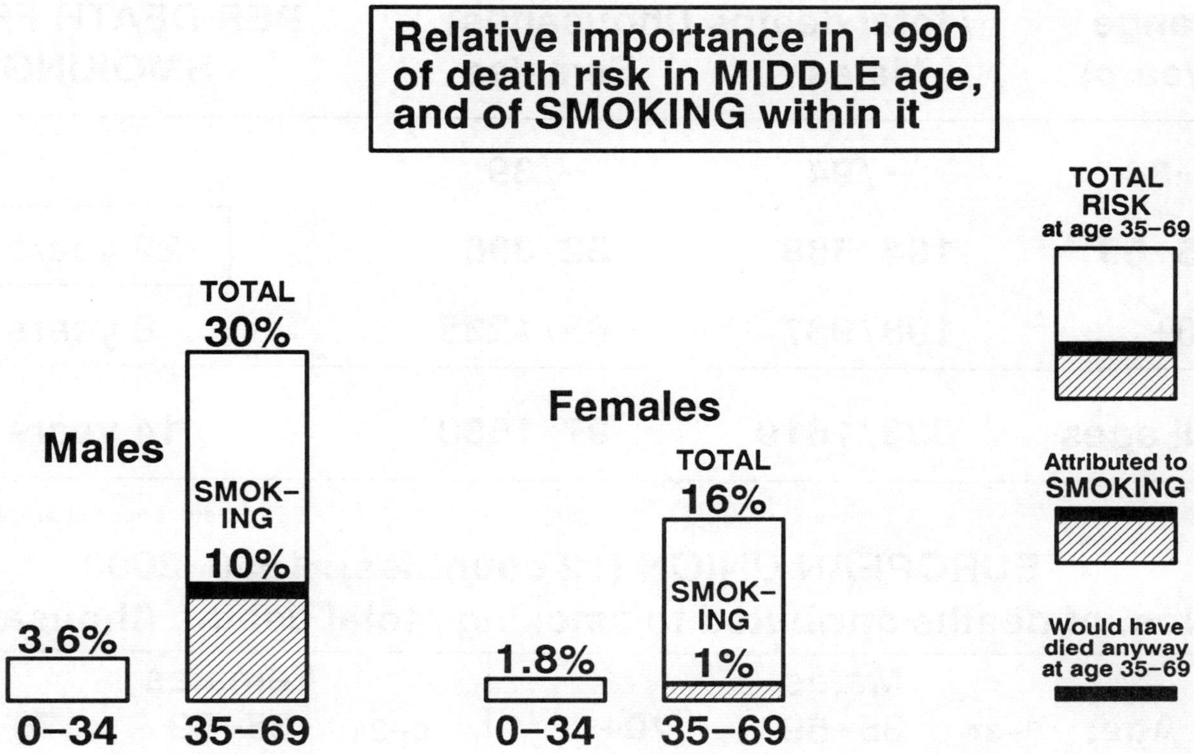

Peto, Lopez et al, 1992, 1994

EUROPEAN UNION (12 countries): 1990 deaths, all ages
Nos. of deaths attributed to smoking / total deaths (thousands)

	Males	Females	Males + Females
All Cancer	191/474 (40%)	26/376 (7%)	217/850 (26%)
All Causes	423/1747 (24%)	90/1753 (5%)	513/3500 (15%)

Peto, Lopez et al, 1992, 1994

EUROPEAN UNION (12 countries): 1995 projections
Relative importance of deaths in MIDDLE age (35–69)

Age range (years)	Deaths attributed to SMOKING / total deaths (thousands) Males	Females	Mean years lost PER DEATH FROM SMOKING
0–34	–/94	–/39	–
35–69	194/588	32/306	22 years
70+	198/937	65/1235	8 years
All ages	393/1619	97/1580	14 years

Peto, Lopez et al, 1992, 1994

EUROPEAN UNION (12 countries): 1950–2000
Nos. of deaths attributed to smoking / total deaths (thousands)

	Males			Females		
Age:	0–34	35–69	70+	0–34	35–69	70+
1955	–/223	143/614 (23%)	41/714 (6%)	–/165	7.5/461 (2%)	2.4/842 (0.3%)
1965	–/175	223/736 (30%)	101/830 (12%)	–/114	17/472 (4%)	11/1041 (1%)
1975	–/127	233/723 (32%)	190/978 (19%)	–/74	22/432 (5%)	25/1237 (2%)
1985	–/91	213/616 (35%)	229/1074 (21%)	–/47	28/341 (8%)	48/1371 (4%)
1995 (projected)	–/94	194/588 (33%)	198/937 (21%)	–/39	32/306 (10%)	65/1235 (5%)
50-year total* (M=millions), mid-1950 to mid-2000: 20/167M						
1950–2000, by age & sex	–/7.1M	10/33M (30%)	7.6/45M (17%)	–/4.4M	1.1/20M (6%)	1.5/57M (3%)

*Estimated as 10 times the sum of the five annual numbers (for 1955, 1965, 1975, 1985 & 1995)

EUROPEAN UNION (12 countries)

Smoking–attributed numbers of deaths per year

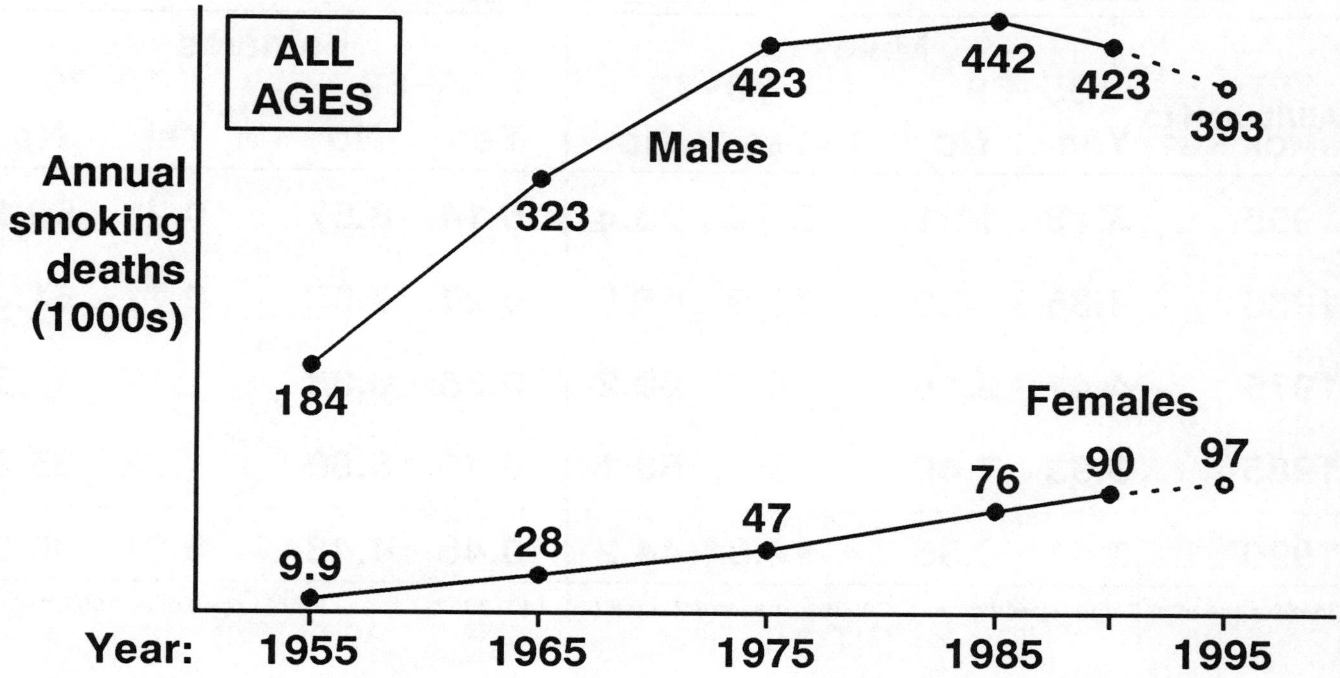

Peto, Lopez et al, 1992, 1994

EUROPEAN UNION (12 countries)

Smoking–attributed numbers of deaths per year

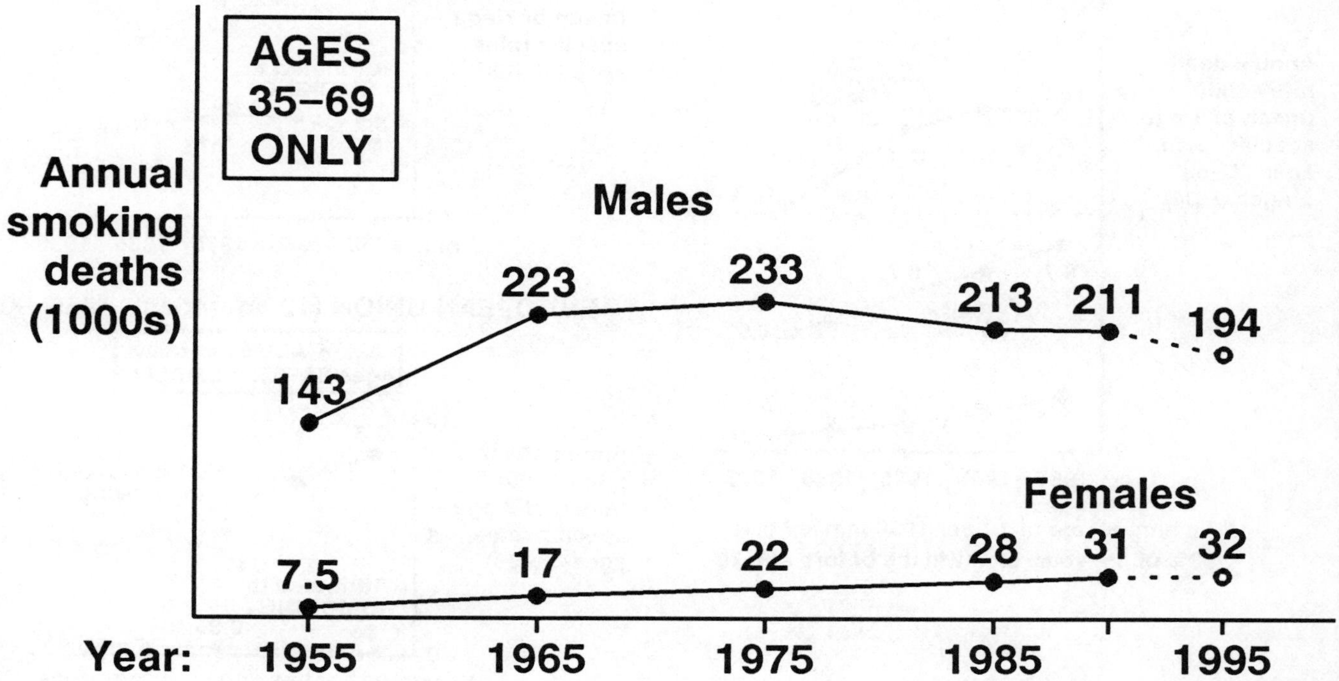

Peto, Lopez et al, 1992, 1994

EUROPEAN UNION (12 countries)
ALL DEATHS (annual rates per 1000):
Trends in mortality attributed to smoking, and in other mortality

	Males				Females			
	35–69		70–79		35–69		70–79	
Attributed to SMOKING?	Yes	No	Yes	No	Yes	No	Yes	No
1955	3.16	11.1	5.16	73.4	0.14	8.57	0.21	59.1
1965	4.36	10.2	10.9	66.5	0.27	7.39	0.71	51.8
1975	4.41	9.16	16.6	60.2	0.35	6.38	1.12	45.5
1985	3.93	7.49	15.7	50.1	0.46	5.00	1.72	35.3
1990	3.51	6.86	14.0	44.2	0.46	4.48	2.01	30.5

35–69 = mean of 7 age-specific rates; 70–79 = mean of 2 rates (70–74 & 75–79) Peto, Lopez et al, 1992, 1994

EUROPEAN UNION (12 countries): 1955–90

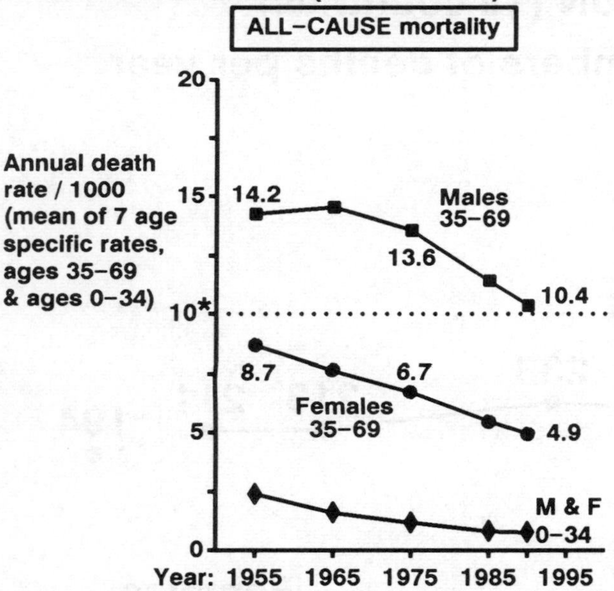

* An annual rate of 10 per 1000 implies that 30% of 35-year-olds will die before age 70

EUROPEAN UNION (12 countries): 1955–90

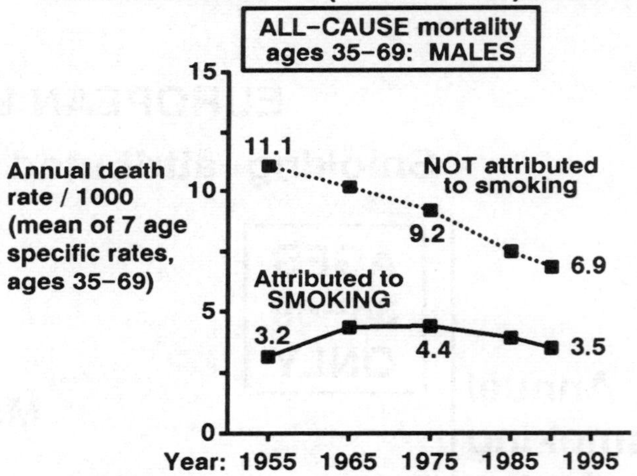

EUROPEAN UNION (12 countries): 1955–90

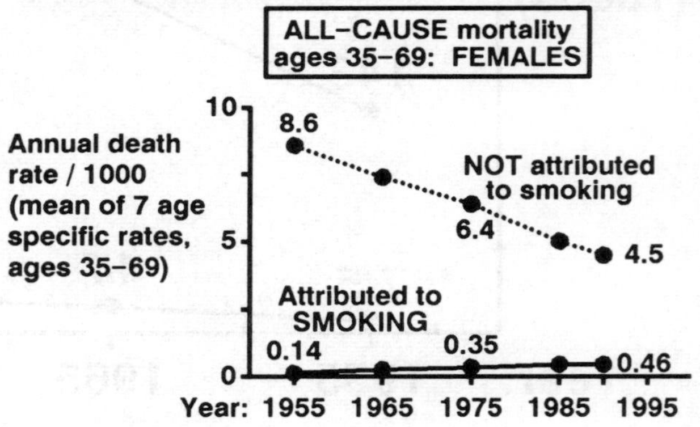

EUROPEAN UNION (12 countries)

ALL CANCER DEATHS (annual rates per 1000): Trends in mortality attributed to smoking, and in other mortality

Attributed to SMOKING?	Males 35–69 Yes	Males 35–69 No	Males 70–79 Yes	Males 70–79 No	Females 35–69 Yes	Females 35–69 No	Females 70–79 Yes	Females 70–79 No
1955	1.00	2.12	1.62	11.0	0.03	2.34	0.03	8.58
1965	1.54	2.08	3.74	11.0	0.07	2.31	0.15	8.63
1975	1.72	2.03	6.00	10.6	0.10	2.20	0.26	8.00
1985	1.84	1.97	6.76	10.4	0.16	2.03	0.50	7.65
1990	1.77	1.98	6.50	10.5	0.18	1.97	0.65	7.38

35–69 = mean of 7 age–specific rates; 70–79 = mean of 2 rates (70–74 & 75–79) Peto, Lopez et al, 1992, 1994

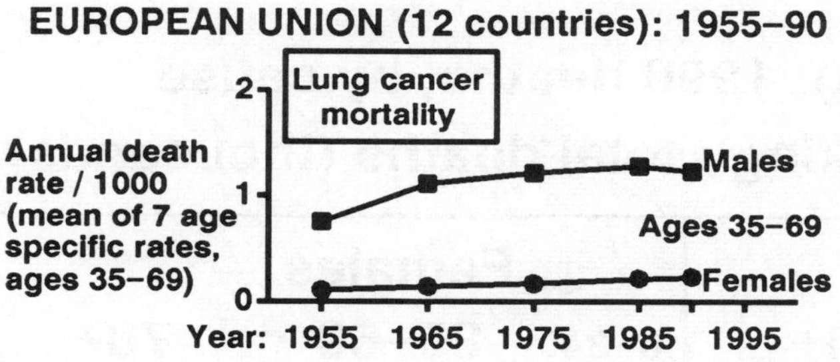

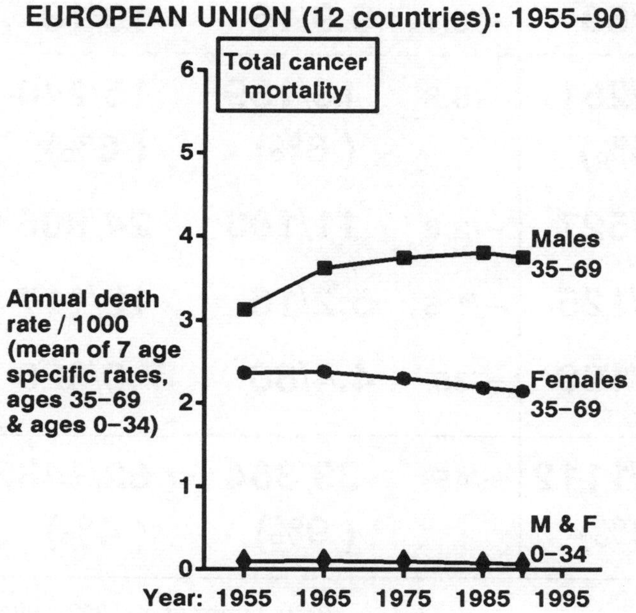

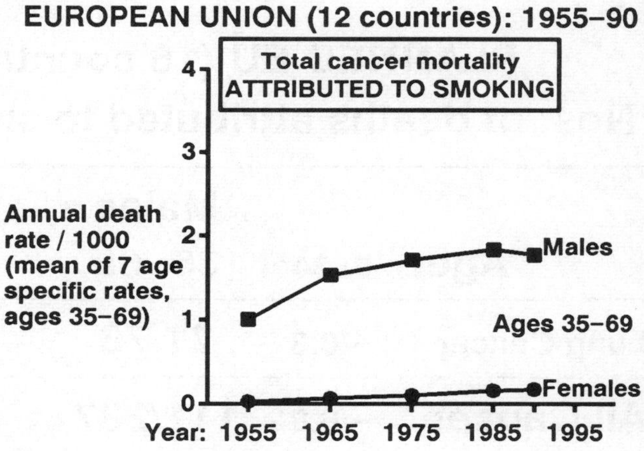

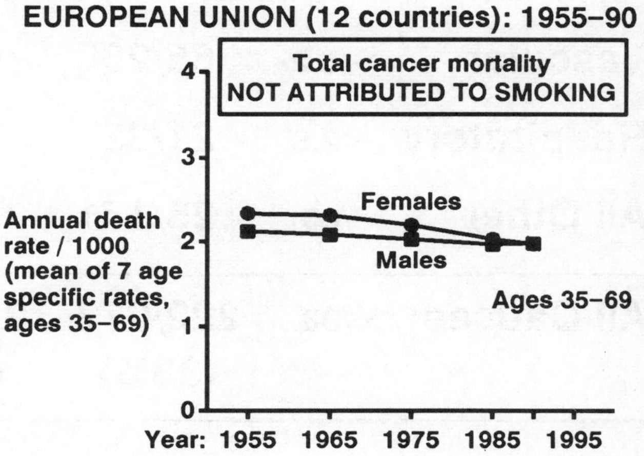

PLANNED EU (16 countries): 1990
Relative importance of deaths in MIDDLE age (35–69)

Age range (years)	Deaths attributed to SMOKING / total deaths (thousands) Males	Females	Mean years lost PER DEATH FROM SMOKING
0–34	–/98	–/45	–
35–69	222/673	33/364	21 years
70+	223/1112	62/1482	8 years
All ages	444/1884	95/1891	14 years

Peto, Lopez et al, 1992, 1994

PLANNED EU (16 countries): 1990 deaths, by cause
Nos. of deaths attributed to smoking / total deaths (thousands)

	Males			Females		
Age:	0–34	35–69	70+	0–34	35–69	70+
Lung Cancer	–/0.3	71/76	57/63	–/0.1	9.9/16	10/18
All Cancer	–/6.8	111/237 (47%)	89/261 (34%)	–/5.8	13/159 (8%)	15/240 (6%)
Vascular	–/5.2	65/230	61/527	–/2.8	11/103	24/806
Respiratory	–/2.6	21/35	56/125	–/1.6	5.2/16	16/117
All Other	–/83	25/171	18/199	–/35	4.4/86	7.0/320
All Causes	–/98	222/673 (33%)	223/1112 (20%)	–/45	33/364 (9%)	62/1482 (4%)

Peto, Lopez et al, 1992, 1994

PLANNED EU (16 countries): 1990
RISKS OF DYING AT AGES 0–34 and 35–69

(Probability that someone entering an age range would die during it, if the death rates in 1990 were to persist unchanged)

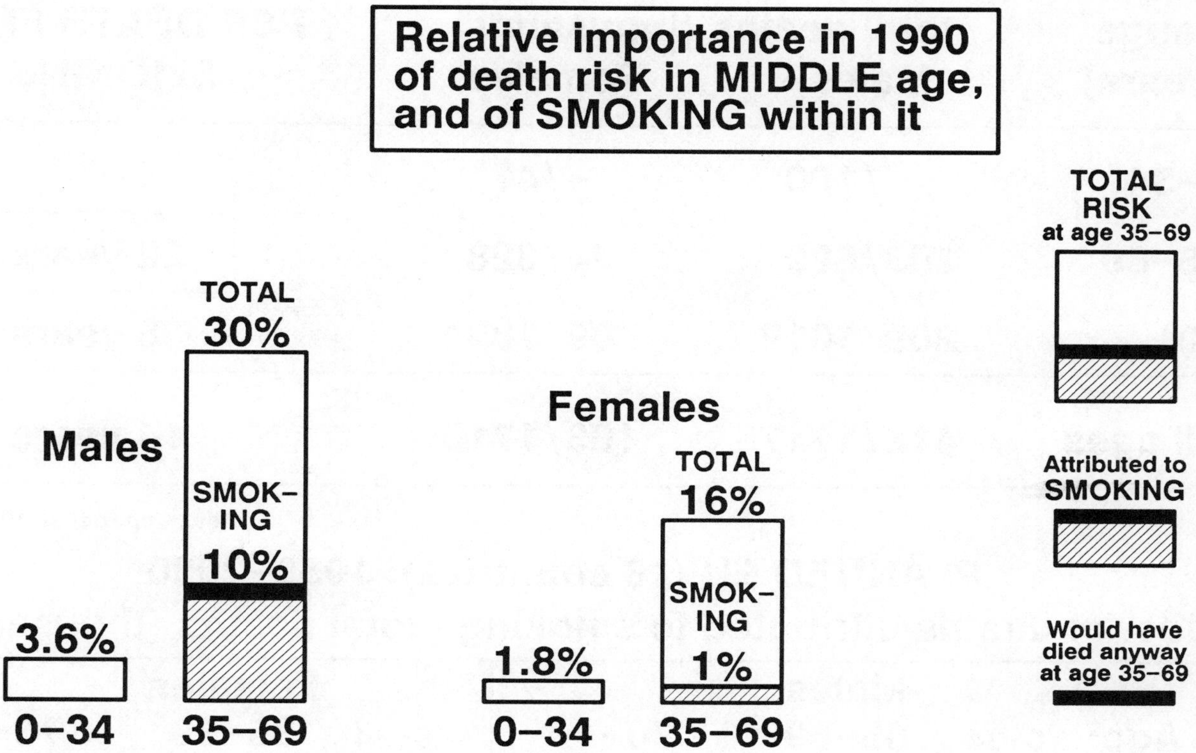

Peto, Lopez et al, 1992, 1994

PLANNED EU (16 countries): 1990 deaths, all ages
Nos. of deaths attributed to smoking / total deaths (thousands)

	Males	Females	Males + Females
All Cancer	200/505 (40%)	28/405 (7%)	228/910 (25%)
All Causes	444/1884 (24%)	95/1891 (5%)	540/3775 (14%)

Peto, Lopez et al, 1992, 1994

PLANNED EU (16 countries): 1995 projections
Relative importance of deaths in MIDDLE age (35–69)

Age range (years)	Deaths attributed to SMOKING / total deaths (thousands) Males	Females	Mean years lost PER DEATH FROM SMOKING
0–34	–/100	–/41	–
35–69	203/629	34/328	22 years
70+	209/1018	69/1344	8 years
All ages	412/1747	103/1713	14 years

Peto, Lopez et al, 1992, 1994

PLANNED EU (16 countries): 1950–2000
Nos. of deaths attributed to smoking / total deaths (thousands)

Age:	Males 0–34	Males 35–69	Males 70+	Females 0–34	Females 35–69	Females 70+
1955	–/236	153/661 (23%)	44/768 (6%)	–/174	7.8/497 (2%)	2.6/906 (0.3%)
1965	–/185	237/792 (30%)	108/896 (12%)	–/121	17/507 (3%)	12/1120 (1%)
1975	–/137	246/777 (32%)	201/1056 (19%)	–/79	23/463 (5%)	26/1329 (2%)
1985	–/97	224/663 (34%)	242/1161 (21%)	–/50	30/366 (8%)	51/1479 (3%)
1995 (projected)	–/100	203/629 (32%)	209/1018 (20%)	–/41	34/328 (10%)	69/1344 (5%)
50-year total* (M=millions), mid-1950 to mid-2000: 21/180M						
1950–2000, by age & sex	–/7.6M	11/35M (31%)	8.0/49M (16%)	–/4.7M	1.1/22M (5%)	1.6/62M (3%)

*Estimated as 10 times the sum of the five annual numbers (for 1955, 1965, 1975, 1985 & 1995)

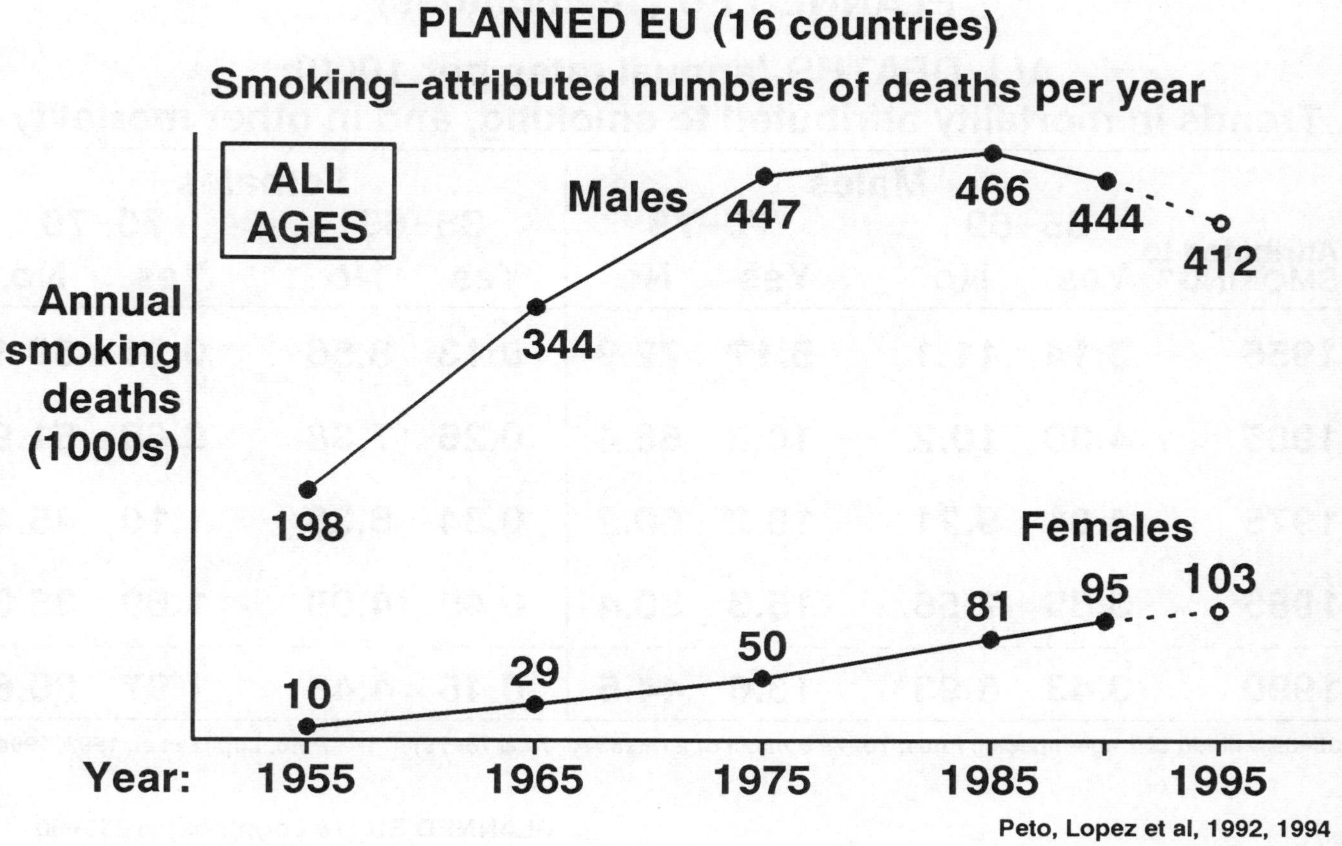
PLANNED EU (16 countries)
Smoking–attributed numbers of deaths per year
ALL AGES
Annual smoking deaths (1000s)
Males
198
344
447
466
444
412
Females
10
29
50
81
95
103
Year:
1955
1965
1975
1985
1995
Peto, Lopez et al, 1992, 1994

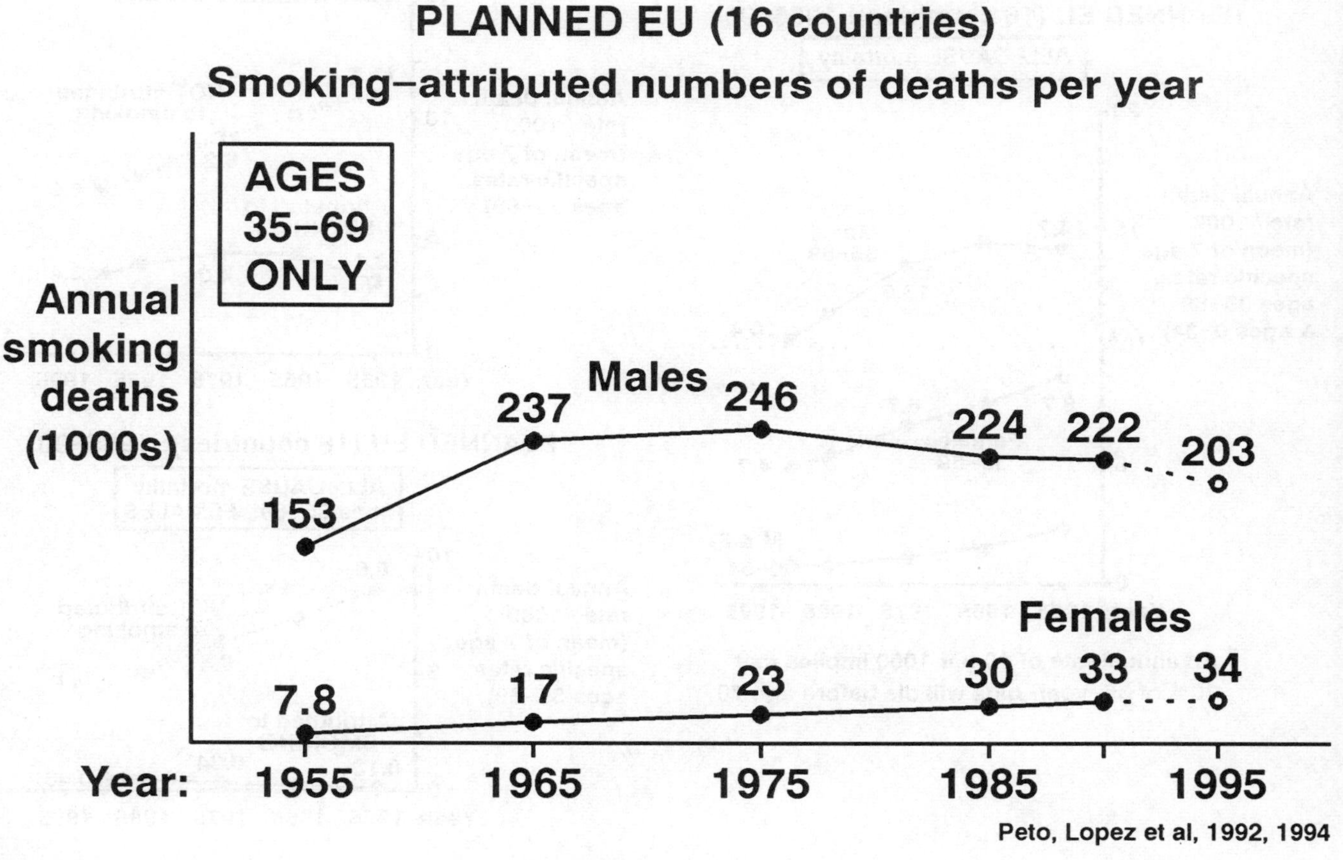
PLANNED EU (16 countries)
Smoking–attributed numbers of deaths per year
AGES 35–69 ONLY
Annual smoking deaths (1000s)
Males
153
237
246
224
222
203
Females
7.8
17
23
30
33
34
Year:
1955
1965
1975
1985
1995
Peto, Lopez et al, 1992, 1994

PLANNED EU (16 countries)

ALL DEATHS (annual rates per 1000): Trends in mortality attributed to smoking, and in other mortality

	Males				Females			
	35–69		70–79		35–69		70–79	
Attributed to SMOKING?	Yes	No	Yes	No	Yes	No	Yes	No
1955	3.14	11.1	5.17	72.9	0.13	8.56	0.21	59.1
1965	4.30	10.2	10.8	66.4	0.26	7.38	0.68	51.9
1975	4.31	9.21	16.2	60.2	0.34	6.36	1.10	45.4
1985	3.85	7.56	15.3	50.4	0.45	4.99	1.69	35.3
1990	3.43	6.93	13.6	44.5	0.46	4.48	1.97	30.6

35–69 = mean of 7 age-specific rates; 70–79 = mean of 2 rates (70–74 & 75–79) Peto, Lopez et al, 1992, 1994

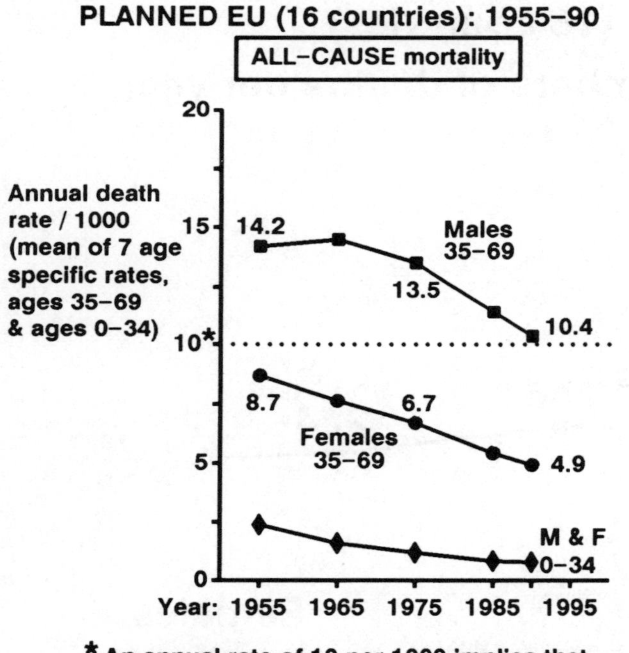

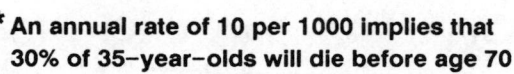

* An annual rate of 10 per 1000 implies that 30% of 35-year-olds will die before age 70

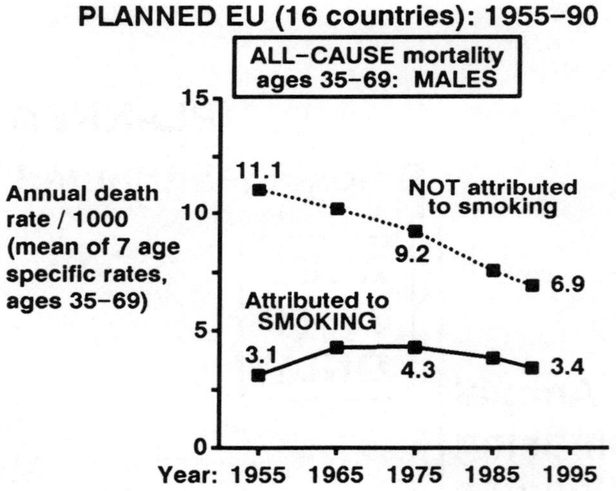

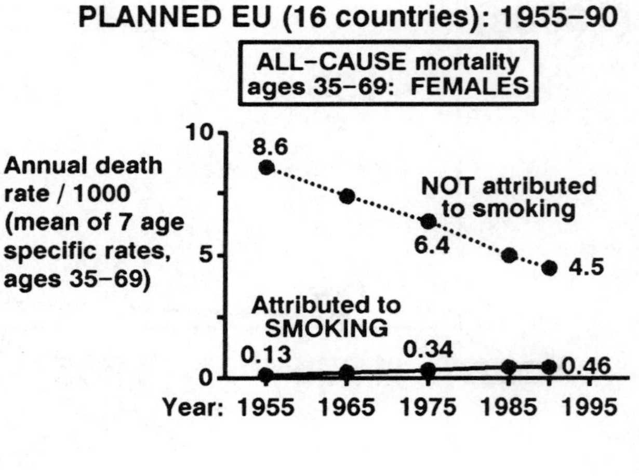

PLANNED EU (16 countries)

ALL CANCER DEATHS (annual rates per 1000): Trends in mortality attributed to smoking, and in other mortality

	Males 35–69		Males 70–79		Females 35–69		Females 70–79	
Attributed to SMOKING?	Yes	No	Yes	No	Yes	No	Yes	No
1955	1.00	2.13	1.65	11.0	0.03	2.35	0.04	8.64
1965	1.51	2.08	3.72	11.1	0.06	2.32	0.14	8.66
1975	1.67	2.02	5.92	10.7	0.10	2.20	0.26	8.04
1985	1.79	1.96	6.58	10.5	0.16	2.03	0.49	7.67
1990	1.73	1.97	6.31	10.5	0.17	1.97	0.63	7.40

35–69 = mean of 7 age-specific rates; 70–79 = mean of 2 rates (70–74 & 75–79) Peto, Lopez et al, 1992, 1994

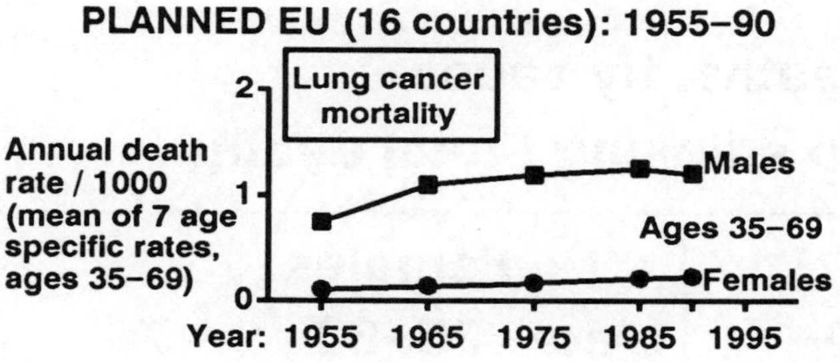

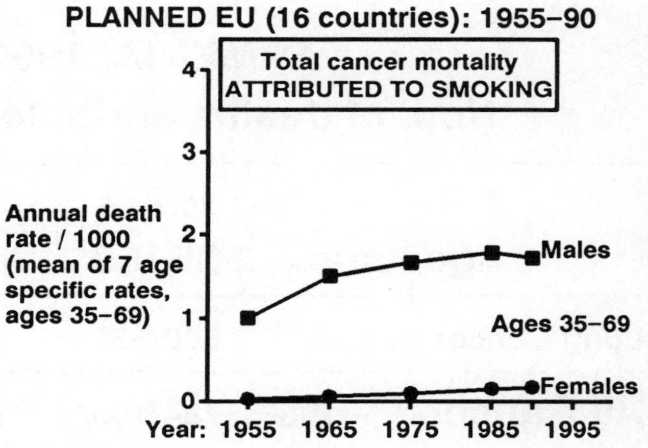

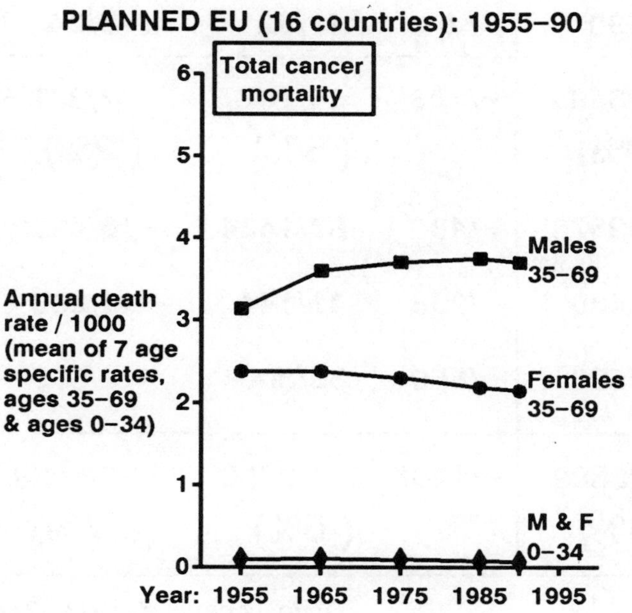

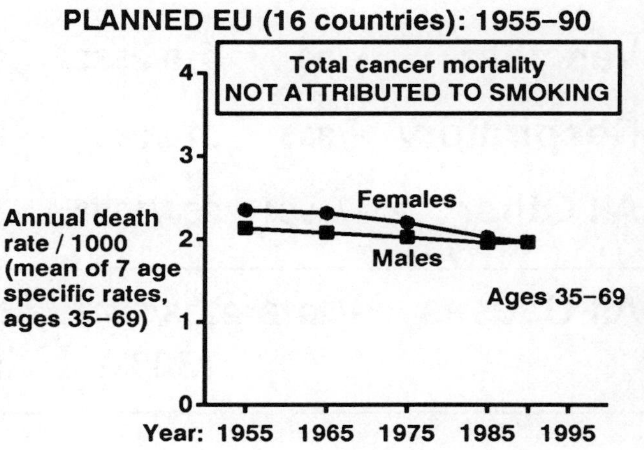

¶ARMENIA: 1990
Relative importance of deaths in MIDDLE age (35–69)

Age range (years)	Deaths attributed to SMOKING / total deaths (thousands) Males	Females	Mean years lost PER DEATH FROM SMOKING
0–34	–/2.1	–/1.3	–
35–69	2.2/5.9	0.2/3.5	21 years
70+	0.5/3.9	0.0/5.4	8 years
All ages	2.8/12	0.3/10	18 years

Peto, Lopez et al, 1992, 1994

ARMENIA: 1990 deaths, by cause
Nos. of deaths attributed to smoking / total deaths

	Males			Females		
Age:	0–34	35–69	70+	0–34	35–69	70+
Lung Cancer	–/ 6	530/562	75/90	–/ 9	41/82	5/24
All Cancer	–/103	784/1505 (52%)	105/359 (29%)	–/103	54/1077 (5%)	7/337 (2%)
Vascular	–/89	919/2562	162/2578	–/48	87/1434	16/4132
Respiratory	–/305	276/360	231/430	–/265	41/144	12/280
All Other	–/1581	254/1520	25/522	–/850	35/800	2/609
All Causes	–/2078	2233/5947 (38%)	523/3889 (13%)	–/1266	217/3455 (6%)	37/5358 (0.7%)

Peto, Lopez et al, 1992, 1994

ARMENIA: 1990

RISKS OF DYING AT AGES 0–34 and 35–69

(Probability that someone entering an age range would die during it, if the death rates in 1990 were to persist unchanged)

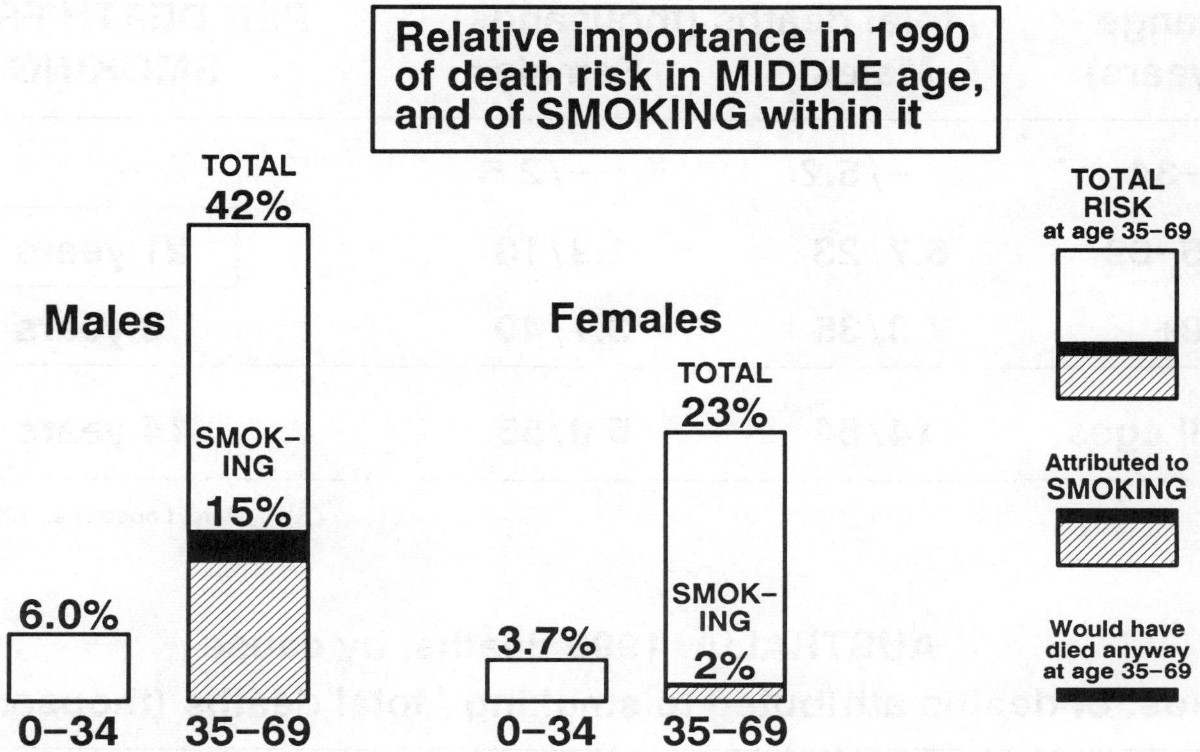

Peto, Lopez et al, 1992, 1994

ARMENIA: 1990 deaths, all ages

Nos. of deaths attributed to smoking / total deaths (thousands)

	Males	Females	Males + Females
All Cancer	0.9/2.0 (45%)	0.1/1.5 (4%)	0.9/3.5 (27%)
All Causes	2.8/12 (23%)	0.3/10 (3%)	3.0/22 (14%)

Peto, Lopez et al, 1992, 1994

AUSTRALIA: 1990

Relative importance of deaths in MIDDLE age (35–69)

Age range (years)	Deaths attributed to SMOKING / total deaths (thousands) Males	Females	Mean years lost PER DEATH FROM SMOKING
0–34	–/5.2	–/2.5	–
35–69	6.7/23	1.9/13	21 years
70+	7.3/35	3.1/40	8 years
All ages	14/64	5.0/55	14 years

Peto, Lopez et al, 1992, 1994

AUSTRALIA: 1990 deaths, by cause

Nos. of deaths attributed to smoking / total deaths (thousands)

	Males			Females		
Age:	0–34	35–69	70+	0–34	35–69	70+
Lung Cancer	–/0.0	2.1/2.3	1.9/2.1	–/0.0	0.6/0.8	0.5/0.8
All Cancer	–/0.4	3.2/8.1 (39%)	2.8/8.7 (33%)	–/0.3	0.7/6.0 (12%)	0.8/6.8 (11%)
Vascular	–/0.2	2.1/9.0	1.9/18	–/0.1	0.5/3.7	1.2/23
Respiratory	–/0.1	0.9/1.5	2.1/3.9	–/0.1	0.4/0.8	0.9/2.6
All Other	–/4.5	0.5/4.9	0.4/5.2	–/2.0	0.2/2.3	0.3/7.0
All Causes	–/5.2	6.7/23 (28%)	7.3/35 (21%)	–/2.5	1.9/13 (15%)	3.1/40 (8%)

Peto, Lopez et al, 1992, 1994

AUSTRALIA: 1990
RISKS OF DYING AT AGES 0–34 and 35–69
(Probability that someone entering an age range would die during it, if the death rates in 1990 were to persist unchanged)

Relative importance in 1990 of death risk in MIDDLE age, and of SMOKING within it

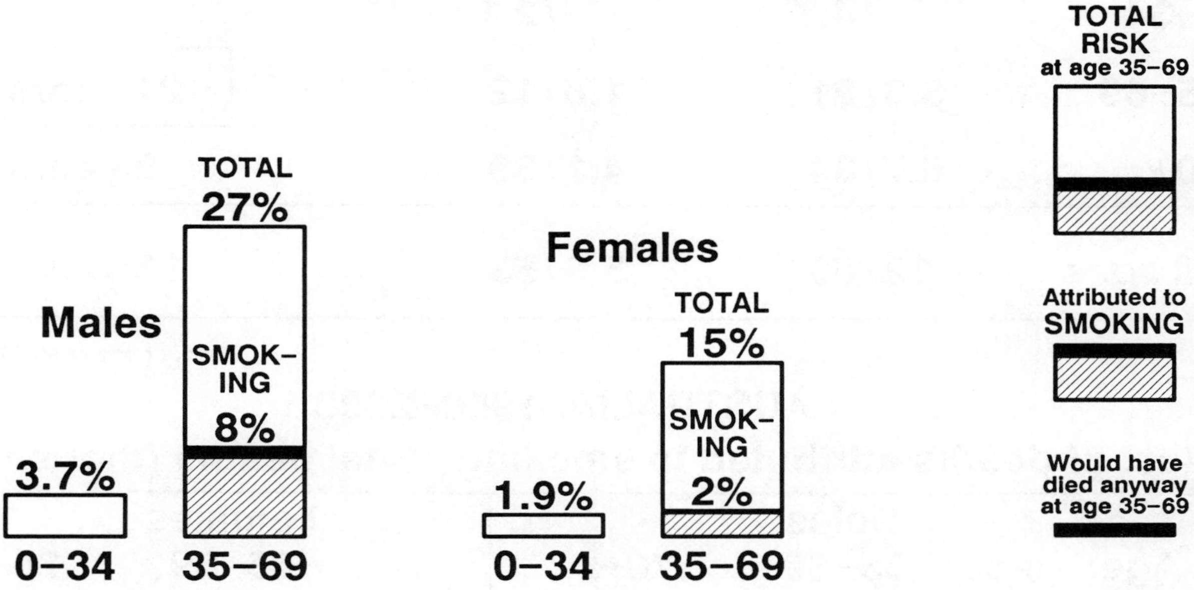

Peto, Lopez et al, 1992, 1994

AUSTRALIA: 1990 deaths, all ages
Nos. of deaths attributed to smoking / total deaths (thousands)

	Males	Females	Males + Females
All Cancer	6.0/17 (35%)	1.5/13 (11%)	7.5/30 (25%)
All Causes	14/64 (22%)	5.0/55 (9%)	19/119 (16%)

Peto, Lopez et al, 1992, 1994

AUSTRALIA: 1995 projections
Relative importance of deaths in MIDDLE age (35–69)

Age range (years)	Deaths attributed to SMOKING / total deaths (thousands) Males	Females	Mean years lost PER DEATH FROM SMOKING
0–34	–/4.7	–/2.1	–
35–69	5.3/21	1.8/12	21 years
70+	6.7/34	4.1/39	8 years
All ages	12/60	5.8/53	13 years

Peto, Lopez et al, 1992, 1994

AUSTRALIA: 1950–2000
Nos. of deaths attributed to smoking / total deaths (thousands)

Age:	Males 0–34	Males 35–69	Males 70+	Females 0–34	Females 35–69	Females 70+
1955	–/6.1	3.4 / 21 (17%)	1.3 / 20 (7%)	–/3.7	0.0 / 12 (0%)	0.0 / 20 (0%)
1965	–/5.9	6.6 / 25 (26%)	3.2 / 25 (13%)	–/3.6	0.1 / 14 (0.9%)	0.1 / 27 (0.2%)
1975	–/6.3	8.6 / 28 (31%)	5.5 / 27 (20%)	–/3.2	1.0 / 15 (7%)	0.6 / 30 (2%)
1985	–/5.6	7.7 / 24 (32%)	7.5 / 34 (22%)	–/2.8	1.8 / 13 (14%)	2.1 / 38 (5%)
1995 (projected)	–/4.7	5.3 / 21 (25%)	6.7 / 34 (20%)	–/2.1	1.8 / 12 (15%)	4.1 / 39 (10%)
50–year total*, mid–1950 to mid–2000: 674/5230						
1950–2000, by age & sex	–/286	316 / 1190 (27%)	242 / 1400 (17%)	–/154	47 / 660 (7%)	69 / 1540 (4%)

*Estimated as 10 times the sum of the five annual numbers (for 1955, 1965, 1975, 1985 & 1995)

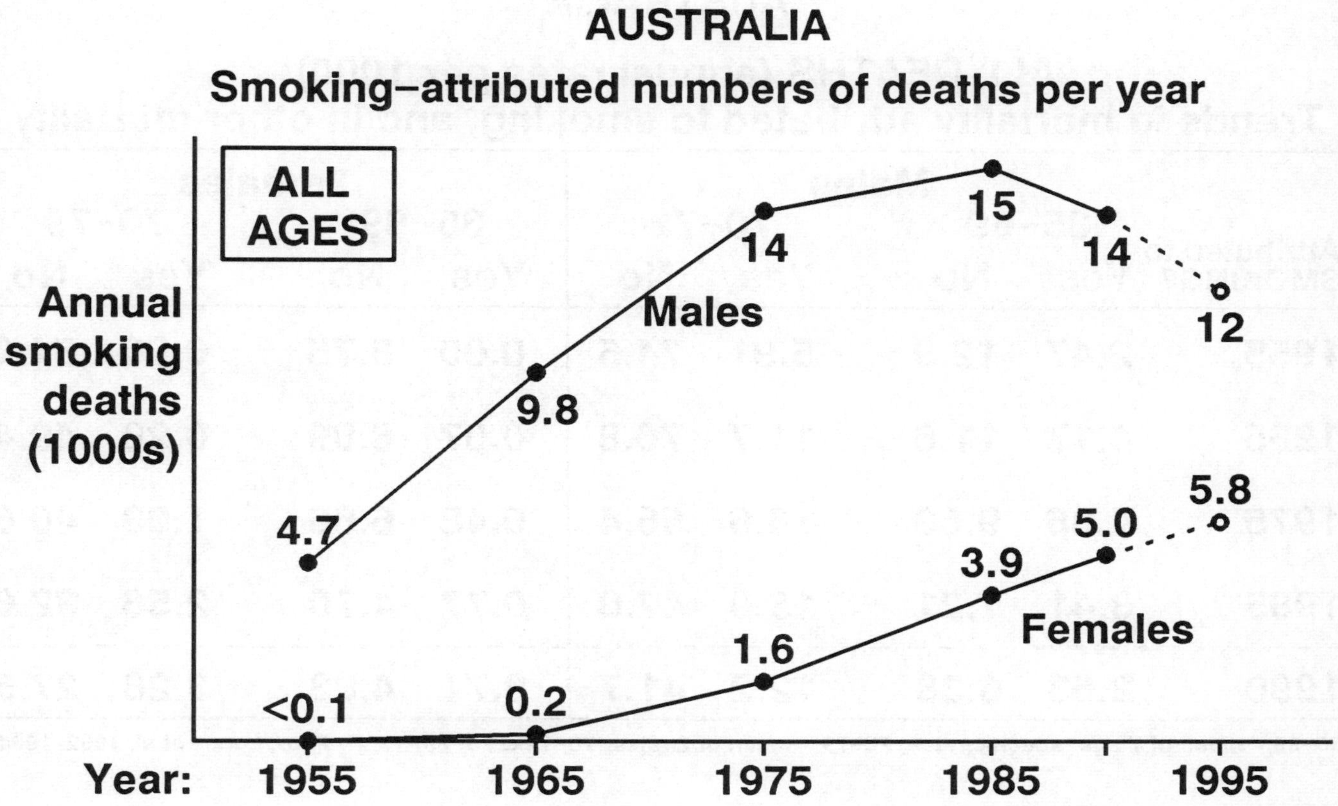

Peto, Lopez et al, 1992, 1994

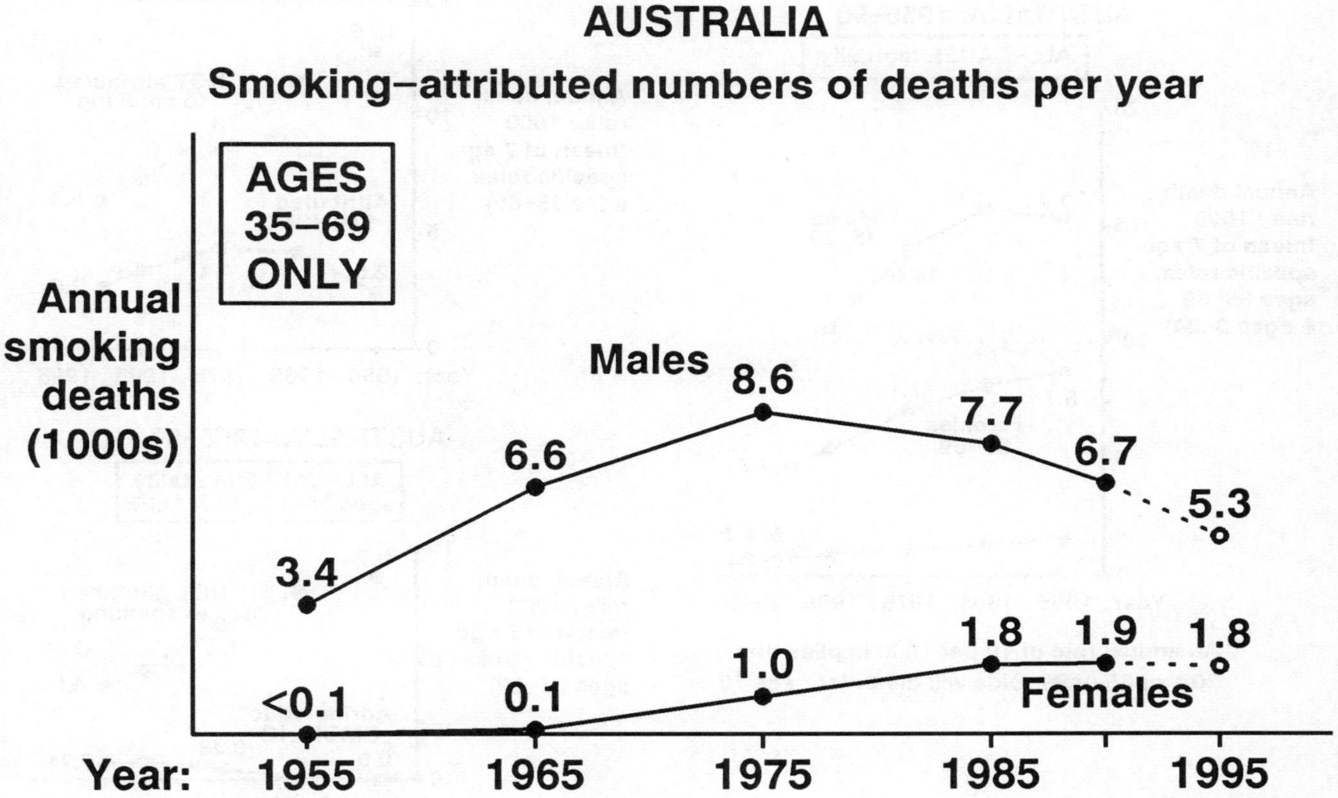

Peto, Lopez et al, 1992, 1994

AUSTRALIA

ALL DEATHS (annual rates per 1000): Trends in mortality attributed to smoking, and in other mortality

	Males				Females			
	35–69		70–79		35–69		70–79	
Attributed to SMOKING?	Yes	No	Yes	No	Yes	No	Yes	No
1955	2.47	12.9	5.91	74.5	0.00	8.75	0.00	54.0
1965	4.17	11.6	11.7	70.8	0.07	8.09	0.20	49.4
1975	4.36	9.63	16.6	56.4	0.48	6.66	1.03	40.6
1985	3.41	7.21	15.0	47.0	0.77	4.70	2.56	32.0
1990	2.63	6.38	12.2	41.7	0.71	4.03	3.26	27.5

35–69 = mean of 7 age-specific rates; 70–79 = mean of 2 rates (70–74 & 75–79) Peto, Lopez et al, 1992, 1994

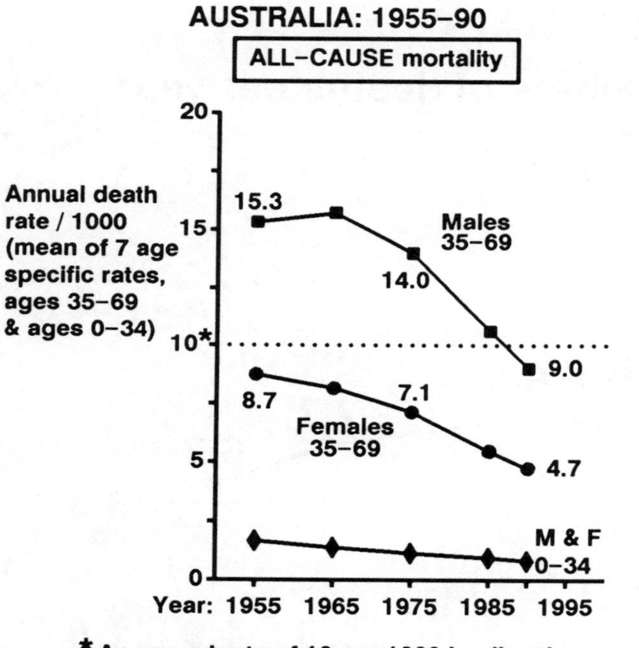

* An annual rate of 10 per 1000 implies that 30% of 35-year-olds will die before age 70

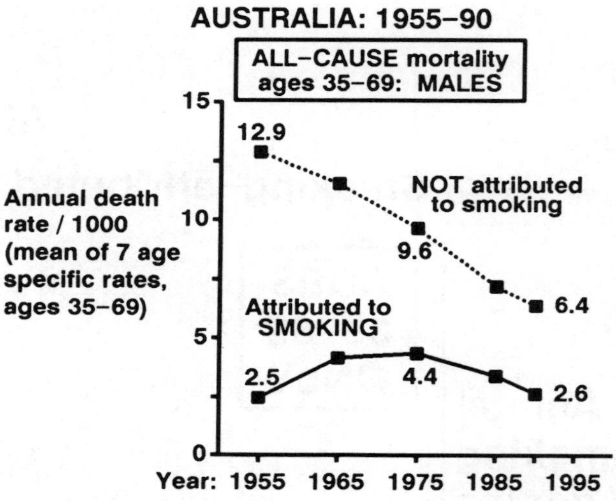

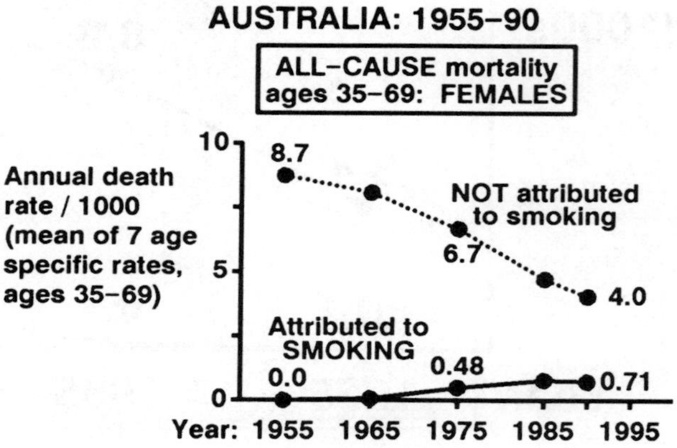

AUSTRALIA

ALL CANCER DEATHS (annual rates per 1000): Trends in mortality attributed to smoking, and in other mortality

	Males				Females			
	35–69		70–79		35–69		70–79	
Attributed to SMOKING?	Yes	No	Yes	No	Yes	No	Yes	No
1955	0.65	1.88	1.84	9.96	0.00	2.10	0.00	7.73
1965	1.17	1.70	3.55	9.49	0.01	1.96	0.04	7.01
1975	1.46	1.76	5.71	9.04	0.12	2.03	0.25	6.87
1985	1.48	1.90	5.97	9.73	0.27	2.01	0.71	6.96
1990	1.27	1.91	5.32	10.0	0.28	1.92	1.02	6.72

35–69 = mean of 7 age-specific rates; 70–79 = mean of 2 rates (70–74 & 75–79) Peto, Lopez et al, 1992, 1994

AUSTRALIA: 1955–90

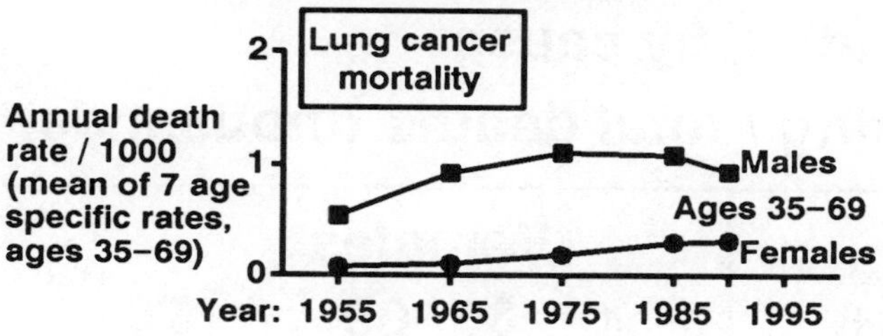

AUSTRALIA: 1955–90

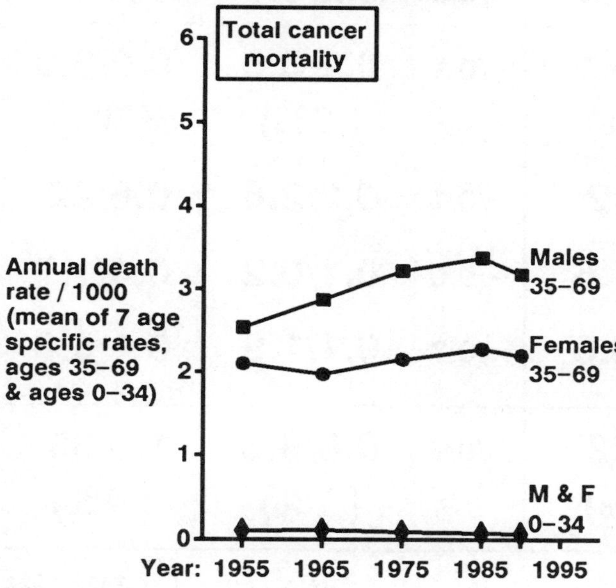

AUSTRALIA: 1955–90

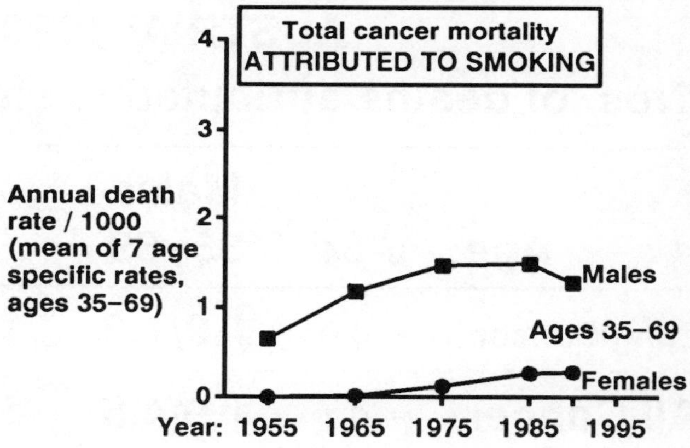

AUSTRALIA: 1955–90

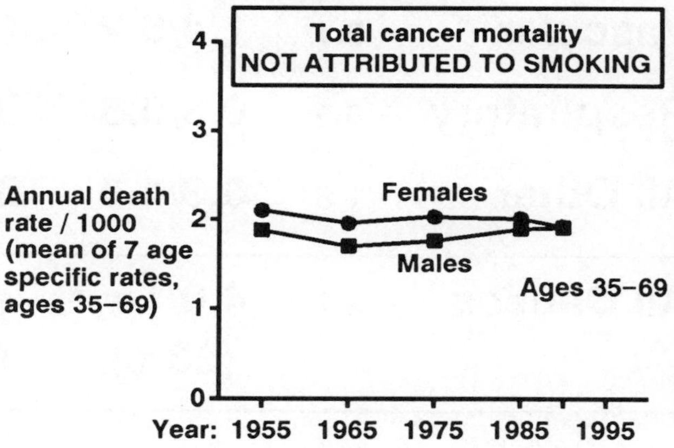

AUSTRIA: 1990
Relative importance of deaths in MIDDLE age (35–69)

Age range (years)	Deaths attributed to SMOKING / total deaths (thousands) Males	Females	Mean years lost PER DEATH FROM SMOKING
0–34	–/2.1	–/0.9	–
35–69	4.0/14	0.6/8.3	21 years
70+	3.6/22	1.5/35	7 years
All ages	7.5/38	2.0/45	14 years

Peto, Lopez et al, 1992, 1994

AUSTRIA: 1990 deaths, by cause
Nos. of deaths attributed to smoking / total deaths (thousands)

	Males			Females		
Age:	0–34	35–69	70+	0–34	35–69	70+
Lung Cancer	–/0.0	1.2/1.3	1.0/1.1	–/0.0	0.2/0.3	0.2/0.4
All Cancer	–/0.1	1.9/4.5 (44%)	1.5/5.1 (29%)	–/0.1	0.2/3.6 (6%)	0.3/6.0 (6%)
Vascular	–/0.1	1.4/5.2	1.2/12	–/0.1	0.2/2.6	0.6/22
Respiratory	–/0.0	0.3/0.5	0.7/1.6	–/0.0	0.1/0.2	0.4/1.7
All Other	–/1.8	0.3/4.0	0.2/3.0	–/0.7	0.1/1.9	0.1/5.3
All Causes	–/2.1	4.0/14 (28%)	3.6/22 (16%)	–/0.9	0.6/8.3 (7%)	1.5/35 (4%)

Peto, Lopez et al, 1992, 1994

AUSTRIA: 1990

RISKS OF DYING AT AGES 0–34 and 35–69

(Probability that someone entering an age range would die during it, if the death rates in 1990 were to persist unchanged)

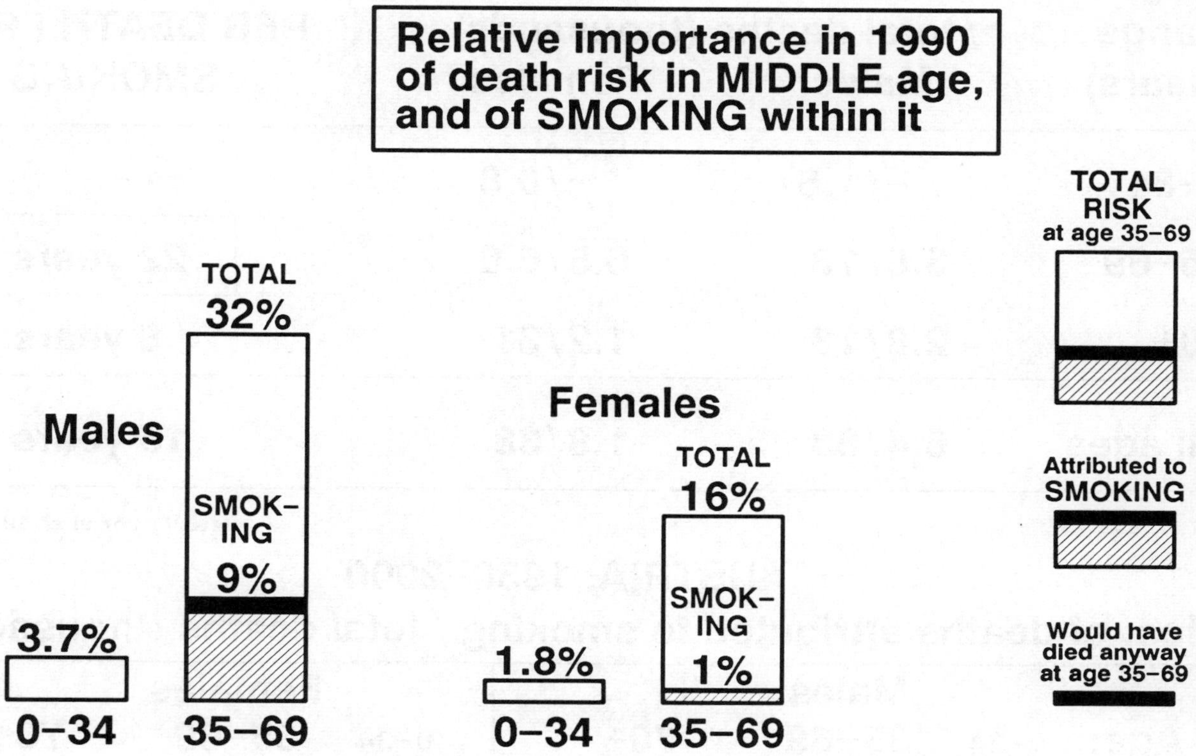

Peto, Lopez et al, 1992, 1994

AUSTRIA: 1990 deaths, all ages

Nos. of deaths attributed to smoking / total deaths (thousands)

	Males	Females	Males + Females
All Cancer	3.4/9.7 (35%)	0.6/9.7 (6%)	4.0/19 (21%)
All Causes	7.5/38 (20%)	2.0/45 (5%)	9.5/83 (12%)

Peto, Lopez et al, 1992, 1994

AUSTRIA: 1995 projections
Relative importance of deaths in MIDDLE age (35–69)

Age range (years)	Deaths attributed to SMOKING / total deaths (thousands) Males	Females	Mean years lost PER DEATH FROM SMOKING
0–34	–/1.6	–/0.8	–
35–69	3.6/13	0.5/6.6	22 years
70+	2.8/18	1.2/31	8 years
All ages	6.4/33	1.8/38	15 years

Peto, Lopez et al, 1992, 1994

AUSTRIA: 1950–2000
Nos. of deaths attributed to smoking / total deaths (thousands)

	Males			Females		
Age:	0–34	35–69	70+	0–34	35–69	70+
1955	–/5.5	5.6 / 18 (31%)	2.1 / 20 (11%)	–/3.6	0.2 / 14 (2%)	0.2 / 24 (0.7%)
1965	–/4.3	6.6 / 20 (32%)	3.9 / 23 (17%)	–/2.7	0.5 / 14 (3%)	0.4 / 30 (1%)
1975	–/3.5	4.7 / 17 (27%)	5.2 / 26 (20%)	–/1.8	0.6 / 12 (5%)	0.8 / 36 (2%)
1985	–/2.6	3.9 / 14 (28%)	4.6 / 25 (18%)	–/1.1	0.5 / 8.4 (5%)	1.5 / 38 (4%)
1995 (projected)	–/1.6	3.6 / 13 (28%)	2.8 / 18 (15%)	–/0.8	0.5 / 6.6 (8%)	1.2 / 31 (4%)
50–year total*, mid–1950 to mid–2000: 494/4355						
1950–2000, by age & sex	–/175	244 / 820 (30%)	186 / 1120 (17%)	–/100	23 / 550 (4%)	41 / 1590 (3%)

*Estimated as 10 times the sum of the five annual numbers (for 1955, 1965, 1975, 1985 & 1995)

AUSTRIA
Smoking–attributed numbers of deaths per year

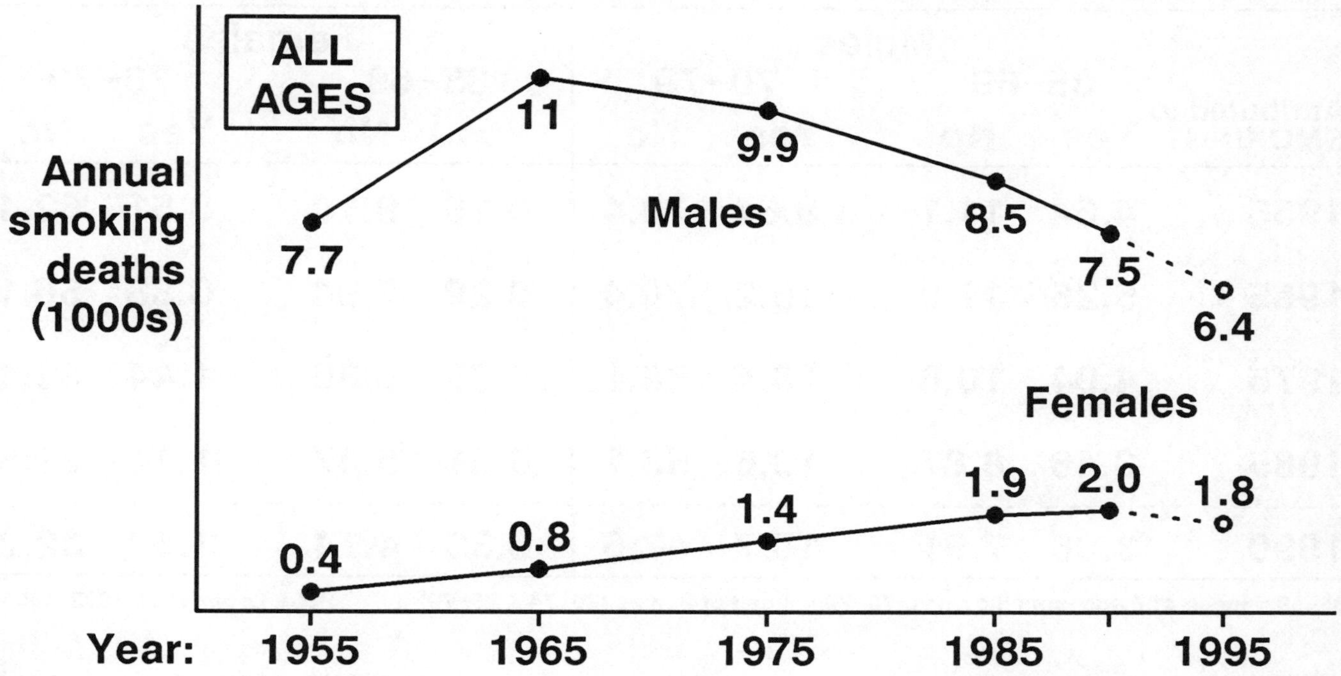

Peto, Lopez et al, 1992, 1994

AUSTRIA
Smoking–attributed numbers of deaths per year

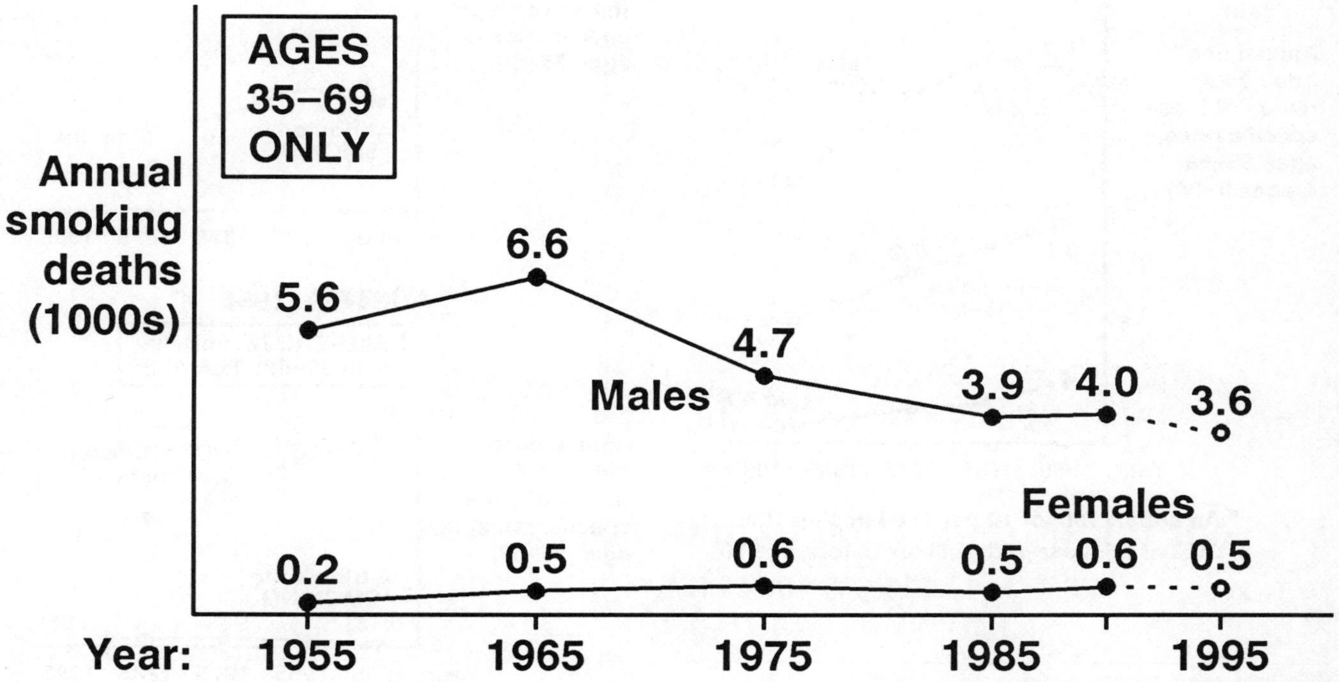

Peto, Lopez et al, 1992, 1994

AUSTRIA

ALL DEATHS (annual rates per 1000): Trends in mortality attributed to smoking, and in other mortality

	Males				Females			
	35–69		70–79		35–69		70–79	
Attributed to SMOKING?	Yes	No	Yes	No	Yes	No	Yes	No
1955	4.64	11.1	9.64	73.4	0.15	9.10	0.51	62.4
1965	5.26	11.0	16.2	70.4	0.29	7.94	0.88	56.1
1975	4.04	10.6	18.4	66.1	0.35	6.86	1.44	49.4
1985	3.46	8.87	13.6	55.1	0.31	5.47	1.74	39.5
1990	3.08	7.91	10.7	47.6	0.35	4.74	1.53	32.2

35–69 = mean of 7 age-specific rates; 70–79 = mean of 2 rates (70–74 & 75–79) Peto, Lopez et al, 1992, 1994

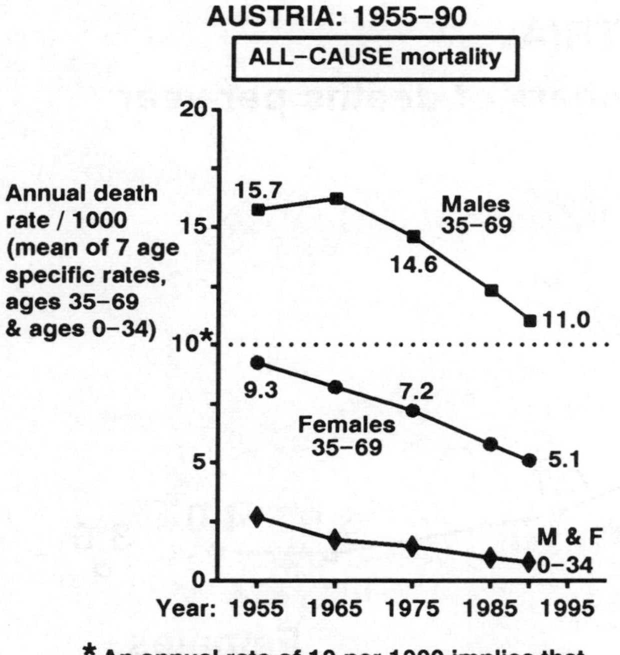

* An annual rate of 10 per 1000 implies that 30% of 35-year-olds will die before age 70

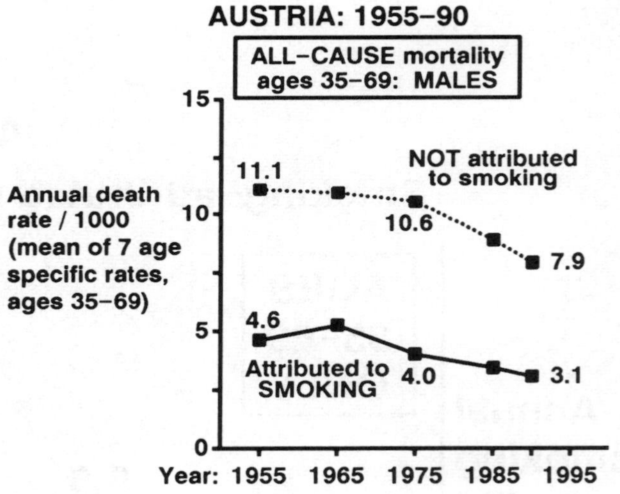

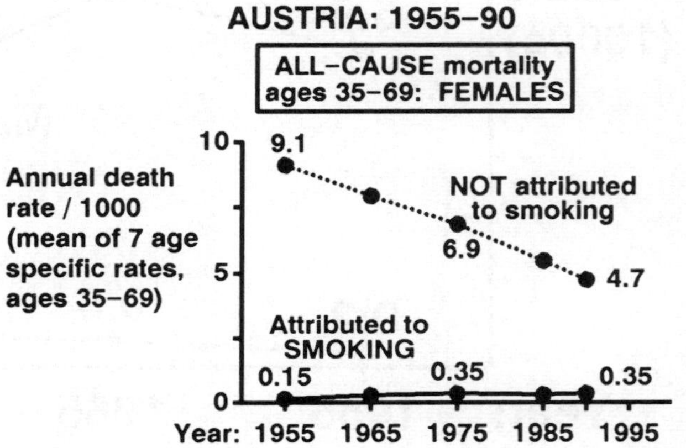

AUSTRIA

ALL CANCER DEATHS (annual rates per 1000): Trends in mortality attributed to smoking, and in other mortality

	Males				Females			
	35–69		70–79		35–69		70–79	
Attributed to SMOKING?	Yes	No	Yes	No	Yes	No	Yes	No
1955	1.71	2.41	3.80	12.7	0.03	2.79	0.10	10.8
1965	1.96	2.30	6.25	12.8	0.07	2.65	0.18	10.3
1975	1.60	2.11	7.45	11.7	0.10	2.47	0.33	9.19
1985	1.51	1.95	5.75	11.0	0.11	2.20	0.47	8.49
1990	1.52	2.00	5.11	10.9	0.14	2.07	0.51	8.05

35–69 = mean of 7 age-specific rates; 70–79 = mean of 2 rates (70–74 & 75–79)   Peto, Lopez et al, 1992, 1994

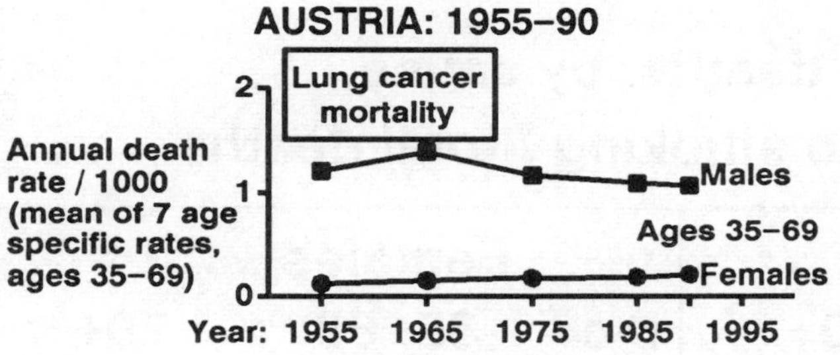

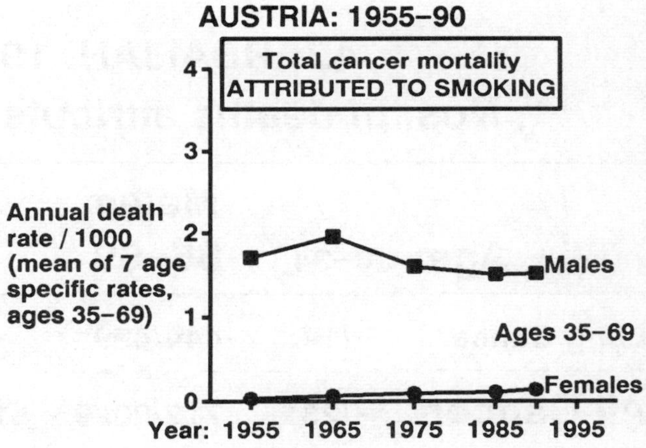

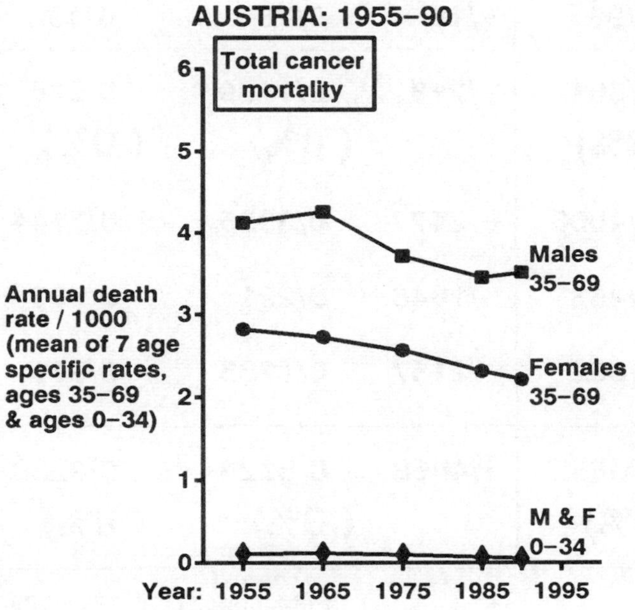

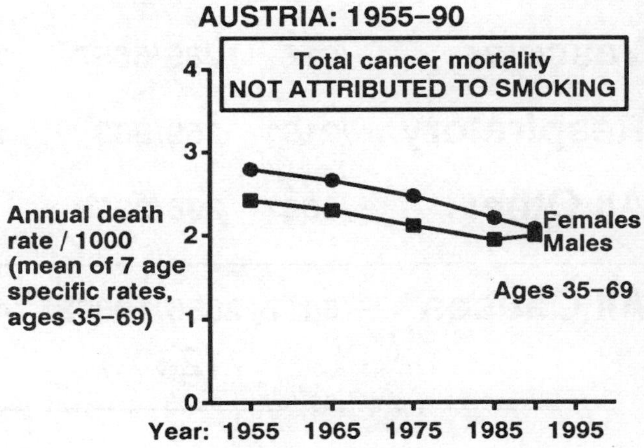

¶AZERBAIJAN: 1990
Relative importance of deaths in MIDDLE age (35–69)

Age range (years)	Deaths attributed to SMOKING / total deaths (thousands) Males	Females	Mean years lost PER DEATH FROM SMOKING
0–34	–/6.4	–/4.5	–
35–69	2.7/11	0.0/6.1	21 years
70+	0.5/5.7	0.0/9.2	8 years
All ages	3.1/23	0.0/20	19 years

Peto, Lopez et al, 1992, 1994

AZERBAIJAN: 1990 deaths, by cause
Nos. of deaths attributed to smoking / total deaths

	Males			Females		
Age:	0–34	35–69	70+	0–34	35–69	70+
Lung Cancer	–/14	444/499	72/96	–/18	0/78	0/43
All Cancer	–/231	712/2029 (35%)	108/561 (19%)	–/218	0/1189 (0%)	0/576 (0%)
Vascular	–/318	1289/5657	154/4006	–/247	0/3356	0/7144
Respiratory	–/2181	359/583	180/453	–/1846	0/291	0/539
All Other	–/3687	296/2629	16/662	–/2157	0/1288	0/971
All Causes	–/6417	2656/10898 (24%)	458/5682 (8%)	–/4468	0/6124 (0%)	0/9230 (0%)

Peto, Lopez et al, 1992, 1994

AZERBAIJAN: 1990

RISKS OF DYING AT AGES 0–34 and 35–69

(Probability that someone entering an age range would die during it, if the death rates in 1990 were to persist unchanged)

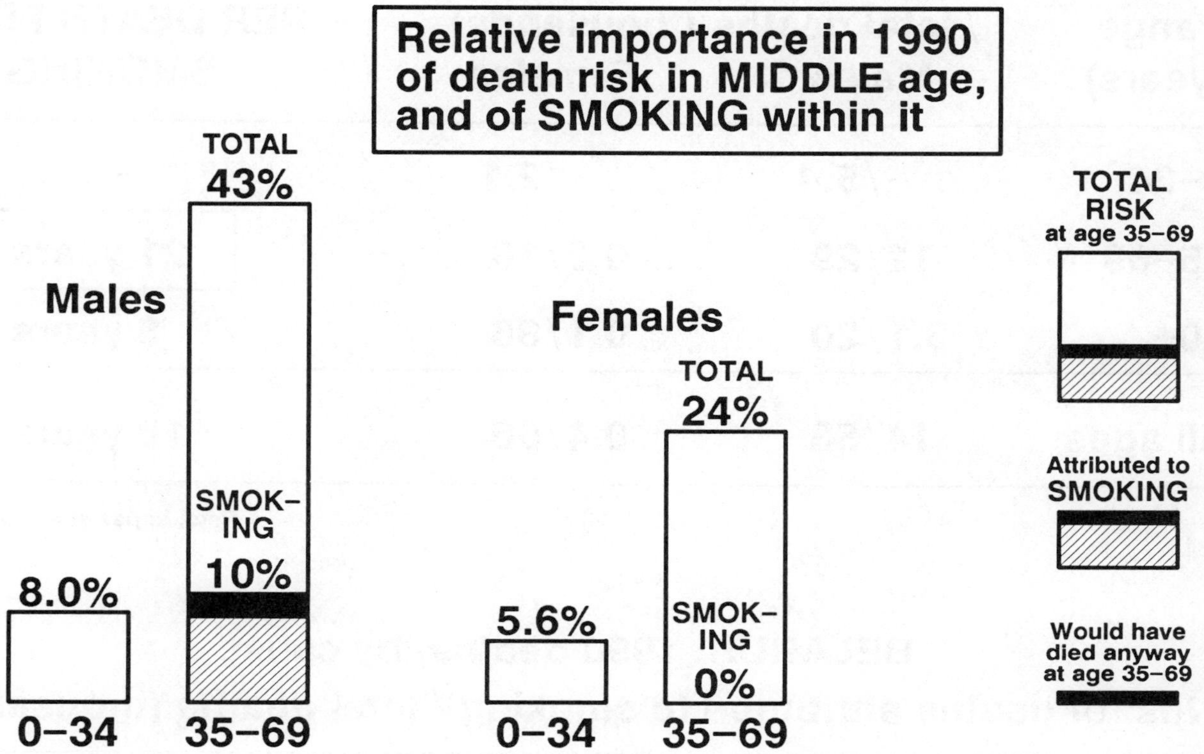

Peto, Lopez et al, 1992, 1994

AZERBAIJAN: 1990 deaths, all ages

Nos. of deaths attributed to smoking / total deaths (thousands)

	Males	Females	Males + Females
All Cancer	0.8/2.8 (29%)	0.0/2.0 (0%)	0.8/4.8 (17%)
All Causes	3.1/23 (14%)	0.0/20 (0%)	3.1/43 (7%)

Peto, Lopez et al, 1992, 1994

¶BELARUS: 1990
Relative importance of deaths in MIDDLE age (35–69)

Age range (years)	Deaths attributed to SMOKING / total deaths (thousands) Males	Females	Mean years lost PER DEATH FROM SMOKING
0–34	–/5.4	–/2.1	–
35–69	11/29	0.3/16	21 years
70+	3.1/20	0.1/38	8 years
All ages	14/53	0.4/56	18 years

Peto, Lopez et al, 1992, 1994

BELARUS: 1990 deaths, by cause
Nos. of deaths attributed to smoking / total deaths (thousands)

	Males			Females		
Age:	0–34	35–69	70+	0–34	35–69	70+
Lung Cancer	–/0.0	2.3/2.4	0.5/0.6	–/0.0	0.0/0.2	0.0/0.2
All Cancer	–/0.3	3.9/7.3 (53%)	0.7/2.4 (30%)	–/0.3	0.1/4.5 (1%)	0.0/2.7 (0.6%)
Vascular	–/0.4	4.8/12	0.9/11	–/0.1	0.1/7.8	0.0/24
Respiratory	–/0.2	1.5/1.9	1.2/2.0	–/0.2	0.1/0.7	0.0/2.5
All Other	–/4.5	0.9/7.1	0.2/4.0	–/1.6	0.0/3.0	0.0/8.8
All Causes	–/5.4	11/29 (39%)	3.1/20 (16%)	–/2.1	0.3/16 (2%)	0.1/38 (0.3%)

Peto, Lopez et al, 1992, 1994

BELARUS: 1990

RISKS OF DYING AT AGES 0–34 and 35–69

(Probability that someone entering an age range would die during it, if the death rates in 1990 were to persist unchanged)

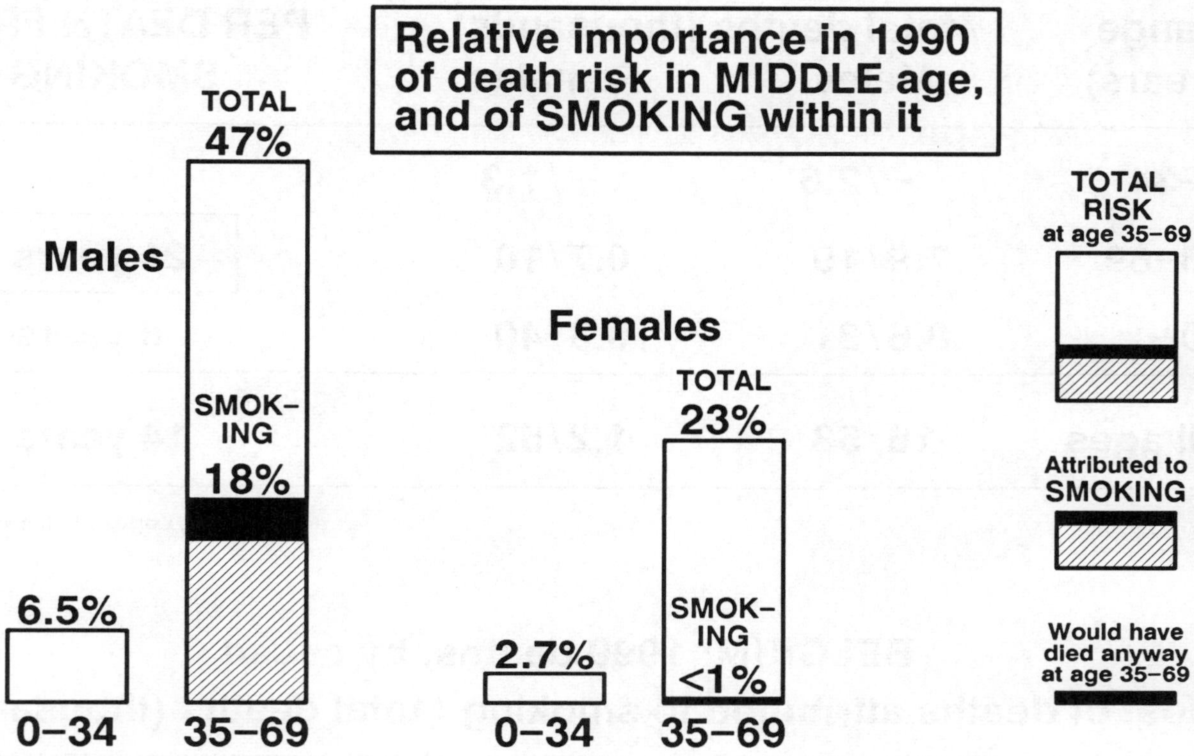

Peto, Lopez et al, 1992, 1994

BELARUS: 1990 deaths, all ages

Nos. of deaths attributed to smoking / total deaths (thousands)

	Males	Females	Males + Females
All Cancer	4.6/10 (46%)	0.1/7.5 (0.9%)	4.7/18 (27%)
All Causes	14/53 (26%)	0.4/56 (0.7%)	14/110 (13%)

Peto, Lopez et al, 1992, 1994

BELGIUM: 1990
Relative importance of deaths in MIDDLE age (35–69)

Age range (years)	Deaths attributed to SMOKING / total deaths (thousands) Males	Females	Mean years lost PER DEATH FROM SMOKING
0–34	–/2.6	–/1.3	–
35–69	7.9/19	0.7/10	21 years
70+	8.6/31	0.6/40	8 years
All ages	16/53	1.2/52	14 years

Peto, Lopez et al, 1992, 1994

BELGIUM: 1990 deaths, by cause
Nos. of deaths attributed to smoking / total deaths (thousands)

	Males			Females		
Age:	0–34	35–69	70+	0–34	35–69	70+
Lung Cancer	–/0.0	2.8/2.9	2.3/2.5	–/0.0	0.2/0.4	0.1/0.3
All Cancer	–/0.2	4.0/7.1 (56%)	3.6/8.1 (44%)	–/0.2	0.3/4.4 (6%)	0.1/6.7 (2%)
Vascular	–/0.1	2.1/6.0	2.1/12	–/0.1	0.2/2.6	0.2/19
Respiratory	–/0.0	0.9/1.5	2.1/4.2	–/0.0	0.1/0.5	0.2/2.8
All Other	–/2.2	0.9/4.6	0.9/6.7	–/1.0	0.1/2.7	0.1/12
All Causes	–/2.6	7.9/19 (41%)	8.6/31 (28%)	–/1.3	0.7/10 (6%)	0.6/40 (1%)

Peto, Lopez et al, 1992, 1994

BELGIUM: 1990

RISKS OF DYING AT AGES 0–34 and 35–69

(Probability that someone entering an age range would die during it, if the death rates in 1990 were to persist unchanged)

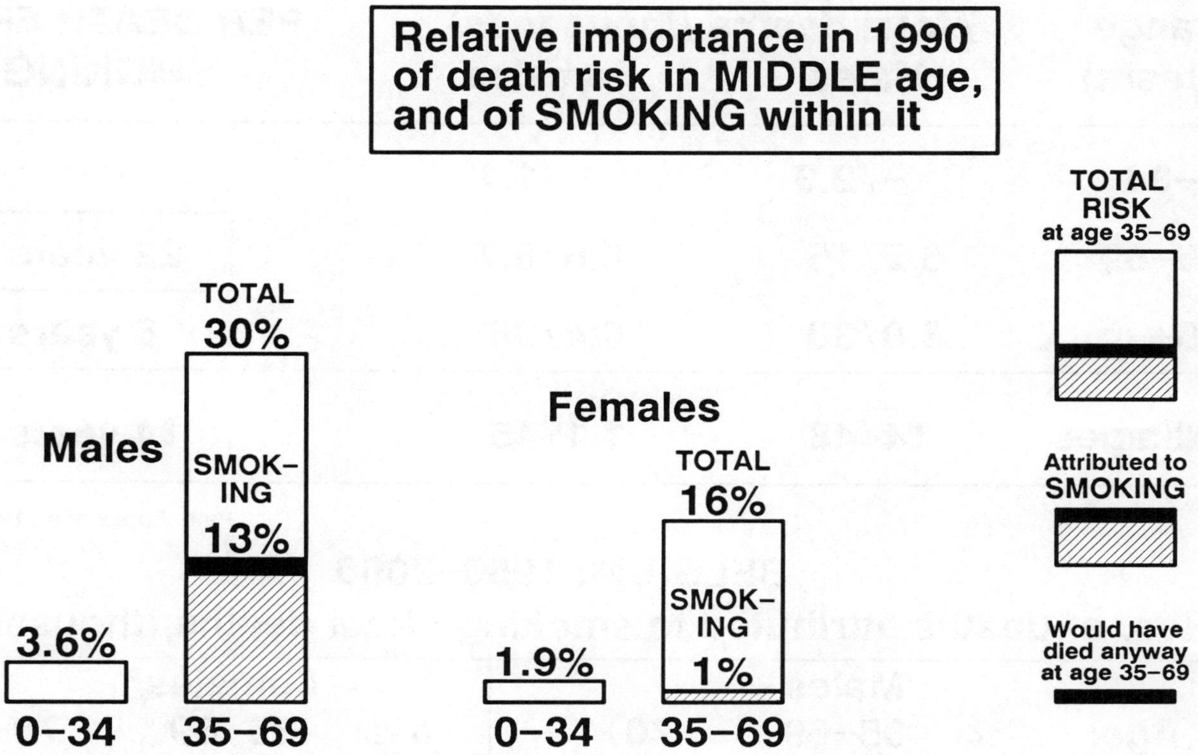

Peto, Lopez et al, 1992, 1994

BELGIUM: 1990 deaths, all ages

Nos. of deaths attributed to smoking / total deaths (thousands)

	Males	Females	Males + Females
All Cancer	7.5/15 (49%)	0.4/11 (4%)	7.9/27 (30%)
All Causes	16/53 (31%)	1.2/52 (2%)	18/105 (17%)

Peto, Lopez et al, 1992, 1994

BELGIUM: 1995 projections
Relative importance of deaths in MIDDLE age (35–69)

Age range (years)	Deaths attributed to SMOKING / total deaths (thousands) Males	Females	Mean years lost PER DEATH FROM SMOKING
0–34	–/2.3	–/1.1	–
35–69	6.2/16	0.6/8.7	22 years
70+	8.0/30	0.4/36	8 years
All ages	14/48	1.1/45	14 years

Peto, Lopez et al, 1992, 1994

BELGIUM: 1950–2000
Nos. of deaths attributed to smoking / total deaths (thousands)

	Males			Females		
Age:	0–34	35–69	70+	0–34	35–69	70+
1955	–/6.2	6.4 / 24 (27%)	1.5 / 28 (6%)	–/4.2	0.0 / 16 (0.1%)	0.0 / 31 (0%)
1965	–/4.6	10 / 27 (38%)	4.3 / 30 (14%)	–/2.9	0.1 / 15 (0.5%)	0.2 / 35 (0.4%)
1975	–/3.6	9.8 / 24 (41%)	8.4 / 35 (24%)	–/1.9	0.4 / 14 (3%)	0.6 / 41 (1%)
1985	–/2.8	8.7 / 20 (44%)	10 / 35 (29%)	–/1.4	0.5 / 10 (5%)	0.8 / 43 (2%)
1995 (projected)	–/2.3	6.2 / 16 (38%)	8.0 / 30 (27%)	–/1.1	0.6 / 8.7 (7%)	0.4 / 36 (1%)
50–year total*, mid–1950 to mid–2000: 769/5497						
1950–2000, by age & sex	–/195	411 / 1110 (37%)	322 / 1580 (20%)	–/115	16 / 637 (3%)	20 / 1860 (1%)

*Estimated as 10 times the sum of the five annual numbers (for 1955, 1965, 1975, 1985 & 1995)

BELGIUM

Smoking–attributed numbers of deaths per year

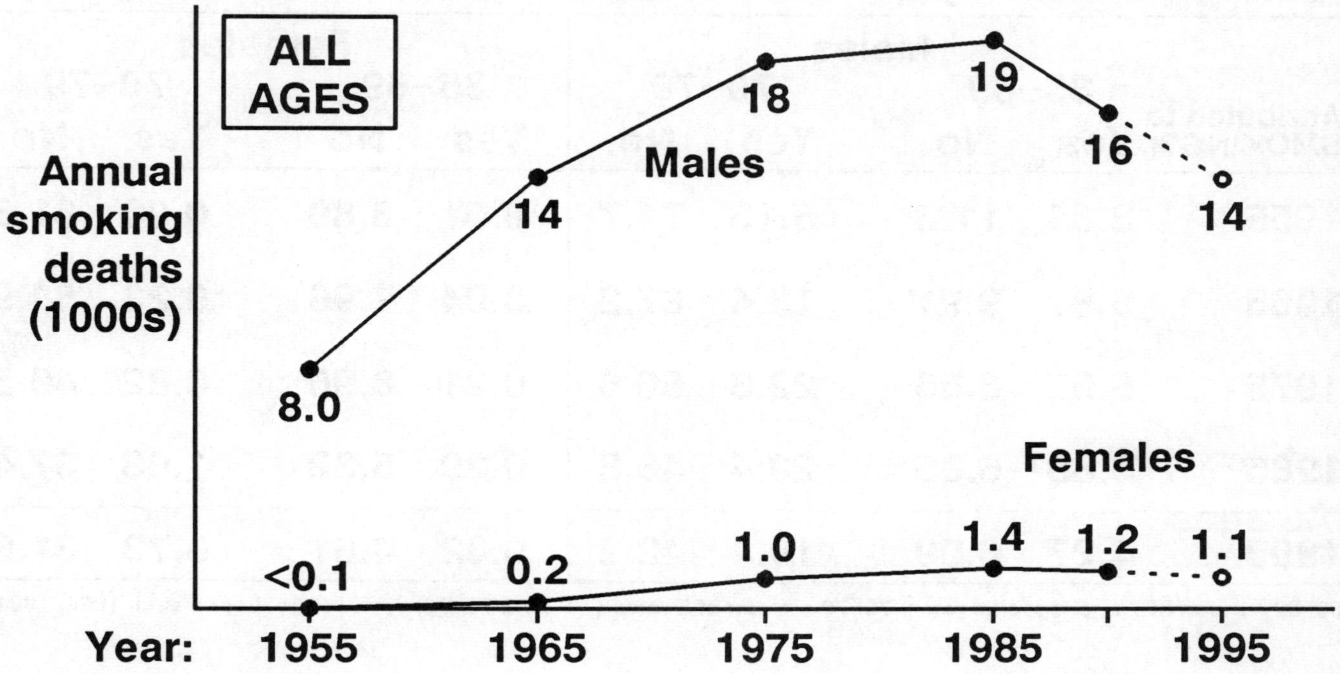

Peto, Lopez et al, 1992, 1994

BELGIUM

Smoking–attributed numbers of deaths per year

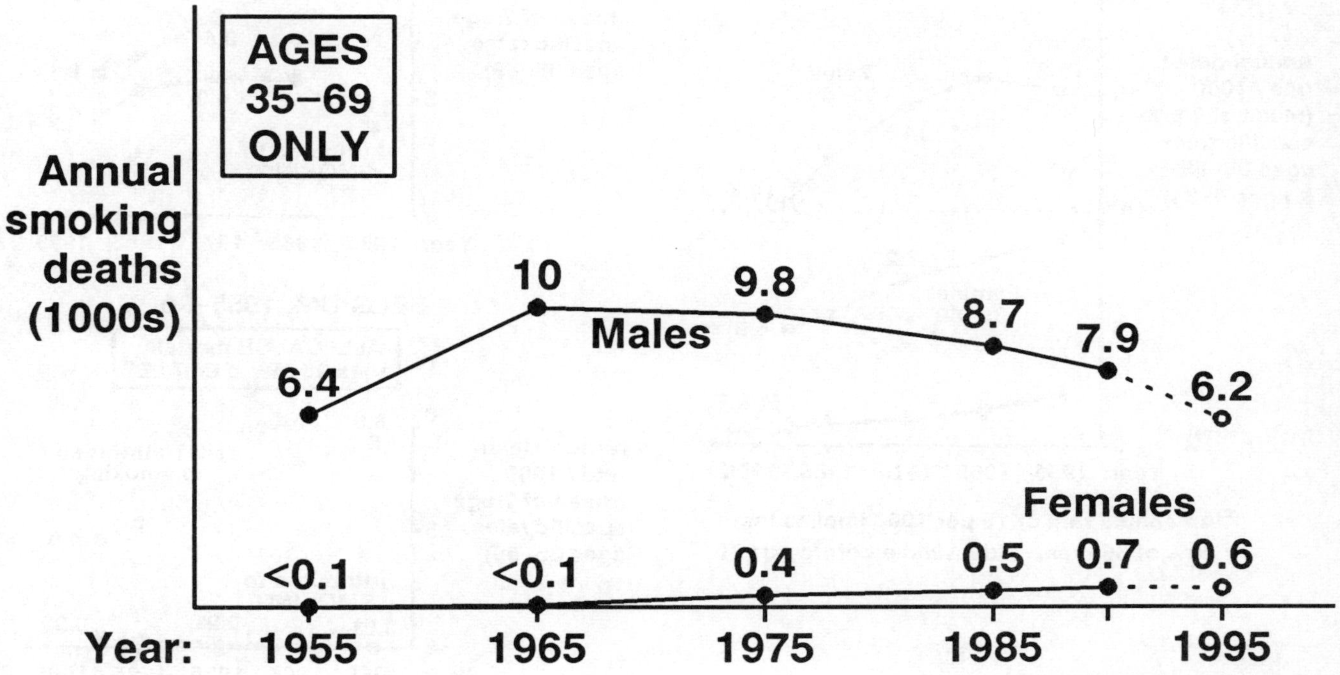

Peto, Lopez et al, 1992, 1994

BELGIUM

ALL DEATHS (annual rates per 1000): Trends in mortality attributed to smoking, and in other mortality

	Males				Females			
	35–69		70–79		35–69		70–79	
Attributed to SMOKING?	Yes	No	Yes	No	Yes	No	Yes	No
1955	3.84	11.3	5.13	74.7	0.01	8.89	0.00	61.6
1965	5.82	9.91	13.4	67.2	0.04	7.96	0.23	54.9
1975	5.97	8.56	22.3	60.6	0.21	6.96	0.82	49.5
1985	5.35	6.85	23.4	48.8	0.29	5.32	1.03	37.4
1990	4.27	6.09	19.4	42.2	0.32	4.61	0.73	31.6

35–69 = mean of 7 age-specific rates; 70–79 = mean of 2 rates (70–74 & 75–79) Peto, Lopez et al, 1992, 1994

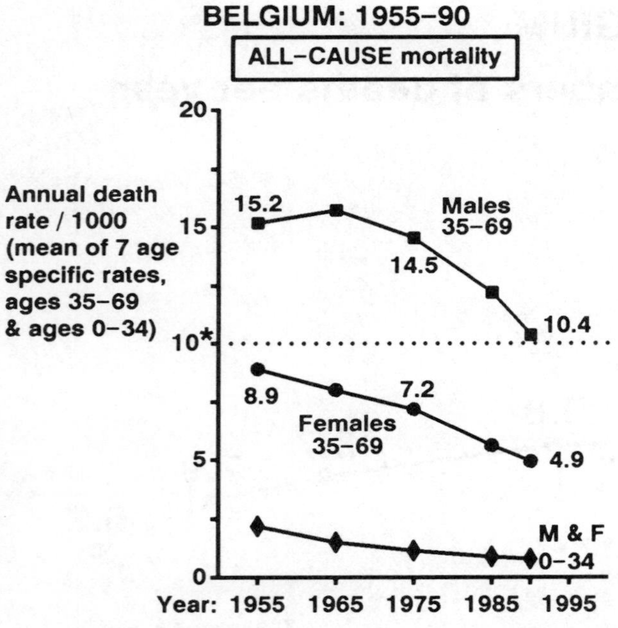

* An annual rate of 10 per 1000 implies that 30% of 35-year-olds will die before age 70

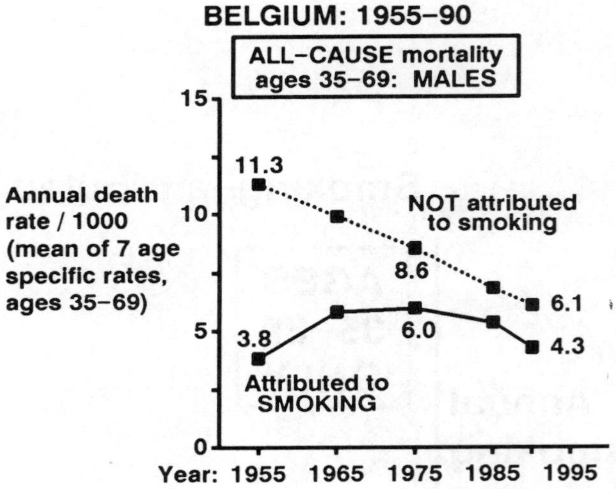

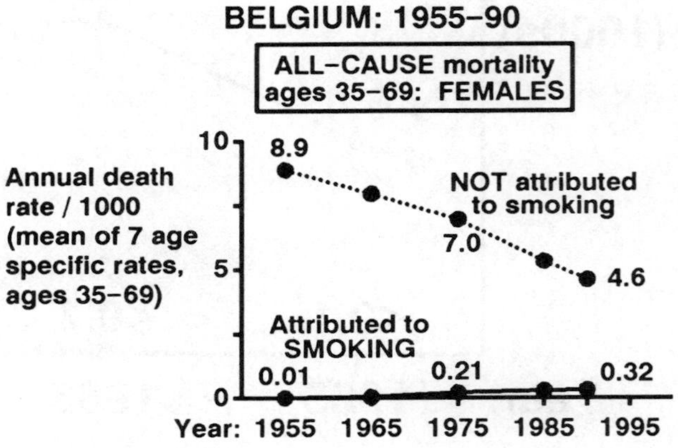

BELGIUM

ALL CANCER DEATHS (annual rates per 1000): Trends in mortality attributed to smoking, and in other mortality

	Males				Females			
	35–69		70–79		35–69		70–79	
Attributed to SMOKING?	Yes	No	Yes	No	Yes	No	Yes	No
1955	1.05	2.17	1.57	11.9	0.00	2.56	0.00	10.2
1965	1.93	2.03	4.55	11.5	0.01	2.44	0.05	9.77
1975	2.31	1.90	8.50	10.5	0.05	2.38	0.18	8.67
1985	2.52	1.75	10.7	10.2	0.10	2.17	0.28	8.38
1990	2.16	1.69	9.23	9.96	0.12	2.01	0.22	7.60

35–69 = mean of 7 age–specific rates; 70–79 = mean of 2 rates (70–74 & 75–79) Peto, Lopez et al, 1992, 1994

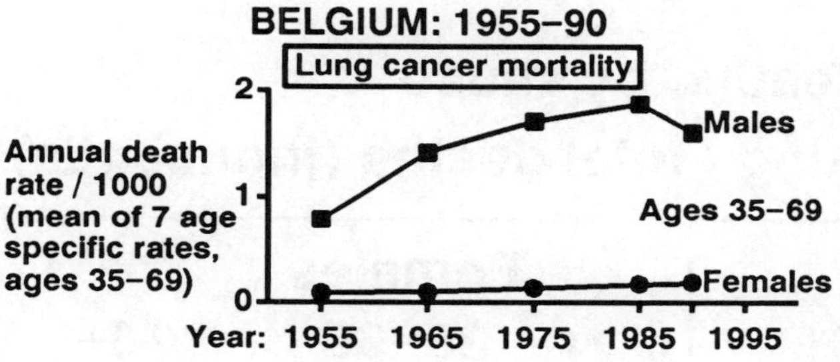

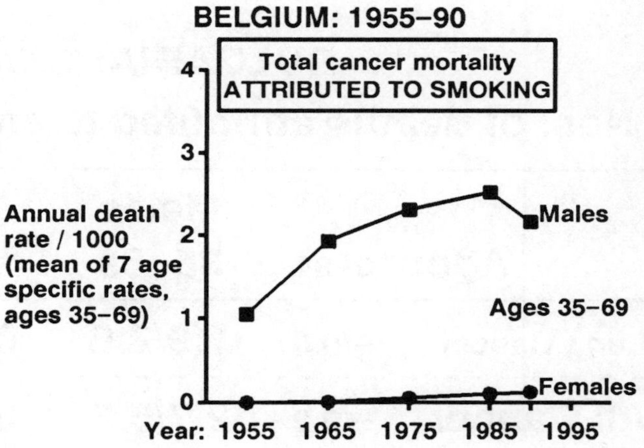

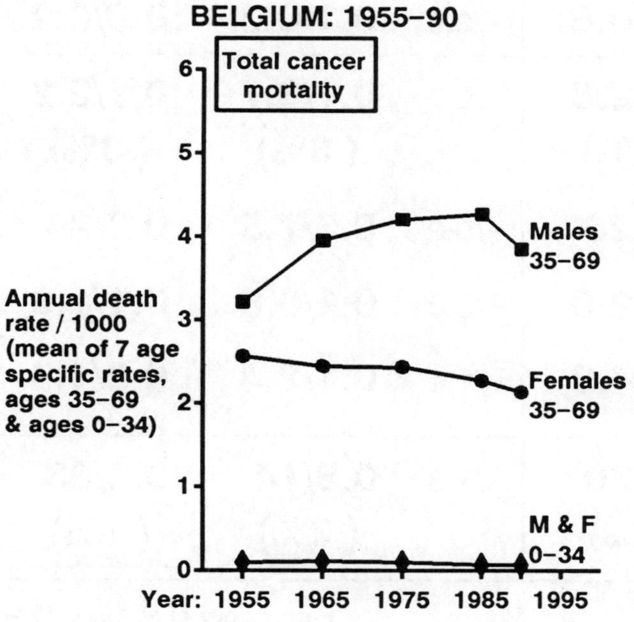

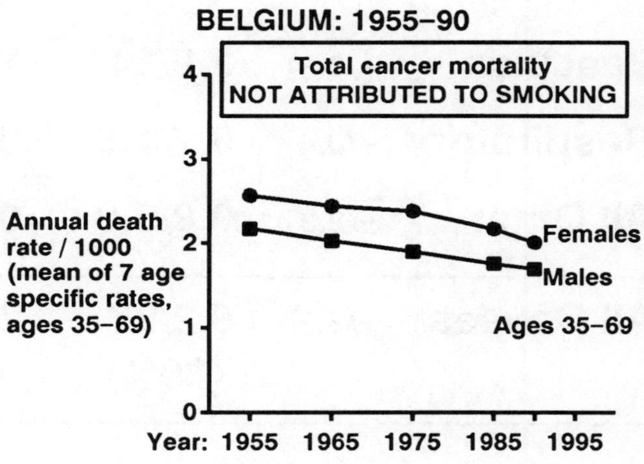

BULGARIA: 1990
Relative importance of deaths in MIDDLE age (35–69)

Age range (years)	Deaths attributed to SMOKING / total deaths (thousands) Males	Females	Mean years lost PER DEATH FROM SMOKING
0–34	–/3.3	–/1.8	–
35–69	8.2/27	0.5/14	20 years
70+	2.2/30	0.4/33	8 years
All ages	10/60	0.9/49	17 years

Peto, Lopez et al, 1992, 1994

BULGARIA: 1990 deaths, by cause
Nos. of deaths attributed to smoking / total deaths (thousands)

	Males			Females		
Age:	0–34	35–69	70+	0–34	35–69	70+
Lung Cancer	–/0.0	1.9/2.0	0.4/0.6	–/0.0	0.1/0.3	0.0/0.2
All Cancer	–/0.2	2.7/5.8 (47%)	0.6/2.8 (21%)	–/0.2	0.1/3.7 (3%)	0.1/2.2 (3%)
Vascular	–/0.3	3.9/14	1.0/20	–/0.2	0.3/7.5	0.2/24
Respiratory	–/0.4	0.7/1.6	0.5/2.0	–/0.3	0.1/0.6	0.1/1.6
All Other	–/2.3	0.8/5.8	0.1/4.2	–/1.1	0.1/2.4	0.0/4.5
All Causes	–/3.3	8.2/27 (30%)	2.2/30 (7%)	–/1.8	0.5/14 (3%)	0.4/33 (1%)

Peto, Lopez et al, 1992, 1994

BULGARIA: 1990

RISKS OF DYING AT AGES 0–34 and 35–69

(Probability that someone entering an age range would die during it, if the death rates in 1990 were to persist unchanged)

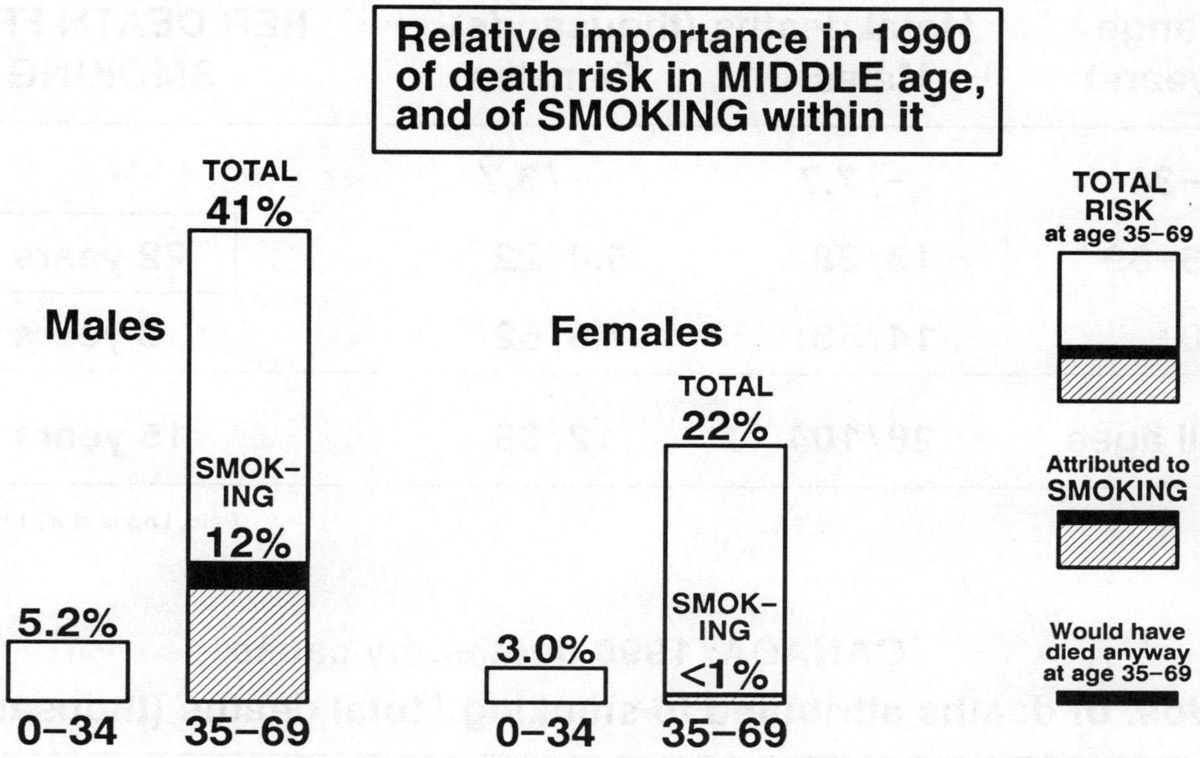

Peto, Lopez et al, 1992, 1994

BULGARIA: 1990 deaths, all ages

Nos. of deaths attributed to smoking / total deaths (thousands)

	Males	Females	Males + Females
All Cancer	3.3/8.9 (38%)	0.2/6.1 (3%)	3.5/15 (23%)
All Causes	10/60 (17%)	0.9/49 (2%)	11/109 (10%)

Peto, Lopez et al, 1992, 1994

CANADA: 1990
Relative importance of deaths in MIDDLE age (35–69)

Age range (years)	Deaths attributed to SMOKING / total deaths (thousands) Males	Females	Mean years lost PER DEATH FROM SMOKING
0–34	–/7.7	–/3.7	–
35–69	13/38	5.0/22	22 years
70+	14/58	7.0/62	8 years
All ages	28/104	12/88	15 years

Peto, Lopez et al, 1992, 1994

CANADA: 1990 deaths, by cause
Nos. of deaths attributed to smoking / total deaths (thousands)

	Males			Females		
Age:	0–34	35–69	70+	0–34	35–69	70+
Lung Cancer	–/0.0	4.7/5.1	4.1/4.5	–/0.0	1.9/2.3	1.5/1.9
All Cancer	–/0.5	6.8/14 (50%)	6.0/15 (40%)	–/0.4	2.4/11 (22%)	2.0/12 (16%)
Vascular	–/0.3	4.0/13	3.5/26	–/0.2	1.3/5.3	2.4/31
Respiratory	–/0.1	1.1/1.8	3.4/7.4	–/0.1	0.6/1.1	1.7/5.8
All Other	–/6.8	1.6/9.8	1.1/10	–/3.0	0.8/4.7	0.9/14
All Causes	–/7.7	13/38 (35%)	14/58 (24%)	–/3.7	5.0/22 (23%)	7.0/62 (11%)

Peto, Lopez et al, 1992, 1994

CANADA: 1990

RISKS OF DYING AT AGES 0–34 and 35–69

(Probability that someone entering an age range would die during it, if the death rates in 1990 were to persist unchanged)

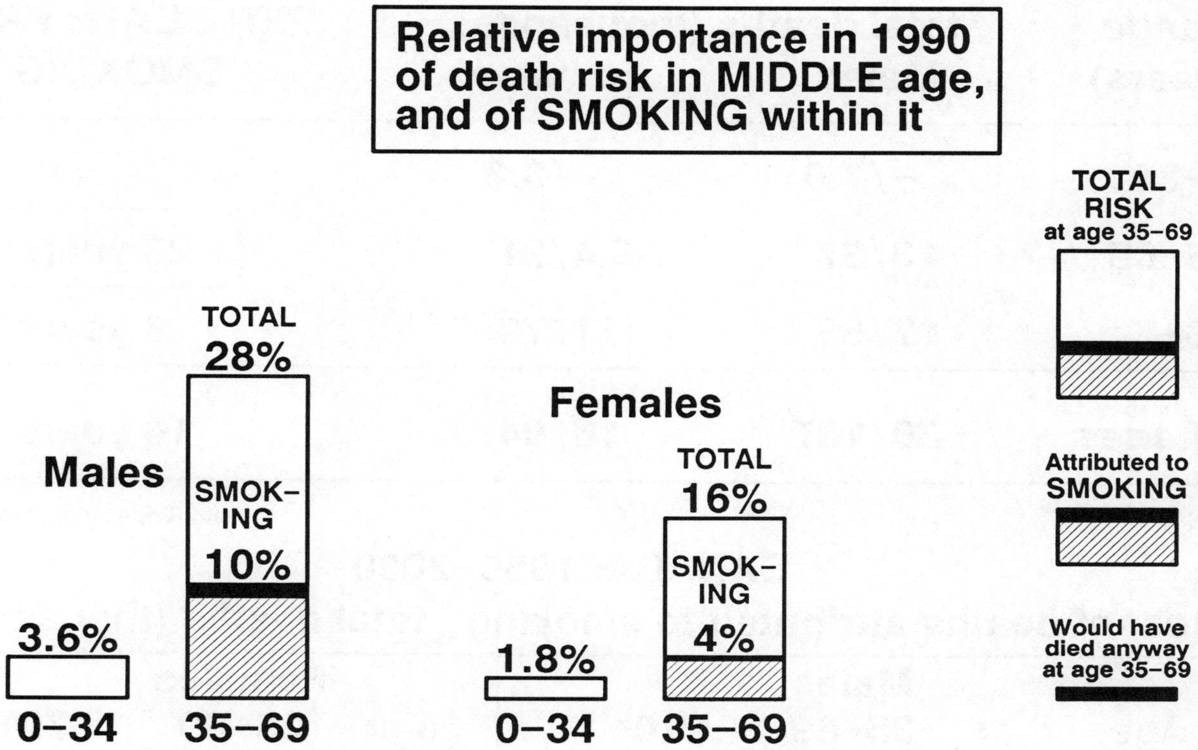

Peto, Lopez et al, 1992, 1994

CANADA: 1990 deaths, all ages

Nos. of deaths attributed to smoking / total deaths (thousands)

	Males	Females	Males + Females
All Cancer	13/29 (44%)	4.4/24 (19%)	17/52 (33%)
All Causes	28/104 (27%)	12/88 (14%)	40/192 (21%)

Peto, Lopez et al, 1992, 1994

CANADA: 1995 projections
Relative importance of deaths in MIDDLE age (35–69)

Age range (years)	Deaths attributed to SMOKING / total deaths (thousands) Males	Females	Mean years lost PER DEATH FROM SMOKING
0–34	–/7.0	–/3.3	–
35–69	13/37	5.4/21	23 years
70+	17/63	11/70	8 years
All ages	30/107	16/94	14 years

Peto, Lopez et al, 1992, 1994

CANADA: 1950–2000
Nos. of deaths attributed to smoking / total deaths (thousands)

Age:	Males 0–34	Males 35–69	Males 70+	Females 0–34	Females 35–69	Females 70+
1955	–/14	4.9/29 (17%)	1.4/32 (4%)	–/9.4	0.1/17 (0.6%)	0.1/27 (0.2%)
1965	–/12	8.4/34 (25%)	3.9/41 (10%)	–/7.5	0.5/19 (3%)	0.1/36 (0.1%)
1975	–/11	12/40 (30%)	8.1/45 (18%)	–/5.7	2.2/22 (10%)	0.7/43 (2%)
1985	–/8.2	13/38 (35%)	12/54 (23%)	–/4.0	4.6/22 (21%)	4.5/55 (8%)
1995 (projected)	–/7.0	13/37 (35%)	17/63 (26%)	–/3.3	5.4/21 (26%)	11/70 (15%)
50–year total*, mid–1950 to mid–2000: 1229/8271						
1950–2000, by age & sex	–/522	513/1780 (29%)	424/2350 (18%)	–/299	128/1010 (13%)	164/2310 (7%)

*Estimated as 10 times the sum of the five annual numbers (for 1955, 1965, 1975, 1985 & 1995)

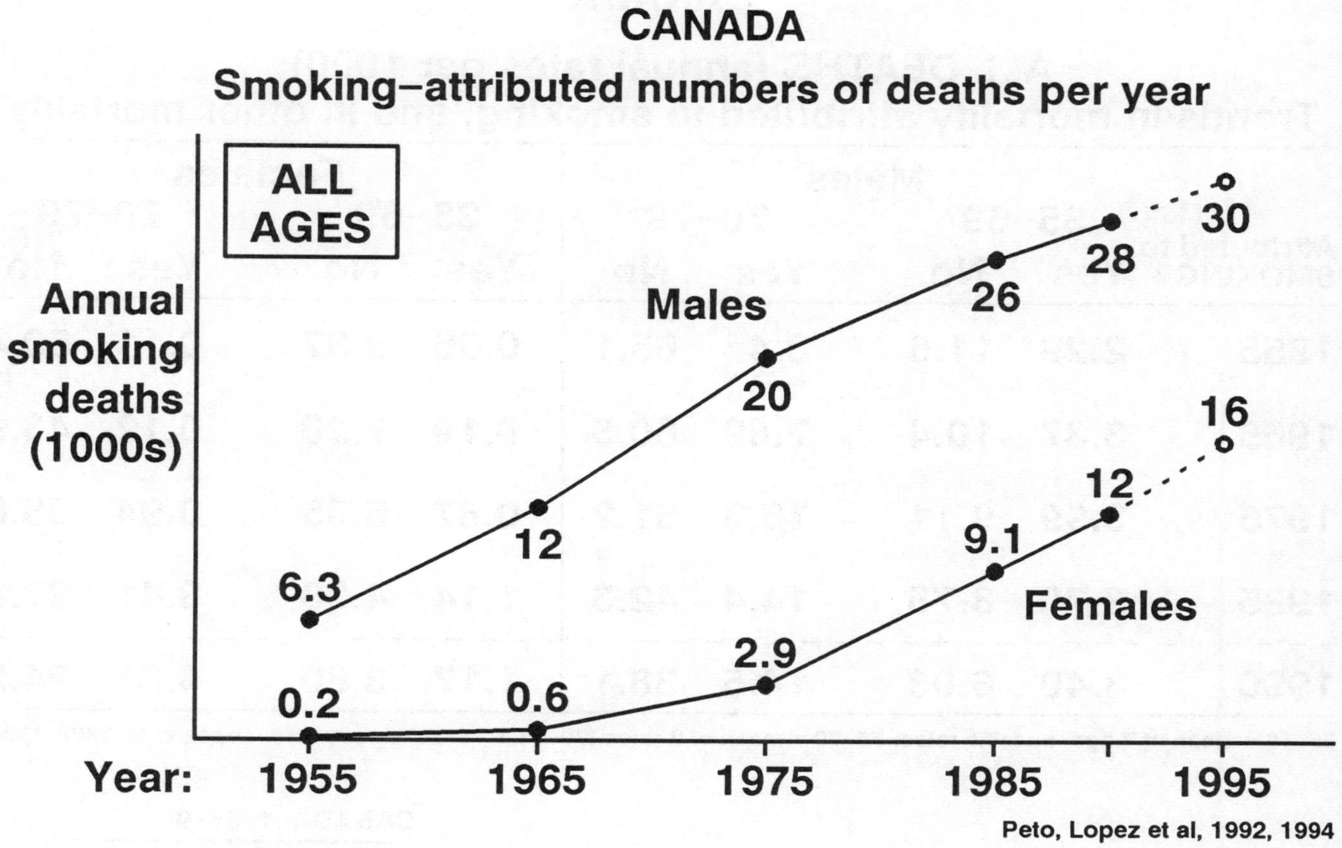
CANADA
Smoking–attributed numbers of deaths per year
ALL AGES
Annual smoking deaths (1000s)
Males
6.3
12
20
26
28
30
Females
0.2
0.6
2.9
9.1
12
16
Year:
1955
1965
1975
1985
1995
Peto, Lopez et al, 1992, 1994

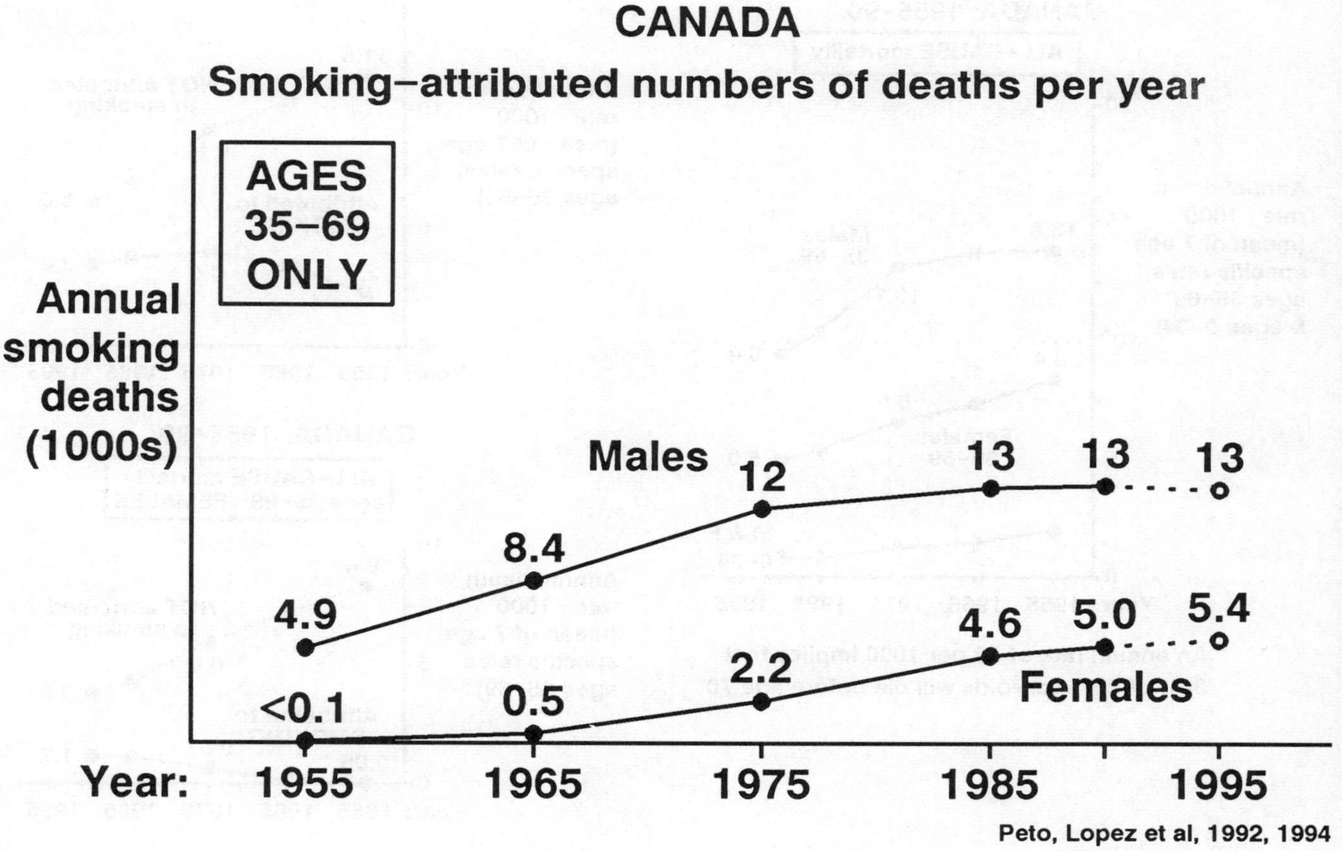
CANADA
Smoking–attributed numbers of deaths per year
AGES 35–69 ONLY
Annual smoking deaths (1000s)
Males
4.9
8.4
12
13
13
13
Females
<0.1
0.5
2.2
4.6
5.0
5.4
Year:
1955
1965
1975
1985
1995
Peto, Lopez et al, 1992, 1994

CANADA

ALL DEATHS (annual rates per 1000): Trends in mortality attributed to smoking, and in other mortality

	Males				Females			
	35–69		70–79		35–69		70–79	
Attributed to SMOKING?	Yes	No	Yes	No	Yes	No	Yes	No
1955	2.29	11.5	3.44	65.1	0.06	8.37	0.11	50.4
1965	3.37	10.4	7.89	60.5	0.19	7.20	0.12	43.9
1975	3.99	9.11	13.3	51.2	0.67	5.95	0.94	35.8
1985	3.70	6.78	14.4	42.3	1.14	4.30	3.41	27.3
1990	3.40	6.03	14.5	38.1	1.17	3.80	4.37	24.2

35–69 = mean of 7 age-specific rates; 70–79 = mean of 2 rates (70–74 & 75–79) Peto, Lopez et al, 1992, 1994

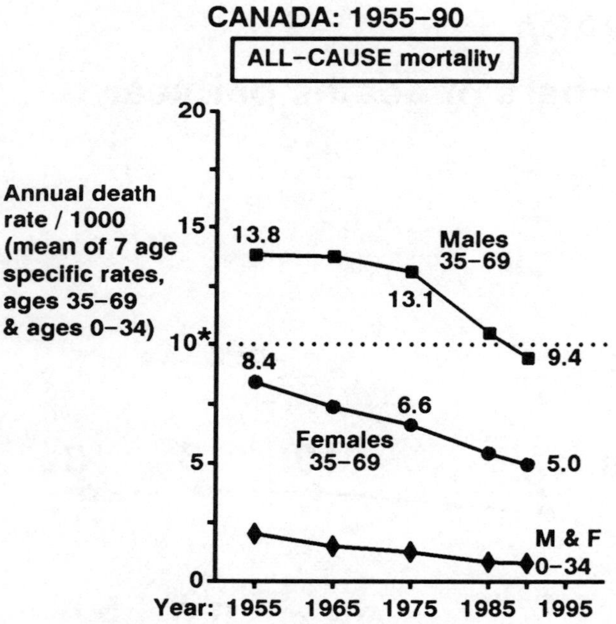

* An annual rate of 10 per 1000 implies that 30% of 35-year-olds will die before age 70

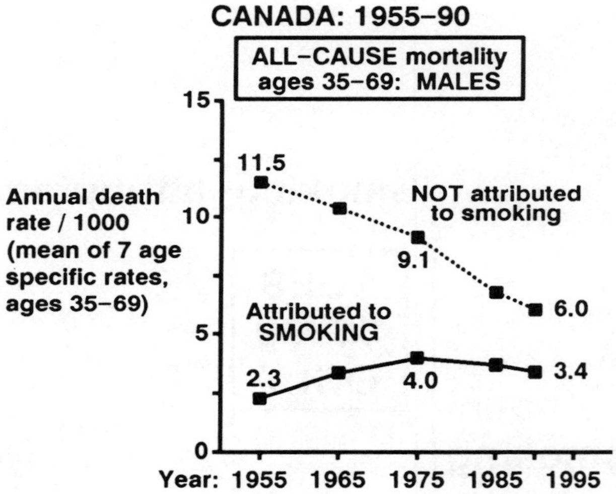

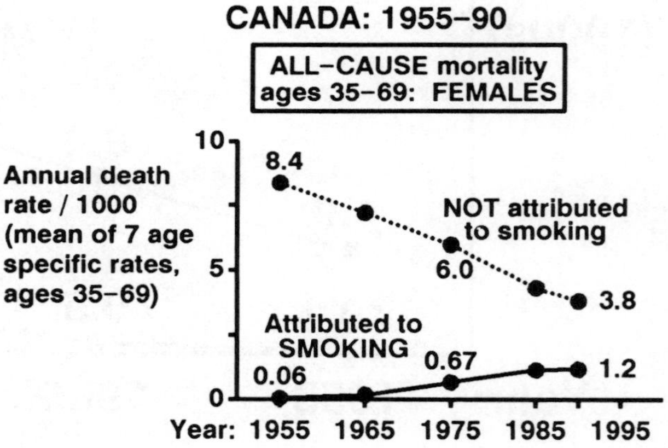

CANADA

ALL CANCER DEATHS (annual rates per 1000): Trends in mortality attributed to smoking, and in other mortality

	Males				Females			
	35–69		70–79		35–69		70–79	
Attributed to SMOKING?	Yes	No	Yes	No	Yes	No	Yes	No
1955	0.71	2.05	1.37	10.7	0.01	2.47	0.03	8.30
1965	1.11	1.82	2.99	9.87	0.05	2.36	0.03	8.00
1975	1.47	1.73	5.35	9.37	0.21	2.14	0.26	7.59
1985	1.72	1.69	6.48	9.13	0.49	1.96	1.21	7.13
1990	1.74	1.72	7.05	9.02	0.55	1.89	1.65	6.94

35–69 = mean of 7 age-specific rates; 70–79 = mean of 2 rates (70–74 & 75–79) Peto, Lopez et al, 1992, 1994

CANADA: 1955–90

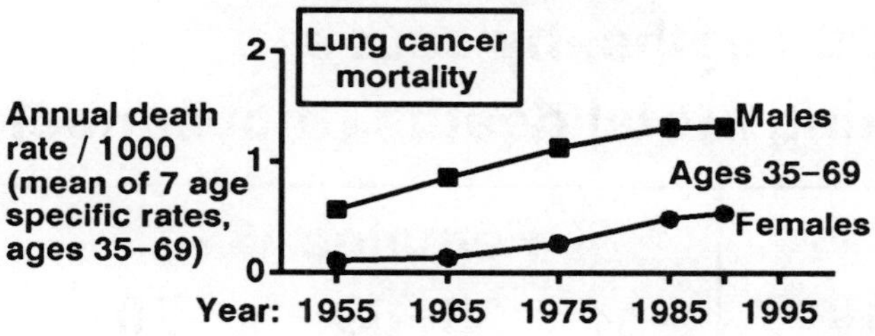

CANADA: 1955–90

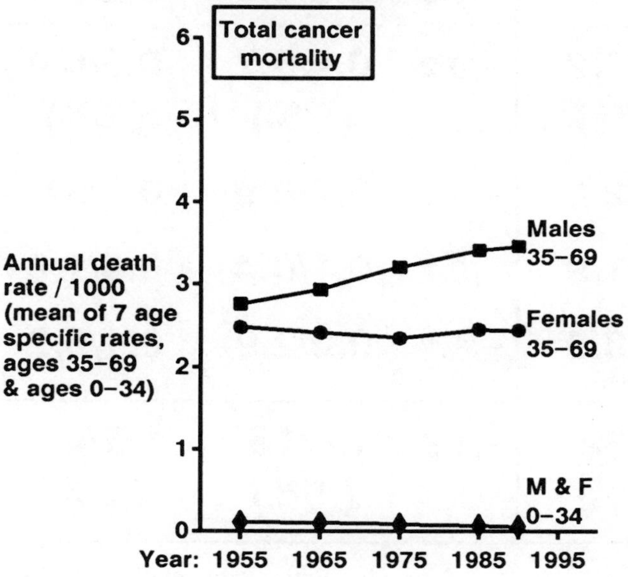

CANADA: 1955–90

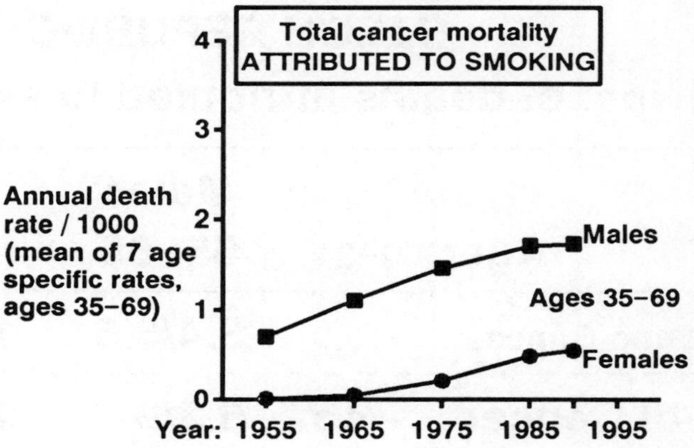

CANADA: 1955–90

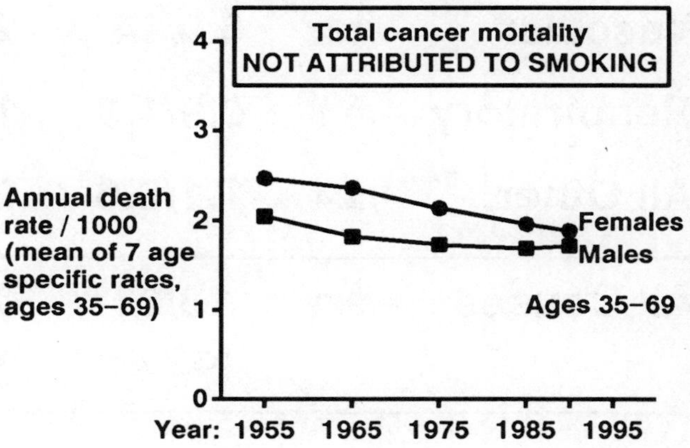

¶CZECH REPUBLIC: 1990
Relative importance of deaths in MIDDLE age (35–69)

Age range (years)	Deaths attributed to SMOKING / total deaths (thousands) Males	Females	Mean years lost PER DEATH FROM SMOKING
0–34	–/3.0	–/1.5	–
35–69	13/31	1.4/16	19 years
70+	6.1/32	1.5/45	7 years
All ages	19/66	2.9/63	15 years

Peto, Lopez et al, 1992, 1994

CZECH REPUBLIC: 1990 deaths, by cause
Nos. of deaths attributed to smoking / total deaths (thousands)

Age:	Males 0–34	Males 35–69	Males 70+	Females 0–34	Females 35–69	Females 70+
Lung Cancer	–/0.0	3.4/3.5	1.3/1.5	–/0.0	0.3/0.5	0.2/0.4
All Cancer	–/0.3	5.3/9.3 (57%)	2.1/6.2 (34%)	–/0.2	0.4/5.7 (7%)	0.3/6.4 (5%)
Vascular	–/0.2	6.0/14	2.6/20	–/0.1	0.7/6.9	0.8/31
Respiratory	–/0.1	0.9/1.3	1.0/1.9	–/0.1	0.1/0.4	0.3/1.6
All Other	–/2.4	1.1/6.6	0.3/3.9	–/1.1	0.2/2.9	0.1/6.2
All Causes	–/3.0	13/31 (42%)	6.1/32 (19%)	–/1.5	1.4/16 (9%)	1.5/45 (3%)

Peto, Lopez et al, 1992, 1994

CZECH REPUBLIC: 1990

RISKS OF DYING AT AGES 0–34 and 35–69

(Probability that someone entering an age range would die during it, if the death rates in 1990 were to persist unchanged)

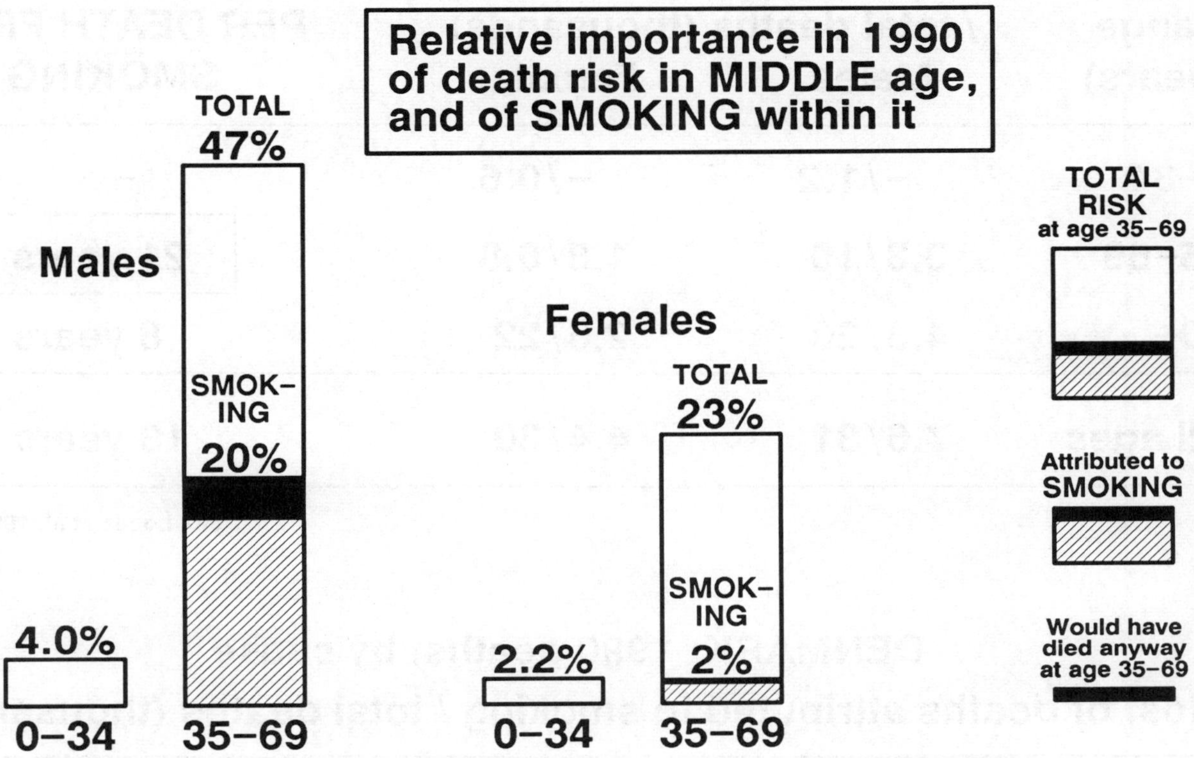

Peto, Lopez et al, 1992, 1994

CZECH REPUBLIC: 1990 deaths, all ages

Nos. of deaths attributed to smoking / total deaths (thousands)

	Males	Females	Males + Females
All Cancer	7.4/16 (47%)	0.7/12 (5%)	8.1/28 (29%)
All Causes	19/66 (29%)	2.9/63 (5%)	22/129 (17%)

Peto, Lopez et al, 1992, 1994

DENMARK: 1990
Relative importance of deaths in MIDDLE age (35–69)

Age range (years)	Deaths attributed to SMOKING / total deaths (thousands) Males	Females	Mean years lost PER DEATH FROM SMOKING
0–34	–/1.2	–/0.6	–
35–69	3.3/10	1.8/6.8	21 years
70+	4.3/20	2.6/22	8 years
All ages	7.6/31	4.4/30	13 years

Peto, Lopez et al, 1992, 1994

DENMARK: 1990 deaths, by cause
Nos. of deaths attributed to smoking / total deaths (thousands)

	Males			Females		
Age:	0–34	35–69	70+	0–34	35–69	70+
Lung Cancer	–/0.0	1.0/1.0	1.1/1.1	–/0.0	0.5/0.6	0.4/0.5
All Cancer	–/0.1	1.4/3.2 (45%)	1.6/4.5 (36%)	–/0.1	0.7/3.0 (23%)	0.6/4.1 (14%)
Vascular	–/0.0	1.0/3.6	1.3/9.8	–/0.0	0.5/1.6	1.0/12
Respiratory	–/0.0	0.4/0.5	1.0/1.9	–/0.0	0.4/0.5	0.6/1.6
All Other	–/1.0	0.5/3.0	0.3/3.2	–/0.5	0.3/1.7	0.3/4.4
All Causes	–/1.2	3.3/10 (32%)	4.3/20 (22%)	–/0.6	1.8/6.8 (27%)	2.6/22 (11%)

Peto, Lopez et al, 1992, 1994

DENMARK: 1990
RISKS OF DYING AT AGES 0–34 and 35–69
(Probability that someone entering an age range would die during it, if the death rates in 1990 were to persist unchanged)

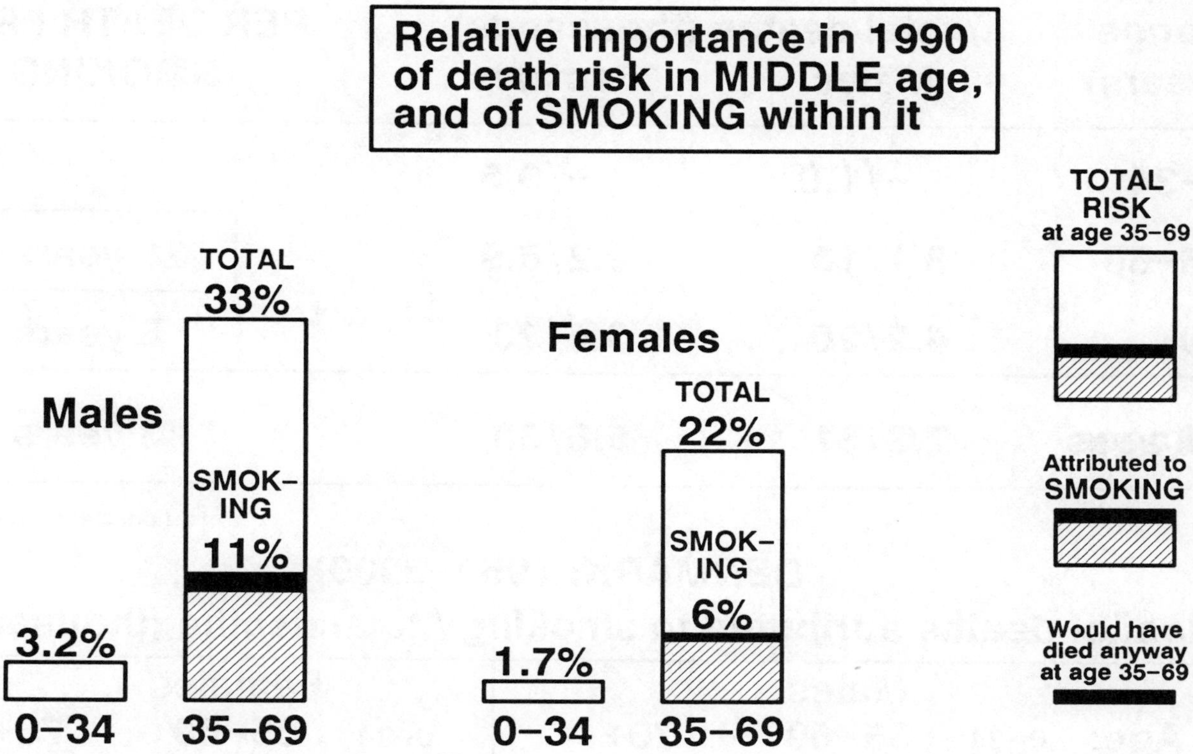

Peto, Lopez et al, 1992, 1994

DENMARK: 1990 deaths, all ages
Nos. of deaths attributed to smoking / total deaths (thousands)

	Males	Females	Males + Females
All Cancer	3.1/7.8 (39%)	1.3/7.2 (18%)	4.3/15 (29%)
All Causes	7.6/31 (25%)	4.4/30 (15%)	12/61 (20%)

Peto, Lopez et al, 1992, 1994

DENMARK: 1995 projections
Relative importance of deaths in MIDDLE age (35–69)

Age range (years)	Deaths attributed to SMOKING / total deaths (thousands) Males	Females	Mean years lost PER DEATH FROM SMOKING
0–34	–/1.0	–/0.5	–
35–69	3.1/10	2.2/6.9	21 years
70+	4.2/20	3.4/23	8 years
All ages	7.3/31	5.6/30	13 years

Peto, Lopez et al, 1992, 1994

DENMARK: 1950–2000
Nos. of deaths attributed to smoking / total deaths (thousands)

	Males			Females		
Age:	0–34	35–69	70+	0–34	35–69	70+
1955	–/2.2	1.4/7.8 (18%)	0.4/10 (4%)	–/1.5	0.0/6.3 (0%)	0.0/11 (0%)
1965	–/2.0	2.9/10 (28%)	1.4/14 (10%)	–/1.3	0.3/6.7 (4%)	0.3/14 (2%)
1975	–/1.5	3.3/10 (31%)	2.7/16 (17%)	–/0.8	0.7/6.5 (10%)	0.6/16 (4%)
1985	–/1.3	3.6/11 (34%)	4.2/18 (23%)	–/0.6	1.5/6.6 (22%)	1.7/21 (8%)
1995 (projected)	–/1.0	3.1/10 (30%)	4.2/20 (21%)	–/0.5	2.2/6.9 (31%)	3.4/23 (15%)
50–year total*, mid–1950 to mid–2000: 379/2575						
1950–2000, by age & sex	–/80	143/488 (29%)	129/780 (17%)	–/47	47/330 (14%)	60/850 (7%)

*Estimated as 10 times the sum of the five annual numbers (for 1955, 1965, 1975, 1985 & 1995)

DENMARK

Smoking–attributed numbers of deaths per year

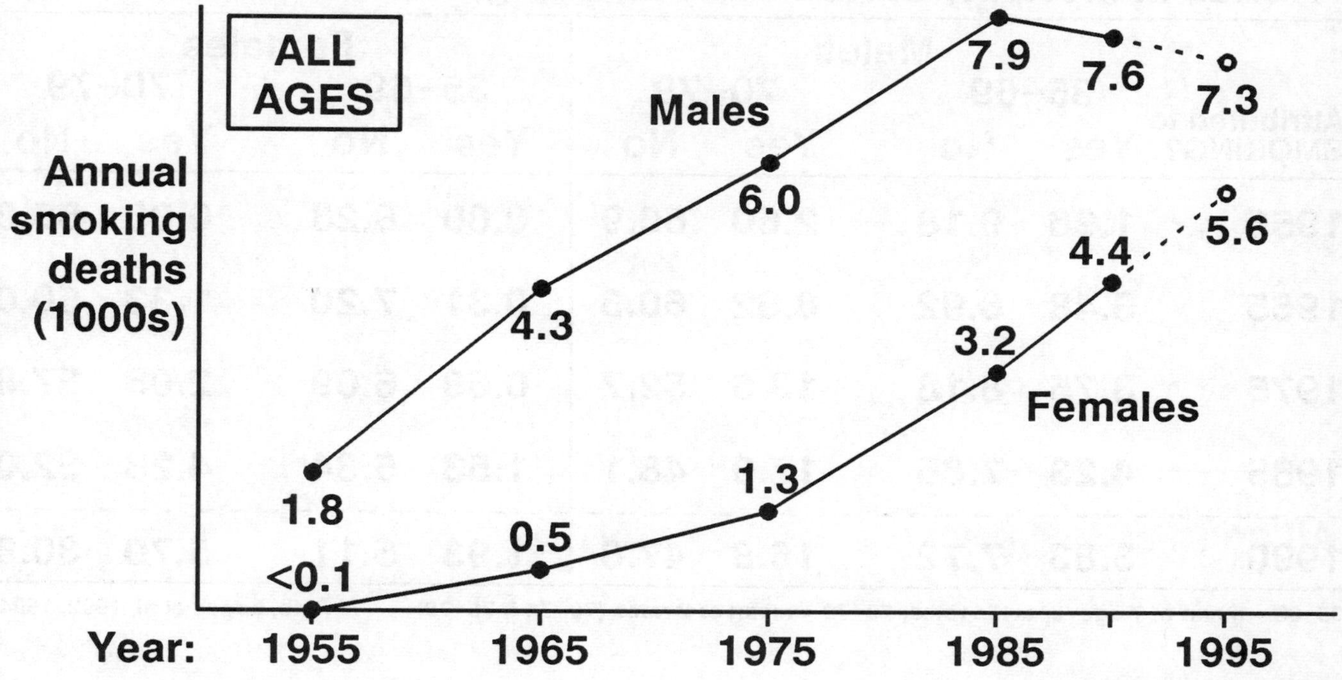

Peto, Lopez et al, 1992, 1994

DENMARK

Smoking–attributed numbers of deaths per year

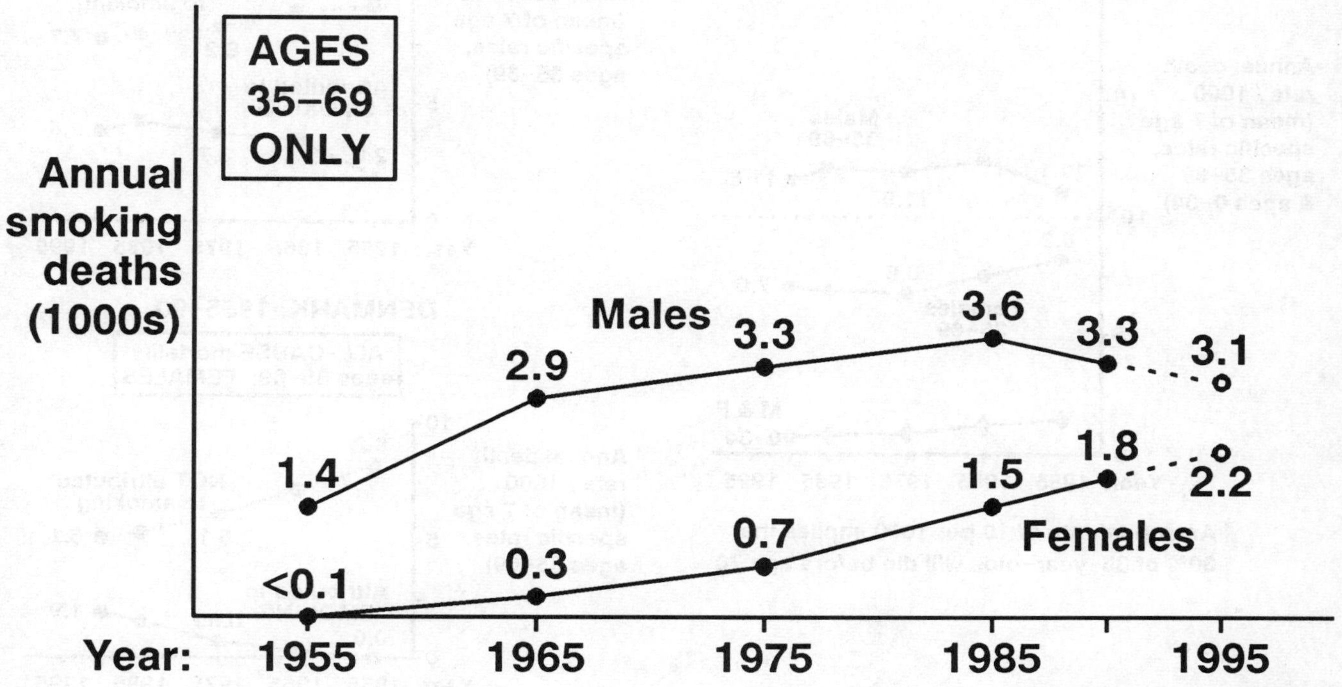

Peto, Lopez et al, 1992, 1994

DENMARK

ALL DEATHS (annual rates per 1000): Trends in mortality attributed to smoking, and in other mortality

	Males				Females			
	35–69		70–79		35–69		70–79	
Attributed to SMOKING?	Yes	No	Yes	No	Yes	No	Yes	No
1955	1.96	9.18	2.60	60.9	0.00	8.23	0.00	55.3
1965	3.48	8.92	8.52	60.3	0.31	7.20	1.33	50.0
1975	3.75	8.18	13.6	52.7	0.69	6.09	2.05	37.8
1985	4.23	7.86	17.0	48.1	1.53	5.34	4.23	32.0
1990	3.83	7.72	16.8	47.8	1.93	5.11	5.70	30.3

35–69 = mean of 7 age–specific rates; 70–79 = mean of 2 rates (70–74 & 75–79) Peto, Lopez et al, 1992, 1994

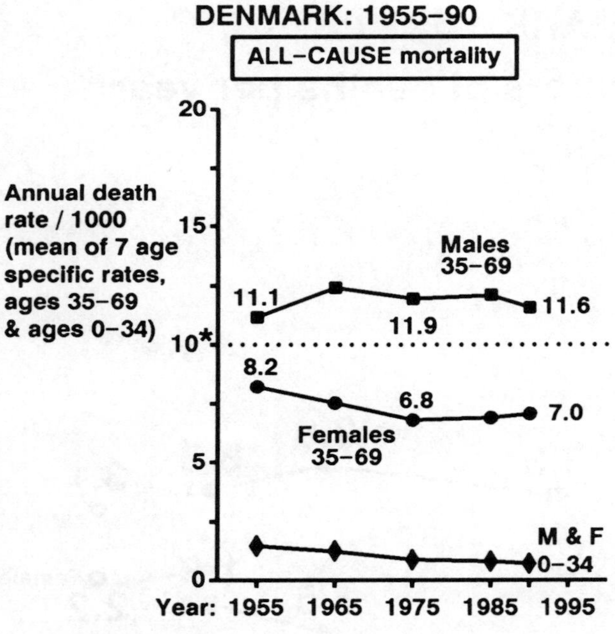

* An annual rate of 10 per 1000 implies that 30% of 35–year–olds will die before age 70

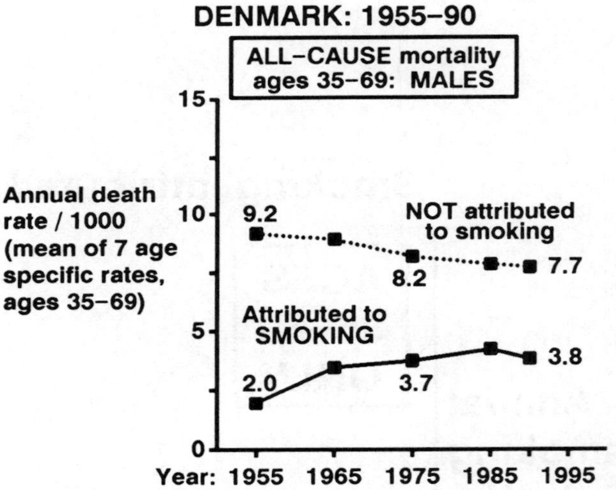

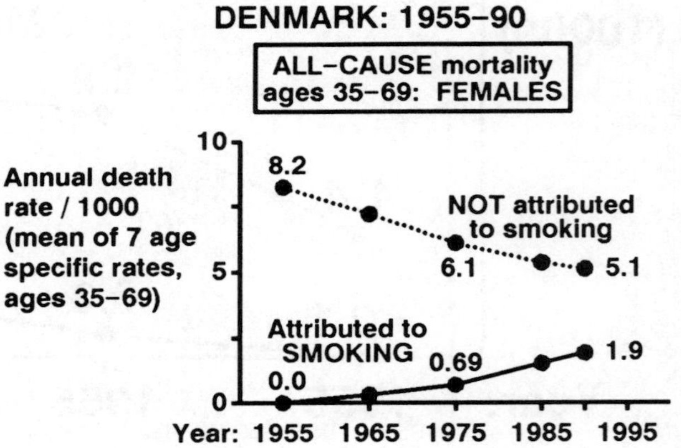

DENMARK

ALL CANCER DEATHS (annual rates per 1000): Trends in mortality attributed to smoking, and in other mortality

	Males				Females			
	35–69		70–79		35–69		70–79	
Attributed to SMOKING?	Yes	No	Yes	No	Yes	No	Yes	No
1955	0.79	2.26	1.19	12.9	0.00	2.93	0.00	11.0
1965	1.33	2.03	3.47	11.8	0.09	2.85	0.34	10.4
1975	1.49	1.85	5.62	10.4	0.24	2.59	0.60	8.89
1985	1.79	1.94	7.27	10.4	0.57	2.43	1.29	8.72
1990	1.69	2.01	7.25	11.0	0.72	2.39	1.85	8.61

35–69 = mean of 7 age-specific rates; 70–79 = mean of 2 rates (70–74 & 75–79) Peto, Lopez et al, 1992, 1994

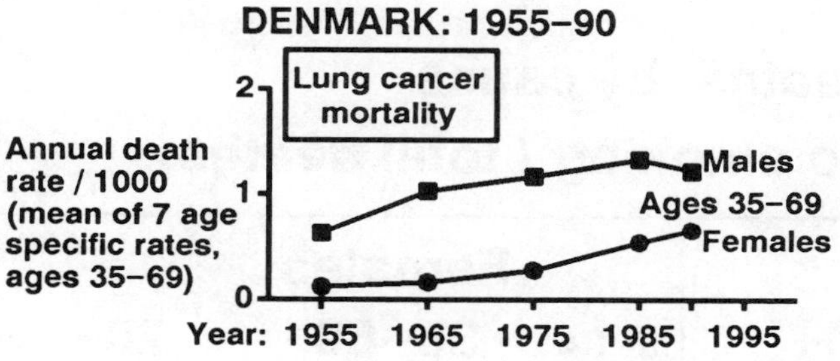

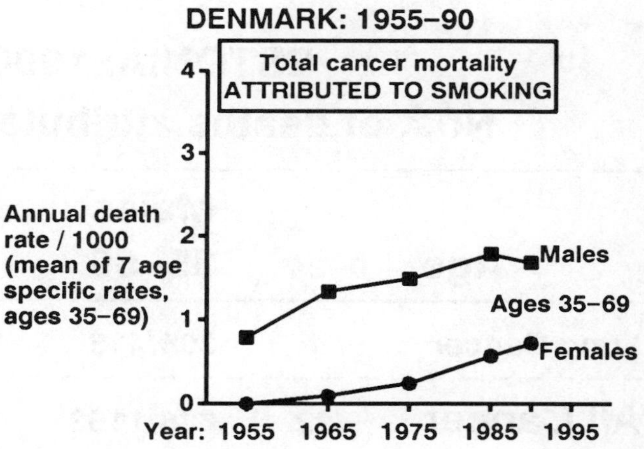

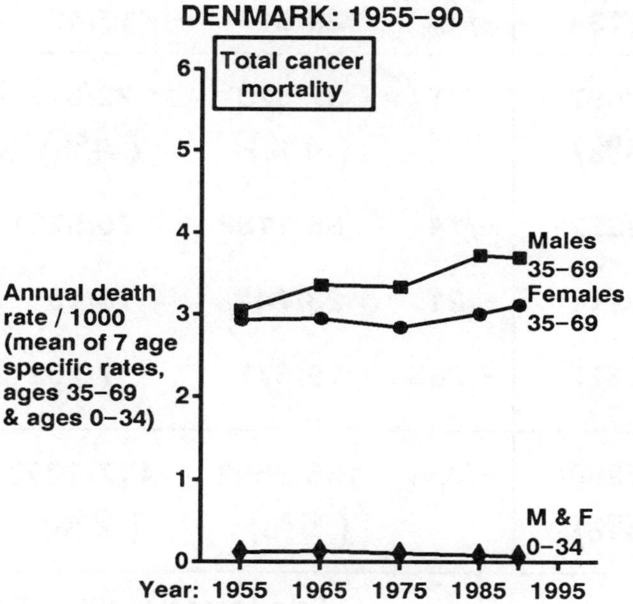

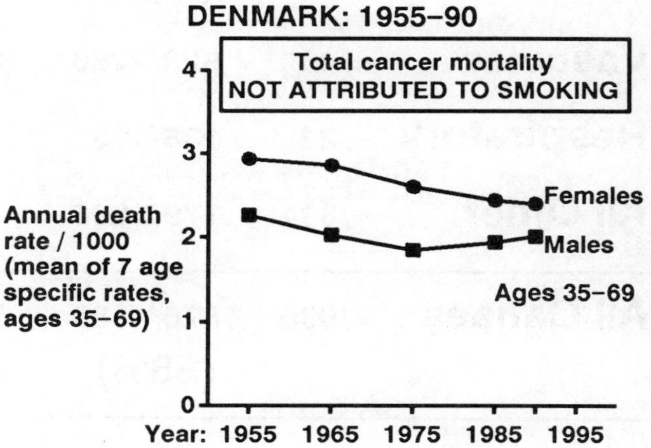

¶ESTONIA: 1990
Relative importance of deaths in MIDDLE age (35–69)

Age range (years)	Deaths attributed to SMOKING / total deaths (thousands) Males	Females	Mean years lost PER DEATH FROM SMOKING
0–34	–/0.9	–/0.4	–
35–69	1.9/4.9	0.2/2.7	20 years
70+	0.5/3.6	0.1/7.1	8 years
All ages	2.4/9.4	0.3/10	17 years

Peto, Lopez et al, 1992, 1994

ESTONIA: 1990 deaths, by cause
Nos. of deaths attributed to smoking / total deaths

Age:	Males 0–34	Males 35–69	Males 70+	Females 0–34	Females 35–69	Females 70+
Lung Cancer	–/1	398/416	120/134	–/0	29/61	17/43
All Cancer	–/32	638/1153 (55%)	174/497 (35%)	–/31	37/823 (4%)	22/612 (4%)
Vascular	–/40	923/2256	279/2621	–/14	86/1188	75/5701
Respiratory	–/24	136/183	68/111	–/21	23/74	13/75
All Other	–/834	179/1296	27/377	–/288	19/577	7/702
All Causes	–/930	1876/4888 (38%)	548/3606 (15%)	–/354	165/2662 (6%)	117/7090 (2%)

Peto, Lopez et al, 1992, 1994

ESTONIA: 1990

RISKS OF DYING AT AGES 0–34 and 35–69

(Probability that someone entering an age range would die during it, if the death rates in 1990 were to persist unchanged)

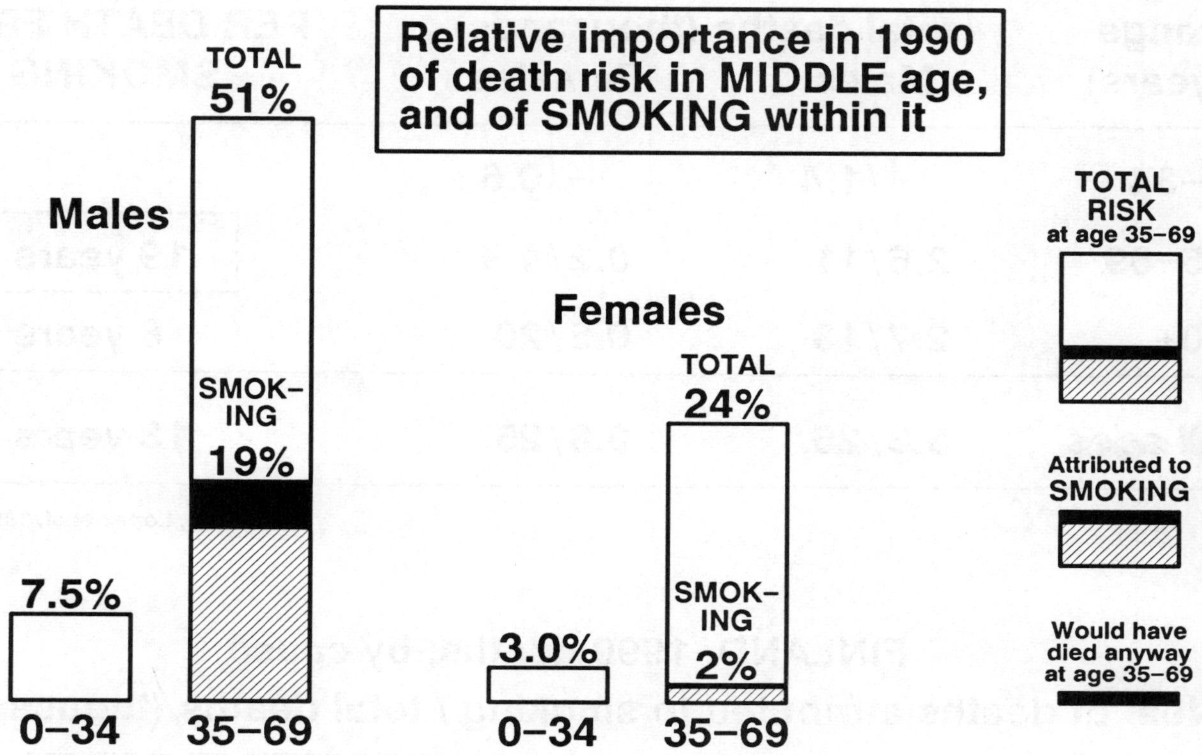

Peto, Lopez et al, 1992, 1994

ESTONIA: 1990 deaths, all ages

Nos. of deaths attributed to smoking / total deaths (thousands)

	Males	Females	Males + Females
All Cancer	0.8/1.7 (48%)	0.1/1.5 (4%)	0.9/3.1 (28%)
All Causes	2.4/9.4 (26%)	0.3/10 (3%)	2.7/20 (14%)

Peto, Lopez et al, 1992, 1994

FINLAND: 1990
Relative importance of deaths in MIDDLE age (35–69)

Age range (years)	Deaths attributed to SMOKING / total deaths (thousands) Males	Females	Mean years lost PER DEATH FROM SMOKING
0–34	–/1.4	–/0.6	–
35–69	2.6/11	0.2/4.9	19 years
70+	2.7/13	0.5/20	8 years
All ages	5.3/25	0.8/25	13 years

Peto, Lopez et al, 1992, 1994

FINLAND: 1990 deaths, by cause
Nos. of deaths attributed to smoking / total deaths (thousands)

	Males			Females		
Age:	0–34	35–69	70+	0–34	35–69	70+
Lung Cancer	–/0.0	0.8/0.8	0.7/0.8	–/0.0	0.1/0.2	0.1/0.2
All Cancer	–/0.1	1.0/2.3 (44%)	1.0/2.7 (39%)	–/0.1	0.1/1.8 (4%)	0.1/2.9 (5%)
Vascular	–/0.1	1.2/4.7	0.9/6.9	–/0.0	0.1/1.7	0.3/11
Respiratory	–/0.0	0.2/0.4	0.5/1.5	–/0.0	0.0/0.2	0.1/1.6
All Other	–/1.3	0.2/3.2	0.2/1.9	–/0.5	0.0/1.2	0.1/3.9
All Causes	–/1.4	2.6/11 (25%)	2.7/13 (21%)	–/0.6	0.2/4.9 (5%)	0.5/20 (3%)

Peto, Lopez et al, 1992, 1994

FINLAND: 1990

RISKS OF DYING AT AGES 0–34 and 35–69

(Probability that someone entering an age range would die during it, if the death rates in 1990 were to persist unchanged)

Relative importance in 1990 of death risk in MIDDLE age, and of SMOKING within it

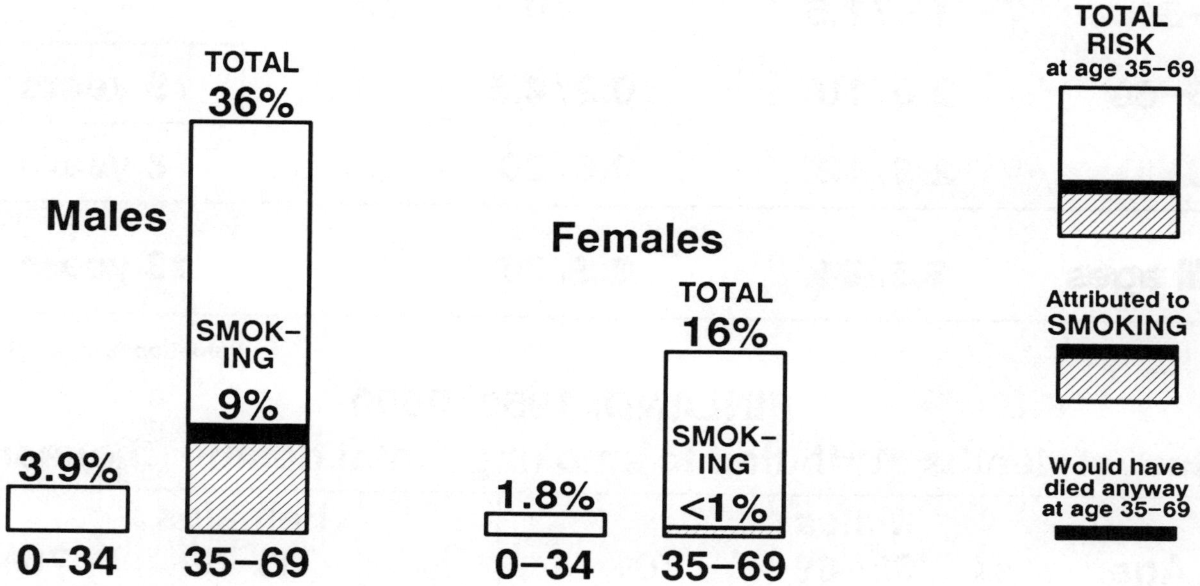

Peto, Lopez et al, 1992, 1994

FINLAND: 1990 deaths, all ages

Nos. of deaths attributed to smoking / total deaths (thousands)

	Males	Females	Males + Females
All Cancer	2.0/5.0 (41%)	0.2/4.8 (5%)	2.3/9.8 (23%)
All Causes	5.3/25 (21%)	0.8/25 (3%)	6.1/50 (12%)

Peto, Lopez et al, 1992, 1994

FINLAND: 1995 projections
Relative importance of deaths in MIDDLE age (35–69)

Age range (years)	Deaths attributed to SMOKING / total deaths (thousands) Males	Females	Mean years lost PER DEATH FROM SMOKING
0–34	–/1.5	–/0.7	–
35–69	2.0/10	0.2/4.8	19 years
70+	2.3/12	0.6/20	8 years
All ages	4.3/24	0.8/25	13 years

Peto, Lopez et al, 1992, 1994

FINLAND: 1950–2000
Nos. of deaths attributed to smoking / total deaths (thousands)

Age:	Males 0–34	Males 35–69	Males 70+	Females 0–34	Females 35–69	Females 70+
1955	–/3.5	3.5/10 (34%)	0.8/6.7 (12%)	–/2.2	0.1/6.6 (2%)	0.0/10 (0%)
1965	–/2.4	4.8/12 (39%)	1.6/8.5 (19%)	–/1.3	0.0/7.0 (0%)	0.0/13 (0%)
1975	–/2.0	4.2/12 (35%)	2.2/9.7 (23%)	–/0.8	0.0/6.1 (0.7%)	0.1/13 (0.5%)
1985	–/1.4	3.4/11 (32%)	3.1/13 (23%)	–/0.6	0.3/4.9 (6%)	0.4/18 (2%)
1995 (projected)	–/1.5	2.0/10 (19%)	2.3/12 (19%)	–/0.7	0.2/4.8 (4%)	0.6/20 (3%)
50–year total*, mid–1950 to mid–2000: 296/2247						
1950–2000, by age & sex	–/108	179/550 (33%)	100/499 (20%)	–/56	6.0/294 (2%)	11/740 (1%)

*Estimated as 10 times the sum of the five annual numbers (for 1955, 1965, 1975, 1985 & 1995)

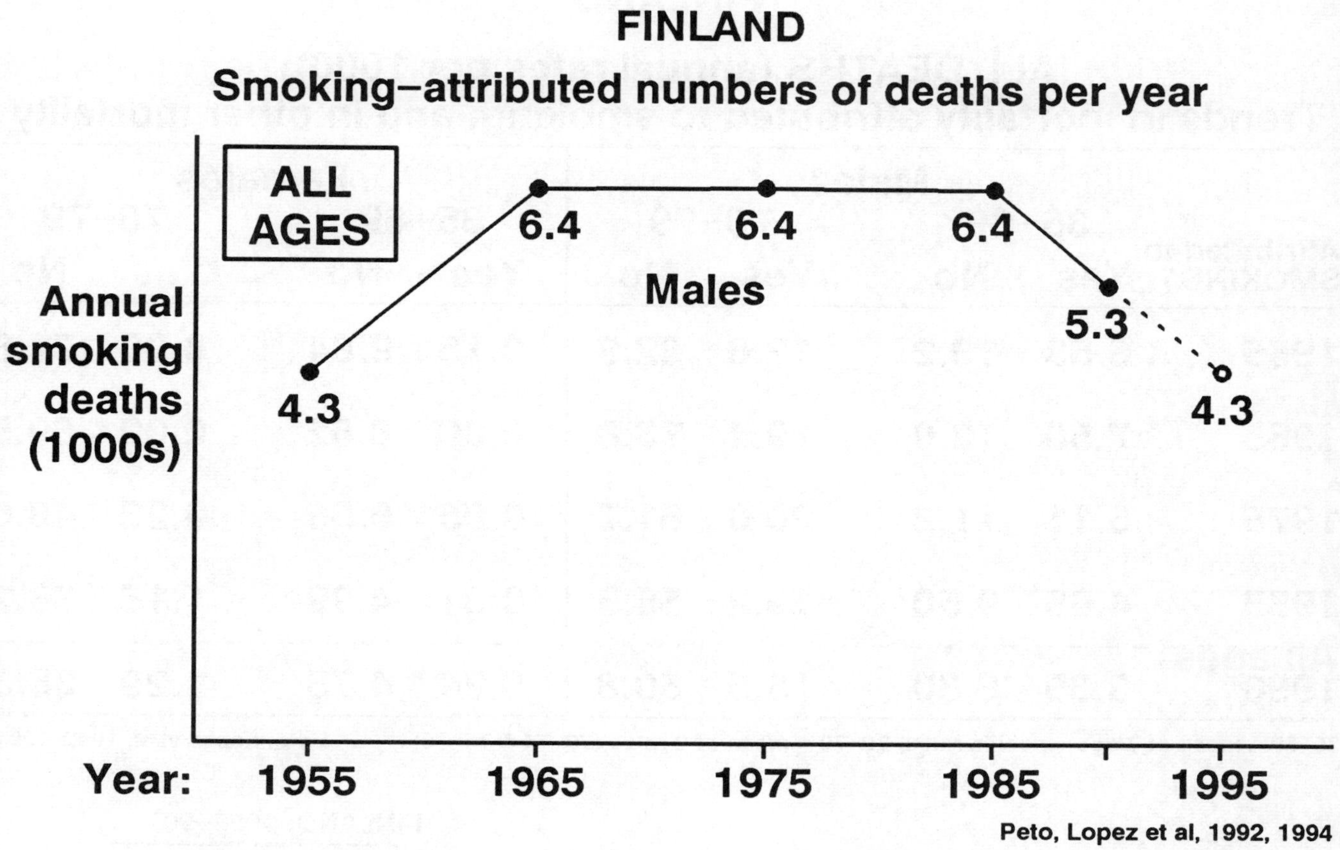
FINLAND
Smoking–attributed numbers of deaths per year
ALL AGES
Annual smoking deaths (1000s)
Males
4.3
6.4
6.4
6.4
5.3
4.3
Year: 1955 1965 1975 1985 1995
Peto, Lopez et al, 1992, 1994

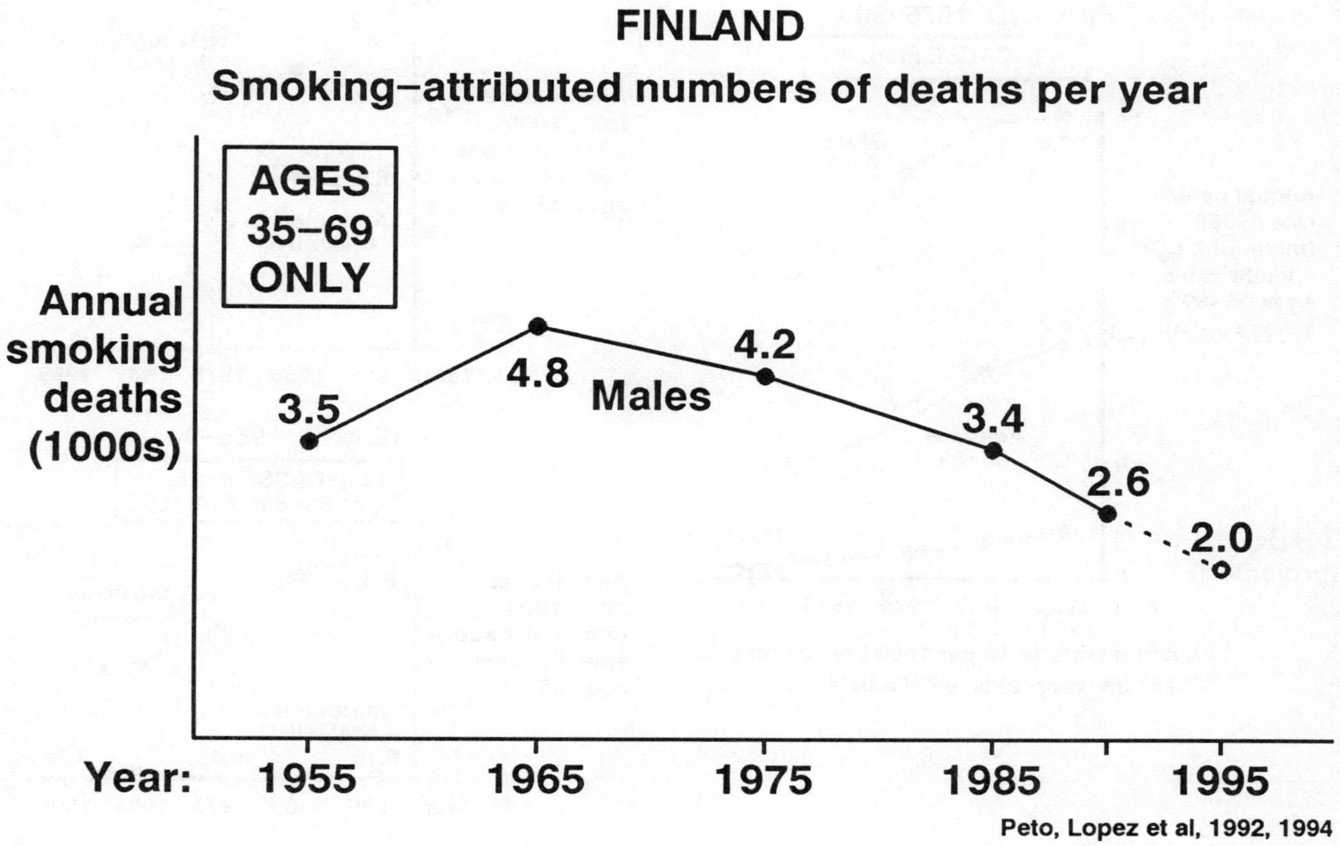
FINLAND
Smoking–attributed numbers of deaths per year
AGES 35–69 ONLY
Annual smoking deaths (1000s)
Males
3.5
4.8
4.2
3.4
2.6
2.0
Year: 1955 1965 1975 1985 1995
Peto, Lopez et al, 1992, 1994

FINLAND

ALL DEATHS (annual rates per 1000): Trends in mortality attributed to smoking, and in other mortality

	Males				Females			
	35–69		70–79		35–69		70–79	
Attributed to SMOKING?	Yes	No	Yes	No	Yes	No	Yes	No
1955	6.53	13.2	12.6	82.5	0.15	9.84	0.00	71.8
1965	7.50	12.0	19.4	73.8	0.00	8.82	0.00	69.5
1975	6.11	11.2	20.0	61.7	0.05	6.65	0.23	48.6
1985	4.65	9.50	19.2	55.5	0.31	4.99	1.15	38.7
1990	3.35	9.30	15.6	50.8	0.24	4.75	1.29	35.3

35–69 = mean of 7 age-specific rates; 70–79 = mean of 2 rates (70–74 & 75–79) Peto, Lopez et al, 1992, 1994

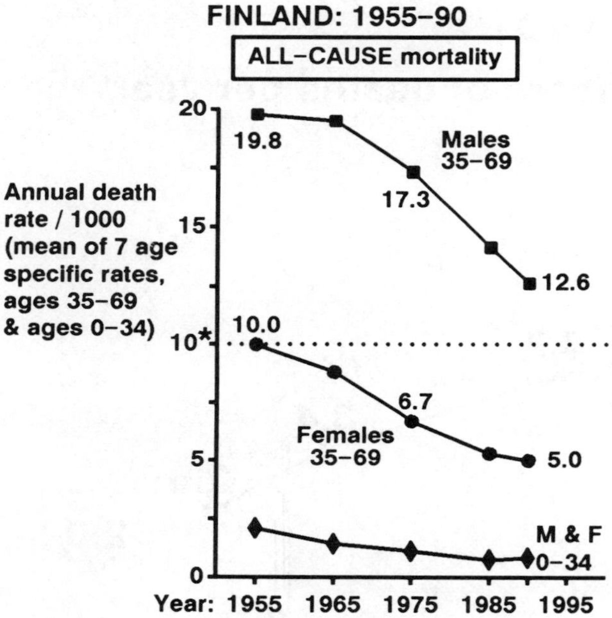

* An annual rate of 10 per 1000 implies that 30% of 35-year-olds will die before age 70

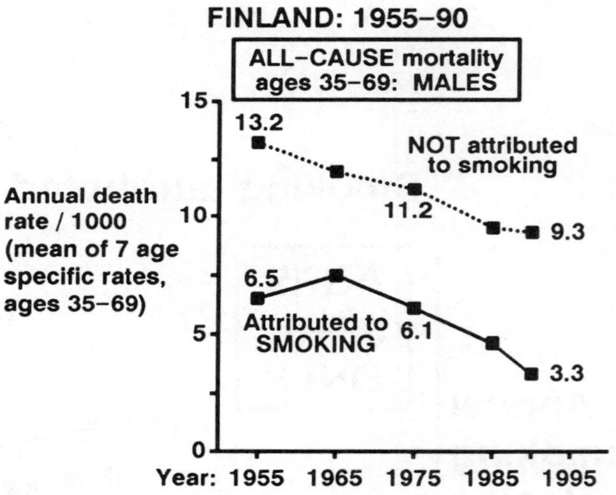

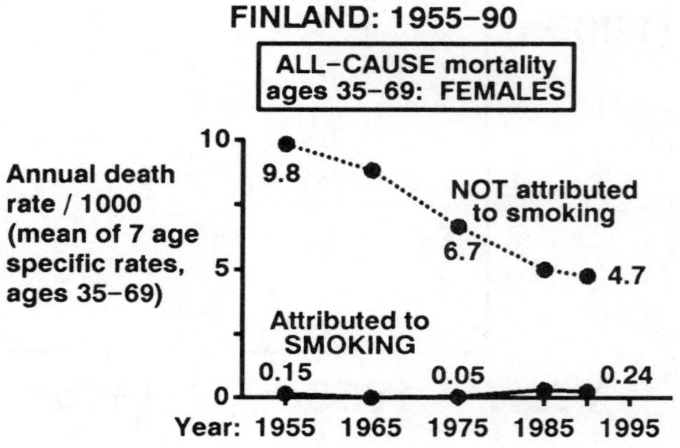

FINLAND

ALL CANCER DEATHS (annual rates per 1000): Trends in mortality attributed to smoking, and in other mortality

	Males				Females			
	35–69		70–79		35–69		70–79	
Attributed to SMOKING?	Yes	No	Yes	No	Yes	No	Yes	No
1955	2.02	2.44	4.50	12.0	0.03	2.35	0.00	9.73
1965	2.25	1.89	6.52	9.91	0.00	2.13	0.00	8.92
1975	1.96	1.78	7.37	9.62	0.01	1.96	0.07	7.88
1985	1.68	1.65	7.43	8.86	0.10	1.73	0.34	7.76
1990	1.33	1.62	6.70	9.12	0.08	1.79	0.43	7.22

35–69 = mean of 7 age-specific rates; 70–79 = mean of 2 rates (70–74 & 75–79) Peto, Lopez et al, 1992, 1994

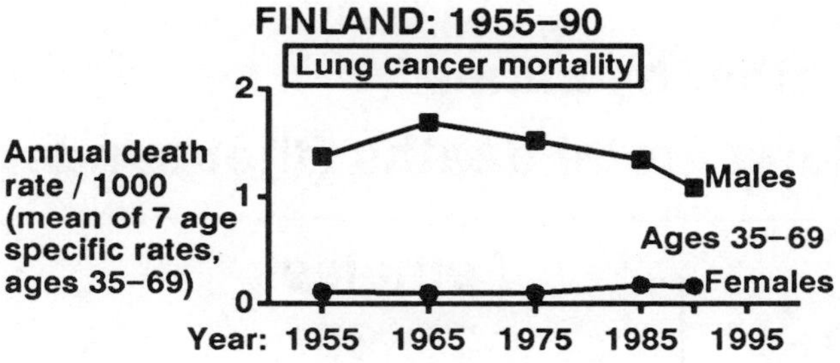

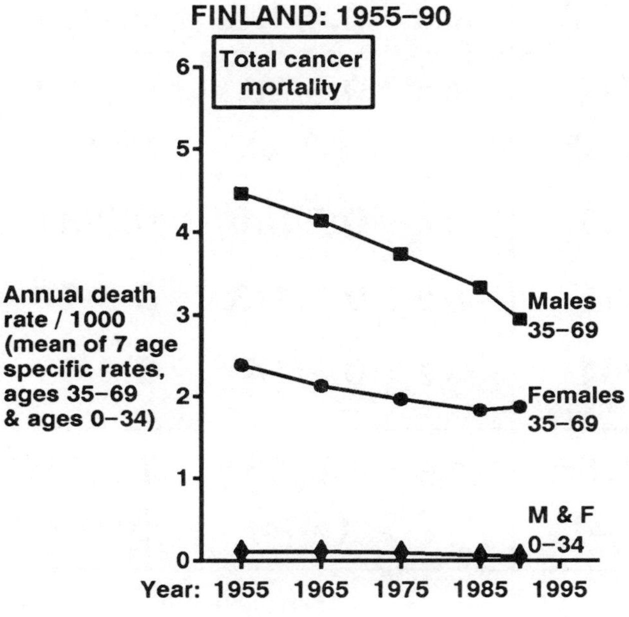

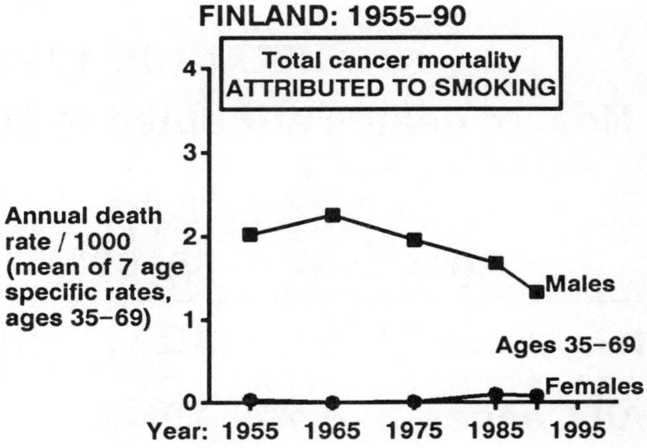

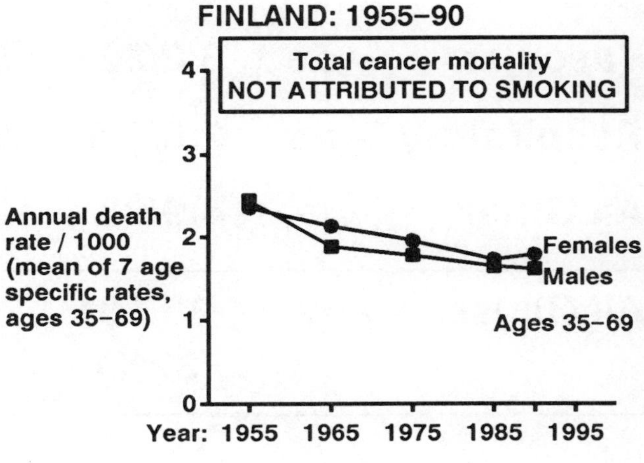

FRANCE: 1990
Relative importance of deaths in MIDDLE age (35–69)

Age range (years)	Deaths attributed to SMOKING / total deaths (thousands) Males	Females	Mean years lost PER DEATH FROM SMOKING
0–34	–/17	–/7.5	–
35–69	33/101	1.0/43	23 years
70+	25/155	1.2/203	7 years
All ages	57/273	2.2/254	16 years

Peto, Lopez et al, 1992, 1994

FRANCE: 1990 deaths, by cause
Nos. of deaths attributed to smoking / total deaths (thousands)

	Males			Females		
Age:	0–34	35–69	70+	0–34	35–69	70+
Lung Cancer	–/0.1	10/11	6.7/7.6	–/0.0	0.4/1.3	0.2/1.5
All Cancer	–/1.0	19/42 (47%)	12/41 (28%)	–/0.8	0.5/20 (2%)	0.3/33 (0.8%)
Vascular	–/0.6	6.2/22	5.0/57	–/0.4	0.2/8.0	0.3/87
Respiratory	–/0.3	2.0/3.9	5.3/16	–/0.2	0.1/1.3	0.5/17
All Other	–/15	4.9/33	2.7/41	–/6.2	0.2/14	0.2/66
All Causes	–/17	33/101 (32%)	25/155 (16%)	–/7.5	1.0/43 (2%)	1.2/203 (0.6%)

Peto, Lopez et al, 1992, 1994

FRANCE: 1990

RISKS OF DYING AT AGES 0–34 and 35–69

(Probability that someone entering an age range would die during it, if the death rates in 1990 were to persist unchanged)

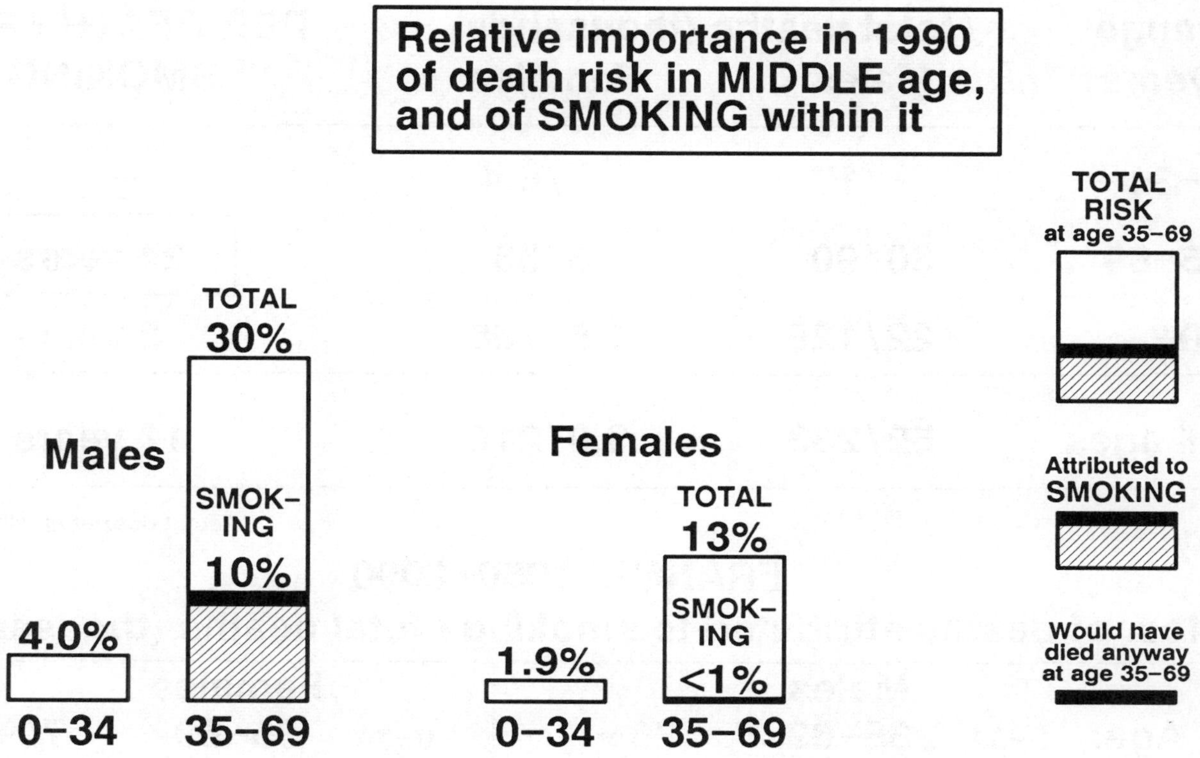

Peto, Lopez et al, 1992, 1994

FRANCE: 1990 deaths, all ages

Nos. of deaths attributed to smoking / total deaths (thousands)

	Males	Females	Males + Females
All Cancer	31/84 (37%)	0.8/54 (1%)	32/138 (23%)
All Causes	57/273 (21%)	2.2/254 (0.9%)	59/526 (11%)

Peto, Lopez et al, 1992, 1994

FRANCE: 1995 projections
Relative importance of deaths in MIDDLE age (35–69)

Age range (years)	Deaths attributed to SMOKING / total deaths (thousands) Males	Females	Mean years lost PER DEATH FROM SMOKING
0–34	–/17	–/6.4	–
35–69	30/90	1.5/38	24 years
70+	22/126	1.5/166	8 years
All ages	52/233	3.0/210	17 years

Peto, Lopez et al, 1992, 1994

FRANCE: 1950–2000
Nos. of deaths attributed to smoking / total deaths (thousands)

	Males			Females		
Age:	0–34	35–69	70+	0–34	35–69	70+
1955	–/31	16/109 (15%)	4.2/126 (3%)	–/21	0.0/74 (0%)	0.0/161 (0%)
1965	–/23	27/124 (22%)	10/132 (8%)	–/14	0.0/66 (0%)	0.0/182 (0%)
1975	–/21	31/115 (27%)	21/155 (14%)	–/11	0.0/55 (0%)	0.0/203 (0%)
1985	–/18	31/100 (32%)	27/169 (16%)	–/8.7	0.3/43 (0.7%)	0.8/214 (0.4%)
1995 (projected)	–/17	30/90 (34%)	22/126 (17%)	–/6.4	1.5/38 (4%)	1.5/166 (0.9%)
50–year total* (M=millions), mid–1950 to mid–2000: 2.2/26M						
1950–2000, by age & sex	–/1.1M	1.4/5.4M (26%)	0.8/7.1M (11%)	–/0.6M	0.02/2.8M (0.7%)	0.02/9.3M (0.2%)

*Estimated as 10 times the sum of the five annual numbers (for 1955, 1965, 1975, 1985 & 1995)

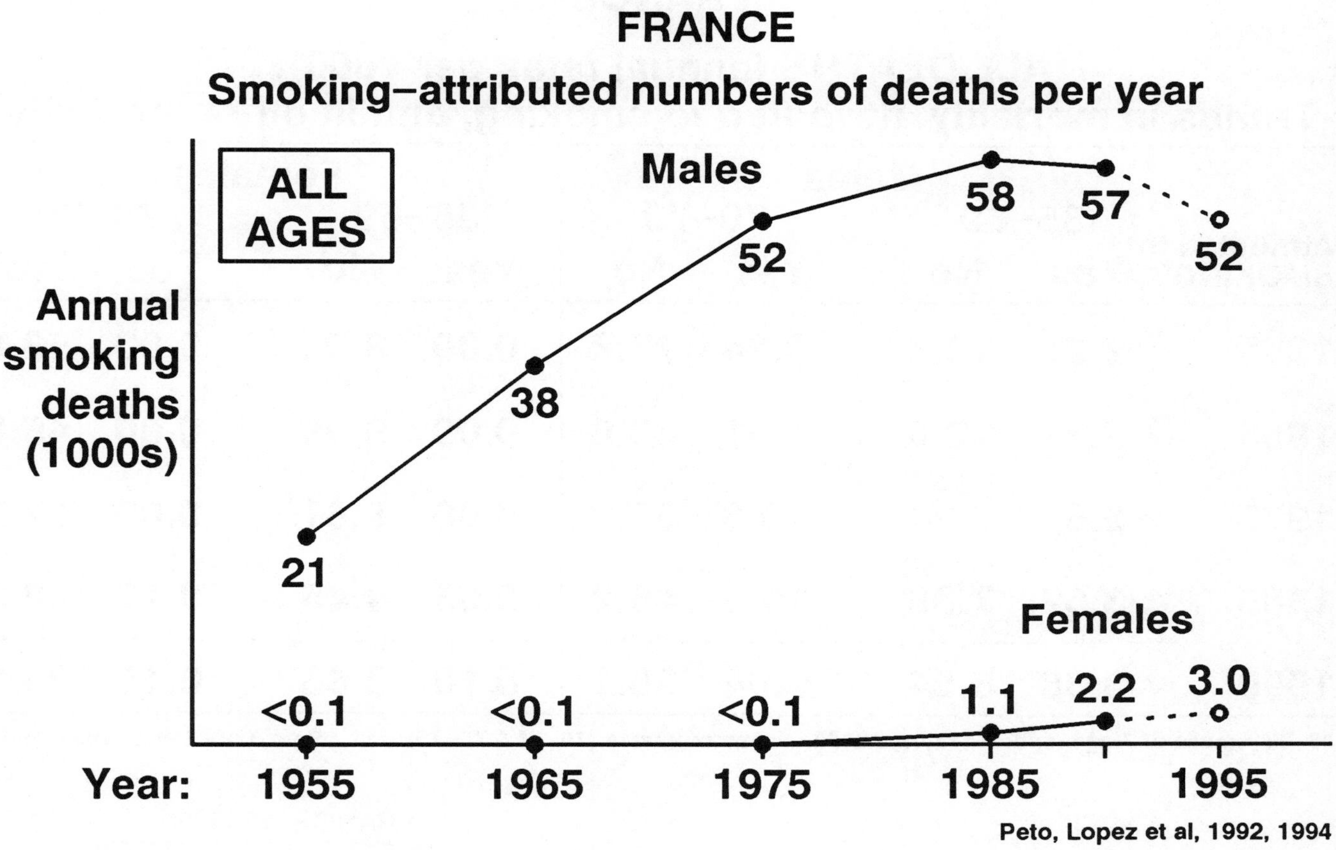
FRANCE
Smoking–attributed numbers of deaths per year
ALL AGES
Males
Annual smoking deaths (1000s)
21
38
52
58
57
52
Females
<0.1
<0.1
<0.1
1.1
2.2
3.0
Year:
1955
1965
1975
1985
1995
Peto, Lopez et al, 1992, 1994

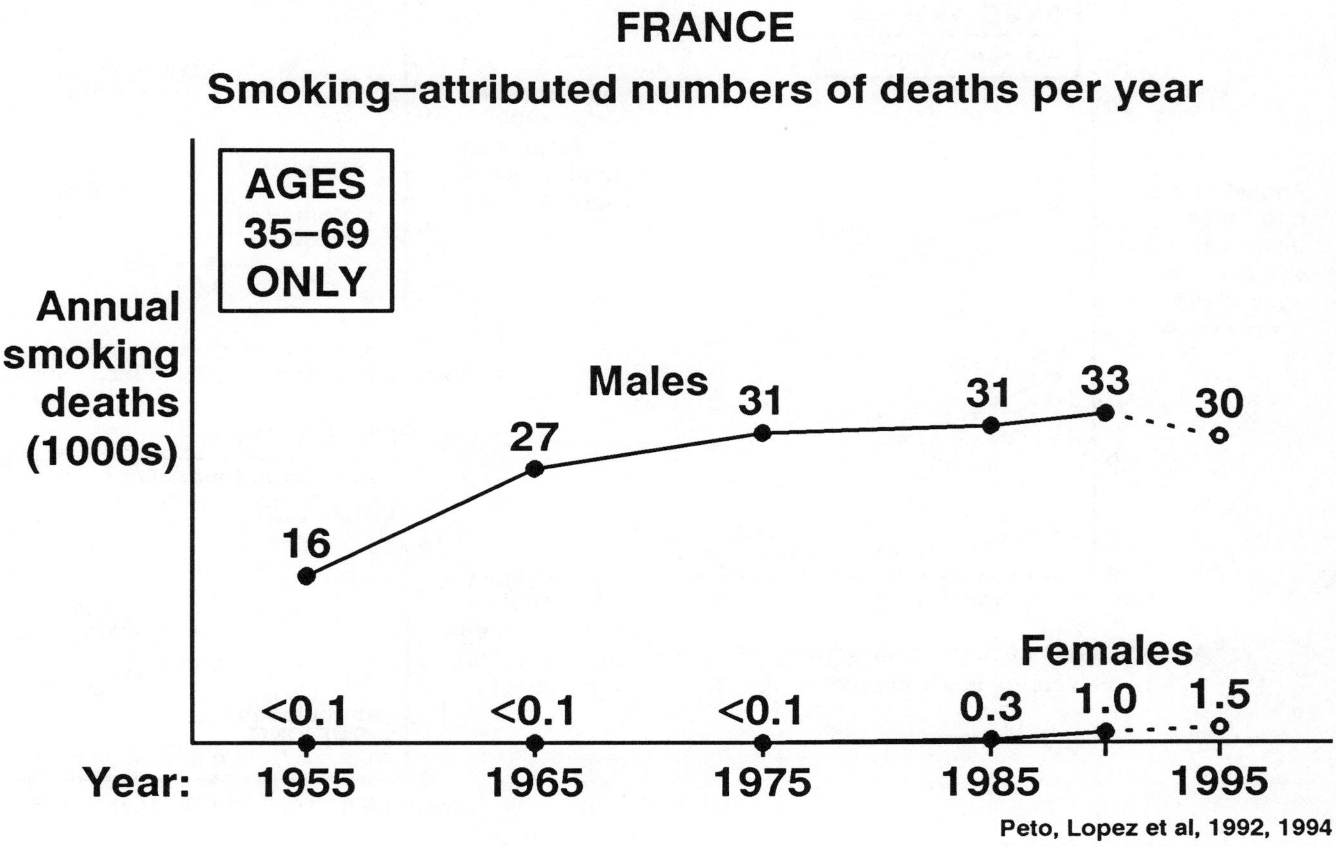
FRANCE
Smoking–attributed numbers of deaths per year
AGES 35–69 ONLY
Annual smoking deaths (1000s)
Males
16
27
31
31
33
30
Females
<0.1
<0.1
<0.1
0.3
1.0
1.5
Year:
1955
1965
1975
1985
1995
Peto, Lopez et al, 1992, 1994

FRANCE

ALL DEATHS (annual rates per 1000): Trends in mortality attributed to smoking, and in other mortality

	Males				Females			
	35–69		70–79		35–69		70–79	
Attributed to SMOKING?	Yes	No	Yes	No	Yes	No	Yes	No
1955	2.22	13.6	3.14	77.8	0.00	8.58	0.00	53.8
1965	3.31	12.0	7.01	68.6	0.00	6.99	0.00	45.0
1975	3.64	9.94	10.3	57.9	0.00	5.81	0.00	37.2
1985	3.52	7.88	10.4	46.2	0.03	4.45	0.15	28.2
1990	3.30	6.84	9.04	38.1	0.10	3.86	0.19	23.3

35–69 = mean of 7 age-specific rates; 70–79 = mean of 2 rates (70–74 & 75–79) Peto, Lopez et al, 1992, 1994

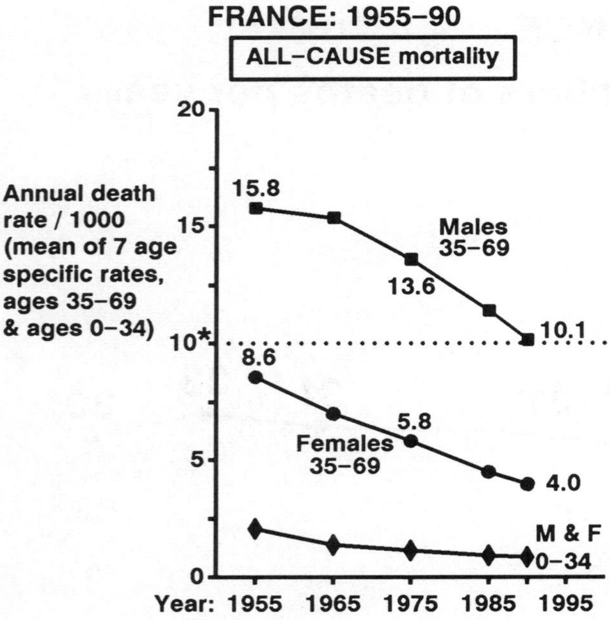

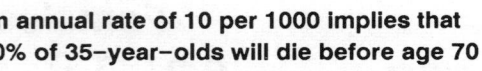

* An annual rate of 10 per 1000 implies that 30% of 35-year-olds will die before age 70

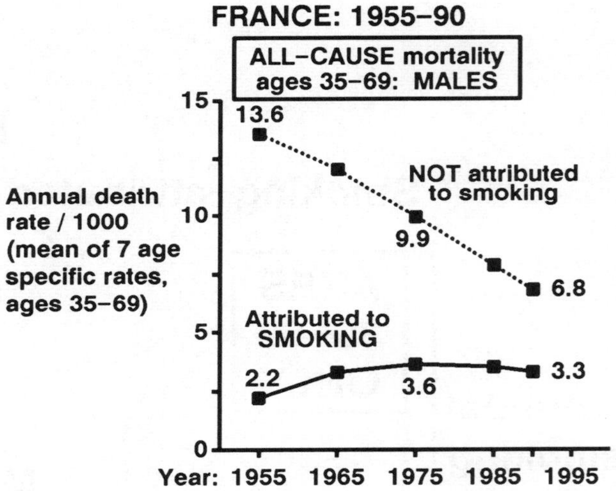

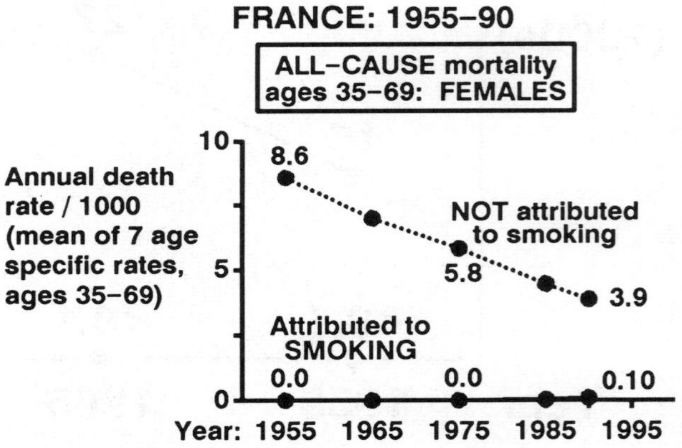

FRANCE

ALL CANCER DEATHS (annual rates per 1000): Trends in mortality attributed to smoking, and in other mortality

	Males				Females			
	35–69		70–79		35–69		70–79	
Attributed to SMOKING?	Yes	No	Yes	No	Yes	No	Yes	No
1955	0.75	2.46	1.10	12.1	0.00	2.21	0.00	8.66
1965	1.39	2.50	2.79	12.5	0.00	2.13	0.00	8.11
1975	1.74	2.40	4.48	12.2	0.00	2.02	0.00	7.45
1985	1.99	2.38	5.42	11.7	0.01	1.82	0.05	6.87
1990	1.99	2.31	5.20	11.3	0.04	1.76	0.07	6.66

35–69 = mean of 7 age–specific rates; 70–79 = mean of 2 rates (70–74 & 75–79) Peto, Lopez et al, 1992, 1994

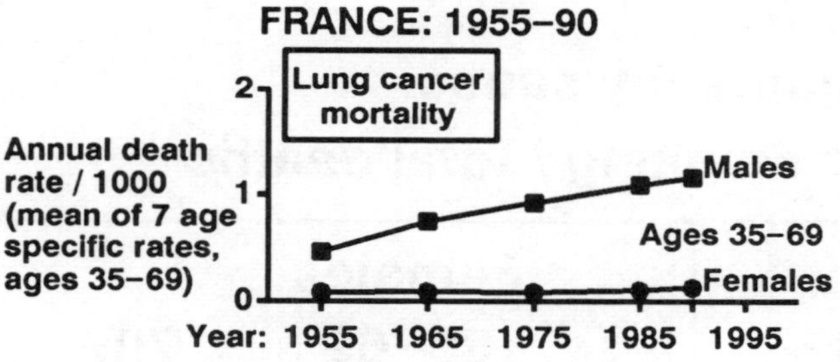

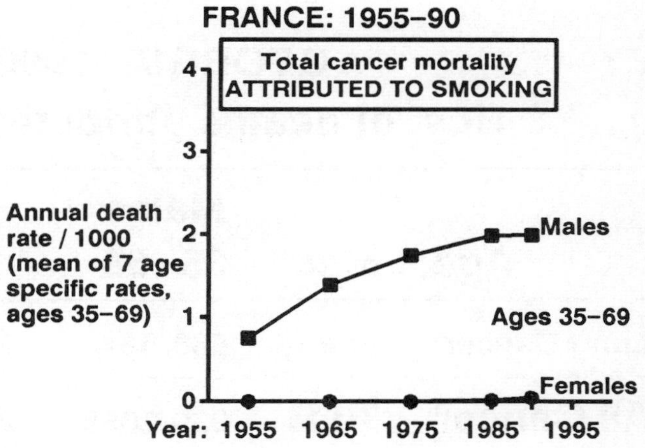

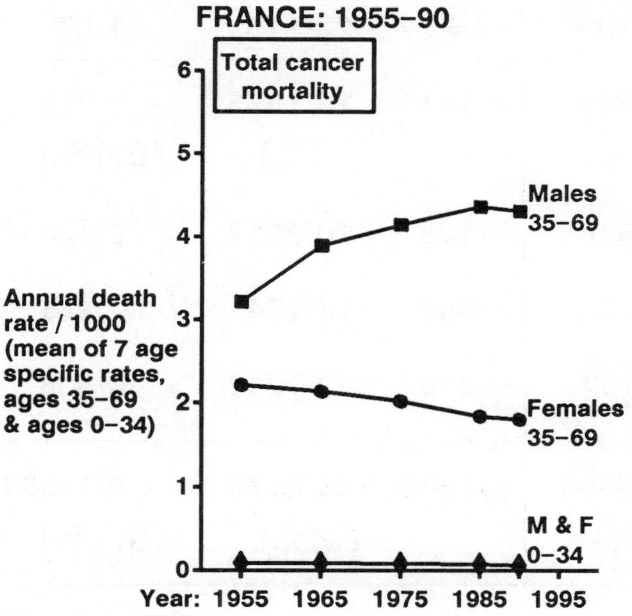

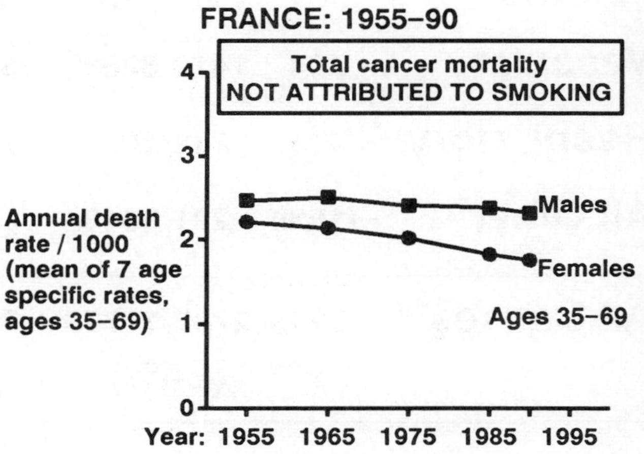

¶GEORGIA: 1990
Relative importance of deaths in MIDDLE age (35–69)

Age range (years)	Deaths attributed to SMOKING / total deaths (thousands) Males	Females	Mean years lost PER DEATH FROM SMOKING
0–34	–/2.6	–/1.4	–
35–69	2.8/12	0.1/7.0	21 years
70+	0.7/8.6	0.0/15	8 years
All ages	3.5/23	0.1/23	18 years

Peto, Lopez et al, 1992, 1994

GEORGIA: 1990 deaths, by cause
Nos. of deaths attributed to smoking / total deaths

	Males			Females		
Age:	0–34	35–69	70+	0–34	35–69	70+
Lung Cancer	–/ 6	568/634	153/190	–/ 6	22/115	1/57
All Cancer	–/134	839/2065 (41%)	205/704 (29%)	–/111	25/1655 (2%)	1/790 (0.1%)
Vascular	–/204	1410/6261	347/6764	–/128	70/3917	5/12441
Respiratory	–/476	242/409	162/375	–/399	18/204	2/485
All Other	–/1835	291/3043	21/707	–/800	10/1200	0/838
All Causes	–/2649	2782/11778 (24%)	735/8550 (9%)	–/1438	123/6976 (2%)	8/14554 (0.1%)

Peto, Lopez et al, 1992, 1994

GEORGIA: 1990

RISKS OF DYING AT AGES 0–34 and 35–69

(Probability that someone entering an age range would die during it, if the death rates in 1990 were to persist unchanged)

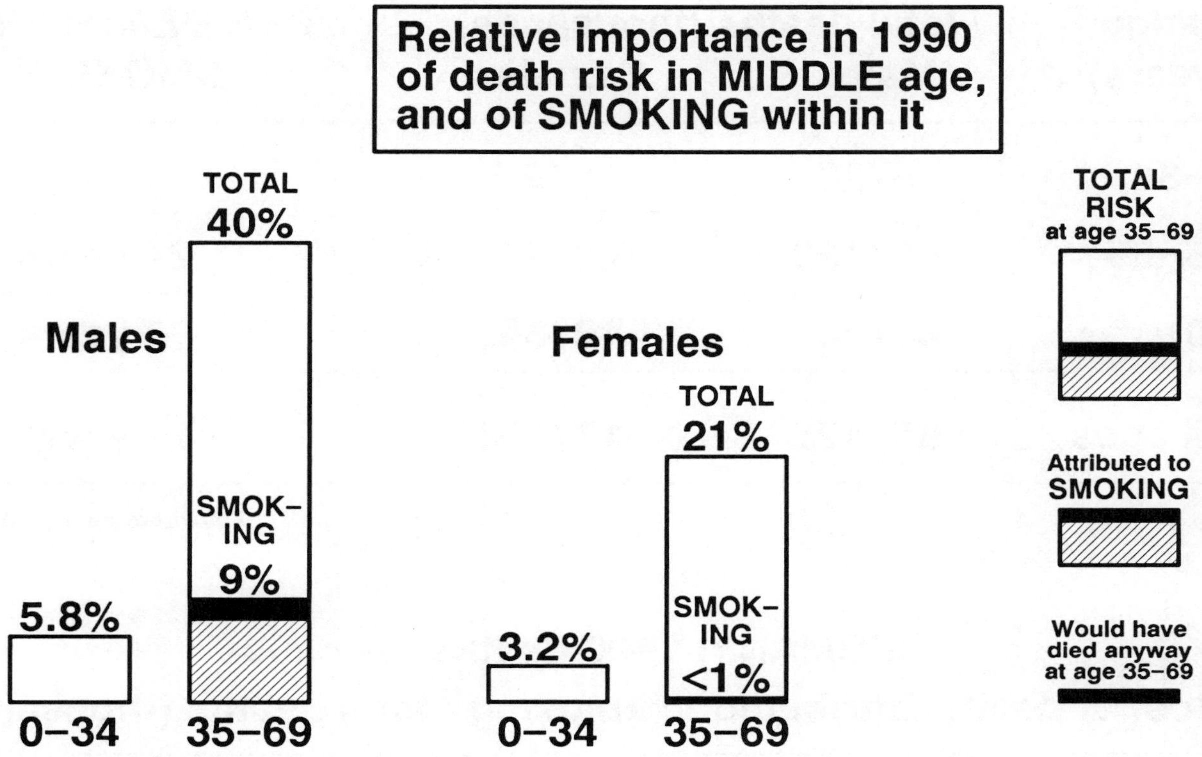

Peto, Lopez et al, 1992, 1994

GEORGIA: 1990 deaths, all ages

Nos. of deaths attributed to smoking / total deaths (thousands)

	Males	Females	Males + Females
All Cancer	1.0/2.9 (36%)	0.0/2.6 (1%)	1.1/5.5 (20%)
All Causes	3.5/23 (15%)	0.1/23 (0.6%)	3.6/46 (8%)

Peto, Lopez et al, 1992, 1994

¶GERMANY: 1990

Relative importance of deaths in MIDDLE age (35–69)

Age range (years)	Deaths attributed to SMOKING / total deaths (thousands) Males	Females	Mean years lost PER DEATH FROM SMOKING
0–34	–/20	–/9.3	–
35–69	52/162	6.2/94	21 years
70+	43/243	10/393	7 years
All ages	95/425	17/496	14 years

Peto, Lopez et al, 1992, 1994

GERMANY: 1990 deaths, by cause

Nos. of deaths attributed to smoking / total deaths (thousands)

	Males			Females		
Age:	0–34	35–69	70+	0–34	35–69	70+
Lung Cancer	–/0.1	15/16	10/11	–/0.0	1.7/3.2	1.7/3.5
All Cancer	–/1.4	23/50 (46%)	16/51 (31%)	–/1.1	2.2/39 (6%)	2.2/62 (4%)
Vascular	–/1.2	17/59	14/133	–/0.6	2.1/29	4.2/240
Respiratory	–/0.4	4.8/7.9	11/23	–/0.3	0.9/3.5	2.9/22
All Other	–/17	7.2/45	2.9/36	–/7.2	1.0/23	1.0/67
All Causes	–/20	52/162 (32%)	43/243 (18%)	–/9.3	6.2/94 (7%)	10/393 (3%)

Peto, Lopez et al, 1992, 1994

GERMANY: 1990

RISKS OF DYING AT AGES 0–34 and 35–69

(Probability that someone entering an age range would die during it, if the death rates in 1990 were to persist unchanged)

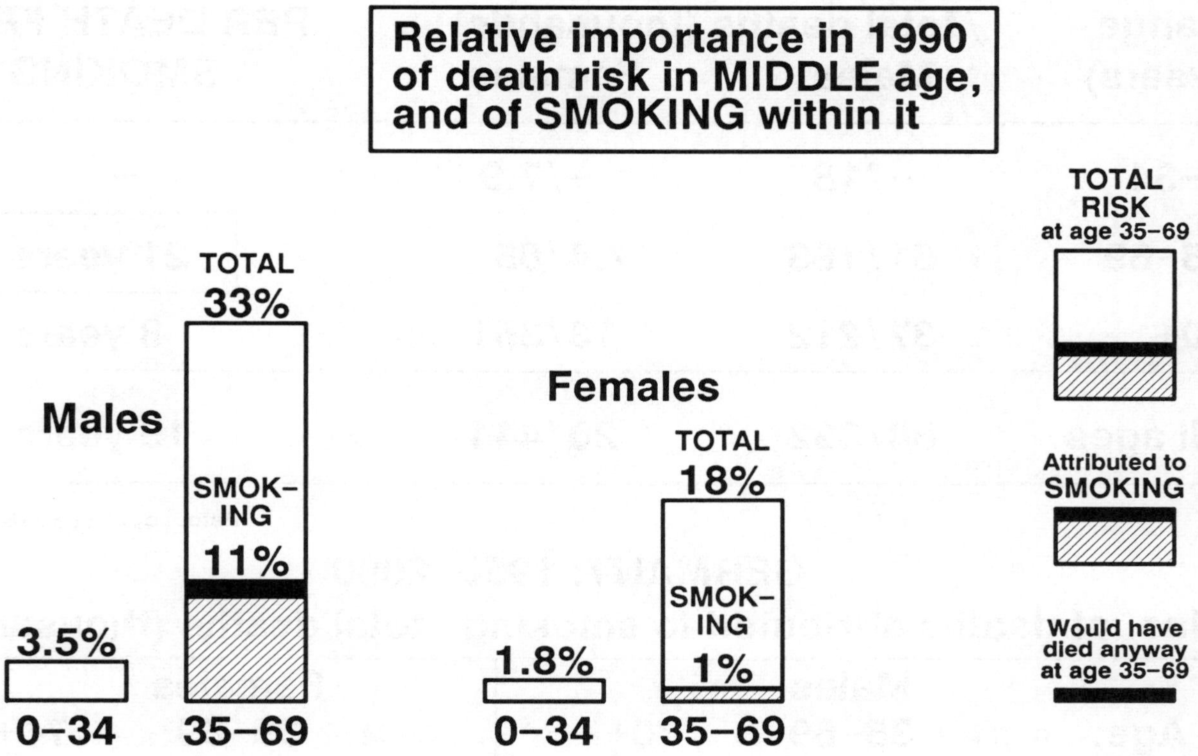

Peto, Lopez et al, 1992, 1994

GERMANY: 1990 deaths, all ages

Nos. of deaths attributed to smoking / total deaths (thousands)

	Males	Females	Males + Females
All Cancer	39/103 (38%)	4.4/102 (4%)	43/205 (21%)
All Causes	95/425 (22%)	17/496 (3%)	112/921 (12%)

Peto, Lopez et al, 1992, 1994

GERMANY: 1995 projections
Relative importance of deaths in MIDDLE age (35–69)

Age range (years)	Deaths attributed to SMOKING / total deaths (thousands) Males	Females	Mean years lost PER DEATH FROM SMOKING
0–34	–/18	–/7.9	–
35–69	51/163	7.4/85	21 years
70+	37/212	13/351	8 years
All ages	88/392	20/444	15 years

Peto, Lopez et al, 1992, 1994

GERMANY: 1950–2000
Nos. of deaths attributed to smoking / total deaths (thousands)

Age:	Males 0–34	Males 35–69	Males 70+	Females 0–34	Females 35–69	Females 70+
1955	–/50	35/153 (23%)	9.4/181 (5%)	–/36	0.9/129 (0.7%)	0.1/207 (0.1%)
1965	–/42	59/201 (29%)	29/234 (13%)	–/26	3.5/148 (2%)	4.1/297 (1%)
1975	–/30	54/180 (30%)	55/271 (20%)	–/16	2.8/129 (2%)	4.3/364 (1%)
1985	–/20	46/141 (33%)	54/272 (20%)	–/10	4.1/89 (5%)	7.2/396 (2%)
1995 (projected)	–/18	51/163 (32%)	37/212 (17%)	–/7.9	7.4/85 (9%)	13/351 (4%)
50–year total* (M=millions), mid–1950 to mid–2000: 4.8/45M						
1950–2000, by age & sex	–/1.6M	2.5/8.4M (30%)	1.8/12M (15%)	–/1.0M	0.2/5.8M (3%)	0.3/16M (2%)

*Estimated as 10 times the sum of the five annual numbers (for 1955, 1965, 1975, 1985 & 1995)

GERMANY
Smoking–attributed numbers of deaths per year

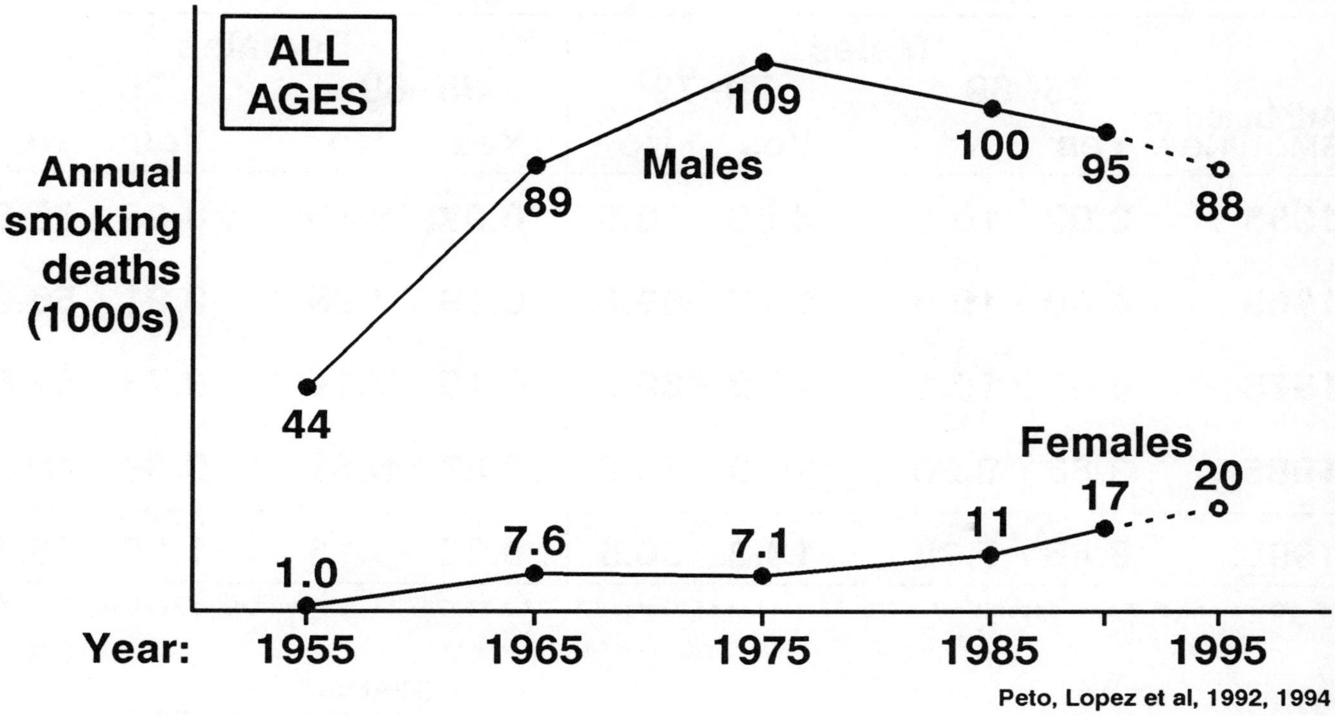

GERMANY
Smoking–attributed numbers of deaths per year

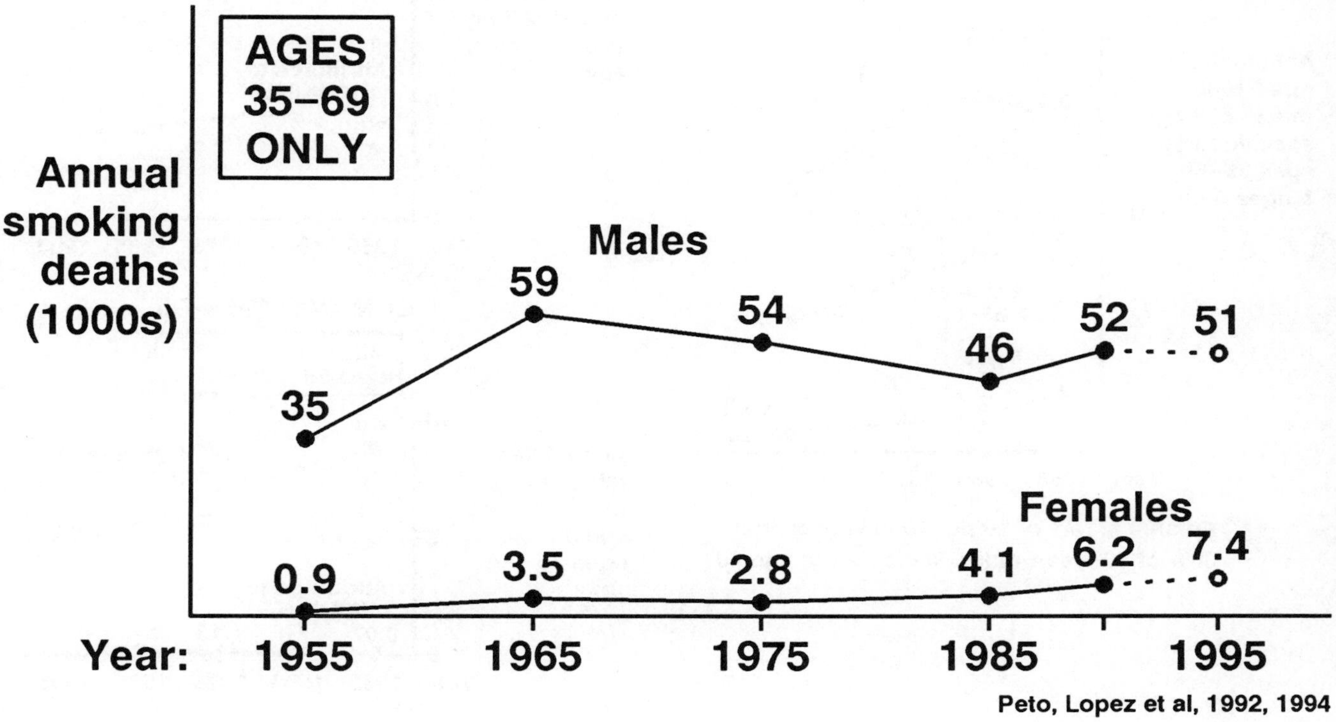

GERMANY

ALL DEATHS (annual rates per 1000): Trends in mortality attributed to smoking, and in other mortality

	Males				Females			
	35–69		70–79		35–69		70–79	
Attributed to SMOKING?	Yes	No	Yes	No	Yes	No	Yes	No
1955	**3.02**	**10.9**	**4.56**	**73.9**	**0.07**	**8.89**	**0.05**	**65.8**
1965	**4.40**	**10.6**	**11.7**	**69.6**	**0.19**	**7.98**	**0.91**	**56.3**
1975	**4.40**	**10.1**	**19.2**	**66.6**	**0.15**	**7.19**	**0.73**	**52.8**
1985	**3.88**	**8.20**	**16.0**	**56.6**	**0.27**	**5.61**	**0.99**	**40.4**
1990	**3.66**	**7.78**	**13.3**	**50.5**	**0.36**	**5.16**	**1.39**	**35.4**

35–69 = mean of 7 age-specific rates; 70–79 = mean of 2 rates (70–74 & 75–79) Peto, Lopez et al, 1992, 1994

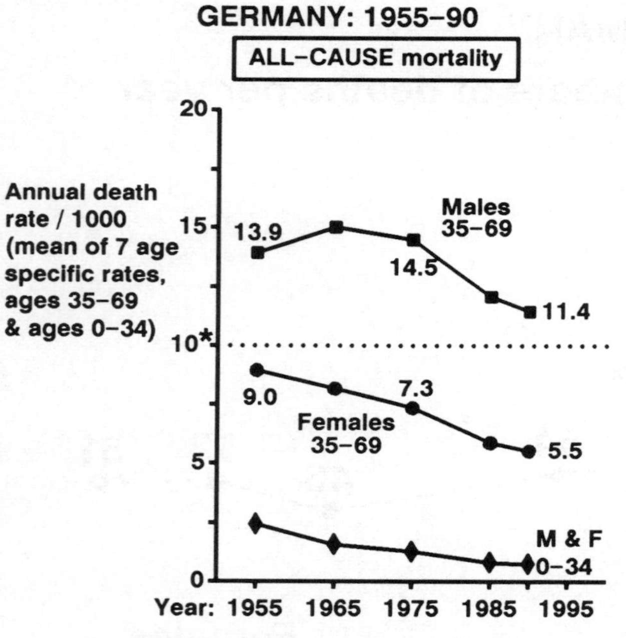

* An annual rate of 10 per 1000 implies that 30% of 35-year-olds will die before age 70

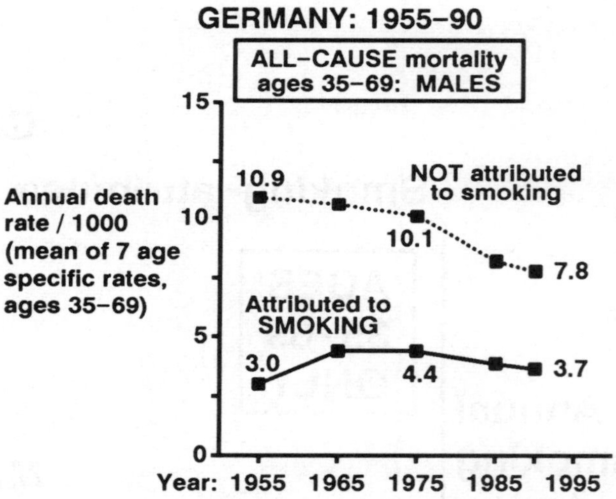

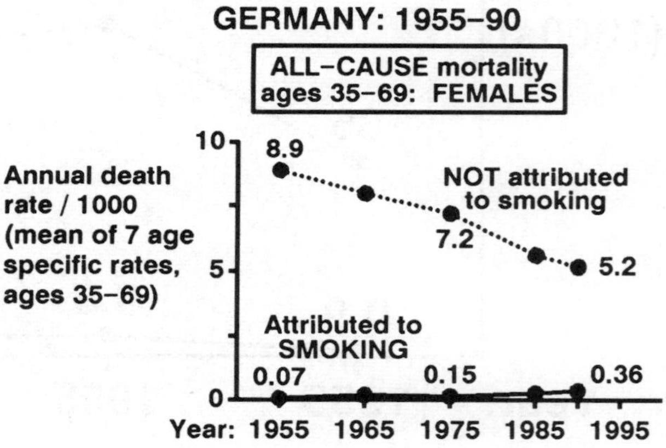

GERMANY

ALL CANCER DEATHS (annual rates per 1000): Trends in mortality attributed to smoking, and in other mortality

	Males				Females			
	35–69		70–79		35–69		70–79	
Attributed to SMOKING?	Yes	No	Yes	No	Yes	No	Yes	No
1955	0.97	2.21	1.55	12.3	0.01	2.65	0.01	10.5
1965	1.50	2.12	4.21	12.2	0.05	2.64	0.20	10.4
1975	1.54	2.08	6.46	11.4	0.04	2.44	0.14	9.22
1985	1.62	1.97	6.25	10.8	0.08	2.19	0.25	8.62
1990	1.63	1.94	5.67	10.8	0.13	2.13	0.39	8.20

35–69 = mean of 7 age-specific rates; 70–79 = mean of 2 rates (70–74 & 75–79) Peto, Lopez et al, 1992, 1994

GERMANY: 1955–90

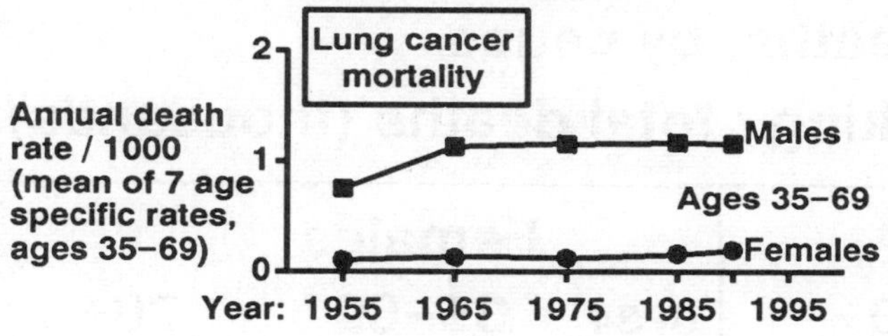

GERMANY: 1955–90

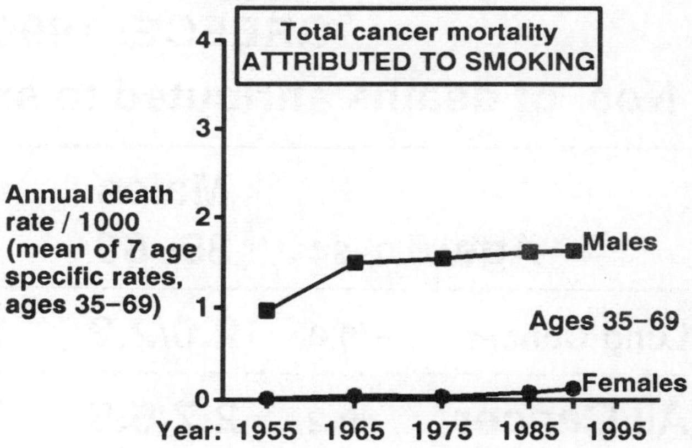

GERMANY: 1955–90

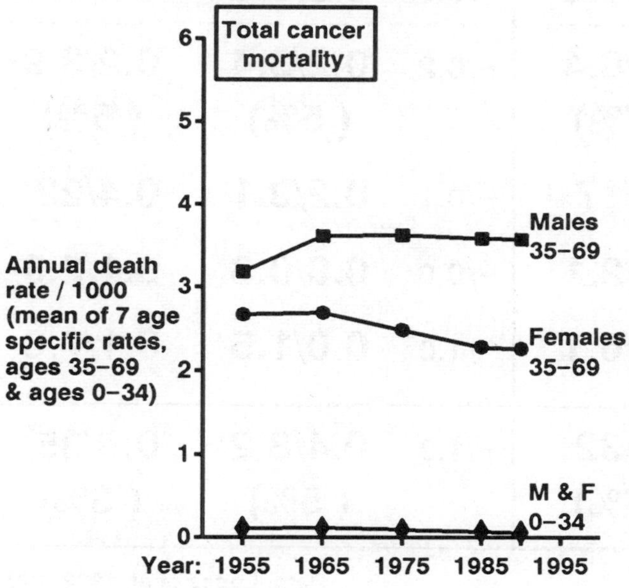

GERMANY: 1955–90

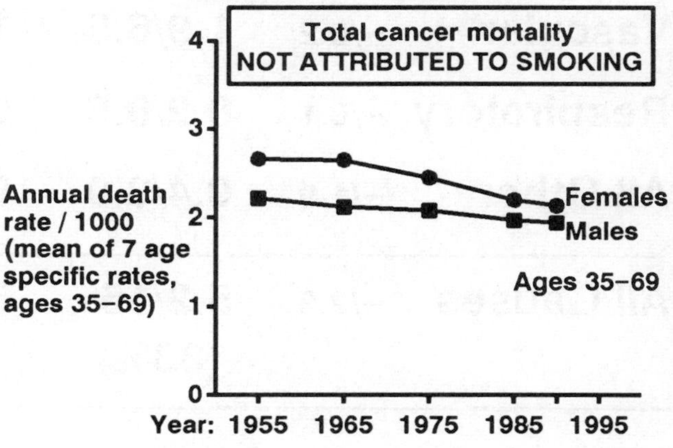

GREECE: 1990
Relative importance of deaths in MIDDLE age (35–69)

Age range (years)	Deaths attributed to SMOKING / total deaths (thousands) Males	Females	Mean years lost PER DEATH FROM SMOKING
0–34	–/2.3	–/1.3	–
35–69	5.2/16	0.4/8.2	22 years
70+	5.2/32	0.9/35	8 years
All ages	10/49	1.3/45	14 years

Peto, Lopez et al, 1992, 1994

GREECE: 1990 deaths, by cause
Nos. of deaths attributed to smoking / total deaths (thousands)

	Males			Females		
Age:	0–34	35–69	70+	0–34	35–69	70+
Lung Cancer	–/0.0	2.0/2.2	1.7/1.8	–/0.0	0.2/0.3	0.2/0.4
All Cancer	–/0.2	2.7/5.5 (49%)	2.4/6.4 (37%)	–/0.2	0.2/3.4 (5%)	0.2/3.9 (6%)
Vascular	–/0.2	1.9/6.5	1.8/17	–/0.1	0.2/3.1	0.4/22
Respiratory	–/0.1	0.2/0.6	0.5/2.1	–/0.0	0.0/0.3	0.1/2.0
All Other	–/1.9	0.4/3.0	0.6/6.1	–/1.0	0.0/1.5	0.1/7.0
All Causes	–/2.3	5.2/16 (33%)	5.2/32 (17%)	–/1.3	0.4/8.2 (5%)	0.9/35 (3%)

Peto, Lopez et al, 1992, 1994

GREECE: 1990

RISKS OF DYING AT AGES 0–34 and 35–69

(Probability that someone entering an age range would die during it, if the death rates in 1990 were to persist unchanged)

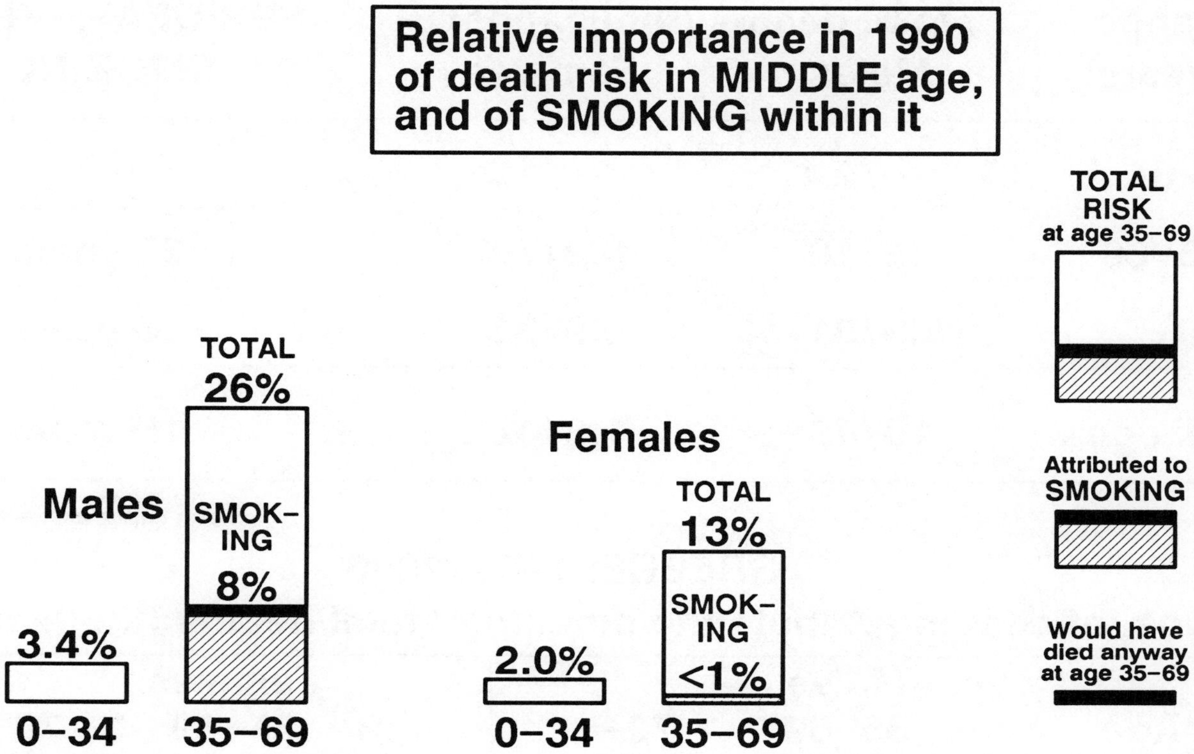

Peto, Lopez et al, 1992, 1994

GREECE: 1990 deaths, all ages

Nos. of deaths attributed to smoking / total deaths (thousands)

	Males	Females	Males + Females
All Cancer	5.0/12 (42%)	0.4/7.4 (5%)	5.4/19 (28%)
All Causes	10/49 (21%)	1.3/45 (3%)	12/94 (12%)

Peto, Lopez et al, 1992, 1994

GREECE: 1995 projections
Relative importance of deaths in MIDDLE age (35–69)

Age range (years)	Deaths attributed to SMOKING / total deaths (thousands) Males	Females	Mean years lost PER DEATH FROM SMOKING
0–34	–/2.1	–/1.2	–
35–69	5.2/16	0.3/7.7	22 years
70+	5.3/31	0.9/33	8 years
All ages	10/48	1.3/42	15 years

Peto, Lopez et al, 1992, 1994

GREECE: 1950–2000
Nos. of deaths attributed to smoking / total deaths (thousands)

	Males			Females		
Age:	0–34	35–69	70+	0–34	35–69	70+
1955	–/6.7	2.0/9.6 (21%)	0.7/11 (6%)	–/5.8	0.5/7.8 (6%)	0.0/13 (0%)
1965	–/5.1	3.1/13 (24%)	1.6/17 (10%)	–/3.8	0.5/9.1 (5%)	0.1/20 (0.3%)
1975	–/3.8	4.2/15 (29%)	3.9/23 (17%)	–/2.5	0.6/9.4 (6%)	0.7/27 (3%)
1985	–/2.9	4.9/15 (33%)	5.3/31 (17%)	–/1.5	0.5/8.8 (5%)	0.7/34 (2%)
1995 (projected)	–/2.1	5.2/16 (34%)	5.3/31 (17%)	–/1.2	0.3/7.7 (4%)	0.9/33 (3%)
50–year total*, mid–1950 to mid–2000: 410/3868						
1950–2000, by age & sex	–/206	194/686 (28%)	168/1130 (15%)	–/148	24/428 (6%)	24/1270 (2%)

*Estimated as 10 times the sum of the five annual numbers (for 1955, 1965, 1975, 1985 & 1995)

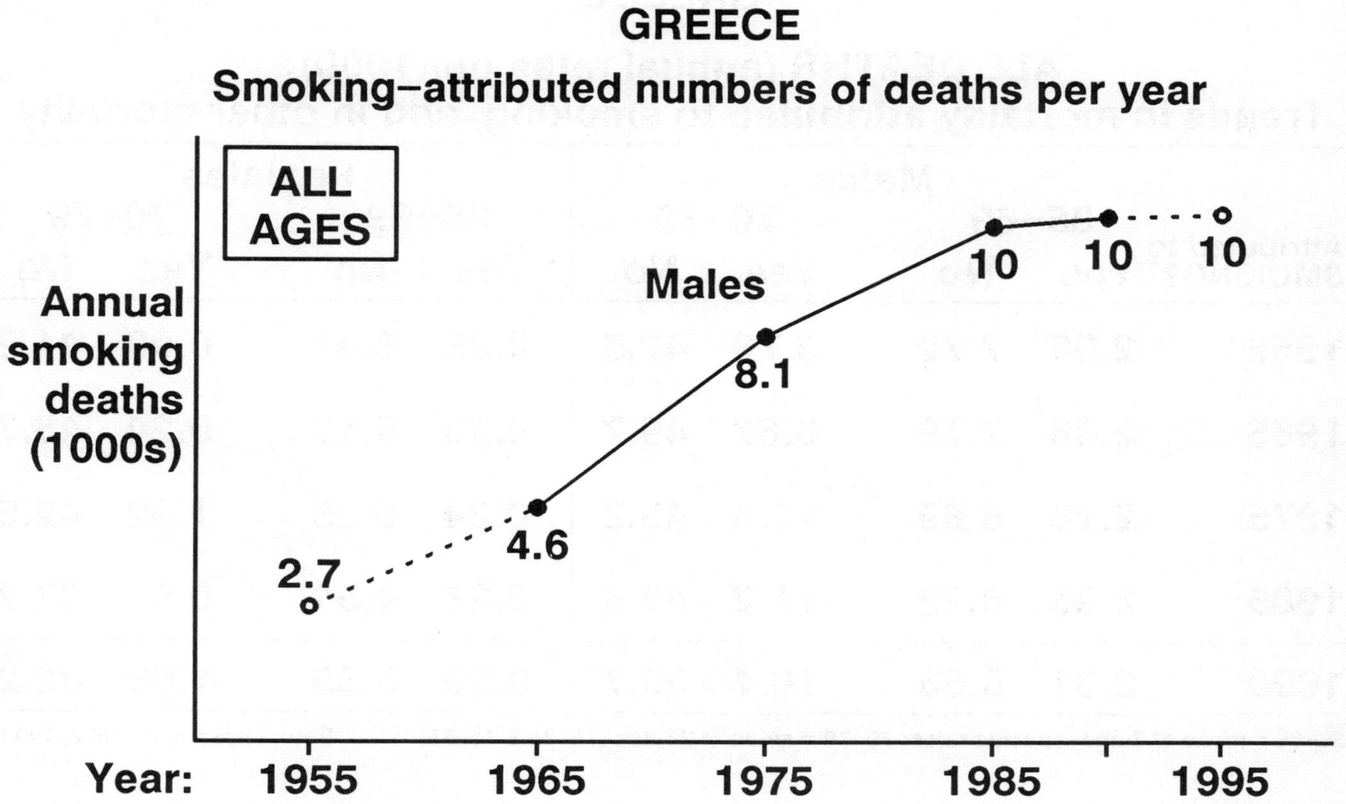

Peto, Lopez et al, 1992, 1994

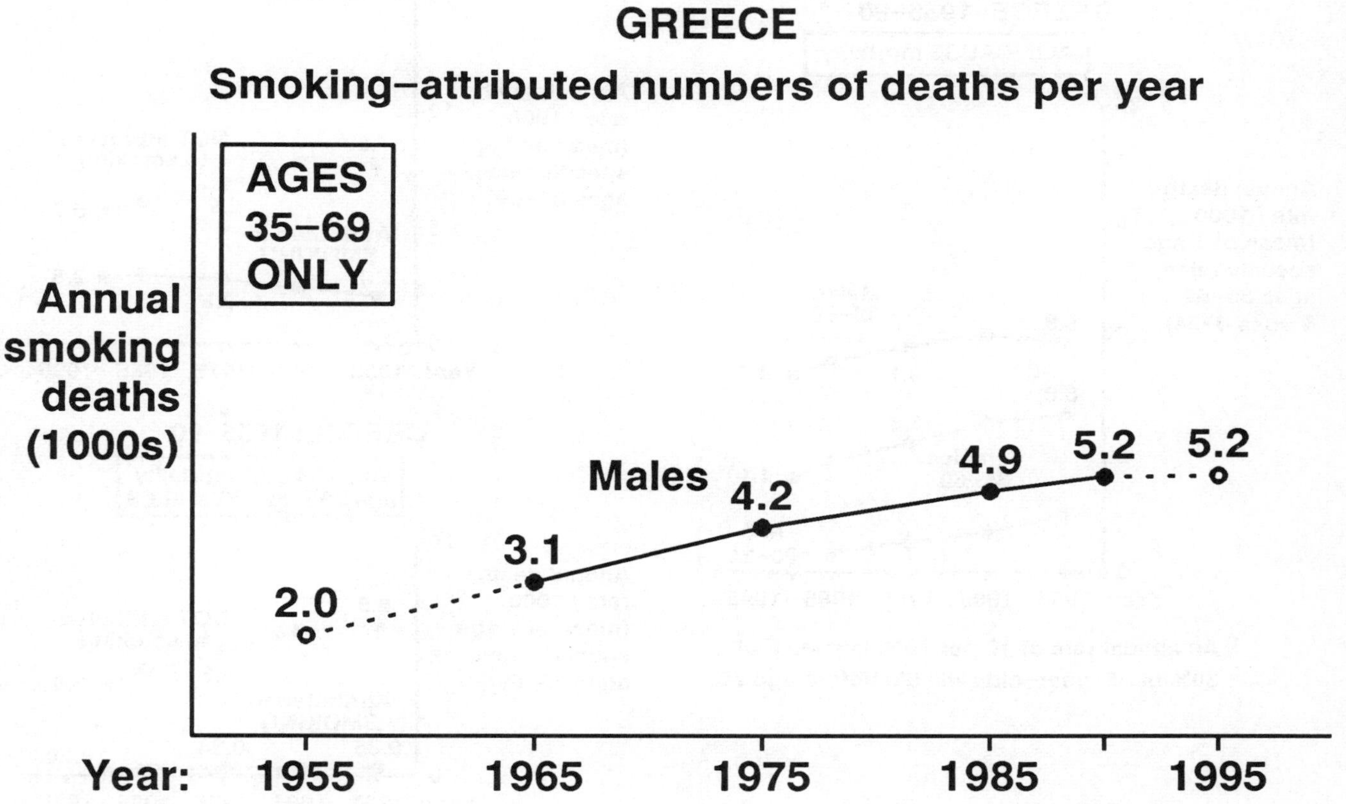

Peto, Lopez et al, 1992, 1994

GREECE

ALL DEATHS (annual rates per 1000): Trends in mortality attributed to smoking, and in other mortality

	Males				Females			
	35–69		70–79		35–69		70–79	
Attributed to SMOKING?	Yes	No	Yes	No	Yes	No	Yes	No
1955	2.06	7.79	3.79	47.5	0.35	6.47	0.00	41.2
1965	2.46	7.78	6.67	49.7	0.33	6.19	0.24	45.7
1975	2.78	6.89	10.9	45.8	0.34	5.25	1.32	42.5
1985	2.96	6.12	11.2	43.5	0.27	4.54	0.84	37.7
1990	2.81	5.66	10.4	39.7	0.20	3.89	1.02	32.2

35–69 = mean of 7 age-specific rates; 70–79 = mean of 2 rates (70–74 & 75–79)   Peto, Lopez et al, 1992, 1994

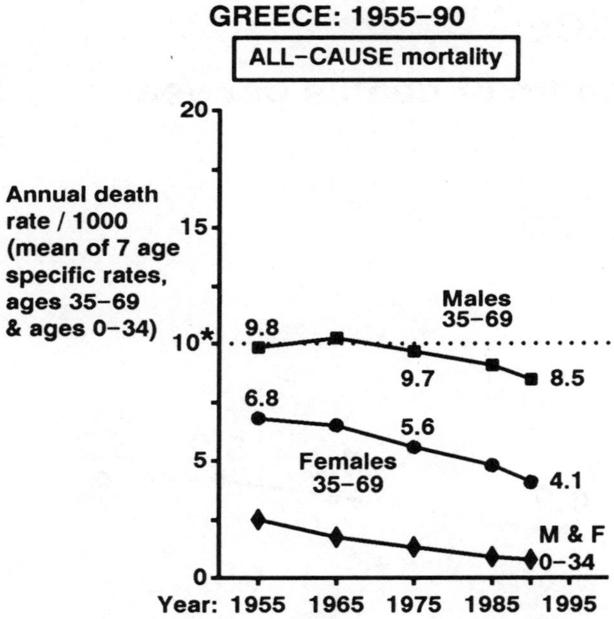

* An annual rate of 10 per 1000 implies that 30% of 35-year-olds will die before age 70

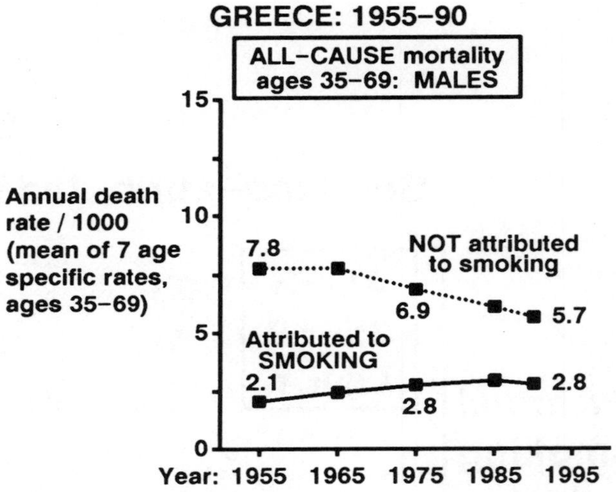

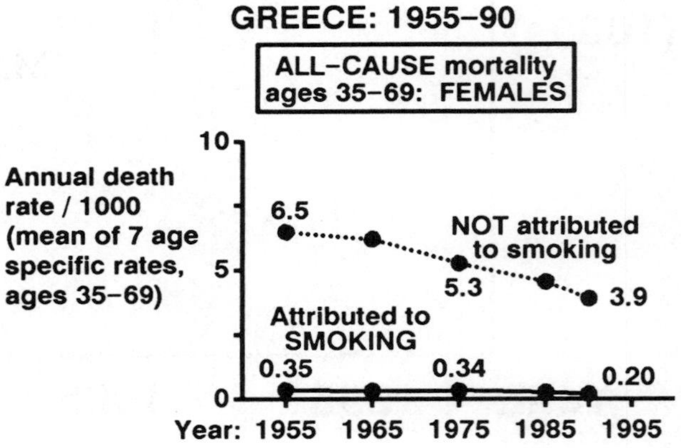

GREECE

ALL CANCER DEATHS (annual rates per 1000): Trends in mortality attributed to smoking, and in other mortality

	Males				Females			
	35–69		70–79		35–69		70–79	
Attributed to SMOKING?	Yes	No	Yes	No	Yes	No	Yes	No
1955	...	...	...	...	...	...	...	...
1965	1.02	1.71	2.70	7.32	0.08	1.67	0.04	4.94
1975	1.21	1.78	4.26	7.94	0.09	1.61	0.22	5.35
1985	1.48	1.58	5.39	8.21	0.10	1.65	0.22	5.81
1990	1.47	1.53	5.55	8.23	0.08	1.54	0.34	5.51

35–69 = mean of 7 age–specific rates; 70–79 = mean of 2 rates (70–74 & 75–79) Peto, Lopez et al, 1992, 1994

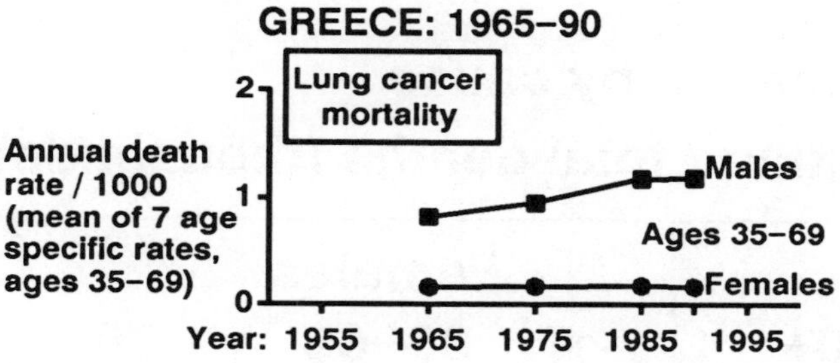

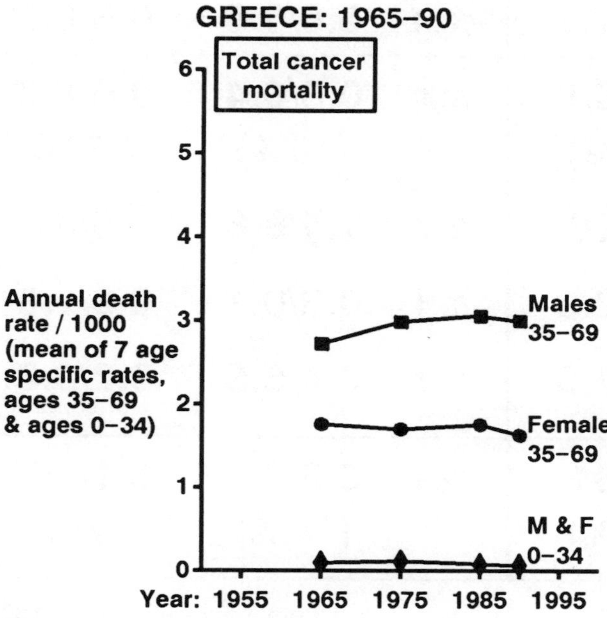

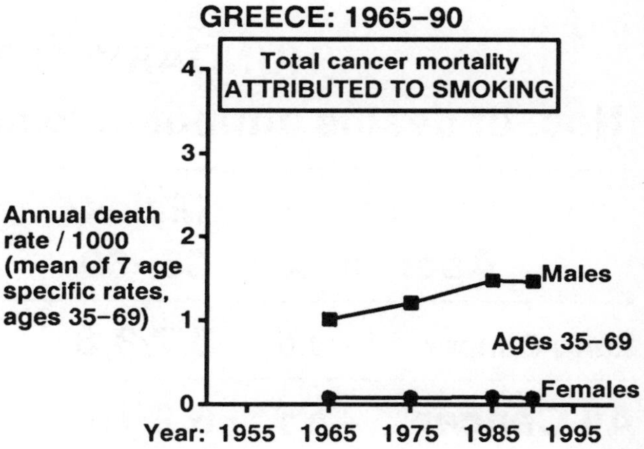

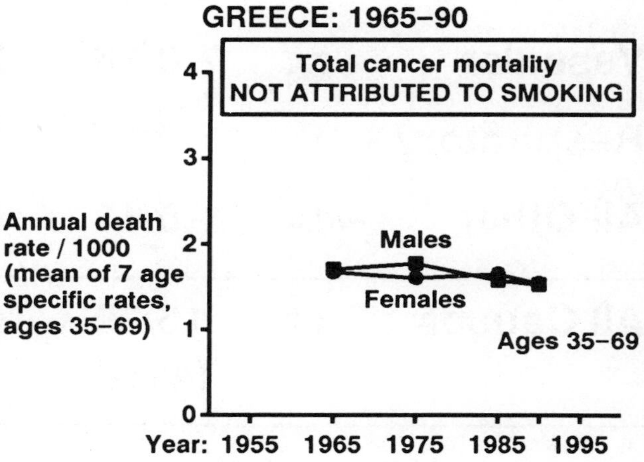

HUNGARY: 1990
Relative importance of deaths in MIDDLE age (35–69)

Age range (years)	Deaths attributed to SMOKING / total deaths (thousands) Males	Females	Mean years lost PER DEATH FROM SMOKING
0–34	–/4.2	–/2.1	–
35–69	16/39	3.0/21	20 years
70+	6.5/34	3.1/46	8 years
All ages	23/77	6.0/69	16 years

Peto, Lopez et al, 1992, 1994

HUNGARY: 1990 deaths, by cause
Nos. of deaths attributed to smoking / total deaths (thousands)

	Males			Females		
Age:	0–34	35–69	70+	0–34	35–69	70+
Lung Cancer	–/0.0	3.7/3.8	1.5/1.6	–/0.0	0.6/0.8	0.5/0.7
All Cancer	–/0.3	6.2/10 (60%)	2.3/6.8 (35%)	–/0.3	0.8/6.4 (13%)	0.6/6.8 (9%)
Vascular	–/0.4	7.0/16	2.4/20	–/0.2	1.4/8.6	1.5/31
Respiratory	–/0.2	1.2/1.6	1.5/2.3	–/0.1	0.3/0.7	0.8/1.8
All Other	–/3.4	1.5/11	0.3/4.5	–/1.6	0.4/5.0	0.2/6.3
All Causes	–/4.2	16/39 (41%)	6.5/34 (19%)	–/2.1	3.0/21 (14%)	3.1/46 (7%)

Peto, Lopez et al, 1992, 1994

HUNGARY: 1990

RISKS OF DYING AT AGES 0–34 and 35–69

(Probability that someone entering an age range would die during it, if the death rates in 1990 were to persist unchanged)

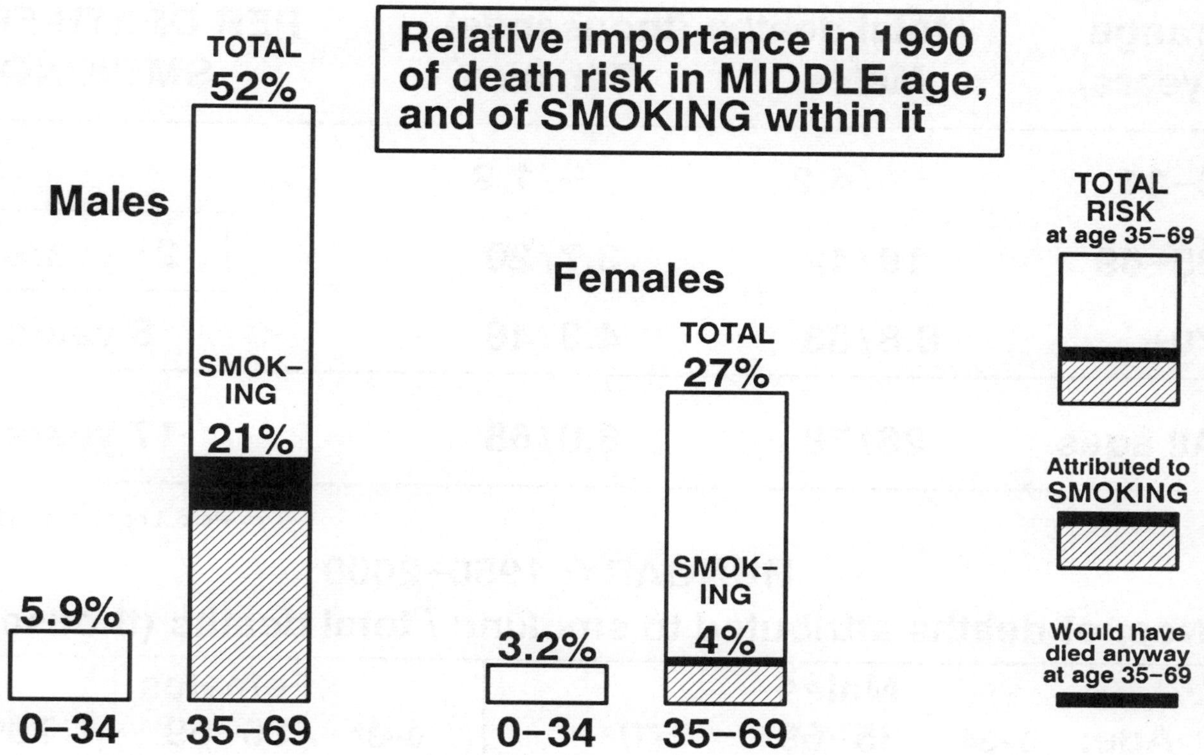

Peto, Lopez et al, 1992, 1994

HUNGARY: 1990 deaths, all ages

Nos. of deaths attributed to smoking / total deaths (thousands)

	Males	Females	Males + Females
All Cancer	8.6/17 (49%)	1.4/13 (11%)	10/31 (32%)
All Causes	23/77 (29%)	6.0/69 (9%)	29/146 (20%)

Peto, Lopez et al, 1992, 1994

HUNGARY: 1995 projections
Relative importance of deaths in MIDDLE age (35–69)

Age range (years)	Deaths attributed to SMOKING / total deaths (thousands) Males	Females	Mean years lost PER DEATH FROM SMOKING
0–34	–/4.2	–/1.9	–
35–69	19/42	3.7/20	21 years
70+	6.8/33	4.3/46	8 years
All ages	26/78	8.0/68	17 years

Peto, Lopez et al, 1992, 1994

HUNGARY: 1950–2000
Nos. of deaths attributed to smoking / total deaths (thousands)

	Males			Females		
Age:	0–34	35–69	70+	0–34	35–69	70+
1955	–/11	3.8 / 20 (20%)	0.7 / 19 (4%)	–/8.2	0.6 / 17 (3%)	0.1 / 23 (0.6%)
1965	–/5.8	6.3 / 24 (26%)	2.8 / 26 (11%)	–/3.8	0.9 / 17 (5%)	0.9 / 31 (3%)
1975	–/6.7	8.0 / 29 (28%)	6.3 / 33 (19%)	–/4.1	1.0 / 19 (5%)	1.8 / 40 (5%)
1985	–/4.8	13 / 34 (38%)	8.0 / 39 (21%)	–/2.5	2.1 / 19 (11%)	2.8 / 48 (6%)
1995 (projected)	–/4.2	19 / 42 (45%)	6.8 / 33 (21%)	–/1.9	3.7 / 20 (18%)	4.3 / 46 (9%)
50–year total*, mid–1950 to mid–2000: 929/6320						
1950–2000, by age & sex	–/325	501 / 1490 (34%)	246 / 1500 (16%)	–/205	83 / 920 (9%)	99 / 1880 (5%)

*Estimated as 10 times the sum of the five annual numbers (for 1955, 1965, 1975, 1985 & 1995)

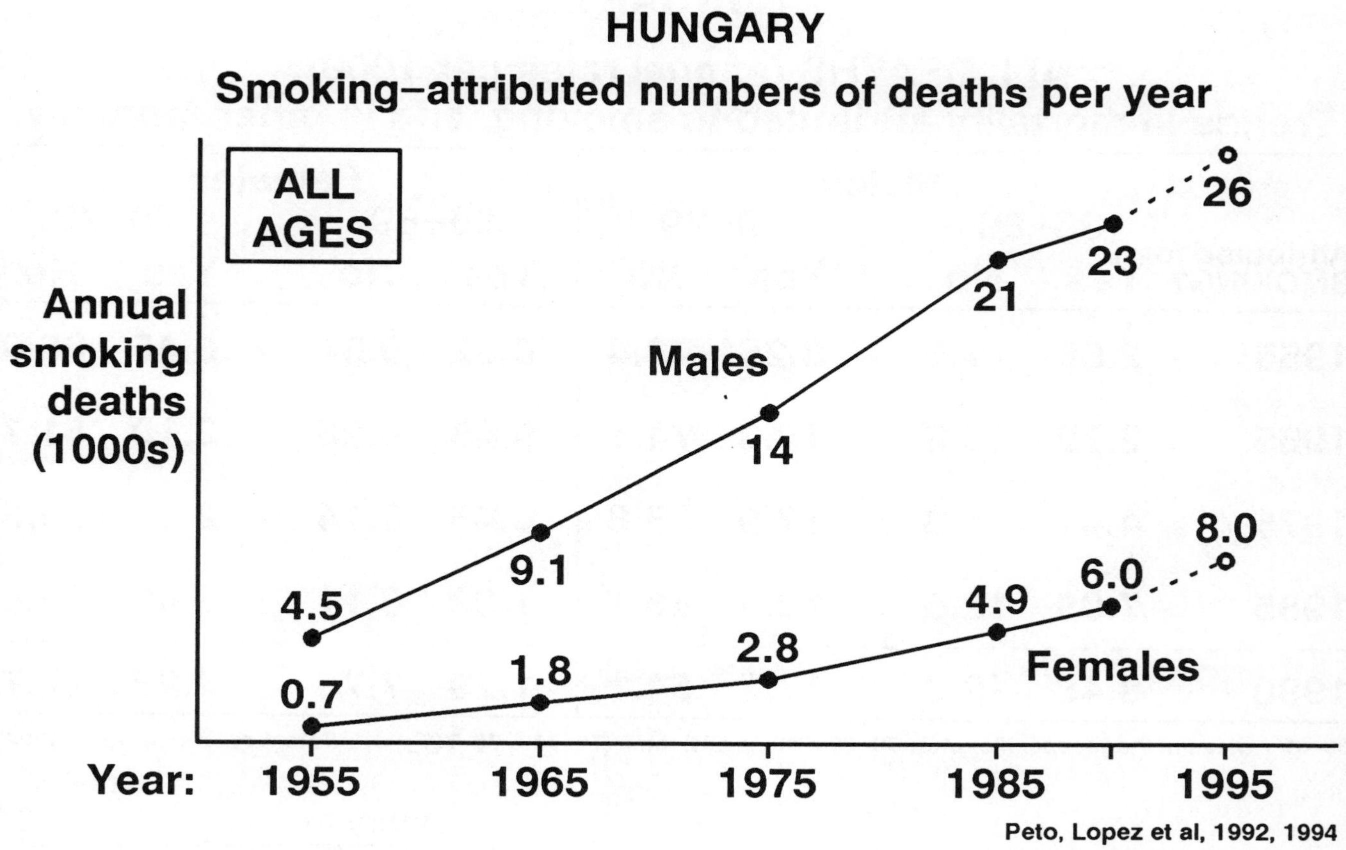
HUNGARY
Smoking–attributed numbers of deaths per year
ALL AGES
Annual smoking deaths (1000s)
Males
4.5
9.1
14
21
23
26
Females
0.7
1.8
2.8
4.9
6.0
8.0
Year:
1955
1965
1975
1985
1995
Peto, Lopez et al, 1992, 1994

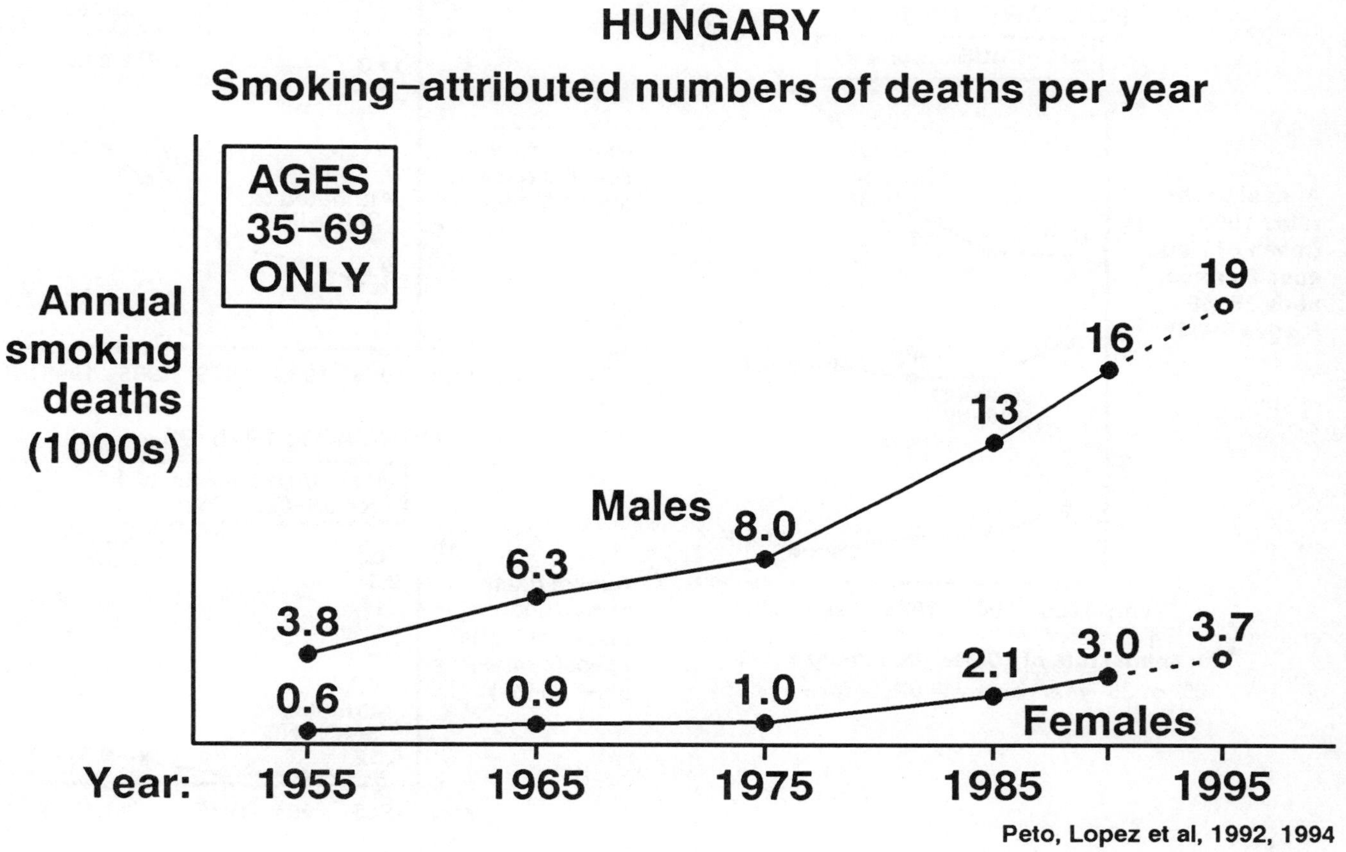
HUNGARY
Smoking–attributed numbers of deaths per year
AGES 35–69 ONLY
Annual smoking deaths (1000s)
Males
3.8
6.3
8.0
13
16
19
Females
0.6
0.9
1.0
2.1
3.0
3.7
Year:
1955
1965
1975
1985
1995
Peto, Lopez et al, 1992, 1994

HUNGARY

ALL DEATHS (annual rates per 1000): Trends in mortality attributed to smoking, and in other mortality

	Males				Females			
	35–69		70–79		35–69		70–79	
Attributed to SMOKING?	Yes	No	Yes	No	Yes	No	Yes	No
1955	2.56	11.3	3.25	73.4	0.32	9.81	0.45	66.0
1965	3.72	10.3	10.3	74.1	0.45	8.26	2.10	61.7
1975	4.41	11.3	17.9	68.8	0.45	8.14	2.95	56.3
1985	7.09	12.5	19.4	68.7	1.02	8.11	3.41	52.0
1990	8.48	12.3	17.8	64.1	1.29	7.76	4.25	47.7

35–69 = mean of 7 age-specific rates; 70–79 = mean of 2 rates (70–74 & 75–79) Peto, Lopez et al, 1992, 1994

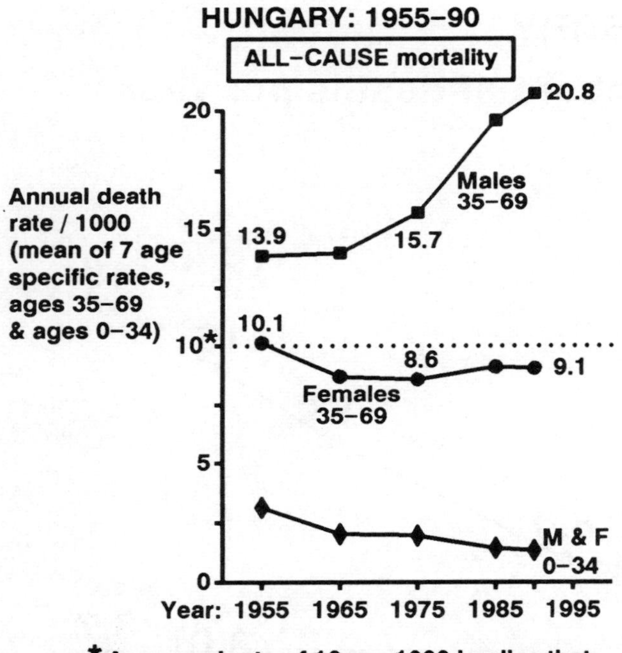

* An annual rate of 10 per 1000 implies that 30% of 35-year-olds will die before age 70

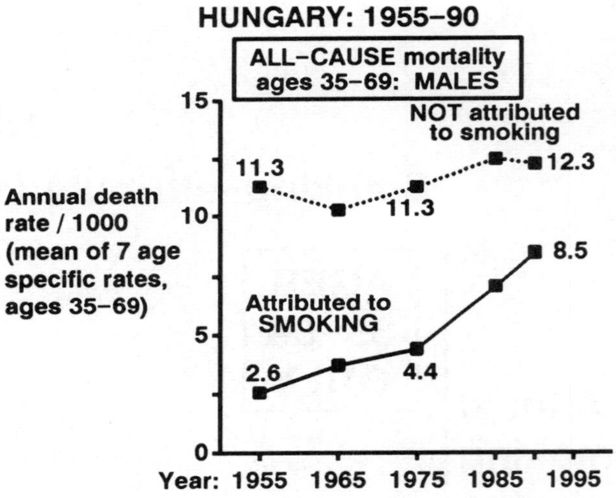

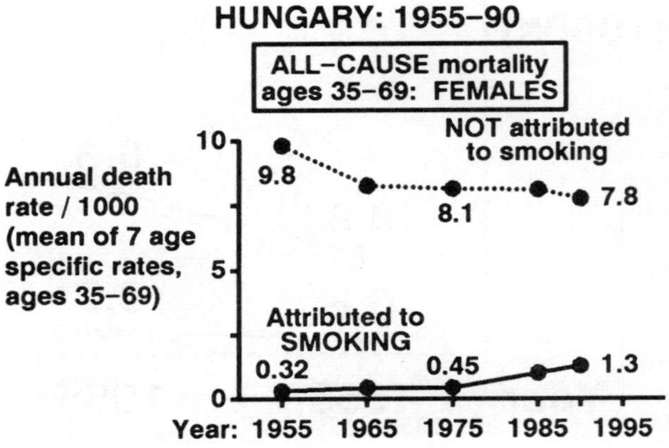

HUNGARY

ALL CANCER DEATHS (annual rates per 1000): Trends in mortality attributed to smoking, and in other mortality

	Males				Females			
	35–69		70–79		35–69		70–79	
Attributed to SMOKING?	Yes	No	Yes	No	Yes	No	Yes	No
1955	0.83	2.24	1.04	9.64	0.06	2.58	0.08	8.23
1965	1.34	2.20	3.58	11.5	0.10	2.46	0.38	9.53
1975	1.62	2.39	6.74	12.1	0.11	2.57	0.61	9.66
1985	2.55	2.25	7.07	11.6	0.25	2.42	0.72	9.08
1990	3.35	2.33	7.16	12.3	0.36	2.43	1.03	9.21

35–69 = mean of 7 age–specific rates; 70–79 = mean of 2 rates (70–74 & 75–79) Peto, Lopez et al, 1992, 1994

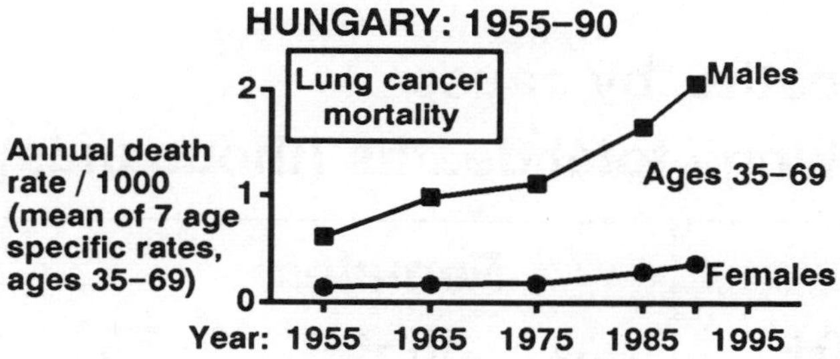

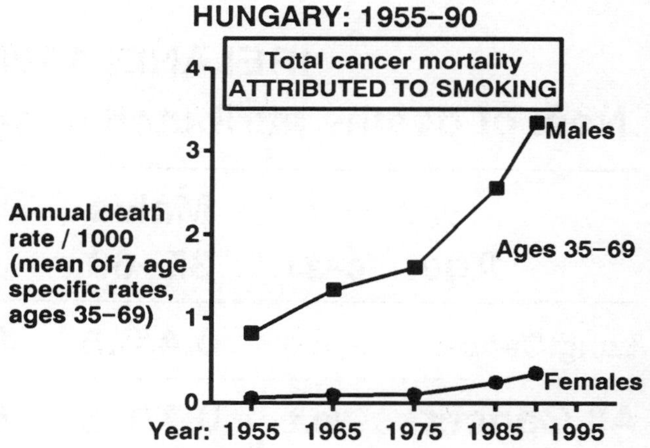

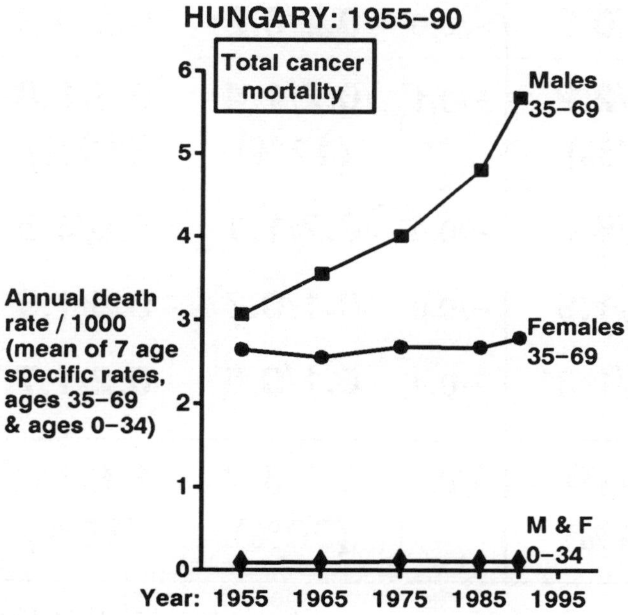

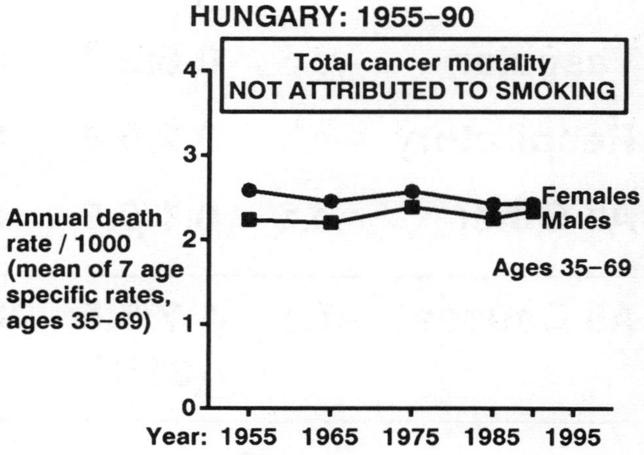

IRELAND: 1990
Relative importance of deaths in MIDDLE age (35–69)

Age range (years)	Deaths attributed to SMOKING / total deaths (thousands) Males	Females	Mean years lost PER DEATH FROM SMOKING
0–34	–/0.9	–/0.5	–
35–69	1.7/5.5	0.7/3.2	20 years
70+	2.5/10	1.6/11	8 years
All ages	4.2/17	2.3/15	12 years

Peto, Lopez et al, 1992, 1994

IRELAND: 1990 deaths, by cause
Nos. of deaths attributed to smoking / total deaths (thousands)

Age:	Males 0–34	Males 35–69	Males 70+	Females 0–34	Females 35–69	Females 70+
Lung Cancer	–/0.0	0.4/0.5	0.5/0.6	–/0.0	0.2/0.2	0.2/0.3
All Cancer	–/0.1	0.7/1.6 (42%)	0.8/2.2 (37%)	–/0.1	0.2/1.4 (17%)	0.3/1.8 (19%)
Vascular	–/0.0	0.6/2.6	0.7/5.0	–/0.0	0.2/1.1	0.6/5.5
Respiratory	–/0.0	0.2/0.4	0.9/1.9	–/0.0	0.1/0.3	0.5/1.8
All Other	–/0.7	0.1/0.9	0.1/1.3	–/0.4	0.1/0.5	0.2/1.7
All Causes	–/0.9	1.7/5.5 (31%)	2.5/10 (24%)	–/0.5	0.7/3.2 (20%)	1.6/11 (15%)

Peto, Lopez et al, 1992, 1994

IRELAND: 1990

RISKS OF DYING AT AGES 0–34 and 35–69

(Probability that someone entering an age range would die during it, if the death rates in 1990 were to persist unchanged)

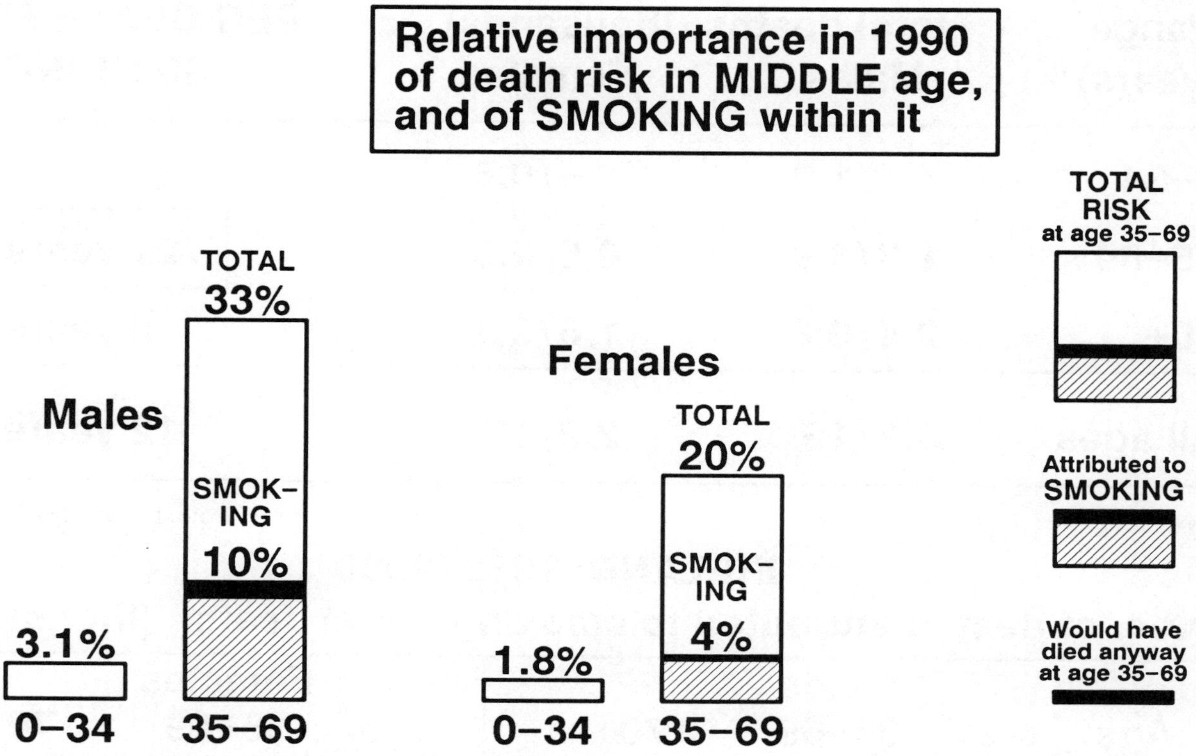

Peto, Lopez et al, 1992, 1994

IRELAND: 1990 deaths, all ages

Nos. of deaths attributed to smoking / total deaths (thousands)

	Males	Females	Males + Females
All Cancer	1.5/3.9 (38%)	0.6/3.3 (18%)	2.1/7.1 (29%)
All Causes	4.2/17 (25%)	2.3/15 (16%)	6.4/31 (20%)

Peto, Lopez et al, 1992, 1994

IRELAND: 1995 projections

Relative importance of deaths in MIDDLE age (35–69)

Age range (years)	Deaths attributed to SMOKING / total deaths (thousands) Males	Females	Mean years lost PER DEATH FROM SMOKING
0–34	–/1.0	–/0.6	–
35–69	1.3/4.9	0.6/2.9	21 years
70+	2.4/9.8	1.6/9.7	8 years
All ages	3.7/16	2.2/13	12 years

Peto, Lopez et al, 1992, 1994

IRELAND: 1950–2000

Nos. of deaths attributed to smoking / total deaths (thousands)

Age:	Males 0–34	Males 35–69	Males 70+	Females 0–34	Females 35–69	Females 70+
1955	–/2.2	1.3/6.6 (20%)	0.2/11 (2%)	–/1.7	0.3/4.9 (7%)	0.0/10 (0%)
1965	–/1.5	1.9/6.5 (30%)	0.8/9.9 (8%)	–/1.1	0.4/4.1 (9%)	0.2/9.9 (2%)
1975	–/1.5	2.3/6.8 (34%)	1.7/9.8 (18%)	–/0.9	0.7/4.0 (18%)	0.6/10 (6%)
1985	–/1.0	2.2/6.2 (35%)	2.5/11 (23%)	–/0.6	0.7/3.6 (20%)	1.4/11 (13%)
1995 (projected)	–/1.0	1.3/4.9 (27%)	2.4/9.8 (24%)	–/0.6	0.6/2.9 (20%)	1.6/9.7 (16%)
50–year total*, mid–1950 to mid–2000: 231/1647						
1950–2000, by age & sex	–/72	90/310 (29%)	76/515 (15%)	–/49	27/195 (14%)	38/506 (8%)

*Estimated as 10 times the sum of the five annual numbers (for 1955, 1965, 1975, 1985 & 1995)

IRELAND

Smoking–attributed numbers of deaths per year

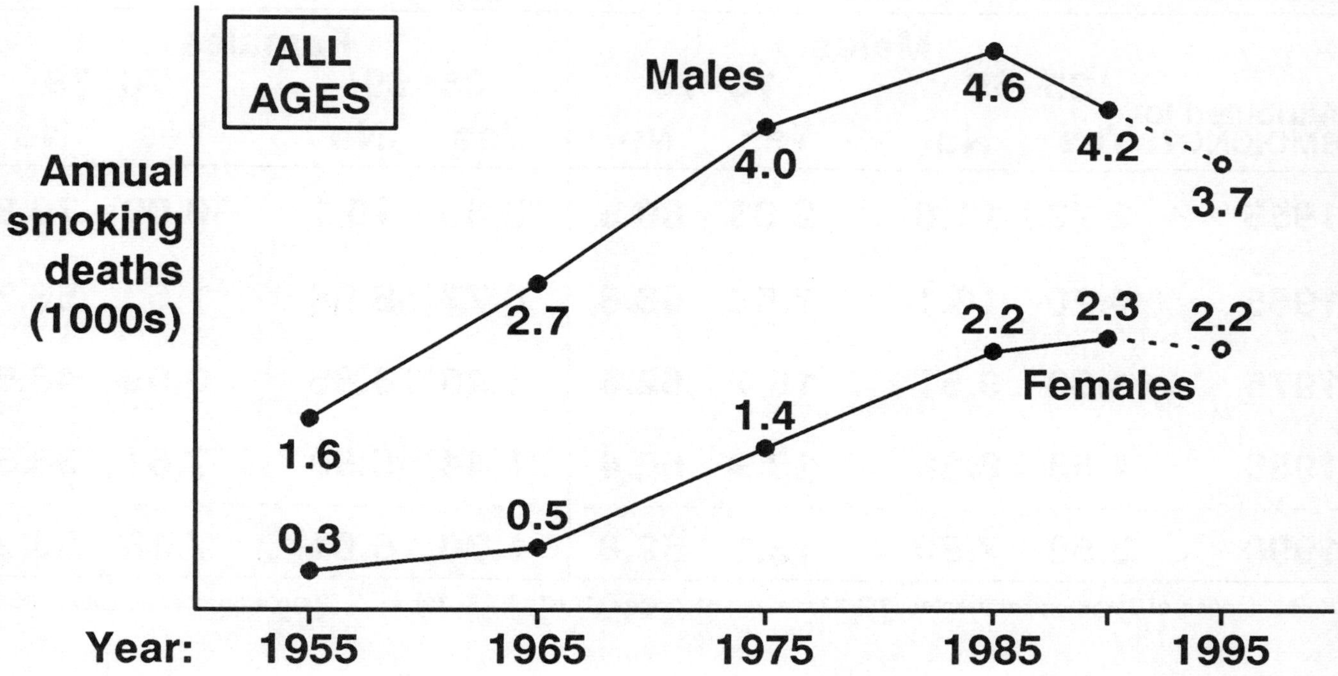

Peto, Lopez et al, 1992, 1994

IRELAND

Smoking–attributed numbers of deaths per year

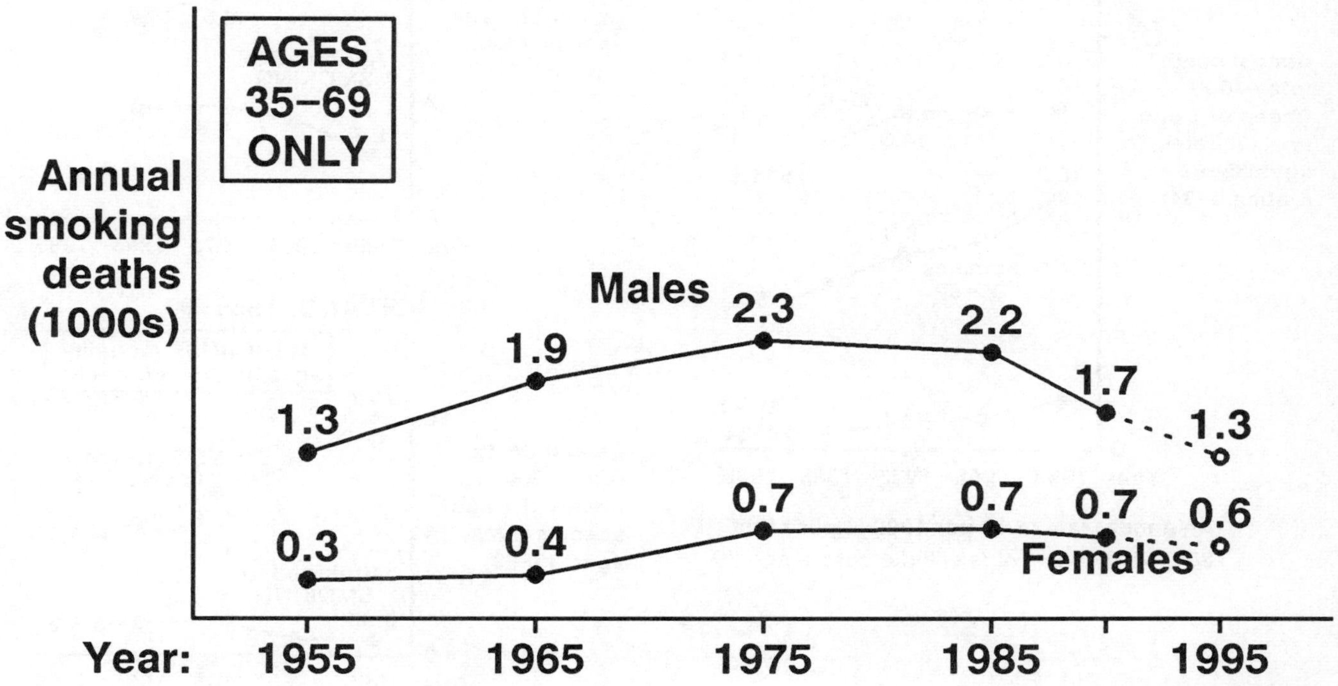

Peto, Lopez et al, 1992, 1994

IRELAND

ALL DEATHS (annual rates per 1000): Trends in mortality attributed to smoking, and in other mortality

	Males				Females			
	35–69		70–79		35–69		70–79	
Attributed to SMOKING?	Yes	No	Yes	No	Yes	No	Yes	No
1955	2.73	11.8	2.03	80.5	0.66	10.1	0.00	70.8
1965	4.20	10.1	7.56	68.8	0.77	8.06	1.63	56.7
1975	4.80	9.51	15.7	62.5	1.46	6.88	3.99	48.5
1985	4.58	8.38	19.9	60.4	1.44	5.59	7.61	38.5
1990	3.59	7.90	18.1	52.8	1.30	5.01	7.38	33.2

35–69 = mean of 7 age–specific rates; 70–79 = mean of 2 rates (70–74 & 75–79) Peto, Lopez et al, 1992, 1994

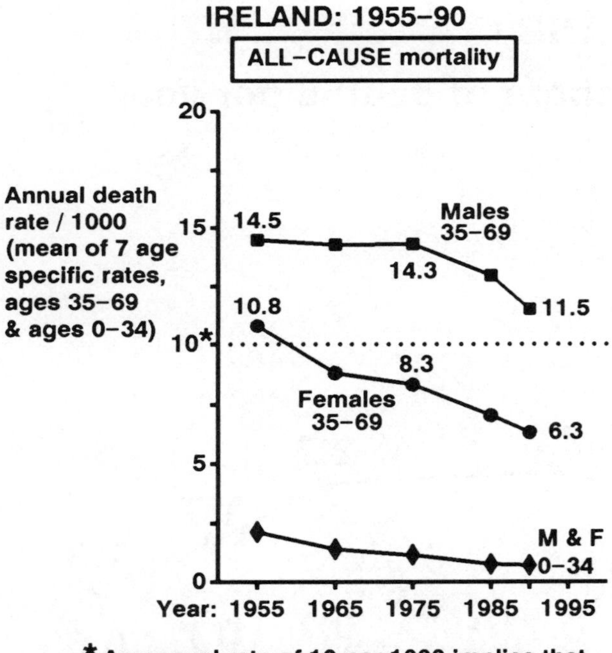

* An annual rate of 10 per 1000 implies that 30% of 35-year-olds will die before age 70

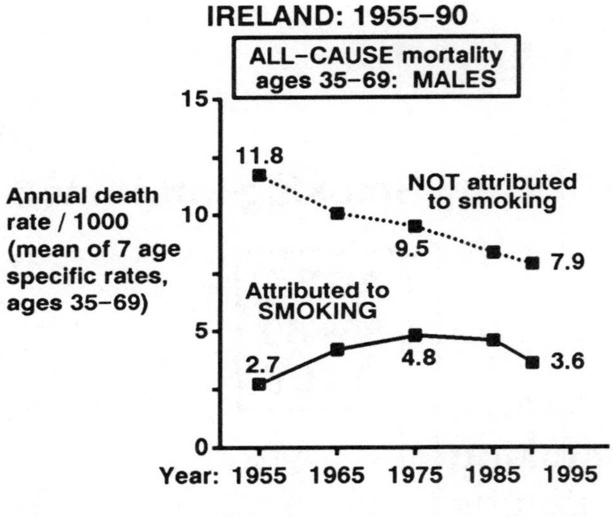

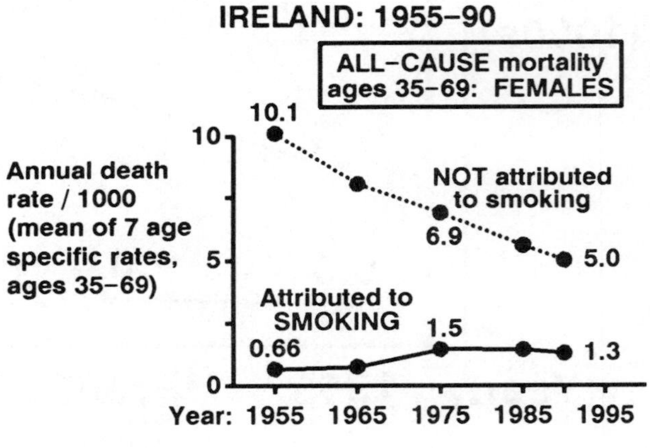

IRELAND

ALL CANCER DEATHS (annual rates per 1000):
Trends in mortality attributed to smoking, and in other mortality

	Males				Females			
	35–69		70–79		35–69		70–79	
Attributed to SMOKING?	Yes	No	Yes	No	Yes	No	Yes	No
1955	0.74	2.10	0.60	10.8	0.13	2.37	0.00	7.75
1965	1.20	1.85	2.22	10.4	0.16	2.27	0.26	7.68
1975	1.57	1.95	5.12	9.14	0.41	2.53	0.87	8.32
1985	1.70	1.90	6.54	9.88	0.45	2.22	1.87	7.35
1990	1.45	1.93	6.69	10.3	0.45	2.19	2.29	7.70

35–69 = mean of 7 age-specific rates; 70–79 = mean of 2 rates (70–74 & 75–79) Peto, Lopez et al, 1992, 1994

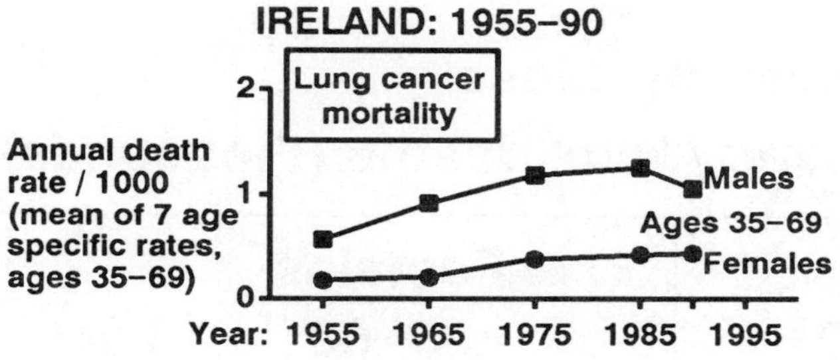

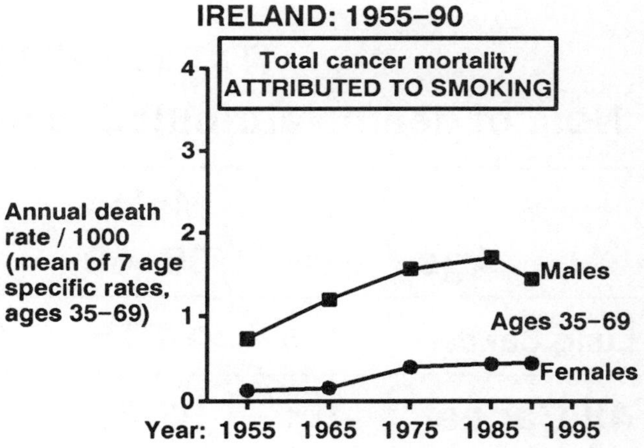

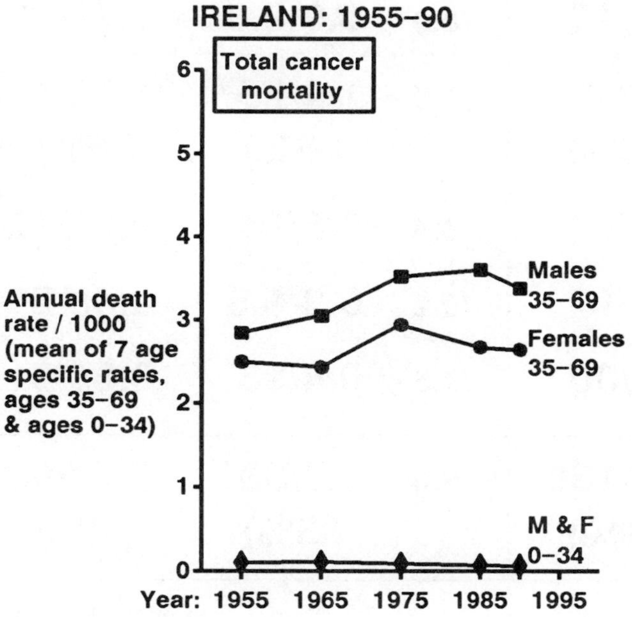

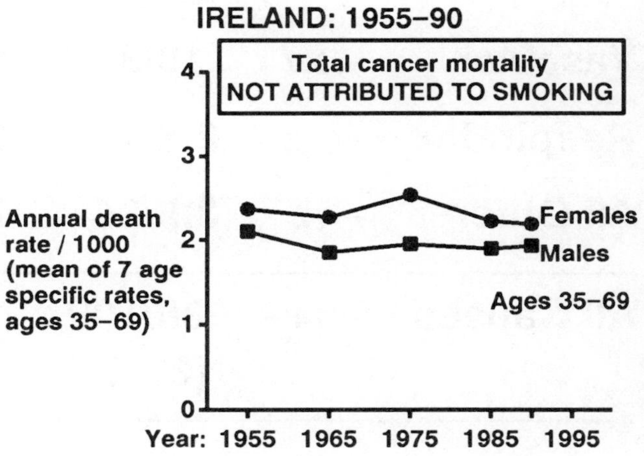

ITALY: 1990
Relative importance of deaths in MIDDLE age (35–69)

Age range (years)	Deaths attributed to SMOKING / total deaths (thousands) Males	Females	Mean years lost PER DEATH FROM SMOKING
0–34	–/14	–/6.0	–
35–69	38/102	2.7/53	21 years
70+	35/166	7.4/203	8 years
All ages	73/282	10/262	14 years

Peto, Lopez et al, 1992, 1994

ITALY: 1990 deaths, by cause
Nos. of deaths attributed to smoking / total deaths (thousands)

	Males			Females		
Age:	0–34	35–69	70+	0–34	35–69	70+
Lung Cancer	–/0.0	14/15	9.1/10	–/0.0	0.9/2.0	1.2/2.4
All Cancer	–/1.1	22/43 (50%)	14/41 (35%)	–/0.9	1.2/25 (5%)	1.7/34 (5%)
Vascular	–/0.7	10/31	9.0/77	–/0.4	0.8/14	2.5/112
Respiratory	–/0.3	2.8/4.4	8.9/17	–/0.2	0.3/1.5	2.4/12
All Other	–/12	3.5/24	2.6/30	–/4.5	0.4/13	0.8/45
All Causes	–/14	38/102 (37%)	35/166 (21%)	–/6.0	2.7/53 (5%)	7.4/203 (4%)

Peto, Lopez et al, 1992, 1994

ITALY: 1990

RISKS OF DYING AT AGES 0–34 and 35–69

(Probability that someone entering an age range would die during it, if the death rates in 1990 were to persist unchanged)

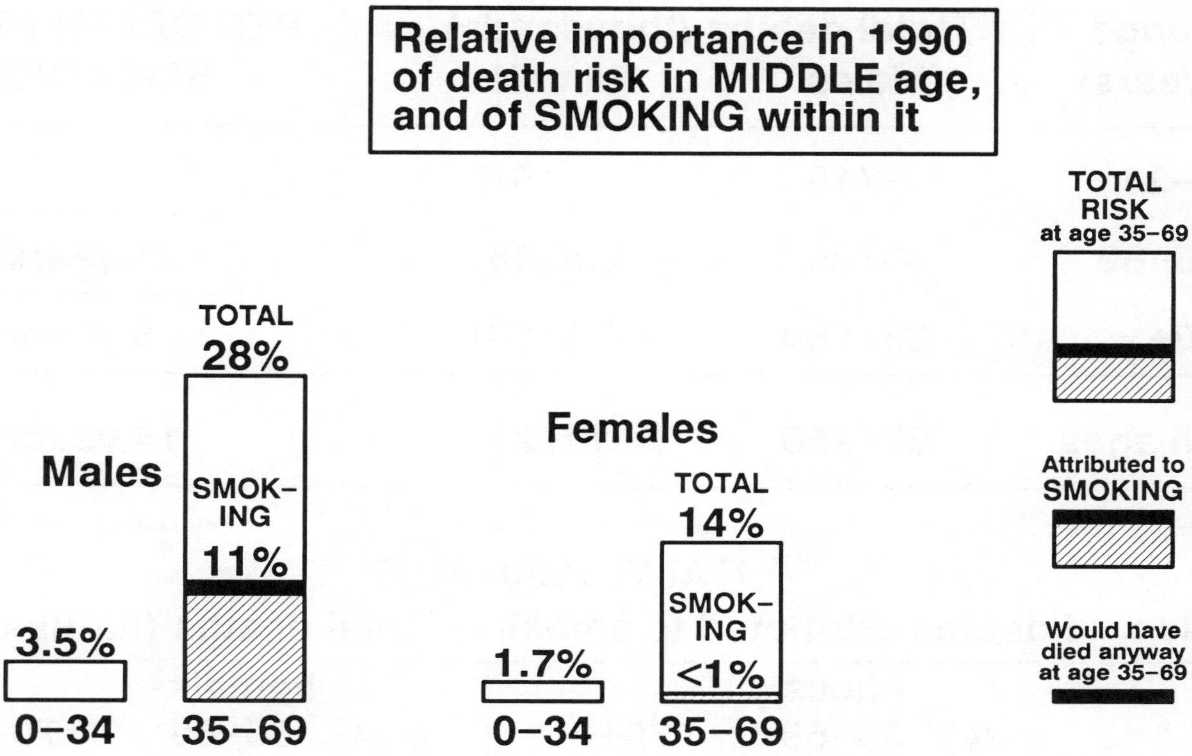

Peto, Lopez et al, 1992, 1994

ITALY: 1990 deaths, all ages

Nos. of deaths attributed to smoking / total deaths (thousands)

	Males	Females	Males + Females
All Cancer	36/85 (42%)	2.8/60 (5%)	39/145 (27%)
All Causes	73/282 (26%)	10/262 (4%)	83/544 (15%)

Peto, Lopez et al, 1992, 1994

ITALY: 1995 projections
Relative importance of deaths in MIDDLE age (35–69)

Age range (years)	Deaths attributed to SMOKING / total deaths (thousands) Males	Females	Mean years lost PER DEATH FROM SMOKING
0–34	–/16	–/5.5	–
35–69	33/89	2.5/46	21 years
70+	35/154	8.1/181	8 years
All ages	68/258	11/232	14 years

Peto, Lopez et al, 1992, 1994

ITALY: 1950–2000
Nos. of deaths attributed to smoking / total deaths (thousands)

	Males			Females		
Age:	0–34	35–69	70+	0–34	35–69	70+
1955	–/45	14/88 (15%)	1.1/102 (1%)	–/34	0.0/67 (0%)	0.0/112 (0%)
1965	–/35	30/113 (26%)	7.7/128 (6%)	–/24	1.1/70 (2%)	0.5/148 (0.3%)
1975	–/22	39/121 (32%)	23/152 (15%)	–/13	1.7/66 (3%)	3.0/180 (2%)
1985	–/13	39/103 (38%)	36/171 (21%)	–/6.8	2.4/53 (5%)	6.3/201 (3%)
1995 (projected)	–/16	33/89 (37%)	35/154 (23%)	–/5.5	2.5/46 (6%)	8.1/181 (4%)
50–year total* (M=millions), mid–1950 to mid–2000: 2.8/26M						
1950–2000, by age & sex	–/1.3M	1.5/5.1M (29%)	1.0/7.1M (14%)	–/0.8M	0.1/3.0M (3%)	0.2/8.2M (2%)

*Estimated as 10 times the sum of the five annual numbers (for 1955, 1965, 1975, 1985 & 1995)

ITALY

Smoking–attributed numbers of deaths per year

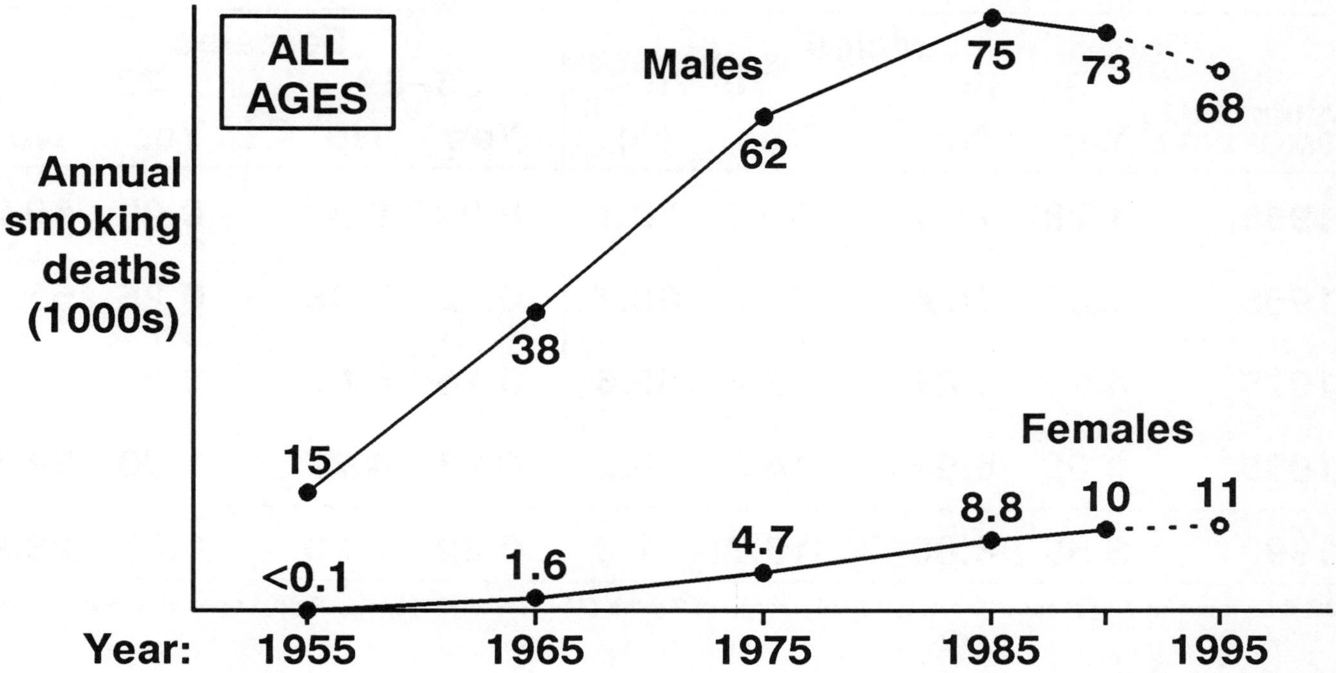

Peto, Lopez et al, 1992, 1994

ITALY

Smoking–attributed numbers of deaths per year

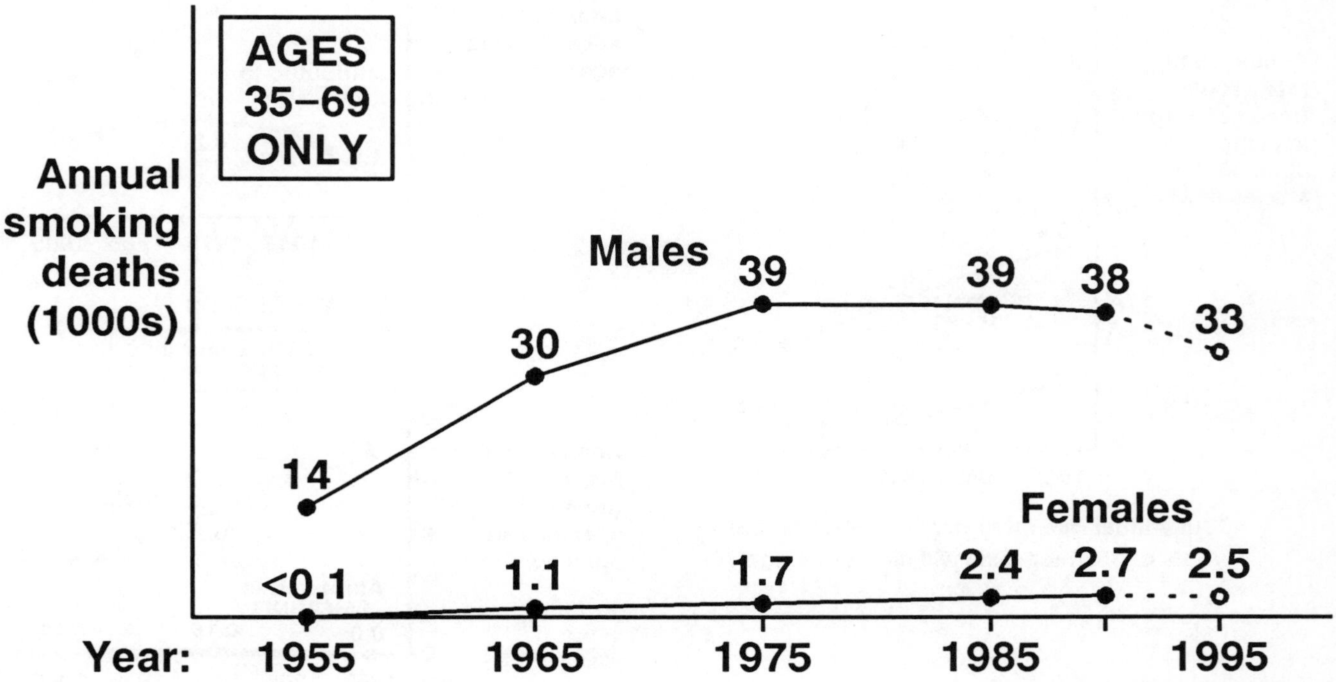

Peto, Lopez et al, 1992, 1994

ITALY

ALL DEATHS (annual rates per 1000): Trends in mortality attributed to smoking, and in other mortality

	Males				Females			
	35–69		70–79		35–69		70–79	
Attributed to SMOKING?	Yes	No	Yes	No	Yes	No	Yes	No
1955	1.78	11.1	0.89	70.1	0.00	8.39	0.00	59.2
1965	3.66	10.6	5.50	68.7	0.12	7.46	0.25	55.7
1975	4.16	8.81	12.6	59.6	0.16	6.08	0.88	44.7
1985	4.09	6.93	14.8	48.9	0.23	4.77	1.30	34.6
1990	3.55	6.00	13.7	41.8	0.22	4.10	1.35	28.9

35–69 = mean of 7 age-specific rates; 70–79 = mean of 2 rates (70–74 & 75–79) Peto, Lopez et al, 1992, 1994

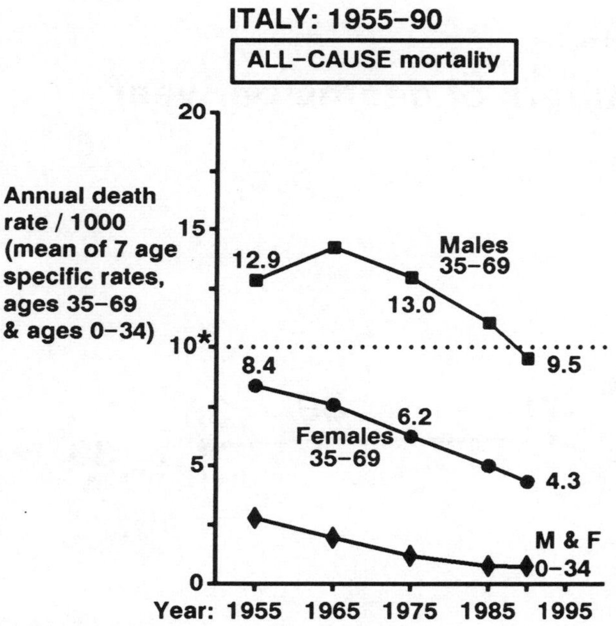

* An annual rate of 10 per 1000 implies that 30% of 35-year-olds will die before age 70

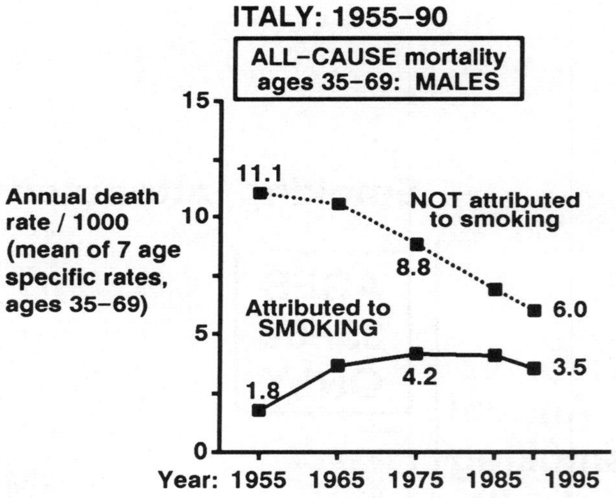

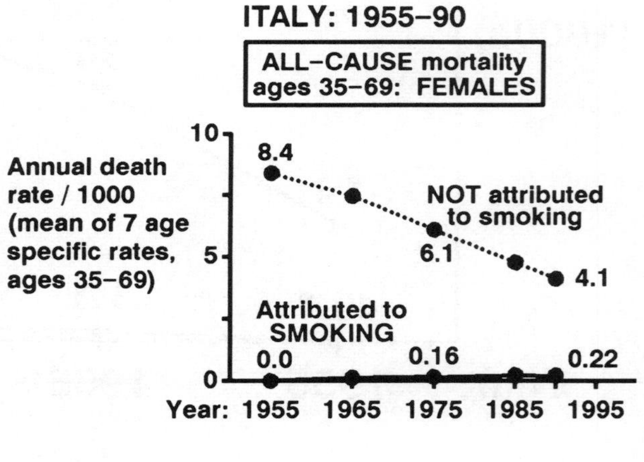

ITALY

ALL CANCER DEATHS (annual rates per 1000): Trends in mortality attributed to smoking, and in other mortality

	Males				Females			
	35–69		70–79		35–69		70–79	
Attributed to SMOKING?	Yes	No	Yes	No	Yes	No	Yes	No
1955	0.57	2.23	0.29	9.61	0.00	2.14	0.00	7.26
1965	1.28	2.26	1.73	10.7	0.03	2.19	0.04	8.08
1975	1.72	2.09	4.46	10.5	0.04	2.09	0.18	7.50
1985	2.14	2.01	6.70	10.9	0.09	1.99	0.38	7.65
1990	2.03	2.00	6.85	10.9	0.09	1.92	0.45	7.45

35–69 = mean of 7 age–specific rates; 70–79 = mean of 2 rates (70–74 & 75–79)   Peto, Lopez et al, 1992, 1994

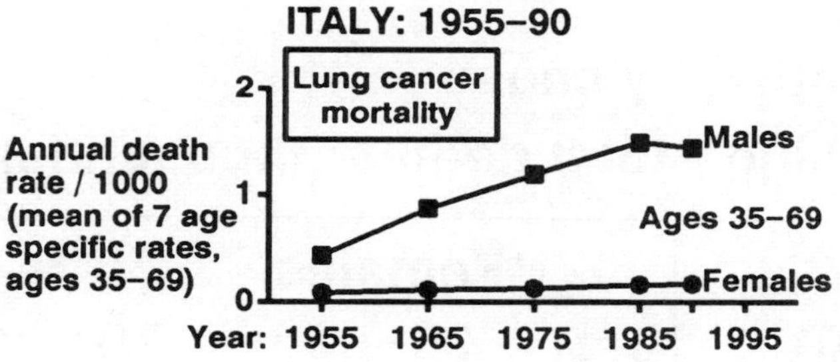

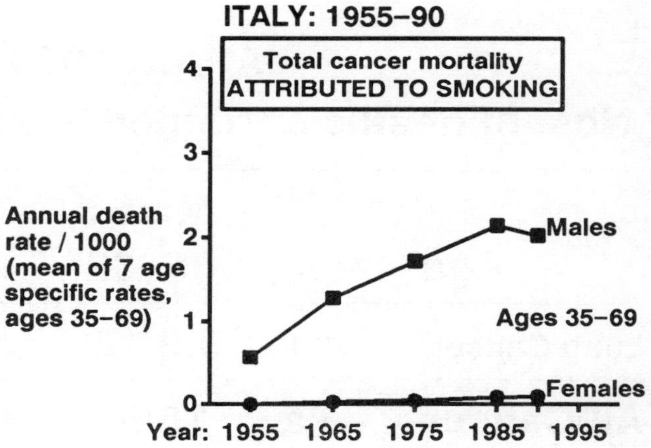

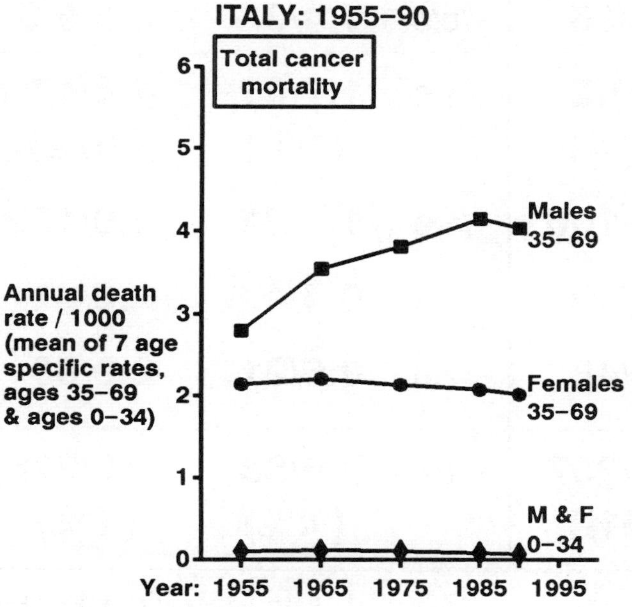

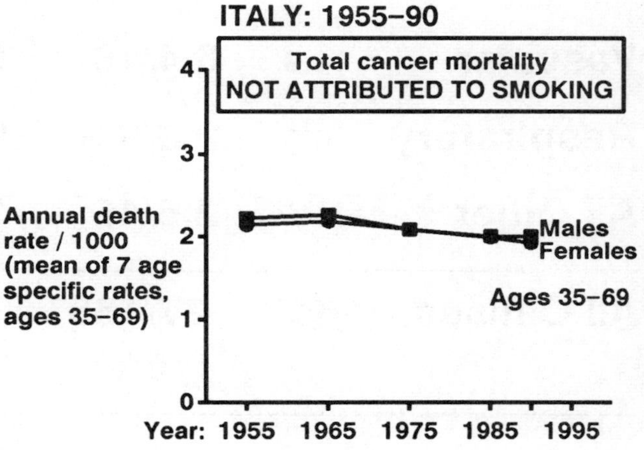

JAPAN: 1990
Relative importance of deaths in MIDDLE age (35–69)

Age range (years)	Deaths attributed to SMOKING / total deaths (thousands) Males	Females	Mean years lost PER DEATH FROM SMOKING
0–34	–/19	–/10	–
35–69	27/168	3.6/88	21 years
70+	42/257	15/278	8 years
All ages	68/444	19/377	12 years

Peto, Lopez et al, 1992, 1994

JAPAN: 1990 deaths, by cause
Nos. of deaths attributed to smoking / total deaths (thousands)

	Males			Females		
Age:	0–34	35–69	70+	0–34	35–69	70+
Lung Cancer	–/0.1	9.9/12	13/15	–/0.0	1.4/3.7	3.8/5.9
All Cancer	–/1.8	16/67 (23%)	20/62 (32%)	–/1.6	1.7/39 (4%)	4.8/47 (10%)
Vascular	–/1.9	6.4/46	9.2/100	–/1.0	1.0/24	5.0/132
Respiratory	–/0.8	2.3/9.9	9.4/48	–/0.5	0.4/4.6	3.6/37
All Other	–/14	2.5/45	3.4/48	–/7.0	0.5/21	2.0/63
All Causes	–/19	27/168 (16%)	42/257 (16%)	–/10	3.6/88 (4%)	15/278 (6%)

Peto, Lopez et al, 1992, 1994

JAPAN: 1990

RISKS OF DYING AT AGES 0–34 and 35–69

(Probability that someone entering an age range would die during it, if the death rates in 1990 were to persist unchanged)

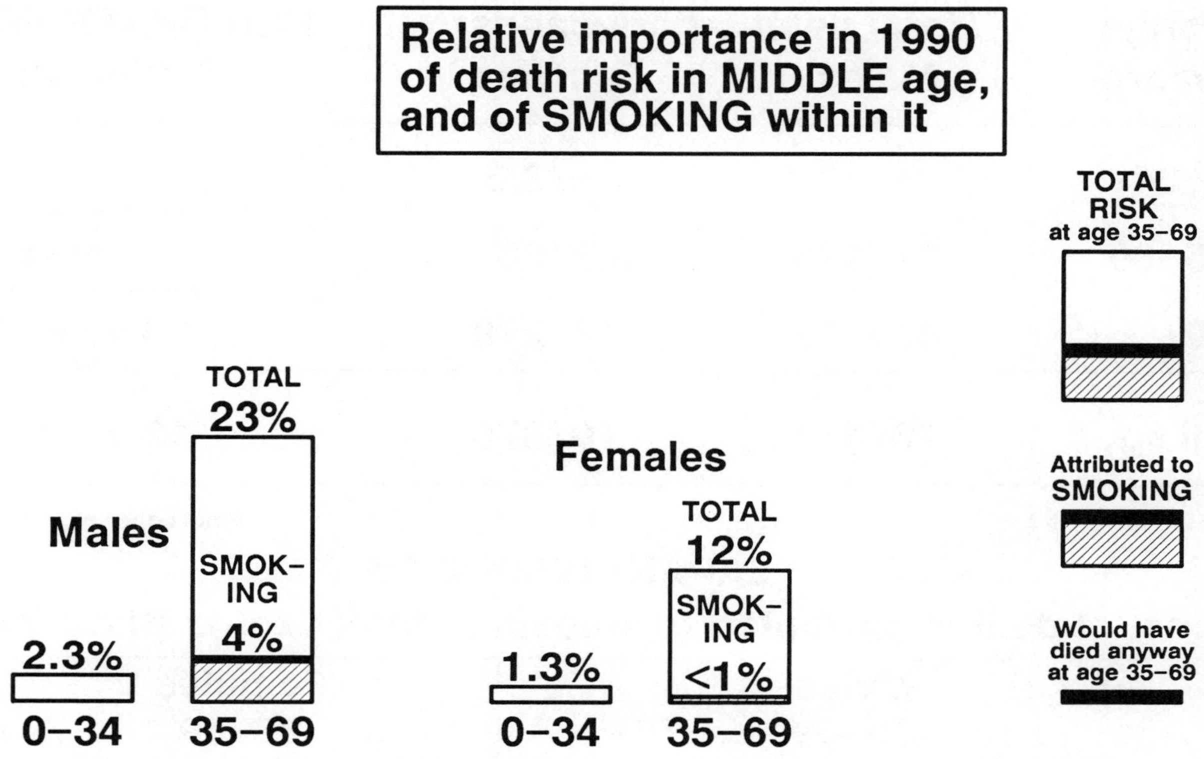

Peto, Lopez et al, 1992, 1994

JAPAN: 1990 deaths, all ages

Nos. of deaths attributed to smoking / total deaths (thousands)

	Males	Females	Males + Females
All Cancer	35/130 (27%)	6.5/87 (7%)	42/217 (19%)
All Causes	68/444 (15%)	19/377 (5%)	87/820 (11%)

Peto, Lopez et al, 1992, 1994

JAPAN: 1995 projections

Relative importance of deaths in MIDDLE age (35–69)

Age range (years)	Deaths attributed to SMOKING / total deaths (thousands) Males	Females	Mean years lost PER DEATH FROM SMOKING
0–34	–/18	–/9.3	–
35–69	31/175	3.3/83	21 years
70+	45/258	16/278	8 years
All ages	76/451	19/370	13 years

Peto, Lopez et al, 1992, 1994

JAPAN: 1950–2000

Nos. of deaths attributed to smoking / total deaths (thousands)

	Males			Females		
Age:	0–34	35–69	70+	0–34	35–69	70+
1955	–/102	2.7/156 (2%)	0.7/107 (0.7%)	–/84	0.0/115 (0%)	0.0/129 (0%)
1965	–/56	13/169 (8%)	6.6/153 (4%)	–/37	1.9/111 (2%)	1.2/174 (0.7%)
1975	–/38	18/156 (11%)	18/184 (10%)	–/24	3.1/101 (3%)	5.2/200 (3%)
1985	–/22	22/157 (14%)	35/229 (15%)	–/12	3.8/90 (4%)	13/242 (5%)
1995 (projected)	–/18	31/175 (18%)	45/258 (17%)	–/9.3	3.3/83 (4%)	16/278 (6%)
50-year total* (M=millions), mid-1950 to mid-2000: 2.4/37M						
1950–2000, by age & sex	–/2.4M	0.9/8.1M (11%)	1.1/9.3M (12%)	–/1.7M	0.1/5.0M (2%)	0.4/10M (4%)

*Estimated as 10 times the sum of the five annual numbers (for 1955, 1965, 1975, 1985 & 1995)

JAPAN
Smoking–attributed numbers of deaths per year

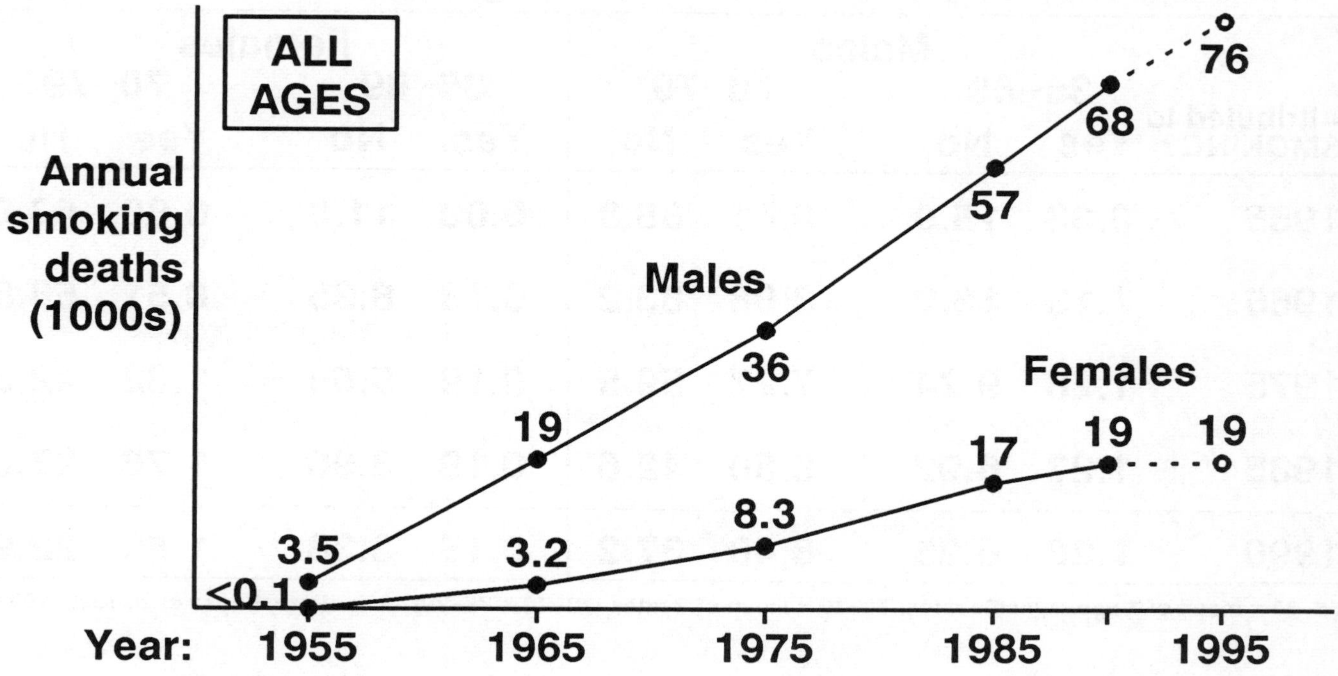

Peto, Lopez et al, 1992, 1994

JAPAN
Smoking–attributed numbers of deaths per year

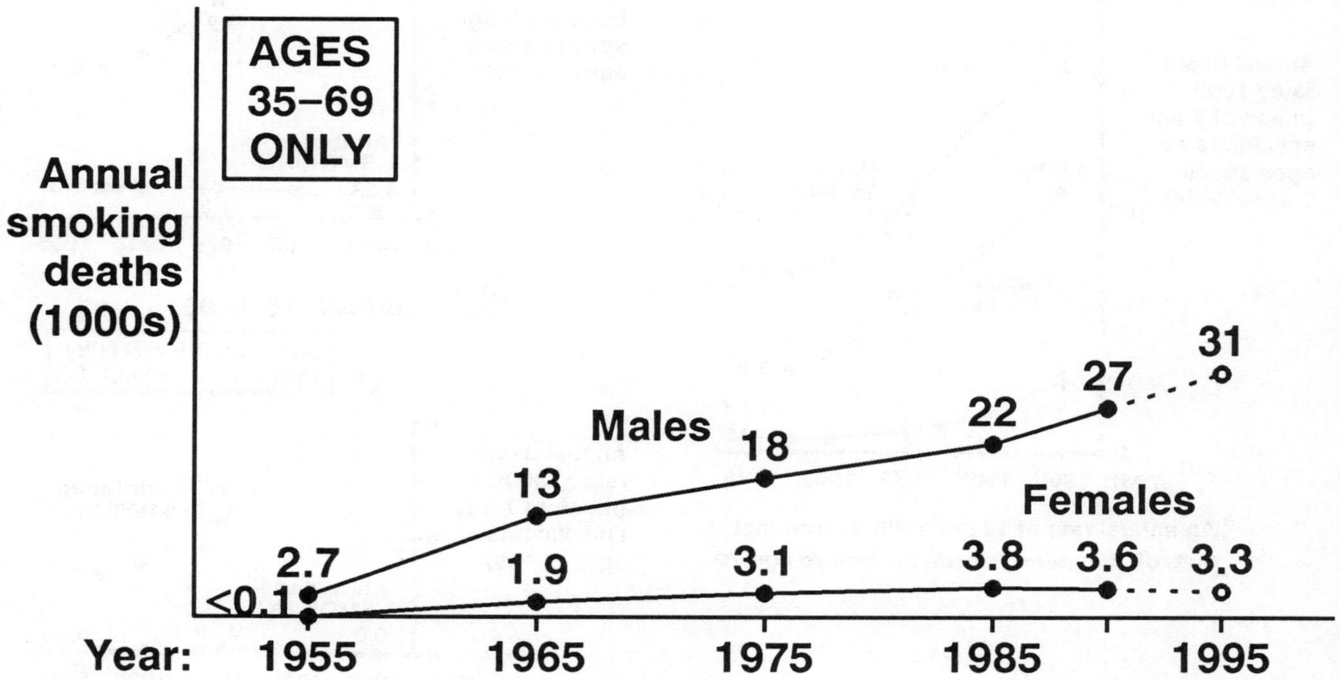

Peto, Lopez et al, 1992, 1994

JAPAN

ALL DEATHS (annual rates per 1000): Trends in mortality attributed to smoking, and in other mortality

	Males				Females			
	35–69		70–79		35–69		70–79	
Attributed to SMOKING?	Yes	No	Yes	No	Yes	No	Yes	No
1955	0.33	15.9	0.61	86.8	0.00	11.0	0.00	63.0
1965	1.13	13.2	3.98	83.2	0.16	8.35	0.51	58.5
1975	1.28	9.24	7.27	59.5	0.19	5.64	1.32	42.3
1985	1.27	6.92	8.80	42.6	0.19	3.90	1.76	27.6
1990	1.28	6.25	8.40	37.2	0.15	3.38	1.60	22.9

35–69 = mean of 7 age-specific rates; 70–79 = mean of 2 rates (70–74 & 75–79) Peto, Lopez et al, 1992, 1994

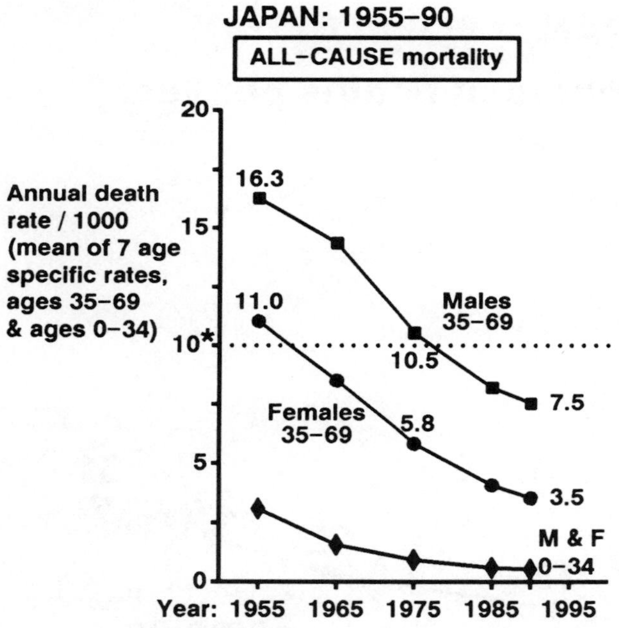

* An annual rate of 10 per 1000 implies that 30% of 35-year-olds will die before age 70

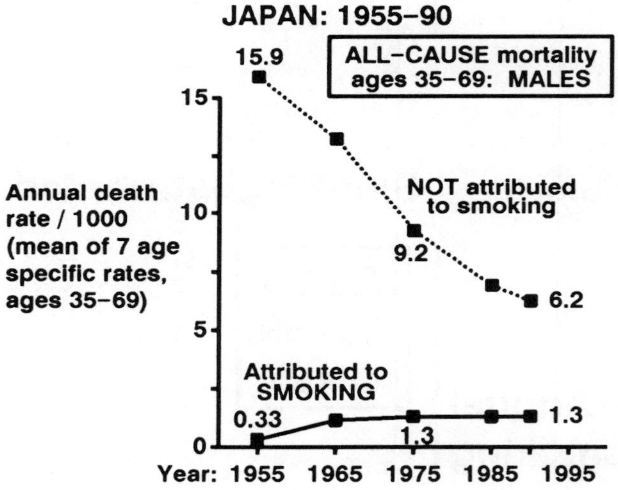

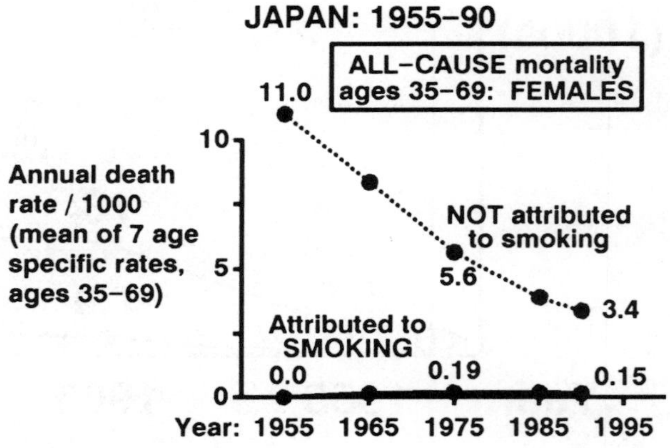

JAPAN

ALL CANCER DEATHS (annual rates per 1000): Trends in mortality attributed to smoking, and in other mortality

	Males				Females			
	35–69		70–79		35–69		70–79	
Attributed to SMOKING?	Yes	No	Yes	No	Yes	No	Yes	No
1955	0.10	2.97	0.17	9.25	0.00	2.30	0.00	5.89
1965	0.40	2.88	1.35	10.9	0.03	2.16	0.11	6.89
1975	0.56	2.49	2.89	10.5	0.06	1.85	0.33	6.71
1985	0.71	2.36	4.50	10.3	0.08	1.57	0.64	6.22
1990	0.76	2.32	4.62	9.58	0.07	1.45	0.66	5.68

35–69 = mean of 7 age-specific rates; 70–79 = mean of 2 rates (70–74 & 75–79) Peto, Lopez et al, 1992, 1994

JAPAN: 1955–90

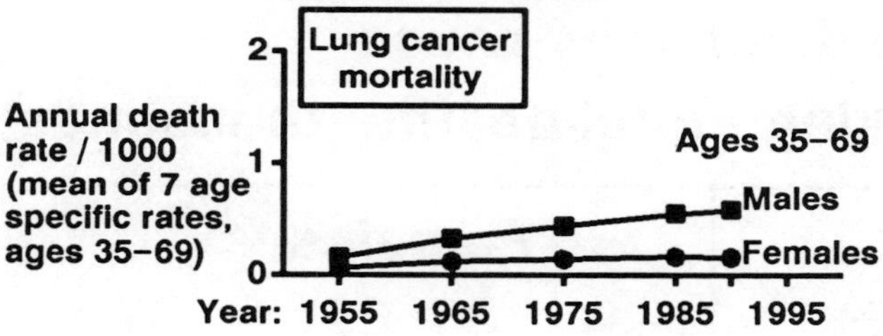

JAPAN: 1955–90

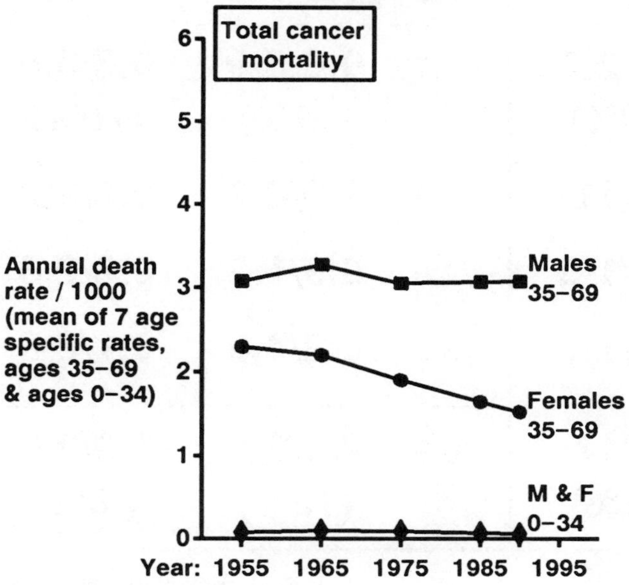

JAPAN: 1955–90

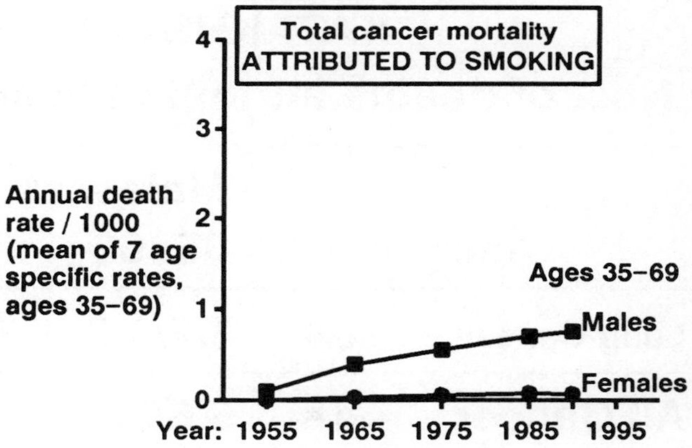

JAPAN: 1955–90

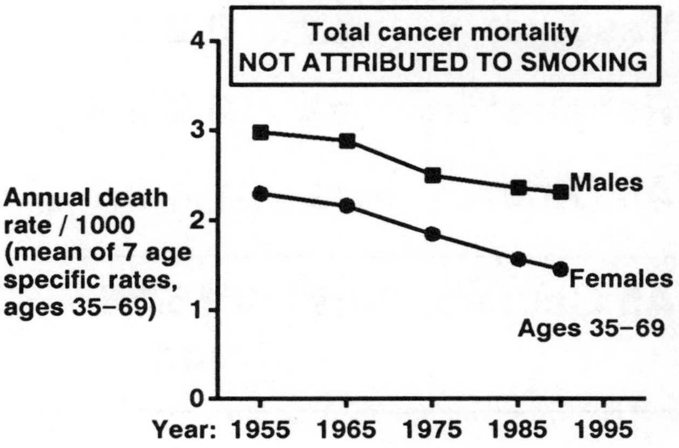

¶KAZAKHSTAN: 1990
Relative importance of deaths in MIDDLE age (35–69)

Age range (years)	Deaths attributed to SMOKING / total deaths (thousands) Males	Females	Mean years lost PER DEATH FROM SMOKING
0–34	–/16	–/8.9	–
35–69	15/35	2.3/20	21 years
70+	3.7/17	1.9/32	8 years
All ages	19/68	4.2/61	18 years

Peto, Lopez et al, 1992, 1994

KAZAKHSTAN: 1990 deaths, by cause
Nos. of deaths attributed to smoking / total deaths (thousands)

	Males			Females		
Age:	0–34	35–69	70+	0–34	35–69	70+
Lung Cancer	–/0.0	3.2/3.3	0.6/0.7	–/0.0	0.3/0.6	0.2/0.3
All Cancer	–/0.6	5.6/9.4 (59%)	1.1/2.7 (40%)	–/0.5	0.6/5.9 (11%)	0.3/3.5 (10%)
Vascular	–/0.7	6.2/14	1.2/11	–/0.4	1.0/8.7	0.6/23
Respiratory	–/2.4	2.0/2.5	1.3/1.9	–/2.0	0.5/1.2	0.8/2.3
All Other	–/12	1.4/9.7	0.1/1.7	–/6.0	0.2/4.3	0.1/2.6
All Causes	–/16	15/35 (43%)	3.7/17 (22%)	–/8.9	2.3/20 (12%)	1.9/32 (6%)

Peto, Lopez et al, 1992, 1994

KAZAKHSTAN: 1990
RISKS OF DYING AT AGES 0–34 and 35–69

(Probability that someone entering an age range would die during it, if the death rates in 1990 were to persist unchanged)

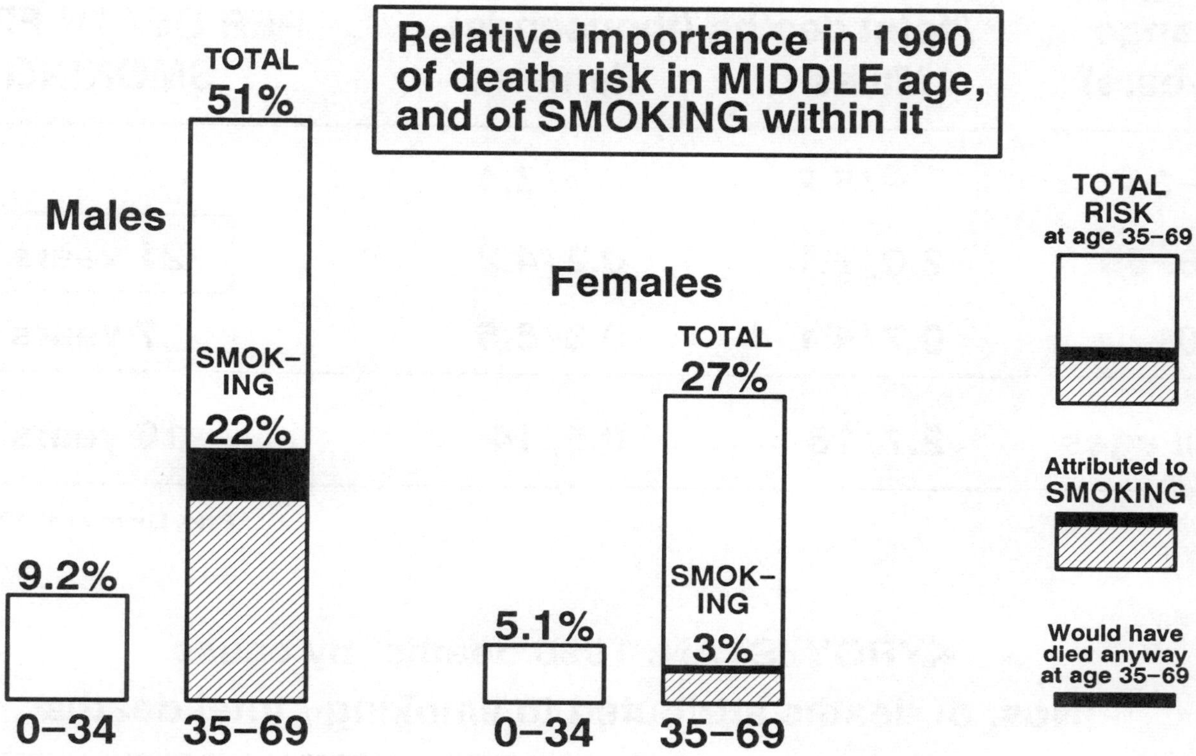

Peto, Lopez et al, 1992, 1994

KAZAKHSTAN: 1990 deaths, all ages
Nos. of deaths attributed to smoking / total deaths (thousands)

	Males	Females	Males + Females
All Cancer	6.6/13 (52%)	1.0/9.9 (10%)	7.6/23 (34%)
All Causes	19/68 (28%)	4.2/61 (7%)	23/129 (18%)

Peto, Lopez et al, 1992, 1994

¶KYRGYZSTAN: 1990
Relative importance of deaths in MIDDLE age (35–69)

Age range (years)	Deaths attributed to SMOKING / total deaths (thousands) Males	Females	Mean years lost PER DEATH FROM SMOKING
0–34	–/5.2	–/3.4	–
35–69	2.0/7.1	0.2/4.2	21 years
70+	0.7/4.1	0.3/6.6	7 years
All ages	2.7/16	0.5/14	16 years

Peto, Lopez et al, 1992, 1994

KYRGYZSTAN: 1990 deaths, by cause
Nos. of deaths attributed to smoking / total deaths

	Males			Females		
Age:	0–34	35–69	70+	0–34	35–69	70+
Lung Cancer	–/ 2	344/375	76/90	–/ 7	20/66	18/47
All Cancer	–/152	570/1365 (42%)	114/371 (31%)	–/99	23/854 (3%)	28/493 (6%)
Vascular	–/174	751/2709	158/2367	–/123	61/1963	65/4348
Respiratory	–/1488	490/695	392/711	–/1245	69/383	232/882
All Other	–/3378	209/2323	28/605	–/1895	15/1035	10/922
All Causes	–/5192	2020/7092 (28%)	692/4054 (17%)	–/3362	168/4235 (4%)	335/6645 (5%)

Peto, Lopez et al, 1992, 1994

KYRGYZSTAN: 1990

RISKS OF DYING AT AGES 0–34 and 35–69

(Probability that someone entering an age range would die during it, if the death rates in 1990 were to persist unchanged)

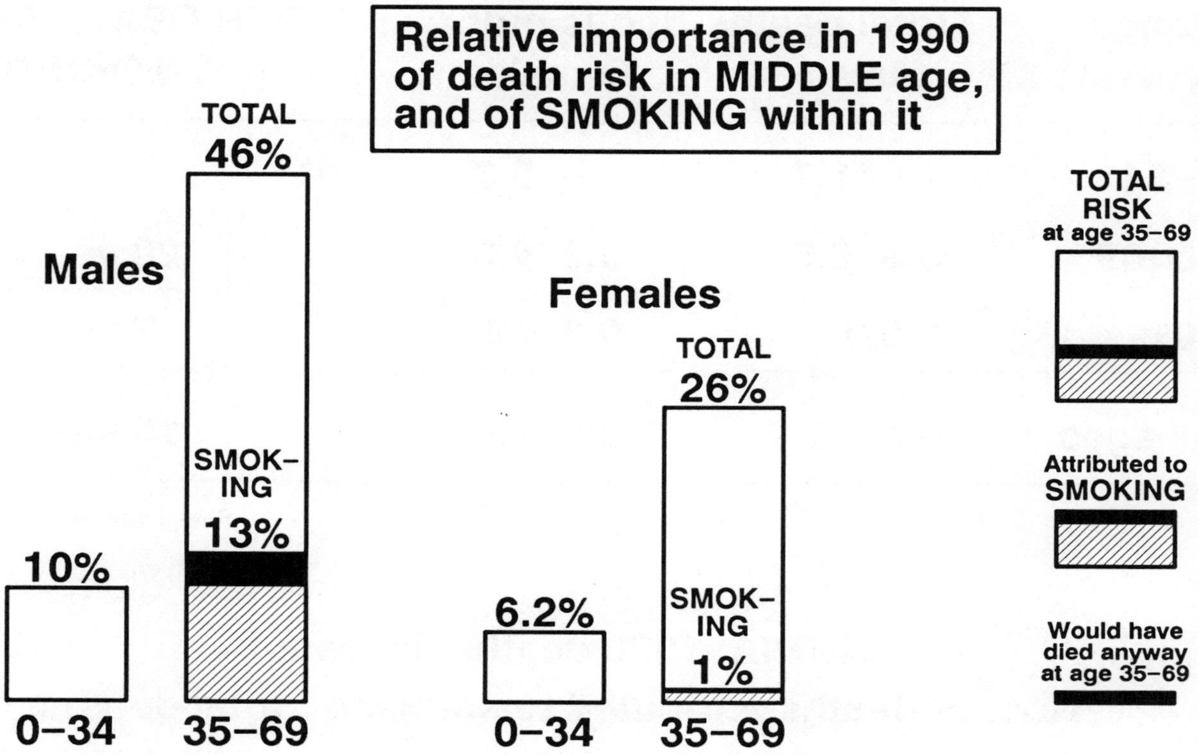

Peto, Lopez et al, 1992, 1994

KYRGYZSTAN: 1990 deaths, all ages

Nos. of deaths attributed to smoking / total deaths (thousands)

	Males	Females	Males + Females
All Cancer	0.7/1.9 (36%)	0.1/1.4 (4%)	0.7/3.3 (22%)
All Causes	2.7/16 (17%)	0.5/14 (4%)	3.2/31 (11%)

Peto, Lopez et al, 1992, 1994

¶LATVIA: 1990
Relative importance of deaths in MIDDLE age (35–69)

Age range (years)	Deaths attributed to SMOKING / total deaths (thousands) Males	Females	Mean years lost PER DEATH FROM SMOKING
0–34	–/1.7	–/0.7	–
35–69	3.3/8.5	0.3/4.8	20 years
70+	1.0/6.7	0.3/12	7 years
All ages	4.3/17	0.6/18	16 years

Peto, Lopez et al, 1992, 1994

LATVIA: 1990 deaths, by cause
Nos. of deaths attributed to smoking / total deaths

	Males			Females		
Age:	0–34	35–69	70+	0–34	35–69	70+
Lung Cancer	–/ 0	680/713	192/215	–/ 1	55/110	28/68
All Cancer	–/86	1082/1955 (55%)	295/920 (32%)	–/76	67/1407 (5%)	39/1053 (4%)
Vascular	–/101	1589/3852	465/4591	–/24	161/2207	142/9523
Respiratory	–/29	305/404	198/323	–/25	39/141	60/259
All Other	–/1486	302/2315	63/889	–/531	33/1061	17/1554
All Causes	–/1702	3278/8526 (38%)	1021/6723 (15%)	–/656	300/4816 (6%)	258/12389 (2%)

Peto, Lopez et al, 1992, 1994

LATVIA: 1990

RISKS OF DYING AT AGES 0–34 and 35–69

(Probability that someone entering an age range would die during it, if the death rates in 1990 were to persist unchanged)

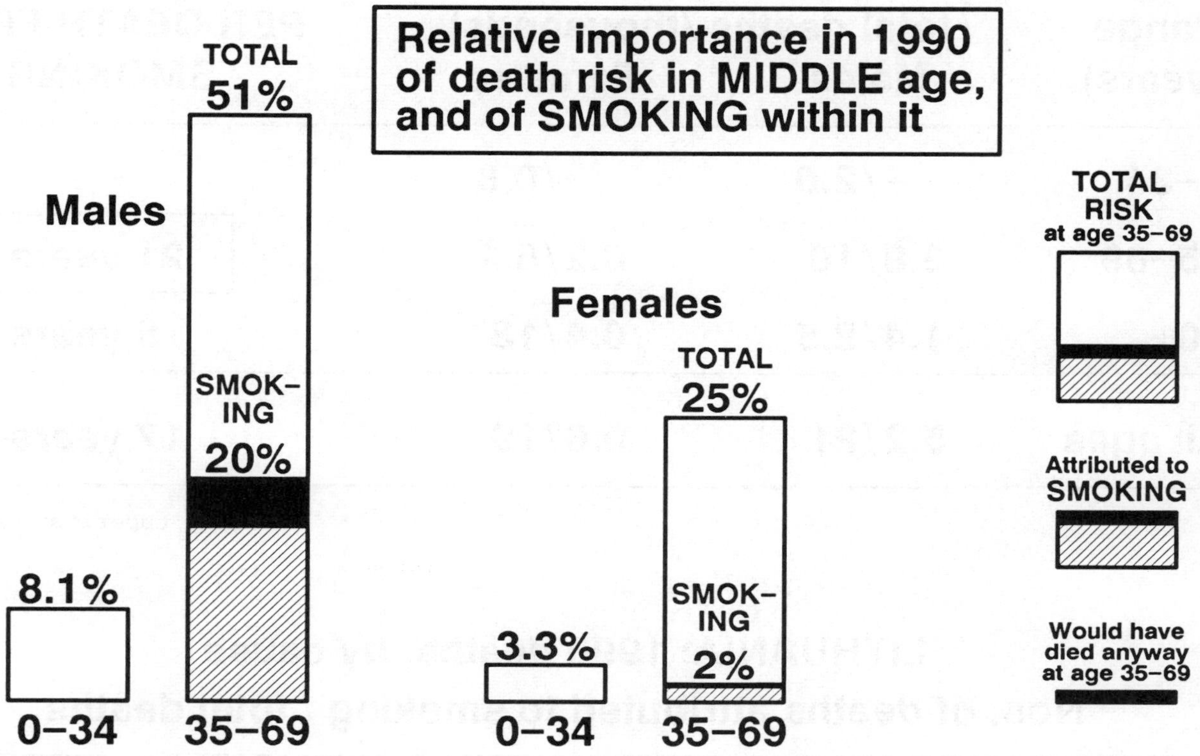

Peto, Lopez et al, 1992, 1994

LATVIA: 1990 deaths, all ages

Nos. of deaths attributed to smoking / total deaths (thousands)

	Males	Females	Males + Females
All Cancer	1.4/3.0 (47%)	0.1/2.5 (4%)	1.5/5.5 (27%)
All Causes	4.3/17 (25%)	0.6/18 (3%)	4.9/35 (14%)

Peto, Lopez et al, 1992, 1994

¶LITHUANIA: 1990
Relative importance of deaths in MIDDLE age (35–69)

Age range (years)	Deaths attributed to SMOKING / total deaths (thousands) Males	Females	Mean years lost PER DEATH FROM SMOKING
0–34	–/2.0	–/0.8	–
35–69	3.8/10	0.2/5.4	21 years
70+	1.4/8.5	0.4/13	8 years
All ages	5.2/21	0.6/19	17 years

Peto, Lopez et al, 1992, 1994

LITHUANIA: 1990 deaths, by cause
Nos. of deaths attributed to smoking / total deaths

	Males			Females		
Age:	0–34	35–69	70+	0–34	35–69	70+
Lung Cancer	–/ 1	865/909	272/303	–/ 3	35/102	46/98
All Cancer	–/95	1399/2555 (55%)	409/1293 (32%)	–/101	45/1709 (3%)	58/1206 (5%)
Vascular	–/114	1658/4159	554/5884	–/40	76/2220	206/10594
Respiratory	–/45	400/505	414/628	–/25	37/198	135/417
All Other	–/1704	364/2965	36/658	–/607	23/1264	11/774
All Causes	–/1958	3821/10184 (38%)	1413/8463 (17%)	–/773	181/5391 (3%)	410/12991 (3%)

Peto, Lopez et al, 1992, 1994

LITHUANIA: 1990

RISKS OF DYING AT AGES 0–34 and 35–69

(Probability that someone entering an age range would die during it, if the death rates in 1990 were to persist unchanged)

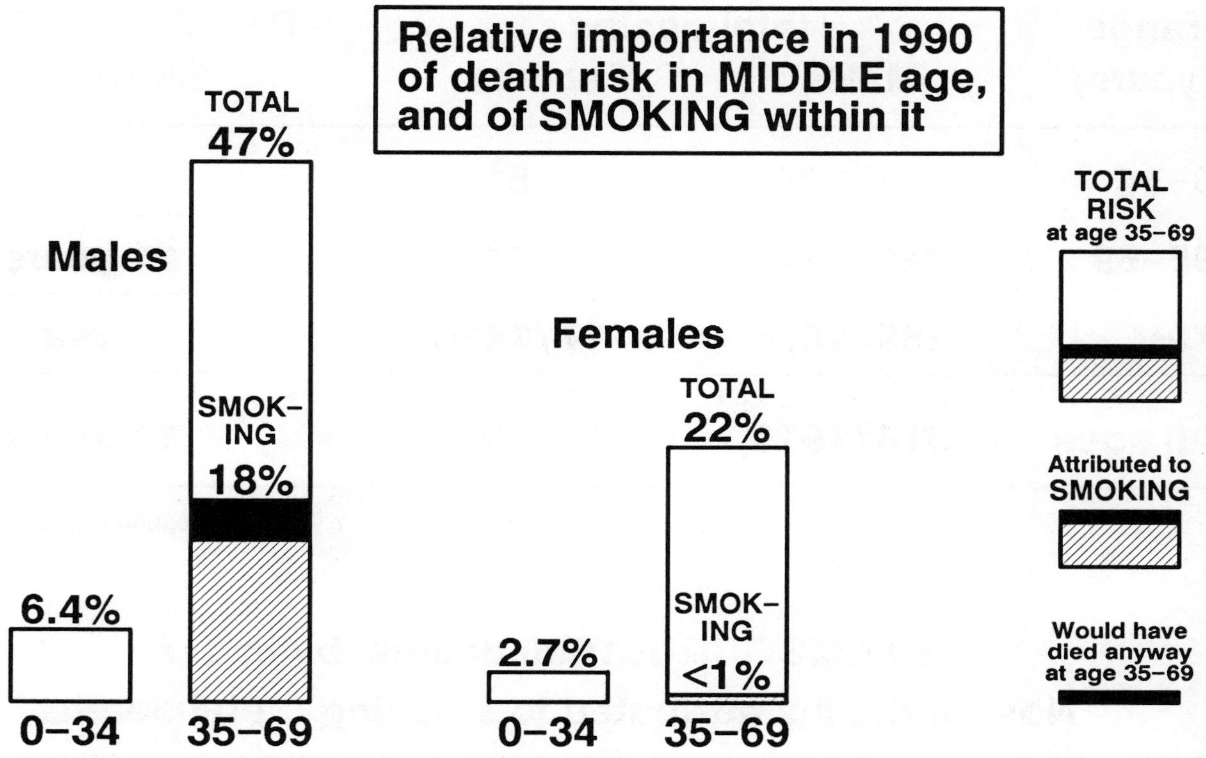

Peto, Lopez et al, 1992, 1994

LITHUANIA: 1990 deaths, all ages

Nos. of deaths attributed to smoking / total deaths (thousands)

	Males	Females	Males + Females
All Cancer	1.8/3.9 (46%)	0.1/3.0 (3%)	1.9/7.0 (27%)
All Causes	5.2/21 (25%)	0.6/19 (3%)	5.8/40 (15%)

Peto, Lopez et al, 1992, 1994

LUXEMBOURG: 1990
Relative importance of deaths in MIDDLE age (35–69)

Age range (years)	Deaths attributed to SMOKING / total deaths Males	Females	Mean years lost PER DEATH FROM SMOKING
0–34	–/108	–/51	–
35–69	249/727	40/443	21 years
70+	269/1078	17/1426	8 years
All ages	518/1913	57/1920	14 years

Peto, Lopez et al, 1992, 1994

LUXEMBOURG: 1990 deaths, by cause
Nos. of deaths attributed to smoking / total deaths

	Males			Females		
Age:	0–34	35–69	70+	0–34	35–69	70+
Lung Cancer	–/0	79/85	71/77	–/0	13/20	2/11
All Cancer	–/2	131/258 (51%)	109/267 (41%)	–/7	17/205 (8%)	3/230 (1%)
Vascular	–/4	74/240	82/550	–/3	13/113	9/869
Respiratory	–/2	21/32	60/110	–/2	6/18	3/71
All Other	–/100	23/197	18/151	–/39	4/107	2/256
All Causes	–/108	249/727 (34%)	269/1078 (25%)	–/51	40/443 (9%)	17/1426 (1%)

Peto, Lopez et al, 1992, 1994

LUXEMBOURG: 1990
RISKS OF DYING AT AGES 0–34 and 35–69
(Probability that someone entering an age range would die during it, if the death rates in 1990 were to persist unchanged)

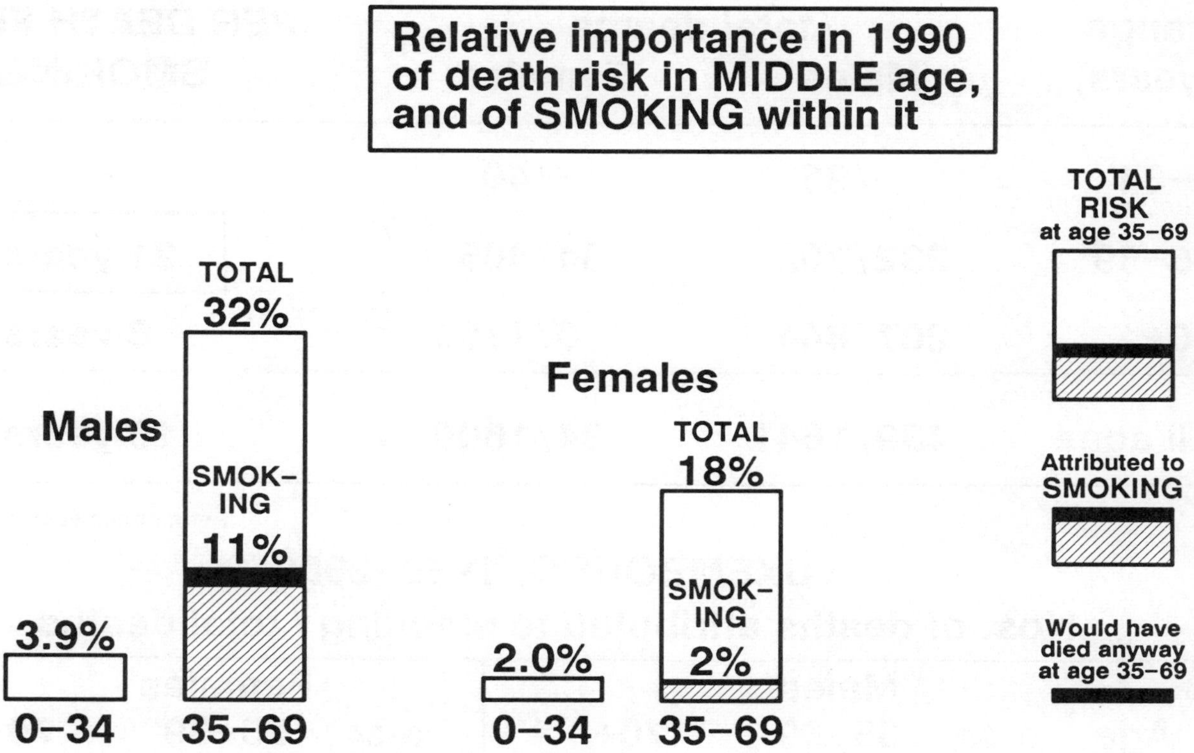

Peto, Lopez et al, 1992, 1994

LUXEMBOURG: 1990 deaths, all ages
Nos. of deaths attributed to smoking / total deaths

	Males	Females	Males + Females
All Cancer	240/527 (46%)	20/442 (5%)	260/969 (27%)
All Causes	518/1913 (27%)	57/1920 (3%)	575/3833 (15%)

Peto, Lopez et al, 1992, 1994

LUXEMBOURG: 1995 projections
Relative importance of deaths in MIDDLE age (35–69)

Age range (years)	Deaths attributed to SMOKING / total deaths: Males	Females	Mean years lost PER DEATH FROM SMOKING
0–34	–/95	–/40	–
35–69	232/702	34/405	21 years
70+	207/844	0/1155	8 years
All ages	439/1641	34/1600	16 years

Peto, Lopez et al, 1992, 1994

LUXEMBOURG: 1950–2000
Nos. of deaths attributed to smoking / total deaths

Age:	Males 0–34	Males 35–69	Males 70+	Females 0–34	Females 35–69	Females 70+
1955	–/223	232/856 (27%)	40/833 (5%)	–/146	0/591 (0%)	0/858 (0%)
1965	–/168	411/1049 (39%)	151/1030 (15%)	–/94	0/593 (0%)	0/1084 (0%)
1975	–/156	403/1032 (39%)	253/1144 (22%)	–/62	3/576 (0.5%)	0/1405 (0%)
1985	–/107	284/766 (37%)	315/1227 (26%)	–/61	41/443 (9%)	0/1476 (0%)
1995 (projected)	–/95	232/702 (33%)	207/844 (25%)	–/40	34/405 (8%)	0/1155 (0%)
50–year total* (thousands), mid–1950 to mid–2000: 26/192						
1950–2000, by age & sex	–/7.5	16/44 (36%)	9.7/51 (19%)	–/4.0	0.8/26 (3%)	0.0/60 (0%)

*Estimated as 10 times the sum of the five annual numbers (for 1955, 1965, 1975, 1985 & 1995)

LUXEMBOURG

Smoking–attributed numbers of deaths per year

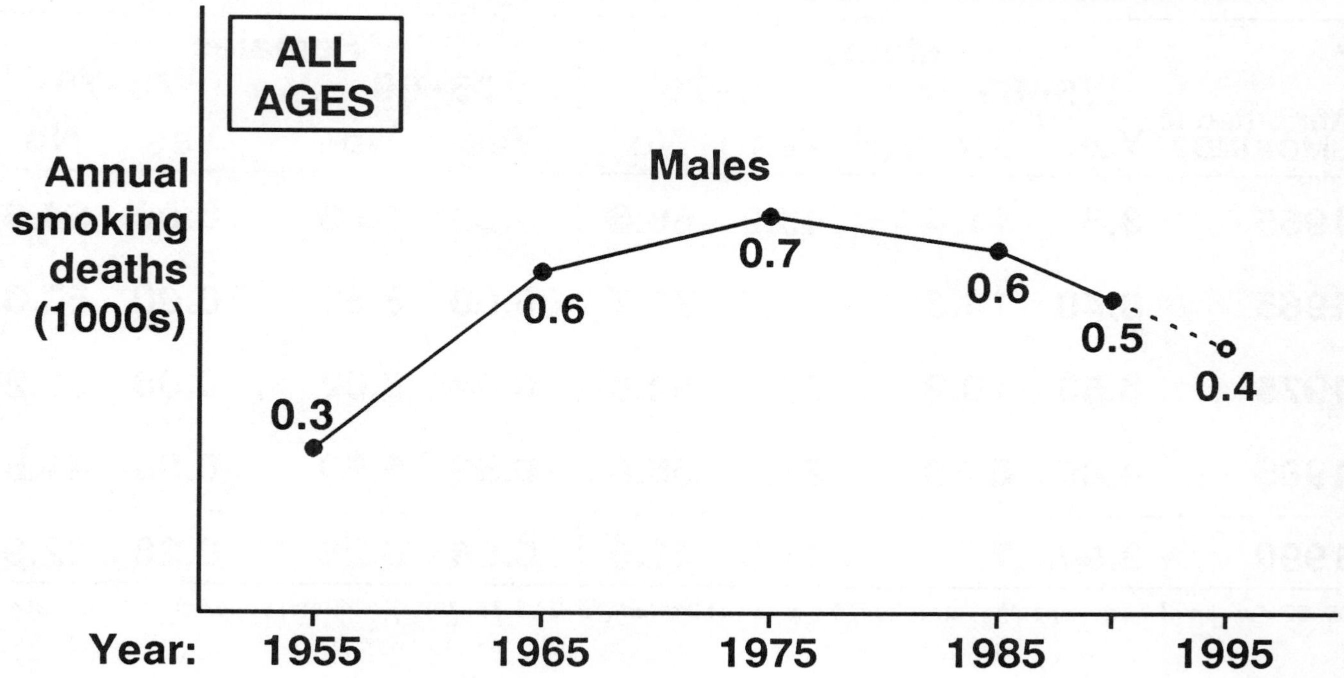

Peto, Lopez et al, 1992, 1994

LUXEMBOURG

Smoking–attributed numbers of deaths per year

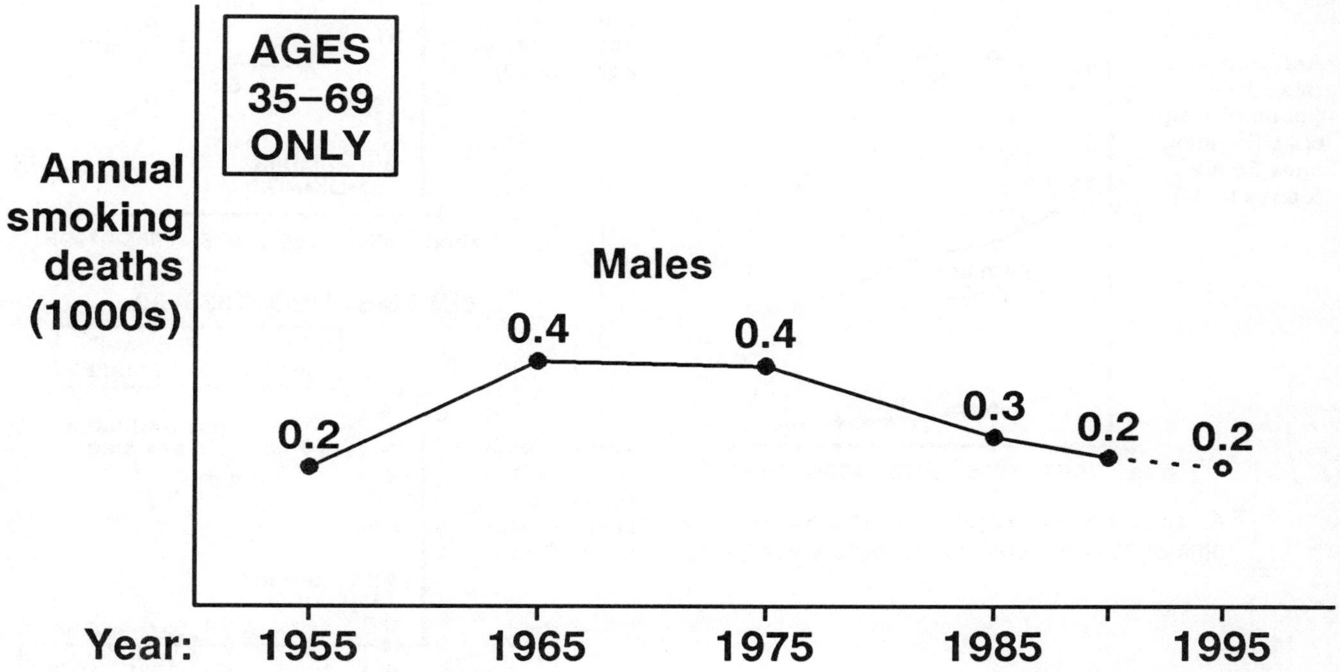

Peto, Lopez et al, 1992, 1994

LUXEMBOURG

ALL DEATHS (annual rates per 1000): Trends in mortality attributed to smoking, and in other mortality

	Males				Females			
	35–69		70–79		35–69		70–79	
Attributed to SMOKING?	Yes	No	Yes	No	Yes	No	Yes	No
1955	3.87	11.4	4.22	66.6	0.00	10.3	0.00	54.3
1965	6.40	10.3	14.5	71.7	0.00	8.61	0.00	57.3
1975	6.53	10.2	20.4	64.6	0.04	8.02	0.00	56.2
1985	4.89	8.30	21.0	55.6	0.59	5.90	0.00	41.5
1990	3.94	7.13	17.9	42.9	0.54	5.25	0.28	32.9

35–69 = mean of 7 age–specific rates; 70–79 = mean of 2 rates (70–74 & 75–79) Peto, Lopez et al, 1992, 1994

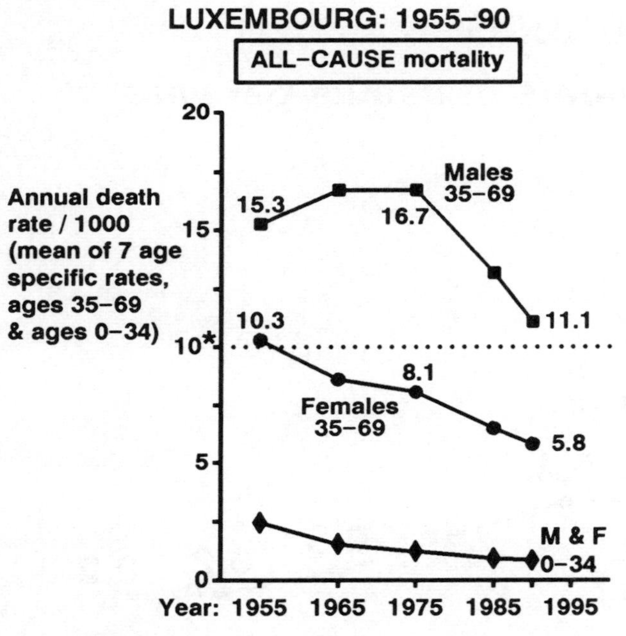

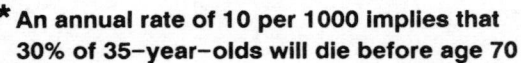

* An annual rate of 10 per 1000 implies that 30% of 35–year–olds will die before age 70

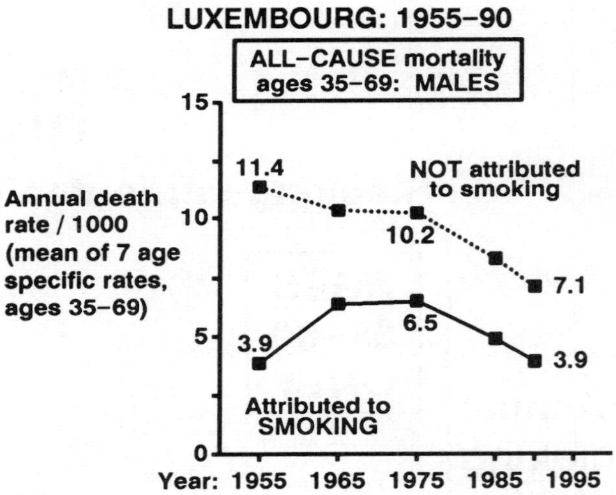

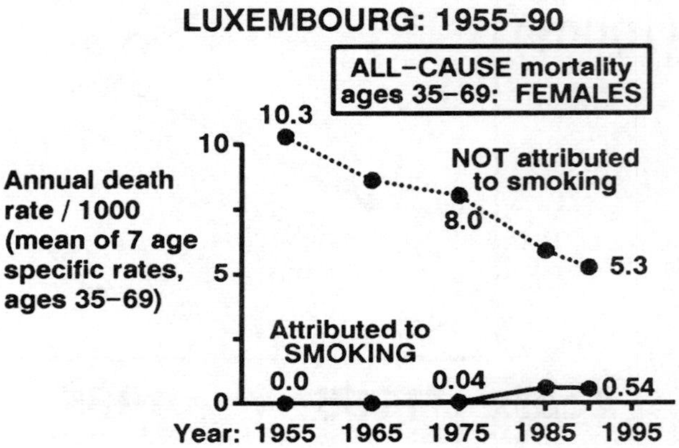

LUXEMBOURG

ALL CANCER DEATHS (annual rates per 1000): Trends in mortality attributed to smoking, and in other mortality

Attributed to SMOKING?	Males 35–69 Yes	Males 35–69 No	Males 70–79 Yes	Males 70–79 No	Females 35–69 Yes	Females 35–69 No	Females 70–79 Yes	Females 70–79 No
1955	1.07	2.15	1.37	10.5	0.00	2.96	0.00	9.02
1965	2.10	2.10	4.67	12.4	0.00	2.60	0.00	10.3
1975	2.53	2.09	8.34	12.0	0.00	2.66	0.00	10.1
1985	2.16	2.08	9.32	11.6	0.18	2.33	0.00	9.76
1990	2.08	1.93	8.08	8.90	0.23	2.46	0.07	7.28

35–69 = mean of 7 age-specific rates; 70–79 = mean of 2 rates (70–74 & 75–79) Peto, Lopez et al, 1992, 1994

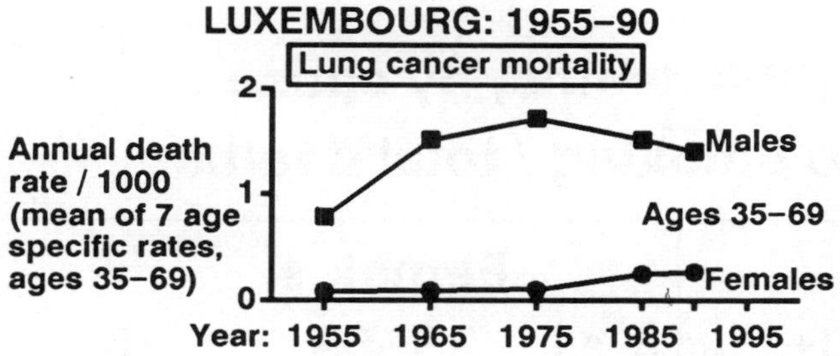

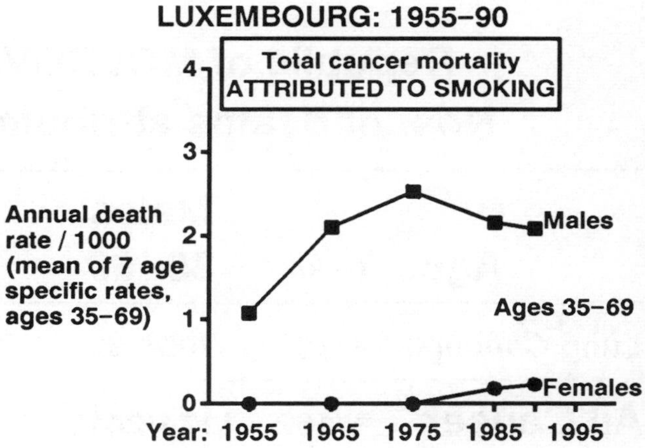

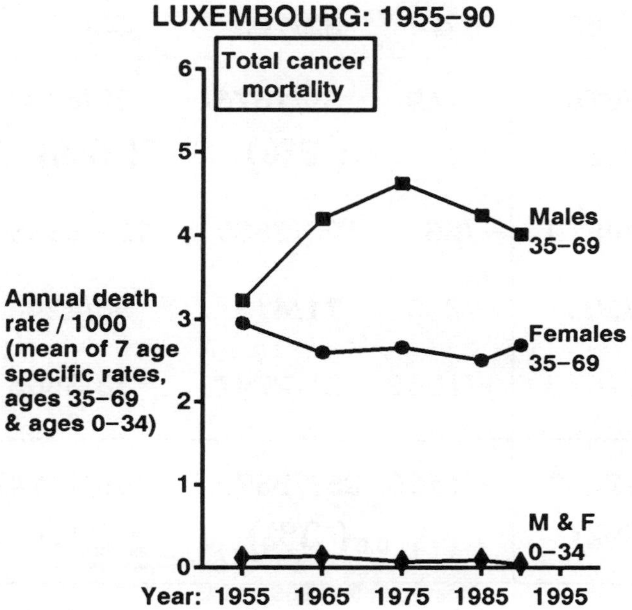

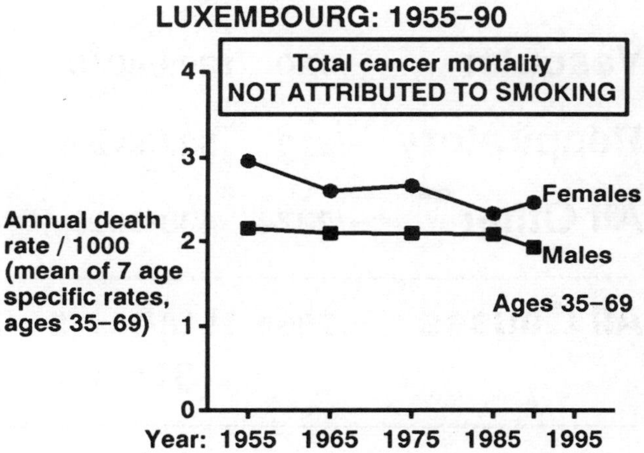

¶Republic of MOLDOVA: 1990
Relative importance of deaths in MIDDLE age (35–69)

Age range (years)	Deaths attributed to SMOKING / total deaths (thousands) Males	Females	Mean years lost PER DEATH FROM SMOKING
0–34	–/3.0	–/1.5	–
35–69	3.5/11	0.3/8.4	20 years
70+	0.7/7.3	0.3/11	8 years
All ages	4.3/21	0.6/21	17 years

Peto, Lopez et al, 1992, 1994

Republic of MOLDOVA: 1990 deaths, by cause
Nos. of deaths attributed to smoking / total deaths

	Males			Females		
Age:	0–34	35–69	70+	0–34	35–69	70+
Lung Cancer	–/10	705/752	132/163	–/ 4	32/103	33/80
All Cancer	–/152	1174/2415 (49%)	181/678 (27%)	–/149	39/1676 (2%)	39/663 (6%)
Vascular	–/120	1309/4018	236/4010	–/55	126/3539	122/6555
Respiratory	–/318	627/919	245/500	–/243	71/413	96/424
All Other	–/2374	408/3820	82/2075	–/1059	21/2747	38/3505
All Causes	–/2964	3518/11172 (31%)	744/7263 (10%)	–/1506	257/8375 (3%)	295/11147 (3%)

Peto, Lopez et al, 1992, 1994

Republic of MOLDOVA: 1990

RISKS OF DYING AT AGES 0–34 and 35–69

(Probability that someone entering an age range would die during it, if the death rates in 1990 were to persist unchanged)

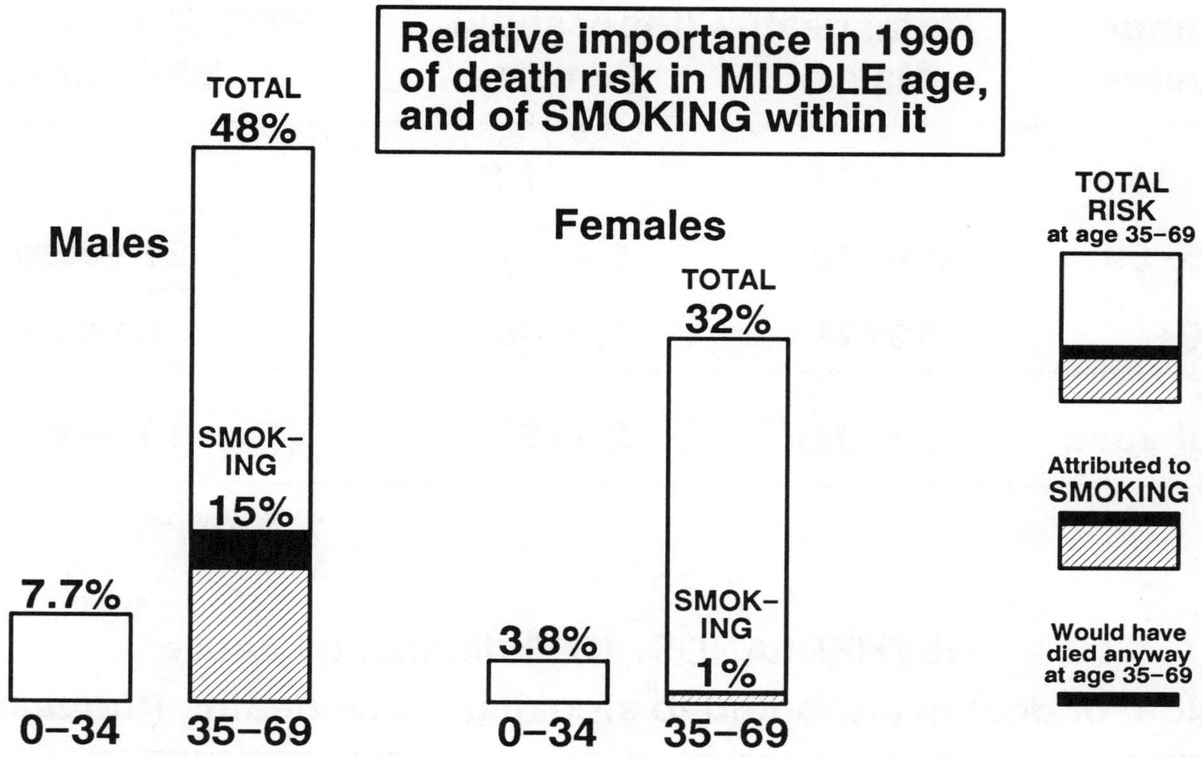

Peto, Lopez et al, 1992, 1994

Republic of MOLDOVA: 1990 deaths, all ages

Nos. of deaths attributed to smoking / total deaths (thousands)

	Males	Females	Males + Females
All Cancer	1.4/3.2 (42%)	0.1/2.5 (3%)	1.4/5.7 (25%)
All Causes	4.3/21 (20%)	0.6/21 (3%)	4.8/42 (11%)

Peto, Lopez et al, 1992, 1994

NETHERLANDS: 1990
Relative importance of deaths in MIDDLE age (35–69)

Age range (years)	Deaths attributed to SMOKING / total deaths (thousands) Males	Females	Mean years lost PER DEATH FROM SMOKING
0–34	–/3.0	–/1.8	–
35–69	8.6/22	1.4/12	21 years
70+	13/41	1.3/48	8 years
All ages	22/67	2.7/62	13 years

Peto, Lopez et al, 1992, 1994

NETHERLANDS: 1990 deaths, by cause
Nos. of deaths attributed to smoking / total deaths (thousands)

	Males			Females		
Age:	0–34	35–69	70+	0–34	35–69	70+
Lung Cancer	–/0.0	3.0/3.2	3.6/3.8	–/0.0	0.5/0.7	0.2/0.5
All Cancer	–/0.2	4.2/8.3 (50%)	5.4/11 (47%)	–/0.2	0.6/6.1 (10%)	0.3/8.9 (4%)
Vascular	–/0.2	2.7/8.4	3.3/17	–/0.1	0.4/3.1	0.4/23
Respiratory	–/0.0	0.7/1.0	3.1/5.2	–/0.0	0.2/0.4	0.4/4.0
All Other	–/2.5	1.1/4.8	1.2/7.3	–/1.4	0.2/2.7	0.2/13
All Causes	–/3.0	8.6/22 (38%)	13/41 (32%)	–/1.8	1.4/12 (11%)	1.3/48 (3%)

Peto, Lopez et al, 1992, 1994

NETHERLANDS: 1990

RISKS OF DYING AT AGES 0–34 and 35–69

(Probability that someone entering an age range would die during it, if the death rates in 1990 were to persist unchanged)

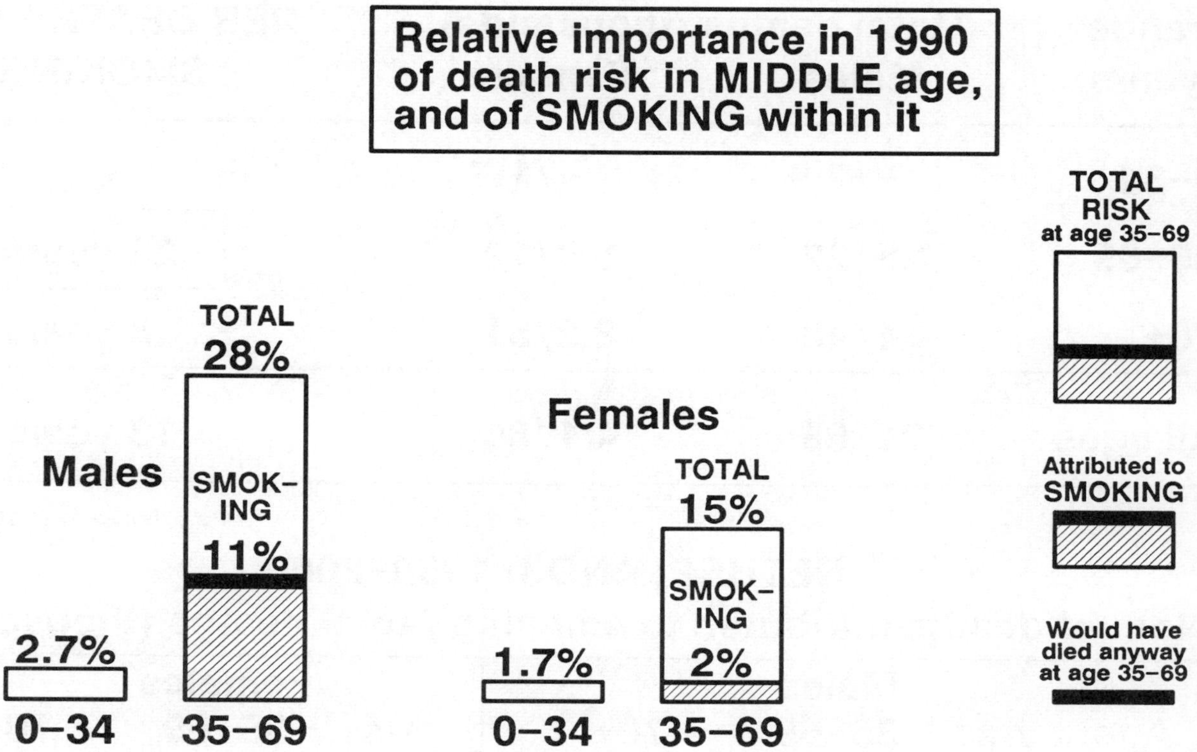

Peto, Lopez et al, 1992, 1994

NETHERLANDS: 1990 deaths, all ages

Nos. of deaths attributed to smoking / total deaths (thousands)

	Males	Females	Males + Females
All Cancer	9.5/20 (48%)	0.9/15 (6%)	10/35 (30%)
All Causes	22/67 (32%)	2.7/62 (4%)	24/129 (19%)

Peto, Lopez et al, 1992, 1994

NETHERLANDS: 1995 projections
Relative importance of deaths in MIDDLE age (35–69)

Age range (years)	Deaths attributed to SMOKING / total deaths (thousands) Males	Females	Mean years lost PER DEATH FROM SMOKING
0–34	–/2.9	–/1.7	–
35–69	7.5/22	1.9/12	22 years
70+	14/43	2.2/51	8 years
All ages	21/68	4.1/65	13 years

Peto, Lopez et al, 1992, 1994

NETHERLANDS: 1950–2000
Nos. of deaths attributed to smoking / total deaths (thousands)

	Males			Females		
Age:	0-34	35–69	70+	0–34	35–69	70+
1955	–/5.4	4.3/16 (27%)	1.5/22 (7%)	–/3.7	0.0/12 (0%)	0.0/22 (0%)
1965	–/4.9	8.2/21 (39%)	4.3/29 (15%)	–/3.1	0.0/13 (0%)	0.0/28 (0%)
1975	–/3.9	10/24 (43%)	9.4/36 (26%)	–/2.3	0.1/13 (0.7%)	0.0/35 (0%)
1985	–/3.1	9.8/23 (43%)	13/40 (32%)	–/1.8	0.9/12 (8%)	0.7/43 (2%)
1995 (projected)	–/2.9	7.5/22 (34%)	14/43 (32%)	–/1.7	1.9/12 (16%)	2.2/51 (4%)
50–year total*, mid–1950 to mid–2000: 878/5498						
1950–2000, by age & sex	–/202	398/1060 (38%)	422/1700 (25%)	–/126	29/620 (5%)	29/1790 (2%)

*Estimated as 10 times the sum of the five annual numbers (for 1955, 1965, 1975, 1985 & 1995)

NETHERLANDS

Smoking–attributed numbers of deaths per year

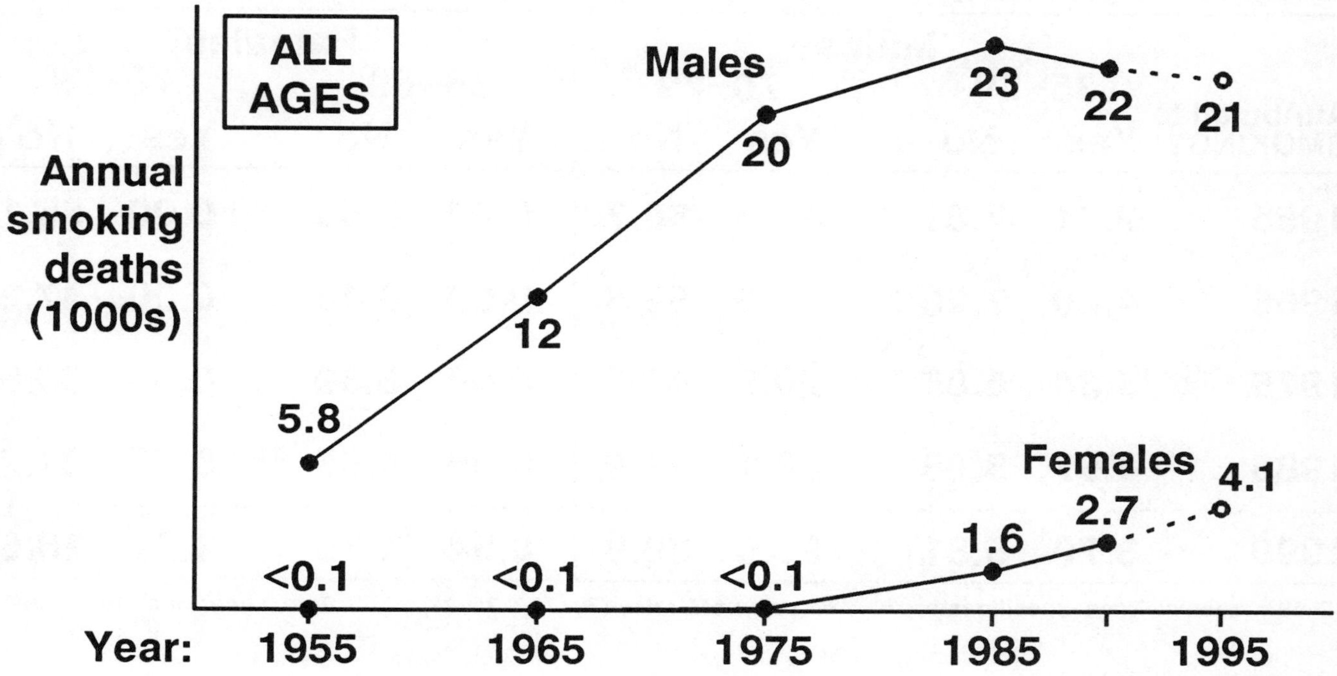

Peto, Lopez et al, 1992, 1994

NETHERLANDS

Smoking–attributed numbers of deaths per year

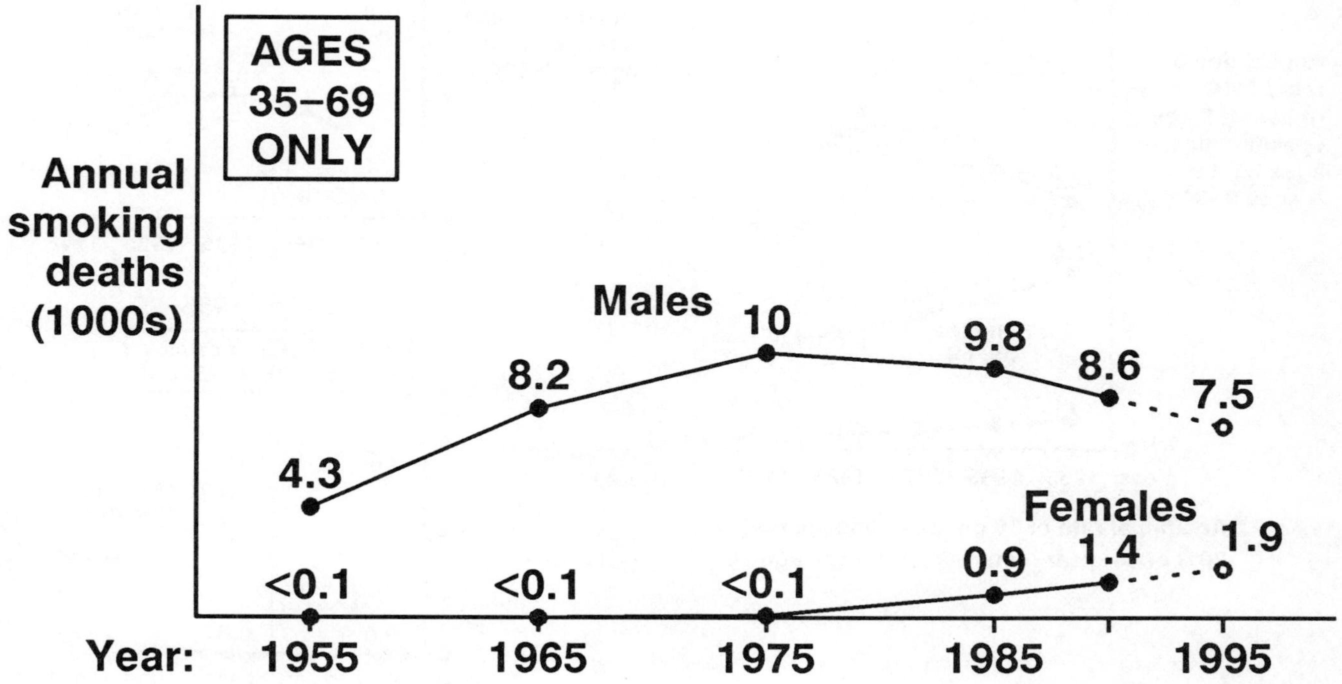

Peto, Lopez et al, 1992, 1994

NETHERLANDS

ALL DEATHS (annual rates per 1000): Trends in mortality attributed to smoking, and in other mortality

	Males				Females			
	35–69		70–79		35–69		70–79	
Attributed to SMOKING?	Yes	No	Yes	No	Yes	No	Yes	No
1955	2.71	7.81	4.95	58.7	0.00	7.49	0.00	55.1
1965	4.60	7.28	11.3	52.5	0.00	6.40	0.00	47.3
1975	5.34	6.85	20.5	47.8	0.04	5.59	0.00	39.6
1985	4.57	5.98	23.1	41.9	0.36	4.55	0.70	31.2
1990	3.70	5.81	21.6	39.8	0.54	4.19	1.21	28.6

35–69 = mean of 7 age-specific rates; 70–79 = mean of 2 rates (70–74 & 75–79) Peto, Lopez et al, 1992, 1994

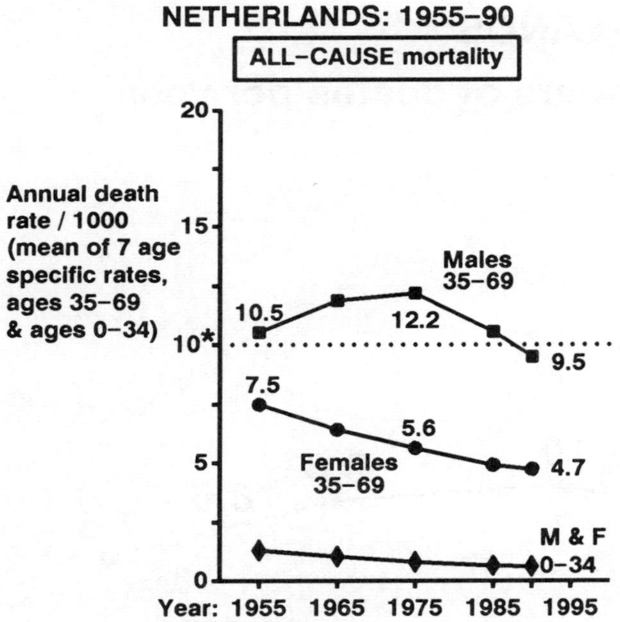

* An annual rate of 10 per 1000 implies that 30% of 35-year-olds will die before age 70

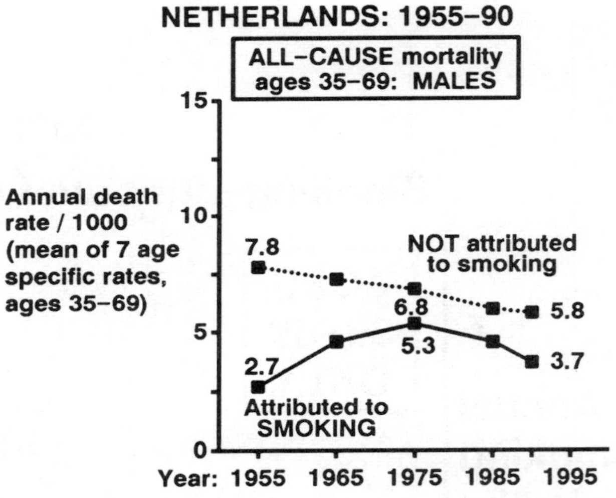

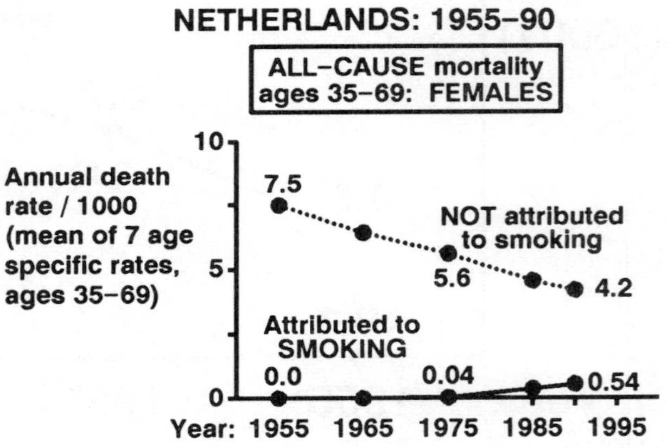

NETHERLANDS

ALL CANCER DEATHS (annual rates per 1000): Trends in mortality attributed to smoking, and in other mortality

	Males				Females			
	35–69		70–79		35–69		70–79	
Attributed to SMOKING?	Yes	No	Yes	No	Yes	No	Yes	No
1955	1.07	1.89	2.03	11.4	0.00	2.52	0.00	10.1
1965	1.85	1.78	4.79	10.7	0.00	2.45	0.00	9.61
1975	2.30	1.77	8.89	10.0	0.01	2.31	0.00	9.04
1985	2.19	1.68	10.9	9.38	0.15	2.12	0.22	8.08
1990	1.82	1.75	10.2	9.73	0.24	2.08	0.38	7.76

35–69 = mean of 7 age-specific rates; 70–79 = mean of 2 rates (70–74 & 75–79) Peto, Lopez et al, 1992, 1994

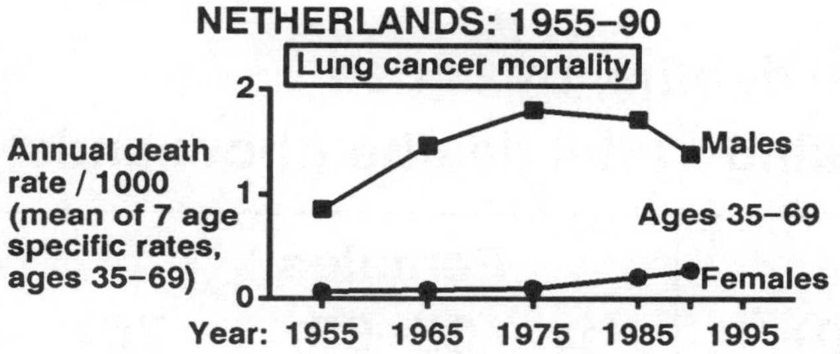

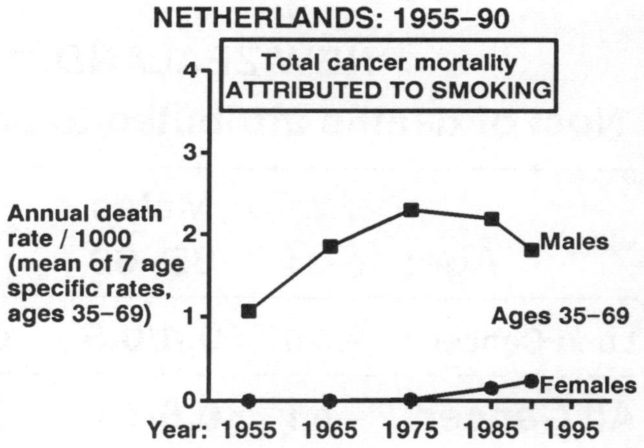

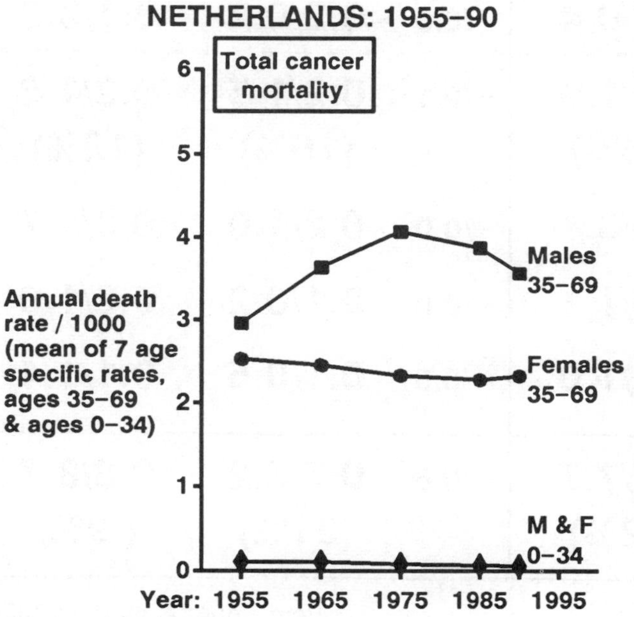

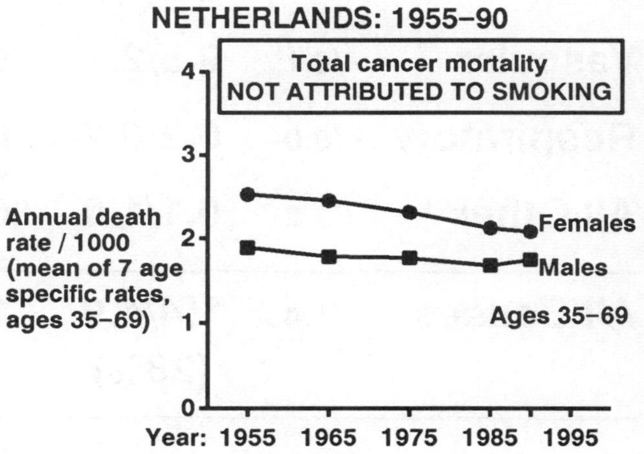

NEW ZEALAND: 1990
Relative importance of deaths in MIDDLE age (35–69)

Age range (years)	Deaths attributed to SMOKING / total deaths (thousands) Males	Females	Mean years lost PER DEATH FROM SMOKING
0–34	–/1.4	–/0.6	–
35–69	1.4/4.9	0.7/3.2	21 years
70+	1.7/7.7	0.8/8.7	8 years
All ages	3.1/14	1.4/13	14 years

Peto, Lopez et al, 1992, 1994

NEW ZEALAND: 1990 deaths, by cause
Nos. of deaths attributed to smoking / total deaths (thousands)

	Males			Females		
Age:	0–34	35–69	70+	0–34	35–69	70+
Lung Cancer	–/0.0	0.4/0.5	0.4/0.4	–/0.0	0.2/0.2	0.1/0.2
All Cancer	–/0.1	0.6/1.6 (39%)	0.6/1.9 (34%)	–/0.1	0.2/1.5 (16%)	0.2/1.6 (12%)
Vascular	–/0.1	0.5/2.1	0.4/3.7	–/0.0	0.2/1.0	0.3/4.7
Respiratory	–/0.0	0.2/0.2	0.5/1.1	–/0.0	0.1/0.2	0.2/1.0
All Other	–/1.2	0.1/1.0	0.1/1.0	–/0.5	0.1/0.5	0.1/1.4
All Causes	–/1.4	1.4/4.9 (28%)	1.7/7.7 (22%)	–/0.6	0.7/3.2 (21%)	0.8/8.7 (9%)

Peto, Lopez et al, 1992, 1994

NEW ZEALAND: 1990
RISKS OF DYING AT AGES 0–34 and 35–69
(Probability that someone entering an age range would die during it, if the death rates in 1990 were to persist unchanged)

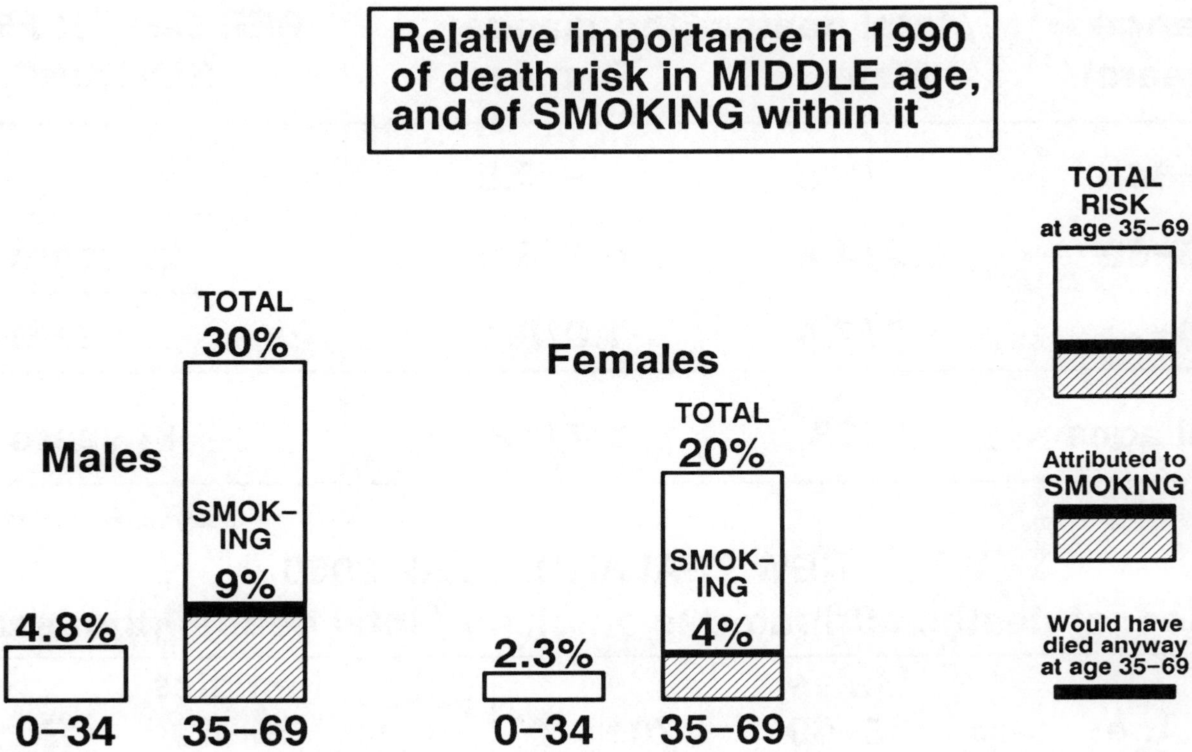

Peto, Lopez et al, 1992, 1994

NEW ZEALAND: 1990 deaths, all ages
Nos. of deaths attributed to smoking / total deaths (thousands)

	Males	Females	Males + Females
All Cancer	1.2/3.5 (35%)	0.4/3.2 (14%)	1.7/6.7 (25%)
All Causes	3.1/14 (22%)	1.4/13 (11%)	4.5/27 (17%)

Peto, Lopez et al, 1992, 1994

NEW ZEALAND: 1995 projections
Relative importance of deaths in MIDDLE age (35–69)

Age range (years)	Deaths attributed to SMOKING / total deaths (thousands) Males	Females	Mean years lost PER DEATH FROM SMOKING
0–34	–/1.5	–/0.5	–
35–69	1.2/4.4	0.7/3.2	22 years
70+	1.6/7.4	1.0/8.1	9 years
All ages	2.8/13	1.7/12	14 years

Peto, Lopez et al, 1992, 1994

NEW ZEALAND: 1950–2000
Nos. of deaths attributed to smoking / total deaths (thousands)

Age:	Males 0–34	Males 35–69	Males 70+	Females 0–34	Females 35–69	Females 70+
1955	–/1.6	0.9 / 4.0 (23%)	0.4 / 5.0 (7%)	–/1.0	0.0 / 2.8 (0%)	0.0 / 4.7 (0%)
1965	–/1.5	1.4 / 5.1 (27%)	0.8 / 6.0 (14%)	–/0.9	0.1 / 3.1 (3%)	0.0 / 6.3 (0%)
1975	–/1.6	1.9 / 5.9 (32%)	1.4 / 6.3 (22%)	–/0.9	0.5 / 3.4 (14%)	0.3 / 7.0 (4%)
1985	–/1.3	1.7 / 5.4 (31%)	1.7 / 7.8 (21%)	–/0.7	0.7 / 3.3 (20%)	0.6 / 8.9 (7%)
1995 (projected)	–/1.5	1.2 / 4.4 (26%)	1.6 / 7.4 (22%)	–/0.5	0.7 / 3.2 (22%)	1.0 / 8.1 (12%)
50–year total*, mid–1950 to mid–2000: 169/1196						
1950–2000, by age & sex	–/75	71 / 248 (29%)	59 / 325 (18%)	–/40	20 / 158 (13%)	19 / 350 (5%)

*Estimated as 10 times the sum of the five annual numbers (for 1955, 1965, 1975, 1985 & 1995)

NEW ZEALAND

Smoking–attributed numbers of deaths per year

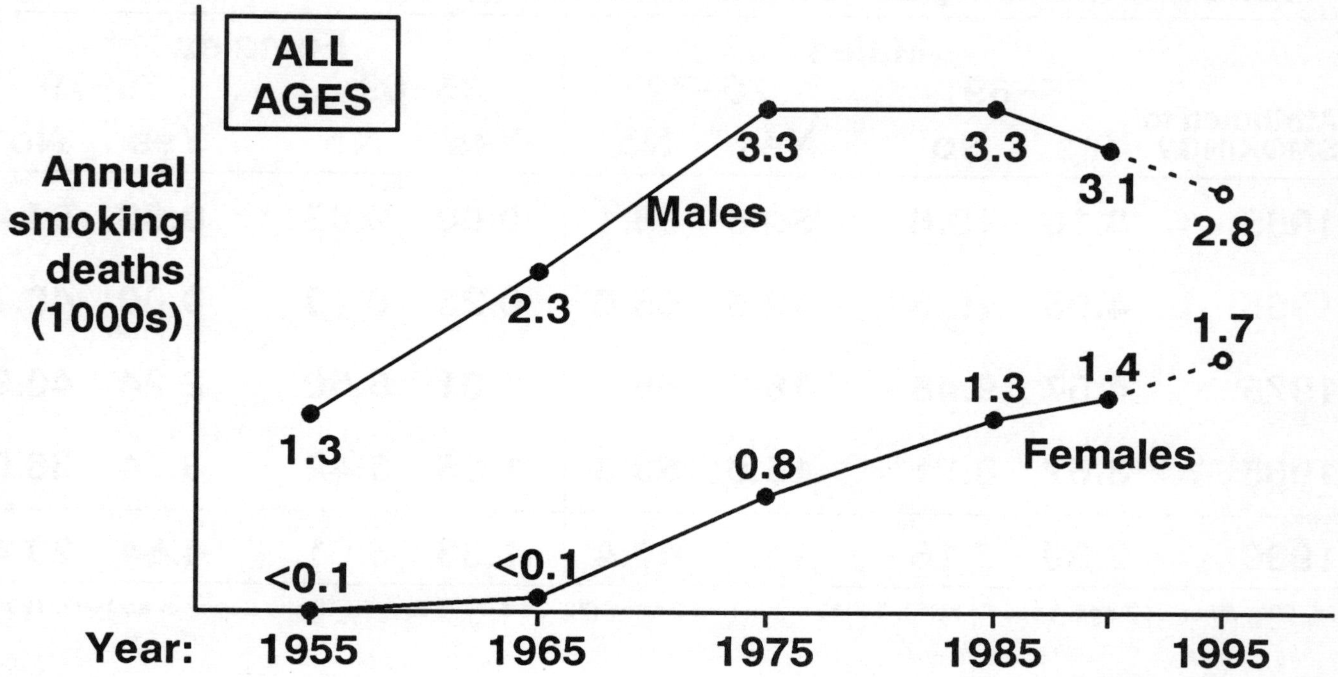

Peto, Lopez et al, 1992, 1994

NEW ZEALAND

Smoking–attributed numbers of deaths per year

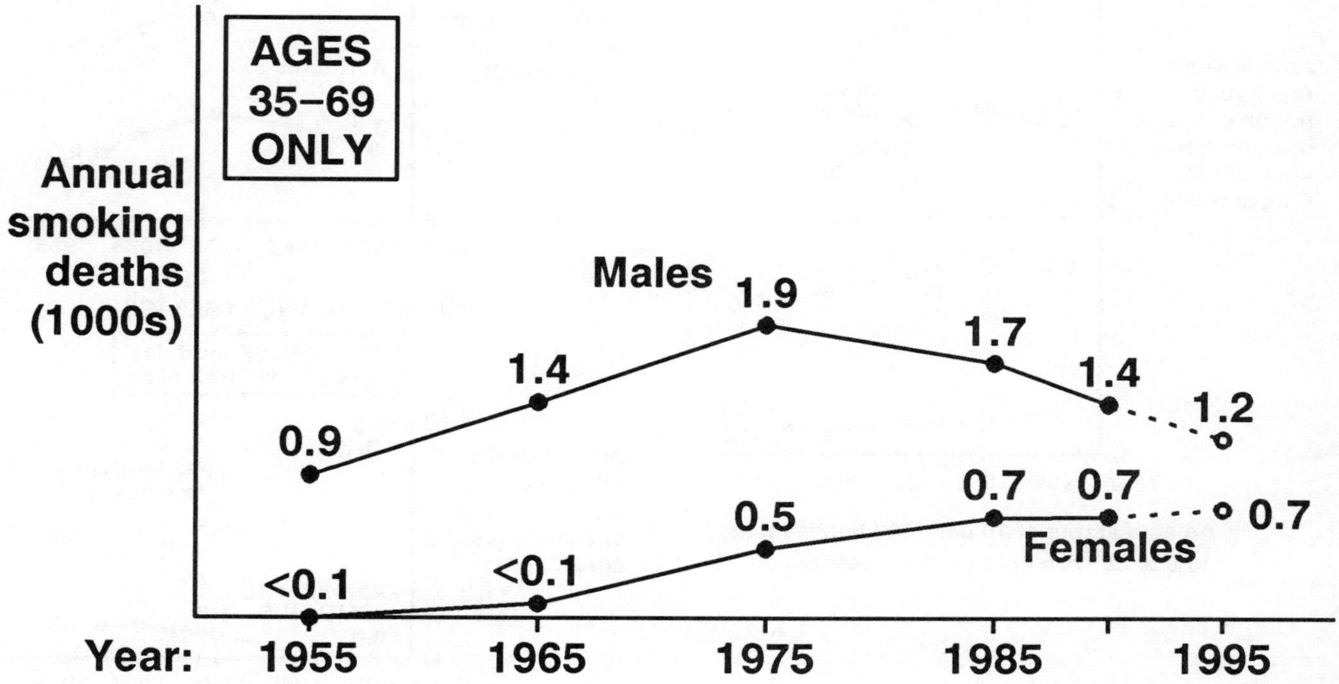

Peto, Lopez et al, 1992, 1994

NEW ZEALAND

ALL DEATHS (annual rates per 1000): Trends in mortality attributed to smoking, and in other mortality

	Males				Females			
	35–69		70–79		35–69		70–79	
Attributed to SMOKING?	Yes	No	Yes	No	Yes	No	Yes	No
1955	3.16	10.6	5.86	68.1	0.00	9.03	0.00	54.2
1965	4.08	10.6	12.5	65.6	0.25	8.13	0.00	48.7
1975	4.57	9.48	18.2	55.1	1.01	6.50	2.24	40.9
1985	3.67	8.21	15.6	53.3	1.35	5.42	3.74	36.0
1990	2.89	7.16	14.7	47.4	1.33	5.01	4.64	29.4

35–69 = mean of 7 age-specific rates; 70–79 = mean of 2 rates (70–74 & 75–79) Peto, Lopez et al, 1992, 1994

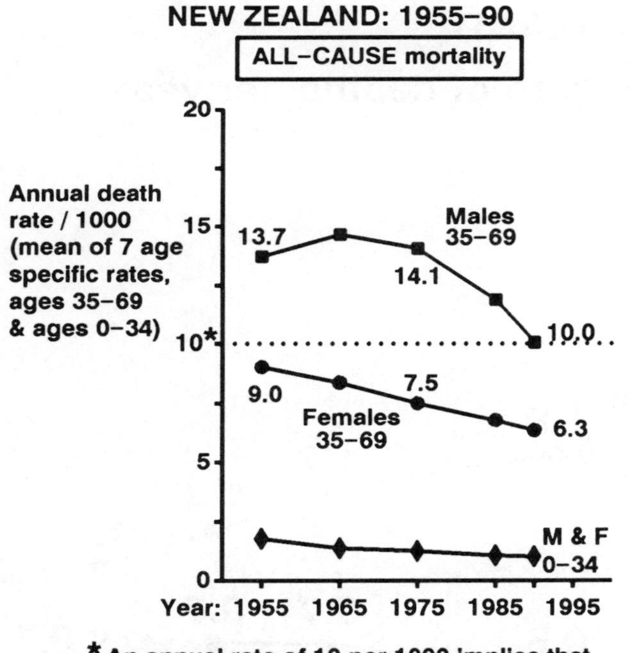

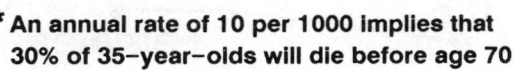

* An annual rate of 10 per 1000 implies that 30% of 35-year-olds will die before age 70

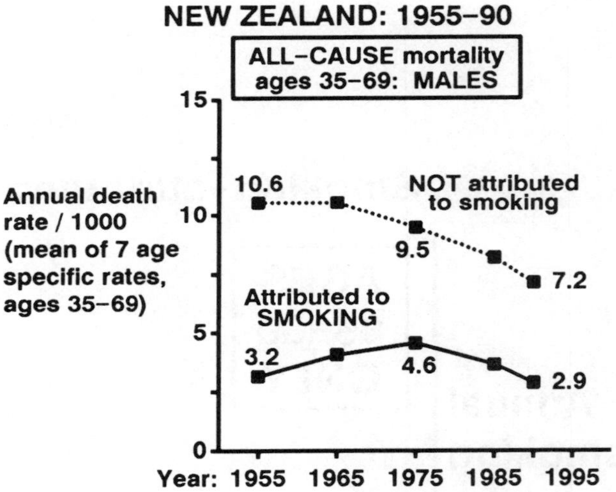

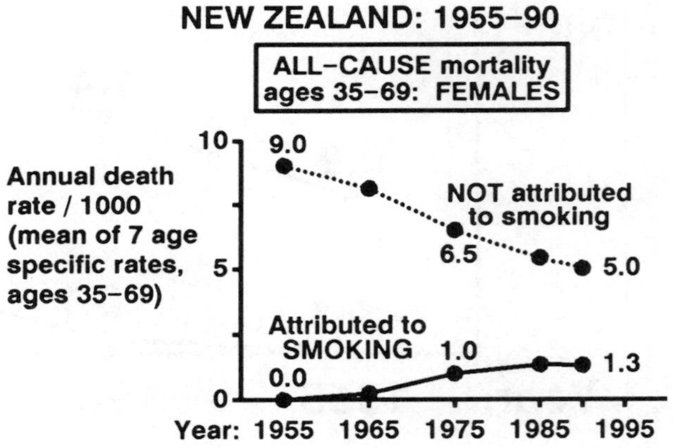

NEW ZEALAND

ALL CANCER DEATHS (annual rates per 1000): Trends in mortality attributed to smoking, and in other mortality

	Males				Females			
	35–69		70–79		35–69		70–79	
Attributed to SMOKING?	Yes	No	Yes	No	Yes	No	Yes	No
1955	0.97	1.97	1.78	10.2	0.00	2.50	0.00	8.97
1965	1.21	1.81	3.87	9.89	0.06	2.44	0.00	7.01
1975	1.56	1.89	6.43	9.52	0.27	2.33	0.54	7.75
1985	1.43	2.13	5.60	10.5	0.42	2.31	0.96	8.01
1990	1.30	2.02	5.96	10.9	0.49	2.45	1.40	7.74

35–69 = mean of 7 age-specific rates; 70–79 = mean of 2 rates (70–74 & 75–79) Peto, Lopez et al, 1992, 1994

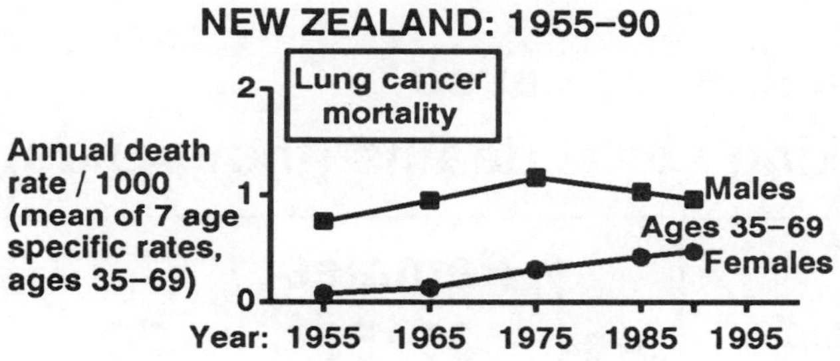

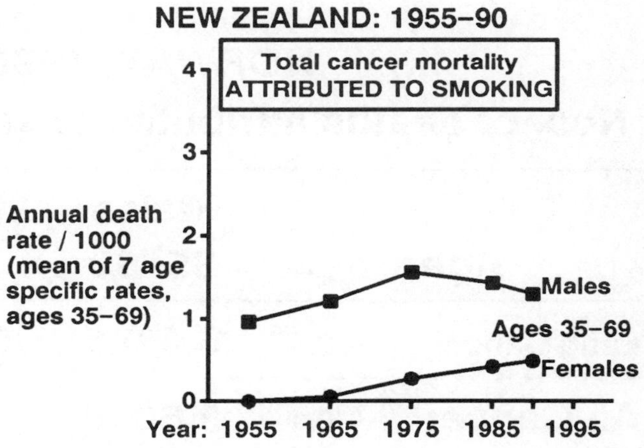

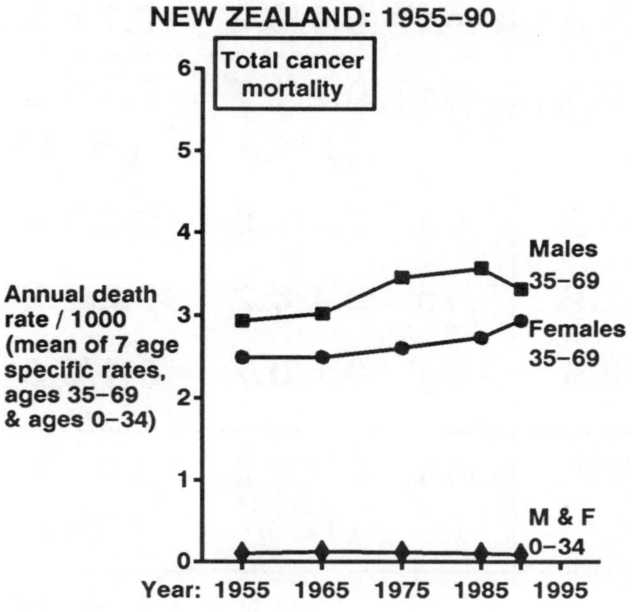

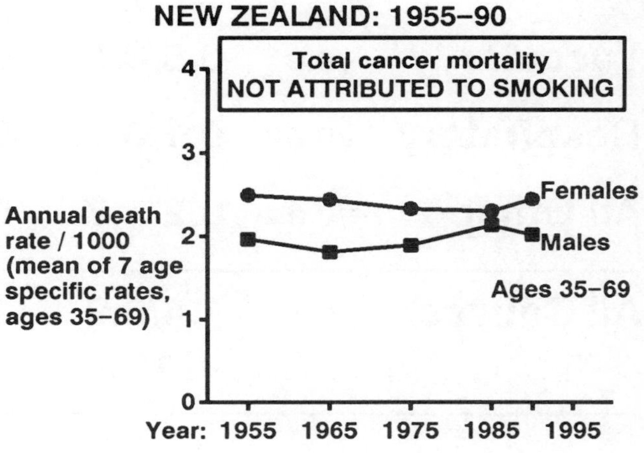

NORWAY: 1990
Relative importance of deaths in MIDDLE age (35–69)

Age range (years)	Deaths attributed to SMOKING / total deaths (thousands) Males	Females	Mean years lost PER DEATH FROM SMOKING
0–34	–/1.1	–/0.5	–
35–69	1.4/6.9	0.4/3.6	20 years
70+	1.9/16	0.6/18	8 years
All ages	3.4/24	1.0/22	13 years

Peto, Lopez et al, 1992, 1994

NORWAY: 1990 deaths, by cause
Nos. of deaths attributed to smoking / total deaths (thousands)

	Males			Females		
Age:	0–34	35–69	70+	0–34	35–69	70+
Lung Cancer	–/0.0	0.4/0.5	0.5/0.5	–/0.0	0.1/0.2	0.1/0.2
All Cancer	–/0.1	0.6/1.9 (32%)	0.7/3.3 (22%)	–/0.1	0.2/1.7 (11%)	0.1/2.8 (5%)
Vascular	–/0.0	0.5/3.0	0.6/8.2	–/0.0	0.1/1.0	0.2/9.4
Respiratory	–/0.0	0.1/0.3	0.4/1.9	–/0.0	0.1/0.2	0.2/2.2
All Other	–/0.9	0.2/1.7	0.1/2.6	–/0.4	0.1/0.7	0.1/3.6
All Causes	–/1.1	1.4/6.9 (21%)	1.9/16 (12%)	–/0.5	0.4/3.6 (12%)	0.6/18 (3%)

Peto, Lopez et al, 1992, 1994

NORWAY: 1990

RISKS OF DYING AT AGES 0–34 and 35–69

(Probability that someone entering an age range would die during it, if the death rates in 1990 were to persist unchanged)

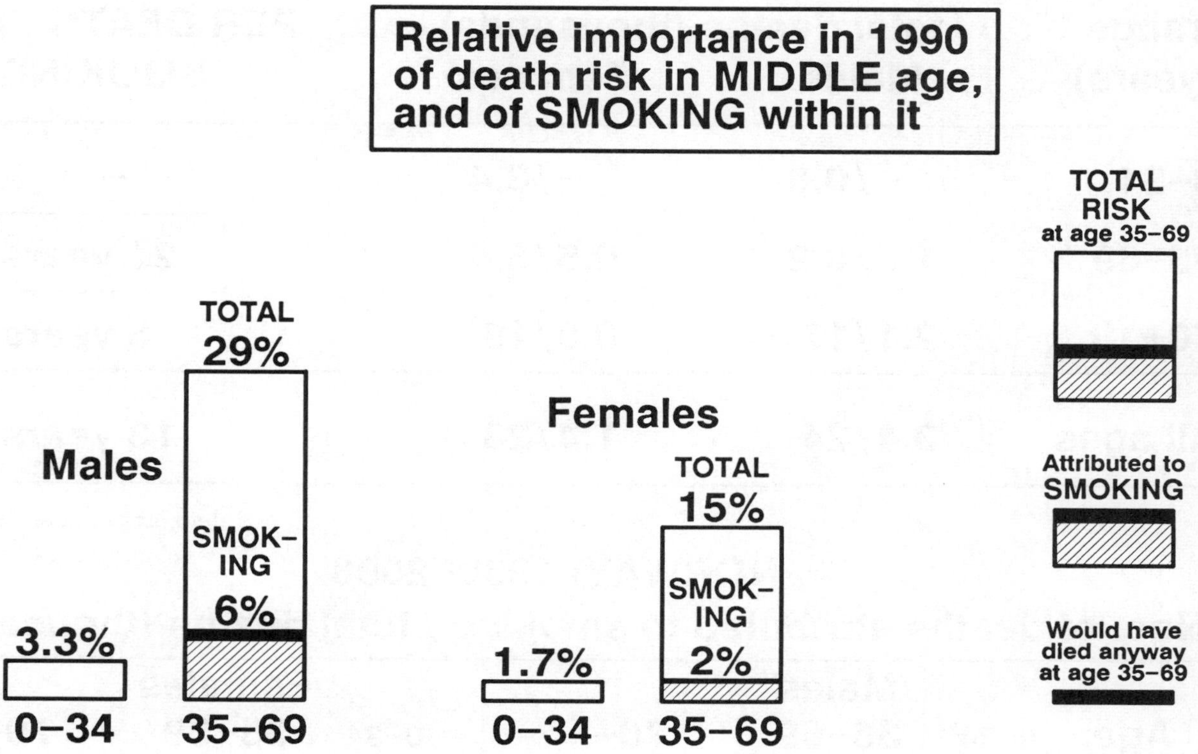

Peto, Lopez et al, 1992, 1994

NORWAY: 1990 deaths, all ages

Nos. of deaths attributed to smoking / total deaths (thousands)

	Males	Females	Males + Females
All Cancer	1.3/5.3 (25%)	0.3/4.6 (7%)	1.6/9.9 (17%)
All Causes	3.4/24 (14%)	1.0/22 (5%)	4.4/46 (10%)

Peto, Lopez et al, 1992, 1994

NORWAY: 1995 projections
Relative importance of deaths in MIDDLE age (35–69)

Age range (years)	Deaths attributed to SMOKING / total deaths (thousands) Males	Females	Mean years lost PER DEATH FROM SMOKING
0–34	–/0.9	–/0.4	–
35–69	1.3/6.2	0.5/3.4	21 years
70+	2.1/17	0.8/19	8 years
All ages	3.4/24	1.4/23	13 years

Peto, Lopez et al, 1992, 1994

NORWAY: 1950–2000
Nos. of deaths attributed to smoking / total deaths (thousands)

	Males			Females		
Age:	0–34	35–69	70+	0–34	35–69	70+
1955	–/1.7	0.4 / 5.4 (7%)	0.0 / 7.7 (0.1%)	–/1.1	0.0 / 4.0 (0%)	0.0 / 9.2 (0%)
1965	–/1.5	0.9 / 7.4 (12%)	0.3 / 10 (3%)	–/0.8	0.0 / 4.2 (0%)	0.0 / 11 (0%)
1975	–/1.3	1.4 / 7.9 (18%)	0.9 / 13 (7%)	–/0.6	0.1 / 4.1 (2%)	0.0 / 13 (0%)
1985	–/1.1	1.6 / 7.5 (22%)	1.8 / 15 (12%)	–/0.5	0.3 / 3.7 (8%)	0.5 / 16 (3%)
1995 (projected)	–/0.9	1.3 / 6.2 (21%)	2.1 / 17 (12%)	–/0.4	0.5 / 3.4 (16%)	0.8 / 19 (4%)
50–year total*, mid–1950 to mid–2000: 129/1946						
1950–2000, by age & sex	–/65	56 / 344 (16%)	51 / 627 (8%)	–/34	9.0 / 194 (5%)	13 / 682 (2%)

*Estimated as 10 times the sum of the five annual numbers (for 1955, 1965, 1975, 1985 & 1995)

NORWAY
Smoking–attributed numbers of deaths per year

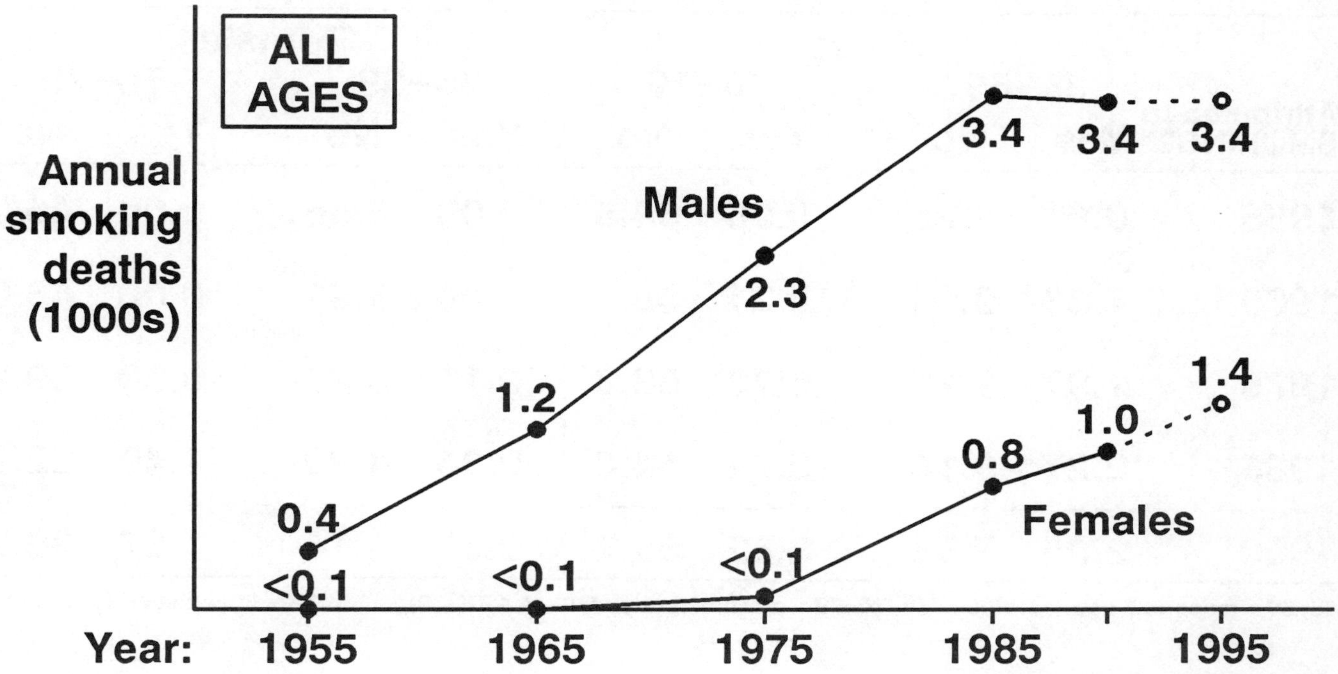

Peto, Lopez et al, 1992, 1994

NORWAY
Smoking–attributed numbers of deaths per year

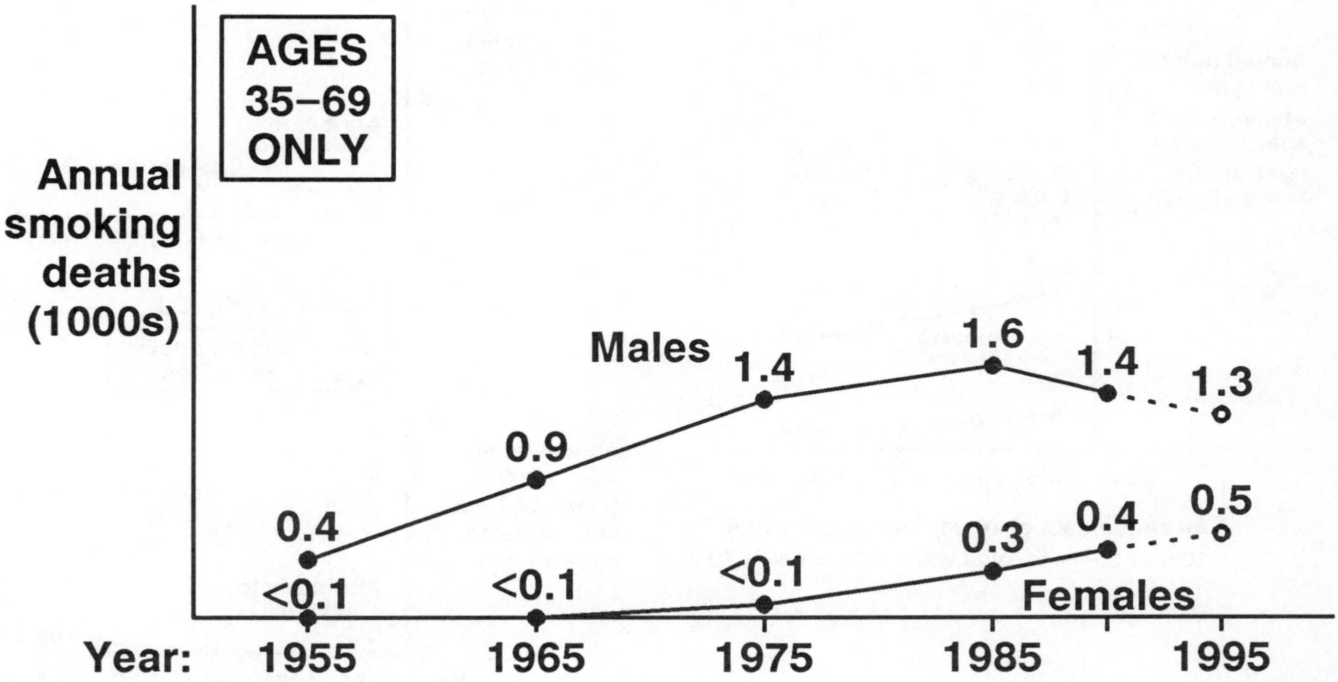

Peto, Lopez et al, 1992, 1994

NORWAY

ALL DEATHS (annual rates per 1000): Trends in mortality attributed to smoking, and in other mortality

	Males				Females			
	35–69		70–79		35–69		70–79	
Attributed to SMOKING?	Yes	No	Yes	No	Yes	No	Yes	No
1955	0.61	9.25	0.06	54.8	0.00	6.66	0.00	46.3
1965	1.33	9.94	2.21	59.1	0.00	5.91	0.00	45.0
1975	1.97	9.21	5.73	58.3	0.11	5.27	0.00	39.2
1985	2.27	8.14	8.74	54.8	0.38	4.39	1.49	32.1
1990	2.06	7.58	8.82	50.7	0.58	4.14	1.67	30.9

35–69 = mean of 7 age-specific rates; 70–79 = mean of 2 rates (70–74 & 75–79)   Peto, Lopez et al, 1992, 1994

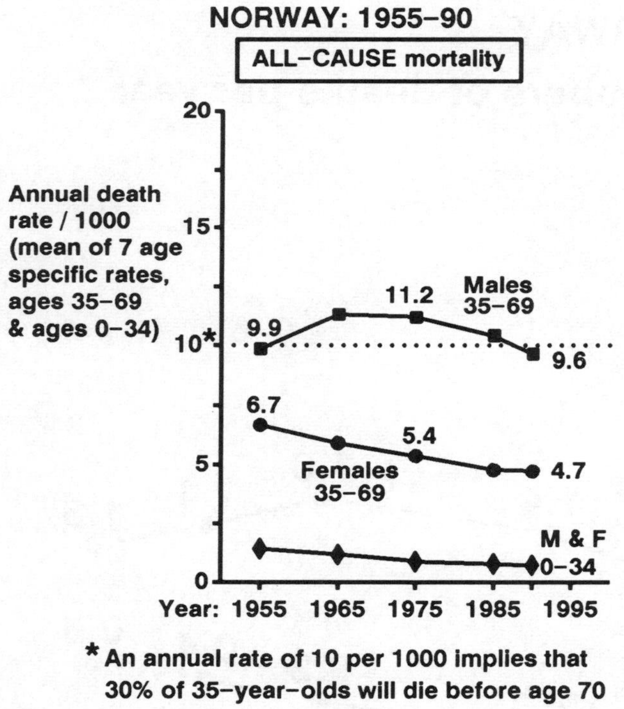

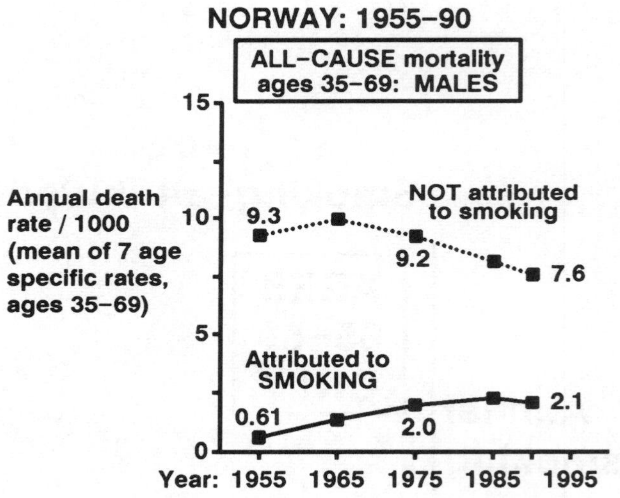

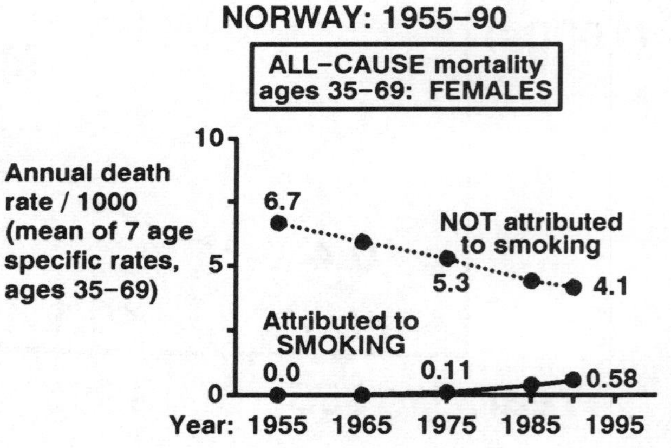

NORWAY

ALL CANCER DEATHS (annual rates per 1000): Trends in mortality attributed to smoking, and in other mortality

	Males				Females			
	35–69		70–79		35–69		70–79	
Attributed to SMOKING?	Yes	No	Yes	No	Yes	No	Yes	No
1955	0.22	2.28	0.02	11.1	0.00	2.26	0.00	8.29
1965	0.47	2.07	0.91	11.4	0.00	2.04	0.00	7.71
1975	0.71	1.94	2.26	11.2	0.04	2.16	0.00	7.26
1985	0.90	1.89	3.56	12.2	0.16	2.01	0.45	7.66
1990	0.88	1.86	3.70	10.9	0.24	1.96	0.53	7.68

35–69 = mean of 7 age–specific rates; 70–79 = mean of 2 rates (70–74 & 75–79) Peto, Lopez et al, 1992, 1994

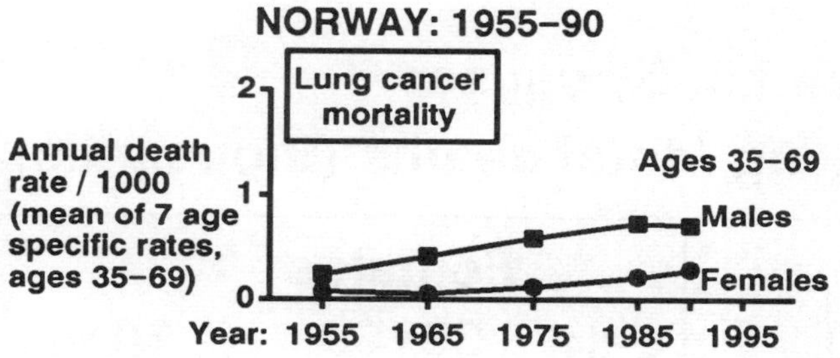

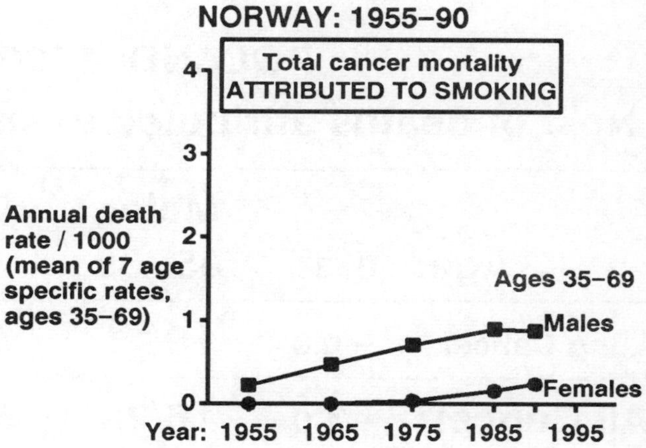

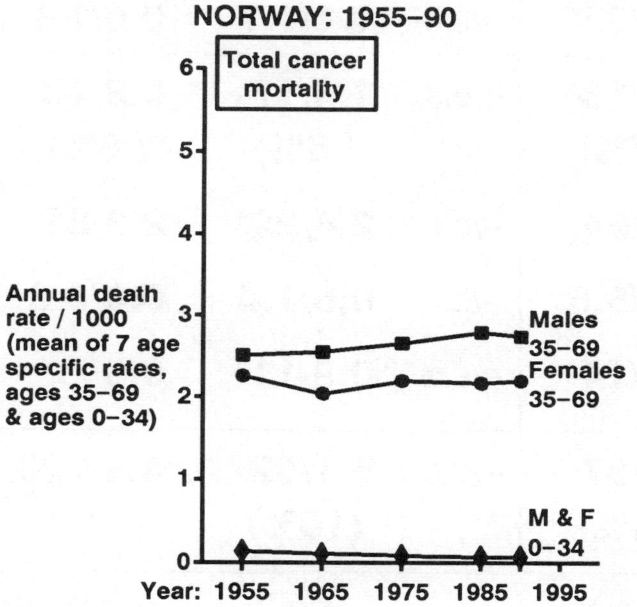

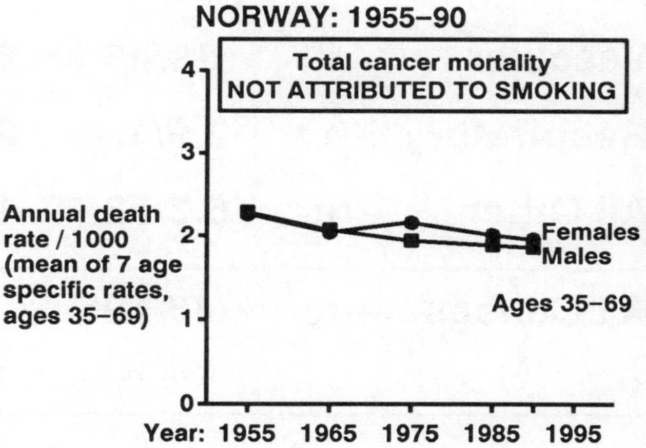

POLAND: 1990
Relative importance of deaths in MIDDLE age (35–69)

Age range (years)	Deaths attributed to SMOKING / total deaths (thousands) Males	Females	Mean years lost PER DEATH FROM SMOKING
0–34	–/18	–/7.8	–
35–69	45/105	5.1/52	21 years
70+	15/87	4.4/120	8 years
All ages	60/209	9.5/179	17 years

Peto, Lopez et al, 1992, 1994

POLAND: 1990 deaths, by cause
Nos. of deaths attributed to smoking / total deaths (thousands)

	Males			Females		
Age:	0–34	35–69	70+	0–34	35–69	70+
Lung Cancer	–/0.0	10/11	3.4/3.7	–/0.0	1.1/1.7	0.6/1.1
All Cancer	–/1.0	16/28 (58%)	5.0/13 (37%)	–/0.8	1.4/17 (8%)	0.8/13 (6%)
Vascular	–/1.4	19/45	6.2/54	–/0.5	2.4/22	2.3/81
Respiratory	–/0.5	2.9/4.1	2.9/5.6	–/0.4	0.5/1.4	0.8/3.8
All Other	–/15	6.3/28	1.3/14	–/6.2	0.9/11	0.5/22
All Causes	–/18	45/105 (42%)	15/87 (18%)	–/7.8	5.1/52 (10%)	4.4/120 (4%)

Peto, Lopez et al, 1992, 1994

POLAND: 1990

RISKS OF DYING AT AGES 0–34 and 35–69

(Probability that someone entering an age range would die during it, if the death rates in 1990 were to persist unchanged)

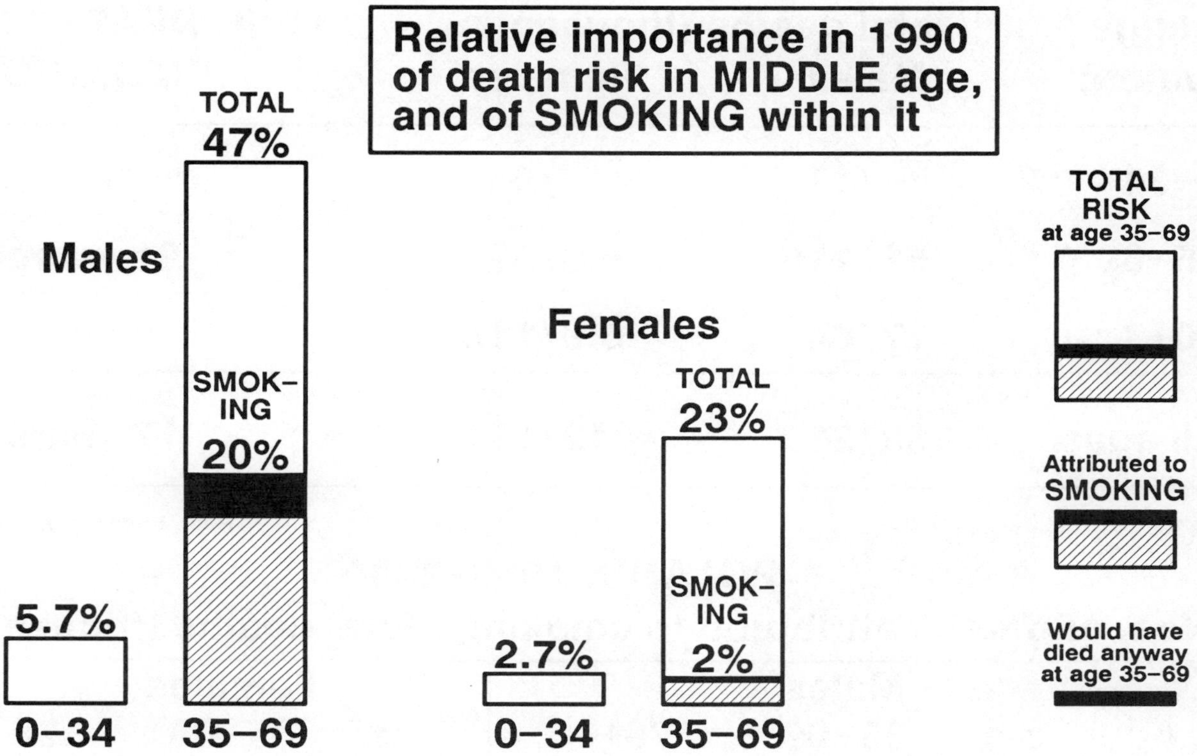

Peto, Lopez et al, 1992, 1994

POLAND: 1990 deaths, all ages

Nos. of deaths attributed to smoking / total deaths (thousands)

	Males	Females	Males + Females
All Cancer	21/42 (50%)	2.2/31 (7%)	23/73 (32%)
All Causes	60/209 (29%)	9.5/179 (5%)	69/388 (18%)

Peto, Lopez et al, 1992, 1994

POLAND: 1995 projections
Relative importance of deaths in MIDDLE age (35–69)

Age range (years)	Deaths attributed to SMOKING / total deaths (thousands) Males	Females	Mean years lost PER DEATH FROM SMOKING
0–34	–/17	–/6.6	–
35–69	51/116	6.3/52	21 years
70+	17/84	5.9/116	8 years
All ages	68/218	12/174	17 years

Peto, Lopez et al, 1992, 1994

POLAND: 1950–2000
Nos. of deaths attributed to smoking / total deaths (thousands)

Age:	Males 0–34	Males 35–69	Males 70+	Females 0–34	Females 35–69	Females 70+
1955	–/54	6.4 / 50 (13%)	1.3 / 32 (4%)	–/40	0.3 / 41 (0.6%)	0.1 / 45 (0.2%)
1965	–/24	13 / 58 (23%)	3.2 / 39 (8%)	–/15	0.5 / 41 (1%)	0.2 / 55 (0.4%)
1975	–/22	22 / 72 (31%)	10 / 64 (16%)	–/11	1.5 / 42 (4%)	1.2 / 85 (1%)
1985	–/20	37 / 89 (42%)	17 / 94 (18%)	–/9.8	3.8 / 46 (8%)	3.3 / 124 (3%)
1995 (projected)	–/17	51 / 116 (44%)	17 / 84 (20%)	–/6.6	6.3 / 52 (12%)	5.9 / 116 (5%)
50–year total* (M=millions), mid–1950 to mid–2000: 2.0/16M						
1950–2000, by age & sex	–/1.4M	1.3 / 3.8M (34%)	0.5 / 3.1M (16%)	–/0.8M	0.1 / 2.2M (5%)	0.1 / 4.3M (2%)

*Estimated as 10 times the sum of the five annual numbers (for 1955, 1965, 1975, 1985 & 1995)

POLAND

Smoking–attributed numbers of deaths per year

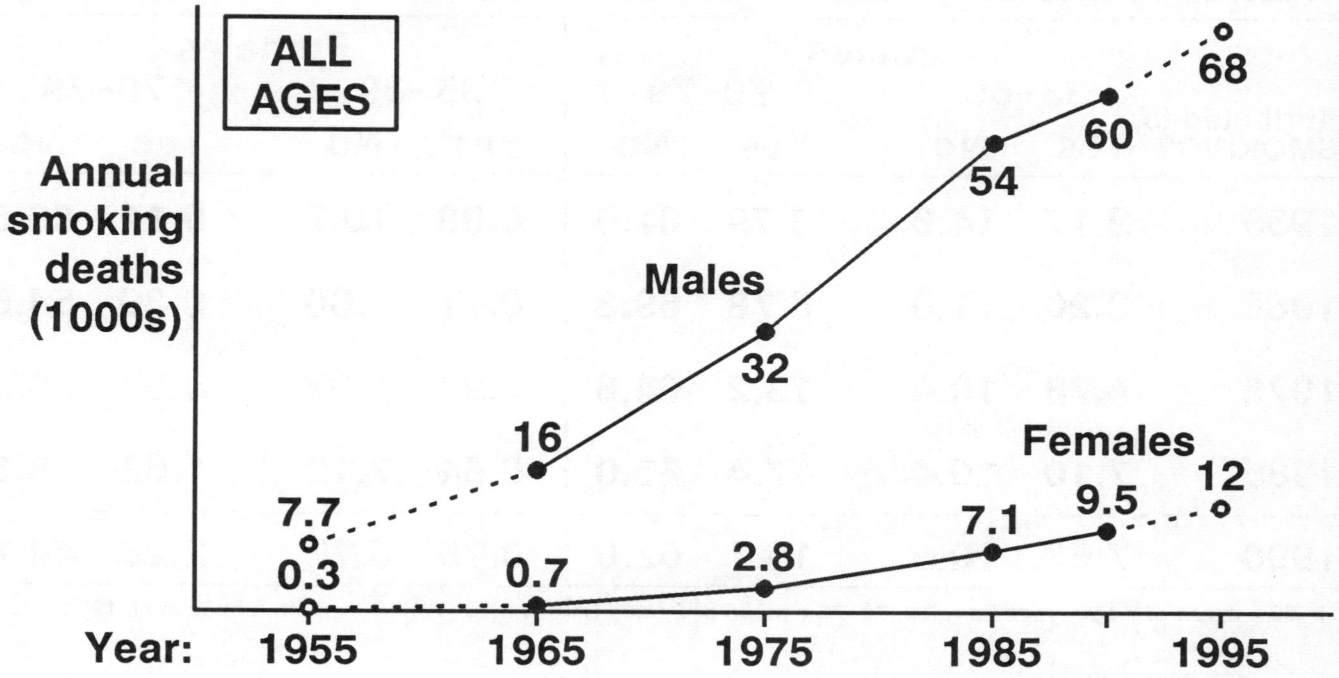

Peto, Lopez et al, 1992, 1994

POLAND

Smoking–attributed numbers of deaths per year

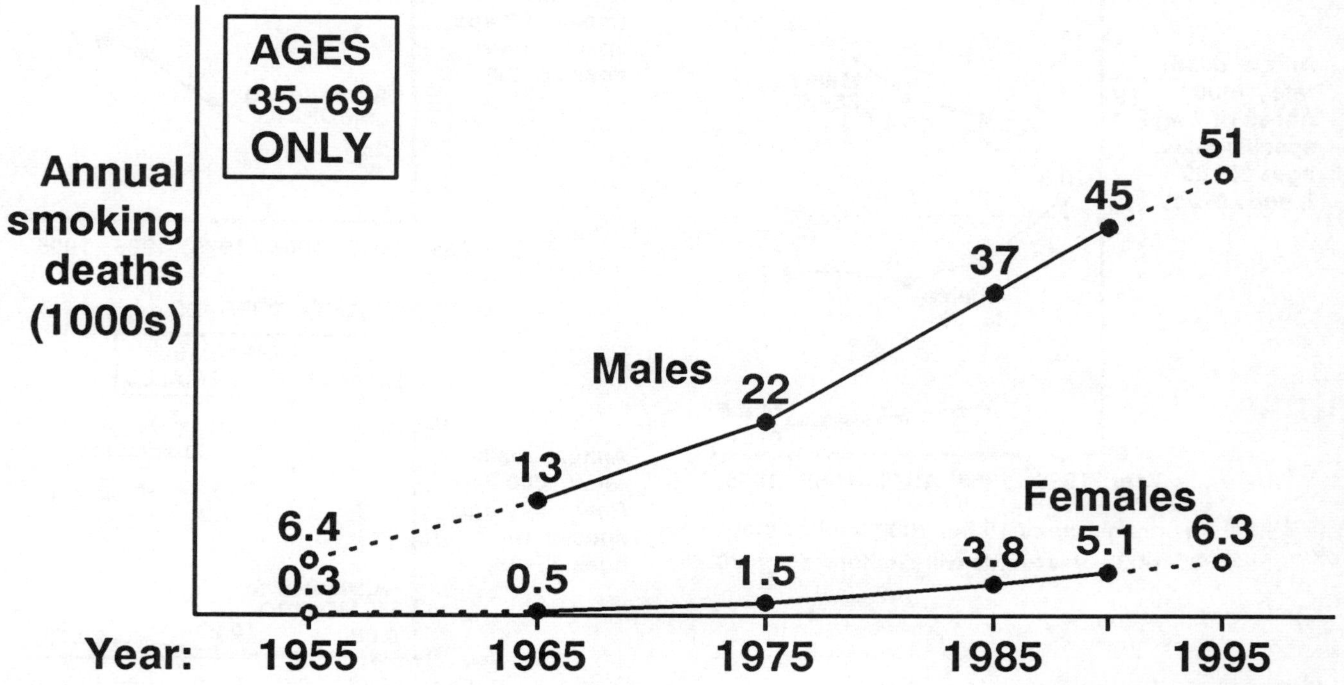

Peto, Lopez et al, 1992, 1994

POLAND

ALL DEATHS (annual rates per 1000): Trends in mortality attributed to smoking, and in other mortality

	Males				Females			
	35–69		70–79		35–69		70–79	
Attributed to SMOKING?	Yes	No	Yes	No	Yes	No	Yes	No
1955	2.17	14.6	3.79	81.0	0.08	10.7	0.17	66.5
1965	3.20	11.0	6.78	69.3	0.11	8.00	0.30	54.6
1975	4.73	10.4	13.2	64.8	0.27	7.02	0.87	49.3
1985	7.10	10.4	17.4	66.0	0.64	7.12	1.62	48.6
1990	7.67	10.5	16.7	62.0	0.75	6.77	2.26	44.7

35–69 = mean of 7 age-specific rates; 70–79 = mean of 2 rates (70–74 & 75–79) Peto, Lopez et al, 1992, 1994

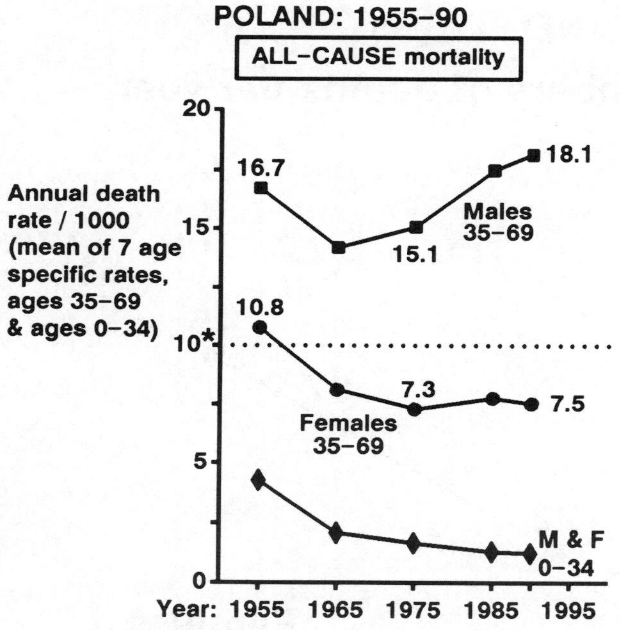

* An annual rate of 10 per 1000 implies that 30% of 35-year-olds will die before age 70

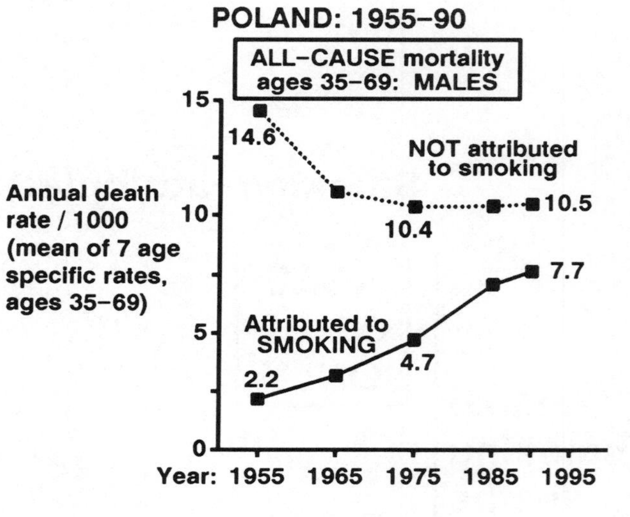

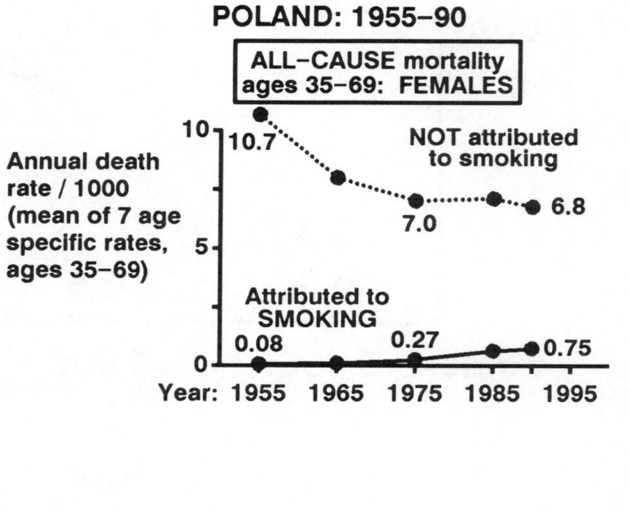

POLAND

ALL CANCER DEATHS (annual rates per 1000): Trends in mortality attributed to smoking, and in other mortality

	Males				Females			
	35–69		70–79		35–69		70–79	
Attributed to SMOKING?	Yes	No	Yes	No	Yes	No	Yes	No
1955	...	...	...	...	...	...	...	...
1965	1.08	2.30	2.24	9.48	0.02	2.37	0.05	7.83
1975	1.68	2.10	4.33	9.24	0.07	2.23	0.17	7.18
1985	2.55	2.09	5.85	9.55	0.16	2.29	0.34	7.23
1990	2.86	2.10	6.30	9.53	0.21	2.25	0.56	7.38

35–69 = mean of 7 age-specific rates; 70–79 = mean of 2 rates (70–74 & 75–79) Peto, Lopez et al, 1992, 1994

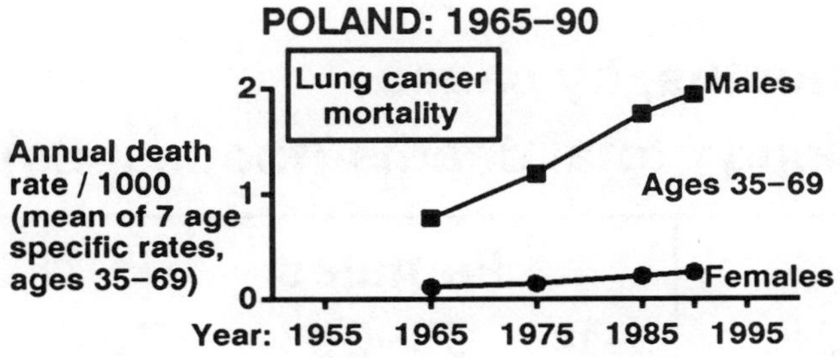

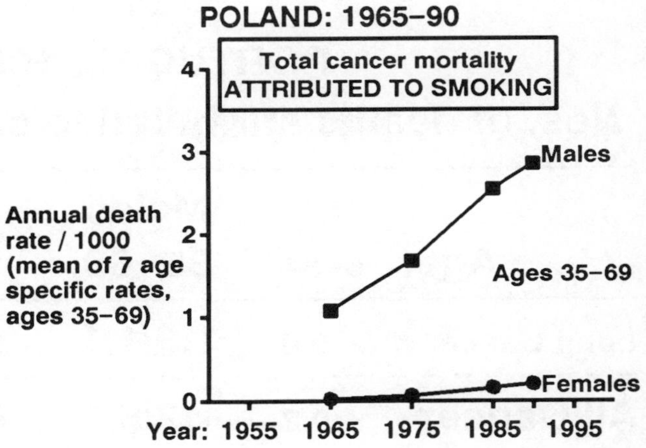

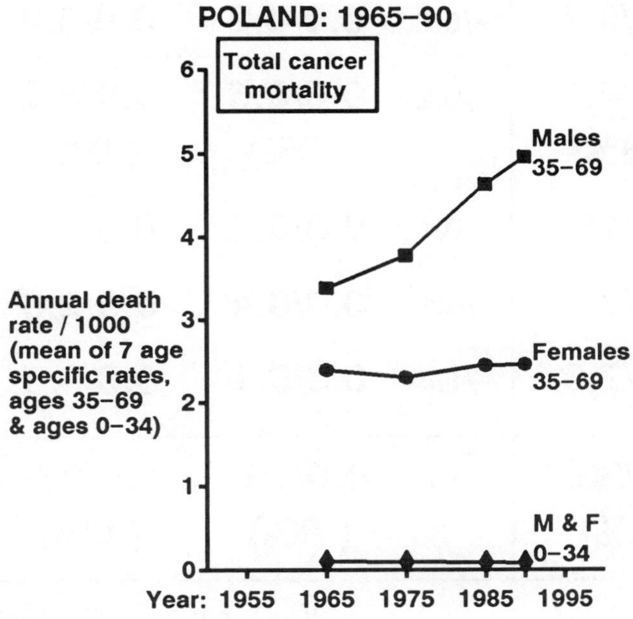

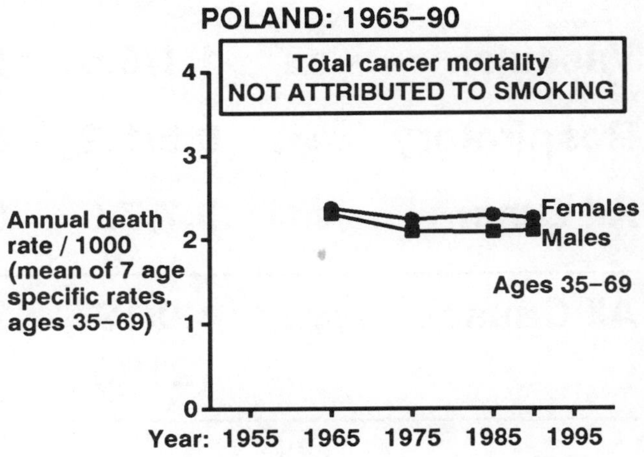

PORTUGAL: 1990
Relative importance of deaths in MIDDLE age (35–69)

Age range (years)	Deaths attributed to SMOKING / total deaths (thousands) Males	Females	Mean years lost PER DEATH FROM SMOKING
0–34	–/4.2	–/1.8	–
35–69	4.0/19	0.0/10	20 years
70+	2.8/30	0.0/37	8 years
All ages	6.8/53	0.0/50	15 years

Peto, Lopez et al, 1992, 1994

PORTUGAL: 1990 deaths, by cause
Nos. of deaths attributed to smoking / total deaths (thousands)

	Males			Females		
Age:	0–34	35–69	70+	0–34	35–69	70+
Lung Cancer	–/0.0	1.0/1.1	0.6/0.7	–/0.0	0.0/0.2	0.0/0.2
All Cancer	–/0.2	1.7/5.1 (33%)	0.9/4.9 (19%)	–/0.2	0.0/3.5 (0%)	0.0/4.2 (0%)
Vascular	–/0.2	1.1/6.0	0.8/15	–/0.1	0.0/3.4	0.0/21
Respiratory	–/0.1	0.5/1.2	0.8/3.0	–/0.1	0.0/0.4	0.0/2.6
All Other	–/3.7	0.7/7.0	0.3/7.3	–/1.4	0.0/3.1	0.0/9.5
All Causes	–/4.2	4.0/19 (21%)	2.8/30 (9%)	–/1.8	0.0/10 (0%)	0.0/37 (0%)

Peto, Lopez et al, 1992, 1994

PORTUGAL: 1990

RISKS OF DYING AT AGES 0–34 and 35–69

(Probability that someone entering an age range would die during it, if the death rates in 1990 were to persist unchanged)

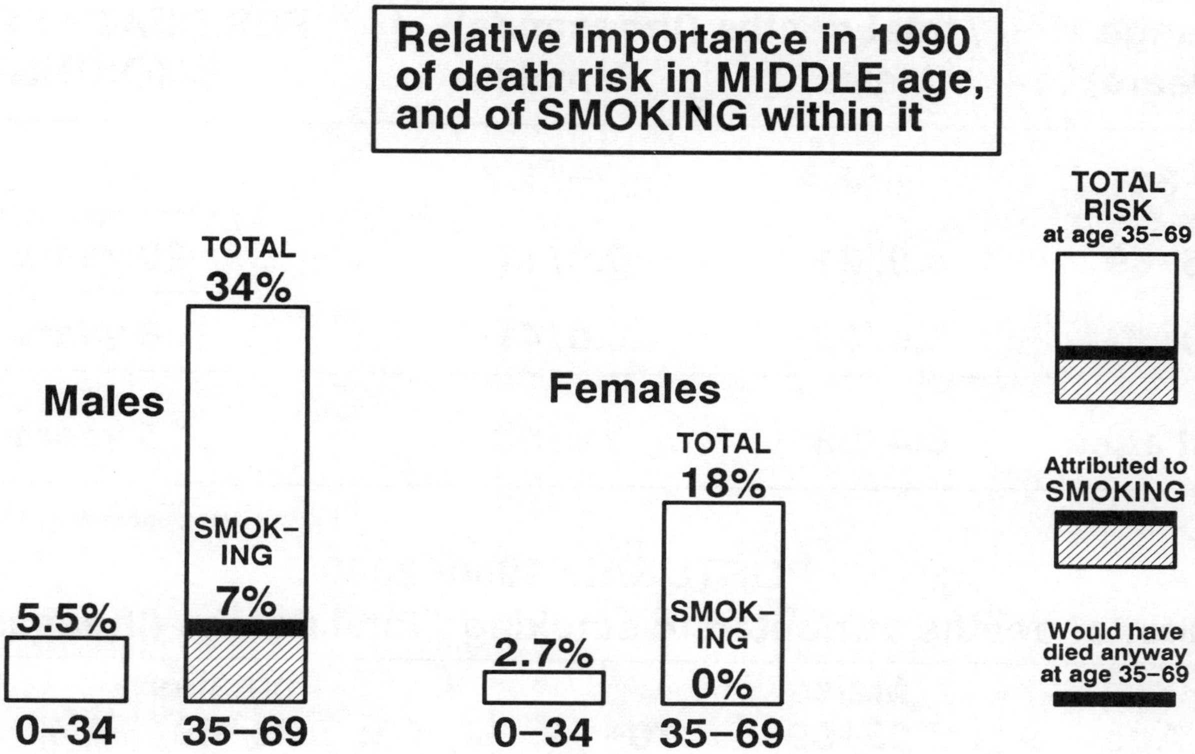

Peto, Lopez et al, 1992, 1994

PORTUGAL: 1990 deaths, all ages

Nos. of deaths attributed to smoking / total deaths (thousands)

	Males	Females	Males + Females
All Cancer	2.6/10 (25%)	0.0/7.9 (0%)	2.6/18 (14%)
All Causes	6.8/53 (13%)	0.0/50 (0%)	6.8/103 (7%)

Peto, Lopez et al, 1992, 1994

PORTUGAL: 1995 projections
Relative importance of deaths in MIDDLE age (35–69)

Age range (years)	Deaths attributed to SMOKING / total deaths (thousands) Males	Females	Mean years lost PER DEATH FROM SMOKING
0–34	–/4.4	–/1.7	–
35–69	4.9/21	0.0/11	20 years
70+	3.5/33	0.0/41	8 years
All ages	8.4/58	0.0/53	15 years

Peto, Lopez et al, 1992, 1994

PORTUGAL: 1950–2000
Nos. of deaths attributed to smoking / total deaths (thousands)

Age:	Males 0–34	Males 35–69	Males 70+	Females 0–34	Females 35–69	Females 70+
1955	–/18	0.8 / 17 (5%)	0.3 / 16 (2%)	–/15	0.0 / 12 (0%)	0.0 / 22 (0%)
1965	–/13	1.5 / 18 (8%)	0.4 / 18 (2%)	–/9.5	0.0 / 12 (0%)	0.0 / 25 (0%)
1975	–/8.0	2.5 / 21 (12%)	1.0 / 22 (4%)	–/5.0	0.0 / 12 (0%)	0.0 / 29 (0%)
1985	–/4.8	3.3 / 19 (18%)	2.3 / 27 (8%)	–/2.3	0.0 / 10 (0%)	0.0 / 34 (0%)
1995 (projected)	–/4.4	4.9 / 21 (24%)	3.5 / 33 (11%)	–/1.7	0.0 / 11 (0%)	0.0 / 41 (0%)
50–year total*, mid–1950 to mid–2000: 205/5017						
1950–2000, by age & sex	–/482	130 / 960 (14%)	75 / 1160 (6%)	–/335	0.0 / 570 (0%)	0.0 / 1510 (0%)

*Estimated as 10 times the sum of the five annual numbers (for 1955, 1965, 1975, 1985 & 1995)

PORTUGAL

Smoking–attributed numbers of deaths per year

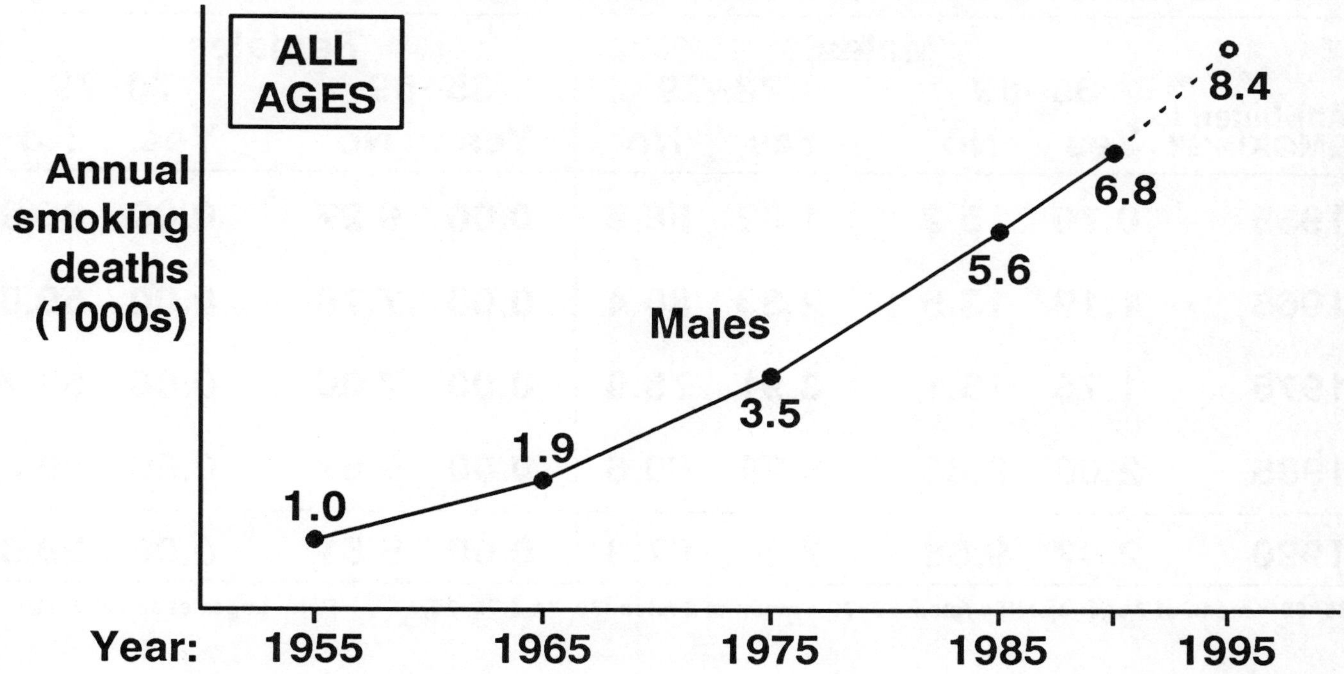

Peto, Lopez et al, 1992, 1994

PORTUGAL

Smoking–attributed numbers of deaths per year

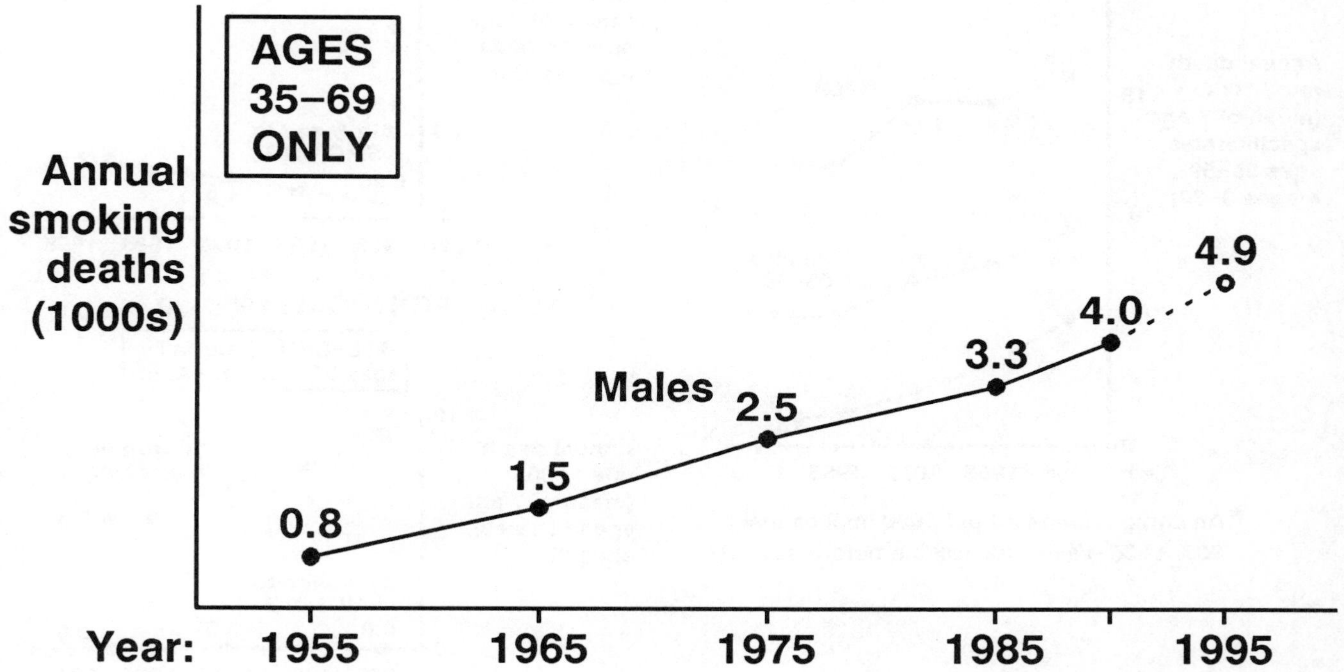

Peto, Lopez et al, 1992, 1994

PORTUGAL

ALL DEATHS (annual rates per 1000): Trends in mortality attributed to smoking, and in other mortality

	Males				Females			
	35–69		70–79		35–69		70–79	
Attributed to SMOKING?	Yes	No	Yes	No	Yes	No	Yes	No
1955	0.70	15.2	1.82	88.9	0.00	9.27	0.00	65.9
1965	1.19	13.5	2.33	80.4	0.00	7.79	0.00	59.8
1975	1.76	13.1	3.91	75.9	0.00	7.06	0.00	53.7
1985	2.06	9.83	6.29	60.6	0.00	5.67	0.00	40.6
1990	2.47	9.58	7.36	57.3	0.00	5.51	0.00	39.0

35–69 = mean of 7 age-specific rates; 70–79 = mean of 2 rates (70–74 & 75–79) Peto, Lopez et al, 1992, 1994

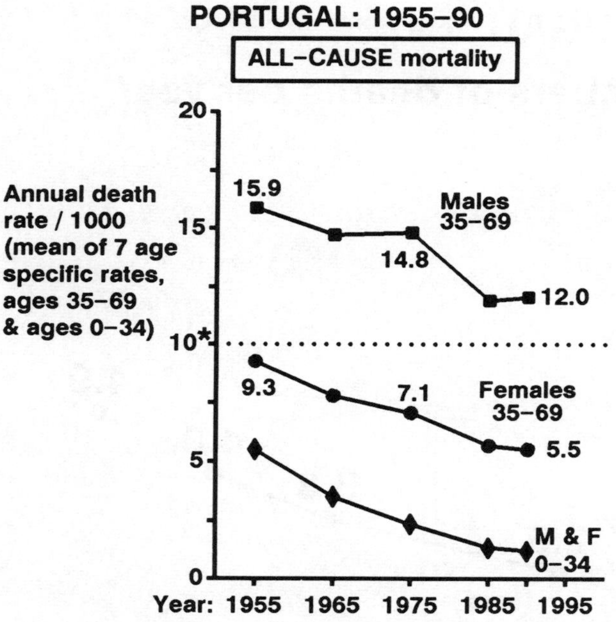

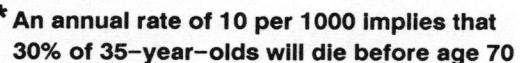

* An annual rate of 10 per 1000 implies that 30% of 35-year-olds will die before age 70

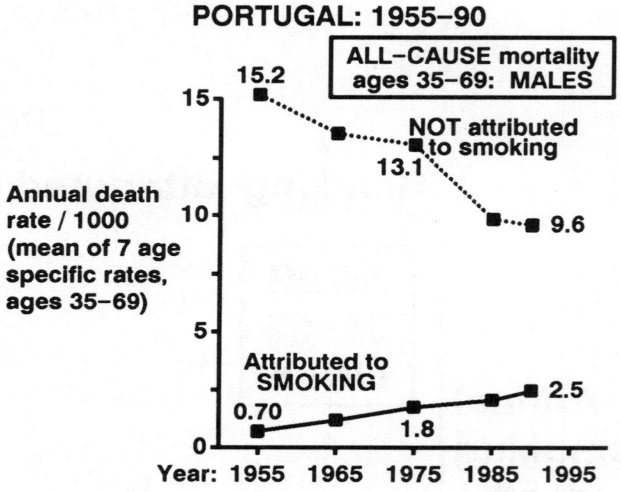

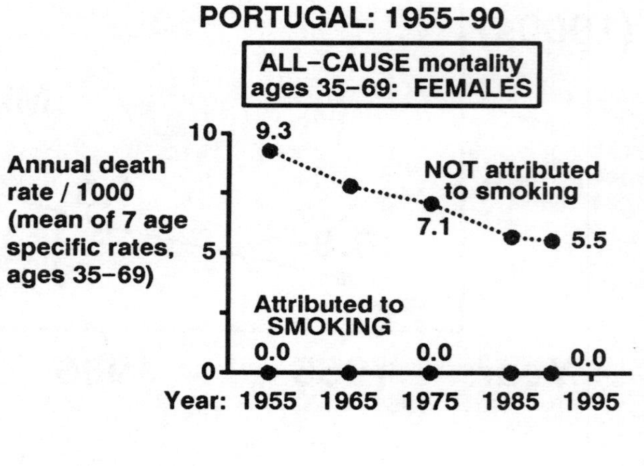

PORTUGAL

ALL CANCER DEATHS (annual rates per 1000): Trends in mortality attributed to smoking, and in other mortality

	Males				Females			
	35–69		70–79		35–69		70–79	
Attributed to SMOKING?	Yes	No	Yes	No	Yes	No	Yes	No
1955	0.18	1.93	0.44	7.23	0.00	1.74	0.00	5.31
1965	0.35	2.12	0.60	8.80	0.00	1.86	0.00	6.27
1975	0.53	2.17	1.08	9.25	0.00	1.77	0.00	6.03
1985	0.83	2.05	2.31	9.75	0.00	1.77	0.00	5.94
1990	1.04	2.17	2.86	10.1	0.00	1.84	0.00	6.69

35–69 = mean of 7 age-specific rates; 70–79 = mean of 2 rates (70–74 & 75–79) Peto, Lopez et al, 1992, 1994

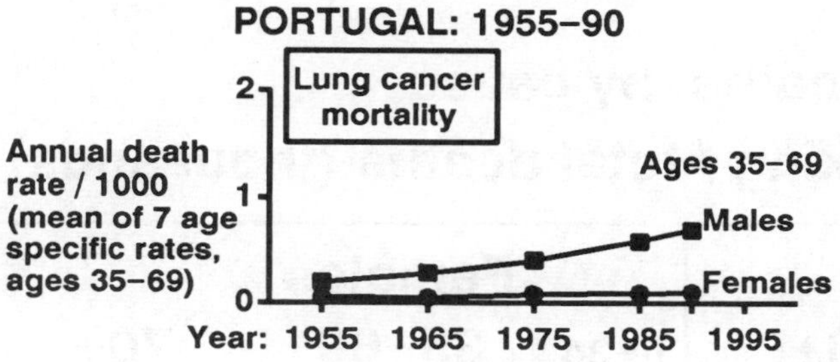

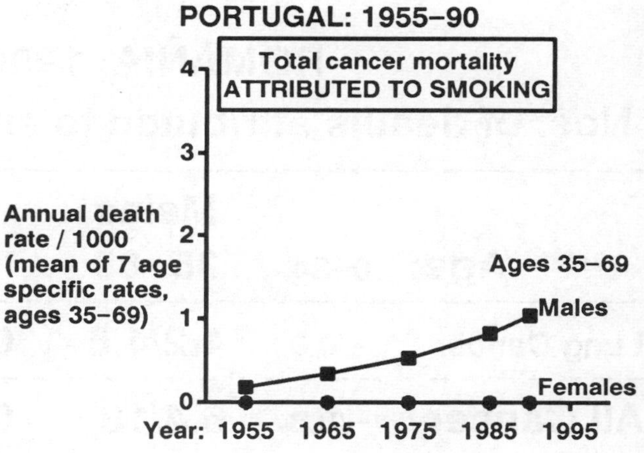

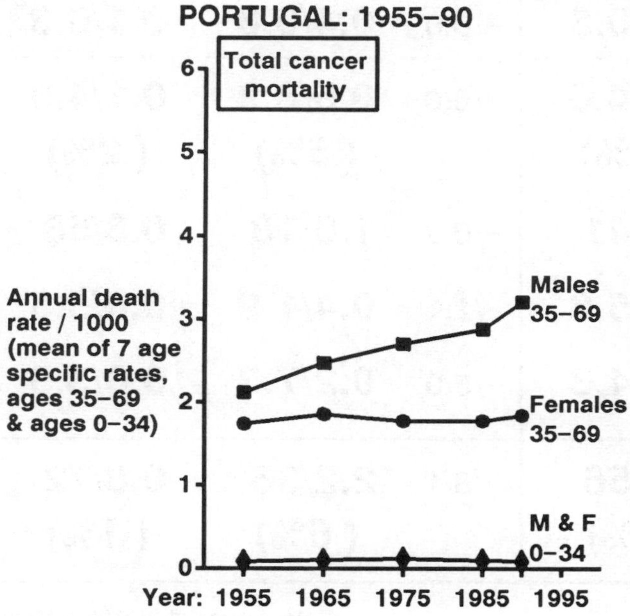

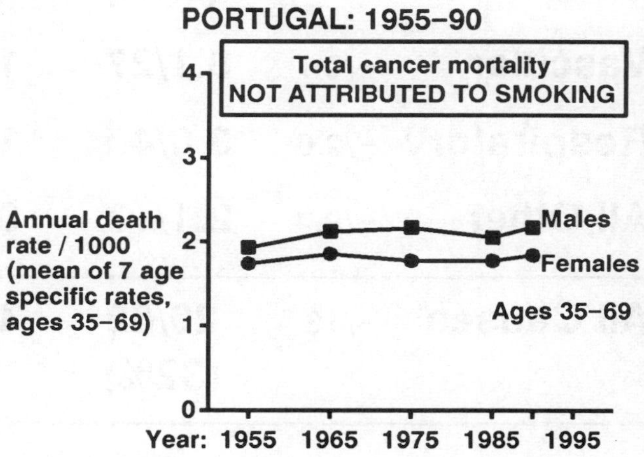

ROMANIA: 1990
Relative importance of deaths in MIDDLE age (35–69)

Age range (years)	Deaths attributed to SMOKING / total deaths (thousands) Males	Females	Mean years lost PER DEATH FROM SMOKING
0–34	–/13	–/8.1	–
35–69	20/62	2.2/36	21 years
70+	4.2/56	0.8/72	8 years
All ages	24/132	2.9/115	19 years

Peto, Lopez et al, 1992, 1994

ROMANIA: 1990 deaths, by cause
Nos. of deaths attributed to smoking / total deaths (thousands)

	Males			Females		
Age:	0–34	35–69	70+	0–34	35–69	70+
Lung Cancer	–/0.0	4.2/4.6	0.6/0.8	–/0.0	0.4/0.8	0.1/0.3
All Cancer	–/0.8	6.4/13 (48%)	0.8/4.6 (18%)	–/0.6	0.5/8.9 (5%)	0.1/4.3 (2%)
Vascular	–/0.7	8.1/27	1.4/41	–/0.3	1.0/18	0.3/58
Respiratory	–/2.6	3.0/4.9	1.9/5.8	–/2.1	0.4/1.9	0.4/5.3
All Other	–/9.4	2.1/17	0.1/4.3	–/5.0	0.2/7.3	0.0/3.5
All Causes	–/13	20/62 (32%)	4.2/56 (8%)	–/8.1	2.2/36 (6%)	0.8/72 (1%)

Peto, Lopez et al, 1992, 1994

ROMANIA: 1990

RISKS OF DYING AT AGES 0–34 and 35–69

(Probability that someone entering an age range would die during it, if the death rates in 1990 were to persist unchanged)

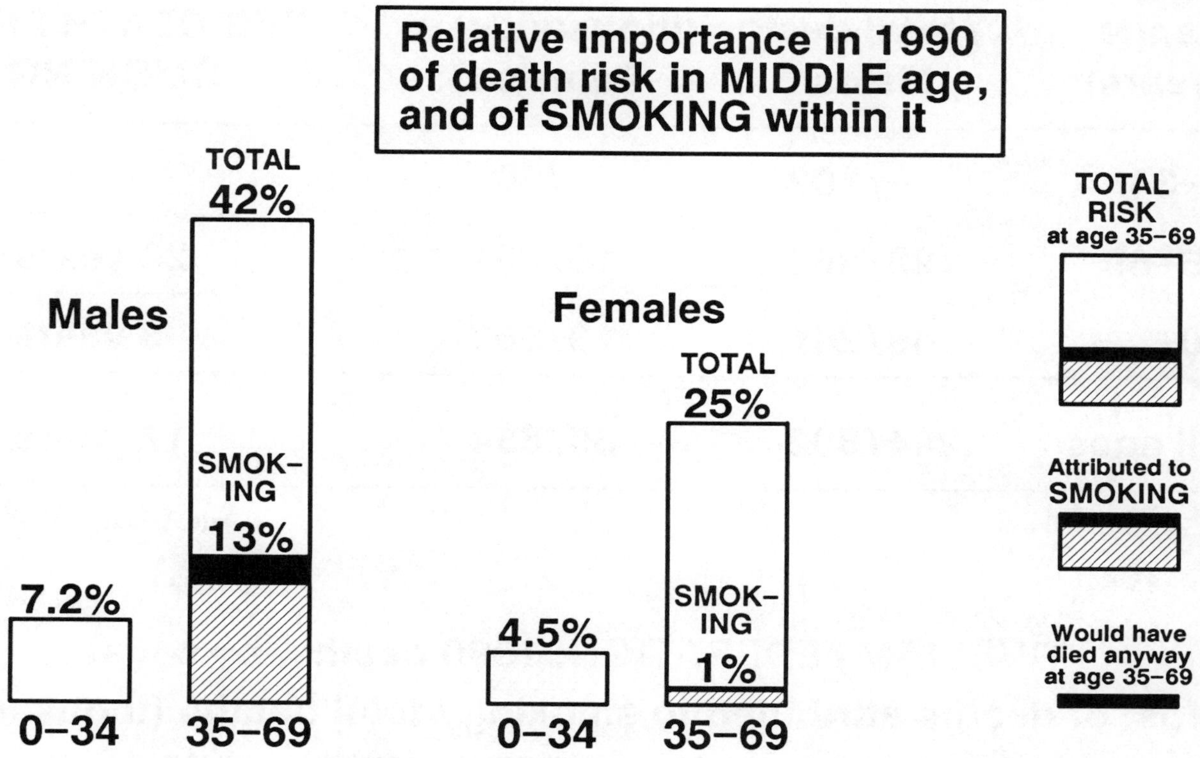

Peto, Lopez et al, 1992, 1994

ROMANIA: 1990 deaths, all ages

Nos. of deaths attributed to smoking / total deaths (thousands)

	Males	Females	Males + Females
All Cancer	7.3/19 (39%)	0.6/14 (4%)	7.8/33 (24%)
All Causes	24/132 (18%)	2.9/115 (3%)	27/247 (11%)

Peto, Lopez et al, 1992, 1994

¶RUSSIAN FEDERATION: 1990
Relative importance of deaths in MIDDLE age (35–69)

Age range (years)	Deaths attributed to SMOKING / total deaths (thousands) Males	Females	Mean years lost PER DEATH FROM SMOKING
0–34	–/102	–/40	–
35–69	192/460	16/251	20 years
70+	49/241	19/563	8 years
All ages	241/802	36/854	17 years

Peto, Lopez et al, 1992, 1994

RUSSIAN FEDERATION: 1990 deaths, by cause
Nos. of deaths attributed to smoking / total deaths (thousands)

	Males			Females		
Age:	0–34	35–69	70+	0–34	35–69	70+
Lung Cancer	–/0.2	41/42	9.4/10	–/0.1	2.7/5.5	2.1/4.3
All Cancer	–/4.4	68/116 (59%)	14/37 (39%)	–/4.0	3.7/72 (5%)	2.9/51 (6%)
Vascular	–/5.7	84/187	19/161	–/1.8	8.1/118	8.9/442
Respiratory	–/5.0	22/28	13/20	–/3.4	3.1/9.5	6.9/23
All Other	–/87	18/129	1.7/23	–/31	1.5/51	0.7/47
All Causes	–/102	192/460 (42%)	49/241 (20%)	–/40	16/251 (7%)	19/563 (3%)

Peto, Lopez et al, 1992, 1994

RUSSIAN FEDERATION: 1990

RISKS OF DYING AT AGES 0–34 and 35–69

(Probability that someone entering an age range would die during it, if the death rates in 1990 were to persist unchanged)

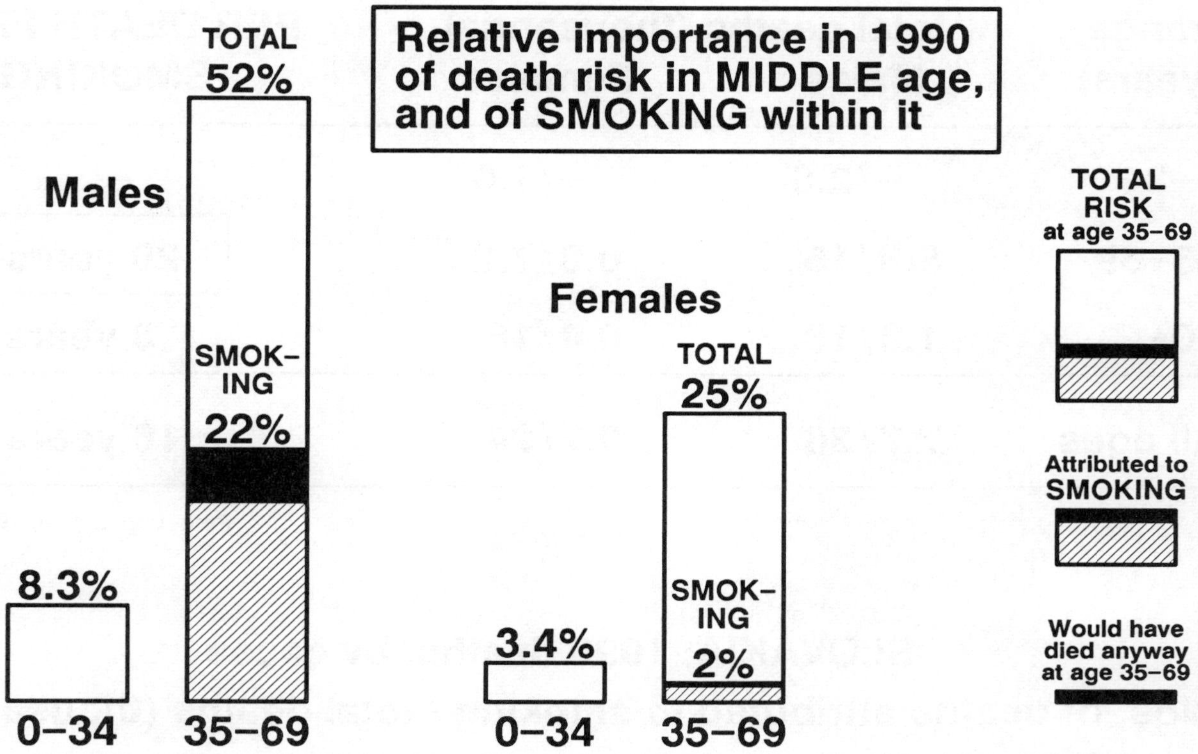

Peto, Lopez et al, 1992, 1994

RUSSIAN FEDERATION: 1990 deaths, all ages

Nos. of deaths attributed to smoking / total deaths (thousands)

	Males	Females	Males + Females
All Cancer	82/157 (52%)	6.5/127 (5%)	89/284 (31%)
All Causes	241/802 (30%)	36/854 (4%)	276/1656 (17%)

Peto, Lopez et al, 1992, 1994

¶SLOVAKIA: 1990
Relative importance of deaths in MIDDLE age (35–69)

Age range (years)	Deaths attributed to SMOKING / total deaths (thousands) Males	Females	Mean years lost PER DEATH FROM SMOKING
0–34	–/2.0	–/1.0	–
35–69	5.8/15	0.3/7.2	20 years
70+	1.9/13	0.4/16	8 years
All ages	7.7/30	0.7/24	16 years

Peto, Lopez et al, 1992, 1994

SLOVAKIA: 1990 deaths, by cause
Nos. of deaths attributed to smoking / total deaths (thousands)

	Males			Females		
Age:	0–34	35–69	70+	0–34	35–69	70+
Lung Cancer	–/0.0	1.3/1.4	0.5/0.5	–/0.0	0.1/0.1	0.1/0.1
All Cancer	–/0.2	2.3/4.0 (58%)	0.7/2.1 (34%)	–/0.1	0.1/2.2 (3%)	0.1/1.7 (5%)
Vascular	–/0.1	2.6/6.5	0.8/8.1	–/0.1	0.2/3.2	0.2/11
Respiratory	–/0.1	0.4/0.8	0.3/1.3	–/0.1	0.0/0.3	0.1/1.4
All Other	–/1.6	0.5/3.9	0.1/1.5	–/0.7	0.0/1.5	0.0/2.0
All Causes	–/2.0	5.8/15 (38%)	1.9/13 (15%)	–/1.0	0.3/7.2 (4%)	0.4/16 (2%)

Peto, Lopez et al, 1992, 1994

SLOVAKIA: 1990

RISKS OF DYING AT AGES 0–34 and 35–69

(Probability that someone entering an age range would die during it, if the death rates in 1990 were to persist unchanged)

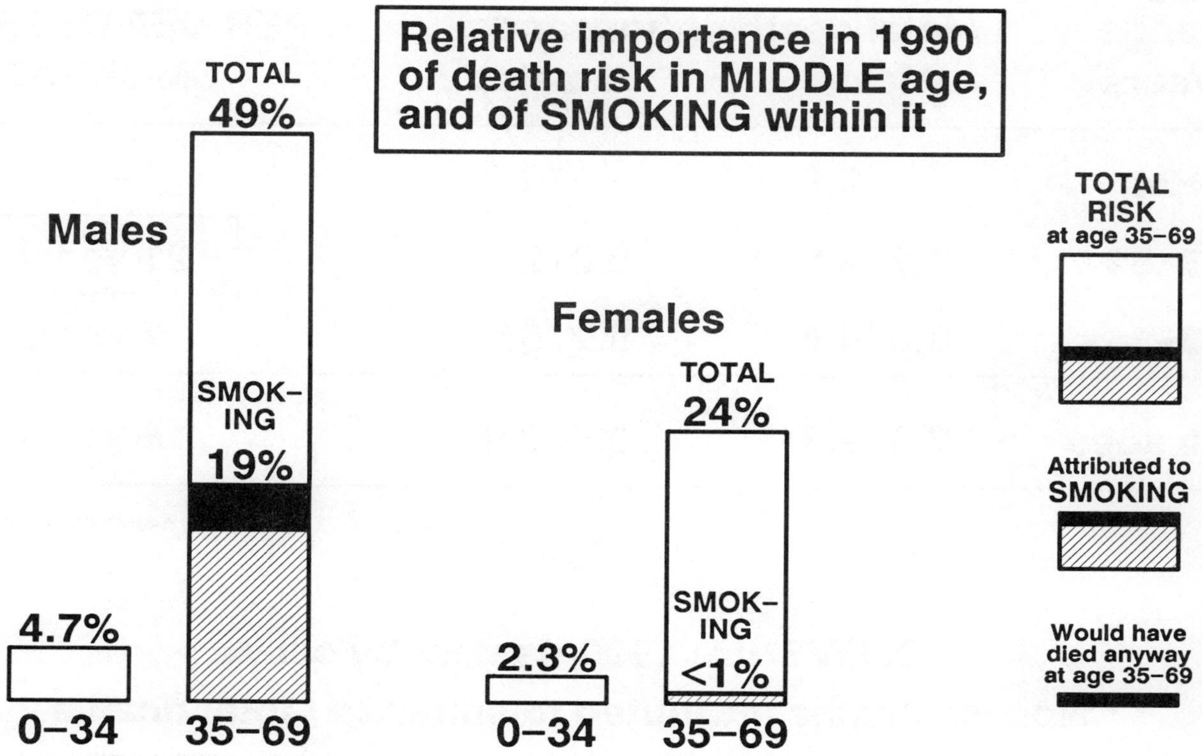

Peto, Lopez et al, 1992, 1994

SLOVAKIA: 1990 deaths, all ages

Nos. of deaths attributed to smoking / total deaths (thousands)

	Males	Females	Males + Females
All Cancer	3.0/6.3 (48%)	0.2/4.0 (4%)	3.2/10 (31%)
All Causes	7.7/30 (26%)	0.7/24 (3%)	8.4/55 (15%)

Peto, Lopez et al, 1992, 1994

¶SLOVENIA: 1990

Relative importance of deaths in MIDDLE age (35–69)

Age range (years)	Deaths attributed to SMOKING / total deaths (thousands) Males	Females	Mean years lost PER DEATH FROM SMOKING
0–34	–/0.6	–/0.2	–
35–69	1.7/4.5	0.2/2.3	21 years
70+	0.8/4.4	0.2/6.5	7 years
All ages	2.5/9.5	0.4/9.0	16 years

Peto, Lopez et al, 1992, 1994

SLOVENIA: 1990 deaths, by cause

Nos. of deaths attributed to smoking / total deaths

	Males			Females		
Age:	0–34	35–69	70+	0–34	35–69	70+
Lung Cancer	–/ 6	517/542	148/166	–/ 0	50/86	25/53
All Cancer	–/43	829/1436 (58%)	240/792 (30%)	–/36	65/889 (7%)	34/892 (4%)
Vascular	–/28	564/1434	232/2413	–/13	61/717	83/4191
Respiratory	–/12	148/212	243/493	–/ 5	19/71	58/372
All Other	–/505	179/1460	43/689	–/194	24/610	15/1048
All Causes	–/588	1720/4542 (38%)	758/4387 (17%)	–/248	169/2287 (7%)	190/6503 (3%)

Peto, Lopez et al, 1992, 1994

SLOVENIA: 1990

RISKS OF DYING AT AGES 0–34 and 35–69

(Probability that someone entering an age range would die during it, if the death rates in 1990 were to persist unchanged)

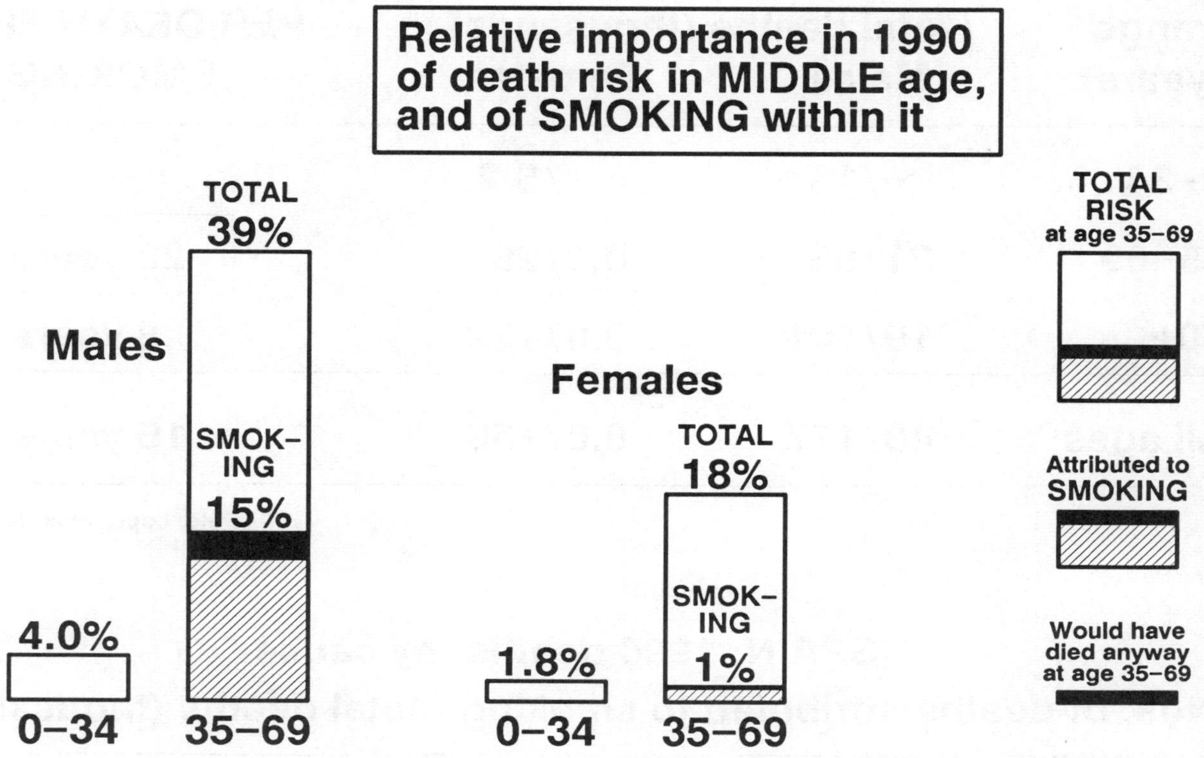

Peto, Lopez et al, 1992, 1994

SLOVENIA: 1990 deaths, all ages

Nos. of deaths attributed to smoking / total deaths (thousands)

	Males	Females	Males + Females
All Cancer	1.1/2.3 (47%)	0.1/1.8 (5%)	1.2/4.1 (29%)
All Causes	2.5/9.5 (26%)	0.4/9.0 (4%)	2.8/19 (15%)

Peto, Lopez et al, 1992, 1994

SPAIN: 1990
Relative importance of deaths in MIDDLE age (35–69)

Age range (years)	Deaths attributed to SMOKING / total deaths (thousands) Males	Females	Mean years lost PER DEATH FROM SMOKING
0–34	–/13	–/5.2	–
35–69	21/63	0.0/29	22 years
70+	19/101	0.0/122	8 years
All ages	40/177	0.0/156	15 years

Peto, Lopez et al, 1992, 1994

SPAIN: 1990 deaths, by cause
Nos. of deaths attributed to smoking / total deaths (thousands)

	Males			Females		
Age:	0–34	35–69	70+	0–34	35–69	70+
Lung Cancer	–/0.1	6.8/7.3	4.7/5.3	–/0.0	0.0/0.5	0.0/0.8
All Cancer	–/0.8	11/23 (47%)	7.4/23 (32%)	–/0.7	0.0/12 (0%)	0.0/17 (0%)
Vascular	–/1.0	4.8/18	4.2/43	–/0.4	0.0/7.6	0.0/66
Respiratory	–/0.5	2.5/4.6	6.2/15	–/0.2	0.0/1.4	0.0/11
All Other	–/10	2.3/17	1.7/21	–/3.9	0.0/7.8	0.0/28
All Causes	–/13	21/63 (33%)	19/101 (19%)	–/5.2	0.0/29 (0%)	0.0/122 (0%)

Peto, Lopez et al, 1992, 1994

SPAIN: 1990

RISKS OF DYING AT AGES 0–34 and 35–69

(Probability that someone entering an age range would die during it, if the death rates in 1990 were to persist unchanged)

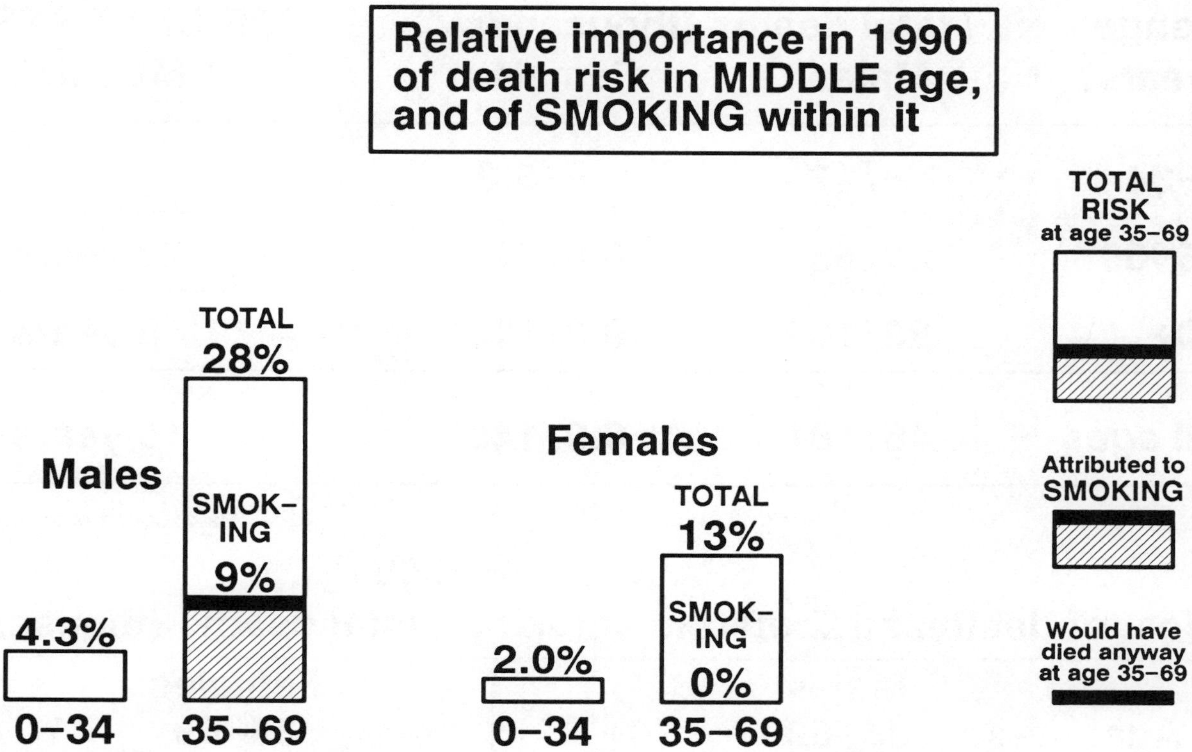

Peto, Lopez et al, 1992, 1994

SPAIN: 1990 deaths, all ages

Nos. of deaths attributed to smoking / total deaths (thousands)

	Males	Females	Males + Females
All Cancer	18/47 (39%)	0.0/30 (0%)	18/77 (24%)
All Causes	40/177 (23%)	0.0/156 (0%)	40/333 (12%)

Peto, Lopez et al, 1992, 1994

SPAIN: 1995 projections
Relative importance of deaths in MIDDLE age (35–69)

Age range (years)	Deaths attributed to SMOKING / total deaths (thousands) Males	Females	Mean years lost PER DEATH FROM SMOKING
0–34	–/17	–/6.0	–
35–69	23/63	0.0/27	23 years
70+	23/102	0.0/115	8 years
All ages	46/181	0.0/148	15 years

Peto, Lopez et al, 1992, 1994

SPAIN: 1950–2000
Nos. of deaths attributed to smoking / total deaths (thousands)

	Males			Females		
Age:	0–34	35–69	70+	0–34	35–69	70+
1955	–/32	5.6 / 52 (11%)	1.6 / 52 (3%)	–/25	0.0 / 40 (0%)	0.0 / 68 (0%)
1965	–/21	8.9 / 55 (16%)	4.7 / 62 (8%)	–/14	0.0 / 38 (0%)	0.0 / 78 (0%)
1975	–/16	14 / 62 (23%)	11 / 78 (13%)	–/9.8	0.0 / 37 (0%)	0.0 / 96 (0%)
1985	–/10	17 / 60 (29%)	16 / 94 (17%)	–/5.1	0.0 / 30 (0%)	0.0 / 113 (0%)
1995 (projected)	–/17	23 / 63 (36%)	23 / 102 (23%)	–/6.0	0.0 / 27 (0%)	0.0 / 115 (0%)

50–year total*, mid–1950 to mid–2000: 1248/14779

1950–2000, by age & sex	–/960	685 / 2920 (23%)	563 / 3880 (15%)	–/599	0.0 / 1720 (0%)	0.0 / 4700 (0%)

*Estimated as 10 times the sum of the five annual numbers (for 1955, 1965, 1975, 1985 & 1995)

SPAIN

Smoking–attributed numbers of deaths per year

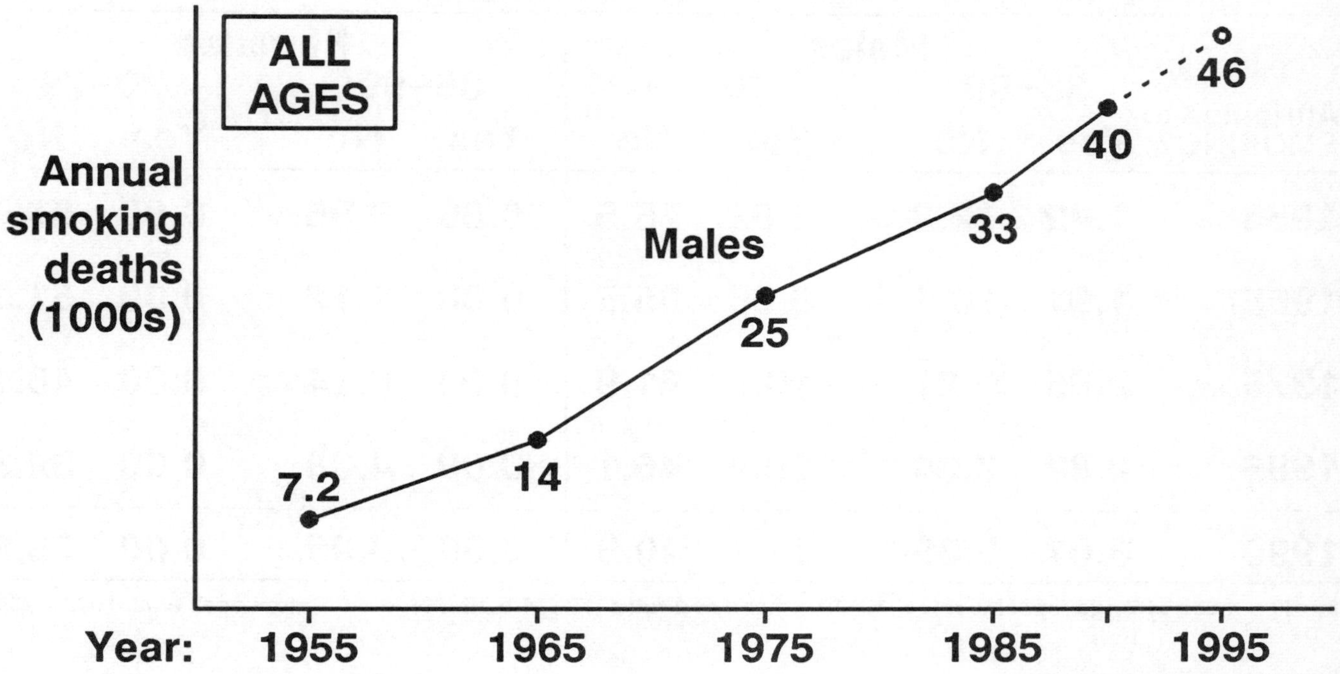

Peto, Lopez et al, 1992, 1994

SPAIN

Smoking–attributed numbers of deaths per year

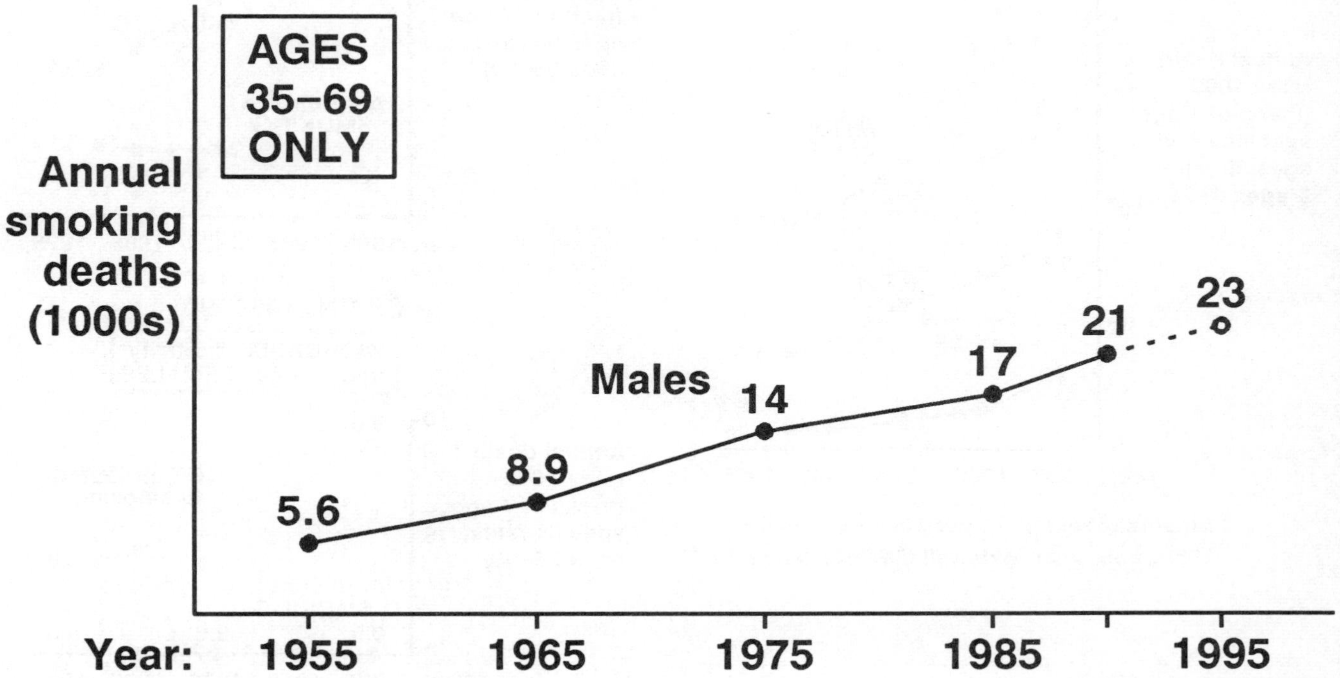

Peto, Lopez et al, 1992, 1994

SPAIN

ALL DEATHS (annual rates per 1000): Trends in mortality attributed to smoking, and in other mortality

	Males				Females			
	35–69		70–79		35–69		70–79	
Attributed to SMOKING?	Yes	No	Yes	No	Yes	No	Yes	No
1955	1.42	12.2	2.62	75.5	0.00	8.96	0.00	57.7
1965	1.91	10.1	6.06	65.5	0.00	7.12	0.00	51.3
1975	2.85	9.27	10.8	61.9	0.00	6.14	0.00	48.1
1985	2.82	7.04	10.9	46.1	0.00	4.38	0.00	32.8
1990	3.07	6.36	11.7	40.5	0.00	3.95	0.00	28.8

35–69 = mean of 7 age-specific rates; 70–79 = mean of 2 rates (70–74 & 75–79) Peto, Lopez et al, 1992, 1994

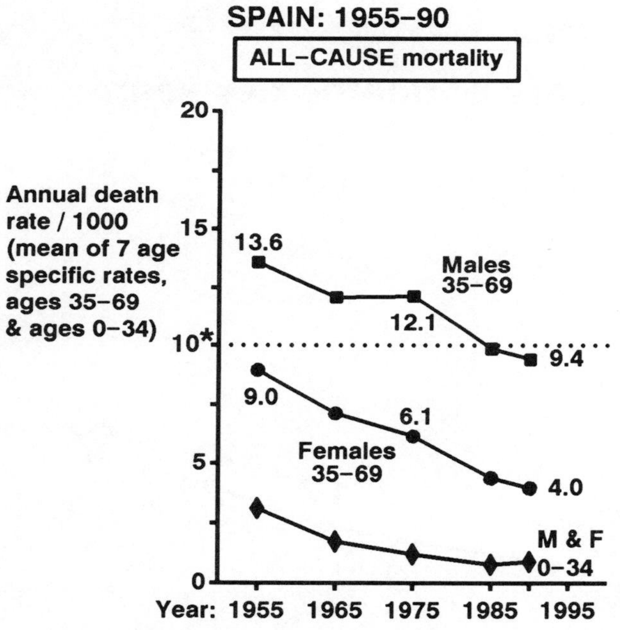

* An annual rate of 10 per 1000 implies that 30% of 35-year-olds will die before age 70

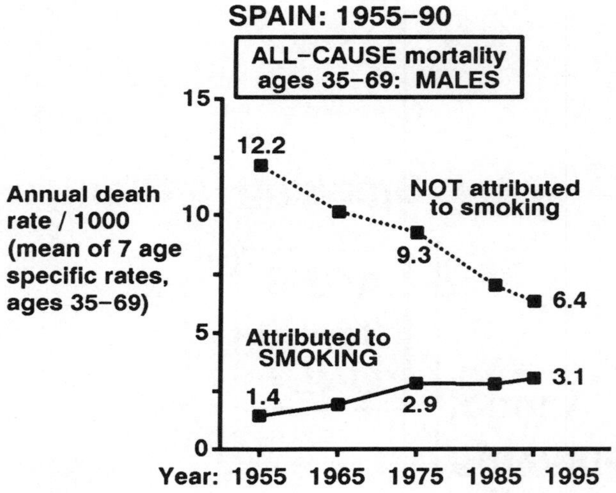

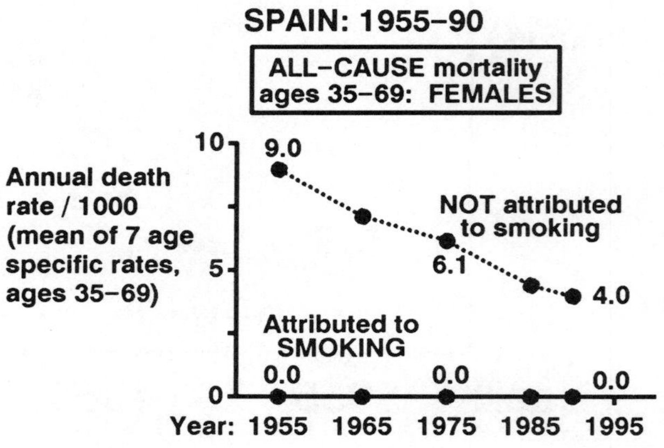

SPAIN

ALL CANCER DEATHS (annual rates per 1000): Trends in mortality attributed to smoking, and in other mortality

	Males				Females			
	35–69		70–79		35–69		70–79	
Attributed to SMOKING?	Yes	No	Yes	No	Yes	No	Yes	No
1955	0.38	1.91	0.64	8.68	0.00	1.74	0.00	6.03
1965	0.64	2.05	1.90	10.5	0.00	1.84	0.00	6.72
1975	1.09	2.08	3.53	10.3	0.00	1.85	0.00	7.14
1985	1.39	1.89	4.72	9.74	0.00	1.59	0.00	6.32
1990	1.63	1.89	5.34	9.99	0.00	1.65	0.00	6.18

35–69 = mean of 7 age–specific rates; 70–79 = mean of 2 rates (70–74 & 75–79) Peto, Lopez et al, 1992, 1994

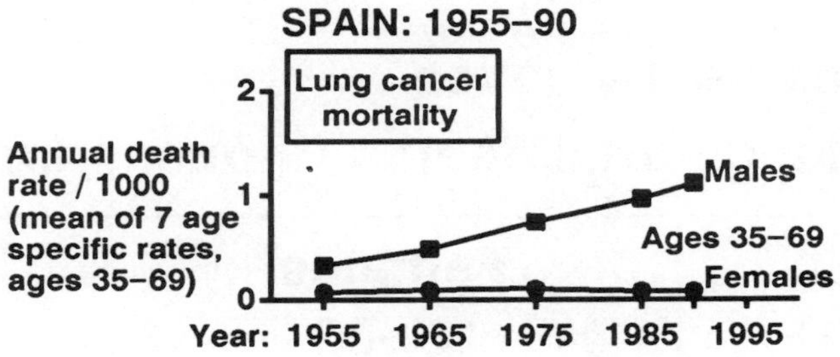

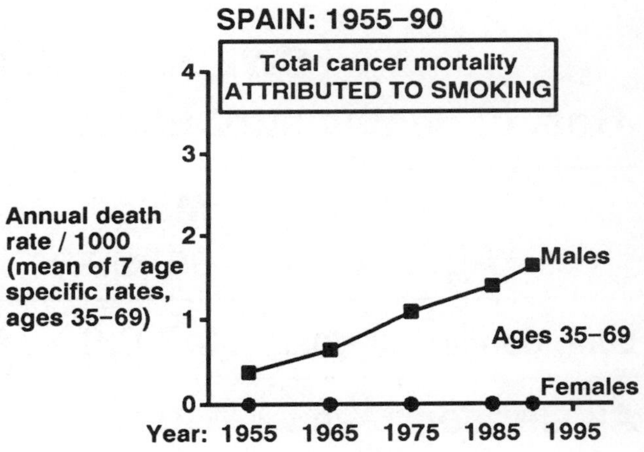

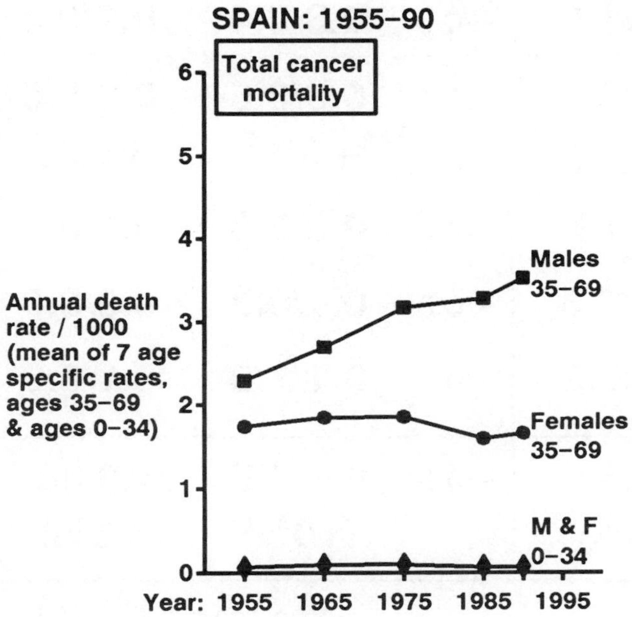

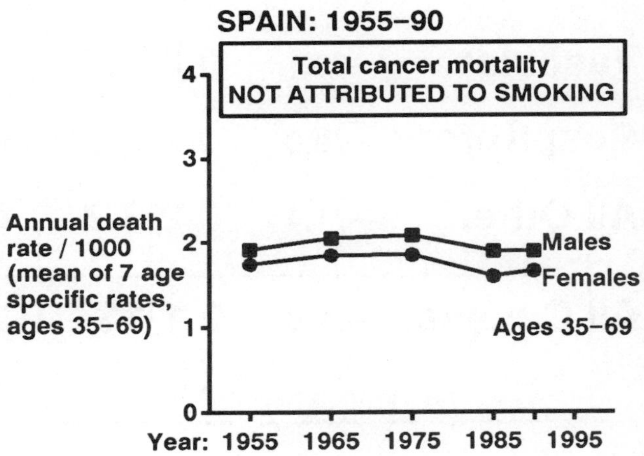

SWEDEN: 1990
Relative importance of deaths in MIDDLE age (35–69)

Age range (years)	Deaths attributed to SMOKING / total deaths (thousands) Males	Females	Mean years lost PER DEATH FROM SMOKING
0–34	–/1.6	–/0.9	–
35–69	2.1/13	0.7/7.5	21 years
70+	3.2/34	1.3/38	8 years
All ages	5.3/49	2.0/46	13 years

Peto, Lopez et al, 1992, 1994

SWEDEN: 1990 deaths, by cause
Nos. of deaths attributed to smoking / total deaths (thousands)

	Males			Females		
Age:	0–34	35–69	70+	0–34	35–69	70+
Lung Cancer	–/0.0	0.7/0.8	0.8/1.0	–/0.0	0.3/0.4	0.2/0.4
All Cancer	–/0.1	1.0/3.7 (26%)	1.3/6.9 (18%)	–/0.1	0.3/3.5 (9%)	0.3/6.0 (5%)
Vascular	–/0.1	0.8/5.6	1.0/19	–/0.0	0.2/2.0	0.5/22
Respiratory	–/0.0	0.2/0.5	0.6/3.3	–/0.0	0.1/0.3	0.3/3.0
All Other	–/1.4	0.2/3.3	0.2/5.2	–/0.7	0.1/1.6	0.1/6.9
All Causes	–/1.6	2.1/13 (16%)	3.2/34 (9%)	–/0.9	0.7/7.5 (10%)	1.3/38 (3%)

Peto, Lopez et al, 1992, 1994

SWEDEN: 1990

RISKS OF DYING AT AGES 0–34 and 35–69

(Probability that someone entering an age range would die during it, if the death rates in 1990 were to persist unchanged)

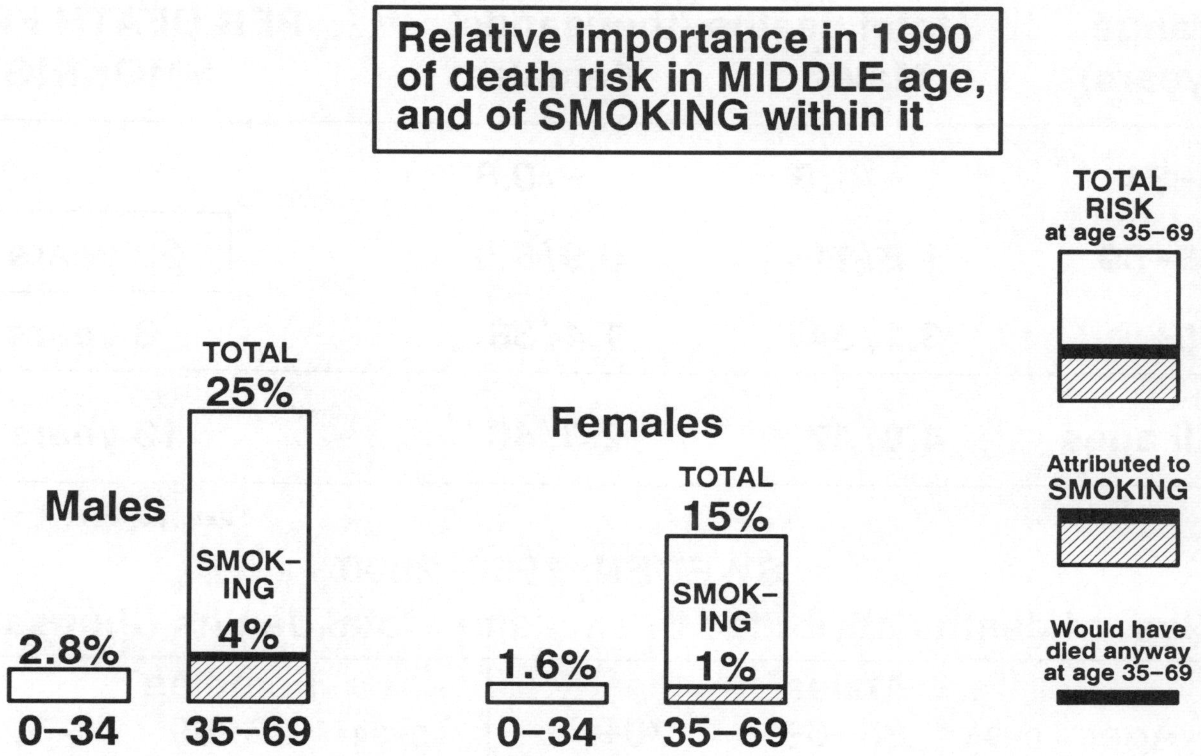

Peto, Lopez et al, 1992, 1994

SWEDEN: 1990 deaths, all ages

Nos. of deaths attributed to smoking / total deaths (thousands)

	Males	Females	Males + Females
All Cancer	2.2/11 (21%)	0.6/9.6 (7%)	2.9/20 (14%)
All Causes	5.3/49 (11%)	2.0/46 (4%)	7.3/95 (8%)

Peto, Lopez et al, 1992, 1994

SWEDEN: 1995 projections
Relative importance of deaths in MIDDLE age (35–69)

Age range (years)	Deaths attributed to SMOKING / total deaths (thousands) Males	Females	Mean years lost PER DEATH FROM SMOKING
0–34	–/1.6	–/0.8	–
35–69	1.8/11	0.9/6.8	22 years
70+	3.1/34	1.4/38	8 years
All ages	4.8/47	2.3/46	13 years

Peto, Lopez et al, 1992, 1994

SWEDEN: 1950–2000
Nos. of deaths attributed to smoking / total deaths (thousands)

Age:	Males 0–34	Males 35–69	Males 70+	Females 0–34	Females 35–69	Females 70+
1955	–/2.8	1.1 / 13 (8%)	0.4 / 19 (2%)	–/1.8	0.0 / 11 (0%)	0.0 / 21 (0%)
1965	–/2.6	1.8 / 15 (12%)	1.2 / 24 (5%)	–/1.5	0.0 / 10 (0%)	0.0 / 25 (0%)
1975	–/2.2	2.6 / 17 (15%)	2.9 / 29 (10%)	–/1.2	0.3 / 9.4 (3%)	0.6 / 29 (2%)
1985	–/1.6	2.6 / 15 (18%)	3.2 / 34 (10%)	–/0.9	0.6 / 7.9 (8%)	0.6 / 35 (2%)
1995 (projected)	–/1.6	1.8 / 11 (16%)	3.1 / 34 (9%)	–/0.8	0.9 / 6.8 (13%)	1.4 / 38 (4%)
50–year total*, mid–1950 to mid–2000: 251 / 4211						
1950–2000, by age & sex	–/108	99 / 710 (14%)	108 / 1400 (8%)	–/62	18 / 451 (4%)	26 / 1480 (2%)

*Estimated as 10 times the sum of the five annual numbers (for 1955, 1965, 1975, 1985 & 1995)

SWEDEN

Smoking–attributed numbers of deaths per year

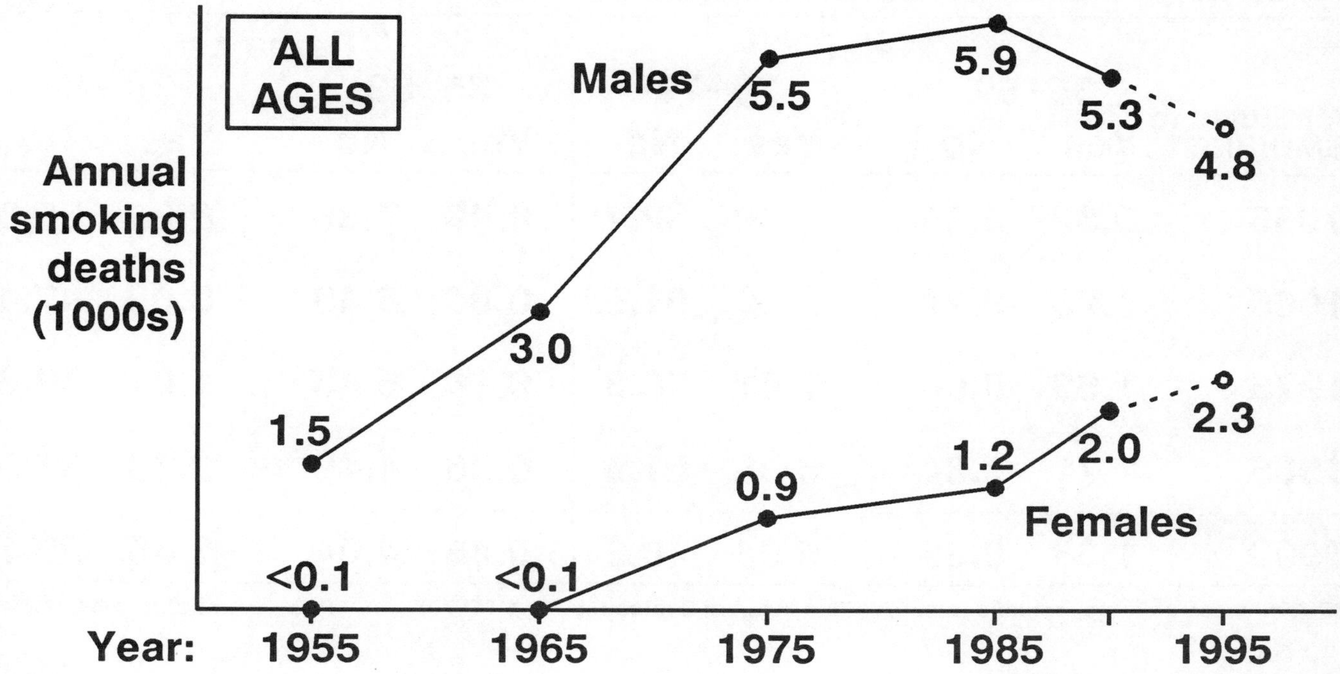

Peto, Lopez et al, 1992, 1994

SWEDEN

Smoking–attributed numbers of deaths per year

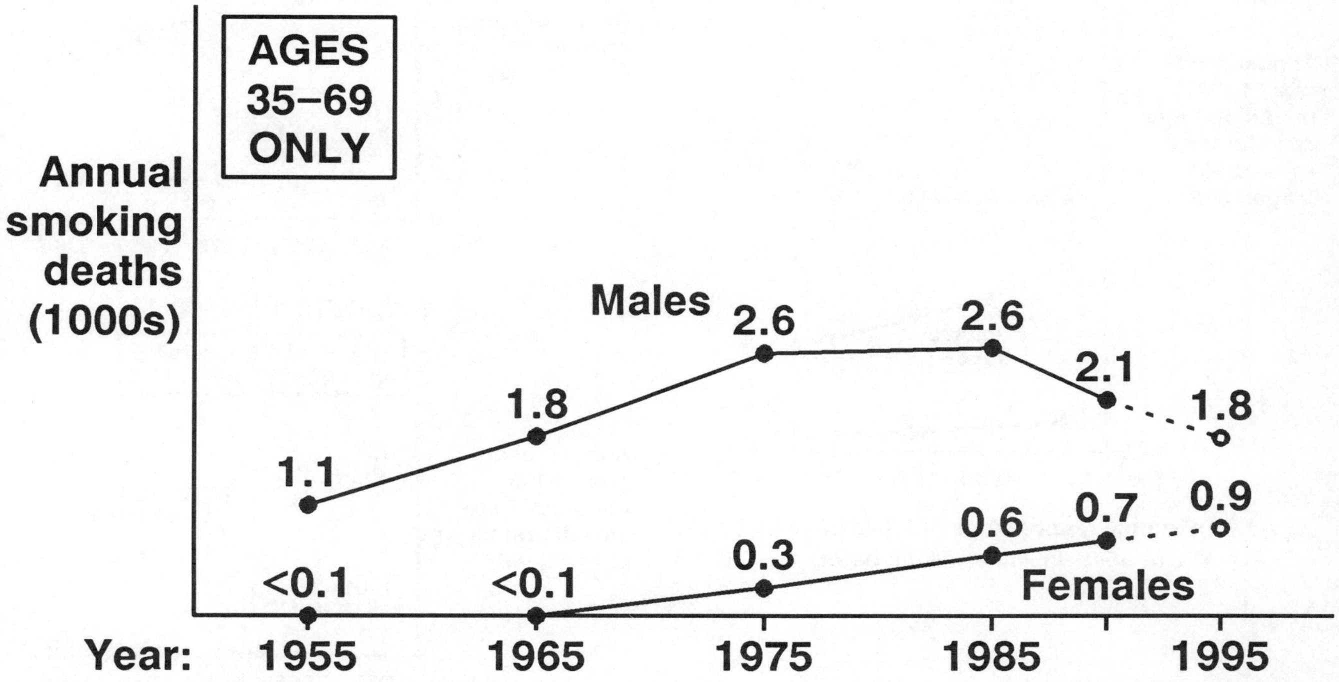

Peto, Lopez et al, 1992, 1994

SWEDEN

ALL DEATHS (annual rates per 1000): Trends in mortality attributed to smoking, and in other mortality

	Males				Females			
	35–69		70–79		35–69		70–79	
Attributed to SMOKING?	Yes	No	Yes	No	Yes	No	Yes	No
1955	0.82	9.84	1.49	62.7	0.00	7.86	0.00	55.0
1965	1.23	9.24	3.89	61.5	0.00	6.46	0.00	47.4
1975	1.63	9.08	7.41	56.8	0.16	5.43	1.01	38.6
1985	1.71	7.84	6.38	51.6	0.36	4.40	0.79	31.5
1990	1.38	6.95	5.94	48.2	0.45	4.04	1.45	28.1

35–69 = mean of 7 age-specific rates; 70–79 = mean of 2 rates (70–74 & 75–79) Peto, Lopez et al, 1992, 1994

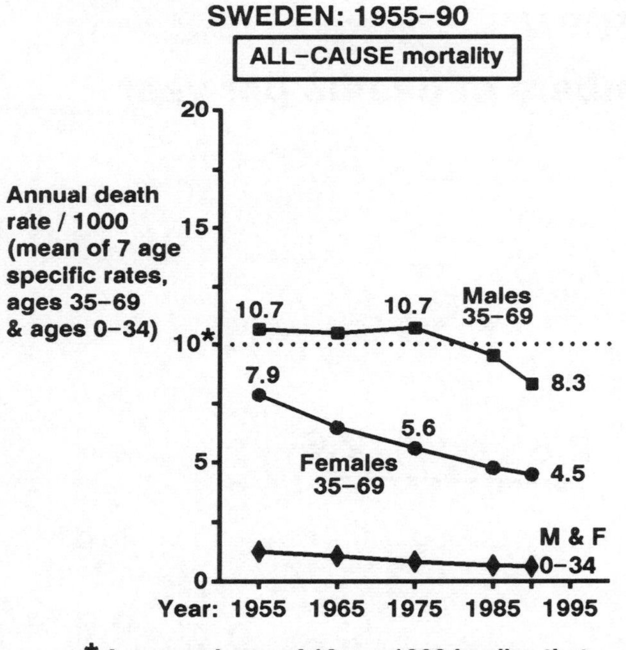

* An annual rate of 10 per 1000 implies that 30% of 35-year-olds will die before age 70

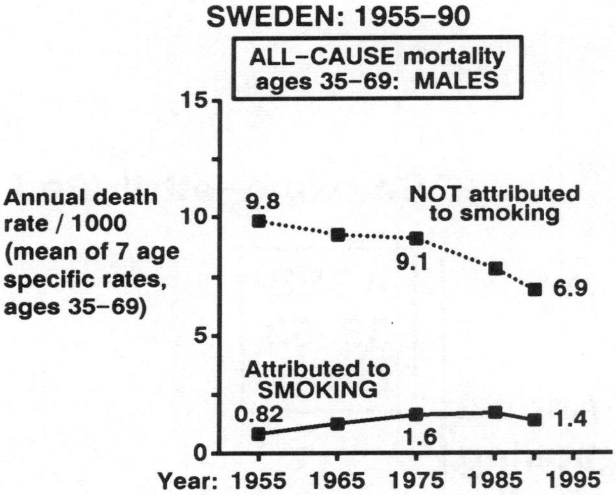

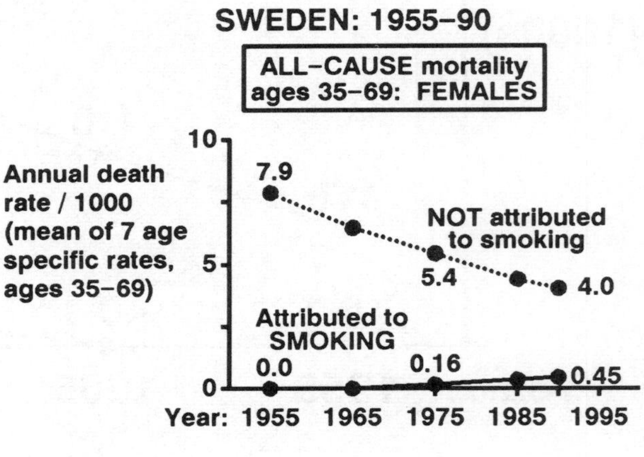

SWEDEN

ALL CANCER DEATHS (annual rates per 1000): Trends in mortality attributed to smoking, and in other mortality

	Males				Females			
	35–69		70–79		35–69		70–79	
Attributed to SMOKING?	Yes	No	Yes	No	Yes	No	Yes	No
1955	0.29	1.99	0.60	11.0	0.00	2.39	0.00	8.39
1965	0.48	1.88	1.59	11.4	0.00	2.22	0.00	8.23
1975	0.64	1.98	3.17	12.0	0.06	2.24	0.32	8.64
1985	0.71	1.79	2.74	10.5	0.14	1.98	0.25	7.46
1990	0.63	1.78	2.69	10.5	0.19	1.91	0.51	7.30

35–69 = mean of 7 age-specific rates; 70–79 = mean of 2 rates (70–74 & 75–79) Peto, Lopez et al, 1992, 1994

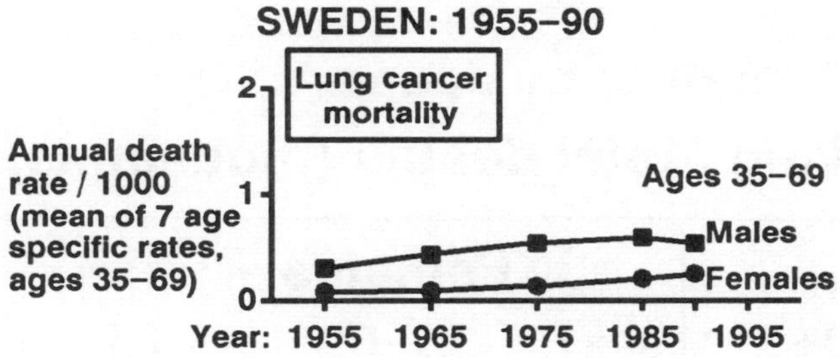

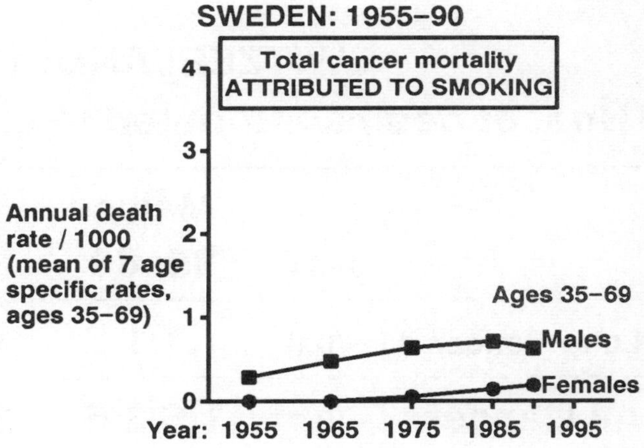

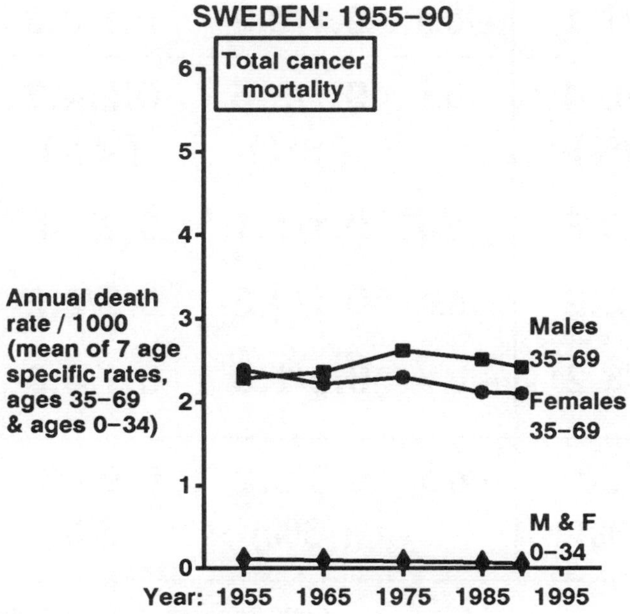

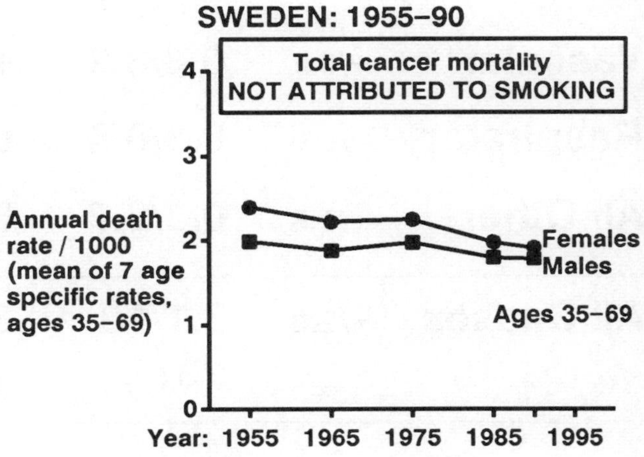

SWITZERLAND: 1990
Relative importance of deaths in MIDDLE age (35–69)

Age range (years)	Deaths attributed to SMOKING / total deaths (thousands) Males	Females	Mean years lost PER DEATH FROM SMOKING
0–34	–/2.0	–/0.9	–
35–69	3.1/10	0.3/5.2	21 years
70+	3.7/20	0.9/25	8 years
All ages	6.8/32	1.2/31	14 years

Peto, Lopez et al, 1992, 1994

SWITZERLAND: 1990 deaths, by cause
Nos. of deaths attributed to smoking / total deaths (thousands)

	Males			Females		
Age:	0–34	35–69	70+	0–34	35–69	70+
Lung Cancer	–/0.0	1.1/1.2	1.0/1.1	–/0.0	0.1/0.2	0.1/0.3
All Cancer	–/0.1	1.6/3.6 (45%)	1.6/5.4 (29%)	–/0.1	0.1/2.5 (6%)	0.2/4.7 (4%)
Vascular	–/0.1	0.8/3.2	1.0/9.8	–/0.0	0.1/1.1	0.3/14
Respiratory	–/0.0	0.3/0.5	0.9/2.2	–/0.0	0.1/0.2	0.2/2.2
All Other	–/1.8	0.3/2.7	0.2/3.2	–/0.7	0.0/1.3	0.1/4.6
All Causes	–/2.0	3.1/10 (31%)	3.7/20 (18%)	–/0.9	0.3/5.2 (6%)	0.9/25 (3%)

Peto, Lopez et al, 1992, 1994

SWITZERLAND: 1990

RISKS OF DYING AT AGES 0–34 and 35–69

(Probability that someone entering an age range would die during it, if the death rates in 1990 were to persist unchanged)

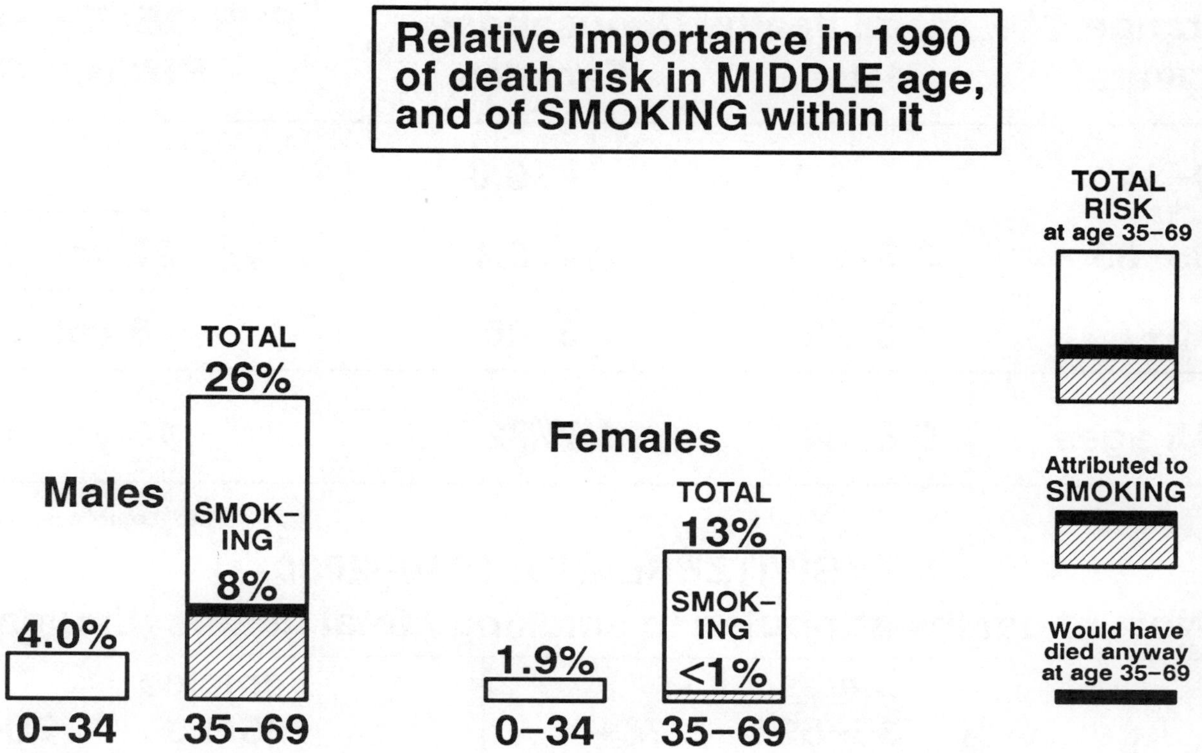

Peto, Lopez et al, 1992, 1994

SWITZERLAND: 1990 deaths, all ages

Nos. of deaths attributed to smoking / total deaths (thousands)

	Males	Females	Males + Females
All Cancer	3.2/9.1 (35%)	0.4/7.3 (5%)	3.5/16 (22%)
All Causes	6.8/32 (21%)	1.2/31 (4%)	7.9/64 (12%)

Peto, Lopez et al, 1992, 1994

SWITZERLAND: 1995 projections
Relative importance of deaths in MIDDLE age (35–69)

Age range (years)	Deaths attributed to SMOKING / total deaths (thousands) Males	Females	Mean years lost PER DEATH FROM SMOKING
0–34	–/2.1	–/0.8	–
35–69	3.0/9.9	0.4/5.1	22 years
70+	3.8/22	1.3/26	8 years
All ages	6.8/34	1.7/32	13 years

Peto, Lopez et al, 1992, 1994

SWITZERLAND: 1950–2000
Nos. of deaths attributed to smoking / total deaths (thousands)

	Males			Females		
Age:	0–34	35–69	70+	0–34	35–69	70+
1955	–/3.0	2.4 / 11 (23%)	0.7 / 12 (6%)	–/1.9	0.0 / 8.1 (0%)	0.0 / 15 (0%)
1965	–/2.7	3.2 / 12 (27%)	1.5 / 14 (10%)	–/1.6	0.0 / 7.7 (0%)	0.0 / 17 (0%)
1975	–/2.1	3.8 / 11 (33%)	2.7 / 16 (17%)	–/1.1	0.1 / 6.3 (2%)	0.0 / 19 (0%)
1985	–/1.7	3.3 / 10 (33%)	3.7 / 19 (19%)	–/0.8	0.2 / 5.3 (5%)	0.3 / 23 (1%)
1995 (projected)	–/2.1	3.0 / 9.9 (30%)	3.8 / 22 (17%)	–/0.8	0.4 / 5.1 (8%)	1.3 / 26 (5%)
50–year total*, mid–1950 to mid–2000: 304/2872						
1950–2000, by age & sex	–/116	157 / 539 (29%)	124 / 830 (15%)	–/62	7.0 / 325 (2%)	16 / 1000 (2%)

*Estimated as 10 times the sum of the five annual numbers (for 1955, 1965, 1975, 1985 & 1995)

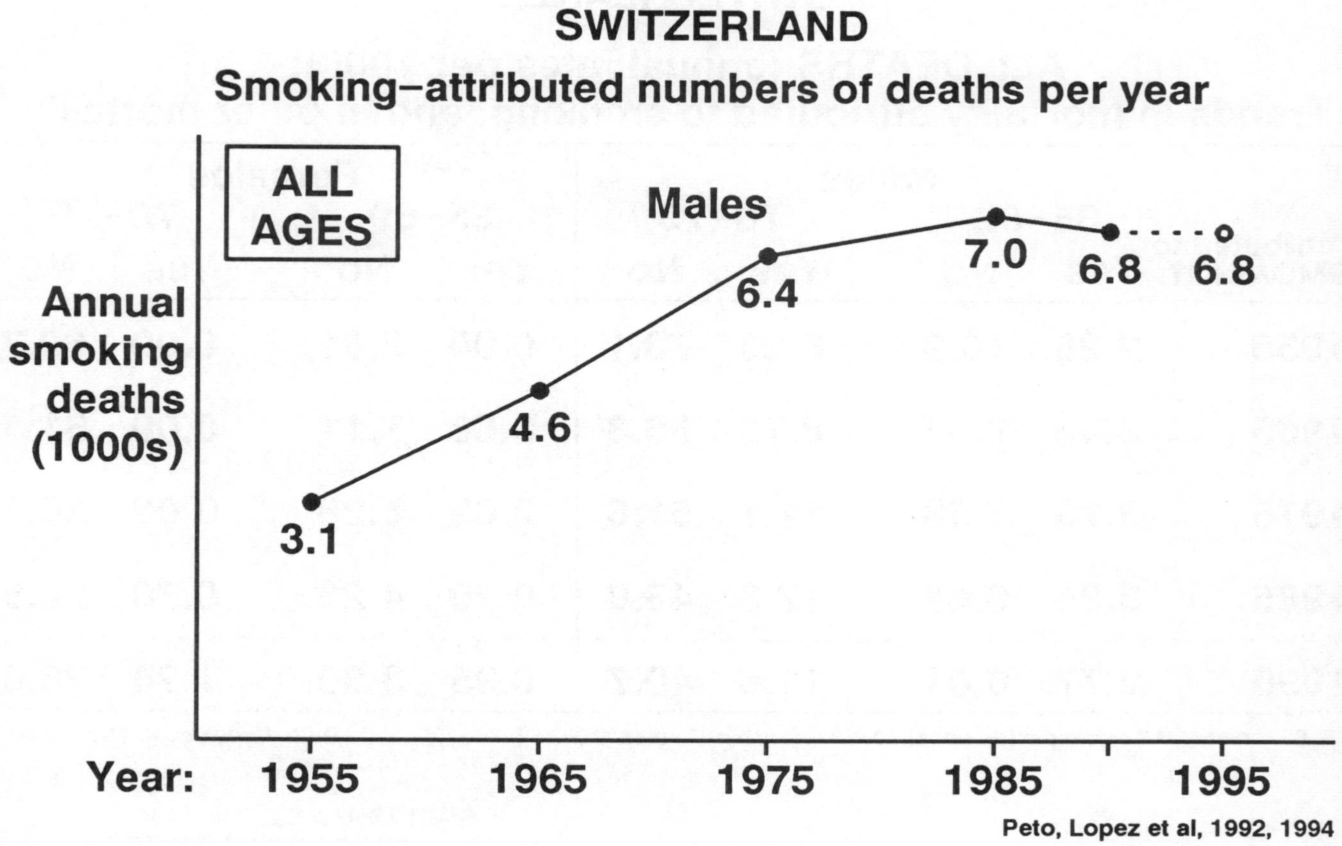
SWITZERLAND
Smoking–attributed numbers of deaths per year
ALL AGES
Males
Annual smoking deaths (1000s)
3.1
4.6
6.4
7.0
6.8
6.8
Year:
1955
1965
1975
1985
1995
Peto, Lopez et al, 1992, 1994

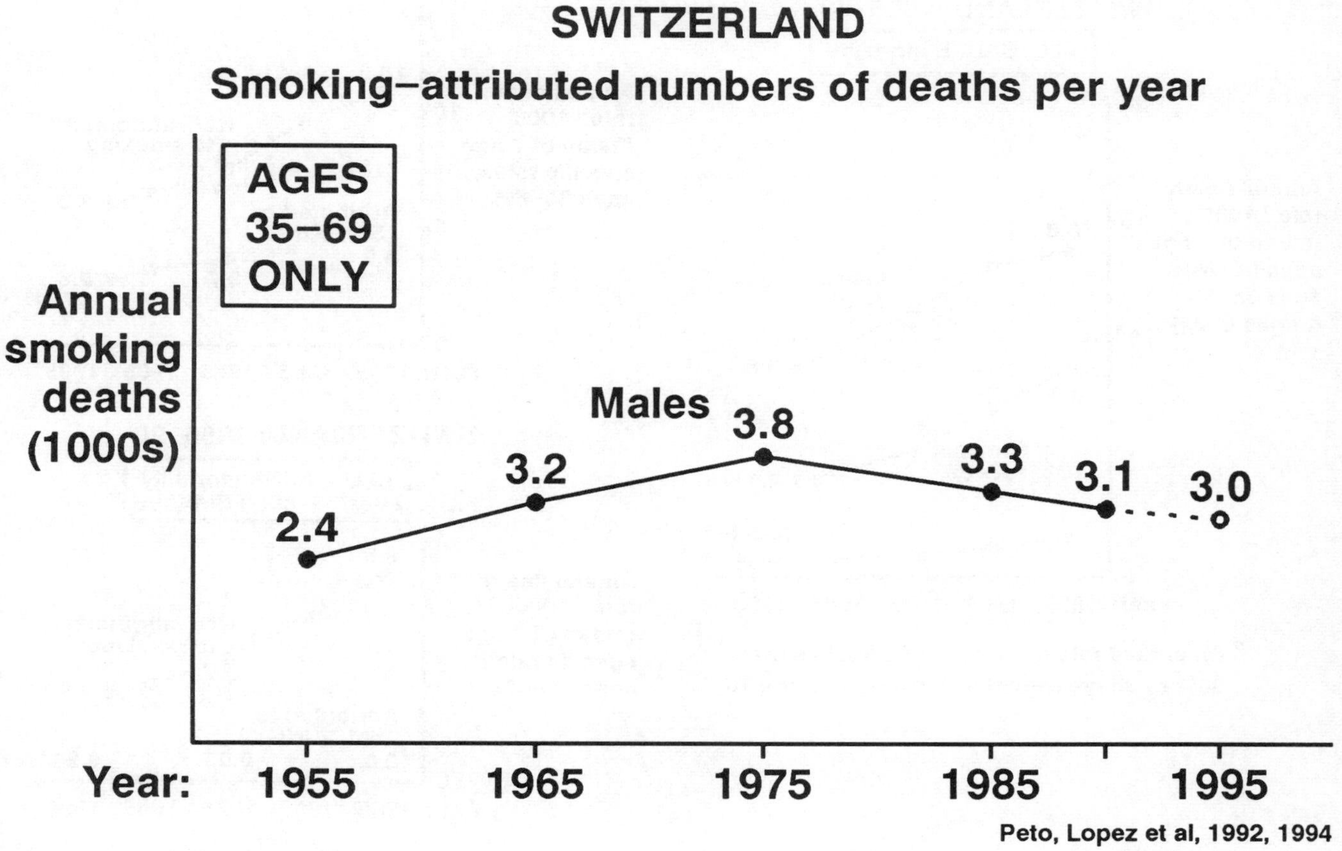
SWITZERLAND
Smoking–attributed numbers of deaths per year
AGES 35–69 ONLY
Males
Annual smoking deaths (1000s)
2.4
3.2
3.8
3.3
3.1
3.0
Year:
1955
1965
1975
1985
1995
Peto, Lopez et al, 1992, 1994

SWITZERLAND

ALL DEATHS (annual rates per 1000): Trends in mortality attributed to smoking, and in other mortality

	Males				Females			
	35–69		70–79		35–69		70–79	
Attributed to SMOKING?	Yes	No	Yes	No	Yes	No	Yes	No
1955	2.95	10.9	5.23	73.1	0.00	8.81	0.00	60.7
1965	3.43	9.67	8.73	66.3	0.00	7.11	0.00	51.3
1975	3.73	7.53	12.1	51.8	0.09	5.28	0.00	38.1
1985	3.24	6.43	12.3	43.0	0.20	4.23	0.70	28.5
1990	2.77	6.01	11.6	40.7	0.25	3.80	1.24	26.0

35–69 = mean of 7 age–specific rates; 70–79 = mean of 2 rates (70–74 & 75–79) Peto, Lopez et al, 1992, 1994

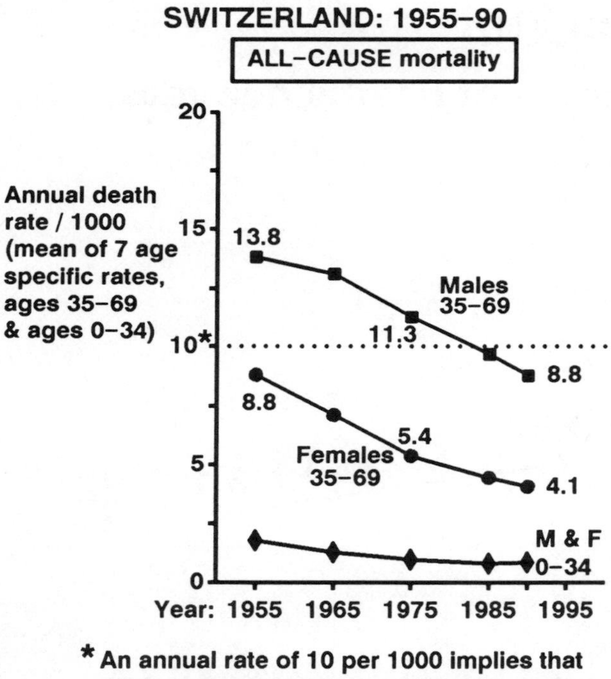

* An annual rate of 10 per 1000 implies that 30% of 35–year–olds will die before age 70

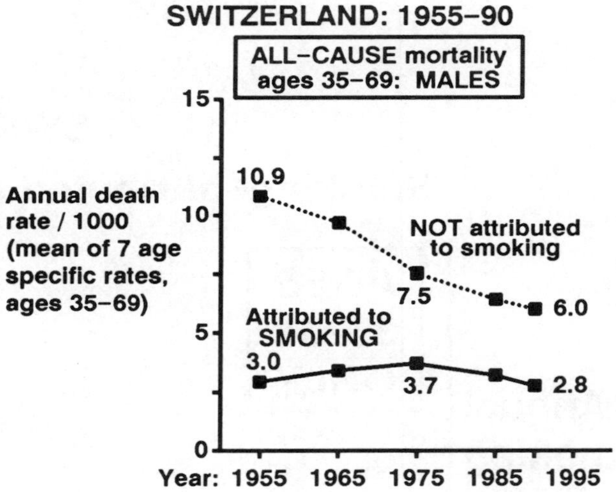

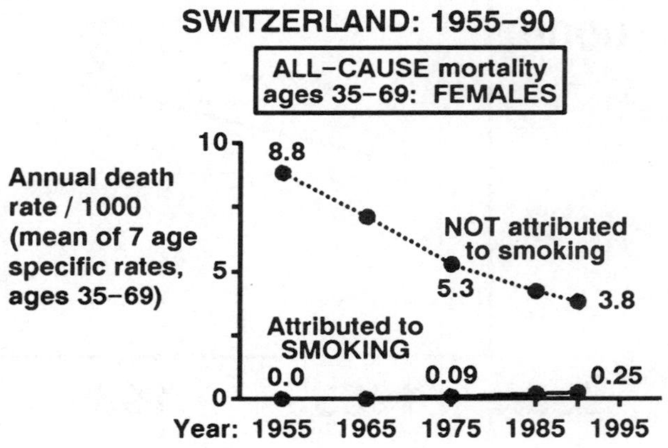

SWITZERLAND

ALL CANCER DEATHS (annual rates per 1000): Trends in mortality attributed to smoking, and in other mortality

	Males				Females			
	35–69		70–79		35–69		70–79	
Attributed to SMOKING?	Yes	No	Yes	No	Yes	No	Yes	No
1955	1.20	2.40	2.24	13.4	0.00	2.50	0.00	9.80
1965	1.45	2.10	3.75	12.2	0.00	2.40	0.00	9.21
1975	1.76	1.85	5.55	11.2	0.03	2.12	0.00	8.60
1985	1.67	1.84	6.23	11.6	0.09	2.01	0.24	7.93
1990	1.46	1.75	5.72	10.9	0.11	1.85	0.46	7.64

35–69 = mean of 7 age-specific rates; 70–79 = mean of 2 rates (70–74 & 75–79) Peto, Lopez et al, 1992, 1994

SWITZERLAND: 1955–90

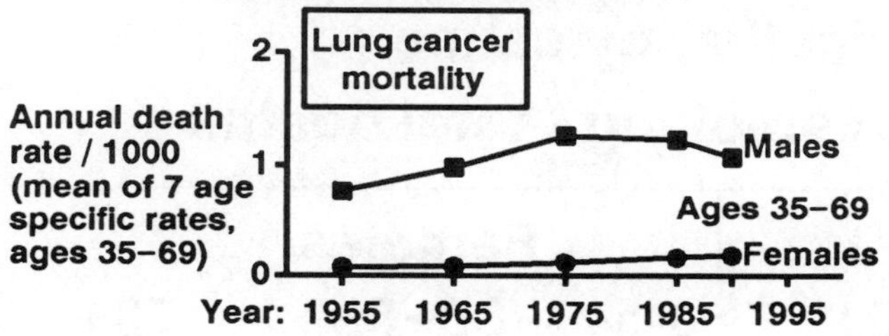

SWITZERLAND: 1955–90

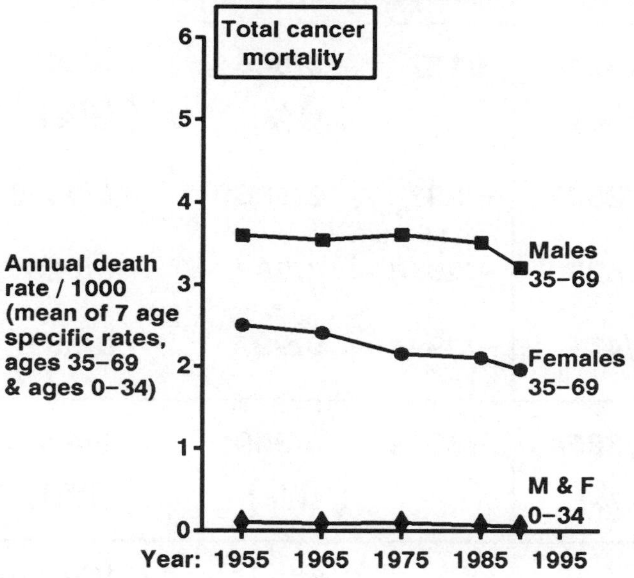

SWITZERLAND: 1955–90

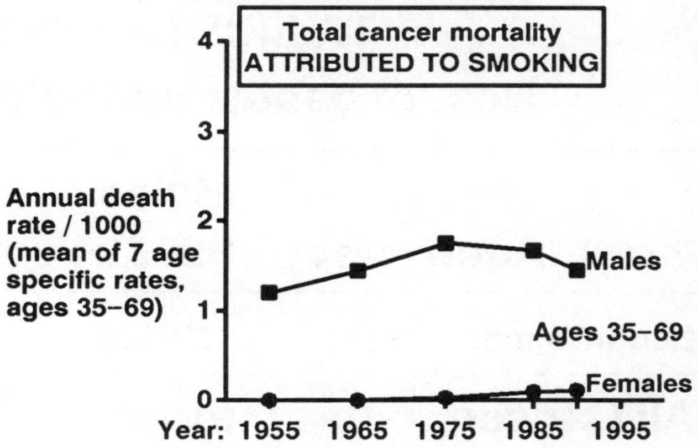

SWITZERLAND: 1955–90

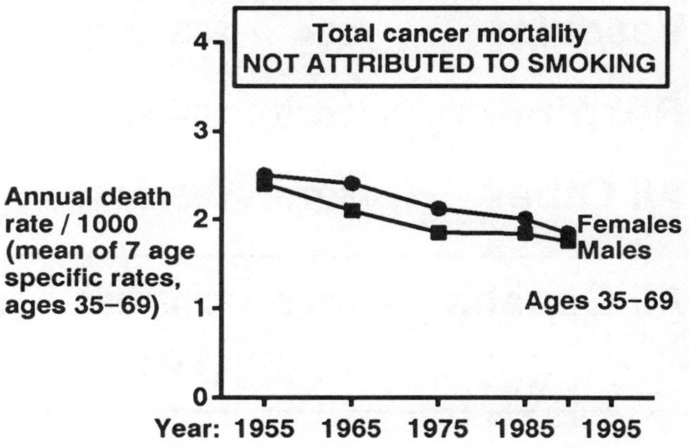

¶TAJIKISTAN: 1990
Relative importance of deaths in MIDDLE age (35–69)

Age range (years)	Deaths attributed to SMOKING / total deaths (thousands) Males	Females	Mean years lost PER DEATH FROM SMOKING
0–34	–/8.6	–/6.9	–
35–69	0.7/5.2	0.0/3.7	22 years
70+	0.2/3.9	0.0/4.8	7 years
All ages	1.0/18	0.0/15	18 years

Peto, Lopez et al, 1992, 1994

TAJIKISTAN: 1990 deaths, by cause
Nos. of deaths attributed to smoking / total deaths

	Males			Females		
Age:	0–34	35–69	70+	0–34	35–69	70+
Lung Cancer	–/11	122/153	28/44	–/ 7	0/40	0/29
All Cancer	–/194	206/987 (21%)	45/324 (14%)	–/137	0/645 (0%)	0/363 (0%)
Vascular	–/134	255/2179	57/2532	–/137	0/1661	0/3330
Respiratory	–/2975	158/424	137/527	–/2614	0/388	0/528
All Other	–/5273	105/1644	8/471	–/3991	0/997	0/565
All Causes	–/8576	724/5234 (14%)	247/3854 (6%)	–/6879	0/3691 (0%)	0/4786 (0%)

Peto, Lopez et al, 1992, 1994

TAJIKISTAN: 1990

RISKS OF DYING AT AGES 0–34 and 35–69

(Probability that someone entering an age range would die during it, if the death rates in 1990 were to persist unchanged)

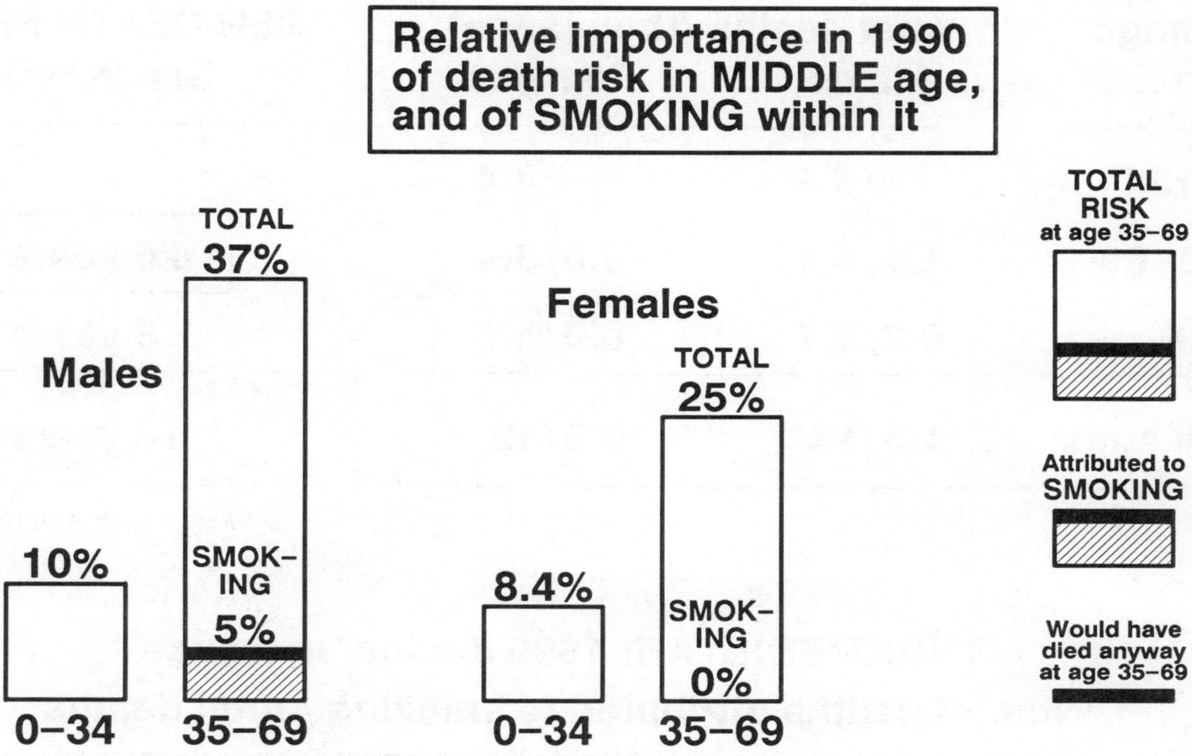

Peto, Lopez et al, 1992, 1994

TAJIKISTAN: 1990 deaths, all ages

Nos. of deaths attributed to smoking / total deaths (thousands)

	Males	Females	Males + Females
All Cancer	0.3/1.5 (17%)	0.0/1.1 (0%)	0.3/2.7 (9%)
All Causes	1.0/18 (5%)	0.0/15 (0%)	1.0/33 (3%)

Peto, Lopez et al, 1992, 1994

¶TURKMENISTAN: 1990
Relative importance of deaths in MIDDLE age (35–69)

Age range (years)	Deaths attributed to SMOKING / total deaths (thousands) Males	Females	Mean years lost PER DEATH FROM SMOKING
0–34	–/6.1	–/4.4	–
35–69	1.1/5.1	0.0/3.4	20 years
70+	0.2/2.7	0.0/4.0	8 years
All ages	1.3/14	0.0/12	18 years

Peto, Lopez et al, 1992, 1994

TURKMENISTAN: 1990 deaths, by cause
Nos. of deaths attributed to smoking / total deaths

	Males			Females		
Age:	0–34	35–69	70+	0–34	35–69	70+
Lung Cancer	–/ 5	146/168	20/30	–/ 2	0/27	0/13
All Cancer	–/119	330/868 (38%)	50/272 (18%)	–/93	0/632 (0%)	0/316 (0%)
Vascular	–/261	490/2520	48/1845	–/211	0/1807	0/2966
Respiratory	–/1961	153/282	63/226	–/1535	0/215	0/319
All Other	–/3798	127/1424	5/314	–/2609	0/714	0/448
All Causes	–/6139	1100/5094 (22%)	166/2657 (6%)	–/4448	0/3368 (0%)	0/4049 (0%)

Peto, Lopez et al, 1992, 1994

TURKMENISTAN: 1990

RISKS OF DYING AT AGES 0–34 and 35–69

(Probability that someone entering an age range would die during it, if the death rates in 1990 were to persist unchanged)

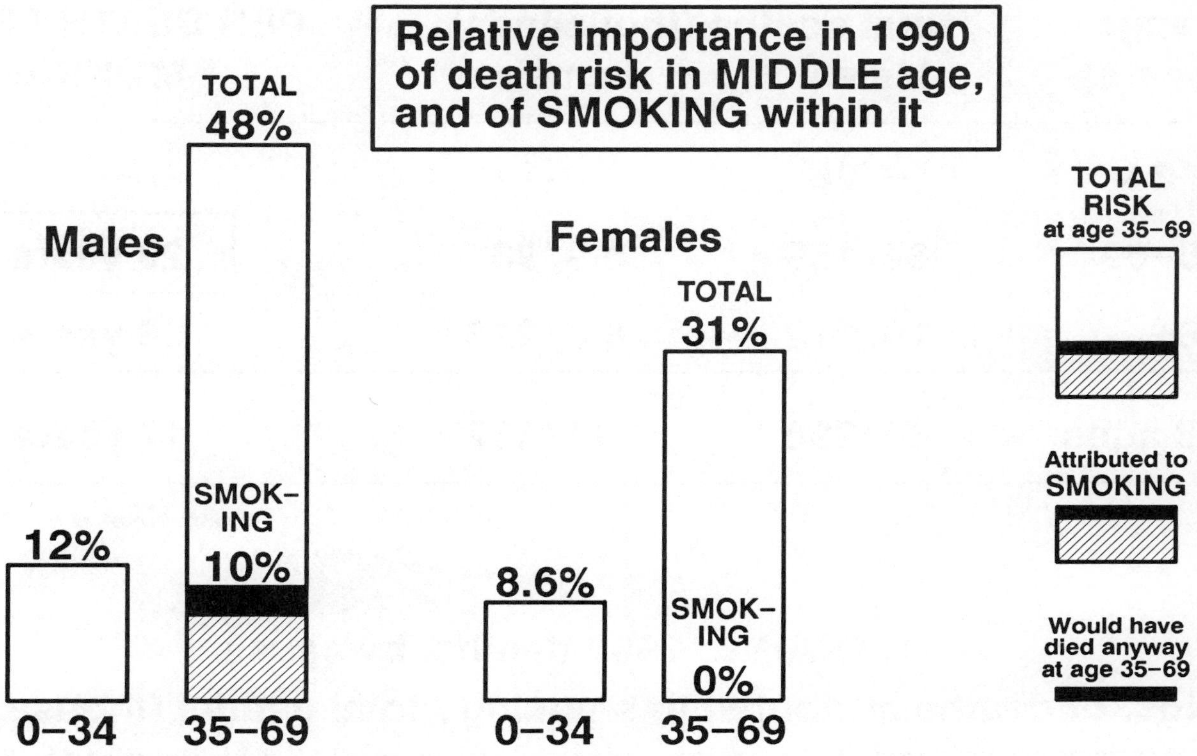

Peto, Lopez et al, 1992, 1994

TURKMENISTAN: 1990 deaths, all ages

Nos. of deaths attributed to smoking / total deaths (thousands)

	Males	Females	Males + Females
All Cancer	0.4/1.3 (30%)	0.0/1.0 (0%)	0.4/2.3 (17%)
All Causes	1.3/14 (9%)	0.0/12 (0%)	1.3/26 (5%)

Peto, Lopez et al, 1992, 1994

¶UKRAINE: 1990

Relative importance of deaths in MIDDLE age (35–69)

Age range (years)	Deaths attributed to SMOKING / total deaths (thousands) Males	Females	Mean years lost PER DEATH FROM SMOKING
0–34	–/26	–/11	–
35–69	64/159	5.9/93	20 years
70+	19/112	8.5/228	8 years
All ages	84/298	14/332	17 years

Peto, Lopez et al, 1992, 1994

UKRAINE: 1990 deaths, by cause

Nos. of deaths attributed to smoking / total deaths (thousands)

	Males			Females		
Age:	0–34	35–69	70+	0–34	35–69	70+
Lung Cancer	–/0.1	14/15	3.4/3.8	–/0.0	1.0/2.1	0.8/1.7
All Cancer	–/1.7	23/42 (56%)	4.9/14 (36%)	–/1.5	1.3/27 (5%)	1.0/16 (6%)
Vascular	–/1.7	26/64	6.5/68	–/0.6	2.9/45	3.3/154
Respiratory	–/1.1	9.1/11	6.7/10	–/0.8	1.3/4.0	3.3/9.9
All Other	–/22	5.9/42	1.4/20	–/8.3	0.5/17	0.8/48
All Causes	–/26	64/159 (40%)	19/112 (17%)	–/11	5.9/93 (6%)	8.5/228 (4%)

Peto, Lopez et al, 1992, 1994

UKRAINE: 1990

RISKS OF DYING AT AGES 0–34 and 35–69

(Probability that someone entering an age range would die during it, if the death rates in 1990 were to persist unchanged)

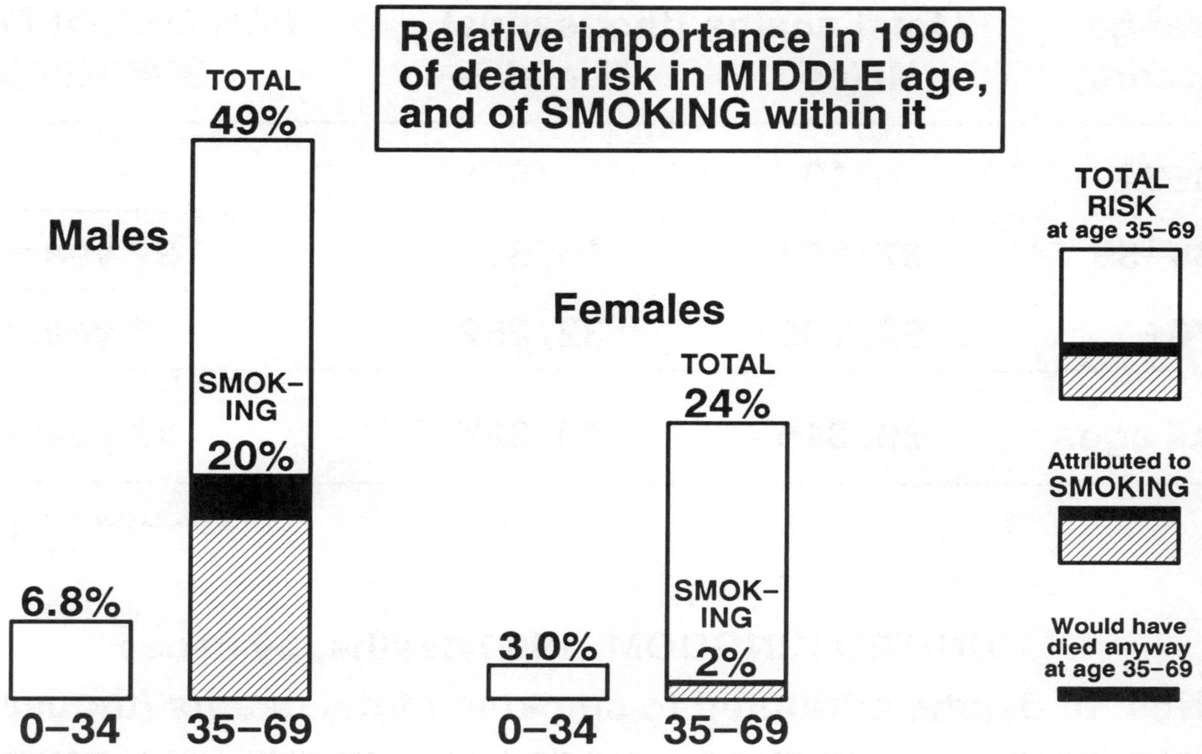

Peto, Lopez et al, 1992, 1994

UKRAINE: 1990 deaths, all ages

Nos. of deaths attributed to smoking / total deaths (thousands)

	Males	Females	Males + Females
All Cancer	28/57 (50%)	2.3/45 (5%)	31/101 (30%)
All Causes	84/298 (28%)	14/332 (4%)	98/630 (16%)

Peto, Lopez et al, 1992, 1994

UNITED KINGDOM: 1990
Relative importance of deaths in MIDDLE age (35–69)

Age range (years)	Deaths attributed to SMOKING / total deaths (thousands) Males	Females	Mean years lost PER DEATH FROM SMOKING
0–34	–/13	–/6.9	–
35–69	37/107	16/68	20 years
70+	52/195	32/252	8 years
All ages	89/315	49/327	13 years

Peto, Lopez et al, 1992, 1994

UNITED KINGDOM: 1990 deaths, by cause
Nos. of deaths attributed to smoking / total deaths (thousands)

	Males			Females		
Age:	0–34	35–69	70+	0–34	35–69	70+
Lung Cancer	–/0.0	11/12	14/15	–/0.0	4.7/5.7	5.5/6.6
All Cancer	–/1.0	16/35 (47%)	21/48 (43%)	–/1.0	6.2/31 (20%)	8.2/45 (18%)
Vascular	–/0.6	14/49	15/93	–/0.4	5.7/22	12/131
Respiratory	–/0.5	4.4/7.1	14/28	–/0.4	2.8/4.8	7.8/31
All Other	–/11	2.4/16	3.4/26	–/5.2	1.7/10	3.8/46
All Causes	–/13	37/107 (35%)	52/195 (27%)	–/6.9	16/68 (24%)	32/252 (13%)

Peto, Lopez et al, 1992, 1994

UNITED KINGDOM: 1990

RISKS OF DYING AT AGES 0–34 and 35–69

(Probability that someone entering an age range would die during it, if the death rates in 1990 were to persist unchanged)

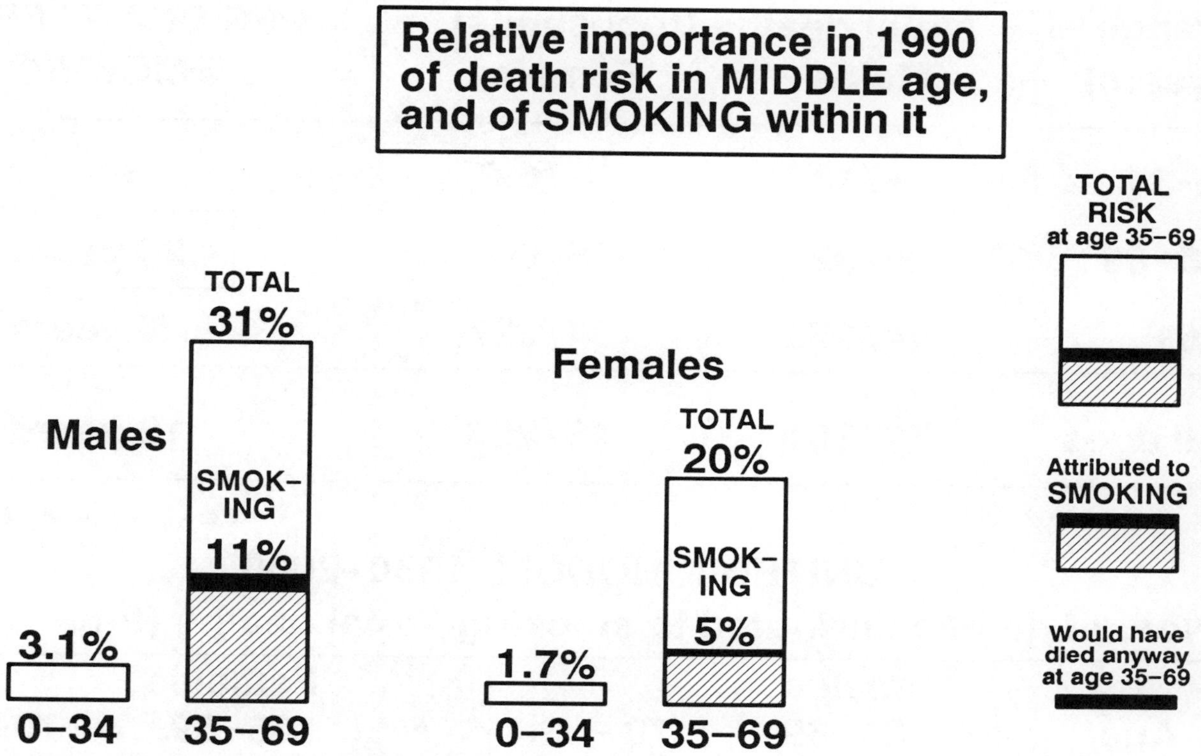

Peto, Lopez et al, 1992, 1994

UNITED KINGDOM: 1990 deaths, all ages

Nos. of deaths attributed to smoking / total deaths (thousands)

	Males	Females	Males + Females
All Cancer	37/84 (44%)	14/77 (19%)	51/161 (32%)
All Causes	89/315 (28%)	49/327 (15%)	138/642 (21%)

Peto, Lopez et al, 1992, 1994

UNITED KINGDOM: 1995 projections
Relative importance of deaths in MIDDLE age (35–69)

Age range (years)	Deaths attributed to SMOKING / total deaths (thousands) Males	Females	Mean years lost PER DEATH FROM SMOKING
0–34	–/13	–/6.2	–
35–69	28/92	15/60	20 years
70+	44/175	34/227	8 years
All ages	73/281	49/293	12 years

Peto, Lopez et al, 1992, 1994

UNITED KINGDOM: 1950–2000
Nos. of deaths attributed to smoking / total deaths (thousands)

	Males			Females		
Age:	0–34	35–69	70+	0–34	35–69	70+
1955	–/23	56/130 (43%)	20/153 (13%)	–/17	5.8/91 (6%)	2.3/183 (1%)
1965	–/23	69/146 (48%)	35/155 (23%)	–/15	11/89 (12%)	6.1/201 (3%)
1975	–/17	62/142 (44%)	52/176 (30%)	–/10	15/85 (18%)	15/232 (6%)
1985	–/13	46/117 (39%)	59/202 (29%)	–/7.5	17/73 (23%)	29/259 (11%)
1995 (projected)	–/13	28/92 (31%)	44/175 (25%)	–/6.2	15/60 (25%)	34/227 (15%)
50–year total* (M=millions), mid–1950 to mid–2000: 6.2/31M						
1950–2000, by age & sex	–/0.9M	2.6/6.3M (41%)	2.1/8.6M (24%)	–/0.6M	0.6/4.0M (15%)	0.9/11M (8%)

*Estimated as 10 times the sum of the five annual numbers (for 1955, 1965, 1975, 1985 & 1995)

UNITED KINGDOM

Smoking–attributed numbers of deaths per year

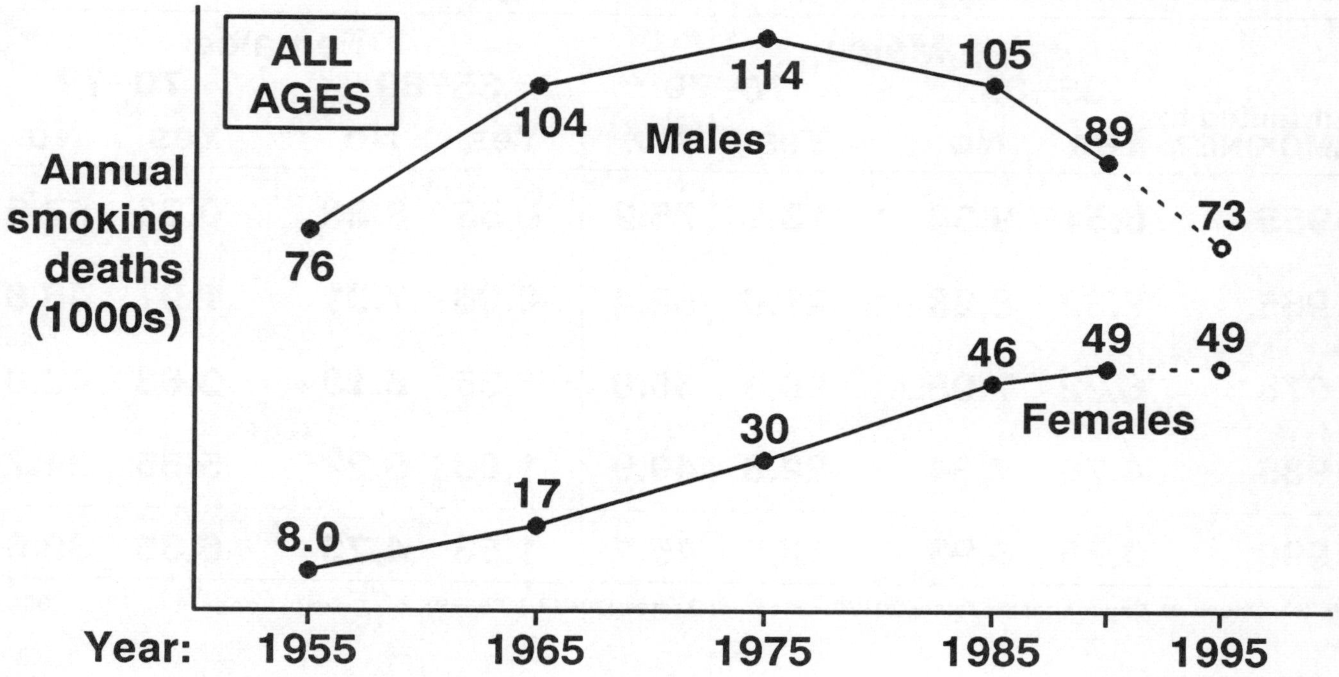

Peto, Lopez et al, 1992, 1994

UNITED KINGDOM

Smoking–attributed numbers of deaths per year

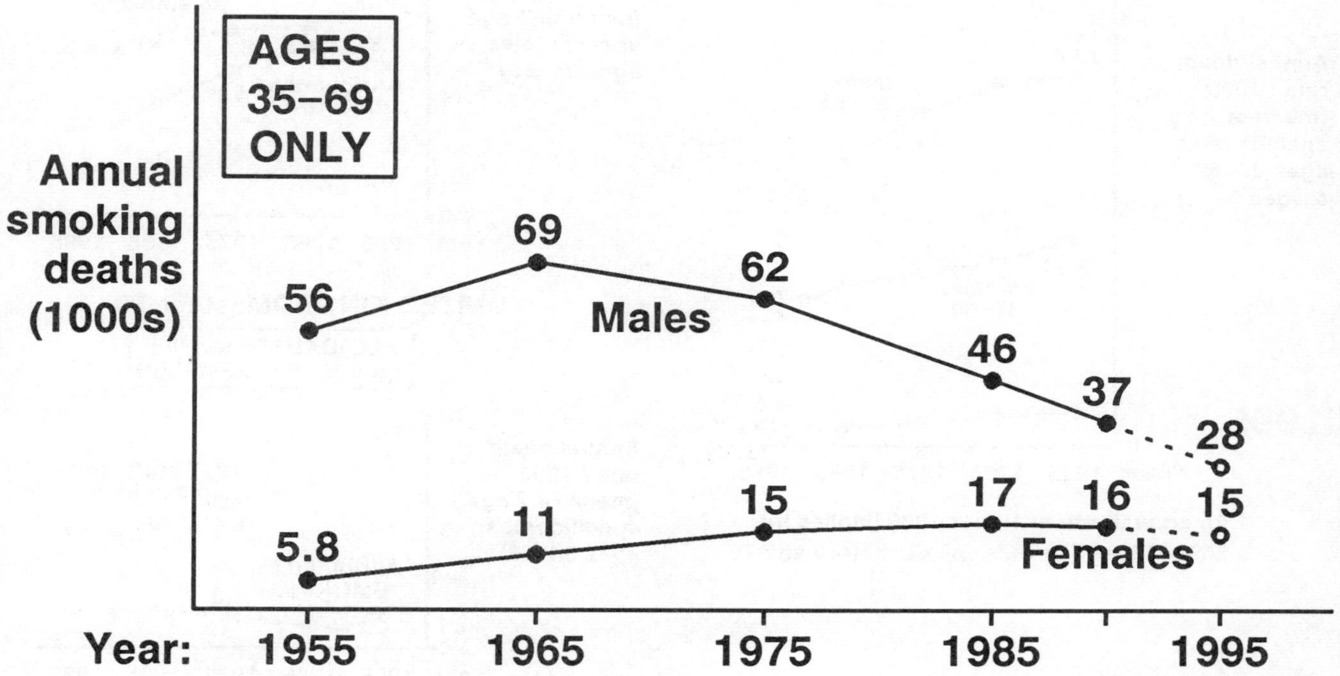

Peto, Lopez et al, 1992, 1994

UNITED KINGDOM

ALL DEATHS (annual rates per 1000): Trends in mortality attributed to smoking, and in other mortality

	Males				Females			
	35–69		70–79		35–69		70–79	
Attributed to SMOKING?	Yes	No	Yes	No	Yes	No	Yes	No
1955	6.51	9.34	13.1	75.2	0.55	8.33	0.93	57.5
1965	7.32	8.23	21.6	62.4	0.96	7.01	1.91	48.8
1975	6.22	7.98	26.4	56.0	1.35	6.13	3.63	42.0
1985	4.78	7.34	22.8	49.9	1.60	5.22	5.85	34.7
1990	3.79	6.93	18.9	45.7	1.53	4.73	6.35	30.6

35–69 = mean of 7 age-specific rates; 70–79 = mean of 2 rates (70–74 & 75–79) Peto, Lopez et al, 1992, 1994

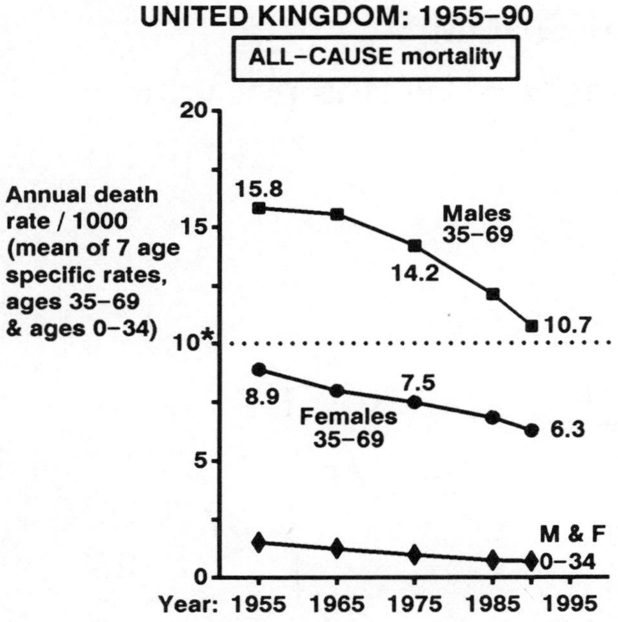

* An annual rate of 10 per 1000 implies that 30% of 35-year-olds will die before age 70

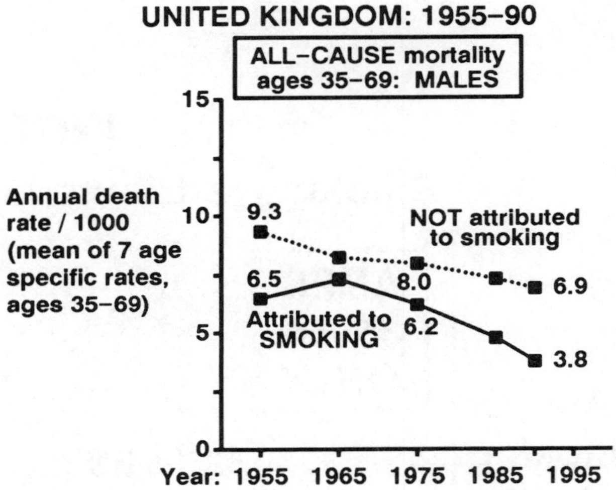

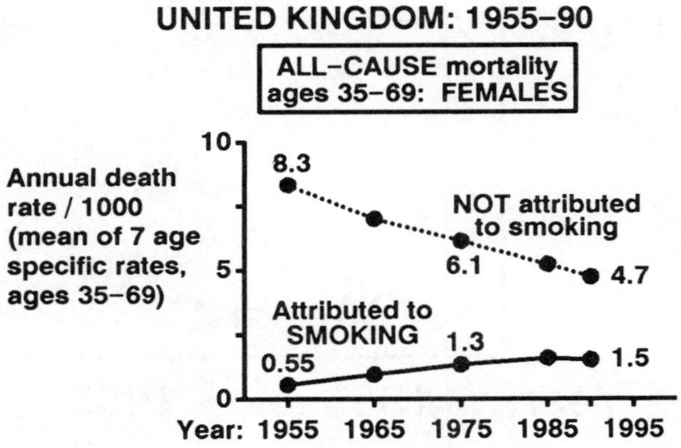

UNITED KINGDOM

ALL CANCER DEATHS (annual rates per 1000): Trends in mortality attributed to smoking, and in other mortality

	Males				Females			
	35–69		70–79		35–69		70–79	
Attributed to SMOKING?	Yes	No	Yes	No	Yes	No	Yes	No
1955	2.00	1.85	3.79	10.6	0.12	2.45	0.16	8.28
1965	2.45	1.66	6.75	9.25	0.25	2.32	0.39	7.76
1975	2.24	1.69	9.41	8.92	0.41	2.32	0.92	7.57
1985	1.94	1.79	9.15	9.54	0.56	2.32	1.77	7.68
1990	1.69	1.89	8.26	10.1	0.57	2.24	2.11	7.58

35–69 = mean of 7 age–specific rates; 70–79 = mean of 2 rates (70–74 & 75–79) Peto, Lopez et al, 1992, 1994

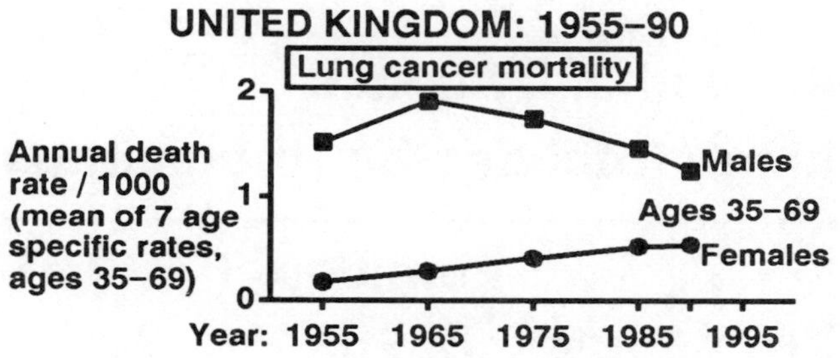

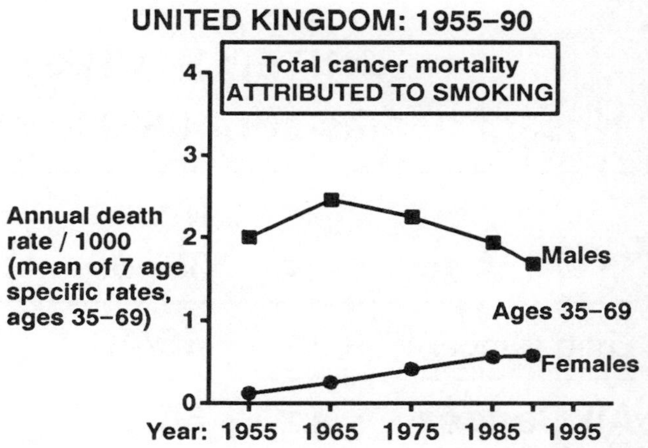

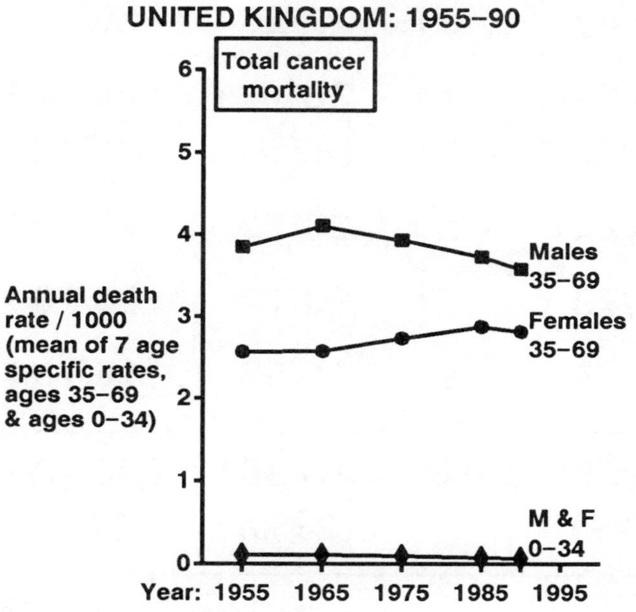

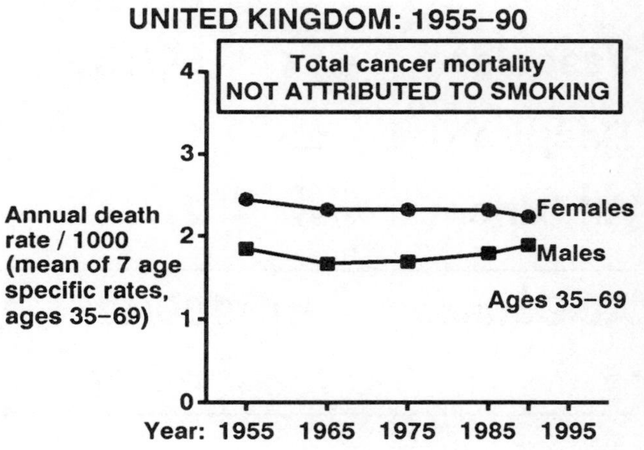

UNITED STATES: 1990
Relative importance of deaths in MIDDLE age (35–69)

Age range (years)	Deaths attributed to SMOKING / total deaths (thousands) Males	Females	Mean years lost PER DEATH FROM SMOKING
0–34	–/103	–/48	–
35–69	150/415	73/257	22 years
70+	136/595	102/730	8 years
All ages	286/1113	175/1035	15 years

Peto, Lopez et al, 1992, 1994

UNITED STATES: 1990 deaths, by cause
Nos. of deaths attributed to smoking / total deaths (thousands)

	Males			Females		
Age:	0–34	35–69	70+	0–34	35–69	70+
Lung Cancer	–/0.2	45/48	39/43	–/0.1	22/26	20/24
All Cancer	–/4.7	64/123 (52%)	56/140 (40%)	–/4.2	28/104 (27%)	26/129 (20%)
Vascular	–/4.6	50/153	39/287	–/3.0	23/78	40/395
Respiratory	–/2.2	15/25	31/73	–/1.7	10/17	24/73
All Other	–/91	21/114	10/95	–/39	11/58	12/134
All Causes	–/103	150/415 (36%)	136/595 (23%)	–/48	73/257 (28%)	102/730 (14%)

Peto, Lopez et al, 1992, 1994

UNITED STATES: 1990

RISKS OF DYING AT AGES 0–34 and 35–69

(Probability that someone entering an age range would die during it, if the death rates in 1990 were to persist unchanged)

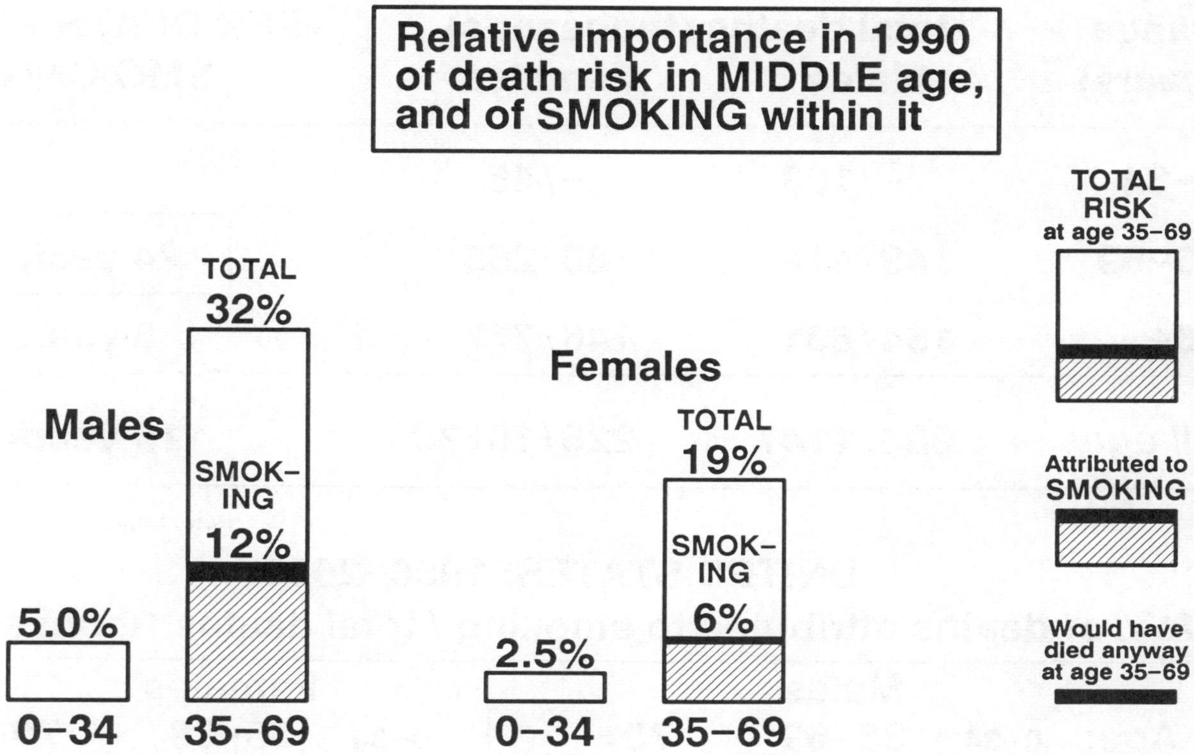

Peto, Lopez et al, 1992, 1994

UNITED STATES: 1990 deaths, all ages

Nos. of deaths attributed to smoking / total deaths (thousands)

	Males	Females	Males + Females
All Cancer	120/268 (45%)	54/237 (23%)	174/505 (34%)
All Causes	286/1113 (26%)	175/1035 (17%)	461/2148 (21%)

Peto, Lopez et al, 1992, 1994

UNITED STATES: 1995 projections
Relative importance of deaths in MIDDLE age (35–69)

Age range (years)	Deaths attributed to SMOKING / total deaths (thousands) Males	Females	Mean years lost PER DEATH FROM SMOKING
0–34	–/103	–/45	–
35–69	149/414	80/255	24 years
70+	154/631	146/777	8 years
All ages	303/1147	226/1077	15 years

Peto, Lopez et al, 1992, 1994

UNITED STATES: 1950–2000
Nos. of deaths attributed to smoking / total deaths (thousands)

	Males			Females		
Age:	0–34	35–69	70+	0–34	35–69	70+
1955	–/119	85/403 (21%)	17/350 (5%)	–/79	1.5/241 (0.6%)	0.0/336 (0%)
1965	–/118	134/460 (29%)	48/458 (10%)	–/74	13/265 (5%)	1.1/454 (0.3%)
1975	–/109	157/457 (34%)	84/485 (17%)	–/56	40/262 (15%)	16/524 (3%)
1985	–/98	154/425 (36%)	123/575 (21%)	–/48	66/261 (25%)	65/680 (10%)
1995 (projected)	–/103	149/414 (36%)	154/631 (24%)	–/45	80/255 (31%)	146/777 (19%)
50–year total* (M=millions), mid–1950 to mid–2000: 15/96M						
1950–2000, by age & sex	–/5.5M	6.8/22M (31%)	4.3/25M (17%)	–/3.0M	2.0/13M (15%)	2.3/28M (8%)

*Estimated as 10 times the sum of the five annual numbers (for 1955, 1965, 1975, 1985 & 1995)

UNITED STATES

Smoking–attributed numbers of deaths per year

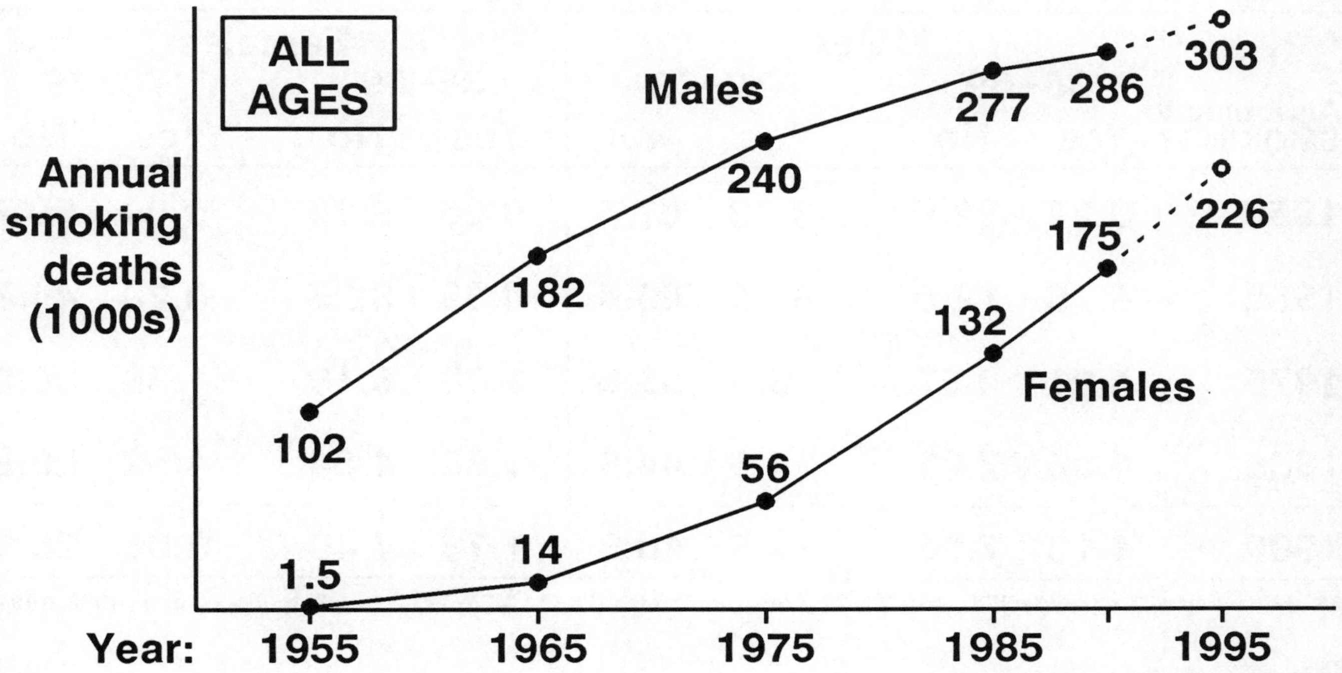

Peto, Lopez et al, 1992, 1994

UNITED STATES

Smoking–attributed numbers of deaths per year

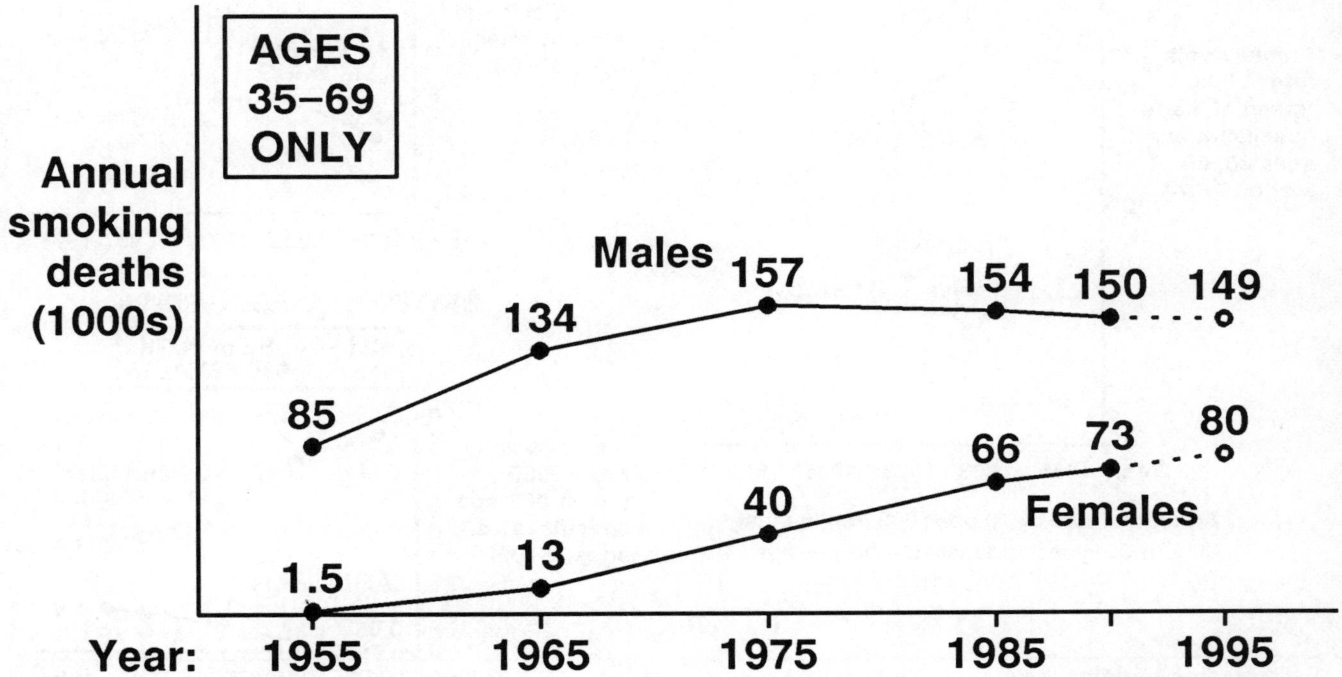

Peto, Lopez et al, 1992, 1994

UNITED STATES

ALL DEATHS (annual rates per 1000): Trends in mortality attributed to smoking, and in other mortality

	Males				Females			
	35–69		70–79		35–69		70–79	
Attributed to SMOKING?	Yes	No	Yes	No	Yes	No	Yes	No
1955	3.27	12.9	3.98	67.5	0.06	9.16	0.00	50.7
1965	4.75	12.0	8.90	63.4	0.39	8.25	0.20	44.7
1975	4.91	9.57	13.5	53.6	1.08	6.10	1.58	36.0
1985	4.36	7.62	14.6	44.9	1.66	4.84	4.52	28.9
1990	4.13	7.06	14.5	40.3	1.78	4.40	6.06	25.5

35–69 = mean of 7 age-specific rates; 70–79 = mean of 2 rates (70–74 & 75–79) Peto, Lopez et al, 1992, 1994

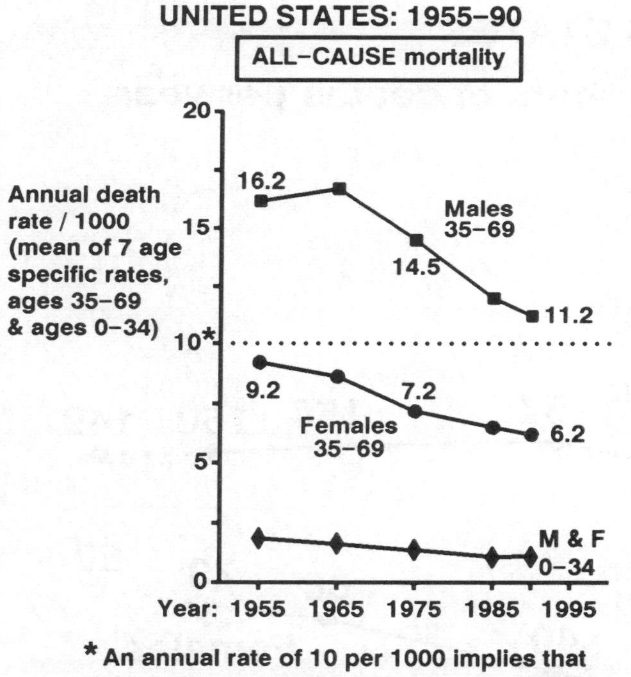

* An annual rate of 10 per 1000 implies that 30% of 35-year-olds will die before age 70

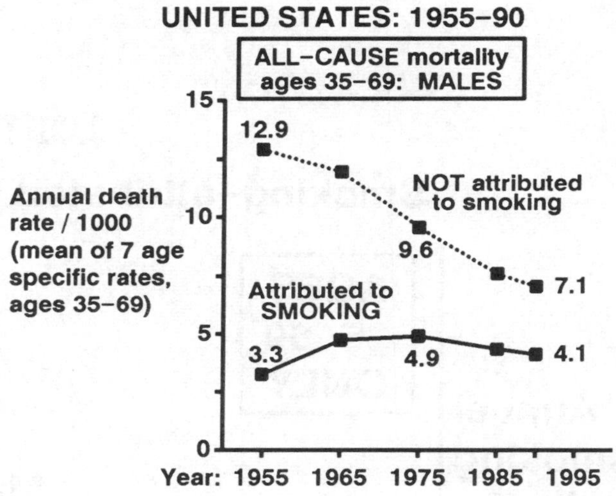

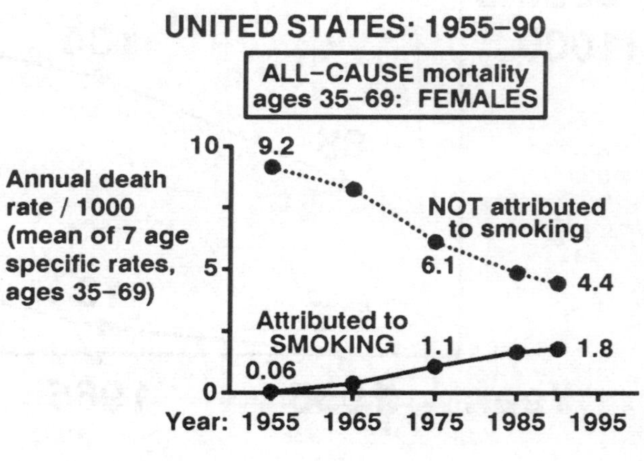

UNITED STATES

ALL CANCER DEATHS (annual rates per 1000): Trends in mortality attributed to smoking, and in other mortality

	Males				Females			
	35–69		70–79		35–69		70–79	
Attributed to SMOKING?	Yes	No	Yes	No	Yes	No	Yes	No
1955	0.94	2.03	1.51	9.71	0.01	2.50	0.00	7.84
1965	1.41	1.89	3.15	9.04	0.10	2.32	0.04	7.12
1975	1.74	1.70	5.22	8.88	0.33	2.04	0.43	6.87
1985	1.81	1.66	6.32	8.60	0.60	1.92	1.43	6.57
1990	1.82	1.67	6.72	8.73	0.69	1.83	2.09	6.47

35–69 = mean of 7 age-specific rates; 70–79 = mean of 2 rates (70–74 & 75–79) Peto, Lopez et al, 1992, 1994

UNITED STATES: 1955-90

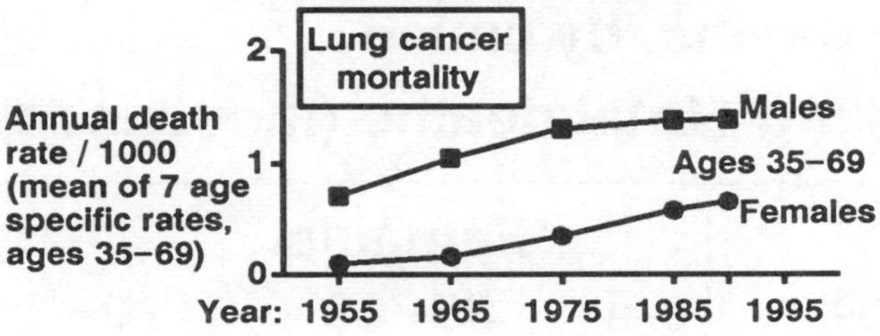

UNITED STATES: 1955-90

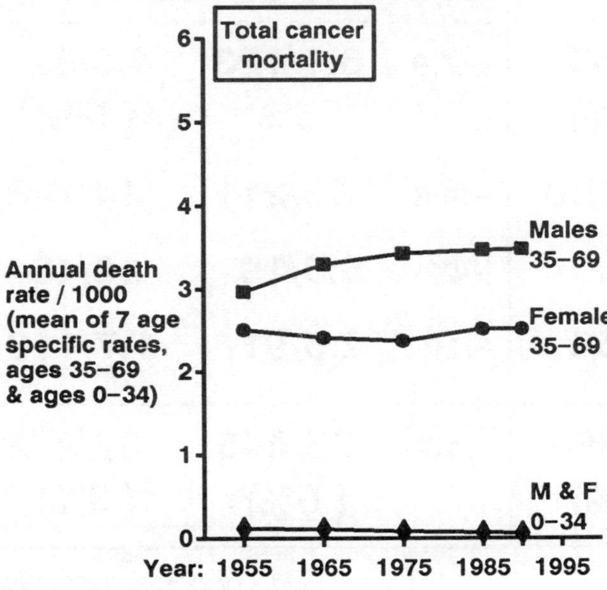

UNITED STATES: 1955-90

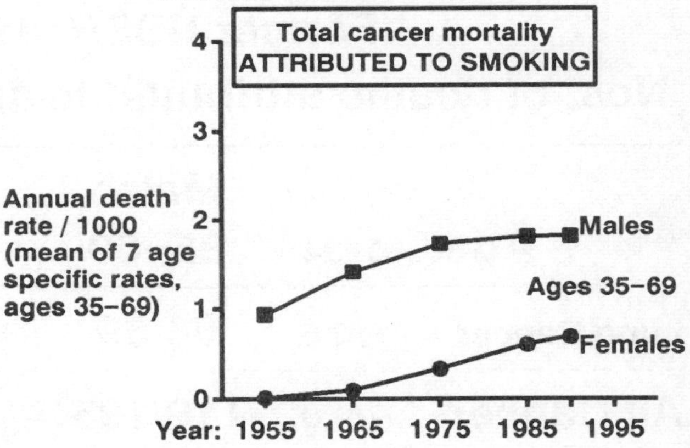

UNITED STATES: 1955-90

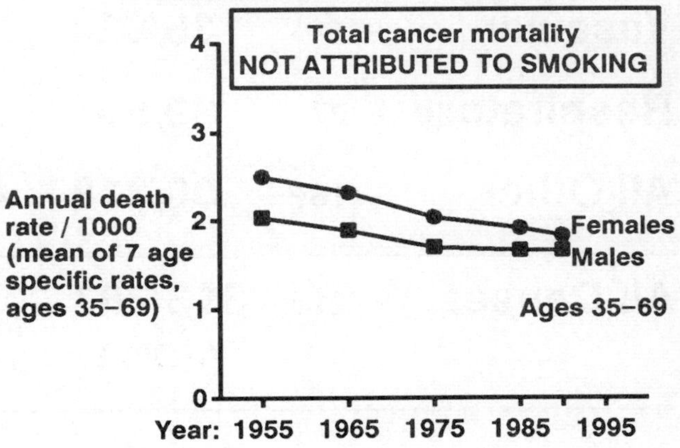

¶Former USSR: 1990
Relative importance of deaths in MIDDLE age (35–69)

Age range (years)	Deaths attributed to SMOKING / total deaths (thousands) Males	Females	Mean years lost PER DEATH FROM SMOKING
0–34	–/215	–/106	–
35–69	313/787	28/445	20 years
70+	84/460	32/972	8 years
All ages	397/1462	60/1523	17 years

Peto, Lopez et al, 1992, 1994

Former USSR: 1990 deaths, by cause
Nos. of deaths attributed to smoking / total deaths (thousands)

	Males			Females		
Age:	0–34	35–69	70+	0–34	35–69	70+
Lung Cancer	–/0.5	66/69	15/17	–/0.2	4.5/9.4	3.2/7.1
All Cancer	–/9.0	110/195 (56%)	23/63 (36%)	–/7.9	6.1/123 (5%)	4.5/82 (5%)
Vascular	–/11	135/324	31/300	–/4.6	13/211	14/728
Respiratory	–/27	39/50	26/39	–/22	5.8/19	13/43
All Other	–/168	30/218	4.0/58	–/72	2.5/91	1.7/119
All Causes	–/215	313/787 (40%)	84/460 (18%)	–/106	28/445 (6%)	32/972 (3%)

Peto, Lopez et al, 1992, 1994

Former USSR: 1990

RISKS OF DYING AT AGES 0–34 and 35–69

(Probability that someone entering an age range would die during it, if the death rates in 1990 were to persist unchanged)

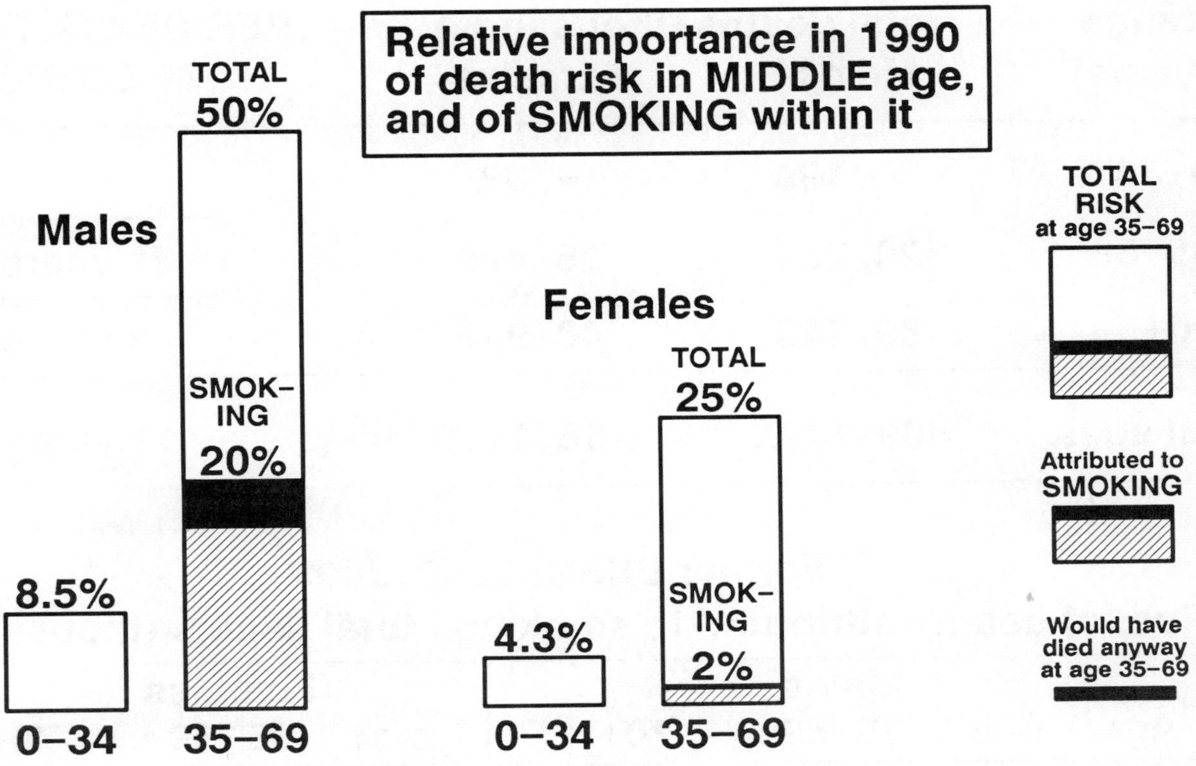

Peto, Lopez et al, 1992, 1994

Former USSR: 1990 deaths, all ages

Nos. of deaths attributed to smoking / total deaths (thousands)

	Males	Females	Males + Females
All Cancer	133/267 (50%)	11/213 (5%)	143/480 (30%)
All Causes	397/1462 (27%)	60/1523 (4%)	457/2985 (15%)

Peto, Lopez et al, 1992, 1994

Former USSR: 1995 projections
Relative importance of deaths in MIDDLE age (35–69)

Age range (years)	Deaths attributed to SMOKING / total deaths (thousands) Males	Females	Mean years lost PER DEATH FROM SMOKING
0–34	–/196	–/89	–
35–69	320/781	28/429	21 years
70+	89/445	40/932	8 years
All ages	409/1422	68/1450	17 years

Peto, Lopez et al, 1992, 1994

Former USSR: 1950–2000
Nos. of deaths attributed to smoking / total deaths (thousands)

Age:	Males 0–34	35–69	70+	Females 0–34	35–69	70+
1955	–/231	72 / 350 (21%)	15 / 207 (7%)	–/165	8.5 / 306 (3%)	0.7 / 399 (0.2%)
1965	–/200	117 / 374 (31%)	29 / 252 (12%)	–/123	14 / 306 (5%)	1.8 / 434 (0.4%)
1975	–/228	185 / 583 (32%)	53 / 364 (15%)	–/125	22 / 395 (6%)	11 / 668 (2%)
1985	–/241	272 / 693 (39%)	87 / 490 (18%)	–/130	25 / 420 (6%)	27 / 973 (3%)
1995 (projected)	–/196	320 / 781 (41%)	89 / 445 (20%)	–/89	28 / 429 (7%)	40 / 932 (4%)
50–year total* (M=millions), mid–1950 to mid–2000: 14/115M						
1950–2000, by age & sex	–/11M	9.7 / 28M (35%)	2.7 / 18M (15%)	–/6.3M	1.0 / 19M (5%)	0.8 / 34M (2%)

*Estimated as 10 times the sum of the five annual numbers (for 1955, 1965, 1975, 1985 & 1995)

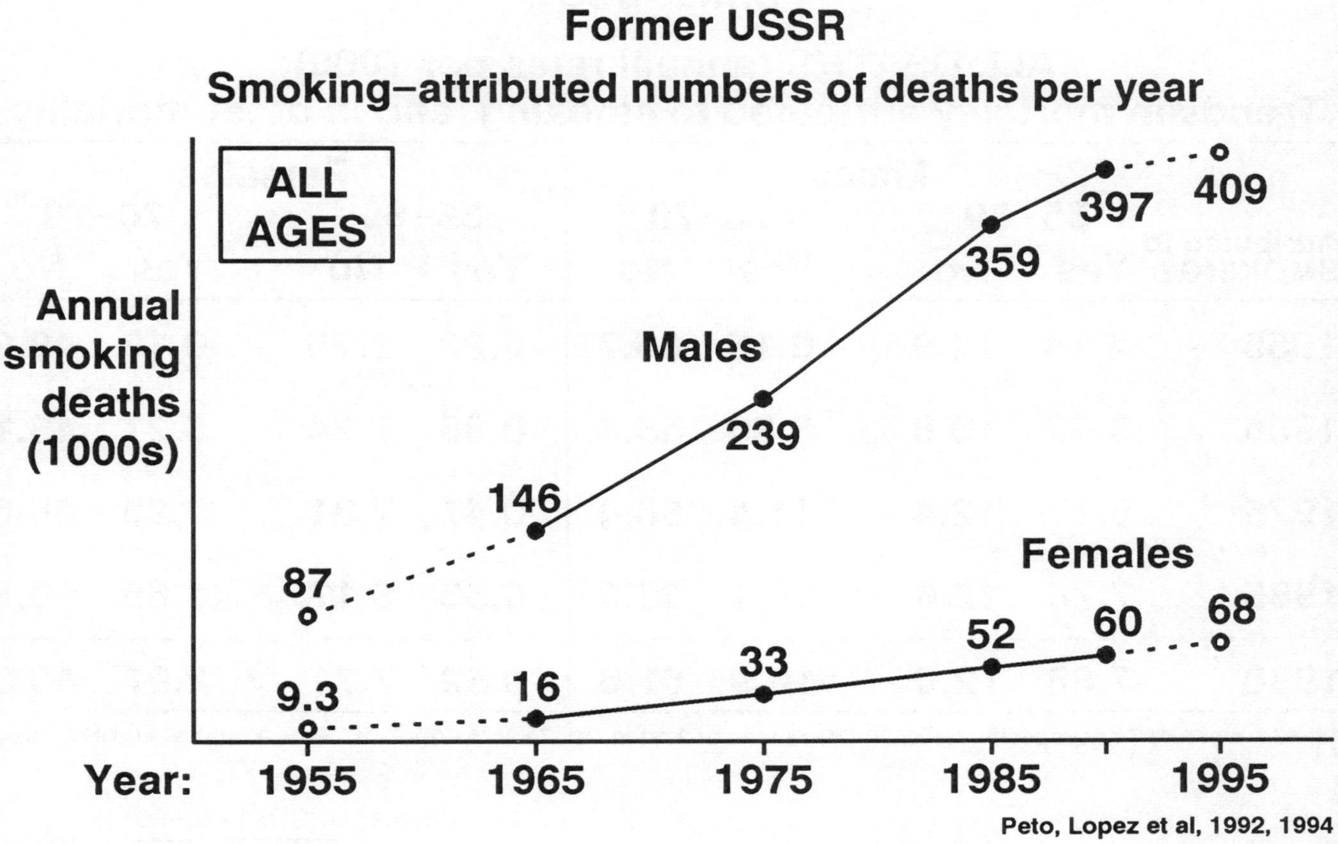
Former USSR
Smoking–attributed numbers of deaths per year
ALL AGES
Annual smoking deaths (1000s)
Males
87
146
239
359
397
409
Females
9.3
16
33
52
60
68
Year:
1955
1965
1975
1985
1995
Peto, Lopez et al, 1992, 1994

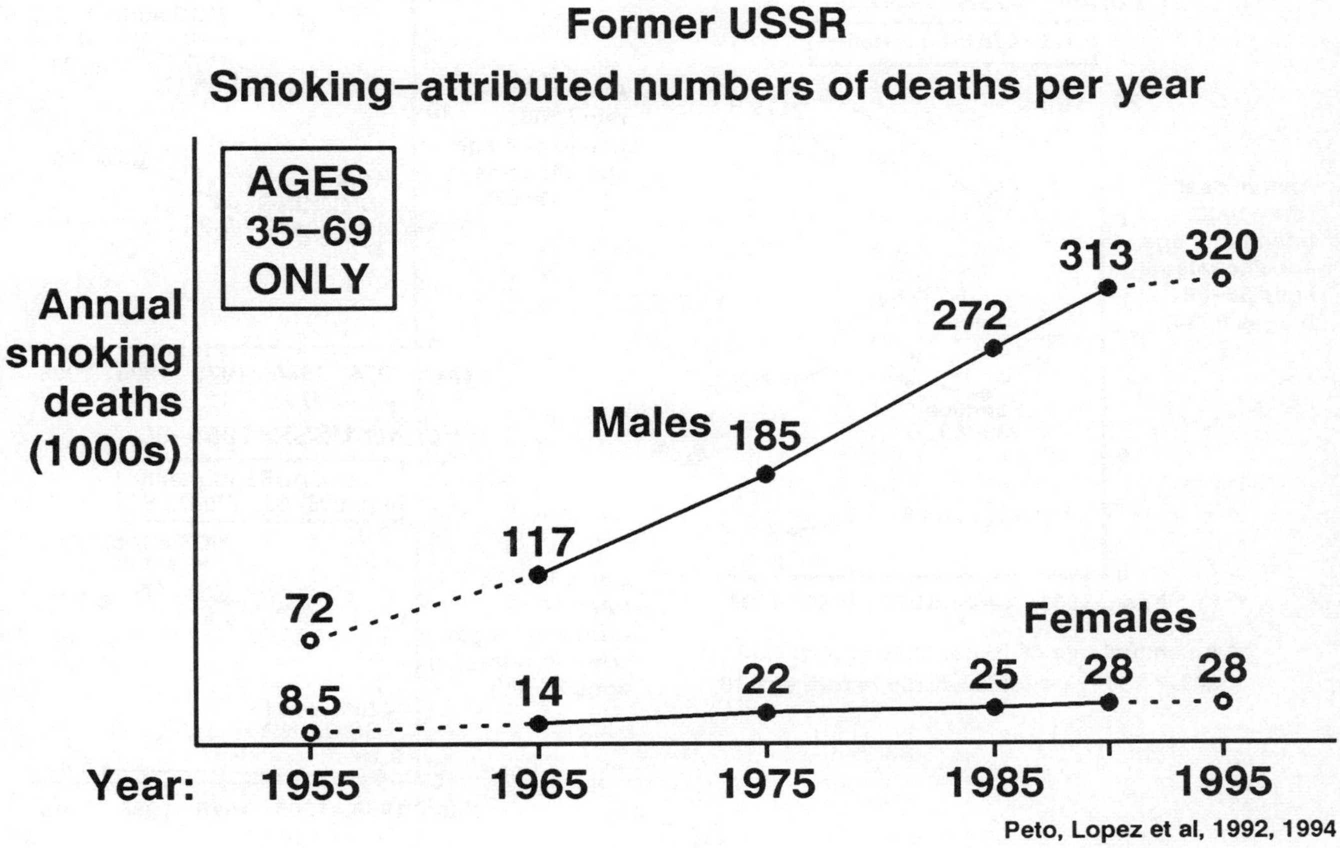
Former USSR
Smoking–attributed numbers of deaths per year
AGES 35–69 ONLY
Annual smoking deaths (1000s)
Males
72
117
185
272
313
320
Females
8.5
14
22
25
28
28
Year:
1955
1965
1975
1985
1995
Peto, Lopez et al, 1992, 1994

Former USSR

ALL DEATHS (annual rates per 1000): Trends in mortality attributed to smoking, and in other mortality

	Males				Females			
	35–69		70–79		35–69		70–79	
Attributed to SMOKING?	Yes	No	Yes	No	Yes	No	Yes	No
1955	4.14	14.9	6.15	66.7	0.28	9.75	0.13	48.9
1965	5.03	10.8	8.36	55.4	0.36	7.24	0.27	43.1
1975	6.17	12.4	11.4	58.4	0.47	7.81	0.93	45.6
1985	7.78	12.6	16.4	68.3	0.53	8.17	1.68	50.5
1990	7.88	12.0	16.9	61.6	0.52	7.71	2.07	46.3

35–69 = mean of 7 age-specific rates; 70–79 = mean of 2 rates (70–74 & 75–79) Peto, Lopez et al, 1992, 1994

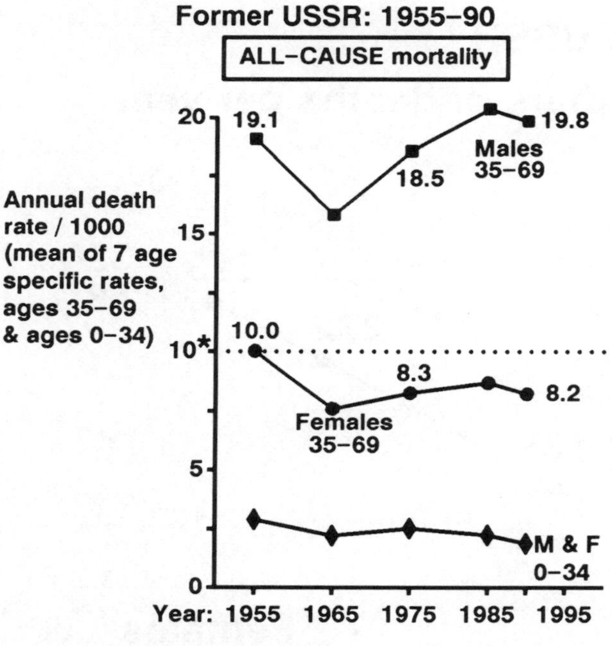

* An annual rate of 10 per 1000 implies that 30% of 35-year-olds will die before age 70

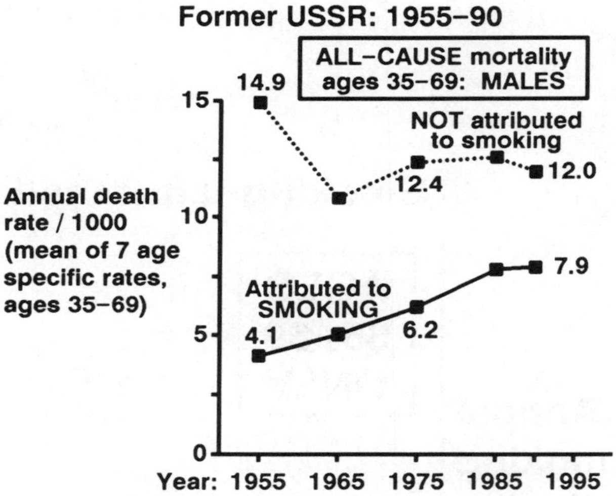

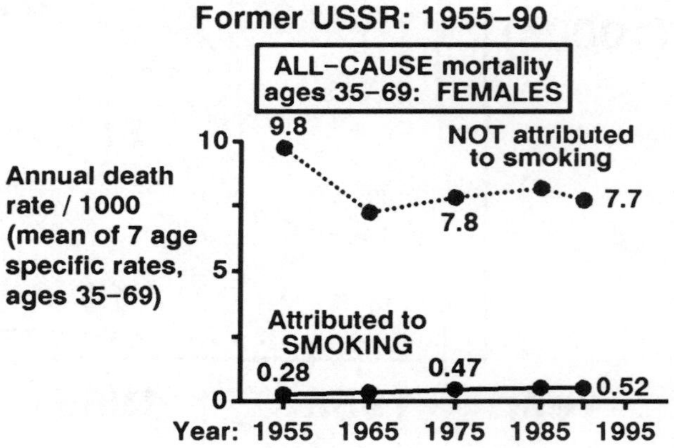

Former USSR

ALL CANCER DEATHS (annual rates per 1000): Trends in mortality attributed to smoking, and in other mortality

	Males				Females			
	35–69		70–79		35–69		70–79	
Attributed to SMOKING?	Yes	No	Yes	No	Yes	No	Yes	No
1955	...	...	...	...	...	...	...	...
1965	1.74	2.57	2.53	8.55	0.08	2.31	0.05	5.68
1975	1.94	2.33	2.98	7.50	0.09	2.16	0.12	5.28
1985	2.49	2.24	4.59	8.49	0.10	2.07	0.25	5.72
1990	2.81	2.27	5.52	8.84	0.11	2.13	0.38	6.16

35–69 = mean of 7 age-specific rates; 70–79 = mean of 2 rates (70–74 & 75–79) Peto, Lopez et al, 1992, 1994

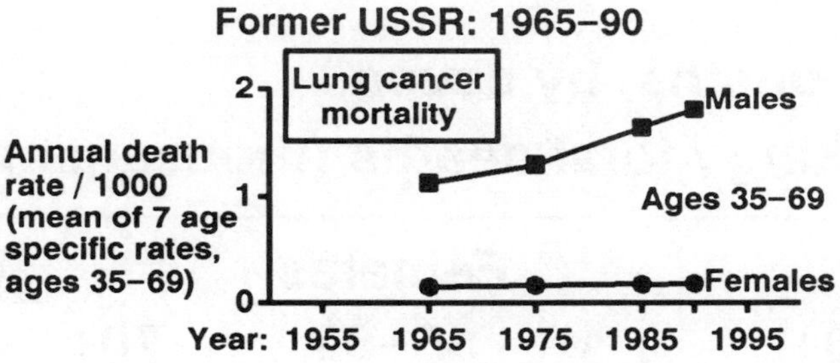

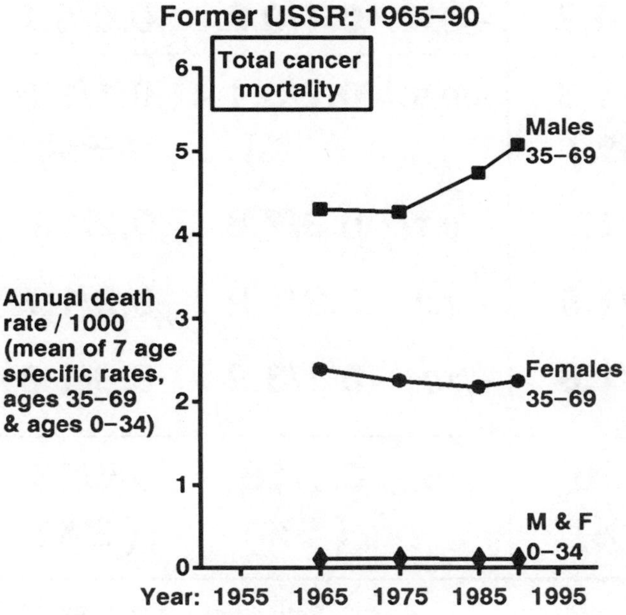

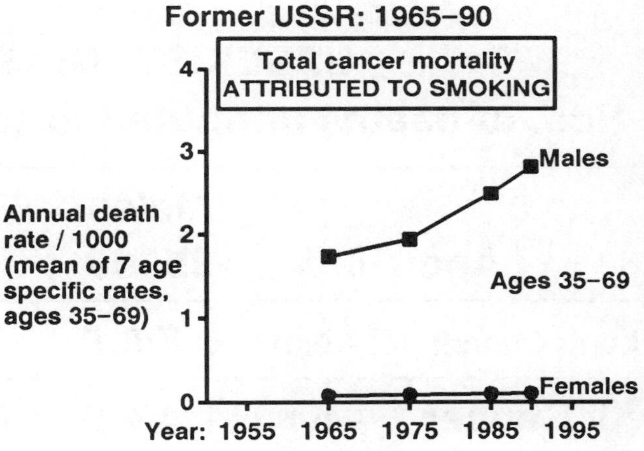

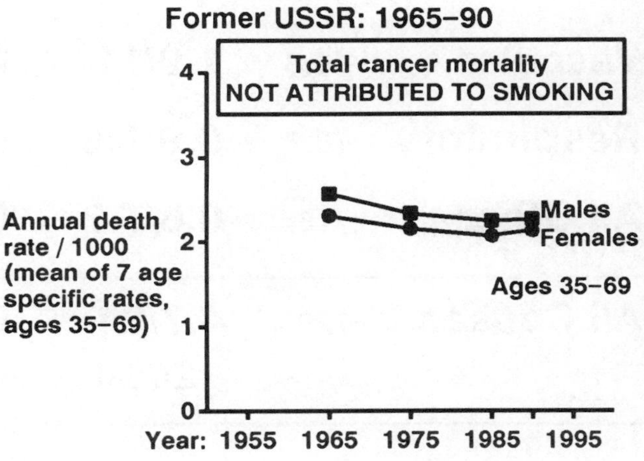

¶UZBEKISTAN: 1990
Relative importance of deaths in MIDDLE age (35–69)

Age range (years)	Deaths attributed to SMOKING / total deaths (thousands) Males	Females	Mean years lost PER DEATH FROM SMOKING
0–34	–/26	–/19	–
35–69	4.7/24	0.7/16	21 years
70+	0.9/16	0.5/23	8 years
All ages	5.6/67	1.3/58	18 years

Peto, Lopez et al, 1992, 1994

UZBEKISTAN: 1990 deaths, by cause
Nos. of deaths attributed to smoking / total deaths (thousands)

	Males			Females		
Age:	0–34	35–69	70+	0–34	35–69	70+
Lung Cancer	–/0.0	0.7/0.9	0.1/0.2	–/0.0	0.1/0.2	0.0/0.1
All Cancer	–/0.7	1.4/4.0 (34%)	0.2/1.3 (16%)	–/0.5	0.2/3.1 (5%)	0.1/1.5 (5%)
Vascular	–/0.8	1.9/11	0.3/12	–/0.7	0.3/7.8	0.2/18
Respiratory	–/8.7	0.9/1.6	0.4/1.5	–/7.2	0.2/1.2	0.3/1.7
All Other	–/16	0.6/7.2	0.0/1.3	–/10	0.1/3.9	0.0/1.6
All Causes	–/26	4.7/24 (20%)	0.9/16 (5%)	–/19	0.7/16 (5%)	0.5/23 (2%)

Peto, Lopez et al, 1992, 1994

UZBEKISTAN: 1990

RISKS OF DYING AT AGES 0–34 and 35–69

(Probability that someone entering an age range would die during it, if the death rates in 1990 were to persist unchanged)

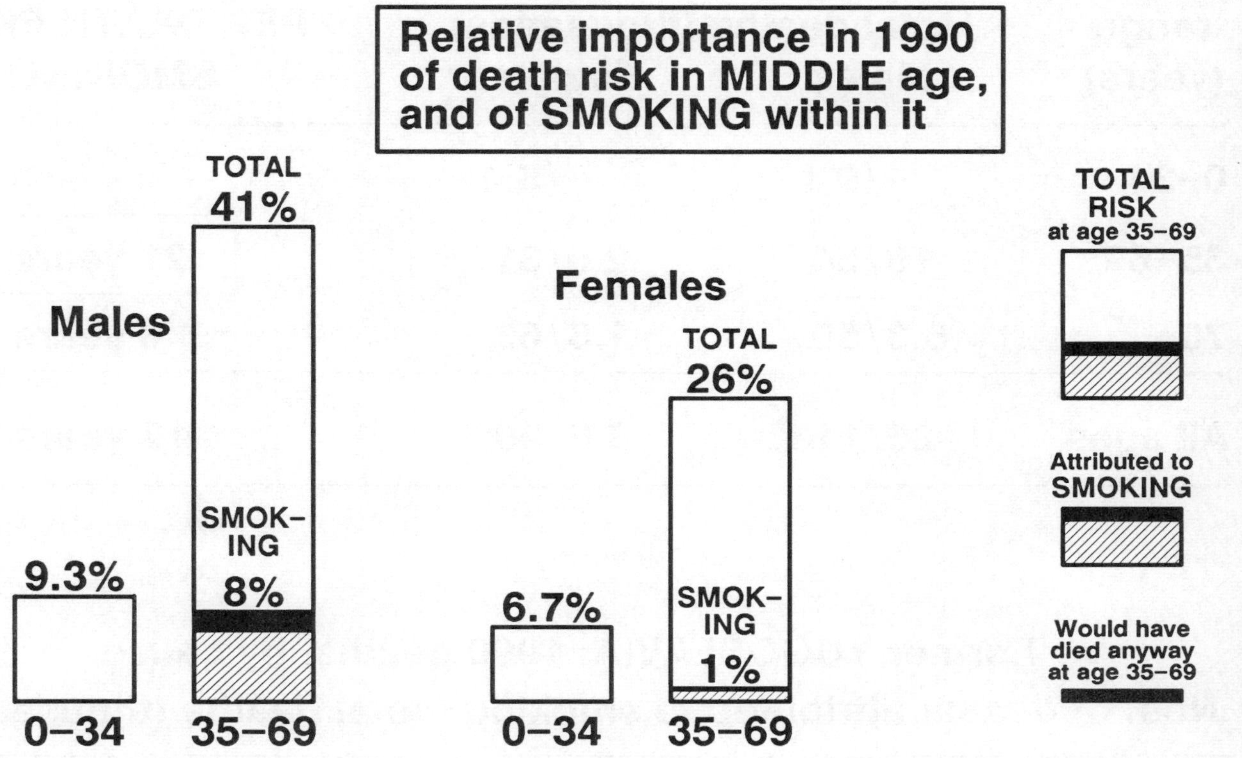

Peto, Lopez et al, 1992, 1994

UZBEKISTAN: 1990 deaths, all ages

Nos. of deaths attributed to smoking / total deaths (thousands)

	Males	Females	Males + Females
All Cancer	1.6/5.9 (26%)	0.2/5.1 (4%)	1.8/11 (16%)
All Causes	5.6/67 (8%)	1.3/58 (2%)	6.9/125 (6%)

Peto, Lopez et al, 1992, 1994

¶Former YUGOSLAVIA: 1990
Relative importance of deaths in MIDDLE age (35–69)

Age range (years)	Deaths attributed to SMOKING / total deaths (thousands) Males	Females	Mean years lost PER DEATH FROM SMOKING
0–34	–/9.1	–/5.4	–
35–69	19/54	2.0/31	21 years
70+	6.3/50	1.6/63	8 years
All ages	26/113	3.6/99	17 years

Peto, Lopez et al, 1992, 1994

Former YUGOSLAVIA: 1990 deaths, by cause
Nos. of deaths attributed to smoking / total deaths (thousands)

	Males			Females		
Age:	0–34	35–69	70+	0–34	35–69	70+
Lung Cancer	–/0.0	5.1/5.4	1.3/1.5	–/0.0	0.4/0.8	0.2/0.4
All Cancer	–/0.5	7.8/15 (53%)	1.9/6.4 (30%)	–/0.5	0.5/9.3 (6%)	0.3/6.0 (4%)
Vascular	–/0.6	7.2/21	2.3/31	–/0.4	0.9/14	0.7/44
Respiratory	–/0.5	1.4/2.0	1.5/3.2	–/0.5	0.3/1.0	0.5/2.5
All Other	–/7.5	3.0/16	0.5/9.0	–/4.1	0.3/7.3	0.1/10
All Causes	–/9.1	19/54 (36%)	6.3/50 (13%)	–/5.4	2.0/31 (6%)	1.6/63 (2%)

Peto, Lopez et al, 1992, 1994

Former YUGOSLAVIA: 1990

RISKS OF DYING AT AGES 0–34 and 35–69

(Probability that someone entering an age range would die during it, if the death rates in 1990 were to persist unchanged)

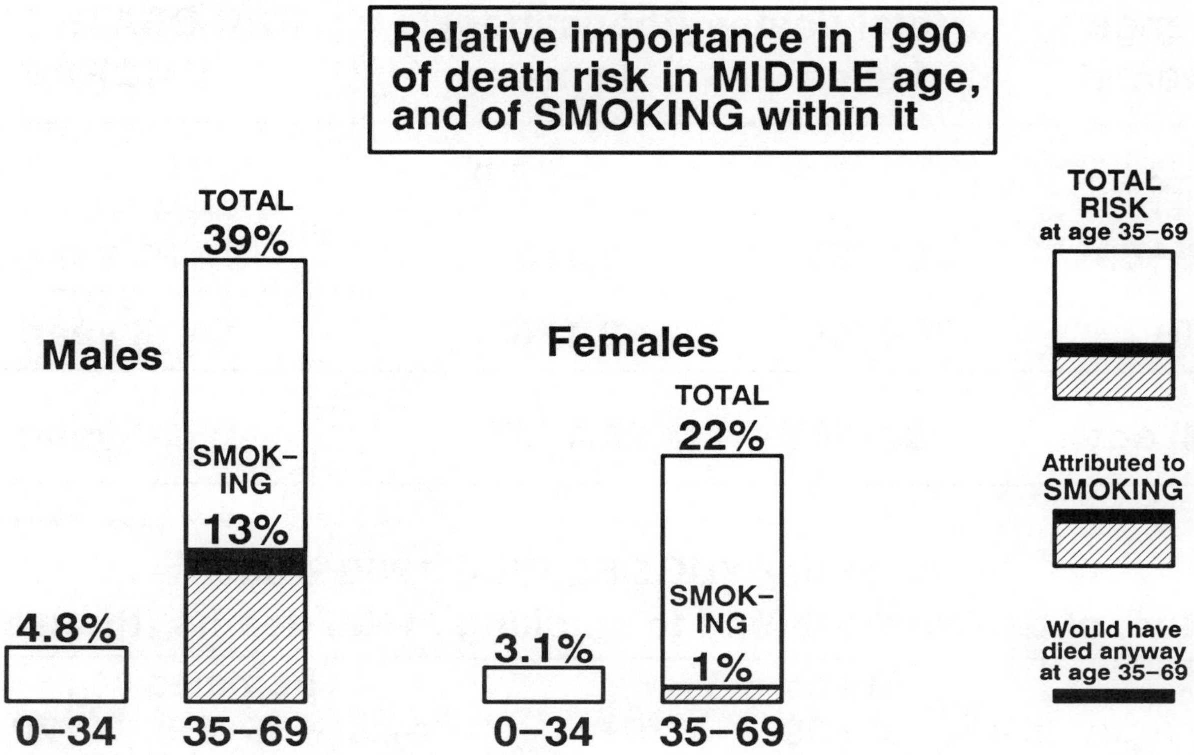

Peto, Lopez et al, 1992, 1994

Former YUGOSLAVIA: 1990 deaths, all ages

Nos. of deaths attributed to smoking / total deaths (thousands)

	Males	Females	Males + Females
All Cancer	9.7/22 (45%)	0.8/16 (5%)	11/38 (28%)
All Causes	26/113 (23%)	3.6/99 (4%)	29/212 (14%)

Peto, Lopez et al, 1992, 1994

Former YUGOSLAVIA: 1995 projections
Relative importance of deaths in MIDDLE age (35–69)

Age range (years)	Deaths attributed to SMOKING / total deaths (thousands) Males	Females	Mean years lost PER DEATH FROM SMOKING
0–34	–/7.3	–/3.9	–
35–69	23/58	2.1/30	21 years
70+	7.4/49	2.1/63	8 years
All ages	30/115	4.1/97	17 years

Peto, Lopez et al, 1992, 1994

Former YUGOSLAVIA: 1950–2000
Nos. of deaths attributed to smoking / total deaths (thousands)

	Males			Females		
Age:	0–34	35–69	70+	0–34	35–69	70+
1955	–/45	3.2/30 (11%)	0.9/25 (3%)	–/41	0.1/28 (0.5%)	0.0/31 (0%)
1965	–/24	6.0/34 (18%)	1.6/28 (6%)	–/20	0.3/26 (1%)	0.0/38 (0%)
1975	–/15	9.4/40 (24%)	4.9/41 (12%)	–/11	0.9/28 (3%)	0.9/50 (2%)
1985	–/12	15/46 (33%)	6.7/55 (12%)	–/7.8	1.7/27 (6%)	1.2/65 (2%)
1995 (projected)	–/7.3	23/58 (39%)	7.4/49 (15%)	–/3.9	2.1/30 (7%)	2.1/63 (3%)
50-year total*, mid-1950 to mid-2000: 874/9790						
1950–2000, by age & sex	–/1033	566/2080 (27%)	215/1980 (11%)	–/837	51/1390 (4%)	42/2470 (2%)

*Estimated as 10 times the sum of the five annual numbers (for 1955, 1965, 1975, 1985 & 1995)

Former YUGOSLAVIA
Smoking–attributed numbers of deaths per year

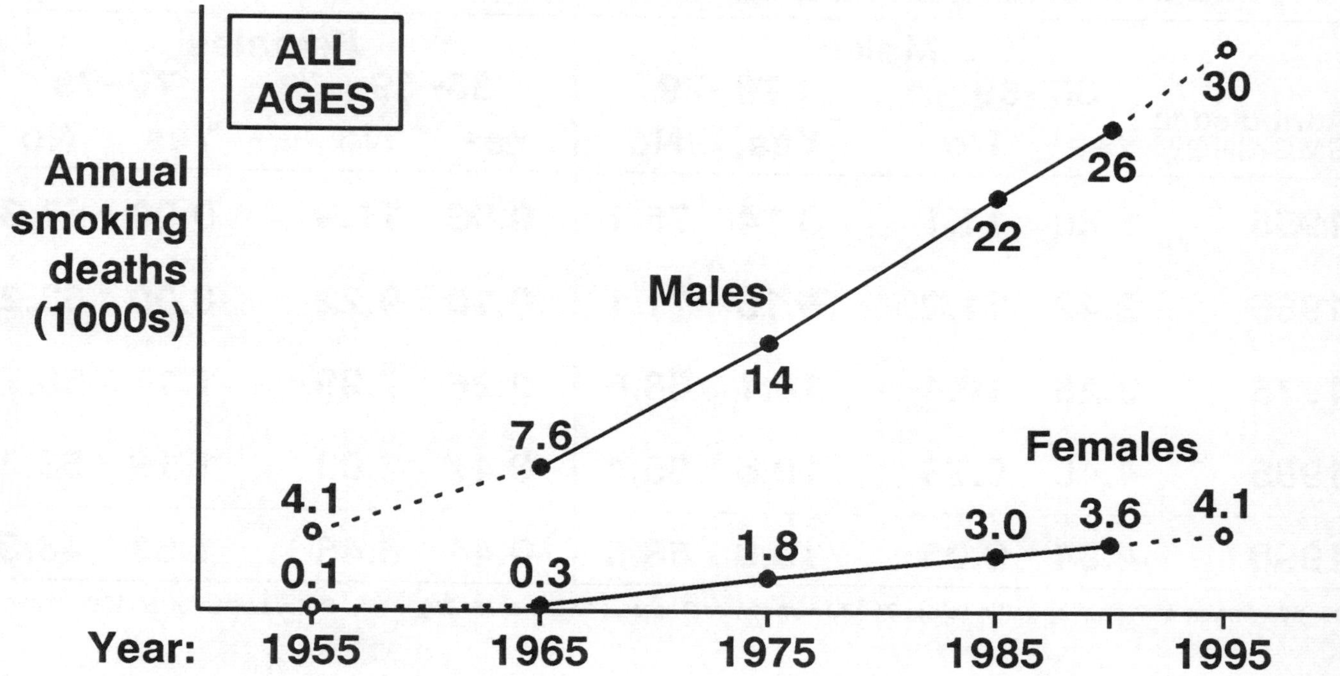

Peto, Lopez et al, 1992, 1994

Former YUGOSLAVIA
Smoking–attributed numbers of deaths per year

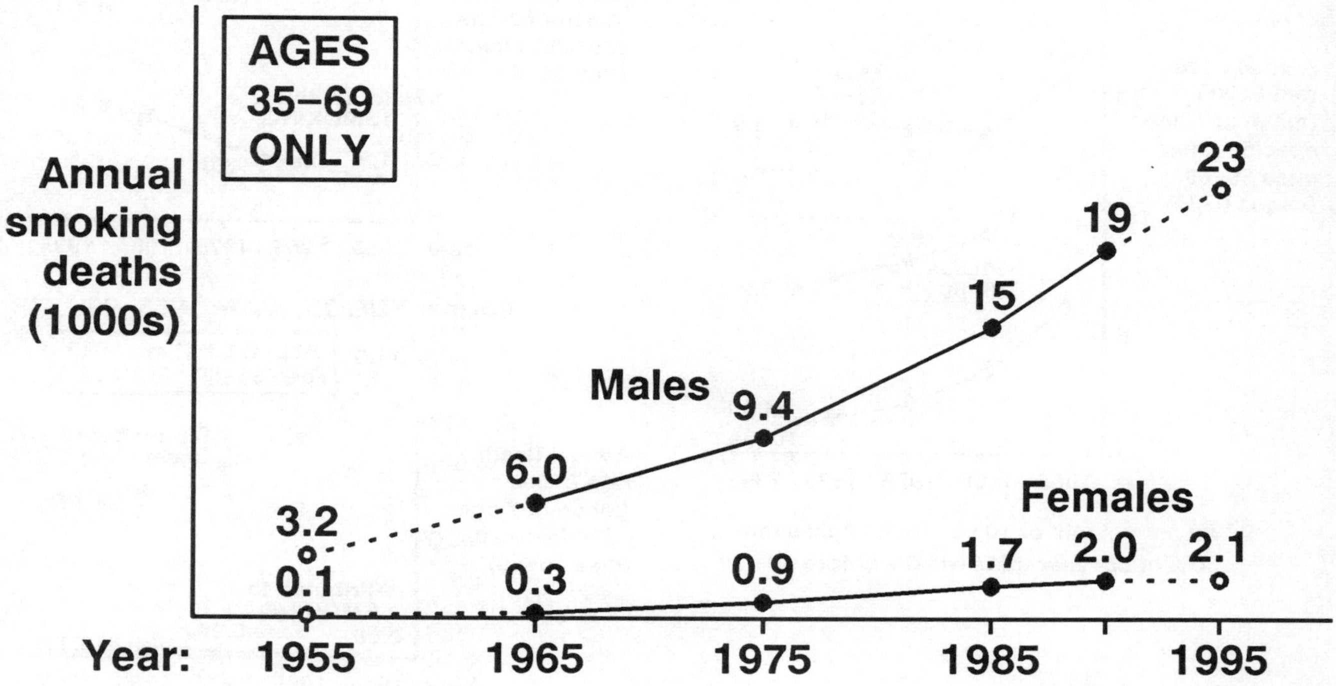

Peto, Lopez et al, 1992, 1994

Former YUGOSLAVIA

ALL DEATHS (annual rates per 1000): Trends in mortality attributed to smoking, and in other mortality

	Males				Females			
	35–69		70–79		35–69		70–79	
Attributed to SMOKING?	Yes	No	Yes	No	Yes	No	Yes	No
1955	1.80	14.1	3.14	75.1	0.06	11.9	0.00	67.3
1965	2.42	11.2	5.15	71.1	0.10	9.22	0.00	63.2
1975	3.28	10.4	10.1	68.6	0.26	7.95	1.17	58.7
1985	4.40	9.78	10.5	65.4	0.47	7.03	1.19	53.2
1990	4.84	9.05	10.6	58.5	0.44	6.48	1.53	46.3

35–69 = mean of 7 age-specific rates; 70–79 = mean of 2 rates (70–74 & 75–79) Peto, Lopez et al, 1992, 1994

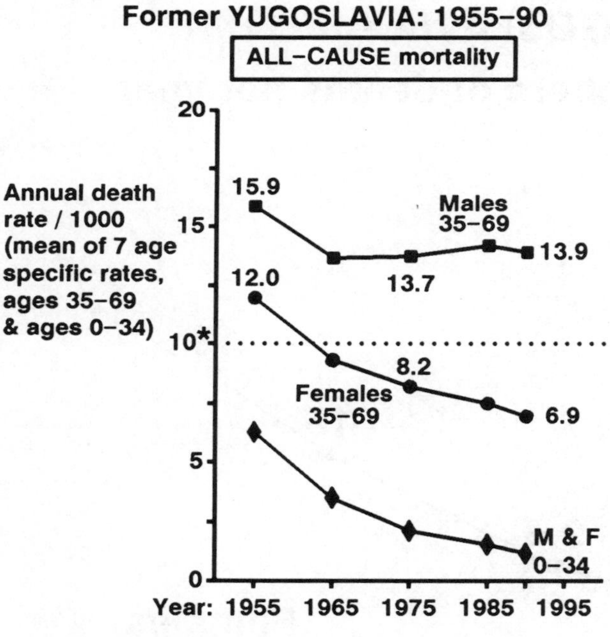

* An annual rate of 10 per 1000 implies that 30% of 35-year-olds will die before age 70

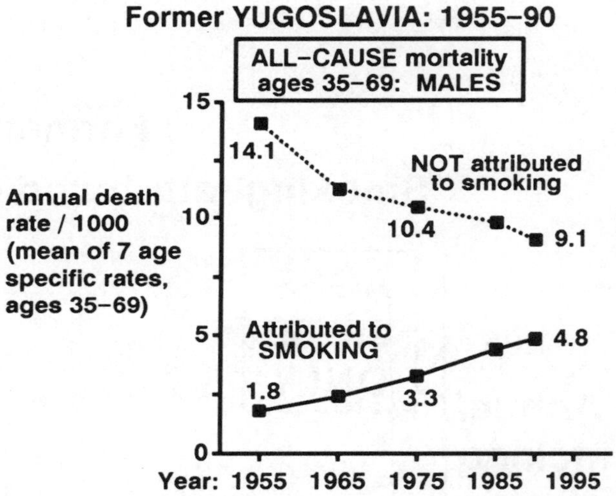

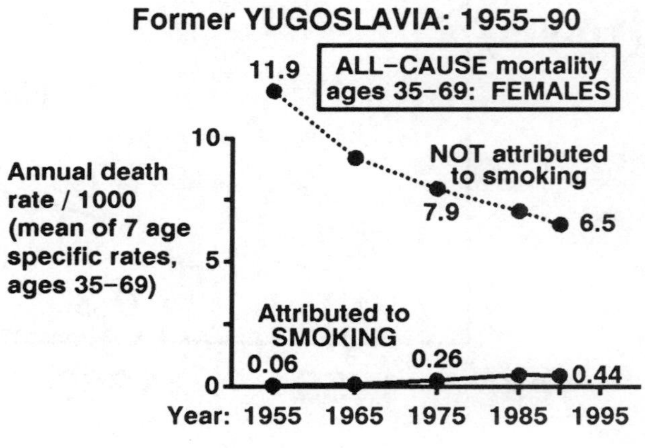

Former YUGOSLAVIA

ALL CANCER DEATHS (annual rates per 1000): Trends in mortality attributed to smoking, and in other mortality

	Males				Females			
	35–69		70–79		35–69		70–79	
Attributed to SMOKING?	Yes	No	Yes	No	Yes	No	Yes	No
1955	...	...	...	...	...	...	...	...
1965	0.74	1.55	1.59	6.65	0.02	1.66	0.00	5.01
1975	1.12	1.74	3.20	7.65	0.05	1.80	0.19	5.87
1985	1.65	1.82	3.72	8.08	0.11	1.84	0.22	6.18
1990	1.99	1.86	3.92	8.14	0.12	1.90	0.31	6.21

35–69 = mean of 7 age–specific rates; 70–79 = mean of 2 rates (70–74 & 75–79)

Peto, Lopez et al, 1992, 1994

Former YUGOSLAVIA: 1965–90

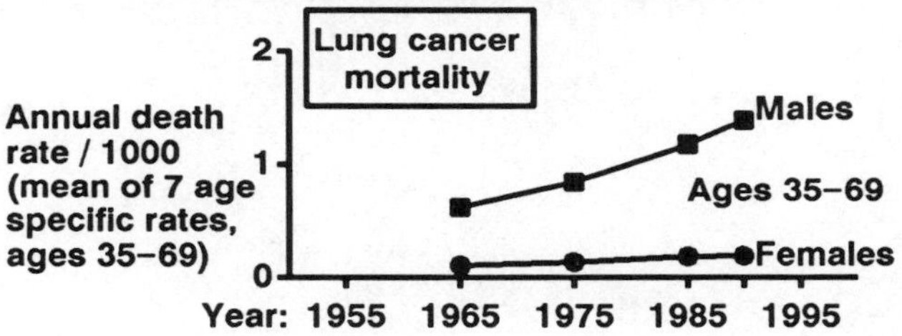

Former YUGOSLAVIA: 1965–90

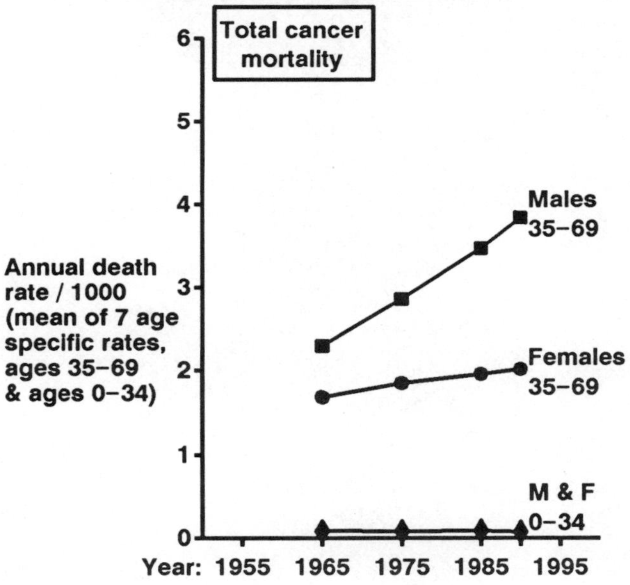

Former YUGOSLAVIA: 1965–90

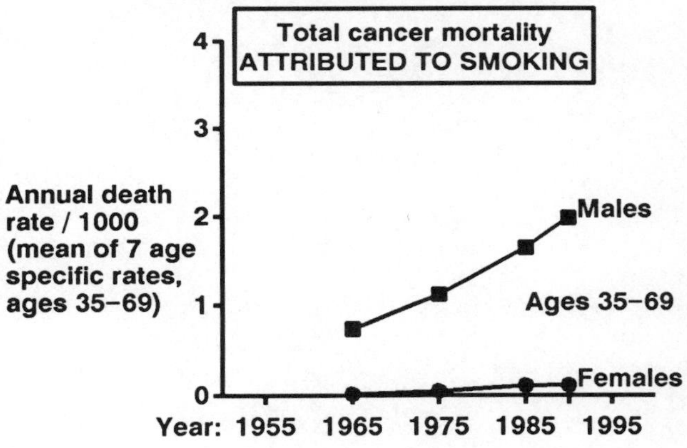

Former YUGOSLAVIA: 1965–90

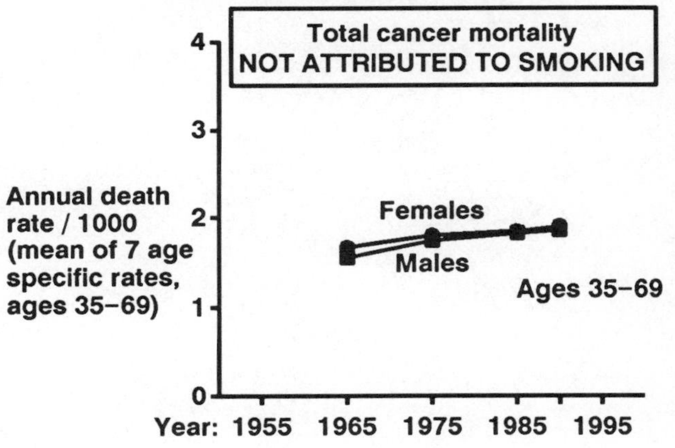

APPENDIX

TABLES

For each population, each set of appendix tables consists of six pages:

First pair	— 1990 cause-specific mortality rates for that population
Second pair	— trends in mortality 1955-1995 (projected) for that population
Third pair	— analyses of smoking-related deaths in 1985, 1990, 1995 and some earlier years

ALL 'DEVELOPED' COUNTRIES: 1990

		No. of deaths			Standardised rates (Defined on p.232)			Annual death rates / 100, 000						
		All ages	0–34	35–69	All ages	0–34	35–69	0–4	5–9	10–14	15–19	20–24	25–29	30–34
ALL CAUSES	M	5812821	504184	2457922	1129.3	157.0	1270.3	365.7	38.7	36.1	103.7	151.9	176.9	226.1
	F	5617860	244415	1375605	666.3	80.1	606.4	286.9	25.2	21.7	41.5	48.9	57.5	78.8
Tuberculosis	M	32504	3102	21803	6.2	0.9	10.1	0.2	0.0	0.0	0.1	0.6	1.8	3.7
	F	9931	1045	4368	1.4	0.3	1.9	0.2	0.0	0.0	0.1	0.4	0.6	0.8
Other infective	M	44507	16680	12652	8.4	5.4	6.3	29.9	1.1	0.7	1.0	1.0	1.6	2.2
and parasitic	F	44102	13224	8737	6.1	4.4	3.8	25.5	0.9	0.6	0.7	1.0	1.2	1.2
ALL CANCER	M	1362438	26602	736143	268.0	8.2	392.1	5.8	5.2	4.5	6.5	7.9	10.5	17.0
	F	1086757	23100	500022	146.0	7.3	218.7	4.8	4.0	3.5	4.5	5.4	9.5	19.2
Mouth and	M	40446	499	30170	7.9	0.2	15.1	0.1	0.1	0.0	0.1	0.2	0.2	0.4
pharynx cancer	F	11290	229	5180	1.5	0.1	2.3	0.0	0.0	0.0	0.1	0.1	0.1	0.2
Oesophagus cancer	M	45596	120	29779	9.0	0.0	15.6	0.0	0.0	0.0	0.0	0.0	0.0	0.2
	F	16249	68	6448	2.1	0.0	2.9	0.0	0.0	0.0	0.0	0.0	0.0	0.1
Stomach cancer	M	142741	1190	80408	28.1	0.4	42.3	0.0	0.0	0.0	0.1	0.2	0.6	1.5
	F	100873	1306	41266	13.1	0.4	18.1	0.0	–	0.0	0.1	0.3	0.7	1.7
Colorectal cancer	M	132923	1125	62656	26.3	0.3	34.0	0.1	0.0	0.0	0.1	0.3	0.6	1.2
	F	140492	860	51928	17.7	0.3	23.1	0.1	0.0	0.0	0.1	0.2	0.4	1.1
Liver cancer	M	37487	345	25007	7.4	0.1	13.3	0.2	0.0	0.0	0.1	0.1	0.1	0.3
	F	17223	222	7828	2.3	0.1	3.5	0.1	0.0	0.0	0.0	0.1	0.1	0.1
Pancreas cancer	M	58338	249	31205	11.5	0.1	16.8	0.0	0.0	0.0	0.0	0.0	0.1	0.4
	F	59501	177	21667	7.5	0.1	9.7	0.0	0.0	0.0	0.0	0.0	0.1	0.2
Larynx cancer	M	30127	77	21497	5.9	0.0	11.1	0.0	0.0	0.0	0.0	0.0	0.0	0.1
	F	2793	28	1542	0.4	0.0	0.7	0.0	–	0.0	0.0	0.0	0.0	0.0
Lung cancer	M	403543	1217	246388	79.6	0.4	132.7	0.1	0.0	0.0	0.1	0.2	0.5	1.6
	F	126486	673	64392	17.4	0.2	28.6	0.0	0.0	0.0	0.1	0.1	0.3	0.8
Malignant melanoma	M	12421	747	7848	2.4	0.2	3.8	0.0	0.0	0.0	0.1	0.2	0.4	0.8
	F	10547	596	5534	1.5	0.2	2.3	–	0.0	0.0	0.0	0.2	0.4	0.6
Female breast cancer	F	176586	2623	104424	25.5	0.8	44.6	0.0	0.0	0.0	0.0	0.1	1.1	4.3
Cervix cancer	F	32508	1407	20241	4.8	0.4	8.5	0.0	–	–	0.0	0.2	0.7	2.1
Other uterine cancer	F	38398	350	18415	5.2	0.1	8.1	0.0	0.0	0.0	0.0	0.1	0.2	0.5
Ovarian cancer	F	59916	854	33518	8.5	0.3	14.6	0.0	0.0	0.1	0.2	0.3	0.5	0.9
Prostate cancer	M	109966	91	24781	22.0	0.0	14.8	0.0	–	0.0	0.0	0.0	0.1	0.1
Bladder cancer	M	44156	83	15808	8.8	0.0	8.9	0.0	0.0	0.0	0.0	0.0	0.0	0.1
	F	18577	41	4441	2.1	0.0	2.0	0.0	0.0	0.0	0.0	0.0	0.0	0.0
Other and ill-defined	M	211385	10792	116074	41.2	3.3	60.7	2.9	2.3	1.8	2.8	3.4	4.2	5.9
cancer sites	F	194824	7197	81480	25.7	2.3	35.8	2.5	1.9	1.8	1.9	1.8	2.5	3.8
Hodgkin's disease	M	4865	1076	2711	0.9	0.3	1.3	0.0	0.0	0.1	0.2	0.5	0.7	0.8
	F	3523	663	1535	0.5	0.2	0.6	0.0	0.0	0.0	0.1	0.3	0.5	0.5
Myeloma and non-	M	47189	2899	23709	9.2	0.9	12.4	0.5	0.7	0.6	0.8	0.9	1.2	1.5
Hodgkin lymphomas	F	41958	1512	16487	5.5	0.5	7.3	0.4	0.3	0.3	0.4	0.6	0.6	0.8
Leukaemia	M	41240	6084	18097	7.9	1.9	9.4	1.9	2.0	1.8	2.1	1.8	1.8	2.0
	F	34997	4282	13688	4.8	1.4	5.9	1.6	1.6	1.2	1.4	1.2	1.2	1.5
ALL VASCULAR	M	2419274	26877	925592	478.9	8.2	495.2	5.3	1.0	1.5	4.0	6.8	12.2	26.4
DISEASE	F	2938437	13383	507672	322.5	4.2	229.1	4.7	0.9	1.3	2.6	3.9	6.0	10.1
Rheumatic heart	M	17113	1336	11920	3.3	0.4	5.7	0.1	0.0	0.1	0.3	0.4	0.8	1.2
disease and fever	F	30102	1186	17503	4.4	0.4	7.6	0.1	0.1	0.1	0.3	0.4	0.7	1.0
Hypertensive disease	M	64924	566	27061	12.8	0.2	14.4	0.1	0.0	0.0	0.1	0.1	0.3	0.7
	F	101929	312	22896	11.6	0.1	10.3	0.0	0.0	0.0	0.0	0.1	0.2	0.3
Ischaemic heart	M	1161928	8142	512089	229.8	2.4	272.8	0.1	0.0	0.1	0.4	1.3	3.5	11.8
disease	F	1146750	1799	212001	127.1	0.6	96.5	0.1	0.0	0.0	0.2	0.5	0.9	2.1
Pulmonary embolism	M	26207	626	10918	5.2	0.2	5.8	0.1	0.0	0.0	0.1	0.2	0.3	0.6
and other venous	F	39002	654	10133	4.6	0.2	4.5	0.0	0.0	0.0	0.1	0.3	0.3	0.6
Cerebrovascular	M	574285	5161	193015	113.8	1.6	104.6	0.9	0.2	0.3	0.9	1.5	2.4	4.7
disease	F	895341	3537	158044	98.7	1.1	71.2	0.7	0.2	0.3	0.7	1.1	1.7	2.9
Other vascular	M	574805	11041	170584	114.0	3.4	91.9	4.1	0.7	0.9	2.3	3.3	4.9	7.5
disease	F	725305	5888	87094	76.3	1.9	39.2	3.8	0.5	0.8	1.3	1.6	2.2	3.1
Chronic obstructive	M	267570	3110	92895	53.0	1.0	51.9	1.5	0.3	0.5	0.8	0.9	1.1	1.6
pulmonary disease	F	167869	2301	42966	19.8	0.7	19.4	1.1	0.2	0.3	0.6	0.8	0.9	1.1
Other respiratory	M	232411	34418	47541	45.7	11.1	25.4	65.9	2.0	1.2	1.4	1.7	2.1	3.3
disease	F	226223	26993	22644	25.7	9.1	10.0	55.7	1.8	1.1	1.0	1.1	1.5	1.6
Peptic ulcer	M	26028	596	12381	5.1	0.2	6.4	0.0	0.0	0.0	0.1	0.1	0.3	0.7
	F	20025	159	4352	2.3	0.0	1.9	0.0	0.0	0.0	0.0	0.1	0.1	0.1
Liver cirrhosis (incl.	M	113315	3521	84422	22.0	1.1	41.6	0.6	0.2	0.2	0.3	0.5	1.4	4.3
USSR other liver)	F	64234	1933	38248	9.3	0.6	16.5	0.4	0.1	0.2	0.3	0.4	0.8	2.0
Renal disease	M	57608	2814	20256	11.3	0.9	10.5	1.0	0.3	0.3	0.5	1.0	1.2	1.8
	F	63173	2199	18231	7.6	0.7	8.0	0.9	0.2	0.3	0.5	0.8	0.9	1.4
Pregnancy and birth	F	3244	2350	894	0.5	0.7	0.3	–	–	–	0.5	1.4	1.4	1.8
Congenital and	M	83526	79795	2694	15.1	25.9	1.2	172.4	2.2	1.4	1.6	1.3	1.1	1.0
perinatal causes	F	62592	58736	2500	11.7	19.9	1.0	132.3	2.0	1.4	1.2	1.0	0.9	0.8
Ill-defined causes	M	146130	21395	41879	28.4	6.7	20.2	26.7	0.7	0.9	2.2	4.2	5.5	7.1
	F	202120	11658	17045	21.3	3.9	7.3	19.3	0.6	0.5	0.9	1.7	1.9	2.3
Other medical causes	M	413048	44973	164589	79.4	13.9	81.6	21.0	5.0	4.6	7.0	9.7	19.7	30.0
	F	478754	24477	115936	56.7	7.9	50.8	16.6	4.2	3.8	4.7	6.4	8.6	11.0
ALL NON-	M	614461	240297	295081	107.7	73.7	127.8	35.2	20.8	20.4	78.2	116.1	118.4	126.9
MEDICAL CAUSES	F	250384	62848	91985	35.5	20.2	37.7	25.3	10.3	8.6	23.8	24.4	23.4	25.5
Motor vehicle	M	158024	82409	61506	26.8	25.3	26.6	5.6	7.9	6.9	36.2	48.6	38.3	33.7
traffic accidents	F	54901	22508	20863	8.4	7.2	8.5	4.0	4.7	3.9	12.3	10.8	7.9	7.0
Fire	M	11938	4430	5419	2.2	1.4	2.4	3.3	0.9	0.5	0.7	1.2	1.4	1.8
	F	7642	2414	2337	1.1	0.8	1.0	2.5	0.8	0.3	0.4	0.5	0.5	0.6
Suicide	M	139006	42703	77377	24.7	12.9	33.8	–	0.1	2.1	12.2	21.1	25.5	29.7
	F	48614	9955	26732	7.4	3.1	11.0	–	0.0	0.6	3.7	5.0	5.5	6.8
Homicide	M	50817	27671	21500	8.4	8.4	8.6	1.7	0.5	1.0	8.8	14.8	16.0	16.1
	F	16389	7124	7396	2.6	2.2	2.9	1.6	0.6	0.7	2.2	2.9	3.7	4.0
POPULATION (thousands):	M=males				583696	318982	230551	43999	43695	43632	45491	45972	48568	47626
	F=females				621017	308170	250618	41988	41779	41740	43405	44342	47649	47267

ALL 'DEVELOPED' COUNTRIES: 1990

Annual death rates / 100, 000 — 9th ICD categories

35–39	40–44	45–49	50–54	55–59	60–64	65–69	70–74	75–79	80+/NK			
292.0	386.9	563.9	940.1	1403.4	2185.7	3119.9	4630.6	7404.4	14529.4	M	ALL CAUSES	001–999
113.7	166.7	256.6	413.1	633.0	1026.1	1635.8	2633.7	4635.7	11560.1	F		
5.5	6.2	7.7	11.9	11.9	13.9	13.8	16.7	22.1	30.0	M	Tuberculosis	010–018, 137
1.0	0.8	1.0	1.6	2.1	2.7	3.7	4.9	6.8	9.8	F		
2.7	3.1	3.7	4.5	6.0	9.3	14.8	24.7	36.1	81.0	M	Other infective	Rest of 001–139
1.2	1.6	2.1	2.7	4.1	5.9	9.0	14.4	23.2	66.4	F	and parasitic	
32.9	68.1	139.0	275.9	469.8	740.9	1018.1	1357.1	1753.6	2305.2	M	ALL CANCER	140–208
38.1	67.2	110.8	174.1	254.6	370.0	515.9	671.2	851.1	1173.3	F		
1.6	4.6	9.7	16.2	21.0	26.0	26.2	26.4	27.6	32.9	M	Mouth and	140–149
0.3	0.7	1.2	1.8	2.8	3.8	5.0	6.5	8.4	13.1	F	pharynx cancer	
0.6	2.4	6.5	13.3	21.2	29.9	35.4	41.3	46.6	51.5	M	Oesophagus cancer	150
0.2	0.4	1.0	2.0	3.4	5.8	7.5	10.7	14.9	20.9	F		
3.9	8.1	15.3	32.6	52.2	82.6	101.4	135.0	186.1	231.3	M	Stomach cancer	151
3.3	5.4	7.8	13.4	19.3	32.1	45.4	63.3	92.2	123.3	F		
2.6	5.1	10.6	21.0	37.2	63.1	98.5	139.0	199.6	292.8	M	Colorectal cancer	153, 154
2.4	4.7	9.1	16.3	25.9	40.7	62.2	87.5	125.2	204.8	F		
0.8	1.7	3.8	8.4	20.2	27.2	30.9	34.4	36.8	35.5	M	Liver cancer	155.0
0.3	0.5	1.0	1.9	3.9	7.1	9.9	12.6	15.5	16.1	F		
1.2	2.8	6.2	11.3	19.2	30.8	45.9	63.4	80.0	98.2	M	Pancreas cancer	157
0.6	1.3	3.0	5.8	10.7	17.9	28.7	41.4	57.5	81.1	F		
0.7	2.3	5.2	10.6	15.5	20.7	22.3	23.5	25.1	27.1	M	Larynx cancer	161
0.1	0.1	0.3	0.5	0.9	1.3	1.6	1.8	2.0	2.1	F		
5.6	16.0	40.5	89.9	163.7	263.5	349.4	430.8	478.8	466.1	M	Lung cancer	162
2.2	5.2	11.4	19.6	33.2	52.9	75.8	99.3	101.8	95.3	F		
1.4	2.0	2.6	3.4	4.4	5.9	7.0	9.3	11.1	14.0	M	Malignant melanoma	172
1.1	1.5	1.9	2.2	2.6	3.2	3.9	5.2	6.3	9.5	F		
11.0	21.5	33.0	46.0	55.7	65.8	79.2	88.0	101.3	143.3	F	Female breast cancer	174
3.9	5.2	6.3	8.0	9.2	12.1	15.0	16.4	18.5	17.5	F	Cervix cancer	180
1.0	1.8	3.2	5.8	10.1	14.6	20.5	25.1	30.9	38.1	F	Other uterine cancer	179, 182
1.8	4.2	8.5	13.5	18.4	24.7	31.2	36.9	41.1	44.9	F	Ovarian cancer	183
0.1	0.2	0.8	3.2	10.0	26.6	62.9	128.5	226.2	441.2	M	Prostate cancer	185
0.2	0.6	1.5	3.9	8.7	17.9	29.8	48.0	80.6	133.0	M	Bladder cancer	188
0.1	0.2	0.4	0.8	1.9	3.9	6.8	10.7	19.4	36.7	F		
8.9	14.8	25.9	45.7	71.3	107.8	150.3	192.1	243.5	328.0	M	Other and ill-defined	Rest of 140–208
6.1	9.9	16.0	26.7	41.6	61.8	88.4	116.0	153.1	237.0	F	cancer sites	
0.9	0.8	0.8	1.1	1.4	1.8	2.1	2.6	3.4	3.7	M	Hodgkin's disease	201
0.4	0.4	0.4	0.4	0.6	0.8	1.4	1.7	2.4	2.4	F		
2.0	3.4	5.3	8.9	13.7	21.7	31.8	47.8	59.6	78.2	M	Myeloma and non-	200, 202–203
1.2	1.7	3.0	4.9	8.0	12.3	20.0	29.5	36.1	49.0	F	Hodgkin lymphomas	
2.3	3.0	4.1	6.5	10.1	15.4	24.3	35.2	48.6	71.8	M	Leukaemia	204–208
2.0	2.4	3.4	4.6	6.3	9.3	13.4	18.6	24.5	38.1	F		
54.4	102.2	175.4	329.5	528.0	904.8	1372.1	2163.6	3764.5	7829.2	M	ALL VASCULAR	390–459
17.6	32.5	59.4	117.6	212.7	413.2	751.1	1373.5	2749.1	7242.5	F	DISEASE	
2.0	2.6	3.7	6.6	7.9	8.6	8.8	9.8	11.0	13.7	M	Rheumatic heart	390–398
1.6	2.3	4.0	8.3	10.2	12.3	14.1	14.7	17.5	22.5	F	disease and fever	
1.5	3.0	5.3	10.0	16.8	25.6	38.6	54.1	96.9	199.1	M	Hypertensive disease	401–405
0.7	1.6	3.1	6.6	11.2	17.6	31.2	50.0	94.0	226.9	F		
28.1	57.3	99.8	191.3	297.4	500.8	735.0	1103.7	1729.9	3113.8	M	Ischaemic heart	410–414
4.4	9.3	19.0	41.4	85.2	181.2	334.7	606.5	1135.2	2657.4	F	disease	
1.0	1.4	2.2	3.5	6.1	10.3	16.2	24.3	41.1	70.5	M	Pulmonary embolism	415.1, 451–453
0.8	1.2	1.9	2.7	4.4	7.4	13.0	19.7	36.9	76.8	F	and other venous	
9.2	17.6	31.4	63.3	108.5	201.8	300.1	506.4	983.4	2053.2	M	Cerebrovascular	430–438
5.5	10.7	19.4	38.5	66.7	129.5	228.1	423.0	876.3	2155.2	F	disease	
12.7	20.4	33.0	54.8	91.2	157.8	273.4	465.3	902.2	2378.8	M	Other vascular	Rest of 390–459
4.7	7.3	12.0	20.0	35.1	65.2	130.0	259.6	589.3	2103.7	F	disease	
2.5	4.5	9.7	25.4	51.8	102.7	166.8	281.1	476.6	835.7	M	Chronic obstructive	490–496
1.6	2.4	4.6	10.2	18.9	35.7	62.3	104.4	167.3	309.9	F	pulmonary disease	
4.8	6.8	10.0	15.3	24.1	40.8	76.0	156.0	314.3	975.9	M	Other respiratory	Rest of 460–519
2.2	2.8	4.1	5.6	9.4	16.0	30.2	65.5	135.6	620.0	F	disease	
1.2	1.9	2.9	5.2	7.3	11.1	15.0	20.9	33.6	67.2	M	Peptic ulcer	531–533
0.2	0.5	0.7	1.2	1.9	3.2	5.8	9.7	17.4	45.9	F		
10.1	16.9	27.7	39.8	55.3	67.7	73.7	70.5	77.3	75.9	M	Liver cirrhosis (incl.	571
4.0	6.3	9.8	14.8	20.8	26.9	33.0	35.4	40.7	39.9	F	USSR other liver)	
2.5	3.2	4.4	7.9	11.3	17.5	26.7	44.4	83.2	199.6	M	Renal disease	580–590
1.8	2.2	3.3	5.9	8.5	13.7	20.5	30.0	49.1	122.3	F		
1.4	0.6	0.1	0.0	0.0	0.0	0.0	–	–	–	F	Pregnancy and birth	630–676
1.0	1.0	1.0	1.2	1.3	1.4	1.7	2.1	2.8	4.7	M	Congenital and	740–779
0.8	0.8	0.9	1.0	1.2	1.2	1.4	1.8	1.8	2.8	F	perinatal causes	
9.4	11.1	13.7	18.9	22.6	28.4	37.0	59.2	135.6	617.2	M	Ill-defined causes	780–799
2.9	3.4	4.4	5.6	7.3	10.4	17.2	36.7	109.6	655.7	F		
37.1	40.7	47.8	60.0	82.1	118.0	185.5	295.5	505.9	1111.1	M	Other medical causes	Rest of 001–799
13.5	16.3	22.8	33.5	51.6	82.7	135.1	218.6	374.0	998.8	F		
127.7	121.1	121.0	144.7	132.0	129.2	118.6	138.6	198.7	396.8	M	ALL NON-	E800–E999
27.3	29.3	32.7	39.3	39.9	44.6	50.6	67.6	109.8	272.9	F	MEDICAL CAUSES	
29.2	25.3	24.2	27.7	27.1	26.3	26.1	30.9	41.8	55.1	M	Motor vehicle	E810–E819
6.9	6.8	7.2	8.4	8.8	10.0	11.5	15.3	20.4	19.9	F	traffic accidents	
2.0	1.9	2.1	2.6	2.6	2.9	3.0	3.5	5.4	10.5	M	Fire	E890–E899
0.6	0.7	0.7	0.8	1.0	1.2	1.7	2.4	4.0	7.3	F		
31.1	31.1	33.7	37.1	35.3	34.8	33.6	40.0	53.9	78.3	M	Suicide	E950–E959
7.4	8.5	10.3	11.6	11.9	13.0	13.9	15.8	19.6	21.9	F		
14.4	11.6	8.7	8.8	6.6	5.9	4.1	3.8	3.9	7.3	M	Homicide	E960–E969
4.0	3.5	2.8	3.0	2.4	2.4	2.0	2.5	2.8	3.7	F		
44753	40909	33201	33812	29551	27670	20654	13347	11114	9703	M	POPULATION (thousands)	
44848	41221	34074	35846	32409	33223	28998	20505	19721	22003	F		

ALL 'DEVELOPED' COUNTRIES: Males

	All ages	0–34	35–69	35–39	40–44	45–49	50–54	55–59	60–64	65–69	70–74	75–79	80+/NK
POPULATION (1000s)													
1955	421171	261104	142589	23333	26377	25598	22384	18453	14643	11801	8563	5316	3599
1965	482051	291922	168568	34776	29439	22551	25053	23253	19231	14265	10057	6537	4968
1975	527484	309386	190844	36579	33578	33159	27485	20140	21445	18459	13100	7850	6304
1985	564989	319588	211744	41425	33891	35060	31290	30222	23494	16364	15203	10275	8180
1990	**583696**	**318982**	**230551**	**44753**	**40909**	**33201**	**33812**	**29551**	**27670**	**20654**	**13347**	**11114**	**9703**
1995 projected	*597949*	*316933*	*244052*	*46654*	*42435*	*38764*	*35487*	*30477*	*28086*	*22150*	*16419*	*10288*	*10257*
NUMBER OF DEATHS													
All causes													
1955	4329060	878103	1809788	77554	121813	182334	253298	321155	386520	467114	514516	494456	632197
1965	4757920	663637	2075528	108971	123634	142609	257808	374278	499323	568905	598934	588034	831787
1975	5342881	604704	2303311	121034	155313	236259	277408	309658	521686	681953	757633	687439	989794
1985	5746048	536200	2303927	111297	131955	229808	310278	464622	523290	532677	793377	844633	1267911
1990	**5812820**	**504184**	**2457923**	**130663**	**158264**	**187229**	**317860**	**414726**	**604785**	**644396**	**618044**	**822937**	**1409732**
1995 projected	*5693586*	*481866*	*2435005*	*139325*	*163225*	*202242*	*307369*	*400723*	*584679*	*637442*	*693934*	*693547*	*1389234*
Lung cancer													
1955	...	...	...	...	...	...	...	...	...	...	...	...	...
1965	185467	1235	133964	1993	4127	7051	17045	28621	37891	37236	26955	15192	8121
1975	271655	1158	174585	2073	5520	14162	21843	27867	47423	55697	48878	29528	17506
1985	364176	1241	215773	2222	5706	15174	28598	51432	58377	54264	62910	48694	35558
1990	**403543**	**1217**	**246388**	**2506**	**6565**	**13455**	**30414**	**48376**	**72913**	**72159**	**57502**	**53214**	**45222**
1995 projected	*436153*	*1252*	*261181*	*2514*	*6742*	*14808*	*30788*	*50115*	*77054*	*79160*	*71594*	*51811*	*50315*
ANNUAL DEATH RATE / 100,000	(*The rates for the age groups 0–34 and 35–69 are the means of seven five-yearly rates, but the all-ages rates are standardised to the conventional "European" age distribution)												
All causes													
1955	1458.9*	306.9*	1568.1*	332.4	461.8	712.3	1131.6	1740.4	2639.7	3958.3	6008.3	9302.1	17564.4
1965	1362.3*	220.6*	1512.7*	313.4	420.0	632.4	1029.1	1609.6	2596.4	3988.2	5955.3	8995.8	16744.1
1975	1304.0*	199.6*	1454.3*	330.9	462.6	712.5	1009.3	1537.6	2432.6	3694.5	5783.5	8757.6	15700.8
1985	1213.3*	168.3*	1332.2*	268.7	389.4	655.5	991.6	1537.4	2227.4	3255.3	5218.5	8220.1	15501.2
1990	**1129.3***	**157.0***	**1270.3***	**292.0**	**386.9**	**563.9**	**940.1**	**1403.4**	**2185.7**	**3119.9**	**4630.6**	**7404.4**	**14529.4**
1995 projected	*1051.9**	*149.7**	*1192.2**	*298.6*	*384.7*	*521.7*	*866.2*	*1314.8*	*2081.7*	*2877.9*	*4226.4*	*6741.4*	*13544.9*
All cancer													
1955	...	...	...	...	...	...	...	...	...	...	...	...	...
1965	233.2*	11.1*	357.5*	38.7	68.5	127.1	244.8	414.7	660.8	947.9	1200.4	1437.5	1673.3
1975	245.1*	10.3*	365.8*	36.6	73.5	150.8	252.9	419.0	671.6	956.0	1302.6	1598.8	1799.6
1985	262.9*	8.9*	382.9*	33.9	70.2	147.4	277.0	478.5	700.2	972.9	1338.4	1743.6	2189.7
1990	**268.0***	**8.2***	**392.1***	**32.9**	**68.1**	**139.0**	**275.9**	**469.8**	**740.9**	**1018.1**	**1357.1**	**1753.6**	**2305.2**
1995 projected	*270.2**	*7.5**	*394.5**	*31.0*	*66.2*	*132.5*	*268.9*	*470.1*	*762.2*	*1030.3*	*1365.0*	*1774.4*	*2381.1*
Lung cancer													
1955	...	...	...	...	...	...	...	...	...	...	...	...	...
1965	52.2*	0.5*	100.0*	5.7	14.0	31.3	68.0	123.1	197.0	261.0	268.0	232.4	163.5
1975	66.0*	0.4*	115.1*	5.7	16.4	42.7	79.5	138.4	221.1	301.7	373.1	376.2	277.7
1985	77.7*	0.4*	129.6*	5.4	16.8	43.3	91.4	170.2	248.5	331.6	413.8	473.9	434.7
1990	**79.6***	**0.4***	**132.7***	**5.6**	**16.0**	**40.5**	**89.9**	**163.7**	**263.5**	**349.4**	**430.8**	**478.8**	**466.1**
1995 projected	*81.3**	*0.4**	*134.6**	*5.4*	*15.9*	*38.2*	*86.8*	*164.4*	*274.3*	*357.4*	*436.0*	*503.6*	*490.6*
Upper aerodigestive cancer (mouth, oesophagus, pharynx and larynx)													
1955	...	...	...	...	...	...	...	...	...	...	...	...	...
1965	19.0*	0.2*	31.2*	2.4	5.4	11.8	22.9	38.5	58.1	79.6	93.9	107.7	127.9
1975	20.1*	0.2*	33.7*	2.4	7.5	17.6	29.2	41.9	59.7	77.8	95.8	112.1	116.2
1985	21.7*	0.2*	38.2*	2.8	8.7	20.1	35.9	55.6	68.0	76.3	90.5	103.8	114.9
1990	**22.9***	**0.2***	**41.7***	**3.0**	**9.4**	**21.4**	**40.0**	**57.7**	**76.6**	**84.0**	**91.2**	**99.4**	**111.5**
1995 projected	*23.9**	*0.2**	*44.7**	*3.1*	*10.7*	*22.9*	*43.2*	*61.9*	*83.6*	*87.8*	*91.6*	*96.7*	*107.4*
Other cancer													
1955	...	...	...	...	...	...	...	...	...	...	...	...	...
1965	161.9*	10.4*	226.2*	30.6	49.1	84.0	153.9	253.1	405.7	607.2	838.5	1097.4	1381.8
1975	159.0*	9.6*	217.0*	28.6	49.6	90.5	144.2	238.8	390.8	576.4	833.7	1110.6	1405.7
1985	163.5*	8.3*	215.1*	25.8	44.7	84.0	149.7	252.7	383.7	565.0	834.1	1165.9	1640.0
1990	**165.5***	**7.6***	**217.7***	**24.3**	**42.6**	**77.1**	**145.9**	**248.4**	**400.8**	**584.8**	**835.2**	**1175.4**	**1727.6**
1995 projected	*165.0**	*6.9**	*215.1**	*22.5*	*39.6*	*71.4*	*138.9*	*243.8*	*404.3*	*585.1*	*837.4*	*1174.1*	*1783.1*
Chronic obstructive pulmonary disease (COPD)													
1955	...	...	...	...	...	...	...	...	...	...	...	...	...
1965	59.3*	1.7*	73.0*	4.8	8.6	16.7	36.5	73.7	141.2	229.2	327.1	467.6	693.6
1975	73.1*	1.7*	78.0*	5.7	11.4	23.1	39.1	72.0	143.1	251.8	431.4	646.9	963.9
1985	62.0*	1.1*	60.8*	3.3	6.8	17.0	34.6	68.5	110.6	185.0	339.3	559.5	937.9
1990	**53.0***	**1.0***	**51.9***	**2.5**	**4.5**	**9.7**	**25.4**	**51.8**	**102.7**	**166.8**	**281.1**	**476.6**	**835.7**
1995 projected	*46.0**	*0.9**	*43.0**	*1.9*	*3.5*	*6.8*	*18.8*	*41.2*	*87.8*	*141.0*	*239.7*	*424.8*	*760.2*
Other respiratory disease													
1955	...	...	...	...	...	...	...	...	...	...	...	...	...
1965	56.9*	22.9*	33.4*	5.3	7.9	12.1	18.6	30.8	56.2	103.1	194.7	369.0	955.7
1975	55.3*	24.7*	31.2*	6.1	9.1	13.5	18.6	30.1	50.5	90.6	182.7	357.3	885.0
1985	50.9*	17.6*	29.4*	5.6	8.0	13.1	19.5	29.0	47.9	82.4	160.5	330.3	955.2
1990	**45.7***	**11.1***	**25.4***	**4.8**	**6.8**	**10.0**	**15.3**	**24.1**	**40.8**	**76.0**	**156.0**	**314.3**	**975.9**
1995 projected	*44.1**	*8.5**	*23.7**	*4.7*	*6.3*	*8.6*	*13.1*	*21.6*	*38.3*	*73.3*	*148.1*	*317.2*	*1012.0*
Vascular disease													
1955	...	...	...	...	...	...	...	...	...	...	...	...	...
1965	620.1*	10.0*	638.1*	58.3	115.9	217.8	387.1	648.3	1140.9	1898.2	3121.1	5012.9	9740.8
1975	602.3*	9.3*	615.6*	64.4	122.0	228.2	385.4	644.8	1090.1	1774.1	2986.5	4864.1	9531.7
1985	548.9*	8.8*	546.5*	55.7	107.1	210.8	358.0	605.8	970.3	1517.4	2651.7	4437.7	8972.9
1990	**478.9***	**8.2***	**495.2***	**54.4**	**102.2**	**175.4**	**329.5**	**528.0**	**904.8**	**1372.1**	**2163.6**	**3764.5**	**7829.2**
1995 projected	*415.0**	*7.4**	*434.8**	*49.8*	*94.6*	*152.2*	*291.3*	*468.1*	*814.0*	*1173.6*	*1834.2*	*3163.4*	*6805.0*
Liver cirrhosis (incl. USSR other liver disease)													
1955	...	...	...	...	...	...	...	...	...	...	...	...	...
1965	22.6*	1.0*	41.2*	8.2	14.9	23.8	37.3	52.0	69.2	83.0	88.3	94.5	86.3
1975	27.1*	1.4*	50.9*	12.1	23.3	36.0	49.9	62.9	79.8	92.5	96.4	97.1	83.3
1985	25.1*	1.3*	47.1*	10.5	19.1	32.0	49.0	62.5	77.2	79.2	86.8	90.5	79.9
1990	**22.0***	**1.1***	**41.6***	**10.1**	**16.9**	**27.7**	**39.8**	**55.3**	**67.7**	**73.7**	**70.5**	**77.3**	**75.9**
1995 projected	*19.5**	*1.0**	*36.8**	*9.6*	*16.0*	*23.9*	*34.2*	*48.7*	*60.3*	*64.9*	*63.8*	*65.4*	*68.8*
Other medical causes													
1955	...	...	...	...	...	...	...	...	...	...	...	...	...
1965	258.8*	97.1*	241.0*	72.7	91.5	120.0	176.9	257.6	389.1	579.3	850.6	1378.7	3138.3
1975	177.9*	69.2*	164.3*	51.9	70.1	97.1	125.0	171.8	254.2	380.1	608.5	962.4	2026.4
1985	157.4*	61.1*	138.5*	48.9	61.6	89.6	113.8	152.3	204.0	299.6	488.1	849.1	1975.9
1990	**153.9***	**53.8***	**136.3***	**59.5**	**67.2**	**81.3**	**109.5**	**142.4**	**199.6**	**294.5**	**463.6**	**819.3**	**2110.8**
1995 projected	*149.9**	*48.1**	*134.5**	*69.5*	*76.4*	*84.6*	*102.8*	*136.2*	*191.6*	*280.4*	*443.7*	*811.0*	*2124.8*
All non-medical causes													
1955	...	...	...	...	...	...	...	...	...	...	...	...	...
1965	111.6*	76.6*	128.6*	125.4	112.7	114.9	128.0	132.5	138.9	147.6	173.1	235.5	456.2
1975	123.3*	83.0*	148.4*	154.0	153.0	163.9	138.4	137.0	143.3	149.4	175.4	231.0	410.8
1985	106.1*	69.6*	127.0*	110.7	116.7	145.5	139.7	140.7	117.2	118.9	153.8	209.4	389.6
1990	**107.7***	**73.7***	**127.8***	**127.7**	**121.1**	**121.0**	**144.7**	**132.0**	**129.2**	**118.6**	**138.6**	**198.7**	**396.8**
1995 projected	*107.1**	*76.2**	*125.0**	*132.0*	*121.8*	*113.1*	*137.0*	*129.1*	*127.7*	*114.4*	*131.8*	*185.2*	*392.9*

ALL 'DEVELOPED' COUNTRIES: Females

	All ages	0–34	35–69	35–39	40–44	45–49	50–54	55–59	60–64	65–69	70–74	75–79	80+/NK
POPULATION (1000s)													
1955	460699	262879	171337	27558	31097	29442	26099	22641	18839	15661	12397	8027	6060
1965	520939	284898	200926	36641	34486	27074	30331	28086	24367	19940	15501	10522	9093
1975	566004	299894	219092	36995	34191	35956	33258	25232	28110	25350	20025	13748	13245
1985	604267	309656	234275	41425	34549	36558	33244	34596	30960	22943	23832	18029	18476
1990	621017	308170	250618	44848	41221	34074	35846	32409	33223	28998	20505	19721	22003
1995 projected	633811	305169	262154	46385	42696	39615	37546	33361	33187	29365	24918	18394	23175
NUMBER OF DEATHS													
All causes													
1955	4011346	651690	1346774	60675	91174	125619	167196	216885	287347	397878	513404	570239	929239
1965	4302004	426403	1379228	60835	82728	97356	164775	224990	316686	431858	560746	675037	1260590
1975	4895907	340230	1421804	53177	72958	119698	167488	191331	335625	481527	660604	793380	1679889
1985	5537698	282686	1339234	48382	60397	105611	148573	243099	340444	392728	706880	928617	2280281
1990	5617855	244415	1375603	50970	68715	87445	148076	205149	340908	474340	540044	914182	2543611
1995 projected	5386830	215171	1311731	50472	67931	93309	142308	194459	318650	444602	596068	774197	2489663
Lung cancer													
1955	...	...	...	...	...	...	...	...	...	...	...	...	...
1965	38000	643	24362	753	1312	2043	3640	4785	5609	6220	5607	4077	3311
1975	62043	561	37957	738	1598	3449	5391	6646	9718	10417	9587	7273	6665
1985	103202	634	55256	899	1689	3690	6261	11219	15515	15983	18247	14600	14465
1990	126486	673	64392	1006	2142	3890	7008	10775	17590	21981	20371	20074	20976
1995 projected	153822	698	72448	1082	2395	4907	8029	12050	18895	25090	28491	24088	28097
ANNUAL DEATH RATE / 100,000 (*The rates for the age groups 0–34 and 35–69 are the means of seven five-yearly rates, but the all-ages rates are standardised to the conventional "European" age distribution)													
All causes													
1955	1039.7*	226.5*	943.5*	220.2	293.2	426.7	640.6	957.9	1525.3	2540.6	4141.3	7104.2	15334.4
1965	880.7*	141.8*	796.5*	166.0	239.9	359.6	543.3	801.1	1299.6	2165.7	3617.5	6415.3	13864.1
1975	794.2*	115.7*	720.8*	143.7	213.4	332.9	503.6	758.3	1194.0	1899.5	3299.0	5770.7	12683.1
1985	725.7*	93.2*	648.8*	116.8	174.8	288.9	446.9	702.7	1099.6	1711.8	2966.2	5150.7	12341.9
1990	666.3*	80.1*	606.4*	113.7	166.7	256.6	413.1	633.0	1026.1	1635.8	2633.7	4635.7	11560.1
1995 projected	612.9*	70.3*	562.8*	108.8	159.1	235.5	379.0	582.9	960.2	1514.1	2392.1	4209.1	10742.8
All cancer													
1955	...	...	...	...	...	...	...	...	...	...	...	...	...
1965	152.9*	9.9*	236.0*	45.5	82.4	134.0	208.1	279.3	383.5	518.9	664.6	854.8	1067.8
1975	145.9*	8.9*	225.7*	40.6	72.6	125.5	195.7	278.0	381.3	486.1	635.6	820.2	1017.9
1985	145.5*	7.9*	220.4*	38.5	66.3	113.0	176.4	266.1	381.8	500.5	657.2	832.5	1127.8
1990	146.0*	7.3*	218.7*	38.1	67.2	110.8	174.1	254.6	370.0	515.9	671.2	851.1	1173.3
1995 projected	145.6*	6.7*	215.1*	37.4	66.7	108.0	168.8	246.7	364.9	512.9	678.7	870.6	1213.1
Lung cancer													
1955	...	...	...	...	...	...	...	...	...	...	...	...	...
1965	7.9*	0.3*	13.8*	2.1	3.8	7.5	12.0	17.0	23.0	31.2	36.2	38.7	36.4
1975	10.8*	0.2*	19.2*	2.0	4.7	9.6	16.2	26.3	34.6	41.1	47.9	52.9	50.3
1985	15.3*	0.2*	26.9*	2.2	4.9	10.1	18.8	32.4	50.1	69.7	76.6	81.0	78.3
1990	17.4*	0.2*	28.6*	2.2	5.2	11.4	19.6	33.2	52.9	75.8	99.3	101.8	95.3
1995 projected	19.9*	0.2*	31.5*	2.3	5.6	12.4	21.4	36.1	56.9	85.4	114.3	131.0	121.2
Upper aerodigestive cancer (mouth, oesophagus, pharynx and larynx)													
1955	...	...	...	...	...	...	...	...	...	...	...	...	...
1965	4.8*	0.1*	6.8*	0.8	1.5	3.0	5.2	8.0	11.9	17.0	23.0	32.8	45.7
1975	4.4*	0.1*	6.5*	0.7	1.6	3.0	5.1	8.3	12.0	14.5	20.2	27.0	38.8
1985	4.0*	0.1*	6.0*	0.5	1.2	2.6	4.5	7.7	10.8	14.8	18.7	24.5	36.4
1990	4.0*	0.1*	5.8*	0.6	1.2	2.5	4.4	7.1	10.9	14.2	19.0	25.3	36.1
1995 projected	4.0*	0.1*	5.8*	0.6	1.3	2.5	4.3	7.0	10.7	14.0	18.5	26.4	36.8
Other cancer													
1955	...	...	...	...	...	...	...	...	...	...	...	...	...
1965	140.2*	9.5*	215.4*	42.6	77.1	123.6	191.0	254.3	348.6	470.7	605.4	783.2	985.7
1975	130.7*	8.6*	200.0*	37.9	66.3	112.9	174.4	243.4	334.8	430.5	567.6	740.3	928.8
1985	126.1*	7.6*	187.5*	35.7	60.3	100.3	153.1	226.0	320.9	416.0	561.9	727.1	1013.1
1990	124.6*	7.0*	184.2*	35.3	60.8	96.9	150.2	214.3	306.2	425.9	552.8	724.0	1041.8
1995 projected	121.7*	6.4*	177.8*	34.5	59.8	93.1	143.2	203.6	297.3	413.4	545.9	713.2	1055.1
Chronic obstructive pulmonary disease (COPD)													
1955	...	...	...	...	...	...	...	...	...	...	...	...	...
1965	22.9*	1.3*	20.0*	1.9	3.1	5.8	10.4	18.4	35.6	64.4	108.8	200.1	399.9
1975	28.1*	1.3*	25.3*	2.9	4.7	8.2	13.6	24.6	45.7	77.5	141.1	237.8	479.0
1985	22.7*	0.9*	22.0*	2.0	3.1	6.7	12.4	23.1	38.6	67.8	116.4	187.7	365.4
1990	19.8*	0.7*	19.4*	1.6	2.4	4.6	10.2	18.9	35.7	62.3	104.4	167.3	309.9
1995 projected	18.4*	0.7*	17.5*	1.3	2.0	3.7	8.7	16.9	32.3	57.7	96.1	161.4	296.3
Other respiratory disease													
1955	...	...	...	...	...	...	...	...	...	...	...	...	...
1965	38.7*	19.5*	16.3*	3.3	4.7	6.3	9.2	14.0	26.2	50.4	107.5	235.2	708.2
1975	36.5*	21.1*	15.0*	3.6	4.5	6.1	8.9	14.8	24.2	43.0	91.9	203.2	626.7
1985	29.4*	14.7*	11.4*	2.4	3.2	4.7	6.9	10.6	18.4	33.6	65.9	149.0	609.3
1990	25.7*	9.1*	10.0*	2.2	2.8	4.1	5.6	9.4	16.0	30.2	65.5	135.6	620.0
1995 projected	24.5*	6.9*	9.4*	2.1	2.7	3.7	5.3	8.8	14.8	28.5	60.8	133.2	643.4
Vascular disease													
1955	...	...	...	...	...	...	...	...	...	...	...	...	...
1965	433.5*	7.8*	331.0*	31.4	53.9	96.2	167.7	294.2	570.7	1103.2	2070.5	3949.7	8687.9
1975	407.2*	5.8*	296.5*	27.2	48.6	86.8	153.1	271.1	517.6	970.8	1922.7	3653.5	8524.3
1985	374.3*	4.7*	258.4*	19.7	36.6	74.6	136.0	251.4	459.3	831.3	1699.9	3257.4	8290.6
1990	322.5*	4.2*	229.1*	17.6	32.5	59.4	117.6	212.7	413.2	751.1	1373.5	2749.1	7242.5
1995 projected	276.6*	3.8*	198.1*	15.2	28.5	49.3	100.0	182.7	364.2	646.9	1142.9	2311.6	6280.4
Liver cirrhosis (incl. USSR other liver disease)													
1955	...	...	...	...	...	...	...	...	...	...	...	...	...
1965	10.1*	0.7*	16.8*	4.3	7.2	11.1	15.1	19.7	26.4	34.1	40.9	49.6	53.0
1975	10.5*	0.7*	18.4*	4.8	8.7	13.1	18.6	24.0	27.9	31.7	38.0	43.4	45.7
1985	10.2*	0.7*	18.1*	4.2	7.2	11.4	17.3	24.5	29.4	32.7	37.3	42.4	41.2
1990	9.3*	0.6*	16.5*	4.0	6.3	9.8	14.8	20.8	26.9	33.0	35.4	40.7	39.9
1995 projected	8.7*	0.6*	15.2*	3.8	6.1	8.7	12.6	18.6	24.9	31.5	34.8	39.1	38.6
Other medical causes													
1955	...	...	...	...	...	...	...	...	...	...	...	...	...
1965	181.4*	80.6*	137.4*	53.0	59.5	72.5	95.1	135.2	211.0	335.3	536.8	968.9	2536.5
1975	122.7*	54.5*	95.1*	32.3	38.5	50.5	69.5	98.9	145.8	230.4	384.0	666.3	1626.0
1985	106.3*	44.2*	78.0*	22.5	27.0	39.8	56.5	82.0	125.8	192.6	315.4	566.7	1617.4
1990	107.5*	38.0*	75.0*	22.9	26.2	35.3	51.5	76.7	119.8	192.7	316.2	582.0	1901.6
1995 projected	105.6*	31.8*	72.6*	23.0	25.9	32.8	47.9	72.6	117.5	189.0	314.2	592.8	2014.8
All non-medical causes													
1955	...	...	...	...	...	...	...	...	...	...	...	...	...
1965	41.2*	22.2*	39.0*	26.7	29.0	33.7	37.7	40.3	46.3	59.3	88.5	157.0	410.7
1975	43.2*	23.4*	44.7*	32.3	35.8	42.6	44.1	47.0	51.5	59.9	85.5	146.3	363.4
1985	37.4*	20.2*	40.5*	27.5	31.5	38.7	41.3	45.0	46.3	53.3	74.1	114.9	290.1
1990	35.5*	20.2*	37.7*	27.3	29.3	32.7	39.3	39.9	44.6	50.6	67.6	109.8	272.9
1995 projected	33.5*	19.8*	34.9*	26.0	27.4	29.4	35.7	36.6	41.5	47.5	64.6	100.4	256.2

ALL 'DEVELOPED' COUNTRIES: 1975

Smoking–attributed deaths (Sm.) and total deaths (Total)

		ALL CAUSES	ALL CANCER	Lung cancer	Upper aero-digestive ca.	Other cancer	COPD	Other respiratory	Vascular disease	Cirrhosis (incl. USSR other liver)	Other medical	Non-medical
Males												
0–34	Sm.	–	–	–	–	–	–	–	–	–	–	–
	Total	604704	30451	1158	604	28689	5122	76536	26186	3772	212600	250037
35–69	Sm.	704015	246766	161571	33304	51891	89806	13856	274061	–	79526	–
	Total	2303311	562462	174585	52853	335024	116005	48494	937190	84787	268376	285997
		(31%)	(44%)	(93%)	(63%)	(15%)	(77%)	(29%)	(29%)		(30%)	
70+	Sm.	414874	130252	85308	14468	30476	108174	11128	137463	–	27857	–
	Total	2434866	409582	95912	28672	284998	168061	107769	1373941	25497	283003	67013
		(17%)	(32%)	(89%)	(50%)	(11%)	(64%)	(10%)	(10%)		(10%)	
Any age	Sm.	1118889	377018	246879	47772	82367	197980	24984	411524	–	107383	–
	Total	5342881	1002495	271655	82129	648711	289188	232799	2337317	114056	763979	603047
		(21%)	(38%)	(91%)	(58%)	(13%)	(68%)	(11%)	(18%)		(14%)	
Females												
0–34	Sm.	–	–	–	–	–	–	–	–	–	–	–
	Total	340230	25340	561	315	24464	3711	62435	16429	1979	160823	69513
35–69	Sm.	98107	27224	20308	2891	4025	15817	2270	40035	–	12761	–
	Total	1421804	450658	37957	12727	399974	48858	29458	568849	37573	190735	95673
		(7%)	(6%)	(54%)	(23%)	(1%)	(32%)	(8%)	(7%)		(7%)	
70+	Sm.	66965	12369	8898	1650	1821	19933	2267	27411	–	4985	–
	Total	3133873	374875	23525	12884	338466	124403	129352	2016358	19634	383875	85376
		(2%)	(3%)	(38%)	(13%)	(1%)	(16%)	(2%)	(1%)		(1%)	
Any age	Sm.	165072	39593	29206	4541	5846	35750	4537	67446	–	17746	–
	Total	4895907	850873	62043	25926	762904	176972	221245	2601636	59186	735433	250562
		(3%)	(5%)	(47%)	(18%)	(1%)	(20%)	(2%)	(3%)		(2%)	
Males+Females												
0–34	Sm.	–	–	–	–	–	–	–	–	–	–	–
	Total	944934	55791	1719	919	53153	8833	138971	42615	5751	373423	319550
35–69	Sm.	802122	273990	181879	36195	55916	105623	16126	314096	–	92287	–
	Total	3725115	1013120	212542	65580	734998	164863	77952	1506039	122360	459111	381670
		(22%)	(27%)	(86%)	(55%)	(8%)	(64%)	(21%)	(21%)		(20%)	
70+	Sm.	481839	142621	94206	16118	32297	128107	13395	164874	–	32842	–
	Total	5568739	784457	119437	41556	623464	292464	237121	3390299	45131	666878	152389
		(9%)	(18%)	(79%)	(39%)	(5%)	(44%)	(6%)	(5%)		(5%)	
Any age	Sm.	1283961	416611	276085	52313	88213	233730	29521	478970	–	125129	–
	Total	10238788	1853368	333698	108055	1411615	466160	454044	4938953	173242	1499412	853609
		(13%)	(22%)	(83%)	(48%)	(6%)	(50%)	(7%)	(10%)		(8%)	

ALL 'DEVELOPED' COUNTRIES: 1985

Smoking–attributed deaths (Sm.) and total deaths (Total)

		ALL CAUSES	ALL CANCER	Lung cancer	Upper aero-digestive ca.	Other cancer	COPD	Other respiratory	Vascular disease	Cirrhosis (incl. USSR other liver)	Other medical	Non-medical
Males												
0–34	Sm.	–	–	–	–	–	–	–	–	–	–	–
	Total	536200	28567	1241	720	26606	3576	54195	28281	4037	190850	226694
35–69	Sm.	805337	311387	201710	45962	63715	79063	16038	309211	–	89638	–
	Total	2303927	644492	215773	67636	361083	97404	49230	904668	87354	251148	269631
		(35%)	(48%)	(93%)	(68%)	(18%)	(81%)	(33%)	(34%)		(36%)	
70+	Sm.	563652	200082	133255	19237	47590	130147	15287	180884	–	37252	–
	Total	2905921	561735	147162	33824	380749	185785	136465	1593069	29032	323068	76767
		(19%)	(36%)	(91%)	(57%)	(12%)	(70%)	(11%)	(11%)		(12%)	
Any age	Sm.	1368989	511469	334965	65199	111305	209210	31325	490095	–	126890	–
	Total	5746048	1234794	364176	102180	768438	286765	239890	2526018	120423	765066	573092
		(24%)	(41%)	(92%)	(64%)	(14%)	(73%)	(13%)	(19%)		(17%)	
Females												
0–34	Sm.	–	–	–	–	–	–	–	–	–	–	–
	Total	282686	24760	634	333	23793	2765	43319	14748	2102	132131	62861
35–69	Sm.	143121	46951	36520	3812	6619	20078	2929	54646	–	18517	–
	Total	1339234	463897	55256	12461	396180	43975	23145	513184	39257	163487	92289
		(11%)	(10%)	(66%)	(31%)	(2%)	(46%)	(13%)	(11%)		(11%)	
70+	Sm.	174321	38219	28242	3978	5999	42332	5916	71715	–	16139	–
	Total	3915778	515084	47312	15587	452185	129091	155136	2524175	24166	476160	91966
		(4%)	(7%)	(60%)	(26%)	(1%)	(33%)	(4%)	(3%)		(3%)	
Any age	Sm.	317442	85170	64762	7790	12618	62410	8845	126361	–	34656	–
	Total	5537698	1003741	103202	28381	872158	175831	221600	3052107	65525	771778	247116
		(6%)	(8%)	(63%)	(27%)	(1%)	(35%)	(4%)	(4%)		(4%)	
Males+Females												
0–34	Sm.	–	–	–	–	–	–	–	–	–	–	–
	Total	818886	53327	1875	1053	50399	6341	97514	43029	6139	322981	289555
35–69	Sm.	948458	358338	238230	49774	70334	99141	18967	363857	–	108155	–
	Total	3643161	1108389	271029	80097	757263	141379	72375	1417852	126611	414635	361920
		(26%)	(32%)	(88%)	(62%)	(9%)	(70%)	(26%)	(26%)		(26%)	
70+	Sm.	737973	238301	161497	23215	53589	172479	21203	252599	–	53391	–
	Total	6821699	1076819	194474	49411	832934	314876	291601	4117244	53198	799228	168733
		(11%)	(22%)	(83%)	(47%)	(6%)	(55%)	(7%)	(6%)		(7%)	
Any age	Sm.	1686431	596639	399727	72989	123923	271620	40170	616456	–	161546	–
	Total	11283746	2238535	467378	130561	1640596	462596	461490	5578125	185948	1536844	820208
		(15%)	(27%)	(86%)	(56%)	(8%)	(59%)	(9%)	(11%)		(11%)	

(To be conservative, no deaths before age 35, and none from liver cirrhosis or non-medical causes, were attributed to smoking.)

ALL 'DEVELOPED' COUNTRIES: 1990

Smoking–attributed deaths (Sm.) and total deaths (Total)

		ALL CAUSES	ALL CANCER	Lung cancer	Upper aero–digestive ca.	Other cancer	COPD	Other respiratory	Vascular disease	Cirrhosis (incl. USSR other liver)	Other medical	Non–medical
Males												
0–34	Sm.	–	–	–	–	–	–	–	–	–	–	–
	Total	504184	26602	1217	696	24689	3110	34418	26877	3521	169359	240297
35–69	Sm.	864710	359606	230509	56011	73086	75760	14574	318020	–	96750	–
	Total	2457923	736143	246388	81445	408310	92895	47541	925592	84422	276249	295081
		(35%)	(49%)	(94%)	(69%)	(18%)	(82%)	(31%)	(34%)		(35%)	
70+	Sm.	554082	212429	141354	19651	51424	122253	16342	163296	–	39762	–
	Total	2850713	599693	155938	34028	409727	171565	150452	1466805	25372	357743	79083
		(19%)	(35%)	(91%)	(58%)	(13%)	(71%)	(11%)	(11%)		(11%)	
Any age	Sm.	1418792	572035	371863	75662	124510	198013	30916	481316	–	136512	–
	Total	5812820	1362438	403543	116169	842726	267570	232411	2419274	113315	803351	614461
		(24%)	(42%)	(92%)	(65%)	(15%)	(74%)	(13%)	(20%)		(17%)	
Females												
0–34	Sm.	–	–	–	–	–	–	–	–	–	–	–
	Total	244415	23100	673	325	22102	2301	26993	13383	1933	113857	62848
35–69	Sm.	159764	55829	43945	4210	7674	21481	3278	57298	–	21878	–
	Total	1375603	500022	64392	13171	422459	42966	22644	507672	38248	172066	91985
		(12%)	(11%)	(68%)	(32%)	(2%)	(50%)	(14%)	(11%)		(13%)	
70+	Sm.	236071	56012	41563	5418	9031	53409	9110	92302	–	25238	–
	Total	3997837	563635	61421	16838	485376	122602	176586	2417382	24053	598028	95551
		(6%)	(10%)	(68%)	(32%)	(2%)	(44%)	(5%)	(4%)		(4%)	
Any age	Sm.	395835	111841	85508	9628	16705	74890	12388	149600	–	47116	–
	Total	5617855	1086757	126486	30334	929937	167869	226223	2938437	64234	883951	250384
		(7%)	(10%)	(68%)	(32%)	(2%)	(45%)	(5%)	(5%)		(5%)	
Males+Females												
0–34	Sm.	–	–	–	–	–	–	–	–	–	–	–
	Total	748599	49702	1890	1021	46791	5411	61411	40260	5454	283216	303145
35–69	Sm.	1024474	415435	274454	60221	80760	97241	17852	375318	–	118628	–
	Total	3833526	1236165	310780	94616	830769	135861	70185	1433264	122670	448315	387066
		(27%)	(34%)	(88%)	(64%)	(10%)	(72%)	(25%)	(26%)		(26%)	
70+	Sm.	790153	268441	182917	25069	60455	175662	25452	255598	–	65000	–
	Total	6848550	1163328	217359	50866	895103	294167	327038	3884187	49425	955771	174634
		(12%)	(23%)	(84%)	(49%)	(7%)	(60%)	(8%)	(7%)		(7%)	
Any age	Sm.	1814627	683876	457371	85290	141215	272903	43304	630916	–	183628	–
	Total	11430675	2449195	530029	146503	1772663	435439	458634	5357711	177549	1687302	864845
		(16%)	(28%)	(86%)	(58%)	(8%)	(63%)	(9%)	(12%)		(11%)	

ALL 'DEVELOPED' COUNTRIES: 1995

Smoking–attributed deaths (Sm.) and total deaths (Total)

		ALL CAUSES	ALL CANCER	Lung cancer	Upper aero–digestive ca.	Other cancer	COPD	Other respiratory	Vascular disease	Cirrhosis (incl. USSR other liver)	Other medical	Non–medical
Males												
0–34	Sm.	–	–	–	–	–	–	–	–	–	–	–
	Total	481866	24274	1252	689	22333	2922	26506	24596	3446	153359	246763
35–69	Sm.	869913	385059	244520	63936	76603	65565	13647	303842	–	101800	–
	Total	2435005	774897	261181	91967	421749	80114	46397	856966	78820	291504	306307
		(36%)	(50%)	(94%)	(70%)	(18%)	(82%)	(29%)	(35%)		(35%)	
70+	Sm.	571618	236396	158031	21304	57061	117070	17957	156434	–	43761	–
	Total	2776715	650891	173720	36008	441163	161022	160753	1324572	24263	374223	80991
		(21%)	(36%)	(91%)	(59%)	(13%)	(73%)	(11%)	(12%)		(12%)	
Any age	Sm.	1441531	621455	402551	85240	133664	182635	31604	460276	–	145561	–
	Total	5693586	1450062	436153	128664	885245	244058	233656	2206134	106529	819086	634061
		(25%)	(43%)	(92%)	(66%)	(15%)	(75%)	(14%)	(21%)		(18%)	
Females												
0–34	Sm.	–	–	–	–	–	–	–	–	–	–	–
	Total	215171	21245	698	317	20230	2139	20638	11900	1880	96240	61129
35–69	Sm.	170586	64630	51442	4576	8612	21748	3572	55649	–	24987	–
	Total	1311731	506018	72448	13405	420165	39525	21776	448081	36258	171354	88719
		(13%)	(13%)	(71%)	(34%)	(2%)	(55%)	(16%)	(12%)		(15%)	
70+	Sm.	304715	79068	59551	6901	12616	65775	12721	110829	–	36322	–
	Total	3859928	610396	80676	17997	511723	122329	188752	2165465	24798	654260	93928
		(8%)	(13%)	(74%)	(38%)	(2%)	(54%)	(7%)	(5%)		(6%)	
Any age	Sm.	475301	143698	110993	11477	21228	87523	16293	166478	–	61309	–
	Total	5386830	1137659	153822	31719	952118	163993	231166	2625446	62936	921854	243776
		(9%)	(13%)	(72%)	(36%)	(2%)	(53%)	(7%)	(6%)		(7%)	
Males+Females												
0–34	Sm.	–	–	–	–	–	–	–	–	–	–	–
	Total	697037	45519	1950	1006	42563	5061	47144	36496	5326	249599	307892
35–69	Sm.	1040499	449689	295962	68512	85215	87313	17219	359491	–	126787	–
	Total	3746736	1280915	333629	105372	841914	119639	68173	1305047	115078	462858	395026
		(28%)	(35%)	(89%)	(65%)	(10%)	(73%)	(25%)	(28%)		(27%)	
70+	Sm.	876333	315464	217582	28205	69677	182845	30678	267263	–	80083	–
	Total	6636643	1261287	254396	54005	952886	283351	349505	3490037	49061	1028483	174919
		(13%)	(25%)	(86%)	(52%)	(7%)	(65%)	(9%)	(8%)		(8%)	
Any age	Sm.	1916832	765153	513544	96717	154892	270158	47897	626754	–	206870	–
	Total	11080416	2587721	589975	160383	1837363	408051	464822	4831580	169465	1740940	877837
		(17%)	(30%)	(87%)	(60%)	(8%)	(66%)	(10%)	(13%)		(12%)	

(To be conservative, no deaths before age 35, and none from liver cirrhosis or non–medical causes, were attributed to smoking.)

¶FORMER SOCIALIST ECONOMIES: 1990

		No. of deaths			Standardised rates (Defined on p.238)			Annual death rates / 100, 000						
		All ages	0–34	35–69	All ages	0–34	35–69	0–4	5–9	10–14	15–19	20–24	25–29	30–34
ALL CAUSES	M	2154134	267906	1123670	1534.7	228.9	1879.1	576.0	61.3	52.6	121.6	200.3	251.4	339.0
	F	2125310	133650	622266	866.3	115.4	805.3	450.0	36.9	28.8	53.6	64.6	72.4	101.5
Tuberculosis	M	22898	2827	17653	14.2	2.5	25.7	0.5	0.1	0.1	0.3	1.8	4.9	9.7
	F	5334	884	2912	2.4	0.8	3.6	0.5	0.1	0.1	0.3	1.2	1.6	1.9
Other infective	M	16198	13286	2298	7.9	10.7	3.5	66.4	2.0	1.4	1.5	1.2	1.2	1.3
and parasitic	F	13835	10994	1850	6.4	9.2	2.3	56.7	1.4	0.9	1.0	1.9	1.5	1.3
ALL CANCER	M	398999	12279	281317	281.3	10.7	483.1	8.6	7.2	5.7	8.6	10.4	13.0	21.4
	F	310178	10663	177029	137.9	9.5	225.4	7.0	5.2	4.4	6.0	7.4	12.4	23.8
Mouth and	M	15797	246	13148	10.6	0.2	21.0	0.1	0.1	0.1	0.2	0.3	0.3	0.5
pharynx cancer	F	3357	135	1668	1.5	0.1	2.1	0.1	0.0	0.0	0.1	0.1	0.2	0.3
Oesophagus cancer	M	14422	55	11015	10.1	0.0	18.5	0.0	0.0	–	0.0	0.1	0.0	0.2
	F	6150	49	2864	2.6	0.0	3.7	0.0	0.0	0.0	0.0	0.0	0.1	0.1
Stomach cancer	M	62906	757	43833	45.0	0.7	75.2	0.0	0.0	0.0	0.2	0.5	1.1	2.8
	F	46234	731	23393	20.0	0.7	30.1	0.0	–	0.0	0.2	0.5	1.2	2.5
Colorectal cancer	M	32739	577	19678	24.4	0.5	35.5	0.3	0.0	0.1	0.2	0.4	0.9	1.7
	F	38579	398	19230	16.6	0.4	24.9	0.2	0.0	0.0	0.1	0.2	0.5	1.4
Liver cancer	M	10881	146	7764	7.8	0.1	13.6	0.2	0.0	0.0	0.1	0.1	0.1	0.3
	F	6919	97	3429	3.0	0.1	4.5	0.1	0.0	0.0	0.0	0.1	0.1	0.2
Pancreas cancer	M	15549	105	9982	11.5	0.1	17.5	0.0	–	0.0	0.0	0.0	0.1	0.5
	F	17390	74	7482	7.3	0.1	9.8	0.0	0.0	0.0	0.0	0.0	0.1	0.2
Larynx cancer	M	14338	55	11846	9.8	0.0	19.5	0.0	–	0.0	0.0	0.0	0.0	0.2
	F	955	19	597	0.4	0.0	0.8	0.0	–	–	0.0	0.0	0.0	0.0
Lung cancer	M	128342	653	100590	89.2	0.6	173.2	0.1	0.0	0.1	0.2	0.5	0.8	2.4
	F	25030	336	14475	11.0	0.3	18.7	0.1	0.0	0.1	0.2	0.2	0.6	1.0
Malignant melanoma	M	3380	252	2374	2.3	0.2	3.7	0.0	0.0	0.0	0.0	0.2	0.4	0.8
	F	3375	210	1893	1.5	0.2	2.3	–	0.0	0.0	0.0	0.2	0.4	0.7
Female breast cancer	F	43403	936	30612	20.4	0.8	38.1	0.0	0.0	0.0	0.0	0.2	1.2	4.3
Cervix cancer	F	16883	672	10956	7.8	0.6	13.7	0.0	–	–	0.0	0.2	0.9	3.0
Other uterine cancer	F	14535	225	8847	6.5	0.2	11.3	0.0	0.0	0.0	0.1	0.1	0.4	0.8
Ovarian cancer	F	18700	341	11788	8.5	0.3	14.9	–	–	0.1	0.2	0.3	0.5	1.0
Prostate cancer	M	15706	48	5988	12.9	0.0	12.1	0.0	–	–	0.0	0.1	0.1	0.1
Bladder cancer	M	11272	39	5385	8.9	0.0	10.2	0.1	0.0	0.0	–	0.0	0.0	0.1
	F	5159	13	1581	2.1	0.0	2.1	–	–	–	0.0	0.0	0.0	0.1
Other and ill-defined	M	52515	4816	37307	35.3	4.2	62.4	3.9	2.7	2.1	3.6	4.4	5.2	7.4
cancer sites	F	46179	3353	28908	21.0	3.0	36.6	3.3	2.2	2.0	2.5	2.4	3.5	5.0
Hodgkin's disease	M	1787	414	1108	1.1	0.4	1.7	0.0	0.1	0.1	0.2	0.5	0.6	1.0
	F	1304	263	640	0.6	0.2	0.8	0.0	0.0	0.1	0.2	0.4	0.5	0.5
Myeloma and non-	M	8505	1431	5489	5.5	1.2	9.1	1.0	1.2	1.0	1.3	1.3	1.4	1.4
Hodgkin lymphomas	F	6547	842	3784	3.0	0.8	4.8	0.8	0.6	0.5	0.7	1.1	0.7	0.9
Leukaemia	M	10849	2681	5806	7.0	2.3	9.8	2.8	3.0	2.2	2.4	1.9	1.9	2.1
	F	9464	1961	4875	4.3	1.7	6.2	2.3	2.2	1.5	1.6	1.4	1.4	1.7
ALL VASCULAR	M	979142	14485	469031	767.5	12.7	828.8	5.1	1.0	1.5	5.6	9.9	19.7	45.8
DISEASE	F	1308654	6246	291202	511.9	5.6	386.5	4.4	1.0	1.3	3.7	5.9	8.4	14.3
Rheumatic heart	M	11225	1162	9053	7.0	1.0	13.6	0.1	0.1	0.2	0.7	1.1	2.0	2.9
disease and fever	F	16378	1004	12701	7.8	0.9	15.8	0.1	0.1	0.2	0.8	1.0	1.6	2.4
Hypertensive disease	M	26677	305	14264	20.5	0.3	25.3	0.1	0.0	0.1	0.1	0.2	0.4	1.0
	F	38909	164	13366	15.9	0.1	17.5	0.1	0.0	0.0	0.1	0.2	0.2	0.5
Ischaemic heart	M	481643	5822	259642	368.8	5.1	449.4	0.0	0.0	0.1	0.8	2.6	7.4	24.6
disease	F	548640	1139	120791	214.2	1.0	161.4	0.1	0.0	0.0	0.4	1.0	1.8	3.8
Pulmonary embolism	M	7551	230	3887	5.8	0.2	6.8	0.1	0.0	0.0	0.1	0.2	0.4	0.6
and other venous	F	12004	221	3861	4.9	0.2	5.0	0.0	–	0.0	0.1	0.3	0.3	0.6
Cerebrovascular	M	266571	2774	119067	212.3	2.4	218.3	1.0	0.2	0.4	1.4	2.4	3.9	7.8
disease	F	447011	1623	105611	175.6	1.5	140.3	0.8	0.3	0.4	1.0	1.7	2.2	3.9
Other vascular	M	185468	4190	63115	153.1	3.7	115.3	3.8	0.6	0.7	2.5	3.4	5.6	8.9
disease	F	245710	2092	34872	93.5	1.9	46.5	3.3	0.6	0.6	1.3	1.7	2.4	3.1
Chronic obstructive	M	106300	1773	52615	82.7	1.5	96.4	2.8	0.4	0.5	1.0	1.3	1.8	3.1
pulmonary disease	F	71145	1350	19980	28.5	1.2	26.2	2.2	0.3	0.4	0.7	1.2	1.6	2.0
Other respiratory	M	53239	29824	13608	31.0	24.0	22.2	151.2	3.9	2.1	2.4	2.3	2.2	3.8
disease	F	40818	23895	5460	18.0	20.0	7.0	127.8	3.5	2.0	1.7	1.7	1.8	1.6
Peptic ulcer	M	10930	429	7467	7.7	0.4	12.4	0.0	0.0	0.0	0.2	0.3	0.7	1.5
	F	5176	99	2173	2.2	0.1	2.8	0.0	0.0	0.0	0.1	0.1	0.1	0.3
Liver cirrhosis (incl.	M	39770	1824	30937	26.7	1.6	50.1	1.3	0.4	0.5	0.8	0.9	2.0	5.2
USSR other liver)	F	26000	1057	16437	11.8	0.9	20.8	0.8	0.3	0.4	0.6	1.0	1.2	2.2
Renal disease	M	18428	2070	10567	12.9	1.8	17.4	1.2	0.6	0.6	1.2	2.6	3.0	3.7
	F	19277	1672	10736	8.6	1.5	13.6	1.1	0.4	0.6	1.3	2.0	2.1	3.1
Pregnancy and birth	F	2410	1718	692	1.1	1.6	0.7	–	–	–	1.0	3.5	2.9	3.7
Congenital and	M	44938	44253	624	20.2	35.4	0.8	238.4	2.8	1.8	1.7	1.3	1.1	1.0
perinatal causes	F	31817	31101	637	14.8	26.0	0.7	173.2	2.7	1.7	1.4	1.2	0.8	0.8
Ill-defined causes	M	60932	6050	18252	48.9	5.1	27.8	14.3	0.8	0.8	2.3	3.9	5.7	8.3
	F	100938	3315	6652	37.5	2.9	8.5	12.2	0.7	0.5	1.1	1.7	1.7	2.2
Other medical causes	M	85381	15466	47018	57.4	13.2	76.4	31.3	7.1	6.2	8.8	9.4	11.3	18.1
	F	86573	11409	39918	37.9	10.0	50.9	24.1	5.8	5.2	6.8	8.2	8.9	11.3
ALL NON-	M	316975	123338	172286	176.5	109.3	234.6	54.9	35.1	31.4	87.3	155.0	184.9	216.3
MEDICAL CAUSES	F	103150	29245	46586	47.2	26.1	56.3	40.1	15.5	11.4	27.8	27.5	27.3	33.1
Motor vehicle	M	69300	34224	31373	37.0	30.6	42.6	6.8	11.6	8.7	29.8	53.5	52.2	51.9
traffic accidents	F	19737	7603	8374	9.1	6.9	10.1	4.7	6.3	4.1	10.1	8.5	6.9	7.6
Fire	M	6299	2455	3133	3.6	2.1	4.4	4.7	1.0	0.7	1.1	1.8	2.3	3.0
	F	3847	1343	1230	1.7	1.2	1.5	3.7	1.0	0.4	0.6	0.8	0.8	0.8
Suicide	M	61169	18846	36996	35.4	16.9	51.3	–	0.1	3.3	14.6	23.4	33.8	42.7
	F	18733	3676	10587	8.7	3.4	12.9	–	0.0	0.8	5.3	5.8	5.3	6.6
Homicide	M	26864	12716	13256	14.1	11.4	16.9	1.0	0.5	0.9	7.7	18.9	23.9	26.9
	F	9016	2973	4876	4.3	2.7	5.7	1.2	0.6	0.7	2.3	3.3	5.0	5.8
POPULATION (thousands): M=males					194921	115123	72326	17902	17440	16660	15787	14578	16102	16655
F=females					213497	111784	84204	17171	16821	16100	15159	14122	15865	16546

FORMER SOCIALIST ECONOMIES: 1990

Annual death rates / 100, 000 — 9th ICD categories

35–39	40–44	45–49	50–54	55–59	60–64	65–69	70–74	75–79	80+/NK			
455.8	670.5	953.4	1461.2	2082.7	3129.5	4400.7	6221.6	9316.7	16925.4	M	ALL CAUSES	001–999
149.1	236.1	344.6	536.5	824.8	1326.0	2220.2	3615.5	6136.4	14038.2	F		
15.0	19.0	24.1	29.7	30.0	31.4	30.3	31.9	31.1	34.8	M	Tuberculosis	010–018, 137
2.6	2.2	2.7	3.3	4.0	4.4	5.8	7.4	8.9	10.1	F		
1.8	2.1	2.5	3.3	4.0	5.0	6.1	6.4	7.5	11.7	M	Other infective	Rest of 001–139
1.1	1.5	1.7	1.9	2.5	3.3	4.1	3.8	5.7	7.6	F	and parasitic	
43.0	97.1	196.4	376.2	605.8	906.6	1156.5	1355.5	1489.1	1383.2	M	ALL CANCER	140–208
44.7	81.7	122.5	184.3	257.5	373.5	513.2	629.8	729.9	737.8	F		
2.4	7.8	15.4	23.4	28.3	34.4	35.1	31.9	31.2	33.7	M	Mouth and	140–149
0.4	0.8	1.2	1.5	2.6	3.4	5.0	5.8	8.6	12.4	F	pharynx cancer	
0.7	3.3	8.8	16.9	25.3	35.9	38.7	41.9	46.2	47.2	M	Oesophagus cancer	150
0.2	0.5	1.5	2.5	4.2	7.3	9.9	14.2	18.5	22.9	F		
6.9	15.5	29.3	58.4	93.3	143.3	180.0	231.6	267.4	234.5	M	Stomach cancer	151
5.1	8.8	12.7	21.4	30.9	53.3	78.3	111.7	138.5	127.8	F		
2.9	5.9	11.4	22.0	37.1	65.4	103.5	140.8	183.8	181.4	M	Colorectal cancer	153, 154
3.0	5.8	9.9	17.8	27.5	43.3	66.8	88.4	113.5	122.8	F		
0.9	1.8	4.1	8.5	19.1	26.7	34.0	38.6	40.4	40.5	M	Liver cancer	155.0
0.4	0.7	1.3	2.5	5.0	8.8	12.4	16.4	20.0	21.8	F		
1.4	3.5	6.8	12.3	20.2	32.3	46.1	61.5	75.5	86.0	M	Pancreas cancer	157
0.7	1.5	3.1	5.8	10.9	18.1	28.4	40.2	55.6	73.2	F		
1.5	5.2	10.6	18.7	27.2	35.4	37.8	37.0	32.9	26.1	M	Larynx cancer	161
0.1	0.3	0.4	0.6	1.0	1.3	1.7	1.9	1.6	2.3	F		
7.9	24.5	62.8	135.7	234.7	342.5	404.3	418.7	377.8	264.7	M	Lung cancer	162
2.1	4.2	8.0	13.2	21.8	33.4	47.9	58.5	63.1	52.9	F		
1.4	1.9	2.7	3.4	4.4	5.7	6.6	8.5	9.6	12.9	M	Malignant melanoma	172
1.1	1.6	2.0	2.2	2.6	3.2	3.8	5.2	6.6	10.1	F		
10.4	21.9	31.8	42.0	45.4	54.0	60.9	62.2	65.9	75.5	F	Female breast cancer	174
5.2	8.3	9.8	11.7	14.6	19.7	26.9	31.1	32.0	26.7	F	Cervix cancer	180
1.7	3.1	5.4	8.6	13.9	19.5	26.9	30.6	33.3	29.6	F	Other uterine cancer	179, 182
2.2	5.0	9.5	14.2	18.8	24.6	30.1	34.7	38.2	39.6	F	Ovarian cancer	183
0.2	0.3	1.2	3.3	9.2	22.6	48.2	84.4	140.0	178.0	M	Prostate cancer	185
0.2	0.7	1.9	4.5	10.1	20.1	34.3	51.9	78.7	114.4	M	Bladder cancer	188
0.1	0.3	0.4	0.9	2.1	3.8	7.1	11.0	18.7	32.0	F		
11.3	19.3	32.0	52.7	72.9	107.5	140.8	151.5	146.2	112.4	M	Other and ill-defined	Rest of 140–208
8.0	13.9	19.1	30.7	43.3	61.1	80.3	88.0	85.9	63.7	F	cancer sites	
1.1	1.1	1.1	1.5	1.9	2.2	2.8	2.8	4.6	3.2	M	Hodgkin's disease	201
0.6	0.6	0.5	0.5	0.8	1.1	1.5	1.9	2.5	2.5	F		
1.7	3.2	3.9	7.9	11.0	16.0	20.0	24.3	21.0	17.2	M	Myeloma and non-	200, 202–203
1.2	1.6	2.2	3.8	5.6	7.8	11.5	12.3	11.2	9.3	F	Hodgkin lymphomas	
2.4	3.2	4.3	6.9	11.1	16.4	24.5	30.0	33.6	31.1	M	Leukaemia	204–208
2.2	2.8	3.8	4.5	6.6	9.8	13.6	15.8	16.2	12.8	F		
96.5	196.6	322.3	550.8	867.0	1468.5	2299.6	3626.6	5962.1	11704.7	M	ALL VASCULAR	390–459
26.4	55.7	99.9	191.0	357.5	673.0	1302.0	2410.8	4452.9	10721.0	F	DISEASE	
5.0	7.7	11.2	16.3	19.4	17.8	17.6	16.2	12.2	11.4	M	Rheumatic heart	390–398
3.9	6.2	11.3	18.3	22.7	23.6	24.3	17.8	15.6	12.2	F	disease and fever	
2.3	5.5	9.7	16.6	29.4	43.0	70.5	93.4	154.9	267.1	M	Hypertensive disease	401–405
1.1	3.1	6.0	11.6	20.1	28.5	52.2	80.6	128.4	229.8	F		
56.5	120.7	195.5	331.7	488.7	796.5	1156.3	1717.6	2635.9	4869.6	M	Ischaemic heart	410–414
7.6	17.7	32.9	66.9	141.4	291.5	571.8	1067.3	1902.6	4446.3	F	disease	
1.1	1.7	2.9	4.0	7.3	11.9	18.9	27.4	45.3	72.5	M	Pulmonary embolism	415.1, 451–453
0.9	1.4	2.2	3.1	4.9	8.2	14.7	21.1	39.0	77.2	F	and other venous	
15.6	33.6	61.3	118.4	215.8	414.2	669.3	1114.2	1812.8	3246.0	M	Cerebrovascular	430–438
7.5	17.8	33.9	68.9	129.8	249.5	474.4	875.9	1577.3	3444.3	F	disease	
15.9	27.5	41.6	63.7	106.3	185.0	367.0	657.8	1301.0	3238.0	M	Other vascular	Rest of 390–459
5.4	9.6	13.6	22.3	38.7	71.6	164.5	348.1	790.1	2511.2	F	disease	
5.0	10.3	22.9	52.9	105.8	188.5	289.1	441.5	679.2	1067.6	M	Chronic obstructive	490–496
2.8	4.5	7.6	14.8	26.5	45.5	82.0	140.5	241.4	481.1	F	pulmonary disease	
6.1	10.0	15.3	19.6	24.6	32.1	47.6	68.8	118.8	234.6	M	Other respiratory	Rest of 460–519
2.1	2.8	4.0	4.7	7.4	10.4	17.7	29.3	49.2	121.0	F	disease	
2.7	4.5	7.0	10.3	13.8	20.7	27.6	32.6	41.5	50.5	M	Peptic ulcer	531–533
0.4	0.8	1.2	2.0	2.9	4.3	8.2	10.8	16.3	22.8	F		
11.1	20.8	33.7	44.5	61.5	81.1	98.0	95.8	95.1	89.3	M	Liver cirrhosis (incl.	571
4.4	7.6	11.8	18.2	26.7	33.3	43.5	44.7	49.6	51.5	F	USSR other liver)	
5.1	7.2	9.6	14.5	19.3	26.5	39.5	52.7	79.6	109.3	M	Renal disease	580–590
3.9	5.2	7.3	10.8	15.2	22.1	30.8	33.6	39.1	45.3	F		
3.2	1.4	0.1	0.0	0.0	0.0	0.0	–	–	–	F	Pregnancy and birth	630–676
0.8	1.0	0.6	1.1	1.0	0.6	0.8	0.5	0.6	1.6	M	Congenital and	740–779
0.8	0.8	0.8	0.9	0.8	0.6	0.6	0.4	0.5	0.5	F	perinatal causes	
13.0	18.1	23.1	27.6	31.5	36.7	44.7	89.7	255.7	1358.5	M	Ill-defined causes	780–799
2.9	4.6	5.3	6.6	9.0	11.2	19.6	59.5	209.4	1339.6	F		
26.2	37.1	48.7	61.5	81.6	113.6	166.2	215.1	307.5	432.0	M	Other medical causes	Rest of 001–799
14.2	19.5	26.9	37.5	55.4	80.7	122.2	154.6	201.8	249.0	F		
229.4	246.6	247.1	269.3	236.9	218.2	194.7	204.5	249.0	447.5	M	ALL NON-	E800–E999
39.8	47.7	53.0	60.4	59.2	63.8	70.6	90.3	131.6	251.0	F	MEDICAL CAUSES	
47.2	45.4	41.6	44.9	42.2	38.0	38.6	38.2	47.0	68.9	M	Motor vehicle	E810–E819
8.0	8.6	8.8	10.4	10.2	11.5	13.2	18.1	22.9	23.5	F	traffic accidents	
3.5	3.9	4.4	4.9	4.7	5.0	4.9	6.0	8.8	15.4	M	Fire	E890–E899
0.9	1.1	1.2	1.2	1.7	1.9	2.6	3.9	6.6	11.6	F		
46.2	50.4	54.9	56.0	51.5	51.5	48.3	57.4	67.7	95.5	M	Suicide	E950–E959
7.9	9.7	12.2	13.5	13.2	16.1	17.8	21.0	24.8	31.1	F		
25.3	23.9	17.8	17.2	13.2	11.9	8.9	8.7	8.4	21.0	M	Homicide	E960–E969
6.9	7.4	5.8	5.9	4.7	4.8	4.3	5.5	5.7	8.9	F		
15356	11974	9238	11974	9520	9098	5167	2796	2666	2010	M	**POPULATION (thousands)**	
15486	12326	9946	13476	11272	12439	9259	5750	6191	5568	F		

FORMER SOCIALIST ECONOMIES: Males

	All ages	0–34	35–69	35–39	40–44	45–49	50–54	55–59	60–64	65–69	70–74	75–79	80+/NK
POPULATION (1000s)													
1955	132457	91081	37644	6061	7490	7338	5878	4632	3532	2713	1923	1097	712
1965	155967	101582	49347	12681	8722	5760	7031	6617	4980	3557	2447	1507	1085
1975	172766	104595	61120	13721	11671	11739	7882	4835	6020	5252	3501	1977	1572
1985	187276	113868	65214	12355	9605	12720	10395	10323	6179	3638	3965	2509	1720
1990	**194921**	**115123**	**72326**	**15356**	**11974**	**9238**	**11974**	**9520**	**9098**	**5167**	**2796**	**2666**	**2010**
1995 projected	*200868*	*117718*	*75202*	*15577*	*12876*	*10277*	*11950*	*9563*	*9384*	*5575*	*3518*	*2360*	*2071*
NUMBER OF DEATHS													
All causes													
1955	1265408	395189	524380	30489	45474	63460	77498	91300	101768	114391	119174	97741	128924
1965	1283269	281849	576814	52171	43485	38981	76939	103712	127395	134131	135226	125550	163830
1975	1740461	299809	826398	70176	77330	113729	98641	90863	169613	206046	208674	174973	230607
1985	2105878	301442	980043	58249	63992	129189	152924	223517	192653	159519	260737	254004	309652
1990	**2154131**	**267907**	**1123669**	**69999**	**80281**	**88072**	**174972**	**198263**	**284712**	**227370**	**173968**	**248386**	**340201**
1995 projected	*2129583*	*245809*	*1143042*	*70015*	*83320*	*95687*	*169761*	*195308*	*291085*	*237866*	*205096*	*206352*	*329284*
Lung cancer													
1955	...	...	...	...	...	...	...	...	...	...	...	...	...
1965	48359	539	37672	834	1314	1882	5535	8635	10243	9229	6021	2859	1268
1975	72269	518	53660	966	2376	6349	7258	7910	14087	14714	10633	5263	2195
1985	106762	684	78920	927	2447	7965	13379	23252	18378	12572	14615	8647	3896
1990	**128342**	**653**	**100590**	**1219**	**2936**	**5801**	**16244**	**22346**	**31157**	**20887**	**11707**	**10072**	**5320**
1995 projected	*145830*	*640*	*112799*	*1184*	*3073*	*6481*	*16712*	*24052*	*35968*	*25329*	*16037*	*10257*	*6097*
ANNUAL DEATH RATE / 100,000													
All causes													
1955	1591.1*	386.0*	1766.0*	503.0	607.2	864.8	1318.4	1971.0	2881.6	4215.7	6198.1	8906.6	18109.2
1965	1337.4*	273.0*	1511.1*	411.4	498.6	676.8	1094.3	1567.3	2558.3	3771.2	5526.2	8332.2	15100.0
1975	1450.0*	293.2*	1716.3*	511.5	662.6	968.8	1251.5	1879.3	2817.5	3923.0	5960.1	8851.1	14665.5
1985	1608.6*	257.3*	1898.9*	471.5	666.3	1015.6	1471.2	2165.2	3118.1	4384.7	6576.2	10122.0	18005.8
1990	**1534.7***	**228.9***	**1879.1***	**455.8**	**670.5**	**953.4**	**1461.2**	**2082.7**	**3129.5**	**4400.7**	**6221.6**	**9316.7**	**16925.3**
1995 projected	*1463.4**	*207.2**	*1837.0**	*449.5*	*647.1*	*931.1*	*1420.5*	*2042.4*	*3102.0*	*4266.7*	*5829.2*	*8745.5*	*15900.2*
All cancer													
1955	...	...	...	...	...	...	...	...	...	...	...	...	...
1965	227.1*	11.2*	390.2*	44.6	79.5	148.1	298.5	459.5	726.0	975.3	1127.8	1179.6	1063.3
1975	231.1*	11.5*	399.7*	44.6	89.9	187.6	296.3	499.2	744.8	935.4	1136.9	1205.5	961.7
1985	262.8*	11.0*	449.2*	44.2	93.7	194.0	353.1	593.4	820.1	1045.7	1258.6	1406.0	1253.8
1990	**281.3***	**10.7***	**483.1***	**43.0**	**97.1**	**196.4**	**376.2**	**605.8**	**906.6**	**1156.5**	**1355.5**	**1489.1**	**1383.2**
1995 projected	*297.0**	*9.8**	*511.5**	*41.9*	*97.1*	*201.5*	*388.5*	*635.9*	*976.2*	*1239.4*	*1422.5*	*1610.2*	*1483.8*
Lung cancer													
1955	...	...	...	...	...	...	...	...	...	...	...	...	...
1965	51.6*	0.6*	104.1*	6.6	15.1	32.7	78.7	130.5	205.7	259.5	246.1	189.7	116.9
1975	62.4*	0.6*	121.6*	7.0	20.4	54.1	92.1	163.6	234.0	280.1	303.7	266.2	139.6
1985	80.7*	0.6*	156.1*	7.5	25.5	62.6	128.7	225.2	297.4	345.6	368.6	344.6	226.5
1990	**89.2***	**0.6***	**173.2***	**7.9**	**24.5**	**62.8**	**135.7**	**234.7**	**342.5**	**404.3**	**418.7**	**377.8**	**264.7**
1995 projected	*97.4**	*0.6**	*189.1**	*7.6*	*23.9*	*63.1*	*139.8*	*251.5*	*383.3*	*454.3*	*455.8*	*434.7*	*294.4*
Upper aerodigestive cancer (mouth, oesophagus, pharynx and larynx)													
1955	...	...	...	...	...	...	...	...	...	...	...	...	...
1965	20.9*	0.3*	34.3*	3.3	6.6	14.8	26.3	39.2	62.7	87.4	108.1	120.8	128.0
1975	20.9*	0.3*	36.2*	3.2	9.3	20.2	32.5	47.4	63.1	77.7	92.9	107.6	103.8
1985	26.2*	0.3*	48.7*	4.6	12.8	26.7	45.4	70.8	85.6	94.9	100.9	109.3	110.2
1990	**30.5***	**0.3***	**59.0***	**4.6**	**16.3**	**34.8**	**59.0**	**80.8**	**105.7**	**111.5**	**110.9**	**110.4**	**106.9**
1995 projected	*35.0**	*0.3**	*69.6**	*5.2*	*20.0*	*43.3*	*72.3*	*95.9*	*124.5*	*126.4*	*114.3*	*117.7*	*106.6*
Other cancer													
1955	...	...	...	...	...	...	...	...	...	...	...	...	...
1965	154.6*	10.3*	251.8*	34.7	57.8	100.7	193.5	289.8	457.6	628.4	773.6	869.1	818.4
1975	147.8*	10.5*	241.9*	34.4	60.2	113.3	171.6	288.2	447.7	577.5	740.3	831.7	718.3
1985	156.0*	10.1*	244.4*	32.1	55.4	104.7	179.0	297.4	437.0	605.2	789.1	952.1	917.0
1990	**161.6***	**9.8***	**250.9***	**30.5**	**56.3**	**98.8**	**181.5**	**290.2**	**458.4**	**640.7**	**825.9**	**1000.9**	**1011.6**
1995 projected	*164.7**	*8.9**	*252.8**	*29.1*	*53.2*	*95.2*	*176.4*	*288.5*	*468.4*	*658.7*	*852.3*	*1057.8*	*1082.8*
Chronic obstructive pulmonary disease (COPD)													
1955	...	...	...	...	...	...	...	...	...	...	...	...	...
1965	88.4*	1.9*	106.9*	8.4	15.2	30.5	60.8	109.2	200.6	323.5	467.1	728.6	1063.5
1975	112.3*	2.2*	126.8*	10.6	22.8	43.8	73.2	132.9	235.0	369.1	616.7	924.9	1457.0
1985	105.3*	1.9*	117.8*	7.9	17.6	36.7	76.5	137.2	217.6	331.3	543.9	871.2	1423.8
1990	**82.7***	**1.5***	**96.4***	**5.0**	**10.3**	**22.9**	**52.9**	**105.8**	**188.5**	**289.1**	**441.5**	**679.2**	**1067.6**
1995 projected	*65.9**	*1.3**	*77.8**	*3.6*	*7.3*	*15.9*	*39.4*	*82.1*	*158.9*	*237.4*	*333.9*	*566.9*	*846.5*
Other respiratory disease													
1955	...	...	...	...	...	...	...	...	...	...	...	...	...
1965	47.3*	42.3*	24.4*	4.5	6.7	9.4	15.4	23.5	43.6	67.6	113.8	175.3	402.0
1975	59.6*	58.0*	31.8*	9.1	13.1	18.4	22.4	33.2	51.2	75.3	129.2	218.7	360.5
1985	47.0*	40.1*	31.3*	10.0	15.0	21.3	28.9	35.1	48.1	60.9	95.6	167.8	318.7
1990	**31.0***	**24.0***	**22.2***	**6.1**	**10.0**	**15.3**	**19.6**	**24.6**	**32.1**	**47.6**	**68.8**	**118.8**	**234.6**
1995 projected	*23.5**	*17.4**	*17.3**	*4.8*	*7.7*	*11.7*	*14.8*	*19.3*	*25.3*	*37.1*	*60.8*	*81.3*	*188.2*
Vascular disease													
1955	...	...	...	...	...	...	...	...	...	...	...	...	...
1965	567.5*	12.1*	535.3*	58.3	99.8	166.1	314.8	511.4	972.8	1624.2	2811.5	4773.7	9633.5
1975	671.3*	13.6*	696.8*	94.1	156.6	277.0	433.3	723.6	1248.8	1944.3	3306.1	5463.6	10262.6
1985	827.0*	13.1*	840.8*	102.3	186.0	330.0	543.5	889.9	1492.7	2341.3	3941.5	6668.9	13296.6
1990	**767.5***	**12.7***	**828.8***	**96.5**	**196.6**	**322.3**	**550.8**	**867.0**	**1468.5**	**2299.6**	**3626.6**	**5962.1**	**11704.7**
1995 projected	*706.5**	*11.4**	*792.6**	*93.4*	*191.0*	*317.9*	*537.8*	*838.2*	*1420.3*	*2149.5*	*3276.2*	*5300.9*	*10471.0*
Liver cirrhosis (incl. USSR other liver disease)													
1955	...	...	...	...	...	...	...	...	...	...	...	...	...
1965	15.4*	1.2*	24.8*	5.7	9.1	12.6	22.2	29.1	42.3	52.8	66.1	74.9	93.6
1975	21.6*	1.6*	38.9*	9.8	16.0	26.0	38.2	51.6	62.1	68.4	76.5	81.3	81.8
1985	29.8*	1.8*	56.6*	13.8	23.2	34.7	52.0	69.3	98.9	104.6	101.6	105.7	93.3
1990	**26.7***	**1.6***	**50.1***	**11.1**	**20.8**	**33.7**	**44.5**	**61.5**	**81.1**	**98.0**	**95.8**	**95.1**	**89.3**
1995 projected	*25.0**	*1.5**	*46.4**	*10.5*	*20.2*	*32.9*	*40.9*	*56.2*	*73.3*	*90.7*	*92.2*	*89.1*	*86.9*
Other medical causes													
1955	...	...	...	...	...	...	...	...	...	...	...	...	...
1965	260.1*	106.7*	269.9*	96.2	121.6	149.0	214.5	286.4	432.6	589.2	797.6	1227.4	2556.9
1975	172.0*	87.9*	178.6*	72.9	92.8	125.9	151.9	201.8	264.2	340.7	500.3	734.3	1235.8
1985	172.0*	92.8*	179.8*	85.7	107.6	140.3	166.9	200.6	246.0	311.3	427.4	647.2	1227.8
1990	**169.1***	**69.1***	**164.0***	**64.7**	**89.1**	**115.6**	**148.1**	**181.1**	**234.5**	**315.2**	**428.8**	**723.4**	**1998.4**
1995 projected	*163.7**	*51.5**	*151.5**	*51.2*	*74.6*	*103.7*	*127.3*	*165.5*	*224.5*	*313.7*	*441.6*	*854.3*	*2341.2*
All non-medical causes													
1955	...	...	...	...	...	...	...	...	...	...	...	...	...
1965	131.6*	97.6*	159.6*	193.7	166.6	161.1	168.1	148.3	140.5	138.5	142.4	172.7	287.1
1975	182.2*	118.4*	243.7*	270.3	271.3	289.9	236.3	237.0	211.3	189.8	194.3	222.7	306.1
1985	164.6*	96.6*	223.3*	207.6	223.1	258.4	250.2	239.6	194.7	189.7	207.7	255.2	391.7
1990	**176.5***	**109.3***	**234.6***	**229.4**	**246.6**	**247.1**	**269.3**	**236.9**	**218.2**	**194.7**	**204.5**	**249.0**	**447.5**
1995 projected	*181.8**	*114.3**	*240.1**	*244.1*	*249.3*	*247.5*	*271.9*	*245.2*	*223.6*	*198.9*	*202.0*	*242.8*	*482.6*

(*The rates for the age groups 0–34 and 35–69 are the means of seven five-yearly rates, but the all-ages rates are standardised to the conventional "European" age distribution)

FORMER SOCIALIST ECONOMIES: Females

	All ages	0–34	35–69	35–39	40–44	45–49	50–54	55–59	60–64	65–69	70–74	75–79	80+/NK
POPULATION (1000s)													
1955	156824	93653	55311	8649	10625	10034	8753	7175	5578	4498	3853	2354	1653
1965	178157	99369	68509	14111	11709	8457	10290	9553	8111	6279	4725	2999	2555
1975	193281	101399	77154	14173	12244	13799	11220	7533	9606	8579	6776	4186	3766
1985	207033	110631	78126	12514	10122	13863	11673	13099	10166	6689	7985	5551	4740
1990	**213497**	**111784**	**84204**	**15486**	**12326**	**9946**	**13476**	**11272**	**12439**	**9259**	**5750**	**6191**	**5568**
1995 projected	*219514*	*114234*	*86818*	*15665*	*13186*	*10938*	*13408*	*11343*	*12648*	*9630*	*6941*	*5774*	*5747*
NUMBER OF DEATHS													
All causes													
1955	1325752	297515	453408	22667	33780	46323	59414	74837	92452	123935	156241	157663	260925
1965	1294192	180752	452079	25090	28982	29200	56027	74349	104224	134207	160651	189639	311071
1975	1699786	170631	548370	25140	30113	51626	63179	64615	131099	182598	243035	263966	473784
1985	2129873	164154	577559	21092	24229	52141	67455	116725	145204	150713	306258	374662	707240
1990	**2125311**	**133653**	**622265**	**23096**	**29107**	**34273**	**72301**	**92969**	**164947**	**205572**	**207905**	**379902**	**781586**
1995 projected	*2033436*	*112995*	*604345*	*21995*	*29145*	*35323*	*66724*	*87006*	*160685*	*203467*	*233626*	*330633*	*751837*
Lung cancer													
1955	...	...	...	...	...	...	...	...	...	...	...	...	...
1965	11862	290	8037	287	428	562	1167	1673	1915	2005	1690	1104	741
1975	16111	257	10092	272	464	1041	1278	1427	2641	2969	2720	1894	1148
1985	21302	283	12122	262	390	1045	1452	2821	3258	2894	3884	2978	2035
1990	**25030**	**336**	**14475**	**330**	**523**	**791**	**1779**	**2460**	**4154**	**4438**	**3366**	**3906**	**2947**
1995 projected	*29154*	*367*	*15980*	*354*	*607*	*975*	*1812*	*2590*	*4464*	*5178*	*4721*	*4424*	*3662*
ANNUAL DEATH RATE / 100,000 (*The rates for the age groups 0–34 and 35–69 are the means of seven five-yearly rates, but the all-ages rates are standardised to the conventional "European" age distribution)													
All causes													
1955	1098.4*	283.0*	1025.2*	262.1	317.9	461.7	678.8	1043.0	1657.6	2755.3	4054.9	6696.8	15786.8
1965	853.2*	174.3*	788.0*	177.8	247.5	345.3	544.5	778.3	1285.0	2137.3	3400.3	6323.2	12174.9
1975	874.7*	166.9*	815.9*	177.4	245.9	374.1	563.1	857.8	1364.8	2128.3	3586.7	6305.8	12581.8
1985	934.9*	142.6*	847.8*	168.5	239.4	376.1	577.9	891.1	1428.3	2253.1	3835.7	6749.3	14920.4
1990	**866.3***	**115.4***	**805.3***	**149.1**	**236.2**	**344.6**	**536.5**	**824.8**	**1326.0**	**2220.2**	**3615.5**	**6136.4**	**14038.3**
1995 projected	*804.4**	*96.1**	*761.8**	*140.4*	*221.0*	*322.9*	*497.6*	*767.1*	*1270.4*	*2112.8*	*3366.0*	*5725.8*	*13082.0*
All cancer													
1955	...	...	...	...	...	...	...	...	...	...	...	...	...
1965	137.7*	9.9*	234.5*	46.2	81.9	131.6	213.5	276.7	386.4	504.9	567.2	684.2	643.6
1975	130.9*	10.1*	223.4*	43.5	73.3	126.8	195.2	276.1	385.9	463.4	549.3	647.2	565.7
1985	132.7*	9.8*	219.6*	46.4	72.6	119.9	179.4	268.4	378.3	472.3	588.8	680.6	667.9
1990	**137.9***	**9.5***	**225.4***	**44.7**	**81.7**	**122.5**	**184.3**	**257.5**	**373.5**	**513.2**	**629.8**	**729.9**	**737.8**
1995 projected	*142.7**	*8.8**	*228.8**	*46.3*	*83.8*	*126.3*	*181.7*	*251.8*	*378.0*	*533.8*	*673.1*	*797.8*	*806.3*
Lung cancer													
1955	...	...	...	...	...	...	...	...	...	...	...	...	...
1965	7.7*	0.3*	13.8*	2.0	3.7	6.6	11.3	17.5	23.6	31.9	35.8	36.8	29.0
1975	8.5*	0.3*	15.1*	1.9	3.8	7.5	11.4	18.9	27.5	34.6	40.1	45.2	30.5
1985	10.0*	0.3*	17.5*	2.1	3.9	7.5	12.4	21.5	32.0	43.3	48.6	53.6	42.9
1990	**11.0***	**0.3***	**18.7***	**2.1**	**4.2**	**8.0**	**13.2**	**21.8**	**33.4**	**47.9**	**58.5**	**63.1**	**52.9**
1995 projected	*12.3**	*0.3**	*20.2**	*2.3*	*4.6*	*8.9*	*13.5*	*22.8*	*35.3*	*53.8*	*68.0*	*76.6*	*63.7*
Upper aerodigestive cancer (mouth, oesophagus, pharynx and larynx)													
1955	...	...	...	...	...	...	...	...	...	...	...	...	...
1965	6.8*	0.2*	10.1*	1.1	2.0	3.9	6.7	11.1	18.6	26.9	33.2	47.4	56.6
1975	5.2*	0.2*	7.9*	1.0	2.4	3.7	5.6	9.5	15.0	18.1	25.5	33.9	38.2
1985	4.6*	0.2*	6.7*	0.7	1.5	3.0	5.5	8.3	11.7	16.2	22.2	28.6	38.6
1990	**4.5***	**0.2***	**6.6***	**0.8**	**1.6**	**3.1**	**4.5**	**7.8**	**11.9**	**16.6**	**21.9**	**28.8**	**37.6**
1995 projected	*4.5**	*0.2**	*6.6**	*0.8*	*1.8*	*3.0*	*4.3*	*7.5*	*12.2*	*16.7*	*20.9*	*29.9*	*37.8*
Other cancer													
1955	...	...	...	...	...	...	...	...	...	...	...	...	...
1965	123.2*	9.4*	210.6*	43.0	76.2	121.0	195.4	248.1	344.2	446.1	498.3	599.9	558.1
1975	117.1*	9.6*	200.4*	40.6	67.1	115.6	178.2	247.6	343.4	410.6	483.7	568.1	497.1
1985	118.2*	9.4*	195.4*	43.6	67.3	109.3	161.5	238.6	334.5	412.8	518.0	598.4	586.3
1990	**122.4***	**9.0***	**200.1***	**41.8**	**75.9**	**111.5**	**166.6**	**227.9**	**328.2**	**448.7**	**549.4**	**638.1**	**647.3**
1995 projected	*125.9**	*8.3**	*202.0**	*43.3*	*77.4*	*114.4*	*163.9*	*221.5*	*330.4*	*463.4*	*584.2*	*691.3*	*704.9*
Chronic obstructive pulmonary disease (COPD)													
1955	...	...	...	...	...	...	...	...	...	...	...	...	...
1965	39.8*	1.2*	34.7*	2.4	4.1	8.8	17.1	31.5	62.3	116.9	198.5	384.6	678.2
1975	51.1*	1.5*	42.2*	4.1	6.4	11.5	20.3	39.7	76.6	136.5	252.7	458.8	947.8
1985	39.5*	1.4*	33.5*	3.9	5.9	10.7	19.7	33.4	56.8	104.3	184.7	333.3	737.8
1990	**28.5***	**1.2***	**26.2***	**2.8**	**4.5**	**7.6**	**14.8**	**26.5**	**45.5**	**82.0**	**140.5**	**241.4**	**481.1**
1995 projected	*21.7**	*1.1**	*20.7**	*2.2*	*3.4*	*5.5*	*11.8*	*21.3*	*36.7*	*63.9*	*101.1*	*183.5*	*356.3*
Other respiratory disease													
1955	...	...	...	...	...	...	...	...	...	...	...	...	...
1965	33.3*	36.1*	11.0*	2.2	3.2	3.8	6.5	9.9	19.0	32.6	62.3	125.4	246.0
1975	42.1*	49.8*	14.2*	4.4	5.3	6.3	9.5	14.7	22.4	36.5	64.4	122.5	239.1
1985	28.6*	33.6*	9.7*	3.2	4.0	5.4	6.9	10.2	15.2	22.9	39.9	77.6	176.0
1990	**18.0***	**20.0***	**7.0***	**2.1**	**2.8**	**4.0**	**4.7**	**7.4**	**10.4**	**17.7**	**29.3**	**49.2**	**121.0**
1995 projected	*13.6**	*14.7**	*5.6**	*1.8*	*2.3*	*3.3*	*3.8*	*6.1*	*8.1*	*13.7*	*25.8*	*33.6*	*94.6*
Vascular disease													
1955	...	...	...	...	...	...	...	...	...	...	...	...	...
1965	439.6*	9.6*	332.0*	33.0	55.0	88.2	166.7	287.6	572.8	1120.5	2066.8	4226.3	8680.4
1975	492.1*	7.7*	378.4*	35.6	61.7	107.0	194.3	350.4	670.9	1228.6	2360.5	4514.9	9780.7
1985	577.9*	6.2*	419.8*	32.0	58.3	115.1	216.9	391.6	748.7	1376.0	2664.7	5139.6	12329.7
1990	**511.9***	**5.6***	**386.5***	**26.4**	**55.7**	**99.9**	**191.0**	**357.5**	**673.0**	**1302.0**	**2410.8**	**4452.9**	**10721.0**
1995 projected	*453.2**	*4.9**	*349.6**	*23.4*	*49.1*	*87.7*	*169.8*	*320.4*	*620.1*	*1176.8*	*2108.6*	*3925.8*	*9426.9*
Liver cirrhosis (incl. USSR other liver disease)													
1955	...	...	...	...	...	...	...	...	...	...	...	...	...
1965	9.2*	0.8*	13.2*	2.7	4.3	5.8	10.1	14.4	22.1	33.3	41.8	60.6	71.0
1975	9.7*	0.8*	15.7*	3.8	6.1	9.2	14.7	21.4	24.7	29.8	38.1	47.3	58.2
1985	12.6*	1.0*	22.4*	5.1	9.5	13.3	20.5	30.3	37.0	41.0	44.2	50.3	54.6
1990	**11.8***	**0.9***	**20.8***	**4.4**	**7.6**	**11.8**	**18.2**	**26.7**	**33.3**	**43.5**	**44.7**	**49.6**	**51.5**
1995 projected	*11.5**	*0.9**	*19.9**	*4.2*	*7.5*	*11.1*	*16.6*	*24.9*	*32.0*	*43.3*	*45.9*	*51.6*	*52.3*
Other medical causes													
1955	...	...	...	...	...	...	...	...	...	...	...	...	...
1965	157.4*	91.6*	124.3*	61.3	65.5	70.1	89.9	119.6	181.3	282.5	404.1	742.6	1678.9
1975	101.6*	70.0*	84.0*	42.2	44.2	52.5	68.8	90.4	120.5	169.3	243.7	393.6	787.1
1985	95.0*	65.3*	82.7*	36.3	39.3	51.5	70.1	90.2	125.7	165.5	225.5	337.9	695.3
1990	**111.0***	**52.1***	**83.1***	**28.9**	**36.1**	**45.9**	**63.0**	**89.8**	**126.6**	**191.3**	**270.0**	**481.7**	**1674.9**
1995 projected	*116.4**	*39.6**	*84.4**	*24.4*	*31.2*	*41.3*	*58.7*	*87.9*	*135.3*	*211.6*	*318.7*	*603.9*	*2096.6*
All non-medical causes													
1955	...	...	...	...	...	...	...	...	...	...	...	...	...
1965	36.2*	25.2*	38.2*	30.1	33.4	37.1	40.6	38.6	41.1	46.6	59.6	99.6	176.8
1975	47.2*	27.0*	58.1*	43.8	48.8	60.8	60.3	65.1	63.7	64.2	78.0	121.5	203.2
1985	48.6*	25.2*	60.1*	41.6	49.8	60.1	64.4	67.0	66.6	71.1	87.9	130.0	259.2
1990	**47.2***	**26.1***	**56.3***	**39.8**	**47.7**	**53.0**	**60.4**	**59.2**	**63.8**	**70.6**	**90.3**	**131.6**	**251.0**
1995 projected	*45.5**	*26.1**	*52.8**	*38.1*	*43.8*	*47.8*	*55.2*	*54.6*	*60.3*	*69.6*	*92.8*	*129.6*	*249.0*

FORMER SOCIALIST ECONOMIES: 1975

Smoking-attributed deaths (Sm.) and total deaths (Total)

		ALL CAUSES	ALL CANCER	Lung cancer	Upper aero-digestive ca.	Other cancer	COPD	Other respiratory	Vascular disease	Cirrhosis (incl. USSR other liver)	Other medical	Non-medical
Males												
0–34	Sm.	–	–	–	–	–	–	–	–	–	–	–
	Total	299809	11130	518	281	10331	2068	64116	11912	1393	94380	114810
35–69	Sm.	256497	80180	49953	11166	19061	43157	4980	96689	–	31491	–
	Total	826398	180100	53660	16646	109794	54994	15355	310148	19106	91134	155561
		(31%)	(45%)	(93%)	(67%)	(17%)	(78%)	(32%)	(31%)		(35%)	
70+	Sm.	93687	23293	15508	3116	4669	35465	1228	29228	–	4473	–
	Total	614254	78758	18091	7013	53654	62788	14516	385134	5573	51464	16021
		(15%)	(30%)	(86%)	(44%)	(9%)	(56%)	(8%)	(8%)		(9%)	
Any age	Sm.	350184	103473	65461	14282	23730	78622	6208	125917	–	35964	–
	Total	1740461	269988	72269	23940	173779	119850	93987	707194	26072	236978	286392
		(20%)	(38%)	(91%)	(60%)	(14%)	(66%)	(7%)	(18%)		(15%)	
Females												
0–34	Sm.	–	–	–	–	–	–	–	–	–	–	–
	Total	170631	9387	257	155	8975	1457	52563	7068	765	72445	26946
35–69	Sm.	27766	5748	4105	826	817	7719	425	11176	–	2698	–
	Total	548370	152155	10092	5290	136773	27296	9619	245411	10746	59283	43860
		(5%)	(4%)	(41%)	(16%)	(1%)	(28%)	(4%)	(5%)		(5%)	
70+	Sm.	17879	2135	1529	328	278	8721	199	6085	–	739	–
	Total	980785	85617	5762	4584	75271	72014	18499	717253	6751	62630	18021
		(2%)	(2%)	(27%)	(7%)	(0%)	(12%)	(1%)	(1%)		(1%)	
Any age	Sm.	45645	7883	5634	1154	1095	16440	624	17261	–	3437	–
	Total	1699786	247159	16111	10029	221019	100767	80681	969732	18262	194358	88827
		(3%)	(3%)	(35%)	(12%)	(0%)	(16%)	(1%)	(2%)		(2%)	
Males+Females												
0–34	Sm.	–	–	–	–	–	–	–	–	–	–	–
	Total	470440	20517	775	436	19306	3525	116679	18980	2158	166825	141756
35–69	Sm.	284263	85928	54058	11992	19878	50876	5405	107865	–	34189	–
	Total	1374768	332255	63752	21936	246567	82290	24974	555559	29852	150417	199421
		(21%)	(26%)	(85%)	(55%)	(8%)	(62%)	(22%)	(19%)		(23%)	
70+	Sm.	111566	25428	17037	3444	4947	44186	1427	35313	–	5212	–
	Total	1595039	164375	23853	11597	128925	134802	33015	1102387	12324	114094	34042
		(7%)	(15%)	(71%)	(30%)	(4%)	(33%)	(4%)	(3%)		(5%)	
Any age	Sm.	395829	111356	71095	15436	24825	95062	6832	143178	–	39401	–
	Total	3440247	517147	88380	33969	394798	220617	174668	1676926	44334	431336	375219
		(12%)	(22%)	(80%)	(45%)	(6%)	(43%)	(4%)	(9%)		(9%)	

FORMER SOCIALIST ECONOMIES: 1985

Smoking-attributed deaths (Sm.) and total deaths (Total)

		ALL CAUSES	ALL CANCER	Lung cancer	Upper aero-digestive ca.	Other cancer	COPD	Other respiratory	Vascular disease	Cirrhosis (incl. USSR other liver)	Other medical	Non-medical
Males												
0–34	Sm.	–	–	–	–	–	–	–	–	–	–	–
	Total	301442	12509	684	367	11458	2202	48955	14791	1989	111110	109886
35–69	Sm.	378643	121185	74933	19261	26991	45884	7221	159184	–	45169	–
	Total	980043	225820	78920	25966	120934	54955	17211	398257	30825	103355	149620
		(39%)	(54%)	(95%)	(74%)	(22%)	(83%)	(42%)	(40%)		(44%)	
70+	Sm.	138138	35949	24010	4529	7410	43459	1240	52026	–	5464	–
	Total	824393	106745	27158	8639	70948	67914	13484	552291	8286	54300	21373
		(17%)	(34%)	(88%)	(52%)	(10%)	(64%)	(9%)	(9%)		(10%)	
Any age	Sm.	516781	157134	98943	23790	34401	89343	8461	211210	–	50633	–
	Total	2105878	345074	106762	34972	203340	125071	79650	965339	41100	268765	280879
		(25%)	(46%)	(93%)	(68%)	(17%)	(71%)	(11%)	(22%)		(19%)	
Females												
0–34	Sm.	–	–	–	–	–	–	–	–	–	–	–
	Total	164154	10928	283	174	10471	1623	39544	6868	1093	75848	28250
35–69	Sm.	36089	7832	5838	873	1121	7369	417	16717	–	3754	–
	Total	577559	155937	12122	4664	139151	21998	6763	270638	16316	59515	46392
		(6%)	(5%)	(48%)	(19%)	(1%)	(33%)	(6%)	(6%)		(6%)	
70+	Sm.	37088	4765	3465	695	605	15276	228	15547	–	1272	–
	Total	1388160	116452	8897	5185	102370	68222	15837	1082501	8905	69721	26522
		(3%)	(4%)	(39%)	(13%)	(1%)	(22%)	(1%)	(1%)		(2%)	
Any age	Sm.	73177	12597	9303	1568	1726	22645	645	32264	–	5026	–
	Total	2129873	283317	21302	10023	251992	91843	62144	1360007	26314	205084	101164
		(3%)	(4%)	(44%)	(16%)	(1%)	(25%)	(1%)	(2%)		(2%)	
Males+Females												
0–34	Sm.	–	–	–	–	–	–	–	–	–	–	–
	Total	465596	23437	967	541	21929	3825	88499	21659	3082	186958	138136
35–69	Sm.	414732	129017	80771	20134	28112	53253	7638	175901	–	48923	–
	Total	1557602	381757	91042	30630	260085	76953	23974	668895	47141	162870	196012
		(27%)	(34%)	(89%)	(66%)	(11%)	(69%)	(32%)	(26%)		(30%)	
70+	Sm.	175226	40714	27475	5224	8015	58735	1468	67573	–	6736	–
	Total	2212553	223197	36055	13824	173318	136136	29321	1634792	17191	124021	47895
		(8%)	(18%)	(76%)	(38%)	(5%)	(43%)	(5%)	(4%)		(5%)	
Any age	Sm.	589958	169731	108246	25358	36127	111988	9106	243474	–	55659	–
	Total	4235751	628391	128064	44995	455332	216914	141794	2325346	67414	473849	382043
		(14%)	(27%)	(85%)	(56%)	(8%)	(52%)	(6%)	(10%)		(12%)	

(To be conservative, no deaths before age 35, and none from liver cirrhosis or non-medical causes, were attributed to smoking.)

FORMER SOCIALIST ECONOMIES: 1990

Smoking–attributed deaths (Sm.) and total deaths (Total)

		ALL CAUSES	ALL CANCER	Lung cancer	Upper aero–digestive ca.	Other cancer	COPD	Other respiratory	Vascular disease	Cirrhosis (incl. USSR other liver)	Other medical	Non–medical
Males												
0–34	Sm.	–	–	–	–	–	–	–	–	–	–	–
	Total	267907	12279	653	356	11270	1773	29824	14485	1824	84384	123338
35–69	Sm.	441175	156874	95828	27184	33862	44359	5685	189183	–	45074	–
	Total	1123669	281317	100590	36008	144719	52615	13608	469031	30937	103875	172286
		(39%)	(56%)	(95%)	(75%)	(23%)	(84%)	(42%)	(40%)		(43%)	
70+	Sm.	126304	36424	24161	4486	7777	34466	882	47788	–	6744	–
	Total	762555	105403	27099	8192	70112	51912	9807	495626	7009	71447	21351
		(17%)	(35%)	(89%)	(55%)	(11%)	(66%)	(9%)	(10%)		(9%)	
Any age	Sm.	567479	193298	119989	31670	41639	78825	6567	236971	–	51818	–
	Total	2154131	398999	128342	44556	226101	106300	53239	979142	39770	259706	316975
		(26%)	(48%)	(93%)	(71%)	(18%)	(74%)	(12%)	(24%)		(20%)	
Females												
0–34	Sm.	–	–	–	–	–	–	–	–	–	–	–
	Total	133653	10663	336	203	10124	1350	23895	6246	1057	61197	29245
35–69	Sm.	42054	9921	7422	1067	1432	7168	377	20038	–	4550	–
	Total	622265	177029	14475	5130	157424	19980	5460	291202	16437	65571	46586
		(7%)	(6%)	(51%)	(21%)	(1%)	(36%)	(7%)	(7%)		(7%)	
70+	Sm.	44448	6710	4876	941	893	15213	228	19609	–	2688	–
	Total	1369393	122486	10219	5131	107136	49815	11463	1011206	8506	138598	27319
		(3%)	(5%)	(48%)	(18%)	(1%)	(31%)	(2%)	(2%)		(2%)	
Any age	Sm.	86502	16631	12298	2008	2325	22381	605	39647	–	7238	–
	Total	2125311	310178	25030	10464	274684	71145	40818	1308654	26000	265366	103150
		(4%)	(5%)	(49%)	(19%)	(1%)	(31%)	(1%)	(3%)		(3%)	
Males+Females												
0–34	Sm.	–	–	–	–	–	–	–	–	–	–	–
	Total	401560	22942	989	559	21394	3123	53719	20731	2881	145581	152583
35–69	Sm.	483229	166795	103250	28251	35294	51527	6062	209221	–	49624	–
	Total	1745934	458346	115065	41138	302143	72595	19068	760233	47374	169446	218872
		(28%)	(36%)	(90%)	(69%)	(12%)	(71%)	(32%)	(28%)		(29%)	
70+	Sm.	170752	43134	29037	5427	8670	49679	1110	67397	–	9432	–
	Total	2131948	227889	37318	13323	177248	101727	21270	1506832	15515	210045	48670
		(8%)	(19%)	(78%)	(41%)	(5%)	(49%)	(5%)	(4%)		(4%)	
Any age	Sm.	653981	209929	132287	33678	43964	101206	7172	276618	–	59056	–
	Total	4279442	709177	153372	55020	500785	177445	94057	2287796	65770	525072	420125
		(15%)	(30%)	(86%)	(61%)	(9%)	(57%)	(8%)	(12%)		(11%)	

FORMER SOCIALIST ECONOMIES: 1995

Smoking–attributed deaths (Sm.) and total deaths (Total)

		ALL CAUSES	ALL CANCER	Lung cancer	Upper aero–digestive ca.	Other cancer	COPD	Other respiratory	Vascular disease	Cirrhosis (incl. USSR other liver)	Other medical	Non–medical
Males												
0–34	Sm.	–	–	–	–	–	–	–	–	–	–	–
	Total	245809	11427	640	349	10438	1511	22127	13202	1751	64266	131525
35–69	Sm.	463158	179403	107862	34150	37391	37431	4763	197983	–	43578	–
	Total	1143042	307673	112799	44367	150507	43831	11012	469343	29801	97822	183560
		(41%)	(58%)	(96%)	(77%)	(25%)	(85%)	(43%)	(42%)		(45%)	
70+	Sm.	135082	44238	29300	5271	9667	29761	823	51137	–	9123	–
	Total	740732	118772	32391	9008	77373	42653	7957	457194	7145	84179	22832
		(18%)	(37%)	(90%)	(59%)	(12%)	(70%)	(10%)	(11%)		(11%)	
Any age	Sm.	598240	223641	137162	39421	47058	67192	5586	249120	–	52701	–
	Total	2129583	437872	145830	53724	238318	87995	41096	939739	38697	246267	337917
		(28%)	(51%)	(94%)	(73%)	(20%)	(76%)	(14%)	(27%)		(21%)	
Females												
0–34	Sm.	–	–	–	–	–	–	–	–	–	–	–
	Total	112995	10085	367	206	9512	1251	17879	5569	1067	47456	29688
35–69	Sm.	44489	11652	8729	1225	1698	6181	353	21070	–	5233	–
	Total	604345	184254	15980	5271	163003	16195	4479	270603	16126	67794	44894
		(7%)	(6%)	(55%)	(23%)	(1%)	(38%)	(8%)	(8%)		(8%)	
70+	Sm.	56202	10005	7270	1315	1420	15050	263	25979	–	4905	–
	Total	1316096	139127	12807	5344	120976	38089	9164	914821	9172	177488	28235
		(4%)	(7%)	(57%)	(25%)	(1%)	(40%)	(3%)	(3%)		(3%)	
Any age	Sm.	100691	21657	15999	2540	3118	21231	616	47049	–	10138	–
	Total	2033436	333466	29154	10821	293491	55535	31522	1190993	26365	292738	102817
		(5%)	(6%)	(55%)	(23%)	(1%)	(38%)	(2%)	(4%)		(3%)	
Males+Females												
0–34	Sm.	–	–	–	–	–	–	–	–	–	–	–
	Total	358804	21512	1007	555	19950	2762	40006	18771	2818	111722	161213
35–69	Sm.	507647	191055	116591	35375	39089	43612	5116	219053	–	48811	–
	Total	1747387	491927	128779	49638	313510	60026	15491	739946	45927	165616	228454
		(29%)	(39%)	(91%)	(71%)	(12%)	(73%)	(33%)	(30%)		(29%)	
70+	Sm.	191284	54243	36570	6586	11087	44811	1086	77116	–	14028	–
	Total	2056828	257899	45198	14352	198349	80742	17121	1372015	16317	261667	51067
		(9%)	(21%)	(81%)	(46%)	(6%)	(55%)	(6%)	(6%)		(5%)	
Any age	Sm.	698931	245298	153161	41961	50176	88423	6202	296169	–	62839	–
	Total	4163019	771338	174984	64545	531809	143530	72618	2130732	65062	539005	440734
		(17%)	(32%)	(88%)	(65%)	(9%)	(62%)	(9%)	(14%)		(12%)	

(To be conservative, no deaths before age 35, and none from liver cirrhosis or non–medical causes, were attributed to smoking.)

OECD DEVELOPED: 1990

		No. of deaths			Standardised rates (Defined on p.244)			Annual death rates / 100, 000						
		All ages	0–34	35–69	All ages	0–34	35–69	0–4	5–9	10–14	15–19	20–24	25–29	30–34
ALL CAUSES	M	3658687	236278	1334252	965.4	114.3	1005.8	221.4	23.7	25.9	94.3	129.4	140.0	165.3
	F	3492550	110765	753339	574.8	57.4	504.3	174.1	17.2	17.2	35.1	41.6	50.1	66.5
Tuberculosis	M	9606	275	4150	2.5	0.1	3.1	0.0	0.0	0.0	0.0	0.1	0.2	0.5
	F	4597	161	1456	0.8	0.1	1.0	0.0	0.0	0.0	0.0	0.1	0.2	0.2
Other infective	M	28309	3394	10354	7.5	1.7	7.5	4.9	0.5	0.3	0.7	0.9	1.8	2.6
and parasitic	F	30267	2230	6887	5.2	1.2	4.6	4.0	0.5	0.4	0.6	0.7	1.0	1.1
ALL CANCER	M	963439	14323	454826	257.4	6.8	351.2	3.9	3.9	3.7	5.5	6.8	9.3	14.6
	F	776579	12437	322993	148.3	6.0	215.4	3.4	3.1	3.0	3.7	4.5	8.0	16.6
Mouth and	M	24649	253	17022	6.8	0.1	12.5	0.0	0.0	0.0	0.1	0.1	0.2	0.4
pharynx cancer	F	7933	94	3512	1.5	0.0	2.3	0.0	0.0	0.0	0.1	0.0	0.1	0.1
Oesophagus cancer	M	31174	65	18764	8.5	0.0	14.3	–	–	0.0	–	0.0	0.0	0.1
	F	10099	19	3584	1.8	0.0	2.4	–	–	–	–	0.0	0.0	0.1
Stomach cancer	M	79835	433	36575	21.3	0.2	28.1	–	–	0.0	0.0	0.1	0.3	0.9
	F	54639	575	17873	9.7	0.3	11.9	0.0	–	–	0.0	0.2	0.5	1.2
Colorectal cancer	M	100184	548	42978	26.7	0.3	33.4	0.0	–	0.0	0.1	0.2	0.4	1.0
	F	101913	462	32698	18.0	0.2	22.1	0.0	–	–	0.0	0.1	0.4	0.9
Liver cancer	M	26606	199	17243	7.3	0.1	13.2	0.1	0.0	0.0	0.1	0.1	0.1	0.2
	F	10304	125	4399	2.0	0.1	3.0	0.1	0.0	0.0	0.0	0.1	0.1	0.1
Pancreas cancer	M	42789	144	21223	11.5	0.1	16.4	0.0	0.0	0.0	0.0	0.0	0.1	0.3
	F	42111	103	14185	7.5	0.0	9.7	0.0	0.0	0.0	0.0	0.0	0.1	0.2
Larynx cancer	M	15789	22	9651	4.3	0.0	7.3	–	0.0	0.0	0.0	0.0	0.0	0.0
	F	1838	9	945	0.4	0.0	0.6	0.0	–	0.0	–	0.0	0.0	0.0
Lung cancer	M	275201	564	145798	74.0	0.3	114.2	0.0	0.0	0.0	0.1	0.1	0.3	1.3
	F	101456	337	49917	20.4	0.2	33.9	0.0	0.0	0.0	0.0	0.1	0.2	0.7
Malignant melanoma	M	9041	495	5474	2.4	0.2	3.9	0.0	–	–	0.1	0.2	0.4	0.9
	F	7172	386	3641	1.5	0.2	2.3	–	0.0	0.0	0.0	0.2	0.4	0.6
Female breast cancer	F	133183	1687	73812	27.8	0.8	48.1	–	–	0.0	0.0	0.1	1.1	4.2
Cervix cancer	F	15625	735	9285	3.4	0.3	5.9	0.0	–	–	0.0	0.1	0.6	1.6
Other uterine cancer	F	23863	125	9568	4.5	0.1	6.5	0.0	–	0.0	0.0	0.0	0.1	0.3
Ovarian cancer	F	41216	513	21730	8.5	0.2	14.5	0.0	0.0	0.1	0.1	0.2	0.4	0.8
Prostate cancer	M	94260	43	18793	24.5	0.0	15.8	0.0	–	0.0	0.0	0.0	0.0	0.0
Bladder cancer	M	32884	44	10423	8.6	0.0	8.4	0.0	0.0	0.0	0.0	0.0	0.0	0.1
	F	13418	28	2860	2.2	0.0	2.0	0.0	0.0	0.0	0.0	0.0	0.0	0.0
Other and ill-defined	M	158870	5976	78767	42.5	2.9	59.7	2.1	2.0	1.6	2.4	3.0	3.7	5.2
cancer sites	F	148645	3844	52572	27.3	1.9	35.3	1.9	1.7	1.6	1.6	1.5	2.0	3.2
Hodgkin's disease	M	3078	662	1603	0.8	0.3	1.1	–	0.0	0.1	0.2	0.4	0.7	0.8
	F	2219	400	895	0.5	0.2	0.6	0.0	0.0	0.0	0.1	0.3	0.4	0.4
Myeloma and non-	M	38684	1468	18220	10.3	0.7	13.8	0.2	0.3	0.4	0.5	0.8	1.1	1.6
Hodgkin lymphomas	F	35411	670	12703	6.5	0.3	8.6	0.2	0.1	0.2	0.3	0.4	0.5	0.7
Leukaemia	M	30391	3403	12291	8.0	1.7	9.2	1.3	1.4	1.6	1.9	1.7	1.7	1.9
	F	25533	2321	8813	4.9	1.2	5.8	1.1	1.2	1.1	1.3	1.1	1.1	1.3
ALL VASCULAR	M	1440132	12392	456561	379.5	5.8	354.4	5.5	1.0	1.4	3.2	5.4	8.4	16.0
DISEASE	F	1629783	7137	216470	242.8	3.5	148.2	4.9	0.8	1.3	2.0	3.0	4.7	7.8
Rheumatic heart	M	5888	174	2867	1.6	0.1	2.2	0.0	0.0	0.0	0.1	0.1	0.1	0.2
disease and fever	F	13724	182	4802	2.5	0.1	3.3	0.0	0.0	0.0	0.1	0.1	0.2	0.2
Hypertensive disease	M	38247	261	12797	10.1	0.1	9.8	0.0	0.0	0.0	0.0	0.1	0.2	0.5
	F	63020	148	9530	9.5	0.1	6.5	0.0	0.0	0.0	0.0	0.0	0.1	0.2
Ischaemic heart	M	680285	2320	252447	180.2	1.1	196.9	0.1	0.0	0.1	0.2	0.6	1.6	4.8
disease	F	598110	660	91210	91.0	0.3	63.1	0.1	0.0	0.0	0.1	0.2	0.5	1.2
Pulmonary embolism	M	18656	396	7031	4.9	0.2	5.4	0.1	0.0	0.0	0.1	0.2	0.3	0.6
and other venous	F	26998	433	6272	4.4	0.2	4.2	0.0	0.0	0.0	0.2	0.3	0.3	0.6
Cerebrovascular	M	307714	2387	73948	80.5	1.1	57.4	0.8	0.2	0.3	0.6	1.1	1.6	3.1
disease	F	448330	1914	52433	65.9	0.9	35.6	0.6	0.2	0.3	0.5	0.8	1.5	2.4
Other vascular	M	389337	6851	107469	102.2	3.3	82.7	4.4	0.7	1.0	2.2	3.3	4.5	6.8
disease	F	479595	3796	52222	69.4	1.9	35.6	4.0	0.5	0.9	1.2	1.5	2.1	3.2
Chronic obstructive	M	161270	1337	40280	42.1	0.6	33.0	0.7	0.2	0.5	0.7	0.7	0.8	0.9
pulmonary disease	F	96724	951	22986	16.1	0.5	15.8	0.4	0.1	0.3	0.5	0.6	0.6	0.7
Other respiratory	M	179172	4594	33933	46.7	2.3	26.4	7.4	0.7	0.6	0.9	1.4	2.1	3.0
disease	F	185405	3098	17184	26.6	1.6	11.6	5.8	0.6	0.6	0.7	0.9	1.3	1.6
Peptic ulcer	M	15098	167	4914	4.0	0.1	3.8	0.0	0.0	0.0	0.0	0.1	0.1	0.3
	F	14849	60	2179	2.2	0.0	1.5	0.0	–	0.0	0.0	0.0	0.1	0.1
Liver cirrhosis	M	73545	1697	53485	20.1	0.8	38.1	0.1	0.0	0.0	0.1	0.2	1.2	3.9
	F	38234	876	21811	8.1	0.4	14.3	0.1	0.0	0.1	0.0	0.2	0.6	1.9
Renal disease	M	39180	744	9689	10.3	0.4	7.5	0.9	0.1	0.1	0.1	0.3	0.4	0.7
	F	43896	527	7495	6.8	0.3	5.1	0.8	0.1	0.1	0.1	0.2	0.3	0.4
Pregnancy and birth	F	834	632	202	0.2	0.3	0.1	–	–	–	0.2	0.5	0.7	0.7
Congenital and	M	38588	35542	2070	11.6	19.3	1.4	127.2	1.8	1.2	1.6	1.4	1.0	1.0
perinatal causes	F	30775	27635	1863	9.4	15.8	1.2	104.1	1.6	1.2	1.0	0.9	0.9	0.8
Ill-defined causes	M	85198	15345	23627	22.7	7.9	16.7	35.2	0.6	0.9	2.1	4.3	5.4	6.5
	F	101182	8343	10393	15.6	4.6	6.8	24.2	0.5	0.5	0.8	1.7	1.9	2.3
Other medical causes	M	327667	29507	117571	85.6	13.9	83.7	14.0	3.6	3.6	6.1	9.9	23.9	36.4
	F	392181	13068	76018	63.2	6.6	50.7	11.3	3.1	2.9	3.6	5.5	8.5	10.9
ALL NON-	M	297486	116959	122795	75.3	54.6	79.1	21.7	11.3	13.6	73.3	98.0	85.3	78.9
MEDICAL CAUSES	F	147234	33603	45399	29.2	16.6	28.2	15.1	6.8	6.8	21.6	22.9	21.4	21.4
Motor vehicle	M	88724	48185	30133	21.9	22.5	19.3	4.8	5.5	5.7	39.6	46.4	31.5	23.9
traffic accidents	F	35164	14905	12489	8.0	7.4	7.7	3.6	3.6	3.8	13.5	11.9	8.4	6.7
Fire	M	5639	1975	2286	1.5	1.0	1.5	2.3	0.7	0.4	0.5	0.9	1.0	1.1
	F	3795	1071	1107	0.8	0.6	0.7	1.7	0.6	0.2	0.3	0.3	0.3	0.5
Suicide	M	77837	23857	40381	19.9	10.9	25.9	–	0.0	1.3	10.9	20.0	21.4	22.7
	F	29881	6279	16145	6.8	2.9	10.0	–	0.0	0.5	2.9	4.7	5.6	6.9
Homicide	M	23953	14955	8244	5.8	6.9	4.8	2.1	0.5	1.0	9.5	13.0	12.0	10.3
	F	7373	4151	2520	1.8	2.0	1.4	2.0	0.6	0.7	2.1	2.8	3.1	3.1
POPULATION (thousands):	M=males				388775	203859	158225	26097	26254	26972	29704	31394	32467	30971
	F=females				407520	196386	166414	24817	24958	25640	28246	30220	31784	30721

OECD DEVELOPED: 1990

Annual death rates / 100, 000 — 9th ICD categories

35–39	40–44	45–49	50–54	55–59	60–64	65–69	70–74	75–79	80+/NK			
206.4	269.5	413.8	654.3	1080.6	1723.3	2692.6	4209.0	6800.9	13903.4	M	**ALL CAUSES**	001–999
94.9	137.1	220.4	338.7	530.7	846.6	1361.6	2251.0	3949.0	10720.6	F		
0.6	0.9	1.4	2.1	3.3	5.4	8.2	12.7	19.3	28.7	M	**Tuberculosis**	010–018, 137
0.2	0.2	0.4	0.5	1.1	1.7	2.8	4.0	5.8	9.8	F		
3.2	3.5	4.2	5.1	7.0	11.5	17.7	29.6	45.2	99.1	M	**Other infective**	Rest of 001–139
1.3	1.7	2.2	3.2	4.9	7.4	11.3	18.6	31.2	86.3	F	**and parasitic**	
27.6	56.1	116.8	221.0	405.2	659.7	972.0	1357.6	1837.0	2546.0	M	**ALL CANCER**	140–208
34.7	61.0	106.0	167.9	253.1	367.9	517.1	687.3	906.5	1320.8	F		
1.3	3.4	7.5	12.2	17.6	21.9	23.3	24.9	26.5	32.6	M	**Mouth and**	140–149
0.3	0.6	1.2	2.1	3.0	4.1	5.1	6.8	8.4	13.3	F	**pharynx cancer**	
0.6	2.1	5.6	11.3	19.2	26.9	34.4	41.1	46.8	52.7	M	**Oesophagus cancer**	150
0.1	0.3	0.8	1.7	2.9	4.8	6.4	9.4	13.2	20.2	F		
2.4	5.0	9.9	18.4	32.7	52.9	75.2	109.3	160.5	230.5	M	**Stomach cancer**	151
2.3	4.0	5.7	8.6	13.1	19.4	30.0	44.4	71.1	121.8	F		
2.4	4.8	10.3	20.5	37.2	61.9	96.8	138.5	204.5	321.9	M	**Colorectal cancer**	153, 154
2.1	4.3	8.8	15.4	25.1	39.1	60.1	87.2	130.6	232.5	F		
0.7	1.6	3.7	8.3	20.7	27.4	29.9	33.3	35.7	34.2	M	**Liver cancer**	155.0
0.2	0.4	0.8	1.5	3.4	6.0	8.6	11.1	13.5	14.1	F		
1.0	2.5	6.0	10.8	18.7	30.1	45.8	63.9	81.4	101.4	M	**Pancreas cancer**	157
0.6	1.2	3.0	5.8	10.6	17.8	28.8	41.8	58.3	83.7	F		
0.2	1.2	3.1	6.1	10.0	13.5	17.2	19.9	22.6	27.4	M	**Larynx cancer**	161
0.0	0.1	0.2	0.5	0.8	1.3	1.6	1.8	2.1	2.0	F		
4.4	12.5	31.9	64.9	129.9	224.8	331.1	434.0	510.7	518.7	M	**Lung cancer**	162
2.3	5.6	12.8	23.4	39.3	64.6	88.9	115.2	119.5	109.7	F		
1.5	2.0	2.6	3.4	4.4	5.9	7.2	9.5	11.5	14.3	M	**Malignant melanoma**	172
1.1	1.5	1.9	2.1	2.6	3.1	3.9	5.2	6.2	9.3	F		
11.3	21.3	33.5	48.5	61.3	72.8	87.8	98.0	117.4	166.3	F	**Female breast cancer**	174
3.2	3.9	4.9	5.7	6.3	7.6	9.5	10.7	12.3	14.4	F	**Cervix cancer**	180
0.7	1.3	2.3	4.0	8.0	11.6	17.5	23.0	29.8	41.0	F	**Other uterine cancer**	179, 182
1.6	3.8	8.1	13.1	18.2	24.8	31.7	37.7	42.4	46.7	F	**Ovarian cancer**	183
0.1	0.2	0.7	3.1	10.4	28.5	67.8	140.1	253.5	509.9	M	**Prostate cancer**	185
0.1	0.6	1.4	3.6	8.0	16.8	28.2	47.0	81.2	137.8	M	**Bladder cancer**	188
0.1	0.2	0.4	0.8	1.9	3.9	6.6	10.6	19.7	38.3	F		
7.7	13.0	23.5	41.8	70.6	108.0	153.5	202.8	274.2	384.3	M	**Other and ill-defined**	Rest of 140–208
5.1	8.2	14.7	24.3	40.6	62.3	92.1	126.9	183.9	295.8	F	**cancer sites**	
0.8	0.7	0.7	0.9	1.2	1.5	1.8	2.5	3.0	3.8	M	**Hodgkin's disease**	201
0.4	0.4	0.3	0.4	0.6	0.7	1.3	1.5	2.3	2.3	F		
2.2	3.5	5.8	9.5	15.0	24.5	35.7	54.0	71.7	94.1	M	**Myeloma and non-**	200, 202–203
1.2	1.7	3.4	5.5	9.3	15.0	24.0	36.2	47.5	62.4	F	**Hodgkin lymphomas**	
2.3	2.9	4.0	6.3	9.6	14.9	24.3	36.5	53.3	82.4	M	**Leukaemia**	204–208
1.9	2.2	3.2	4.6	6.2	9.0	13.3	19.7	28.2	46.7	F		
32.4	63.2	118.7	208.1	366.9	628.7	1062.7	1775.9	3071.0	6816.5	M	**ALL VASCULAR**	390–459
12.9	22.6	42.7	73.3	135.5	257.6	492.7	969.2	1969.5	6064.2	F	**DISEASE**	
0.4	0.5	0.8	1.3	2.4	4.0	5.8	8.1	10.6	14.3	M	**Rheumatic heart**	390–398
0.4	0.6	1.1	2.2	3.5	5.5	9.4	13.5	18.4	25.9	F	**disease and fever**	
1.0	1.9	3.5	6.4	10.9	17.1	28.0	43.6	78.6	181.3	M	**Hypertensive disease**	401–405
0.5	0.9	2.0	3.6	6.4	11.0	21.3	38.1	78.2	226.0	F		
13.2	31.1	62.9	114.2	206.5	355.9	594.4	941.0	1444.0	2655.0	M	**Ischaemic heart**	410–414
2.6	5.8	13.3	26.1	55.2	115.3	223.4	426.9	784.0	2051.5	F	**disease**	
0.9	1.3	1.9	3.2	5.6	9.5	15.3	23.5	39.8	70.0	M	**Pulmonary embolism**	415.1, 451–453
0.8	1.2	1.8	2.5	4.1	6.9	12.2	19.1	36.0	76.7	F	**and other venous**	
5.8	11.0	19.8	33.1	57.6	97.7	177.0	345.4	721.6	1741.6	M	**Cerebrovascular**	430–438
4.4	7.7	13.3	20.2	33.0	57.6	112.6	246.5	555.5	1718.5	F	**disease**	
11.0	17.4	29.7	49.9	84.0	144.5	242.1	414.2	776.4	2154.3	M	**Other vascular**	Rest of 390–459
4.3	6.4	11.3	18.7	33.2	61.3	113.7	225.0	497.5	1965.6	F	**disease**	
1.2	2.0	4.5	10.3	26.2	60.6	126.0	238.5	412.6	775.1	M	**Chronic obstructive**	490–496
1.0	1.6	3.4	7.3	14.8	29.8	53.0	90.3	133.4	251.9	F	**pulmonary disease**	
4.1	5.5	8.0	12.9	23.8	45.1	85.4	179.1	376.1	1169.7	M	**Other respiratory**	Rest of 460–519
2.2	2.8	4.1	6.2	10.5	19.3	36.1	79.6	175.2	789.0	F	**disease**	
0.5	0.8	1.4	2.3	4.2	6.4	10.8	17.8	31.1	71.6	M	**Peptic ulcer**	531–533
0.1	0.3	0.5	0.8	1.4	2.5	4.7	9.3	17.9	53.7	F		
9.6	15.3	25.3	37.3	52.4	61.1	65.6	63.8	71.7	72.4	M	**Liver cirrhosis**	571
3.7	5.7	9.0	12.7	17.6	23.1	28.1	31.8	36.6	36.0	F		
1.1	1.6	2.4	4.2	7.5	13.1	22.4	42.3	84.3	223.1	M	**Renal disease**	580–590
0.7	0.9	1.7	2.9	4.9	8.8	15.7	28.6	53.7	148.3	F		
0.5	0.2	0.0	–	–	–	–	–	–	–	F	**Pregnancy and birth**	630–676
1.1	1.0	1.1	1.3	1.4	1.7	2.0	2.5	3.5	5.5	M	**Congenital and**	740–779
0.8	0.8	0.9	1.1	1.4	1.5	1.7	2.4	2.5	3.6	F	**perinatal causes**	
7.5	8.2	10.1	14.2	18.4	24.3	34.5	51.1	97.7	423.5	M	**Ill-defined causes**	780–799
3.0	2.9	4.0	5.1	6.3	10.0	16.0	27.8	63.9	424.0	F		
42.7	42.2	47.4	59.1	82.3	120.1	191.9	316.8	568.6	1288.6	M	**Other medical causes**	Rest of 001–799
13.2	15.0	21.1	31.1	49.6	83.8	141.1	243.5	452.8	1252.7	F		
74.7	69.2	72.4	76.4	82.2	85.6	93.3	121.1	182.9	383.5	M	**ALL NON-**	E800–E999
20.7	21.5	24.4	26.6	29.6	33.1	41.2	58.7	99.8	280.3	F	**MEDICAL CAUSES**	
19.8	17.0	17.5	18.3	19.9	20.6	21.9	28.9	40.1	51.5	M	**Motor vehicle**	E810–E819
6.3	6.0	6.6	7.2	8.0	9.1	10.7	14.2	19.2	18.7	F	**traffic accidents**	
1.2	1.2	1.2	1.4	1.6	1.9	2.4	2.9	4.3	9.2	M	**Fire**	E890–E899
0.4	0.5	0.6	0.6	0.7	0.7	1.3	1.9	2.9	5.8	F		
23.2	23.1	25.6	26.7	27.6	26.6	28.7	35.4	49.6	73.8	M	**Suicide**	E950–E959
7.2	8.0	9.6	10.5	11.2	11.1	12.1	13.7	17.3	18.8	F		
8.8	6.5	5.2	4.2	3.4	3.0	2.5	2.5	2.4	3.7	M	**Homicide**	E960–E969
2.4	1.8	1.6	1.2	1.2	1.0	1.0	1.3	1.4	2.0	F		
29397	28935	23963	21838	20031	18573	15488	10551	8448	7693	M	**POPULATION (thousands)**	
29362	28895	24128	22370	21136	20784	19739	14755	13530	16436	F		

OECD DEVELOPED: Males

	All ages	0–34	35–69	35–39	40–44	45–49	50–54	55–59	60–64	65–69	70–74	75–79	80+/NK
POPULATION (1000s)													
1955	288715	170024	104944	17272	18888	18260	16506	13821	11111	9088	6641	4218	2887
1965	326084	190340	119221	22095	20717	16791	18022	16636	14252	10708	7610	5030	3883
1975	354718	204791	129724	22858	21906	21420	19604	15305	15426	13206	9599	5873	4732
1985	377714	205720	146530	29070	24286	22340	20895	19899	17315	12726	11238	7766	6460
1990	**388775**	**203859**	**158225**	**29397**	**28935**	**23963**	**21838**	**20031**	**18573**	**15488**	**10551**	**8448**	**7693**
1995 projected	*397081*	*199215*	*168851*	*31077*	*29559*	*28487*	*23536*	*20914*	*18703*	*16575*	*12901*	*7928*	*8186*
NUMBER OF DEATHS													
All causes													
1955	3063652	482914	1285408	47065	76339	118874	175800	229855	284752	352723	395342	396715	503273
1965	3474651	381788	1498714	56800	80149	103628	180869	270566	371928	434774	463708	462484	667957
1975	3602420	304895	1476913	50858	77983	122530	178767	218795	352073	475907	548959	512466	759187
1985	3640170	234758	1323884	53048	67963	100619	157354	241105	330637	373158	532640	590629	958259
1990	**3658689**	**236277**	**1334254**	**60664**	**77983**	**99157**	**142888**	**216463**	**320073**	**417026**	**444076**	**574551**	**1069531**
1995 projected	*3564003*	*236057*	*1291963*	*69310*	*79905*	*106555*	*137608*	*205415*	*293594*	*399576*	*488838*	*487195*	*1059950*
Lung cancer													
1955	74709	566	57036	691	1981	4770	9162	13103	14291	13038	9386	5199	2522
1965	137108	696	96292	1159	2813	5169	11510	19986	27648	28007	20934	12333	6853
1975	199386	640	120925	1107	3144	7813	14585	19957	33336	40983	38245	24265	15311
1985	257414	557	136853	1295	3259	7209	15219	28180	39999	41692	48295	40047	31662
1990	**275201**	**564**	**145798**	**1287**	**3629**	**7654**	**14170**	**26030**	**41756**	**51272**	**45795**	**43142**	**39902**
1995 projected	*290323*	*612*	*148382*	*1330*	*3669*	*8327*	*14076*	*26063*	*41086*	*53831*	*55557*	*41554*	*44218*
ANNUAL DEATH RATE / 100,000 (*The rates for the age groups 0–34 and 35–69 are the means of seven five-yearly rates, but the all-ages rates are standardised to the conventional "European" age distribution)													
All causes													
1955	1405.4*	264.2*	1500.0*	272.5	404.2	651.0	1065.1	1663.1	2562.8	3881.4	5953.3	9405.0	17430.1
1965	1360.4*	192.3*	1508.7*	257.1	386.9	617.2	1003.6	1626.4	2609.7	4060.3	6093.3	9194.6	17203.6
1975	1234.0*	152.3*	1339.7*	222.5	356.0	572.0	911.9	1429.6	2282.4	3603.6	5719.0	8726.2	16044.8
1985	1051.8*	114.7*	1102.8*	182.5	279.8	450.4	753.1	1211.7	1909.5	2932.4	4739.5	7605.5	14834.4
1990	**965.4***	**114.3***	**1005.8***	**206.4**	**269.5**	**413.8**	**654.3**	**1080.6**	**1723.4**	**2692.6**	**4209.0**	**6800.9**	**13903.4**
1995 projected	*889.5**	*115.3**	*916.4**	*223.0*	*270.3*	*374.0*	*584.7*	*982.2*	*1569.8*	*2410.7*	*3789.2*	*6145.0*	*12949.0*
All cancer													
1955	207.2*	10.2*	306.7*	31.6	58.6	117.6	220.1	368.3	562.6	788.3	1052.8	1343.3	1593.9
1965	233.7*	11.1*	345.2*	35.3	63.9	119.8	223.9	396.9	638.0	938.8	1223.7	1514.7	1843.7
1975	248.6*	9.7*	351.9*	31.8	64.8	130.6	235.4	393.7	643.0	964.2	1363.0	1731.2	2078.0
1985	258.3*	7.7*	354.1*	29.5	60.9	120.9	239.1	418.9	657.4	952.1	1366.5	1852.7	2438.8
1990	**257.4***	**6.8***	**351.2***	**27.6**	**56.1**	**116.8**	**221.0**	**405.2**	**659.7**	**972.0**	**1357.6**	**1837.0**	**2546.0**
1995 projected	*254.5**	*6.2**	*343.3**	*25.6*	*52.7*	*107.7*	*208.1*	*394.3*	*654.8*	*960.0*	*1349.4*	*1823.3*	*2608.1*
Lung cancer													
1955	33.2*	0.4*	66.1*	4.0	10.5	26.1	55.5	94.8	128.6	143.5	141.3	123.3	87.3
1965	52.2*	0.4*	98.5*	5.2	13.6	30.8	63.9	120.1	194.0	261.6	275.1	245.2	176.5
1975	67.0*	0.3*	112.4*	4.8	14.4	36.5	74.4	130.4	216.1	310.3	398.4	413.2	323.6
1985	74.9*	0.3*	117.6*	4.5	13.4	32.3	72.8	141.6	231.0	327.6	429.7	515.7	490.1
1990	**74.0***	**0.3***	**114.2***	**4.4**	**12.5**	**31.9**	**64.9**	**129.9**	**224.8**	**331.1**	**434.0**	**510.7**	**518.7**
1995 projected	*73.2**	*0.3**	*110.7**	*4.3*	*12.4*	*29.2*	*59.8*	*124.6*	*219.7*	*324.8*	*430.7*	*524.1*	*540.2*
Upper aerodigestive cancer (mouth, oesophagus, pharynx and larynx)													
1955	17.3*	0.2*	26.5*	1.3	3.7	9.3	19.8	34.5	49.6	67.1	86.2	113.1	136.4
1965	18.3*	0.2*	30.1*	1.8	4.9	10.8	21.5	38.2	56.5	77.1	89.3	103.7	127.9
1975	19.8*	0.2*	32.7*	1.8	6.5	16.2	27.9	40.2	58.3	77.9	96.8	113.6	120.4
1985	19.8*	0.2*	33.9*	2.0	7.0	16.4	31.2	47.7	61.7	71.0	86.9	102.0	116.1
1990	**19.6***	**0.2***	**34.1***	**2.2**	**6.6**	**16.2**	**29.6**	**46.8**	**62.4**	**74.8**	**85.9**	**95.9**	**112.7**
1995 projected	*19.2**	*0.2**	*33.8**	*2.1*	*6.6*	*15.5*	*28.4*	*46.3*	*63.0*	*74.8*	*85.4*	*90.4*	*107.6*
Other cancer													
1955	156.6*	9.7*	214.1*	26.3	44.4	82.2	144.7	239.0	384.3	577.8	825.2	1106.9	1370.2
1965	163.2*	10.5*	216.7*	28.2	45.5	78.3	138.5	238.6	387.6	600.2	859.3	1165.8	1539.3
1975	161.9*	9.2*	206.8*	25.1	43.9	77.9	133.1	223.1	368.6	576.0	867.7	1204.4	1634.1
1985	163.6*	7.3*	202.6*	23.1	40.4	72.2	135.1	229.6	364.7	553.4	849.9	1235.0	1832.5
1990	**163.9***	**6.4***	**202.9***	**21.1**	**36.9**	**68.7**	**126.5**	**228.5**	**372.5**	**566.1**	**837.6**	**1230.5**	**1914.6**
1995 projected	*162.1**	*5.7**	*198.8**	*19.2*	*33.7*	*62.9*	*119.9*	*223.3*	*372.1*	*560.4*	*833.3*	*1208.7*	*1960.3*
Chronic obstructive pulmonary disease (COPD)													
1955	37.7*	2.6*	46.8*	2.8	5.8	13.3	30.4	55.1	88.2	132.2	183.2	269.0	439.8
1965	49.8*	1.6*	60.8*	2.7	5.8	12.0	26.9	59.6	120.5	197.8	282.1	389.4	590.2
1975	58.7*	1.5*	58.6*	2.8	5.4	11.7	25.4	52.7	107.3	205.2	363.8	553.4	800.1
1985	46.6*	0.7*	38.8*	1.3	2.5	5.8	13.7	32.9	72.4	143.2	267.1	458.7	808.5
1990	**42.1***	**0.6***	**33.0***	**1.2**	**2.0**	**4.5**	**10.3**	**26.2**	**60.6**	**126.0**	**238.5**	**412.6**	**775.1**
1995 projected	*38.5**	*0.7**	*28.3**	*1.1*	*1.8*	*3.5*	*8.4*	*22.5*	*52.1*	*108.5*	*214.0*	*382.5*	*738.4*
Other respiratory disease													
1955	64.0*	23.1*	41.7*	6.8	9.6	16.0	26.2	42.4	69.9	121.2	222.6	442.1	1039.5
1965	57.4*	13.0*	36.6*	5.7	8.4	13.0	19.8	33.7	60.6	114.9	220.8	427.0	1110.4
1975	49.6*	6.2*	30.7*	4.3	7.0	10.7	17.1	29.1	50.2	96.7	202.2	403.9	1059.3
1985	46.8*	2.7*	27.8*	3.7	5.2	8.4	14.8	25.8	47.9	88.5	183.4	382.7	1124.7
1990	**46.7***	**2.3***	**26.4***	**4.1**	**5.5**	**8.0**	**12.9**	**23.8**	**45.1**	**85.4**	**179.1**	**376.1**	**1169.7**
1995 projected	*47.5**	*2.2**	*26.1**	*4.7*	*5.6*	*7.5*	*12.3*	*22.6*	*44.8*	*85.4*	*172.0*	*387.3*	*1220.5*
Vascular disease													
1955	623.4*	11.8*	655.7*	58.5	112.5	215.7	400.8	694.9	1181.8	1926.0	3137.5	5103.4	9416.8
1965	638.1*	8.9*	674.8*	58.3	122.6	235.5	415.2	702.7	1199.7	1989.2	3220.6	5084.6	9770.7
1975	575.9*	7.4*	581.7*	46.5	103.5	201.4	366.1	619.9	1028.2	1706.3	2870.0	4662.3	9288.8
1985	454.3*	6.5*	435.0*	35.9	75.8	143.0	265.8	458.5	783.9	1281.9	2196.7	3716.7	7821.9
1990	**379.5***	**5.8***	**354.4***	**32.4**	**63.2**	**118.7**	**208.1**	**366.9**	**628.7**	**1062.7**	**1775.9**	**3071.0**	**6816.5**
1995 projected	*315.0**	*5.4**	*284.7**	*28.0*	*52.5*	*92.4*	*166.1*	*298.8*	*509.8*	*845.4*	*1441.0*	*2527.3*	*5877.5*
Liver cirrhosis													
1955	18.7*	0.7*	35.1*	5.8	12.5	21.6	33.9	44.9	57.3	69.7	74.4	72.3	57.1
1965	25.2*	1.0*	47.2*	9.6	17.3	27.7	43.2	61.0	78.6	93.0	95.4	100.4	84.2
1975	29.5*	1.3*	56.0*	13.5	27.2	41.5	54.7	66.5	86.8	102.1	103.6	102.5	83.8
1985	23.4*	1.0*	43.5*	9.2	17.5	30.4	47.5	58.9	69.4	71.9	81.5	85.6	76.4
1990	**20.1***	**0.8***	**38.1***	**9.6**	**15.3**	**25.3**	**37.3**	**52.4**	**61.1**	**65.6**	**63.8**	**71.7**	**72.4**
1995 projected	*17.4**	*0.8**	*32.9**	*9.2*	*14.1*	*20.7*	*30.9*	*45.3*	*53.8*	*56.2*	*56.0*	*58.4*	*64.3*
Other medical causes													
1955	352.3*	147.9*	299.5*	85.2	115.0	165.2	238.5	333.4	466.8	692.3	1094.3	1913.4	4386.1
1965	255.8*	91.9*	229.5*	59.2	78.8	110.1	162.2	246.2	373.9	576.0	867.7	1424.1	3300.8
1975	176.8*	59.3*	157.3*	39.3	58.0	81.3	114.3	162.3	250.3	395.8	647.9	1039.2	2289.2
1985	144.1*	41.5*	119.6*	33.3	43.4	60.8	87.4	127.2	189.0	296.3	509.5	914.4	2175.0
1990	**144.1***	**43.4***	**123.6***	**56.7**	**58.2**	**68.0**	**88.3**	**123.9**	**182.5**	**287.6**	**472.8**	**849.6**	**2140.1**
1995 projected	*143.7**	*44.7**	*127.3**	*78.6*	*77.2*	*77.7*	*90.3*	*122.8*	*175.0*	*269.2*	*444.3*	*798.2*	*2070.0*
All non-medical causes													
1955	102.1*	67.8*	114.4*	81.8	90.2	101.5	115.2	124.0	136.4	151.7	188.5	261.5	496.9
1965	100.5*	64.8*	114.7*	86.3	90.0	99.1	112.4	126.1	138.4	150.6	183.0	254.4	503.5
1975	95.0*	66.8*	103.4*	84.3	90.0	94.8	99.0	105.5	116.7	133.3	168.5	233.8	445.6
1985	78.3*	54.7*	83.9*	69.5	74.6	81.2	84.7	89.5	89.5	98.6	134.8	194.6	389.1
1990	**75.3***	**54.6***	**79.1***	**74.7**	**69.2**	**72.4**	**76.4**	**82.2**	**85.6**	**93.3**	**121.1**	**182.9**	**383.5**
1995 projected	*72.8**	*55.5**	*73.8**	*75.9*	*66.3*	*64.6*	*68.5*	*75.9*	*79.5*	*86.1*	*112.6*	*168.0*	*370.3*

OECD DEVELOPED: Females

	All ages	0–34	35–69	35–39	40–44	45–49	50–54	55–59	60–64	65–69	70–74	75–79	80+/NK
POPULATION (1000s)													
1955	303875	169226	116026	18909	20472	19408	17346	15466	13262	11163	8544	5672	4407
1965	342782	185528	132417	22530	22778	18617	20041	18533	16257	13661	10777	7523	6538
1975	372723	198494	141938	22822	21948	22157	22039	17699	18504	16770	13249	9562	9480
1985	397235	199026	156148	28911	24427	22695	21571	21497	20794	16253	15847	12478	13736
1990	407520	196386	166414	29362	28895	24128	22370	21136	20784	19739	14755	13530	16436
1995 projected	414296	190935	175336	30720	29510	28677	24138	22019	20539	19735	17978	12619	17428
NUMBER OF DEATHS													
All causes													
1955	2685594	354175	893366	38008	57394	79296	107782	142048	194895	273943	357163	412576	668314
1965	3007812	245651	927149	35745	53746	68156	108748	150641	212462	297651	400095	485398	949519
1975	3196121	169599	873434	28037	42845	68072	104309	126716	204526	298929	417569	529414	1206105
1985	3407825	118532	761675	27290	36168	53470	81118	126374	195240	242015	400622	553955	1573041
1990	3492544	110762	753338	27874	39608	53172	75775	112180	175961	268768	332139	534280	1762025
1995 projected	3353394	102176	707386	28477	38786	57986	75584	107453	157965	241135	362442	443564	1737826
Lung cancer													
1955	15100	380	9685	306	576	997	1336	1855	2130	2485	2202	1703	1130
1965	26138	353	16325	466	884	1481	2473	3112	3694	4215	3917	2973	2570
1975	45932	304	27865	466	1134	2408	4113	5219	7077	7448	6867	5379	5517
1985	81900	351	43134	637	1299	2645	4809	8398	12257	13089	14363	11622	12430
1990	101456	337	49917	676	1619	3099	5229	8315	13436	17543	17005	16168	18029
1995 projected	124668	331	56468	728	1788	3932	6217	9460	14431	19912	23770	19664	24435

ANNUAL DEATH RATE / 100,000 (*The rates for the age groups 0–34 and 35–69 are the means of seven five-yearly rates, but the all-ages rates are standardised to the conventional "European" age distribution)

	All ages	0–34	35–69	35–39	40–44	45–49	50–54	55–59	60–64	65–69	70–74	75–79	80+/NK
All causes													
1955	1010.2*	194.6*	907.6*	201.0	280.4	408.6	621.4	918.5	1469.6	2454.0	4180.2	7273.3	15164.8
1965	889.7*	124.9*	800.3*	158.7	236.0	366.1	542.6	812.8	1306.9	2178.8	3712.7	6452.1	14524.2
1975	752.5*	88.1*	671.8*	122.9	195.2	307.2	473.3	715.9	1105.3	1782.5	3151.8	5536.5	12723.4
1985	627.4*	61.6*	552.8*	94.4	148.1	235.6	376.0	587.9	938.9	1489.0	2528.0	4439.5	11452.1
1990	574.8*	57.4*	504.3*	94.9	137.1	220.4	338.7	530.7	846.6	1361.6	2251.0	3949.0	10720.6
1995 projected	526.3*	53.5*	459.8*	92.7	131.4	202.2	313.1	488.0	769.1	1221.9	2016.1	3515.0	9971.4
All cancer													
1955	159.5*	9.8*	240.6*	49.8	89.5	138.8	206.0	282.8	387.4	529.9	707.0	932.9	1166.4
1965	159.0*	9.9*	236.6*	45.0	82.6	135.2	205.4	280.7	382.0	525.4	707.3	922.8	1233.6
1975	152.2*	8.4*	226.8*	38.8	72.2	124.8	196.0	278.8	379.0	497.8	679.8	895.9	1197.6
1985	150.2*	6.8*	220.4*	35.0	63.7	108.8	174.7	264.7	383.5	512.1	691.6	900.1	1286.6
1990	148.3*	6.0*	215.4*	34.7	61.0	106.0	167.9	253.1	367.9	517.1	687.3	906.5	1320.8
1995 projected	145.6*	5.5*	208.3*	32.9	59.0	101.0	161.7	244.1	356.9	502.7	680.9	903.9	1347.3
Lung cancer													
1955	5.6*	0.2*	9.7*	1.6	2.8	5.1	7.7	12.0	16.1	22.3	25.8	30.0	25.6
1965	8.0*	0.2*	13.8*	2.1	3.9	8.0	12.3	16.8	22.7	30.9	36.3	39.5	39.3
1975	12.0*	0.2*	21.3*	2.0	5.2	10.9	18.7	29.5	38.2	44.4	51.8	56.3	58.2
1985	17.9*	0.2*	31.4*	2.2	5.3	11.7	22.3	39.1	58.9	80.5	90.6	93.1	90.5
1990	20.4*	0.2*	33.9*	2.3	5.6	12.8	23.4	39.3	64.6	88.9	115.2	119.5	109.7
1995 projected	23.4*	0.2*	37.4*	2.4	6.1	13.7	25.8	43.0	70.3	100.9	132.2	155.8	140.2
Upper aerodigestive cancer (mouth, oesophagus, pharynx and larynx)													
1955	4.0*	0.1*	5.1*	0.8	1.4	2.5	3.8	5.8	8.7	12.9	20.4	30.1	42.2
1965	3.9*	0.1*	5.2*	0.6	1.2	2.5	4.4	6.4	8.6	12.5	18.6	27.0	41.5
1975	4.0*	0.1*	5.7*	0.5	1.2	2.6	4.8	7.7	10.4	12.7	17.4	24.0	39.1
1985	3.8*	0.1*	5.7*	0.5	1.1	2.3	4.0	7.3	10.4	14.2	16.9	22.6	35.7
1990	3.7*	0.1*	5.4*	0.4	1.1	2.2	4.3	6.7	10.2	13.0	17.9	23.7	35.6
1995 projected	3.7*	0.1*	5.3*	0.5	1.1	2.3	4.3	6.7	9.7	12.7	17.5	24.9	36.5
Other cancer													
1955	149.9*	9.5*	225.8*	47.4	85.2	131.2	194.4	265.0	362.7	494.7	660.9	872.8	1098.5
1965	147.1*	9.6*	217.6*	42.3	77.5	124.7	188.7	257.5	350.8	482.0	652.4	856.3	1152.8
1975	136.3*	8.1*	199.8*	36.3	65.9	111.3	172.5	241.6	330.3	440.7	610.5	815.7	1100.3
1985	128.5*	6.6*	183.3*	32.3	57.4	94.8	148.5	218.4	314.2	417.4	584.1	784.3	1160.4
1990	124.2*	5.8*	176.1*	31.9	54.4	90.9	140.3	207.1	293.1	415.2	554.2	763.3	1175.5
1995 projected	118.4*	5.3*	165.6*	30.1	51.9	85.0	131.6	194.4	276.9	389.1	531.1	723.2	1170.6
Chronic obstructive pulmonary disease (COPD)													
1955	16.0*	2.0*	11.8*	1.7	2.3	3.4	5.9	10.4	20.3	38.5	72.3	136.2	293.0
1965	15.7*	1.3*	12.9*	1.7	2.6	4.4	6.9	11.7	22.3	40.3	69.5	126.6	291.2
1975	17.8*	1.2*	16.8*	2.2	3.7	6.1	10.3	18.1	29.7	47.3	84.0	141.1	292.8
1985	15.6*	0.6*	16.5*	1.2	1.9	4.2	8.5	16.9	29.8	52.8	81.9	122.9	237.0
1990	16.1*	0.5*	15.8*	1.0	1.6	3.4	7.3	14.8	29.8	53.0	90.3	133.4	251.9
1995 projected	17.0*	0.5*	15.9*	0.9	1.4	3.0	7.0	14.7	29.7	54.7	94.2	151.4	276.6
Other respiratory disease													
1955	49.3*	20.8*	23.9*	5.5	6.5	8.4	13.0	20.7	38.2	74.7	159.8	339.2	892.2
1965	39.9*	11.0*	18.9*	4.1	5.5	7.5	10.6	16.2	29.7	58.6	127.3	279.0	888.9
1975	31.9*	5.1*	15.4*	3.1	4.0	5.9	8.5	14.8	25.2	46.4	106.0	238.5	780.7
1985	26.5*	2.0*	12.1*	2.0	2.8	4.2	7.0	10.8	20.0	38.0	78.9	180.8	758.8
1990	26.6*	1.6*	11.6*	2.2	2.8	4.1	6.2	10.5	19.3	36.1	79.6	175.2	789.0
1995 projected	27.1*	1.5*	11.4*	2.2	2.8	3.9	6.1	10.2	19.0	35.7	74.3	178.7	824.4
Vascular disease													
1955	461.5*	10.9*	386.8*	39.0	64.9	115.6	209.2	358.2	664.1	1256.2	2316.7	4164.5	8414.2
1965	430.9*	6.8*	330.6*	30.4	53.4	99.8	168.1	297.5	569.7	1095.2	2072.1	3839.5	8690.9
1975	368.0*	4.9*	254.9*	22.0	41.3	74.3	132.2	237.4	438.0	838.9	1698.8	3276.4	8025.2
1985	287.7*	3.9*	182.1*	14.4	27.6	49.8	92.3	165.9	317.7	607.2	1213.9	2420.1	6896.8
1990	242.8*	3.5*	148.2*	12.9	22.6	42.7	73.3	135.5	257.6	492.7	969.2	1969.5	6064.2
1995 projected	202.4*	3.2*	119.0*	11.0	19.3	34.7	61.2	111.7	206.6	388.3	770.1	1572.9	5242.8
Liver cirrhosis													
1955	8.9*	0.6*	15.8*	4.1	6.8	10.8	16.1	20.1	24.1	28.5	33.1	36.3	35.6
1965	10.7*	0.6*	18.7*	5.3	8.7	13.6	17.6	22.4	28.5	34.5	40.5	45.2	46.0
1975	11.0*	0.7*	19.9*	5.4	10.1	15.6	20.5	25.1	29.5	32.7	38.0	41.7	40.7
1985	9.0*	0.5*	16.0*	3.9	6.2	10.3	15.6	21.0	25.7	29.3	33.9	38.9	36.6
1990	8.1*	0.4*	14.3*	3.7	5.7	9.0	12.7	17.6	23.1	28.1	31.8	36.6	36.0
1995 projected	7.3*	0.4*	12.7*	3.5	5.4	7.8	10.5	15.4	20.5	25.8	30.4	33.4	34.1
Other medical causes													
1955	273.6*	128.8*	193.1*	80.0	87.0	104.4	137.8	188.2	289.9	464.5	793.9	1482.3	3884.7
1965	190.5*	74.7*	143.4*	47.8	56.5	73.6	97.7	143.2	225.7	359.6	594.9	1059.1	2871.6
1975	130.9*	46.2*	100.5*	26.1	35.3	49.2	69.9	102.5	158.9	261.7	455.8	785.6	1959.3
1985	107.1*	30.8*	75.3*	16.6	21.9	32.7	49.1	77.0	125.8	203.7	360.7	668.5	1935.5
1990	103.6*	28.8*	70.8*	19.7	22.0	30.9	44.6	69.7	115.7	193.4	334.2	627.9	1978.4
1995 projected	99.7*	26.6*	66.6*	22.2	23.5	29.5	41.8	64.7	106.5	178.0	312.4	587.7	1987.8
All non-medical causes													
1955	41.5*	21.5*	35.7*	20.9	23.3	27.1	33.3	38.0	45.6	61.6	97.4	181.9	478.7
1965	43.0*	20.5*	39.3*	24.5	26.8	32.1	36.3	41.1	48.9	65.2	101.1	179.9	502.2
1975	40.6*	21.6*	37.6*	25.2	28.6	31.2	35.9	39.2	45.1	57.6	89.4	157.1	427.0
1985	31.2*	17.0*	30.5*	21.4	23.9	25.6	28.8	31.6	36.4	46.0	67.1	108.1	300.8
1990	29.2*	16.6*	28.2*	20.7	21.5	24.4	26.6	29.6	33.1	41.2	58.7	99.8	280.3
1995 projected	27.2*	16.0*	25.9*	19.9	20.0	22.3	24.9	27.2	30.0	36.7	53.7	87.1	258.6

OECD DEVELOPED: 1975

Smoking-attributed deaths (Sm.) and total deaths (Total)

		ALL CAUSES	ALL CANCER	Lung cancer	Upper aero-digestive ca.	Other cancer	COPD	Other respiratory	Vascular disease	Liver cirrhosis	Other medical	Non-medical
Males												
0-34	Sm.	–	–	–	–	–	–	–	–	–	–	–
	Total	304895	19321	640	323	18358	3054	12420	14274	2379	118220	135227
35-69	Sm.	447518	166586	111618	22138	32830	46649	8876	177372	–	48035	–
	Total	1476913	382362	120925	36207	225230	61011	33139	627042	65681	177242	130436
		(30%)	(44%)	(92%)	(61%)	(15%)	(76%)	(27%)	(28%)		(27%)	
70+	Sm.	321187	106959	69800	11352	25807	72709	9900	108235	–	23384	–
	Total	1820612	330824	77821	21659	231344	105273	93253	988807	19924	231539	50992
		(18%)	(32%)	(90%)	(52%)	(11%)	(69%)	(11%)	(11%)		(10%)	
Any age	Sm.	768705	273545	181418	33490	58637	119358	18776	285607	–	71419	–
	Total	3602420	732507	199386	58189	474932	169338	138812	1630123	87984	527001	316655
		(21%)	(37%)	(91%)	(58%)	(12%)	(70%)	(14%)	(18%)		(14%)	
Females												
0-34	Sm.	–	–	–	–	–	–	–	–	–	–	–
	Total	169599	15953	304	160	15489	2254	9872	9361	1214	88378	42567
35-69	Sm.	70341	21476	16203	2065	3208	8098	1845	28859	–	10063	–
	Total	873434	298503	27865	7437	263201	21562	19839	323438	26827	131452	51813
		(8%)	(7%)	(58%)	(28%)	(1%)	(38%)	(9%)	(9%)		(8%)	
70+	Sm.	49086	10234	7369	1322	1543	11212	2068	21326	–	4246	–
	Total	2153088	289258	17763	8300	263195	52389	110853	1299105	12883	321245	67355
		(2%)	(4%)	(41%)	(16%)	(1%)	(21%)	(2%)	(2%)		(1%)	
Any age	Sm.	119427	31710	23572	3387	4751	19310	3913	50185	–	14309	–
	Total	3196121	603714	45932	15897	541885	76205	140564	1631904	40924	541075	161735
		(4%)	(5%)	(51%)	(21%)	(1%)	(25%)	(3%)	(3%)		(3%)	
Males+Females												
0-34	Sm.	–	–	–	–	–	–	–	–	–	–	–
	Total	474494	35274	944	483	33847	5308	22292	23635	3593	206598	177794
35-69	Sm.	517859	188062	127821	24203	36038	54747	10721	206231	–	58098	–
	Total	2350347	680865	148790	43644	488431	82573	52978	950480	92508	308694	182249
		(22%)	(28%)	(86%)	(55%)	(7%)	(66%)	(20%)	(22%)		(19%)	
70+	Sm.	370273	117193	77169	12674	27350	83921	11968	129561	–	27630	–
	Total	3973700	620082	95584	29959	494539	157662	204106	2287912	32807	552784	118347
		(9%)	(19%)	(81%)	(42%)	(6%)	(53%)	(6%)	(6%)		(5%)	
Any age	Sm.	888132	305255	204990	36877	63388	138668	22689	335792	–	85728	–
	Total	6798541	1336221	245318	74086	1016817	245543	279376	3262027	128908	1068076	478390
		(13%)	(23%)	(84%)	(50%)	(6%)	(56%)	(8%)	(10%)		(8%)	

OECD DEVELOPED: 1985

Smoking-attributed deaths (Sm.) and total deaths (Total)

		ALL CAUSES	ALL CANCER	Lung cancer	Upper aero-digestive ca.	Other cancer	COPD	Other respiratory	Vascular disease	Liver cirrhosis	Other medical	Non-medical
Males												
0-34	Sm.	–	–	–	–	–	–	–	–	–	–	–
	Total	234758	16058	557	353	15148	1374	5240	13490	2048	79740	116808
35-69	Sm.	426694	190202	126777	26701	36724	33179	8817	150027	–	44469	–
	Total	1323884	418672	136853	41670	240149	42449	32019	506411	56529	147793	120011
		(32%)	(45%)	(93%)	(64%)	(15%)	(78%)	(28%)	(30%)		(30%)	
70+	Sm.	425514	164133	109245	14708	40180	86688	14047	128858	–	31788	–
	Total	2081528	454990	120004	25185	309801	117871	122981	1040778	20746	268768	55394
		(20%)	(36%)	(91%)	(58%)	(13%)	(74%)	(11%)	(12%)		(12%)	
Any age	Sm.	852208	354335	236022	41409	76904	119867	22864	278885	–	76257	–
	Total	3640170	889720	257414	67208	565098	161694	160240	1560679	79323	496301	292213
		(23%)	(40%)	(92%)	(62%)	(14%)	(74%)	(14%)	(18%)		(15%)	
Females												
0-34	Sm.	–	–	–	–	–	–	–	–	–	–	–
	Total	118532	13832	351	159	13322	1142	3775	7880	1009	56283	34611
35-69	Sm.	107032	39119	30682	2939	5498	12709	2512	37929	–	14763	–
	Total	761675	307960	43134	7797	257029	21977	16382	242546	22941	103972	45897
		(14%)	(13%)	(71%)	(38%)	(2%)	(58%)	(15%)	(16%)		(14%)	
70+	Sm.	137233	33454	24777	3283	5394	27056	5688	56168	–	14867	–
	Total	2527618	398632	38415	10402	349815	60869	139299	1441674	15261	406439	65444
		(5%)	(8%)	(64%)	(32%)	(2%)	(44%)	(4%)	(4%)		(4%)	
Any age	Sm.	244265	72573	55459	6222	10892	39765	8200	94097	–	29630	–
	Total	3407825	720424	81900	18358	620166	83988	159456	1692100	39211	566694	145952
		(7%)	(10%)	(68%)	(34%)	(2%)	(47%)	(5%)	(6%)		(5%)	
Males+Females												
0-34	Sm.	–	–	–	–	–	–	–	–	–	–	–
	Total	353290	29890	908	512	28470	2516	9015	21370	3057	136023	151419
35-69	Sm.	533726	229321	157459	29640	42222	45888	11329	187956	–	59232	–
	Total	2085559	726632	179987	49467	497178	64426	48401	748957	79470	251765	165908
		(26%)	(32%)	(87%)	(60%)	(8%)	(71%)	(23%)	(25%)		(24%)	
70+	Sm.	562747	197587	134022	17991	45574	113744	19735	185026	–	46655	–
	Total	4609146	853622	158419	35587	659616	178740	262280	2482452	36007	675207	120838
		(12%)	(23%)	(85%)	(51%)	(7%)	(64%)	(8%)	(7%)		(7%)	
Any age	Sm.	1096473	426908	291481	47631	87796	159632	31064	372982	–	105887	–
	Total	7047995	1610144	339314	85566	1185264	245682	319696	3252779	118534	1062995	438165
		(16%)	(27%)	(86%)	(56%)	(7%)	(65%)	(10%)	(11%)		(10%)	

(To be conservative, no deaths before age 35, and none from liver cirrhosis or non-medical causes, were attributed to smoking.)

OECD DEVELOPED: 1990

Smoking–attributed deaths (Sm.) and total deaths (Total)

		ALL CAUSES	ALL CANCER	Lung cancer	Upper aero-digestive ca.	Other cancer	COPD	Other respiratory	Vascular disease	Liver cirrhosis	Other medical	Non-medical
Males												
0–34	Sm.	–	–	–	–	–	–	–	–	–	–	–
	Total	236277	14323	564	340	13419	1337	4594	12392	1697	84975	116959
35–69	Sm.	423535	202732	134681	28827	39224	31401	8889	128837	–	51676	–
	Total	1334254	454826	145798	45437	263591	40280	33933	456561	53485	172374	122795
		(32%)	(45%)	(92%)	(63%)	(15%)	(78%)	(26%)	(28%)		(30%)	
70+	Sm.	427778	176005	117193	15165	43647	87787	15460	115508	–	33018	–
	Total	2088158	494290	128839	25836	339615	119653	140645	971179	18363	286296	57732
		(20%)	(36%)	(91%)	(59%)	(13%)	(73%)	(11%)	(12%)		(12%)	
Any age	Sm.	851313	378737	251874	43992	82871	119188	24349	244345	–	84694	–
	Total	3658689	963439	275201	71613	616625	161270	179172	1440132	73545	543645	297486
		(23%)	(39%)	(92%)	(61%)	(13%)	(74%)	(14%)	(17%)		(16%)	
Females												
0–34	Sm.	–	–	–	–	–	–	–	–	–	–	–
	Total	110762	12437	337	122	11978	951	3098	7137	876	52660	33603
35–69	Sm.	117710	45908	36523	3143	6242	14313	2901	37260	–	17328	–
	Total	753338	322993	49917	8041	265035	22986	17184	216470	21811	106495	45399
		(16%)	(14%)	(73%)	(39%)	(2%)	(62%)	(17%)	(17%)		(16%)	
70+	Sm.	191623	49302	36687	4477	8138	38196	8882	72693	–	22550	–
	Total	2628444	441149	51202	11707	378240	72787	165123	1406176	15547	459430	68232
		(7%)	(11%)	(72%)	(38%)	(2%)	(52%)	(5%)	(5%)		(5%)	
Any age	Sm.	309333	95210	73210	7620	14380	52509	11783	109953	–	39878	–
	Total	3492544	776579	101456	19870	655253	96724	185405	1629783	38234	618585	147234
		(9%)	(12%)	(72%)	(38%)	(2%)	(54%)	(6%)	(7%)		(6%)	
Males+Females												
0–34	Sm.	–	–	–	–	–	–	–	–	–	–	–
	Total	347039	26760	901	462	25397	2288	7692	19529	2573	137635	150562
35–69	Sm.	541245	248640	171204	31970	45466	45714	11790	166097	–	69004	–
	Total	2087592	777819	195715	53478	528626	63266	51117	673031	75296	278869	168194
		(26%)	(32%)	(87%)	(60%)	(9%)	(72%)	(23%)	(25%)		(25%)	
70+	Sm.	619401	225307	153880	19642	51785	125983	24342	188201	–	55568	–
	Total	4716602	935439	180041	37543	717855	192440	305768	2377355	33910	745726	125964
		(13%)	(24%)	(85%)	(52%)	(7%)	(65%)	(8%)	(8%)		(7%)	
Any age	Sm.	1160646	473947	325084	51612	97251	171697	36132	354298	–	124572	–
	Total	7151233	1740018	376657	91483	1271878	257994	364577	3069915	111779	1162230	444720
		(16%)	(27%)	(86%)	(56%)	(8%)	(67%)	(10%)	(12%)		(11%)	

OECD DEVELOPED: 1995

Smoking–attributed deaths (Sm.) and total deaths (Total)

		ALL CAUSES	ALL CANCER	Lung cancer	Upper aero-digestive ca.	Other cancer	COPD	Other respiratory	Vascular disease	Liver cirrhosis	Other medical	Non-medical
Males												
0–34	Sm.	–	–	–	–	–	–	–	–	–	–	–
	Total	236057	12847	612	340	11895	1411	4379	11394	1695	89093	115238
35–69	Sm.	406755	205656	136658	29786	39212	28134	8884	105859	–	58222	–
	Total	1291963	467224	148382	47600	271242	36283	35385	387623	49019	193682	122747
		(31%)	(44%)	(92%)	(63%)	(14%)	(78%)	(25%)	(27%)		(30%)	
70+	Sm.	436536	192158	128731	16033	47394	87309	17134	105297	–	34638	–
	Total	2035983	532119	141329	27000	363790	118369	152796	867378	17118	290044	58159
		(21%)	(36%)	(91%)	(59%)	(13%)	(74%)	(11%)	(12%)		(12%)	
Any age	Sm.	843291	397814	265389	45819	86606	115443	26018	211156	–	92860	–
	Total	3564003	1012190	290323	74940	646927	156063	192560	1266395	67832	572819	296144
		(24%)	(39%)	(91%)	(61%)	(13%)	(74%)	(14%)	(17%)		(16%)	
Females												
0–34	Sm.	–	–	–	–	–	–	–	–	–	–	–
	Total	102176	11160	331	111	10718	888	2759	6331	813	48784	31441
35–69	Sm.	126097	52978	42713	3351	6914	15567	3219	34579	–	19754	–
	Total	707386	321764	56468	8134	257162	23330	17297	177478	20132	103560	43825
		(18%)	(16%)	(76%)	(41%)	(3%)	(67%)	(19%)	(19%)		(19%)	
70+	Sm.	248513	69063	52281	5586	11196	50725	12458	84850	–	31417	–
	Total	2543832	471269	67869	12653	390747	84240	179588	1250644	15626	476772	65693
		(10%)	(15%)	(77%)	(44%)	(3%)	(60%)	(7%)	(7%)		(7%)	
Any age	Sm.	374610	122041	94994	8937	18110	66292	15677	119429	–	51171	–
	Total	3353394	804193	124668	20898	658627	108458	199644	1434453	36571	629116	140959
		(11%)	(15%)	(76%)	(43%)	(3%)	(61%)	(8%)	(8%)		(8%)	
Males+Females												
0–34	Sm.	–	–	–	–	–	–	–	–	–	–	–
	Total	338233	24007	943	451	22613	2299	7138	17725	2508	137877	146679
35–69	Sm.	532852	258634	179371	33137	46126	43701	12103	140438	–	77976	–
	Total	1999349	788988	204850	55734	528404	59613	52682	565101	69151	297242	166572
		(27%)	(33%)	(88%)	(59%)	(9%)	(73%)	(23%)	(25%)		(26%)	
70+	Sm.	685049	261221	181012	21619	58590	138034	29592	190147	–	66055	–
	Total	4579815	1003388	209198	39653	754537	202609	332384	2118022	32744	766816	123852
		(15%)	(26%)	(87%)	(55%)	(8%)	(68%)	(9%)	(9%)		(9%)	
Any age	Sm.	1217901	519855	360383	54756	104716	181735	41695	330585	–	144031	–
	Total	6917397	1816383	414991	95838	1305554	264521	392204	2700848	104403	1201935	437103
		(18%)	(29%)	(87%)	(57%)	(8%)	(69%)	(11%)	(12%)		(12%)	

(To be conservative, no deaths before age 35, and none from liver cirrhosis or non-medical causes, were attributed to smoking.)

EUROPEAN UNION (12 countries): 1990

		No. of deaths			Standardised rates (Defined on p.250)			Annual death rates / 100, 000						
		All ages	0–34	35–69	All ages	0–34	35–69	0–4	5–9	10–14	15–19	20–24	25–29	30–34
ALL CAUSES	M	1746893	91634	628399	997.3	105.1	1037.0	209.8	23.0	25.3	82.9	120.2	128.2	146.2
	F	1752901	42245	340051	588.7	53.0	494.2	162.8	17.3	17.3	31.1	38.4	45.2	59.1
Tuberculosis	M	4022	140	1809	2.3	0.2	2.9	0.0	0.0	0.0	0.1	0.1	0.3	0.5
	F	2070	66	577	0.8	0.1	0.8	0.0	–	0.0	0.0	0.1	0.2	0.2
Other infective	M	9169	1098	3120	5.3	1.3	5.0	4.5	0.4	0.3	0.7	0.8	1.1	1.5
and parasitic	F	10247	724	2035	3.7	0.9	2.9	3.5	0.6	0.3	0.6	0.4	0.6	0.7
ALL CANCER	M	474406	6390	224762	274.4	7.2	375.1	4.2	4.4	4.1	6.1	7.1	9.5	14.8
	F	375926	5403	148400	150.3	6.3	214.8	3.7	3.5	3.2	4.1	4.6	8.1	16.7
Mouth and	M	14916	123	10828	9.0	0.1	17.0	0.1	0.0	0.0	0.1	0.1	0.1	0.5
pharynx cancer	F	3592	40	1657	1.5	0.0	2.4	0.0	0.0	0.0	0.1	0.0	0.1	0.1
Oesophagus cancer	M	15700	33	9773	9.3	0.0	15.9	–	–	0.0	–	0.0	0.1	0.2
	F	5406	11	1741	2.0	0.0	2.5	–	–	–	–	0.0	0.0	0.1
Stomach cancer	M	36166	166	15425	20.8	0.2	25.9	–	–	0.0	0.0	0.1	0.3	0.9
	F	27498	189	7444	9.8	0.2	10.8	0.0	–	–	0.1	0.1	0.3	0.9
Colorectal cancer	M	48195	210	19815	27.6	0.2	33.5	0.0	–	0.0	0.1	0.1	0.4	0.9
	F	51842	177	15374	18.8	0.2	22.5	0.0	–	–	0.0	0.1	0.4	0.9
Liver cancer	M	9115	68	5309	5.3	0.1	9.0	0.1	0.0	0.0	0.0	0.1	0.1	0.1
	F	3814	41	1467	1.5	0.0	2.2	0.1	0.1	0.0	0.0	0.0	0.1	0.1
Pancreas cancer	M	18953	74	9544	11.0	0.1	15.9	0.0	0.0	0.0	0.0	0.0	0.1	0.3
	F	18663	43	6090	7.0	0.0	8.9	0.0	0.0	–	0.0	0.1	0.1	0.2
Larynx cancer	M	10895	14	6894	6.5	0.0	11.2	–	0.0	–	0.0	0.0	0.0	0.1
	F	866	6	415	0.4	0.0	0.6	0.0	–	0.0	–	0.0	–	0.0
Lung cancer	M	132920	262	72944	77.6	0.3	122.8	0.1	0.0	0.0	0.1	0.1	0.3	1.4
	F	32481	128	15326	13.7	0.1	22.4	0.0	–	–	0.1	0.1	0.2	0.6
Malignant melanoma	M	3447	189	2156	2.0	0.2	3.3	–	–	–	0.1	0.2	0.5	0.7
	F	3384	167	1706	1.5	0.2	2.4	–	0.0	–	0.0	0.2	0.4	0.6
Female breast cancer	F	69653	746	37796	31.2	0.8	54.0	–	–	0.0	0.1	0.1	1.1	4.5
Cervix cancer	F	7484	291	4309	3.5	0.3	6.1	0.0	–	–	–	0.1	0.6	1.6
Other uterine cancer	F	12909	67	5130	5.1	0.1	7.5	0.0	–	0.0	0.0	0.0	0.1	0.4
Ovarian cancer	F	20594	233	10917	9.1	0.3	15.8	0.0	0.0	0.0	0.2	0.2	0.4	0.9
Prostate cancer	M	46334	26	8853	25.7	0.0	16.0	0.0	–	0.0	0.0	0.0	0.1	0.1
Bladder cancer	M	20985	18	6921	11.9	0.0	12.0	–	0.0	–	0.0	0.0	0.0	0.1
	F	7687	16	1613	2.6	0.0	2.4	0.0	–	0.0	0.0	0.0	0.0	0.1
Other and ill-defined	M	85502	2853	42360	49.6	3.2	69.7	2.3	2.4	1.8	2.8	3.4	4.2	5.7
cancer sites	F	81566	1742	27489	31.2	2.1	40.0	2.1	1.9	1.6	1.7	1.7	2.3	3.4
Hodgkin's disease	M	1724	318	942	1.0	0.3	1.4	–	0.0	0.1	0.2	0.5	0.7	0.8
	F	1251	202	527	0.6	0.2	0.7	0.0	–	0.0	0.2	0.3	0.5	0.6
Myeloma and non-	M	15559	578	7531	9.0	0.6	12.4	0.2	0.3	0.4	0.6	0.7	1.0	1.2
Hodgkin lymphomas	F	14980	281	5382	5.9	0.3	7.8	0.2	0.1	0.2	0.3	0.3	0.5	0.7
Leukaemia	M	13989	1448	5465	8.0	1.7	9.0	1.4	1.6	1.6	2.0	1.7	1.7	1.8
	F	12244	1015	4012	4.9	1.2	5.8	1.3	1.4	1.2	1.3	1.1	1.1	1.3
ALL VASCULAR	M	696818	4924	211665	392.7	5.4	357.9	4.0	1.0	1.3	3.0	5.5	7.9	15.2
DISEASE	F	839446	2668	96059	252.5	3.1	141.7	3.5	0.8	1.4	2.2	2.9	4.3	6.7
Rheumatic heart	M	3042	79	1548	1.8	0.1	2.6	0.0	0.0	0.0	0.1	0.1	0.1	0.2
disease and fever	F	7378	74	2689	2.9	0.1	3.9	0.0	0.0	0.0	0.0	0.1	0.2	0.2
Hypertensive disease	M	18736	74	5742	10.6	0.1	9.7	0.0	0.0	0.0	0.0	0.1	0.1	0.3
	F	34058	48	4488	10.4	0.1	6.6	0.0	0.0	–	0.0	0.0	0.1	0.1
Ischaemic heart	M	311580	1043	121407	177.9	1.1	204.9	0.1	0.0	0.0	0.2	0.6	1.7	5.2
disease	F	265658	250	39888	83.6	0.3	59.1	0.1	–	0.0	0.1	0.3	0.5	1.0
Pulmonary embolism	M	10919	180	3918	6.2	0.2	6.5	0.1	0.0	0.0	0.1	0.2	0.3	0.6
and other venous	F	17066	201	3529	5.7	0.2	5.1	0.0	–	0.0	0.2	0.3	0.3	0.6
Cerebrovascular	M	165860	1079	35452	92.2	1.2	60.7	0.6	0.3	0.4	0.8	1.3	1.6	3.2
disease	F	255974	855	24667	75.7	1.0	36.3	0.5	0.3	0.5	0.7	0.9	1.5	2.4
Other vascular	M	186675	2464	43596	104.1	2.7	73.5	3.1	0.6	0.8	1.9	3.1	4.0	5.7
disease	F	259307	1237	20798	74.1	1.5	30.6	2.8	0.4	0.9	1.1	1.3	1.7	2.3
Chronic obstructive	M	85311	527	20385	47.7	0.6	35.9	0.7	0.1	0.4	0.6	0.6	0.8	1.0
pulmonary disease	F	45015	374	8925	14.9	0.4	13.2	0.4	0.1	0.2	0.5	0.6	0.5	0.7
Other respiratory	M	67161	1915	12888	37.4	2.3	21.8	7.0	0.5	0.6	1.1	1.6	2.3	2.9
disease	F	79503	1134	6038	22.9	1.5	8.8	5.7	0.5	0.4	0.7	0.7	1.2	1.1
Peptic ulcer	M	8450	79	2701	4.8	0.1	4.5	0.0	–	0.0	0.0	0.1	0.2	0.3
	F	8138	23	1180	2.5	0.0	1.7	0.0	–	0.0	0.0	0.0	0.0	0.1
Liver cirrhosis	M	40090	924	28513	24.0	1.0	44.8	0.1	0.0	0.0	0.0	0.3	1.5	5.0
	F	21361	421	12277	9.9	0.5	17.6	0.1	0.0	0.1	0.1	0.2	0.7	2.1
Renal disease	M	17357	300	4107	9.7	0.3	6.9	0.7	0.1	0.1	0.2	0.3	0.4	0.7
	F	19363	182	3030	6.2	0.2	4.4	0.5	0.1	0.1	0.1	0.2	0.2	0.4
Pregnancy and birth	F	334	254	80	0.2	0.3	0.1	–	–	–	0.1	0.4	0.6	0.8
Congenital and	M	14639	13489	839	10.9	18.3	1.2	120.1	1.8	1.3	1.7	1.3	1.1	0.9
perinatal causes	F	11502	10309	751	8.8	14.8	1.0	96.8	1.7	1.4	1.1	0.9	0.9	0.7
Ill-defined causes	M	53910	7574	16504	31.3	9.3	25.9	36.6	1.2	1.5	3.1	6.2	7.6	8.7
	F	66149	3779	7045	20.9	5.1	10.1	25.2	0.9	0.9	1.1	2.3	2.3	2.7
Other medical causes	M	154192	12065	50324	87.4	13.4	80.8	13.8	3.6	4.3	7.2	11.8	23.9	29.3
	F	202869	5383	34496	66.5	6.5	50.2	11.5	3.1	3.1	3.9	5.8	8.5	9.4
ALL NON-	M	121357	42204	50779	69.5	45.7	74.2	18.0	9.9	11.2	59.1	84.6	71.7	65.5
MEDICAL CAUSES	F	70970	11519	19155	28.7	13.4	26.8	11.9	6.0	6.2	16.7	19.3	17.0	16.8
Motor vehicle	M	38966	20518	13539	22.0	22.1	19.6	4.1	5.1	5.8	38.0	48.0	31.3	22.5
traffic accidents	F	13759	5418	4855	7.0	6.3	6.7	3.0	3.5	3.8	10.8	10.6	7.0	5.4
Fire	M	1819	549	789	1.1	0.6	1.2	1.3	0.4	0.2	0.4	0.7	0.8	0.7
	F	1426	274	417	0.6	0.3	0.6	1.1	0.3	0.1	0.1	0.3	0.3	0.3
Suicide	M	30892	8070	16490	17.9	8.5	23.9	–	0.0	0.8	6.4	14.9	17.4	20.1
	F	12730	2271	6902	6.3	2.5	9.6	–	0.1	0.2	1.9	4.0	5.0	6.2
Homicide	M	3189	1460	1590	1.8	1.6	2.2	0.7	0.3	0.3	1.4	2.3	2.9	3.2
	F	1178	520	489	0.7	0.6	0.7	0.8	0.3	0.2	0.6	0.8	0.8	0.8
POPULATION (thousands):	M=males				167849	85895	69740	10392	10478	11171	12477	14081	14355	12941
	F=females				176872	82349	73127	9851	9925	10601	11869	13526	13898	12679

EUROPEAN UNION (12 countries): 1990

Annual death rates / 100, 000 — 9th ICD categories

35–39	40–44	45–49	50–54	55–59	60–64	65–69	70–74	75–79	80+/NK			
186.0	260.8	415.8	670.9	1111.4	1782.7	2831.2	4413.1	7208.0	14539.0	M	ALL CAUSES	001–999
91.1	133.5	214.7	323.9	513.7	824.1	1358.7	2301.8	4208.8	11403.7	F		
0.6	1.0	1.4	2.0	3.0	5.1	7.5	11.5	16.8	23.8	M	Tuberculosis	010–018, 137
0.2	0.2	0.3	0.4	0.9	1.3	2.6	3.5	5.7	10.0	F		
1.9	2.1	2.7	3.4	4.7	8.0	12.2	20.5	31.9	74.1	M	Other infective	Rest of 001–139
0.7	1.0	1.3	1.9	3.2	4.9	7.5	11.7	22.3	63.6	F	and parasitic	
29.8	64.5	132.6	240.6	428.6	693.9	1035.6	1441.0	1958.2	2694.0	M	ALL CANCER	140–208
36.7	63.5	108.3	167.4	252.3	363.6	511.8	678.2	927.6	1409.7	F		
2.1	5.7	12.0	18.2	24.8	28.1	28.3	30.3	31.3	36.4	M	Mouth and	140–149
0.4	0.9	1.7	2.3	3.0	4.0	4.5	5.6	7.2	12.7	F	pharynx cancer	
0.9	3.0	7.5	13.5	21.9	29.2	35.6	42.1	48.2	55.7	M	Oesophagus cancer	150
0.2	0.4	1.0	1.9	2.9	5.0	6.4	10.3	14.7	24.3	F		
2.2	4.5	8.5	15.7	27.6	47.5	75.4	111.6	165.7	240.3	M	Stomach cancer	151
1.7	2.8	4.4	6.8	11.8	17.7	30.7	47.7	77.9	140.3	F		
2.2	4.6	9.9	19.9	36.0	61.4	100.3	146.3	219.5	344.8	M	Colorectal cancer	153, 154
2.2	4.3	8.6	14.7	25.1	39.6	62.7	91.5	141.6	253.5	F		
0.4	0.7	2.0	4.8	10.1	18.9	26.3	31.1	32.0	28.4	M	Liver cancer	155.0
0.2	0.4	0.8	1.0	2.2	4.0	6.5	8.6	11.4	12.0	F		
1.0	2.7	6.1	10.9	18.5	28.4	43.7	61.1	77.0	94.4	M	Pancreas cancer	157
0.6	1.3	2.7	5.3	9.6	16.5	26.6	37.6	55.1	77.8	F		
0.5	2.3	5.7	9.6	15.6	20.1	24.8	29.1	32.2	37.4	M	Larynx cancer	161
0.0	0.1	0.3	0.6	0.8	1.1	1.2	1.4	2.0	2.6	F		
5.3	15.5	37.2	71.5	142.6	239.9	347.8	446.2	517.0	510.1	M	Lung cancer	162
1.9	4.7	8.8	14.2	24.4	42.6	60.1	76.6	82.2	79.8	F		
1.3	1.8	2.2	3.1	3.9	5.1	6.0	6.9	9.3	11.3	M	Malignant melanoma	172
1.2	1.6	2.1	2.3	2.7	3.2	3.8	4.9	6.3	9.3	F		
12.4	23.5	37.9	55.8	70.2	81.9	96.3	107.7	128.5	188.7	F	Female breast cancer	174
3.5	4.0	4.9	5.4	6.2	8.0	10.3	12.0	13.5	14.6	F	Cervix cancer	180
1.0	1.7	2.7	4.6	9.5	13.4	19.4	25.7	33.1	46.5	F	Other uterine cancer	179, 182
1.6	4.1	8.4	14.5	20.1	27.5	34.4	39.4	43.4	48.4	F	Ovarian cancer	183
0.1	0.2	0.9	3.2	10.5	28.7	68.2	144.5	272.4	540.0	M	Prostate cancer	185
0.1	0.7	2.1	5.2	11.5	23.7	40.8	68.1	110.4	176.8	M	Bladder cancer	188
0.2	0.2	0.5	0.9	2.4	4.6	7.9	13.2	23.7	43.9	F		
8.8	15.8	28.3	49.1	81.9	125.1	179.0	237.4	321.1	451.3	M	Other and ill-defined	Rest of 140–208
6.1	9.4	17.1	27.0	45.9	70.8	103.7	142.2	211.7	351.5	F	cancer sites	
1.0	0.9	1.0	1.2	1.4	1.8	2.5	3.2	3.8	4.5	M	Hodgkin's disease	201
0.5	0.5	0.5	0.5	0.7	0.9	1.6	2.0	2.8	2.5	F		
1.9	3.3	5.4	8.9	13.0	21.9	32.3	46.8	62.6	76.4	M	Myeloma and non-	200, 202–203
1.2	1.7	3.1	5.2	8.6	13.6	21.6	32.0	42.8	53.2	F	Hodgkin lymphomas	
2.1	3.0	3.7	5.9	9.3	14.1	24.6	36.4	55.7	86.4	M	Leukaemia	204–208
1.8	2.0	2.8	4.6	6.0	9.1	14.1	19.7	29.7	47.9	F		
30.9	59.4	108.4	198.5	362.6	640.2	1104.9	1859.0	3290.0	7135.0	M	ALL VASCULAR	390–459
11.9	18.8	35.1	61.4	121.9	244.3	498.5	1027.1	2159.6	6426.1	F	DISEASE	
0.4	0.5	0.9	1.8	2.8	5.0	6.5	9.1	12.2	13.9	M	Rheumatic heart	390–398
0.4	0.6	1.3	2.6	4.1	6.9	11.6	17.0	20.0	26.4	F	disease and fever	
0.6	1.2	2.7	5.9	10.5	17.7	29.3	47.3	89.8	193.8	M	Hypertensive disease	401–405
0.3	0.6	1.3	3.2	6.0	11.1	23.9	43.5	93.7	247.9	F		
14.5	33.0	63.1	117.3	215.9	373.5	617.0	955.0	1452.0	2371.0	M	Ischaemic heart	410–414
2.4	5.1	10.9	22.0	49.2	108.0	216.2	420.7	779.3	1773.0	F	disease	
0.9	1.6	2.2	3.9	6.6	12.2	18.2	31.1	51.2	90.8	M	Pulmonary embolism	415.1, 451–453
0.9	1.3	2.1	2.9	4.8	8.7	15.4	26.1	47.7	102.5	F	and other venous	
5.2	9.3	16.8	28.8	54.9	103.8	206.0	413.9	865.3	2048.9	M	Cerebrovascular	430–438
4.5	6.6	11.1	16.7	31.3	58.3	125.3	296.1	673.5	2016.3	F	disease	
9.3	13.8	22.8	40.8	71.9	128.0	227.8	402.5	819.5	2416.6	M	Other vascular	Rest of 390–459
3.5	4.6	8.4	14.0	26.4	51.3	106.1	223.7	545.4	2259.9	F	disease	
1.3	2.2	4.8	11.4	28.6	65.9	137.0	264.3	461.9	916.3	M	Chronic obstructive	490–496
1.0	1.3	3.3	5.8	12.2	24.6	43.9	76.4	120.0	275.9	F	pulmonary disease	
3.6	4.5	6.9	10.8	19.7	35.4	71.6	136.8	288.9	933.3	M	Other respiratory	Rest of 460–519
1.4	2.3	3.0	4.7	7.7	14.7	28.2	63.5	146.2	708.9	F	disease	
0.6	0.9	1.6	2.7	4.9	7.5	13.4	21.8	39.0	84.3	M	Peptic ulcer	531–533
0.2	0.4	0.6	0.9	1.6	2.9	5.7	11.0	19.8	59.4	F		
10.9	16.8	28.3	43.6	59.5	72.6	82.2	81.8	91.8	88.8	M	Liver cirrhosis	571
4.6	7.7	12.4	16.3	21.1	27.7	33.0	37.1	41.6	42.2	F		
0.8	1.4	2.0	3.9	7.4	11.8	21.2	38.9	79.7	215.7	M	Renal disease	580–590
0.5	0.7	1.4	2.5	4.5	7.7	13.8	26.1	48.9	135.7	F		
0.5	0.2	0.0	–	–	–	–	–	–	–	F	Pregnancy and birth	630–676
0.9	0.9	1.1	1.4	1.3	1.6	1.6	1.8	2.6	3.4	M	Congenital and	740–779
0.8	0.8	0.8	1.0	1.2	1.3	1.4	1.8	1.8	2.5	F	perinatal causes	
10.0	12.1	16.4	22.6	28.7	38.2	53.4	81.5	140.1	553.9	M	Ill-defined causes	780–799
4.1	4.0	6.2	7.6	9.3	15.3	24.2	42.6	93.6	561.7	F		
30.4	32.0	41.6	56.3	82.6	122.2	200.2	337.2	620.4	1395.1	M	Other medical causes	Rest of 001–799
10.9	13.2	19.2	28.5	49.1	83.6	146.9	262.1	511.8	1356.0	F		
64.4	62.9	68.1	73.7	79.8	80.4	90.4	117.0	186.8	421.1	M	ALL NON-	E800–E999
17.5	19.4	22.8	25.5	28.6	32.3	41.2	60.6	109.9	352.1	F	MEDICAL CAUSES	
19.2	17.4	17.6	18.9	21.3	20.8	22.2	30.4	41.8	50.3	M	Motor vehicle	E810–E819
5.3	5.2	5.7	6.4	7.2	8.0	9.4	13.2	17.9	17.4	F	traffic accidents	
0.8	0.9	1.1	1.1	1.3	1.2	1.9	2.0	3.3	6.9	M	Fire	E890–E899
0.3	0.4	0.5	0.5	0.7	0.6	1.1	1.5	2.6	5.6	F		
21.2	21.4	23.4	25.1	25.5	24.1	26.6	32.3	48.6	79.0	M	Suicide	E950–E959
6.6	7.4	9.2	10.0	10.7	11.1	12.3	13.3	17.4	18.6	F		
3.2	2.8	2.2	2.3	2.0	1.5	1.1	1.0	1.1	1.4	M	Homicide	E960–E969
0.9	0.7	0.7	0.8	0.6	0.5	0.5	0.7	0.7	0.9	F		
11996	11909	10268	10309	9394	8623	7242	4489	4017	3709	M	**POPULATION (thousands)**	
11850	11743	10180	10440	9841	9689	9385	6446	6707	8243	F		

EUROPEAN UNION (12 countries): Males

	All ages	0–34	35–69	35–39	40–44	45–49	50–54	55–59	60–64	65–69	70–74	75–79	80+/NK
POPULATION (1000s)													
1955	136865	77511	52069	7434	9317	9400	8732	7095	5508	4584	3473	2294	1518
1965	151303	84476	58482	10457	9919	7254	8939	8699	7605	5609	3809	2541	1995
1975	159902	88017	61543	10877	10313	10043	9300	6617	7612	6782	5109	2970	2263
1985	164768	86948	65423	11935	10403	10528	9796	9245	8126	5390	5411	3874	3112
1990	**167849**	**85895**	**69741**	**11996**	**11909**	**10268**	**10309**	**9394**	**8623**	**7242**	**4489**	**4017**	**3709**
1995 projected	*168689*	*83565*	*72267*	*12803*	*11870*	*11568*	*9999*	*9758*	*8681*	*7587*	*5946*	*3222*	*3688*
NUMBER OF DEATHS													
All causes													
1955	1551156	222925	613845	18307	33754	56106	86948	112284	135176	171270	206355	223948	284083
1965	1740687	174602	736137	24428	35034	40037	82301	134945	195206	224186	231493	238926	359529
1975	1828126	127439	722504	22509	35218	56256	84236	93417	175831	255037	305142	278295	394746
1985	1780740	90622	615993	20431	28383	47808	75313	116087	162054	165917	271922	315490	486713
1990	**1746889**	**91632**	**628399**	**22317**	**31058**	**42695**	**69160**	**104400**	**153731**	**205038**	**198080**	**289526**	**539252**
1995 projected	*1619246*	*94114*	*588155*	*24713*	*29986*	*42937*	*59401*	*97645*	*140866*	*192607*	*232487*	*209324*	*495166*
Lung cancer													
1955	42822	307	33042	325	1142	2725	5596	7936	8116	7202	5279	2918	1276
1965	78459	391	55930	562	1351	2328	6110	11766	17078	16735	11639	6769	3730
1975	106816	325	63323	566	1518	3798	7262	9146	17819	23214	22083	13505	7580
1985	129520	294	67575	633	1589	3805	8005	14397	20190	18956	24678	21103	15870
1990	**132920**	**262**	**72944**	**633**	**1847**	**3820**	**7367**	**13396**	**20690**	**25191**	**20027**	**20768**	**18919**
1995 projected	*132496*	*292*	*72012*	*707*	*1906*	*4059*	*6543*	*13005*	*20182*	*25610*	*25303*	*16389*	*18500*
ANNUAL DEATH RATE / 100,000 (*The rates for the age groups 0–34 and 35–69 are the means of seven five-yearly rates, but the all-ages rates are standardised to the conventional "European" age distribution)													
All causes													
1955	1414.9*	274.1*	1424.9*	246.3	362.3	596.9	995.8	1582.6	2454.1	3736.0	5942.0	9763.2	18715.1
1965	1358.1*	193.2*	1453.5*	233.6	353.2	551.9	920.7	1551.2	2566.9	3996.9	6077.5	9404.0	18018.0
1975	1284.5*	148.6*	1356.6*	206.9	341.5	560.2	905.8	1411.8	2310.1	3760.3	5973.2	9370.4	17444.8
1985	1095.9*	106.2*	1142.1*	171.2	272.8	454.1	768.8	1255.7	1994.2	3078.1	5025.6	8143.9	15639.3
1990	**997.3***	**105.1***	**1037.0***	**186.0**	**260.8**	**415.8**	**670.9**	**1111.4**	**1782.7**	**2831.2**	**4413.1**	**7208.0**	**14538.9**
1995 projected	*911.8**	*107.8**	*939.0**	*193.0*	*252.6*	*371.2*	*594.0*	*1000.6*	*1622.7*	*2538.6*	*3909.8*	*6496.0*	*13425.0*
All cancer													
1955	212.7*	10.0*	312.8*	30.1	57.9	118.1	225.0	383.3	575.6	799.9	1097.2	1419.1	1622.7
1965	248.0*	11.5*	362.1*	34.5	64.5	120.4	227.1	415.1	677.6	995.3	1308.1	1647.7	2013.3
1975	265.0*	10.5*	374.5*	32.4	68.2	138.1	251.1	413.4	683.7	1035.0	1442.0	1882.0	2210.8
1985	277.0*	8.3*	380.3*	31.4	67.1	132.0	259.0	448.8	703.8	1020.1	1460.4	1980.2	2612.3
1990	**274.4***	**7.2***	**375.1***	**29.8**	**64.5**	**132.6**	**240.6**	**428.6**	**693.9**	**1035.6**	**1441.0**	**1958.2**	**2694.0**
1995 projected	*270.1**	*6.4**	*365.0**	*28.2*	*63.0*	*126.5*	*228.5*	*410.2*	*682.6*	*1015.7*	*1416.1*	*1945.7*	*2744.5*
Lung cancer													
1955	37.0*	0.4*	75.1*	4.4	12.3	29.0	64.1	111.9	147.3	157.1	152.0	127.2	84.1
1965	58.1*	0.5*	111.1*	5.4	13.6	32.1	68.4	135.3	224.6	298.4	305.6	266.4	186.9
1975	72.2*	0.4*	121.5*	5.2	14.7	37.8	78.1	138.2	234.1	342.3	432.3	454.7	335.0
1985	80.5*	0.3*	127.8*	5.3	15.3	36.1	81.7	155.7	248.5	351.7	456.1	544.7	509.9
1990	**77.6***	**0.3***	**122.8***	**5.3**	**15.5**	**37.2**	**71.5**	**142.6**	**239.9**	**347.8**	**446.2**	**517.0**	**510.1**
1995 projected	*74.8**	*0.3**	*117.9**	*5.5*	*16.1*	*35.1*	*65.4*	*133.3*	*232.5*	*337.5*	*425.5*	*508.6*	*501.6*
Upper aerodigestive cancer (mouth, oesophagus, pharynx and larynx)													
1955	19.0*	0.2*	28.6*	1.4	4.0	10.7	21.9	39.1	53.4	69.5	95.0	128.8	150.8
1965	21.3*	0.2*	34.7*	2.5	6.1	12.8	25.0	43.3	64.6	88.5	101.3	121.7	153.6
1975	24.0*	0.2*	39.9*	2.6	9.6	22.5	36.4	49.4	68.1	90.5	111.6	137.2	142.4
1985	25.3*	0.2*	44.4*	3.1	11.2	23.8	45.0	63.3	78.1	85.9	102.6	118.4	137.1
1990	**24.8***	**0.2***	**44.2***	**3.4**	**10.9**	**25.2**	**41.3**	**62.3**	**77.3**	**88.7**	**101.4**	**111.7**	**129.5**
1995 projected	*24.3**	*0.2**	*43.8**	*3.3*	*11.3*	*25.0*	*41.6*	*60.9*	*77.7*	*87.0*	*99.1*	*106.4*	*122.6*
Other cancer													
1955	156.7*	9.4*	209.1*	24.3	41.6	78.4	139.0	232.3	374.8	573.3	850.2	1163.1	1387.9
1965	168.7*	10.8*	216.3*	26.7	44.8	75.5	133.8	236.6	388.4	608.4	901.2	1259.6	1672.9
1975	168.8*	9.8*	213.2*	24.6	43.9	77.7	136.7	225.7	381.5	602.3	898.1	1290.1	1733.4
1985	171.2*	7.7*	208.2*	23.0	40.6	72.1	132.3	229.8	377.3	582.5	901.7	1317.0	1965.2
1990	**172.0***	**6.7***	**208.1***	**21.1**	**38.1**	**70.2**	**127.8**	**223.7**	**376.6**	**599.0**	**893.3**	**1329.4**	**2054.5**
1995 projected	*171.0**	*6.0**	*203.2**	*19.4*	*35.7*	*66.4*	*121.4*	*216.0*	*372.4*	*591.2*	*891.5*	*1330.7*	*2120.3*
Chronic obstructive pulmonary disease (COPD)													
1955	55.8*	2.8*	71.0*	4.3	8.6	20.3	46.6	84.6	135.6	197.2	265.9	387.0	664.2
1965	65.7*	1.6*	79.0*	3.5	7.8	16.0	34.6	77.4	158.0	255.5	371.6	515.6	812.3
1975	74.5*	1.7*	72.0*	3.3	6.6	15.2	32.0	65.6	128.9	252.5	449.0	707.3	1076.8
1985	53.6*	0.7*	43.7*	1.5	3.1	6.7	15.9	37.5	81.5	159.4	295.8	523.3	965.8
1990	**47.7***	**0.6***	**35.9***	**1.3**	**2.2**	**4.8**	**11.4**	**28.6**	**65.9**	**137.0**	**264.3**	**461.9**	**916.3**
1995 projected	*43.4**	*0.6**	*30.6**	*1.0*	*1.7*	*3.4*	*8.9*	*23.3*	*56.1*	*119.9*	*231.0*	*431.1*	*873.6*
Other respiratory disease													
1955	76.4*	28.1*	46.8*	6.7	9.1	15.8	28.6	47.6	80.1	139.8	261.5	533.4	1288.0
1965	58.9*	15.0*	33.8*	4.6	7.0	11.2	16.6	30.2	58.0	108.7	216.9	432.6	1182.2
1975	54.8*	7.7*	31.5*	3.9	6.5	10.2	16.3	29.4	51.0	103.4	213.9	441.3	1217.3
1985	41.9*	2.8*	25.2*	3.2	4.3	7.5	13.5	24.3	43.9	79.5	160.4	335.2	1004.7
1990	**37.4***	**2.3***	**21.8***	**3.6**	**4.5**	**6.9**	**10.8**	**19.7**	**35.4**	**71.6**	**136.8**	**288.9**	**933.3**
1995 projected	*33.5**	*2.3**	*19.2**	*4.3*	*4.6*	*6.2*	*9.5*	*16.7*	*31.7*	*61.5*	*115.1*	*255.2*	*852.4*
Vascular disease													
1955	554.5*	11.7*	528.9*	42.3	75.1	151.0	296.7	535.8	960.2	1641.2	2868.7	4944.0	8916.2
1965	571.0*	8.4*	568.9*	47.7	96.2	176.5	319.5	569.8	1031.9	1741.0	2907.8	4777.9	9192.2
1975	563.4*	6.9*	543.8*	39.8	89.4	178.6	331.3	553.5	955.8	1658.0	2830.4	4730.5	9417.8
1985	467.7*	6.0*	435.6*	33.2	69.1	134.3	255.3	455.5	791.0	1310.5	2304.0	3973.0	8117.2
1990	**392.7***	**5.4***	**357.9***	**30.9**	**59.4**	**108.4**	**198.5**	**362.6**	**640.2**	**1104.9**	**1859.0**	**3290.0**	**7135.0**
1995 projected	*328.6**	*5.1**	*290.5**	*27.6*	*49.4*	*82.1*	*152.8*	*292.9*	*527.8*	*900.7*	*1497.4*	*2746.8*	*6216.6*
Liver cirrhosis													
1955	21.1*	0.7*	40.4*	4.9	11.6	21.9	37.4	53.3	71.1	82.3	88.3	78.6	59.8
1965	30.1*	0.9*	55.8*	8.9	16.7	27.7	46.6	72.1	97.7	120.8	125.7	133.8	109.3
1975	34.4*	1.3*	64.4*	12.8	26.8	43.7	59.2	75.9	103.5	129.0	130.5	136.1	111.1
1985	28.3*	1.1*	52.5*	10.0	19.4	33.9	52.7	69.9	86.9	94.6	107.6	111.2	95.5
1990	**24.0***	**1.0***	**44.8***	**10.9**	**16.8**	**28.3**	**43.6**	**59.5**	**72.6**	**82.2**	**81.8**	**91.8**	**88.8**
1995 projected	*20.6**	*1.1**	*38.2**	*10.6*	*15.7*	*23.8*	*37.2*	*51.3*	*61.1*	*67.7*	*68.4*	*74.0*	*78.5*
Other medical causes													
1955	403.9*	166.3*	320.3*	88.1	119.3	175.8	254.2	361.0	506.9	736.5	1182.3	2151.4	5683.4
1965	293.9*	102.0*	251.1*	62.3	85.5	117.6	176.1	268.7	413.4	634.4	970.7	1637.6	4164.6
1975	205.9*	66.0*	176.1*	42.0	64.1	90.0	126.6	179.7	277.7	452.9	738.3	1225.0	2900.5
1985	156.5*	42.7*	128.3*	31.8	45.2	66.7	95.3	137.7	202.4	318.8	561.5	1021.5	2419.2
1990	**151.7***	**42.9***	**127.3***	**45.2**	**50.4**	**66.7**	**92.3**	**132.4**	**194.4**	**309.5**	**513.3**	**930.4**	**2350.5**
1995 projected	*147.0**	*43.7**	*124.9**	*56.4*	*57.4*	*65.2*	*87.6*	*129.4*	*187.2*	*291.3*	*472.8*	*874.2*	*2249.3*
All non-medical causes													
1955	90.5*	54.5*	104.7*	69.8	80.7	94.0	107.3	117.0	124.6	139.2	178.0	249.8	480.7
1965	90.4*	53.8*	102.8*	72.1	75.5	82.4	100.1	118.0	130.4	141.2	176.7	258.8	544.2
1975	86.5*	54.5*	94.2*	72.8	79.9	84.5	89.3	94.2	109.6	129.4	169.1	248.3	510.5
1985	70.9*	44.7*	76.6*	60.0	64.7	72.9	77.0	82.0	84.6	95.1	135.9	199.5	424.7
1990	**69.5***	**45.7***	**74.2***	**64.4**	**62.9**	**68.1**	**73.7**	**79.8**	**80.4**	**90.4**	**117.0**	**186.8**	**421.1**
1995 projected	*68.7**	*48.6**	*70.6**	*64.9*	*60.9*	*63.9*	*69.5*	*76.8*	*76.3*	*81.8*	*108.9*	*169.0*	*410.1*

EUROPEAN UNION (12 countries): Females

	All ages	0–34	35–69	35–39	40–44	45–49	50–54	55–59	60–64	65–69	70–74	75–79	80+/NK
POPULATION (1000s)													
1955	147739	76898	60411	8278	10386	10307	9476	8525	7291	6149	4776	3224	2431
1965	162067	81491	66905	10656	11039	8225	10290	10048	8988	7659	5946	4137	3589
1975	169637	84505	67826	10643	10232	10381	10561	7789	9391	8828	7280	5150	4878
1985	174475	83547	69561	11723	10272	10543	10027	10000	9916	7079	7941	6512	6915
1990	176872	82349	73127	11850	11743	10180	10440	9841	9689	9385	6446	6707	8243
1995 projected	176604	79794	74732	12545	11750	11507	10120	10174	9502	9134	8517	5333	8229
NUMBER OF DEATHS													
All causes													
1955	1468304	165240	461271	15272	26616	38944	54597	73335	103555	148952	203973	244862	392958
1965	1627549	114435	472313	15369	23910	27444	51686	76790	113835	163279	225731	277652	537418
1975	1743407	74377	431999	12253	18851	30600	48874	54331	103469	163621	239538	310854	686639
1985	1759006	46660	341195	10845	14694	24071	36439	57332	91782	106032	209619	309606	851926
1990	1752900	42243	340051	10792	15676	21858	33812	50554	79846	127513	148367	282290	939949
1995 projected	1580434	38834	306141	10935	14941	22341	29721	47590	70908	109705	171920	199423	864116
Lung cancer													
1955	8828	220	5707	152	317	585	783	1138	1253	1479	1314	1007	580
1965	14288	188	8590	196	365	600	1189	1627	2101	2512	2295	1746	1469
1975	19549	139	10624	147	347	746	1479	1702	2867	3336	3378	2762	2646
1985	28155	146	13093	209	355	753	1314	2549	3947	3966	5226	4647	5043
1990	32481	128	15326	224	556	894	1481	2402	4132	5637	4936	5516	6575
1995 projected	36219	130	16597	282	675	1146	1516	2672	4343	5963	6984	5078	7430
ANNUAL DEATH RATE / 100,000 (*The rates for the age groups 0–34 and 35–69 are the means of seven five-yearly rates, but the all-ages rates are standardised to the conventional "European" age distribution)													
All causes													
1955	1031.8*	207.4*	871.1*	184.5	256.3	377.9	576.2	860.3	1420.4	2422.2	4271.2	7595.8	16162.7
1965	894.7*	129.0*	765.6*	144.2	216.6	333.7	502.3	764.3	1266.6	2131.8	3796.5	6711.6	14973.3
1975	794.0*	90.5*	672.8*	115.1	184.2	294.8	462.8	697.5	1101.8	1853.4	3290.6	6036.4	14076.9
1985	650.2*	59.2*	546.3*	92.5	143.0	228.3	363.4	573.3	925.6	1497.8	2639.9	4754.4	12320.3
1990	588.7*	53.0*	494.2*	91.1	133.5	214.7	323.9	513.7	824.1	1358.7	2301.8	4208.8	11403.7
1995 projected	533.1*	48.5*	445.3*	87.2	127.2	194.2	293.7	467.8	746.2	1201.1	2018.6	3739.5	10501.3
All cancer													
1955	160.7*	9.7*	236.8*	46.4	84.7	132.8	198.1	273.3	385.2	537.2	736.0	987.5	1229.6
1965	164.8*	9.7*	238.3*	43.9	82.2	133.7	203.9	279.0	387.4	537.8	748.5	1006.4	1366.0
1975	157.6*	8.6*	230.2*	38.7	72.8	124.7	199.8	278.7	383.3	513.1	694.3	958.4	1318.3
1985	152.8*	7.1*	218.6*	37.1	65.4	109.5	172.8	262.2	377.1	506.3	699.4	931.1	1392.4
1990	150.3*	6.3*	214.8*	36.7	63.5	108.3	167.4	252.3	363.6	511.8	678.2	927.6	1409.7
1995 projected	146.6*	5.6*	207.4*	35.3	61.9	103.3	160.6	243.6	354.3	492.5	660.7	910.7	1420.9
Lung cancer													
1955	6.0*	0.3*	10.5*	1.8	3.1	5.7	8.3	13.3	17.2	24.1	27.5	31.2	23.9
1965	8.1*	0.2*	13.8*	1.8	3.3	7.3	11.6	16.2	23.4	32.8	38.6	42.2	40.9
1975	9.8*	0.2*	16.6*	1.4	3.4	7.2	14.0	21.9	30.5	37.8	46.4	53.6	54.2
1985	12.5*	0.2*	21.0*	1.8	3.5	7.1	13.1	25.5	39.8	56.0	65.8	71.4	72.9
1990	13.7*	0.1*	22.4*	1.9	4.7	8.8	14.2	24.4	42.6	60.1	76.6	82.2	79.8
1995 projected	15.0*	0.1*	24.3*	2.2	5.7	10.0	15.0	26.3	45.7	65.3	82.0	95.2	90.3
Upper aerodigestive cancer (mouth, oesophagus, pharynx and larynx)													
1955	4.0*	0.1*	4.9*	0.9	1.2	2.5	3.5	5.4	8.3	12.5	20.7	32.7	46.1
1965	3.8*	0.1*	4.6*	0.6	1.1	2.2	3.4	5.1	7.7	11.8	18.4	29.6	48.1
1975	3.7*	0.1*	4.9*	0.5	1.3	2.2	3.9	5.9	8.4	11.6	17.0	25.1	44.3
1985	3.8*	0.1*	5.5*	0.7	1.2	2.4	4.0	7.2	9.8	13.0	16.5	23.1	39.8
1990	3.9*	0.1*	5.5*	0.5	1.4	3.0	4.8	6.7	10.0	12.2	17.4	24.0	39.6
1995 projected	4.0*	0.1*	5.7*	0.6	1.6	3.6	5.2	7.0	9.8	12.0	16.7	26.4	40.7
Other cancer													
1955	150.7*	9.3*	221.4*	43.6	80.4	124.6	186.4	254.6	359.7	500.7	687.7	923.6	1159.7
1965	152.9*	9.4*	219.9*	41.4	77.8	124.2	188.9	257.7	356.3	493.3	691.5	934.6	1276.9
1975	144.0*	8.3*	208.7*	36.8	68.2	115.3	181.9	250.9	344.4	463.7	630.9	879.7	1219.8
1985	136.5*	6.8*	192.2*	34.7	60.8	99.9	155.7	229.5	327.5	437.3	617.1	836.6	1279.7
1990	132.7*	6.1*	186.9*	34.3	57.3	96.4	148.5	221.1	311.0	439.6	584.3	821.3	1290.3
1995 projected	127.5*	5.4*	177.4*	32.4	54.5	89.8	140.5	210.3	298.8	415.2	562.0	789.1	1289.9
Chronic obstructive pulmonary disease (COPD)													
1955	22.9*	2.3*	17.0*	2.3	3.1	4.7	7.9	14.5	29.8	56.6	104.6	198.5	431.7
1965	21.3*	1.2*	16.4*	2.0	2.9	5.0	8.2	14.1	28.9	54.1	97.7	181.8	416.7
1975	22.3*	1.2*	18.2*	2.3	3.9	6.5	10.5	18.8	31.2	54.3	101.1	186.4	422.9
1985	15.7*	0.6*	14.7*	1.4	2.0	4.1	8.1	15.2	26.0	46.2	74.8	118.0	280.2
1990	14.9*	0.4*	13.2*	1.0	1.3	3.3	5.8	12.2	24.6	43.9	76.4	120.0	275.9
1995 projected	14.6*	0.4*	12.3*	0.8	1.0	2.4	4.8	11.1	23.5	42.6	73.7	120.9	279.3
Other respiratory disease													
1955	59.5*	25.2*	26.7*	5.2	6.1	8.5	13.2	22.4	44.2	87.3	196.0	419.2	1099.5
1965	42.6*	12.7*	17.6*	3.0	4.1	5.9	9.2	14.6	27.8	58.9	135.8	303.2	965.2
1975	37.2*	6.3*	16.3*	2.8	3.4	5.5	8.6	15.4	26.2	52.2	119.0	278.7	947.1
1985	25.1*	2.0*	10.1*	1.6	1.9	3.4	5.5	8.5	16.7	33.0	70.1	168.4	748.8
1990	22.9*	1.5*	8.8*	1.4	2.3	3.0	4.7	7.7	14.7	28.2	63.5	146.2	708.9
1995 projected	21.0*	1.3*	7.9*	1.5	2.2	2.7	4.2	6.8	13.1	24.9	52.1	132.0	667.0
Vascular disease													
1955	436.1*	11.2*	342.9*	33.8	52.2	92.3	168.1	300.1	588.9	1164.7	2263.6	4158.7	8059.9
1965	401.5*	6.2*	289.5*	24.8	43.1	77.7	134.8	249.5	503.8	992.5	1995.7	3769.2	8183.7
1975	372.5*	4.6*	242.0*	18.9	34.9	65.8	114.9	211.2	410.8	837.8	1717.9	3446.5	8327.9
1985	298.6*	3.6*	175.8*	12.8	23.1	42.0	80.4	152.2	307.2	612.8	1287.2	2624.3	7280.9
1990	252.5*	3.1*	141.7*	11.9	18.8	35.1	61.4	121.9	244.3	498.5	1027.1	2159.6	6426.1
1995 projected	211.8*	2.8*	112.7*	10.3	16.1	26.7	48.2	98.5	196.5	392.9	810.7	1775.5	5598.8
Liver cirrhosis													
1955	9.6*	0.5*	17.5*	3.5	6.2	11.0	17.5	23.4	28.3	32.9	35.3	38.3	35.6
1965	11.9*	0.5*	20.4*	4.6	7.9	11.8	17.3	24.1	34.9	42.0	51.6	57.5	56.6
1975	12.4*	0.7*	21.6*	5.9	10.9	16.3	21.5	26.4	31.4	38.4	45.7	53.4	52.6
1985	10.7*	0.5*	19.1*	4.9	7.7	12.6	18.9	25.0	30.9	33.9	39.9	45.8	43.3
1990	9.9*	0.5*	17.6*	4.6	7.7	12.4	16.3	21.1	27.7	33.0	37.1	41.6	42.2
1995 projected	9.2*	0.5*	16.2*	4.6	7.9	11.8	14.5	19.1	24.8	30.4	35.1	37.7	39.7
Other medical causes													
1955	306.1*	143.1*	197.1*	76.9	84.4	104.0	139.7	190.5	300.4	484.0	839.0	1608.6	4846.1
1965	211.3*	82.3*	148.0*	46.6	55.2	73.3	96.7	144.7	236.9	382.3	659.2	1190.6	3400.6
1975	150.8*	51.4*	109.1*	25.8	35.4	49.7	73.0	109.0	173.0	297.9	516.2	927.2	2439.2
1985	116.1*	31.5*	78.2*	16.0	21.8	33.3	50.6	78.4	130.4	217.1	397.2	745.7	2190.0
1990	109.5*	27.8*	71.4*	17.9	20.6	29.9	42.7	69.8	116.9	202.0	358.9	703.9	2188.8
1995 projected	103.6*	24.8*	64.8*	18.4	20.1	25.9	37.5	62.8	106.3	182.9	331.8	668.7	2171.1
All non-medical causes													
1955	36.9*	15.4*	33.1*	16.5	19.6	24.6	31.7	36.1	43.5	59.5	96.6	185.2	460.3
1965	41.4*	16.4*	35.5*	19.2	21.3	26.3	32.2	38.3	46.8	64.1	108.0	203.0	584.6
1975	41.1*	17.7*	35.4*	20.8	22.8	26.4	34.5	38.0	45.8	59.7	96.3	185.9	568.8
1985	31.2*	13.8*	29.7*	18.7	21.2	23.5	27.1	31.8	37.3	48.4	71.3	121.1	384.7
1990	28.7*	13.4*	26.8*	17.5	19.4	22.8	25.5	28.6	32.3	41.2	60.6	109.9	352.1
1995 projected	26.4*	13.1*	24.0*	16.3	18.0	21.3	23.9	25.8	27.6	34.9	54.5	93.9	324.5

EUROPEAN UNION (12 countries): 1975

Smoking-attributed deaths (Sm.) and total deaths (Total)

		ALL CAUSES	ALL CANCER	Lung cancer	Upper aero-digestive ca.	Other cancer	COPD	Other respiratory	Vascular disease	Liver cirrhosis	Other medical	Non-medical
Males												
0-34	Sm.	–	–	–	–	–	–	–	–	–	–	–
	Total	127439	8914	325	184	8405	1427	6680	5723	1040	56837	46818
35-69	Sm.	233007	90115	58812	13281	18022	28426	4650	82945	–	26871	–
	Total	722504	197364	63323	21503	112538	36809	16471	284124	35703	95734	56299
		(32%)	(46%)	(93%)	(62%)	(16%)	(77%)	(28%)	(29%)		(28%)	
70+	Sm.	190118	60983	39116	6898	14969	47908	6297	59910	–	15020	–
	Total	978183	179586	43168	12997	123421	68307	51578	498194	13221	139731	27566
		(19%)	(34%)	(91%)	(53%)	(12%)	(70%)	(12%)	(12%)		(11%)	
Any age	Sm.	423125	151098	97928	20179	32991	76334	10947	142855	–	41891	–
	Total	1828126	385864	106816	34684	244364	106543	74729	788041	49964	292302	130683
		(23%)	(39%)	(92%)	(58%)	(14%)	(72%)	(15%)	(18%)		(14%)	
Females												
0-34	Sm.	–	–	–	–	–	–	–	–	–	–	–
	Total	74377	6960	139	76	6745	1015	5155	3715	564	42290	14678
35-69	Sm.	22329	6576	4921	615	1040	3122	803	8969	–	2859	–
	Total	431999	148627	10624	3114	134889	11615	10395	153535	14106	70264	23457
		(5%)	(4%)	(46%)	(20%)	(1%)	(27%)	(8%)	(6%)		(4%)	
70+	Sm.	24853	4723	3258	715	750	6676	1380	10097	–	1977	–
	Total	1237031	164199	8786	4691	150722	37589	69213	708753	8644	204304	44329
		(2%)	(3%)	(37%)	(15%)	(0%)	(18%)	(2%)	(1%)		(1%)	
Any age	Sm.	47182	11299	8179	1330	1790	9798	2183	19066	–	4836	–
	Total	1743407	319786	19549	7881	292356	50219	84763	866003	23314	316858	82464
		(3%)	(4%)	(42%)	(17%)	(1%)	(20%)	(3%)	(2%)		(2%)	
Males+Females												
0-34	Sm.	–	–	–	–	–	–	–	–	–	–	–
	Total	201816	15874	464	260	15150	2442	11835	9438	1604	99127	61496
35-69	Sm.	255336	96691	63733	13896	19062	31548	5453	91914	–	29730	–
	Total	1154503	345991	73947	24617	247427	48424	26866	437659	49809	165998	79756
		(22%)	(28%)	(86%)	(56%)	(8%)	(65%)	(20%)	(21%)		(18%)	
70+	Sm.	214971	65706	42374	7613	15719	54584	7677	70007	–	16997	–
	Total	2215214	343785	51954	17688	274143	105896	120791	1206947	21865	344035	71895
		(10%)	(19%)	(82%)	(43%)	(6%)	(52%)	(6%)	(6%)		(5%)	
Any age	Sm.	470307	162397	106107	21509	34781	86132	13130	161921	–	46727	–
	Total	3571533	705650	126365	42565	536720	156762	159492	1654044	73278	609160	213147
		(13%)	(23%)	(84%)	(51%)	(6%)	(55%)	(8%)	(10%)		(8%)	

EUROPEAN UNION (12 countries): 1985

Smoking-attributed deaths (Sm.) and total deaths (Total)

		ALL CAUSES	ALL CANCER	Lung cancer	Upper aero-digestive ca.	Other cancer	COPD	Other respiratory	Vascular disease	Liver cirrhosis	Other medical	Non-medical
Males												
0-34	Sm.	–	–	–	–	–	–	–	–	–	–	–
	Total	90622	7258	294	193	6771	632	2228	5274	915	33620	40695
35-69	Sm.	212634	98671	63035	16717	18919	16951	3922	70650	–	22440	–
	Total	615993	203675	67575	25294	110806	21447	13043	227338	30560	71225	48705
		(35%)	(48%)	(93%)	(66%)	(17%)	(79%)	(30%)	(31%)		(32%)	
70+	Sm.	229298	86880	56430	8485	21965	49270	6592	68889	–	17667	–
	Total	1074125	237029	61651	14406	160972	66331	52934	531192	13103	145238	28298
		(21%)	(37%)	(92%)	(59%)	(14%)	(74%)	(12%)	(13%)		(12%)	
Any age	Sm.	441932	185551	119465	25202	40884	66221	10514	139539	–	40107	–
	Total	1780740	447962	129520	39893	278549	88410	68205	763804	44578	250083	117698
		(25%)	(41%)	(92%)	(63%)	(15%)	(75%)	(15%)	(18%)		(16%)	
Females												
0-34	Sm.	–	–	–	–	–	–	–	–	–	–	–
	Total	46660	5978	146	77	5755	519	1519	3032	449	23368	11795
35-69	Sm.	28032	9894	7489	908	1497	3998	560	10059	–	3521	–
	Total	341195	139404	13093	3471	122840	8979	6143	105428	12536	48833	19872
		(8%)	(7%)	(57%)	(26%)	(1%)	(45%)	(9%)	(10%)		(7%)	
70+	Sm.	48330	11074	7747	1425	1902	10594	2139	19401	–	5122	–
	Total	1371151	212451	14916	5565	191970	33007	68307	776569	9141	231533	40143
		(4%)	(5%)	(52%)	(26%)	(1%)	(32%)	(3%)	(2%)		(2%)	
Any age	Sm.	76362	20968	15236	2333	3399	14592	2699	29460	–	8643	–
	Total	1759006	357833	28155	9113	320565	42505	75969	885029	22126	303734	71810
		(4%)	(6%)	(54%)	(26%)	(1%)	(34%)	(4%)	(3%)		(3%)	
Males+Females												
0-34	Sm.	–	–	–	–	–	–	–	–	–	–	–
	Total	137282	13236	440	270	12526	1151	3747	8306	1364	56988	52490
35-69	Sm.	240666	108565	70524	17625	20416	20949	4482	80709	–	25961	–
	Total	957188	343079	80668	28765	233646	30426	19186	332766	43096	120058	68577
		(25%)	(32%)	(87%)	(61%)	(9%)	(69%)	(23%)	(24%)		(22%)	
70+	Sm.	277628	97954	64177	9910	23867	59864	8731	88290	–	22789	–
	Total	2445276	449480	76567	19971	352942	99338	121241	1307761	22244	376771	68441
		(11%)	(22%)	(84%)	(50%)	(7%)	(60%)	(7%)	(7%)		(6%)	
Any age	Sm.	518294	206519	134701	27535	44283	80813	13213	168999	–	48750	–
	Total	3539746	805795	157675	49006	599114	130915	144174	1648833	66704	553817	189508
		(15%)	(26%)	(85%)	(56%)	(7%)	(62%)	(9%)	(10%)		(9%)	

(To be conservative, no deaths before age 35, and none from liver cirrhosis or non-medical causes, were attributed to smoking.)

EUROPEAN UNION (12 countries): 1990

Smoking-attributed deaths (Sm.) and total deaths (Total)

		ALL CAUSES	ALL CANCER	Lung cancer	Upper aero-digestive ca.	Other cancer	COPD	Other respiratory	Vascular disease	Liver cirrhosis	Other medical	Non-medical
Males												
0–34	Sm.	–	–	–	–	–	–	–	–	–	–	–
	Total	91632	6390	262	170	5958	527	1915	4924	924	34748	42204
35–69	Sm.	211469	106276	67816	18051	20409	15968	3678	61424	–	24123	–
	Total	628399	224762	72944	27496	124322	20385	12888	211665	28513	79407	50779
		(34%)	(47%)	(93%)	(66%)	(16%)	(78%)	(29%)	(29%)		(30%)	
70+	Sm.	211489	84608	54410	8116	22082	47241	5977	56876	–	16787	–
	Total	1026858	243254	59714	13843	169697	64399	52358	480229	10653	147591	28374
		(21%)	(35%)	(91%)	(59%)	(13%)	(73%)	(11%)	(12%)		(11%)	
Any age	Sm.	422958	190884	122226	26167	42491	63209	9655	118300	–	40910	–
	Total	1746889	474406	132920	41509	299977	85311	67161	696818	40090	261746	121357
		(24%)	(40%)	(92%)	(63%)	(14%)	(74%)	(14%)	(17%)		(16%)	
Females												
0–34	Sm.	–	–	–	–	–	–	–	–	–	–	–
	Total	42243	5403	128	57	5218	374	1134	2668	421	20724	11519
35–69	Sm.	31321	12015	9207	1068	1740	4355	613	10189	–	4149	–
	Total	340051	148400	15326	3814	129260	8925	6038	96059	12277	49197	19155
		(9%)	(8%)	(60%)	(28%)	(1%)	(49%)	(10%)	(11%)		(8%)	
70+	Sm.	58221	14058	9769	1797	2492	12842	2636	22045	–	6640	–
	Total	1370606	222123	17027	5994	199102	35716	72331	740719	8663	250758	40296
		(4%)	(6%)	(57%)	(30%)	(1%)	(36%)	(4%)	(3%)		(3%)	
Any age	Sm.	89542	26073	18976	2865	4232	17197	3249	32234	–	10789	–
	Total	1752900	375926	32481	9865	333580	45015	79503	839446	21361	320679	70970
		(5%)	(7%)	(58%)	(29%)	(1%)	(38%)	(4%)	(4%)		(3%)	
Males+Females												
0–34	Sm.	–	–	–	–	–	–	–	–	–	–	–
	Total	133875	11793	390	227	11176	901	3049	7592	1345	55472	53723
35–69	Sm.	242790	118291	77023	19119	22149	20323	4291	71613	–	28272	–
	Total	968450	373162	88270	31310	253582	29310	18926	307724	40790	128604	69934
		(25%)	(32%)	(87%)	(61%)	(9%)	(69%)	(23%)	(23%)		(22%)	
70+	Sm.	269710	98666	64179	9913	24574	60083	8613	78921	–	23427	–
	Total	2397464	465377	76741	19837	368799	100115	124689	1220948	19316	398349	68670
		(11%)	(21%)	(84%)	(50%)	(7%)	(60%)	(7%)	(6%)		(6%)	
Any age	Sm.	512500	216957	141202	29032	46723	80406	12904	150534	–	51699	–
	Total	3499789	850332	165401	51374	633557	130326	146664	1536264	61451	582425	192327
		(15%)	(26%)	(85%)	(57%)	(7%)	(62%)	(9%)	(10%)		(9%)	

EUROPEAN UNION (12 countries): 1995

Smoking-attributed deaths (Sm.) and total deaths (Total)

		ALL CAUSES	ALL CANCER	Lung cancer	Upper aero-digestive ca.	Other cancer	COPD	Other respiratory	Vascular disease	Liver cirrhosis	Other medical	Non-medical
Males												
0–34	Sm.	–	–	–	–	–	–	–	–	–	–	–
	Total	94114	5718	292	170	5256	478	1978	4712	1046	36818	43364
35–69	Sm.	194477	104605	66705	18217	19683	13835	3255	48731	–	24051	–
	Total	588155	224926	72012	28104	124810	17860	11798	176919	25135	81308	50209
		(33%)	(47%)	(93%)	(65%)	(16%)	(77%)	(28%)	(28%)		(30%)	
70+	Sm.	198237	85024	54716	8121	22187	43760	5232	48081	–	16140	–
	Total	936977	248129	60192	13841	174096	59851	46509	406845	9348	139247	27048
		(21%)	(34%)	(91%)	(59%)	(13%)	(73%)	(11%)	(12%)		(12%)	
Any age	Sm.	392714	189629	121421	26338	41870	57595	8487	96812	–	40191	–
	Total	1619246	478773	132496	42115	304162	78189	60285	588476	35529	257373	120621
		(24%)	(40%)	(92%)	(63%)	(14%)	(74%)	(14%)	(16%)		(16%)	
Females												
0–34	Sm.	–	–	–	–	–	–	–	–	–	–	–
	Total	38834	4878	130	50	4698	310	999	2393	439	18981	10834
35–69	Sm.	32017	13557	10474	1209	1874	4332	598	9118	–	4412	–
	Total	306141	143286	16597	3953	122736	8236	5390	75718	11416	44633	17462
		(10%)	(9%)	(63%)	(31%)	(2%)	(53%)	(11%)	(12%)		(10%)	
70+	Sm.	65171	17204	12107	2091	3006	14274	2780	22960	–	7953	–
	Total	1235459	221758	19492	6174	196092	35713	66372	624431	8265	242570	36350
		(5%)	(8%)	(62%)	(34%)	(2%)	(40%)	(4%)	(4%)		(3%)	
Any age	Sm.	97188	30761	22581	3300	4880	18606	3378	32078	–	12365	–
	Total	1580434	369922	36219	10177	323526	44259	72761	702542	20120	306184	64646
		(6%)	(8%)	(62%)	(32%)	(2%)	(42%)	(5%)	(5%)		(4%)	
Males+Females												
0–34	Sm.	–	–	–	–	–	–	–	–	–	–	–
	Total	132948	10596	422	220	9954	788	2977	7105	1485	55799	54198
35–69	Sm.	226494	118162	77179	19426	21557	18167	3853	57849	–	28463	–
	Total	894296	368212	88609	32057	247546	26096	17188	252637	36551	125941	67671
		(25%)	(32%)	(87%)	(61%)	(9%)	(70%)	(22%)	(23%)		(23%)	
70+	Sm.	263408	102228	66823	10212	25193	58034	8012	71041	–	24093	–
	Total	2172436	469887	79684	20015	370188	95564	112881	1031276	17613	381817	63398
		(12%)	(22%)	(84%)	(51%)	(7%)	(61%)	(7%)	(7%)		(6%)	
Any age	Sm.	489902	220390	144002	29638	46750	76201	11865	128890	–	52556	–
	Total	3199680	848695	168715	52292	627688	122448	133046	1291018	55649	563557	185267
		(15%)	(26%)	(85%)	(57%)	(7%)	(62%)	(9%)	(10%)		(9%)	

(To be conservative, no deaths before age 35, and none from liver cirrhosis or non-medical causes, were attributed to smoking.)

PLANNED EU (16 countries): 1990

		No. of deaths			Standardised rates (Defined on p.256)			Annual death rates / 100, 000						
		All ages	0–34	35–69	All ages	0–34	35–69	0–4	5–9	10–14	15–19	20–24	25–29	30–34
ALL CAUSES	M	1883522	97894	673252	996.7	104.6	1035.5	208.1	22.9	25.0	83.1	119.8	127.2	146.1
	F	1891044	45174	364300	588.6	52.8	493.4	161.9	17.1	17.1	31.2	38.2	45.0	58.8
Tuberculosis	M	4335	143	1933	2.3	0.1	2.9	0.0	0.0	0.0	0.1	0.1	0.3	0.5
	F	2308	67	634	0.8	0.1	0.9	0.0	–	0.0	0.0	0.1	0.2	0.2
Other infective and parasitic	M	9717	1162	3290	5.2	1.3	4.9	4.5	0.4	0.3	0.7	0.8	1.0	1.4
	F	10844	769	2154	3.6	0.9	2.9	3.5	0.6	0.3	0.6	0.4	0.5	0.7
ALL CANCER	M	505142	6766	237194	270.9	7.1	369.3	4.1	4.4	4.0	6.0	7.0	9.4	14.6
	F	404631	5763	158984	150.1	6.2	214.5	3.8	3.5	3.1	4.1	4.5	8.1	16.6
Mouth and pharynx cancer	M	15606	135	11287	8.8	0.1	16.6	0.1	0.0	0.0	0.1	0.1	0.1	0.5
	F	3859	43	1736	1.5	0.0	2.3	0.0	0.0	0.0	0.1	0.0	0.1	0.1
Oesophagus cancer	M	16301	36	10091	9.0	0.0	15.4	–	–	0.0	–	0.0	0.1	0.2
	F	5675	11	1808	2.0	0.0	2.5	–	–	–	–	0.0	0.0	0.1
Stomach cancer	M	38703	181	16375	20.6	0.2	25.7	–	–	0.0	0.0	0.1	0.3	0.9
	F	29521	203	7992	9.8	0.2	10.8	0.0	–	–	0.0	0.1	0.3	0.9
Colorectal cancer	M	51830	231	21176	27.5	0.2	33.3	0.0	–	0.0	0.1	0.2	0.4	0.9
	F	55883	186	16503	18.8	0.2	22.5	0.0	–	–	0.0	0.1	0.4	0.8
Liver cancer	M	9645	75	5567	5.2	0.1	8.8	0.1	0.0	0.0	0.1	0.1	0.1	0.1
	F	4188	42	1613	1.5	0.0	2.2	0.0	0.0	0.0	0.0	0.0	0.1	0.1
Pancreas cancer	M	20627	75	10294	11.1	0.1	16.0	0.0	0.0	0.0	0.0	0.0	0.1	0.3
	F	20702	49	6682	7.2	0.1	9.1	0.0	0.0	–	0.0	0.1	0.1	0.2
Larynx cancer	M	11229	15	7079	6.2	0.0	10.7	–	0.0	–	0.0	0.0	0.0	0.1
	F	898	6	429	0.4	0.0	0.6	0.0	–	0.0	–	0.0	–	0.0
Lung cancer	M	139839	267	76427	75.8	0.3	120.1	0.1	0.0	0.0	0.1	0.1	0.3	1.3
	F	34831	142	16426	13.6	0.1	22.4	0.0	–	–	0.1	0.1	0.2	0.6
Malignant melanoma	M	3928	202	2436	2.2	0.2	3.5	0.0	–	–	0.1	0.2	0.5	0.7
	F	3765	183	1901	1.6	0.2	2.5	–	0.0	–	0.0	0.2	0.4	0.6
Female breast cancer	F	74382	788	40190	31.0	0.8	53.5	–	–	0.0	0.1	0.1	1.1	4.4
Cervix cancer	F	8076	307	4614	3.5	0.3	6.0	0.0	–	–	–	0.1	0.6	1.5
Other uterine cancer	F	13921	71	5504	5.1	0.1	7.5	0.0	–	0.0	0.0	0.0	0.1	0.4
Ovarian cancer	F	22466	245	11844	9.2	0.3	16.0	0.0	0.0	0.0	0.2	0.2	0.4	0.9
Prostate cancer	M	51131	26	9694	26.2	0.0	16.3	0.0	–	0.0	0.0	0.0	0.1	0.1
Bladder cancer	M	22110	18	7203	11.6	0.0	11.6	–	0.0	–	0.0	0.0	0.0	0.1
	F	8226	16	1730	2.6	0.0	2.4	0.0	–	0.0	0.0	0.0	0.0	0.1
Other and ill-defined cancer sites	M	90327	3020	44560	48.7	3.2	68.4	2.2	2.4	1.8	2.8	3.3	4.1	5.7
	F	87256	1870	29333	31.0	2.1	39.8	2.1	1.9	1.6	1.7	1.7	2.3	3.4
Hodgkin's disease	M	1846	331	1005	1.0	0.3	1.4	–	0.0	0.1	0.2	0.5	0.7	0.8
	F	1355	211	562	0.6	0.2	0.7	0.0	–	0.0	0.1	0.3	0.5	0.5
Myeloma and non-Hodgkin lymphomas	M	17050	612	8167	9.2	0.6	12.5	0.2	0.3	0.4	0.6	0.7	0.9	1.2
	F	16502	298	5855	6.0	0.3	8.0	0.2	0.1	0.2	0.3	0.3	0.5	0.7
Leukaemia	M	14964	1537	5829	8.0	1.7	8.9	1.4	1.6	1.6	1.9	1.7	1.7	1.8
	F	13106	1083	4254	4.9	1.2	5.7	1.3	1.4	1.2	1.3	1.1	1.1	1.3
ALL VASCULAR DISEASE	M	762179	5211	230196	397.9	5.3	362.9	3.9	1.0	1.3	3.0	5.3	7.9	15.1
	F	911760	2818	103418	254.0	3.1	142.1	3.4	0.7	1.4	2.1	2.9	4.3	6.6
Rheumatic heart disease and fever	M	3235	82	1618	1.7	0.1	2.5	0.0	0.0	0.0	0.1	0.1	0.1	0.2
	F	7874	76	2779	2.8	0.1	3.8	0.0	0.0	0.0	0.0	0.1	0.2	0.2
Hypertensive disease	M	19780	77	6022	10.3	0.1	9.5	0.0	0.0	0.0	0.0	0.1	0.1	0.3
	F	35809	51	4685	10.1	0.1	6.5	0.0	0.0	–	0.0	0.0	0.1	0.1
Ischaemic heart disease	M	348624	1095	133807	184.4	1.1	210.7	0.1	0.0	0.0	0.2	0.6	1.6	5.1
	F	296155	260	43657	86.2	0.3	60.3	0.1	–	0.0	0.1	0.2	0.5	1.0
Pulmonary embolism and other venous	M	12105	191	4223	6.4	0.2	6.6	0.1	0.0	0.0	0.1	0.2	0.3	0.6
	F	18984	212	3838	6.0	0.2	5.3	0.0	–	0.0	0.2	0.4	0.3	0.6
Cerebrovascular disease	M	178911	1166	38144	92.1	1.2	60.8	0.7	0.3	0.4	0.8	1.3	1.7	3.3
	F	276112	910	26414	75.6	1.0	36.1	0.5	0.3	0.5	0.7	0.9	1.5	2.4
Other vascular disease	M	199516	2598	46378	103.0	2.7	72.8	2.9	0.6	0.8	1.9	3.1	4.0	5.6
	F	276820	1307	22043	73.3	1.5	30.2	2.7	0.4	0.8	1.1	1.3	1.7	2.3
Chronic obstructive pulmonary disease	M	89502	565	21378	46.3	0.6	35.1	0.6	0.2	0.4	0.6	0.6	0.8	0.9
	F	47320	389	9455	14.6	0.4	13.0	0.4	0.1	0.2	0.5	0.5	0.5	0.7
Other respiratory disease	M	73195	1991	13675	37.7	2.2	21.5	6.8	0.5	0.5	1.1	1.5	2.2	2.8
	F	86716	1191	6441	23.1	1.4	8.8	5.5	0.5	0.4	0.7	0.7	1.1	1.1
Peptic ulcer	M	9254	89	2968	4.8	0.1	4.6	0.0	–	0.0	0.0	0.1	0.2	0.3
	F	8922	23	1290	2.6	0.0	1.8	0.0	–	0.0	0.0	0.0	0.0	0.1
Liver cirrhosis	M	42538	966	30398	23.7	1.0	44.5	0.1	0.0	0.0	0.1	0.3	1.5	4.9
	F	22488	446	12945	9.7	0.5	17.3	0.1	0.0	0.1	0.1	0.2	0.7	2.1
Renal disease	M	18271	308	4303	9.5	0.3	6.8	0.7	0.1	0.1	0.1	0.3	0.3	0.7
	F	20556	196	3184	6.1	0.2	4.4	0.5	0.1	0.1	0.1	0.2	0.2	0.4
Pregnancy and birth	F	350	266	84	0.2	0.3	0.1	–	–	–	0.1	0.4	0.6	0.7
Congenital and perinatal causes	M	15751	14507	904	10.8	18.3	1.3	119.6	1.9	1.4	1.7	1.4	1.1	0.9
	F	12416	11108	821	8.8	14.8	1.1	96.6	1.7	1.4	1.1	0.9	1.0	0.7
Ill-defined causes	M	55790	7906	16962	30.0	9.0	24.8	36.3	1.1	1.4	2.9	5.9	7.2	8.3
	F	68395	3979	7191	20.1	5.0	9.6	25.0	0.9	0.8	1.0	2.2	2.2	2.6
Other medical causes	M	164551	12612	53534	86.5	13.1	80.0	13.6	3.5	4.2	7.0	11.5	23.1	28.5
	F	217261	5666	36665	66.0	6.3	49.7	11.2	3.0	3.1	3.8	5.7	8.4	9.2
ALL NON-MEDICAL CAUSES	M	133281	45661	56509	71.0	46.1	76.9	17.7	9.8	11.2	59.8	85.1	72.2	67.1
	F	77072	12485	21034	29.1	13.6	27.4	11.8	6.0	6.2	17.1	19.5	17.1	17.2
Motor vehicle traffic accidents	M	41207	21677	14306	21.6	21.8	19.3	4.0	5.1	5.7	37.9	47.2	30.6	22.3
	F	14642	5766	5142	6.9	6.3	6.7	2.9	3.4	3.7	11.0	10.5	7.0	5.2
Fire	M	2036	596	897	1.1	0.6	1.2	1.3	0.4	0.2	0.4	0.7	0.7	0.8
	F	1515	290	442	0.6	0.3	0.6	1.1	0.3	0.1	0.1	0.3	0.2	0.3
Suicide	M	34885	9275	18658	18.8	9.1	25.2	–	0.0	0.9	7.1	16.0	18.5	21.3
	F	14216	2575	7754	6.6	2.6	10.0	–	0.0	0.2	2.1	4.3	5.1	6.6
Homicide	M	3487	1577	1752	1.9	1.6	2.2	0.8	0.3	0.3	1.4	2.4	2.9	3.2
	F	1324	588	553	0.7	0.6	0.7	0.8	0.3	0.2	0.6	0.8	0.8	0.9
POPULATION (thousands):	M=males				180312	92118	74951	11208	11263	11955	13350	15077	15369	13897
	F=females				189964	88292	78531	10626	10673	11347	12700	14474	14868	13603

PLANNED EU (16 countries): 1990

Annual death rates / 100, 000

9th ICD categories

35–39	40–44	45–49	50–54	55–59	60–64	65–69	70–74	75–79	80+/NK			
186.2	262.7	416.5	668.4	1110.2	1780.7	2823.9	4410.0	7208.8	14548.5	M	**ALL CAUSES**	001–999
90.5	134.1	214.7	323.4	513.4	821.3	1356.1	2299.6	4211.3	11422.0	F		
0.6	1.0	1.4	2.0	3.0	5.1	7.5	11.6	16.9	23.9	M	**Tuberculosis**	010–018, 137
0.2	0.2	0.4	0.4	0.9	1.3	2.7	3.7	5.8	10.4	F		
1.8	2.1	2.7	3.3	4.6	7.9	11.9	20.3	31.1	72.8	M	**Other infective**	Rest of 001–139
0.7	1.0	1.3	2.0	3.2	4.8	7.4	11.5	21.8	62.3	F	**and parasitic**	
29.3	63.1	129.7	235.9	421.7	684.0	1021.3	1422.6	1937.5	2679.1	M	**ALL CANCER**	140–208
36.4	63.4	108.1	166.9	252.3	362.9	511.8	677.8	928.8	1407.3	F		
2.0	5.4	11.7	17.7	24.0	27.4	27.7	29.3	30.6	35.4	M	**Mouth and**	140–149
0.4	0.8	1.6	2.2	3.0	3.9	4.4	5.5	7.4	13.0	F	**pharynx cancer**	
0.9	2.8	7.1	13.0	21.2	28.2	34.3	40.8	46.5	53.8	M	**Oesophagus cancer**	150
0.2	0.4	0.9	1.9	2.8	4.8	6.3	10.0	14.5	23.6	F		
2.1	4.4	8.2	15.3	27.3	47.1	75.2	110.4	164.3	239.7	M	**Stomach cancer**	151
1.6	2.8	4.4	6.7	11.8	17.9	30.7	47.4	77.4	139.5	F		
2.2	4.6	9.8	19.7	36.2	61.3	99.7	145.3	219.5	343.7	M	**Colorectal cancer**	153, 154
2.2	4.3	8.6	14.7	25.3	39.6	62.8	91.5	141.8	253.3	F		
0.4	0.7	2.0	4.7	9.9	18.3	25.9	30.0	31.6	29.0	M	**Liver cancer**	155.0
0.2	0.4	0.8	1.1	2.3	4.1	6.6	8.8	11.6	12.1	F		
1.0	2.6	6.2	10.9	18.5	28.7	44.2	62.3	77.5	95.9	M	**Pancreas cancer**	157
0.6	1.3	2.8	5.4	9.8	16.8	27.2	39.2	56.7	80.1	F		
0.4	2.2	5.4	9.2	15.0	19.3	23.7	27.7	30.9	35.8	M	**Larynx cancer**	161
0.0	0.1	0.3	0.5	0.8	1.0	1.2	1.4	2.0	2.5	F		
5.1	15.0	36.3	69.8	139.4	235.1	339.7	435.0	503.5	498.8	M	**Lung cancer**	162
1.9	4.8	8.9	14.3	24.5	42.4	59.8	75.5	81.8	79.3	F		
1.2	1.9	2.5	3.3	4.0	5.3	6.4	7.7	10.0	12.0	M	**Malignant melanoma**	172
1.2	1.6	2.1	2.3	2.8	3.3	4.0	5.1	6.6	9.5	F		
12.3	23.3	37.7	55.0	69.8	81.1	95.5	106.7	128.1	187.3	F	**Female breast cancer**	174
3.4	3.9	4.9	5.5	6.2	8.1	10.3	12.1	13.7	14.8	F	**Cervix cancer**	180
1.0	1.7	2.7	4.6	9.5	13.4	19.4	25.4	33.3	46.7	F	**Other uterine cancer**	179, 182
1.6	4.2	8.6	14.6	20.4	27.8	34.8	40.1	44.1	49.2	F	**Ovarian cancer**	183
0.1	0.2	0.9	3.2	10.9	29.2	69.6	148.2	278.1	550.4	M	**Prostate cancer**	185
0.1	0.7	2.0	5.0	11.2	23.2	39.4	65.7	108.3	173.8	M	**Bladder cancer**	188
0.2	0.2	0.5	0.9	2.4	4.6	7.9	13.0	23.6	43.5	F		
8.8	15.5	27.5	48.2	80.3	122.7	175.9	232.4	314.3	442.0	M	**Other and ill-defined**	Rest of 140–208
6.1	9.4	16.7	26.9	45.7	70.4	103.2	141.5	210.1	347.8	F	**cancer sites**	
1.0	0.9	1.0	1.2	1.5	1.8	2.5	3.3	3.8	4.5	M	**Hodgkin's disease**	201
0.5	0.5	0.5	0.5	0.7	0.9	1.6	2.0	2.9	2.7	F		
1.9	3.4	5.4	8.9	13.1	22.2	32.7	48.2	63.2	79.0	M	**Myeloma and non–**	200, 202–203
1.2	1.7	3.1	5.2	8.6	13.8	22.1	33.0	43.8	54.7	F	**Hodgkin lymphomas**	
2.1	2.9	3.7	5.9	9.1	14.1	24.5	36.2	55.3	85.3	M	**Leukaemia**	204–208
1.8	2.0	2.8	4.6	5.9	9.0	13.9	19.7	29.5	47.9	F		
30.9	60.0	109.9	200.3	368.2	650.6	1120.8	1892.9	3338.1	7209.6	M	**ALL VASCULAR**	390–459
11.9	19.0	35.3	61.3	122.4	244.8	500.0	1033.4	2174.0	6475.3	F	**DISEASE**	
0.4	0.4	0.8	1.8	2.8	4.7	6.6	8.9	12.2	14.3	M	**Rheumatic heart**	390–398
0.4	0.6	1.2	2.5	4.0	6.7	11.3	16.9	20.3	26.6	F	**disease and fever**	
0.6	1.2	2.7	5.7	10.3	17.3	28.6	46.3	88.2	189.2	M	**Hypertensive disease**	401–405
0.3	0.6	1.2	3.2	5.9	10.8	23.1	42.1	90.7	242.4	F		
14.4	33.3	64.4	119.5	221.5	385.0	637.1	995.5	1509.0	2480.3	M	**Ischaemic heart**	410–414
2.4	5.2	11.2	22.2	50.1	109.7	221.1	433.2	802.6	1842.0	F	**disease**	
0.9	1.6	2.3	4.0	6.7	12.4	18.6	32.5	54.3	95.6	M	**Pulmonary embolism**	415.1, 451–453
0.9	1.3	2.1	2.9	5.1	8.8	16.1	26.8	50.4	108.0	F	**and other venous**	
5.3	9.6	17.0	29.0	55.3	104.0	205.4	412.8	865.0	2040.2	M	**Cerebrovascular**	430–438
4.6	6.6	11.0	16.8	31.2	58.2	124.6	294.8	672.8	2018.0	F	**disease**	
9.2	13.8	22.7	40.4	71.6	127.3	224.8	397.4	810.1	2391.0	M	**Other vascular**	Rest of 390–459
3.5	4.7	8.5	13.8	26.2	50.8	104.1	220.1	537.9	2239.5	F	**disease**	
1.2	2.2	4.7	11.2	28.2	64.6	133.3	255.6	447.8	887.7	M	**Chronic obstructive**	490–496
1.0	1.3	3.1	5.8	12.1	24.2	43.4	74.0	117.0	267.9	F	**pulmonary disease**	
3.5	4.5	6.8	11.0	19.8	34.9	70.2	136.1	292.7	951.2	M	**Other respiratory**	Rest of 460–519
1.4	2.3	3.0	4.7	7.6	14.3	28.1	62.9	147.4	720.0	F	**disease**	
0.6	1.0	1.6	2.8	5.0	7.7	13.7	22.1	38.4	85.9	M	**Peptic ulcer**	531–533
0.2	0.4	0.6	0.9	1.6	3.0	5.7	11.2	20.1	60.4	F		
10.7	17.0	28.6	43.2	59.3	72.1	80.7	78.8	89.2	85.9	M	**Liver cirrhosis**	571
4.5	7.5	12.2	16.1	20.8	27.3	32.3	35.9	40.6	41.0	F		
0.7	1.3	2.0	3.9	7.1	11.5	20.7	37.9	77.4	210.4	M	**Renal disease**	580–590
0.5	0.7	1.3	2.4	4.4	7.5	13.5	25.6	48.4	133.6	F		
0.4	0.2	0.0	–	–	–	–	–	–	–	F	**Pregnancy and birth**	630–676
0.9	0.9	1.1	1.3	1.3	1.6	1.7	1.8	2.5	3.6	M	**Congenital and**	740–779
0.8	0.8	0.8	1.0	1.3	1.4	1.4	1.8	1.9	2.5	F	**perinatal causes**	
9.5	11.5	15.4	21.7	27.7	36.7	51.2	77.4	133.8	531.6	M	**Ill-defined causes**	780–799
3.8	3.8	5.8	7.2	8.9	14.6	22.9	40.4	89.0	539.3	F		
30.1	32.0	41.3	55.7	82.0	120.9	198.0	333.1	613.5	1382.7	M	**Other medical causes**	Rest of 001–799
10.8	13.2	19.2	28.5	48.5	82.3	145.4	260.0	506.5	1350.1	F		
66.3	66.2	71.2	76.0	82.2	83.1	93.0	119.6	190.0	424.0	M	**ALL NON–**	E800–E999
17.8	20.4	23.6	26.0	29.4	33.0	41.4	61.4	110.0	351.9	F	**MEDICAL CAUSES**	
18.7	17.0	17.5	18.5	21.0	20.5	22.0	29.8	41.3	49.2	M	**Motor vehicle**	E810–E819
5.1	5.1	5.6	6.3	7.3	7.9	9.2	13.1	17.7	17.2	F	**traffic accidents**	
0.9	1.0	1.1	1.1	1.3	1.2	2.0	2.1	3.5	7.2	M	**Fire**	E890–E899
0.3	0.4	0.5	0.5	0.7	0.6	1.1	1.5	2.5	5.6	F		
22.4	23.0	24.9	26.2	26.4	25.3	28.1	33.3	50.0	78.6	M	**Suicide**	E950–E959
6.9	8.0	9.7	10.4	11.1	11.6	12.6	13.6	17.6	18.6	F		
3.2	2.9	2.4	2.4	2.1	1.5	1.2	1.0	1.2	1.5	M	**Homicide**	E960–E969
0.9	0.8	0.7	0.7	0.7	0.5	0.5	0.6	0.7	0.9	F		
12917	12889	11116	11002	10005	9227	7795	4887	4345	4012	M	**POPULATION (thousands)**	
12742	12687	11006	11134	10479	10369	10114	7010	7241	8890	F		

PLANNED EU (16 countries): Males

	All ages	0–34	35–69	35–39	40–44	45–49	50–54	55–59	60–64	65–69	70–74	75–79	80+/NK
POPULATION (1000s)													
1955	147470	83276	56325	8092	10064	10147	9420	7679	5969	4953	3746	2476	1648
1965	162637	90582	63023	11184	10665	7889	9644	9380	8195	6066	4127	2747	2158
1975	171812	94531	66093	11608	10985	10748	10007	7200	8224	7321	5512	3222	2456
1985	176926	93157	70360	12920	11262	11239	10435	9893	8746	5866	5850	4189	3370
1990	**180312**	**92118**	**74951**	**12917**	**12889**	**11116**	**11002**	**10005**	**9227**	**7795**	**4887**	**4345**	**4012**
1995 projected	*181124*	*89520*	*77672*	*13742*	*12777*	*12527*	*10827*	*10422*	*9251*	*8126*	*6405*	*3520*	*4006*
NUMBER OF DEATHS													
All causes													
1955	1665723	236474	661286	19870	36333	60190	93325	121186	145866	184516	221559	240143	306261
1965	1872841	185359	791809	26369	37720	43345	88561	144829	209489	241496	250066	257618	387989
1975	1969355	136554	777070	24231	37774	60341	90363	101067	189191	274103	327834	300680	427217
1985	1921702	97275	663013	22329	30945	51116	80323	124144	174064	180092	293408	340645	527361
1990	**1883517**	**97892**	**673250**	**24052**	**33859**	**46295**	**73544**	**111079**	**164296**	**220125**	**215496**	**313249**	**583630**
1995 projected	*1747175*	*99761*	*629029*	*26446*	*32458*	*46538*	*63866*	*103938*	*149827*	*205956*	*250696*	*228970*	*538719*
Lung cancer													
1955	46311	320	35663	345	1200	2896	6000	8601	8808	7813	5733	3212	1383
1965	83808	412	59582	594	1423	2463	6493	12453	18201	17955	12532	7297	3985
1975	113423	339	66940	589	1583	3975	7634	9687	18810	24662	23565	14451	8128
1985	136620	301	71134	657	1675	3951	8359	15105	21293	20094	26066	22293	16826
1990	**139839**	**267**	**76427**	**658**	**1937**	**4032**	**7679**	**13950**	**21691**	**26480**	**21255**	**21879**	**20011**
1995 projected	*139113*	*299*	*75277*	*732*	*2006*	*4276*	*6869*	*13532*	*21031*	*26831*	*26663*	*17315*	*19559*
ANNUAL DEATH RATE / 100,000 (*The rates for the age groups 0–34 and 35–69 are the means of seven five-yearly rates, but the all-ages rates are standardised to the conventional "European" age distribution)													
All causes													
1955	1406.4*	270.9*	1419.6*	245.5	361.0	593.2	990.7	1578.2	2443.8	3725.1	5915.2	9699.8	18581.6
1965	1353.7*	191.9*	1448.4*	235.8	353.7	549.5	918.3	1544.0	2556.4	3980.9	6059.2	9378.5	17975.6
1975	1280.4*	148.4*	1352.2*	208.7	343.9	561.4	903.0	1403.7	2300.3	3744.2	5948.0	9333.4	17398.3
1985	1095.4*	106.3*	1141.1*	172.8	274.8	454.8	769.8	1254.8	1990.3	3070.2	5015.2	8131.9	15650.8
1990	**996.7***	**104.6***	**1035.5***	**186.2**	**262.7**	**416.5**	**668.4**	**1110.2**	**1780.7**	**2823.9**	**4410.0**	**7208.8**	**14548.5**
1995 projected	*911.3**	*106.8**	*937.0**	*192.4*	*254.0*	*371.5*	*589.9*	*997.3*	*1619.6*	*2534.5*	*3914.0*	*6504.2*	*13448.1*
All cancer													
1955	213.7*	10.1*	313.8*	30.1	57.7	116.8	224.1	384.5	578.3	805.0	1103.8	1428.9	1636.4
1965	247.3*	11.5*	359.5*	34.7	63.9	118.8	224.3	410.7	673.1	990.9	1308.7	1652.9	2018.8
1975	263.7*	10.4*	369.9*	32.0	67.4	136.2	247.0	406.2	674.9	1025.3	1436.6	1883.7	2240.6
1985	273.8*	8.2*	374.3*	30.9	66.1	129.6	254.7	441.2	692.5	1005.0	1442.2	1967.0	2605.4
1990	**270.9***	**7.1***	**369.3***	**29.3**	**63.1**	**129.7**	**235.9**	**421.7**	**684.0**	**1021.3**	**1422.6**	**1937.5**	**2679.1**
1995 projected	*266.2**	*6.3**	*359.3**	*27.7*	*61.7*	*123.3*	*222.8*	*403.2*	*672.9*	*1003.3*	*1398.9*	*1915.9*	*2717.9*
Lung cancer													
1955	37.1*	0.4*	75.1*	4.3	11.9	28.5	63.7	112.0	147.6	157.7	153.1	129.7	83.9
1965	57.5*	0.5*	109.7*	5.3	13.3	31.2	67.3	132.8	222.1	296.0	303.7	265.6	184.6
1975	70.9*	0.4*	119.0*	5.1	14.4	37.0	76.3	134.5	228.7	336.9	427.6	448.6	331.0
1985	78.7*	0.3*	124.8*	5.1	14.9	35.2	80.1	152.7	243.5	342.6	445.5	532.2	499.4
1990	**75.8***	**0.3***	**120.1***	**5.1**	**15.0**	**36.3**	**69.8**	**139.4**	**235.1**	**339.7**	**435.0**	**503.5**	**498.8**
1995 projected	*72.9**	*0.3**	*115.1**	*5.3*	*15.7*	*34.1*	*63.4*	*129.8*	*227.3*	*330.2*	*416.3*	*491.9*	*488.3*
Upper aerodigestive cancer (mouth, oesophagus, pharynx and larynx)													
1955	18.6*	0.2*	27.9*	1.4	3.9	10.2	21.0	38.0	52.2	68.3	93.5	125.9	150.1
1965	20.6*	0.2*	33.5*	2.4	5.9	12.2	23.8	41.9	62.7	85.9	98.8	119.0	149.7
1975	23.1*	0.2*	38.2*	2.5	9.2	21.6	34.7	46.9	65.5	87.1	107.6	132.6	139.4
1985	24.3*	0.2*	42.6*	3.0	10.8	23.0	43.2	60.8	74.9	82.7	98.8	114.7	133.4
1990	**23.9***	**0.2***	**42.7***	**3.3**	**10.3**	**24.2**	**39.9**	**60.3**	**74.9**	**85.7**	**97.8**	**108.0**	**125.0**
1995 projected	*23.6**	*0.2**	*42.5**	*3.2*	*10.7*	*24.1*	*40.2*	*59.2*	*75.6*	*84.5*	*96.1*	*102.2*	*117.7*
Other cancer													
1955	158.0*	9.5*	210.8*	24.4	41.9	78.1	139.4	234.5	378.5	579.0	857.3	1173.3	1402.4
1965	169.2*	10.8*	216.2*	27.0	44.6	75.3	133.2	236.1	388.3	609.1	906.3	1268.2	1684.4
1975	169.7*	9.8*	212.7*	24.4	43.8	77.6	136.0	224.7	380.7	601.4	901.5	1302.5	1770.1
1985	170.8*	7.7*	206.8*	22.9	40.5	71.5	131.4	227.7	374.1	579.7	897.9	1320.1	1972.7
1990	**171.2***	**6.6***	**206.6***	**20.9**	**37.7**	**69.2**	**126.1**	**222.0**	**374.0**	**595.9**	**889.8**	**1326.0**	**2055.2**
1995 projected	*169.8**	*5.9**	*201.6**	*19.2*	*35.2*	*65.0*	*119.2*	*214.1*	*370.0*	*588.5*	*886.5*	*1321.8*	*2112.0*
Chronic obstructive pulmonary disease (COPD)													
1955	52.9*	2.7*	67.1*	4.0	8.1	19.1	44.0	80.1	127.5	186.5	252.5	366.8	631.2
1965	63.3*	1.6*	75.9*	3.4	7.5	15.2	33.0	74.2	152.2	245.9	355.9	495.5	794.1
1975	71.3*	1.6*	69.1*	3.2	6.5	14.7	30.7	62.6	123.5	242.5	429.9	676.5	1028.1
1985	52.3*	0.7*	42.7*	1.5	3.1	6.6	15.6	37.0	80.2	154.8	288.2	509.7	941.9
1990	**46.3***	**0.6***	**35.1***	**1.2**	**2.2**	**4.7**	**11.2**	**28.2**	**64.6**	**133.3**	**255.6**	**447.8**	**887.7**
1995 projected	*41.9**	*0.6**	*29.8**	*1.0*	*1.7*	*3.4*	*8.7*	*22.8*	*54.7*	*116.4*	*223.8*	*413.9*	*839.1*
Other respiratory disease													
1955	75.8*	27.5*	46.1*	6.6	8.9	15.6	28.1	46.9	79.0	138.0	260.7	531.1	1291.2
1965	59.2*	14.5*	33.7*	4.7	6.9	11.0	16.4	30.0	57.8	109.1	218.9	441.4	1203.2
1975	54.8*	7.5*	31.2*	3.9	6.6	10.3	16.1	28.9	50.4	102.3	213.9	440.8	1224.6
1985	42.3*	2.7*	24.9*	3.2	4.3	7.5	13.6	24.0	43.3	78.2	159.7	338.7	1029.6
1990	**37.7***	**2.2***	**21.5***	**3.5**	**4.5**	**6.8**	**11.0**	**19.8**	**34.9**	**70.2**	**136.1**	**292.7**	**951.2**
1995 projected	*33.9**	*2.2**	*19.0**	*4.1*	*4.5*	*6.2*	*9.7*	*16.8*	*31.3*	*60.6*	*114.9*	*259.3*	*868.8*
Vascular disease													
1955	556.5*	11.6*	532.8*	42.3	75.8	152.5	298.4	541.5	967.2	1652.2	2873.2	4943.7	8945.8
1965	574.6*	8.4*	573.4*	48.3	97.2	177.9	323.7	575.3	1039.2	1752.4	2922.9	4793.1	9250.0
1975	566.8*	6.8*	548.8*	40.0	90.3	180.5	334.1	558.4	964.9	1673.5	2843.5	4751.9	9459.6
1985	473.5*	6.0*	442.6*	33.5	69.6	135.6	259.3	462.8	803.6	1333.7	2336.5	4013.9	8198.7
1990	**397.9***	**5.3***	**362.9***	**30.9**	**60.0**	**109.9**	**200.3**	**368.2**	**650.6**	**1120.8**	**1892.9**	**3338.1**	**7209.6**
1995 projected	*333.3**	*5.1**	*294.2**	*27.5*	*49.7*	*83.3*	*154.0*	*296.4*	*535.0*	*913.2*	*1527.3*	*2800.8*	*6291.2*
Liver cirrhosis													
1955	20.4*	0.6*	38.9*	4.7	11.1	21.0	36.0	51.6	68.1	79.9	86.0	76.7	57.5
1965	29.2*	0.9*	54.0*	8.7	16.2	26.4	45.1	69.7	95.2	116.9	121.8	129.6	107.3
1975	33.6*	1.3*	63.1*	12.6	26.8	43.1	58.2	73.8	101.1	125.8	127.1	132.5	108.6
1985	27.7*	1.1*	51.5*	10.0	19.2	33.8	52.1	69.0	85.4	91.1	103.8	108.1	92.1
1990	**23.7***	**1.0***	**44.5***	**10.7**	**17.0**	**28.6**	**43.2**	**59.3**	**72.1**	**80.7**	**78.8**	**89.2**	**85.9**
1995 projected	*20.5**	*1.0**	*38.3**	*10.4*	*16.1*	*24.4*	*37.0*	*51.5*	*61.3*	*67.3*	*66.9*	*71.6*	*75.9*
Other medical causes													
1955	395.4*	162.9*	314.7*	87.0	117.0	172.4	250.8	354.6	497.6	723.7	1160.1	2102.4	5539.6
1965	288.2*	100.6*	246.7*	61.6	84.3	114.8	173.3	263.6	406.4	622.8	953.2	1605.9	4062.2
1975	201.7*	65.0*	172.9*	41.8	63.7	88.5	124.7	176.2	272.6	442.4	724.4	1197.7	2823.6
1985	153.2*	42.2*	125.9*	31.3	44.9	65.8	94.4	135.9	198.4	310.9	547.3	993.5	2355.2
1990	**149.2***	**42.3***	**125.3***	**44.3**	**49.8**	**65.5**	**90.8**	**130.8**	**191.5**	**304.7**	**504.3**	**913.5**	**2311.0**
1995 projected	*145.5**	*42.9**	*123.2**	*55.0*	*56.4*	*63.7*	*85.8*	*127.6*	*185.1*	*288.7*	*469.9*	*869.1*	*2240.6*
All non-medical causes													
1955	91.7*	55.6*	106.2*	70.9	82.4	95.8	109.2	119.0	126.1	139.8	178.8	250.2	480.0
1965	91.8*	54.6*	105.1*	74.4	77.8	85.4	102.5	120.5	132.4	142.9	177.7	260.1	540.1
1975	88.5*	55.7*	97.3*	75.2	82.6	88.1	92.1	97.7	113.0	132.5	172.5	250.4	513.2
1985	72.5*	45.4*	79.2*	62.3	67.5	75.9	80.1	84.9	86.9	96.5	137.5	201.0	428.0
1990	**71.0***	**46.1***	**76.9***	**66.3**	**66.2**	**71.2**	**76.0**	**82.2**	**83.1**	**93.0**	**119.6**	**190.0**	**424.0**
1995 projected	*70.1**	*48.7**	*73.3**	*66.8*	*64.0*	*67.2*	*71.8*	*79.0*	*79.2*	*85.0*	*112.2*	*173.6*	*414.5*

PLANNED EU (16 countries): Females

	All ages	0–34	35–69	35–39	40–44	45–49	50–54	55–59	60–64	65–69	70–74	75–79	80+/NK
POPULATION (1000s)													
1955	159050	82579	65240	9000	11205	11124	10229	9198	7858	6627	5140	3472	2620
1965	174055	87337	72023	11391	11874	8929	11079	10822	9681	8248	6395	4449	3851
1975	182208	90719	72839	11352	10894	11107	11373	8464	10129	9520	7848	5556	5245
1985	187330	89509	74763	12665	11101	11243	10675	10700	10684	7695	8568	7029	7460
1990	**189964**	**88292**	**78531**	**12742**	**12687**	**11006**	**11134**	**10479**	**10369**	**10114**	**7010**	**7241**	**8890**
1995 projected	*189632*	*85497*	*80223*	*13462*	*12634*	*12438*	*10937*	*10854*	*10119*	*9779*	*9181*	*5815*	*8916*
NUMBER OF DEATHS													
All causes													
1955	1576477	173949	496658	16485	28574	41803	58848	78960	111384	160604	219403	263633	422834
1965	1748148	120733	507333	16285	25568	29543	55329	82469	122238	175901	242847	299293	577942
1975	1870873	78844	463382	13011	20012	32565	52294	58602	111066	175832	257381	334637	736629
1985	1894914	49758	366152	11711	15884	25575	38687	61142	98481	114672	225740	334324	918940
1990	**1891046**	**45171**	**364302**	**11525**	**17010**	**23632**	**36006**	**53799**	**85167**	**137163**	**161201**	**304933**	**1015439**
1995 projected	*1712926*	*41491*	*327771*	*11647*	*16174*	*24261*	*32137*	*50756*	*75374*	*117422*	*185519*	*217933*	*940212*
Lung cancer													
1955	9494	236	6111	158	332	618	847	1221	1359	1576	1414	1097	636
1965	15163	197	9082	206	379	632	1253	1723	2222	2667	2439	1866	1579
1975	20916	144	11303	151	368	791	1559	1809	3060	3565	3625	2970	2874
1985	30202	154	14004	229	385	809	1407	2723	4223	4228	5565	4978	5501
1990	**34831**	**142**	**16426**	**239**	**605**	**980**	**1587**	**2568**	**4394**	**6053**	**5294**	**5921**	**7048**
1995 projected	*38823*	*141*	*17815*	*303*	*729*	*1255*	*1653*	*2861*	*4623*	*6391*	*7484*	*5449*	*7934*
ANNUAL DEATH RATE / 100,000 (*The rates for the age groups 0–34 and 35–69 are the means of seven five-yearly rates, but the all-ages rates are standardised to the conventional "European" age distribution)													
All causes													
1955	1028.4*	203.3*	869.8*	183.2	255.0	375.8	575.3	858.4	1417.5	2423.4	4269.0	7593.5	16141.5
1965	894.0*	127.4*	763.7*	143.0	215.3	330.9	499.4	762.0	1262.6	2132.8	3797.6	6726.9	15006.0
1975	790.9*	89.5*	669.6*	114.6	183.7	293.2	459.8	692.4	1096.5	1847.0	3279.5	6022.9	14045.8
1985	649.1*	58.8*	544.1*	92.5	143.1	227.5	362.4	571.4	921.7	1490.3	2634.6	4756.7	12317.9
1990	**588.6***	**52.8***	**493.4***	**90.4**	**134.1**	**214.7**	**323.4**	**513.4**	**821.3**	**1356.1**	**2299.6**	**4211.3**	**11422.0**
1995 projected	*534.1**	*48.4**	*445.2**	*86.5*	*128.0*	*195.1*	*293.8*	*467.6*	*744.9*	*1200.8*	*2020.6*	*3747.6*	*10545.5*
All cancer													
1955	161.7*	9.8*	238.0*	46.9	84.9	132.7	199.6	274.5	386.8	540.4	741.1	994.7	1239.6
1965	164.9*	9.7*	238.1*	43.6	82.0	133.5	203.1	278.5	387.1	538.5	750.5	1008.9	1369.3
1975	157.9*	8.6*	230.2*	38.4	72.8	124.1	199.1	278.8	383.5	514.8	695.9	963.7	1330.2
1985	152.6*	7.1*	218.2*	36.7	65.1	109.1	172.7	261.6	377.5	504.9	699.3	932.6	1393.9
1990	**150.1***	**6.2***	**214.5***	**36.4**	**63.4**	**108.1**	**166.9**	**252.3**	**362.9**	**511.8**	**677.8**	**928.8**	**1407.3**
1995 projected	*146.3**	*5.6**	*207.1**	*35.0*	*62.0*	*103.3*	*160.1*	*243.3*	*353.9*	*492.4*	*660.4*	*909.6*	*1415.8*
Lung cancer													
1955	6.0*	0.3*	10.4*	1.8	3.0	5.6	8.3	13.3	17.3	23.8	27.5	31.6	24.3
1965	8.0*	0.2*	13.5*	1.8	3.2	7.1	11.3	15.9	23.0	32.3	38.1	41.9	41.0
1975	9.7*	0.2*	16.4*	1.3	3.4	7.1	13.7	21.4	30.2	37.4	46.2	53.5	54.8
1985	12.4*	0.2*	20.8*	1.8	3.5	7.2	13.2	25.4	39.5	54.9	64.9	70.8	73.7
1990	**13.6***	**0.1***	**22.4***	**1.9**	**4.8**	**8.9**	**14.3**	**24.5**	**42.4**	**59.8**	**75.5**	**81.8**	**79.3**
1995 projected	*15.0**	*0.1**	*24.4**	*2.3*	*5.8*	*10.1*	*15.1*	*26.4*	*45.7*	*65.4*	*81.5*	*93.7*	*89.0*
Upper aerodigestive cancer (mouth, oesophagus, pharynx and larynx)													
1955	4.1*	0.1*	5.0*	0.9	1.2	2.4	3.6	5.5	8.5	12.8	21.3	33.4	46.6
1965	3.8*	0.1*	4.6*	0.6	1.1	2.1	3.4	5.2	7.7	11.9	18.6	30.0	48.2
1975	3.7*	0.1*	4.8*	0.5	1.3	2.2	3.9	5.8	8.4	11.5	16.9	25.4	44.3
1985	3.8*	0.1*	5.3*	0.6	1.2	2.4	3.9	7.1	9.6	12.6	16.3	23.1	39.4
1990	**3.8***	**0.1***	**5.4***	**0.5**	**1.4**	**2.9**	**4.6**	**6.5**	**9.7**	**11.9**	**17.0**	**23.9**	**39.1**
1995 projected	*3.9**	*0.1**	*5.5**	*0.6*	*1.6*	*3.5*	*5.0*	*6.8*	*9.5*	*11.7*	*16.4*	*26.3*	*40.0*
Other cancer													
1955	151.6*	9.4*	222.6*	44.2	80.7	124.8	187.7	255.8	361.0	503.8	692.2	929.8	1168.7
1965	153.1*	9.4*	220.0*	41.2	77.7	124.4	188.4	257.5	356.4	494.3	693.8	936.9	1280.1
1975	144.5*	8.3*	209.1*	36.6	68.2	114.8	181.5	251.6	344.9	465.8	632.8	884.9	1231.0
1985	136.5*	6.8*	192.1*	34.2	60.5	99.5	155.7	229.0	328.4	437.3	618.1	838.7	1280.8
1990	**132.7***	**6.0***	**186.8***	**33.9**	**57.2**	**96.3**	**148.0**	**221.2**	**310.9**	**440.1**	**585.3**	**823.1**	**1289.0**
1995 projected	*127.4**	*5.4**	*177.2**	*32.1*	*54.6*	*89.7*	*140.0*	*210.1*	*298.7*	*415.3*	*562.5*	*789.6*	*1286.8*
Chronic obstructive pulmonary disease (COPD)													
1955	21.8*	2.2*	16.1*	2.1	2.9	4.5	7.6	13.8	28.4	53.6	99.5	189.2	413.4
1965	20.6*	1.2*	15.8*	1.9	2.8	4.8	7.8	13.6	27.7	52.2	93.8	175.9	408.5
1975	21.6*	1.2*	17.7*	2.2	3.9	6.3	10.4	18.4	30.3	52.6	97.3	178.9	405.9
1985	15.4*	0.6*	14.5*	1.4	2.0	4.1	8.0	15.0	25.8	45.4	73.6	116.6	275.3
1990	**14.6***	**0.4***	**13.0***	**1.0**	**1.3**	**3.1**	**5.8**	**12.1**	**24.2**	**43.4**	**74.0**	**117.0**	**267.9**
1995 projected	*14.1**	*0.4**	*12.1**	*0.8*	*1.0*	*2.3*	*4.9*	*10.9*	*23.1*	*41.8*	*71.3*	*117.0*	*268.2*
Other respiratory disease													
1955	59.2*	24.5*	26.6*	5.2	6.2	8.5	13.1	22.0	43.7	87.4	196.2	422.3	1104.7
1965	43.0*	12.2*	17.8*	3.0	4.0	5.8	9.0	14.7	28.1	60.2	138.6	311.9	983.7
1975	37.2*	6.1*	16.1*	2.8	3.4	5.4	8.5	15.1	25.9	51.5	118.5	281.8	952.8
1985	25.3*	2.0*	10.0*	1.6	1.9	3.5	5.4	8.4	16.5	32.8	70.2	170.2	762.4
1990	**23.1***	**1.4***	**8.8***	**1.4**	**2.3**	**3.0**	**4.7**	**7.6**	**14.3**	**28.1**	**62.9**	**147.4**	**720.0**
1995 projected	*21.2**	*1.2**	*7.9**	*1.5*	*2.2*	*2.8*	*4.3*	*6.8*	*12.8*	*25.0*	*51.6*	*133.4*	*676.3*
Vascular disease													
1955	439.2*	10.9*	344.6*	33.2	51.9	92.5	168.3	300.9	591.9	1173.7	2277.0	4189.5	8144.8
1965	404.3*	6.1*	290.2*	24.6	42.9	77.0	135.0	249.9	504.2	997.7	2004.6	3798.9	8277.7
1975	373.1*	4.5*	241.7*	18.7	34.8	65.4	114.4	209.5	410.4	838.9	1720.1	3451.6	8360.4
1985	300.0*	3.5*	175.7*	12.9	23.0	41.9	80.1	151.8	306.4	613.9	1293.5	2642.3	7325.9
1990	**254.0***	**3.1***	**142.1***	**11.9**	**19.0**	**35.3**	**61.3**	**122.4**	**244.8**	**500.0**	**1033.4**	**2174.0**	**6475.3**
1995 projected	*213.4**	*2.8**	*113.3**	*10.3*	*16.3*	*27.0*	*48.4*	*99.2*	*197.2*	*394.5*	*816.8*	*1789.9*	*5648.7*
Liver cirrhosis													
1955	9.3*	0.5*	16.8*	3.2	5.8	10.5	16.6	22.5	27.1	32.0	34.9	38.0	35.4
1965	11.5*	0.5*	19.6*	4.5	7.6	11.2	16.6	23.1	33.8	40.6	50.3	56.1	55.8
1975	12.0*	0.7*	20.9*	5.7	10.7	15.9	20.9	25.4	30.6	37.2	44.5	52.3	52.1
1985	10.5*	0.5*	18.7*	4.8	7.6	12.3	18.7	24.6	30.2	32.7	38.4	44.4	42.4
1990	**9.7***	**0.5***	**17.3***	**4.5**	**7.5**	**12.2**	**16.1**	**20.8**	**27.3**	**32.3**	**35.9**	**40.6**	**41.0**
1995 projected	*9.0**	*0.5**	*15.9**	*4.5*	*7.8*	*11.6*	*14.3*	*18.8*	*24.5*	*30.0*	*34.4*	*36.6*	*38.4*
Other medical causes													
1955	300.0*	139.8*	194.4*	75.6	83.4	102.5	138.3	188.5	296.1	476.7	823.6	1574.7	4736.5
1965	208.1*	81.2*	146.5*	46.0	54.2	72.0	95.3	143.6	235.2	379.3	652.8	1173.0	3328.8
1975	147.7*	50.5*	107.1*	25.3	34.8	49.0	71.8	106.7	169.9	292.2	506.8	908.5	2375.6
1985	113.7*	31.2*	76.7*	15.8	21.5	32.9	49.8	77.3	127.7	212.0	388.0	728.9	2130.9
1990	**108.1***	**27.6***	**70.3***	**17.5**	**20.3**	**29.4**	**42.5**	**68.8**	**114.9**	**199.1**	**354.2**	**693.6**	**2158.7**
1995 projected	*103.3**	*24.7**	*64.2**	*17.9*	*19.7*	*25.7*	*37.4*	*62.0*	*105.0*	*181.8*	*330.9*	*667.0*	*2175.4*
All non-medical causes													
1955	37.2*	15.6*	33.2*	17.0	19.9	24.6	31.9	36.1	43.6	59.7	96.6	185.0	467.2
1965	41.5*	16.5*	35.7*	19.4	21.8	26.7	32.5	38.6	46.5	64.3	107.0	202.4	582.2
1975	41.5*	17.9*	35.9*	21.5	23.3	27.1	34.8	38.5	46.0	59.9	96.4	186.0	568.7
1985	31.6*	13.9*	30.2*	19.3	22.0	23.7	27.7	32.7	37.6	48.6	71.6	121.6	387.0
1990	**29.1***	**13.6***	**27.4***	**17.8**	**20.4**	**23.6**	**26.0**	**29.4**	**33.0**	**41.4**	**61.4**	**110.0**	**351.9**
1995 projected	*26.8**	*13.2**	*24.7**	*16.5*	*19.1*	*22.4*	*24.5*	*26.6*	*28.4*	*35.4*	*55.1*	*94.2*	*322.7*

PLANNED EU (16 countries): 1975

Smoking–attributed deaths (Sm.) and total deaths (Total)

		ALL CAUSES	ALL CANCER	Lung cancer	Upper aero–digestive ca.	Other cancer	COPD	Other respiratory	Vascular disease	Liver cirrhosis	Other medical	Non–medical
Males												
0–34	Sm.	–	–	–	–	–	–	–	–	–	–	–
	Total	136554	9559	339	194	9026	1477	6971	6088	1118	59940	51401
35–69	Sm.	245970	94813	62075	13697	19041	29381	4922	88708	–	28146	–
	Total	777070	210285	66940	22234	121111	38142	17609	309474	37701	101342	62517
		(32%)	(45%)	(93%)	(62%)	(16%)	(77%)	(28%)	(29%)		(28%)	
70+	Sm.	201433	65084	41753	7217	16114	49537	6714	64285	–	15813	–
	Total	1055731	194882	46144	13624	135114	70735	56063	542087	13941	147845	30178
		(19%)	(33%)	(90%)	(53%)	(12%)	(70%)	(12%)	(12%)		(11%)	
Any age	Sm.	447403	159897	103828	20914	35155	78918	11636	152993	–	43959	–
	Total	1969355	414726	113423	36052	265251	110354	80643	857649	52760	309127	144096
		(23%)	(39%)	(92%)	(58%)	(13%)	(72%)	(14%)	(18%)		(14%)	
Females												
0–34	Sm.	–	–	–	–	–	–	–	–	–	–	–
	Total	78844	7463	144	78	7241	1056	5347	3924	600	44494	15960
35–69	Sm.	23316	6864	5146	631	1087	3242	826	9383	–	3001	–
	Total	463382	160176	11303	3315	145558	12179	11054	165359	14738	74321	25555
		(5%)	(4%)	(46%)	(19%)	(1%)	(27%)	(7%)	(6%)		(4%)	
70+	Sm.	26384	5063	3499	752	812	6962	1433	10812	–	2114	–
	Total	1328647	177918	9469	5058	163391	38869	74930	765231	9129	214843	47727
		(2%)	(3%)	(37%)	(15%)	(0%)	(18%)	(2%)	(1%)		(1%)	
Any age	Sm.	49700	11927	8645	1383	1899	10204	2259	20195	–	5115	–
	Total	1870873	345557	20916	8451	316190	52104	91331	934514	24467	333658	89242
		(3%)	(3%)	(41%)	(16%)	(1%)	(20%)	(2%)	(2%)		(2%)	
Males+Females												
0–34	Sm.	–	–	–	–	–	–	–	–	–	–	–
	Total	215398	17022	483	272	16267	2533	12318	10012	1718	104434	67361
35–69	Sm.	269286	101677	67221	14328	20128	32623	5748	98091	–	31147	–
	Total	1240452	370461	78243	25549	266669	50321	28663	474833	52439	175663	88072
		(22%)	(27%)	(86%)	(56%)	(8%)	(65%)	(20%)	(21%)		(18%)	
70+	Sm.	227817	70147	45252	7969	16926	56499	8147	75097	–	17927	–
	Total	2384378	372800	55613	18682	298505	109604	130993	1307318	23070	362688	77905
		(10%)	(19%)	(81%)	(43%)	(6%)	(52%)	(6%)	(6%)		(5%)	
Any age	Sm.	497103	171824	112473	22297	37054	89122	13895	173188	–	49074	–
	Total	3840228	760283	134339	44503	581441	162458	171974	1792163	77227	642785	233338
		(13%)	(23%)	(84%)	(50%)	(6%)	(55%)	(8%)	(10%)		(8%)	

PLANNED EU (16 countries): 1985

Smoking–attributed deaths (Sm.) and total deaths (Total)

		ALL CAUSES	ALL CANCER	Lung cancer	Upper aero–digestive ca.	Other cancer	COPD	Other respiratory	Vascular disease	Liver cirrhosis	Other medical	Non–medical
Males												
0–34	Sm.	–	–	–	–	–	–	–	–	–	–	–
	Total	97275	7709	301	197	7211	677	2337	5622	981	35654	44295
35–69	Sm.	224197	103276	66246	17191	19839	17832	4116	75553	–	23420	–
	Total	663013	215752	71134	26115	118503	22675	13916	248752	32334	75384	54200
		(34%)	(48%)	(93%)	(66%)	(17%)	(79%)	(30%)	(30%)		(31%)	
70+	Sm.	242007	91568	59533	8820	23215	51664	7006	73422	–	18347	–
	Total	1161414	254561	65185	15076	174300	69948	58227	581096	13700	152998	30884
		(21%)	(36%)	(91%)	(59%)	(13%)	(74%)	(12%)	(13%)		(12%)	
Any age	Sm.	466204	194844	125779	26011	43054	69496	11122	148975	–	41767	–
	Total	1921702	478022	136620	41388	300014	93300	74480	835470	47015	264036	129379
		(24%)	(41%)	(92%)	(63%)	(14%)	(74%)	(15%)	(18%)		(16%)	
Females												
0–34	Sm.	–	–	–	–	–	–	–	–	–	–	–
	Total	49758	6368	154	81	6133	563	1592	3193	476	24796	12770
35–69	Sm.	29655	10501	7966	947	1588	4226	588	10624	–	3716	–
	Total	366152	149743	14004	3650	132089	9577	6560	113671	13200	51630	21771
		(8%)	(7%)	(57%)	(26%)	(1%)	(44%)	(9%)	(9%)		(7%)	
70+	Sm.	51350	11774	8266	1487	2021	11296	2242	20687	–	5351	–
	Total	1479004	229456	16044	5955	207457	35040	74853	843073	9578	243451	43553
		(3%)	(5%)	(52%)	(25%)	(1%)	(32%)	(3%)	(2%)		(2%)	
Any age	Sm.	81005	22275	16232	2434	3609	15522	2830	31311	–	9067	–
	Total	1894914	385567	30202	9686	345679	45180	83005	959937	23254	319877	78094
		(4%)	(6%)	(54%)	(25%)	(1%)	(34%)	(3%)	(3%)		(3%)	
Males+Females												
0–34	Sm.	–	–	–	–	–	–	–	–	–	–	–
	Total	147033	14077	455	278	13344	1240	3929	8815	1457	60450	57065
35–69	Sm.	253852	113777	74212	18138	21427	22058	4704	86177	–	27136	–
	Total	1029165	365495	85138	29765	250592	32252	20476	362423	45534	127014	75971
		(25%)	(31%)	(87%)	(61%)	(9%)	(68%)	(23%)	(24%)		(21%)	
70+	Sm.	293357	103342	67799	10307	25236	62960	9248	94109	–	23698	–
	Total	2640418	484017	81229	21031	381757	104988	133080	1424169	23278	396449	74437
		(11%)	(21%)	(83%)	(49%)	(7%)	(60%)	(7%)	(7%)		(6%)	
Any age	Sm.	547209	217119	142011	28445	46663	85018	13952	180286	–	50834	–
	Total	3816616	863589	166822	51074	645693	138480	157485	1795407	70269	583913	207473
		(14%)	(25%)	(85%)	(56%)	(7%)	(61%)	(9%)	(10%)		(9%)	

(To be conservative, no deaths before age 35, and none from liver cirrhosis or non–medical causes, were attributed to smoking.)

PLANNED EU (16 countries): 1990

Smoking–attributed deaths (Sm.) and total deaths (Total)

		ALL CAUSES	ALL CANCER	Lung cancer	Upper aero–digestive ca.	Other cancer	COPD	Other respiratory	Vascular disease	Liver cirrhosis	Other medical	Non–medical
Males												
0–34	Sm.	–	–	–	–	–	–	–	–	–	–	–
	Total	97892	6766	267	186	6313	565	1991	5211	966	36732	45661
35–69	Sm.	221656	110819	70929	18591	21299	16659	3849	65266	–	25063	–
	Total	673250	237194	76427	28456	132311	21378	13675	230196	30398	83900	56509
		(33%)	(47%)	(93%)	(65%)	(16%)	(78%)	(28%)	(28%)		(30%)	
70+	Sm.	222830	89095	57385	8430	23280	49245	6353	60625	–	17512	–
	Total	1112375	261182	63145	14491	183546	67559	57529	526772	11174	157048	31111
		(20%)	(34%)	(91%)	(58%)	(13%)	(73%)	(11%)	(12%)		(11%)	
Any age	Sm.	444486	199914	128314	27021	44579	65904	10202	125891	–	42575	–
	Total	1883517	505142	139839	43133	322170	89502	73195	762179	42538	277680	133281
		(24%)	(40%)	(92%)	(63%)	(14%)	(74%)	(14%)	(17%)		(15%)	
Females												
0–34	Sm.	–	–	–	–	–	–	–	–	–	–	–
	Total	45171	5763	142	60	5561	389	1191	2818	446	22079	12485
35–69	Sm.	33292	12813	9851	1111	1851	4594	649	10831	–	4405	–
	Total	364302	158984	16426	3974	138584	9455	6441	103418	12945	52025	21034
		(9%)	(8%)	(60%)	(28%)	(1%)	(49%)	(10%)	(10%)		(8%)	
70+	Sm.	62089	14999	10451	1889	2659	13576	2786	23687	–	7041	–
	Total	1481573	239884	18263	6399	215222	37476	79084	805524	9097	266955	43553
		(4%)	(6%)	(57%)	(30%)	(1%)	(36%)	(4%)	(3%)		(3%)	
Any age	Sm.	95381	27812	20302	3000	4510	18170	3435	34518	–	11446	–
	Total	1891046	404631	34831	10433	359367	47320	86716	911760	22488	341059	77072
		(5%)	(7%)	(58%)	(29%)	(1%)	(38%)	(4%)	(4%)		(3%)	
Males+Females												
0–34	Sm.	–	–	–	–	–	–	–	–	–	–	–
	Total	143063	12529	409	246	11874	954	3182	8029	1412	58811	58146
35–69	Sm.	254948	123632	80780	19702	23150	21253	4498	76097	–	29468	–
	Total	1037552	396178	92853	32430	270895	30833	20116	333614	43343	135925	77543
		(25%)	(31%)	(87%)	(61%)	(9%)	(69%)	(22%)	(23%)		(22%)	
70+	Sm.	284919	104094	67836	10319	25939	62821	9139	84312	–	24553	–
	Total	2593948	501066	81408	20890	398768	105035	136613	1332296	20271	424003	74664
		(11%)	(21%)	(83%)	(49%)	(7%)	(60%)	(7%)	(6%)		(6%)	
Any age	Sm.	539867	227726	148616	30021	49089	84074	13637	160409	–	54021	–
	Total	3774563	909773	174670	53566	681537	136822	159911	1673939	65026	618739	210353
		(14%)	(25%)	(85%)	(56%)	(7%)	(61%)	(9%)	(10%)		(9%)	

PLANNED EU (16 countries): 1995

Smoking–attributed deaths (Sm.) and total deaths (Total)

		ALL CAUSES	ALL CANCER	Lung cancer	Upper aero–digestive ca.	Other cancer	COPD	Other respiratory	Vascular disease	Liver cirrhosis	Other medical	Non–medical
Males												
0–34	Sm.	–	–	–	–	–	–	–	–	–	–	–
	Total	99761	6032	299	184	5549	511	2046	4954	1082	38636	46500
35–69	Sm.	203133	108887	69589	18819	20479	14356	3401	51572	–	24917	–
	Total	629029	237041	75277	29210	132554	18629	12548	191830	27061	85910	56010
		(32%)	(46%)	(92%)	(64%)	(15%)	(77%)	(27%)	(27%)		(29%)	
70+	Sm.	208516	89333	57593	8420	23320	45402	5569	51271	–	16941	–
	Total	1018385	265924	63537	14467	187920	62522	51288	448446	9847	150452	29906
		(20%)	(34%)	(91%)	(58%)	(12%)	(73%)	(11%)	(11%)		(11%)	
Any age	Sm.	411649	198220	127182	27239	43799	59758	8970	102843	–	41858	–
	Total	1747175	508997	139113	43861	326023	81662	65882	645230	37990	274998	132416
		(24%)	(39%)	(91%)	(62%)	(13%)	(73%)	(14%)	(16%)		(15%)	
Females												
0–34	Sm.	–	–	–	–	–	–	–	–	–	–	–
	Total	41491	5215	141	52	5022	325	1049	2533	460	20170	11739
35–69	Sm.	34120	14510	11248	1258	2004	4548	636	9717	–	4709	–
	Total	327771	153264	17815	4115	131334	8661	5773	81382	12053	47311	19327
		(10%)	(9%)	(63%)	(31%)	(2%)	(53%)	(11%)	(12%)		(10%)	
70+	Sm.	69270	18297	12908	2199	3190	14943	2939	24577	–	8514	–
	Total	1343664	239760	20867	6602	212291	37261	72788	682705	8714	263125	39311
		(5%)	(8%)	(62%)	(33%)	(2%)	(40%)	(4%)	(4%)		(3%)	
Any age	Sm.	103390	32807	24156	3457	5194	19491	3575	34294	–	13223	–
	Total	1712926	398239	38823	10769	348647	46247	79610	766620	21227	330606	70377
		(6%)	(8%)	(62%)	(32%)	(1%)	(42%)	(4%)	(4%)		(4%)	
Males+Females												
0–34	Sm.	–	–	–	–	–	–	–	–	–	–	–
	Total	141252	11247	440	236	10571	836	3095	7487	1542	58806	58239
35–69	Sm.	237253	123397	80837	20077	22483	18904	4037	61289	–	29626	–
	Total	956800	390305	93092	33325	263888	27290	18321	273212	39114	133221	75337
		(25%)	(32%)	(87%)	(60%)	(9%)	(69%)	(22%)	(22%)		(22%)	
70+	Sm.	277786	107630	70501	10619	26510	60345	8508	75848	–	25455	–
	Total	2362049	505684	84404	21069	400211	99783	124076	1131151	18561	413577	69217
		(12%)	(21%)	(84%)	(50%)	(7%)	(60%)	(7%)	(7%)		(6%)	
Any age	Sm.	515039	231027	151338	30696	48993	79249	12545	137137	–	55081	–
	Total	3460101	907236	177936	54630	674670	127909	145492	1411850	59217	605604	202793
		(15%)	(25%)	(85%)	(56%)	(7%)	(62%)	(9%)	(10%)		(9%)	

(To be conservative, no deaths before age 35, and none from liver cirrhosis or non–medical causes, were attributed to smoking.)

¶ARMENIA: 1990

Cause	Sex	No. of deaths: All ages	No. of deaths: 0–34	No. of deaths: 35–69	Standardised rates (Defined on p.262): All ages	Standardised rates: 0–34	Standardised rates: 35–69	Annual death rates / 100, 000: 0–4	5–9	10–14	15–19	20–24	25–29	30–34
ALL CAUSES	M	11914	2078	5947	1298.2	178.0	1531.9	572.3	49.9	42.0	72.7	123.8	162.8	222.4
	F	10079	1266	3455	814.2	108.3	765.0	460.8	28.7	18.6	43.7	48.5	56.6	101.0
Tuberculosis	M	85	13	67	7.7	1.2	15.3	0.5	–	–	–	0.8	1.9	5.4
	F	12	1	9	1.0	0.1	2.0	–	–	–	–	0.7	–	–
Other infective and parasitic	M	206	194	10	9.6	14.8	2.4	101.6	1.1	–	–	–	–	0.7
	F	159	150	6	7.6	12.1	1.3	78.9	2.4	–	0.8	1.5	–	1.3
ALL CANCER	M	1967	103	1505	209.0	9.6	381.8	5.9	5.1	2.0	5.8	9.0	13.4	26.3
	F	1517	103	1077	123.8	9.6	225.6	3.4	3.6	2.1	5.7	7.5	10.3	35.0
Mouth and pharynx cancer	M	36	2	28	3.8	0.2	7.2	–	–	–	–	1.5	–	–
	F	7	1	4	0.6	0.1	1.2	–	0.6	–	–	–	–	–
Oesophagus cancer	M	38	–	29	4.2	–	6.1	–	–	–	–	–	–	–
	F	26	1	11	2.4	0.1	2.5	–	–	–	–	–	–	0.6
Stomach cancer	M	299	9	218	33.7	0.9	56.1	–	–	–	–	0.8	0.6	4.7
	F	203	7	134	17.0	0.6	29.1	–	–	–	–	–	1.8	2.6
Colorectal cancer	M	131	6	93	14.6	0.6	23.5	–	–	–	–	0.8	0.6	2.7
	F	136	5	87	11.4	0.5	19.9	–	–	–	–	–	–	3.2
Liver cancer	M	...	...	...	...	...	...	...	...	...	...	...	...	...
	F	...	...	...	...	...	...	...	...	...	...	...	...	...
Pancreas cancer	M	...	...	...	...	...	...	...	...	...	...	...	...	...
	F	...	...	...	...	...	...	...	...	...	...	...	...	...
Larynx cancer	M	86	–	73	9.0	–	17.4	–	–	–	–	–	–	–
	F	6	–	4	0.6	–	0.8	–	–	–	–	–	–	–
Lung cancer	M	658	6	562	68.8	0.6	141.3	–	–	–	0.7	1.5	1.3	0.7
	F	115	9	82	9.6	0.9	17.8	–	–	–	–	2.2	1.2	2.6
Malignant melanoma	M	...	...	...	...	...	...	...	...	...	...	...	...	...
	F	...	...	...	...	...	...	...	...	...	...	...	...	...
Female breast cancer	F	312	13	253	26.1	1.2	51.5	–	–	–	–	–	0.6	7.8
Cervix cancer	F	92	7	76	7.2	0.6	13.8	–	–	–	–	–	–	4.5
Other uterine cancer	F	82	3	64	6.8	0.3	13.6	–	–	–	–	–	0.6	1.3
Ovarian cancer	F	...	...	...	...	...	...	...	...	...	...	...	...	...
Prostate cancer	M	40	1	22	4.5	0.1	5.2	0.5	–	–	–	–	–	–
Bladder cancer	M	...	...	...	...	...	...	...	...	...	...	...	...	...
	F	...	...	...	...	...	...	...	...	...	...	...	...	...
Other and ill-defined cancer sites	M	538	33	392	59.0	3.1	104.8	1.6	1.1	0.7	3.6	1.5	5.1	8.1
	F	437	24	302	35.1	2.3	62.6	–	–	–	4.0	2.2	3.6	6.5
Hodgkin's disease	M	...	...	...	...	...	...	...	...	...	...	...	...	...
	F	...	...	...	...	...	...	...	...	...	...	...	...	...
Myeloma and all lymphomas	M	81	22	56	6.6	2.1	12.9	0.5	1.7	0.7	–	1.5	2.6	7.4
	F	37	9	23	2.5	0.8	4.1	0.6	0.6	–	–	1.5	1.2	1.9
Leukaemia	M	60	24	32	4.8	2.1	7.3	3.2	2.3	0.7	1.5	1.5	3.2	2.7
	F	64	24	37	4.5	2.2	8.8	2.8	2.4	2.1	1.6	1.5	1.2	3.9
ALL VASCULAR DISEASE	M	5229	89	2562	672.1	8.5	689.0	2.1	1.1	0.7	6.5	5.3	7.0	37.1
	F	5614	48	1434	484.2	4.6	338.4	2.8	–	0.7	7.3	6.0	7.9	7.8
Rheumatic heart disease and fever	M	90	12	76	7.6	1.2	16.4	–	–	0.7	1.5	2.3	1.3	2.7
	F	120	16	95	9.1	1.6	18.2	–	–	0.7	4.9	1.5	3.0	1.3
Hypertensive disease	M	–	–	–	–	–	–	–	–	–	–	–	–	–
	F	3	–	–	0.2	–	–	–	–	–	–	–	–	–
Ischaemic heart disease	M	3633	46	1839	463.2	4.4	484.9	–	–	–	–	2.3	3.2	25.6
	F	3495	16	747	302.2	1.5	180.7	0.6	–	–	–	1.5	3.6	4.5
Pulmonary embolism and other venous	M	...	...	...	...	...	...	...	...	...	...	...	...	...
	F	...	...	...	...	...	...	...	...	...	...	...	...	...
Cerebrovascular disease	M	1220	18	501	165.9	1.7	147.1	1.1	1.1	–	3.6	0.8	1.3	4.0
	F	1743	11	521	151.2	1.1	123.7	1.7	–	–	1.6	2.2	0.6	1.3
Other vascular disease, incl. venous	M	286	13	146	35.4	1.2	40.6	1.1	–	–	1.5	–	1.3	4.7
	F	253	5	71	21.4	0.5	15.8	0.6	–	–	0.8	0.7	0.6	0.6
Chronic obstructive pulmonary disease	M	733	8	322	99.4	0.8	94.2	–	–	1.3	0.7	0.8	1.9	0.7
	F	376	7	115	32.4	0.7	26.1	–	–	–	0.8	0.7	1.2	1.9
Other respiratory disease	M	362	297	38	20.8	22.8	9.5	151.1	2.3	2.0	0.7	0.8	1.3	1.3
	F	313	258	29	16.5	20.9	6.1	136.6	1.2	2.8	2.4	2.2	0.6	0.6
Peptic ulcer	M	103	7	71	11.4	0.7	18.7	–	–	–	–	–	1.9	2.7
	F	37	–	22	3.4	–	5.1	–	–	–	–	–	–	–
Liver cirrhosis and other liver disease	M	245	12	192	25.8	1.2	48.5	–	–	2.0	0.7	2.3	1.3	2.0
	F	139	7	74	11.5	0.7	15.6	–	–	–	0.8	–	1.8	1.9
Renal disease	M	163	23	100	17.1	2.3	24.5	0.5	–	1.3	0.7	7.5	4.5	1.3
	F	131	21	79	10.2	1.9	18.0	1.1	1.8	2.1	0.8	1.5	4.3	1.9
Pregnancy and birth	F	32	22	10	1.7	2.1	1.3	–	–	–	1.6	3.7	3.6	5.8
Congenital and perinatal causes	M	421	414	7	18.3	31.5	1.6	218.6	0.6	0.7	–	0.8	–	–
	F	298	295	3	13.5	23.6	0.5	164.6	–	–	0.8	–	–	–
Ill-defined causes	M	294	55	75	35.0	4.7	17.3	15.4	1.1	1.3	0.7	5.3	4.5	4.7
	F	358	43	42	28.7	3.7	9.1	17.9	0.6	–	0.8	3.7	0.6	1.9
Other medical causes	M	623	102	361	66.7	9.2	96.2	13.3	5.7	3.9	8.7	6.0	11.5	15.5
	F	604	89	357	47.8	8.2	77.8	10.6	7.8	1.4	6.5	7.5	6.7	16.8
ALL NON-MEDICAL CAUSES	M	1483	761	637	105.5	70.7	132.8	63.3	32.9	26.9	48.0	85.5	113.7	124.7
	F	489	222	198	32.1	20.0	38.1	44.8	11.4	9.7	15.4	13.4	19.5	25.9
Motor vehicle traffic accidents	M	475	245	206	34.1	23.2	45.2	6.4	13.0	8.5	13.1	27.8	44.1	49.2
	F	157	58	82	11.0	5.5	16.9	4.5	4.2	4.1	6.5	5.2	3.6	10.4
Fire	M	18	10	7	1.1	0.9	1.3	2.1	1.1	–	–	0.8	1.3	0.7
	F	18	6	7	1.2	0.5	1.2	1.7	–	–	–	1.5	0.6	–
Suicide	M	64	26	36	4.6	2.6	6.9	–	–	–	4.4	3.0	3.8	6.7
	F	29	7	19	2.2	0.7	3.4	–	–	–	0.8	1.5	1.2	1.3
Homicide	M	177	103	66	11.8	10.1	12.4	–	1.1	0.7	6.5	21.8	18.5	22.2
	F	26	13	12	1.6	1.2	1.9	–	–	–	–	1.5	3.6	3.2
POPULATION (thousands): M=males					1624.9	1092.4	492.8	188.0	176.4	152.2	137.5	133.3	156.6	148.4
F=females					1685.4	1067.0	546.3	178.6	167.2	144.8	123.7	133.9	164.4	154.4

ARMENIA: 1990

Annual death rates / 100, 000

9th ICD categories

35–39	40–44	45–49	50–54	55–59	60–64	65–69	70–74	75–79	80+/NK			
299.6	505.6	658.2	1002.2	1615.7	2598.5	4043.5	5700.8	8323.7	15328.2	M	ALL CAUSES	001–999
149.8	218.8	253.8	503.7	756.9	1289.8	2182.3	3384.0	5711.4	13239.5	F		
4.5	6.9	16.4	19.1	18.2	16.5	25.4	7.9	14.4	15.3	M	Tuberculosis	010–018, 137
0.8	–	–	3.1	2.6	–	7.2	4.2	–	4.2	F		
0.9	–	3.6	1.1	2.8	4.5	3.6	7.9	7.2	–	M	Other infective	Rest of 001–139
–	–	1.7	1.0	2.6	1.3	2.4	8.4	4.1	–	F	and parasitic	
45.7	87.5	160.0	268.8	469.8	709.8	931.2	992.1	1115.1	595.4	M	ALL CANCER	140–208
62.3	100.4	131.9	193.7	241.8	352.5	496.4	485.2	479.7	437.0	F		
0.9	1.4	5.5	6.7	7.0	10.5	18.1	15.7	21.6	7.6	M	Mouth and	140–149
–	–	–	1.0	–	–	7.2	4.2	–	4.2	F	pharynx cancer	
–	–	5.5	10.1	8.4	15.0	3.6	31.5	21.6	15.3	M	Oesophagus cancer	150
–	1.3	1.7	2.1	1.3	3.9	7.2	25.3	16.3	16.8	F		
5.4	15.3	23.6	33.7	74.3	99.2	141.3	196.9	251.8	91.6	M	Stomach cancer	151
5.1	6.4	5.0	24.1	26.3	57.4	79.1	101.3	65.0	92.4	F		
3.6	8.3	5.5	15.7	23.8	49.6	58.0	86.6	71.9	84.0	M	Colorectal cancer	153, 154
1.7	3.9	6.7	12.6	14.5	37.9	62.4	50.6	65.0	67.2	F		
...	...	...	...	...	...	...	...	...	...	M	Liver cancer	Not given separately
...	...	...	...	...	...	...	...	...	...	F		
...	...	...	...	...	...	...	...	...	...	M	Pancreas cancer	Not given separately
...	...	...	...	...	...	...	...	...	...	F		
2.7	2.8	1.8	16.9	26.6	34.6	36.2	55.1	7.2	38.2	M	Larynx cancer	161
–	–	1.7	–	–	3.9	–	8.4	–	–	F		
5.4	22.2	56.4	104.6	186.5	291.7	322.5	299.2	251.8	129.8	M	Lung cancer	162
3.4	6.4	10.0	13.6	21.0	24.8	45.6	46.4	20.3	33.6	F		
...	...	...	...	...	...	...	...	...	...	M	Malignant melanoma	Not given
...	...	...	...	...	...	...	...	...	...	F		separately
17.7	30.9	51.8	57.6	59.1	49.6	93.5	84.4	73.2	33.6	F	Female breast cancer	174
6.7	15.4	8.3	19.9	22.3	14.4	9.6	21.1	16.3	–	F	Cervix cancer	180
2.5	3.9	15.0	9.4	17.1	20.9	26.4	16.9	32.5	12.6	F	Other uterine cancer	179, 182
...	...	...	...	...	...	...	...	...	...	F	Ovarian cancer	Not given separately
–	–	1.8	2.2	8.4	16.5	7.2	7.9	71.9	45.8	M	Prostate cancer	185
...	...	...	...	...	...	...	...	...	...	M	Bladder cancer	Not given separately
...	...	...	...	...	...	...	...	...	...	F		
17.9	25.0	50.9	60.7	109.4	165.4	304.3	267.7	402.9	175.6	M	Other and ill-defined	Rest of 140–208,
16.8	28.3	26.7	48.2	68.3	120.1	129.5	109.7	182.9	168.1	F	cancer sites	incl. 155, 157, 172, 183, 188
...	...	...	...	...	...	...	...	...	...	M	Hodgkin's disease	Not given separately
...	...	...	...	...	...	...	...	...	...	F		
5.4	8.3	3.6	11.2	12.6	24.1	25.4	15.7	–	7.6	M	Myeloma and all	200–203,
5.9	1.3	–	2.1	5.3	9.1	4.8	8.4	4.1	8.4	F	lymphomas	incl. 201
4.5	4.2	5.5	6.7	12.6	3.0	14.5	15.7	14.4	–	M	Leukaemia	204–208
2.5	2.6	5.0	3.1	6.6	10.4	31.2	8.4	4.1	–	F		
73.5	162.5	238.2	418.4	711.1	1194.0	2025.4	3267.7	5129.5	11068.7	M	ALL VASCULAR	390–459
26.9	39.9	55.1	149.7	282.5	639.7	1175.1	2236.3	4280.5	10710.1	F	DISEASE	
4.5	9.7	10.9	19.1	22.4	30.1	18.1	–	–	15.3	M	Rheumatic heart	390–398
9.3	12.9	15.0	23.0	22.3	20.9	24.0	4.2	16.3	16.8	F	disease and fever	
–	–	–	–	–	–	–	–	–	–	M	Hypertensive disease	401–405
–	–	–	–	–	–	–	–	4.1	8.4	F		
53.8	119.4	189.1	325.1	533.0	822.6	1351.4	2173.2	3467.6	7557.3	M	Ischaemic heart	410–414
7.6	14.2	21.7	61.8	144.5	348.6	666.7	1354.4	2817.1	7218.5	F	disease	
...	...	...	...	...	...	...	...	...	...	M	Pulmonary embolism	Not given
...	...	...	...	...	...	...	...	...	...	F	and other venous	separately
8.1	26.4	29.1	59.6	113.6	267.7	525.4	937.0	1417.3	2938.9	M	Cerebrovascular	430–438
7.6	10.3	16.7	56.5	101.2	235.0	438.8	793.2	1296.7	2958.0	F	disease	
7.2	6.9	9.1	14.6	42.1	73.7	130.4	157.5	244.6	557.3	M	Other vascular	Rest of 390–459,
2.5	2.6	1.7	8.4	14.5	35.2	45.6	84.4	146.3	508.4	F	disease, incl. venous	incl. 415, 451–3
1.8	6.9	25.5	28.1	88.4	186.5	322.5	622.0	827.3	1595.4	M	Chronic obstructive	490–496
0.8	2.6	3.3	16.8	36.8	43.1	79.1	173.0	268.3	617.6	F	pulmonary disease	
4.5	1.4	9.1	10.1	5.6	10.5	25.4	47.2	71.9	84.0	M	Other respiratory	Rest of 460–519
0.8	1.3	5.0	1.0	11.8	13.1	9.6	33.8	20.3	54.6	F	disease	
5.4	4.2	12.7	6.7	21.0	30.1	50.7	47.2	71.9	68.7	M	Peptic ulcer	531–533
–	1.3	5.0	4.2	5.3	5.2	14.4	25.3	16.3	21.0	F		
7.2	20.8	27.3	39.4	57.5	67.7	119.6	78.7	122.3	106.9	M	Liver cirrhosis and	570–573, 576,
4.2	3.9	–	9.4	15.8	37.9	38.4	71.7	89.4	79.8	F	other liver disease	575.2–579.9
1.8	12.5	9.1	23.6	28.1	42.1	54.3	70.9	100.7	129.8	M	Renal disease	580–590
2.5	3.9	5.0	11.5	22.3	23.5	57.6	25.3	56.9	46.2	F		
7.6	1.3	–	–	–	–	–	–	–	–	F	Pregnancy and birth	630–676
0.9	4.2	–	1.1	1.4	–	3.6	–	–	–	M	Congenital and	740–779
–	1.3	–	2.1	–	–	–	–	–	–	F	perinatal causes	
8.1	5.6	10.9	16.9	11.2	36.1	32.6	102.4	230.2	908.4	M	Ill-defined causes	780–799
1.7	3.9	8.3	7.3	7.9	13.1	21.6	42.2	178.9	920.2	F		
17.9	37.5	47.3	55.1	68.7	171.4	275.4	315.0	424.5	465.6	M	Other medical causes	Rest of 001–799
11.8	27.0	18.4	60.7	92.0	124.0	211.0	215.2	215.4	226.9	F		
127.4	155.6	98.2	113.6	131.8	129.3	173.9	141.7	208.6	290.1	M	ALL NON–	E800–E999
30.3	32.2	20.0	42.9	35.5	36.6	69.5	63.3	101.6	121.8	F	MEDICAL CAUSES	
40.4	54.2	23.6	34.9	35.1	45.1	83.3	63.0	57.6	61.1	M	Motor vehicle	E810–E819
7.6	14.2	13.4	14.7	14.5	18.3	36.0	12.7	28.5	29.4	F	traffic accidents	
2.7	–	1.8	–	1.4	3.0	–	–	–	7.6	M	Fire	E890–E899
3.4	–	–	–	1.3	1.3	2.4	–	16.3	4.2	F		
7.2	15.3	3.6	4.5	8.4	6.0	3.6	–	14.4	–	M	Suicide	E950–E959
2.5	3.9	1.7	8.4	1.3	1.3	4.8	8.4	4.1	–	F		
22.4	13.9	18.2	9.0	9.8	6.0	7.2	–	7.2	53.4	M	Homicide	E960–E969
2.5	1.3	1.7	6.3	–	1.3	–	–	4.1	–	F		
111.5	72.0	55.0	88.9	71.3	66.5	27.6	12.7	13.9	13.1	M	POPULATION (thousands)	
118.8	77.7	59.9	95.5	76.1	76.6	41.7	23.7	24.6	23.8	F		

ARMENIA: Males

	All ages	0–34	35–69	35–39	40–44	45–49	50–54	55–59	60–64	65–69	70–74	75–79	80+/NK
POPULATION (1000s)													
1985–90	1606.2	1099.9	461.7	95.4	58.1	80.0	81.3	76.5	50.3	20.1	16.4	14.6	13.6
1985	1571.9	1090.6	432.6	77.4	58.7	95.2	77.2	74.6	33.0	16.5	20.3	14.9	13.5
1990	**1624.9**	**1092.4**	**492.8**	**111.5**	**72.0**	**55.0**	**88.9**	**71.3**	**66.5**	**27.6**	**12.7**	**13.9**	**13.1**
1995 projected	*1830.9*	*1231.0*	*555.2*	*125.6*	*81.1*	*62.0*	*100.2*	*80.3*	*74.9*	*31.1*	*14.3*	*15.7*	*14.7*
NUMBER OF DEATHS													
All causes													
1985–90	11601	2804	4934	304	265	492	798	1086	1250	739	802	1104	1957
1985	9977	2297	3931	199	189	550	684	990	781	538	925	1049	1775
1990	**11914**	**2078**	**5947**	**334**	**364**	**362**	**891**	**1152**	**1728**	**1116**	**724**	**1157**	**2008**
1995 projected	*15520*	*2259*	*8011*	*505*	*519*	*496*	*1178*	*1479*	*2311*	*1523*	*993*	*1639*	*2618*
Lung cancer													
1985–90	541	8	447	7	12	40	75	128	130	55	37	33	16
1985	452	10	358	5	13	45	70	101	85	39	48	27	9
1990	**658**	**6**	**562**	**6**	**16**	**31**	**93**	**133**	**194**	**89**	**38**	**35**	**17**
1995 projected	*926*	*6*	*780*	*7*	*20*	*40*	*130*	*179*	*279*	*125*	*58*	*55*	*27*
ANNUAL DEATH RATE / 100,000 (*The rates for the age groups 0–34 and 35–69 are the means of seven five-yearly rates, but the all-ages rates are standardised to the conventional "European" age distribution)													
All causes													
1985–90	1232.3*	237.5*	1421.8*	318.7	456.1	615.0	981.5	1419.6	2485.1	3676.6	4890.2	7561.6	14389.7
1985	1115.3*	195.2*	1285.3*	257.1	322.0	577.7	886.0	1327.1	2366.7	3260.6	4556.7	7040.3	13148.1
1990	**1298.2***	**178.0***	**1531.9***	**299.6**	**505.6**	**658.2**	**1002.2**	**1615.7**	**2598.5**	**4043.5**	**5700.8**	**8323.7**	**15328.2**
1995 projected	*1536.5**	*177.6**	*1834.6**	*402.1*	*640.0*	*800.0*	*1175.6*	*1841.8*	*3085.4*	*4897.1*	*6944.1*	*10439.5*	*17809.5*
All cancer													
1985–90	191.4*	9.4*	351.5*	39.8	75.7	137.5	258.3	415.7	668.0	865.7	823.2	958.9	705.9
1985	182.9*	10.4*	337.9*	34.9	68.1	143.9	251.3	379.4	693.9	793.9	763.5	859.1	674.1
1990	**209.0***	**9.6***	**381.8***	**45.7**	**87.5**	**160.0**	**268.8**	**469.8**	**709.8**	**931.2**	**992.1**	**1115.1**	**595.4**
1995 projected	*245.1**	*10.8**	*438.1**	*60.5*	*103.6*	*177.4*	*308.4*	*513.1*	*817.1*	*1086.8*	*1265.7*	*1401.3*	*659.9*
Lung cancer													
1985–90	59.8*	0.8*	124.2*	7.3	20.7	50.0	92.3	167.3	258.4	273.6	225.6	226.0	117.6
1985	54.6*	1.0*	113.7*	6.5	22.1	47.3	90.7	135.4	257.6	236.4	236.5	181.2	66.7
1990	**68.8***	**0.6***	**141.3***	**5.4**	**22.2**	**56.4**	**104.6**	**186.5**	**291.7**	**322.5**	**299.2**	**251.8**	**129.8**
1995 projected	*86.9**	*0.5**	*174.5**	*5.6*	*24.7*	*64.5*	*129.7*	*222.9*	*372.5*	*401.9*	*405.6*	*350.3*	*183.7*
Upper aerodigestive cancer (mouth, oesophagus, pharynx and larynx)													
1985–90	16.1*	0.2*	30.2*	3.1	3.4	12.5	25.8	39.2	57.7	69.7	73.2	68.5	66.2
1985	14.3*	0.2*	26.8*	1.3	–	10.5	20.7	40.2	60.6	54.5	59.1	73.8	51.9
1990	**17.1***	**0.2***	**30.6***	**3.6**	**4.2**	**12.7**	**33.7**	**42.1**	**60.2**	**58.0**	**102.4**	**50.4**	**61.1**
1995 projected	*20.1**	*0.4**	*36.3**	*5.6*	*6.2*	*17.7*	*40.9*	*47.3*	*62.8*	*74.0*	*118.9*	*70.1*	*54.4*
Other cancer													
1985–90	115.4*	8.4*	197.1*	29.4	51.6	75.0	140.2	209.2	351.9	522.4	524.4	664.4	522.1
1985	113.9*	9.3*	197.4*	27.1	46.0	86.1	139.9	203.8	375.8	503.0	468.0	604.0	555.6
1990	**123.2***	**8.8***	**209.9***	**36.8**	**61.1**	**90.9**	**130.5**	**241.2**	**357.9**	**550.7**	**590.6**	**812.9**	**404.6**
1995 projected	*138.1**	*9.9**	*227.2**	*49.4*	*72.7*	*95.2*	*137.7*	*242.8*	*381.8*	*610.9*	*741.3*	*980.9*	*421.8*
Chronic obstructive pulmonary disease (COPD)													
1985–90	97.5*	0.9*	97.5*	3.1	6.9	20.0	46.7	79.7	192.8	333.3	554.9	869.9	1492.6
1985	100.6*	1.9*	105.1*	2.6	10.2	21.0	71.2	76.4	197.0	357.6	576.4	838.9	1474.1
1990	**99.4***	**0.8***	**94.2***	**1.8**	**6.9**	**25.5**	**28.1**	**88.4**	**186.5**	**322.5**	**622.0**	**827.3**	**1595.4**
1995 projected	*100.2**	*0.7**	*89.4**	*1.6*	*7.4*	*17.7*	*23.0*	*77.2*	*177.6*	*321.5*	*629.4*	*885.4*	*1673.5*
Other respiratory disease													
1985–90	27.0*	33.6*	10.0*	4.2	5.2	6.3	8.6	5.2	15.9	24.9	36.6	61.6	110.3
1985	36.3*	48.5*	11.3*	2.6	5.1	4.2	11.7	4.0	15.2	36.4	44.3	33.6	170.4
1990	**20.8***	**22.8***	**9.5***	**4.5**	**1.4**	**9.1**	**10.1**	**5.6**	**10.5**	**25.4**	**47.2**	**71.9**	**84.0**
1995 projected	*15.7**	*14.1**	*8.9**	*4.0*	*1.2*	*9.7*	*12.0*	*5.0*	*8.0*	*22.5*	*62.9*	*57.3*	*68.0*
Vascular disease													
1985–90	606.1*	9.3*	611.0*	65.0	130.8	220.0	367.8	575.2	1107.4	1810.9	2786.6	4678.1	10360.3
1985	566.5*	8.6*	567.9*	73.6	92.0	209.0	314.8	561.7	1081.8	1642.4	2581.3	4570.5	9585.2
1990	**672.1***	**8.5***	**689.0***	**73.5**	**162.5**	**238.2**	**418.4**	**711.1**	**1194.0**	**2025.4**	**3267.7**	**5129.5**	**11068.7**
1995 projected	*806.0**	*8.4**	*841.7**	*107.5*	*208.4*	*317.7*	*515.0*	*838.1*	*1432.6*	*2472.7*	*3916.1*	*6490.4*	*12666.7*
Liver cirrhosis and other liver disease													
1985–90	22.0*	0.9*	36.8*	5.2	10.3	20.0	29.5	44.4	63.6	84.6	85.4	109.6	147.1
1985	23.9*	1.2*	38.2*	11.6	11.9	22.1	28.5	50.9	51.5	90.9	88.7	147.7	163.0
1990	**25.8***	**1.2***	**48.5***	**7.2**	**20.8**	**27.3**	**39.4**	**57.5**	**67.7**	**119.6**	**78.7**	**122.3**	**106.9**
1995 projected	*28.7**	*1.2**	*59.3**	*8.0*	*25.9*	*38.7*	*46.9*	*72.2*	*85.4*	*138.3*	*76.9*	*89.2*	*74.8*
Other medical causes													
1985–90	143.4*	70.3*	152.5*	51.4	58.5	73.8	116.9	147.7	256.5	363.2	426.8	609.6	1147.1
1985	142.6*	79.7*	152.1*	62.0	63.0	91.4	139.9	168.9	266.7	272.7	403.9	516.8	903.7
1990	**165.7***	**64.4***	**176.0***	**39.5**	**70.8**	**100.0**	**123.7**	**151.5**	**300.8**	**445.7**	**551.2**	**848.9**	**1587.8**
1995 projected	*195.4**	*50.5**	*208.6**	*32.6*	*70.3*	*100.0*	*113.8*	*150.7*	*381.8*	*610.9*	*790.2*	*1216.6*	*2251.7*
All non-medical causes													
1985–90	144.9*	113.1*	162.3*	149.9	168.7	137.5	153.8	151.6	180.9	194.0	176.8	274.0	426.5
1985	62.4*	44.9*	72.7*	69.8	71.6	86.1	68.7	85.8	60.6	66.7	98.5	73.8	177.8
1990	**105.5***	**70.7***	**132.8***	**127.4**	**155.6**	**98.2**	**113.6**	**131.8**	**129.3**	**173.9**	**141.7**	**208.6**	**290.1**
1995 projected	*145.3**	*91.8**	*188.5**	*187.9*	*223.2*	*138.7*	*156.7*	*185.6*	*182.9*	*244.4*	*202.8*	*299.4*	*415.0*

ARMENIA: Females

	All ages	0–34	35–69	35–39	40–44	45–49	50–54	55–59	60–64	65–69	70–74	75–79	80+/NK
POPULATION (1000s)													
1985–90	1673.9	1082.9	514.2	101.7	62.5	86.1	85.9	82.0	63.3	32.7	28.6	24.5	23.7
1985	1643.6	1077.3	484.9	82.2	63.5	100.7	80.0	82.0	47.7	28.8	33.9	24.4	23.1
1990	1685.4	1067.0	546.3	118.8	77.7	59.9	95.5	76.1	76.6	41.7	23.7	24.6	23.8
1995 projected	1899.1	1202.3	615.6	133.9	87.6	67.5	107.6	85.7	86.3	47.0	26.7	27.7	26.8
NUMBER OF DEATHS													
All causes													
1985–90	11287	2553	3369	238	191	294	474	645	848	679	933	1463	2969
1985	9604	1858	2467	99	126	280	325	528	603	506	1006	1428	2845
1990	10079	1266	3455	178	170	152	481	576	988	910	802	1405	3151
1995 projected	12016	1173	4420	238	201	190	618	715	1285	1173	962	1692	3769
Lung cancer													
1985–90	101	4	68	3	3	8	12	13	16	13	14	9	6
1985	92	3	63	6	2	10	16	15	6	8	15	6	5
1990	115	9	82	4	5	6	13	16	19	19	11	5	8
1995 projected	152	12	109	5	5	6	13	21	30	29	14	6	11
ANNUAL DEATH RATE / 100,000													
All causes													
1985–90	881.2*	222.1*	805.1*	234.0	305.6	341.5	551.8	786.6	1339.7	2076.5	3262.2	5971.4	12527.4
1985	780.0*	158.4*	666.9*	120.4	198.4	278.1	406.3	643.9	1264.2	1756.9	2967.6	5852.5	12316.0
1990	814.2*	108.3*	765.0*	149.8	218.8	253.8	503.7	756.9	1289.8	2182.3	3384.0	5711.4	13239.5
1995 projected	871.9*	90.5*	868.9*	177.7	229.5	281.5	574.3	834.3	1489.0	2495.7	3603.0	6108.3	14063.4
All cancer													
1985–90	110.8*	9.3*	198.0*	45.2	75.2	115.0	175.8	220.7	341.2	412.8	430.1	477.6	405.1
1985	106.3*	9.5*	181.9*	45.0	77.2	128.1	163.8	191.5	320.8	347.2	392.3	500.0	467.5
1990	123.8*	9.6*	225.6*	62.3	100.4	131.9	193.7	241.8	352.5	496.4	485.2	479.7	437.0
1995 projected	142.8*	10.6*	270.1*	84.4	114.2	151.1	226.8	280.0	434.5	600.0	561.8	469.3	421.6
Lung cancer													
1985–90	8.9*	0.4*	16.0*	2.9	4.8	9.3	14.0	15.9	25.3	39.8	49.0	36.7	25.3
1985	8.1*	0.3*	14.1*	7.3	3.1	9.9	20.0	18.3	12.6	27.8	44.2	24.6	21.6
1990	9.6*	0.9*	17.8*	3.4	6.4	10.0	13.6	21.0	24.8	45.6	46.4	20.3	33.6
1995 projected	11.1*	1.0*	21.6*	3.7	5.7	8.9	12.1	24.5	34.8	61.7	52.4	21.7	41.0
Upper aerodigestive cancer (mouth, oesophagus, pharynx and larynx)													
1985–90	3.4*	0.1*	4.7*	1.0	1.6	1.2	3.5	3.7	9.5	12.2	21.0	24.5	25.3
1985	2.6*	0.1*	2.5*	–	1.6	1.0	5.0	1.2	2.1	6.9	11.8	20.5	39.0
1990	3.6*	0.2*	4.5*	–	1.3	3.3	3.1	1.3	7.8	14.4	38.0	16.3	21.0
1995 projected	4.3*	0.1*	5.8*	–	2.3	3.0	3.7	2.3	10.4	19.1	52.4	14.4	14.9
Other cancer													
1985–90	98.5*	8.8*	177.4*	41.3	68.8	104.5	158.3	201.2	306.5	360.9	360.1	416.3	354.4
1985	95.6*	9.2*	165.2*	37.7	72.4	117.2	138.8	172.0	306.1	312.5	336.3	454.9	406.9
1990	110.7*	8.6*	203.3*	58.9	92.7	118.5	177.0	219.4	319.8	436.5	400.8	443.1	382.4
1995 projected	127.4*	9.5*	242.7*	80.7	106.2	139.3	211.0	253.2	389.3	519.1	456.9	433.2	365.7
Chronic obstructive pulmonary disease (COPD)													
1985–90	42.5*	0.7*	30.3*	2.0	4.8	5.8	14.0	28.0	50.6	107.0	202.8	424.5	860.8
1985	45.4*	0.9*	37.4*	3.6	6.3	5.0	16.3	25.6	73.4	131.9	174.0	442.6	909.1
1990	32.4*	0.7*	26.1*	0.8	2.6	3.3	16.8	36.8	43.1	79.1	173.0	268.3	617.6
1995 projected	23.9*	0.6*	20.9*	0.7	2.3	3.0	20.4	30.3	30.1	59.6	119.9	187.7	436.6
Other respiratory disease													
1985–90	24.5*	35.6*	5.6*	1.0	1.6	2.3	2.3	7.3	12.6	12.2	28.0	32.7	59.1
1985	35.2*	53.5*	6.0*	1.2	3.1	–	3.8	9.8	10.5	13.9	32.4	36.9	82.3
1990	16.5*	20.9*	6.1*	0.8	1.3	5.0	1.0	11.8	13.1	9.6	33.8	20.3	54.6
1995 projected	12.1*	13.8*	6.3*	0.7	2.3	5.9	0.9	12.8	12.7	8.5	26.2	18.1	41.0
Vascular disease													
1985–90	462.5*	5.3*	321.6*	22.6	46.4	66.2	147.8	284.1	595.6	1088.7	2087.4	4342.9	10012.7
1985	454.7*	6.8*	310.6*	20.7	56.7	67.5	121.3	264.6	643.6	1000.0	2005.9	4307.4	9917.7
1990	484.2*	4.6*	338.4*	26.9	39.9	55.1	149.7	282.5	639.7	1175.1	2236.3	4280.5	10710.1
1995 projected	511.6*	4.5*	361.4*	20.9	32.0	54.8	158.9	291.7	692.9	1278.7	2314.6	4610.1	11287.3
Liver cirrhosis and other liver disease													
1985–90	11.0*	0.6*	14.4*	2.0	1.6	3.5	8.1	15.9	30.0	39.8	52.4	81.6	122.4
1985	12.3*	0.9*	13.3*	2.4	1.6	3.0	5.0	23.2	23.1	34.7	59.0	102.5	164.5
1990	11.5*	0.7*	15.6*	4.2	3.9	–	9.4	15.8	37.9	38.4	71.7	89.4	79.8
1995 projected	11.6*	0.8*	18.0*	6.0	4.6	–	7.4	18.7	42.9	46.8	71.2	72.2	59.7
Other medical causes													
1985–90	98.4*	56.0*	102.3*	25.6	38.4	47.6	76.8	106.1	167.5	253.8	262.2	375.5	725.7
1985	95.9*	63.5*	91.3*	30.4	34.6	58.6	73.8	101.2	153.0	187.5	253.7	368.9	571.4
1990	113.8*	51.8*	115.1*	24.4	38.6	38.4	90.1	132.7	167.1	314.1	320.7	471.5	1218.5
1995 projected	133.0*	39.6*	141.8*	23.2	30.8	38.5	99.4	156.4	229.4	414.9	430.7	664.3	1723.9
All non-medical causes													
1985–90	131.5*	114.6*	132.8*	135.7	137.6	101.0	126.9	124.4	142.2	162.1	199.3	236.7	341.8
1985	30.2*	23.3*	26.3*	17.0	18.9	15.9	22.5	28.0	39.8	41.7	50.1	94.3	203.5
1990	32.1*	20.0*	38.1*	30.3	32.2	20.0	42.9	35.5	36.6	69.5	63.3	101.6	121.8
1995 projected	37.0*	20.6*	50.2*	41.8	43.4	28.1	60.4	44.3	46.3	87.2	78.7	86.6	93.3

(*The rates for the age groups 0–34 and 35–69 are the means of seven five-yearly rates, but the all-ages rates are standardised to the conventional "European" age distribution)

ARMENIA: 1985–1990

Smoking-attributed deaths (Sm.) and total deaths (Total)

		ALL CAUSES	ALL CANCER	Lung cancer	Upper aero-digestive ca.	Other cancer	COPD	Other respiratory	Vascular disease	Cirrhosis/ other liver	Other medical	Non-medical
Males												
0–34	Sm.	–	–	–	–	–	–	–	–	–	–	–
	Total	2804	101	8	2	91	10	442	94	10	890	1257
35–69	Sm.	1725	615	419	74	122	227	13	673	–	197	–
	Total	4934	1230	447	109	674	286	36	1974	134	552	722
		(35%)	(50%)	(94%)	(68%)	(18%)	(79%)	(36%)	(34%)		(36%)	
70+	Sm.	473	96	70	12	14	224	1	135	–	17	–
	Total	3863	371	86	31	254	421	30	2549	50	315	127
		(12%)	(26%)	(81%)	(39%)	(6%)	(53%)	(3%)	(5%)		(5%)	
Any age	Sm.	2198	711	489	86	136	451	14	808	–	214	–
	Total	11601	1702	541	142	1019	717	508	4617	194	1757	2106
		(19%)	(42%)	(90%)	(61%)	(13%)	(63%)	(3%)	(18%)		(12%)	
Females												
0–34	Sm.	–	–	–	–	–	–	–	–	–	–	–
	Total	2553	98	4	1	93	8	447	56	6	682	1256
35–69	Sm.	157	38	29	4	5	35	0	61	–	23	–
	Total	3369	875	68	19	788	112	24	1202	58	433	665
		(5%)	(4%)	(43%)	(21%)	(1%)	(31%)	(0%)	(5%)		(5%)	
70+	Sm.	54	8	6	1	1	22	0	21	–	3	–
	Total	5365	336	29	18	289	366	30	4034	64	339	196
		(1%)	(2%)	(21%)	(6%)	(0%)	(6%)	(0%)	(1%)		(1%)	
Any age	Sm.	211	46	35	5	6	57	0	82	–	26	–
	Total	11287	1309	101	38	1170	486	501	5292	128	1454	2117
		(2%)	(4%)	(35%)	(13%)	(1%)	(12%)	(0%)	(2%)		(2%)	
Males+Females												
0–34	Sm.	–	–	–	–	–	–	–	–	–	–	–
	Total	5357	199	12	3	184	18	889	150	16	1572	2513
35–69	Sm.	1882	653	448	78	127	262	13	734	–	220	–
	Total	8303	2105	515	128	1462	398	60	3176	192	985	1387
		(23%)	(31%)	(87%)	(61%)	(9%)	(66%)	(22%)	(23%)		(22%)	
70+	Sm.	527	104	76	13	15	246	1	156	–	20	–
	Total	9228	707	115	49	543	787	60	6583	114	654	323
		(6%)	(15%)	(66%)	(27%)	(3%)	(31%)	(2%)	(2%)		(3%)	
Any age	Sm.	2409	757	524	91	142	508	14	890	–	240	–
	Total	22888	3011	642	180	2189	1203	1009	9909	322	3211	4223
		(11%)	(25%)	(82%)	(51%)	(6%)	(42%)	(1%)	(9%)		(7%)	

ARMENIA: 1985

Smoking-attributed deaths (Sm.) and total deaths (Total)

		ALL CAUSES	ALL CANCER	Lung cancer	Upper aero-digestive ca.	Other cancer	COPD	Other respiratory	Vascular disease	Cirrhosis/ other liver	Other medical	Non-medical
Males												
0–34	Sm.	–	–	–	–	–	–	–	–	–	–	–
	Total	2297	108	10	2	96	20	619	84	11	963	492
35–69	Sm.	1425	491	333	58	100	207	11	527	–	189	–
	Total	3931	1041	358	86	597	264	32	1600	129	539	326
		(36%)	(47%)	(93%)	(67%)	(17%)	(78%)	(34%)	(33%)		(35%)	
70+	Sm.	445	91	67	10	14	216	1	121	–	16	–
	Total	3749	374	84	30	260	441	37	2499	62	281	55
		(12%)	(24%)	(80%)	(33%)	(5%)	(49%)	(3%)	(5%)		(6%)	
Any age	Sm.	1870	582	400	68	114	423	12	648	–	205	–
	Total	9977	1523	452	118	953	725	688	4183	202	1783	873
		(19%)	(38%)	(88%)	(58%)	(12%)	(58%)	(2%)	(15%)		(11%)	
Females												
0–34	Sm.	–	–	–	–	–	–	–	–	–	–	–
	Total	1858	101	3	1	97	9	651	70	9	751	267
35–69	Sm.	115	34	28	1	5	20	1	39	–	21	–
	Total	2467	756	63	10	683	119	23	1030	50	375	114
		(5%)	(4%)	(44%)	(10%)	(1%)	(17%)	(4%)	(4%)		(6%)	
70+	Sm.	0	0	0	0	0	0	0	0	–	0	–
	Total	5279	363	26	18	319	377	39	4022	83	308	87
		(0%)	(0%)	(0%)	(0%)	(0%)	(0%)	(0%)	(0%)		(0%)	
Any age	Sm.	115	34	28	1	5	20	1	39	–	21	–
	Total	9604	1220	92	29	1099	505	713	5122	142	1434	468
		(1%)	(3%)	(30%)	(3%)	(0%)	(4%)	(0%)	(1%)		(1%)	
Males+Females												
0–34	Sm.	–	–	–	–	–	–	–	–	–	–	–
	Total	4155	209	13	3	193	29	1270	154	20	1714	759
35–69	Sm.	1540	525	361	59	105	227	12	566	–	210	–
	Total	6398	1797	421	96	1280	383	55	2630	179	914	440
		(24%)	(29%)	(86%)	(61%)	(8%)	(59%)	(22%)	(22%)		(23%)	
70+	Sm.	445	91	67	10	14	216	1	121	–	16	–
	Total	9028	737	110	48	579	818	76	6521	145	589	142
		(5%)	(12%)	(61%)	(21%)	(2%)	(26%)	(1%)	(2%)		(3%)	
Any age	Sm.	1985	616	428	69	119	443	13	687	–	226	–
	Total	19581	2743	544	147	2052	1230	1401	9305	344	3217	1341
		(10%)	(22%)	(79%)	(47%)	(6%)	(36%)	(1%)	(7%)		(7%)	

(To be conservative, no deaths before age 35, and none from liver cirrhosis or non-medical causes, were attributed to smoking.)

ARMENIA: 1990

Smoking–attributed deaths (Sm.) and total deaths (Total)

		ALL CAUSES	ALL CANCER	Lung cancer	Upper aero–digestive ca.	Other cancer	COPD	Other respiratory	Vascular disease	Cirrhosis/ other liver	Other medical	Non–medical
Males												
0–34	Sm.	–	–	–	–	–	–	–	–	–	–	–
	Total	2078	103	6	2	95	8	297	89	12	808	761
35–69	Sm.	2233	784	530	93	161	262	14	919	–	254	–
	Total	5947	1505	562	130	813	322	38	2562	192	691	637
		(38%)	(52%)	(94%)	(72%)	(20%)	(81%)	(37%)	(36%)		(37%)	
70+	Sm.	523	105	75	13	17	230	1	162	–	25	–
	Total	3889	359	90	28	241	403	27	2578	41	396	85
		(13%)	(29%)	(83%)	(46%)	(7%)	(57%)	(4%)	(6%)		(6%)	
Any age	Sm.	2756	889	605	106	178	492	15	1081	–	279	–
	Total	11914	1967	658	160	1149	733	362	5229	245	1895	1483
		(23%)	(45%)	(92%)	(66%)	(15%)	(67%)	(4%)	(21%)		(15%)	
Females												
0–34	Sm.	–	–	–	–	–	–	–	–	–	–	–
	Total	1266	103	9	2	92	7	258	48	7	621	222
35–69	Sm.	217	54	41	3	10	40	1	87	–	35	–
	Total	3455	1077	82	19	976	115	29	1434	74	528	198
		(6%)	(5%)	(50%)	(16%)	(1%)	(35%)	(3%)	(6%)		(7%)	
70+	Sm.	37	7	5	1	1	12	0	16	–	2	–
	Total	5358	337	24	18	295	254	26	4132	58	482	69
		(1%)	(2%)	(21%)	(6%)	(0%)	(5%)	(0%)	(0%)		(0%)	
Any age	Sm.	254	61	46	4	11	52	1	103	–	37	–
	Total	10079	1517	115	39	1363	376	313	5614	139	1631	489
		(3%)	(4%)	(40%)	(10%)	(1%)	(14%)	(0%)	(2%)		(2%)	
Males+Females												
0–34	Sm.	–	–	–	–	–	–	–	–	–	–	–
	Total	3344	206	15	4	187	15	555	137	19	1429	983
35–69	Sm.	2450	838	571	96	171	302	15	1006	–	289	–
	Total	9402	2582	644	149	1789	437	67	3996	266	1219	835
		(26%)	(32%)	(89%)	(64%)	(10%)	(69%)	(22%)	(25%)		(24%)	
70+	Sm.	560	112	80	14	18	242	1	178	–	27	–
	Total	9247	696	114	46	536	657	53	6710	99	878	154
		(6%)	(16%)	(70%)	(30%)	(3%)	(37%)	(2%)	(3%)		(3%)	
Any age	Sm.	3010	950	651	110	189	544	16	1184	–	316	–
	Total	21993	3484	773	199	2512	1109	675	10843	384	3526	1972
		(14%)	(27%)	(84%)	(55%)	(8%)	(49%)	(2%)	(11%)		(9%)	

ARMENIA: 1995

Smoking–attributed deaths (Sm.) and total deaths (Total)

		ALL CAUSES	ALL CANCER	Lung cancer	Upper aero–digestive ca.	Other cancer	COPD	Other respiratory	Vascular disease	Cirrhosis/ other liver	Other medical	Non–medical
Males												
0–34	Sm.	–	–	–	–	–	–	–	–	–	–	–
	Total	2259	128	6	4	118	8	207	99	14	717	1086
35–69	Sm.	3207	1103	743	129	231	285	17	1447	–	355	–
	Total	8011	1941	780	172	989	337	41	3532	267	871	1022
		(40%)	(57%)	(95%)	(75%)	(23%)	(85%)	(41%)	(41%)		(41%)	
70+	Sm.	846	175	125	18	32	312	3	300	–	56	–
	Total	5250	498	140	36	322	475	28	3441	36	635	137
		(16%)	(35%)	(89%)	(50%)	(10%)	(66%)	(11%)	(9%)		(9%)	
Any age	Sm.	4053	1278	868	147	263	597	20	1747	–	411	–
	Total	15520	2567	926	212	1429	820	276	7072	317	2223	2245
		(26%)	(50%)	(94%)	(69%)	(18%)	(73%)	(7%)	(25%)		(18%)	
Females												
0–34	Sm.	–	–	–	–	–	–	–	–	–	–	–
	Total	1173	128	12	1	115	7	191	52	10	534	251
35–69	Sm.	342	82	62	6	14	46	2	151	–	61	–
	Total	4420	1456	109	28	1319	107	34	1713	95	718	297
		(8%)	(6%)	(57%)	(21%)	(1%)	(43%)	(6%)	(9%)		(8%)	
70+	Sm.	50	11	7	3	1	11	0	24	–	4	–
	Total	6423	393	31	22	340	201	23	4920	55	761	70
		(1%)	(3%)	(23%)	(14%)	(0%)	(5%)	(0%)	(0%)		(1%)	
Any age	Sm.	392	93	69	9	15	57	2	175	–	65	–
	Total	12016	1977	152	51	1774	315	248	6685	160	2013	618
		(3%)	(5%)	(45%)	(18%)	(1%)	(18%)	(1%)	(3%)		(3%)	
Males+Females												
0–34	Sm.	–	–	–	–	–	–	–	–	–	–	–
	Total	3432	256	18	5	233	15	398	151	24	1251	1337
35–69	Sm.	3549	1185	805	135	245	331	19	1598	–	416	–
	Total	12431	3397	889	200	2308	444	75	5245	362	1589	1319
		(29%)	(35%)	(91%)	(68%)	(11%)	(75%)	(25%)	(30%)		(26%)	
70+	Sm.	896	186	132	21	33	323	3	324	–	60	–
	Total	11673	891	171	58	662	676	51	8361	91	1396	207
		(8%)	(21%)	(77%)	(36%)	(5%)	(48%)	(6%)	(4%)		(4%)	
Any age	Sm.	4445	1371	937	156	278	654	22	1922	–	476	–
	Total	27536	4544	1078	263	3203	1135	524	13757	477	4236	2863
		(16%)	(30%)	(87%)	(59%)	(9%)	(58%)	(4%)	(14%)		(11%)	

(To be conservative, no deaths before age 35, and none from liver cirrhosis or non–medical causes, were attributed to smoking.)

AUSTRALIA: 1990

		No. of deaths			Standardised rates (Defined on p.268)			Annual death rates / 100, 000						
		All ages	0–34	35–69	All ages	0–34	35–69	0–4	5–9	10–14	15–19	20–24	25–29	30–34
ALL CAUSES	M	64056	5185	23492	898.1	108.3	901.1	214.2	22.6	20.2	90.2	135.9	137.9	137.2
	F	54859	2511	12735	549.3	55.2	474.2	171.5	13.8	15.3	39.3	44.3	46.0	56.5
Tuberculosis	M	58	–	22	0.8	–	0.8	–	–	–	–	–	–	–
	F	33	1	13	0.4	0.0	0.5	–	–	–	–	–	0.1	–
Other infective and parasitic	M	377	67	129	5.1	1.4	4.3	4.2	0.5	0.2	1.1	0.7	1.3	2.0
	F	344	36	84	3.5	0.8	3.2	2.8	0.2	0.7	0.4	0.6	0.6	0.4
ALL CANCER	M	17218	358	8128	242.7	7.4	318.0	5.9	4.0	2.4	5.4	7.1	10.5	16.6
	F	13089	288	5984	147.8	6.1	220.1	2.8	3.1	4.0	3.9	4.2	9.2	15.6
Mouth and pharynx cancer	M	464	5	317	6.6	0.1	12.1	–	0.2	–	–	0.1	–	0.4
	F	175	4	80	2.0	0.1	3.1	–	–	–	0.1	0.1	–	0.3
Oesophagus cancer	M	501	3	286	7.1	0.1	11.5	–	–	–	–	0.1	–	0.3
	F	224	–	78	2.4	–	3.0	–	–	–	–	–	–	–
Stomach cancer	M	781	4	336	11.1	0.1	13.1	–	–	–	–	–	0.1	0.4
	F	485	8	160	5.1	0.2	6.0	–	–	–	–	–	0.1	1.0
Colorectal cancer	M	2189	11	1080	30.9	0.2	42.5	–	–	–	0.1	–	0.7	0.7
	F	1943	14	788	21.4	0.3	29.7	–	–	–	–	0.6	0.3	1.2
Liver cancer	M	184	1	106	2.6	0.0	4.0	–	–	–	–	–	–	0.1
	F	51	–	28	0.6	–	1.0	–	–	–	–	–	–	–
Pancreas cancer	M	709	4	366	10.0	0.1	14.4	–	–	–	–	–	0.1	0.4
	F	657	2	258	7.2	0.0	10.0	–	–	–	–	–	0.1	0.1
Larynx cancer	M	229	1	152	3.3	0.0	6.1	–	–	–	–	–	0.1	–
	F	22	–	12	0.2	–	0.5	–	–	–	–	–	–	–
Lung cancer	M	4447	4	2332	62.7	0.1	93.6	–	–	–	–	0.1	0.1	0.3
	F	1593	6	818	18.4	0.1	31.0	–	0.2	–	–	–	0.3	0.4
Malignant melanoma	M	512	29	315	7.1	0.6	11.3	0.2	–	–	0.1	0.4	1.3	2.1
	F	317	23	156	3.6	0.5	5.2	–	–	0.2	–	0.4	1.3	1.4
Female breast cancer	F	2421	33	1433	29.1	0.7	50.9	–	–	–	–	–	1.0	3.7
Cervix cancer	F	339	24	221	4.0	0.5	7.2	–	–	–	–	0.1	1.3	2.0
Other uterine cancer	F	217	2	86	2.4	0.0	3.3	–	–	–	–	–	–	0.3
Ovarian cancer	F	732	12	390	8.7	0.3	14.4	–	–	0.2	–	0.3	0.3	1.0
Prostate cancer	M	2078	–	435	30.0	–	18.6	–	–	–	–	–	–	–
Bladder cancer	M	479	1	151	6.9	0.0	6.1	0.2	–	–	–	–	–	–
	F	233	–	65	2.3	–	2.5	–	–	–	–	–	–	–
Other and ill-defined cancer sites	M	3083	165	1565	43.0	3.4	59.3	2.9	2.0	1.6	2.6	3.2	5.2	6.4
	F	2420	92	978	26.7	2.0	36.1	1.8	2.1	2.3	1.9	1.5	2.3	2.2
Hodgkin's disease	M	40	8	21	0.5	0.2	0.7	–	–	–	–	0.1	0.4	0.6
	F	32	4	11	0.3	0.1	0.4	–	–	–	–	0.1	0.1	0.3
Myeloma and non-Hodgkin lymphomas	M	922	45	429	12.8	0.9	15.9	0.5	–	0.2	1.1	1.2	1.4	2.1
	F	779	13	281	8.5	0.3	10.7	0.2	0.2	0.2	0.3	–	0.6	0.6
Leukaemia	M	600	77	237	8.2	1.6	8.8	2.2	1.9	0.6	1.4	1.7	1.0	2.6
	F	449	51	141	4.8	1.1	5.0	0.8	0.7	1.2	1.6	0.9	1.6	1.0
ALL VASCULAR DISEASE	M	26795	209	8979	385.8	4.3	355.3	1.9	0.3	1.3	3.5	5.4	7.7	10.0
	F	26972	106	3660	251.3	2.2	141.6	1.8	0.3	0.8	1.3	1.9	3.8	5.6
Rheumatic heart disease and fever	M	125	8	57	1.8	0.2	2.2	0.2	–	0.2	–	0.1	0.3	0.4
	F	228	6	74	2.4	0.1	2.8	–	–	–	–	0.3	0.1	0.4
Hypertensive disease	M	398	5	107	5.8	0.1	4.2	–	–	–	–	0.3	0.3	0.1
	F	637	1	71	5.8	0.0	2.8	–	–	–	–	–	0.1	–
Ischaemic heart disease	M	17008	58	6373	243.7	1.2	252.3	–	–	–	0.6	1.3	2.0	4.4
	F	13867	14	2177	131.3	0.3	85.1	–	–	–	0.1	0.1	0.4	1.3
Pulmonary embolism and other venous	M	134	1	59	1.9	0.0	2.3	–	–	–	–	–	0.1	–
	F	178	2	61	1.9	0.0	2.3	–	–	–	–	–	0.1	0.1
Cerebrovascular disease	M	4777	43	1134	69.6	0.9	45.1	0.3	–	0.3	0.6	1.6	2.1	1.3
	F	7204	26	789	65.9	0.5	30.0	–	–	0.3	0.6	0.6	0.8	1.4
Other vascular disease	M	4353	94	1249	63.1	1.9	49.2	1.4	0.3	0.8	2.4	2.0	2.9	3.7
	F	4858	57	488	44.0	1.2	18.7	1.8	0.3	0.5	0.6	0.9	2.1	2.3
Chronic obstructive pulmonary disease	M	3986	51	1105	57.1	1.1	45.4	0.5	0.8	0.8	1.3	1.5	1.7	1.0
	F	2073	53	639	21.7	1.1	24.6	0.3	0.2	0.7	1.6	1.9	1.3	1.9
Other respiratory disease	M	1437	63	345	20.9	1.3	13.4	4.6	0.6	0.5	0.3	1.0	1.0	1.4
	F	1393	35	155	12.8	0.8	5.8	4.2	0.2	–	–	0.4	0.1	0.6
Peptic ulcer	M	381	1	127	5.6	0.0	5.1	–	–	–	–	0.1	–	–
	F	436	–	46	4.0	–	1.8	–	–	–	–	–	–	–
Liver cirrhosis	M	783	35	609	10.8	0.7	21.9	0.2	–	–	–	0.3	1.1	3.4
	F	318	13	207	3.9	0.3	7.4	–	–	–	–	–	0.7	1.2
Renal disease	M	627	4	104	9.3	0.1	4.0	–	–	–	–	0.3	0.3	–
	F	834	8	144	8.0	0.2	5.5	0.2	–	–	–	0.3	0.1	0.6
Pregnancy and birth	F	17	15	2	0.2	0.3	0.0	–	–	–	–	0.6	0.8	0.7
Congenital and perinatal causes	M	903	827	46	11.2	18.2	1.5	119.9	1.9	1.1	1.7	1.7	0.4	1.0
	F	759	700	38	9.7	16.2	1.3	104.4	1.5	1.2	1.8	1.8	2.0	0.9
Ill-defined causes	M	462	329	71	5.9	7.2	2.4	46.8	–	–	0.8	1.0	1.1	0.9
	F	349	209	34	4.0	4.8	1.1	31.5	–	0.2	0.7	0.3	0.4	0.7
Other medical causes	M	5561	572	1785	77.8	11.8	65.8	10.5	3.1	2.1	6.3	11.2	21.0	28.5
	F	5969	252	1042	57.4	5.4	38.8	9.1	2.0	1.7	5.0	6.7	6.5	7.1
ALL NON-MEDICAL CAUSES	M	5468	2669	2042	65.0	54.7	63.2	19.7	11.4	12.0	69.8	105.6	91.9	72.4
	F	2273	795	687	24.6	16.9	22.4	14.4	6.5	6.2	24.5	25.5	20.2	21.3
Motor vehicle traffic accidents	M	1661	1052	441	18.8	21.6	13.6	5.6	7.3	6.2	35.7	43.7	30.7	21.9
	F	706	355	228	8.0	7.6	7.5	3.1	4.6	3.2	15.5	13.7	7.1	5.9
Fire	M	66	21	32	0.8	0.4	1.1	0.2	0.2	0.2	0.3	0.6	1.7	–
	F	26	5	8	0.3	0.1	0.3	0.2	–	–	–	0.1	0.3	0.1
Suicide	M	1758	797	812	20.7	16.2	24.7	–	–	0.8	17.1	36.5	33.5	25.5
	F	444	173	211	5.2	3.6	6.7	–	–	–	4.2	5.2	6.2	9.4
Homicide	M	236	123	105	2.7	2.5	3.1	1.7	0.5	0.5	2.5	4.9	4.3	3.3
	F	138	78	48	1.6	1.7	1.3	1.5	1.0	0.5	1.2	2.4	2.8	2.3
POPULATION (thousands):	**M=males**				8511.4	4747.5	3269.1	645.3	647.3	634.0	717.4	688.5	715.8	699.2
	F=females				8553.8	4584.4	3233.2	612.9	615.0	600.5	685.0	669.8	706.8	694.4

AUSTRALIA: 1990

9th ICD categories

Annual death rates / 100, 000

35–39	40–44	45–49	50–54	55–59	60–64	65–69	70–74	75–79	80+/NK			
147.8	208.7	313.2	528.7	938.9	1581.6	2588.9	4082.6	6704.9	13173.2	M	ALL CAUSES	001–999
73.9	110.7	183.7	323.3	490.1	802.3	1335.6	2272.4	3888.5	10160.1	F		
0.2	0.2	0.6	0.2	0.5	1.9	2.2	3.7	8.4	12.3	M	Tuberculosis	010–018, 137
–	–	0.4	0.2	0.6	1.1	1.1	2.2	1.8	3.7	F		
2.4	3.1	2.8	3.6	2.2	9.0	7.3	14.7	36.2	76.0	M	Other infective	Rest of 001–139
0.6	0.5	1.0	2.7	1.7	4.3	11.2	10.7	17.7	63.7	F	and parasitic	
25.1	50.9	96.9	183.9	359.8	593.0	916.2	1274.9	1789.6	2605.4	M	ALL CANCER	140–208
34.0	62.7	102.4	181.8	261.5	373.6	525.0	684.8	863.2	1249.1	F		
0.8	1.2	6.8	8.3	17.4	23.4	27.1	25.2	26.5	37.6	M	Mouth and	140–149
0.2	0.3	0.6	2.7	4.7	4.3	8.6	10.0	11.3	15.9	F	pharynx cancer	
0.6	0.9	1.6	6.9	14.2	20.9	35.1	36.7	43.4	53.1	M	Oesophagus cancer	150
–	0.2	1.3	0.7	3.3	6.5	9.2	12.2	17.7	30.2	F		
0.9	2.2	5.6	7.1	14.2	22.8	38.9	63.8	85.4	138.9	M	Stomach cancer	151
1.2	0.5	1.5	4.5	7.8	12.1	14.6	23.7	36.7	70.2	F		
1.7	6.9	12.7	23.8	46.6	80.8	125.2	161.5	234.3	313.7	M	Colorectal cancer	153, 154
2.0	4.8	10.4	27.4	33.1	52.6	77.7	104.2	134.6	229.5	F		
0.6	0.8	2.0	2.4	4.9	7.3	10.2	16.1	16.8	13.1	M	Liver cancer	155.0
0.2	0.2	0.2	0.5	0.8	4.0	1.4	3.7	3.2	2.4	F		
0.9	2.0	4.4	8.1	15.3	27.7	42.4	52.8	68.0	97.2	M	Pancreas cancer	157
0.6	0.2	1.7	6.7	15.6	17.8	27.5	36.2	48.5	78.4	F		
0.2	0.3	0.6	3.1	9.8	11.4	17.5	16.1	11.0	19.6	M	Larynx cancer	161
–	–	–	–	0.3	0.5	2.6	1.5	2.3	0.4	F		
1.5	6.4	21.8	47.3	107.9	186.5	283.6	355.7	463.4	506.5	M	Lung cancer	162
2.3	5.7	9.6	18.2	34.8	62.6	83.8	102.7	113.7	98.0	F		
3.2	4.4	7.5	11.7	13.4	16.3	22.3	27.5	37.5	40.8	M	Malignant melanoma	172
3.0	4.0	3.3	4.2	5.0	8.9	7.7	15.9	18.1	22.5	F		
9.4	23.3	35.7	56.9	61.5	73.1	96.4	97.6	112.8	180.5	F	Female breast cancer	174
5.0	5.5	7.7	4.5	6.7	8.9	12.0	10.7	15.4	12.7	F	Cervix cancer	180
–	0.5	0.6	2.0	3.1	6.7	10.3	12.9	13.6	26.1	F	Other uterine cancer	179, 182
2.1	2.3	8.8	12.5	19.2	25.9	30.1	44.7	42.6	47.0	F	Ovarian cancer	183
–	0.2	0.4	2.9	9.5	31.8	85.4	179.4	315.2	625.0	M	Prostate cancer	185
0.3	0.2	1.0	3.3	7.4	11.4	19.1	35.3	67.3	119.3	M	Bladder cancer	188
0.3	0.5	0.8	0.7	2.5	3.2	9.2	10.7	20.4	38.4	F		
8.4	16.2	20.9	43.5	69.8	107.9	148.2	204.2	268.0	403.6	M	Other and ill-defined	Rest of 140–208
5.0	11.0	14.0	30.2	43.4	59.9	89.2	119.7	177.6	258.9	F	cancer sites	
0.6	0.6	–	0.5	0.3	1.9	1.0	0.9	1.3	5.7	M	Hodgkin's disease	201
0.2	0.2	0.2	–	0.3	0.3	1.7	2.6	1.4	2.9	F		
3.2	5.2	8.3	9.8	18.5	28.8	37.6	58.7	97.7	138.1	M	Myeloma and non-	200, 202–203
0.6	1.5	3.3	6.0	14.2	18.6	31.0	53.2	63.4	82.1	F	Hodgkin lymphomas	
2.3	3.4	3.4	5.2	10.6	13.9	22.6	40.8	53.7	93.1	M	Leukaemia	204–208
1.8	2.3	2.5	4.0	5.0	7.6	11.8	22.5	29.9	53.1	F		
23.5	49.5	99.3	194.1	361.7	639.7	1119.2	1901.8	3327.5	6799.0	M	ALL VASCULAR	390–459
9.1	13.6	29.9	63.4	117.5	250.6	507.2	1071.3	2132.3	6370.4	F	DISEASE	
0.5	0.2	1.4	1.2	2.5	4.1	5.4	10.1	8.4	20.4	M	Rheumatic heart	390–398
0.8	0.2	0.8	2.2	3.9	3.8	7.7	11.1	25.4	25.3	F	disease and fever	
0.6	0.3	0.8	3.3	4.1	7.1	13.4	28.5	49.2	120.9	M	Hypertensive disease	401–405
–	0.3	0.2	2.0	2.2	5.1	9.5	22.9	43.5	166.2	F		
14.2	35.1	69.5	136.8	274.7	450.5	785.5	1277.2	2078.3	3744.3	M	Ischaemic heart	410–414
3.0	6.1	13.2	29.4	66.3	155.7	322.1	656.7	1183.5	2975.5	F	disease	
0.2	0.6	0.8	0.5	2.2	5.7	6.1	6.4	16.2	28.6	M	Pulmonary embolism	415.1, 451–453
0.8	0.5	0.2	1.7	1.7	3.0	8.0	12.9	11.3	22.5	F	and other venous	
3.0	6.6	11.1	23.8	39.2	83.5	148.2	317.6	653.1	1551.5	M	Cerebrovascular	430–438
3.0	4.2	9.2	19.2	25.9	50.2	98.4	234.3	551.4	1853.0	F	disease	
5.0	6.7	15.7	28.6	39.0	88.9	160.6	262.0	522.3	1333.3	M	Other vascular	Rest of 390–459
1.5	2.3	6.3	8.7	17.5	32.9	61.4	133.4	317.2	1327.9	F	disease	
2.0	3.1	6.0	13.3	34.1	86.2	173.4	328.1	537.9	1049.0	M	Chronic obstructive	490–496
1.5	3.1	4.0	12.7	22.6	48.8	79.7	125.6	184.4	258.9	F	pulmonary disease	
2.3	2.8	5.0	6.7	9.8	22.0	45.3	86.3	150.8	496.7	M	Other respiratory	Rest of 460–519
0.9	1.0	2.3	3.7	4.7	9.2	18.9	38.1	73.9	382.6	F	disease	
0.3	0.6	1.0	2.1	4.6	11.1	15.6	23.4	32.4	124.2	M	Peptic ulcer	531–533
–	–	0.2	0.7	3.1	2.7	6.0	19.6	37.2	104.1	F		
4.9	8.6	14.5	20.2	28.6	34.8	41.7	32.1	31.1	17.2	M	Liver cirrhosis	571
2.7	2.4	3.3	7.2	9.7	10.5	15.8	16.3	13.1	10.2	F		
0.3	1.6	1.8	1.4	1.4	7.3	14.3	25.7	82.8	273.7	M	Renal disease	580–590
0.5	0.6	1.3	4.0	7.2	10.0	14.9	31.4	64.3	185.8	F		
0.3	–	–	–	–	–	–	–	–	–	F	Pregnancy and birth	630–676
1.2	0.9	1.0	1.2	0.8	2.7	2.9	5.0	6.5	7.4	M	Congenital and	740–779
0.6	1.0	1.0	1.7	0.8	1.9	1.7	2.2	1.8	4.5	F	perinatal causes	
1.5	1.6	1.8	2.4	2.5	2.7	4.1	3.2	9.1	33.5	M	Ill-defined causes	780–799
0.9	0.6	1.3	1.0	0.8	0.5	2.6	1.5	2.7	39.2	F		
20.9	25.3	27.2	43.1	64.3	101.4	178.1	293.3	568.3	1378.3	M	Other medical causes	Rest of 001–799
7.0	8.7	14.6	24.2	40.7	60.4	116.2	221.4	415.0	1290.3	F		
63.2	60.6	55.4	56.4	68.7	69.6	68.5	90.4	124.3	300.7	M	ALL NON-	E800–E999
15.7	16.5	21.9	19.7	19.2	28.6	35.3	47.3	81.1	197.6	F	MEDICAL CAUSES	
12.0	14.8	12.9	12.6	13.1	14.1	15.6	24.8	38.8	44.1	M	Motor vehicle	E810–E819
5.3	4.8	7.1	7.0	5.6	11.6	10.9	14.4	22.2	14.3	F	traffic accidents	
0.8	0.6	0.4	1.4	1.6	0.8	1.9	2.3	1.9	4.1	M	Fire	E890–E899
–	–	0.4	0.2	–	0.3	1.1	1.1	1.8	2.4	F		
27.3	25.1	22.6	22.6	28.3	23.9	22.6	28.5	23.3	41.7	M	Suicide	E950–E959
5.3	6.0	7.9	6.5	6.4	6.7	7.7	8.5	8.2	7.8	F		
4.4	3.3	3.2	1.9	3.3	3.5	1.9	1.8	1.9	0.8	M	Homicide	E960–E969
2.4	1.9	2.3	1.0	0.6	0.3	0.6	1.8	1.8	1.2	F		
656.3	640.5	503.5	420.3	366.9	367.8	313.8	217.9	154.5	122.4	M	**POPULATION (thousands)**	
656.5	618.8	478.6	400.9	359.1	370.7	348.6	270.6	220.7	244.9	F		

AUSTRALIA: Males

	All ages	0–34	35–69	35–39	40–44	45–49	50–54	55–59	60–64	65–69	70–74	75–79	80+/NK
POPULATION (1000s)													
1955	4656.3	2732.0	1726.9	326.0	332.4	292.2	245.4	205.4	177.8	147.7	98.0	56.7	42.7
1965	5714.5	3389.4	2077.1	398.2	393.1	329.0	321.5	268.8	209.0	157.5	115.4	78.2	54.4
1975	6913.5	4224.3	2394.8	419.8	385.9	409.5	385.2	308.9	275.9	209.6	143.0	83.8	67.6
1985	7860.8	4557.6	2879.6	620.5	496.1	415.4	374.8	379.9	341.4	251.5	204.6	124.7	94.3
1990	**8511.4**	**4747.5**	**3269.1**	**656.3**	**640.5**	**503.5**	**420.3**	**366.9**	**367.8**	**313.8**	**217.9**	**154.5**	**122.4**
1995 projected	*8939.7*	*4828.1*	*3556.4*	*713.4*	*659.4*	*612.6*	*497.4*	*403.1*	*346.0*	*324.5*	*254.7*	*164.2*	*136.3*
NUMBER OF DEATHS													
All causes													
1955	46188	6096	20551	749	1163	1748	2520	3438	4686	6247	6317	5459	7765
1965	55770	5901	24928	998	1465	1999	3480	4507	5748	6731	7659	7714	9568
1975	60738	6308	27531	869	1285	2398	3712	4746	6659	7862	8450	7272	11177
1985	63579	5600	24351	886	1110	1552	2461	4345	6449	7548	9725	9542	14361
1990	**64056**	**5185**	**23492**	**970**	**1337**	**1577**	**2222**	**3445**	**5817**	**8124**	**8896**	**10359**	**16124**
1995 projected	*60018*	*4703*	*21001*	*1042*	*1246*	*1608*	*2153*	*3129*	*4634*	*7189*	*9026*	*9552*	*15736*
Lung cancer													
1955	1013	4	719	10	21	59	115	149	189	176	167	84	39
1965	2099	11	1395	19	36	73	173	315	357	422	333	225	135
1975	3392	15	2120	17	42	152	257	405	607	640	612	388	257
1985	4396	3	2440	15	35	103	263	502	755	767	835	624	494
1990	**4447**	**4**	**2332**	**10**	**41**	**110**	**199**	**396**	**686**	**890**	**775**	**716**	**620**
1995 projected	*4195*	*3*	*2025*	*9*	*35*	*96*	*179*	*346*	*558*	*802*	*814*	*699*	*654*
ANNUAL DEATH RATE / 100,000	(*The rates for the age groups 0–34 and 35–69 are the means of seven five-yearly rates, but the all-ages rates are standardised to the conventional "European" age distribution)												
All causes													
1955	1412.6*	205.6*	1534.8*	229.8	349.9	598.2	1026.9	1673.8	2635.5	4229.5	6445.9	9627.9	18185.0
1965	1406.7*	168.7*	1573.4*	250.6	372.7	607.6	1082.4	1676.7	2750.2	4273.7	6636.9	9864.5	17588.2
1975	1267.3*	148.9*	1398.6*	207.0	333.0	585.6	963.7	1536.4	2413.6	3751.0	5909.1	8677.8	16534.0
1985	1044.4*	123.6*	1061.5*	142.8	223.7	373.6	656.6	1143.7	1889.0	3001.2	4753.2	7652.0	15229.1
1990	**898.1***	**108.3***	**901.1***	**147.8**	**208.7**	**313.2**	**528.7**	**938.9**	**1581.6**	**2588.9**	**4082.6**	**6704.9**	**13173.2**
1995 projected	*776.7**	*96.2**	*765.9**	*146.1*	*189.0*	*262.5*	*432.9*	*776.2*	*1339.3*	*2215.4*	*3543.8*	*5817.3*	*11545.1*
All cancer													
1955	194.0*	11.0*	253.5*	28.8	48.7	95.5	179.3	273.1	471.9	677.0	1002.0	1358.0	1974.2
1965	210.5*	11.9*	287.0*	35.2	53.4	96.0	193.8	306.9	509.1	814.6	1130.8	1477.0	1906.3
1975	240.5*	9.7*	322.3*	25.0	60.6	123.3	215.2	367.4	582.8	881.7	1311.9	1639.6	2369.8
1985	253.3*	7.9*	337.9*	28.0	44.7	106.2	222.8	379.8	653.2	930.8	1292.3	1847.6	2644.8
1990	**242.7***	**7.4***	**318.0***	**25.1**	**50.9**	**96.9**	**183.9**	**359.8**	**593.0**	**916.2**	**1274.9**	**1789.6**	**2605.4**
1995 projected	*231.2**	*6.9**	*296.8**	*26.6*	*47.3*	*84.1*	*164.3*	*322.5*	*557.2*	*875.5*	*1235.6*	*1738.7*	*2557.6*
Lung cancer													
1955	29.8*	0.2*	53.5*	3.1	6.3	20.2	46.9	72.5	106.3	119.2	170.4	148.1	91.3
1965	52.2*	0.4*	92.3*	4.8	9.2	22.2	53.8	117.2	170.8	267.9	288.6	287.7	248.2
1975	69.3*	0.4*	110.7*	4.0	10.9	37.1	66.7	131.1	220.0	305.3	428.0	463.0	380.2
1985	71.3*	0.1*	109.0*	2.4	7.1	24.8	70.2	132.1	221.1	305.0	408.1	500.4	523.9
1990	**62.7***	**0.1***	**93.6***	**1.5**	**6.4**	**21.8**	**47.3**	**107.9**	**186.5**	**283.6**	**355.7**	**463.4**	**506.5**
1995 projected	*54.9**	*0.1**	*78.9**	*1.3*	*5.3*	*15.7*	*36.0*	*85.8*	*161.3*	*247.1*	*319.6*	*425.7*	*479.8*
Upper aerodigestive cancer (mouth, oesophagus, pharynx and larynx)													
1955	14.5*	0.2*	17.7*	1.2	1.5	5.8	9.4	18.0	38.2	49.4	69.4	118.2	187.4
1965	12.7*	–	20.0*	1.8	4.1	5.5	11.5	26.4	35.4	55.2	71.9	67.8	102.9
1975	16.5*	0.1*	26.1*	1.0	5.2	11.7	25.2	35.9	40.2	63.5	79.7	94.3	124.3
1985	17.7*	0.2*	29.0*	1.3	3.2	8.2	22.9	34.7	60.6	72.0	84.6	101.8	126.2
1990	**16.9***	**0.2***	**29.7***	**1.5**	**2.5**	**8.9**	**18.3**	**41.4**	**55.7**	**79.7**	**78.0**	**80.9**	**110.3**
1995 projected	*16.0**	*0.1**	*29.3**	*1.4*	*2.4*	*7.5*	*18.7*	*39.7*	*58.1*	*77.0*	*71.1*	*74.9*	*92.4*
Other cancer													
1955	149.7*	10.6*	182.3*	24.5	40.9	69.5	123.1	182.6	327.3	508.5	762.2	1091.7	1695.6
1965	145.6*	11.5*	174.8*	28.6	40.2	68.4	128.5	163.3	302.9	491.4	770.4	1121.5	1555.1
1975	154.7*	9.2*	185.5*	20.0	44.6	74.5	123.3	200.4	322.6	512.9	804.2	1082.3	1865.4
1985	164.4*	7.6*	200.0*	24.3	34.5	73.2	129.7	213.0	371.4	553.9	799.6	1245.4	1994.7
1990	**163.1***	**7.1***	**194.6***	**22.1**	**42.0**	**66.1**	**118.2**	**210.4**	**350.7**	**552.9**	**841.2**	**1245.3**	**1988.6**
1995 projected	*160.3**	*6.7**	*188.6**	*24.0*	*39.6*	*60.9*	*109.6*	*197.0*	*337.9*	*551.3*	*844.9*	*1238.1*	*1985.3*
Chronic obstructive pulmonary disease (COPD)													
1955	43.0*	1.9*	45.0*	1.5	4.5	9.2	19.2	47.7	83.8	149.0	213.3	345.7	660.4
1965	63.1*	1.5*	70.1*	1.8	4.3	12.5	30.2	58.8	146.4	236.8	371.8	539.6	832.7
1975	77.7*	2.2*	71.3*	4.0	4.7	13.2	32.5	68.6	132.3	243.8	479.7	731.5	1161.2
1985	71.6*	1.4*	58.1*	2.1	4.4	8.9	16.3	50.0	104.9	220.3	399.8	695.3	1285.3
1990	**57.1***	**1.1***	**45.4***	**2.0**	**3.1**	**6.0**	**13.3**	**34.1**	**86.2**	**173.4**	**328.1**	**537.9**	**1049.0**
1995 projected	*45.1**	*0.9**	*35.5**	*1.4*	*2.1*	*4.4*	*9.2*	*26.0*	*66.5*	*138.7*	*256.4*	*426.9*	*841.5*
Other respiratory disease													
1955	54.7*	11.1*	43.3*	3.7	13.8	15.7	21.2	50.6	76.5	121.2	181.6	382.7	1002.3
1965	55.7*	8.8*	33.5*	5.5	7.1	15.2	20.8	33.9	61.2	90.8	195.0	409.2	1237.1
1975	29.1*	3.9*	19.0*	2.9	6.7	9.8	12.5	20.7	30.1	50.6	80.4	218.4	664.2
1985	26.8*	1.7*	16.8*	3.1	4.2	5.8	9.6	15.0	29.9	49.7	95.8	175.6	675.5
1990	**20.9***	**1.3***	**13.4***	**2.3**	**2.8**	**5.0**	**6.7**	**9.8**	**22.0**	**45.3**	**86.3**	**150.8**	**496.7**
1995 projected	*16.5**	*1.0**	*10.8**	*1.5*	*2.1*	*3.6*	*4.6*	*6.9*	*17.6*	*39.1*	*75.0*	*124.8*	*377.8*
Vascular disease													
1955	760.8*	10.0*	831.4*	55.5	113.7	264.9	517.9	902.1	1464.0	2501.7	3957.1	5841.3	11316.2
1965	795.9*	7.0*	890.8*	62.8	152.6	283.3	578.5	970.6	1632.5	2554.9	4133.4	6209.7	11336.4
1975	682.6*	5.7*	743.9*	57.4	113.2	272.0	477.9	805.1	1338.9	2142.7	3435.0	5146.8	10418.6
1985	489.4*	5.1*	471.2*	26.9	69.5	136.5	275.6	501.4	838.3	1450.1	2417.9	4025.7	8411.5
1990	**385.8***	**4.3***	**355.3***	**23.5**	**49.5**	**99.3**	**194.1**	**361.7**	**639.7**	**1119.2**	**1901.8**	**3327.5**	**6799.0**
1995 projected	*303.3**	*3.9**	*265.2**	*17.0*	*35.0*	*68.2*	*135.9*	*263.5*	*478.9*	*858.2*	*1512.8*	*2662.6*	*5537.8*
Liver cirrhosis													
1955	8.2*	0.3*	15.7*	3.7	5.4	11.0	14.3	21.4	30.4	23.7	16.3	38.8	32.8
1965	7.9*	0.4*	16.5*	3.5	5.1	10.0	19.0	18.6	23.9	35.6	23.4	25.6	7.4
1975	15.1*	0.4*	32.2*	7.6	15.0	23.0	42.8	46.0	43.1	48.2	35.0	31.0	11.8
1985	12.8*	0.7*	25.4*	5.0	8.7	16.6	27.5	37.1	42.5	40.2	43.5	30.5	29.7
1990	**10.8***	**0.7***	**21.9***	**4.9**	**8.6**	**14.5**	**20.2**	**28.6**	**34.8**	**41.7**	**32.1**	**31.1**	**17.2**
1995 projected	*8.9**	*0.7**	*18.1**	*4.8*	*7.6*	*11.4*	*15.5*	*22.1*	*30.1*	*35.4*	*29.1*	*22.5*	*13.2*
Other medical causes													
1955	242.3*	93.6*	227.4*	52.1	72.2	105.7	164.2	242.0	366.1	589.7	878.6	1379.2	2669.8
1965	166.0*	64.8*	155.0*	37.4	48.1	78.7	119.1	163.7	244.5	393.7	589.3	959.1	1805.1
1975	126.8*	51.8*	111.7*	23.6	35.2	54.5	93.5	121.7	183.0	270.5	427.3	714.8	1486.7
1985	118.0*	43.7*	81.5*	19.8	21.4	32.0	43.0	84.2	139.4	231.0	396.4	756.2	1895.0
1990	**115.8***	**38.8***	**83.9***	**26.8**	**33.3**	**36.1**	**54.0**	**76.3**	**136.2**	**224.7**	**369.0**	**743.7**	**1905.2**
1995 projected	*113.6**	*35.4**	*84.8**	*36.7*	*41.9*	*44.7*	*55.1*	*75.2*	*128.9*	*210.8*	*352.6*	*715.6*	*1903.9*
All non-medical causes													
1955	109.6*	77.6*	118.5*	84.4	91.5	96.2	110.8	136.8	142.9	167.2	196.9	282.2	529.3
1965	107.6*	74.4*	120.5*	104.5	102.0	111.9	121.0	124.3	132.5	147.3	193.2	244.2	463.2
1975	95.3*	75.2*	98.1*	86.5	97.4	89.9	89.3	106.8	103.3	113.5	139.9	195.7	421.6
1985	72.5*	63.2*	70.6*	57.9	70.8	67.6	61.9	76.1	80.8	79.1	107.5	121.1	287.4
1990	**65.0***	**54.7***	**63.2***	**63.2**	**60.6**	**55.4**	**56.4**	**68.7**	**69.6**	**68.5**	**90.4**	**124.3**	**300.7**
1995 projected	*57.9**	*47.4**	*54.7**	*58.0*	*52.9*	*46.0*	*48.3*	*60.0*	*60.1*	*57.6*	*82.4*	*126.1*	*313.3*

AUSTRALIA: Females

	All ages	0–34	35–69	35–39	40–44	45–49	50–54	55–59	60–64	65–69	70–74	75–79	80+/NK
POPULATION (1000s)													
1955	4543.4	2576.6	1706.7	316.6	315.6	265.3	229.1	215.1	199.0	166.0	118.8	77.1	64.2
1965	5626.4	3212.7	2044.6	367.2	376.5	323.6	313.1	257.2	215.3	191.7	160.0	113.0	96.1
1975	6858.2	4034.1	2364.4	396.7	362.1	381.0	375.6	315.0	297.0	237.0	182.1	135.0	142.6
1985	7897.6	4395.1	2860.8	600.8	475.9	395.7	360.3	371.5	362.6	294.0	258.8	183.7	199.2
1990	**8553.8**	**4584.4**	**3233.2**	**656.5**	**618.8**	**478.6**	**400.9**	**359.1**	**370.7**	**348.6**	**270.6**	**220.7**	**244.9**
1995 projected	*8962.0*	*4597.0*	*3538.5*	*699.0*	*651.2*	*601.7*	*482.1*	*397.2*	*354.3*	*353.0*	*310.9*	*241.0*	*274.6*
NUMBER OF DEATHS													
All causes													
1955	35848	3748	12461	503	790	1062	1355	1898	2874	3979	4763	5228	9648
1965	43945	3601	13731	584	866	1286	1760	2184	2894	4157	5987	6988	13638
1975	48283	3249	14773	518	732	1244	1858	2423	3513	4485	5709	7010	17542
1985	54227	2795	13328	496	594	937	1357	2262	3324	4358	6662	7975	23467
1990	**54859**	**2511**	**12735**	**485**	**685**	**879**	**1296**	**1760**	**2974**	**4656**	**6149**	**8582**	**24882**
1995 projected	*52560*	*2136*	*11577*	*466*	*597*	*924*	*1271*	*1654*	*2484*	*4181*	*6306*	*8163*	*24378*
Lung cancer													
1955	165	4	103	3	6	14	11	14	21	34	25	16	17
1965	296	1	173	7	7	18	32	31	34	44	53	32	37
1975	610	2	384	8	13	35	66	58	108	96	83	73	68
1985	1252	8	715	15	19	39	70	154	190	228	220	152	157
1990	**1593**	**6**	**818**	**15**	**35**	**46**	**73**	**125**	**232**	**292**	**278**	**251**	**240**
1995 projected	*1971*	*3*	*887*	*17*	*37*	*56*	*75*	*137*	*230*	*335*	*384*	*344*	*353*
ANNUAL DEATH RATE / 100,000													
All causes													
1955	942.2*	125.7*	874.9*	158.9	250.3	400.3	591.4	882.4	1444.2	2397.0	4009.3	6780.8	15028.0
1965	874.2*	104.7*	815.8*	159.0	230.0	397.4	562.1	849.1	1344.2	2168.5	3741.9	6184.1	14191.5
1975	747.3*	79.2*	714.1*	130.6	202.2	326.5	494.7	769.2	1182.8	1892.4	3135.1	5192.6	12301.5
1985	632.8*	65.0*	547.0*	82.6	124.8	236.8	376.6	608.9	916.7	1482.3	2574.2	4341.3	11780.6
1990	**549.3***	**55.2***	**474.2***	**73.9**	**110.7**	**183.7**	**323.3**	**490.1**	**802.3**	**1335.6**	**2272.4**	**3888.5**	**10160.1**
1995 projected	*478.3**	*47.0**	*411.1**	*66.7*	*91.7*	*153.6*	*263.6*	*416.4*	*701.1*	*1184.4*	*2028.3*	*3387.1*	*8877.6*
All cancer													
1955	147.4*	9.9*	210.3*	38.9	71.6	126.3	186.8	245.5	318.6	484.3	673.4	872.9	1255.5
1965	138.9*	9.9*	197.3*	40.3	70.1	124.8	165.8	232.5	314.9	432.4	642.5	767.3	1214.4
1975	144.8*	8.2*	215.3*	39.3	65.5	120.2	182.6	269.5	366.0	463.7	617.2	807.4	1225.1
1985	152.5*	7.5*	228.0*	34.8	60.1	116.2	193.2	288.0	370.4	533.0	672.7	861.7	1293.7
1990	**147.8***	**6.1***	**220.1***	**34.0**	**62.7**	**102.4**	**181.8**	**261.5**	**373.6**	**525.0**	**684.8**	**863.2**	**1249.1**
1995 projected	*141.5**	*5.1**	*208.7**	*31.9*	*56.1*	*92.9*	*160.8*	*244.0*	*357.6*	*517.6*	*680.0*	*848.5*	*1225.4*
Lung cancer													
1955	4.3*	0.2*	7.2*	0.9	1.9	5.3	4.8	6.5	10.6	20.5	21.0	20.8	26.5
1965	6.1*	0.0*	10.0*	1.9	1.9	5.6	10.2	12.1	15.8	23.0	33.1	28.3	38.5
1975	10.2*	0.1*	18.2*	2.0	3.6	9.2	17.6	18.4	36.4	40.5	45.6	54.1	47.7
1985	16.6*	0.2*	29.6*	2.5	4.0	9.9	19.4	41.5	52.4	77.6	85.0	82.7	78.8
1990	**18.4***	**0.1***	**31.0***	**2.3**	**5.7**	**9.6**	**18.2**	**34.8**	**62.6**	**83.8**	**102.7**	**113.7**	**98.0**
1995 projected	*20.6**	*0.1**	*32.5**	*2.4*	*5.7*	*9.3*	*15.6*	*34.5*	*64.9*	*94.9*	*123.5*	*142.7*	*128.6*
Upper aerodigestive cancer (mouth, oesophagus, pharynx and larynx)													
1955	3.9*	0.2*	4.2*	–	–	2.6	2.2	6.5	4.5	13.9	21.0	29.8	51.4
1965	4.1*	–	5.0*	0.3	1.1	0.9	3.2	8.6	9.3	12.0	22.5	26.5	55.2
1975	4.8*	0.1*	6.2*	–	1.7	1.8	4.3	6.7	11.4	17.7	21.4	31.1	63.1
1985	5.3*	0.0*	7.6*	0.7	0.6	3.5	4.2	10.2	13.2	20.4	27.4	31.0	54.2
1990	**4.6***	**0.1***	**6.6***	**0.2**	**0.5**	**1.9**	**3.5**	**8.4**	**11.3**	**20.4**	**23.7**	**31.3**	**46.5**
1995 projected	*4.0**	*0.0**	*5.6**	*0.1*	*0.3*	*1.3*	*2.5*	*6.8*	*10.2*	*18.1*	*22.2*	*28.2*	*42.2*
Other cancer													
1955	139.2*	9.5*	198.8*	37.9	69.7	118.4	179.8	232.5	303.5	450.0	631.3	822.3	1177.6
1965	128.6*	9.9*	182.2*	38.1	67.2	118.4	152.3	211.9	289.8	397.5	586.9	712.4	1120.7
1975	129.8*	8.1*	190.8*	37.3	60.2	109.2	160.8	244.4	318.2	405.5	550.2	722.2	1114.3
1985	130.6*	7.3*	190.8*	31.6	55.5	102.9	169.6	236.3	304.7	435.0	560.3	748.0	1160.6
1990	**124.8***	**5.9***	**182.6***	**31.5**	**56.6**	**90.9**	**160.1**	**218.3**	**299.7**	**420.8**	**558.4**	**718.2**	**1104.5**
1995 projected	*116.9**	*5.0**	*170.6**	*29.3*	*50.1*	*82.3*	*142.7*	*202.7*	*282.5*	*404.5*	*534.3*	*677.6*	*1054.6*
Chronic obstructive pulmonary disease (COPD)													
1955	12.3*	1.2*	7.8*	1.3	2.2	2.6	3.1	10.7	11.6	22.9	38.7	79.1	308.4
1965	11.1*	1.4*	10.7*	2.5	1.9	3.1	8.0	12.8	20.4	26.1	47.5	57.5	195.6
1975	17.6*	1.8*	21.5*	3.8	7.7	8.9	12.2	20.6	35.0	62.4	80.2	109.6	215.3
1985	22.7*	1.3*	26.8*	2.5	3.4	9.1	17.5	29.3	47.2	78.9	127.1	164.4	270.6
1990	**21.7***	**1.1***	**24.6***	**1.5**	**3.1**	**4.0**	**12.7**	**22.6**	**48.8**	**79.7**	**125.6**	**184.4**	**258.9**
1995 projected	*21.0**	*0.9**	*22.7**	*1.1*	*2.0*	*2.7*	*8.7*	*19.6*	*46.6*	*78.2*	*129.9*	*185.1*	*263.7*
Other respiratory disease													
1955	34.6*	9.9*	16.4*	3.5	5.4	9.0	10.5	18.6	24.6	43.4	107.7	199.7	799.1
1965	31.3*	7.3*	15.1*	4.6	5.6	8.3	9.3	11.3	24.6	42.3	84.4	218.6	745.1
1975	16.9*	2.6*	9.1*	2.3	2.2	6.8	6.1	6.7	14.1	25.3	42.3	105.9	437.6
1985	17.3*	1.4*	8.3*	1.0	1.9	3.3	5.0	8.6	16.3	21.8	51.4	90.4	508.5
1990	**12.8***	**0.8***	**5.8***	**0.9**	**1.0**	**2.3**	**3.7**	**4.7**	**9.2**	**18.9**	**38.1**	**73.9**	**382.6**
1995 projected	*9.6**	*0.6**	*4.1**	*0.6*	*0.6*	*1.5*	*2.5*	*3.3*	*6.5*	*13.6*	*29.9*	*54.8*	*291.3*
Vascular disease													
1955	531.8*	7.1*	453.3*	36.6	72.9	138.3	254.5	415.2	811.1	1444.6	2563.1	4572.0	10076.3
1965	513.1*	5.4*	412.8*	35.9	65.3	135.4	233.2	402.8	715.7	1301.0	2445.6	4359.3	10249.7
1975	428.6*	4.4*	333.7*	31.3	58.0	103.9	188.8	310.8	565.0	1078.1	1975.3	3517.0	9003.5
1985	313.9*	3.2*	189.8*	13.6	24.4	49.5	88.8	177.9	340.6	634.0	1338.5	2552.5	7782.6
1990	**251.3***	**2.2***	**141.6***	**9.1**	**13.6**	**29.9**	**63.4**	**117.5**	**250.6**	**507.2**	**1071.3**	**2132.3**	**6370.4**
1995 projected	*201.1**	*1.6**	*105.6**	*6.3*	*9.1*	*20.4*	*43.4*	*81.3*	*186.6*	*392.1*	*863.3*	*1707.9*	*5239.6*
Liver cirrhosis													
1955	3.8*	0.4*	7.3*	1.9	3.2	5.7	7.9	10.2	13.1	9.0	10.1	13.0	7.8
1965	4.2*	0.6*	7.1*	3.5	1.9	6.2	7.3	7.8	10.7	12.5	16.9	12.4	14.6
1975	5.1*	0.2*	10.7*	3.0	4.4	8.4	10.4	17.8	17.5	13.1	11.5	13.3	4.9
1985	4.5*	0.2*	8.7*	2.0	4.2	6.1	7.8	13.2	14.1	13.6	15.8	13.6	11.0
1990	**3.9***	**0.3***	**7.4***	**2.7**	**2.4**	**3.3**	**7.2**	**9.7**	**10.5**	**15.8**	**16.3**	**13.1**	**10.2**
1995 projected	*3.4**	*0.3**	*6.1**	*2.3*	*1.5*	*2.3*	*5.2*	*7.6*	*9.0*	*15.0*	*16.7*	*12.0*	*9.5*
Other medical causes													
1955	169.9*	79.3*	145.8*	57.2	76.4	90.8	94.7	145.0	221.1	335.5	525.3	867.7	1923.7
1965	126.1*	56.9*	119.8*	37.9	45.9	69.8	85.3	126.4	192.3	281.2	402.5	600.0	1300.7
1975	93.9*	39.6*	83.2*	22.2	29.5	39.9	56.7	95.9	140.1	197.9	330.0	499.3	1069.4
1985	93.3*	32.7*	58.5*	8.2	12.6	26.0	39.7	60.8	96.8	165.6	310.7	574.3	1674.2
1990	**87.2***	**27.8***	**52.2***	**9.9**	**11.5**	**19.8**	**34.7**	**54.9**	**80.9**	**153.8**	**289.0**	**540.6**	**1691.3**
1995 projected	*80.8**	*23.5**	*45.6**	*9.9*	*9.5*	*16.1*	*29.0*	*46.1*	*71.1*	*137.4*	*265.7*	*509.1*	*1678.4*
All non-medical causes													
1955	42.4*	18.0*	34.1*	19.6	18.7	27.5	34.0	37.2	44.2	57.2	90.9	176.4	657.3
1965	49.5*	23.4*	53.0*	34.3	39.3	49.8	53.3	55.6	65.5	73.0	102.5	169.0	471.4
1975	40.3*	22.4*	40.7*	28.7	34.8	38.3	37.8	47.9	45.1	51.9	78.5	140.0	345.7
1985	28.7*	18.6*	26.8*	20.5	18.3	26.5	24.7	31.0	31.4	35.4	58.0	84.4	240.0
1990	**24.6***	**16.9***	**22.4***	**15.7**	**16.5**	**21.9**	**19.7**	**19.2**	**28.6**	**35.3**	**47.3**	**81.1**	**197.6**
1995 projected	*20.9**	*14.9**	*18.3**	*14.6*	*12.9*	*17.6*	*14.1*	*14.6*	*23.7*	*30.6*	*42.8*	*69.7*	*169.7*

(*The rates for the age groups 0–34 and 35–69 are the means of seven five-yearly rates, but the all-ages rates are standardised to the conventional "European" age distribution)

AUSTRALIA: 1975

Smoking-attributed deaths (Sm.) and total deaths (Total)

		ALL CAUSES	ALL CANCER	Lung cancer	Upper aero-digestive ca.	Other cancer	COPD	Other respiratory	Vascular disease	Liver cirrhosis	Other medical	Non-medical
Males												
0–34	Sm.	–	–	–	–	–	–	–	–	–	–	–
	Total	6308	392	15	3	374	94	170	219	16	2316	3101
35–69	Sm.	8573	2828	1955	333	540	998	108	3985	–	654	–
	Total	27531	6264	2120	524	3620	1302	379	14305	711	2266	2304
		(31%)	(45%)	(92%)	(64%)	(15%)	(77%)	(28%)	(28%)		(29%)	
70+	Sm.	5511	1706	1138	162	406	1500	79	1964	–	262	–
	Total	26899	4852	1257	277	3318	2084	747	16268	84	2215	649
		(20%)	(35%)	(91%)	(58%)	(12%)	(72%)	(11%)	(12%)		(12%)	
Any age	Sm.	14084	4534	3093	495	946	2498	187	5949	–	916	–
	Total	60738	11508	3392	804	7312	3480	1296	30792	811	6797	6054
		(23%)	(39%)	(91%)	(62%)	(13%)	(72%)	(14%)	(19%)		(13%)	
Females												
0–34	Sm.	–	–	–	–	–	–	–	–	–	–	–
	Total	3249	314	2	4	308	74	110	163	7	1683	898
35–69	Sm.	1000	257	195	25	37	161	14	447	–	121	–
	Total	14773	4572	384	126	4062	440	189	6651	238	1747	936
		(7%)	(6%)	(51%)	(20%)	(1%)	(37%)	(7%)	(7%)		(7%)	
70+	Sm.	599	121	82	22	17	147	9	282	–	40	–
	Total	30261	3961	224	171	3566	601	844	21184	46	2800	825
		(2%)	(3%)	(37%)	(13%)	(0%)	(24%)	(1%)	(1%)		(1%)	
Any age	Sm.	1599	378	277	47	54	308	23	729	–	161	–
	Total	48283	8847	610	301	7936	1115	1143	27998	291	6230	2659
		(3%)	(4%)	(45%)	(16%)	(1%)	(28%)	(2%)	(3%)		(3%)	
Males+Females												
0–34	Sm.	–	–	–	–	–	–	–	–	–	–	–
	Total	9557	706	17	7	682	168	280	382	23	3999	3999
35–69	Sm.	9573	3085	2150	358	577	1159	122	4432	–	775	–
	Total	42304	10836	2504	650	7682	1742	568	20956	949	4013	3240
		(23%)	(28%)	(86%)	(55%)	(8%)	(67%)	(21%)	(21%)		(19%)	
70+	Sm.	6110	1827	1220	184	423	1647	88	2246	–	302	–
	Total	57160	8813	1481	448	6884	2685	1591	37452	130	5015	1474
		(11%)	(21%)	(82%)	(41%)	(6%)	(61%)	(6%)	(6%)		(6%)	
Any age	Sm.	15683	4912	3370	542	1000	2806	210	6678	–	1077	–
	Total	109021	20355	4002	1105	15248	4595	2439	58790	1102	13027	8713
		(14%)	(24%)	(84%)	(49%)	(7%)	(61%)	(9%)	(11%)		(8%)	

AUSTRALIA: 1985

Smoking-attributed deaths (Sm.) and total deaths (Total)

		ALL CAUSES	ALL CANCER	Lung cancer	Upper aero-digestive ca.	Other cancer	COPD	Other respiratory	Vascular disease	Liver cirrhosis	Other medical	Non-medical
Males												
0–34	Sm.	–	–	–	–	–	–	–	–	–	–	–
	Total	5600	361	3	9	349	66	74	231	30	1911	2927
35–69	Sm.	7735	3339	2246	421	672	942	104	2829	–	521	–
	Total	24351	7686	2440	664	4582	1235	384	10526	633	1900	1987
		(32%)	(43%)	(92%)	(63%)	(15%)	(76%)	(27%)	(27%)		(27%)	
70+	Sm.	7479	2658	1771	248	639	2108	121	2175	–	417	–
	Total	33628	7442	1953	419	5070	2897	1052	17899	155	3541	642
		(22%)	(36%)	(91%)	(59%)	(13%)	(73%)	(12%)	(12%)		(12%)	
Any age	Sm.	15214	5997	4017	669	1311	3050	225	5004	–	938	–
	Total	63579	15489	4396	1092	10001	4198	1510	28656	818	7352	5556
		(24%)	(39%)	(91%)	(61%)	(13%)	(73%)	(15%)	(17%)		(13%)	
Females												
0–34	Sm.	–	–	–	–	–	–	–	–	–	–	–
	Total	2795	332	8	2	322	60	60	142	9	1366	826
35–69	Sm.	1839	647	492	65	90	360	27	611	–	194	–
	Total	13328	5631	715	182	4734	642	201	4474	224	1419	737
		(14%)	(11%)	(69%)	(36%)	(2%)	(56%)	(13%)	(14%)		(14%)	
70+	Sm.	2055	467	329	69	69	551	41	815	–	181	–
	Total	38104	5901	529	236	5136	1170	1312	23656	88	5194	783
		(5%)	(8%)	(62%)	(29%)	(1%)	(47%)	(3%)	(3%)		(3%)	
Any age	Sm.	3894	1114	821	134	159	911	68	1426	–	375	–
	Total	54227	11864	1252	420	10192	1872	1573	28272	321	7979	2346
		(7%)	(9%)	(66%)	(32%)	(2%)	(49%)	(4%)	(5%)		(5%)	
Males+Females												
0–34	Sm.	–	–	–	–	–	–	–	–	–	–	–
	Total	8395	693	11	11	671	126	134	373	39	3277	3753
35–69	Sm.	9574	3986	2738	486	762	1302	131	3440	–	715	–
	Total	37679	13317	3155	846	9316	1877	585	15000	857	3319	2724
		(25%)	(30%)	(87%)	(57%)	(8%)	(69%)	(22%)	(23%)		(22%)	
70+	Sm.	9534	3125	2100	317	708	2659	162	2990	–	598	–
	Total	71732	13343	2482	655	10206	4067	2364	41555	243	8735	1425
		(13%)	(23%)	(85%)	(48%)	(7%)	(65%)	(7%)	(7%)		(7%)	
Any age	Sm.	19108	7111	4838	803	1470	3961	293	6430	–	1313	–
	Total	117806	27353	5648	1512	20193	6070	3083	56928	1139	15331	7902
		(16%)	(26%)	(86%)	(53%)	(7%)	(65%)	(10%)	(11%)		(9%)	

(To be conservative, no deaths before age 35, and none from liver cirrhosis or non-medical causes, were attributed to smoking.)

AUSTRALIA: 1990

Smoking–attributed deaths (Sm.) and total deaths (Total)

		ALL CAUSES	ALL CANCER	Lung cancer	Upper aero–digestive ca.	Other cancer	COPD	Other respiratory	Vascular disease	Liver cirrhosis	Other medical	Non–medical
Males												
0–34	Sm.	–	–	–	–	–	–	–	–	–	–	–
	Total	5185	358	4	9	345	51	63	209	35	1800	2669
35–69	Sm.	6682	3186	2114	441	631	813	79	2065	–	539	–
	Total	23492	8128	2332	755	5041	1105	345	8979	609	2284	2042
		(28%)	(39%)	(91%)	(58%)	(13%)	(74%)	(23%)	(23%)		(24%)	
70+	Sm.	7302	2846	1893	242	711	2000	108	1899	–	449	–
	Total	35379	8732	2111	430	6191	2830	1029	17607	139	4285	757
		(21%)	(33%)	(90%)	(56%)	(11%)	(71%)	(10%)	(11%)		(10%)	
Any age	Sm.	13984	6032	4007	683	1342	2813	187	3964	–	988	–
	Total	64056	17218	4447	1194	11577	3986	1437	26795	783	8369	5468
		(22%)	(35%)	(90%)	(57%)	(12%)	(71%)	(13%)	(15%)		(12%)	
Females												
0–34	Sm.	–	–	–	–	–	–	–	–	–	–	–
	Total	2511	288	6	4	278	53	35	106	13	1221	795
35–69	Sm.	1863	737	575	65	97	371	22	536	–	197	–
	Total	12735	5984	818	170	4996	639	155	3660	207	1403	687
		(15%)	(12%)	(70%)	(38%)	(2%)	(58%)	(14%)	(15%)		(14%)	
70+	Sm.	3096	760	546	96	118	800	58	1168	–	310	–
	Total	39613	6817	769	247	5801	1381	1203	23206	98	6117	791
		(8%)	(11%)	(71%)	(39%)	(2%)	(58%)	(5%)	(5%)		(5%)	
Any age	Sm.	4959	1497	1121	161	215	1171	80	1704	–	507	–
	Total	54859	13089	1593	421	11075	2073	1393	26972	318	8741	2273
		(9%)	(11%)	(70%)	(38%)	(2%)	(56%)	(6%)	(6%)		(6%)	
Males+Females												
0–34	Sm.	–	–	–	–	–	–	–	–	–	–	–
	Total	7696	646	10	13	623	104	98	315	48	3021	3464
35–69	Sm.	8545	3923	2689	506	728	1184	101	2601	–	736	–
	Total	36227	14112	3150	925	10037	1744	500	12639	816	3687	2729
		(24%)	(28%)	(85%)	(55%)	(7%)	(68%)	(20%)	(21%)		(20%)	
70+	Sm.	10398	3606	2439	338	829	2800	166	3067	–	759	–
	Total	74992	15549	2880	677	11992	4211	2232	40813	237	10402	1548
		(14%)	(23%)	(85%)	(50%)	(7%)	(66%)	(7%)	(8%)		(7%)	
Any age	Sm.	18943	7529	5128	844	1557	3984	267	5668	–	1495	–
	Total	118915	30307	6040	1615	22652	6059	2830	53767	1101	17110	7741
		(16%)	(25%)	(85%)	(52%)	(7%)	(66%)	(9%)	(11%)		(9%)	

AUSTRALIA: 1995

Smoking–attributed deaths (Sm.) and total deaths (Total)

		ALL CAUSES	ALL CANCER	Lung cancer	Upper aero–digestive ca.	Other cancer	COPD	Other respiratory	Vascular disease	Liver cirrhosis	Other medical	Non–medical
Males												
0–34	Sm.	–	–	–	–	–	–	–	–	–	–	–
	Total	4703	344	3	7	334	42	50	195	35	1677	2360
35–69	Sm.	5256	2736	1795	411	530	613	56	1353	–	498	–
	Total	21001	7903	2025	776	5102	882	286	6950	539	2519	1922
		(25%)	(35%)	(89%)	(53%)	(10%)	(70%)	(20%)	(19%)		(20%)	
70+	Sm.	6695	2879	1923	232	724	1715	88	1564	–	449	–
	Total	34314	9488	2167	430	6891	2501	911	15773	129	4668	844
		(20%)	(30%)	(89%)	(54%)	(11%)	(69%)	(10%)	(10%)		(10%)	
Any age	Sm.	11951	5615	3718	643	1254	2328	144	2917	–	947	–
	Total	60018	17735	4195	1213	12327	3425	1247	22918	703	8864	5126
		(20%)	(32%)	(89%)	(53%)	(10%)	(68%)	(12%)	(13%)		(11%)	
Females												
0–34	Sm.	–	–	–	–	–	–	–	–	–	–	–
	Total	2136	245	3	2	240	43	25	77	17	1035	694
35–69	Sm.	1783	786	627	59	100	358	15	436	–	188	–
	Total	11577	5985	887	150	4948	598	113	2803	180	1288	610
		(15%)	(13%)	(71%)	(39%)	(2%)	(60%)	(13%)	(16%)		(15%)	
70+	Sm.	4054	1111	828	115	168	1022	66	1412	–	443	–
	Total	38847	7524	1081	253	6190	1574	1025	21188	107	6662	767
		(10%)	(15%)	(77%)	(45%)	(3%)	(65%)	(6%)	(7%)		(7%)	
Any age	Sm.	5837	1897	1455	174	268	1380	81	1848	–	631	–
	Total	52560	13754	1971	405	11378	2215	1163	24068	304	8985	2071
		(11%)	(14%)	(74%)	(43%)	(2%)	(62%)	(7%)	(8%)		(7%)	
Males+Females												
0–34	Sm.	–	–	–	–	–	–	–	–	–	–	–
	Total	6839	589	6	9	574	85	75	272	52	2712	3054
35–69	Sm.	7039	3522	2422	470	630	971	71	1789	–	686	–
	Total	32578	13888	2912	926	10050	1480	399	9753	719	3807	2532
		(22%)	(25%)	(83%)	(51%)	(6%)	(66%)	(18%)	(18%)		(18%)	
70+	Sm.	10749	3990	2751	347	892	2737	154	2976	–	892	–
	Total	73161	17012	3248	683	13081	4075	1936	36961	236	11330	1611
		(15%)	(23%)	(85%)	(51%)	(7%)	(67%)	(8%)	(8%)		(8%)	
Any age	Sm.	17788	7512	5173	817	1522	3708	225	4765	–	1578	–
	Total	112578	31489	6166	1618	23705	5640	2410	46986	1007	17849	7197
		(16%)	(24%)	(84%)	(50%)	(6%)	(66%)	(9%)	(10%)		(9%)	

(To be conservative, no deaths before age 35, and none from liver cirrhosis or non–medical causes, were attributed to smoking.)

AUSTRIA: 1990

		No. of deaths			Standardised rates (Defined on p.274)			Annual death rates / 100, 000						
		All ages	0–34	35–69	All ages	0–34	35–69	0–4	5–9	10–14	15–19	20–24	25–29	30–34
ALL CAUSES	M	38386	2113	14197	1016.9	106.7	1099.7	211.4	20.4	19.5	99.3	131.0	113.8	151.4
	F	44566	932	8263	613.3	52.4	509.0	177.8	13.8	12.2	31.3	36.2	41.1	54.4
Tuberculosis	M	119	3	61	3.2	0.1	4.5	–	–	–	–	0.3	0.3	0.3
	F	59	1	14	0.9	0.0	0.9	–	–	–	–	–	0.3	–
Other infective	M	71	11	34	2.1	0.7	2.4	4.0	–	–	–	0.3	–	0.3
and parasitic	F	75	13	25	1.5	0.8	1.6	3.2	0.4	0.5	0.4	0.3	0.3	0.3
ALL CANCER	M	9666	115	4458	261.3	5.6	351.6	1.3	1.7	4.0	5.2	5.1	7.6	14.1
	F	9664	109	3571	158.4	5.5	221.4	6.5	2.2	1.4	2.0	4.4	6.3	15.8
Mouth and	M	323	3	257	9.1	0.1	18.6	–	–	–	–	–	–	1.0
pharynx cancer	F	75	–	28	1.2	–	1.8	–	–	–	–	–	–	–
Oesophagus cancer	M	191	1	128	5.3	0.0	9.8	–	–	–	–	–	–	0.3
	F	44	–	12	0.7	–	0.8	–	–	–	–	–	–	–
Stomach cancer	M	973	5	376	26.1	0.2	30.4	–	–	–	–	–	0.6	1.0
	F	864	5	229	12.6	0.2	14.3	–	–	–	–	–	0.6	1.0
Colorectal cancer	M	1285	5	535	34.5	0.2	42.9	–	–	–	–	–	0.3	1.3
	F	1465	2	417	22.1	0.1	25.9	–	–	–	–	–	–	0.7
Liver cancer	M	190	2	103	5.2	0.1	8.5	–	–	–	0.7	–	–	–
	F	74	–	32	1.2	–	2.0	–	–	–	–	–	–	–
Pancreas cancer	M	485	–	236	13.3	–	18.4	–	–	–	–	–	–	–
	F	602	3	175	9.1	0.1	10.9	–	–	–	–	–	0.3	0.7
Larynx cancer	M	209	1	130	5.9	0.0	9.8	–	–	–	–	0.3	–	–
	F	15	–	7	0.2	–	0.4	–	–	–	–	–	–	–
Lung cancer	M	2427	1	1349	66.9	0.0	106.7	–	–	–	–	–	–	0.3
	F	752	3	327	12.8	0.1	20.2	–	–	–	–	–	–	1.0
Malignant melanoma	M	120	4	78	3.3	0.2	5.6	–	–	–	–	–	0.6	0.7
	F	118	5	60	2.2	0.2	3.7	–	–	–	–	0.3	0.6	0.7
Female breast cancer	F	1736	11	871	31.9	0.5	53.9	–	–	–	–	–	0.6	3.0
Cervix cancer	F	199	4	121	4.0	0.2	7.4	–	–	–	–	–	–	1.3
Other uterine cancer	F	448	2	180	7.4	0.1	11.2	–	–	–	–	–	–	0.7
Ovarian cancer	F	655	4	308	11.7	0.2	19.1	–	–	–	–	0.3	0.3	0.7
Prostate cancer	M	1110	–	190	28.3	–	16.2	–	–	–	–	–	–	–
Bladder cancer	M	358	–	112	9.3	–	9.1	–	–	–	–	–	–	–
	F	186	–	44	2.6	–	2.7	–	–	–	–	–	–	–
Other and ill–defined	M	1344	48	683	36.6	2.4	53.7	0.9	0.8	1.8	3.0	2.4	2.3	5.4
cancer sites	F	1728	36	539	27.1	1.9	33.5	3.7	0.9	1.4	0.8	1.6	1.8	3.4
Hodgkin's disease	M	63	7	33	1.7	0.3	2.4	–	0.4	–	–	0.3	1.2	0.3
	F	66	5	18	1.0	0.2	1.1	–	–	–	–	0.6	0.3	0.7
Myeloma and non–	M	296	10	138	8.1	0.5	10.8	–	–	0.4	–	0.3	0.6	2.0
Hodgkin lymphomas	F	342	7	107	5.3	0.3	6.6	0.5	–	–	–	0.6	0.6	0.7
Leukaemia	M	292	28	110	7.7	1.4	8.8	0.4	0.4	1.8	1.5	1.8	2.0	1.7
	F	295	22	96	5.1	1.2	6.0	2.3	1.3	–	1.2	1.0	1.2	1.3
ALL VASCULAR	M	17672	109	5226	460.8	5.1	419.3	2.6	0.4	0.4	4.5	5.4	9.7	12.8
DISEASE	F	24957	61	2599	302.5	2.9	159.3	1.9	–	–	1.6	3.5	3.9	9.7
Rheumatic heart	M	56	1	25	1.5	0.0	2.0	–	–	–	–	0.3	–	–
disease and fever	F	194	–	46	2.8	–	2.8	–	–	–	–	–	–	–
Hypertensive disease	M	464	2	133	12.1	0.1	10.5	–	–	–	–	–	–	0.7
	F	956	3	122	12.0	0.1	7.6	–	–	–	–	0.3	–	0.7
Ischaemic heart	M	7956	16	2990	211.3	0.7	240.6	–	–	–	–	0.3	1.8	3.0
disease	F	8304	2	1119	104.6	0.1	68.5	–	–	–	–	–	0.3	0.3
Pulmonary embolism	M	514	3	150	13.4	0.1	11.8	–	–	–	–	–	0.3	0.7
and other venous	F	1047	8	185	13.7	0.4	11.4	–	–	–	0.4	1.3	0.6	0.3
Cerebrovascular	M	4118	34	876	105.7	1.7	70.6	2.2	–	0.4	1.5	1.8	2.3	3.4
disease	F	7081	21	598	83.9	1.0	36.3	0.5	–	–	–	1.3	0.9	4.4
Other vascular	M	4564	53	1052	116.7	2.5	83.7	0.4	0.4	–	3.0	3.0	5.3	5.0
disease	F	7375	27	529	85.4	1.3	32.6	1.4	–	–	1.2	0.6	2.1	4.0
Chronic obstructive	M	1355	14	335	34.8	0.7	27.6	0.4	0.4	0.9	0.7	0.6	0.9	1.0
pulmonary disease	F	890	5	144	11.4	0.2	8.8	0.5	–	–	–	–	0.6	0.7
Other respiratory	M	834	31	194	21.5	1.7	14.6	7.0	–	0.4	0.4	0.6	1.8	1.7
disease	F	1119	24	94	13.6	1.4	5.7	6.5	0.4	–	0.8	–	0.9	1.3
Peptic ulcer	M	245	7	88	6.5	0.3	7.0	–	–	–	–	–	0.6	1.7
	F	269	–	45	3.5	–	2.8	–	–	–	–	–	–	–
Liver cirrhosis	M	1486	22	1136	41.9	1.0	83.2	–	–	–	0.4	0.6	1.5	4.7
	F	658	12	397	13.2	0.6	24.5	–	–	–	0.4	0.3	1.2	2.0
Renal disease	M	300	4	94	7.8	0.2	7.6	–	–	–	–	0.6	–	0.7
	F	436	6	76	5.9	0.3	4.7	0.5	–	–	0.8	–	–	1.0
Pregnancy and birth	F	6	4	2	0.1	0.2	0.1	–	–	–	–	0.3	0.9	–
Congenital and	M	301	293	7	10.3	18.2	0.5	120.0	3.4	0.9	1.1	1.8	–	0.3
perinatal causes	F	263	248	9	9.4	16.3	0.6	108.6	1.8	0.9	–	1.6	–	1.0
Ill–defined causes	M	256	95	19	7.3	5.9	1.3	39.6	–	0.4	–	0.3	–	1.0
	F	451	54	17	6.3	3.5	1.0	24.1	–	–	–	–	0.6	–
Other medical causes	M	2471	185	922	65.2	9.4	70.1	15.8	3.0	4.4	5.6	7.8	10.8	18.1
	F	3753	91	709	52.1	4.9	43.3	11.6	2.2	1.9	4.4	2.5	6.6	5.4
ALL NON–	M	3610	1224	1623	94.2	57.8	110.0	20.7	11.5	8.0	81.3	107.5	80.7	94.7
MEDICAL CAUSES	F	1966	304	561	34.5	15.6	34.3	14.4	6.7	7.5	21.0	23.2	19.5	17.1
Motor vehicle	M	1046	576	358	26.4	27.2	23.9	3.1	6.4	4.9	52.8	56.0	33.6	33.9
traffic accidents	F	362	127	111	7.6	6.5	6.7	3.7	3.1	1.4	14.3	11.8	7.5	3.7
Fire	M	25	8	7	0.7	0.4	0.5	1.3	–	–	–	–	–	1.7
	F	17	2	3	0.3	0.1	0.2	0.5	–	0.5	–	–	–	–
Suicide	M	1284	360	682	33.8	16.4	46.3	–	–	0.4	17.6	31.0	30.1	35.6
	F	541	86	281	11.5	4.0	17.2	–	–	0.9	2.8	7.6	7.8	9.1
Homicide	M	69	35	30	1.9	1.8	1.8	3.5	0.8	–	1.5	2.1	1.5	3.0
	F	56	25	25	1.4	1.4	1.5	1.9	0.9	1.9	0.8	1.0	1.5	1.7
POPULATION (thousands):	M=males				3693.8	1927.9	1510.0	227.5	235.5	226.2	266.9	332.1	341.9	297.8
	F=females				4024.6	1852.5	1655.0	215.4	225.2	213.6	252.3	314.7	333.6	297.7

AUSTRIA: 1990

9th ICD categories

Annual death rates / 100, 000

35–39	40–44	45–49	50–54	55–59	60–64	65–69	70–74	75–79	80+/NK			
183.8	312.6	491.4	674.0	1183.2	1903.8	2949.5	4341.0	7320.6	14268.8	M	ALL CAUSES	001–999
88.5	158.2	231.1	343.9	549.3	800.6	1391.3	2243.1	4495.6	12124.4	F		
0.8	1.2	5.1	2.7	4.2	7.1	10.6	12.0	17.9	34.6	M	Tuberculosis	010–018, 137
–	–	0.4	0.9	1.5	1.4	2.0	3.4	5.9	14.4	F		
0.4	1.6	1.6	2.2	4.2	4.9	2.0	10.8	6.7	13.1	M	Other infective	Rest of 001–139
–	0.8	0.4	2.2	1.5	2.7	3.3	5.5	6.5	8.9	F	and parasitic	
27.3	58.7	127.3	215.4	394.9	665.0	972.7	1321.7	1870.0	2781.4	M	ALL CANCER	140–208
35.4	70.9	107.6	171.7	274.6	363.1	526.3	665.3	1047.0	1604.1	F		
2.8	5.1	19.1	17.9	25.9	28.8	30.6	22.9	24.7	26.3	M	Mouth and	140–149
–	0.8	0.8	1.3	2.0	4.1	3.3	6.2	8.8	11.4	F	pharynx cancer	
1.2	0.8	6.2	7.6	13.8	16.9	21.9	21.7	28.0	22.7	M	Oesophagus cancer	150
–	0.4	–	–	2.0	2.3	0.8	3.4	3.5	10.4	F		
4.3	4.7	6.2	12.1	30.7	57.6	97.1	154.2	213.0	327.4	M	Stomach cancer	151
2.8	3.6	1.5	6.6	22.0	22.8	40.8	52.3	106.4	184.8	F		
2.0	5.5	10.5	25.1	54.5	75.6	127.0	180.7	278.0	414.6	M	Colorectal cancer	153, 154
2.0	5.6	10.8	22.1	34.5	40.6	66.1	99.2	171.7	302.3	F		
–	0.8	1.2	4.5	9.5	14.7	28.6	24.1	35.9	39.4	M	Liver cancer	155.0
–	0.4	–	–	3.0	4.6	6.1	4.1	12.9	6.9	F		
1.2	2.4	9.0	13.4	18.5	37.0	47.2	74.7	78.5	139.8	M	Pancreas cancer	157
0.8	2.8	2.7	4.0	12.0	23.3	30.6	51.7	66.4	116.9	F		
–	3.9	4.7	9.9	13.2	17.4	19.3	27.7	32.5	31.1	M	Larynx cancer	161
–	–	0.4	–	1.0	–	1.6	0.7	0.6	3.0	F		
4.0	15.8	38.2	61.4	121.2	218.6	287.9	357.8	415.9	488.6	M	Lung cancer	162
2.8	5.6	11.2	13.7	20.5	37.0	50.6	55.1	86.4	96.6	F		
0.8	3.9	4.3	5.4	6.4	9.8	8.6	9.6	17.9	16.7	M	Malignant melanoma	172
0.8	3.2	3.1	3.1	4.0	4.1	7.3	7.6	12.3	10.4	F		
13.0	22.3	37.4	50.3	74.0	73.9	106.5	110.2	151.1	216.6	F	Female breast cancer	174
2.8	2.8	7.3	9.7	6.5	10.5	12.2	11.0	15.3	15.9	F	Cervix cancer	180
2.0	5.6	3.9	5.7	14.0	20.5	26.5	26.2	53.5	67.9	F	Other uterine cancer	179, 182
0.4	5.2	12.3	16.3	24.0	33.8	42.0	52.3	62.3	79.8	F	Ovarian cancer	183
–	0.4	1.6	3.6	13.2	29.4	65.2	144.6	317.3	617.7	M	Prostate cancer	185
–	0.4	3.1	0.9	9.5	23.9	25.9	38.6	97.5	151.7	M	Bladder cancer	188
0.4	0.4	0.8	1.8	1.5	4.6	9.4	9.6	21.2	45.6	F		
7.1	10.6	16.7	39.0	58.2	91.9	152.3	172.3	201.8	346.5	M	Other and ill-defined	Rest of 140–208
5.5	9.6	10.4	23.8	40.0	60.7	84.5	117.8	194.0	323.1	F	cancer sites	
1.2	2.0	–	1.8	3.2	4.4	4.7	9.6	7.8	9.6	M	Hodgkin's disease	201
0.8	0.8	0.4	1.3	0.5	0.9	2.9	3.4	9.4	10.9	F		
0.8	2.0	4.3	7.6	8.5	23.9	28.6	48.2	58.3	66.9	M	Myeloma and non–	200, 202–203
0.4	–	2.7	3.5	6.0	9.6	23.7	32.4	40.6	55.5	F	Hodgkin lymphomas	
2.0	0.4	2.3	5.4	8.5	15.2	27.9	34.9	62.8	82.4	M	Leukaemia	204–208
1.2	2.0	1.9	8.4	7.0	10.0	11.4	22.0	30.6	46.1	F		
32.4	68.2	130.8	206.4	415.6	771.6	1309.8	2166.3	3913.7	8420.5	M	ALL VASCULAR	390–459
14.6	27.9	49.0	64.5	140.1	266.0	553.2	1109.5	2537.9	8111.5	F	DISEASE	
–	–	0.4	0.9	5.3	1.1	6.6	7.2	7.8	20.3	M	Rheumatic heart	390–398
0.4	0.8	1.2	0.9	2.0	5.9	8.6	15.8	28.8	37.7	F	disease and fever	
0.8	0.8	3.9	6.7	14.8	18.5	27.9	54.2	105.4	227.0	M	Hypertensive disease	401–405
0.8	0.4	1.2	4.4	9.5	16.0	21.2	48.2	89.9	301.3	F		
14.2	35.9	70.1	115.1	239.3	462.2	747.3	1095.2	1761.2	2951.0	M	Ischaemic heart	410–414
2.8	8.0	17.7	21.6	59.0	114.1	256.6	475.9	938.3	2426.2	F	disease	
1.2	1.2	6.2	6.7	10.1	24.5	32.6	71.1	136.8	215.1	M	Pulmonary embolism	415.1, 451–453
0.8	1.2	3.5	5.7	13.0	17.8	37.9	44.1	133.5	279.0	F	and other venous	
7.5	12.6	21.8	36.3	60.9	114.7	240.7	492.8	1011.2	2266.4	M	Cerebrovascular	430–438
7.1	9.6	12.3	17.7	23.5	54.7	129.3	284.4	755.4	2360.8	F	disease	
8.7	17.7	28.4	40.8	85.2	150.6	254.7	445.8	891.3	2740.7	M	Other vascular	Rest of 390–459
2.8	8.0	13.1	14.1	33.0	57.5	99.6	241.0	592.0	2706.6	F	disease	
0.8	2.8	5.1	11.6	28.1	47.3	97.7	144.6	317.3	720.4	M	Chronic obstructive	490–496
0.4	2.0	1.9	6.6	7.5	13.2	30.2	39.3	89.4	263.6	F	pulmonary disease	
2.0	5.5	7.0	13.4	22.8	18.5	33.2	72.3	171.5	473.1	M	Other respiratory	Rest of 460–519
2.0	3.2	3.1	5.3	4.5	7.3	14.7	30.3	89.4	398.9	F	disease	
–	2.0	1.9	3.6	6.9	14.7	19.9	26.5	22.4	129.0	M	Peptic ulcer	531–533
0.4	0.8	1.2	1.8	3.5	4.6	7.3	11.7	21.8	84.2	F		
14.6	38.2	61.9	71.2	113.8	132.7	149.6	125.3	135.7	123.1	M	Liver cirrhosis	571
5.9	10.0	20.1	23.0	30.0	36.5	46.1	43.4	53.5	47.1	F		
–	2.0	2.3	5.4	5.8	11.4	25.9	34.9	53.8	149.3	M	Renal disease	580–590
1.2	0.4	1.2	3.1	6.0	6.8	14.3	26.2	50.0	114.5	F		
0.8	–	–	–	–	–	–	–	–	–	F	Pregnancy and birth	630–676
0.4	–	0.8	0.4	–	1.1	0.7	–	–	1.2	M	Congenital and	740–779
0.4	–	0.8	0.4	1.0	0.5	0.8	0.7	0.6	2.0	F	perinatal causes	
0.4	1.6	0.8	0.9	0.5	3.8	1.3	8.4	26.9	132.6	M	Ill-defined causes	780–799
–	0.4	0.4	1.8	1.0	0.9	2.9	5.5	16.5	170.5	F		
21.7	27.6	37.8	36.3	79.4	106.0	182.2	253.0	507.8	837.5	M	Other medical causes	Rest of 001–799
7.1	13.5	17.4	29.1	38.0	56.1	141.6	221.8	432.7	939.0	F		
83.0	103.3	109.0	104.3	106.9	119.6	143.6	165.1	276.9	452.8	M	ALL NON–	E800–E999
20.5	28.3	27.8	33.6	40.0	41.5	48.6	80.6	144.6	365.7	F	MEDICAL CAUSES	
22.1	24.4	26.1	19.7	21.2	25.6	27.9	31.3	51.6	47.8	M	Motor vehicle	E810–E819
5.5	5.6	5.4	6.2	6.5	7.8	10.2	19.3	29.4	22.8	F	traffic accidents	
0.4	0.8	–	–	–	1.1	1.3	2.4	3.4	6.0	M	Fire	E890–E899
–	–	0.4	0.4	–	–	0.4	1.4	0.6	4.5	F		
32.8	41.8	48.3	47.0	43.4	44.6	66.5	67.5	98.7	117.1	M	Suicide	E950–E959
11.4	16.3	14.7	18.5	20.0	21.4	18.0	28.9	31.7	38.7	F		
0.8	3.9	2.3	3.1	1.6	1.1	–	–	2.2	2.4	M	Homicide	E960–E969
0.8	2.0	1.5	–	3.0	0.9	2.4	–	0.6	2.5	F		
253.0	253.7	256.8	223.3	188.9	183.9	150.4	83.0	89.2	83.7	M	**POPULATION (thousands)**	
254.1	251.0	259.2	226.5	199.9	219.2	245.1	145.2	170.1	201.8	F		

AUSTRIA: Males

	All ages	0–34	35–69	35–39	40–44	45–49	50–54	55–59	60–64	65–69	70–74	75–79	80+/NK
POPULATION (1000s)													
1955	3227.8	1712.1	1319.9	141.6	214.1	237.7	243.2	203.8	154.3	125.2	94.7	61.0	40.1
1965	3390.7	1849.5	1329.4	223.4	206.2	134.5	199.3	212.6	201.7	151.7	99.1	63.8	48.9
1975	3543.2	1973.6	1313.8	234.8	208.9	217.3	195.5	123.5	171.6	162.2	129.1	75.1	51.6
1985	3583.3	1898.1	1406.2	253.7	259.8	228.5	197.9	198.4	169.0	98.9	119.5	89.4	70.1
1990	**3693.8**	**1927.9**	**1510.0**	**253.0**	**253.7**	**256.8**	**223.3**	**188.9**	**183.9**	**150.4**	**83.0**	**89.2**	**83.7**
1995 projected	*3647.4*	*1799.3*	*1586.0*	*294.4*	*250.2*	*248.1*	*247.9*	*210.4*	*173.3*	*161.7*	*122.7*	*58.5*	*80.9*
NUMBER OF DEATHS													
All causes													
1955	43523	5523	18308	348	809	1460	2604	3601	4173	5313	6117	6185	7390
1965	47415	4269	20451	658	820	810	1824	3569	5822	6948	6758	6710	9227
1975	46821	3542	17288	608	922	1403	1877	1844	4129	6505	8418	7804	9769
1985	41873	2570	13893	552	965	1192	1797	2751	3532	3104	6130	7698	11582
1990	**38386**	**2113**	**14197**	**465**	**793**	**1262**	**1505**	**2235**	**3501**	**4436**	**3603**	**6530**	**11943**
1995 projected	*32744*	*1592*	*12938*	*471*	*695*	*1001*	*1394*	*2136*	*3009*	*4232*	*4610*	*3654*	*9950*
Lung cancer													
1955	1925	5	1431	3	25	88	219	377	368	351	259	172	58
1965	2611	11	1754	13	24	35	144	314	595	629	441	277	128
1975	2670	7	1344	13	27	76	126	158	360	584	671	430	218
1985	2461	1	1188	6	44	61	155	268	372	282	454	435	383
1990	**2427**	**1**	**1349**	**10**	**40**	**98**	**137**	**229**	**402**	**433**	**297**	**371**	**409**
1995 projected	*2296*	*2*	*1332*	*12*	*49*	*89*	*138*	*232*	*365*	*447*	*400*	*216*	*346*
ANNUAL DEATH RATE / 100,000 (*The rates for the age groups 0–34 and 35–69 are the means of seven five-yearly rates, but the all-ages rates are standardised to the conventional "European" age distribution)													
All causes													
1955	1510.0*	324.5*	1574.8*	245.8	377.9	614.2	1070.7	1766.9	2704.5	4243.6	6459.3	10139.3	18428.9
1965	1487.1*	213.2*	1622.1*	294.5	397.7	602.2	915.2	1678.7	2886.5	4580.1	6819.4	10517.2	18869.1
1975	1411.6*	189.0*	1459.4*	258.9	441.4	645.7	960.1	1493.1	2406.2	4010.5	6520.5	10391.5	18932.2
1985	1180.0*	134.4*	1233.4*	217.6	371.4	521.7	908.0	1386.6	2089.9	3138.5	5129.7	8610.7	16522.1
1990	**1016.9***	**106.7***	**1099.7***	**183.8**	**312.6**	**491.4**	**674.0**	**1183.2**	**1903.8**	**2949.5**	**4341.0**	**7320.6**	**14268.8**
1995 projected	*877.4**	*84.9**	*967.5**	*160.0*	*277.8*	*403.5*	*562.3*	*1015.2*	*1736.3*	*2617.2*	*3757.1*	*6246.2*	*12299.1*
All cancer													
1955	275.9*	10.7*	412.4*	31.1	58.4	130.8	261.9	512.3	770.6	1121.4	1477.3	1816.4	2099.8
1965	295.7*	11.8*	425.6*	44.3	61.6	127.1	212.7	473.7	810.6	1249.2	1698.3	2108.2	2329.2
1975	282.2*	10.7*	371.6*	29.8	68.9	129.8	232.7	405.7	674.2	1059.8	1603.4	2233.0	2569.8
1985	265.5*	7.0*	345.4*	33.5	74.3	117.7	241.5	416.8	616.6	917.1	1356.5	1993.3	2811.7
1990	**261.3***	**5.6***	**351.6***	**27.3**	**58.7**	**127.3**	**215.4**	**394.9**	**665.0**	**972.7**	**1321.7**	**1870.0**	**2781.4**
1995 projected	*255.7**	*4.5**	*351.6**	*22.1*	*56.8*	*119.3*	*204.1*	*393.1*	*684.4*	*981.4*	*1275.5*	*1793.2*	*2705.8*
Lung cancer													
1955	61.0*	0.3*	120.7*	2.1	11.7	37.0	90.0	185.0	238.5	280.4	273.5	282.0	144.6
1965	75.9*	0.6*	139.0*	5.8	11.6	26.0	72.3	147.7	295.0	414.6	445.0	434.2	261.8
1975	76.5*	0.4*	116.5*	5.5	12.9	35.0	64.5	127.9	209.8	360.0	519.8	572.6	422.5
1985	71.3*	0.0*	109.2*	2.4	16.9	26.7	78.3	135.1	220.1	285.1	379.9	486.6	546.4
1990	**66.9***	**0.0***	**106.7***	**4.0**	**15.8**	**38.2**	**61.4**	**121.2**	**218.6**	**287.9**	**357.8**	**415.9**	**488.6**
1995 projected	*62.0**	*0.1**	*101.8**	*4.1*	*19.6*	*35.9*	*55.7*	*110.3*	*210.6*	*276.4*	*326.0*	*369.2*	*427.7*
Upper aerodigestive cancer (mouth, oesophagus, pharynx and larynx)													
1955	18.0*	0.1*	24.1*	3.5	1.9	5.9	14.8	30.9	49.3	62.3	95.0	108.2	214.5
1965	17.4*	0.1*	26.0*	2.2	1.5	8.2	10.0	32.0	54.5	73.8	92.8	117.6	155.4
1975	16.1*	0.3*	25.8*	2.1	8.1	14.3	21.5	29.1	47.2	58.0	68.2	81.2	131.8
1985	17.9*	0.1*	31.2*	3.2	14.6	24.1	30.8	43.3	49.1	53.6	72.0	74.9	97.0
1990	**20.3***	**0.2***	**38.1***	**4.0**	**9.9**	**30.0**	**35.4**	**52.9**	**63.1**	**71.8**	**72.3**	**85.2**	**80.0**
1995 projected	*23.2**	*0.3**	*45.0**	*3.1*	*10.4*	*32.2*	*42.0*	*64.2*	*79.6*	*83.5*	*81.5*	*87.2*	*76.6*
Other cancer													
1955	196.9*	10.3*	267.6*	25.4	44.8	87.9	157.1	296.4	482.8	778.8	1108.8	1426.2	1740.6
1965	202.4*	11.1*	260.6*	36.3	48.5	92.9	130.5	294.0	461.1	760.7	1160.4	1556.4	1912.1
1975	189.7*	10.1*	229.3*	22.1	47.9	80.5	146.8	248.6	417.2	641.8	1015.5	1579.2	2015.5
1985	176.2*	6.8*	204.9*	28.0	42.7	67.0	132.4	238.4	347.3	578.4	904.6	1431.8	2168.3
1990	**174.0***	**5.3***	**206.8***	**19.4**	**33.1**	**59.2**	**118.7**	**220.8**	**383.4**	**613.0**	**891.6**	**1368.8**	**2212.7**
1995 projected	*170.5**	*4.1**	*204.8**	*14.9*	*26.8*	*51.2*	*106.5*	*218.6*	*394.1*	*621.5*	*868.0*	*1336.8*	*2201.5*
Chronic obstructive pulmonary disease (COPD)													
1955	28.5*	1.8*	27.5*	0.7	2.8	4.6	21.0	46.1	44.1	73.5	119.3	195.1	503.7
1965	61.9*	1.0*	61.7*	2.2	3.9	5.9	15.1	48.4	125.9	230.1	289.6	413.8	1206.5
1975	38.0*	1.1*	34.0*	1.7	3.8	8.3	11.8	34.0	53.0	125.2	213.8	375.5	600.8
1985	46.6*	0.8*	35.8*	2.4	5.0	4.4	14.1	35.3	66.3	123.4	225.9	425.1	935.8
1990	**34.8***	**0.7***	**27.6***	**0.8**	**2.8**	**5.1**	**11.6**	**28.1**	**47.3**	**97.7**	**144.6**	**317.3**	**720.4**
1995 projected	*26.0**	*0.6**	*20.2**	*0.7*	*2.0*	*4.0*	*9.7*	*20.9*	*35.8*	*68.0*	*103.5*	*235.9*	*548.8*
Other respiratory disease													
1955	85.4*	31.4*	50.6*	2.8	7.9	16.0	37.0	52.0	85.5	152.6	315.7	600.0	1428.9
1965	58.9*	12.5*	42.3*	12.1	8.2	8.2	16.6	41.4	73.9	135.8	275.5	528.2	924.3
1975	66.9*	8.6*	39.7*	6.8	14.4	15.6	21.0	31.6	65.3	123.3	280.4	552.6	1434.1
1985	27.7*	2.6*	20.6*	3.9	5.4	10.1	16.2	23.2	21.9	63.7	95.4	209.2	589.2
1990	**21.5***	**1.7***	**14.6***	**2.0**	**5.5**	**7.0**	**13.4**	**22.8**	**18.5**	**33.2**	**72.3**	**171.5**	**473.1**
1995 projected	*17.0**	*1.3**	*11.2**	*1.4*	*4.0*	*5.6*	*11.7*	*20.0*	*12.7*	*22.9*	*53.8*	*133.3*	*382.0*
Vascular disease													
1955	586.5*	12.2*	573.7*	38.8	76.1	149.3	296.5	573.6	1060.9	1820.3	3021.1	5118.0	9394.0
1965	614.2*	7.9*	618.2*	49.7	102.8	177.7	310.1	578.1	1128.4	1980.9	3214.9	5253.9	9681.0
1975	648.0*	7.4*	593.9*	46.4	107.2	184.5	348.3	576.5	1010.5	1883.5	3267.2	5603.2	11286.8
1985	564.7*	6.1*	506.9*	41.8	89.7	149.2	292.6	525.7	945.0	1504.6	2715.5	4850.1	10204.0
1990	**460.8***	**5.1***	**419.3***	**32.4**	**68.2**	**130.8**	**206.4**	**415.6**	**771.6**	**1309.8**	**2166.3**	**3913.7**	**8420.5**
1995 projected	*371.9**	*4.4**	*336.6**	*24.5*	*55.6*	*98.8*	*158.5*	*323.2*	*637.0*	*1058.8*	*1743.3*	*3114.5*	*6898.6*
Liver cirrhosis													
1955	24.2*	0.7*	44.4*	3.5	8.9	20.6	37.0	58.4	71.9	110.2	125.7	116.4	64.8
1965	42.3*	0.9*	76.9*	9.0	19.9	40.9	59.2	91.3	144.8	173.4	188.7	191.2	184.0
1975	53.4*	2.5*	99.3*	14.1	51.7	66.7	94.1	115.8	155.6	197.3	193.6	217.0	180.2
1985	47.8*	2.2*	91.2*	21.3	33.5	64.8	95.5	123.5	159.2	140.5	154.0	176.7	127.0
1990	**41.9***	**1.0***	**83.2***	**14.6**	**38.2**	**61.9**	**71.2**	**113.8**	**132.7**	**149.6**	**125.3**	**135.7**	**123.1**
1995 projected	*36.4**	*0.7**	*73.2**	*12.6*	*36.4*	*54.0*	*60.9*	*94.1*	*122.3*	*132.3*	*107.6*	*112.8*	*105.1*
Other medical causes													
1955	376.9*	177.8*	318.5*	75.6	100.0	151.5	268.1	349.4	506.8	778.0	1169.0	1929.5	4336.7
1965	281.9*	103.2*	239.4*	56.0	88.3	101.1	157.0	255.9	408.0	609.8	919.3	1641.1	3832.3
1975	182.4*	71.3*	157.1*	43.0	64.1	81.0	108.4	156.3	256.4	390.3	670.8	1037.3	2199.6
1985	116.7*	45.9*	105.0*	24.8	38.5	48.6	95.5	124.0	163.9	239.6	376.6	692.4	1336.7
1990	**102.4***	**34.8***	**93.4***	**23.7**	**35.9**	**50.2**	**51.5**	**101.1**	**149.0**	**242.7**	**345.8**	**635.7**	**1297.5**
1995 projected	*90.7**	*26.6**	*82.1**	*23.1*	*34.8*	*37.5*	*38.3*	*78.4*	*136.8*	*225.7*	*319.5*	*608.5*	*1236.1*
All non-medical causes													
1955	132.6*	89.8*	147.9*	93.2	123.8	141.4	149.3	175.2	164.6	187.7	231.3	363.9	601.0
1965	132.2*	75.9*	158.0*	121.3	113.0	141.3	144.5	190.0	194.8	201.1	233.1	380.9	711.7
1975	140.6*	87.5*	163.9*	117.1	131.2	159.7	143.7	173.3	191.1	231.2	291.2	372.8	660.9
1985	111.1*	69.9*	128.5*	89.9	125.1	126.9	152.6	138.1	117.2	149.6	205.9	264.0	517.8
1990	**94.2***	**57.8***	**110.0***	**83.0**	**103.3**	**109.0**	**104.3**	**106.9**	**119.6**	**143.6**	**165.1**	**276.9**	**452.8**
1995 projected	*79.7**	*46.9**	*92.6**	*75.7*	*88.3*	*84.2*	*79.1*	*85.6*	*107.3*	*128.0*	*154.0*	*247.9*	*422.7*

AUSTRIA: Females

	All ages	0–34	35–69	35–39	40–44	45–49	50–54	55–59	60–64	65–69	70–74	75–79	80+/NK
POPULATION (1000s)													
1955	3719.2	1749.2	1676.3	190.4	273.7	288.3	277.4	252.7	213.6	180.2	137.8	92.5	63.4
1965	3864.1	1781.0	1706.3	236.2	282.7	183.8	261.7	271.2	252.6	218.1	166.6	115.5	94.7
1975	3976.6	1902.3	1605.0	230.9	207.7	234.5	274.7	175.8	243.2	238.2	201.9	143.5	123.9
1985	3974.3	1850.2	1579.6	249.1	258.9	227.7	202.5	224.7	258.3	158.4	202.5	170.9	171.1
1990	**4024.6**	**1852.5**	**1655.0**	**254.1**	**251.0**	**259.2**	**226.5**	**199.9**	**219.2**	**245.1**	**145.2**	**170.1**	**201.8**
1995 projected	*3953.5*	*1738.9*	*1666.6*	*296.9*	*252.7*	*247.0*	*253.9*	*220.2*	*191.5*	*204.4*	*219.8*	*118.8*	*209.4*
NUMBER OF DEATHS													
All causes													
1955	41472	3637	14121	378	746	1109	1752	2244	3208	4684	6182	7489	10043
1965	46858	2672	13740	338	624	618	1391	2254	3367	5148	6795	8453	15198
1975	49220	1809	11720	290	413	714	1282	1296	2919	4806	7260	9444	18987
1985	47705	1103	8416	267	463	568	795	1358	2539	2426	5791	9212	23183
1990	**44566**	**932**	**8263**	**225**	**397**	**599**	**779**	**1098**	**1755**	**3410**	**3257**	**7647**	**24467**
1995 projected	*38307*	*750*	*6607*	*226*	*355*	*509*	*788*	*1035*	*1348*	*2346*	*4097*	*4477*	*22376*
Lung cancer													
1955	304	6	180	2	4	16	33	40	38	47	52	36	30
1965	417	4	239	5	7	9	26	47	63	82	78	48	48
1975	544	1	272	1	7	13	31	30	85	105	112	82	77
1985	692	4	260	4	12	15	23	55	85	66	110	136	182
1990	**752**	**3**	**327**	**7**	**14**	**29**	**31**	**41**	**81**	**124**	**80**	**147**	**195**
1995 projected	*770*	*4*	*338*	*11*	*19*	*37*	*37*	*46*	*76*	*112*	*129*	*100*	*199*
ANNUAL DEATH RATE / 100,000 (*The rates for the age groups 0–34 and 35–69 are the means of seven five-yearly rates, but the all-ages rates are standardised to the conventional "European" age distribution)													
All causes													
1955	1063.9*	212.8*	925.2*	198.5	272.6	384.7	631.6	888.0	1501.9	2599.3	4486.2	8096.2	15840.7
1965	958.1*	133.2*	822.3*	143.1	220.7	336.2	531.5	831.1	1332.9	2360.4	4078.6	7318.6	16048.6
1975	861.1*	101.2*	721.5*	125.6	198.8	304.5	466.7	737.2	1200.2	2017.6	3595.8	6581.2	15324.5
1985	709.0*	62.6*	578.1*	107.2	178.8	249.5	392.6	604.4	983.0	1531.6	2859.8	5390.3	13549.4
1990	**613.3***	**52.4***	**509.0***	**88.5**	**158.2**	**231.1**	**343.9**	**549.3**	**800.6**	**1391.3**	**2243.1**	**4495.6**	**12124.4**
1995 projected	*528.7**	*44.0**	*436.4**	*76.1*	*140.5*	*206.1*	*310.4*	*470.0*	*703.9*	*1147.7*	*1864.0*	*3768.5*	*10685.8*
All cancer													
1955	195.3*	11.6*	282.0*	62.5	105.2	144.3	246.6	303.9	446.6	664.8	906.4	1263.8	1541.0
1965	192.3*	12.3*	272.1*	45.7	93.7	146.9	223.2	313.1	442.2	640.1	878.8	1220.8	1661.0
1975	177.2*	9.1*	256.0*	38.5	84.7	129.2	202.4	312.9	434.2	590.3	785.5	1118.5	1538.3
1985	164.6*	6.9*	231.1*	30.9	72.2	114.6	183.2	276.8	422.4	517.7	769.4	1022.2	1557.0
1990	**158.4***	**5.5***	**221.4***	**35.4**	**70.9**	**107.6**	**171.7**	**274.6**	**363.1**	**526.3**	**665.3**	**1047.0**	**1604.1**
1995 projected	*151.2**	*5.2**	*204.9**	*33.7*	*68.1*	*102.4*	*164.2*	*249.8*	*344.6*	*471.6*	*630.6*	*989.9*	*1649.0*
Lung cancer													
1955	7.3*	0.3*	11.4*	1.1	1.5	5.5	11.9	15.8	17.8	26.1	37.7	38.9	47.3
1965	8.5*	0.3*	14.2*	2.1	2.5	4.9	9.9	17.3	24.9	37.6	46.8	41.6	50.7
1975	10.1*	0.1*	16.7*	0.4	3.4	5.5	11.3	17.1	35.0	44.1	55.5	57.1	62.1
1985	11.9*	0.2*	17.6*	1.6	4.6	6.6	11.4	24.5	32.9	41.7	54.3	79.6	106.4
1990	**12.8***	**0.1***	**20.2***	**2.8**	**5.6**	**11.2**	**13.7**	**20.5**	**37.0**	**50.6**	**55.1**	**86.4**	**96.6**
1995 projected	*13.7**	*0.2**	*22.3**	*3.7*	*7.5*	*15.0*	*14.6*	*20.9*	*39.7*	*54.8*	*58.7*	*84.2*	*95.0*
Upper aerodigestive cancer (mouth, oesophagus, pharynx and larynx)													
1955	3.4*	0.2*	3.5*	1.1	1.8	0.3	3.6	3.6	6.1	8.3	11.6	33.5	48.9
1965	2.8*	0.1*	3.3*	0.4	1.1	1.1	2.3	5.9	5.1	6.9	11.4	24.2	33.8
1975	2.1*	0.1*	2.6*	0.4	1.4	1.7	2.5	3.4	3.3	5.0	6.4	15.3	26.6
1985	2.1*	0.1*	2.8*	0.4	0.4	1.8	1.5	4.9	6.6	3.8	7.9	16.4	19.9
1990	**2.2***	–	**3.0***	–	**1.2**	**1.2**	**1.3**	**5.0**	**6.4**	**5.7**	**10.3**	**12.9**	**24.8**
1995 projected	*2.3**	–	*3.2**	–	*1.2*	*1.2*	*1.2*	*5.0*	*7.3*	*6.8*	*10.5*	*13.5*	*25.8*
Other cancer													
1955	184.6*	11.1*	267.1*	60.4	101.9	138.4	231.1	284.5	422.8	630.4	857.0	1191.4	1444.8
1965	181.0*	11.9*	254.7*	43.2	90.2	140.9	210.9	289.8	412.1	595.6	820.5	1155.0	1576.6
1975	165.1*	9.0*	236.8*	37.7	79.9	122.0	188.6	292.4	396.0	541.1	723.6	1046.0	1449.6
1985	150.6*	6.6*	210.8*	28.9	67.2	106.3	170.4	247.4	382.9	472.2	707.2	926.3	1430.7
1990	**143.5***	**5.4***	**198.3***	**32.7**	**64.1**	**95.3**	**156.7**	**249.1**	**319.8**	**470.0**	**599.9**	**947.7**	**1482.7**
1995 projected	*135.2**	*5.0**	*179.4**	*30.0*	*59.4*	*86.2*	*148.5*	*223.9*	*297.7*	*410.0*	*561.4*	*892.3*	*1528.2*
Chronic obstructive pulmonary disease (COPD)													
1955	14.1*	2.3*	6.9*	–	0.4	1.4	4.7	7.9	12.2	21.6	47.9	130.8	318.6
1965	22.2*	0.8*	13.1*	1.3	1.8	4.9	6.5	11.4	17.8	47.7	69.6	154.1	606.1
1975	13.7*	0.7*	12.2*	1.7	4.3	3.8	6.2	16.5	19.3	33.6	56.5	112.2	249.4
1985	15.6*	1.1*	9.5*	1.6	3.1	4.4	4.0	7.6	15.9	30.3	62.7	134.6	354.8
1990	**11.4***	**0.2***	**8.8***	**0.4**	**2.0**	**1.9**	**6.6**	**7.5**	**13.2**	**30.2**	**39.3**	**89.4**	**263.6**
1995 projected	*8.6**	*0.2**	*7.4**	*0.3*	*1.2*	*1.6*	*6.7*	*7.3*	*12.5*	*22.5*	*27.3*	*62.3*	*190.1*
Other respiratory disease													
1955	56.3*	22.7*	24.8*	4.2	9.1	9.0	10.5	17.0	41.2	82.7	194.5	438.9	1026.8
1965	40.2*	10.2*	21.5*	3.0	4.2	6.0	8.4	17.7	34.0	77.0	168.1	377.5	737.1
1975	42.6*	6.7*	19.6*	1.7	3.9	6.8	9.1	18.2	37.0	60.5	146.6	365.9	1021.0
1985	15.3*	1.9*	6.6*	1.6	2.7	3.5	3.0	5.8	11.6	18.3	46.4	110.6	414.4
1990	**13.6***	**1.4***	**5.7***	**2.0**	**3.2**	**3.1**	**5.3**	**4.5**	**7.3**	**14.7**	**30.3**	**89.4**	**398.9**
1995 projected	*12.1**	*1.1**	*4.8**	*2.0*	*3.2*	*3.6*	*5.5*	*3.6*	*5.2*	*10.3*	*22.7*	*74.1*	*371.1*
Vascular disease													
1955	469.5*	8.8*	355.4*	29.4	47.9	92.3	169.1	296.0	611.9	1241.4	2365.7	4601.1	9022.1
1965	437.7*	4.5*	300.7*	19.5	40.0	67.5	136.0	266.2	511.5	1064.2	2120.6	4161.9	9304.1
1975	431.9*	5.1*	263.3*	19.1	30.3	64.4	117.2	217.3	445.3	949.6	1967.8	3921.3	10121.1
1985	369.0*	3.6*	194.4*	16.9	28.2	52.7	93.3	154.0	331.0	685.0	1518.5	3358.1	9397.4
1990	**302.5***	**2.9***	**159.3***	**14.6**	**27.9**	**49.0**	**64.5**	**140.1**	**266.0**	**553.2**	**1109.5**	**2537.9**	**8111.5**
1995 projected	*243.8**	*2.6**	*124.8**	*13.8*	*25.3*	*39.3*	*54.0*	*113.1*	*215.1*	*412.9*	*818.5*	*1957.9*	*6771.3*
Liver cirrhosis													
1955	7.9*	0.6*	11.5*	1.6	1.1	8.0	7.9	15.8	16.4	30.0	47.9	45.4	50.5
1965	11.5*	0.6*	18.0*	2.1	7.1	6.5	16.0	20.3	32.5	41.3	54.6	62.3	81.3
1975	14.2*	1.0*	23.7*	4.8	10.1	18.3	23.3	29.0	37.4	42.8	60.9	53.7	75.1
1985	14.4*	0.7*	26.7*	9.2	12.7	18.0	29.1	40.9	39.1	37.9	40.5	45.1	57.3
1990	**13.2***	**0.6***	**24.5***	**5.9**	**10.0**	**20.1**	**23.0**	**30.0**	**36.5**	**46.1**	**43.4**	**53.5**	**47.1**
1995 projected	*12.3**	*0.5**	*22.4**	*4.0*	*8.7*	*17.4*	*18.9*	*24.5*	*34.5*	*48.4*	*49.1*	*54.7*	*46.3*
Other medical causes													
1955	268.9*	142.4*	196.6*	66.7	80.4	96.1	147.1	198.3	308.1	479.5	800.4	1388.1	3293.4
1965	201.9*	85.4*	149.0*	48.7	40.7	62.6	94.0	154.5	243.9	398.4	653.7	1074.5	2968.3
1975	127.3*	53.4*	100.1*	23.8	34.2	49.5	70.6	95.6	166.9	260.3	454.2	764.5	1603.7
1985	87.0*	31.1*	67.0*	15.3	23.6	31.6	43.0	70.8	113.8	171.1	316.0	551.8	1237.9
1990	**79.6***	**26.1***	**54.9***	**9.8**	**15.9**	**21.6**	**39.3**	**52.5**	**73.0**	**172.2**	**274.8**	**533.8**	**1333.5**
1995 projected	*73.3**	*21.4**	*44.3**	*7.4*	*11.1*	*16.6*	*30.3*	*37.7*	*60.6*	*146.3*	*253.4*	*521.9*	*1391.1*
All non-medical causes													
1955	51.8*	24.5*	48.0*	34.1	28.5	33.6	45.8	49.1	65.5	79.4	123.4	228.1	588.3
1965	52.4*	19.6*	48.0*	22.9	33.3	41.9	47.4	47.9	51.1	91.7	133.3	267.5	690.6
1975	54.3*	25.1*	46.6*	35.9	31.3	32.4	37.9	47.8	60.0	80.6	124.3	245.3	715.9
1985	43.1*	17.3*	42.7*	31.7	36.3	24.6	37.0	48.5	49.2	71.3	106.2	167.9	530.7
1990	**34.5***	**15.6***	**34.3***	**20.5**	**28.3**	**27.8**	**33.6**	**40.0**	**41.5**	**48.6**	**80.6**	**144.6**	**365.7**
1995 projected	*27.4**	*13.0**	*27.8**	*14.8*	*23.0*	*25.1*	*30.7*	*34.1*	*31.3*	*35.7*	*62.3*	*107.7*	*267.0*

AUSTRIA: 1975

Smoking-attributed deaths (Sm.) and total deaths (Total)

		ALL CAUSES	ALL CANCER	Lung cancer	Upper aero-digestive ca.	Other cancer	COPD	Other respiratory	Vascular disease	Liver cirrhosis	Other medical	Non-medical
Males												
0–34	Sm.	–	–	–	–	–	–	–	–	–	–	–
	Total	3542	205	7	5	193	20	160	139	46	1300	1672
35–69	Sm.	4721	1860	1245	197	418	303	129	1893	–	536	–
	Total	17288	4328	1344	306	2678	389	472	6916	1200	1889	2094
		(27%)	(43%)	(93%)	(64%)	(16%)	(78%)	(27%)	(27%)		(28%)	
70+	Sm.	5226	1882	1217	138	527	661	210	2066	–	407	–
	Total	25991	5073	1319	217	3537	868	1517	14250	506	2780	997
		(20%)	(37%)	(92%)	(64%)	(15%)	(76%)	(14%)	(14%)		(15%)	
Any age	Sm.	9947	3742	2462	335	945	964	339	3959	–	943	–
	Total	46821	9606	2670	528	6408	1277	2149	21305	1752	5969	4763
		(21%)	(39%)	(92%)	(63%)	(15%)	(75%)	(16%)	(19%)		(16%)	
Females												
0–34	Sm.	–	–	–	–	–	–	–	–	–	–	–
	Total	1809	169	1	1	167	13	118	93	18	930	468
35–69	Sm.	585	157	124	6	27	63	19	256	–	90	–
	Total	11720	4136	272	41	3823	195	319	4307	383	1630	750
		(5%)	(4%)	(46%)	(15%)	(1%)	(32%)	(6%)	(6%)		(6%)	
70+	Sm.	823	159	118	10	31	166	34	388	–	76	–
	Total	35691	5097	271	68	4758	584	2086	22140	293	4001	1490
		(2%)	(3%)	(44%)	(15%)	(1%)	(28%)	(2%)	(2%)		(2%)	
Any age	Sm.	1408	316	242	16	58	229	53	644	–	166	–
	Total	49220	9402	544	110	8748	792	2523	26540	694	6561	2708
		(3%)	(3%)	(44%)	(15%)	(1%)	(29%)	(2%)	(2%)		(3%)	
Males+Females												
0–34	Sm.	–	–	–	–	–	–	–	–	–	–	–
	Total	5351	374	8	6	360	33	278	232	64	2230	2140
35–69	Sm.	5306	2017	1369	203	445	366	148	2149	–	626	–
	Total	29008	8464	1616	347	6501	584	791	11223	1583	3519	2844
		(18%)	(24%)	(85%)	(59%)	(7%)	(63%)	(19%)	(19%)		(18%)	
70+	Sm.	6049	2041	1335	148	558	827	244	2454	–	483	–
	Total	61682	10170	1590	285	8295	1452	3603	36390	799	6781	2487
		(10%)	(20%)	(84%)	(52%)	(7%)	(57%)	(7%)	(7%)		(7%)	
Any age	Sm.	11355	4058	2704	351	1003	1193	392	4603	–	1109	–
	Total	96041	19008	3214	638	15156	2069	4672	47845	2446	12530	7471
		(12%)	(21%)	(84%)	(55%)	(7%)	(58%)	(8%)	(10%)		(9%)	

AUSTRIA: 1985

Smoking-attributed deaths (Sm.) and total deaths (Total)

		ALL CAUSES	ALL CANCER	Lung cancer	Upper aero-digestive ca.	Other cancer	COPD	Other respiratory	Vascular disease	Liver cirrhosis	Other medical	Non-medical
Males												
0–34	Sm.	–	–	–	–	–	–	–	–	–	–	–
	Total	2570	136	1	2	133	15	48	117	40	773	1441
35–69	Sm.	3903	1677	1097	245	335	277	66	1518	–	365	–
	Total	13893	3801	1188	384	2229	361	225	5387	1131	1223	1765
		(28%)	(44%)	(92%)	(64%)	(15%)	(77%)	(29%)	(28%)		(30%)	
70+	Sm.	4646	1745	1148	128	469	939	77	1658	–	227	–
	Total	25410	5374	1272	221	3881	1306	714	14734	431	2006	845
		(18%)	(32%)	(90%)	(58%)	(12%)	(72%)	(11%)	(11%)		(11%)	
Any age	Sm.	8549	3422	2245	373	804	1216	143	3176	–	592	–
	Total	41873	9311	2461	607	6243	1682	987	20238	1602	4002	4051
		(20%)	(37%)	(91%)	(61%)	(13%)	(72%)	(14%)	(16%)		(15%)	
Females												
0–34	Sm.	–	–	–	–	–	–	–	–	–	–	–
	Total	1103	128	4	2	122	21	32	67	13	506	336
35–69	Sm.	455	163	128	9	26	48	6	175	–	63	–
	Total	8416	3429	260	43	3126	136	97	2710	409	982	653
		(5%)	(5%)	(49%)	(21%)	(1%)	(35%)	(6%)	(6%)		(6%)	
70+	Sm.	1487	307	233	18	56	400	26	653	–	101	–
	Total	38186	5969	428	78	5463	964	992	24893	257	3701	1410
		(4%)	(5%)	(54%)	(23%)	(1%)	(41%)	(3%)	(3%)		(3%)	
Any age	Sm.	1942	470	361	27	82	448	32	828	–	164	–
	Total	47705	9526	692	123	8711	1121	1121	27670	679	5189	2399
		(4%)	(5%)	(52%)	(22%)	(1%)	(40%)	(3%)	(3%)		(3%)	
Males+Females												
0–34	Sm.	–	–	–	–	–	–	–	–	–	–	–
	Total	3673	264	5	4	255	36	80	184	53	1279	1777
35–69	Sm.	4358	1840	1225	254	361	325	72	1693	–	428	–
	Total	22309	7230	1448	427	5355	497	322	8097	1540	2205	2418
		(20%)	(25%)	(85%)	(59%)	(7%)	(65%)	(22%)	(21%)		(19%)	
70+	Sm.	6133	2052	1381	146	525	1339	103	2311	–	328	–
	Total	63596	11343	1700	299	9344	2270	1706	39627	688	5707	2255
		(10%)	(18%)	(81%)	(49%)	(6%)	(59%)	(6%)	(6%)		(6%)	
Any age	Sm.	10491	3892	2606	400	886	1664	175	4004	–	756	–
	Total	89578	18837	3153	730	14954	2803	2108	47908	2281	9191	6450
		(12%)	(21%)	(83%)	(55%)	(6%)	(59%)	(8%)	(8%)		(8%)	

(To be conservative, no deaths before age 35, and none from liver cirrhosis or non-medical causes, were attributed to smoking.)

AUSTRIA: 1990

Smoking–attributed deaths (Sm.) and total deaths (Total)

		ALL CAUSES	ALL CANCER	Lung cancer	Upper aero–digestive ca.	Other cancer	COPD	Other respiratory	Vascular disease	Liver cirrhosis	Other medical	Non–medical
Males												
0–34	Sm.	–	–	–	–	–	–	–	–	–	–	–
	Total	2113	115	1	5	109	14	31	109	22	598	1224
35–69	Sm.	3956	1940	1241	322	377	253	56	1371	–	336	–
	Total	14197	4458	1349	515	2594	335	194	5226	1136	1225	1623
		(28%)	(44%)	(92%)	(63%)	(15%)	(76%)	(29%)	(26%)		(27%)	
70+	Sm.	3558	1471	958	111	402	689	56	1159	–	183	–
	Total	22076	5093	1077	203	3813	1006	609	12337	328	1940	763
		(16%)	(29%)	(89%)	(55%)	(11%)	(68%)	(9%)	(9%)		(9%)	
Any age	Sm.	7514	3411	2199	433	779	942	112	2530	–	519	–
	Total	38386	9666	2427	723	6516	1355	834	17672	1486	3763	3610
		(20%)	(35%)	(91%)	(60%)	(12%)	(70%)	(13%)	(14%)		(14%)	
Females												
0–34	Sm.	–	–	–	–	–	–	–	–	–	–	–
	Total	932	109	3	0	106	5	24	61	12	417	304
35–69	Sm.	568	225	180	12	33	59	9	205	–	70	–
	Total	8263	3571	327	47	3197	144	94	2599	397	897	561
		(7%)	(6%)	(55%)	(26%)	(1%)	(41%)	(10%)	(8%)		(8%)	
70+	Sm.	1459	334	246	22	66	336	29	643	–	117	–
	Total	35371	5984	422	87	5475	741	1001	22297	249	3998	1101
		(4%)	(6%)	(58%)	(25%)	(1%)	(45%)	(3%)	(3%)		(3%)	
Any age	Sm.	2027	559	426	34	99	395	38	848	–	187	–
	Total	44566	9664	752	134	8778	890	1119	24957	658	5312	1966
		(5%)	(6%)	(57%)	(25%)	(1%)	(44%)	(3%)	(3%)		(4%)	
Males+Females												
0–34	Sm.	–	–	–	–	–	–	–	–	–	–	–
	Total	3045	224	4	5	215	19	55	170	34	1015	1528
35–69	Sm.	4524	2165	1421	334	410	312	65	1576	–	406	–
	Total	22460	8029	1676	562	5791	479	288	7825	1533	2122	2184
		(20%)	(27%)	(85%)	(59%)	(7%)	(65%)	(23%)	(20%)		(19%)	
70+	Sm.	5017	1805	1204	133	468	1025	85	1802	–	300	–
	Total	57447	11077	1499	290	9288	1747	1610	34634	577	5938	1864
		(9%)	(16%)	(80%)	(46%)	(5%)	(59%)	(5%)	(5%)		(5%)	
Any age	Sm.	9541	3970	2625	467	878	1337	150	3378	–	706	–
	Total	82952	19330	3179	857	15294	2245	1953	42629	2144	9075	5576
		(12%)	(21%)	(83%)	(54%)	(6%)	(60%)	(8%)	(8%)		(8%)	

AUSTRIA: 1995

Smoking–attributed deaths (Sm.) and total deaths (Total)

		ALL CAUSES	ALL CANCER	Lung cancer	Upper aero–digestive ca.	Other cancer	COPD	Other respiratory	Vascular disease	Liver cirrhosis	Other medical	Non–medical
Males												
0–34	Sm.	–	–	–	–	–	–	–	–	–	–	–
	Total	1592	91	2	6	83	11	23	88	15	450	914
35–69	Sm.	3584	1969	1219	383	367	191	43	1091	–	290	–
	Total	12938	4609	1332	627	2650	257	158	4345	1037	1110	1422
		(28%)	(43%)	(92%)	(61%)	(14%)	(74%)	(27%)	(25%)		(26%)	
70+	Sm.	2820	1304	845	112	347	466	39	855	–	156	–
	Total	18214	4803	962	213	3628	709	453	9542	283	1748	676
		(15%)	(27%)	(88%)	(53%)	(10%)	(66%)	(9%)	(9%)		(9%)	
Any age	Sm.	6404	3273	2064	495	714	657	82	1946	–	446	–
	Total	32744	9503	2296	846	6361	977	634	13975	1335	3308	3012
		(20%)	(34%)	(90%)	(59%)	(11%)	(67%)	(13%)	(14%)		(13%)	
Females												
0–34	Sm.	–	–	–	–	–	–	–	–	–	–	–
	Total	750	99	4	0	95	4	19	54	10	333	231
35–69	Sm.	537	250	201	14	35	49	8	169	–	61	–
	Total	6607	3116	338	48	2730	111	76	1844	344	666	450
		(8%)	(8%)	(59%)	(29%)	(1%)	(44%)	(11%)	(9%)		(9%)	
70+	Sm.	1235	332	245	24	63	235	24	524	–	120	–
	Total	30950	6015	428	93	5494	532	915	18304	270	4090	824
		(4%)	(6%)	(57%)	(26%)	(1%)	(44%)	(3%)	(3%)		(3%)	
Any age	Sm.	1772	582	446	38	98	284	32	693	–	181	–
	Total	38307	9230	770	141	8319	647	1010	20202	624	5089	1505
		(5%)	(6%)	(58%)	(27%)	(1%)	(44%)	(3%)	(3%)		(4%)	
Males+Females												
0–34	Sm.	–	–	–	–	–	–	–	–	–	–	–
	Total	2342	190	6	6	178	15	42	142	25	783	1145
35–69	Sm.	4121	2219	1420	397	402	240	51	1260	–	351	–
	Total	19545	7725	1670	675	5380	368	234	6189	1381	1776	1872
		(21%)	(29%)	(85%)	(59%)	(7%)	(65%)	(22%)	(20%)		(20%)	
70+	Sm.	4055	1636	1090	136	410	701	63	1379	–	276	–
	Total	49164	10818	1390	306	9122	1241	1368	27846	553	5838	1500
		(8%)	(15%)	(78%)	(44%)	(4%)	(56%)	(5%)	(5%)		(5%)	
Any age	Sm.	8176	3855	2510	533	812	941	114	2639	–	627	–
	Total	71051	18733	3066	987	14680	1624	1644	34177	1959	8397	4517
		(12%)	(21%)	(82%)	(54%)	(6%)	(58%)	(7%)	(8%)		(7%)	

(To be conservative, no deaths before age 35, and none from liver cirrhosis or non–medical causes, were attributed to smoking.)

¶AZERBAIJAN: 1990

		No. of deaths			Standardised rates (Defined on p.280)			Annual death rates / 100, 000						
		All ages	0–34	35–69	All ages	0–34	35–69	0–4	5–9	10–14	15–19	20–24	25–29	30–34
ALL CAUSES	M	22997	6417	10898	1314.9	236.8	1625.8	935.8	56.8	42.9	81.3	127.9	176.2	236.6
	F	19822	4468	6124	774.3	163.9	775.2	796.2	45.9	28.0	40.3	55.1	81.8	99.7
Tuberculosis	M	397	77	285	20.4	3.6	34.4	–	–	0.6	0.3	2.4	11.4	10.4
	F	128	39	66	4.9	1.7	7.4	1.0	–	0.3	1.0	2.3	2.7	4.3
Other infective	M	773	737	26	15.9	24.2	3.7	162.8	1.3	0.9	0.9	1.5	1.5	0.4
and parasitic	F	598	574	20	12.2	20.0	2.2	133.4	1.3	0.6	2.2	0.3	0.5	1.7
ALL CANCER	M	2821	231	2029	177.6	9.9	302.0	9.1	5.1	3.5	6.1	8.7	14.1	22.6
	F	1983	218	1189	86.7	9.2	142.1	6.3	5.4	3.7	5.1	8.8	12.1	23.3
Mouth and	M	60	4	45	3.7	0.2	5.9	–	–	–	–	0.9	–	0.4
pharynx cancer	F	22	3	14	0.9	0.1	1.5	–	–	–	–	–	0.5	0.3
Oesophagus cancer	M	185	3	133	12.6	0.1	20.7	–	–	–	0.3	0.3	0.3	–
	F	149	2	85	6.8	0.1	10.5	–	–	–	–	–	0.3	0.3
Stomach cancer	M	577	23	420	39.0	1.1	66.3	0.5	–	–	0.9	0.3	1.5	4.3
	F	388	8	212	17.8	0.4	25.8	–	–	–	–	0.6	–	2.0
Colorectal cancer	M	139	17	101	8.2	0.8	14.8	–	–	–	0.3	0.6	1.8	2.9
	F	136	12	78	6.1	0.5	9.2	–	–	–	0.3	0.6	0.3	2.7
Liver cancer	M	...	...	...	...	...	...	...	...	...	...	...	...	...
	F	...	...	...	...	...	...	...	...	...	...	...	...	...
Pancreas cancer	M	...	...	...	...	...	...	...	...	...	...	...	...	...
	F	...	...	...	...	...	...	...	...	...	...	...	...	...
Larynx cancer	M	50	–	44	3.0	–	6.3	–	–	–	–	–	–	–
	F	19	–	15	0.9	–	2.0	–	–	–	–	–	–	–
Lung cancer	M	609	14	499	38.1	0.6	71.3	–	0.3	0.3	0.3	0.6	1.2	1.8
	F	139	18	78	6.2	0.8	10.2	–	–	0.3	0.6	0.6	1.4	2.7
Malignant melanoma	M	...	...	...	...	...	...	...	...	...	...	...	...	...
	F	...	...	...	...	...	...	...	...	...	...	...	...	...
Female breast cancer	F	231	11	181	10.6	0.5	20.7	–	0.3	–	–	–	0.8	2.3
Cervix cancer	F	49	6	30	2.2	0.3	3.3	–	–	–	–	0.3	0.3	1.3
Other uterine cancer	F	80	9	53	3.5	0.4	5.8	0.2	–	–	–	0.9	0.8	0.7
Ovarian cancer	F	...	...	...	...	...	...	...	...	...	...	...	...	...
Prostate cancer	M	127	5	51	10.4	0.2	10.0	–	–	–	–	–	0.9	0.7
Bladder cancer	M	...	...	...	...	...	...	...	...	...	...	...	...	...
	F	...	...	...	...	...	...	...	...	...	...	...	...	...
Other and ill-defined	M	875	61	649	55.2	2.8	95.2	0.9	0.8	0.3	1.5	2.4	5.5	7.9
cancer sites	F	610	55	392	27.0	2.4	47.8	–	0.3	0.9	1.6	2.1	4.1	8.0
Hodgkin's disease	M	...	...	...	...	...	...	...	...	...	...	...	...	...
	F	...	...	...	...	...	...	...	...	...	...	...	...	...
Myeloma and all	M	191	98	85	7.3	3.9	11.2	6.8	4.1	2.6	2.6	3.6	2.8	4.7
lymphomas	F	157	91	51	4.8	3.6	5.3	5.8	4.6	2.4	2.5	3.5	3.6	3.0
Leukaemia	M	8	6	2	0.2	0.2	0.2	0.9	–	0.3	0.3	–	–	–
	F	3	3	–	0.1	0.1	–	0.2	0.3	–	–	0.3	–	–
ALL VASCULAR	M	9981	318	5657	737.1	14.6	888.3	4.1	2.5	1.7	7.8	13.5	22.8	49.6
DISEASE	F	10747	247	3356	471.2	10.4	443.5	5.1	2.7	2.1	7.6	9.1	22.5	24.0
Rheumatic heart	M	77	13	47	4.6	0.6	7.1	–	–	0.3	0.6	0.3	1.2	1.8
disease and fever	F	115	23	41	4.5	1.0	4.7	0.5	–	0.3	0.3	0.6	2.5	2.7
Hypertensive disease	M	565	15	290	43.8	0.6	48.8	0.9	–	–	0.3	0.3	1.2	1.8
	F	897	14	312	40.1	0.6	42.4	0.5	0.5	0.3	0.3	0.9	1.1	0.3
Ischaemic heart	M	7206	171	4150	533.5	8.1	645.2	0.5	0.3	–	3.2	7.5	11.4	34.1
disease	F	7018	105	2060	307.3	4.5	273.0	1.2	0.5	0.6	2.5	5.6	8.2	13.0
Pulmonary embolism	M	...	...	...	...	...	...	...	...	...	...	...	...	...
and other venous	F	...	...	...	...	...	...	...	...	...	...	...	...	...
Cerebrovascular	M	1869	64	1020	139.8	2.8	165.7	1.4	1.0	1.2	2.6	2.1	5.5	5.7
disease	F	2467	55	834	109.4	2.3	110.5	1.2	1.3	0.9	2.9	0.9	5.2	3.7
Other vascular	M	264	55	150	15.4	2.4	21.6	1.4	1.3	0.3	1.2	3.3	3.4	6.1
disease, incl. venous	F	250	50	109	9.9	2.1	13.1	1.7	0.3	–	1.6	1.2	5.5	4.3
Chronic obstructive	M	952	45	496	71.9	1.8	80.5	3.9	0.5	1.2	0.9	2.1	2.2	1.8
pulmonary disease	F	777	48	237	33.2	1.9	30.8	3.6	1.9	0.3	0.3	1.5	2.7	3.0
Other respiratory	M	2265	2136	87	48.2	70.3	13.1	463.2	11.2	4.9	3.8	2.4	4.3	2.2
disease	F	1899	1798	54	39.2	62.8	6.0	408.3	12.9	6.7	2.9	3.5	3.0	2.3
Peptic ulcer	M	152	13	110	9.4	0.6	16.4	–	–	–	–	0.6	1.5	2.2
	F	62	3	30	2.8	0.1	4.0	–	–	0.3	–	–	0.3	0.3
Liver cirrhosis and	M	744	50	523	47.7	2.2	76.2	0.9	1.8	0.3	1.5	1.5	3.1	6.5
other liver disease	F	716	39	343	31.1	1.6	43.4	1.2	1.1	0.3	1.0	1.5	2.2	4.3
Renal disease	M	228	63	117	12.3	2.5	16.1	5.2	1.3	0.6	1.7	0.9	3.4	4.7
	F	192	58	84	7.3	2.3	9.9	5.1	0.8	0.6	1.3	3.2	2.2	3.0
Pregnancy and birth	F	17	13	4	0.5	0.6	0.4	–	–	–	–	0.9	1.1	2.0
Congenital and	M	713	708	3	13.3	23.3	0.5	154.4	1.0	2.0	2.3	1.2	1.8	0.4
perinatal causes	F	527	522	1	10.3	18.2	0.1	122.3	1.1	0.9	1.3	0.9	0.3	0.3
Ill-defined causes	M	403	143	125	22.7	5.5	15.7	19.1	0.3	1.4	2.6	2.7	3.4	8.6
	F	402	93	56	14.8	3.4	7.2	16.4	0.3	0.6	0.6	1.8	1.9	2.3
Other medical causes	M	1137	501	501	51.4	18.7	71.9	62.4	9.4	5.2	11.0	15.0	14.8	12.9
	F	999	395	412	35.6	15.0	48.9	51.5	7.6	5.8	4.8	8.8	14.5	12.3
ALL NON-	M	2431	1395	939	87.0	59.7	107.1	50.6	22.4	20.6	42.4	75.2	91.9	114.5
MEDICAL CAUSES	F	775	421	272	24.5	16.5	29.2	42.1	10.8	5.8	12.4	12.6	15.6	16.3
Motor vehicle	M	796	415	348	30.0	18.6	38.8	3.4	5.9	8.1	9.6	21.1	34.7	47.8
traffic accidents	F	176	68	91	6.3	2.9	9.5	1.5	3.8	1.2	3.8	2.1	2.7	5.0
Fire	M	148	114	27	4.3	4.2	2.9	15.9	1.5	0.6	0.3	3.9	3.7	3.6
	F	140	97	27	3.9	3.6	2.9	14.5	1.9	1.2	1.6	1.5	2.5	2.3
Suicide	M	89	36	51	3.7	1.6	6.1	–	0.3	–	2.6	2.1	2.5	3.9
	F	25	11	11	0.9	0.5	1.5	–	–	–	0.6	0.6	1.4	0.7
Homicide	M	345	213	114	12.0	9.6	11.9	0.2	0.5	0.9	8.4	17.8	18.8	20.8
	F	79	39	32	2.7	1.6	3.8	1.0	0.3	0.3	1.9	3.5	2.5	2.0
POPULATION (thousands):	M=males				3378.6	2457.0	857.5	439.1	392.6	345.0	344.3	332.3	325.2	278.5
	F=females				3542.0	2433.4	963.7	413.7	370.7	328.5	314.9	341.3	364.5	299.8

AZERBAIJAN: 1990

Annual death rates / 100, 000

9th ICD categories

35–39	40–44	45–49	50–54	55–59	60–64	65–69	70–74	75–79	80+/NK			
328.4	582.0	734.8	1154.9	1824.8	2776.1	3979.3	5373.8	7528.0	13713.6	M	**ALL CAUSES**	001–999
131.5	217.0	293.8	531.5	828.6	1346.7	2077.0	3286.0	5388.1	9868.3	F		
14.9	33.5	41.3	44.9	38.1	35.8	32.2	60.7	46.7	56.3	M	**Tuberculosis**	010–018, 137
7.7	3.0	6.4	5.5	4.9	10.2	13.8	19.1	11.4	16.7	F		
2.0	–	2.0	3.1	5.3	4.0	9.2	9.3	14.0	23.5	M	**Other infective**	Rest of 001–139
0.5	2.3	0.9	2.2	3.5	3.4	2.8	–	2.3	5.6	F	**and parasitic**	
35.9	75.1	139.5	235.4	359.5	558.2	710.3	822.4	906.5	896.7	M	**ALL CANCER**	140–208
35.8	61.0	89.1	121.2	163.1	227.4	297.1	375.0	415.5	402.6	F		
–	3.3	4.9	5.5	10.7	10.0	6.9	18.7	18.7	14.1	M	**Mouth and**	140–149
0.5	–	3.7	2.7	2.1	–	1.4	–	4.6	5.6	F	**pharynx cancer**	
1.0	0.8	6.9	12.9	26.7	43.8	52.9	56.1	88.8	84.5	M	**Oesophagus cancer**	150
1.0	3.0	3.7	8.8	10.5	23.0	23.4	36.0	41.1	50.1	F		
5.6	12.2	27.5	38.7	71.6	131.3	177.0	205.6	215.0	206.6	M	**Stomach cancer**	151
2.4	8.3	9.2	21.4	36.4	45.1	57.8	97.5	134.7	116.9	F		
2.0	4.1	4.9	15.4	16.8	23.9	36.8	28.0	28.0	42.3	M	**Colorectal cancer**	153, 154
2.4	4.5	5.5	8.2	11.9	13.6	17.9	33.9	38.8	24.1	F		
...	...	...	...	...	...	...	...	...	...	M	**Liver cancer**	Not given separately
...	...	...	...	...	...	...	...	...	...	F		
...	...	...	...	...	...	...	...	...	...	M	**Pancreas cancer**	Not given separately
...	...	...	...	...	...	...	...	...	...	F		
–	0.8	5.9	6.1	6.9	12.9	11.5	–	4.7	23.5	M	**Larynx cancer**	161
0.5	–	0.9	1.1	3.5	0.9	6.9	–	4.6	3.7	F		
7.2	15.5	34.4	61.5	96.0	142.3	142.5	191.6	158.9	98.6	M	**Lung cancer**	162
1.5	3.0	3.7	3.8	9.8	22.1	27.5	36.0	25.1	27.8	F		
...	...	...	...	...	...	...	...	...	...	M	**Malignant melanoma**	Not given
...	...	...	...	...	...	...	...	...	...	F		separately
10.6	13.6	24.8	20.3	17.5	21.3	37.1	25.4	27.4	27.8	F	**Female breast cancer**	174
0.5	0.8	2.8	4.4	4.9	6.0	4.1	14.8	6.8	5.6	F	**Cervix cancer**	180
0.5	5.3	2.8	7.7	8.4	9.4	6.9	16.9	9.1	11.1	F	**Other uterine cancer**	179, 182
...	...	...	...	...	...	...	...	...	...	F	**Ovarian cancer**	Not given separately
–	–	2.9	1.2	6.9	19.9	39.1	42.1	126.2	164.3	M	**Prostate cancer**	185
...	...	...	...	...	...	...	...	...	...	M	**Bladder cancer**	Not given separately
...	...	...	...	...	...	...	...	...	...	F		
14.9	34.3	46.2	79.3	108.9	162.2	220.7	266.4	247.7	258.2	M	**Other and ill-defined**	Rest of 140–208,
12.1	15.8	30.3	37.3	50.4	80.1	108.7	101.7	121.0	115.0	F	**cancer sites**	incl. 155, 157, 172, 183, 188
...	...	...	...	...	...	...	...	...	...	M	**Hodgkin's disease**	Not given separately
...	...	...	...	...	...	...	...	...	...	F		
5.1	4.1	5.9	14.1	14.5	11.9	23.0	14.0	18.7	4.7	M	**Myeloma and all**	200–203,
3.9	6.8	1.8	5.5	7.7	6.0	5.5	12.7	2.3	14.8	F	**lymphomas**	incl. 201
–	–	–	0.6	0.8	–	–	–	–	–	M	**Leukaemia**	204–208
–	–	–	–	–	–	–	–	–	–	F		
90.2	210.6	314.3	559.3	999.2	1616.9	2427.6	3448.6	5196.3	10122.1	M	**ALL VASCULAR**	390–459
35.3	81.4	108.4	254.5	454.9	816.9	1353.5	2362.3	4153.0	7810.8	F	**DISEASE**	
0.5	4.1	3.9	6.8	6.9	9.0	18.4	9.3	23.4	46.9	M	**Rheumatic heart**	390–398
1.0	4.5	0.9	3.3	8.4	7.7	6.9	16.9	27.4	57.5	F	**disease and fever**	
3.6	9.0	9.8	28.9	43.4	88.6	158.6	210.3	317.8	690.1	M	**Hypertensive disease**	401–405
1.9	5.3	7.3	19.2	52.5	67.3	143.1	237.3	276.3	627.1	F		
65.6	157.6	246.6	421.0	745.6	1160.2	1719.5	2537.4	3724.3	7253.5	M	**Ischaemic heart**	410–414
19.3	37.7	63.4	156.3	270.8	532.4	830.8	1525.4	2792.2	5398.9	F	**disease**	
...	...	...	...	...	...	...	...	...	...	M	**Pulmonary embolism**	Not given
...	...	...	...	...	...	...	...	...	...	F	**and other venous**	separately
12.8	24.5	44.2	91.0	179.0	325.4	482.8	649.5	1060.7	1967.1	M	**Cerebrovascular**	430–438
8.2	24.9	29.4	66.4	109.9	190.8	343.9	559.3	1006.8	1619.7	F	**disease**	
7.7	15.5	9.8	11.7	24.4	33.8	48.3	42.1	70.1	164.3	M	**Other vascular**	Rest of 390–459,
4.8	9.0	7.3	9.3	13.3	18.7	28.9	23.3	50.2	107.6	F	**disease, incl. venous**	incl. 415, 451–3
4.1	10.6	25.5	41.8	91.4	160.2	229.9	401.9	588.8	934.3	M	**Chronic obstructive**	490–496
3.9	6.0	10.1	19.7	30.8	54.5	90.8	154.7	271.7	556.6	F	**pulmonary disease**	
5.6	9.0	3.9	4.9	12.2	21.9	34.5	32.7	46.7	117.4	M	**Other respiratory**	Rest of 460–519
1.9	2.3	4.6	7.1	7.7	10.2	8.3	8.5	13.7	68.6	F	**disease**	
5.1	6.5	5.9	10.4	17.5	27.9	41.4	28.0	56.1	51.6	M	**Peptic ulcer**	531–533
1.5	2.3	1.8	1.6	4.2	2.6	13.8	10.6	27.4	22.3	F		
14.3	40.8	40.3	50.4	96.7	120.4	170.1	177.6	238.3	385.0	M	**Liver cirrhosis and**	570–573, 576,
5.8	11.3	13.8	32.4	55.3	63.9	121.0	108.1	200.9	361.8	F	**other liver disease**	575.2–579.9
8.2	5.7	9.8	14.1	17.5	22.9	34.5	32.7	65.4	126.8	M	**Renal disease**	580–590
3.9	5.3	7.3	9.3	9.8	11.9	22.0	27.5	18.3	53.8	F		
0.5	0.8	0.9	–	0.7	–	–	–	–	–	F	**Pregnancy and birth**	630–676
0.5	0.8	–	–	–	–	2.3	–	–	9.4	M	**Congenital and**	740–779
–	–	–	0.5	–	–	–	–	4.6	3.7	F	**perinatal causes**	
9.7	13.1	11.8	16.6	12.9	24.9	20.7	74.8	93.5	464.8	M	**Ill-defined causes**	780–799
2.4	3.8	1.8	4.4	6.3	8.5	23.4	53.0	86.8	352.5	F		
26.1	35.1	38.3	54.7	86.1	90.5	172.4	158.9	172.9	300.5	M	**Other medical causes**	Rest of 001–799
12.1	10.6	26.6	40.0	63.7	94.5	94.9	120.8	123.3	150.3	F		
111.7	141.2	102.2	119.2	88.3	92.5	94.3	126.2	102.8	225.4	M	**ALL NON–**	E800–E999
20.3	27.1	22.0	32.9	23.8	42.6	35.8	46.6	59.4	63.1	F	**MEDICAL CAUSES**	
45.1	54.7	39.3	43.6	30.5	28.9	29.9	46.7	28.0	79.8	M	**Motor vehicle**	E810–E819
7.7	8.3	7.3	12.6	9.1	10.2	11.0	14.8	11.4	9.3	F	**traffic accidents**	
4.1	2.4	–	3.1	4.6	4.0	2.3	18.7	9.3	4.7	M	**Fire**	E890–E899
3.4	1.5	1.8	0.5	2.8	7.7	2.8	10.6	9.1	13.0	F		
1.5	12.2	6.9	9.8	1.5	6.0	4.6	4.7	4.7	–	M	**Suicide**	E950–E959
0.5	2.3	1.8	–	0.7	0.9	4.1	2.1	–	3.7	F		
16.9	21.2	6.9	13.5	11.4	9.0	4.6	14.0	28.0	42.3	M	**Homicide**	E960–E969
1.0	1.5	5.5	4.4	2.8	4.3	6.9	4.2	6.8	5.6	F		
195.2	122.5	101.8	162.7	131.3	100.5	43.5	21.4	21.4	21.3	M	**POPULATION (thousands)**	
206.8	132.7	108.9	182.3	142.9	117.4	72.7	47.2	43.8	53.9	F		

AZERBAIJAN: Males

	All ages	0–34	35–69	35–39	40–44	45–49	50–54	55–59	60–64	65–69	70–74	75–79	80+/NK
POPULATION (1000s)													
1985–90	3312.8	2416.9	824.5	169.8	102.5	148.9	159.2	131.1	77.8	35.2	27.0	22.2	22.2
1985	3220.2	2363.8	779.2	134.1	109.3	179.9	149.8	120.9	55.4	29.8	32.8	21.5	22.9
1990	3378.6	2457.0	857.5	195.2	122.5	101.8	162.7	131.3	100.5	43.5	21.4	21.4	21.3
1995 projected	3635.3	2643.8	922.6	210.0	131.8	109.5	175.1	141.3	108.1	46.8	23.0	23.0	22.9
NUMBER OF DEATHS													
All causes													
1985–90	23497	6812	9971	516	508	1017	1843	2398	2251	1438	1592	1925	3197
1985	23286	6761	9028	441	432	1307	1747	2312	1568	1221	2044	1970	3483
1990	22997	6417	10898	641	713	748	1879	2396	2790	1731	1150	1611	2921
1995 projected	23396	6283	11716	856	870	870	1974	2513	2915	1718	1070	1569	2758
Lung cancer													
1985–90	730	14	584	10	16	55	120	168	143	72	61	42	29
1985	658	10	505	7	12	61	97	159	114	55	70	44	29
1990	609	14	499	14	19	35	100	126	143	62	41	34	21
1995 projected	537	16	434	21	23	38	89	100	111	52	36	33	18
ANNUAL DEATH RATE / 100,000 (*The rates for the age groups 0–34 and 35–69 are the means of seven five-yearly rates, but the all-ages rates are standardised to the conventional "European" age distribution)													
All causes													
1985–90	1376.0*	253.2*	1635.4*	303.9	495.6	683.0	1157.7	1829.1	2893.3	4085.2	5896.3	8671.2	14400.9
1985	1417.2*	260.3*	1636.7*	328.9	395.2	726.5	1166.2	1912.3	2830.3	4097.3	6231.7	9162.8	15209.6
1990	1314.9*	236.8*	1625.8*	328.4	582.0	734.8	1154.9	1824.8	2776.1	3979.3	5373.8	7528.0	13713.6
1995 projected	1230.7*	222.2*	1590.8*	407.6	660.1	794.5	1127.4	1778.5	2696.6	3670.9	4652.2	6821.7	12043.7
All cancer													
1985–90	201.8*	10.9*	343.7*	38.3	74.1	135.7	265.7	431.0	642.7	818.2	981.5	1058.6	955.0
1985	202.3*	10.5*	339.1*	39.5	58.6	124.0	235.0	432.6	635.4	849.0	1073.2	1116.3	943.2
1990	177.6*	9.9*	302.0*	35.9	75.1	139.5	235.4	359.5	558.2	710.3	822.4	906.5	896.7
1995 projected	158.3*	9.7*	271.3*	43.3	85.0	150.7	219.9	319.9	482.0	598.3	678.3	756.5	790.4
Lung cancer													
1985–90	47.9*	0.6*	92.9*	5.9	15.6	36.9	75.4	128.1	183.8	204.5	225.9	189.2	130.6
1985	46.9*	0.5*	91.0*	5.2	11.0	33.9	64.8	131.5	205.8	184.6	213.4	204.7	126.6
1990	38.1*	0.6*	71.3*	7.2	15.5	34.4	61.5	96.0	142.3	142.5	191.6	158.9	98.6
1995 projected	31.2*	0.7*	56.8*	10.0	17.5	34.7	50.8	70.8	102.7	111.1	156.5	143.5	78.6
Upper aerodigestive cancer (mouth, oesophagus, pharynx and larynx)													
1985–90	27.1*	0.5*	47.5*	4.1	7.8	20.1	36.4	58.7	86.1	119.3	122.2	148.6	139.6
1985	28.8*	0.4*	52.2*	8.9	4.6	17.8	39.4	60.4	83.0	151.0	149.4	144.2	122.3
1990	19.3*	0.3*	32.9*	1.0	4.9	17.7	24.6	44.2	66.7	71.3	74.8	112.1	122.1
1995 projected	14.4*	0.3*	23.4*	1.0	3.8	13.7	17.7	32.6	46.3	49.1	52.2	91.3	104.8
Other cancer													
1985–90	126.8*	9.7*	203.2*	28.3	50.7	78.6	153.9	244.1	372.8	494.3	633.3	720.7	684.7
1985	126.6*	9.5*	196.0*	25.4	43.0	72.3	130.8	240.7	346.6	513.4	710.4	767.4	694.3
1990	120.2*	9.0*	197.8*	27.7	54.7	87.4	149.4	219.3	349.3	496.6	556.1	635.5	676.1
1995 projected	112.7*	8.7*	191.1*	32.4	63.7	102.3	151.3	216.6	333.0	438.0	469.6	521.7	607.0
Chronic obstructive pulmonary disease (COPD)													
1985–90	72.9*	2.2*	83.9*	5.3	12.7	22.2	47.7	90.8	155.5	252.8	348.1	572.1	1018.0
1985	88.7*	2.5*	98.6*	6.7	11.0	23.9	60.1	118.3	194.9	275.2	445.1	711.6	1244.5
1990	71.9*	1.8*	80.5*	4.1	10.6	25.5	41.8	91.4	160.2	229.9	401.9	588.8	934.3
1995 projected	59.3*	1.4*	66.2*	2.9	9.9	21.0	32.6	70.8	129.5	196.6	339.1	530.4	729.3
Other respiratory disease													
1985–90	56.5*	82.9*	13.4*	3.5	5.9	7.4	9.4	16.0	20.6	31.3	44.4	58.6	139.6
1985	61.7*	90.2*	13.1*	4.5	2.7	8.3	10.0	18.2	14.4	33.6	73.2	46.5	170.3
1990	48.2*	70.3*	13.1*	5.6	9.0	3.9	4.9	12.2	21.9	34.5	32.7	46.7	117.4
1995 projected	38.2*	54.7*	12.1*	8.1	10.6	3.7	3.4	11.3	22.2	25.6	26.1	34.8	87.3
Vascular disease													
1985–90	775.5*	13.6*	874.1*	86.6	182.4	279.4	541.5	939.7	1637.5	2451.7	3855.6	6085.6	10941.4
1985	777.1*	13.1*	841.0*	91.7	135.4	295.7	549.4	956.2	1536.1	2322.1	3801.8	6325.6	11397.4
1990	737.1*	14.6*	888.3*	90.2	210.6	314.3	559.3	999.2	1616.9	2427.6	3448.6	5196.3	10122.1
1995 projected	697.9*	15.4*	902.9*	117.6	239.8	343.4	574.0	1030.4	1668.8	2346.2	3052.2	4769.6	8751.1
Liver cirrhosis and other liver disease													
1985–90	40.9*	2.0*	61.2*	10.0	24.4	32.9	52.1	77.0	106.7	125.0	151.9	247.7	355.9
1985	47.8*	1.9*	68.0*	11.9	15.6	40.6	73.4	72.8	113.7	147.7	207.3	288.4	449.8
1990	47.7*	2.2*	76.2*	14.3	40.8	40.3	50.4	96.7	120.4	170.1	177.6	238.3	385.0
1995 projected	47.8*	2.5*	81.5*	20.5	55.4	40.2	49.7	98.4	137.8	168.8	160.9	204.3	327.5
Other medical causes													
1985–90	148.9*	87.6*	160.1*	60.1	85.9	103.4	145.1	180.0	239.1	306.8	396.3	518.0	824.3
1985	167.5*	98.7*	183.3*	91.7	91.5	126.7	154.9	209.3	263.5	345.6	490.9	534.9	834.1
1990	145.4*	78.4*	158.6*	66.6	94.7	109.0	143.8	177.5	206.0	312.6	364.5	448.6	1032.9
1995 projected	126.4*	62.8*	132.6*	55.7	79.7	100.5	124.5	147.2	173.0	247.9	295.7	426.1	1117.9
All non-medical causes													
1985–90	79.5*	54.1*	99.1*	100.1	110.2	102.1	96.1	94.6	91.3	99.4	118.5	130.6	166.7
1985	72.0*	43.3*	93.6*	82.8	80.5	107.3	83.4	105.0	72.2	124.2	140.2	139.5	170.3
1990	87.0*	59.7*	107.1*	111.7	141.2	102.2	119.2	88.3	92.5	94.3	126.2	102.8	225.4
1995 projected	102.8*	75.7*	124.2*	159.5	179.8	135.2	123.4	100.5	83.3	87.6	100.0	100.0	240.2

AZERBAIJAN: Females

	All ages	0–34	35–69	35–39	40–44	45–49	50–54	55–59	60–64	65–69	70–74	75–79	80+/NK
POPULATION (1000s)													
1985–90	3485.1	2396.9	933.8	180.0	109.8	162.3	170.1	143.3	103.3	65.0	53.9	45.7	54.8
1985	3391.5	2339.2	892.0	143.2	115.8	196.3	154.2	134.0	88.1	60.4	60.8	45.6	53.9
1990	**3542.0**	**2433.4**	**963.7**	**206.8**	**132.7**	**108.9**	**182.3**	**142.9**	**117.4**	**72.7**	**47.2**	**43.8**	**53.9**
1995 projected	*3811.3*	*2618.4*	*1037.0*	*222.5*	*142.8*	*117.2*	*196.2*	*153.8*	*126.3*	*78.2*	*50.8*	*47.1*	*58.0*
NUMBER OF DEATHS													
All causes													
1985–90	21631	5179	5990	259	233	516	928	1220	1441	1393	1909	2598	5955
1985	21893	5209	5633	219	232	687	820	1184	1180	1311	2333	2603	6115
1990	**19822**	**4468**	**6124**	**272**	**288**	**320**	**969**	**1184**	**1581**	**1510**	**1551**	**2360**	**5319**
1995 projected	*19159*	*3860*	*6276*	*298*	*283*	*332*	*978*	*1252*	*1648*	*1485*	*1531*	*2293*	*5199*
Lung cancer													
1985–90	154	10	85	4	3	8	12	17	22	19	19	17	23
1985	136	5	69	2	2	7	11	12	15	20	23	17	22
1990	**139**	**18**	**78**	**3**	**4**	**4**	**7**	**14**	**26**	**20**	**17**	**11**	**15**
1995 projected	*147*	*27*	*85*	*4*	*5*	*4*	*7*	*16*	*28*	*21*	*15*	*8*	*12*
ANNUAL DEATH RATE / 100,000 (*The rates for the age groups 0–34 and 35–69 are the means of seven five-yearly rates, but the all-ages rates are standardised to the conventional "European" age distribution)													
All causes													
1985–90	833.8*	193.7*	801.3*	143.9	212.2	317.9	545.6	851.4	1395.0	2143.1	3541.7	5684.9	10866.8
1985	859.0*	202.0*	804.1*	152.9	200.3	350.0	531.8	883.6	1339.4	2170.5	3837.2	5708.3	11345.1
1990	**774.3***	**163.9***	**775.2***	**131.5**	**217.0**	**293.8**	**531.5**	**828.6**	**1346.7**	**2077.0**	**3286.0**	**5388.1**	**9868.3**
1995 projected	*706.2**	*132.9**	*733.1**	*133.9*	*198.2*	*283.3*	*498.5*	*814.0*	*1304.8*	*1899.0*	*3013.8*	*4868.4*	*8963.8*
All cancer													
1985–90	101.3*	9.8*	166.1*	39.4	64.7	98.0	148.1	191.9	277.8	343.1	439.7	514.2	467.2
1985	104.4*	9.0*	169.9*	38.4	62.2	104.9	155.6	220.9	271.3	336.1	472.0	546.1	462.0
1990	**86.7***	**9.2***	**142.1***	**35.8**	**61.0**	**89.1**	**121.2**	**163.1**	**227.4**	**297.1**	**375.0**	**415.5**	**402.6**
1995 projected	*72.1**	*8.9**	*118.2**	*35.5*	*53.9*	*75.9*	*93.3*	*128.1*	*192.4*	*248.1*	*299.2*	*339.7*	*329.3*
Lung cancer													
1985–90	7.0*	0.5*	11.3*	2.2	2.7	4.9	7.1	11.9	21.3	29.2	35.3	37.2	42.0
1985	6.5*	0.2*	10.4*	1.4	1.7	3.6	7.1	9.0	17.0	33.1	37.8	37.3	40.8
1990	**6.2***	**0.8***	**10.2***	**1.5**	**3.0**	**3.7**	**3.8**	**9.8**	**22.1**	**27.5**	**36.0**	**25.1**	**27.8**
1995 projected	*5.8**	*1.1**	*10.2**	*1.8*	*3.5*	*3.4*	*3.6*	*10.4*	*22.2*	*26.9*	*29.5*	*17.0*	*20.7*
Upper aerodigestive cancer (mouth, oesophagus, pharynx and larynx)													
1985–90	9.6*	0.3*	14.9*	2.2	3.6	8.0	14.1	17.4	23.2	35.4	51.9	59.1	56.6
1985	9.3*	0.4*	13.0*	2.1	5.2	10.2	14.9	20.9	15.9	21.5	52.6	59.2	59.4
1990	**8.6***	**0.2***	**13.9***	**1.9**	**3.0**	**8.3**	**12.6**	**16.1**	**23.9**	**31.6**	**36.0**	**50.2**	**59.4**
1995 projected	*8.2**	*0.2**	*14.0**	*1.3*	*2.1*	*6.8*	*10.2*	*16.3*	*29.3*	*32.0*	*31.5*	*46.7*	*53.4*
Other cancer													
1985–90	84.7*	9.0*	140.0*	35.0	58.3	85.0	127.0	162.6	233.3	278.5	352.5	417.9	368.6
1985	88.6*	8.5*	146.5*	34.9	55.3	91.2	133.6	191.0	238.4	281.5	381.6	449.6	361.8
1990	**72.0***	**8.2***	**118.0***	**32.4**	**55.0**	**77.1**	**104.8**	**137.2**	**181.4**	**238.0**	**303.0**	**340.2**	**315.4**
1995 projected	*58.0**	*7.6**	*93.9**	*32.4*	*48.3*	*65.7*	*79.5*	*101.4*	*140.9*	*189.3*	*238.2*	*276.0*	*255.2*
Chronic obstructive pulmonary disease (COPD)													
1985–90	34.7*	2.2*	31.0*	5.0	5.5	11.1	20.0	30.0	53.2	92.3	157.7	267.0	624.1
1985	39.6*	1.8*	33.9*	5.6	3.5	12.2	21.4	36.6	52.2	106.0	195.7	304.8	732.8
1990	**33.2***	**1.9***	**30.8***	**3.9**	**6.0**	**10.1**	**19.7**	**30.8**	**54.5**	**90.8**	**154.7**	**271.7**	**556.6**
1995 projected	*27.7**	*1.7**	*27.2**	*4.5*	*5.6*	*9.4*	*16.8*	*28.6*	*49.1*	*76.7*	*129.9*	*212.3*	*444.8*
Other respiratory disease													
1985–90	49.2*	78.4*	6.1*	2.2	2.7	3.1	5.3	6.3	10.6	12.3	24.1	35.0	91.2
1985	53.6*	84.9*	5.4*	2.8	1.7	3.6	5.2	5.2	7.9	11.6	32.9	50.4	109.5
1990	**39.2***	**62.8***	**6.0***	**1.9**	**2.3**	**4.6**	**7.1**	**7.7**	**10.2**	**8.3**	**8.5**	**13.7**	**68.6**
1995 projected	*29.6**	*45.8**	*6.8**	*2.2*	*2.1*	*6.0*	*9.7*	*10.4*	*11.1*	*6.4*	*5.9*	*10.6*	*50.0*
Vascular disease													
1985–90	507.7*	10.8*	454.9*	39.4	67.4	121.4	249.3	457.1	834.5	1415.4	2564.0	4402.6	8906.9
1985	512.7*	9.5*	444.3*	34.2	64.8	135.5	230.2	431.3	782.1	1432.1	2718.8	4337.7	9246.8
1990	**471.2***	**10.4***	**443.5***	**35.3**	**81.4**	**108.4**	**254.5**	**454.9**	**816.9**	**1353.5**	**2362.3**	**4153.0**	**7810.8**
1995 projected	*433.5**	*11.1**	*427.3**	*40.4*	*76.3*	*111.8*	*257.4*	*471.4*	*802.1*	*1231.5*	*2169.3*	*3685.8*	*6879.3*
Liver cirrhosis and other liver disease													
1985–90	26.2*	1.7*	33.4*	5.0	8.2	15.4	27.6	41.2	55.2	81.5	111.3	157.5	323.0
1985	28.6*	1.5*	31.7*	4.2	4.3	18.3	25.9	50.7	42.0	76.2	153.0	162.3	410.0
1990	**31.1***	**1.6***	**43.4***	**5.8**	**11.3**	**13.8**	**32.4**	**55.3**	**63.9**	**121.0**	**108.1**	**200.9**	**361.8**
1995 projected	*34.3**	*1.7**	*51.2**	*8.1*	*12.6*	*16.2*	*34.1*	*68.9*	*89.5*	*129.2*	*118.1*	*201.7*	*355.2*
Other medical causes													
1985–90	87.7*	70.8*	81.0*	34.4	37.3	46.8	67.0	97.7	126.8	156.9	183.7	238.5	377.7
1985	92.7*	76.4*	88.2*	50.3	40.6	48.4	68.1	105.2	136.2	168.9	205.6	232.5	304.3
1990	**88.4***	**61.3***	**80.1***	**28.5**	**27.9**	**45.9**	**63.6**	**93.1**	**131.2**	**170.6**	**230.9**	**274.0**	**604.8**
1995 projected	*86.6**	*48.6**	*74.9**	*19.8*	*20.3*	*40.1*	*57.6*	*85.2*	*125.1*	*176.5*	*253.9*	*367.3*	*855.2*
All non-medical causes													
1985–90	26.9*	20.0*	28.7*	18.3	26.4	22.2	28.2	27.2	36.8	41.5	61.2	70.0	76.6
1985	27.3*	19.0*	30.6*	17.5	23.3	27.0	25.3	33.6	47.7	39.7	59.2	74.6	79.8
1990	**24.5***	**16.5***	**29.2***	**20.3**	**27.1**	**22.0**	**32.9**	**23.8**	**42.6**	**35.8**	**46.6**	**59.4**	**63.1**
1995 projected	*22.4**	*15.1**	*27.4**	*23.4*	*27.3*	*23.9*	*29.6*	*21.5*	*35.6*	*30.7*	*37.4*	*51.0*	*50.0*

AZERBAIJAN: 1985–1990

Smoking-attributed deaths (Sm.) and total deaths (Total)

Age		ALL CAUSES	ALL CANCER	Lung cancer	Upper aero-digestive ca.	Other cancer	COPD	Other respiratory	Vascular disease	Cirrhosis/ other liver	Other medical	Non-medical
Males												
0–34	Sm.	–	–	–	–	–	–	–	–	–	–	–
	Total	6812	249	14	10	225	54	2461	286	43	2460	1259
35–69	Sm.	2998	887	535	177	175	342	26	1404	–	339	–
	Total	9971	2119	584	289	1246	460	86	4981	402	1105	818
		(30%)	(42%)	(92%)	(61%)	(14%)	(74%)	(30%)	(28%)		(31%)	
70+	Sm.	644	164	105	33	26	219	2	237	–	22	–
	Total	6714	712	132	97	483	447	56	4821	175	405	98
		(10%)	(23%)	(80%)	(34%)	(5%)	(49%)	(4%)	(5%)		(5%)	
Any age	Sm.	3642	1051	640	210	201	561	28	1641	–	361	–
	Total	23497	3080	730	396	1954	961	2603	10088	620	3970	2175
		(15%)	(34%)	(88%)	(53%)	(10%)	(58%)	(1%)	(16%)		(9%)	
Females												
0–34	Sm.	–	–	–	–	–	–	–	–	–	–	–
	Total	5179	223	10	7	206	53	2206	246	38	1909	504
35–69	Sm.	112	23	15	6	2	26	0	55	–	8	–
	Total	5990	1338	85	117	1136	225	49	3203	259	666	250
		(2%)	(2%)	(18%)	(5%)	(0%)	(12%)	(0%)	(2%)		(1%)	
70+	Sm.	52	7	5	2	0	22	0	22	–	1	–
	Total	10462	728	59	86	583	549	79	8275	309	415	107
		(0%)	(1%)	(8%)	(2%)	(0%)	(4%)	(0%)	(0%)		(0%)	
Any age	Sm.	164	30	20	8	2	48	0	77	–	9	–
	Total	21631	2289	154	210	1925	827	2334	11724	606	2990	861
		(1%)	(1%)	(13%)	(4%)	(0%)	(6%)	(0%)	(1%)		(0%)	
Males+Females												
0–34	Sm.	–	–	–	–	–	–	–	–	–	–	–
	Total	11991	472	24	17	431	107	4667	532	81	4369	1763
35–69	Sm.	3110	910	550	183	177	368	26	1459	–	347	–
	Total	15961	3457	669	406	2382	685	135	8184	661	1771	1068
		(19%)	(26%)	(82%)	(45%)	(7%)	(54%)	(19%)	(18%)		(20%)	
70+	Sm.	696	171	110	35	26	241	2	259	–	23	–
	Total	17176	1440	191	183	1066	996	135	13096	484	820	205
		(4%)	(12%)	(58%)	(19%)	(2%)	(24%)	(1%)	(2%)		(3%)	
Any age	Sm.	3806	1081	660	218	203	609	28	1718	–	370	–
	Total	45128	5369	884	606	3879	1788	4937	21812	1226	6960	3036
		(8%)	(20%)	(75%)	(36%)	(5%)	(34%)	(1%)	(8%)		(5%)	

AZERBAIJAN: 1985

Smoking-attributed deaths (Sm.) and total deaths (Total)

Age		ALL CAUSES	ALL CANCER	Lung cancer	Upper aero-digestive ca.	Other cancer	COPD	Other respiratory	Vascular disease	Cirrhosis/ other liver	Other medical	Non-medical
Males												
0–34	Sm.	–	–	–	–	–	–	–	–	–	–	–
	Total	6761	225	10	7	208	58	2563	256	39	2614	1006
35–69	Sm.	2736	768	461	164	143	360	23	1226	–	359	–
	Total	9028	1820	505	272	1043	487	79	4325	411	1185	721
		(30%)	(42%)	(91%)	(60%)	(14%)	(74%)	(29%)	(28%)		(30%)	
70+	Sm.	784	186	115	40	31	297	4	271	–	26	–
	Total	7497	808	143	108	557	584	73	5217	233	467	115
		(10%)	(23%)	(80%)	(37%)	(6%)	(51%)	(5%)	(5%)		(6%)	
Any age	Sm.	3520	954	576	204	174	657	27	1497	–	385	–
	Total	23286	2853	658	387	1808	1129	2715	9798	683	4266	1842
		(15%)	(33%)	(88%)	(53%)	(10%)	(58%)	(1%)	(15%)		(9%)	
Females												
0–34	Sm.	–	–	–	–	–	–	–	–	–	–	–
	Total	5209	202	5	7	190	43	2288	205	31	1972	468
35–69	Sm.	0	0	0	0	0	0	0	0	–	0	–
	Total	5633	1311	69	107	1135	228	42	2877	238	682	255
		(0%)	(0%)	(0%)	(0%)	(0%)	(0%)	(0%)	(0%)		(0%)	
70+	Sm.	0	0	0	0	0	0	0	0	–	0	–
	Total	11051	785	62	91	632	653	102	8615	388	395	113
		(0%)	(0%)	(0%)	(0%)	(0%)	(0%)	(0%)	(0%)		(0%)	
Any age	Sm.	0	0	0	0	0	0	0	0	–	0	–
	Total	21893	2298	136	205	1957	924	2432	11697	657	3049	836
		(0%)	(0%)	(0%)	(0%)	(0%)	(0%)	(0%)	(0%)		(0%)	
Males+Females												
0–34	Sm.	–	–	–	–	–	–	–	–	–	–	–
	Total	11970	427	15	14	398	101	4851	461	70	4586	1474
35–69	Sm.	2736	768	461	164	143	360	23	1226	–	359	–
	Total	14661	3131	574	379	2178	715	121	7202	649	1867	976
		(19%)	(25%)	(80%)	(43%)	(7%)	(50%)	(19%)	(17%)		(19%)	
70+	Sm.	784	186	115	40	31	297	4	271	–	26	–
	Total	18548	1593	205	199	1189	1237	175	13832	621	862	228
		(4%)	(12%)	(56%)	(20%)	(3%)	(24%)	(2%)	(2%)		(3%)	
Any age	Sm.	3520	954	576	204	174	657	27	1497	–	385	–
	Total	45179	5151	794	592	3765	2053	5147	21495	1340	7315	2678
		(8%)	(19%)	(73%)	(34%)	(5%)	(32%)	(1%)	(7%)		(5%)	

(To be conservative, no deaths before age 35, and none from liver cirrhosis or non-medical causes, were attributed to smoking.)

AZERBAIJAN: 1990

Smoking-attributed deaths (Sm.) and total deaths (Total)

		ALL CAUSES	ALL CANCER	Lung cancer	Upper aero-digestive ca.	Other cancer	COPD	Other respiratory	Vascular disease	Cirrhosis/ other liver	Other medical	Non-medical
Males												
0–34	Sm.	–	–	–	–	–	–	–	–	–	–	–
	Total	6417	231	14	7	210	45	2136	318	50	2242	1395
35–69	Sm.	2656	712	444	123	145	339	20	1289	–	296	–
	Total	10898	2029	499	222	1308	496	87	5657	523	1167	939
		(24%)	(35%)	(89%)	(55%)	(11%)	(68%)	(23%)	(23%)		(25%)	
70+	Sm.	458	108	72	19	17	179	1	154	–	16	–
	Total	5682	561	96	66	399	411	42	4006	171	394	97
		(8%)	(19%)	(75%)	(29%)	(4%)	(44%)	(2%)	(4%)		(4%)	
Any age	Sm.	3114	820	516	142	162	518	21	1443	–	312	–
	Total	22997	2821	609	295	1917	952	2265	9981	744	3803	2431
		(14%)	(29%)	(85%)	(48%)	(8%)	(54%)	(1%)	(14%)		(8%)	
Females												
0–34	Sm.	–	–	–	–	–	–	–	–	–	–	–
	Total	4468	218	18	5	195	48	1798	247	39	1697	421
35–69	Sm.	0	0	0	0	0	0	0	0	–	0	–
	Total	6124	1189	78	114	997	237	54	3356	343	673	272
		(0%)	(0%)	(0%)	(0%)	(0%)	(0%)	(0%)	(0%)		(0%)	
70+	Sm.	0	0	0	0	0	0	0	0	–	0	–
	Total	9230	576	43	71	462	492	47	7144	334	555	82
		(0%)	(0%)	(0%)	(0%)	(0%)	(0%)	(0%)	(0%)		(0%)	
Any age	Sm.	0	0	0	0	0	0	0	0	–	0	–
	Total	19822	1983	139	190	1654	777	1899	10747	716	2925	775
		(0%)	(0%)	(0%)	(0%)	(0%)	(0%)	(0%)	(0%)		(0%)	
Males+Females												
0–34	Sm.	–	–	–	–	–	–	–	–	–	–	–
	Total	10885	449	32	12	405	93	3934	565	89	3939	1816
35–69	Sm.	2656	712	444	123	145	339	20	1289	–	296	–
	Total	17022	3218	577	336	2305	733	141	9013	866	1840	1211
		(16%)	(22%)	(77%)	(37%)	(6%)	(46%)	(14%)	(14%)		(16%)	
70+	Sm.	458	108	72	19	17	179	1	154	–	16	–
	Total	14912	1137	139	137	861	903	89	11150	505	949	179
		(3%)	(9%)	(52%)	(14%)	(2%)	(20%)	(1%)	(1%)		(2%)	
Any age	Sm.	3114	820	516	142	162	518	21	1443	–	312	–
	Total	42819	4804	748	485	3571	1729	4164	20728	1460	6728	3206
		(7%)	(17%)	(69%)	(29%)	(5%)	(30%)	(1%)	(7%)		(5%)	

AZERBAIJAN: 1995

Smoking-attributed deaths (Sm.) and total deaths (Total)

		ALL CAUSES	ALL CANCER	Lung cancer	Upper aero-digestive ca.	Other cancer	COPD	Other respiratory	Vascular disease	Cirrhosis/ other liver	Other medical	Non-medical
Males												
0–34	Sm.	–	–	–	–	–	–	–	–	–	–	–
	Total	6283	242	16	8	218	38	1778	363	59	1943	1860
35–69	Sm.	2315	587	376	85	126	268	19	1211	–	230	–
	Total	11716	2006	434	172	1400	431	93	6302	614	1061	1209
		(20%)	(29%)	(87%)	(49%)	(9%)	(62%)	(20%)	(19%)		(22%)	
70+	Sm.	373	91	63	15	13	145	0	124	–	13	–
	Total	5397	511	87	57	367	367	34	3803	159	422	101
		(7%)	(18%)	(72%)	(26%)	(4%)	(40%)	(0%)	(3%)		(3%)	
Any age	Sm.	2688	678	439	100	139	413	19	1335	–	243	–
	Total	23396	2759	537	237	1985	836	1905	10468	832	3426	3170
		(11%)	(25%)	(82%)	(42%)	(7%)	(49%)	(1%)	(13%)		(7%)	
Females												
0–34	Sm.	–	–	–	–	–	–	–	–	–	–	–
	Total	3860	223	27	4	192	47	1403	284	45	1453	405
35–69	Sm.	0	0	0	0	0	0	0	0	–	0	–
	Total	6276	1062	85	121	856	228	69	3536	442	660	279
		(0%)	(0%)	(0%)	(0%)	(0%)	(0%)	(0%)	(0%)		(0%)	
70+	Sm.	0	0	0	0	0	0	0	0	–	0	–
	Total	9023	503	35	69	399	424	37	6828	361	798	72
		(0%)	(0%)	(0%)	(0%)	(0%)	(0%)	(0%)	(0%)		(0%)	
Any age	Sm.	0	0	0	0	0	0	0	0	–	0	–
	Total	19159	1788	147	194	1447	699	1509	10648	848	2911	756
		(0%)	(0%)	(0%)	(0%)	(0%)	(0%)	(0%)	(0%)		(0%)	
Males+Females												
0–34	Sm.	–	–	–	–	–	–	–	–	–	–	–
	Total	10143	465	43	12	410	85	3181	647	104	3396	2265
35–69	Sm.	2315	587	376	85	126	268	19	1211	–	230	–
	Total	17992	3068	519	293	2256	659	162	9838	1056	1721	1488
		(13%)	(19%)	(72%)	(29%)	(6%)	(41%)	(12%)	(12%)		(13%)	
70+	Sm.	373	91	63	15	13	145	0	124	–	13	–
	Total	14420	1014	122	126	766	791	71	10631	520	1220	173
		(3%)	(9%)	(52%)	(12%)	(2%)	(18%)	(0%)	(1%)		(1%)	
Any age	Sm.	2688	678	439	100	139	413	19	1335	–	243	–
	Total	42555	4547	684	431	3432	1535	3414	21116	1680	6337	3926
		(6%)	(15%)	(64%)	(23%)	(4%)	(27%)	(1%)	(6%)		(4%)	

(To be conservative, no deaths before age 35, and none from liver cirrhosis or non-medical causes, were attributed to smoking.)

¶BELARUS: 1990

		No. of deaths			Standardised rates (Defined on p.286)			Annual death rates / 100, 000						
		All ages	0–34	35–69	All ages	0–34	35–69	0–4	5–9	10–14	15–19	20–24	25–29	30–34
ALL CAUSES	M	53453	5381	28530	1467.5	191.4	1818.7	318.7	47.5	41.1	121.3	229.9	256.0	325.3
	F	56129	2130	15990	799.3	77.3	745.0	231.9	29.5	27.3	48.6	56.0	57.6	89.9
Tuberculosis	M	341	27	276	8.4	0.9	15.6	–	0.2	–	–	0.6	0.9	4.7
	F	106	4	50	1.7	0.1	2.3	0.3	–	–	0.3	–	0.2	0.2
Other infective	M	125	82	37	2.7	2.8	2.3	17.3	–	0.3	0.8	0.3	0.7	0.5
and parasitic	F	154	91	47	2.9	3.3	2.2	20.2	0.3	0.3	0.6	0.6	1.0	0.2
ALL CANCER	M	10060	332	7343	270.7	11.9	476.5	7.7	11.0	4.3	9.9	14.6	16.1	19.8
	F	7484	290	4470	122.8	10.4	205.9	7.6	6.3	7.2	7.8	8.3	12.2	23.6
Mouth and	M	378	9	331	9.5	0.3	19.9	–	0.5	–	0.3	0.6	0.5	0.5
pharynx cancer	F	87	2	38	1.3	0.1	1.8	–	–	–	–	–	0.2	0.2
Oesophagus cancer	M	281	1	230	7.4	0.0	14.9	–	–	–	–	–	–	0.2
	F	39	–	10	0.6	–	0.5	–	–	–	–	–	–	–
Stomach cancer	M	1998	22	1433	54.7	0.8	92.8	–	–	–	–	1.8	0.9	2.8
	F	1509	30	791	23.8	1.1	36.9	–	–	0.3	0.6	1.4	1.7	3.5
Colorectal cancer	M	777	10	492	22.2	0.3	33.8	–	–	–	–	0.3	0.5	1.6
	F	993	9	505	15.7	0.3	23.7	–	–	0.3	0.3	0.6	–	1.2
Liver cancer	M	...	...	...	...	...	...	...	...	...	...	...	...	...
	F	...	...	...	...	...	...	...	...	...	...	...	...	...
Pancreas cancer	M	...	...	...	...	...	...	...	...	...	...	...	...	...
	F	...	...	...	...	...	...	...	...	...	...	...	...	...
Larynx cancer	M	413	–	363	10.5	–	22.7	–	–	–	–	–	–	–
	F	11	1	6	0.2	0.0	0.3	–	–	–	–	–	–	0.2
Lung cancer	M	3024	10	2438	80.4	0.4	156.8	–	–	–	0.6	0.3	0.5	1.2
	F	411	1	237	6.6	0.0	11.0	–	–	–	–	–	0.2	–
Malignant melanoma	M	...	...	...	...	...	...	...	...	...	...	...	...	...
	F	...	...	...	...	...	...	...	...	...	...	...	...	...
Female breast cancer	F	1024	23	785	18.1	0.8	35.7	–	–	–	–	0.3	1.2	4.0
Cervix cancer	F	360	10	230	6.1	0.3	10.7	–	–	–	–	–	0.7	1.6
Other uterine cancer	F	337	3	228	5.5	0.1	10.4	–	–	–	–	–	0.2	0.5
Ovarian cancer	F	...	...	...	...	...	...	...	...	...	...	...	...	...
Prostate cancer	M	370	2	163	11.4	0.1	11.7	–	–	–	0.3	–	–	0.2
Bladder cancer	M	...	...	...	...	...	...	...	...	...	...	...	...	...
	F	...	...	...	...	...	...	...	...	...	...	...	...	...
Other and ill–defined	M	2244	152	1559	59.9	5.5	102.5	4.1	2.9	2.1	4.4	7.6	8.5	8.6
cancer sites	F	2202	120	1363	36.4	4.3	62.3	5.3	2.5	3.3	3.1	2.6	4.8	8.7
Hodgkin's disease	M	...	...	...	...	...	...	...	...	...	...	...	...	...
	F	...	...	...	...	...	...	...	...	...	...	...	...	...
Myeloma and all	M	263	46	170	6.7	1.6	10.6	0.2	1.5	1.1	1.9	1.2	2.6	3.0
lymphomas	F	226	33	128	3.8	1.2	5.8	0.5	1.0	0.3	1.4	1.4	1.4	2.3
Leukaemia	M	312	80	164	7.9	2.9	10.8	3.4	6.1	1.1	2.5	2.9	2.6	1.6
	F	285	58	149	4.9	2.2	6.9	1.8	2.8	3.0	2.5	2.0	1.7	1.4
ALL VASCULAR	M	23748	356	12232	692.7	12.2	812.5	1.9	0.5	2.1	3.9	7.0	21.8	48.4
DISEASE	F	31987	118	7815	439.5	4.2	368.8	3.3	0.8	1.1	3.6	4.6	5.0	11.2
Rheumatic heart	M	389	31	341	9.2	1.1	19.1	–	–	–	–	0.6	2.1	4.7
disease and fever	F	456	18	393	8.2	0.6	17.5	–	–	–	–	1.4	0.7	2.3
Hypertensive disease	M	312	10	250	7.9	0.4	14.9	–	–	–	0.3	0.6	0.5	1.2
	F	367	3	203	5.8	0.1	9.2	–	–	–	0.3	–	–	0.5
Ischaemic heart	M	15342	144	7629	451.4	4.9	509.5	–	–	–	0.8	1.8	7.6	24.0
disease	F	19149	27	3765	256.4	0.9	179.9	–	–	0.3	–	1.1	1.4	3.7
Pulmonary embolism	M	...	...	...	...	...	...	...	...	...	...	...	...	...
and other venous	F	...	...	...	...	...	...	...	...	...	...	...	...	...
Cerebrovascular	M	5682	58	2931	167.2	2.0	200.0	–	0.2	0.5	0.8	0.9	4.3	7.2
disease	F	9480	32	2822	133.9	1.1	132.8	0.8	0.3	0.6	0.6	1.4	1.2	3.3
Other vascular	M	2023	113	1081	57.0	4.0	69.0	1.9	0.2	1.6	1.9	3.2	7.3	11.4
disease, incl. venous	F	2535	38	632	35.2	1.4	29.5	2.5	0.5	0.3	2.8	0.6	1.7	1.4
Chronic obstructive	M	3732	41	1724	111.1	1.4	121.8	1.7	0.5	0.5	0.3	0.6	1.9	4.4
pulmonary disease	F	3028	24	635	41.1	0.9	30.0	0.5	0.5	–	0.8	0.9	1.7	1.6
Other respiratory	M	439	199	171	10.4	6.9	10.5	43.2	0.5	0.5	0.8	0.3	1.4	1.2
disease	F	319	138	85	5.4	5.0	3.8	29.2	1.3	0.6	1.4	1.4	1.0	0.2
Peptic ulcer	M	214	4	151	5.8	0.1	9.4	–	–	–	–	–	0.2	0.7
	F	94	1	35	1.4	0.0	1.7	–	–	–	–	0.3	–	–
Liver cirrhosis and	M	466	17	362	12.3	0.6	22.8	0.5	–	–	–	0.3	0.7	2.6
other liver disease	F	311	17	192	5.1	0.6	8.8	–	0.3	0.6	0.8	0.9	0.5	1.4
Renal disease	M	424	45	267	11.3	1.6	17.2	0.7	0.7	–	1.7	2.0	2.6	3.5
	F	506	34	323	8.5	1.2	14.9	0.3	0.3	1.1	1.4	1.7	1.4	2.6
Pregnancy and birth	F	31	22	9	0.6	0.8	0.4	–	–	–	–	0.9	1.0	3.5
Congenital and	M	826	812	14	15.9	28.0	0.8	182.5	1.9	1.9	2.2	3.5	2.1	1.9
perinatal causes	F	552	529	22	11.1	19.1	1.0	125.8	2.3	1.7	1.4	1.1	0.7	0.7
Ill–defined causes	M	3175	92	357	100.7	3.2	21.4	7.9	0.5	0.3	1.9	2.0	4.7	5.1
	F	7299	28	144	86.7	1.0	6.8	3.5	0.5	–	0.6	1.4	0.2	0.9
Other medical causes	M	1888	289	1039	50.0	10.3	64.5	19.9	4.1	5.1	9.1	8.2	11.4	14.2
	F	2013	240	932	32.0	8.8	43.0	14.9	4.5	5.5	8.1	9.2	6.7	12.6
ALL NON–	M	8015	3085	4557	175.5	111.4	243.4	35.3	27.5	26.2	90.7	190.5	191.3	218.4
MEDICAL CAUSES	F	2245	594	1231	40.5	21.7	55.6	26.5	12.6	9.4	21.9	24.7	25.9	30.9
Motor vehicle	M	1845	916	844	39.6	33.7	45.7	4.8	10.2	6.4	35.9	73.2	54.3	51.2
traffic accidents	F	496	176	227	8.9	6.6	10.1	5.5	4.3	3.3	10.3	10.1	5.0	7.5
Fire	M	127	56	58	2.9	2.1	3.4	3.8	0.5	1.3	1.4	3.8	1.7	1.9
	F	78	20	22	1.2	0.7	1.0	2.8	1.0	–	0.6	–	0.5	0.2
Suicide	M	1650	499	1064	37.0	17.7	57.2	–	–	2.1	11.6	26.3	37.9	46.3
	F	435	72	277	7.7	2.6	12.4	–	–	0.8	2.8	4.0	5.3	5.4
Homicide	M	483	251	216	10.0	9.1	11.2	0.2	–	0.3	8.5	18.1	18.3	18.4
	F	229	73	129	4.3	2.6	6.0	0.5	0.3	0.3	2.2	3.2	5.8	6.1
POPULATION (thousands):	**M=males**				4783.8	2757.8	1834.5	416.4	410.3	374.5	362.6	342.7	421.9	429.4
	F=females				5427.6	2708.2	2230.6	396.7	396.0	363.0	360.2	348.2	417.0	427.1

BELARUS: 1990
9th ICD categories

Annual death rates / 100, 000

35–39	40–44	45–49	50–54	55–59	60–64	65–69	70–74	75–79	80+/NK			
462.3	674.8	988.5	1472.3	2033.7	2979.9	4119.5	6115.9	8457.9	16513.2	M	**ALL CAUSES**	001–999
130.2	217.1	358.6	505.5	772.9	1199.7	2031.0	3541.4	5553.4	13472.7	F		
7.9	10.1	19.2	16.5	22.1	17.5	15.8	18.3	18.4	23.1	M	**Tuberculosis**	010–018, 137
0.5	0.7	2.8	1.9	2.1	3.4	5.0	10.3	10.7	10.9	F		
1.1	2.1	1.3	1.9	2.2	2.1	5.3	3.0	4.6	1.7	M	**Other infective**	Rest of 001–139
1.1	1.7	2.0	1.4	1.8	3.4	3.8	3.4	4.2	2.3	F	**and parasitic**	
38.6	97.5	211.6	376.3	601.2	926.1	1084.2	1390.2	1252.7	1080.9	M	**ALL CANCER**	140–208
43.6	77.4	128.6	168.4	232.1	327.0	464.3	596.9	567.7	514.1	F		
1.6	5.9	14.5	26.6	28.4	30.9	31.6	22.9	18.4	18.2	M	**Mouth and**	140–149
0.3	–	0.8	1.4	2.7	2.3	5.0	8.9	11.3	8.6	F	**pharynx cancer**	
1.4	1.0	7.3	13.3	23.9	22.1	35.3	30.5	32.2	14.9	M	**Oesophagus cancer**	150
–	–	–	0.3	0.6	0.9	1.5	4.8	4.2	8.6	F		
9.8	21.7	41.8	74.2	113.0	177.5	211.3	291.2	312.4	244.2	M	**Stomach cancer**	151
6.8	12.5	18.5	26.0	35.3	59.1	100.1	134.2	166.9	121.1	F		
1.6	6.6	9.8	21.4	31.1	69.8	96.2	150.9	157.7	120.5	M	**Colorectal cancer**	153, 154
3.5	6.1	11.8	14.9	27.3	34.2	68.0	99.9	96.2	98.1	F		
...	...	...	...	...	...	...	...	...	...	M	**Liver cancer**	Not given separately
...	...	...	...	...	...	...	...	...	...	F		
...	...	...	...	...	...	...	...	...	...	M	**Pancreas cancer**	Not given separately
...	...	...	...	...	...	...	...	...	...	F		
1.4	4.9	11.1	22.0	28.4	49.3	42.1	36.6	23.0	18.2	M	**Larynx cancer**	161
–	–	–	–	0.3	0.6	1.1	–	0.6	1.7	F		
6.3	22.7	64.0	124.1	218.1	332.1	330.1	426.8	280.2	186.5	M	**Lung cancer**	162
1.4	2.4	7.5	9.7	11.0	16.8	28.7	36.3	30.3	39.6	F		
...	...	...	...	...	...	...	...	...	...	M	**Malignant melanoma**	Not given
...	...	...	...	...	...	...	...	...	...	F		separately
11.6	22.3	36.2	34.0	46.0	50.8	48.9	50.7	49.9	33.3	F	**Female breast cancer**	174
3.0	6.1	9.0	7.7	11.6	15.4	21.8	26.7	24.9	22.4	F	**Cervix cancer**	180
2.2	0.7	3.5	10.0	12.2	18.0	26.4	26.7	22.0	17.2	F	**Other uterine cancer**	179, 182
...	...	...	...	...	...	...	...	...	...	F	**Ovarian cancer**	Not given separately
–	–	1.7	5.2	11.2	26.7	36.8	93.0	96.5	133.7	M	**Prostate cancer**	185
...	...	...	...	...	...	...	...	...	...	M	**Bladder cancer**	Not given separately
...	...	...	...	...	...	...	...	...	...	F		
13.1	24.4	53.3	72.3	123.1	179.2	251.9	265.2	274.1	297.0	M	**Other and ill-defined**	Rest of 140–208,
10.8	22.3	33.8	57.0	72.9	105.6	133.4	165.6	136.6	141.7	F	**cancer sites**	incl. 155, 157, 172, 183, 188
...	...	...	...	...	...	...	...	...	...	M	**Hodgkin's disease**	Not given separately
...	...	...	...	...	...	...	...	...	...	F		
1.9	5.6	5.5	8.8	12.3	19.6	20.3	33.5	24.5	14.9	M	**Myeloma and all**	200–203,
1.9	2.0	3.5	3.9	6.8	10.6	12.2	19.2	10.7	10.9	F	**lymphomas**	incl. 201
1.4	4.5	2.6	8.4	11.6	18.8	28.6	39.6	33.7	33.0	M	**Leukaemia**	204–208
2.2	3.0	3.9	3.6	5.6	12.8	17.2	24.0	14.3	10.9	F		
107.8	230.2	352.8	606.8	859.0	1398.5	2132.3	3408.5	4961.7	9379.5	M	**ALL VASCULAR**	390–459
20.8	51.1	108.1	190.3	360.8	635.7	1214.7	2332.0	3741.1	8231.2	F	**DISEASE**	
7.4	10.1	14.5	26.9	33.7	22.1	18.8	13.7	9.2	3.3	M	**Rheumatic heart**	390–398
2.7	8.5	13.0	22.4	27.9	27.4	20.6	16.4	9.5	2.9	F	**disease and fever**	
4.6	7.3	7.7	17.2	17.2	26.3	24.1	21.3	30.6	29.7	M	**Hypertensive disease**	401–405
0.8	2.0	4.7	10.0	11.0	17.1	18.7	27.4	29.7	40.7	F		
62.9	145.0	224.0	372.4	534.2	863.8	1363.9	2181.4	3291.0	6582.5	M	**Ischaemic heart**	410–414
6.2	13.5	39.7	63.9	158.9	312.7	664.1	1346.3	2304.6	5455.5	F	**disease**	
...	...	...	...	...	...	...	...	...	...	M	**Pulmonary embolism**	Not given
...	...	...	...	...	...	...	...	...	...	F	**and other venous**	separately
17.2	37.0	67.8	133.2	197.2	380.1	567.7	937.5	1254.2	2077.6	M	**Cerebrovascular**	430–438
7.6	17.6	36.6	71.6	133.7	231.7	430.6	782.3	1130.0	2053.9	F	**disease**	
15.6	30.7	38.8	57.1	76.7	106.1	157.9	254.6	376.7	686.5	M	**Other vascular**	Rest of 390–459,
3.5	9.5	14.2	22.4	29.4	46.8	80.6	159.5	267.2	678.1	F	**disease, incl. venous**	incl. 415, 451–3
5.5	9.4	26.9	60.6	140.7	226.0	383.5	568.6	972.4	1582.5	M	**Chronic obstructive**	490–496
2.4	5.1	9.8	16.9	31.4	47.1	97.1	206.0	397.3	802.6	F	**pulmonary disease**	
3.3	5.6	9.4	8.4	8.6	20.1	18.0	27.4	27.6	54.5	M	**Other respiratory**	Rest of 460–519
0.3	0.7	1.6	3.9	7.1	6.6	6.5	7.5	17.8	31.6	F	**disease**	
2.7	3.1	5.5	5.8	15.0	15.0	18.8	21.3	27.6	44.6	M	**Peptic ulcer**	531–533
–	0.3	0.4	0.6	1.2	3.4	5.7	13.0	8.9	13.8	F		
2.2	7.0	11.5	25.6	26.2	39.3	48.1	64.0	42.9	28.1	M	**Liver cirrhosis and**	570–573, 576,
1.9	3.7	5.1	8.3	11.9	12.8	17.6	16.4	17.8	27.5	F	**other liver disease**	575.2–579.9
4.9	5.9	8.5	15.6	16.5	26.7	42.1	57.9	62.8	54.5	M	**Renal disease**	580–590
3.0	5.7	11.4	12.2	15.1	25.1	31.7	33.5	32.7	25.8	F		
1.6	0.7	–	0.3	–	–	–	–	–	–	F	**Pregnancy and birth**	630–676
0.5	1.4	1.3	0.3	0.4	0.8	0.8	–	–	–	M	**Congenital and**	740–779
1.6	2.0	0.4	0.8	0.9	0.3	0.8	–	0.6	–	F	**perinatal causes**	
11.2	11.2	20.9	26.3	19.8	19.2	41.4	166.2	611.0	3660.1	M	**Ill-defined causes**	780–799
1.6	2.0	2.8	6.4	5.3	8.6	20.6	121.8	507.7	3496.3	F		
25.7	31.4	36.7	54.5	71.5	95.2	136.8	221.0	291.0	371.3	M	**Other medical causes**	Rest of 001–799
12.2	15.2	24.0	34.0	42.7	69.6	103.2	127.3	160.3	220.9	F		
250.8	259.9	282.8	273.6	250.7	193.4	192.5	169.2	185.3	232.7	M	**ALL NON-**	E800–E999
39.5	50.7	61.7	60.3	60.5	56.8	60.0	73.2	86.7	95.8	F	**MEDICAL CAUSES**	
45.4	53.4	46.9	48.3	45.6	35.1	45.1	42.7	38.3	52.8	M	**Motor vehicle**	E810–E819
7.3	8.1	9.8	13.0	10.1	12.3	10.3	17.8	17.2	21.8	F	**traffic accidents**	
2.2	2.1	6.0	2.6	3.4	2.9	4.5	3.0	7.7	9.9	M	**Fire**	E890–E899
0.8	0.7	0.4	0.6	1.5	1.4	1.5	3.4	11.3	6.9	F		
55.8	53.8	75.1	63.2	59.5	48.9	44.4	42.7	39.8	54.5	M	**Suicide**	E950–E959
9.5	9.8	11.8	13.8	12.7	15.1	14.1	17.1	17.2	18.4	F		
17.0	12.9	11.1	11.0	8.6	10.0	7.5	6.1	4.6	14.9	M	**Homicide**	E960–E969
5.1	8.1	10.2	5.3	5.3	3.1	4.6	5.5	3.6	7.5	F		
365.6	286.3	234.4	308.5	267.3	239.4	133.0	65.6	65.3	60.6	M	**POPULATION (thousands)**	
369.5	295.7	254.3	361.6	337.3	350.5	261.7	146.1	168.4	174.3	F		

BELARUS: Males

	All ages	0–34	35–69	35–39	40–44	45–49	50–54	55–59	60–64	65–69	70–74	75–79	80+/NK
POPULATION (1000s)													
1985–90	4703.8	2750.6	1750.9	342.7	240.5	292.4	292.4	280.4	197.6	104.9	78.0	66.4	57.9
1985	4628.4	2746.7	1665.0	294.8	244.5	327.1	290.7	267.0	157.0	83.9	94.3	66.4	56.0
1990	**4783.8**	**2757.8**	**1834.5**	**365.6**	**286.3**	**234.4**	**308.5**	**267.3**	**239.4**	**133.0**	**65.6**	**65.3**	**60.6**
1995 projected	*4830.1*	*2784.5*	*1852.3*	*369.1*	*289.1*	*236.7*	*311.5*	*269.9*	*241.7*	*134.3*	*66.2*	*65.9*	*61.2*
NUMBER OF DEATHS													
All causes													
1985–90	49669	5239	24723	1407	1545	2664	3958	5335	5612	4202	4462	5773	9472
1985	50922	5560	23807	1361	1723	3206	4141	5399	4554	3423	5692	6192	9671
1990	**53453**	**5381**	**28530**	**1690**	**1932**	**2317**	**4542**	**5436**	**7134**	**5479**	**4012**	**5523**	**10007**
1995 projected	*53250*	*5350*	*29141*	*1658*	*1931*	*2361*	*4656*	*5608*	*7309*	*5618*	*3892*	*5313*	*9554*
Lung cancer													
1985–90	2691	12	2142	24	53	169	372	588	583	353	256	186	95
1985	2323	10	1821	19	71	171	358	536	403	263	281	143	68
1990	**3024**	**10**	**2438**	**23**	**65**	**150**	**383**	**583**	**795**	**439**	**280**	**183**	**113**
1995 projected	*3541*	*7*	*2765*	*18*	*67*	*152*	*410*	*672*	*903*	*543*	*347*	*264*	*158*
ANNUAL DEATH RATE / 100,000 (*The rates for the age groups 0–34 and 35–69 are the means of seven five-yearly rates, but the all-ages rates are standardised to the conventional "European" age distribution)													
All causes													
1985–90	1416.1*	185.9*	1723.7*	410.6	642.4	911.1	1353.6	1902.6	2840.1	4005.7	5720.5	8694.3	16359.2
1985	1494.2*	199.0*	1796.2*	461.7	704.7	980.1	1424.5	2022.1	2900.6	4079.9	6036.1	9325.3	17269.6
1990	**1467.5***	**191.4***	**1818.7***	**462.3**	**674.8**	**988.5**	**1472.3**	**2033.7**	**2979.9**	**4119.5**	**6115.9**	**8457.9**	**16513.2**
1995 projected	*1441.1**	*189.8**	*1842.0**	*449.2*	*667.9*	*997.5*	*1494.7*	*2077.8*	*3024.0*	*4183.2*	*5879.2*	*8062.2*	*15611.1*
All cancer													
1985–90	254.6*	11.7*	459.3*	42.0	101.5	202.1	371.4	581.7	845.6	1070.5	1150.0	1210.8	993.1
1985	236.2*	11.9*	429.9*	43.1	106.7	186.5	350.5	555.8	757.3	1009.5	1087.0	1054.2	846.4
1990	**270.7***	**11.9***	**476.5***	**38.6**	**97.5**	**211.6**	**376.3**	**601.2**	**926.1**	**1084.2**	**1390.2**	**1252.7**	**1080.9**
1995 projected	*308.4**	*10.7**	*533.7**	*33.3*	*96.9*	*221.8*	*407.4*	*680.3*	*1031.4*	*1265.1*	*1616.3*	*1590.3*	*1330.1*
Lung cancer													
1985–90	74.7*	0.4*	150.8*	7.0	22.0	57.8	127.2	209.7	295.0	336.5	328.2	280.1	164.1
1985	68.0*	0.4*	140.3*	6.4	29.0	52.3	123.2	200.7	256.7	313.5	298.0	215.4	121.4
1990	**80.4***	**0.4***	**156.8***	**6.3**	**22.7**	**64.0**	**124.1**	**218.1**	**332.1**	**330.1**	**426.8**	**280.2**	**186.5**
1995 projected	*94.5**	*0.2**	*178.7**	*4.9*	*23.2*	*64.2*	*131.6*	*249.0*	*373.6*	*404.3*	*524.2*	*400.6*	*258.2*
Upper aerodigestive cancer (mouth, oesophagus, pharynx and larynx)													
1985–90	24.5*	0.3*	49.9*	4.7	14.6	29.8	49.9	66.0	86.5	98.2	82.1	75.3	63.9
1985	20.9*	0.3*	42.4*	5.1	13.1	25.1	35.4	57.7	73.2	87.0	73.2	66.3	55.4
1990	**27.5***	**0.4***	**57.6***	**4.4**	**11.9**	**32.8**	**61.9**	**80.8**	**102.3**	**109.0**	**89.9**	**73.5**	**51.2**
1995 projected	*35.3**	*0.4**	*76.2**	*3.8*	*13.1*	*45.2*	*86.0*	*112.3*	*135.3*	*137.8*	*105.7*	*75.9*	*53.9*
Other cancer													
1985–90	155.3*	10.9*	258.6*	30.3	64.9	114.6	194.3	306.0	464.1	635.8	739.7	855.4	765.1
1985	147.3*	11.3*	247.3*	31.5	64.6	109.1	192.0	297.4	427.4	609.1	715.8	772.6	669.6
1990	**162.8***	**11.2***	**262.1***	**27.9**	**62.9**	**114.8**	**190.3**	**302.3**	**491.6**	**645.1**	**873.5**	**898.9**	**843.2**
1995 projected	*178.5**	*10.1**	*278.8**	*24.7*	*60.5*	*112.4*	*189.7*	*319.0*	*522.5*	*723.0*	*986.4*	*1113.8*	*1018.0*
Chronic obstructive pulmonary disease (COPD)													
1985–90	132.1*	1.4*	128.2*	7.3	16.6	35.6	70.5	141.2	242.9	383.2	646.2	1158.1	2193.4
1985	161.2*	1.6*	150.5*	9.2	26.2	47.4	94.9	168.5	307.0	400.5	846.2	1441.3	2612.5
1990	**111.1***	**1.4***	**121.8***	**5.5**	**9.4**	**26.9**	**60.6**	**140.7**	**226.0**	**383.5**	**568.6**	**972.4**	**1582.5**
1995 projected	*81.0**	*1.2**	*92.9**	*3.8*	*6.6*	*18.6*	*43.7*	*103.4*	*190.7*	*283.7*	*398.8*	*695.0*	*1119.3*
Other respiratory disease													
1985–90	11.3*	10.3*	9.1*	3.5	5.0	6.8	8.9	10.3	13.7	15.3	21.8	25.6	41.5
1985	14.2*	14.6*	11.6*	5.4	6.1	7.3	11.7	13.1	13.4	23.8	20.1	21.1	32.1
1990	**10.4***	**6.9***	**10.5***	**3.3**	**5.6**	**9.4**	**8.4**	**8.6**	**20.1**	**18.0**	**27.4**	**27.6**	**54.5**
1995 projected	*9.4**	*4.5**	*9.9**	*2.2*	*5.2*	*8.4*	*6.7*	*8.2*	*18.2*	*20.1*	*30.2*	*33.4*	*76.8*
Vascular disease													
1985–90	736.2*	12.4*	779.7*	103.0	212.9	328.7	544.1	808.8	1364.4	2096.3	3401.3	5588.9	11626.9
1985	805.3*	13.4*	825.3*	118.0	219.6	358.6	569.7	879.0	1422.3	2209.8	3625.7	6274.1	13182.1
1990	**692.7***	**12.2***	**812.5***	**107.8**	**230.2**	**352.8**	**606.8**	**859.0**	**1398.5**	**2132.3**	**3408.5**	**4961.7**	**9379.5**
1995 projected	*597.2**	*10.4**	*778.6**	*102.1*	*220.0*	*355.7*	*599.7*	*841.8*	*1340.1*	*1991.1*	*2897.3*	*4018.2*	*6913.4*
Liver cirrhosis and other liver disease													
1985–90	12.9*	0.6*	25.0*	4.7	8.3	14.4	21.2	27.1	45.0	54.3	46.2	48.2	38.0
1985	16.9*	0.9*	35.3*	12.6	11.9	25.4	31.0	36.7	63.1	66.7	36.1	48.2	37.5
1990	**12.3***	**0.6***	**22.8***	**2.2**	**7.0**	**11.5**	**25.6**	**26.2**	**39.3**	**48.1**	**64.0**	**42.9**	**28.1**
1995 projected	*10.0**	*0.3**	*17.2**	*1.4*	*4.8*	*8.0*	*17.7*	*18.2*	*27.3*	*43.2*	*65.0*	*53.1*	*22.9*
Other medical causes													
1985–90	119.1*	53.8*	117.3*	47.3	63.2	82.4	105.7	135.2	162.4	225.0	310.3	484.9	1248.7
1985	111.5*	66.9*	134.1*	66.5	88.8	105.8	124.5	158.4	163.7	231.2	269.4	310.2	380.4
1990	**194.8***	**47.0***	**131.3***	**54.2**	**65.3**	**93.4**	**120.9**	**147.4**	**176.7**	**260.9**	**487.8**	**1015.3**	**4155.1**
1995 projected	*236.7**	*34.0**	*137.4**	*36.6*	*51.2*	*79.8*	*110.4*	*144.1*	*184.1*	*355.2*	*676.7*	*1450.7*	*5875.8*
All non-medical causes													
1985–90	149.9*	95.7*	205.2*	202.8	234.9	241.1	231.9	198.3	166.0	161.1	144.9	177.7	217.6
1985	148.8*	89.6*	209.5*	206.9	245.4	249.2	242.2	210.5	173.9	138.3	151.6	176.2	178.6
1990	**175.5***	**111.4***	**243.4***	**250.8**	**259.9**	**282.8**	**273.6**	**250.7**	**193.4**	**192.5**	**169.2**	**185.3**	**232.7**
1995 projected	*198.3**	*128.6**	*272.3**	*269.8*	*283.3*	*305.0*	*309.1*	*282.0*	*232.1*	*224.9*	*194.9*	*221.5*	*272.9*

BELARUS: Females

	All ages	0–34	35–69	35–39	40–44	45–49	50–54	55–59	60–64	65–69	70–74	75–79	80+/NK
POPULATION (1000s)													
1985–90	5364.8	2694.8	2164.4	346.5	251.3	325.2	345.9	360.6	328.0	206.9	178.0	163.6	164.0
1985	5300.6	2682.1	2096.4	298.6	258.8	371.8	346.9	365.6	286.0	168.7	212.1	155.8	154.2
1990	5427.6	2708.2	2230.6	369.5	295.7	254.3	361.6	337.3	350.5	261.7	146.1	168.4	174.3
1995 projected	5480.1	2734.3	2252.3	373.1	298.6	256.8	365.1	340.6	353.9	264.2	147.5	170.0	176.0
NUMBER OF DEATHS													
All causes													
1985–90	53452	2286	14590	456	540	1040	1697	2698	3929	4230	5910	9183	21483
1985	54768	2570	14225	448	578	1355	1786	2897	3568	3593	7253	9221	21499
1990	56129	2130	15990	481	642	912	1828	2607	4205	5315	5174	9352	23483
1995 projected	54186	1784	15753	445	621	902	1807	2554	4077	5347	5069	9177	22403
Lung cancer													
1985–90	410	3	221	4	6	16	28	44	63	60	67	65	54
1985	376	5	186	4	4	31	17	39	43	48	82	63	40
1990	411	1	237	5	7	19	35	37	59	75	53	51	69
1995 projected	434	1	258	6	7	25	41	45	60	74	48	54	73
ANNUAL DEATH RATE / 100,000 (*The rates for the age groups 0–34 and 35–69 are the means of seven five-yearly rates, but the all-ages rates are standardised to the conventional "European" age distribution)													
All causes													
1985–90	784.8*	82.9*	735.3*	131.6	214.9	319.8	490.6	748.2	1197.9	2044.5	3320.2	5613.1	13099.4
1985	832.1*	94.4*	774.6*	150.0	223.3	364.4	514.8	792.4	1247.6	2129.8	3419.6	5918.5	13942.3
1990	799.3*	77.3*	745.0*	130.2	217.1	358.6	505.5	772.9	1199.7	2031.0	3541.4	5553.4	13472.7
1995 projected	764.5*	64.3*	728.4*	119.3	208.0	351.2	494.9	749.9	1152.0	2023.8	3436.6	5398.2	12729.0
All cancer													
1985–90	116.5*	10.4*	201.7*	43.3	72.4	112.2	169.1	232.7	333.2	449.0	506.7	533.6	451.8
1985	110.7*	11.5*	193.8*	45.2	61.8	118.9	159.4	225.7	326.2	419.7	468.6	491.7	372.9
1990	122.8*	10.4*	205.9*	43.6	77.4	128.6	168.4	232.1	327.0	464.3	596.9	567.7	514.1
1995 projected	136.8*	9.3*	219.7*	46.4	84.4	139.8	175.3	235.5	335.1	521.6	709.8	757.1	639.8
Lung cancer													
1985–90	6.6*	0.1*	11.0*	1.2	2.4	4.9	8.1	12.2	19.2	29.0	37.6	39.7	32.9
1985	6.2*	0.2*	10.0*	1.3	1.5	8.3	4.9	10.7	15.0	28.5	38.7	40.4	25.9
1990	6.6*	0.0*	11.0*	1.4	2.4	7.5	9.7	11.0	16.8	28.7	36.3	30.3	39.6
1995 projected	7.0*	0.0*	11.9*	1.6	2.3	9.7	11.2	13.2	17.0	28.0	32.5	31.8	41.5
Upper aerodigestive cancer (mouth, oesophagus, pharynx and larynx)													
1985–90	2.1*	0.1*	3.0*	0.3	0.8	0.9	1.4	3.3	6.1	8.2	10.1	13.4	17.1
1985	1.7*	0.1*	2.7*	–	0.4	1.3	2.3	3.3	5.6	5.9	9.0	8.3	11.7
1990	2.1*	0.1*	2.5*	0.3	–	0.8	1.7	3.6	3.7	7.6	13.7	16.0	18.9
1995 projected	2.5*	0.1*	2.5*	0.3	–	0.4	1.4	2.9	3.7	9.1	19.7	23.5	26.7
Other cancer													
1985–90	107.8*	10.2*	187.7*	41.8	69.2	106.4	159.6	217.1	307.9	411.8	459.0	480.4	401.8
1985	102.7*	11.2*	181.1*	43.9	59.9	109.2	152.2	211.7	305.6	385.3	421.0	442.9	335.3
1990	114.2*	10.3*	192.3*	41.9	75.1	120.3	157.1	217.6	306.4	428.0	546.9	521.4	455.5
1995 projected	127.3*	9.2*	205.3*	44.5	82.0	129.7	162.7	219.3	314.5	484.5	657.6	701.8	571.6
Chronic obstructive pulmonary disease (COPD)													
1985–90	52.3*	1.0*	33.2*	2.9	6.4	9.2	16.5	29.7	54.6	113.1	238.2	470.0	1188.4
1985	65.6*	1.8*	43.2*	2.7	5.8	13.2	21.6	36.9	67.8	154.7	295.6	570.0	1483.1
1990	41.1*	0.9*	30.0*	2.4	5.1	9.8	16.9	31.4	47.1	97.1	206.0	397.3	802.6
1995 projected	29.5*	0.6*	21.4*	1.9	4.0	7.4	13.4	23.5	32.5	67.4	146.4	292.9	567.0
Other respiratory disease													
1985–90	6.3*	7.6*	2.9*	0.9	1.2	1.8	2.3	3.3	4.3	6.3	9.0	14.1	22.6
1985	8.1*	11.0*	2.8*	0.7	1.5	1.9	3.2	3.6	4.5	4.1	9.0	14.1	17.5
1990	5.4*	5.0*	3.8*	0.3	0.7	1.6	3.9	7.1	6.6	6.5	7.5	17.8	31.6
1995 projected	5.4*	3.4*	4.9*	0.3	0.3	1.6	5.5	10.0	9.0	7.6	8.8	26.5	44.3
Vascular disease													
1985–90	491.8*	4.3*	374.0*	24.0	50.1	99.0	190.5	347.2	644.2	1262.9	2318.5	4213.3	10342.1
1985	543.2*	4.3*	404.6*	26.5	55.6	111.9	206.7	381.6	694.8	1355.1	2446.0	4607.2	11786.6
1990	439.5*	4.2*	368.8*	20.8	51.1	108.1	190.3	360.8	635.7	1214.7	2332.0	3741.1	8231.2
1995 projected	361.9*	3.9*	334.9*	18.0	46.6	99.3	177.2	330.6	562.6	1109.8	2029.2	3129.4	6011.4
Liver cirrhosis and other liver disease													
1985–90	5.3*	0.5*	9.4*	1.7	3.6	5.5	7.5	12.2	15.5	19.8	18.0	22.0	22.6
1985	6.5*	0.5*	12.3*	3.7	6.2	10.0	10.1	18.3	16.8	20.7	18.9	22.5	20.1
1990	5.1*	0.6*	8.8*	1.9	3.7	5.1	8.3	11.9	12.8	17.6	16.4	17.8	27.5
1995 projected	4.2*	0.7*	6.5*	1.3	2.7	3.5	5.8	8.5	9.3	14.4	13.6	19.4	29.5
Other medical causes													
1985–90	75.7*	38.7*	64.3*	22.5	30.6	39.1	52.3	69.1	95.7	140.6	171.3	284.2	968.9
1985	57.8*	43.3*	62.2*	26.8	35.5	45.5	59.1	67.3	82.5	118.6	123.1	147.6	161.5
1990	144.9*	34.4*	72.1*	21.7	28.4	43.6	57.5	69.1	113.8	170.8	309.4	725.1	3769.9
1995 projected	186.0*	25.5*	85.6*	17.2	24.1	39.7	56.4	78.7	146.1	237.3	439.3	1068.8	5331.8
All non-medical causes													
1985–90	36.9*	20.4*	49.9*	36.4	50.5	52.9	52.3	54.1	50.3	52.7	58.4	75.8	103.0
1985	40.1*	22.0*	55.7*	44.5	56.8	63.2	54.8	59.1	54.9	56.9	58.5	65.5	100.5
1990	40.5*	21.7*	55.6*	39.5	50.7	61.7	60.3	60.5	56.8	60.0	73.2	86.7	95.8
1995 projected	40.8*	21.0*	55.4*	34.3	45.9	60.0	61.4	63.1	57.4	65.9	89.5	104.1	105.1

BELARUS: 1985–1990

Smoking–attributed deaths (Sm.) and total deaths (Total)

		ALL CAUSES	ALL CANCER	Lung cancer	Upper aero–digestive ca.	Other cancer	COPD	Other respiratory	Vascular disease	Cirrhosis/ other liver	Other medical	Non–medical
Males												
0–34	Sm.	–	–	–	–	–	–	–	–	–	–	–
	Total	5239	324	12	9	303	38	300	348	17	1544	2668
35–69	Sm.	9598	3335	2027	542	766	1367	60	4090	–	746	–
	Total	24723	6490	2142	743	3605	1653	142	10580	362	1800	3696
		(39%)	(51%)	(95%)	(73%)	(21%)	(83%)	(42%)	(39%)		(41%)	
70+	Sm.	3250	664	461	72	131	1527	5	961	–	93	–
	Total	19707	2276	537	151	1588	2543	58	13096	90	1287	357
		(16%)	(29%)	(86%)	(48%)	(8%)	(60%)	(9%)	(7%)		(7%)	
Any age	Sm.	12848	3999	2488	614	897	2894	65	5051	–	839	–
	Total	49669	9090	2691	903	5496	4234	500	24024	469	4631	6721
		(26%)	(44%)	(92%)	(68%)	(16%)	(68%)	(13%)	(21%)		(18%)	
Females												
0–34	Sm.	–	–	–	–	–	–	–	–	–	–	–
	Total	2286	286	3	4	279	28	212	118	13	1073	556
35–69	Sm.	251	43	35	2	6	74	0	117	–	17	–
	Total	14590	4143	221	60	3862	633	59	7168	195	1317	1075
		(2%)	(1%)	(16%)	(3%)	(0%)	(12%)	(0%)	(2%)		(1%)	
70+	Sm.	408	39	32	3	4	240	0	120	–	9	–
	Total	36576	2516	186	68	2262	3142	76	27981	105	2359	397
		(1%)	(2%)	(17%)	(4%)	(0%)	(8%)	(0%)	(0%)		(0%)	
Any age	Sm.	659	82	67	5	10	314	0	237	–	26	–
	Total	53452	6945	410	132	6403	3803	347	35267	313	4749	2028
		(1%)	(1%)	(16%)	(4%)	(0%)	(8%)	(0%)	(1%)		(1%)	
Males+Females												
0–34	Sm.	–	–	–	–	–	–	–	–	–	–	–
	Total	7525	610	15	13	582	66	512	466	30	2617	3224
35–69	Sm.	9849	3378	2062	544	772	1441	60	4207	–	763	–
	Total	39313	10633	2363	803	7467	2286	201	17748	557	3117	4771
		(25%)	(32%)	(87%)	(68%)	(10%)	(63%)	(30%)	(24%)		(24%)	
70+	Sm.	3658	703	493	75	135	1767	5	1081	–	102	–
	Total	56283	4792	723	219	3850	5685	134	41077	195	3646	754
		(6%)	(15%)	(68%)	(34%)	(4%)	(31%)	(4%)	(3%)		(3%)	
Any age	Sm.	13507	4081	2555	619	907	3208	65	5288	–	865	–
	Total	103121	16035	3101	1035	11899	8037	847	59291	782	9380	8749
		(13%)	(25%)	(82%)	(60%)	(8%)	(40%)	(8%)	(9%)		(9%)	

BELARUS: 1985

Smoking–attributed deaths (Sm.) and total deaths (Total)

		ALL CAUSES	ALL CANCER	Lung cancer	Upper aero–digestive ca.	Other cancer	COPD	Other respiratory	Vascular disease	Cirrhosis/ other liver	Other medical	Non–medical
Males												
0–34	Sm.	–	–	–	–	–	–	–	–	–	–	–
	Total	5560	328	10	8	310	44	414	366	25	1885	2498
35–69	Sm.	9039	2779	1721	413	645	1469	67	3889	–	835	–
	Total	23807	5537	1821	574	3142	1790	165	10148	492	1995	3680
		(38%)	(50%)	(95%)	(72%)	(21%)	(82%)	(41%)	(38%)		(42%)	
70+	Sm.	3309	586	413	62	111	1742	4	927	–	50	–
	Total	21555	2199	492	144	1563	3218	51	14967	87	673	360
		(15%)	(27%)	(84%)	(43%)	(7%)	(54%)	(8%)	(6%)		(7%)	
Any age	Sm.	12348	3365	2134	475	756	3211	71	4816	–	885	–
	Total	50922	8064	2323	726	5015	5052	630	25481	604	4553	6538
		(24%)	(42%)	(92%)	(65%)	(15%)	(64%)	(11%)	(19%)		(19%)	
Females												
0–34	Sm.	–	–	–	–	–	–	–	–	–	–	–
	Total	2570	311	5	4	302	48	303	117	13	1185	593
35–69	Sm.	114	16	13	1	2	43	0	51	–	4	–
	Total	14225	3756	186	52	3518	737	57	7024	249	1228	1174
		(1%)	(0%)	(7%)	(2%)	(0%)	(6%)	(0%)	(1%)		(0%)	
70+	Sm.	550	41	35	2	4	346	0	157	–	6	–
	Total	37973	2335	185	50	2100	3802	68	30541	106	740	381
		(1%)	(2%)	(19%)	(4%)	(0%)	(9%)	(0%)	(1%)		(1%)	
Any age	Sm.	664	57	48	3	6	389	0	208	–	10	–
	Total	54768	6402	376	106	5920	4587	428	37682	368	3153	2148
		(1%)	(1%)	(13%)	(3%)	(0%)	(8%)	(0%)	(1%)		(0%)	
Males+Females												
0–34	Sm.	–	–	–	–	–	–	–	–	–	–	–
	Total	8130	639	15	12	612	92	717	483	38	3070	3091
35–69	Sm.	9153	2795	1734	414	647	1512	67	3940	–	839	–
	Total	38032	9293	2007	626	6660	2527	222	17172	741	3223	4854
		(24%)	(30%)	(86%)	(66%)	(10%)	(60%)	(30%)	(23%)		(26%)	
70+	Sm.	3859	627	448	64	115	2088	4	1084	–	56	–
	Total	59528	4534	677	194	3663	7020	119	45508	193	1413	741
		(6%)	(14%)	(66%)	(33%)	(3%)	(30%)	(3%)	(2%)		(4%)	
Any age	Sm.	13012	3422	2182	478	762	3600	71	5024	–	895	–
	Total	105690	14466	2699	832	10935	9639	1058	63163	972	7706	8686
		(12%)	(24%)	(81%)	(57%)	(7%)	(37%)	(7%)	(8%)		(12%)	

(To be conservative, no deaths before age 35, and none from liver cirrhosis or non–medical causes, were attributed to smoking.)

BELARUS: 1990

Smoking-attributed deaths (Sm.) and total deaths (Total)

		ALL CAUSES	ALL CANCER	Lung cancer	Upper aero-digestive ca.	Other cancer	COPD	Other respiratory	Vascular disease	Cirrhosis/ other liver	Other medical	Non-medical
Males												
0–34	Sm.	–	–	–	–	–	–	–	–	–	–	–
	Total	5381	332	10	10	312	41	199	356	17	1351	3085
35–69	Sm.	11005	3863	2312	681	870	1428	71	4755	–	888	–
	Total	28530	7343	2438	924	3981	1724	171	12232	362	2141	4557
		(39%)	(53%)	(95%)	(74%)	(22%)	(83%)	(42%)	(39%)		(41%)	
70+	Sm.	3067	724	502	69	153	1200	6	903	–	234	–
	Total	19542	2385	576	138	1671	1967	69	11160	87	3501	373
		(16%)	(30%)	(87%)	(50%)	(9%)	(61%)	(9%)	(8%)		(7%)	
Any age	Sm.	14072	4587	2814	750	1023	2628	77	5658	–	1122	–
	Total	53453	10060	3024	1072	5964	3732	439	23748	466	6993	8015
		(26%)	(46%)	(93%)	(70%)	(17%)	(70%)	(18%)	(24%)		(16%)	
Females												
0–34	Sm.	–	–	–	–	–	–	–	–	–	–	–
	Total	2130	290	1	3	286	24	138	118	17	949	594
35–69	Sm.	282	53	43	3	7	77	0	127	–	25	–
	Total	15990	4470	237	54	4179	635	85	7815	192	1562	1231
		(2%)	(1%)	(18%)	(6%)	(0%)	(12%)	(0%)	(2%)		(2%)	
70+	Sm.	120	17	13	2	2	48	0	49	–	6	–
	Total	38009	2724	173	80	2471	2369	96	24054	102	8244	420
		(0%)	(1%)	(8%)	(3%)	(0%)	(2%)	(0%)	(0%)		(0%)	
Any age	Sm.	402	70	56	5	9	125	0	176	–	31	–
	Total	56129	7484	411	137	6936	3028	319	31987	311	10755	2245
		(1%)	(1%)	(14%)	(4%)	(0%)	(4%)	(0%)	(1%)		(0%)	
Males+Females												
0–34	Sm.	–	–	–	–	–	–	–	–	–	–	–
	Total	7511	622	11	13	598	65	337	474	34	2300	3679
35–69	Sm.	11287	3916	2355	684	877	1505	71	4882	–	913	–
	Total	44520	11813	2675	978	8160	2359	256	20047	554	3703	5788
		(25%)	(33%)	(88%)	(70%)	(11%)	(64%)	(28%)	(24%)		(25%)	
70+	Sm.	3187	741	515	71	155	1248	6	952	–	240	–
	Total	57551	5109	749	218	4142	4336	165	35214	189	11745	793
		(6%)	(15%)	(69%)	(33%)	(4%)	(29%)	(4%)	(3%)		(2%)	
Any age	Sm.	14474	4657	2870	755	1032	2753	77	5834	–	1153	–
	Total	109582	17544	3435	1209	12900	6760	758	55735	777	17748	10260
		(13%)	(27%)	(84%)	(62%)	(8%)	(41%)	(10%)	(10%)		(6%)	

BELARUS: 1995

Smoking-attributed deaths (Sm.) and total deaths (Total)

		ALL CAUSES	ALL CANCER	Lung cancer	Upper aero-digestive ca.	Other cancer	COPD	Other respiratory	Vascular disease	Cirrhosis/ other liver	Other medical	Non-medical
Males												
0–34	Sm.	–	–	–	–	–	–	–	–	–	–	–
	Total	5350	301	7	11	283	36	133	306	10	988	3576
35–69	Sm.	11681	4589	2640	944	1005	1131	68	4986	–	907	–
	Total	29141	8225	2765	1242	4218	1334	157	11908	266	2127	5124
		(40%)	(56%)	(95%)	(76%)	(24%)	(85%)	(43%)	(42%)		(43%)	
70+	Sm.	3445	1026	695	89	242	975	9	973	–	462	–
	Total	18759	2932	769	153	2010	1407	89	8797	92	5000	442
		(18%)	(35%)	(90%)	(58%)	(12%)	(69%)	(10%)	(11%)		(9%)	
Any age	Sm.	15126	5615	3335	1033	1247	2106	77	5959	–	1369	–
	Total	53250	11458	3541	1406	6511	2777	379	21011	368	8115	9142
		(28%)	(49%)	(94%)	(73%)	(19%)	(76%)	(20%)	(28%)		(17%)	
Females												
0–34	Sm.	–	–	–	–	–	–	–	–	–	–	–
	Total	1784	262	1	4	257	16	93	108	19	709	577
35–69	Sm.	348	80	64	4	12	71	2	155	–	40	–
	Total	15753	4790	258	54	4478	460	112	7157	143	1856	1235
		(2%)	(2%)	(25%)	(7%)	(0%)	(15%)	(2%)	(2%)		(2%)	
70+	Sm.	63	11	8	1	2	22	0	25	–	5	–
	Total	36649	3460	175	116	3169	1712	136	18893	105	11849	494
		(0%)	(0%)	(5%)	(1%)	(0%)	(1%)	(0%)	(0%)		(0%)	
Any age	Sm.	411	91	72	5	14	93	2	180	–	45	–
	Total	54186	8512	434	174	7904	2188	341	26158	267	14414	2306
		(1%)	(1%)	(17%)	(3%)	(0%)	(4%)	(1%)	(1%)		(0%)	
Males+Females												
0–34	Sm.	–	–	–	–	–	–	–	–	–	–	–
	Total	7134	563	8	15	540	52	226	414	29	1697	4153
35–69	Sm.	12029	4669	2704	948	1017	1202	70	5141	–	947	–
	Total	44894	13015	3023	1296	8696	1794	269	19065	409	3983	6359
		(27%)	(36%)	(89%)	(73%)	(12%)	(67%)	(26%)	(27%)		(24%)	
70+	Sm.	3508	1037	703	90	244	997	9	998	–	467	–
	Total	55408	6392	944	269	5179	3119	225	27690	197	16849	936
		(6%)	(16%)	(74%)	(33%)	(5%)	(32%)	(4%)	(4%)		(3%)	
Any age	Sm.	15537	5706	3407	1038	1261	2199	79	6139	–	1414	–
	Total	107436	19970	3975	1580	14415	4965	720	47169	635	22529	11448
		(14%)	(29%)	(86%)	(66%)	(9%)	(44%)	(11%)	(13%)		(6%)	

(To be conservative, no deaths before age 35, and none from liver cirrhosis or non-medical causes, were attributed to smoking.)

BELGIUM: 1990 (estimated)

		No. of deaths			Standardised rates (Defined on p.292)			Annual death rates / 100, 000						
		All ages	0–34	35–69	All ages	0–34	35–69	0–4	5–9	10–14	15–19	20–24	25–29	30–34
ALL CAUSES	M	53059	2616	19169	1031.5	104.2	1036.0	191.8	23.8	23.4	94.4	134.7	122.6	138.8
	F	51557	1261	10111	589.9	54.3	492.8	146.7	20.9	18.5	34.8	48.5	45.0	65.5
Tuberculosis	M	82	1	34	1.6	0.0	1.8	–	–	–	–	–	0.2	–
	F	36	1	8	0.4	0.0	0.4	–	–	–	–	–	0.3	–
Other infective	M	404	24	161	7.9	1.0	8.6	1.6	–	1.0	0.9	0.5	0.5	2.3
and parasitic	F	511	27	99	5.9	1.2	4.8	3.4	0.3	0.3	0.9	0.3	2.0	0.8
ALL CANCER	M	15357	190	7072	299.6	7.4	385.0	3.3	4.9	4.2	7.4	6.1	9.0	16.8
	F	11198	159	4377	152.1	6.3	213.4	2.4	5.5	1.0	2.8	7.2	8.6	16.6
Mouth and	M	328	9	238	6.7	0.4	12.3	1.0	–	0.3	–	–	–	1.3
pharynx cancer	F	95	1	47	1.4	0.0	2.3	–	–	–	–	–	–	0.3
Oesophagus cancer	M	352	5	218	7.0	0.2	11.6	–	–	0.3	–	0.3	–	0.8
	F	118	–	41	1.6	–	2.0	–	–	–	–	–	–	–
Stomach cancer	M	799	3	301	15.5	0.1	16.5	–	–	–	–	–	–	0.8
	F	653	4	129	7.4	0.1	6.3	–	–	–	–	0.3	0.3	0.5
Colorectal cancer	M	1459	9	582	28.3	0.3	31.9	–	–	0.3	0.3	0.3	0.5	1.0
	F	1657	4	486	20.2	0.1	23.8	–	–	–	–	–	0.5	0.5
Liver cancer	M	160	2	84	3.1	0.1	4.6	–	–	–	–	0.3	–	0.3
	F	121	1	33	1.5	0.0	1.6	–	–	–	–	–	0.3	–
Pancreas cancer	M	569	–	281	11.1	–	15.4	–	–	–	–	–	–	–
	F	548	3	163	6.8	0.1	8.0	–	–	–	–	0.3	–	0.5
Larynx cancer	M	393	2	230	7.9	0.1	12.3	–	–	–	–	0.3	–	0.3
	F	47	–	19	0.7	–	0.9	–	–	–	–	–	–	–
Lung cancer	M	5416	3	2918	105.8	0.1	159.5	–	–	–	–	–	–	0.8
	F	720	3	380	10.6	0.1	18.5	–	–	–	–	0.3	0.3	0.3
Malignant melanoma	M	90	5	56	1.8	0.2	2.9	–	–	–	–	0.3	0.5	0.5
	F	102	5	56	1.6	0.2	2.7	–	–	–	0.3	0.6	0.5	–
Female breast cancer	F	2337	31	1322	36.4	1.1	64.1	–	–	–	–	0.6	1.3	6.2
Cervix cancer	F	208	1	116	3.3	0.0	5.6	–	–	–	–	–	0.3	–
Other uterine cancer	F	340	3	122	4.4	0.1	6.0	–	–	–	–	–	0.3	0.5
Ovarian cancer	F	631	5	333	9.5	0.2	16.3	–	–	–	0.3	0.3	0.3	0.5
Prostate cancer	M	1577	2	297	30.0	0.1	17.0	–	–	–	–	–	0.5	–
Bladder cancer	M	636	–	194	12.3	–	10.7	–	–	–	–	–	–	–
	F	229	2	41	2.6	0.1	2.0	–	–	–	–	0.3	–	0.3
Other and ill-defined	M	2658	85	1267	52.1	3.4	68.5	0.7	3.9	2.2	3.9	2.9	2.9	7.0
cancer sites	F	2532	59	815	32.7	2.4	39.8	1.4	3.4	–	1.9	3.3	2.3	4.7
Hodgkin's disease	M	43	7	21	0.8	0.3	1.1	–	–	–	–	0.5	0.5	0.8
	F	32	6	14	0.5	0.2	0.7	–	–	–	–	0.3	0.8	0.5
Myeloma and non-	M	427	22	206	8.3	0.8	11.2	–	–	–	0.9	0.3	1.9	2.5
Hodgkin lymphomas	F	435	10	136	5.7	0.4	6.6	0.7	–	0.3	–	0.6	0.5	0.8
Leukaemia	M	450	36	179	8.8	1.5	9.6	1.6	1.0	1.0	2.4	1.1	2.2	1.0
	F	393	21	124	5.2	0.9	6.0	0.3	2.1	0.7	0.3	0.6	1.3	1.0
ALL VASCULAR	M	18376	138	5965	354.0	5.2	327.8	2.0	1.6	1.6	4.7	5.6	5.8	15.3
DISEASE	F	21593	97	2592	222.1	3.8	127.3	1.4	1.4	0.7	3.7	3.1	6.8	9.6
Rheumatic heart	M	13	–	6	0.3	–	0.3	–	–	–	–	–	–	–
disease and fever	F	42	–	8	0.5	–	0.4	–	–	–	–	–	–	–
Hypertensive disease	M	255	3	117	5.0	0.1	6.4	–	–	–	–	0.3	0.2	0.3
	F	397	2	70	4.4	0.1	3.4	–	–	–	–	–	0.5	–
Ischaemic heart	M	6502	35	2862	126.3	1.3	156.2	–	–	–	0.3	0.3	1.5	6.8
disease	F	5034	8	872	56.0	0.3	42.9	–	–	–	0.6	0.3	0.8	0.5
Pulmonary embolism	M	310	3	109	6.0	0.1	6.1	–	–	–	–	–	0.5	0.3
and other venous	F	546	9	113	6.3	0.3	5.5	–	–	–	–	0.3	0.5	1.6
Cerebrovascular	M	3888	39	926	74.4	1.5	51.3	0.3	0.7	0.6	2.1	1.6	1.2	4.0
disease	F	6100	34	662	61.7	1.3	32.4	–	0.7	–	1.2	1.4	1.8	4.1
Other vascular	M	7408	58	1945	142.0	2.3	107.5	1.6	1.0	1.0	2.4	3.5	2.4	4.0
disease	F	9474	44	867	93.2	1.8	42.7	1.4	0.7	0.7	1.9	1.1	3.3	3.4
Chronic obstructive	M	3034	16	876	58.3	0.6	48.9	0.3	–	0.3	0.3	0.3	1.5	1.5
pulmonary disease	F	1145	7	280	13.5	0.3	13.7	–	–	–	0.3	–	0.5	1.0
Other respiratory	M	2684	30	627	51.2	1.3	35.2	3.9	1.3	0.3	0.3	1.1	0.5	1.5
disease	F	2160	26	189	21.2	1.1	9.3	3.8	–	0.3	0.3	1.1	0.8	1.6
Peptic ulcer	M	175	2	44	3.3	0.1	2.4	–	–	–	–	0.3	0.2	–
	F	185	2	20	1.9	0.1	1.0	0.3	–	–	–	–	–	0.3
Liver cirrhosis	M	695	12	501	14.3	0.4	25.9	–	–	–	–	–	0.5	2.5
	F	507	11	297	8.2	0.4	14.3	–	–	–	–	–	0.3	2.6
Renal disease	M	695	5	165	13.3	0.2	9.2	–	–	–	0.3	–	0.2	0.8
	F	861	1	121	9.0	0.0	5.9	–	–	–	–	–	–	0.3
Pregnancy and birth	F	8	4	4	0.2	0.2	0.2	–	–	–	–	0.8	0.3	–
Congenital and	M	347	331	11	8.8	15.3	0.6	101.8	0.7	1.9	0.9	0.5	1.2	0.3
perinatal causes	F	252	237	6	6.7	11.6	0.3	78.7	1.0	0.7	0.3	0.6	–	–
Ill-defined causes	M	3194	256	891	62.9	10.9	47.4	48.9	0.7	0.6	2.7	5.6	7.5	10.3
	F	4407	136	416	45.0	6.4	20.2	34.0	1.7	0.7	1.2	4.2	1.5	1.3
Other medical causes	M	3957	149	1145	76.5	6.1	61.8	11.1	3.9	3.5	5.6	4.8	5.1	8.5
	F	6348	103	901	67.9	4.4	44.1	8.6	1.7	2.7	5.0	3.3	3.5	6.0
ALL NON-	M	4059	1462	1677	79.8	55.7	81.5	18.9	10.7	10.0	71.2	109.9	90.2	79.3
MEDICAL CAUSES	F	2346	450	801	35.7	18.5	37.9	14.1	9.2	12.1	20.2	28.0	20.5	25.6
Motor vehicle	M	1346	759	437	26.3	29.1	21.1	4.6	4.9	6.4	46.9	66.7	46.2	28.0
traffic accidents	F	488	215	174	9.1	9.0	8.2	4.8	5.8	7.1	12.1	15.5	8.1	9.3
Fire	M	52	25	17	1.1	1.0	0.9	2.0	0.3	–	0.9	1.1	1.0	1.8
	F	44	11	14	0.7	0.5	0.7	2.1	0.3	–	0.6	–	–	0.5
Suicide	M	1343	356	706	26.4	13.1	34.0	–	–	1.3	11.3	22.7	26.3	30.3
	F	569	94	346	10.2	3.6	16.4	–	–	0.7	1.9	5.8	7.1	9.6
Homicide	M	76	38	33	1.5	1.4	1.5	0.3	–	–	0.3	2.4	4.1	2.5
	F	60	30	23	1.2	1.2	1.0	1.4	0.3	0.7	1.9	1.4	1.3	1.8
POPULATION (thousands):	M=males				4870.3	2448.1	2071.8	306.6	307.1	311.5	337.0	374.9	411.2	399.8
	F=females				5097.0	2345.2	2136.5	291.0	292.5	297.5	322.3	360.5	395.4	386.0

BELGIUM: 1990 (estimated)

Annual death rates / 100, 000

9th ICD categories

Cause	Sex	35–39	40–44	45–49	50–54	55–59	60–64	65–69	70–74	75–79	80+/NK	ICD
ALL CAUSES	M	170.9	271.1	404.6	632.7	1059.8	1777.6	2935.4	4599.2	7713.3	15644.2	001–999
	F	106.2	163.8	243.6	341.7	524.7	779.1	1290.9	2214.6	4258.1	11417.1	
Tuberculosis	M	0.3	0.6	0.4	2.5	1.4	3.4	4.2	10.1	11.9	19.2	010–018, 137
	F	–	–	–	–	1.3	0.3	1.1	4.0	2.1	6.5	
Other infective and parasitic	M	3.8	2.5	4.7	5.7	8.4	8.7	26.2	24.9	46.6	126.9	Rest of 001–139
	F	0.8	1.4	1.8	2.5	4.0	6.1	17.2	18.8	43.8	108.8	
ALL CANCER	M	25.5	69.0	141.8	242.4	427.9	738.4	1050.3	1564.2	2274.0	3273.1	140–208
	F	34.3	73.8	114.6	177.9	269.0	351.8	472.6	650.0	913.4	1526.3	
Mouth and pharynx cancer	M	2.1	6.4	9.4	12.9	16.5	22.6	16.1	16.3	22.1	32.7	140–149
	F	0.6	0.6	2.2	2.8	3.0	3.7	3.2	5.7	6.7	9.8	
Oesophagus cancer	M	1.1	2.5	7.6	11.8	16.9	18.1	23.2	20.2	36.5	57.7	150
	F	–	–	1.1	2.5	3.0	4.1	3.5	9.7	7.7	18.3	
Stomach cancer	M	1.1	1.4	5.8	11.8	17.2	32.0	46.0	72.4	139.1	228.8	151
	F	0.8	2.9	1.5	3.5	9.1	8.8	17.2	34.1	66.5	134.8	
Colorectal cancer	M	2.1	4.2	6.2	19.7	34.5	62.5	94.2	152.5	223.9	392.3	153, 154
	F	2.2	4.9	10.3	14.8	26.8	40.8	67.0	90.5	139.1	300.6	
Liver cancer	M	0.8	–	0.7	3.2	3.2	10.2	14.4	20.2	16.1	27.9	155.0
	F	–	–	1.5	1.1	3.0	1.7	4.2	9.1	14.9	17.1	
Pancreas cancer	M	0.5	2.0	7.3	10.4	16.5	28.6	42.2	59.1	88.2	103.8	157
	F	–	1.2	2.9	3.9	8.7	15.6	23.9	35.3	57.7	84.7	
Larynx cancer	M	0.3	4.5	8.7	11.8	13.4	21.5	25.8	43.6	38.2	57.7	161
	F	0.3	0.3	0.7	1.1	1.3	2.0	0.7	2.3	5.7	5.3	
Lung cancer	M	5.6	24.0	47.9	86.5	186.5	326.3	439.8	611.7	774.4	765.4	162
	F	2.5	6.4	7.7	13.8	24.2	33.3	41.8	46.7	48.9	65.2	
Malignant melanoma	M	0.8	2.0	1.8	3.2	2.8	4.1	5.5	7.8	10.2	6.7	172
	F	1.1	1.2	1.8	2.1	3.4	4.8	4.6	5.1	5.2	9.0	
Female breast cancer	F	14.5	31.5	45.0	67.4	88.9	88.4	113.3	117.2	149.4	198.8	174
Cervix cancer	F	1.4	3.5	5.5	5.3	5.4	9.2	9.1	12.0	14.4	17.1	180
Other uterine cancer	F	0.8	1.4	2.2	3.5	6.7	11.2	15.8	23.3	27.8	48.9	179, 182
Ovarian cancer	F	2.2	3.5	10.7	15.5	22.8	25.8	33.7	34.7	47.9	56.6	183
Prostate cancer	M	–	–	0.4	1.8	13.0	29.7	73.9	161.1	302.0	687.5	185
Bladder cancer	M	0.3	0.8	2.9	4.7	10.2	24.8	31.3	77.0	128.1	184.6	188
	F	–	–	–	1.4	2.3	3.4	7.0	16.5	22.7	46.0	
Other and ill-defined cancer sites	M	7.2	15.4	31.5	48.5	74.2	123.8	178.7	244.4	366.4	538.5	Rest of 140–208
	F	4.5	11.3	14.7	30.4	46.6	77.2	94.0	152.0	221.5	391.4	
Hodgkin's disease	M	0.8	0.8	1.1	0.7	1.1	0.4	2.5	2.3	4.2	6.7	201
	F	0.6	0.6	–	0.7	1.0	0.3	1.4	0.6	3.1	2.0	
Myeloma and non-Hodgkin lymphomas	M	1.3	2.5	7.3	6.5	9.9	21.1	29.6	38.9	55.1	80.8	200, 202–203
	F	2.2	2.0	3.7	3.9	5.7	9.9	18.9	34.7	41.7	59.9	
Leukaemia	M	1.3	2.5	3.3	8.6	12.0	12.8	27.0	36.6	69.6	101.9	204–208
	F	0.6	2.6	2.9	4.2	7.0	11.6	13.3	20.5	32.5	60.7	
ALL VASCULAR DISEASE	M	22.5	60.0	98.3	179.2	323.4	564.9	1046.0	1642.0	2992.4	6379.8	390–459
	F	12.3	24.3	33.5	61.1	108.4	207.3	444.6	894.7	1987.1	5488.8	
Rheumatic heart disease and fever	M	–	–	0.4	–	0.7	0.8	0.4	0.8	1.7	3.8	390–398
	F	0.3	0.3	–	0.4	–	0.7	1.1	3.4	4.6	7.7	
Hypertensive disease	M	0.3	1.1	2.2	3.9	8.1	9.8	19.4	29.6	39.0	49.0	401–405
	F	0.6	1.2	1.5	0.7	4.4	5.4	10.2	22.8	42.2	82.7	
Ischaemic heart disease	M	8.9	32.7	55.1	95.9	171.4	275.5	453.7	625.7	976.3	1586.5	410–414
	F	2.2	4.6	7.0	23.3	39.2	76.8	147.4	323.3	546.1	1028.9	
Pulmonary embolism and other venous	M	–	1.1	1.1	3.9	4.6	8.7	23.2	35.0	46.6	94.2	415.1, 451–453
	F	1.1	1.4	2.6	2.1	4.4	10.9	16.1	28.5	54.6	109.2	
Cerebrovascular disease	M	4.8	8.7	13.1	24.1	40.8	85.8	181.7	330.7	689.6	1620.2	430–438
	F	5.3	8.1	12.2	14.1	28.2	50.3	108.8	208.3	570.8	1600.8	
Other vascular disease	M	8.6	16.5	26.5	51.3	97.8	184.4	367.6	620.2	1239.2	3026.0	Rest of 390–459
	F	2.8	8.7	10.3	20.5	32.2	63.2	161.1	308.5	768.7	2659.5	
Chronic obstructive pulmonary disease	M	1.9	2.2	6.5	17.6	42.6	102.4	169.4	340.9	547.1	1018.3	490–496
	F	2.0	2.3	4.8	8.5	16.1	26.2	36.1	64.3	104.1	221.2	
Other respiratory disease	M	2.1	3.9	3.6	8.3	27.8	59.5	141.5	228.8	437.7	1170.2	Rest of 460–519
	F	0.3	2.6	2.9	4.2	9.4	13.6	31.9	60.9	148.4	631.4	
Peptic ulcer	M	0.5	0.6	0.4	0.4	2.5	3.0	9.7	17.9	30.5	67.3	531–533
	F	–	1.2	–	0.4	0.7	1.7	2.8	7.4	18.5	46.4	
Liver cirrhosis	M	6.7	13.1	27.6	27.3	34.5	29.4	42.7	49.8	51.7	54.8	571
	F	5.9	9.0	15.1	12.7	16.1	21.1	20.4	29.0	33.0	34.2	
Renal disease	M	0.3	1.1	2.2	5.0	7.4	17.7	30.4	49.0	103.5	326.9	580–590
	F	–	1.4	1.1	4.6	5.7	10.5	18.2	35.3	73.2	217.9	
Pregnancy and birth	F	0.8	0.3	–	–	–	–	–	–	–	–	630–676
Congenital and perinatal causes	M	0.3	0.6	0.4	–	1.1	0.4	1.3	0.8	2.5	1.0	740–779
	F	–	0.3	0.7	–	0.3	–	0.7	1.1	0.5	2.4	
Ill-defined causes	M	11.5	20.4	21.8	31.6	45.7	77.5	122.9	211.7	357.9	1301.0	780–799
	F	10.3	4.1	10.7	14.5	17.4	29.2	55.1	104.2	246.3	1301.0	
Other medical causes	M	15.6	16.8	27.6	36.6	57.7	90.0	188.4	308.2	632.7	1462.5	Rest of 001–799
	F	8.6	10.4	19.5	21.2	40.3	72.1	136.5	262.9	568.8	1538.9	
ALL NON-MEDICAL CAUSES	M	80.0	80.4	69.6	76.1	79.5	82.4	102.2	151.0	224.8	443.3	E800–E999
	F	30.9	32.7	38.7	34.2	35.9	39.1	53.7	82.0	119.0	293.3	
Motor vehicle traffic accidents	M	23.1	19.0	17.4	24.4	22.9	18.8	22.0	35.0	41.6	53.8	E810–E819
	F	7.0	8.4	9.2	7.1	9.4	7.5	8.8	14.8	18.0	15.5	
Fire	M	0.5	–	0.7	0.7	1.1	1.5	1.7	3.1	2.5	2.9	E890–E899
	F	0.3	0.6	0.4	0.7	0.3	2.0	0.4	–	1.5	6.5	
Suicide	M	32.7	40.2	31.9	28.4	30.6	35.0	39.3	52.9	79.7	114.4	E950–E959
	F	14.8	13.3	17.7	18.4	14.8	17.3	18.2	23.3	24.7	16.3	
Homicide	M	1.3	2.8	1.1	2.5	1.8	1.1	–	1.6	2.5	–	E960–E969
	F	2.2	1.2	1.8	1.4	0.3	0.3	–	0.6	1.5	1.2	
POPULATION (thousands)	M	372.7	358.2	275.8	278.5	284.2	265.7	236.7	128.5	117.9	104.0	
	F	358.9	345.6	271.4	283.3	298.1	294.2	285.0	175.7	194.1	245.5	

BELGIUM: Males

	All ages	0–34	35–69	35–39	40–44	45–49	50–54	55–59	60–64	65–69	70–74	75–79	80+/NK
POPULATION (1000s)													
1955	4358.4	2266.4	1813.4	237.1	310.6	318.2	309.5	263.2	206.8	168.0	132.6	87.1	58.9
1965	4636.2	2434.5	1902.7	329.5	333.5	222.2	285.1	279.7	255.1	197.6	135.8	89.9	73.3
1975	4798.7	2561.8	1895.7	300.0	317.0	316.3	313.1	200.4	239.2	209.7	163.1	101.5	76.6
1985	4811.8	2496.6	1941.7	362.6	281.4	286.7	297.3	286.9	269.0	157.8	162.7	113.9	96.9
1990	**4870.3**	**2448.1**	**2071.8**	**372.7**	**358.2**	**275.8**	**278.5**	**284.2**	**265.7**	**236.7**	**128.5**	**117.9**	**104.0**
1995 projected	*4813.1*	*2267.8*	*2154.3*	*395.7*	*371.1*	*358.4*	*273.3*	*264.1*	*258.3*	*233.4*	*190.4*	*94.4*	*106.2*
NUMBER OF DEATHS													
All causes													
1955	57913	6190	23728	557	1180	2128	3340	4538	5387	6598	8072	8599	11324
1965	61623	4565	26631	775	1191	1324	2948	4895	7099	8399	8551	8817	13059
1975	62609	3562	23927	579	996	1662	2824	3077	6024	8765	10793	10100	14227
1985	57424	2820	19868	670	842	1234	2223	3666	5802	5431	8955	10188	15593
1990	**53059**	**2616**	**19169**	**637**	**971**	**1116**	**1762**	**3012**	**4723**	**6948**	**5910**	**9094**	**16270**
1995 projected	*48158*	*2273*	*16242*	*626*	*931*	*1285*	*1476*	*2322*	*3856*	*5746*	*7461*	*6482*	*15700*
Lung cancer													
1955	1636	9	1273	11	40	99	255	314	290	264	202	107	45
1965	3326	10	2397	15	57	83	280	530	723	709	486	289	144
1975	4780	14	2743	21	62	149	283	387	762	1079	1061	617	345
1985	5923	12	3002	27	61	131	335	599	991	858	1141	1010	758
1990 estimated	**5416**	**3**	**2918**	**21**	**86**	**132**	**241**	**530**	**867**	**1041**	**786**	**913**	**796**
1995 projected	*4827*	*2*	*2449*	*22*	*91*	*146*	*201*	*418*	*705*	*866*	*982*	*644*	*750*
ANNUAL DEATH RATE / 100,000 (*The rates for the age groups 0–34 and 35–69 are the means of seven five-yearly rates, but the all-ages rates are standardised to the conventional "European" age distribution)													
All causes													
1955	1457.6*	256.0*	1517.0*	234.9	379.9	668.8	1079.2	1724.2	2604.9	3927.4	6087.5	9872.6	19225.8
1965	1405.6*	180.5*	1572.2*	235.2	357.1	595.9	1034.0	1750.1	2782.8	4250.5	6296.8	9807.6	17815.8
1975	1364.4*	144.4*	1452.6*	193.0	314.2	525.5	901.9	1535.4	2518.4	4179.8	6617.4	9950.7	18573.1
1985	1162.3*	113.1*	1219.8*	184.8	299.2	430.4	747.7	1277.8	2156.9	3441.7	5504.0	8944.7	16091.8
1990	**1031.5***	**104.2***	**1036.0***	**170.9**	**271.1**	**404.6**	**632.7**	**1059.8**	**1777.6**	**2935.4**	**4599.2**	**7713.3**	**15644.2**
1995 projected	*917.1**	*97.3**	*877.4**	*158.2*	*250.9*	*358.5*	*540.1*	*879.2*	*1492.8*	*2461.9*	*3918.6*	*6866.5*	*14783.4*
All cancer													
1955	228.7*	9.6*	321.7*	30.8	67.3	135.8	238.8	399.3	559.5	820.2	1135.7	1567.2	2032.3
1965	271.8*	11.0*	395.4*	34.3	64.8	122.0	253.6	476.2	739.3	1077.9	1353.5	1853.2	2341.1
1975	303.0*	11.0*	420.6*	34.0	70.0	137.8	245.6	468.1	773.8	1215.1	1733.9	2071.9	2727.2
1985	322.1*	8.2*	427.1*	28.7	70.7	132.9	271.4	471.2	801.5	1212.9	1756.0	2428.4	3233.2
1990 estimated	**299.6***	**7.4***	**385.0***	**25.5**	**69.0**	**141.8**	**242.4**	**427.9**	**738.4**	**1050.3**	**1564.2**	**2274.0**	**3273.1**
1995 projected	*275.9**	*6.2**	*344.0**	*24.0*	*70.9*	*134.8*	*221.7*	*383.2*	*650.0*	*923.7*	*1395.5*	*2123.9*	*3224.1*
Lung cancer													
1955	38.4*	0.4*	78.2*	4.6	12.9	31.1	82.4	119.3	140.2	157.1	152.3	122.8	76.4
1965	72.2*	0.4*	141.3*	4.6	17.1	37.4	98.2	189.5	283.4	358.8	357.9	321.5	196.5
1975	100.6*	0.6*	170.0*	7.0	19.6	47.1	90.4	193.1	318.6	514.5	650.5	607.9	450.4
1985	120.5*	0.4*	186.9*	7.4	21.7	45.7	112.7	208.8	368.4	543.7	701.3	886.7	782.2
1990 estimated	**105.8***	**0.1***	**159.5***	**5.6**	**24.0**	**47.9**	**86.5**	**186.5**	**326.3**	**439.8**	**611.7**	**774.4**	**765.4**
1995 projected	*91.4**	*0.1**	*135.2**	*5.6*	*24.5*	*40.7*	*73.5*	*158.3*	*272.9*	*371.0*	*515.8*	*682.2*	*706.2*
Upper aerodigestive cancer (mouth, oesophagus, pharynx and larynx)													
1955	13.8*	0.0*	19.8*	0.8	1.9	6.6	16.2	28.5	39.7	45.2	71.6	98.7	120.5
1965	16.8*	0.2*	25.2*	2.1	3.9	7.7	20.3	31.1	51.7	59.2	87.6	101.2	140.5
1975	17.9*	0.2*	28.4*	3.0	5.0	9.8	17.6	40.4	53.5	69.6	86.5	103.4	139.7
1985	20.4*	0.2*	32.8*	1.9	8.5	20.9	27.6	45.3	61.0	64.6	84.8	109.7	152.7
1990 estimated	**21.7***	**0.6***	**36.2***	**3.5**	**13.4**	**25.7**	**36.6**	**46.8**	**62.1**	**65.1**	**80.2**	**96.7**	**148.1**
1995 projected	*22.5**	*0.5**	*38.9**	*4.8*	*17.8*	*33.2*	*41.3*	*49.6*	*62.3*	*63.4*	*73.5*	*93.2*	*137.5*
Other cancer													
1955	176.5*	9.1*	223.6*	25.3	52.5	98.1	140.2	251.5	379.6	617.9	911.8	1345.6	1835.3
1965	182.8*	10.3*	229.0*	27.6	43.8	77.0	135.0	255.6	404.2	659.9	908.0	1430.5	2004.1
1975	184.5*	10.2*	222.2*	24.0	45.4	80.9	137.7	234.5	401.8	630.9	996.9	1360.6	2137.1
1985	181.3*	7.6*	207.3*	19.3	40.5	66.3	131.2	217.1	372.1	604.6	969.9	1432.0	2298.2
1990 estimated	**172.2***	**6.6***	**189.3***	**16.4**	**31.5**	**68.2**	**119.2**	**194.6**	**350.0**	**545.4**	**872.4**	**1402.9**	**2359.6**
1995 projected	*162.0**	*5.6**	*169.9**	*13.6*	*28.6*	*60.8*	*106.8*	*175.3*	*314.8*	*489.3*	*806.2*	*1348.5*	*2380.4*
Chronic obstructive pulmonary disease (COPD)													
1955	75.1*	3.0*	120.4*	5.1	17.1	47.1	90.5	164.5	247.6	270.8	305.4	397.2	602.7
1965	77.3*	1.5*	110.9*	5.8	12.0	31.1	66.6	133.0	221.1	306.7	451.4	520.6	660.3
1975	73.8*	1.3*	85.9*	3.3	6.9	14.5	43.4	90.8	171.4	270.9	451.3	629.6	868.1
1985	55.4*	1.3*	55.4*	1.7	7.1	7.0	19.8	43.6	103.3	205.3	314.1	510.1	830.8
1990 estimated	**58.3***	**0.6***	**48.9***	**1.9**	**2.2**	**6.5**	**17.6**	**42.6**	**102.4**	**169.4**	**340.9**	**547.1**	**1018.3**
1995 projected	*61.6**	*0.5**	*45.6**	*1.3*	*1.6*	*5.0*	*16.1*	*40.5*	*89.8*	*164.5*	*344.5*	*600.6*	*1189.3*
Other respiratory disease													
1955	57.8*	23.6*	34.2*	3.4	5.2	9.7	22.3	35.3	61.9	101.8	174.2	414.5	955.9
1965	38.3*	5.9*	28.6*	2.4	4.8	13.1	16.1	27.9	46.6	89.1	134.0	291.4	758.5
1975	42.8*	3.2*	25.9*	2.7	3.2	5.7	10.2	24.0	40.1	95.4	183.9	405.9	930.8
1985	56.5*	1.3*	47.5*	2.2	2.1	9.1	17.5	45.0	96.7	159.7	262.4	516.2	1077.4
1990 estimated	**51.2***	**1.3***	**35.2***	**2.1**	**3.9**	**3.6**	**8.3**	**27.8**	**59.5**	**141.5**	**228.8**	**437.7**	**1170.2**
1995 projected	*47.1**	*1.2**	*27.6**	*2.8*	*2.7*	*2.5*	*5.9*	*19.3*	*44.5*	*115.7*	*193.8*	*402.5*	*1180.8*
Vascular disease													
1955	551.5*	8.8*	595.2*	38.0	89.5	181.0	369.3	629.9	1075.4	1783.3	2905.0	4632.6	7847.2
1965	637.7*	7.4*	658.1*	50.7	115.7	208.4	399.5	691.5	1200.7	1940.3	3212.8	5218.0	9994.5
1975	566.0*	7.4*	571.7*	38.7	84.9	191.0	352.0	574.4	1012.1	1749.2	2900.1	4647.3	9031.3
1985	450.3*	5.4*	436.7*	37.5	70.0	126.3	231.4	454.5	815.2	1321.9	2312.2	3905.2	7335.4
1990 estimated	**354.0***	**5.2***	**327.8***	**22.5**	**60.0**	**98.3**	**179.2**	**323.4**	**564.9**	**1046.0**	**1642.0**	**2992.4**	**6379.8**
1995 projected	*274.9**	*4.4**	*237.6**	*17.7*	*45.5*	*75.1*	*128.8*	*224.9*	*415.4*	*755.8*	*1218.5*	*2327.3*	*5320.2*
Liver cirrhosis													
1955	10.9*	0.2*	18.3*	3.4	5.5	8.8	14.2	25.1	31.9	39.3	49.0	64.3	57.7
1965	14.0*	0.2*	24.9*	3.6	3.9	11.3	19.3	35.4	45.5	55.2	57.4	80.1	66.8
1975	18.2*	0.4*	31.4*	6.3	12.3	19.6	24.3	44.9	45.6	66.8	79.7	89.7	88.8
1985	17.5*	1.1*	31.0*	10.5	18.1	16.7	28.3	36.2	41.6	65.3	65.2	76.4	74.3
1990 estimated	**14.3***	**0.4***	**25.9***	**6.7**	**13.1**	**27.6**	**27.3**	**34.5**	**29.4**	**42.7**	**49.8**	**51.7**	**54.8**
1995 projected	*12.1**	*0.3**	*22.4**	*4.5*	*13.5*	*28.7*	*29.3*	*28.8*	*21.7*	*30.0*	*34.7*	*39.2*	*38.6*
Other medical causes													
1955	436.3*	161.2*	313.1*	83.1	101.4	192.0	239.7	343.8	487.9	743.5	1288.8	2448.9	7135.8
1965	264.1*	92.8*	239.0*	53.4	82.2	114.8	170.8	258.5	387.3	605.8	901.3	1547.3	3347.9
1975	265.0*	62.0*	216.1*	40.3	62.1	83.1	134.1	229.5	338.6	624.7	1046.0	1772.4	4321.1
1985	177.4*	42.2*	129.2*	27.6	42.6	57.2	84.8	130.0	204.8	357.4	639.2	1278.3	3128.0
1990 estimated	**174.3***	**33.6***	**131.7***	**32.2**	**42.4**	**57.3**	**81.9**	**124.2**	**200.6**	**383.2**	**622.6**	**1185.8**	**3304.8**
1995 projected	*169.5**	*26.8**	*129.7**	*33.1*	*43.1*	*54.7*	*77.2*	*117.8*	*202.1*	*380.0*	*590.9*	*1154.7*	*3369.1*
All non-medical causes													
1955	97.3*	49.7*	114.2*	71.3	94.0	94.3	104.4	126.1	140.7	168.5	229.3	347.9	594.2
1965	102.3*	61.8*	115.4*	85.0	73.8	95.4	108.0	127.6	142.3	175.6	186.3	297.0	646.7
1975	95.7*	59.0*	101.0*	67.7	74.8	73.7	92.3	103.8	136.7	157.8	222.6	334.0	605.7
1985	83.1*	53.6*	93.0*	76.7	88.5	81.3	94.5	97.2	93.7	119.1	154.9	230.0	412.8
1990 estimated	**79.8***	**55.7***	**81.5***	**80.0**	**80.4**	**69.6**	**76.1**	**79.5**	**82.4**	**102.2**	**151.0**	**224.8**	**443.3**
1995 projected	*76.2**	*58.0**	*70.5**	*74.8*	*73.6*	*57.8*	*61.1*	*64.7*	*69.3*	*92.1*	*140.8*	*218.2*	*461.4*

BELGIUM: Females

	All ages	0–34	35–69	35–39	40–44	45–49	50–54	55–59	60–64	65–69	70–74	75–79	80+/NK
POPULATION (1000s)													
1955	4509.8	2204.9	1935.0	231.6	310.1	323.0	322.2	293.5	248.5	206.1	166.4	114.0	89.5
1965	4811.8	2336.0	2033.3	326.6	336.0	226.5	297.4	303.1	292.5	251.2	192.4	132.0	118.1
1975	5002.3	2442.2	2010.9	295.3	316.6	321.2	324.6	215.1	273.4	264.7	232.7	167.5	149.0
1985	5046.4	2390.6	2016.9	347.7	274.6	288.6	305.3	305.4	302.5	192.8	229.0	193.2	216.7
1990	**5097.0**	**2345.2**	**2136.5**	**358.9**	**345.6**	**271.4**	**283.3**	**298.1**	**294.2**	**285.0**	**175.7**	**194.1**	**245.5**
1995 projected	*5031.9*	*2184.5*	*2197.1*	*381.9*	*358.2*	*347.0*	*271.7*	*275.5*	*284.0*	*278.8*	*257.4*	*151.0*	*241.9*
NUMBER OF DEATHS													
All causes													
1955	50830	4223	15647	397	773	1217	1819	2679	3602	5160	7398	8981	14581
1965	53422	2931	15474	450	687	802	1564	2408	3905	5658	7647	9302	18068
1975	56816	1931	13621	349	620	999	1576	1631	3153	5293	8309	10882	22073
1985	54188	1430	10238	360	489	795	1158	1749	2819	2868	6242	9595	26683
1990	**51557**	**1261**	**10111**	**381**	**566**	**661**	**968**	**1564**	**2292**	**3679**	**3891**	**8265**	**28029**
1995 projected	*45310*	*1059*	*8708*	*391*	*541*	*761*	*838*	*1263*	*1918*	*2996*	*4821*	*5468*	*25254*
Lung cancer													
1955	273	5	158	2	8	17	21	36	31	43	39	50	21
1965	366	6	185	6	8	12	18	35	45	61	55	54	66
1975	513	13	245	3	12	16	28	44	65	77	87	85	83
1985	697	4	315	5	14	23	41	60	99	73	121	101	156
1990 *estimated*	**720**	**3**	**380**	**9**	**22**	**21**	**39**	**72**	**98**	**119**	**82**	**95**	**160**
1995 projected	*720*	*3*	*392*	*12*	*26*	*28*	*41*	*70*	*102*	*113*	*114*	*66*	*145*
ANNUAL DEATH RATE / 100,000													
All causes													
1955	1036.4*	180.6*	889.7*	171.4	249.3	376.8	564.6	912.8	1449.5	2503.6	4445.9	7878.1	16291.6
1965	918.8*	117.9*	800.6*	137.8	204.5	354.1	525.9	794.5	1335.0	2252.4	3974.5	7047.0	15298.9
1975	838.2*	83.5*	717.4*	118.2	195.8	311.0	485.5	758.3	1153.3	1999.6	3570.7	6496.7	14814.1
1985	665.9*	62.5*	561.2*	103.5	178.1	275.5	379.3	572.7	931.9	1487.6	2725.8	4966.4	12313.3
1990	**589.9***	**54.3***	**492.8***	**106.2**	**163.8**	**243.6**	**341.7**	**524.7**	**779.1**	**1290.9**	**2214.6**	**4258.1**	**11417.1**
1995 projected	*520.9**	*47.9**	*427.1**	*102.4*	*151.0*	*219.3*	*308.4*	*458.4*	*675.4*	*1074.6*	*1873.0*	*3621.2*	*10439.9*
All cancer													
1955	182.8*	10.2*	256.3*	48.8	93.2	147.4	202.4	307.0	415.3	579.8	822.7	1210.5	1604.5
1965	179.1*	10.9*	244.4*	37.4	80.1	147.5	205.8	301.6	397.9	540.6	804.6	1158.3	1690.1
1975	170.3*	8.4*	243.3*	37.9	79.9	128.6	206.7	309.2	408.6	532.3	709.5	1059.7	1583.2
1985	161.3*	6.1*	227.1*	35.4	76.1	125.1	180.8	274.7	374.5	523.3	741.9	991.2	1541.8
1990 *estimated*	**152.1***	**6.3***	**213.4***	**34.3**	**73.8**	**114.6**	**177.9**	**269.0**	**351.8**	**472.6**	**650.0**	**913.4**	**1526.3**
1995 projected	*141.0**	*6.1**	*196.1**	*33.3*	*69.2*	*108.6*	*170.0*	*251.9*	*321.8*	*417.5*	*579.6*	*828.5*	*1471.3*
Lung cancer													
1955	5.4*	0.2*	8.7*	0.9	2.6	5.3	6.5	12.3	12.5	20.9	23.4	43.9	23.5
1965	6.4*	0.3*	9.5*	1.8	2.4	5.3	6.1	11.5	15.4	24.3	28.6	40.9	55.9
1975	8.4*	0.5*	13.1*	1.0	3.8	5.0	8.6	20.5	23.8	29.1	37.4	50.7	55.7
1985	10.4*	0.2*	16.9*	1.4	5.1	8.0	13.4	19.6	32.7	37.9	52.8	52.3	72.0
1990 *estimated*	**10.6***	**0.1***	**18.5***	**2.5**	**6.4**	**7.7**	**13.8**	**24.2**	**33.3**	**41.8**	**46.7**	**48.9**	**65.2**
1995 projected	*10.8**	*0.1**	*19.3**	*3.1*	*7.3*	*8.1*	*15.1*	*25.4*	*35.9*	*40.5*	*44.3*	*43.7*	*59.9*
Upper aerodigestive cancer (mouth, oesophagus, pharynx and larynx)													
1955	3.4*	0.1*	3.6*	0.9	–	1.5	3.1	3.7	5.2	10.7	19.8	30.7	43.6
1965	3.0*	0.0*	4.0*	0.6	0.3	0.9	3.4	4.9	7.2	10.7	12.0	19.7	39.8
1975	2.8*	0.1*	3.4*	1.0	0.9	1.6	1.8	3.3	6.9	7.9	15.0	23.3	29.5
1985	3.7*	0.0*	5.6*	0.9	2.2	3.5	3.6	7.9	7.9	13.5	14.0	20.2	35.5
1990 *estimated*	**3.7***	**0.0***	**5.2***	**0.8**	**0.9**	**4.1**	**6.4**	**7.4**	**9.9**	**7.4**	**17.6**	**20.1**	**33.4**
1995 projected	*3.7**	*0.0**	*5.4**	*0.5*	*0.8*	*4.9*	*7.4*	*8.7*	*8.1*	*7.2*	*16.3*	*19.2*	*32.2*
Other cancer													
1955	174.0*	9.9*	244.0*	47.1	90.6	140.6	192.7	291.0	397.6	548.3	779.4	1136.0	1537.4
1965	169.6*	10.6*	230.8*	34.9	77.4	141.3	196.4	285.1	375.4	505.6	764.0	1097.7	1594.4
1975	159.1*	7.7*	226.8*	35.9	75.2	122.0	196.2	285.4	377.8	495.3	657.1	985.7	1498.0
1985	147.2*	5.9*	204.6*	33.1	68.8	113.7	163.8	247.2	333.9	472.0	675.1	918.7	1434.2
1990 *estimated*	**137.7***	**6.1***	**189.7***	**30.9**	**66.6**	**102.8**	**157.8**	**237.5**	**308.6**	**423.5**	**585.7**	**844.4**	**1427.7**
1995 projected	*126.5**	*5.9**	*171.3**	*29.6*	*61.1*	*95.7*	*147.6*	*217.8*	*277.8*	*369.8*	*519.0*	*765.6*	*1379.1*
Chronic obstructive pulmonary disease (COPD)													
1955	19.7*	2.8*	14.2*	1.7	1.3	5.9	7.1	10.2	20.9	51.9	72.1	200.0	357.5
1965	19.0*	1.3*	15.7*	2.8	2.4	6.2	8.4	12.5	24.3	53.3	89.9	150.0	355.6
1975	19.6*	1.0*	18.2*	2.7	2.8	6.2	12.6	23.7	28.9	50.2	83.4	147.5	351.7
1985	13.1*	1.1*	11.9*	1.7	2.9	6.2	8.2	13.4	17.9	33.2	65.9	102.0	207.2
1990 *estimated*	**13.5***	**0.3***	**13.7***	**2.0**	**2.3**	**4.8**	**8.5**	**16.1**	**26.2**	**36.1**	**64.3**	**104.1**	**221.2**
1995 projected	*14.2**	*0.2**	*15.1**	*1.6*	*2.0*	*4.3*	*8.8*	*20.0*	*31.0*	*38.4*	*64.5*	*102.0*	*232.7*
Other respiratory disease													
1955	42.2*	18.0*	17.1*	3.5	4.5	5.6	6.2	15.3	26.2	58.7	149.0	308.8	784.4
1965	24.2*	4.7*	10.3*	2.1	3.0	3.5	5.0	9.2	16.4	33.0	72.8	181.1	606.3
1975	25.1*	2.2*	12.6*	3.0	3.2	4.4	6.2	14.9	15.7	40.8	76.1	200.0	657.0
1985	20.2*	1.3*	10.5*	1.7	2.9	2.8	3.9	11.5	14.9	35.8	62.4	176.5	524.2
1990 *estimated*	**21.2***	**1.1***	**9.3***	**0.3**	**2.6**	**2.9**	**4.2**	**9.4**	**13.6**	**31.9**	**60.9**	**148.4**	**631.4**
1995 projected	*21.7**	*1.0**	*8.3**	*0.3*	*2.0*	*2.9*	*3.7*	*8.3*	*11.6*	*29.4*	*52.8*	*135.8*	*702.8*
Vascular disease													
1955	402.8*	7.5*	346.6*	31.5	49.7	91.6	176.0	323.0	612.1	1142.2	2268.6	3900.0	6650.3
1965	432.8*	6.6*	312.6*	24.8	40.8	82.6	140.2	259.3	555.6	1085.2	2108.6	4001.5	8962.7
1975	354.6*	4.7*	243.0*	17.3	31.3	69.1	116.1	214.8	406.0	846.6	1766.7	3323.6	7464.4
1985	276.1*	4.3*	170.0*	13.2	25.9	50.6	86.1	137.9	313.4	562.8	1269.4	2509.3	6348.9
1990 *estimated*	**222.1***	**3.8***	**127.3***	**12.3**	**24.3**	**33.5**	**61.1**	**108.4**	**207.3**	**444.6**	**894.7**	**1987.1**	**5488.8**
1995 projected	*177.2**	*3.5**	*91.4**	*11.3*	*18.7*	*24.2*	*44.5*	*74.4*	*152.1*	*314.6*	*677.2*	*1548.3*	*4633.3*
Liver cirrhosis													
1955	5.4*	0.2*	8.1*	1.7	1.9	3.7	5.0	9.9	12.9	21.3	26.4	39.5	39.1
1965	6.6*	0.2*	10.1*	2.1	2.4	6.2	10.8	9.6	18.1	21.5	31.2	39.4	45.7
1975	8.8*	0.3*	14.0*	1.0	6.3	10.6	17.3	13.9	21.6	27.6	36.1	45.4	60.4
1985	8.8*	0.5*	14.5*	3.7	5.5	13.9	19.0	15.4	22.5	21.3	38.4	32.1	46.1
1990 *estimated*	**8.2***	**0.4***	**14.3***	**5.9**	**9.0**	**15.1**	**12.7**	**16.1**	**21.1**	**20.4**	**29.0**	**33.0**	**34.2**
1995 projected	*7.8**	*0.5**	*13.8**	*8.1*	*11.4*	*14.4*	*11.4*	*13.8*	*20.1*	*17.2*	*25.6*	*26.5*	*29.4*
Other medical causes													
1955	343.9*	127.5*	207.3*	63.5	74.2	95.4	132.8	195.2	304.6	585.2	1014.4	2017.5	6387.7
1965	208.0*	73.1*	163.9*	38.0	49.7	77.7	111.6	161.0	266.0	443.5	747.9	1277.3	3003.4
1975	206.8*	46.2*	135.7*	26.4	37.9	52.3	84.1	133.9	207.4	407.6	786.9	1481.2	3981.2
1985	144.9*	30.3*	80.1*	14.7	19.7	35.0	42.9	76.0	138.5	233.9	454.6	1016.0	3286.6
1990 *estimated*	**137.1***	**23.9***	**76.9***	**20.6**	**19.1**	**33.9**	**43.1**	**69.8**	**120.0**	**231.6**	**433.7**	**953.1**	**3222.0**
1995 projected	*128.6**	*19.1**	*71.8**	*21.5*	*20.1*	*32.9*	*40.5*	*61.3*	*110.2*	*215.9*	*406.8*	*882.8*	*3127.3*
All non-medical causes													
1955	39.5*	14.4*	40.3*	20.7	24.5	27.2	35.1	52.1	57.5	64.5	92.5	201.8	468.2
1965	49.3*	21.1*	43.5*	30.6	26.2	30.5	44.0	41.2	56.8	75.2	119.5	239.4	635.1
1975	53.0*	20.7*	50.6*	29.8	34.4	39.9	42.5	47.9	65.1	94.4	112.2	239.4	716.1
1985	41.5*	18.9*	47.1*	33.1	45.2	41.9	38.3	43.9	50.2	77.3	93.0	139.2	358.6
1990 *estimated*	**35.7***	**18.5***	**37.9***	**30.9**	**32.7**	**38.7**	**34.2**	**35.9**	**39.1**	**53.7**	**82.0**	**119.0**	**293.3**
1995 projected	*30.4**	*17.5**	*30.6**	*26.4*	*27.6*	*32.0*	*29.4*	*28.7*	*28.5*	*41.6*	*66.4*	*97.4*	*243.1*

(*The rates for the age groups 0–34 and 35–69 are the means of seven five-yearly rates, but the all-ages rates are standardised to the conventional "European" age distribution)

BELGIUM: 1975

Smoking-attributed deaths (Sm.) and total deaths (Total)

		ALL CAUSES	ALL CANCER	Lung cancer	Upper aero-digestive ca.	Other cancer	COPD	Other respiratory	Vascular disease	Liver cirrhosis	Other medical	Non-medical
Males												
0–34	Sm.	–	–	–	–	–	–	–	–	–	–	–
	Total	3562	275	14	5	256	33	77	179	9	1487	1502
35–69	Sm.	9766	3736	2604	340	792	1152	147	3405	–	1326	–
	Total	23927	6866	2743	466	3657	1374	412	9331	535	3581	1828
		(41%)	(54%)	(95%)	(73%)	(22%)	(84%)	(36%)	(36%)		(37%)	
70+	Sm.	8410	2892	1887	235	770	1600	214	2642	–	1062	–
	Total	35120	7020	2023	353	4644	2040	1425	16365	289	6815	1166
		(24%)	(41%)	(93%)	(67%)	(17%)	(78%)	(15%)	(16%)		(16%)	
Any age	Sm.	18176	6628	4491	575	1562	2752	361	6047	–	2388	–
	Total	62609	14161	4780	824	8557	3447	1914	25875	833	11883	4496
		(29%)	(47%)	(94%)	(70%)	(18%)	(80%)	(19%)	(23%)		(20%)	
Females												
0–34	Sm.	–	–	–	–	–	–	–	–	–	–	–
	Total	1931	196	13	3	180	24	50	109	6	1045	501
35–69	Sm.	398	103	78	7	18	70	6	139	–	80	–
	Total	13621	4640	245	64	4331	341	236	4562	275	2573	994
		(3%)	(2%)	(32%)	(11%)	(0%)	(21%)	(3%)	(3%)		(3%)	
70+	Sm.	611	106	75	11	20	188	14	204	–	99	–
	Total	41264	5785	255	118	5412	965	1491	20800	250	10244	1729
		(1%)	(2%)	(29%)	(9%)	(0%)	(19%)	(1%)	(1%)		(1%)	
Any age	Sm.	1009	209	153	18	38	258	20	343	–	179	–
	Total	56816	10621	513	185	9923	1330	1777	25471	531	13862	3224
		(2%)	(2%)	(30%)	(10%)	(0%)	(19%)	(1%)	(1%)		(1%)	
Males+Females												
0–34	Sm.	–	–	–	–	–	–	–	–	–	–	–
	Total	5493	471	27	8	436	57	127	288	15	2532	2003
35–69	Sm.	10164	3839	2682	347	810	1222	153	3544	–	1406	–
	Total	37548	11506	2988	530	7988	1715	648	13893	810	6154	2822
		(27%)	(33%)	(90%)	(65%)	(10%)	(71%)	(24%)	(26%)		(23%)	
70+	Sm.	9021	2998	1962	246	790	1788	228	2846	–	1161	–
	Total	76384	12805	2278	471	10056	3005	2916	37165	539	17059	2895
		(12%)	(23%)	(86%)	(52%)	(8%)	(60%)	(8%)	(8%)		(7%)	
Any age	Sm.	19185	6837	4644	593	1600	3010	381	6390	–	2567	–
	Total	119425	24782	5293	1009	18480	4777	3691	51346	1364	25745	7720
		(16%)	(28%)	(88%)	(59%)	(9%)	(63%)	(10%)	(12%)		(10%)	

BELGIUM: 1985

Smoking-attributed deaths (Sm.) and total deaths (Total)

		ALL CAUSES	ALL CANCER	Lung cancer	Upper aero-digestive ca.	Other cancer	COPD	Other respiratory	Vascular disease	Liver cirrhosis	Other medical	Non-medical
Males												
0–34	Sm.	–	–	–	–	–	–	–	–	–	–	–
	Total	2820	214	12	5	197	34	31	142	29	945	1425
35–69	Sm.	8691	4074	2863	427	784	709	286	2765	–	857	–
	Total	19868	6913	3002	569	3342	832	733	6966	540	2124	1760
		(44%)	(59%)	(95%)	(75%)	(23%)	(85%)	(39%)	(40%)		(40%)	
70+	Sm.	10193	4177	2753	297	1127	1573	394	3001	–	1048	–
	Total	34736	8756	2909	411	5436	1897	2059	15318	265	5527	914
		(29%)	(48%)	(95%)	(72%)	(21%)	(83%)	(19%)	(20%)		(19%)	
Any age	Sm.	18884	8251	5616	724	1911	2282	680	5766	–	1905	–
	Total	57424	15883	5923	985	8975	2763	2823	22426	834	8596	4099
		(33%)	(52%)	(95%)	(74%)	(21%)	(83%)	(24%)	(26%)		(22%)	
Females												
0–34	Sm.	–	–	–	–	–	–	–	–	–	–	–
	Total	1430	152	4	1	147	26	28	106	13	638	467
35–69	Sm.	543	198	149	20	29	72	9	178	–	86	–
	Total	10238	4226	315	104	3807	216	183	2980	282	1439	912
		(5%)	(5%)	(47%)	(19%)	(1%)	(33%)	(5%)	(6%)		(6%)	
70+	Sm.	813	193	142	19	32	192	19	285	–	124	–
	Total	42520	6955	378	148	6429	797	1620	21513	250	10126	1259
		(2%)	(3%)	(38%)	(13%)	(0%)	(24%)	(1%)	(1%)		(1%)	
Any age	Sm.	1356	391	291	39	61	264	28	463	–	210	–
	Total	54188	11333	697	253	10383	1039	1831	24599	545	12203	2638
		(3%)	(3%)	(42%)	(15%)	(1%)	(25%)	(2%)	(2%)		(2%)	
Males+Females												
0–34	Sm.	–	–	–	–	–	–	–	–	–	–	–
	Total	4250	366	16	6	344	60	59	248	42	1583	1892
35–69	Sm.	9234	4272	3012	447	813	781	295	2943	–	943	–
	Total	30106	11139	3317	673	7149	1048	916	9946	822	3563	2672
		(31%)	(38%)	(91%)	(66%)	(11%)	(75%)	(32%)	(30%)		(26%)	
70+	Sm.	11006	4370	2895	316	1159	1765	413	3286	–	1172	–
	Total	77256	15711	3287	559	11865	2694	3679	36831	515	15653	2173
		(14%)	(28%)	(88%)	(57%)	(10%)	(66%)	(11%)	(9%)		(7%)	
Any age	Sm.	20240	8642	5907	763	1972	2546	708	6229	–	2115	–
	Total	111612	27216	6620	1238	19358	3802	4654	47025	1379	20799	6737
		(18%)	(32%)	(89%)	(62%)	(10%)	(67%)	(15%)	(13%)		(10%)	

(To be conservative, no deaths before age 35, and none from liver cirrhosis or non-medical causes, were attributed to smoking.)

BELGIUM: 1990

Smoking-attributed deaths (Sm.) and total deaths (Total)

		ALL CAUSES	ALL CANCER	Lung cancer	Upper aero-digestive ca.	Other cancer	COPD	Other respiratory	Vascular disease	Liver cirrhosis	Other medical	Non-medical
Males												
0–34	Sm.	–	–	–	–	–	–	–	–	–	–	–
	Total	2616	190	3	16	171	16	30	138	12	768	1462
35–69	Sm.	7858	3970	2761	492	717	727	208	2079	–	874	–
	Total	19169	7072	2918	686	3468	876	627	5965	501	2451	1677
		(41%)	(56%)	(95%)	(72%)	(21%)	(83%)	(33%)	(35%)		(36%)	
70+	Sm.	8604	3565	2342	257	966	1729	333	2052	–	925	–
	Total	31274	8095	2495	371	5229	2142	2027	12273	182	5635	920
		(28%)	(44%)	(94%)	(69%)	(18%)	(81%)	(16%)	(17%)		(16%)	
Any age	Sm.	16462	7535	5103	749	1683	2456	541	4131	–	1799	–
	Total	53059	15357	5416	1073	8868	3034	2684	18376	695	8854	4059
		(31%)	(49%)	(94%)	(70%)	(19%)	(81%)	(20%)	(22%)		(20%)	
Females												
0–34	Sm.	–	–	–	–	–	–	–	–	–	–	–
	Total	1261	159	3	1	155	7	26	97	11	511	450
35–69	Sm.	653	256	196	25	35	105	13	172	–	107	–
	Total	10111	4377	380	107	3890	280	189	2592	297	1575	801
		(6%)	(6%)	(52%)	(23%)	(1%)	(38%)	(7%)	(7%)		(7%)	
70+	Sm.	593	142	104	16	22	166	16	174	–	95	–
	Total	40185	6662	337	152	6173	858	1945	18904	199	10522	1095
		(1%)	(2%)	(31%)	(11%)	(0%)	(19%)	(1%)	(1%)		(1%)	
Any age	Sm.	1246	398	300	41	57	271	29	346	–	202	–
	Total	51557	11198	720	260	10218	1145	2160	21593	507	12608	2346
		(2%)	(4%)	(42%)	(16%)	(1%)	(24%)	(1%)	(2%)		(2%)	
Males+Females												
0–34	Sm.	–	–	–	–	–	–	–	–	–	–	–
	Total	3877	349	6	17	326	23	56	235	23	1279	1912
35–69	Sm.	8511	4226	2957	517	752	832	221	2251	–	981	–
	Total	29280	11449	3298	793	7358	1156	816	8557	798	4026	2478
		(29%)	(37%)	(90%)	(65%)	(10%)	(72%)	(27%)	(26%)		(24%)	
70+	Sm.	9197	3707	2446	273	988	1895	349	2226	–	1020	–
	Total	71459	14757	2832	523	11402	3000	3972	31177	381	16157	2015
		(13%)	(25%)	(86%)	(52%)	(9%)	(63%)	(9%)	(7%)		(6%)	
Any age	Sm.	17708	7933	5403	790	1740	2727	570	4477	–	2001	–
	Total	104616	26555	6136	1333	19086	4179	4844	39969	1202	21462	6405
		(17%)	(30%)	(88%)	(59%)	(9%)	(65%)	(12%)	(11%)		(9%)	

BELGIUM: 1995

Smoking-attributed deaths (Sm.) and total deaths (Total)

		ALL CAUSES	ALL CANCER	Lung cancer	Upper aero-digestive ca.	Other cancer	COPD	Other respiratory	Vascular disease	Liver cirrhosis	Other medical	Non-medical
Males												
0–34	Sm.	–	–	–	–	–	–	–	–	–	–	–
	Total	2273	150	2	14	134	12	26	108	8	593	1376
35–69	Sm.	6248	3362	2293	516	553	639	140	1335	–	772	–
	Total	16242	6294	2449	757	3088	796	482	4291	453	2418	1508
		(38%)	(53%)	(94%)	(68%)	(18%)	(80%)	(29%)	(31%)		(32%)	
70+	Sm.	8006	3330	2209	247	874	1950	300	1556	–	870	–
	Total	29643	8086	2376	374	5336	2486	2003	10167	144	5793	964
		(27%)	(41%)	(93%)	(66%)	(16%)	(78%)	(15%)	(15%)		(15%)	
Any age	Sm.	14254	6692	4502	763	1427	2589	440	2891	–	1642	–
	Total	48158	14530	4827	1145	8558	3294	2511	14566	605	8804	3848
		(30%)	(46%)	(93%)	(67%)	(17%)	(79%)	(18%)	(20%)		(19%)	
Females												
0–34	Sm.	–	–	–	–	–	–	–	–	–	–	–
	Total	1059	146	3	1	142	5	22	84	14	395	393
35–69	Sm.	639	271	210	26	35	120	12	130	–	106	–
	Total	8708	3986	392	109	3485	302	166	1829	296	1462	667
		(7%)	(7%)	(54%)	(24%)	(1%)	(40%)	(7%)	(7%)		(7%)	
70+	Sm.	423	112	83	13	16	127	12	105	–	67	–
	Total	35543	6302	325	149	5828	883	2041	15289	177	9945	906
		(1%)	(2%)	(26%)	(9%)	(0%)	(14%)	(1%)	(1%)		(1%)	
Any age	Sm.	1062	383	293	39	51	247	24	235	–	173	–
	Total	45310	10434	720	259	9455	1190	2229	17202	487	11802	1966
		(2%)	(4%)	(41%)	(15%)	(1%)	(21%)	(1%)	(1%)		(1%)	
Males+Females												
0–34	Sm.	–	–	–	–	–	–	–	–	–	–	–
	Total	3332	296	5	15	276	17	48	192	22	988	1769
35–69	Sm.	6887	3633	2503	542	588	759	152	1465	–	878	–
	Total	24950	10280	2841	866	6573	1098	648	6120	749	3880	2175
		(28%)	(35%)	(88%)	(63%)	(9%)	(69%)	(23%)	(24%)		(23%)	
70+	Sm.	8429	3442	2292	260	890	2077	312	1661	–	937	–
	Total	65186	14388	2701	523	11164	3369	4044	25456	321	15738	1870
		(13%)	(24%)	(85%)	(50%)	(8%)	(62%)	(8%)	(7%)		(6%)	
Any age	Sm.	15316	7075	4795	802	1478	2836	464	3126	–	1815	–
	Total	93468	24964	5547	1404	18013	4484	4740	31768	1092	20606	5814
		(16%)	(28%)	(86%)	(57%)	(8%)	(63%)	(10%)	(10%)		(9%)	

(To be conservative, no deaths before age 35, and none from liver cirrhosis or non-medical causes, were attributed to smoking.)

BULGARIA: 1990

		No. of deaths			Standardised rates (Defined on p.298)			Annual death rates / 100, 000						
		All ages	0–34	35–69	All ages	0–34	35–69	0–4	5–9	10–14	15–19	20–24	25–29	30–34
ALL CAUSES	M	59780	3300	26966	1352.7	153.4	1509.7	392.2	43.4	49.3	99.5	139.1	152.4	198.1
	F	48828	1774	14234	872.0	86.4	727.1	292.9	36.0	26.9	48.1	52.1	58.5	90.7
Tuberculosis	M	162	6	126	3.5	0.3	6.8	–	–	–	–	0.6	0.3	1.0
	F	47	3	25	0.9	0.1	1.3	–	–	–	0.3	–	0.3	0.3
Other infective	M	186	78	69	4.5	3.7	3.8	18.1	1.3	0.9	1.2	1.3	1.3	1.9
and parasitic	F	135	56	49	3.0	2.8	2.4	12.5	1.7	0.3	0.3	2.0	0.7	1.9
ALL CANCER	M	8898	248	5811	195.3	11.3	324.5	9.2	3.9	7.9	9.7	13.0	15.2	20.0
	F	6144	212	3703	116.1	10.0	187.1	5.4	4.1	2.8	5.3	9.8	13.9	28.6
Mouth and	M	214	3	167	4.8	0.1	9.1	–	–	–	–	0.3	0.3	0.3
pharynx cancer	F	44	2	18	0.9	0.1	0.9	0.4	–	–	–	–	–	0.3
Oesophagus cancer	M	200	–	154	4.4	–	8.5	–	–	–	–	–	–	–
	F	72	2	39	1.3	0.1	1.9	–	–	0.3	–	–	–	0.3
Stomach cancer	M	1321	6	788	28.9	0.3	44.6	–	–	–	–	0.3	1.7	–
	F	950	12	449	17.3	0.6	22.8	–	–	–	0.9	0.3	1.4	1.3
Colorectal cancer	M	999	10	578	22.0	0.5	32.5	–	–	–	0.3	0.6	0.3	1.9
	F	819	10	445	15.0	0.5	22.6	0.4	–	–	–	0.3	0.3	2.3
Liver cancer	M	534	5	364	11.5	0.2	20.4	0.7	0.3	–	–	–	0.3	0.3
	F	363	7	204	6.6	0.3	10.4	–	–	–	0.6	–	0.7	1.0
Pancreas cancer	M	421	3	279	9.3	0.1	15.6	–	–	–	–	–	0.3	0.6
	F	266	1	152	4.8	0.0	7.8	–	–	0.3	–	–	–	–
Larynx cancer	M	296	3	231	6.5	0.1	12.8	–	–	–	–	–	–	1.0
	F	14	1	9	0.2	0.0	0.5	–	–	–	–	0.3	–	–
Lung cancer	M	2583	22	2010	56.3	1.0	111.6	0.3	–	0.6	0.3	1.6	2.3	1.9
	F	448	13	266	8.3	0.6	13.5	0.4	0.3	0.6	–	0.3	1.0	1.6
Malignant melanoma	M	45	2	28	1.0	0.1	1.5	–	–	0.3	–	0.3	–	–
	F	29	2	14	0.5	0.1	0.7	–	–	–	–	–	–	0.6
Female breast cancer	F	1068	21	762	21.1	1.0	38.3	–	–	–	–	–	1.7	5.1
Cervix cancer	F	260	21	187	5.2	1.0	9.3	–	–	–	–	0.7	1.0	5.1
Other uterine cancer	F	416	11	280	8.0	0.5	14.1	–	–	–	–	0.7	0.7	2.3
Ovarian cancer	F	279	10	210	5.5	0.5	10.6	–	–	–	0.3	0.3	1.4	1.3
Prostate cancer	M	613	2	184	13.8	0.1	10.9	–	–	–	–	0.3	0.3	–
Bladder cancer	M	286	4	149	6.2	0.2	8.6	0.3	–	0.3	–	–	0.3	0.3
	F	84	1	33	1.5	0.0	1.7	–	–	–	–	–	–	0.3
Other and ill-defined	M	934	102	609	20.7	4.7	33.6	4.8	2.6	1.2	4.4	4.9	6.9	7.9
cancer sites	F	748	57	455	14.3	2.7	23.0	2.5	2.1	1.2	2.5	3.0	2.7	4.8
Hodgkin's disease	M	52	14	32	1.2	0.6	1.7	0.3	0.3	–	–	0.6	1.0	2.2
	F	23	–	17	0.4	–	0.8	–	–	–	–	–	–	–
Myeloma and non-	M	158	25	103	3.5	1.1	5.6	0.3	–	1.2	1.8	1.0	1.0	2.5
Hodgkin lymphomas	F	96	13	64	1.9	0.6	3.3	1.1	0.3	–	0.3	1.7	1.0	–
Leukaemia	M	242	47	135	5.3	2.1	7.6	2.4	0.6	4.4	3.0	2.9	0.3	1.0
	F	165	28	99	3.3	1.3	4.9	0.7	1.4	0.3	0.6	2.0	2.0	2.3
ALL VASCULAR	M	34649	341	13815	784.0	15.6	785.1	15.4	2.6	5.9	10.0	11.7	22.1	41.7
DISEASE	F	32182	180	7518	557.9	8.5	387.1	12.5	3.4	3.7	5.9	7.1	10.1	17.1
Rheumatic heart	M	178	9	142	3.9	0.4	7.7	–	–	0.3	0.6	0.3	1.0	0.6
disease and fever	F	272	11	223	5.4	0.5	11.2	–	–	0.3	0.3	1.0	0.3	1.6
Hypertensive disease	M	1558	7	780	34.5	0.3	44.1	–	–	–	0.3	–	0.7	1.3
	F	1644	7	515	28.8	0.3	26.4	–	–	–	–	0.3	0.3	1.6
Ischaemic heart	M	12321	109	5317	278.5	5.0	300.2	–	–	–	0.6	4.5	8.6	21.3
disease	F	9918	20	2098	170.5	0.9	108.4	–	–	–	–	1.0	2.4	3.2
Pulmonary embolism	M	...	...	...	...	...	...	...	...	...	...	...	...	...
and other venous	F	...	...	...	...	...	...	...	...	...	...	...	...	...
Cerebrovascular	M	11196	93	4458	251.9	4.3	255.5	8.2	0.3	2.3	3.0	3.2	4.6	8.3
disease	F	11198	56	2986	194.5	2.7	154.0	4.3	1.4	1.2	2.2	1.7	2.7	5.1
Other vascular	M	9396	123	3118	215.2	5.6	177.6	7.2	2.3	3.2	5.6	3.6	7.3	10.2
disease, incl. venous	F	9150	86	1696	158.7	4.1	87.1	8.2	2.1	2.2	3.4	3.0	4.4	5.5
Chronic obstructive	M	1430	8	608	31.9	0.4	34.8	0.7	–	0.3	–	–	0.3	1.3
pulmonary disease	F	786	2	239	13.7	0.1	12.3	–	–	0.3	–	–	–	0.3
Other respiratory	M	2515	372	945	58.2	17.8	52.8	95.9	6.8	2.1	3.0	5.5	5.3	6.4
disease	F	1721	270	367	32.7	13.6	18.8	75.5	4.8	2.2	2.2	3.7	2.0	4.5
Peptic ulcer	M	272	4	156	6.0	0.2	8.8	–	–	–	–	0.3	0.3	0.6
	F	108	1	41	1.9	0.0	2.1	–	–	–	–	–	–	0.3
Liver cirrhosis	M	1201	27	942	26.4	1.2	51.4	1.4	0.3	0.3	0.3	0.6	0.3	5.4
	F	360	11	230	6.6	0.5	11.8	–	–	0.3	0.3	1.0	0.3	1.6
Renal disease	M	847	38	402	18.8	1.8	22.8	2.0	0.3	0.9	0.3	1.3	3.6	3.8
	F	633	31	321	11.7	1.5	16.3	0.7	–	0.6	0.6	1.7	2.7	3.9
Pregnancy and birth	F	22	12	10	0.5	0.6	0.4	–	–	–	0.9	1.7	1.4	–
Congenital and	M	540	530	10	14.6	25.8	0.5	176.5	1.3	0.9	0.9	–	–	1.0
perinatal causes	F	383	382	1	10.9	19.5	0.0	130.7	3.4	1.2	0.9	–	–	–
Ill-defined causes	M	2406	68	513	59.0	3.2	28.4	7.8	0.6	0.3	3.2	3.2	2.3	4.5
	F	2979	43	243	51.9	2.1	12.4	6.4	1.0	0.6	1.9	1.0	1.0	2.6
Other medical causes	M	2402	226	1282	53.8	10.5	71.0	26.6	5.5	5.6	8.0	7.1	9.3	11.1
	F	2033	187	912	37.6	9.0	46.5	20.1	6.2	5.9	7.4	5.4	7.8	10.0
ALL NON-	M	4272	1354	2287	96.6	61.7	119.1	38.6	20.7	24.4	62.9	94.2	91.9	99.5
MEDICAL CAUSES	F	1295	384	575	26.7	18.3	28.4	29.0	11.3	9.0	22.0	18.6	18.2	19.6
Motor vehicle	M	1092	457	533	24.7	20.8	27.5	6.5	9.1	5.3	22.1	40.6	33.1	29.3
traffic accidents	F	317	124	139	6.7	5.8	6.7	3.2	5.8	2.5	8.7	9.1	6.4	5.1
Fire	M	99	24	42	2.3	1.1	2.2	2.7	–	0.3	0.6	1.6	1.7	1.0
	F	51	13	19	1.0	0.6	0.9	2.9	0.7	–	0.3	–	0.3	0.3
Suicide	M	920	210	484	20.7	9.5	25.8	–	–	4.1	10.9	17.2	16.2	18.1
	F	403	58	209	7.8	2.7	10.5	–	–	0.6	5.0	3.4	4.4	5.5
Homicide	M	224	96	116	5.1	4.4	5.9	1.0	0.3	0.6	3.2	8.1	9.9	7.6
	F	68	28	27	1.5	1.3	1.3	0.4	1.4	0.6	0.9	0.3	2.0	3.5
POPULATION (thousands):	M=males				4435.4	2205.7	1940.1	293.0	308.7	340.5	338.7	307.8	302.5	314.5
	F=females				4555.4	2119.8	2046.5	279.3	291.9	323.9	322.2	295.8	295.9	310.8

BULGARIA: 1990

Annual death rates / 100, 000

9th ICD categories

35-39	40-44	45-49	50-54	55-59	60-64	65-69	70-74	75-79	80+/NK			
287.3	484.4	740.5	1139.3	1633.3	2512.2	3771.2	5787.1	9314.8	17680.1	M	ALL CAUSES	001-999
123.4	186.4	294.5	447.4	731.0	1210.0	2096.8	3692.7	6895.4	15811.0	F		
3.7	3.7	4.1	3.1	10.3	10.8	11.6	8.2	11.7	11.7	M	Tuberculosis	010-018, 137
–	–	2.5	0.7	0.7	1.4	3.8	2.9	6.6	5.2	F		
0.6	2.4	2.6	5.0	3.6	5.4	6.7	10.0	7.8	26.0	M	Other infective	Rest of 001-139
1.9	1.2	2.9	2.2	2.7	2.4	3.8	3.6	7.4	12.9	F	and parasitic	
44.7	88.1	158.0	278.3	402.4	562.7	737.1	916.7	1049.9	979.2	M	ALL CANCER	140-208
40.3	79.6	113.6	162.0	219.2	308.9	386.1	492.7	616.1	616.8	F		
0.3	4.9	8.2	11.2	11.0	15.4	12.5	15.4	18.6	10.4	M	Mouth and	140-149
–	1.2	0.7	1.5	1.0	0.3	1.5	5.8	4.4	8.6	F	pharynx cancer	
0.6	3.4	4.5	9.3	13.5	12.7	15.2	13.6	15.6	19.5	M	Oesophagus cancer	150
0.9	0.6	0.7	1.5	3.4	3.5	3.0	5.8	8.8	9.5	F		
5.9	8.3	14.5	33.2	50.6	83.0	116.4	181.2	203.3	154.7	M	Stomach cancer	151
4.7	6.4	9.8	15.6	26.2	39.8	57.3	101.5	129.0	150.3	F		
4.7	7.6	11.9	25.1	38.1	57.1	83.3	125.9	158.4	143.0	M	Colorectal cancer	153, 154
2.2	7.6	12.4	14.5	29.3	38.1	54.2	76.6	103.2	102.2	F		
5.3	2.4	8.2	10.8	27.1	39.0	50.2	56.2	65.5	46.8	M	Liver cancer	155.0
0.9	0.9	3.6	5.9	12.8	22.0	26.7	32.1	47.2	37.8	F		
0.6	4.6	11.5	12.7	20.0	24.7	34.9	41.7	47.9	57.2	M	Pancreas cancer	157
0.9	1.2	2.9	5.2	8.4	16.8	18.8	29.2	38.3	18.0	F		
1.9	4.3	8.2	15.4	14.6	21.6	23.3	19.9	23.5	20.8	M	Larynx cancer	161
–	–	–	0.7	0.3	0.3	1.9	–	2.9	–	F		
12.4	29.7	52.8	108.5	153.6	199.2	225.3	220.1	187.7	150.8	M	Lung cancer	162
2.2	5.1	5.1	10.0	12.4	26.9	32.8	36.5	49.4	44.7	F		
1.2	0.9	0.7	1.2	2.1	1.9	2.2	2.7	3.9	10.4	M	Malignant melanoma	172
0.3	0.3	0.4	0.4	1.0	1.4	1.1	1.5	5.9	2.6	F		
9.3	20.9	30.9	47.1	49.8	52.8	57.3	66.4	72.2	82.5	F	Female breast cancer	174
3.4	10.6	6.6	10.0	9.1	10.1	15.1	10.2	16.2	13.7	F	Cervix cancer	180
3.1	5.4	10.6	12.6	17.5	24.5	25.2	32.1	34.6	29.2	F	Other uterine cancer	179, 182
2.2	4.2	10.6	11.1	11.4	15.7	19.2	13.9	16.9	14.6	F	Ovarian cancer	183
–	0.3	0.4	2.7	6.4	22.8	43.9	95.1	154.4	213.3	M	Prostate cancer	185
0.3	0.9	3.3	5.4	7.8	15.4	26.9	36.2	58.7	42.9	M	Bladder cancer	188
0.6	0.6	0.7	1.1	1.3	1.7	5.6	10.2	16.9	11.2	F		
6.8	15.0	21.2	30.1	42.4	47.5	72.1	77.9	76.2	76.7	M	Other and ill-defined	Rest of 140-208
6.8	9.7	13.1	18.9	24.2	40.2	47.8	53.3	55.3	75.6	F	cancer sites	
1.2	0.9	2.2	2.3	1.1	1.5	2.7	–	3.9	2.6	M	Hodgkin's disease	201
0.9	0.3	–	0.7	0.7	1.4	1.9	1.5	1.5	1.7	F		
1.6	3.1	5.2	5.4	7.8	5.8	10.3	12.7	10.8	6.5	M	Myeloma and non-	200, 202-203
–	0.9	1.8	3.0	3.0	5.2	9.0	4.4	5.2	5.2	F	Hodgkin lymphomas	
1.9	1.8	5.2	5.0	6.1	15.1	17.9	18.1	21.5	23.4	M	Leukaemia	204-208
1.9	3.6	3.6	2.2	7.4	8.0	7.5	11.7	8.1	9.5	F		
81.4	181.0	309.7	510.6	817.9	1345.4	2249.9	3737.3	6623.7	12472.0	M	ALL VASCULAR	390-459
31.9	52.6	103.4	183.8	363.5	663.9	1310.7	2631.4	5294.0	11765.5	F	DISEASE	
2.5	4.9	4.5	9.3	9.3	10.8	12.5	9.1	15.6	1.3	M	Rheumatic heart	390-398
4.0	4.2	5.1	13.7	14.8	20.6	15.8	13.9	12.5	1.7	F	disease and fever	
1.6	10.1	20.1	25.1	57.7	76.4	117.8	163.9	288.4	383.6	M	Hypertensive disease	401-405
1.2	4.5	6.2	15.2	29.6	50.0	78.0	156.9	272.7	461.3	F		
35.4	81.3	133.1	211.5	330.4	499.8	810.1	1273.6	2185.7	4230.2	M	Ischaemic heart	410-414
6.8	10.6	24.8	39.3	93.1	185.2	399.2	781.0	1662.5	3843.6	F	disease	
...	...	...	...	...	...	...	...	...	...	M	Pulmonary embolism	Not given
...	...	...	...	...	...	...	...	...	...	F	and other venous	separately
22.0	41.3	82.2	152.1	250.5	457.7	782.8	1364.1	2263.0	3672.3	M	Cerebrovascular	430-438
10.2	18.5	33.9	67.5	140.2	266.6	541.2	1083.2	1960.9	3445.9	F	disease	
19.9	43.4	69.9	112.7	170.0	300.7	526.6	926.6	1871.0	4184.7	M	Other vascular	Rest of 390-459,
9.6	14.8	33.5	48.2	85.7	141.5	276.5	596.4	1385.4	4012.9	F	disease, incl. venous	incl. 415, 451-3
1.9	3.7	8.9	20.5	38.8	69.1	100.8	171.2	294.2	421.3	M	Chronic obstructive	490-496
1.2	1.2	3.3	8.2	11.1	23.1	38.0	60.6	125.3	250.9	F	pulmonary disease	
12.7	22.0	27.5	36.7	48.8	87.2	134.3	243.7	384.2	697.0	M	Other respiratory	Rest of 460-519
3.1	4.2	8.0	10.4	16.8	31.1	58.0	121.9	241.0	506.9	F	disease	
1.2	2.1	4.5	5.8	9.3	14.3	24.6	24.5	36.2	62.4	M	Peptic ulcer	531-533
0.3	0.6	0.4	1.9	2.7	3.1	5.6	10.2	14.7	27.5	F		
14.6	19.0	33.1	54.0	68.8	86.8	83.3	83.3	87.0	66.3	M	Liver cirrhosis	571
0.9	2.7	4.0	8.9	11.8	20.3	33.9	29.2	34.6	27.5	F		
3.4	5.8	10.4	13.1	19.2	42.5	65.4	106.0	154.4	171.7	M	Renal disease	580-590
3.4	4.2	6.9	10.4	19.5	26.2	43.7	54.7	66.3	99.7	F		
2.5	0.6	–	–	–	–	–	–	–	–	F	Pregnancy and birth	630-676
1.6	0.3	1.5	–	–	–	–	–	–	–	M	Congenital and	740-779
–	0.3	–	–	–	–	–	–	–	–	F	perinatal causes	
7.1	11.0	17.5	25.9	28.9	47.1	61.4	87.0	150.5	2048.1	M	Ill-defined causes	780-799
3.7	3.3	9.1	9.6	10.1	18.2	32.8	50.4	120.9	2113.4	F		
19.3	27.2	42.8	57.1	73.1	118.5	159.4	231.9	315.7	409.6	M	Other medical causes	Rest of 001-799
10.5	11.8	21.1	24.1	47.4	75.8	134.8	174.5	272.7	279.2	F		
95.0	118.0	120.1	129.3	112.3	122.3	136.6	167.6	199.4	314.7	M	ALL NON-	E800-E999
23.6	23.9	19.3	25.2	25.6	35.6	45.6	60.6	95.8	105.7	F	MEDICAL CAUSES	
23.6	29.1	24.9	31.3	31.0	28.2	24.2	35.3	25.4	48.1	M	Motor vehicle	E810-E819
6.8	8.5	6.6	5.6	5.7	7.3	6.8	9.5	21.4	10.3	F	traffic accidents	
2.2	1.2	3.0	1.5	2.9	2.7	1.8	5.4	12.7	18.2	M	Fire	E890-E899
0.6	1.2	0.4	0.4	0.7	1.0	2.3	2.9	4.4	7.7	F		
16.8	18.3	24.5	23.9	24.6	30.9	41.6	47.1	70.4	132.6	M	Suicide	E950-E959
7.4	5.4	6.9	9.3	9.1	14.3	20.7	27.7	35.4	43.0	F		
6.5	8.0	7.1	7.3	2.9	5.8	3.6	1.8	5.9	5.2	M	Homicide	E960-E969
1.2	2.1	1.5	1.9	0.7	0.7	1.1	2.9	1.5	6.0	F		
322.0	327.0	269.0	259.1	280.6	259.1	223.3	110.4	102.3	76.9	M	**POPULATION (thousands)**	
322.4	330.5	274.7	269.8	297.4	286.2	265.5	137.0	135.7	116.4	F		

BULGARIA: Males

	All ages	0–34	35–69	35–39	40–44	45–49	50–54	55–59	60–64	65–69	70–74	75–79	80+/NK
POPULATION (1000s)													
1955	3743.1	2339.6	1263.8	200.3	252.1	240.7	211.6	162.1	116.9	80.1	68.4	42.4	28.9
1965	4101.0	2267.7	1654.7	329.7	323.4	196.5	248.7	233.2	187.4	135.8	80.0	52.4	46.2
1975	4354.4	2276.4	1826.7	288.1	323.3	321.9	307.6	178.1	221.8	185.9	130.1	71.3	49.9
1985	4452.7	2187.4	1941.4	346.6	285.5	273.2	312.2	305.2	276.2	142.5	157.7	101.7	64.5
1990	**4435.4**	**2205.7**	**1940.1**	**322.0**	**327.0**	**269.0**	**259.1**	**280.6**	**259.1**	**223.3**	**110.4**	**102.3**	**76.9**
1995 projected	*4465.9*	*2153.1*	*1967.7*	*307.5*	*318.4*	*325.6*	*265.0*	*250.0*	*266.3*	*234.9*	*181.9*	*75.0*	*88.2*
NUMBER OF DEATHS													
All causes													
1955	35752	11594	12162	474	859	1274	1705	2220	2302	3328	4035	3261	4700
1965	35145	4716	14913	696	924	833	1768	2593	3688	4411	4113	4500	6903
1975	48494	4379	20148	699	1108	1780	2619	2373	4822	6747	7899	7171	8897
1985	59345	3439	24102	986	1216	1925	3161	4752	6735	5327	9171	9948	12685
1990	**59780**	**3300**	**26966**	**925**	**1584**	**1992**	**2952**	**4583**	**6509**	**8421**	**6389**	**9529**	**13596**
1995 projected	*62864*	*3110*	*28562*	*941*	*1648*	*2661*	*3240*	*4308*	*6848*	*8916*	*10274*	*6557*	*14361*
Lung cancer													
1955	...	...	...	...	...	...	...	...	...	...	...	...	...
1965	1739	12	1205	17	30	47	152	258	336	365	252	160	110
1975	2008	14	1389	17	57	143	205	181	362	424	344	174	87
1985	2484	22	1812	47	54	164	275	417	547	308	334	205	111
1990	**2583**	**22**	**2010**	**40**	**97**	**142**	**281**	**431**	**516**	**503**	**243**	**192**	**116**
1995 projected	*2839*	*23*	*2163*	*46*	*96*	*196*	*315*	*416*	*553*	*541*	*400*	*133*	*120*
ANNUAL DEATH RATE / 100,000													
All causes													
1955	1392.9*	472.7*	1343.7*	236.6	340.7	529.3	805.8	1369.5	1969.2	4154.8	5899.1	7691.0	16263.0
1965	1144.6*	209.0*	1137.1*	211.1	285.7	423.9	710.9	1111.9	1968.0	3248.2	5141.3	8587.8	14941.6
1975	1311.8*	188.3*	1303.6*	242.6	342.7	553.0	851.4	1332.4	2174.0	3629.4	6071.5	10057.5	17829.7
1985	1381.8*	161.5*	1451.6*	284.5	425.9	704.6	1012.5	1557.0	2438.5	3738.2	5815.5	9781.7	19666.7
1990	**1352.7***	**153.4***	**1509.7***	**287.3**	**484.4**	**740.5**	**1139.3**	**1633.3**	**2512.2**	**3771.2**	**5787.1**	**9314.8**	**17680.1**
1995 projected	*1329.5**	*146.6**	*1564.8**	*306.0*	*517.6*	*817.3*	*1222.6*	*1723.2*	*2571.5*	*3795.7*	*5648.2*	*8742.7*	*16282.3*
All cancer													
1955	...	...	...	...	...	...	...	...	...	...	...	...	...
1965	198.7*	11.3*	303.1*	27.0	56.9	96.2	194.2	339.6	549.1	858.6	1107.5	1341.6	1233.8
1975	178.6*	10.9*	281.5*	35.1	65.3	123.0	199.0	322.9	500.0	725.1	939.3	1133.2	969.9
1985	185.8*	12.3*	304.1*	45.0	65.1	153.4	230.6	379.8	549.2	705.3	850.3	1027.5	1024.8
1990	**195.3***	**11.3***	**324.5***	**44.7**	**88.1**	**158.0**	**278.3**	**402.4**	**562.7**	**737.1**	**916.7**	**1049.9**	**979.2**
1995 projected	*205.3**	*10.7**	*346.4**	*50.1*	*97.7*	*181.2*	*305.3*	*432.0*	*586.2*	*772.7*	*953.3*	*1072.0*	*969.4*
Lung cancer													
1955	...	...	...	...	...	...	...	...	...	...	...	...	...
1965	53.9*	0.5*	94.0*	5.2	9.3	23.9	61.1	110.6	179.3	268.8	315.0	305.3	238.1
1975	49.4*	0.7*	89.6*	5.9	17.6	44.4	66.6	101.6	163.2	228.1	264.4	244.0	174.3
1985	53.7*	1.0*	104.5*	13.6	18.9	60.0	88.1	136.6	198.0	216.1	211.8	201.6	172.1
1990	**56.3***	**1.0***	**111.6***	**12.4**	**29.7**	**52.8**	**108.5**	**153.6**	**199.2**	**225.3**	**220.1**	**187.7**	**150.8**
1995 projected	*58.7**	*1.0**	*118.4**	*15.0*	*30.2*	*60.2*	*118.9*	*166.4*	*207.7*	*230.3*	*219.9*	*177.3*	*136.1*
Upper aerodigestive cancer (mouth, oesophagus, pharynx and larynx)													
1955	...	...	...	...	...	...	...	...	...	...	...	...	...
1965	10.6*	0.1*	17.2*	2.1	3.1	9.7	13.3	21.0	34.7	36.8	50.0	66.8	62.8
1975	10.4*	0.4*	18.1*	3.8	4.9	9.0	19.2	20.2	28.9	40.9	46.1	47.7	52.1
1985	11.8*	0.3*	22.0*	4.6	7.7	12.8	18.6	30.1	37.7	42.8	38.0	58.0	45.0
1990	**15.7***	**0.3***	**30.3***	**2.8**	**12.5**	**20.8**	**35.9**	**39.2**	**49.8**	**51.1**	**48.9**	**57.7**	**50.7**
1995 projected	*20.1**	*0.2**	*40.3**	*3.3*	*17.6*	*29.5*	*50.2*	*55.2*	*62.7*	*63.9*	*55.0*	*62.7*	*53.3*
Other cancer													
1955	...	...	...	...	...	...	...	...	...	...	...	...	...
1965	134.3*	10.7*	191.8*	19.7	44.5	62.6	119.8	208.0	335.1	553.0	742.5	969.5	932.9
1975	118.7*	9.8*	173.7*	25.3	42.7	69.6	113.1	201.0	307.9	456.2	628.7	841.5	743.5
1985	120.2*	11.0*	177.5*	26.8	38.5	80.5	124.0	213.0	313.5	446.3	600.5	767.9	807.8
1990	**123.3***	**10.0***	**182.5***	**29.5**	**45.9**	**84.4**	**133.9**	**209.6**	**313.8**	**460.8**	**647.6**	**804.5**	**777.6**
1995 projected	*126.5**	*9.4**	*187.8**	*31.9*	*49.9*	*91.5*	*136.2*	*210.4*	*315.8*	*478.5*	*678.4*	*832.0*	*780.0*
Chronic obstructive pulmonary disease (COPD)													
1955	...	...	...	...	...	...	...	...	...	...	...	...	...
1965	68.2*	0.3*	84.9*	4.5	11.4	23.4	43.0	78.5	147.3	286.5	372.5	639.3	740.3
1975	74.1*	0.4*	81.3*	4.9	8.7	18.9	39.0	82.5	152.4	262.5	455.8	680.2	927.9
1985	44.4*	0.6*	47.5*	0.9	5.3	12.8	28.2	50.8	85.1	149.5	254.3	398.2	598.4
1990	**31.9***	**0.4***	**34.8***	**1.9**	**3.7**	**8.9**	**20.5**	**38.8**	**69.1**	**100.8**	**171.2**	**294.2**	**421.3**
1995 projected	*23.1**	*0.4**	*25.3**	*1.6*	*2.8*	*6.4*	*15.1*	*30.0*	*50.3*	*70.7*	*120.4*	*216.0*	*301.6*
Other respiratory disease													
1955	...	...	...	...	...	...	...	...	...	...	...	...	...
1965	81.4*	47.5*	49.2*	5.8	9.0	13.7	28.1	38.2	93.4	156.1	295.0	494.3	956.7
1975	113.9*	38.9*	87.5*	8.0	13.0	26.1	47.8	99.4	144.7	273.3	483.5	868.2	1493.0
1985	71.5*	20.8*	61.6*	13.3	20.0	32.9	45.2	64.2	91.2	164.2	258.1	518.2	967.4
1990	**58.2***	**17.8***	**52.8***	**12.7**	**22.0**	**27.5**	**36.7**	**48.8**	**87.2**	**134.3**	**243.7**	**384.2**	**697.0**
1995 projected	*47.2**	*15.3**	*46.0**	*12.0*	*20.7*	*24.3*	*29.1*	*41.6*	*73.2*	*120.9*	*196.3*	*290.7*	*507.9*
Vascular disease													
1955	...	...	...	...	...	...	...	...	...	...	...	...	...
1965	483.6*	10.1*	415.6*	35.8	61.8	112.0	215.9	363.2	766.8	1353.5	2538.8	4765.3	8153.7
1975	637.5*	10.0*	573.3*	59.4	93.7	183.3	311.8	528.4	1006.3	1830.0	3471.9	6077.1	10316.6
1985	788.2*	11.2*	735.0*	79.1	145.4	279.3	438.8	738.2	1291.1	2173.3	3739.4	6827.9	13606.2
1990	**784.0***	**15.6***	**785.1***	**81.4**	**181.0**	**309.7**	**510.6**	**817.9**	**1345.4**	**2249.9**	**3737.3**	**6623.7**	**12472.0**
1995 projected	*778.4**	*18.9**	*826.7**	*94.6*	*204.5*	*358.1*	*569.8*	*880.4*	*1405.2*	*2274.2*	*3675.1*	*6278.7*	*11657.6*
Liver cirrhosis													
1955	...	...	...	...	...	...	...	...	...	...	...	...	...
1965	7.9*	0.7*	12.4*	2.7	3.7	2.0	9.2	14.6	20.8	33.9	46.3	36.3	43.3
1975	12.2*	0.6*	22.7*	3.5	7.4	13.0	22.1	34.3	32.5	46.3	46.9	58.9	30.1
1985	25.8*	1.1*	50.9*	8.9	18.9	31.1	47.7	68.5	84.0	96.8	82.4	90.5	68.2
1990	**26.4***	**1.2***	**51.4***	**14.6**	**19.0**	**33.1**	**54.0**	**68.8**	**86.8**	**83.3**	**83.3**	**87.0**	**66.3**
1995 projected	*26.9**	*1.2**	*52.2**	*17.6*	*21.4*	*35.9*	*56.6*	*71.6*	*82.6*	*79.6*	*78.1*	*90.7*	*64.6*
Other medical causes													
1955	...	...	...	...	...	...	...	...	...	...	...	...	...
1965	229.0*	84.4*	186.9*	60.7	67.4	103.8	139.1	195.1	294.0	448.5	643.8	1131.7	3549.8
1975	206.5*	70.0*	150.6*	47.9	61.6	86.7	119.3	164.0	223.2	351.8	512.7	1005.6	3797.6
1985	168.5*	56.0*	134.8*	39.2	57.1	75.4	108.9	142.5	210.7	309.5	459.1	675.5	2998.4
1990	**160.2***	**45.3***	**142.1***	**37.0**	**52.6**	**83.3**	**110.0**	**144.3**	**238.5**	**329.2**	**467.4**	**676.4**	**2729.5**
1995 projected	*153.5**	*37.5**	*148.0**	*32.5*	*52.8*	*84.5*	*112.8*	*152.8*	*255.0*	*345.7*	*473.9*	*636.0*	*2530.6*
All non-medical causes													
1955	...	...	...	...	...	...	...	...	...	...	...	...	...
1965	75.8*	54.7*	84.9*	74.6	75.4	72.8	81.2	82.8	96.6	111.2	137.5	179.4	264.1
1975	88.8*	57.6*	106.8*	84.0	93.1	101.9	112.5	101.1	115.0	140.4	161.4	234.2	294.6
1985	97.5*	59.5*	117.8*	98.1	114.2	119.7	113.1	113.0	127.1	139.6	171.8	243.9	403.1
1990	**96.6***	**61.7***	**119.1***	**95.0**	**118.0**	**120.1**	**129.3**	**112.3**	**122.3**	**136.6**	**167.6**	**199.4**	**314.7**
1995 projected	*95.2**	*62.6**	*120.3**	*97.6*	*117.8*	*126.8*	*134.0*	*114.8*	*119.0*	*132.0*	*151.2*	*158.7*	*250.6*

(*The rates for the age groups 0–34 and 35–69 are the means of seven five-yearly rates, but the all-ages rates are standardised to the conventional "European" age distribution)

BULGARIA: Females

	All ages	0–34	35–69	35–39	40–44	45–49	50–54	55–59	60–64	65–69	70–74	75–79	80+/NK
POPULATION (1000s)													
1955	3756.3	2222.8	1347.5	202.9	268.0	256.4	209.5	165.6	136.7	108.4	91.9	55.0	39.1
1965	4100.5	2197.7	1667.1	324.2	323.7	197.2	242.5	236.4	192.5	150.6	99.2	75.0	61.5
1975	4367.7	2194.4	1860.8	288.0	323.3	318.8	316.6	181.0	229.6	203.5	149.9	90.1	72.5
1985	4506.2	2102.9	2002.0	344.9	284.9	279.5	319.1	309.6	296.2	167.8	178.6	130.2	92.5
1990	**4555.4**	**2119.8**	**2046.5**	**322.4**	**330.5**	**274.7**	**269.8**	**297.4**	**286.2**	**265.5**	**137.0**	**135.7**	**116.4**
1995 projected	*4570.2*	*2049.9*	*2058.3*	*303.4*	*320.4*	*331.1*	*273.9*	*268.5*	*293.3*	*267.7*	*229.0*	*105.8*	*127.2*
NUMBER OF DEATHS													
All causes													
1955	32208	9331	10067	409	613	936	1157	1571	1968	3413	4061	3640	5109
1965	31825	3114	10549	449	601	588	1195	1725	2457	3534	4207	5526	8429
1975	41480	2691	12440	326	550	928	1444	1353	3016	4823	6608	7444	12297
1985	48140	1999	12642	393	493	777	1442	2316	3718	3503	7288	9820	16391
1990	**48828**	**1774**	**14234**	**398**	**616**	**809**	**1207**	**2174**	**3463**	**5567**	**5059**	**9357**	**18404**
1995 projected	*48214*	*1507*	*13972*	*408*	*637*	*1003*	*1220*	*1909*	*3503*	*5292*	*7823*	*6662*	*18250*
Lung cancer													
1955	...	...	...	...	...	...	...	...	...	...	...	...	...
1965	346	5	220	9	14	16	24	54	53	50	59	35	27
1975	358	7	225	6	6	28	33	39	57	56	47	49	30
1985	506	8	298	6	13	22	38	72	73	74	76	83	41
1990	**448**	**13**	**266**	**7**	**17**	**14**	**27**	**37**	**77**	**87**	**50**	**67**	**52**
1995 projected	*392*	*11*	*219*	*8*	*14*	*14*	*19*	*27*	*62*	*75*	*65*	*47*	*50*
ANNUAL DEATH RATE / 100,000 (*The rates for the age groups 0–34 and 35–69 are the means of seven five-yearly rates, but the all-ages rates are standardised to the conventional "European" age distribution)													
All causes													
1955	1094.4*	402.9*	983.5*	201.6	228.7	365.1	552.3	948.7	1439.6	3148.5	4418.9	6618.2	13066.5
1965	905.1*	143.6*	781.1*	138.5	185.7	298.2	492.8	729.7	1276.4	2346.6	4240.9	7368.0	13705.7
1975	978.2*	120.0*	780.2*	113.2	170.1	291.1	456.1	747.5	1313.6	2370.0	4408.3	8261.9	16961.4
1985	942.2*	99.0*	729.7*	113.9	173.0	278.0	451.9	748.1	1255.2	2087.6	4080.6	7542.2	17720.0
1990	**872.0***	**86.4***	**727.1***	**123.4**	**186.4**	**294.5**	**447.4**	**731.0**	**1210.0**	**2096.8**	**3692.7**	**6895.4**	**15811.0**
1995 projected	*812.0**	*75.9**	*709.1**	*134.5*	*198.8*	*302.9*	*445.4*	*711.0*	*1194.3*	*1976.8*	*3416.2*	*6296.8*	*14347.5*
All cancer													
1955	...	...	...	...	...	...	...	...	...	...	...	...	...
1965	122.8*	9.2*	185.1*	34.5	52.2	88.7	151.3	205.2	302.3	461.5	633.1	748.0	775.6
1975	112.2*	11.1*	177.6*	34.7	53.8	111.0	148.5	215.5	298.3	381.3	508.3	636.0	561.4
1985	121.4*	11.8*	191.2*	42.9	70.2	112.0	171.1	238.4	327.5	376.0	539.2	652.8	640.0
1990	**116.1***	**10.0***	**187.1***	**40.3**	**79.6**	**113.6**	**162.0**	**219.2**	**308.9**	**386.1**	**492.7**	**616.1**	**616.8**
1995 projected	*111.2**	*8.4**	*180.6**	*42.5*	*82.1*	*113.9*	*154.8*	*205.6*	*299.4*	*365.7*	*468.6*	*586.0*	*591.2*
Lung cancer													
1955	...	...	...	...	...	...	...	...	...	...	...	...	...
1965	9.5*	0.2*	15.5*	2.8	4.3	8.1	9.9	22.8	27.5	33.2	59.5	46.7	43.9
1975	8.3*	0.3*	13.9*	2.1	1.9	8.8	10.4	21.5	24.8	27.5	31.4	54.4	41.4
1985	9.8*	0.4*	16.9*	1.7	4.6	7.9	11.9	23.3	24.6	44.1	42.6	63.7	44.3
1990	**8.3***	**0.6***	**13.5***	**2.2**	**5.1**	**5.1**	**10.0**	**12.4**	**26.9**	**32.8**	**36.5**	**49.4**	**44.7**
1995 projected	*6.8**	*0.5**	*11.1**	*2.6*	*4.4*	*4.2*	*6.9*	*10.1*	*21.1*	*28.0*	*28.4*	*44.4*	*39.3*
Upper aerodigestive cancer (mouth, oesophagus, pharynx and larynx)													
1955	...	...	...	...	...	...	...	...	...	...	...	...	...
1965	2.4*	0.2*	3.3*	0.6	0.6	1.0	1.6	4.2	5.2	10.0	14.1	13.3	22.8
1975	2.3*	0.2*	3.4*	1.4	0.6	1.6	3.2	4.4	7.0	5.9	8.7	12.2	20.7
1985	1.9*	0.2*	2.2*	0.3	1.1	1.1	1.9	3.6	4.7	3.0	10.6	13.8	14.1
1990	**2.5***	**0.2***	**3.3***	**0.9**	**1.8**	**1.5**	**3.7**	**4.7**	**4.2**	**6.4**	**11.7**	**16.2**	**18.0**
1995 projected	*3.1**	*0.3**	*4.4**	*1.3*	*2.5*	*2.1*	*5.1*	*6.0*	*5.8*	*7.8*	*14.4*	*18.9*	*22.0*
Other cancer													
1955	...	...	...	...	...	...	...	...	...	...	...	...	...
1965	110.9*	8.8*	166.3*	31.2	47.3	79.6	139.8	178.1	269.6	418.3	559.5	688.0	708.9
1975	101.6*	10.6*	160.3*	31.3	51.3	100.7	134.9	189.5	266.6	347.9	468.3	569.4	499.3
1985	109.6*	11.2*	172.1*	40.9	64.6	103.0	157.3	211.6	298.1	329.0	486.0	575.3	581.6
1990	**105.4***	**9.1***	**170.3***	**37.2**	**72.6**	**107.0**	**148.3**	**202.1**	**277.8**	**346.9**	**444.5**	**550.5**	**554.1**
1995 projected	*101.3**	*7.6**	*165.1**	*38.6*	*75.2*	*107.5*	*142.8*	*189.6*	*272.4*	*329.8*	*425.8*	*522.7*	*529.9*
Chronic obstructive pulmonary disease (COPD)													
1955	...	...	...	...	...	...	...	...	...	...	...	...	...
1965	36.3*	0.1*	34.7*	2.2	3.1	5.6	21.0	33.0	64.4	113.5	205.6	342.7	559.3
1975	34.7*	0.3*	30.3*	1.7	4.0	5.0	14.8	26.5	55.3	104.7	188.8	341.8	584.8
1985	20.1*	0.2*	14.7*	0.6	1.8	0.7	8.8	12.9	28.4	50.1	106.4	179.0	413.0
1990	**13.7***	**0.1***	**12.3***	**1.2**	**1.2**	**3.3**	**8.2**	**11.1**	**23.1**	**38.0**	**60.6**	**125.3**	**250.9**
1995 projected	*10.1**	*0.0**	*9.8**	*1.3*	*1.6*	*3.6*	*8.0*	*9.3*	*18.1*	*26.5*	*42.4*	*87.9*	*177.7*
Other respiratory disease													
1955	...	...	...	...	...	...	...	...	...	...	...	...	...
1965	67.2*	40.7*	33.5*	5.6	5.3	10.1	12.8	30.0	53.5	117.5	219.8	448.0	873.2
1975	87.8*	33.3*	51.6*	4.5	8.0	15.4	24.6	43.6	88.4	176.9	357.6	694.8	1349.0
1985	46.8*	19.5*	25.9*	4.3	7.7	11.1	11.6	22.3	37.5	87.0	170.8	325.7	773.0
1990	**32.7***	**13.6***	**18.8***	**3.1**	**4.2**	**8.0**	**10.4**	**16.8**	**31.1**	**58.0**	**121.9**	**241.0**	**506.9**
1995 projected	*23.5**	*9.8**	*13.8**	*2.6*	*3.1*	*6.0*	*8.0*	*13.8*	*22.2*	*41.1*	*87.3*	*170.1*	*358.5*
Vascular disease													
1955	...	...	...	...	...	...	...	...	...	...	...	...	...
1965	483.1*	10.8*	375.9*	40.7	57.2	103.4	191.8	313.9	623.9	1300.1	2662.3	5012.0	8406.5
1975	550.5*	7.1*	389.7*	26.0	48.9	90.3	172.1	312.7	675.5	1402.0	2905.9	5730.3	10652.4
1985	594.0*	6.7*	385.9*	27.8	48.8	93.7	176.4	339.8	673.5	1341.5	2852.7	5732.0	12924.3
1990	**557.9***	**8.5***	**387.1***	**31.9**	**52.6**	**103.4**	**183.8**	**363.5**	**663.9**	**1310.7**	**2631.4**	**5294.0**	**11765.5**
1995 projected	*522.8**	*10.3**	*378.2**	*33.6*	*57.7*	*109.6*	*195.0*	*368.3*	*655.6*	*1227.5*	*2431.0*	*4885.6*	*10761.0*
Liver cirrhosis													
1955	...	...	...	...	...	...	...	...	...	...	...	...	...
1965	4.3*	0.9*	6.1*	0.9	1.9	2.5	5.8	5.9	6.2	19.3	24.2	29.3	17.9
1975	4.8*	0.5*	8.3*	1.4	2.8	4.4	5.7	10.5	14.4	18.7	16.7	32.2	17.9
1985	7.0*	0.3*	11.1*	2.3	2.1	3.6	7.5	14.5	20.6	26.8	30.2	43.8	49.7
1990	**6.6***	**0.5***	**11.8***	**0.9**	**2.7**	**4.0**	**8.9**	**11.8**	**20.3**	**33.9**	**29.2**	**34.6**	**27.5**
1995 projected	*6.4**	*0.6**	*12.2**	*1.0*	*2.5*	*4.8*	*8.4*	*11.2*	*21.5*	*35.9*	*27.9*	*27.4*	*19.7*
Other medical causes													
1955	...	...	...	...	...	...	...	...	...	...	...	...	...
1965	165.7*	66.5*	119.6*	39.5	50.4	68.5	84.1	116.3	191.2	287.5	427.4	694.7	2905.7
1975	159.2*	50.7*	92.8*	26.0	32.8	39.8	65.7	101.7	145.5	237.8	366.9	705.9	3611.0
1985	123.5*	41.0*	72.7*	16.5	23.2	32.9	48.9	86.2	131.7	169.2	305.7	513.8	2736.2
1990	**118.4***	**35.5***	**81.6***	**22.3**	**22.1**	**43.0**	**48.9**	**83.1**	**127.2**	**224.5**	**296.4**	**488.6**	**2537.8**
1995 projected	*113.7**	*30.1**	*87.0**	*25.7*	*26.5*	*46.5*	*50.7*	*80.4*	*142.2*	*237.2*	*300.4*	*469.8*	*2363.2*
All non-medical causes													
1955	...	...	...	...	...	...	...	...	...	...	...	...	...
1965	25.7*	15.3*	26.2*	15.1	15.8	19.3	26.0	25.4	34.8	47.1	68.5	93.3	167.5
1975	28.8*	17.0*	30.0*	18.8	19.8	25.1	24.6	37.0	36.1	48.6	64.0	121.0	184.8
1985	29.4*	19.5*	28.2*	19.4	19.3	24.0	27.6	33.9	36.1	36.9	75.6	95.2	183.8
1990	**26.7***	**18.3***	**28.4***	**23.6**	**23.9**	**19.3**	**25.2**	**25.6**	**35.6**	**45.6**	**60.6**	**95.8**	**105.7**
1995 projected	*24.3**	*16.5**	*27.5**	*27.7*	*25.3*	*18.4*	*20.4*	*22.3*	*35.5*	*43.0*	*58.5*	*69.9*	*76.3*

BULGARIA: 1975

Smoking–attributed deaths (Sm.) and total deaths (Total)

		ALL CAUSES	ALL CANCER	Lung cancer	Upper aero–digestive ca.	Other cancer	COPD	Other respiratory	Vascular disease	Liver cirrhosis	Other medical	Non–medical
Males												
0–34	Sm.	–	–	–	–	–	–	–	–	–	–	–
	Total	4379	242	14	8	220	9	931	219	14	1655	1309
35–69	Sm.	5513	1763	1257	172	334	860	301	1971	–	618	–
	Total	20148	4352	1389	291	2672	1196	1302	8598	363	2424	1913
		(27%)	(41%)	(90%)	(59%)	(13%)	(72%)	(23%)	(23%)		(25%)	
70+	Sm.	2899	688	509	52	127	886	139	983	–	203	–
	Total	23967	2514	605	120	1789	1541	1993	13998	118	3279	524
		(12%)	(27%)	(84%)	(43%)	(7%)	(57%)	(7%)	(7%)		(6%)	
Any age	Sm.	8412	2451	1766	224	461	1746	440	2954	–	821	–
	Total	48494	7108	2008	419	4681	2746	4226	22815	495	7358	3746
		(17%)	(34%)	(88%)	(53%)	(10%)	(64%)	(10%)	(13%)		(11%)	
Females												
0–34	Sm.	–	–	–	–	–	–	–	–	–	–	–
	Total	2691	240	7	4	229	7	759	152	10	1147	376
35–69	Sm.	505	106	84	8	14	102	29	207	–	61	–
	Total	12440	2949	225	57	2667	469	808	6036	135	1518	525
		(4%)	(4%)	(37%)	(14%)	(1%)	(22%)	(4%)	(3%)		(4%)	
70+	Sm.	455	40	33	2	5	196	20	161	–	38	–
	Total	26349	1742	126	39	1577	1015	2140	17242	67	3804	339
		(2%)	(2%)	(26%)	(5%)	(0%)	(19%)	(1%)	(1%)		(1%)	
Any age	Sm.	960	146	117	10	19	298	49	368	–	99	–
	Total	41480	4931	358	100	4473	1491	3707	23430	212	6469	1240
		(2%)	(3%)	(33%)	(10%)	(0%)	(20%)	(1%)	(2%)		(2%)	
Males+Females												
0–34	Sm.	–	–	–	–	–	–	–	–	–	–	–
	Total	7070	482	21	12	449	16	1690	371	24	2802	1685
35–69	Sm.	6018	1869	1341	180	348	962	330	2178	–	679	–
	Total	32588	7301	1614	348	5339	1665	2110	14634	498	3942	2438
		(18%)	(26%)	(83%)	(52%)	(7%)	(58%)	(16%)	(15%)		(17%)	
70+	Sm.	3354	728	542	54	132	1082	159	1144	–	241	–
	Total	50316	4256	731	159	3366	2556	4133	31240	185	7083	863
		(7%)	(17%)	(74%)	(34%)	(4%)	(42%)	(4%)	(4%)		(3%)	
Any age	Sm.	9372	2597	1883	234	480	2044	489	3322	–	920	–
	Total	89974	12039	2366	519	9154	4237	7933	46245	707	13827	4986
		(10%)	(22%)	(80%)	(45%)	(5%)	(48%)	(6%)	(7%)		(7%)	

BULGARIA: 1985

Smoking–attributed deaths (Sm.) and total deaths (Total)

		ALL CAUSES	ALL CANCER	Lung cancer	Upper aero–digestive ca.	Other cancer	COPD	Other respiratory	Vascular disease	Liver cirrhosis	Other medical	Non–medical
Males												
0–34	Sm.	–	–	–	–	–	–	–	–	–	–	–
	Total	3439	269	22	7	240	13	433	245	24	1168	1287
35–69	Sm.	7342	2386	1675	252	459	563	307	3369	–	717	–
	Total	24102	5162	1812	388	2962	744	1016	11738	898	2303	2241
		(30%)	(46%)	(92%)	(65%)	(15%)	(76%)	(30%)	(29%)		(31%)	
70+	Sm.	2714	701	520	55	126	610	83	1152	–	168	–
	Total	31804	3047	650	148	2249	1192	1558	21617	266	3345	779
		(9%)	(23%)	(80%)	(37%)	(6%)	(51%)	(5%)	(5%)		(5%)	
Any age	Sm.	10056	3087	2195	307	585	1173	390	4521	–	885	–
	Total	59345	8478	2484	543	5451	1949	3007	33600	1188	6816	4307
		(17%)	(36%)	(88%)	(57%)	(11%)	(60%)	(13%)	(13%)		(13%)	
Females												
0–34	Sm.	–	–	–	–	–	–	–	–	–	–	–
	Total	1999	250	8	5	237	3	385	143	6	811	401
35–69	Sm.	702	167	137	8	22	80	24	356	–	75	–
	Total	12642	3546	298	43	3205	245	431	6358	199	1312	551
		(6%)	(5%)	(46%)	(19%)	(1%)	(33%)	(6%)	(6%)		(6%)	
70+	Sm.	857	103	82	8	13	243	25	423	–	63	–
	Total	33499	2405	200	50	2155	805	1444	24513	157	3746	429
		(3%)	(4%)	(41%)	(16%)	(1%)	(30%)	(2%)	(2%)		(2%)	
Any age	Sm.	1559	270	219	16	35	323	49	779	–	138	–
	Total	48140	6201	506	98	5597	1053	2260	31014	362	5869	1381
		(3%)	(4%)	(43%)	(16%)	(1%)	(31%)	(2%)	(3%)		(2%)	
Males+Females												
0–34	Sm.	–	–	–	–	–	–	–	–	–	–	–
	Total	5438	519	30	12	477	16	818	388	30	1979	1688
35–69	Sm.	8044	2553	1812	260	481	643	331	3725	–	792	–
	Total	36744	8708	2110	431	6167	989	1447	18096	1097	3615	2792
		(22%)	(29%)	(86%)	(60%)	(8%)	(65%)	(23%)	(21%)		(22%)	
70+	Sm.	3571	804	602	63	139	853	108	1575	–	231	–
	Total	65303	5452	850	198	4404	1997	3002	46130	423	7091	1208
		(5%)	(15%)	(71%)	(32%)	(3%)	(43%)	(4%)	(3%)		(3%)	
Any age	Sm.	11615	3357	2414	323	620	1496	439	5300	–	1023	–
	Total	107485	14679	2990	641	11048	3002	5267	64614	1550	12685	5688
		(11%)	(23%)	(81%)	(50%)	(6%)	(50%)	(8%)	(8%)		(8%)	

(To be conservative, no deaths before age 35, and none from liver cirrhosis or non–medical causes, were attributed to smoking.)

BULGARIA: 1990

Smoking–attributed deaths (Sm.) and total deaths (Total)

Age		ALL CAUSES	ALL CANCER	Lung cancer	Upper aero-digestive ca.	Other cancer	COPD	Other respiratory	Vascular disease	Liver cirrhosis	Other medical	Non-medical
Males												
0–34	Sm.	–	–	–	–	–	–	–	–	–	–	–
	Total	3300	248	22	6	220	8	372	341	27	950	1354
35–69	Sm.	8205	2737	1860	363	514	462	282	3938	–	786	–
	Total	26966	5811	2010	552	3249	608	945	13815	942	2558	2287
		(30%)	(47%)	(93%)	(66%)	(16%)	(76%)	(30%)	(29%)		(31%)	
70+	Sm.	2176	601	436	53	112	396	60	972	–	147	–
	Total	29514	2839	551	152	2136	814	1198	20493	232	3307	631
		(7%)	(21%)	(79%)	(35%)	(5%)	(49%)	(5%)	(5%)		(4%)	
Any age	Sm.	10381	3338	2296	416	626	858	342	4910	–	933	–
	Total	59780	8898	2583	710	5605	1430	2515	34649	1201	6815	4272
		(17%)	(38%)	(89%)	(59%)	(11%)	(60%)	(14%)	(14%)		(14%)	
Females												
0–34	Sm.	–	–	–	–	–	–	–	–	–	–	–
	Total	1774	212	13	5	194	2	270	180	11	715	384
35–69	Sm.	494	109	89	6	14	54	13	263	–	55	–
	Total	14234	3703	266	66	3371	239	367	7518	230	1602	575
		(3%)	(3%)	(33%)	(9%)	(0%)	(23%)	(4%)	(3%)		(3%)	
70+	Sm.	408	58	46	5	7	99	8	210	–	33	–
	Total	32820	2229	169	59	2001	545	1084	24484	119	4023	336
		(1%)	(3%)	(27%)	(8%)	(0%)	(18%)	(1%)	(1%)		(1%)	
Any age	Sm.	902	167	135	11	21	153	21	473	–	88	–
	Total	48828	6144	448	130	5566	786	1721	32182	360	6340	1295
		(2%)	(3%)	(30%)	(8%)	(0%)	(19%)	(1%)	(1%)		(1%)	
Males+Females												
0–34	Sm.	–	–	–	–	–	–	–	–	–	–	–
	Total	5074	460	35	11	414	10	642	521	38	1665	1738
35–69	Sm.	8699	2846	1949	369	528	516	295	4201	–	841	–
	Total	41200	9514	2276	618	6620	847	1312	21333	1172	4160	2862
		(21%)	(30%)	(86%)	(60%)	(8%)	(61%)	(22%)	(20%)		(20%)	
70+	Sm.	2584	659	482	58	119	495	68	1182	–	180	–
	Total	62334	5068	720	211	4137	1359	2282	44977	351	7330	967
		(4%)	(13%)	(67%)	(27%)	(3%)	(36%)	(3%)	(3%)		(2%)	
Any age	Sm.	11283	3505	2431	427	647	1011	363	5383	–	1021	–
	Total	108608	15042	3031	840	11171	2216	4236	66831	1561	13155	5567
		(10%)	(23%)	(80%)	(51%)	(6%)	(46%)	(9%)	(8%)		(8%)	

BULGARIA: 1995

Smoking–attributed deaths (Sm.) and total deaths (Total)

Age		ALL CAUSES	ALL CANCER	Lung cancer	Upper aero-digestive ca.	Other cancer	COPD	Other respiratory	Vascular disease	Liver cirrhosis	Other medical	Non-medical
Males												
0–34	Sm.	–	–	–	–	–	–	–	–	–	–	–
	Total	3110	233	23	5	205	8	306	406	26	754	1377
35–69	Sm.	9012	3084	2010	507	567	346	261	4462	–	859	–
	Total	28562	6320	2163	750	3407	450	842	14903	975	2715	2357
		(32%)	(49%)	(93%)	(68%)	(17%)	(77%)	(31%)	(30%)		(32%)	
70+	Sm.	2418	732	521	71	140	316	56	1142	–	172	–
	Total	31192	3393	653	194	2546	647	1023	21676	267	3571	615
		(8%)	(22%)	(80%)	(37%)	(5%)	(49%)	(5%)	(5%)		(5%)	
Any age	Sm.	11430	3816	2531	578	707	662	317	5604	–	1031	–
	Total	62864	9946	2839	949	6158	1105	2171	36985	1268	7040	4349
		(18%)	(38%)	(89%)	(61%)	(11%)	(60%)	(15%)	(15%)		(15%)	
Females												
0–34	Sm.	–	–	–	–	–	–	–	–	–	–	–
	Total	1507	175	11	6	158	1	186	210	12	583	340
35–69	Sm.	235	50	41	4	5	23	4	130	–	28	–
	Total	13972	3602	219	87	3296	192	272	7382	239	1724	561
		(2%)	(1%)	(19%)	(5%)	(0%)	(12%)	(1%)	(2%)		(2%)	
70+	Sm.	191	27	22	3	2	42	3	101	–	18	–
	Total	32735	2445	162	81	2202	416	836	24424	118	4191	305
		(1%)	(1%)	(14%)	(4%)	(0%)	(10%)	(0%)	(0%)		(0%)	
Any age	Sm.	426	77	63	7	7	65	7	231	–	46	–
	Total	48214	6222	392	174	5656	609	1294	32016	369	6498	1206
		(1%)	(1%)	(16%)	(4%)	(0%)	(11%)	(1%)	(1%)		(1%)	
Males+Females												
0–34	Sm.	–	–	–	–	–	–	–	–	–	–	–
	Total	4617	408	34	11	363	9	492	616	38	1337	1717
35–69	Sm.	9247	3134	2051	511	572	369	265	4592	–	887	–
	Total	42534	9922	2382	837	6703	642	1114	22285	1214	4439	2918
		(22%)	(32%)	(86%)	(61%)	(9%)	(57%)	(24%)	(21%)		(20%)	
70+	Sm.	2609	759	543	74	142	358	59	1243	–	190	–
	Total	63927	5838	815	275	4748	1063	1859	46100	385	7762	920
		(4%)	(13%)	(67%)	(27%)	(3%)	(34%)	(3%)	(3%)		(2%)	
Any age	Sm.	11856	3893	2594	585	714	727	324	5835	–	1077	–
	Total	111078	16168	3231	1123	11814	1714	3465	69001	1637	13538	5555
		(11%)	(24%)	(80%)	(52%)	(6%)	(42%)	(9%)	(8%)		(8%)	

(To be conservative, no deaths before age 35, and none from liver cirrhosis or non–medical causes, were attributed to smoking.)

CANADA: 1990

		No. of deaths			Standardised rates (Defined on p.304)			Annual death rates / 100, 000						
		All ages	0–34	35–69	All ages	0–34	35–69	0–4	5–9	10–14	15–19	20–24	25–29	30–34
ALL CAUSES	M	103968	7700	38196	910.7	104.8	943.0	196.6	23.2	28.2	95.9	121.1	122.9	145.7
	F	88005	3723	21850	538.7	53.2	496.6	157.2	18.3	18.5	34.3	39.0	43.2	62.1
Tuberculosis	M	94	2	40	0.8	0.0	1.0	0.1	–	–	–	–	–	0.1
	F	70	1	17	0.4	0.0	0.4	–	–	–	–	–	–	0.1
Other infective	M	565	78	197	4.9	1.1	4.7	2.4	0.2	0.1	0.8	1.3	0.8	1.8
and parasitic	F	544	54	153	3.5	0.8	3.4	1.5	0.6	0.9	0.9	0.5	0.4	0.8
ALL CANCER	M	28866	467	13577	256.7	6.2	346.4	3.4	3.9	3.5	4.8	7.7	7.3	12.9
	F	23560	437	10748	162.4	5.8	243.9	3.4	2.7	3.5	3.4	3.4	7.4	16.6
Mouth and	M	687	9	455	6.2	0.1	11.3	–	–	0.1	–	0.5	0.2	0.1
pharynx cancer	F	273	7	130	1.9	0.1	3.0	–	–	–	–	0.1	0.3	0.3
Oesophagus cancer	M	736	2	412	6.6	0.0	10.6	–	–	–	–	–	–	0.2
	F	273	3	122	1.9	0.0	2.9	–	–	–	–	–	–	0.3
Stomach cancer	M	1305	5	600	11.6	0.1	15.2	–	–	–	–	–	0.1	0.3
	F	795	6	244	5.0	0.1	5.7	–	–	–	–	0.1	0.3	0.2
Colorectal cancer	M	2993	13	1379	26.7	0.2	34.9	–	–	–	0.2	–	0.2	0.8
	F	2792	12	1011	18.2	0.1	23.4	–	–	–	0.1	–	0.3	0.6
Liver cancer	M	247	9	154	2.2	0.1	3.9	–	–	0.1	0.1	0.1	0.2	0.3
	F	129	8	58	0.9	0.1	1.3	0.1	–	0.2	–	0.1	0.2	0.2
Pancreas cancer	M	1329	3	644	11.9	0.0	16.5	–	–	–	–	–	0.1	0.2
	F	1282	3	467	8.4	0.0	10.9	–	–	–	–	–	0.1	0.2
Larynx cancer	M	434	–	255	3.9	–	6.4	–	–	–	–	–	–	–
	F	79	–	49	0.6	–	1.2	–	–	–	–	–	–	–
Lung cancer	M	9536	12	5059	85.2	0.2	131.2	0.1	–	–	–	0.2	–	0.8
	F	4168	26	2292	30.3	0.3	53.1	0.1	0.1	–	–	–	0.3	1.8
Malignant melanoma	M	318	19	192	2.8	0.2	4.2	–	–	–	–	–	0.3	1.4
	F	179	13	95	1.3	0.2	2.0	–	–	–	–	0.2	0.2	0.8
Female breast cancer	F	4712	66	2690	34.1	0.8	59.1	–	–	–	–	0.1	0.8	4.6
Cervix cancer	F	443	31	251	3.2	0.4	5.1	–	–	–	–	0.6	0.6	1.5
Other uterine cancer	F	606	4	238	4.0	0.1	5.6	–	–	–	–	0.1	–	0.3
Ovarian cancer	F	1222	20	639	8.8	0.2	14.5	–	–	0.1	0.1	–	0.6	0.9
Prostate cancer	M	3212	–	705	28.5	–	19.5	–	–	–	–	–	–	–
Bladder cancer	M	821	2	257	7.3	0.0	6.7	–	–	–	–	–	–	0.2
	F	366	–	57	2.1	–	1.3	–	–	–	–	–	–	–
Other and ill–defined	M	4706	228	2329	41.5	3.1	58.0	2.2	2.0	1.4	2.9	4.1	3.6	5.2
cancer sites	F	4094	125	1624	27.4	1.7	37.1	1.7	1.2	2.1	1.5	0.7	1.6	3.3
Hodgkin's disease	M	98	19	49	0.8	0.2	1.1	–	–	0.1	–	0.5	0.7	0.4
	F	64	18	19	0.4	0.2	0.4	–	–	–	0.1	0.1	0.7	0.7
Myeloma and non–	M	1439	42	678	12.8	0.5	16.7	0.1	0.3	–	0.3	0.9	0.9	1.3
Hodgkin lymphomas	F	1271	26	467	8.5	0.3	10.8	0.4	0.1	–	0.2	0.3	0.6	0.8
Leukaemia	M	1005	104	409	8.7	1.4	10.2	1.0	1.6	1.8	1.3	1.4	1.2	1.9
	F	812	69	295	5.4	1.0	6.5	1.0	1.2	1.0	1.3	0.9	1.0	0.6
ALL VASCULAR	M	38825	276	12991	346.3	3.5	332.5	1.6	0.8	0.4	1.9	3.4	5.9	10.7
DISEASE	F	36266	172	5324	204.6	2.3	125.7	2.6	0.3	0.8	1.7	1.7	3.4	5.5
Rheumatic heart	M	171	4	76	1.5	0.0	1.9	–	–	–	–	–	0.3	0.1
disease and fever	F	366	4	134	2.4	0.0	3.1	–	–	–	–	–	0.3	–
Hypertensive disease	M	480	2	133	4.3	0.0	3.5	–	–	–	–	0.1	–	0.1
	F	744	2	79	4.1	0.0	1.9	0.1	–	–	–	–	–	0.1
Ischaemic heart	M	24500	86	9217	218.6	1.1	235.8	0.1	–	–	0.2	0.7	1.9	4.5
disease	F	19331	22	3109	110.5	0.3	74.3	–	–	0.1	0.4	0.2	0.1	1.2
Pulmonary embolism	M	470	7	191	4.2	0.1	4.9	–	–	–	–	–	0.2	0.4
and other venous	F	554	12	139	3.4	0.2	3.2	–	–	–	0.1	0.2	0.3	0.4
Cerebrovascular	M	6070	67	1424	54.1	0.9	36.2	0.1	0.5	0.2	0.3	1.1	1.3	2.5
disease	F	7951	69	997	44.0	0.9	22.9	0.5	0.2	0.2	0.3	0.9	1.6	2.4
Other vascular	M	7134	110	1950	63.6	1.4	50.2	1.4	0.3	0.2	1.4	1.6	2.3	3.0
disease	F	7320	63	866	40.2	0.9	20.4	2.0	0.1	0.4	0.8	0.4	1.0	1.4
Chronic obstructive	M	5035	27	1055	44.7	0.4	28.8	0.1	0.2	0.4	0.6	0.5	0.3	0.4
pulmonary disease	F	2690	32	631	16.4	0.4	15.2	0.2	–	0.3	0.6	0.6	0.6	0.8
Other respiratory	M	4317	86	794	38.7	1.2	20.3	3.4	0.6	0.4	0.5	0.8	0.8	1.7
disease	F	4231	70	437	23.0	1.0	10.0	3.3	0.6	0.3	0.4	0.3	0.8	1.3
Peptic ulcer	M	331	1	127	3.0	0.0	3.2	–	–	–	–	–	0.1	–
	F	312	3	54	1.8	0.0	1.2	0.1	–	–	–	–	0.1	0.1
Liver cirrhosis	M	1483	20	1067	13.3	0.2	25.9	–	–	–	–	0.1	0.5	1.1
	F	672	19	397	5.0	0.2	8.8	–	–	–	0.1	–	0.3	1.2
Renal disease	M	1069	14	248	9.6	0.2	6.4	0.3	0.1	0.1	0.1	0.1	0.2	0.4
	F	1153	22	193	6.6	0.3	4.5	0.5	0.1	0.2	0.3	0.1	0.7	0.2
Pregnancy and birth	F	10	8	2	0.1	0.1	0.0	–	–	–	–	0.2	0.2	0.3
Congenital and	M	1400	1296	71	11.6	19.2	1.5	125.9	1.7	0.9	2.3	1.6	1.2	1.1
perinatal causes	F	1122	1005	60	9.5	15.6	1.3	103.0	2.0	1.3	0.3	0.7	0.8	0.9
Ill–defined causes	M	2738	654	1111	23.2	9.1	25.0	28.4	0.6	1.1	6.4	8.6	7.7	10.7
	F	2176	347	499	13.7	5.0	10.9	21.6	0.9	0.6	2.1	2.0	3.9	4.3
Other medical causes	M	10180	715	3370	88.4	9.4	77.7	11.0	2.7	2.9	5.5	6.1	14.2	23.2
	F	11204	374	2037	65.2	5.2	46.1	9.5	3.1	2.7	2.3	5.5	5.4	8.0
ALL NON–	M	9065	4064	3548	69.5	54.3	69.6	20.0	12.2	18.3	73.0	91.0	83.8	81.7
MEDICAL CAUSES	F	3995	1179	1298	26.6	16.4	25.1	11.4	8.1	7.9	22.2	23.9	19.2	22.2
Motor vehicle	M	2543	1523	793	18.8	20.7	15.7	5.4	6.1	8.4	35.2	37.7	28.7	23.2
traffic accidents	F	1102	523	408	8.0	7.4	7.9	2.9	4.2	4.6	12.5	13.5	7.5	6.9
Fire	M	213	92	84	1.7	1.3	1.7	2.5	0.8	0.6	0.8	1.4	1.1	1.6
	F	124	52	46	0.9	0.8	0.9	1.7	0.7	0.4	0.6	0.8	0.7	0.4
Suicide	M	2673	1210	1233	20.0	15.8	23.3	–	–	2.5	19.1	29.7	29.1	30.1
	F	706	255	391	5.1	3.4	7.0	–	0.1	0.7	4.7	5.2	5.3	7.6
Homicide	M	355	197	143	2.6	2.6	2.6	1.6	0.5	0.4	2.9	4.0	4.6	4.1
	F	199	116	69	1.4	1.6	1.2	1.2	0.8	0.3	1.9	1.6	2.4	2.8
POPULATION (thousands):	M=males				13097	7184	5114	959	949	933	954	1017	1190	1182
	F=females				13483	6991	5281	916	903	895	907	981	1191	1198

CANADA: 1990

Annual death rates / 100, 000

9th ICD categories

35–39	40–44	45–49	50–54	55–59	60–64	65–69	70–74	75–79	80+/NK			
175.8	225.9	357.3	592.3	989.8	1664.0	2595.9	4117.3	6407.5	13234.3	M	ALL CAUSES	001–999
83.9	124.3	208.0	339.6	539.7	838.1	1342.7	2152.5	3565.9	9711.9	F		
0.4	–	0.6	–	1.7	1.3	2.9	3.2	6.5	11.6	M	Tuberculosis	010–018, 137
–	0.1	–	0.2	1.1	0.3	1.1	3.2	3.7	6.0	F		
1.3	1.7	2.3	3.3	4.7	7.6	12.0	21.5	29.4	67.5	M	Other infective	Rest of 001–139
1.0	1.1	1.2	3.1	3.6	5.9	7.9	11.8	18.4	53.0	F	and parasitic	
24.3	45.2	107.5	210.3	384.0	663.1	990.5	1400.6	1812.6	2623.2	M	ALL CANCER	140–208
33.1	61.5	113.2	192.1	300.1	420.0	587.3	764.3	952.7	1356.1	F		
0.9	2.3	3.7	7.9	15.2	23.6	25.4	22.4	26.1	38.7	M	Mouth and	140–149
0.5	0.5	1.3	2.3	3.6	7.0	5.5	7.7	12.2	14.2	F	pharynx cancer	
0.3	1.2	3.1	7.4	11.3	20.3	30.5	34.8	45.3	43.3	M	Oesophagus cancer	150
–	0.4	0.4	1.9	3.4	6.2	7.9	9.0	10.2	17.3	F		
1.2	2.3	5.2	9.9	15.7	28.8	43.5	62.8	84.5	130.4	M	Stomach cancer	151
0.7	0.7	2.2	3.3	6.6	9.2	16.9	26.0	41.0	68.7	F		
2.5	5.2	12.4	22.3	41.4	64.1	96.5	147.4	195.2	290.2	M	Colorectal cancer	153, 154
1.5	4.5	8.8	16.1	27.7	43.7	61.4	88.4	130.4	220.9	F		
0.6	0.4	1.4	1.6	6.0	4.9	12.4	10.9	11.8	8.4	M	Liver cancer	155.0
0.3	0.1	0.9	0.9	1.0	2.5	3.5	3.8	6.8	5.3	F		
0.4	2.2	5.4	10.4	18.7	29.4	49.4	68.7	79.2	118.8	M	Pancreas cancer	157
0.5	1.9	3.8	5.0	12.3	18.7	34.2	53.8	58.9	88.2	F		
0.2	0.6	2.2	4.4	8.8	15.3	13.5	18.3	22.5	28.9	M	Larynx cancer	161
–	–	0.3	0.8	1.5	2.7	3.0	2.7	3.1	1.7	F		
3.6	10.2	34.0	75.6	148.0	262.7	384.4	514.4	579.8	605.5	M	Lung cancer	162
2.6	9.4	20.7	42.4	65.1	97.4	134.1	160.1	161.0	138.0	F		
2.4	1.9	2.6	5.3	4.2	7.4	5.7	11.2	11.0	19.6	M	Malignant melanoma	172
1.1	1.2	1.2	3.0	2.5	1.8	3.0	4.5	5.7	7.5	F		
13.7	22.5	37.4	51.5	75.7	97.9	114.9	125.3	151.4	208.9	F	Female breast cancer	174
2.9	3.4	4.1	4.8	6.6	5.5	8.6	10.4	10.8	18.5	F	Cervix cancer	180
0.4	1.0	1.2	3.4	6.2	9.4	17.5	21.3	27.2	41.9	F	Other uterine cancer	179, 182
1.4	3.4	7.1	14.2	18.0	24.9	32.6	37.1	49.0	54.4	F	Ovarian cancer	183
0.2	0.1	1.2	4.4	11.8	37.3	81.4	164.5	277.3	591.5	M	Prostate cancer	185
0.4	0.6	1.4	2.5	7.3	13.3	21.4	34.8	67.4	129.9	M	Bladder cancer	188
–	0.2	0.3	0.8	1.3	3.2	3.7	12.7	20.1	43.8	F		
7.1	11.7	24.0	38.8	62.1	106.4	155.6	204.0	256.0	386.6	M	Other and ill-defined	Rest of 140–208
5.2	8.3	13.6	28.3	48.0	59.6	97.1	126.4	169.5	286.0	F	cancer sites	
0.6	0.8	0.1	0.8	0.8	2.3	2.3	1.5	5.3	5.6	M	Hodgkin's disease	201
0.1	0.1	0.1	0.3	0.3	0.5	1.6	2.0	2.3	2.4	F		
2.4	3.1	7.7	12.3	20.7	30.3	40.2	66.0	88.2	129.9	M	Myeloma and non–	200, 202–203
0.8	1.2	5.7	7.8	13.4	19.2	27.4	50.4	62.0	80.9	F	Hodgkin lymphomas	
1.6	2.4	3.1	6.8	12.0	16.9	28.4	38.9	62.9	95.9	M	Leukaemia	204–208
1.4	2.7	4.3	5.2	6.9	10.7	14.3	22.4	31.4	57.3	F		
23.4	51.4	101.3	189.2	343.5	607.1	1011.4	1699.3	2772.6	6056.8	M	ALL VASCULAR	390–459
9.4	15.1	28.9	61.8	113.1	223.0	428.8	825.8	1625.1	5149.6	F	DISEASE	
0.4	0.2	0.5	1.1	1.8	4.7	4.6	9.7	11.0	14.4	M	Rheumatic heart	390–398
0.4	0.6	1.3	3.0	3.1	4.9	8.3	10.2	21.2	26.0	F	disease and fever	
0.1	0.5	0.5	1.3	3.8	7.2	10.9	17.1	40.0	88.0	M	Hypertensive disease	401–405
0.1	0.1	0.4	0.8	2.1	2.7	7.1	18.3	32.8	112.3	F		
13.4	35.1	75.1	139.3	250.5	434.5	702.5	1126.8	1748.1	3304.1	M	Ischaemic heart	410–414
2.1	5.2	15.0	31.4	68.2	137.5	261.0	497.9	929.3	2581.3	F	disease	
0.6	0.6	1.7	3.3	5.7	6.8	15.3	16.5	36.7	58.7	M	Pulmonary embolism	415.1, 451–453
0.5	0.8	0.9	2.2	2.3	6.4	9.4	16.1	31.4	53.2	F	and other venous	
4.5	6.8	11.1	17.9	34.4	63.7	115.2	236.4	450.0	1245.9	M	Cerebrovascular	430–438
3.6	5.7	7.8	14.5	18.2	38.8	71.3	157.0	324.6	1215.1	F	disease	
4.4	8.2	12.4	26.4	47.2	90.0	162.7	292.7	486.7	1345.6	M	Other vascular	Rest of 390–459
2.7	2.6	3.5	9.9	19.2	32.8	71.8	126.4	285.8	1161.6	F	disease	
0.8	0.9	2.6	7.9	19.5	52.2	117.7	241.5	466.3	927.8	M	Chronic obstructive	490–496
0.5	1.0	2.3	5.2	13.1	29.1	54.9	104.7	140.9	256.8	F	pulmonary disease	
2.3	4.0	4.6	12.1	18.2	36.4	64.1	131.5	287.5	1065.2	M	Other respiratory	Rest of 460–519
1.5	2.0	4.7	5.2	9.2	18.1	29.6	64.0	142.0	708.0	F	disease	
0.4	0.6	1.0	1.4	4.0	6.8	8.0	10.6	19.2	55.9	M	Peptic ulcer	531–533
0.2	0.3	0.4	0.3	1.1	2.7	3.7	8.1	18.1	37.3	F		
4.6	4.6	12.4	24.5	31.4	47.0	57.0	52.5	48.6	46.1	M	Liver cirrhosis	571
1.3	3.8	5.4	7.8	10.2	13.7	19.2	21.0	24.1	18.8	F		
0.7	0.5	1.5	2.8	5.8	12.4	21.2	39.2	69.8	234.3	M	Renal disease	580–590
0.5	0.4	1.6	2.2	3.8	6.7	16.8	24.2	48.1	159.2	F		
0.1	0.1	–	–	–	–	–	–	–	–	F	Pregnancy and birth	630–676
1.4	0.5	1.4	1.7	1.8	2.0	1.5	2.4	6.5	4.2	M	Congenital and	740–779
0.2	0.5	1.3	1.3	2.5	2.2	1.2	4.1	5.4	4.8	F	perinatal causes	
11.5	12.3	14.4	21.2	30.4	36.6	48.8	67.2	102.9	229.6	M	Ill-defined causes	780–799
4.0	4.1	6.1	8.1	11.1	14.9	27.9	39.1	60.0	227.7	F		
31.4	38.0	43.0	52.2	72.2	117.6	189.7	344.0	648.8	1555.2	M	Other medical causes	Rest of 001–799
10.0	10.4	21.9	27.8	47.0	75.3	130.6	236.6	458.7	1475.8	F		
73.2	66.1	64.4	65.5	72.7	74.0	71.1	103.8	136.8	356.8	M	ALL NON–	E800–E999
22.4	23.9	21.2	24.6	23.8	26.3	33.7	45.5	68.8	258.7	F	MEDICAL CAUSES	
16.8	14.4	13.1	14.1	14.5	20.0	16.6	23.3	28.6	36.3	M	Motor vehicle	E810–E819
6.4	7.7	7.2	7.4	7.7	9.0	10.1	12.0	17.5	13.5	F	traffic accidents	
1.6	1.6	0.9	1.6	1.8	2.0	2.5	1.8	4.9	8.8	M	Fire	E890–E899
0.9	0.8	0.1	0.9	1.1	1.2	1.2	1.1	2.0	3.4	F		
28.0	25.4	24.6	21.8	24.7	20.3	18.5	23.9	30.2	34.9	M	Suicide	E950–E959
9.5	8.4	7.5	7.4	6.2	4.5	5.8	6.1	3.7	4.8	F		
3.8	2.6	3.7	2.0	2.7	1.4	2.1	2.7	1.2	1.4	M	Homicide	E960–E969
1.4	2.1	1.4	1.1	1.1	0.3	1.1	1.8	1.1	0.5	F		
1083	988	776	636	600	555	476	339	245	215	M	POPULATION (thousands)	
1101	993	773	639	610	598	567	442	353	415	F		

CANADA: Males

	All ages	0–34	35–69	35–39	40–44	45–49	50–54	55–59	60–64	65–69	70–74	75–79	80+/NK
POPULATION (1000s)													
1955	7883	4850	2661	541	500	437	373	315	266	231	180	112	79
1965	9863	6150	3257	644	613	537	487	406	320	250	193	141	122
1975	11349	7077	3755	663	647	628	587	478	429	326	235	146	137
1985	12540	7262	4566	991	785	649	622	591	527	402	322	207	183
1990	13097	7184	5114	1083	988	776	636	600	555	476	339	245	215
1995 projected	13635	6952	5774	1206	1092	1007	791	625	555	498	398	263	250
NUMBER OF DEATHS													
All causes													
1955	74701	13983	28660	1177	1771	2506	3654	4769	6328	8455	9729	9337	12992
1965	87208	12138	34188	1448	2161	2986	4763	6118	7768	8944	10569	11523	18790
1975	96925	11195	40289	1485	2211	3476	5374	6906	9611	11226	12106	11298	22037
1985	100460	8213	38214	1541	1918	2549	4273	6710	9520	11703	14543	14098	25392
1990	103968	7700	38196	1903	2233	2772	3768	5934	9240	12346	13966	15692	28414
1995 projected	107132	7045	37353	2161	2362	3193	4101	5532	8276	11728	15073	16021	31640
Lung cancer													
1955	1621	8	1144	20	29	79	165	264	278	309	247	126	96
1965	3077	13	2055	18	78	136	290	406	538	589	489	327	193
1975	5485	18	3342	24	100	210	408	675	933	992	953	628	544
1985	8278	18	4607	42	92	187	492	993	1309	1492	1542	1096	1015
1990	9536	12	5059	39	101	264	481	887	1459	1828	1745	1420	1300
1995 projected	10837	8	5347	35	112	331	546	891	1444	1988	2161	1668	1653
ANNUAL DEATH RATE / 100,000 (*The rates for the age groups 0–34 and 35–69 are the means of seven five-yearly rates, but the all-ages rates are standardised to the conventional "European" age distribution)													
All causes													
1955	1289.6*	242.1*	1383.1*	217.7	354.5	574.0	979.4	1515.9	2381.6	3658.6	5393.0	8321.7	16424.8
1965	1236.1*	186.4*	1375.1*	224.8	352.4	555.8	978.6	1506.9	2426.7	3580.5	5484.7	8195.6	15389.0
1975	1195.4*	163.8*	1310.2*	224.1	341.9	553.7	916.3	1446.3	2242.4	3446.7	5155.9	7749.0	16120.7
1985	983.9*	110.6*	1048.2*	155.5	244.5	392.8	686.6	1135.7	1807.1	2914.8	4517.9	6810.6	13860.3
1990	910.7*	104.8*	943.0*	175.8	225.9	357.3	592.3	989.8	1664.0	2595.9	4117.3	6407.5	13234.3
1995 projected	848.2*	100.2*	851.7*	179.2	216.3	317.1	518.7	885.4	1491.4	2353.6	3791.9	6094.0	12681.4
All cancer													
1955	201.6*	10.9*	275.7*	30.2	48.6	99.2	190.8	328.0	505.5	727.4	1041.0	1375.2	1876.1
1965	212.0*	11.0*	293.0*	30.3	53.6	102.6	191.7	325.9	536.4	810.6	1117.8	1454.5	1931.2
1975	240.5*	9.4*	320.6*	27.5	57.1	116.1	214.3	371.7	583.1	874.7	1268.3	1677.0	2438.2
1985	253.2*	7.3*	341.4*	23.7	50.7	101.2	210.2	418.6	632.9	952.7	1366.9	1755.6	2578.1
1990	256.7*	6.2*	346.4*	24.3	45.2	107.5	210.3	384.0	663.1	990.5	1400.6	1812.6	2623.2
1995 projected	257.9*	5.3*	344.5*	21.7	42.8	104.1	198.3	376.0	661.9	1007.0	1427.7	1860.0	2680.2
Lung cancer													
1955	29.5*	0.2*	56.3*	3.7	5.8	18.1	44.2	83.9	104.6	133.7	136.9	112.3	121.4
1965	46.4*	0.3*	86.3*	2.8	12.7	25.3	59.6	100.0	168.1	235.8	253.8	232.6	158.1
1975	69.0*	0.3*	112.2*	3.6	15.5	33.5	69.6	141.4	217.7	304.6	405.9	430.7	398.0
1985	82.2*	0.2*	130.3*	4.2	11.7	28.8	79.1	168.1	248.5	371.6	479.0	529.5	554.0
1990	85.2*	0.2*	131.2*	3.6	10.2	34.0	75.6	148.0	262.7	384.4	514.4	579.8	605.5
1995 projected	87.9*	0.1*	131.0*	2.9	10.3	32.9	69.1	142.6	260.2	399.0	543.6	634.5	662.5
Upper aerodigestive cancer (mouth, oesophagus, pharynx and larynx)													
1955	14.7*	0.1*	17.5*	–	2.6	7.1	12.1	16.8	35.0	48.9	80.9	122.1	174.5
1965	14.1*	0.2*	19.1*	1.1	2.9	6.0	12.3	24.9	35.0	51.2	66.9	98.2	158.9
1975	15.9*	0.1*	24.7*	1.8	3.6	13.5	24.2	29.3	39.7	60.5	68.1	92.6	139.7
1985	16.6*	0.2*	27.4*	1.1	3.8	9.7	20.4	41.1	53.7	61.8	78.0	85.0	118.4
1990	16.7*	0.1*	28.3*	1.4	4.1	9.0	19.6	35.4	59.2	69.4	75.5	93.9	110.9
1995 projected	16.7*	0.1*	28.3*	1.4	3.8	8.4	17.3	34.4	60.9	71.8	79.0	92.4	111.4
Other cancer													
1955	157.4*	10.6*	201.9*	26.5	40.2	74.0	134.5	227.3	365.8	544.8	823.2	1140.8	1580.3
1965	151.5*	10.5*	187.6*	26.4	38.0	71.3	119.8	201.0	333.3	523.6	797.1	1123.8	1614.3
1975	155.6*	9.0*	183.7*	22.0	38.0	69.1	120.5	201.0	325.7	509.7	794.3	1153.6	1900.5
1985	154.4*	6.9*	183.8*	18.4	35.2	62.7	110.7	209.4	330.7	519.3	809.9	1141.1	1905.6
1990	154.8*	5.9*	186.9*	19.3	30.9	64.4	115.1	200.7	341.1	536.8	810.7	1138.8	1906.8
1995 projected	153.4*	5.1*	185.2*	17.4	28.7	62.8	111.9	198.9	340.8	536.2	805.0	1133.1	1906.2
Chronic obstructive pulmonary disease (COPD)													
1955	17.2*	2.0*	22.3*	1.3	3.8	7.3	14.2	24.8	43.7	61.0	71.0	100.7	199.7
1965	31.8*	1.4*	39.2*	2.0	4.4	7.1	24.2	38.4	80.6	117.7	184.7	248.9	344.0
1975	51.1*	1.7*	52.6*	2.9	4.5	9.2	22.5	52.8	98.9	177.5	287.5	462.3	719.8
1985	47.2*	0.5*	34.3*	1.0	2.0	3.7	10.9	24.7	55.4	142.0	283.9	471.0	890.3
1990	44.7*	0.4*	28.8*	0.8	0.9	2.6	7.9	19.5	52.2	117.7	241.5	466.3	927.8
1995 projected	42.7*	0.3*	24.0*	0.6	0.6	1.8	5.8	16.8	43.8	98.7	219.1	459.1	950.3
Other respiratory disease													
1955	50.9*	21.3*	27.6*	4.1	7.2	10.3	14.5	26.1	47.4	83.5	146.3	324.4	924.1
1965	45.8*	10.0*	25.8*	3.7	5.9	10.2	14.2	26.1	43.4	76.9	156.7	317.2	1003.3
1975	45.9*	4.5*	24.5*	3.5	3.9	9.1	16.0	25.3	39.9	74.0	155.5	356.7	1145.6
1985	39.7*	1.7*	21.0*	3.0	3.6	6.0	11.6	14.9	36.6	71.2	150.7	300.0	1050.2
1990	38.7*	1.2*	20.3*	2.3	4.0	4.6	12.1	18.2	36.4	64.1	131.5	287.5	1065.2
1995 projected	38.0*	0.9*	19.0*	2.2	3.3	4.4	12.8	18.9	34.6	56.6	120.0	292.1	1066.9
Vascular disease													
1955	686.9*	9.9*	751.1*	59.2	135.7	260.9	494.5	831.2	1342.5	2133.7	3296.0	5197.9	10513.3
1965	669.8*	7.3*	740.3*	56.8	145.4	264.7	503.4	822.7	1354.6	2034.4	3269.3	5069.0	10014.7
1975	593.9*	5.9*	634.7*	46.8	108.1	218.4	404.9	690.7	1141.6	1832.4	2754.7	4321.0	9782.7
1985	422.5*	4.0*	433.6*	30.7	68.5	136.4	270.0	447.7	778.7	1303.4	2061.5	3262.3	7003.3
1990	346.3*	3.5*	332.5*	23.4	51.4	101.3	189.2	343.5	607.1	1011.4	1699.3	2772.6	6056.8
1995 projected	283.2*	3.0*	253.6*	16.9	36.3	70.4	137.6	256.9	462.1	795.3	1386.9	2365.2	5209.2
Liver cirrhosis													
1955	8.9*	0.5*	16.2*	2.0	6.6	10.1	16.9	20.7	24.1	33.3	30.5	36.5	36.7
1965	11.7*	0.5*	21.6*	7.5	9.6	14.5	22.8	27.6	33.1	36.0	44.6	46.2	31.9
1975	22.4*	1.0*	44.4*	11.2	23.0	34.4	49.6	58.8	64.4	69.4	77.9	43.9	43.9
1985	14.6*	0.5*	28.4*	4.3	9.6	16.2	26.7	38.3	43.8	60.3	55.9	53.1	39.8
1990	13.3*	0.2*	25.9*	4.6	4.6	12.4	24.5	31.4	47.0	57.0	52.5	48.6	46.1
1995 projected	12.2*	0.2*	23.4*	3.2	3.1	9.4	20.2	29.1	43.8	54.8	48.3	51.4	46.9
Other medical causes													
1955	219.0*	118.2*	181.4*	43.8	63.9	87.5	135.9	186.6	284.9	467.3	636.9	1058.8	2326.2
1965	159.0*	74.6*	138.3*	30.3	36.2	61.1	104.0	146.1	232.7	357.5	565.1	859.9	1650.3
1975	133.3*	54.6*	117.4*	29.4	42.7	62.1	92.9	124.4	192.7	277.6	465.5	703.0	1567.7
1985	130.5*	37.9*	111.1*	26.4	37.1	52.1	82.0	113.2	172.6	294.6	471.6	815.9	1933.4
1990	141.4*	38.9*	119.5*	47.1	53.7	64.4	82.7	120.6	184.2	284.1	488.2	883.2	2158.4
1995 projected	151.9*	40.5*	126.9*	63.9	71.6	73.0	87.6	124.8	183.5	284.2	503.9	943.3	2388.0
All non-medical causes													
1955	105.2*	79.2*	108.8*	77.1	88.7	98.7	112.6	98.5	133.6	152.3	171.3	228.2	548.7
1965	106.1*	81.6*	117.0*	94.2	97.2	95.7	118.3	120.2	145.9	147.3	146.3	199.9	413.6
1975	108.4*	86.7*	115.9*	102.9	102.7	104.3	115.9	122.5	121.8	141.2	146.5	185.2	422.8
1985	76.3*	58.7*	78.3*	66.3	73.0	77.2	75.4	78.4	87.1	90.7	127.4	152.7	365.2
1990	69.5*	54.3*	69.6*	73.2	66.1	64.4	65.5	72.7	74.0	71.1	103.8	136.8	356.8
1995 projected	62.4*	49.9*	60.2*	70.7	58.6	54.0	56.3	62.9	61.8	57.0	86.0	122.9	339.9

CANADA: Females

	All ages	0–34	35–69	35–39	40–44	45–49	50–54	55–59	60–64	65–69	70–74	75–79	80+/NK
POPULATION (1000s)													
1955	7690	4733	2575	545	487	409	350	306	260	219	175	115	92
1965	9708	5931	3253	634	625	537	477	395	320	265	216	162	146
1975	11377	6845	3808	638	620	620	610	504	455	362	282	206	235
1985	12818	7058	4709	988	775	644	619	615	593	476	408	295	348
1990	**13483**	**6991**	**5281**	**1101**	**993**	**773**	**639**	**610**	**598**	**567**	**442**	**353**	**415**
1995 projected	*13922*	*6645*	*5886*	*1204*	*1101*	*1006*	*789*	*639*	*585*	*562*	*516*	*390*	*484*
NUMBER OF DEATHS													
All causes													
1955	53453	9366	16834	835	1146	1521	1935	2734	3645	5018	6609	7245	13399
1965	61731	7546	18602	840	1273	1764	2504	3016	3962	5243	7203	8872	19508
1975	70251	5664	21590	786	1222	2002	2758	3595	4945	6282	7850	9412	25735
1985	80863	3982	21802	807	1097	1540	2335	3652	5415	6956	9354	11392	34333
1990	**88005**	**3723**	**21850**	**924**	**1235**	**1608**	**2171**	**3293**	**5010**	**7609**	**9516**	**12602**	**40314**
1995 projected	*94172*	*3261*	*21098*	*960*	*1232*	*1856*	*2406*	*3141*	*4492*	*7011*	*10303*	*13310*	*46200*
Lung cancer													
1955	336	7	198	8	13	21	26	31	45	54	48	46	37
1965	515	11	332	18	20	38	57	57	71	71	67	56	49
1975	1248	11	845	12	41	84	139	164	213	192	148	99	145
1985	3164	14	1929	30	83	139	250	393	510	524	514	358	349
1990	**4168**	**26**	**2292**	**29**	**93**	**160**	**271**	**397**	**582**	**760**	**708**	**569**	**573**
1995 projected	*5428*	*25*	*2635*	*30*	*94*	*205*	*336*	*438*	*636*	*896*	*1027*	*838*	*903*
ANNUAL DEATH RATE / 100,000 (*The rates for the age groups 0–34 and 35–69 are the means of seven five-yearly rates, but the all-ages rates are standardised to the conventional "European" age distribution)													
All causes													
1955	923.3*	159.8*	842.9*	153.3	235.4	372.3	552.4	892.9	1404.6	2289.2	3783.1	6327.5	14532.5
1965	806.2*	113.0*	738.4*	132.6	203.6	328.2	524.6	763.7	1239.7	1976.3	3340.9	5473.2	13325.1
1975	683.3*	88.5*	661.8*	123.1	197.2	323.0	452.1	713.7	1086.3	1736.8	2782.7	4566.7	10941.8
1985	571.8*	57.3*	544.0*	81.7	141.6	239.2	377.5	594.2	913.2	1460.7	2290.4	3856.5	9880.0
1990	**538.7***	**53.2***	**496.6***	**83.9**	**124.3**	**208.0**	**339.6**	**539.7**	**838.1**	**1342.7**	**2152.5**	**3565.9**	**9711.9**
1995 projected	*510.1**	*49.5**	*455.4**	*79.7*	*111.9*	*184.4*	*304.9*	*491.5*	*768.1*	*1247.3*	*1997.9*	*3409.3*	*9539.5*
All cancer													
1955	167.5*	10.8*	247.8*	47.0	92.6	143.9	208.7	301.8	398.8	541.5	728.1	938.0	1365.5
1965	161.8*	9.1*	241.1*	47.0	84.5	142.2	214.7	285.4	386.4	527.3	687.4	918.0	1325.1
1975	155.2*	7.6*	234.7*	36.0	73.6	136.5	191.1	291.2	391.9	522.8	700.8	869.5	1219.4
1985	162.1*	6.7*	244.9*	30.5	67.5	118.0	202.4	305.7	413.0	577.5	736.0	932.0	1332.7
1990	**162.4***	**5.8***	**243.9***	**33.1**	**61.5**	**113.2**	**192.1**	**300.1**	**420.0**	**587.3**	**764.3**	**952.7**	**1356.1**
1995 projected	*161.9**	*5.2**	*240.4**	*31.2*	*58.5*	*105.4*	*183.4*	*291.5*	*418.1*	*594.6*	*776.2*	*977.5*	*1387.2*
Lung cancer													
1955	6.1*	0.2*	9.8*	1.5	2.7	5.1	7.4	10.1	17.3	24.6	27.5	40.2	40.1
1965	7.2*	0.2*	12.6*	2.8	3.2	7.1	11.9	14.4	22.2	26.8	31.1	34.5	33.5
1975	13.4*	0.2*	25.3*	1.9	6.6	13.6	22.8	32.6	46.8	53.1	52.5	48.0	61.6
1985	26.1*	0.2*	48.0*	3.0	10.7	21.6	40.4	63.9	86.0	110.0	125.9	121.2	100.4
1990	**30.3***	**0.3***	**53.1***	**2.6**	**9.4**	**20.7**	**42.4**	**65.1**	**97.4**	**134.1**	**160.1**	**161.0**	**138.0**
1995 projected	*35.3**	*0.3**	*58.7**	*2.5*	*8.5*	*20.4*	*42.6*	*68.5*	*108.8*	*159.4*	*199.1*	*214.7*	*186.5*
Upper aerodigestive cancer (mouth, oesophagus, pharynx and larynx)													
1955	3.8*	0.1*	4.2*	0.4	1.8	1.5	3.1	6.5	6.2	10.0	22.9	27.1	46.6
1965	4.0*	0.0*	4.7*	–	0.6	3.2	3.4	6.1	6.3	13.2	20.9	27.8	53.3
1975	4.3*	0.1*	5.5*	0.6	0.3	2.7	3.3	8.7	11.6	11.1	21.6	28.6	48.0
1985	4.4*	0.1*	6.3*	0.2	1.0	2.0	5.2	8.3	12.1	15.1	18.6	33.2	41.4
1990	**4.4***	**0.1***	**7.0***	**0.5**	**0.9**	**1.9**	**5.0**	**8.5**	**15.9**	**16.4**	**19.5**	**25.5**	**33.2**
1995 projected	*4.3**	*0.2**	*7.7**	*0.6*	*0.9*	*1.8*	*4.9*	*9.5*	*18.0*	*18.1*	*17.5*	*20.2*	*26.2*
Other cancer													
1955	157.5*	10.5*	233.7*	45.2	88.1	137.3	198.1	285.1	375.3	506.8	677.7	870.7	1278.7
1965	150.6*	8.9*	223.8*	44.2	80.6	131.9	199.5	264.9	357.9	487.4	635.4	855.6	1238.4
1975	137.5*	7.3*	203.9*	33.5	66.7	120.2	165.1	250.0	333.5	458.7	626.7	792.8	1109.7
1985	131.6*	6.5*	190.7*	27.2	55.7	94.4	156.8	233.5	314.8	452.3	591.6	777.6	1190.8
1990	**127.8***	**5.3***	**183.8***	**30.0**	**51.2**	**90.6**	**144.7**	**226.5**	**306.8**	**436.7**	**584.7**	**766.3**	**1184.8**
1995 projected	*122.3**	*4.8**	*174.0**	*28.2*	*49.1*	*83.3*	*135.9*	*213.4*	*291.4*	*417.0*	*559.6*	*742.6*	*1174.5*
Chronic obstructive pulmonary disease (COPD)													
1955	6.9*	1.4*	6.2*	0.9	1.0	2.7	5.4	5.6	8.9	18.7	25.2	35.8	121.5
1965	8.2*	0.9*	9.1*	1.4	1.9	5.6	5.7	11.4	15.6	22.2	44.1	42.6	110.0
1975	12.8*	1.3*	15.6*	1.6	3.6	6.0	10.0	19.1	28.8	40.1	67.0	84.4	139.0
1985	13.9*	0.4*	14.9*	0.6	1.8	3.7	6.3	16.1	24.6	51.4	78.6	121.9	188.8
1990	**16.4***	**0.4***	**15.2***	**0.5**	**1.0**	**2.3**	**5.2**	**13.1**	**29.1**	**54.9**	**104.7**	**140.9**	**256.8**
1995 projected	*19.4**	*0.4**	*16.5**	*0.3*	*0.7*	*1.7*	*4.1*	*13.0*	*30.1*	*65.5*	*121.8*	*177.0*	*328.9*
Other respiratory disease													
1955	38.5*	18.1*	17.4*	4.6	6.8	6.1	11.1	17.3	26.6	49.3	92.2	202.6	771.1
1965	30.1*	8.6*	14.0*	2.7	4.5	8.0	9.0	11.6	22.8	39.2	81.2	164.7	726.8
1975	25.9*	3.7*	13.8*	2.7	4.2	5.3	8.7	10.3	20.0	45.3	73.7	178.6	659.4
1985	22.8*	1.2*	10.9*	1.9	2.7	4.8	4.7	9.9	19.1	33.0	62.9	140.1	679.1
1990	**23.0***	**1.0***	**10.0***	**1.5**	**2.0**	**4.7**	**5.2**	**9.2**	**18.1**	**29.6**	**64.0**	**142.0**	**708.0**
1995 projected	*23.3**	*0.8**	*9.3**	*1.3*	*1.7*	*4.5*	*4.9*	*8.6*	*16.2*	*28.1*	*62.2*	*147.5*	*734.7*
Vascular disease													
1955	493.9*	6.4*	398.7*	28.5	56.1	118.5	198.4	386.7	705.2	1297.9	2338.3	4206.1	9901.3
1965	434.4*	4.6*	318.2*	24.9	42.2	80.6	166.6	287.2	569.5	1056.2	2026.0	3583.0	9486.3
1975	338.6*	3.5*	251.4*	18.0	38.3	73.9	121.8	239.4	440.5	827.8	1505.5	2784.1	7442.2
1985	243.0*	2.6*	161.5*	11.0	18.7	44.3	80.3	146.3	293.9	535.7	997.3	1962.1	5843.5
1990	**204.6***	**2.3***	**125.7***	**9.4**	**15.1**	**28.9**	**61.8**	**113.1**	**223.0**	**428.8**	**825.8**	**1625.1**	**5149.6**
1995 projected	*170.5**	*2.0**	*97.1**	*7.6*	*10.7*	*21.0*	*45.7*	*84.7*	*171.2*	*338.7*	*663.6*	*1353.0*	*4469.8*
Liver cirrhosis													
1955	4.4*	0.3*	7.2*	1.8	3.1	7.1	7.7	9.8	11.6	9.6	15.5	18.3	24.9
1965	5.8*	0.8*	10.5*	3.0	5.6	7.8	10.7	12.9	16.6	16.6	16.2	19.7	17.1
1975	9.2*	0.7*	18.5*	5.2	8.9	16.5	19.5	20.8	30.5	27.9	21.6	22.3	16.2
1985	6.1*	0.3*	11.1*	1.7	4.0	7.5	11.8	14.0	20.2	18.7	23.0	24.0	19.9
1990	**5.0***	**0.2***	**8.8***	**1.3**	**3.8**	**5.4**	**7.8**	**10.2**	**13.7**	**19.2**	**21.0**	**24.1**	**18.8**
1995 projected	*4.1**	*0.2**	*6.8**	*1.2*	*3.0*	*4.0*	*5.4*	*7.0*	*10.9*	*16.4*	*20.0*	*24.1*	*18.4*
Other medical causes													
1955	171.8*	100.0*	134.7*	51.6	52.8	69.5	92.5	137.5	213.1	326.2	502.0	783.4	1811.3
1965	123.3*	62.6*	105.7*	29.5	36.5	49.1	72.9	107.9	180.9	263.1	421.6	609.5	1254.8
1975	97.1*	43.0*	81.9*	22.1	26.6	43.1	57.7	80.4	128.1	215.6	336.8	523.5	1138.6
1985	94.1*	28.2*	70.7*	13.7	23.2	31.8	42.7	69.6	112.0	201.8	339.1	593.1	1556.8
1990	**100.7***	**27.1***	**67.9***	**15.9**	**17.0**	**32.3**	**43.0**	**70.3**	**107.9**	**189.2**	**327.1**	**612.3**	**1963.9**
1995 projected	*107.4**	*25.8**	*64.2**	*15.0*	*16.0*	*30.1*	*42.8*	*67.9*	*101.2*	*176.7*	*317.4*	*672.4*	*2353.3*
All non-medical causes													
1955	40.3*	22.8*	30.8*	18.9	23.0	24.5	28.5	34.3	40.5	46.1	81.9	143.2	536.9
1965	42.6*	26.2*	39.9*	24.0	28.5	35.0	45.0	47.4	47.9	51.6	64.5	135.7	405.1
1975	44.6*	28.6*	45.9*	37.6	42.1	41.8	43.3	52.4	46.6	57.2	77.3	104.3	327.0
1985	29.8*	17.8*	30.0*	22.3	23.6	29.0	29.3	32.5	30.4	42.6	53.4	83.3	259.3
1990	**26.6***	**16.4***	**25.1***	**22.4**	**23.9**	**21.2**	**24.6**	**23.8**	**26.3**	**33.7**	**45.5**	**68.8**	**258.7**
1995 projected	*23.6**	*15.1**	*21.0**	*23.1*	*21.3*	*17.8*	*18.5*	*18.8*	*20.3*	*27.4*	*36.6*	*57.9*	*247.4*

CANADA: 1975

Smoking–attributed deaths (Sm.) and total deaths (Total)

		ALL CAUSES	ALL CANCER	Lung cancer	Upper aero–digestive ca.	Other cancer	COPD	Other respiratory	Vascular disease	Liver cirrhosis	Other medical	Non–medical
Males												
0–34	Sm.	–	–	–	–	–	–	–	–	–	–	–
	Total	11195	641	18	7	616	110	290	381	60	3517	6196
35–69	Sm.	12243	4425	3087	494	844	1147	209	5359	–	1103	–
	Total	40289	9660	3342	769	5549	1492	732	18914	1513	3730	4248
		(30%)	(46%)	(92%)	(64%)	(15%)	(77%)	(29%)	(28%)		(30%)	
70+	Sm.	8076	2883	1909	273	701	1640	245	2841	–	467	–
	Total	45441	8756	2125	486	6145	2333	2451	26141	307	4261	1192
		(18%)	(33%)	(90%)	(56%)	(11%)	(70%)	(10%)	(11%)		(11%)	
Any age	Sm.	20319	7308	4996	767	1545	2787	454	8200	–	1570	–
	Total	96925	19057	5485	1262	12310	3935	3473	45436	1880	11508	11636
		(21%)	(38%)	(91%)	(61%)	(13%)	(71%)	(13%)	(18%)		(14%)	
Females												
0–34	Sm.	–	–	–	–	–	–	–	–	–	–	–
	Total	5664	485	11	5	469	84	231	220	46	2644	1954
35–69	Sm.	2201	716	550	58	108	255	48	866	–	316	–
	Total	21590	7840	845	180	6815	502	436	7758	654	2693	1707
		(10%)	(9%)	(65%)	(32%)	(2%)	(51%)	(11%)	(11%)		(12%)	
70+	Sm.	744	188	135	26	27	150	21	323	–	62	–
	Total	42997	6637	392	233	6012	690	2127	27489	145	4707	1202
		(2%)	(3%)	(34%)	(11%)	(0%)	(22%)	(1%)	(1%)		(1%)	
Any age	Sm.	2945	904	685	84	135	405	69	1189	–	378	–
	Total	70251	14962	1248	418	13296	1276	2794	35467	845	10044	4863
		(4%)	(6%)	(55%)	(20%)	(1%)	(32%)	(2%)	(3%)		(4%)	
Males+Females												
0–34	Sm.	–	–	–	–	–	–	–	–	–	–	–
	Total	16859	1126	29	12	1085	194	521	601	106	6161	8150
35–69	Sm.	14444	5141	3637	552	952	1402	257	6225	–	1419	–
	Total	61879	17500	4187	949	12364	1994	1168	26672	2167	6423	5955
		(23%)	(29%)	(87%)	(58%)	(8%)	(70%)	(22%)	(23%)		(22%)	
70+	Sm.	8820	3071	2044	299	728	1790	266	3164	–	529	–
	Total	88438	15393	2517	719	12157	3023	4578	53630	452	8968	2394
		(10%)	(20%)	(81%)	(42%)	(6%)	(59%)	(6%)	(6%)		(6%)	
Any age	Sm.	23264	8212	5681	851	1680	3192	523	9389	–	1948	–
	Total	167176	34019	6733	1680	25606	5211	6267	80903	2725	21552	16499
		(14%)	(24%)	(84%)	(51%)	(7%)	(61%)	(8%)	(12%)		(9%)	

CANADA: 1985

Smoking–attributed deaths (Sm.) and total deaths (Total)

		ALL CAUSES	ALL CANCER	Lung cancer	Upper aero–digestive ca.	Other cancer	COPD	Other respiratory	Vascular disease	Liver cirrhosis	Other medical	Non–medical
Males												
0–34	Sm.	–	–	–	–	–	–	–	–	–	–	–
	Total	8213	547	18	13	516	37	121	306	34	2645	4523
35–69	Sm.	13355	6125	4301	679	1145	897	224	4773	–	1336	–
	Total	38214	12230	4607	1005	6618	1126	736	15386	1088	4162	3486
		(35%)	(50%)	(93%)	(68%)	(17%)	(80%)	(30%)	(31%)		(32%)	
70+	Sm.	12172	4899	3344	396	1159	2619	368	3424	–	862	–
	Total	54033	12757	3653	644	8460	3520	3030	26219	363	6749	1395
		(23%)	(38%)	(92%)	(61%)	(14%)	(74%)	(12%)	(13%)		(13%)	
Any age	Sm.	25527	11024	7645	1075	2304	3516	592	8197	–	2198	–
	Total	100460	25534	8278	1662	15594	4683	3887	41911	1485	13556	9404
		(25%)	(43%)	(92%)	(65%)	(15%)	(75%)	(15%)	(20%)		(16%)	
Females												
0–34	Sm.	–	–	–	–	–	–	–	–	–	–	–
	Total	3982	495	14	7	474	31	83	195	22	1862	1294
35–69	Sm.	4554	1977	1565	132	280	402	99	1416	–	660	–
	Total	21802	9914	1929	250	7735	573	431	6229	464	2837	1354
		(21%)	(20%)	(81%)	(53%)	(4%)	(70%)	(23%)	(23%)		(23%)	
70+	Sm.	4502	1250	908	132	210	815	162	1756	–	519	–
	Total	55079	10390	1221	318	8851	1337	3031	30175	234	8547	1365
		(8%)	(12%)	(74%)	(42%)	(2%)	(61%)	(5%)	(6%)		(6%)	
Any age	Sm.	9056	3227	2473	264	490	1217	261	3172	–	1179	–
	Total	80863	20799	3164	575	17060	1941	3545	36599	720	13246	4013
		(11%)	(16%)	(78%)	(46%)	(3%)	(63%)	(7%)	(9%)		(9%)	
Males+Females												
0–34	Sm.	–	–	–	–	–	–	–	–	–	–	–
	Total	12195	1042	32	20	990	68	204	501	56	4507	5817
35–69	Sm.	17909	8102	5866	811	1425	1299	323	6189	–	1996	–
	Total	60016	22144	6536	1255	14353	1699	1167	21615	1552	6999	4840
		(30%)	(37%)	(90%)	(65%)	(10%)	(76%)	(28%)	(29%)		(29%)	
70+	Sm.	16674	6149	4252	528	1369	3434	530	5180	–	1381	–
	Total	109112	23147	4874	962	17311	4857	6061	56394	597	15296	2760
		(15%)	(27%)	(87%)	(55%)	(8%)	(71%)	(9%)	(9%)		(9%)	
Any age	Sm.	34583	14251	10118	1339	2794	4733	853	11369	–	3377	–
	Total	181323	46333	11442	2237	32654	6624	7432	78510	2205	26802	13417
		(19%)	(31%)	(88%)	(60%)	(9%)	(71%)	(11%)	(14%)		(13%)	

(To be conservative, no deaths before age 35, and none from liver cirrhosis or non–medical causes, were attributed to smoking.)

CANADA: 1990

Smoking–attributed deaths (Sm.) and total deaths (Total)

	Age		ALL CAUSES	ALL CANCER	Lung cancer	Upper aero–digestive ca.	Other cancer	COPD	Other respiratory	Vascular disease	Liver cirrhosis	Other medical	Non–medical
Males	0–34	Sm.	–	–	–	–	–	–	–	–	–	–	–
		Total	7700	467	12	11	444	27	86	276	20	2760	4064
	35–69	Sm.	13469	6758	4723	756	1279	844	243	3975	–	1649	–
		Total	38196	13577	5059	1122	7396	1055	794	12991	1067	5164	3548
			(35%)	(50%)	(93%)	(67%)	(17%)	(80%)	(31%)	(31%)		(32%)	
	70+	Sm.	14113	5996	4115	459	1422	3004	441	3530	–	1142	–
		Total	58072	14822	4465	724	9633	3953	3437	25558	396	8453	1453
			(24%)	(40%)	(92%)	(63%)	(15%)	(76%)	(13%)	(14%)		(14%)	
	Any age	Sm.	27582	12754	8838	1215	2701	3848	684	7505	–	2791	–
		Total	103968	28866	9536	1857	17473	5035	4317	38825	1483	16377	9065
			(27%)	(44%)	(93%)	(65%)	(15%)	(76%)	(16%)	(19%)		(17%)	
Females	0–34	Sm.	–	–	–	–	–	–	–	–	–	–	–
		Total	3723	437	26	10	401	32	70	172	19	1814	1179
	35–69	Sm.	5042	2385	1894	168	323	461	109	1329	–	758	–
		Total	21850	10748	2292	301	8155	631	437	5324	397	3015	1298
			(23%)	(22%)	(83%)	(56%)	(4%)	(73%)	(25%)	(25%)		(25%)	
	70+	Sm.	7031	1983	1485	159	339	1403	277	2432	–	936	–
		Total	62432	12375	1850	314	10211	2027	3724	30770	256	11762	1518
			(11%)	(16%)	(80%)	(51%)	(3%)	(69%)	(7%)	(8%)		(8%)	
	Any age	Sm.	12073	4368	3379	327	662	1864	386	3761	–	1694	–
		Total	88005	23560	4168	625	18767	2690	4231	36266	672	16591	3995
			(14%)	(19%)	(81%)	(52%)	(4%)	(69%)	(9%)	(10%)		(10%)	
Males+Females	0–34	Sm.	–	–	–	–	–	–	–	–	–	–	–
		Total	11423	904	38	21	845	59	156	448	39	4574	5243
	35–69	Sm.	18511	9143	6617	924	1602	1305	352	5304	–	2407	–
		Total	60046	24325	7351	1423	15551	1686	1231	18315	1464	8179	4846
			(31%)	(38%)	(90%)	(65%)	(10%)	(77%)	(29%)	(29%)		(29%)	
	70+	Sm.	21144	7979	5600	618	1761	4407	718	5962	–	2078	–
		Total	120504	27197	6315	1038	19844	5980	7161	56328	652	20215	2971
			(18%)	(29%)	(89%)	(60%)	(9%)	(74%)	(10%)	(11%)		(10%)	
	Any age	Sm.	39655	17122	12217	1542	3363	5712	1070	11266	–	4485	–
		Total	191973	52426	13704	2482	36240	7725	8548	75091	2155	32968	13060
			(21%)	(33%)	(89%)	(62%)	(9%)	(74%)	(13%)	(15%)		(14%)	

CANADA: 1995

Smoking–attributed deaths (Sm.) and total deaths (Total)

	Age		ALL CAUSES	ALL CANCER	Lung cancer	Upper aero–digestive ca.	Other cancer	COPD	Other respiratory	Vascular disease	Liver cirrhosis	Other medical	Non–medical
Males	0–34	Sm.	–	–	–	–	–	–	–	–	–	–	–
		Total	7045	391	8	8	375	23	64	224	17	2760	3566
	35–69	Sm.	13260	7125	4987	800	1338	734	243	3193	–	1965	–
		Total	37353	14385	5347	1192	7846	918	800	10529	1025	6194	3502
			(35%)	(50%)	(93%)	(67%)	(17%)	(80%)	(30%)	(30%)		(32%)	
	70+	Sm.	16524	7365	5084	546	1735	3451	538	3658	–	1512	–
		Total	62734	17252	5482	835	10935	4449	3907	24728	444	10441	1513
			(26%)	(43%)	(93%)	(65%)	(16%)	(78%)	(14%)	(15%)		(14%)	
	Any age	Sm.	29784	14490	10071	1346	3073	4185	781	6851	–	3477	–
		Total	107132	32028	10837	2035	19156	5390	4771	35481	1486	19395	8581
			(28%)	(45%)	(93%)	(66%)	(16%)	(78%)	(16%)	(19%)		(18%)	
Females	0–34	Sm.	–	–	–	–	–	–	–	–	–	–	–
		Total	3261	380	25	12	343	31	54	138	17	1615	1026
	35–69	Sm.	5386	2772	2217	200	355	521	116	1159	–	818	–
		Total	21098	11178	2635	342	8201	688	427	4228	331	3016	1230
			(26%)	(25%)	(84%)	(58%)	(4%)	(76%)	(27%)	(27%)		(27%)	
	70+	Sm.	10548	3044	2349	174	521	2207	448	3209	–	1640	–
		Total	69813	14537	2768	296	11473	2912	4455	30351	286	15659	1613
			(15%)	(21%)	(85%)	(59%)	(5%)	(76%)	(10%)	(11%)		(10%)	
	Any age	Sm.	15934	5816	4566	374	876	2728	564	4368	–	2458	–
		Total	94172	26095	5428	650	20017	3631	4936	34717	634	20290	3869
			(17%)	(22%)	(84%)	(58%)	(4%)	(75%)	(11%)	(13%)		(12%)	
Males+Females	0–34	Sm.	–	–	–	–	–	–	–	–	–	–	–
		Total	10306	771	33	20	718	54	118	362	34	4375	4592
	35–69	Sm.	18646	9897	7204	1000	1693	1255	359	4352	–	2783	–
		Total	58451	25563	7982	1534	16047	1606	1227	14757	1356	9210	4732
			(32%)	(39%)	(90%)	(65%)	(11%)	(78%)	(29%)	(29%)		(30%)	
	70+	Sm.	27072	10409	7433	720	2256	5658	986	6867	–	3152	–
		Total	132547	31789	8250	1131	22408	7361	8362	55079	730	26100	3126
			(20%)	(33%)	(90%)	(64%)	(10%)	(77%)	(12%)	(12%)		(12%)	
	Any age	Sm.	45718	20306	14637	1720	3949	6913	1345	11219	–	5935	–
		Total	201304	58123	16265	2685	39173	9021	9707	70198	2120	39685	12450
			(23%)	(35%)	(90%)	(64%)	(10%)	(77%)	(14%)	(16%)		(15%)	

(To be conservative, no deaths before age 35, and none from liver cirrhosis or non–medical causes, were attributed to smoking.)

¶CZECH REPUBLIC: 1990

		No. of deaths			Standardised rates (Defined on p.310)			Annual death rates / 100, 000						
		All ages	0–34	35–69	All ages	0–34	35–69	0–4	5–9	10–14	15–19	20–24	25–29	30–34
ALL CAUSES	M	66468	2954	31434	1520.5	118.0	1809.5	285.3	31.2	25.2	73.0	126.0	123.6	161.6
	F	62698	1479	15953	857.0	62.2	765.1	211.3	18.6	16.4	40.0	38.1	39.3	71.4
Tuberculosis	M	127	1	80	2.9	0.0	4.4	–	–	–	–	–	–	0.3
	F	80	1	20	1.1	0.0	1.0	–	–	–	0.2	–	–	–
Other infective	M	95	15	54	2.1	0.6	3.0	1.8	0.6	0.2	–	0.3	0.6	0.8
and parasitic	F	138	13	50	2.1	0.6	2.3	3.5	–	–	–	–	0.3	0.3
ALL CANCER	M	15797	276	9294	358.1	10.6	544.1	7.8	7.6	6.0	9.5	12.8	13.9	16.9
	F	12378	234	5711	188.5	9.5	272.6	9.4	4.7	4.9	5.8	6.3	11.9	23.5
Mouth and	M	377	1	310	8.4	0.0	16.7	–	–	–	–	–	0.3	–
pharynx cancer	F	91	2	36	1.4	0.1	1.7	–	–	–	–	–	–	0.6
Oesophagus cancer	M	275	1	201	6.1	0.0	11.3	–	–	–	–	0.3	–	–
	F	57	–	18	0.8	–	0.9	–	–	–	–	–	–	–
Stomach cancer	M	1261	10	613	28.9	0.4	36.4	–	–	–	–	–	0.9	1.9
	F	938	8	316	13.5	0.3	15.0	–	–	–	–	–	0.9	1.4
Colorectal cancer	M	2294	9	1152	52.7	0.4	68.8	–	–	–	–	–	1.4	1.1
	F	1894	8	695	27.3	0.3	33.6	–	–	–	0.2	–	0.9	1.1
Liver cancer	M	–	–	–	–	–	–	–	–	–	–	–	–	–
	F	–	–	–	–	–	–	–	–	–	–	–	–	–
Pancreas cancer	M	764	1	466	17.3	0.0	27.2	–	–	–	–	–	–	0.3
	F	656	6	284	9.6	0.2	13.7	–	–	–	0.2	0.3	0.3	0.9
Larynx cancer	M	319	–	235	7.1	–	13.0	–	–	–	–	–	–	–
	F	27	1	15	0.4	0.0	0.7	–	–	–	–	–	–	0.3
Lung cancer	M	4979	5	3511	112.4	0.2	206.7	–	–	–	–	0.3	–	1.1
	F	851	3	485	13.5	0.1	23.3	–	–	–	–	–	0.6	0.3
Malignant melanoma	M	170	4	120	3.8	0.2	6.5	–	–	–	–	0.3	0.3	0.6
	F	173	6	86	2.7	0.3	3.9	–	–	–	–	0.6	0.3	0.9
Female breast cancer	F	1907	21	1080	30.7	0.9	51.5	–	–	–	–	0.3	0.6	5.2
Cervix cancer	F	417	24	248	6.8	1.0	11.2	–	–	–	–	–	2.1	4.9
Other uterine cancer	F	575	3	270	8.6	0.1	13.0	–	–	–	–	–	0.3	0.6
Ovarian cancer	F	794	11	499	13.2	0.5	23.6	–	–	–	0.2	0.6	0.6	1.7
Prostate cancer	M	1074	1	283	25.0	0.0	17.9	–	–	–	–	–	0.3	–
Bladder cancer	M	583	1	265	13.5	0.0	16.5	0.3	–	–	–	–	–	–
	F	172	–	49	2.4	–	2.4	–	–	–	–	–	–	–
Other and ill–defined	M	2758	133	1625	62.1	5.1	93.5	4.8	2.5	2.5	5.8	5.7	8.0	6.6
cancer sites	F	2993	74	1265	44.6	3.0	60.8	6.3	2.1	2.6	2.7	1.5	2.1	3.7
Hodgkin's disease	M	90	13	56	2.0	0.5	3.0	–	–	0.2	0.5	0.6	0.6	1.7
	F	66	8	31	1.1	0.3	1.4	–	–	0.2	0.2	1.2	0.3	0.3
Myeloma and non–	M	378	21	219	8.5	0.8	12.9	–	1.7	0.4	0.7	1.7	0.6	0.6
Hodgkin lymphomas	F	381	12	169	5.8	0.5	8.0	0.6	0.6	0.2	0.7	0.3	0.3	0.6
Leukaemia	M	475	76	238	10.3	2.9	13.8	2.7	3.4	2.9	2.5	4.0	1.7	3.0
	F	386	47	165	6.0	1.9	7.7	2.5	2.1	1.9	1.5	1.5	2.7	1.1
ALL VASCULAR	M	34421	157	14240	800.5	6.2	845.1	1.5	0.3	0.9	1.6	6.8	8.8	23.5
DISEASE	F	37975	63	6857	487.9	2.6	333.2	1.9	–	0.2	1.7	2.4	3.6	8.3
Rheumatic heart	M	283	8	200	6.5	0.3	11.2	–	–	–	–	0.3	0.9	1.1
disease and fever	F	417	1	260	6.8	0.0	12.7	–	–	–	–	–	0.3	–
Hypertensive disease	M	293	2	156	6.7	0.1	8.9	–	–	–	–	0.3	–	0.3
	F	372	–	110	5.2	–	5.4	–	–	–	–	–	–	–
Ischaemic heart	M	18473	55	8867	425.9	2.2	524.6	–	–	–	0.2	1.4	1.7	11.9
disease	F	16173	9	3207	210.2	0.4	156.4	–	–	–	0.2	0.3	0.9	1.1
Pulmonary embolism	M	344	3	163	7.9	0.1	9.4	–	–	–	–	–	–	0.8
and other venous	F	495	3	158	6.8	0.1	7.6	–	–	–	–	–	–	0.9
Cerebrovascular	M	9640	27	3130	226.6	1.0	189.3	–	0.3	0.7	0.5	1.7	1.4	2.8
disease	F	13552	22	2155	171.8	0.9	104.6	0.3	–	–	0.7	0.9	0.9	3.4
Other vascular	M	5388	62	1724	126.9	2.5	101.7	1.5	–	0.2	0.9	3.1	4.8	6.6
disease	F	6966	28	967	87.1	1.2	46.6	1.6	–	0.2	0.7	1.2	1.5	2.9
Chronic obstructive	M	2046	26	858	47.5	1.0	51.1	0.6	0.3	0.2	0.5	1.4	2.0	2.2
pulmonary disease	F	905	8	268	12.5	0.3	12.9	0.3	0.3	–	0.7	0.3	–	0.6
Other respiratory	M	1277	67	448	29.9	2.7	25.5	11.1	0.8	0.9	1.2	0.6	1.7	2.8
disease	F	1195	47	175	15.6	2.0	8.3	8.5	0.9	1.2	0.7	0.6	0.9	1.1
Peptic ulcer	M	442	4	241	10.0	0.2	13.6	–	–	–	0.2	–	0.6	0.3
	F	231	–	70	3.1	–	3.3	–	–	–	–	–	–	–
Liver cirrhosis	M	1596	39	1303	34.8	1.6	68.6	–	–	–	–	0.6	2.3	8.0
	F	585	12	356	9.7	0.5	16.7	–	–	–	0.2	0.3	0.3	2.6
Renal disease	M	935	16	446	21.3	0.6	25.3	0.3	0.3	0.2	0.2	1.4	0.9	1.1
	F	1059	13	385	15.0	0.5	18.7	0.6	0.3	0.2	0.5	0.3	0.6	1.1
Pregnancy and birth	F	11	6	5	0.2	0.3	0.2	–	–	–	–	0.9	0.3	0.6
Congenital and	M	744	742	2	17.6	31.6	0.1	213.4	1.7	1.8	1.6	0.9	0.6	1.1
perinatal causes	F	503	499	4	12.5	22.3	0.1	150.6	1.5	1.2	1.0	0.6	0.3	0.9
Ill–defined causes	M	290	25	107	6.9	1.0	5.7	3.9	0.3	–	0.2	1.1	0.3	1.4
	F	410	17	28	5.1	0.7	1.3	4.4	–	–	0.2	–	0.3	0.3
Other medical causes	M	3316	234	1629	74.6	9.3	90.2	18.3	4.2	2.9	5.6	9.1	11.4	13.5
	F	3561	189	1208	51.9	7.7	57.6	15.1	4.1	4.4	6.6	4.5	6.9	12.3
ALL NON–	M	5382	1352	2732	114.3	52.5	132.9	26.7	15.2	12.1	52.4	91.0	80.7	89.8
MEDICAL CAUSES	F	3667	377	816	51.6	15.2	36.9	17.0	6.8	4.2	22.3	22.0	14.0	19.8
Motor vehicle	M	951	390	452	19.3	14.9	21.8	3.0	5.6	3.6	21.8	32.1	21.9	16.6
traffic accidents	F	342	114	113	5.8	4.4	5.1	1.6	2.9	1.4	11.9	8.3	2.1	2.6
Fire	M	86	20	38	1.9	0.8	2.0	–	1.1	0.2	1.2	0.6	0.6	1.7
	F	45	3	10	0.6	0.1	0.5	0.6	–	–	–	0.3	–	–
Suicide	M	1434	280	883	30.3	10.9	42.6	–	–	1.1	8.6	17.6	20.7	28.5
	F	563	88	304	9.6	3.6	13.6	–	–	0.2	3.2	6.3	5.7	9.8
Homicide	M	102	33	57	2.0	1.3	2.6	0.9	0.3	0.2	1.4	0.9	2.8	2.5
	F	95	42	41	1.8	1.7	1.7	2.5	0.6	0.7	1.7	2.7	2.1	1.7
POPULATION (thousands):	**M=males**				5036.5	2634.7	2125.0	333.7	356.2	447.9	431.4	351.6	352.0	361.9
	F=females				5326.1	2517.6	2293.8	318.0	339.5	428.0	412.1	335.8	335.6	348.6

CZECH REPUBLIC: 1990

Annual death rates / 100, 000

9th ICD categories

35–39	40–44	45–49	50–54	55–59	60–64	65–69	70–74	75–79	80+/NK			
275.0	450.5	783.3	1257.4	1962.2	3148.9	4789.3	6891.4	10788.5	18848.7	M	ALL CAUSES	001–999
103.4	176.6	291.1	447.7	786.6	1293.7	2256.3	3850.0	6789.1	14982.2	F		
0.7	1.9	2.7	4.8	6.4	6.2	8.0	9.2	15.3	28.1	M	Tuberculosis	010–018, 137
0.2	–	0.3	–	2.1	2.0	2.0	5.3	9.2	18.9	F		
1.0	0.2	2.4	2.0	4.4	4.2	7.1	4.1	9.6	16.1	M	Other infective	Rest of 001–139
0.2	1.7	1.2	2.6	1.4	3.7	5.5	6.0	13.5	22.8	F	and parasitic	
45.0	92.8	199.3	404.8	655.4	1002.1	1409.6	1816.6	2339.7	2689.4	M	ALL CANCER	140–208
42.5	78.5	140.5	189.6	332.3	467.2	657.8	878.0	1240.7	1569.5	F		
1.9	8.3	13.8	20.7	22.7	24.5	25.1	20.5	23.0	29.5	M	Mouth and	140–149
0.5	0.5	0.9	2.6	2.1	3.4	2.0	4.7	9.7	15.6	F	pharynx cancer	
1.4	2.6	6.6	10.0	18.3	22.0	18.0	12.3	34.4	33.5	M	Oesophagus cancer	150
–	0.2	0.6	0.4	1.8	1.7	1.4	2.0	8.1	11.7	F		
2.4	5.9	11.1	20.7	40.9	64.1	109.8	171.1	236.4	299.9	M	Stomach cancer	151
3.2	4.8	6.8	11.3	15.0	22.8	41.2	76.0	103.8	171.3	F		
4.6	5.7	21.3	47.0	73.1	131.9	198.4	290.0	425.8	542.2	M	Colorectal cancer	153, 154
2.2	5.0	14.8	18.5	41.2	59.1	94.4	146.7	222.8	310.9	F		
–	–	–	–	–	–	–	–	–	–	M	Liver cancer	155.0
–	–	–	–	–	–	–	–	–	–	F		
2.2	5.7	7.8	20.3	29.4	62.0	63.0	87.1	114.8	123.2	M	Pancreas cancer	157
0.5	2.4	4.7	7.2	12.2	24.8	44.3	49.3	83.3	76.8	F		
1.9	5.5	9.0	13.1	16.3	16.6	28.4	30.7	30.6	29.5	M	Larynx cancer	161
–	0.2	0.9	–	1.1	0.7	2.0	1.3	1.1	3.9	F		
8.2	28.9	74.0	166.5	269.5	382.7	517.0	543.0	552.2	476.6	M	Lung cancer	162
1.2	5.5	12.4	14.4	32.2	45.5	52.1	60.7	79.5	69.5	F		
1.9	2.6	5.1	4.8	8.7	11.6	10.4	13.3	14.4	24.1	M	Malignant melanoma	172
2.0	2.9	3.3	3.4	2.9	6.1	6.8	12.0	16.2	18.4	F		
7.6	16.8	33.4	51.8	64.4	90.3	96.5	113.3	156.3	193.0	F	Female breast cancer	174
5.9	9.4	7.7	7.2	12.9	17.3	18.1	22.0	28.7	32.8	F	Cervix cancer	180
2.5	1.9	5.3	6.0	16.5	17.3	41.2	46.0	55.7	72.3	F	Other uterine cancer	179, 182
5.4	8.9	14.8	18.5	32.6	40.4	44.6	54.0	59.0	52.3	F	Ovarian cancer	183
–	–	0.6	3.2	13.1	38.3	70.1	159.8	314.8	408.3	M	Prostate cancer	185
–	0.7	1.2	5.2	17.5	31.2	59.7	98.4	107.2	145.9	M	Bladder cancer	188
0.2	0.2	–	1.9	2.9	2.7	8.9	14.0	23.8	32.3	F		
14.9	20.2	39.3	73.3	108.9	167.2	230.6	298.2	359.8	445.8	M	Other and ill-defined	Rest of 140–208
8.6	12.2	24.9	36.3	76.6	105.6	161.6	210.7	315.8	419.4	F	cancer sites	
1.0	1.9	0.9	5.2	4.0	1.7	6.6	5.1	9.6	8.0	M	Hodgkin's disease	201
0.2	1.2	1.5	1.5	1.8	1.7	2.0	6.7	3.8	5.6	F		
2.4	2.1	1.8	7.6	16.3	25.8	34.1	47.1	48.8	54.9	M	Myeloma and non-	200, 202–203
1.0	2.2	5.0	4.5	8.2	15.3	20.1	34.0	38.4	43.4	F	Hodgkin lymphomas	
2.2	2.6	6.9	7.2	16.7	22.5	38.4	40.0	67.9	68.3	M	Leukaemia	204–208
1.5	4.1	3.6	4.2	7.9	12.6	20.4	24.7	34.6	40.6	F		
56.1	139.0	281.4	496.4	854.9	1547.8	2539.8	3921.1	6548.3	12522.1	M	ALL VASCULAR	390–459
16.7	36.0	67.2	148.8	304.3	570.1	1189.2	2294.0	4399.1	10834.3	F	DISEASE	
1.7	2.4	7.2	12.4	16.3	18.3	20.4	35.9	22.0	22.8	M	Rheumatic heart	390–398
0.5	1.2	4.4	11.7	17.2	22.1	32.0	30.0	34.1	26.7	F	disease and fever	
1.2	2.4	3.9	6.4	11.5	17.5	19.4	30.7	45.0	77.6	M	Hypertensive disease	401–405
0.2	1.0	0.6	4.2	7.9	6.8	17.0	30.0	41.1	78.4	F		
33.7	84.9	182.2	329.9	563.2	966.3	1511.8	2097.3	3219.1	5542.2	M	Ischaemic heart	410–414
3.4	10.8	28.7	58.2	146.4	284.6	562.4	1079.3	1907.0	4344.8	F	disease	
1.2	2.4	4.5	5.6	8.3	17.9	26.0	43.0	66.0	89.7	M	Pulmonary embolism	415.1, 451–453
0.5	1.9	2.1	3.8	7.5	13.9	23.5	30.7	61.7	96.8	F	and other venous	
7.7	25.4	49.4	80.5	164.9	354.4	642.5	1158.8	2093.8	4235.6	M	Cerebrovascular	430–438
6.4	11.3	18.6	41.2	84.9	173.9	395.7	804.7	1653.3	3954.9	F	disease	
10.6	21.6	34.2	61.8	90.6	173.5	319.6	555.3	1102.4	2554.2	M	Other vascular	Rest of 390–459
5.6	9.8	12.7	29.8	40.5	68.9	158.5	319.3	702.0	2332.6	F	disease	
3.6	7.1	15.3	29.9	53.7	95.7	152.5	238.7	383.7	706.8	M	Chronic obstructive	490–496
1.7	2.4	5.9	7.9	14.0	24.8	33.4	58.0	91.4	207.5	F	pulmonary disease	
5.3	7.1	13.5	16.3	30.2	32.9	73.4	125.0	219.1	550.2	M	Other respiratory	Rest of 460–519
1.2	3.1	3.8	3.8	5.7	16.0	24.2	66.0	117.9	364.8	F	disease	
2.4	3.6	8.4	9.6	14.3	25.0	32.2	48.2	75.6	95.0	M	Peptic ulcer	531–533
0.7	1.2	0.6	1.5	2.9	6.1	10.2	14.0	24.9	52.3	F		
19.0	40.1	58.7	72.5	89.0	99.8	100.9	88.1	99.5	85.7	M	Liver cirrhosis	571
3.2	9.6	11.2	15.5	19.3	26.5	31.4	39.3	48.7	37.8	F		
6.0	6.4	12.9	20.7	27.0	40.3	63.4	86.1	171.3	281.1	M	Renal disease	580–590
2.5	2.2	3.8	11.3	17.2	35.0	58.6	74.7	129.3	172.4	F		
1.0	0.2	–	–	–	–	–	–	–	–	F	Pregnancy and birth	630–676
0.2	–	–	–	–	–	0.5	–	–	–	M	Congenital and	740–779
0.5	0.2	0.3	–	–	–	–	–	–	–	F	perinatal causes	
1.7	3.3	3.9	5.6	8.3	8.7	8.0	10.2	21.1	168.7	M	Ill-defined causes	780–799
0.5	0.2	0.9	1.9	1.4	1.4	3.1	10.0	19.5	174.6	F		
26.9	33.9	55.1	65.3	91.8	131.0	227.3	303.3	512.9	831.3	M	Other medical causes	Rest of 001–799
11.3	14.2	26.9	35.5	54.4	91.3	169.4	249.3	385.1	599.6	F		
107.1	115.1	129.8	129.5	126.8	155.2	166.7	240.8	392.3	874.2	M	ALL NON-	E800–E999
21.1	27.1	28.4	29.1	31.5	49.6	71.6	155.3	309.9	927.7	F	MEDICAL CAUSES	
18.5	19.7	21.6	21.1	19.5	25.4	27.0	28.7	36.4	57.6	M	Motor vehicle	E810–E819
4.9	3.1	4.7	7.2	3.6	6.5	5.5	17.3	23.8	25.0	F	traffic accidents	
1.2	0.9	0.9	1.6	1.2	4.2	4.3	9.2	5.7	17.4	M	Fire	E890–E899
–	–	0.3	–	0.4	1.0	1.7	2.7	2.7	12.8	F		
34.4	39.1	44.7	45.4	37.8	40.8	56.3	74.8	80.4	152.6	M	Suicide	E950–E959
8.1	10.8	13.3	10.2	12.9	18.7	21.5	28.0	24.9	46.2	F		
3.4	3.6	1.8	1.6	2.8	2.9	1.9	2.0	4.8	6.7	M	Homicide	E960–E969
1.7	3.4	0.3	1.9	0.7	2.0	2.0	2.0	2.2	2.8	F		
415.6	421.5	333.7	251.0	251.6	240.4	211.2	97.6	104.5	74.7	M	POPULATION (thousands)	
407.2	416.7	338.0	264.7	279.3	294.5	293.4	150.0	184.9	179.8	F		

CZECH REPUBLIC: Males

	All ages	0–34	35–69	35–39	40–44	45–49	50–54	55–59	60–64	65–69	70–74	75–79	80+/NK
POPULATION (1000s)													
1955	4562.1	2557.6	1794.6	212.6	339.5	349.0	319.8	250.0	185.4	138.3	102.8	62.4	44.7
1965	4747.4	2578.8	1943.4	328.6	343.7	200.7	316.3	313.1	260.0	181.0	111.9	66.4	46.9
1975	4876.6	2729.3	1861.2	276.6	293.9	308.6	315.1	177.1	261.2	228.7	155.0	82.2	48.9
1985	5016.3	2720.8	1964.4	428.6	343.2	262.9	271.4	272.0	256.5	129.8	161.5	106.5	63.1
1990	**5036.5**	**2634.7**	**2125.0**	**415.6**	**421.5**	**333.7**	**251.0**	**251.6**	**240.4**	**211.2**	**97.6**	**104.5**	**74.7**
1995 projected	*5126.0*	*2620.6*	*2206.8*	*388.5*	*440.9*	*402.3*	*298.3*	*234.0*	*236.6*	*206.2*	*160.4*	*63.3*	*74.9*
NUMBER OF DEATHS													
All causes													
1955	48954	5910	23012	521	1221	2242	3403	4582	5156	5887	6531	6066	7435
1965	55424	4872	27208	791	1295	1119	3060	5153	7394	8396	7768	6759	8817
1975	64619	4870	28893	751	1228	2015	3543	3106	7555	10695	11573	9271	10012
1985	66589	3256	27104	1064	1512	1898	3246	5264	8190	5930	11814	11971	12444
1990	**66468**	**2954**	**31434**	**1143**	**1899**	**2614**	**3156**	**4937**	**7570**	**10115**	**6726**	**11274**	**14080**
1995 projected	*66162*	*2901*	*32401*	*1109*	*2125*	*3327*	*3896*	*4624*	*7606*	*9714*	*10740*	*6468*	*13652*
Lung cancer													
1955	2187	16	1740	10	38	116	295	459	458	364	266	126	39
1965	4124	18	2958	24	65	69	283	584	944	989	688	292	168
1975	5024	14	3075	22	67	184	389	402	877	1134	1044	607	284
1985	4974	8	3072	41	107	199	425	707	1024	569	888	640	366
1990	**4979**	**5**	**3511**	**34**	**122**	**247**	**418**	**678**	**920**	**1092**	**530**	**577**	**356**
1995 projected	*5141*	*4*	*3645*	*29*	*120*	*300*	*511*	*626*	*957*	*1102*	*875*	*307*	*310*
ANNUAL DEATH RATE / 100,000 (*The rates for the age groups 0–34 and 35–69 are the means of seven five-yearly rates, but the all-ages rates are standardised to the conventional "European" age distribution)													
All causes													
1955	1412.7*	217.3*	1597.4*	245.1	359.6	642.4	1064.1	1832.8	2781.0	4256.7	6353.1	9721.2	16633.1
1965	1466.9*	195.8*	1610.1*	240.7	376.8	557.5	967.4	1645.8	2843.8	4638.7	6941.9	10179.2	18799.6
1975	1557.0*	169.1*	1684.2*	271.5	417.8	652.9	1124.4	1753.8	2892.4	4676.4	7466.5	11278.6	20474.4
1985	1543.6*	124.1*	1757.7*	248.3	440.6	721.9	1196.0	1935.3	3193.0	4568.6	7315.2	11240.4	19721.1
1990	**1520.5***	**118.0***	**1809.5***	**275.0**	**450.5**	**783.3**	**1257.4**	**1962.2**	**3148.9**	**4789.3**	**6891.4**	**10788.5**	**18848.7**
1995 projected	*1499.1**	*114.2**	*1828.9**	*285.5*	*482.0*	*827.0*	*1306.1*	*1976.1*	*3214.7*	*4711.0*	*6695.8*	*10218.0*	*18227.0*
All cancer													
1955	254.7*	12.5*	413.8*	35.7	66.6	145.6	292.4	513.2	769.7	1073.8	1299.6	1588.1	1382.6
1965	315.5*	13.0*	479.4*	40.5	80.3	130.0	269.7	500.2	911.5	1423.8	1866.0	2042.2	2162.0
1975	336.7*	11.8*	481.4*	40.1	89.8	165.9	319.9	553.4	872.1	1328.4	1897.4	2356.4	2689.2
1985	344.2*	10.9*	508.5*	47.1	105.5	202.7	395.7	613.2	971.5	1223.4	1786.4	2208.5	2705.2
1990	**358.1***	**10.6***	**544.1***	**45.0**	**92.8**	**199.3**	**404.8**	**655.4**	**1002.1**	**1409.6**	**1816.6**	**2339.7**	**2689.4**
1995 projected	*372.8**	*10.4**	*571.4**	*39.6*	*88.7*	*196.4*	*419.7*	*678.2*	*1087.9*	*1489.3*	*1920.2*	*2369.7*	*2790.4*
Lung cancer													
1955	57.7*	0.6*	119.3*	4.7	11.2	33.2	92.2	183.6	247.0	263.2	258.8	201.9	87.2
1965	96.5*	0.8*	178.0*	7.3	18.9	34.4	89.5	186.5	363.1	546.4	614.8	439.8	358.2
1975	112.1*	0.5*	181.8*	8.0	22.8	59.6	123.5	227.0	335.8	495.8	673.5	738.4	580.8
1985	112.5*	0.3*	195.8*	9.6	31.2	75.7	156.6	259.9	399.2	438.4	549.8	600.9	580.0
1990	**112.4***	**0.2***	**206.7***	**8.2**	**28.9**	**74.0**	**166.5**	**269.5**	**382.7**	**517.0**	**543.0**	**552.2**	**476.6**
1995 projected	*111.7**	*0.2**	*212.4**	*7.5*	*27.2*	*74.6*	*171.3*	*267.5*	*404.5*	*534.4*	*545.5*	*485.0*	*413.9*
Upper aerodigestive cancer (mouth, oesophagus, pharynx and larynx)													
1955	15.1*	0.2*	20.9*	0.5	1.5	8.3	13.4	29.2	36.1	57.1	86.6	110.6	132.0
1965	14.3*	0.1*	20.8*	2.1	1.7	3.5	10.1	24.3	35.0	69.1	74.2	90.4	151.4
1975	15.3*	0.3*	22.0*	1.8	5.4	10.7	22.5	24.3	37.9	51.6	68.4	107.1	135.0
1985	18.9*	0.2*	32.5*	4.9	13.7	22.8	38.3	43.8	47.6	56.2	63.2	98.6	106.2
1990	**21.6***	**0.1***	**41.0***	**5.3**	**16.4**	**29.4**	**43.8**	**57.2**	**63.2**	**71.5**	**63.5**	**88.0**	**92.4**
1995 projected	*25.0**	*0.1**	*50.3**	*5.9*	*20.0*	*34.6*	*54.0*	*71.8*	*81.6*	*84.4*	*64.2*	*82.1*	*81.4*
Other cancer													
1955	182.0*	11.6*	273.6*	30.6	53.9	104.0	186.7	300.4	486.5	753.4	954.3	1275.6	1163.3
1965	204.7*	12.1*	280.6*	31.0	59.6	92.2	170.1	289.4	513.5	808.3	1176.9	1512.0	1652.5
1975	209.4*	11.0*	277.6*	30.4	61.6	95.6	173.9	302.1	498.5	780.9	1155.5	1510.9	1973.4
1985	212.8*	10.5*	280.2*	32.7	60.6	104.2	200.8	309.6	524.8	728.8	1173.4	1508.9	2019.0
1990	**224.1***	**10.4***	**296.5***	**31.5**	**47.4**	**95.9**	**194.4**	**328.7**	**556.2**	**821.0**	**1210.0**	**1699.5**	**2120.5**
1995 projected	*236.0**	*10.2**	*308.7**	*26.3*	*41.5*	*87.2*	*194.4*	*338.9*	*601.9*	*870.5*	*1310.5*	*1802.5*	*2295.1*
Chronic obstructive pulmonary disease (COPD)													
1955	29.1*	0.9*	29.7*	1.9	3.8	6.0	20.6	36.4	53.4	86.0	134.2	258.0	445.2
1965	98.8*	0.8*	110.5*	4.6	8.7	14.0	38.9	94.5	208.8	403.9	563.0	859.9	1368.9
1975	94.5*	1.1*	82.9*	5.8	7.8	20.7	43.2	69.5	149.3	284.2	561.3	835.8	1599.2
1985	60.6*	0.9*	55.7*	3.0	5.0	18.3	33.9	66.9	109.6	153.3	307.7	554.9	1000.0
1990	**47.5***	**1.0***	**51.1***	**3.6**	**7.1**	**15.3**	**29.9**	**53.7**	**95.7**	**152.5**	**238.7**	**383.7**	**706.8**
1995 projected	*37.2**	*1.3**	*44.5**	*5.1*	*7.0*	*13.7*	*24.5*	*45.3*	*86.6*	*129.5*	*180.2*	*267.0*	*500.7*
Other respiratory disease													
1955	74.1*	16.9*	51.4*	4.7	8.2	16.6	24.4	58.4	95.5	151.8	334.6	591.3	1241.6
1965	49.4*	9.5*	32.9*	2.7	4.4	11.0	21.5	21.4	53.5	116.0	193.9	375.0	978.7
1975	49.4*	6.4*	27.1*	3.6	7.5	8.4	11.1	17.5	45.9	95.3	200.0	435.5	1098.2
1985	42.4*	4.2*	33.1*	5.1	6.7	12.9	22.8	33.1	56.5	94.8	161.0	349.3	824.1
1990	**29.9***	**2.7***	**25.5***	**5.3**	**7.1**	**13.5**	**16.3**	**30.2**	**32.9**	**73.4**	**125.0**	**219.1**	**550.2**
1995 projected	*21.8**	*2.1**	*19.5**	*4.9*	*7.3*	*11.7*	*14.1*	*20.9*	*24.1*	*53.8*	*87.3*	*153.2*	*388.5*
Vascular disease													
1955	638.9*	13.8*	676.2*	48.0	92.8	213.5	377.1	732.4	1213.1	2056.4	3315.2	5405.4	9319.9
1965	654.9*	9.2*	645.1*	54.2	121.6	205.8	367.1	644.8	1161.2	1960.8	3239.5	5265.1	11014.9
1975	757.0*	6.5*	771.6*	74.1	133.0	250.2	484.9	778.1	1377.1	2303.9	3801.9	6146.0	12157.5
1985	816.7*	6.5*	850.3*	57.2	141.3	272.0	494.1	891.5	1611.7	2484.6	4128.8	6713.6	12721.1
1990	**800.5***	**6.2***	**845.1***	**56.1**	**139.0**	**281.4**	**496.4**	**854.9**	**1547.8**	**2539.8**	**3921.1**	**6548.3**	**12522.1**
1995 projected	*777.9**	*5.8**	*822.6**	*55.6*	*138.8*	*280.4*	*485.1*	*817.9*	*1521.6*	*2458.8*	*3791.1*	*6241.7*	*12287.0*
Liver cirrhosis													
1955	10.6*	0.2*	18.5*	1.9	4.7	9.2	17.8	19.2	28.6	48.4	63.2	49.7	38.0
1965	17.8*	0.6*	30.7*	2.7	11.1	12.0	17.7	39.3	58.1	74.0	81.3	82.8	104.5
1975	25.5*	1.3*	47.6*	10.5	20.4	29.8	36.8	56.5	82.7	96.2	104.5	76.6	102.2
1985	26.4*	1.0*	50.3*	11.2	28.3	33.1	47.9	54.4	73.3	104.0	88.5	96.7	88.7
1990	**34.8***	**1.6***	**68.6***	**19.0**	**40.1**	**58.7**	**72.5**	**89.0**	**99.8**	**100.9**	**88.1**	**99.5**	**85.7**
1995 projected	*44.1**	*2.2**	*89.0**	*26.5*	*55.8*	*81.8*	*101.9*	*124.4*	*123.8*	*109.1*	*87.3*	*102.7*	*85.4*
Other medical causes													
1955	294.1*	102.2*	285.6*	61.1	83.1	136.1	207.6	343.2	485.4	682.6	1014.6	1479.2	3608.5
1965	211.2*	90.3*	179.2*	32.0	49.5	68.3	118.9	196.7	306.5	482.9	759.6	1206.3	2471.2
1975	176.7*	77.5*	148.4*	39.4	52.4	70.3	114.2	146.8	220.5	394.8	628.4	1019.5	1993.9
1985	143.9*	49.1*	136.6*	31.0	49.0	68.5	89.5	146.3	239.4	332.8	590.1	901.4	1542.0
1990	**135.4***	**43.3***	**142.3***	**39.0**	**49.3**	**85.4**	**108.0**	**152.2**	**215.5**	**346.6**	**461.1**	**805.7**	**1420.3**
1995 projected	*127.4**	*39.1**	*140.5**	*39.1*	*56.9*	*98.7*	*121.7*	*150.9*	*212.6*	*303.6*	*404.0*	*704.6*	*1293.7*
All non-medical causes													
1955	111.2*	70.9*	122.1*	91.7	100.4	115.5	124.1	130.0	135.4	157.6	191.6	349.4	597.3
1965	119.3*	72.4*	132.3*	104.1	101.3	116.6	133.7	148.8	144.2	177.3	238.6	347.9	699.4
1975	117.1*	64.7*	125.3*	98.0	106.8	107.6	114.2	132.1	144.7	173.6	272.9	408.8	834.4
1985	109.4*	51.6*	123.1*	93.6	104.9	114.5	112.0	129.8	131.0	175.7	252.6	416.0	839.9
1990	**114.3***	**52.5***	**132.9***	**107.1**	**115.1**	**129.8**	**129.5**	**126.8**	**155.2**	**166.7**	**240.8**	**392.3**	**874.2**
1995 projected	*118.0**	*53.3**	*141.3**	*114.5*	*127.5*	*144.4*	*139.1*	*138.5*	*158.1*	*166.8*	*225.7*	*379.1*	*881.2*

CZECH REPUBLIC: Females

	All ages	0–34	35–69	35–39	40–44	45–49	50–54	55–59	60–64	65–69	70–74	75–79	80+/NK
POPULATION (1000s)													
1955	4804.0	2513.7	2000.1	222.2	349.8	366.2	339.5	298.7	236.1	187.6	141.9	87.0	61.3
1965	5037.8	2488.3	2167.5	339.9	367.7	216.1	341.1	343.7	306.5	252.5	179.4	114.4	88.2
1975	5185.7	2615.6	2061.5	276.2	299.0	328.2	350.9	204.1	309.0	294.1	234.1	157.7	116.8
1985	5320.4	2607.9	2125.8	419.8	342.2	269.8	288.3	310.3	320.6	174.8	241.3	188.0	157.4
1990	**5326.1**	**2517.6**	**2293.8**	**407.2**	**416.7**	**338.0**	**264.7**	**279.3**	**294.5**	**293.4**	**150.0**	**184.9**	**179.8**
1995 projected	*5395.6*	*2503.5*	*2343.1*	*380.3*	*435.8*	*399.7*	*308.1*	*258.1*	*282.0*	*279.1*	*251.1*	*115.5*	*182.4*
NUMBER OF DEATHS													
All causes													
1955	44341	3816	16328	379	891	1414	2066	2793	3568	5217	6739	7386	10072
1965	49684	2694	16770	438	761	685	1785	2799	4136	6166	7724	8740	13756
1975	59695	2726	16292	306	555	995	1831	1624	4105	6876	9963	11985	18729
1985	65052	1643	14187	440	586	763	1448	2503	4422	4025	9989	13897	25336
1990	**62698**	**1479**	**15953**	**421**	**736**	**984**	**1185**	**2197**	**3810**	**6620**	**5775**	**12553**	**26938**
1995 projected	*58252*	*1418*	*15027*	*413*	*787*	*1114*	*1321*	*1910*	*3525*	*5957*	*9010*	*7199*	*25598*
Lung cancer													
1955	411	11	270	2	14	26	38	54	54	82	72	34	24
1965	476	2	275	5	7	11	42	59	65	86	92	51	56
1975	532	2	250	6	5	19	36	37	63	84	96	114	70
1985	723	3	368	7	9	36	50	65	111	90	136	110	106
1990	**851**	**3**	**485**	**5**	**23**	**42**	**38**	**90**	**134**	**153**	**91**	**147**	**125**
1995 projected	*978*	*3*	*549*	*7*	*26*	*48*	*50*	*104*	*154*	*160*	*174*	*102*	*150*
ANNUAL DEATH RATE / 100,000 (*The rates for the age groups 0–34 and 35–69 are the means of seven five-yearly rates, but the all-ages rates are standardised to the conventional "European" age distribution)													
All causes													
1955	1058.1*	141.4*	949.6*	170.6	254.7	386.1	608.5	935.1	1511.2	2780.9	4749.1	8489.7	16430.7
1965	950.0*	112.1*	826.0*	128.9	207.0	317.0	523.3	814.4	1349.4	2442.0	4305.5	7639.9	15596.4
1975	938.8*	98.1*	797.6*	110.8	185.6	303.2	521.8	795.7	1328.5	2338.0	4255.9	7599.9	16035.1
1985	912.4*	65.9*	792.8*	104.8	171.2	282.8	502.3	806.6	1379.3	2302.6	4139.7	7392.0	16096.6
1990	**857.0***	**62.2***	**765.1***	**103.4**	**176.6**	**291.1**	**447.7**	**786.6**	**1293.7**	**2256.3**	**3850.0**	**6789.1**	**14982.2**
1995 projected	*805.6**	*58.8**	*731.6**	*108.6*	*180.6*	*278.7*	*428.8*	*740.0*	*1250.0*	*2134.4*	*3588.2*	*6232.9*	*14034.0*
All cancer													
1955	183.0*	12.8*	280.5*	48.6	96.6	145.0	222.4	324.4	460.4	665.8	878.8	1131.0	1132.1
1965	184.2*	9.8*	269.5*	48.2	89.2	123.6	219.6	308.1	441.1	657.0	906.9	1140.7	1441.0
1975	178.0*	10.4*	253.5*	41.3	69.6	131.6	226.8	287.1	428.5	589.6	805.6	1162.3	1513.7
1985	179.3*	8.0*	264.7*	44.8	74.8	131.2	217.8	307.8	459.5	616.7	856.2	1080.3	1454.3
1990	**188.5***	**9.5***	**272.6***	**42.5**	**78.5**	**140.5**	**189.6**	**332.3**	**467.2**	**657.8**	**878.0**	**1240.7**	**1569.5**
1995 projected	*197.6**	*10.8**	*277.9**	*43.9*	*81.0*	*134.6*	*189.5*	*332.4*	*488.3*	*675.7*	*940.7*	*1320.3*	*1739.6*
Lung cancer													
1955	8.9*	0.5*	15.4*	0.9	4.0	7.1	11.2	18.1	22.9	43.7	50.7	39.1	39.2
1965	8.6*	0.1*	13.3*	1.5	1.9	5.1	12.3	17.2	21.2	34.1	51.3	44.6	63.5
1975	8.6*	0.1*	12.4*	2.2	1.7	5.8	10.3	18.1	20.4	28.6	41.0	72.3	59.9
1985	11.8*	0.1*	20.3*	1.7	2.6	13.3	17.3	20.9	34.6	51.5	56.4	58.5	67.3
1990	**13.5***	**0.1***	**23.3***	**1.2**	**5.5**	**12.4**	**14.4**	**32.2**	**45.5**	**52.1**	**60.7**	**79.5**	**69.5**
1995 projected	*15.5**	*0.1**	*26.9**	*1.8*	*6.0*	*12.0*	*16.2*	*40.3*	*54.6*	*57.3*	*69.3*	*88.3*	*82.2*
Upper aerodigestive cancer (mouth, oesophagus, pharynx and larynx)													
1955	2.9*	0.1*	3.8*	1.8	2.0	1.6	2.4	6.0	5.1	8.0	9.9	21.8	31.0
1965	2.3*	0.1*	2.1*	–	0.8	1.4	0.6	1.7	3.9	5.9	15.6	21.0	34.0
1975	2.2*	0.0*	2.7*	0.4	–	1.8	2.0	4.4	3.9	6.5	12.4	13.3	25.7
1985	2.1*	0.1*	2.6*	0.2	0.9	0.7	2.1	3.2	5.3	5.7	6.6	13.8	33.0
1990	**2.6***	**0.1***	**3.3***	**0.5**	**1.0**	**2.4**	**3.0**	**5.0**	**5.8**	**5.5**	**8.0**	**18.9**	**31.1**
1995 projected	*3.0**	*0.2**	*4.0**	*0.8*	*1.4*	*3.3*	*4.2*	*6.6*	*6.4*	*5.7*	*9.6*	*19.0*	*33.4*
Other cancer													
1955	171.2*	12.3*	261.2*	45.9	90.6	136.3	208.8	300.3	432.4	614.1	818.2	1070.1	1062.0
1965	173.2*	9.6*	254.2*	46.8	86.5	117.1	206.7	289.2	416.0	617.0	840.0	1075.2	1343.5
1975	167.2*	10.3*	238.4*	38.7	67.9	124.0	214.6	264.6	404.2	554.6	752.2	1076.7	1428.1
1985	165.4*	7.8*	241.8*	42.9	71.3	117.1	198.4	283.6	419.5	559.5	793.2	1008.0	1353.9
1990	**172.4***	**9.3***	**246.0***	**40.8**	**72.0**	**125.7**	**172.3**	**295.0**	**416.0**	**600.2**	**809.3**	**1142.2**	**1468.9**
1995 projected	*179.1**	*10.5**	*247.0**	*41.3*	*73.7*	*119.3*	*169.1*	*285.5*	*427.3*	*612.7*	*861.8*	*1213.0*	*1623.9*
Chronic obstructive pulmonary disease (COPD)													
1955	15.5*	0.6*	8.3*	0.9	2.0	1.1	1.8	6.4	12.7	33.0	68.4	155.2	367.0
1965	32.2*	0.5*	20.9*	0.9	2.7	4.6	10.0	19.2	34.9	73.7	165.6	313.8	680.3
1975	26.7*	0.7*	17.8*	0.4	2.3	5.5	11.4	20.1	28.8	56.4	123.5	226.4	594.2
1985	16.4*	0.2*	17.6*	2.1	2.9	5.2	15.3	17.4	26.2	53.8	65.1	118.6	287.2
1990	**12.5***	**0.3***	**12.9***	**1.7**	**2.4**	**5.9**	**7.9**	**14.0**	**24.8**	**33.4**	**58.0**	**91.4**	**207.5**
1995 projected	*9.4**	*0.3**	*9.9**	*1.6*	*2.3*	*4.3*	*5.8*	*10.8*	*18.1*	*26.5*	*43.8*	*65.8*	*153.0*
Other respiratory disease													
1955	57.3*	15.2*	30.7*	4.1	6.0	11.5	13.8	25.4	46.2	108.2	229.0	503.4	1066.9
1965	34.6*	6.3*	15.6*	2.6	3.5	5.1	9.7	12.5	24.8	50.7	127.6	269.2	820.9
1975	36.4*	4.9*	15.4*	2.9	4.3	5.8	5.7	17.1	21.7	50.3	134.1	321.5	890.4
1985	26.8*	3.0*	12.5*	1.7	3.5	2.2	6.6	11.0	19.0	43.5	95.3	227.1	676.0
1990	**15.6***	**2.0***	**8.3***	**1.2**	**3.1**	**3.8**	**3.8**	**5.7**	**16.0**	**24.2**	**66.0**	**117.9**	**364.8**
1995 projected	*11.2**	*1.5**	*6.0**	*1.1*	*3.4*	*3.3*	*2.6*	*3.9*	*11.0*	*16.8*	*45.8*	*81.4*	*258.2*
Vascular disease													
1955	520.3*	12.8*	400.7*	38.3	58.6	109.0	202.9	342.1	649.7	1404.6	2661.0	5121.8	9693.3
1965	474.4*	4.7*	324.2*	22.4	46.0	82.4	153.9	288.6	540.9	1135.0	2275.4	4573.4	10062.4
1975	506.4*	3.5*	350.8*	23.2	42.8	83.5	157.0	309.2	601.3	1238.4	2493.4	4769.2	10742.3
1985	523.4*	2.5*	348.3*	14.8	35.7	68.6	156.4	319.4	636.3	1207.1	2512.2	4945.2	11470.1
1990	**487.9***	**2.6***	**333.2***	**16.7**	**36.0**	**67.2**	**148.8**	**304.3**	**570.1**	**1189.2**	**2294.0**	**4399.1**	**10834.3**
1995 projected	*448.3**	*2.7**	*310.1**	*17.9*	*36.0*	*64.5*	*141.2*	*276.6*	*537.9*	*1096.7*	*2056.2*	*3932.5*	*10054.3*
Liver cirrhosis													
1955	6.7*	0.4*	9.8*	0.5	1.7	3.5	6.8	13.1	15.2	27.7	25.4	40.2	71.8
1965	7.9*	0.3*	11.1*	2.4	1.9	4.2	5.6	7.6	18.6	37.2	49.6	61.2	59.0
1975	8.2*	0.3*	11.4*	1.4	3.3	5.2	8.0	11.8	16.2	33.7	47.0	57.7	65.1
1985	8.7*	0.3*	13.7*	2.4	5.0	6.3	11.8	19.0	27.8	24.0	37.3	52.1	53.4
1990	**9.7***	**0.5***	**16.7***	**3.2**	**9.6**	**11.2**	**15.5**	**19.3**	**26.5**	**31.4**	**39.3**	**48.7**	**37.8**
1995 projected	*10.7**	*0.6**	*19.4**	*4.5*	*13.5*	*15.8*	*19.1*	*20.1*	*28.7*	*34.0*	*40.6*	*44.2*	*30.7*
Other medical causes													
1955	227.2*	79.9*	176.5*	59.9	58.6	83.0	120.2	172.7	277.8	463.2	744.9	1269.0	3551.4
1965	164.5*	69.7*	141.1*	29.1	36.7	62.0	82.4	137.9	231.0	408.3	627.6	980.8	1850.3
1975	126.6*	58.4*	104.1*	20.3	31.4	42.0	73.2	106.3	168.9	286.3	483.1	726.7	1371.6
1985	101.7*	37.4*	96.9*	18.1	21.6	41.5	64.9	93.8	160.0	278.6	402.8	614.4	1100.4
1990	**91.1***	**32.1***	**84.5***	**16.9**	**19.9**	**34.0**	**52.9**	**79.5**	**139.6**	**248.8**	**359.3**	**581.4**	**1040.6**
1995 projected	*81.1**	*27.3**	*73.5**	*17.9*	*17.2*	*28.3*	*43.5*	*67.0*	*121.3*	*219.3*	*325.0*	*526.4*	*984.1*
All non-medical causes													
1955	48.0*	19.8*	43.1*	18.5	31.2	33.0	40.6	50.9	49.1	78.4	141.6	269.0	548.1
1965	52.2*	20.8*	43.7*	23.2	26.9	35.2	42.2	40.4	58.1	80.0	152.7	300.7	682.5
1975	56.7*	19.9*	44.7*	21.4	31.8	29.6	39.6	44.1	63.1	83.3	169.2	336.1	857.9
1985	56.1*	14.5*	39.1*	21.0	27.8	27.8	29.5	38.3	50.5	78.9	170.7	354.3	1055.3
1990	**51.6***	**15.2***	**36.9***	**21.1**	**27.1**	**28.4**	**29.1**	**31.5**	**49.6**	**71.6**	**155.3**	**309.9**	**927.7**
1995 projected	*47.3**	*15.7**	*34.7**	*21.8*	*27.1*	*28.0*	*26.9*	*29.1*	*44.7*	*65.2*	*136.2*	*262.3*	*814.1*

CZECH REPUBLIC: 1975

Smoking–attributed deaths (Sm.) and total deaths (Total)

		ALL CAUSES	ALL CANCER	Lung cancer	Upper aero–digestive ca.	Other cancer	COPD	Other respiratory	Vascular disease	Liver cirrhosis	Other medical	Non–medical
Males												
0–34	Sm.	–	–	–	–	–	–	–	–	–	–	–
	Total	4870	326	14	7	305	31	189	177	34	2315	1798
35–69	Sm.	11707	4314	2930	290	1094	1188	172	5013	–	1020	–
	Total	28893	8191	3075	385	4731	1402	462	13140	833	2579	2286
		(41%)	(53%)	(95%)	(75%)	(23%)	(85%)	(37%)	(38%)		(40%)	
70+	Sm.	8558	2756	1820	181	755	1892	212	3174	–	524	–
	Total	30856	6193	1935	260	3998	2339	1205	16890	275	2787	1167
		(28%)	(45%)	(94%)	(70%)	(19%)	(81%)	(18%)	(19%)		(19%)	
Any age	Sm.	20265	7070	4750	471	1849	3080	384	8187	–	1544	–
	Total	64619	14710	5024	652	9034	3772	1856	30207	1142	7681	5251
		(31%)	(48%)	(95%)	(72%)	(20%)	(82%)	(21%)	(27%)		(20%)	
Females												
0–34	Sm.	–	–	–	–	–	–	–	–	–	–	–
	Total	2726	272	2	1	269	17	137	93	9	1664	534
35–69	Sm.	400	93	71	5	17	63	8	179	–	57	–
	Total	16292	5194	250	54	4890	362	310	7148	232	2126	920
		(2%)	(2%)	(28%)	(9%)	(0%)	(17%)	(3%)	(3%)		(3%)	
70+	Sm.	1289	179	127	14	38	463	38	530	–	79	–
	Total	40677	5487	280	80	5127	1340	1861	25905	277	3879	1928
		(3%)	(3%)	(45%)	(18%)	(1%)	(35%)	(2%)	(2%)		(2%)	
Any age	Sm.	1689	272	198	19	55	526	46	709	–	136	–
	Total	59695	10953	532	135	10286	1719	2308	33146	518	7669	3382
		(3%)	(2%)	(37%)	(14%)	(1%)	(31%)	(2%)	(2%)		(2%)	
Males+Females												
0–34	Sm.	–	–	–	–	–	–	–	–	–	–	–
	Total	7596	598	16	8	574	48	326	270	43	3979	2332
35–69	Sm.	12107	4407	3001	295	1111	1251	180	5192	–	1077	–
	Total	45185	13385	3325	439	9621	1764	772	20288	1065	4705	3206
		(27%)	(33%)	(90%)	(67%)	(12%)	(71%)	(23%)	(26%)		(23%)	
70+	Sm.	9847	2935	1947	195	793	2355	250	3704	–	603	–
	Total	71533	11680	2215	340	9125	3679	3066	42795	552	6666	3095
		(14%)	(25%)	(88%)	(57%)	(9%)	(64%)	(8%)	(9%)		(9%)	
Any age	Sm.	21954	7342	4948	490	1904	3606	430	8896	–	1680	–
	Total	124314	25663	5556	787	19320	5491	4164	63353	1660	15350	8633
		(18%)	(29%)	(89%)	(62%)	(10%)	(66%)	(10%)	(14%)		(11%)	

CZECH REPUBLIC: 1985

Smoking–attributed deaths (Sm.) and total deaths (Total)

		ALL CAUSES	ALL CANCER	Lung cancer	Upper aero–digestive ca.	Other cancer	COPD	Other respiratory	Vascular disease	Liver cirrhosis	Other medical	Non–medical
Males												
0–34	Sm.	–	–	–	–	–	–	–	–	–	–	–
	Total	3256	299	8	5	286	24	109	175	28	1256	1365
35–69	Sm.	11770	4480	2945	426	1109	718	218	5383	–	971	–
	Total	27104	7919	3072	546	4301	832	499	12570	833	2168	2283
		(43%)	(57%)	(96%)	(78%)	(26%)	(86%)	(44%)	(43%)		(45%)	
70+	Sm.	7957	2679	1754	177	748	1325	166	3338	–	449	–
	Total	36229	6944	1894	274	4776	1719	1152	21845	302	2886	1381
		(22%)	(39%)	(93%)	(65%)	(16%)	(77%)	(14%)	(15%)		(16%)	
Any age	Sm.	19727	7159	4699	603	1857	2043	384	8721	–	1420	–
	Total	66589	15162	4974	825	9363	2575	1760	34590	1163	6310	5029
		(30%)	(47%)	(94%)	(73%)	(20%)	(79%)	(22%)	(25%)		(23%)	
Females												
0–34	Sm.	–	–	–	–	–	–	–	–	–	–	–
	Total	1643	214	3	2	209	4	74	64	9	909	369
35–69	Sm.	1030	262	204	10	48	128	18	481	–	141	–
	Total	14187	4932	368	49	4515	309	215	5961	268	1740	762
		(7%)	(5%)	(55%)	(20%)	(1%)	(41%)	(8%)	(8%)		(8%)	
70+	Sm.	1181	212	156	15	41	246	28	615	–	80	–
	Total	49222	6386	352	94	5940	832	1721	33413	272	3859	2739
		(2%)	(3%)	(44%)	(16%)	(1%)	(30%)	(2%)	(2%)		(2%)	
Any age	Sm.	2211	474	360	25	89	374	46	1096	–	221	–
	Total	65052	11532	723	145	10664	1145	2010	39438	549	6508	3870
		(3%)	(4%)	(50%)	(17%)	(1%)	(33%)	(2%)	(3%)		(3%)	
Males+Females												
0–34	Sm.	–	–	–	–	–	–	–	–	–	–	–
	Total	4899	513	11	7	495	28	183	239	37	2165	1734
35–69	Sm.	12800	4742	3149	436	1157	846	236	5864	–	1112	–
	Total	41291	12851	3440	595	8816	1141	714	18531	1101	3908	3045
		(31%)	(37%)	(92%)	(73%)	(13%)	(74%)	(33%)	(32%)		(28%)	
70+	Sm.	9138	2891	1910	192	789	1571	194	3953	–	529	–
	Total	85451	13330	2246	368	10716	2551	2873	55258	574	6745	4120
		(11%)	(22%)	(85%)	(52%)	(7%)	(62%)	(7%)	(7%)		(8%)	
Any age	Sm.	21938	7633	5059	628	1946	2417	430	9817	–	1641	–
	Total	131641	26694	5697	970	20027	3720	3770	74028	1712	12818	8899
		(17%)	(29%)	(89%)	(65%)	(10%)	(65%)	(11%)	(13%)		(13%)	

(To be conservative, no deaths before age 35, and none from liver cirrhosis or non–medical causes, were attributed to smoking.)

CZECH REPUBLIC: 1990

Smoking–attributed deaths (Sm.) and total deaths (Total)

		ALL CAUSES	ALL CANCER	Lung cancer	Upper aero–digestive ca.	Other cancer	COPD	Other respiratory	Vascular disease	Liver cirrhosis	Other medical	Non–medical
Males												
0–34	Sm.	–	–	–	–	–	–	–	–	–	–	–
	Total	2954	276	5	2	269	26	67	157	39	1037	1352
35–69	Sm.	13319	5255	3368	585	1302	741	196	5980	–	1147	–
	Total	31434	9294	3511	746	5037	858	448	14240	1303	2559	2732
		(42%)	(57%)	(96%)	(78%)	(26%)	(86%)	(44%)	(42%)		(45%)	
70+	Sm.	6074	2142	1346	140	656	876	98	2647	–	311	–
	Total	32080	6227	1463	223	4541	1162	762	20024	254	2353	1298
		(19%)	(34%)	(92%)	(63%)	(14%)	(75%)	(13%)	(13%)		(13%)	
Any age	Sm.	19393	7397	4714	725	1958	1617	294	8627	–	1458	–
	Total	66468	15797	4979	971	9847	2046	1277	34421	1596	5949	5382
		(29%)	(47%)	(95%)	(75%)	(20%)	(79%)	(23%)	(25%)		(25%)	
Females												
0–34	Sm.	–	–	–	–	–	–	–	–	–	–	–
	Total	1479	234	3	3	228	8	47	63	12	738	377
35–69	Sm.	1362	384	296	20	68	127	17	659	–	175	–
	Total	15953	5711	485	69	5157	268	175	6857	356	1770	816
		(9%)	(7%)	(61%)	(29%)	(1%)	(47%)	(10%)	(10%)		(10%)	
70+	Sm.	1520	293	202	26	65	265	26	838	–	98	–
	Total	45266	6433	363	103	5967	629	973	31055	217	3485	2474
		(3%)	(5%)	(56%)	(25%)	(1%)	(42%)	(3%)	(3%)		(3%)	
Any age	Sm.	2882	677	498	46	133	392	43	1497	–	273	–
	Total	62698	12378	851	175	11352	905	1195	37975	585	5993	3667
		(5%)	(5%)	(59%)	(26%)	(1%)	(43%)	(4%)	(4%)		(5%)	
Males+Females												
0–34	Sm.	–	–	–	–	–	–	–	–	–	–	–
	Total	4433	510	8	5	497	34	114	220	51	1775	1729
35–69	Sm.	14681	5639	3664	605	1370	868	213	6639	–	1322	–
	Total	47387	15005	3996	815	10194	1126	623	21097	1659	4329	3548
		(31%)	(38%)	(92%)	(74%)	(13%)	(77%)	(34%)	(31%)		(31%)	
70+	Sm.	7594	2435	1548	166	721	1141	124	3485	–	409	–
	Total	77346	12660	1826	326	10508	1791	1735	51079	471	5838	3772
		(10%)	(19%)	(85%)	(51%)	(7%)	(64%)	(7%)	(7%)		(7%)	
Any age	Sm.	22275	8074	5212	771	2091	2009	337	10124	–	1731	–
	Total	129166	28175	5830	1146	21199	2951	2472	72396	2181	11942	9049
		(17%)	(29%)	(89%)	(67%)	(10%)	(68%)	(14%)	(14%)		(14%)	

CZECH REPUBLIC: 1995

Smoking–attributed deaths (Sm.) and total deaths (Total)

		ALL CAUSES	ALL CANCER	Lung cancer	Upper aero–digestive ca.	Other cancer	COPD	Other respiratory	Vascular disease	Liver cirrhosis	Other medical	Non–medical
Males												
0–34	Sm.	–	–	–	–	–	–	–	–	–	–	–
	Total	2901	272	4	2	266	33	51	145	52	944	1404
35–69	Sm.	13682	5621	3499	744	1378	656	161	6014	–	1230	–
	Total	32401	9819	3645	946	5228	757	357	13987	1791	2645	3045
		(42%)	(57%)	(96%)	(79%)	(26%)	(87%)	(45%)	(43%)		(47%)	
70+	Sm.	5843	2208	1373	134	701	619	69	2663	–	284	–
	Total	30860	6670	1492	216	4962	833	528	19235	269	2063	1262
		(19%)	(33%)	(92%)	(62%)	(14%)	(74%)	(13%)	(14%)		(14%)	
Any age	Sm.	19525	7829	4872	878	2079	1275	230	8677	–	1514	–
	Total	66162	16761	5141	1164	10456	1623	936	33367	2112	5652	5711
		(30%)	(47%)	(95%)	(75%)	(20%)	(79%)	(25%)	(26%)		(27%)	
Females												
0–34	Sm.	–	–	–	–	–	–	–	–	–	–	–
	Total	1418	261	3	4	254	8	35	65	13	627	409
35–69	Sm.	1509	480	364	30	86	106	16	724	–	183	–
	Total	15027	5763	549	86	5128	204	128	6210	426	1517	779
		(10%)	(8%)	(66%)	(35%)	(2%)	(52%)	(13%)	(12%)		(12%)	
70+	Sm.	1722	373	258	30	85	219	24	985	–	121	–
	Total	41807	7060	426	107	6527	465	680	28044	209	3219	2130
		(4%)	(5%)	(61%)	(28%)	(1%)	(47%)	(4%)	(4%)		(4%)	
Any age	Sm.	3231	853	622	60	171	325	40	1709	–	304	–
	Total	58252	13084	978	197	11909	677	843	34319	648	5363	3318
		(6%)	(7%)	(64%)	(30%)	(1%)	(48%)	(5%)	(5%)		(6%)	
Males+Females												
0–34	Sm.	–	–	–	–	–	–	–	–	–	–	–
	Total	4319	533	7	6	520	41	86	210	65	1571	1813
35–69	Sm.	15191	6101	3863	774	1464	762	177	6738	–	1413	–
	Total	47428	15582	4194	1032	10356	961	485	20197	2217	4162	3824
		(32%)	(39%)	(92%)	(75%)	(14%)	(79%)	(36%)	(33%)		(34%)	
70+	Sm.	7565	2581	1631	164	786	838	93	3648	–	405	–
	Total	72667	13730	1918	323	11489	1298	1208	47279	478	5282	3392
		(10%)	(19%)	(85%)	(51%)	(7%)	(65%)	(8%)	(8%)		(8%)	
Any age	Sm.	22756	8682	5494	938	2250	1600	270	10386	–	1818	–
	Total	124414	29845	6119	1361	22365	2300	1779	67686	2760	11015	9029
		(18%)	(29%)	(90%)	(69%)	(10%)	(70%)	(15%)	(15%)		(17%)	

(To be conservative, no deaths before age 35, and none from liver cirrhosis or non-medical causes, were attributed to smoking.)

¶Former CZECHOSLOVAKIA: 1990

		No. of deaths			Standardised rates (Defined on p.316)			Annual death rates / 100, 000						
		All ages	**0–34**	**35–69**	**All ages**	**0–34**	**35–69**	**0–4**	**5–9**	**10–14**	**15–19**	**20–24**	**25–29**	**30–34**
ALL CAUSES	**M**	96731	4957	46674	1515.3	124.8	1850.5	295.1	30.9	25.9	76.9	127.7	132.6	184.2
	F	87054	2439	23180	845.9	64.0	768.2	218.9	19.5	18.4	38.9	39.1	43.0	70.3
Tuberculosis	**M**	174	2	113	2.7	0.0	4.3	–	–	–	–	–	–	0.3
	F	109	1	29	1.1	0.0	1.0	–	–	–	0.2	–	–	–
Other infective and parasitic	**M**	124	21	68	1.9	0.5	2.6	1.8	0.5	0.1	0.2	0.2	0.4	0.5
	F	164	17	61	1.8	0.5	2.0	2.7	–	0.2	–	–	0.2	0.2
ALL CANCER	**M**	22073	429	13318	344.6	10.5	537.4	7.9	8.0	5.1	9.1	11.4	13.5	18.7
	F	16408	354	7917	176.7	9.1	260.6	7.3	3.6	4.9	5.4	7.1	12.8	22.5
Mouth and pharynx cancer	**M**	813	3	693	12.6	0.1	25.6	–	–	–	–	–	0.4	0.2
	F	128	5	54	1.3	0.1	1.8	–	–	–	–	–	0.4	0.5
Oesophagus cancer	**M**	457	2	347	7.0	0.1	13.4	–	–	–	–	0.2	–	0.2
	F	79	1	29	0.8	0.0	1.0	–	–	–	–	0.2	–	–
Stomach cancer	**M**	1853	15	957	29.2	0.4	39.3	–	–	–	–	–	1.1	1.6
	F	1355	11	498	13.9	0.3	16.3	–	–	–	–	–	0.9	1.1
Colorectal cancer	**M**	2988	14	1537	47.1	0.4	63.3	–	–	–	–	–	1.1	1.4
	F	2478	14	968	25.5	0.4	32.4	–	–	–	0.3	–	0.8	1.4
Liver cancer	**M**	453	7	278	7.1	0.2	11.2	0.4	–	–	–	0.2	–	0.7
	F	284	5	159	3.1	0.1	5.3	0.4	–	–	–	–	–	0.5
Pancreas cancer	**M**	1032	6	641	16.1	0.2	25.8	–	–	–	–	0.2	0.4	0.5
	F	872	7	403	9.0	0.2	13.5	–	–	–	0.2	0.2	0.4	0.5
Larynx cancer	**M**	514	1	392	7.9	0.0	15.0	–	–	–	–	–	–	0.2
	F	39	1	23	0.5	0.0	0.8	–	–	–	–	–	–	0.2
Lung cancer	**M**	6909	13	4900	108.0	0.3	199.6	–	–	–	–	0.2	0.2	1.9
	F	1125	4	628	12.4	0.1	20.9	–	–	–	–	–	0.4	0.4
Malignant melanoma	**M**	223	9	152	3.4	0.2	5.7	–	–	–	–	0.4	0.5	0.7
	F	211	10	105	2.3	0.3	3.3	–	–	–	–	0.6	0.2	1.1
Female breast cancer	**F**	2521	33	1476	28.6	0.9	48.3	–	–	–	–	0.4	0.6	5.0
Cervix cancer	**F**	604	37	382	7.0	1.0	11.9	–	–	–	–	–	1.7	5.0
Other uterine cancer	**F**	787	5	403	8.4	0.1	13.3	–	–	–	–	–	0.4	0.5
Ovarian cancer	**F**	1014	18	664	11.8	0.5	21.7	–	–	0.2	0.3	0.8	0.8	1.3
Prostate cancer	**M**	1417	1	398	22.7	0.0	17.4	–	–	–	–	–	0.2	–
Bladder cancer	**M**	778	1	369	12.4	0.0	15.8	0.2	–	–	–	–	–	–
	F	219	1	69	2.2	0.0	2.3	–	–	–	–	–	–	0.2
Other and ill–defined cancer sites	**M**	3411	205	2007	52.6	5.0	79.5	5.3	2.7	2.2	5.5	5.7	7.6	6.2
	F	3652	114	1590	38.5	2.9	52.8	4.6	1.8	2.6	2.1	2.7	3.4	3.2
Hodgkin's disease	**M**	110	16	68	1.6	0.4	2.5	–	–	0.1	0.3	0.4	0.4	1.6
	F	81	9	37	1.0	0.2	1.2	–	–	0.2	0.2	0.8	0.4	0.2
Myeloma and non–Hodgkin lymphomas	**M**	474	34	270	7.3	0.8	10.9	–	1.7	0.3	1.1	1.1	0.7	0.9
	F	464	15	209	5.0	0.4	6.9	0.4	0.4	0.3	0.8	0.2	0.2	0.4
Leukaemia	**M**	641	102	309	9.6	2.5	12.3	2.0	3.6	2.5	2.1	3.1	1.1	2.8
	F	495	64	220	5.4	1.6	7.1	1.9	1.4	1.7	1.6	1.3	2.5	0.9
ALL VASCULAR DISEASE	**M**	49156	300	20750	785.5	7.5	850.6	1.3	0.5	1.2	2.8	7.6	11.4	27.7
	F	52368	121	10094	481.4	3.1	339.8	2.5	0.4	0.3	2.2	3.3	4.5	8.8
Rheumatic heart disease and fever	**M**	345	12	249	5.4	0.3	9.6	–	–	0.1	0.2	0.4	0.5	0.9
	F	492	2	315	5.6	0.1	10.6	–	–	–	–	–	0.2	0.2
Hypertensive disease	**M**	625	2	340	9.8	0.1	13.6	–	–	–	–	0.2	–	0.2
	F	781	1	243	7.7	0.0	8.2	–	–	–	–	–	–	0.2
Ischaemic heart disease	**M**	26685	118	12635	424.4	2.9	516.9	–	–	–	0.3	1.8	3.4	15.1
	F	23407	17	4719	216.2	0.4	159.5	–	–	–	0.2	0.4	0.9	1.6
Pulmonary embolism and other venous	**M**	384	3	190	6.0	0.1	7.6	–	–	–	–	–	–	0.5
	F	538	3	174	5.3	0.1	5.8	–	–	–	–	–	–	0.5
Cerebrovascular disease	**M**	12752	49	4395	205.3	1.2	183.0	–	0.2	0.4	0.9	2.0	1.8	3.1
	F	17175	31	3018	156.5	0.8	101.5	0.6	–	–	0.8	0.6	0.9	2.7
Other vascular disease	**M**	8365	116	2941	134.5	2.9	119.8	1.3	0.3	0.6	1.4	3.1	5.6	8.0
	F	9975	67	1625	90.0	1.7	54.1	1.9	0.4	0.3	1.3	2.3	2.5	3.6
Chronic obstructive pulmonary disease	**M**	2466	32	1029	39.3	0.8	42.5	0.4	0.2	0.3	0.5	0.9	1.6	1.7
	F	1103	10	315	10.7	0.2	10.5	0.4	0.2	0.2	0.5	0.2	–	0.4
Other respiratory disease	**M**	3052	209	1035	48.6	5.2	40.6	21.1	2.2	2.5	3.4	1.1	2.0	4.3
	F	2781	156	449	26.0	4.1	14.9	19.1	1.4	2.0	0.6	1.2	2.6	2.0
Peptic ulcer	**M**	561	7	311	8.7	0.2	12.1	0.2	–	–	0.2	–	0.4	0.5
	F	297	1	93	2.9	0.0	3.1	0.2	–	–	–	–	–	–
Liver cirrhosis	**M**	2867	85	2370	43.2	2.1	86.6	0.2	–	–	–	0.6	3.6	10.6
	F	997	26	658	11.8	0.7	21.2	0.2	0.2	–	0.3	0.2	0.8	3.1
Renal disease	**M**	1371	32	685	21.4	0.8	26.8	0.9	0.2	0.1	0.5	0.9	0.9	2.1
	F	1502	29	610	15.5	0.7	20.4	1.1	0.5	0.3	0.6	0.6	0.8	1.3
Pregnancy and birth	**F**	16	8	8	0.2	0.2	0.2	–	–	–	–	0.6	0.4	0.5
Congenital and perinatal causes	**M**	1209	1207	2	17.7	31.6	0.1	215.7	1.5	1.2	1.1	0.7	0.4	0.7
	F	821	817	4	12.4	22.2	0.1	150.4	1.8	1.4	1.0	0.4	0.2	0.5
Ill–defined causes	**M**	755	59	232	12.2	1.5	8.4	4.6	0.2	–	0.5	1.1	1.4	2.8
	F	1024	36	83	9.0	1.0	2.6	4.2	–	–	0.5	0.6	0.9	0.5
Other medical causes	**M**	4637	359	2379	71.1	8.9	90.3	15.3	4.8	3.0	5.4	7.2	10.6	16.3
	F	4760	268	1691	49.0	6.9	55.7	12.8	3.8	4.3	5.6	4.6	5.7	11.3
ALL NON–MEDICAL CAUSES	**M**	8286	2215	4382	118.4	55.0	148.2	25.7	12.8	12.4	53.6	96.0	86.4	98.0
	F	4704	595	1168	47.3	15.2	36.3	18.0	7.7	5.0	22.0	20.4	14.1	19.2
Motor vehicle traffic accidents	**M**	1582	694	730	21.5	17.2	24.4	4.4	5.3	4.0	21.9	38.9	23.6	21.8
	F	545	197	181	6.3	4.9	5.6	2.1	3.9	1.7	12.2	7.5	3.8	3.2
Fire	**M**	130	26	62	1.9	0.6	2.3	–	0.7	0.1	0.8	1.1	0.7	1.0
	F	71	7	16	0.7	0.2	0.5	0.6	0.2	–	0.2	0.4	–	–
Suicide	**M**	2082	441	1298	29.8	11.0	43.4	–	–	1.2	8.6	16.6	21.8	28.7
	F	716	121	398	8.4	3.1	12.3	–	–	0.5	3.0	5.8	4.3	8.3
Homicide	**M**	176	60	96	2.4	1.5	3.0	1.3	0.2	0.1	1.1	1.5	3.4	2.9
	F	130	53	56	1.6	1.4	1.6	1.9	0.5	0.5	1.3	1.7	1.9	1.8
POPULATION (thousands):	**M=males**				7627.1	4146.1	3079.2	543.9	585.2	691.8	651.7	541.8	554.2	577.5
	F=females				8033.5	3970.1	3345.7	522.7	558.9	658.8	624.1	519.2	530.2	556.2

Former CZECHOSLOVAKIA: 1990

Annual death rates / 100, 000

9th ICD categories

35–39	40–44	45–49	50–54	55–59	60–64	65–69	70–74	75–79	80+/NK			
298.7	491.0	842.5	1356.7	2031.6	3189.8	4743.3	6705.9	10371.0	18112.5	M	ALL CAUSES	001–999
111.7	183.0	298.6	470.3	800.2	1282.4	2231.0	3747.3	6625.2	14578.4	F		
0.5	1.9	3.2	5.2	5.2	5.5	8.9	9.2	12.7	24.3	M	Tuberculosis	010–018, 137
0.2	–	0.2	0.3	2.2	2.6	1.4	4.7	8.6	18.7	F		
0.8	0.3	2.6	1.6	3.5	4.0	5.3	5.0	7.4	15.3	M	Other infective	Rest of 001–139
0.3	1.4	1.5	1.8	1.5	2.8	4.5	5.7	11.0	18.3	F	and parasitic	
46.6	100.0	207.6	422.0	656.8	973.7	1354.9	1700.9	2163.1	2421.2	M	ALL CANCER	140–208
44.7	78.3	133.8	190.2	315.3	442.8	619.1	809.2	1141.7	1399.3	F		
3.5	13.0	24.4	36.2	34.9	32.0	35.5	29.1	24.1	36.0	M	Mouth and	140–149
0.6	0.5	0.6	1.8	2.2	3.3	3.3	3.8	8.6	15.5	F	pharynx cancer	
1.4	3.9	8.6	13.9	20.2	24.2	21.7	15.6	37.4	27.0	M	Oesophagus cancer	150
–	0.2	0.4	0.5	1.7	2.3	1.7	1.4	7.5	10.7	F		
2.4	6.2	11.8	26.1	45.5	69.0	114.4	162.3	229.9	277.2	M	Stomach cancer	151
3.7	5.4	7.1	11.9	17.4	25.4	43.5	78.4	110.7	158.4	F		
4.9	5.9	20.3	45.1	66.8	120.6	179.8	253.7	381.7	457.2	M	Colorectal cancer	153, 154
2.7	5.2	12.9	19.7	40.9	55.9	89.1	136.0	207.2	270.7	F		
1.4	2.7	2.8	9.2	12.5	19.3	30.6	39.0	38.8	49.5	M	Liver cancer	155.0
0.8	0.5	1.0	2.5	6.8	12.0	13.6	17.0	18.1	15.1	F		
2.2	5.9	8.6	21.2	28.6	54.0	59.8	76.5	107.6	104.4	M	Pancreas cancer	157
0.6	2.5	4.6	6.1	12.1	26.3	42.0	42.0	77.3	70.1	F		
1.9	5.7	11.1	15.5	18.8	21.9	30.2	27.6	34.8	27.0	M	Larynx cancer	161
0.2	0.2	0.6	1.0	1.2	0.5	1.7	1.4	0.8	4.0	F		
7.3	29.0	70.8	162.0	265.5	371.3	491.0	518.8	504.7	458.1	M	Lung cancer	162
1.8	5.1	9.5	13.1	28.6	38.8	49.2	57.6	76.1	70.5	F		
1.6	2.5	3.9	4.9	7.1	11.0	8.9	12.8	13.4	21.6	M	Malignant melanoma	172
1.5	2.2	2.9	2.8	2.7	4.9	6.2	9.0	13.0	17.5	F		
7.7	18.1	35.7	48.0	60.3	81.0	87.2	99.2	146.0	171.2	F	Female breast cancer	174
6.9	9.6	8.3	9.1	13.3	17.6	18.2	21.7	25.9	29.1	F	Cervix cancer	180
2.7	2.2	5.6	7.3	15.7	21.1	38.7	43.5	53.8	59.7	F	Other uterine cancer	179, 182
4.4	8.5	13.5	18.9	29.1	35.7	41.8	45.8	47.5	45.4	F	Ovarian cancer	183
–	–	0.9	3.3	13.4	34.9	69.7	146.7	276.7	357.3	M	Prostate cancer	185
0.2	1.0	1.7	4.9	16.6	29.4	56.9	84.3	94.9	132.3	M	Bladder cancer	188
0.5	0.5	0.2	1.8	2.9	2.1	8.1	13.7	19.6	27.9	F		
14.5	18.3	34.0	60.6	95.1	141.4	192.2	243.8	298.1	368.1	M	Other and ill-defined	Rest of 140–208
7.1	11.3	22.8	36.1	64.9	90.0	137.3	177.6	263.7	358.3	F	cancer sites	
0.9	1.5	1.3	3.5	3.3	2.0	4.9	3.5	8.7	7.2	M	Hodgkin's disease	201
0.5	0.8	1.2	1.0	1.7	1.4	1.4	6.6	3.9	4.4	F		
2.1	1.7	1.9	8.4	13.1	22.5	26.6	41.1	45.5	39.6	M	Myeloma and non-	200, 202–203
0.8	2.0	4.2	3.8	7.0	12.9	17.4	29.8	33.4	36.6	F	Hodgkin lymphomas	
2.4	2.7	5.6	7.1	15.3	20.2	32.9	46.1	66.8	58.5	M	Leukaemia	204–208
2.1	3.4	2.7	4.8	6.8	11.5	18.6	24.6	28.6	34.2	F		
60.2	145.4	295.4	518.8	876.2	1547.6	2510.4	3815.7	6274.1	12003.6	M	ALL VASCULAR	390–459
18.4	38.9	73.0	159.6	313.8	576.0	1198.5	2248.5	4334.8	10488.9	F	DISEASE	
1.3	3.0	5.6	10.1	15.5	14.4	17.4	25.5	17.4	19.8	M	Rheumatic heart	390–398
0.3	1.5	4.4	9.9	14.0	17.9	26.3	24.1	27.9	21.1	F	disease and fever	
1.3	3.0	6.4	10.6	15.5	23.9	34.5	45.4	70.9	101.7	M	Hypertensive disease	401–405
0.2	0.8	1.0	5.8	12.3	11.7	25.8	39.7	59.3	120.2	F		
33.5	86.7	184.1	330.1	561.3	954.4	1468.0	2067.3	3159.8	5659.8	M	Ischaemic heart	410–414
4.0	12.3	28.2	59.6	149.9	289.9	572.2	1084.6	1939.6	4551.4	F	disease	
0.9	1.7	4.1	4.4	7.1	13.8	21.4	30.5	50.8	64.8	M	Pulmonary embolism	415.1, 451–453
0.3	1.7	1.5	3.0	5.3	10.3	18.4	25.0	47.9	74.0	F	and other venous	
9.6	26.8	53.3	86.5	163.8	337.0	604.3	1065.9	1869.0	3607.6	M	Cerebrovascular	430–438
6.9	11.2	20.5	43.2	85.7	168.2	374.7	746.3	1514.9	3457.8	F	disease	
13.6	24.2	42.0	77.2	112.9	204.0	364.8	581.1	1106.3	2550.0	M	Other vascular	Rest of 390–459
6.6	11.3	17.4	38.1	46.5	78.0	181.0	328.8	745.3	2264.3	F	disease	
2.5	6.2	12.8	23.7	44.2	81.4	126.5	197.7	317.5	586.0	M	Chronic obstructive	490–496
1.3	2.0	5.0	5.8	11.1	19.7	28.2	51.5	78.5	186.7	F	pulmonary disease	
8.1	14.3	18.2	28.3	41.4	67.2	106.8	204.1	378.3	858.7	M	Other respiratory	Rest of 460–519
1.6	4.1	5.8	7.8	10.2	26.1	48.5	102.0	197.0	580.4	F	disease	
2.4	3.9	8.1	8.2	12.3	21.6	27.9	41.1	64.2	80.1	M	Peptic ulcer	531–533
0.6	0.8	0.4	1.0	3.1	5.6	9.8	12.8	23.9	45.8	F		
27.2	45.3	72.8	92.7	112.1	134.4	121.9	106.3	104.3	95.4	M	Liver cirrhosis	571
5.5	11.2	16.2	21.5	31.0	28.7	34.6	41.6	44.3	44.6	F		
6.6	7.1	12.8	21.8	31.1	39.5	69.0	82.9	167.8	257.4	M	Renal disease	580–590
2.6	3.4	5.4	12.6	21.5	38.3	58.8	79.4	118.9	156.1	F		
1.0	0.2	0.2	–	–	–	–	–	–	–	F	Pregnancy and birth	630–676
0.2	–	–	–	–	–	0.3	–	–	–	M	Congenital and	740–779
0.3	0.2	0.2	–	–	–	–	–	–	–	F	perinatal causes	
3.6	4.5	6.4	8.2	8.5	14.4	13.5	15.6	50.1	330.3	M	Ill-defined causes	780–799
1.3	1.4	2.5	2.3	1.7	4.5	4.8	17.9	38.1	306.5	F		
28.5	38.4	56.9	70.7	89.7	133.6	214.6	294.1	463.9	711.1	M	Other medical causes	Rest of 001–799
12.4	13.7	24.9	36.9	55.4	88.6	157.9	237.1	356.4	553.7	F		
111.5	123.7	145.5	155.8	150.8	166.8	183.4	233.2	367.6	729.1	M	ALL NON-	E800–E999
21.5	27.6	29.5	30.6	33.4	46.7	65.0	137.0	272.0	779.5	F	MEDICAL CAUSES	
19.1	23.2	21.8	27.2	24.0	28.6	26.9	34.0	37.4	48.6	M	Motor vehicle	E810–E819
5.0	3.9	4.4	7.1	4.6	7.8	6.2	17.9	24.7	26.3	F	traffic accidents	
1.6	1.2	0.6	1.9	1.4	4.3	4.9	7.8	8.0	17.1	M	Fire	E890–E899
–	–	0.4	0.3	0.2	0.9	1.9	2.8	4.3	12.3	F		
33.8	38.2	47.3	50.8	43.6	38.4	51.3	60.9	80.9	122.4	M	Suicide	E950–E959
7.6	10.2	12.5	9.9	12.1	15.5	18.2	22.7	21.2	37.8	F		
3.8	3.7	2.4	1.6	3.0	3.5	3.3	2.8	4.0	9.0	M	Homicide	E960–E969
1.8	2.9	0.2	1.8	1.0	2.3	1.4	1.9	2.4	4.4	F		
632.4	594.1	467.2	367.8	366.8	346.6	304.3	141.1	149.6	111.1	M	**POPULATION (thousands)**	
619.4	591.1	481.9	395.9	413.0	425.7	418.7	211.7	254.8	251.2	F		

Former CZECHOSLOVAKIA: Males

	All ages	0–34	35–69	35–39	40–44	45–49	50–54	55–59	60–64	65–69	70–74	75–79	80+/NK
POPULATION (1000s)													
1955	6377.7	3724.2	2379.8	294.7	453.6	463.3	419.8	329.8	239.5	179.1	132.9	82.3	58.5
1965	6910.9	3892.1	2712.7	475.1	492.5	283.8	434.3	425.8	352.5	248.7	151.8	89.7	64.6
1975	7211.4	4141.7	2667.1	407.7	432.0	446.7	452.4	250.9	362.1	315.3	215.5	117.5	69.6
1985	7547.9	4255.7	2819.3	604.9	481.9	386.8	397.2	393.0	369.1	186.4	227.6	151.4	93.9
1990	**7627.1**	**4146.1**	**3079.2**	**632.4**	**594.1**	**467.2**	**367.8**	**366.8**	**346.6**	**304.3**	**141.1**	**149.6**	**111.1**
1995 projected	*7746.0*	*4120.0*	*3192.2*	*591.2*	*621.4*	*563.2*	*437.1*	*341.1*	*341.1*	*297.1*	*231.9*	*90.6*	*111.3*
NUMBER OF DEATHS													
All causes													
1955	65871	10279	29542	715	1679	2933	4438	5830	6561	7386	8239	7843	9968
1965	74399	7819	35705	1182	1834	1568	4041	6641	9517	10922	10048	8872	11955
1975	89642	7878	39813	1187	1947	3060	5152	4322	10021	14124	15333	12846	13772
1985	95202	5622	39450	1618	2248	3013	5053	7613	11616	8289	15992	16351	17787
1990	**96731**	**4957**	**46674**	**1889**	**2917**	**3936**	**4990**	**7452**	**11056**	**14434**	**9462**	**15515**	**20123**
1995 projected	*98010*	*4755*	*49284*	*1873*	*3300*	*5077*	*6313*	*7185*	*11393*	*14143*	*15257*	*8962*	*19752*
Lung cancer													
1955	2435	24	1948	13	51	134	342	509	507	392	287	133	43
1965	4883	26	3547	35	80	87	348	705	1115	1177	791	334	185
1975	6198	21	3856	36	99	254	509	497	1050	1411	1276	727	318
1985	6723	14	4245	56	155	293	638	947	1374	782	1163	836	465
1990	**6909**	**13**	**4900**	**46**	**172**	**331**	**596**	**974**	**1287**	**1494**	**732**	**755**	**509**
1995 projected	*7258*	*11*	*5146*	*38*	*162*	*386*	*733*	*926*	*1371*	*1530*	*1210*	*416*	*475*
ANNUAL DEATH RATE / 100,000 (*The rates for the age groups 0–34 and 35–69 are the means of seven five-yearly rates, but the all-ages rates are standardised to the conventional "European" age distribution)													
All causes													
1955	1418.5*	250.2*	1562.0*	242.6	370.1	633.1	1057.2	1767.7	2739.5	4124.0	6199.4	9529.8	17039.3
1965	1425.5*	205.0*	1536.5*	248.8	372.4	552.5	930.5	1559.7	2699.9	4391.6	6619.2	9890.7	18506.2
1975	1523.5*	182.1*	1647.9*	291.1	450.7	685.0	1138.8	1722.6	2767.5	4479.5	7115.1	10932.8	19787.4
1985	1521.7*	134.9*	1759.5*	267.5	466.5	779.0	1272.2	1937.2	3147.1	4446.9	7026.4	10799.9	18942.5
1990	**1515.3***	**124.8***	**1850.5***	**298.7**	**491.0**	**842.5**	**1356.7**	**2031.6**	**3189.8**	**4743.3**	**6705.9**	**10371.0**	**18112.5**
1995 projected	*1517.9**	*118.2**	*1914.4**	*316.8*	*531.1*	*901.5*	*1444.3*	*2106.4*	*3340.1*	*4760.4*	*6579.1*	*9891.8*	*17746.6*
All cancer													
1955	235.0*	11.6*	385.5*	33.9	65.9	140.1	281.3	471.5	725.3	980.5	1195.6	1397.3	1254.7
1965	291.1*	12.8*	444.5*	39.1	76.5	124.7	258.3	466.9	848.8	1297.1	1702.2	1878.5	1941.2
1975	314.4*	12.1*	458.4*	43.9	92.6	166.8	311.5	526.1	817.5	1250.2	1738.3	2171.1	2366.4
1985	325.7*	10.9*	495.2*	46.6	108.1	208.1	402.3	586.8	930.9	1183.5	1674.0	2035.7	2335.5
1990	**344.6***	**10.5***	**537.4***	**46.6**	**100.0**	**207.6**	**422.0**	**656.8**	**973.7**	**1354.9**	**1700.9**	**2163.1**	**2421.2**
1995 projected	*363.1**	*10.1**	*571.8**	*43.5*	*98.8*	*211.6*	*453.7*	*698.6*	*1067.4*	*1429.1*	*1787.0*	*2197.6*	*2573.2*
Lung cancer													
1955	48.9*	0.7*	101.6*	4.4	11.2	28.9	81.5	154.3	211.7	218.9	216.0	161.6	73.5
1965	83.3*	0.8*	155.6*	7.4	16.2	30.7	80.1	165.6	316.3	473.3	521.1	372.4	286.4
1975	97.9*	0.6*	162.4*	8.8	22.9	56.9	112.5	198.1	290.0	447.5	592.1	618.7	456.9
1985	105.7*	0.3*	187.2*	9.3	32.2	75.7	160.6	241.0	372.3	419.5	511.0	552.2	495.2
1990	**108.0***	**0.3***	**199.6***	**7.3**	**29.0**	**70.8**	**162.0**	**265.5**	**371.3**	**491.0**	**518.8**	**504.7**	**458.1**
1995 projected	*109.3**	*0.3**	*208.2**	*6.4*	*26.1*	*68.5*	*167.7*	*271.5*	*401.9*	*515.0*	*521.8*	*459.2*	*426.8*
Upper aerodigestive cancer (mouth, oesophagus, pharynx and larynx)													
1955	14.8*	0.2*	20.5*	1.0	2.2	8.4	13.6	27.6	35.1	55.8	84.3	105.7	135.0
1965	13.9*	0.1*	20.4*	1.7	3.2	5.3	11.7	22.5	33.5	65.1	69.2	94.8	134.7
1975	16.7*	0.3*	24.7*	2.5	7.6	14.3	24.3	32.7	39.5	51.7	72.4	110.6	135.1
1985	22.2*	0.2*	39.6*	5.8	17.0	30.2	51.1	53.4	58.0	61.7	74.7	99.7	99.0
1990	**27.5***	**0.2***	**54.1***	**6.8**	**22.6**	**44.1**	**65.5**	**73.9**	**78.2**	**87.4**	**72.3**	**96.3**	**90.0**
1995 projected	*33.8**	*0.2**	*69.6**	*8.5*	*29.4*	*56.5*	*86.5*	*97.3*	*104.1*	*105.0*	*76.8*	*89.4*	*85.4*
Other cancer													
1955	171.2*	10.8*	263.4*	28.5	52.5	102.7	186.3	289.6	478.5	705.8	895.4	1130.0	1046.2
1965	193.9*	11.9*	268.4*	30.1	57.1	88.8	166.5	278.8	499.0	758.7	1112.0	1411.4	1520.1
1975	199.9*	11.2*	271.3*	32.6	62.0	95.6	174.6	295.3	488.0	751.0	1073.8	1441.7	1774.4
1985	197.8*	10.4*	268.4*	31.6	58.9	102.1	190.6	292.4	500.7	702.3	1088.3	1383.8	1741.2
1990	**209.1***	**10.1***	**283.7***	**32.6**	**48.5**	**92.7**	**194.4**	**317.3**	**524.2**	**776.5**	**1109.9**	**1562.2**	**1873.1**
1995 projected	*220.0**	*9.7**	*294.1**	*28.6*	*43.3*	*86.6*	*199.5*	*329.8*	*561.4*	*809.2*	*1188.4*	*1649.0*	*2061.1*
Chronic obstructive pulmonary disease (COPD)													
1955	31.3*	1.1*	34.5*	2.7	5.1	7.3	25.0	41.5	62.6	97.2	152.7	261.2	429.1
1965	99.5*	0.8*	107.4*	4.6	7.1	12.3	38.7	95.3	207.4	386.0	555.3	901.9	1422.6
1975	103.8*	0.9*	91.6*	5.6	10.4	23.5	48.2	77.7	157.1	318.4	611.1	956.6	1722.7
1985	60.7*	0.8*	49.7*	2.3	5.2	15.3	28.4	57.3	97.5	142.2	310.2	581.2	1092.7
1990	**39.3***	**0.8***	**42.5***	**2.5**	**6.2**	**12.8**	**23.7**	**44.2**	**81.4**	**126.5**	**197.7**	**317.5**	**586.0**
1995 projected	*30.1**	*0.9**	*35.7**	*3.6*	*5.8*	*11.0*	*19.0*	*36.1*	*70.4*	*104.0*	*146.6*	*219.6*	*415.1*
Other respiratory disease													
1955	79.9*	27.4*	52.9*	5.4	10.1	16.0	24.1	58.8	97.7	158.0	347.6	575.9	1210.3
1965	54.3*	13.6*	33.9*	3.2	4.9	10.6	19.3	21.8	57.0	120.2	205.5	385.7	1066.6
1975	62.3*	13.2*	35.1*	5.4	8.8	12.8	14.4	28.7	58.3	117.7	244.5	541.3	1232.8
1985	65.1*	8.7*	54.2*	8.3	10.0	22.2	39.5	52.7	93.2	153.4	250.0	519.2	1150.2
1990	**48.6***	**5.2***	**40.6***	**8.1**	**14.3**	**18.2**	**28.3**	**41.4**	**67.2**	**106.8**	**204.1**	**378.3**	**858.7**
1995 projected	*37.0**	*3.9**	*30.8**	*8.8*	*14.3*	*15.4*	*21.5*	*29.9*	*47.5*	*78.4*	*148.8*	*290.3*	*660.4*
Vascular disease													
1955	605.1*	16.9*	647.4*	46.5	93.0	203.1	363.0	691.0	1169.1	1965.9	3175.3	5002.4	8666.7
1965	624.3*	10.8*	603.7*	56.4	115.1	200.1	340.1	592.5	1080.6	1840.8	3063.9	5073.6	10626.9
1975	724.7*	7.8*	729.7*	76.3	134.5	248.3	467.9	738.5	1292.5	2149.7	3592.1	5864.7	11801.7
1985	782.3*	7.2*	824.1*	64.0	146.1	280.2	506.3	870.5	1548.1	2353.5	3903.8	6360.0	12042.6
1990	**785.5***	**7.5***	**850.6***	**60.2**	**145.4**	**295.4**	**518.8**	**876.2**	**1547.6**	**2510.4**	**3815.7**	**6274.1**	**12003.6**
1995 projected	*780.0**	*7.2**	*857.9**	*58.7*	*146.9*	*298.8*	*526.2*	*873.9*	*1589.0*	*2511.9*	*3753.8*	*6030.9*	*11936.2*
Liver cirrhosis													
1955	10.1*	0.2*	17.1*	2.0	4.9	8.6	17.2	17.6	27.1	42.4	55.7	52.2	42.7
1965	16.3*	0.7*	27.9*	2.9	9.1	16.2	19.3	34.8	48.5	64.7	75.8	74.7	86.7
1975	28.8*	1.6*	53.4*	12.8	28.9	38.3	46.4	63.0	81.5	103.1	103.0	91.9	114.9
1985	31.8*	1.3*	61.3*	15.7	32.8	46.3	60.7	70.5	93.5	110.0	99.7	107.7	91.6
1990	**43.2***	**2.1***	**86.6***	**27.2**	**45.3**	**72.8**	**92.7**	**112.1**	**134.4**	**121.9**	**106.3**	**104.3**	**95.4**
1995 projected	*55.9**	*2.9**	*115.4**	*37.7*	*63.2*	*100.9*	*129.7*	*156.0*	*176.2*	*144.1*	*109.5*	*109.3*	*94.3*
Other medical causes													
1955	352.1*	123.0*	308.5*	65.5	92.2	147.4	227.5	363.3	525.3	738.7	1099.3	1944.1	4926.5
1965	224.2*	93.2*	189.4*	34.3	55.6	73.6	127.6	205.7	316.0	513.1	799.1	1262.0	2738.4
1975	170.1*	78.2*	145.1*	41.7	54.9	73.9	116.7	151.5	210.7	366.6	572.6	938.7	1837.6
1985	145.0*	52.3*	141.6*	35.2	53.1	76.8	101.5	155.2	240.9	328.9	547.9	825.0	1525.0
1990	**135.7***	**43.6***	**144.7***	**42.5**	**56.1**	**90.1**	**115.6**	**150.2**	**218.7**	**339.5**	**447.9**	**766.0**	**1418.5**
1995 projected	*127.0**	*37.0**	*141.4**	*44.3*	*63.4*	*101.0*	*122.4*	*144.8*	*211.4*	*302.6*	*404.1*	*686.5*	*1323.5*
All non-medical causes													
1955	105.0*	70.0*	116.1*	86.5	99.0	110.5	119.1	124.0	132.4	141.3	173.1	296.5	509.4
1965	115.9*	73.2*	129.7*	108.2	104.0	114.9	127.1	142.6	141.6	169.7	217.4	314.4	623.8
1975	119.4*	68.3*	134.6*	105.5	120.6	121.6	133.7	137.1	150.0	173.8	253.4	368.5	711.2
1985	111.2*	53.8*	133.3*	95.4	111.2	130.0	133.4	144.3	143.1	175.4	240.8	371.2	705.0
1990	**118.4***	**55.0***	**148.2***	**111.5**	**123.7**	**145.5**	**155.8**	**150.8**	**166.8**	**183.4**	**233.2**	**367.6**	**729.1**
1995 projected	*124.7**	*56.2**	*161.3**	*120.3*	*138.6*	*162.6*	*171.8*	*167.1*	*178.2*	*190.2*	*229.4*	*357.6*	*743.9*

Former CZECHOSLOVAKIA: Females

	All ages	0–34	35–69	35–39	40–44	45–49	50–54	55–59	60–64	65–69	70–74	75–79	80+/NK
POPULATION (1000s)													
1955	6715.0	3673.7	2661.6	309.3	474.4	488.5	448.8	392.9	304.2	243.5	182.5	112.5	84.7
1965	7247.8	3765.8	2981.9	489.8	521.7	302.2	463.2	461.4	408.6	335.0	234.5	149.4	116.2
1975	7590.3	3981.2	2930.1	412.9	442.1	473.7	499.4	284.4	421.3	396.3	314.0	210.9	154.1
1985	7950.7	4080.9	3065.2	595.8	488.0	403.7	426.4	448.5	457.1	245.7	330.4	256.9	217.3
1990	**8033.5**	**3970.1**	**3345.7**	**619.4**	**591.1**	**481.9**	**395.9**	**413.0**	**425.7**	**418.7**	**211.7**	**254.8**	**251.2**
1995 projected	*8127.9*	*3944.7*	*3415.0*	*578.5*	*618.2*	*569.9*	*460.8*	*381.6*	*407.7*	*398.3*	*354.4*	*159.1*	*254.7*
NUMBER OF DEATHS													
All causes													
1955	60346	6891	21632	542	1248	1901	2784	3668	4730	6759	8784	9576	13463
1965	66619	4544	22380	632	1088	963	2387	3684	5487	8139	10067	11430	18198
1975	79920	4358	22313	484	814	1459	2591	2277	5596	9092	13030	15709	24510
1985	88903	2837	20309	666	867	1225	2166	3690	6181	5514	13401	18405	33951
1990	**87054**	**2439**	**23180**	**692**	**1082**	**1439**	**1862**	**3305**	**5459**	**9341**	**7933**	**16881**	**36621**
1995 projected	*81521*	*2247*	*21985*	*675*	*1135*	*1638*	*2081*	*2908*	*5107*	*8441*	*12445*	*9728*	*35116*
Lung cancer													
1955	491	14	330	2	19	36	51	64	65	93	82	38	27
1965	620	8	355	6	9	16	53	77	82	112	115	70	72
1975	700	4	345	6	12	24	52	51	90	110	132	132	87
1985	958	8	491	14	18	44	62	91	143	119	176	142	141
1990	**1125**	**4**	**628**	**11**	**30**	**46**	**52**	**118**	**165**	**206**	**122**	**194**	**177**
1995 projected	*1288*	*4*	*690*	*11*	*31*	*52*	*67*	*131*	*185*	*213*	*235*	*139*	*220*
ANNUAL DEATH RATE / 100,000 (*The rates for the age groups 0–34 and 35–69 are the means of seven five-yearly rates, but the all-ages rates are standardised to the conventional "European" age distribution)													
All causes													
1955	1068.6*	168.8*	958.9*	175.2	263.1	389.2	620.3	933.6	1554.9	2775.8	4813.2	8512.0	15894.9
1965	954.4*	121.9*	820.3*	129.0	208.5	318.7	515.3	798.4	1342.9	2429.6	4293.0	7650.6	15660.9
1975	932.1*	103.6*	793.0*	117.2	184.1	308.0	518.8	800.6	1328.3	2294.2	4149.7	7448.6	15905.3
1985	898.8*	71.0*	788.6*	111.8	177.7	303.4	508.0	822.7	1352.2	2244.2	4056.0	7164.3	15624.0
1990	**845.9***	**64.0***	**768.2***	**111.7**	**183.0**	**298.6**	**470.3**	**800.2**	**1282.4**	**2231.0**	**3747.3**	**6625.2**	**14578.4**
1995 projected	*799.6**	*58.3**	*739.0**	*116.7*	*183.6*	*287.4*	*451.6*	*762.1*	*1252.6*	*2119.3*	*3511.6*	*6114.4*	*13787.2*
All cancer													
1955	170.2*	11.8*	267.3*	46.6	95.1	140.4	216.8	308.7	447.4	616.4	822.5	1006.2	950.4
1965	174.4*	10.1*	257.0*	44.3	85.3	124.4	207.9	291.1	417.5	628.4	854.2	1081.0	1315.8
1975	169.9*	10.0*	245.1*	39.2	66.3	128.1	215.9	286.9	414.0	565.0	775.8	1092.9	1390.0
1985	169.8*	8.7*	252.9*	45.3	73.8	132.8	202.9	309.5	433.4	572.6	802.4	1007.0	1316.2
1990	**176.7***	**9.1***	**260.6***	**44.7**	**78.3**	**133.8**	**190.2**	**315.3**	**442.8**	**619.1**	**809.2**	**1141.7**	**1399.3**
1995 projected	*183.6**	*9.7**	*264.5**	*46.3*	*79.1*	*129.7*	*186.4*	*313.2*	*461.1*	*635.5*	*860.9*	*1200.5*	*1536.7*
Lung cancer													
1955	8.1*	0.4*	14.2*	0.6	4.0	7.4	11.4	16.3	21.4	38.2	44.9	33.8	31.9
1965	8.5*	0.2*	12.8*	1.2	1.7	5.3	11.4	16.7	20.1	33.4	49.0	46.9	62.0
1975	8.3*	0.1*	12.4*	1.5	2.7	5.1	10.4	17.9	21.4	27.8	42.0	62.6	56.5
1985	11.0*	0.2*	18.8*	2.3	3.7	10.9	14.5	20.3	31.3	48.4	53.3	55.3	64.9
1990	**12.4***	**0.1***	**20.9***	**1.8**	**5.1**	**9.5**	**13.1**	**28.6**	**38.8**	**49.2**	**57.6**	**76.1**	**70.5**
1995 projected	*14.1**	*0.1**	*23.4**	*1.9*	*5.0*	*9.1*	*14.5*	*34.3*	*45.4*	*53.5*	*66.3*	*87.4*	*86.4*
Upper aerodigestive cancer (mouth, oesophagus, pharynx and larynx)													
1955	2.9*	0.1*	3.9*	1.6	1.7	1.8	2.7	5.9	4.9	8.6	11.5	20.4	27.2
1965	2.4*	0.1*	2.5*	–	1.5	1.0	1.1	1.7	4.4	8.1	13.2	18.7	35.3
1975	2.2*	0.0*	2.8*	0.5	–	1.9	1.6	5.3	3.6	6.8	11.5	15.6	25.3
1985	2.4*	0.2*	2.7*	0.2	1.4	1.0	2.3	4.0	5.3	4.9	9.4	15.6	32.2
1990	**2.6***	**0.2***	**3.5***	**0.8**	**0.8**	**1.7**	**3.3**	**5.1**	**6.1**	**6.7**	**6.6**	**16.9**	**30.3**
1995 projected	*2.8**	*0.1**	*4.0**	*0.9*	*1.1*	*2.3*	*3.9*	*6.3*	*7.4*	*6.3*	*7.3*	*15.7*	*30.2*
Other cancer													
1955	159.2*	11.3*	249.3*	44.3	89.4	131.2	202.8	286.6	421.1	569.6	766.0	952.0	891.4
1965	163.5*	9.8*	241.6*	43.1	82.0	118.1	195.4	272.6	393.0	586.9	791.9	1015.4	1218.6
1975	159.3*	9.8*	229.9*	37.3	63.6	121.2	203.8	263.7	389.0	530.4	722.3	1014.7	1308.2
1985	156.5*	8.3*	231.4*	42.8	68.6	120.9	186.0	285.2	396.8	519.3	739.7	936.2	1219.1
1990	**161.8***	**8.8***	**236.2***	**42.1**	**72.4**	**122.6**	**173.8**	**281.6**	**397.9**	**563.2**	**744.9**	**1048.7**	**1298.6**
1995 projected	*166.7**	*9.4**	*237.1**	*43.6*	*73.0*	*118.3*	*168.0*	*272.5*	*408.4*	*575.7*	*787.2*	*1097.4*	*1420.1*
Chronic obstructive pulmonary disease (COPD)													
1955	16.2*	0.9*	10.7*	1.0	2.3	2.3	3.8	8.7	17.4	39.4	82.7	153.8	324.7
1965	36.4*	0.5*	24.4*	1.0	2.5	6.3	9.9	20.6	39.2	91.6	191.0	367.5	738.4
1975	32.6*	0.7*	20.6*	0.7	3.6	6.8	11.4	22.5	35.1	63.8	146.2	277.4	752.1
1985	17.9*	0.3*	15.8*	1.8	2.3	5.9	13.6	14.0	24.5	48.4	70.2	142.5	354.8
1990	**10.7***	**0.2***	**10.5***	**1.3**	**2.0**	**5.0**	**5.8**	**11.1**	**19.7**	**28.2**	**51.5**	**78.5**	**186.7**
1995 projected	*7.9**	*0.2**	*7.9**	*1.2*	*1.8*	*3.5*	*4.3*	*8.4*	*14.2*	*21.8*	*38.1*	*55.9*	*136.2*
Other respiratory disease													
1955	63.7*	24.4*	34.8*	5.2	7.6	12.1	14.9	28.8	53.6	121.6	260.3	512.9	1005.9
1965	40.3*	10.8*	16.6*	3.1	3.5	5.3	10.8	12.8	27.7	53.4	151.4	312.6	887.3
1975	44.9*	10.2*	19.4*	2.9	5.0	6.1	7.6	18.3	29.9	66.1	163.4	368.9	1016.2
1985	38.2*	5.6*	19.5*	3.7	4.3	3.5	11.3	17.8	28.9	66.7	148.6	325.4	875.3
1990	**26.0***	**4.1***	**14.9***	**1.6**	**4.1**	**5.8**	**7.8**	**10.2**	**26.1**	**48.5**	**102.0**	**197.0**	**580.4**
1995 projected	*19.2**	*3.2**	*11.1**	*1.2*	*4.0*	*5.3*	*5.6*	*7.6*	*19.9*	*34.4*	*70.3*	*140.2*	*429.9*
Vascular disease													
1955	498.7*	14.6*	409.7*	40.4	63.2	111.4	209.7	351.2	681.5	1410.3	2696.4	4876.4	8585.6
1965	474.4*	5.8*	327.4*	24.9	50.0	84.4	153.9	290.4	555.3	1133.1	2296.4	4545.5	9964.7
1975	499.0*	3.6*	348.1*	25.2	43.9	87.8	161.6	305.2	603.6	1209.7	2418.8	4684.7	10586.6
1985	510.9*	2.9*	350.0*	17.8	39.1	82.7	165.6	323.1	628.1	1193.3	2458.5	4755.5	11035.9
1990	**481.4***	**3.1***	**339.8***	**18.4**	**38.9**	**73.0**	**159.6**	**313.8**	**576.0**	**1198.5**	**2248.5**	**4334.8**	**10488.9**
1995 projected	*447.3**	*3.0**	*319.4**	*18.5*	*36.4*	*68.3*	*151.5*	*290.4*	*555.8*	*1115.0*	*2046.0*	*3910.1*	*9863.0*
Liver cirrhosis													
1955	5.9*	0.4*	8.9*	0.3	1.9	3.5	6.9	10.9	13.1	25.5	23.0	33.8	55.5
1965	7.6*	0.3*	11.1*	2.4	2.1	4.0	6.9	8.5	18.1	35.8	44.8	54.9	55.1
1975	9.0*	0.4*	13.4*	2.9	3.6	7.2	12.6	14.8	19.5	33.1	43.3	56.9	67.5
1985	9.5*	0.4*	16.0*	4.0	7.6	8.4	17.8	21.2	28.4	24.8	36.0	45.9	49.2
1990	**11.8***	**0.7***	**21.2***	**5.5**	**11.2**	**16.2**	**21.5**	**31.0**	**28.7**	**34.6**	**41.6**	**44.3**	**44.6**
1995 projected	*14.3**	*0.8**	*26.6**	*7.1*	*15.5*	*21.8*	*28.4*	*38.3*	*34.3*	*40.9*	*47.1*	*44.6*	*46.3*
Other medical causes													
1955	271.2*	98.0*	189.1*	65.6	65.6	89.5	130.6	181.0	297.2	494.5	803.3	1697.8	4507.7
1965	173.4*	74.8*	143.4*	31.6	39.9	62.2	86.4	138.7	232.5	412.2	622.6	1024.1	2076.6
1975	124.5*	59.3*	103.5*	22.0	32.3	44.5	73.1	108.6	168.5	275.0	452.2	672.4	1343.3
1985	102.7*	39.3*	97.1*	18.1	23.4	43.1	65.9	98.8	162.8	267.4	394.7	584.3	1123.8
1990	**91.8***	**31.5***	**85.0***	**18.7**	**21.0**	**35.3**	**54.8**	**85.5**	**142.4**	**237.2**	**357.6**	**556.9**	**1099.1**
1995 projected	*82.2**	*25.4**	*74.1**	*19.4*	*18.3*	*29.1*	*45.8*	*72.6*	*123.9*	*209.9*	*324.8*	*522.3*	*1069.5*
All non-medical causes													
1955	42.7*	18.7*	38.4*	16.2	27.4	30.1	37.7	44.3	44.7	68.2	124.9	231.1	465.2
1965	47.8*	19.5*	40.4*	21.6	25.3	32.1	39.5	36.4	52.6	74.9	132.6	265.1	623.1
1975	52.3*	19.5*	43.0*	24.2	29.4	27.4	36.6	44.3	57.7	81.5	150.0	295.4	749.5
1985	49.7*	13.9*	37.4*	21.0	27.3	27.0	31.0	38.4	46.2	70.8	145.6	303.6	868.8
1990	**47.3***	**15.2***	**36.3***	**21.5**	**27.6**	**29.5**	**30.6**	**33.4**	**46.7**	**65.0**	**137.0**	**272.0**	**779.5**
1995 projected	*45.0**	*16.1**	*35.4**	*23.0*	*28.5*	*29.8*	*29.5*	*31.7*	*43.4*	*61.8*	*124.4*	*240.7*	*705.5*

Former CZECHOSLOVAKIA: 1975

Smoking–attributed deaths (Sm.) and total deaths (Total)

		ALL CAUSES	ALL CANCER	Lung cancer	Upper aero–digestive ca.	Other cancer	COPD	Other respiratory	Vascular disease	Liver cirrhosis	Other medical	Non–medical
Males												
0–34	Sm.	–	–	–	–	–	–	–	–	–	–	–
	Total	7878	499	21	12	466	37	594	308	62	3536	2842
35–69	Sm.	15100	5460	3651	440	1369	1793	293	6220	–	1334	–
	Total	39813	10955	3856	605	6494	2159	836	17429	1336	3564	3534
		(38%)	(50%)	(95%)	(73%)	(21%)	(83%)	(35%)	(36%)		(37%)	
70+	Sm.	10762	3277	2161	251	865	2843	312	3737	–	593	–
	Total	41951	7944	2321	380	5243	3640	2021	22846	410	3616	1474
		(26%)	(41%)	(93%)	(66%)	(16%)	(78%)	(15%)	(16%)		(16%)	
Any age	Sm.	25862	8737	5812	691	2234	4636	605	9957	–	1927	–
	Total	89642	19398	6198	997	12203	5836	3451	40583	1808	10716	7850
		(29%)	(45%)	(94%)	(69%)	(18%)	(79%)	(18%)	(25%)		(18%)	
Females												
0–34	Sm.	–	–	–	–	–	–	–	–	–	–	–
	Total	4358	385	4	1	380	27	438	140	14	2565	789
35–69	Sm.	565	126	97	7	22	102	14	244	–	79	–
	Total	22313	6939	345	76	6518	573	541	9726	380	2919	1235
		(3%)	(2%)	(28%)	(9%)	(0%)	(18%)	(3%)	(3%)		(3%)	
70+	Sm.	1545	199	143	17	39	649	47	565	–	85	–
	Total	53249	6883	351	108	6424	2203	2857	33789	360	4908	2249
		(3%)	(3%)	(41%)	(16%)	(1%)	(29%)	(2%)	(2%)		(2%)	
Any age	Sm.	2110	325	240	24	61	751	61	809	–	164	–
	Total	79920	14207	700	185	13322	2803	3836	43655	754	10392	4273
		(3%)	(2%)	(34%)	(13%)	(0%)	(27%)	(2%)	(2%)		(2%)	
Males+Females												
0–34	Sm.	–	–	–	–	–	–	–	–	–	–	–
	Total	12236	884	25	13	846	64	1032	448	76	6101	3631
35–69	Sm.	15665	5586	3748	447	1391	1895	307	6464	–	1413	–
	Total	62126	17894	4201	681	13012	2732	1377	27155	1716	6483	4769
		(25%)	(31%)	(89%)	(66%)	(11%)	(69%)	(22%)	(24%)		(22%)	
70+	Sm.	12307	3476	2304	268	904	3492	359	4302	–	678	–
	Total	95200	14827	2672	488	11667	5843	4878	56635	770	8524	3723
		(13%)	(23%)	(86%)	(55%)	(8%)	(60%)	(7%)	(8%)		(8%)	
Any age	Sm.	27972	9062	6052	715	2295	5387	666	10766	–	2091	–
	Total	169562	33605	6898	1182	25525	8639	7287	84238	2562	21108	12123
		(16%)	(27%)	(88%)	(60%)	(9%)	(62%)	(9%)	(13%)		(10%)	

Former CZECHOSLOVAKIA: 1985

Smoking–attributed deaths (Sm.) and total deaths (Total)

		ALL CAUSES	ALL CANCER	Lung cancer	Upper aero–digestive ca.	Other cancer	COPD	Other respiratory	Vascular disease	Liver cirrhosis	Other medical	Non–medical
Males												
0–34	Sm.	–	–	–	–	–	–	–	–	–	–	–
	Total	5622	465	14	8	443	32	361	306	58	2167	2233
35–69	Sm.	16596	6297	4063	756	1478	909	500	7439	–	1451	–
	Total	39450	11154	4245	976	5933	1061	1178	17708	1500	3281	3568
		(42%)	(56%)	(96%)	(77%)	(25%)	(86%)	(42%)	(42%)		(44%)	
70+	Sm.	10517	3432	2268	260	904	1970	328	4222	–	565	–
	Total	50130	9085	2464	414	6207	2612	2435	29822	476	3928	1772
		(21%)	(38%)	(92%)	(63%)	(15%)	(75%)	(13%)	(14%)		(14%)	
Any age	Sm.	27113	9729	6331	1016	2382	2879	828	11661	–	2016	–
	Total	95202	20704	6723	1398	12583	3705	3974	47836	2034	9376	7573
		(28%)	(47%)	(94%)	(73%)	(19%)	(78%)	(21%)	(24%)		(22%)	
Females												
0–34	Sm.	–	–	–	–	–	–	–	–	–	–	–
	Total	2837	357	8	6	343	13	224	117	15	1553	558
35–69	Sm.	1292	324	253	16	55	152	33	606	–	177	–
	Total	20309	6807	491	76	6240	398	481	8589	457	2521	1056
		(6%)	(5%)	(52%)	(21%)	(1%)	(38%)	(7%)	(7%)		(7%)	
70+	Sm.	1476	253	188	20	45	361	50	717	–	95	–
	Total	65757	8098	459	141	7498	1369	3229	44321	344	5247	3149
		(2%)	(3%)	(41%)	(14%)	(1%)	(26%)	(2%)	(2%)		(2%)	
Any age	Sm.	2768	577	441	36	100	513	83	1323	–	272	–
	Total	88903	15262	958	223	14081	1780	3934	53027	816	9321	4763
		(3%)	(4%)	(46%)	(16%)	(1%)	(29%)	(2%)	(2%)		(3%)	
Males+Females												
0–34	Sm.	–	–	–	–	–	–	–	–	–	–	–
	Total	8459	822	22	14	786	45	585	423	73	3720	2791
35–69	Sm.	17888	6621	4316	772	1533	1061	533	8045	–	1628	–
	Total	59759	17961	4736	1052	12173	1459	1659	26297	1957	5802	4624
		(30%)	(37%)	(91%)	(73%)	(13%)	(73%)	(32%)	(31%)		(28%)	
70+	Sm.	11993	3685	2456	280	949	2331	378	4939	–	660	–
	Total	115887	17183	2923	555	13705	3981	5664	74143	820	9175	4921
		(10%)	(21%)	(84%)	(50%)	(7%)	(59%)	(7%)	(7%)		(7%)	
Any age	Sm.	29881	10306	6772	1052	2482	3392	911	12984	–	2288	–
	Total	184105	35966	7681	1621	26664	5485	7908	100863	2850	18697	12336
		(16%)	(29%)	(88%)	(65%)	(9%)	(62%)	(12%)	(13%)		(12%)	

(To be conservative, no deaths before age 35, and none from liver cirrhosis or non–medical causes, were attributed to smoking.)

Former CZECHOSLOVAKIA: 1990

Smoking–attributed deaths (Sm.) and total deaths (Total)

		ALL CAUSES	ALL CANCER	Lung cancer	Upper aero–digestive ca.	Other cancer	COPD	Other respiratory	Vascular disease	Liver cirrhosis	Other medical	Non–medical
Males												
0–34	Sm.	–	–	–	–	–	–	–	–	–	–	–
	Total	4957	429	13	6	410	32	209	300	85	1687	2215
35–69	Sm.	19157	7567	4693	1114	1760	884	445	8582	–	1679	–
	Total	46674	13318	4900	1432	6986	1029	1035	20750	2370	3790	4382
		(41%)	(57%)	(96%)	(78%)	(25%)	(86%)	(43%)	(41%)		(44%)	
70+	Sm.	7970	2841	1825	209	807	1036	216	3465	–	412	–
	Total	45100	8326	1996	346	5984	1405	1808	28106	412	3354	1689
		(18%)	(34%)	(91%)	(60%)	(13%)	(74%)	(12%)	(12%)		(12%)	
Any age	Sm.	27127	10408	6518	1323	2567	1920	661	12047	–	2091	–
	Total	96731	22073	6909	1784	13380	2466	3052	49156	2867	8831	8286
		(28%)	(47%)	(94%)	(74%)	(19%)	(78%)	(22%)	(25%)		(24%)	
Females												
0–34	Sm.	–	–	–	–	–	–	–	–	–	–	–
	Total	2439	354	4	7	343	10	156	121	26	1177	595
35–69	Sm.	1679	461	355	25	81	134	37	830	–	217	–
	Total	23180	7917	628	106	7183	315	449	10094	658	2579	1168
		(7%)	(6%)	(57%)	(24%)	(1%)	(43%)	(8%)	(8%)		(8%)	
70+	Sm.	1915	370	265	31	74	313	53	1051	–	128	–
	Total	61435	8137	493	133	7511	778	2176	42153	313	4937	2941
		(3%)	(5%)	(54%)	(23%)	(1%)	(40%)	(2%)	(2%)		(3%)	
Any age	Sm.	3594	831	620	56	155	447	90	1881	–	345	–
	Total	87054	16408	1125	246	15037	1103	2781	52368	997	8693	4704
		(4%)	(5%)	(55%)	(23%)	(1%)	(41%)	(3%)	(4%)		(4%)	
Males+Females												
0–34	Sm.	–	–	–	–	–	–	–	–	–	–	–
	Total	7396	783	17	13	753	42	365	421	111	2864	2810
35–69	Sm.	20836	8028	5048	1139	1841	1018	482	9412	–	1896	–
	Total	69854	21235	5528	1538	14169	1344	1484	30844	3028	6369	5550
		(30%)	(38%)	(91%)	(74%)	(13%)	(76%)	(32%)	(31%)		(30%)	
70+	Sm.	9885	3211	2090	240	881	1349	269	4516	–	540	–
	Total	106535	16463	2489	479	13495	2183	3984	70259	725	8291	4630
		(9%)	(20%)	(84%)	(50%)	(7%)	(62%)	(7%)	(6%)		(7%)	
Any age	Sm.	30721	11239	7138	1379	2722	2367	751	13928	–	2436	–
	Total	183785	38481	8034	2030	28417	3569	5833	101524	3864	17524	12990
		(17%)	(29%)	(89%)	(68%)	(10%)	(66%)	(13%)	(14%)		(14%)	

Former CZECHOSLOVAKIA: 1995

Smoking–attributed deaths (Sm.) and total deaths (Total)

		ALL CAUSES	ALL CANCER	Lung cancer	Upper aero–digestive ca.	Other cancer	COPD	Other respiratory	Vascular disease	Liver cirrhosis	Other medical	Non–medical
Males												
0–34	Sm.	–	–	–	–	–	–	–	–	–	–	–
	Total	4755	412	11	6	395	37	155	286	111	1442	2312
35–69	Sm.	20267	8337	4938	1514	1885	756	369	9015	–	1790	–
	Total	49284	14316	5146	1928	7242	874	819	21107	3312	3874	4982
		(41%)	(58%)	(96%)	(79%)	(26%)	(86%)	(45%)	(43%)		(46%)	
70+	Sm.	7960	3022	1923	217	882	733	167	3639	–	399	–
	Total	43971	8999	2101	354	6544	1001	1343	27454	458	3032	1684
		(18%)	(34%)	(92%)	(61%)	(13%)	(73%)	(12%)	(13%)		(13%)	
Any age	Sm.	28227	11359	6861	1731	2767	1489	536	12654	–	2189	–
	Total	98010	23727	7258	2288	14181	1912	2317	48847	3881	8348	8978
		(29%)	(48%)	(95%)	(76%)	(20%)	(78%)	(23%)	(26%)		(26%)	
Females												
0–34	Sm.	–	–	–	–	–	–	–	–	–	–	–
	Total	2247	371	4	4	363	9	120	114	28	952	653
35–69	Sm.	1821	553	422	35	96	111	34	901	–	222	–
	Total	21985	7961	690	122	7149	235	335	9234	841	2220	1159
		(8%)	(7%)	(61%)	(29%)	(1%)	(47%)	(10%)	(10%)		(10%)	
70+	Sm.	2290	493	355	36	102	263	52	1314	–	168	–
	Total	57289	8875	594	128	8153	571	1567	38593	356	4706	2621
		(4%)	(6%)	(60%)	(28%)	(1%)	(46%)	(3%)	(3%)		(4%)	
Any age	Sm.	4111	1046	777	71	198	374	86	2215	–	390	–
	Total	81521	17207	1288	254	15665	815	2022	47941	1225	7878	4433
		(5%)	(6%)	(60%)	(28%)	(1%)	(46%)	(4%)	(5%)		(5%)	
Males+Females												
0–34	Sm.	–	–	–	–	–	–	–	–	–	–	–
	Total	7002	783	15	10	758	46	275	400	139	2394	2965
35–69	Sm.	22088	8890	5360	1549	1981	867	403	9916	–	2012	–
	Total	71269	22277	5836	2050	14391	1109	1154	30341	4153	6094	6141
		(31%)	(40%)	(92%)	(76%)	(14%)	(78%)	(35%)	(33%)		(33%)	
70+	Sm.	10250	3515	2278	253	984	996	219	4953	–	567	–
	Total	101260	17874	2695	482	14697	1572	2910	66047	814	7738	4305
		(10%)	(20%)	(85%)	(52%)	(7%)	(63%)	(8%)	(7%)		(7%)	
Any age	Sm.	32338	12405	7638	1802	2965	1863	622	14869	–	2579	–
	Total	179531	40934	8546	2542	29846	2727	4339	96788	5106	16226	13411
		(18%)	(30%)	(89%)	(71%)	(10%)	(68%)	(14%)	(15%)		(16%)	

(To be conservative, no deaths before age 35, and none from liver cirrhosis or non–medical causes, were attributed to smoking.)

DENMARK: 1990

		No. of deaths			Standardised rates (Defined on p.322)			Annual death rates / 100, 000						
		All ages	0–34	35–69	All ages	0–34	35–69	0–4	5–9	10–14	15–19	20–24	25–29	30–34
ALL CAUSES	M	30944	1158	10283	1083.4	93.3	1155.7	220.6	25.7	25.3	51.5	88.1	102.0	139.7
	F	29645	569	6767	687.5	50.2	704.3	160.1	16.8	17.4	27.2	36.9	38.0	54.7
Tuberculosis	M	32	–	9	1.1	–	0.9	–	–	–	–	–	–	–
	F	20	–	11	0.6	–	1.2	–	–	–	–	–	–	–
Other infective and parasitic	M	234	63	115	8.8	4.9	10.0	8.7	0.7	–	0.5	1.5	9.7	13.1
	F	127	15	34	3.5	1.4	3.3	5.6	0.8	–	0.6	–	1.5	1.1
ALL CANCER	M	7814	98	3192	277.3	7.8	369.6	7.4	7.3	3.1	5.3	9.4	6.8	15.2
	F	7211	75	2999	200.9	6.1	311.4	4.2	3.8	2.6	5.0	5.7	5.7	16.0
Mouth and pharynx cancer	M	161	2	94	6.1	0.2	10.4	–	–	–	–	–	–	1.1
	F	72	–	28	1.9	–	2.9	–	–	–	–	–	–	–
Oesophagus cancer	M	211	–	119	7.8	–	13.6	–	–	–	–	–	–	–
	F	74	–	32	2.1	–	3.5	–	–	–	–	–	–	–
Stomach cancer	M	340	–	136	11.9	–	15.6	–	–	–	–	–	–	–
	F	241	4	68	5.9	0.3	7.0	–	–	–	–	–	0.5	1.7
Colorectal cancer	M	1032	6	388	35.9	0.4	45.6	–	–	–	–	–	0.5	2.6
	F	1076	5	294	26.4	0.4	31.0	–	–	–	–	–	0.5	2.2
Liver cancer	M	85	–	35	3.0	–	4.1	–	–	–	–	–	–	–
	F	63	3	27	1.8	0.3	2.7	–	0.8	–	–	–	0.5	0.6
Pancreas cancer	M	349	1	150	12.5	0.1	17.3	–	–	–	–	–	–	0.5
	F	396	–	128	10.3	–	13.7	–	–	–	–	–	–	–
Larynx cancer	M	96	–	54	3.6	–	6.3	–	–	–	–	–	–	–
	F	25	–	13	0.8	–	1.4	–	–	–	–	–	–	–
Lung cancer	M	2180	3	1030	78.7	0.2	121.8	–	–	–	0.5	–	0.5	0.5
	F	1118	2	614	34.3	0.2	64.8	–	–	–	–	–	–	1.1
Malignant melanoma	M	119	3	82	4.6	0.2	8.6	–	–	–	–	–	0.5	1.1
	F	106	5	61	3.4	0.4	5.7	–	–	–	0.6	1.6	–	0.6
Female breast cancer	F	1285	11	657	38.5	0.9	66.9	–	–	–	–	–	1.5	4.4
Cervix cancer	F	230	3	122	7.0	0.2	12.3	–	–	–	–	0.5	0.5	0.6
Other uterine cancer	F	196	–	70	5.2	–	7.6	–	–	–	–	–	–	–
Ovarian cancer	F	449	1	246	14.0	0.1	25.4	–	–	–	–	0.5	–	–
Prostate cancer	M	951	–	189	31.6	–	23.2	–	–	–	–	–	–	–
Bladder cancer	M	447	–	131	15.3	–	15.9	–	–	–	–	–	–	–
	F	137	–	44	3.3	–	4.8	–	–	–	–	–	–	–
Other and ill-defined cancer sites	M	1165	46	524	42.1	3.6	58.3	3.3	3.7	1.2	3.7	5.4	3.4	4.7
	F	1219	22	438	32.5	1.9	45.7	3.5	0.8	1.9	0.6	1.6	0.5	4.4
Hodgkin's disease	M	37	8	17	1.3	0.6	1.7	–	0.7	–	–	1.5	1.0	1.1
	F	18	2	10	0.6	0.1	1.0	–	–	–	–	–	1.0	–
Myeloma and non-Hodgkin lymphomas	M	371	9	149	13.2	0.7	16.6	–	–	0.6	–	1.0	1.0	2.1
	F	313	6	91	7.9	0.5	9.5	–	0.8	–	1.7	0.5	–	0.6
Leukaemia	M	270	20	94	9.6	1.8	10.6	4.0	2.9	1.2	1.1	1.5	–	1.6
	F	193	11	56	5.0	1.0	5.5	0.7	1.5	0.6	2.2	1.0	0.5	–
ALL VASCULAR DISEASE	M	13461	37	3598	459.1	2.7	420.0	–	–	0.6	1.6	5.9	2.4	8.4
	F	13735	31	1609	272.3	2.4	172.4	0.7	–	0.6	2.2	1.0	3.1	9.4
Rheumatic heart disease and fever	M	88	–	32	3.1	–	3.7	–	–	–	–	–	–	–
	F	153	–	36	3.4	–	3.9	–	–	–	–	–	–	–
Hypertensive disease	M	157	–	68	5.6	–	7.9	–	–	–	–	–	–	–
	F	208	–	50	4.8	–	5.3	–	–	–	–	–	–	–
Ischaemic heart disease	M	8325	11	2437	286.1	0.8	285.5	–	–	–	0.5	1.0	1.5	2.6
	F	7272	5	847	143.9	0.4	91.6	–	–	–	0.6	–	–	2.2
Pulmonary embolism and other venous	M	207	–	65	7.2	–	7.3	–	–	–	–	–	–	–
	F	231	4	44	5.1	0.3	4.5	–	–	–	0.6	0.5	–	1.1
Cerebrovascular disease	M	2371	10	505	79.3	0.7	58.1	–	–	–	0.5	1.5	0.5	2.6
	F	3196	14	380	64.1	1.1	39.8	–	–	0.6	1.1	–	1.5	4.4
Other vascular disease	M	2313	16	491	77.8	1.2	57.5	–	–	0.6	0.5	3.4	0.5	3.2
	F	2675	8	252	51.0	0.6	27.3	0.7	–	–	–	0.5	1.5	1.7
Chronic obstructive pulmonary disease	M	1746	18	455	59.1	1.4	55.3	2.0	0.7	1.2	1.1	1.0	1.5	2.6
	F	1201	4	437	31.5	0.3	47.4	–	0.8	–	0.6	1.0	–	–
Other respiratory disease	M	733	10	87	24.0	0.9	9.7	2.7	–	1.2	–	0.5	–	1.6
	F	950	5	56	17.3	0.5	5.7	2.8	–	–	–	0.5	–	–
Peptic ulcer	M	242	1	56	8.1	0.1	6.7	–	–	–	–	–	–	0.5
	F	309	–	58	6.6	–	6.2	–	–	–	–	–	–	–
Liver cirrhosis	M	486	12	396	19.3	0.9	40.1	0.7	–	–	–	–	–	5.8
	F	226	4	156	7.8	0.3	15.4	–	–	0.6	–	–	–	1.7
Renal disease	M	38	–	12	1.3	–	1.3	–	–	–	–	–	–	–
	F	22	1	14	0.7	0.1	1.4	–	–	–	–	–	0.5	–
Pregnancy and birth	F	1	–	1	0.0	–	0.1	–	–	–	–	–	–	–
Congenital and perinatal causes	M	247	207	30	12.3	19.5	3.0	127.0	1.5	1.9	1.1	1.5	2.4	1.1
	F	191	164	20	9.8	16.1	1.9	98.7	1.5	4.5	1.7	2.6	1.5	2.2
Ill-defined causes	M	1450	83	615	53.2	7.6	68.0	45.5	–	0.6	–	1.5	3.4	2.1
	F	1328	44	316	32.2	4.3	33.2	26.8	–	–	0.6	0.5	–	2.2
Other medical causes	M	2270	90	778	79.9	7.3	83.5	16.0	2.2	4.9	3.2	2.0	8.7	14.2
	F	2727	60	560	61.5	5.2	57.7	12.0	4.6	0.6	1.7	5.2	5.1	7.2
ALL NON-MEDICAL CAUSES	M	2191	539	940	80.0	40.2	87.7	10.7	13.2	11.7	38.8	65.0	67.0	75.1
	F	1597	166	496	42.7	13.4	47.0	9.2	5.3	8.4	15.0	20.3	20.6	14.9
Motor vehicle traffic accidents	M	424	195	124	15.6	14.7	12.3	2.0	8.1	6.2	23.9	25.1	24.3	13.1
	F	193	70	63	6.6	5.8	6.0	2.1	5.3	7.7	8.9	9.9	4.6	2.2
Fire	M	28	7	11	1.1	0.6	1.1	1.3	0.7	0.6	0.5	–	0.5	0.5
	F	30	4	10	0.9	0.3	0.9	1.4	–	–	–	0.5	0.5	–
Suicide	M	815	164	504	30.7	11.9	46.5	–	–	1.9	7.4	20.2	20.4	33.6
	F	426	41	280	14.8	3.1	26.5	–	–	–	2.2	5.7	7.2	6.6
Homicide	M	24	13	10	0.9	1.0	0.9	1.3	–	–	0.5	2.0	1.9	1.1
	F	27	14	11	1.1	1.1	1.0	2.1	–	–	1.7	1.0	2.1	1.1
POPULATION (thousands):	M=males				2532.8	1235.7	1077.2	149.6	136.4	162.0	188.2	203.2	205.9	190.4
	F=females				2607.1	1175.9	1090.4	141.8	130.9	154.9	180.2	192.5	194.6	181.0

DENMARK: 1990
9th ICD categories

Annual death rates / 100, 000

35–39	40–44	45–49	50–54	55–59	60–64	65–69	70–74	75–79	80+/NK			
188.3	306.4	431.7	728.7	1253.8	1979.6	3201.6	5024.6	7898.2	15433.6	M	**ALL CAUSES**	001–999
106.0	177.5	294.0	517.5	840.4	1209.1	1786.0	2744.3	4453.1	11550.4	F		
0.5	1.4	0.5	–	0.8	0.9	1.8	5.6	13.3	14.4	M	**Tuberculosis**	010–018, 137
–	–	0.6	1.4	–	3.9	2.3	2.6	2.0	3.1	F		
14.9	13.0	11.9	9.8	8.8	6.8	4.5	15.6	8.8	57.6	M	**Other infective**	Rest of 001–139
2.8	2.5	2.2	1.4	3.9	6.3	3.8	9.7	17.2	39.1	F	**and parasitic**	
20.7	66.5	94.8	211.3	399.5	682.0	1112.5	1552.5	2094.4	2740.8	M	**ALL CANCER**	140–208
37.0	81.0	144.2	260.1	410.9	545.8	700.5	937.6	1154.4	1505.9	F		
–	1.4	6.5	13.2	10.4	18.7	22.5	24.6	33.9	32.0	M	**Mouth and**	140–149
–	1.0	2.2	2.1	4.6	3.9	6.2	7.0	11.1	19.5	F	**pharynx cancer**	
1.6	1.9	4.9	6.3	17.6	28.1	35.1	39.1	32.4	56.0	M	**Oesophagus cancer**	150
–	0.5	–	3.5	6.2	7.8	6.2	10.5	12.1	14.1	F		
1.1	3.9	4.9	9.8	16.8	17.9	54.9	59.2	87.0	147.2	M	**Stomach cancer**	151
1.1	3.0	2.8	4.9	6.9	16.4	13.9	25.5	45.4	74.3	F		
2.7	8.2	8.1	21.6	39.2	79.1	160.2	181.9	300.9	433.6	M	**Colorectal cancer**	153, 154
0.6	5.0	12.3	25.2	42.4	54.0	77.8	151.1	189.7	326.0	F		
–	0.5	1.6	1.4	4.0	6.8	14.4	17.9	31.0	20.8	M	**Liver cancer**	155.0
1.1	1.0	1.1	2.1	2.3	3.9	7.7	7.9	8.1	12.5	F		
–	3.4	4.9	11.9	20.0	34.0	46.8	74.8	79.6	123.2	M	**Pancreas cancer**	157
1.1	2.0	2.2	9.1	17.7	36.0	27.7	67.7	66.6	97.7	F		
–	1.0	–	6.3	8.8	12.8	15.3	13.4	16.2	30.4	M	**Larynx cancer**	161
–	–	0.6	1.4	3.1	2.3	2.3	1.8	6.1	3.1	F		
1.6	11.1	23.3	58.6	140.1	235.5	382.5	526.8	551.6	481.6	M	**Lung cancer**	162
3.3	10.0	25.2	47.6	90.2	107.3	170.1	158.2	182.6	110.2	F		
2.7	4.8	3.8	9.1	12.0	16.2	11.7	16.7	13.3	16.0	M	**Malignant melanoma**	172
2.2	5.0	6.7	7.7	6.2	7.8	4.6	9.7	12.1	13.3	F		
13.2	26.5	36.3	66.4	90.2	121.4	113.9	133.6	168.5	233.0	F	**Female breast cancer**	174
3.3	5.5	7.3	9.1	17.0	19.6	24.6	33.4	24.2	33.6	F	**Cervix cancer**	180
0.6	–	1.7	3.5	6.9	13.3	26.9	36.0	42.4	33.6	F	**Other uterine cancer**	179, 182
2.2	4.5	17.3	23.1	37.0	43.9	50.0	71.2	54.5	52.4	F	**Ovarian cancer**	183
–	1.0	–	6.3	16.8	49.3	89.1	176.3	358.4	577.6	M	**Prostate cancer**	185
–	0.5	1.1	4.9	13.6	36.6	54.9	100.4	134.2	216.0	M	**Bladder cancer**	188
–	–	1.1	1.4	4.6	9.4	16.9	12.3	22.2	44.6	F		
5.9	18.8	24.9	44.6	64.9	102.0	146.7	184.2	269.9	395.2	M	**Other and ill-defined**	Rest of 140–208
5.0	11.0	19.0	36.4	63.2	77.5	107.8	140.6	207.9	307.3	F	**cancer sites**	
1.1	1.9	1.1	–	1.6	0.9	5.4	6.7	4.4	4.8	M	**Hodgkin's disease**	201
–	–	1.1	0.7	0.8	1.6	3.1	1.8	3.0	0.8	F		
1.6	5.3	6.0	13.2	20.0	29.8	40.5	73.7	116.5	108.8	M	**Myeloma and non-**	200, 202–203
2.2	3.0	1.7	9.1	9.3	10.2	30.8	51.8	61.6	75.1	F	**Hodgkin lymphomas**	
2.7	2.9	3.8	4.2	13.6	14.5	32.4	56.9	64.9	97.6	M	**Leukaemia**	204–208
1.1	3.0	5.6	7.0	2.3	9.4	10.0	17.6	36.3	54.7	F		
20.7	50.6	107.8	229.4	462.0	764.5	1305.1	2293.5	3818.6	8291.2	M	**ALL VASCULAR**	390–459
13.2	16.0	38.6	85.3	165.0	309.3	579.7	1076.4	2128.2	6849.9	F	**DISEASE**	
–	–	1.6	1.4	4.8	11.1	7.2	19.0	28.0	32.0	M	**Rheumatic heart**	390–398
–	–	0.6	2.1	2.3	5.5	16.9	16.7	26.2	56.3	F	**disease and fever**	
0.5	1.0	2.2	3.5	10.4	14.5	23.4	30.1	38.3	57.6	M	**Hypertensive disease**	401–405
0.6	0.5	1.7	4.2	6.2	6.3	17.7	23.7	39.4	71.9	F		
12.2	28.4	68.8	156.2	327.5	519.6	885.7	1484.4	2346.6	4729.6	M	**Ischaemic heart**	410–414
3.9	4.0	18.4	29.4	95.6	174.6	315.6	584.4	1146.3	3611.4	F	**disease**	
0.5	1.0	4.9	4.2	10.4	11.1	18.9	40.2	67.8	96.0	M	**Pulmonary embolism**	415.1, 451–453
1.1	2.0	1.7	2.8	2.3	2.3	19.2	22.0	48.4	86.0	F	**and other venous**	
3.7	12.0	20.0	28.6	57.6	102.0	182.7	363.8	746.3	1638.4	M	**Cerebrovascular**	430–438
5.0	9.0	13.4	31.5	33.2	72.8	113.9	254.8	519.7	1561.4	F	**disease**	
3.7	8.2	10.3	35.6	51.2	106.3	187.2	356.0	591.4	1737.6	M	**Other vascular**	Rest of 390–459
2.8	0.5	2.8	15.4	25.4	47.8	96.2	174.9	348.1	1462.9	F	**disease**	
1.1	3.4	3.3	14.6	52.8	94.4	217.8	359.4	591.4	880.0	M	**Chronic obstructive**	490–496
0.6	4.0	4.5	20.3	55.5	103.4	144.0	171.4	224.0	268.2	F	**pulmonary disease**	
3.2	3.4	3.3	5.6	6.4	17.0	28.8	41.3	197.6	744.0	M	**Other respiratory**	Rest of 460–519
1.1	3.0	2.8	2.8	5.4	7.0	17.7	46.6	117.1	562.9	F	**disease**	
–	1.4	–	2.8	4.8	11.9	26.1	31.3	61.9	184.0	M	**Peptic ulcer**	531–533
0.6	1.5	1.1	2.8	7.7	11.0	18.5	22.0	51.5	136.8	F		
16.5	22.2	35.8	40.4	52.8	58.7	54.0	46.9	31.0	24.0	M	**Liver cirrhosis**	571
5.5	6.5	12.3	19.6	23.1	17.2	23.9	23.7	13.1	20.3	F		
–	1.4	–	–	0.8	2.6	4.5	8.9	13.3	14.4	M	**Renal disease**	580–590
0.6	–	1.1	2.1	1.5	2.3	2.3	–	3.0	3.1	F		
0.6	–	–	–	–	–	–	–	–	–	F	**Pregnancy and birth**	630–676
1.1	2.4	2.7	2.8	2.4	6.0	3.6	2.2	5.9	6.4	M	**Congenital and**	740–779
0.6	1.5	1.1	3.5	1.5	2.3	3.1	3.5	1.0	1.6	F	**perinatal causes**	
9.6	20.7	32.0	52.3	77.7	117.3	166.5	215.4	293.5	576.0	M	**Ill-defined causes**	780–799
3.9	6.0	13.4	19.6	38.6	68.9	82.4	143.2	205.9	469.9	F		
21.8	34.7	46.6	68.3	103.3	125.0	184.5	303.6	529.5	1233.6	M	**Other medical causes**	Rest of 001–799
14.9	16.0	25.2	49.7	67.8	80.7	149.3	218.8	382.4	1156.4	F		
78.2	85.3	93.2	91.4	81.7	92.7	91.8	148.4	238.9	667.2	M	**ALL NON-**	E800–E999
24.8	39.5	47.0	49.0	59.4	50.9	58.5	88.8	153.4	533.2	F	**MEDICAL CAUSES**	
10.1	7.2	9.8	11.2	12.8	17.9	17.1	37.9	48.7	60.8	M	**Motor vehicle**	E810–E819
3.3	6.0	3.4	8.4	6.9	6.3	7.7	12.3	21.2	19.5	F	**traffic accidents**	
1.1	1.0	–	0.7		3.4	1.8	1.1	2.9	11.2	M	**Fire**	E890–E899
0.6	0.5	2.2	0.7	0.8	1.6	–	1.8	5.0	7.0	F		
39.4	49.1	53.1	53.0	39.2	48.5	43.2	52.5	54.6	100.8	M	**Suicide**	E950–E959
13.8	22.5	26.3	28.7	32.4	30.5	31.6	28.1	35.3	29.7	F		
0.5	1.0	1.1	2.8	–	0.9		1.1	–	–	M	**Homicide**	E960–E969
1.7	1.0	0.6	1.4	1.5	–	0.8	–	1.0	0.8	F		
188.0	207.6	184.6	143.4	124.9	117.6	111.1	89.6	67.8	62.5	M	**POPULATION (thousands)**	
181.2	200.0	178.9	143.0	129.7	127.7	129.9	113.8	99.1	127.9	F		

DENMARK: Males

	All ages	0–34	35–69	35–39	40–44	45–49	50–54	55–59	60–64	65–69	70–74	75–79	80+/NK
POPULATION (1000s)													
1955	2202.6	1205.9	870.4	150.9	154.4	148.3	130.8	114.4	94.6	77.0	59.0	39.3	28.0
1965	2358.8	1275.1	932.4	141.9	152.8	146.6	147.1	136.8	114.7	92.5	68.2	45.7	37.4
1975	2504.3	1374.0	950.5	151.0	138.3	139.9	148.4	133.7	130.1	109.1	80.3	53.2	46.3
1985	2518.9	1266.3	1040.5	209.7	188.0	147.8	131.3	127.7	127.2	108.8	92.2	64.0	55.9
1990	**2532.8**	**1235.7**	**1077.2**	**188.0**	**207.6**	**184.6**	**143.4**	**124.9**	**117.6**	**111.1**	**89.6**	**67.8**	**62.5**
1995 projected	*2550.5*	*1203.2*	*1122.3*	*189.9*	*188.3*	*205.2*	*180.8*	*137.4*	*116.1*	*104.6*	*93.0*	*66.2*	*65.8*
NUMBER OF DEATHS													
All causes													
1955	20368	2158	7825	257	383	658	992	1386	1766	2383	2787	3134	4464
1965	25847	1983	10039	247	433	643	1136	1872	2527	3181	3608	3871	6346
1975	27574	1530	10467	274	400	628	1201	1693	2644	3627	4230	4257	7090
1985	30328	1305	10584	373	483	681	1052	1676	2690	3629	4655	5109	8675
1990	**30944**	**1158**	**10283**	**354**	**636**	**797**	**1045**	**1566**	**2328**	**3557**	**4502**	**5355**	**9646**
1995 projected	*31144*	*1047*	*10142*	*394*	*598*	*857*	*1234*	*1615*	*2188*	*3256*	*4605*	*5200*	*10150*
Lung cancer													
1955	583	2	443	2	11	27	79	105	114	105	67	44	27
1965	1228	3	828	6	17	43	87	186	245	244	218	109	70
1975	1728	4	1007	7	17	31	113	161	286	392	365	222	130
1985	2266	1	1126	10	15	37	108	201	336	419	448	394	297
1990	**2180**	**3**	**1030**	**3**	**23**	**43**	**84**	**175**	**277**	**425**	**472**	**374**	**301**
1995 projected	*2068*	*2*	*960*	*3*	*19*	*37*	*86*	*163*	*253*	*399*	*478*	*343*	*285*
ANNUAL DEATH RATE / 100,000 (*The rates for the age groups 0–34 and 35–69 are the means of seven five-yearly rates, but the all-ages rates are standardised to the conventional "European" age distribution)													
All causes													
1955	1115.2*	173.9*	1113.4*	170.3	248.1	443.7	758.4	1211.5	1866.8	3094.8	4723.7	7974.6	15942.9
1965	1193.5*	150.7*	1239.8*	174.1	283.4	438.6	772.3	1368.4	2203.1	3438.9	5290.3	8470.5	16967.9
1975	1114.3*	113.2*	1193.1*	181.5	289.2	448.9	809.3	1266.3	2032.3	3324.5	5267.7	8001.9	15313.2
1985	1112.3*	106.2*	1208.5*	177.9	256.9	460.8	801.2	1312.5	2114.8	3335.5	5048.8	7982.8	15518.8
1990	**1083.4***	**93.3***	**1155.7***	**188.3**	**306.4**	**431.7**	**728.7**	**1253.8**	**1979.6**	**3201.6**	**5024.6**	**7898.2**	**15433.6**
1995 projected	*1061.4**	*85.5**	*1114.0**	*207.5*	*317.6*	*417.6*	*682.5*	*1175.4*	*1884.6*	*3112.8*	*4951.6*	*7855.0*	*15425.5*
All cancer													
1955	227.8*	11.8*	304.5*	29.2	56.3	101.8	204.1	338.3	538.1	863.6	1159.3	1653.9	2246.4
1965	251.8*	13.5*	335.5*	32.4	58.2	113.9	201.9	400.6	612.9	928.6	1303.5	1759.3	2521.4
1975	247.6*	10.9*	333.4*	33.1	55.7	100.1	226.4	344.1	621.1	953.3	1399.8	1802.6	2259.2
1985	277.9*	8.9*	372.3*	30.5	54.8	90.7	232.3	422.9	700.5	1074.4	1468.5	2057.8	2815.7
1990	**277.3***	**7.8***	**369.6***	**20.7**	**66.5**	**94.8**	**211.3**	**399.5**	**682.0**	**1112.5**	**1552.5**	**2094.4**	**2740.8**
1995 projected	*275.9**	*6.9**	*366.4**	*21.6*	*66.4*	*91.1*	*198.6*	*376.3*	*675.3*	*1135.8*	*1592.5*	*2081.6*	*2743.2*
Lung cancer													
1955	30.7*	0.2*	62.2*	1.3	7.1	18.2	60.4	91.8	120.5	136.4	113.6	112.0	96.4
1965	54.9*	0.2*	102.5*	4.2	11.1	29.3	59.1	136.0	213.6	263.8	319.6	238.5	187.2
1975	68.4*	0.3*	116.4*	4.6	12.3	22.2	76.1	120.4	219.8	359.3	454.5	417.3	280.8
1985	84.0*	0.1*	132.4*	4.8	8.0	25.0	82.3	157.4	264.2	385.1	485.9	615.6	531.3
1990	**78.7***	**0.2***	**121.8***	**1.6**	**11.1**	**23.3**	**58.6**	**140.1**	**235.5**	**382.5**	**526.8**	**551.6**	**481.6**
1995 projected	*73.2**	*0.1**	*113.6**	*1.6*	*10.1*	*18.0*	*47.6*	*118.6*	*217.9*	*381.5*	*514.0*	*518.1*	*433.1*
Upper aerodigestive cancer (mouth, oesophagus, pharynx and larynx)													
1955	10.4*	0.1*	12.3*	0.7	1.9	4.7	7.6	17.5	25.4	28.6	40.7	106.9	125.0
1965	9.8*	0.1*	14.7*	0.7	3.9	8.2	5.4	11.0	31.4	42.2	30.8	54.7	128.3
1975	9.8*	–	14.7*	2.0	1.4	5.7	10.8	14.2	25.4	43.1	51.1	69.5	79.9
1985	14.5*	–	25.2*	0.5	4.3	12.2	18.3	25.8	57.4	57.9	69.4	76.6	85.9
1990	**17.5***	**0.2***	**30.3***	**1.6**	**4.3**	**11.4**	**25.8**	**36.8**	**59.5**	**72.9**	**77.0**	**82.6**	**118.4**
1995 projected	*20.6**	*0.2**	*35.4**	*2.1*	*4.2*	*13.2*	*32.6*	*43.7*	*70.6*	*81.3*	*87.1*	*96.7*	*147.4*
Other cancer													
1955	186.7*	11.5*	229.9*	27.2	47.3	78.9	136.1	229.0	392.2	698.7	1005.1	1435.1	2025.0
1965	187.1*	13.2*	218.4*	27.5	43.2	76.4	137.3	253.7	367.9	622.7	953.1	1466.1	2205.9
1975	169.4*	10.6*	202.3*	26.5	41.9	72.2	139.5	209.4	375.9	550.9	894.1	1315.8	1898.5
1985	179.3*	8.8*	214.7*	25.3	42.6	53.5	131.8	239.6	378.9	631.4	913.2	1365.6	2198.6
1990	**181.1***	**7.4***	**217.5***	**17.6**	**51.1**	**60.1**	**126.9**	**222.6**	**386.9**	**657.1**	**948.7**	**1460.2**	**2140.8**
1995 projected	*182.1**	*6.5**	*217.4**	*17.9*	*52.0*	*59.9*	*118.4*	*214.0*	*386.7*	*673.0*	*991.4*	*1466.8*	*2162.6*
Chronic obstructive pulmonary disease (COPD)													
1955	9.6*	1.1*	11.0*	2.0	2.6	4.0	9.9	12.2	18.0	28.6	30.5	53.4	150.0
1965	28.4*	0.6*	38.8*	–	2.0	7.5	19.0	38.7	85.4	118.9	145.2	199.1	320.9
1975	42.7*	0.9*	48.4*	2.0	2.2	11.4	24.3	47.1	80.7	171.4	292.7	357.1	490.3
1985	60.5*	0.6*	61.7*	1.0	3.2	9.5	24.4	52.5	120.3	221.5	339.5	576.6	887.3
1990	**59.1***	**1.4***	**55.3***	**1.1**	**3.4**	**3.3**	**14.6**	**52.8**	**94.4**	**217.8**	**359.4**	**591.4**	**880.0**
1995 projected	*58.2**	*1.9**	*51.1**	*1.6*	*2.1*	*1.9*	*11.6*	*42.2*	*86.1*	*212.2*	*366.7*	*598.2*	*884.5*
Other respiratory disease													
1955	30.1*	8.9*	16.8*	1.3	–	6.7	10.7	21.0	28.5	49.4	96.6	190.8	621.4
1965	28.8*	4.0*	14.8*	2.1	2.0	3.4	10.9	11.7	26.2	47.6	89.4	203.5	735.3
1975	40.2*	2.2*	20.4*	2.0	5.1	5.0	6.7	20.9	27.7	75.2	132.0	360.9	1045.4
1985	29.3*	1.3*	9.5*	2.4	0.5	2.7	7.6	6.3	15.7	31.3	82.4	223.4	915.9
1990	**24.0***	**0.9***	**9.7***	**3.2**	**3.4**	**3.3**	**5.6**	**6.4**	**17.0**	**28.8**	**41.3**	**197.6**	**744.0**
1995 projected	*19.9**	*0.8**	*8.5**	*4.2*	*4.8*	*3.4*	*5.0*	*5.8*	*16.4*	*20.1*	*32.3*	*152.6*	*614.0*
Vascular disease													
1955	548.8*	5.2*	500.0*	28.5	52.5	151.0	295.1	528.0	861.5	1583.1	2591.5	4737.9	9935.7
1965	615.9*	5.6*	587.3*	30.3	81.2	162.3	328.3	633.0	1088.1	1788.1	2992.7	5074.4	10788.8
1975	559.7*	3.2*	548.1*	29.8	70.9	166.5	330.2	581.2	976.9	1681.0	2803.2	4582.7	9477.3
1985	497.5*	2.8*	487.6*	25.8	53.7	136.0	294.0	519.2	888.4	1496.3	2455.5	4051.6	8517.0
1990	**459.1***	**2.7***	**420.0***	**20.7**	**50.6**	**107.8**	**229.4**	**462.0**	**764.5**	**1305.1**	**2293.5**	**3818.6**	**8291.2**
1995 projected	*423.7**	*2.6**	*362.1**	*18.4*	*40.4*	*82.4*	*186.9*	*387.2*	*657.2*	*1162.5*	*2108.6*	*3696.4*	*7984.8*
Liver cirrhosis													
1955	5.9*	0.3*	9.6*	0.7	2.6	5.4	6.9	14.0	18.0	19.5	32.2	43.3	17.9
1965	7.6*	0.3*	12.9*	1.4	6.5	3.4	11.6	15.4	21.8	30.3	35.2	43.8	34.8
1975	13.7*	0.7*	27.0*	6.6	20.2	29.3	27.0	34.4	37.7	33.9	33.6	30.1	32.4
1985	16.9*	1.5*	34.5*	11.0	12.2	30.4	37.3	44.6	55.0	50.6	38.0	32.8	30.4
1990	**19.3***	**0.9***	**40.1***	**16.5**	**22.2**	**35.8**	**40.4**	**52.8**	**58.7**	**54.0**	**46.9**	**31.0**	**24.0**
1995 projected	*21.8**	*1.0**	*45.7**	*23.2*	*29.2*	*41.9*	*44.8*	*57.5*	*63.7*	*59.3*	*50.5*	*31.7*	*21.3*
Other medical causes													
1955	194.9*	91.8*	153.0*	36.4	48.6	82.9	116.2	163.5	244.2	379.2	630.5	1073.8	2357.1
1965	171.3*	81.2*	142.5*	32.4	45.2	64.8	87.7	158.6	241.5	367.6	570.4	932.2	1933.2
1975	127.1*	46.0*	119.9*	31.1	47.7	58.6	86.9	137.6	176.0	301.6	452.1	672.9	1514.0
1985	141.0*	37.4*	143.3*	28.1	45.7	86.6	102.1	164.4	228.8	347.4	516.3	795.3	1787.1
1990	**164.8***	**39.3***	**173.3***	**47.9**	**75.1**	**93.7**	**136.0**	**198.6**	**270.4**	**391.5**	**582.6**	**926.3**	**2086.4**
1995 projected	*190.3**	*42.1**	*204.1**	*66.9*	*97.2*	*116.0*	*159.8*	*238.0*	*310.1*	*440.7*	*662.4*	*1046.8*	*2433.1*
All non-medical causes													
1955	98.0*	54.8*	118.5*	72.2	85.5	91.7	115.4	134.6	158.6	171.4	183.1	221.4	614.3
1965	89.6*	45.5*	107.9*	75.4	88.4	83.2	112.8	110.4	127.3	157.8	154.0	258.2	633.7
1975	83.3*	49.4*	95.9*	76.8	87.5	77.9	107.8	101.0	112.2	108.2	154.4	195.5	494.6
1985	89.3*	53.7*	99.6*	79.2	86.7	104.9	103.6	102.6	106.1	114.0	148.6	245.3	565.3
1990	**80.0***	**40.2***	**87.7***	**78.2**	**85.3**	**93.2**	**91.4**	**81.7**	**92.7**	**91.8**	**148.4**	**238.9**	**667.2**
1995 projected	*71.5**	*30.1**	*76.0**	*71.6*	*77.5*	*80.9*	*75.8*	*68.4*	*75.8*	*82.2*	*138.7*	*247.7*	*744.7*

DENMARK: Females

	All ages	0–34	35–69	35–39	40–44	45–49	50–54	55–59	60–64	65–69	70–74	75–79	80+/NK
POPULATION (1000s)													
1955	2236.6	1178.7	914.5	153.1	156.9	152.1	137.8	124.5	103.9	86.2	66.5	43.6	33.3
1965	2399.3	1227.7	982.5	144.5	157.0	149.5	151.4	144.1	127.3	108.7	83.2	57.2	48.7
1975	2550.1	1305.0	991.1	147.4	138.7	142.6	153.9	139.7	141.2	127.6	104.3	76.8	72.9
1985	2594.8	1208.6	1061.6	200.5	180.8	145.9	133.9	134.2	140.3	126.0	117.7	96.5	110.4
1990	**2607.1**	**1175.9**	**1090.4**	**181.2**	**200.0**	**178.9**	**143.0**	**129.7**	**127.7**	**129.9**	**113.8**	**99.1**	**127.9**
1995 projected	*2607.6*	*1136.7*	*1124.3*	*182.2*	*181.6*	*198.3*	*176.5*	*139.8*	*125.1*	*120.8*	*118.8*	*96.5*	*131.3*
NUMBER OF DEATHS													
All causes													
1955	18423	1485	6280	222	361	519	720	1030	1434	1994	2650	3086	4922
1965	22037	1255	6712	223	315	466	754	1115	1552	2287	3067	3766	7237
1975	23065	821	6533	183	285	500	782	1061	1527	2195	2975	3936	8800
1985	27750	624	6597	240	332	476	740	1098	1642	2069	3314	4274	12941
1990	**29645**	**569**	**6767**	**192**	**355**	**526**	**740**	**1090**	**1544**	**2320**	**3123**	**4413**	**14773**
1995 projected	*30029*	*508*	*6884*	*175*	*297*	*543*	*889*	*1185*	*1597*	*2198*	*3297*	*4211*	*15129*
Lung cancer													
1955	140	3	85	3	3	5	7	14	24	29	19	14	19
1965	257	3	142	2	3	10	26	24	29	48	51	28	33
1975	459	3	263	–	13	20	39	63	59	69	75	61	57
1985	881	4	504	7	5	38	67	103	144	140	153	123	97
1990	**1118**	**2**	**614**	**6**	**20**	**45**	**68**	**117**	**137**	**221**	**180**	**181**	**141**
1995 projected	*1406*	*2*	*724*	*8*	*21*	*52*	*89*	*133*	*167*	*254*	*257*	*227*	*196*
ANNUAL DEATH RATE / 100,000													
All causes													
1955	919.7*	122.4*	822.8*	145.0	230.1	341.2	522.5	827.3	1380.2	2313.2	3985.0	7078.0	14780.8
1965	865.1*	99.2*	751.7*	154.3	200.6	311.7	498.0	773.8	1219.2	2104.0	3686.3	6583.9	14860.4
1975	714.8*	64.3*	678.5*	124.2	205.5	350.6	508.1	759.5	1081.4	1720.2	2852.3	5125.0	12071.3
1985	692.6*	55.9*	687.5*	119.7	183.6	326.3	552.7	818.2	1170.3	1642.1	2815.6	4429.0	11721.9
1990	**687.5***	**50.2***	**704.3***	**106.0**	**177.5**	**294.0**	**517.5**	**840.4**	**1209.1**	**1786.0**	**2744.3**	**4453.1**	**11550.4**
1995 projected	*685.1**	*46.0**	*711.6**	*96.0*	*163.5*	*273.8*	*503.7*	*847.6*	*1276.6*	*1819.5*	*2775.3*	*4363.7*	*11522.5*
All cancer													
1955	207.0*	12.1*	293.0*	57.5	105.2	160.4	233.7	341.4	487.0	665.9	900.8	1302.8	1873.9
1965	207.4*	12.5*	294.5*	69.2	92.4	152.5	258.9	351.1	454.8	682.6	896.6	1258.7	1891.2
1975	189.8*	9.9*	283.7*	41.4	79.3	169.7	248.2	378.0	468.8	600.3	779.5	1118.5	1565.2
1985	199.8*	7.7*	300.3*	39.9	61.4	156.3	260.6	409.1	551.7	623.0	883.6	1118.1	1687.5
1990	**200.9***	**6.1***	**311.4***	**37.0**	**81.0**	**144.2**	**260.1**	**410.9**	**545.8**	**700.5**	**937.6**	**1154.4**	**1505.9**
1995 projected	*202.6**	*4.8**	*318.9**	*38.4*	*80.9*	*144.2*	*255.0*	*408.4*	*566.7*	*738.4*	*992.4*	*1162.7*	*1425.7*
Lung cancer													
1955	6.8*	0.3*	11.5*	2.0	1.9	3.3	5.1	11.2	23.1	33.6	28.6	32.1	57.1
1965	10.1*	0.3*	15.8*	1.4	1.9	6.7	17.2	16.7	22.8	44.2	61.3	49.0	67.8
1975	15.8*	0.2*	27.1*	–	9.4	14.0	25.3	45.1	41.8	54.1	71.9	79.4	78.2
1985	28.3*	0.3*	53.3*	3.5	2.8	26.0	50.0	76.8	102.6	111.1	130.0	127.5	87.9
1990	**34.3***	**0.2***	**64.8***	**3.3**	**10.0**	**25.2**	**47.6**	**90.2**	**107.3**	**170.1**	**158.2**	**182.6**	**110.2**
1995 projected	*41.5**	*0.1**	*75.9**	*4.4*	*11.6*	*26.2*	*50.4*	*95.1*	*133.5*	*210.3*	*216.3*	*235.2*	*149.3*
Upper aerodigestive cancer (mouth, oesophagus, pharynx and larynx)													
1955	4.1*	–	5.2*	–	0.6	1.3	2.2	1.6	9.6	20.9	22.6	55.0	33.0
1965	4.2*	–	5.3*	–	–	0.7	4.6	6.2	6.3	19.3	18.0	29.7	59.5
1975	3.8*	0.1*	4.7*	–	–	1.4	3.2	7.2	8.5	12.5	12.5	26.0	59.0
1985	4.1*	–	5.5*	–	2.2	2.1	5.2	6.0	11.4	11.9	17.8	22.8	50.7
1990	**4.8***	**–**	**7.7***	**–**	**1.5**	**2.8**	**7.0**	**13.9**	**14.1**	**14.6**	**19.3**	**29.3**	**36.7**
1995 projected	*5.8**	*–*	*10.0**	*–*	*1.7*	*3.0*	*9.6*	*19.3*	*20.0*	*16.6*	*22.7*	*33.2*	*33.5*
Other cancer													
1955	196.0*	11.8*	276.4*	55.5	102.6	155.8	226.4	328.5	454.3	611.4	849.6	1215.6	1783.8
1965	193.1*	12.2*	273.4*	67.8	90.4	145.2	237.1	328.2	425.8	619.1	817.3	1180.1	1763.9
1975	170.2*	9.6*	251.9*	41.4	69.9	154.3	219.6	325.7	418.6	533.7	695.1	1013.0	1428.0
1985	167.4*	7.4*	241.5*	36.4	56.4	128.2	205.4	326.4	437.6	500.0	735.8	967.9	1548.9
1990	**161.8***	**6.0***	**238.9***	**33.7**	**69.5**	**116.3**	**205.6**	**306.9**	**424.4**	**515.8**	**760.1**	**942.5**	**1358.9**
1995 projected	*155.2**	*4.6**	*232.9**	*34.0*	*67.7*	*115.0*	*194.9*	*294.0*	*413.3*	*511.6*	*753.4*	*894.3*	*1243.0*
Chronic obstructive pulmonary disease (COPD)													
1955	4.5*	0.7*	3.0*	–	0.6	0.7	2.2	5.6	3.8	8.1	16.5	41.3	87.1
1965	9.0*	0.4*	8.1*	1.4	1.3	2.0	5.3	10.4	14.1	22.1	36.1	80.4	160.2
1975	14.3*	0.6*	17.7*	1.4	2.2	7.7	20.1	20.8	29.7	42.3	70.0	99.0	164.6
1985	26.7*	0.8*	37.7*	2.5	2.2	8.2	25.4	55.1	66.3	104.0	138.5	177.2	256.3
1990	**31.5***	**0.3***	**47.4***	**0.6**	**4.0**	**4.5**	**20.3**	**55.5**	**103.4**	**144.0**	**171.4**	**224.0**	**268.2**
1995 projected	*38.1**	*0.3**	*59.9**	*0.5*	*2.8*	*3.5*	*18.1*	*67.2*	*136.7*	*190.4*	*217.2*	*254.9*	*303.9*
Other respiratory disease													
1955	28.7*	8.9*	14.0*	2.0	3.8	2.6	8.0	15.3	22.1	44.1	70.7	169.7	669.7
1965	22.6*	3.2*	7.5*	0.7	1.9	3.3	4.6	8.3	8.6	24.8	80.5	131.1	655.0
1975	28.3*	1.8*	11.0*	2.7	2.9	4.2	6.5	7.2	17.7	36.1	76.7	235.7	818.9
1985	21.6*	0.7*	7.6*	1.0	1.7	2.7	3.7	7.5	13.5	23.0	51.0	137.8	712.0
1990	**17.3***	**0.5***	**5.7***	**1.1**	**3.0**	**2.8**	**2.8**	**5.4**	**7.0**	**17.7**	**46.6**	**117.1**	**562.9**
1995 projected	*14.1**	*0.3**	*4.7**	*1.6*	*3.9*	*3.0*	*2.3*	*3.6*	*4.8*	*14.1*	*39.6*	*95.3*	*450.9*
Vascular disease													
1955	457.8*	3.2*	319.0*	20.9	31.9	54.6	132.1	239.4	557.3	1197.2	2305.3	4412.8	9594.6
1965	426.4*	3.9*	262.4*	14.5	35.0	50.2	104.4	213.7	454.0	965.0	2037.3	4005.2	9739.2
1975	334.1*	2.3*	214.4*	21.7	37.5	57.5	105.3	191.1	359.1	728.8	1445.8	2933.6	7842.2
1985	282.7*	2.1*	174.8*	11.0	26.5	44.6	100.8	155.7	308.6	576.2	1233.6	2203.1	6998.2
1990	**272.3***	**2.4***	**172.4***	**13.2**	**16.0**	**38.6**	**85.3**	**165.0**	**309.3**	**579.7**	**1076.4**	**2128.2**	**6849.9**
1995 projected	*259.8**	*2.7**	*161.5**	*9.9*	*13.2*	*30.8*	*81.6*	*161.7*	*308.6*	*524.8*	*1000.0*	*1961.7*	*6683.9*
Liver cirrhosis													
1955	7.7*	0.2*	11.7*	0.7	3.2	4.6	7.3	13.7	22.1	30.2	45.1	57.3	45.0
1965	7.4*	0.5*	9.4*	1.4	1.3	3.3	6.6	11.8	17.3	23.9	39.7	59.4	67.8
1975	7.6*	0.4*	10.8*	1.4	7.9	10.5	11.7	12.2	17.7	14.1	33.6	32.6	70.0
1985	7.7*	0.5*	14.3*	3.5	7.7	7.5	17.2	20.9	20.0	23.0	20.4	28.0	27.2
1990	**7.8***	**0.3***	**15.4***	**5.5**	**6.5**	**12.3**	**19.6**	**23.1**	**17.2**	**23.9**	**23.7**	**13.1**	**20.3**
1995 projected	*8.0**	*0.3**	*16.4**	*4.9*	*8.3*	*14.1*	*23.2*	*23.6*	*16.8*	*24.0*	*20.2*	*11.4*	*14.5*
Other medical causes													
1955	158.8*	80.1*	138.7*	44.4	59.9	72.3	100.9	156.6	232.9	303.9	473.7	786.7	1633.6
1965	134.9*	59.8*	121.4*	39.4	43.3	61.5	71.3	115.9	205.8	312.8	447.1	792.0	1406.6
1975	94.6*	32.2*	82.5*	15.6	28.8	45.6	53.3	83.8	130.3	220.2	354.7	569.0	1231.8
1985	104.4*	26.5*	95.1*	17.5	27.1	50.7	79.9	111.0	148.3	231.0	393.4	626.9	1501.8
1990	**115.0***	**27.1***	**104.9***	**23.7**	**27.5**	**44.7**	**80.4**	**121.0**	**175.4**	**261.7**	**399.8**	**663.0**	**1810.0**
1995 projected	*125.0**	*27.3**	*111.8**	*24.7*	*27.0*	*42.9*	*81.6*	*133.0*	*196.6*	*276.5*	*416.7*	*723.3*	*2102.8*
All non-medical causes													
1955	55.2*	17.1*	43.4*	19.6	25.5	46.0	38.5	55.4	54.9	63.8	172.9	307.3	876.9
1965	57.5*	18.8*	48.3*	27.7	25.5	38.8	46.9	62.5	64.4	72.7	149.0	257.0	940.5
1975	46.0*	17.1*	58.3*	40.0	46.9	55.4	63.0	66.6	58.1	78.4	92.0	136.7	378.6
1985	49.8*	17.5*	57.9*	44.4	57.0	56.2	65.0	58.9	62.0	61.9	95.2	137.8	538.9
1990	**42.7***	**13.4***	**47.0***	**24.8**	**39.5**	**47.0**	**49.0**	**59.4**	**50.9**	**58.5**	**88.8**	**153.4**	**533.2**
1995 projected	*37.5**	*10.3**	*38.3**	*15.9*	*27.5*	*35.3*	*41.9*	*50.1*	*46.4*	*51.3*	*89.2*	*154.4*	*540.7*

(*The rates for the age groups 0–34 and 35–69 are the means of seven five-yearly rates, but the all-ages rates are standardised to the conventional "European" age distribution)

DENMARK: 1975

Smoking–attributed deaths (Sm.) and total deaths (Total)

		ALL CAUSES	ALL CANCER	Lung cancer	Upper aero–digestive ca.	Other cancer	COPD	Other respiratory	Vascular disease	Liver cirrhosis	Other medical	Non–medical
Males												
0–34	Sm.	–	–	–	–	–	–	–	–	–	–	–
	Total	1530	151	4	0	147	12	29	44	9	604	681
35–69	Sm.	3268	1288	931	83	274	320	47	1310	–	303	–
	Total	10467	2911	1007	128	1776	413	173	4748	251	1066	905
		(31%)	(44%)	(92%)	(65%)	(15%)	(77%)	(27%)	(28%)		(28%)	
70+	Sm.	2692	982	648	66	268	463	77	1011	–	159	–
	Total	15577	3129	717	115	2297	652	782	9077	58	1422	457
		(17%)	(31%)	(90%)	(57%)	(12%)	(71%)	(10%)	(11%)		(11%)	
Any age	Sm.	5960	2270	1579	149	542	783	124	2321	–	462	–
	Total	27574	6191	1728	243	4220	1077	984	13869	318	3092	2043
		(22%)	(37%)	(91%)	(61%)	(13%)	(73%)	(13%)	(17%)		(15%)	
Females												
0–34	Sm.	–	–	–	–	–	–	–	–	–	–	–
	Total	821	130	3	2	125	8	23	29	5	403	223
35–69	Sm.	674	236	177	15	44	91	14	233	–	100	–
	Total	6533	2751	263	45	2443	172	105	2032	106	792	575
		(10%)	(9%)	(67%)	(33%)	(2%)	(53%)	(13%)	(11%)		(13%)	
70+	Sm.	650	162	113	20	29	117	23	292	–	56	–
	Total	15711	2813	193	76	2544	269	858	9478	111	1705	477
		(4%)	(6%)	(59%)	(26%)	(1%)	(43%)	(3%)	(3%)		(3%)	
Any age	Sm.	1324	398	290	35	73	208	37	525	–	156	–
	Total	23065	5694	459	123	5112	449	986	11539	222	2900	1275
		(6%)	(7%)	(63%)	(28%)	(1%)	(46%)	(4%)	(5%)		(5%)	
Males+Females												
0–34	Sm.	–	–	–	–	–	–	–	–	–	–	–
	Total	2351	281	7	2	272	20	52	73	14	1007	904
35–69	Sm.	3942	1524	1108	98	318	411	61	1543	–	403	–
	Total	17000	5662	1270	173	4219	585	278	6780	357	1858	1480
		(23%)	(27%)	(87%)	(57%)	(8%)	(70%)	(22%)	(23%)		(22%)	
70+	Sm.	3342	1144	761	86	297	580	100	1303	–	215	–
	Total	31288	5942	910	191	4841	921	1640	18555	169	3127	934
		(11%)	(19%)	(84%)	(45%)	(6%)	(63%)	(6%)	(7%)		(7%)	
Any age	Sm.	7284	2668	1869	184	615	991	161	2846	–	618	–
	Total	50639	11885	2187	366	9332	1526	1970	25408	540	5992	3318
		(14%)	(22%)	(85%)	(50%)	(7%)	(65%)	(8%)	(11%)		(10%)	

DENMARK: 1985

Smoking–attributed deaths (Sm.) and total deaths (Total)

		ALL CAUSES	ALL CANCER	Lung cancer	Upper aero–digestive ca.	Other cancer	COPD	Other respiratory	Vascular disease	Liver cirrhosis	Other medical	Non–medical
Males												
0–34	Sm.	–	–	–	–	–	–	–	–	–	–	–
	Total	1305	113	1	0	112	8	14	38	19	391	722
35–69	Sm.	3647	1528	1051	150	327	413	25	1272	–	409	–
	Total	10584	3206	1126	220	1860	515	82	4163	322	1286	1010
		(34%)	(48%)	(93%)	(68%)	(18%)	(80%)	(30%)	(31%)		(32%)	
70+	Sm.	4243	1598	1051	102	445	904	95	1364	–	282	–
	Total	18439	4245	1139	161	2945	1178	731	9618	73	1984	610
		(23%)	(38%)	(92%)	(63%)	(15%)	(77%)	(13%)	(14%)		(14%)	
Any age	Sm.	7890	3126	2102	252	772	1317	120	2636	–	691	–
	Total	30328	7564	2266	381	4917	1701	827	13819	414	3661	2342
		(26%)	(41%)	(93%)	(66%)	(16%)	(77%)	(15%)	(19%)		(19%)	
Females												
0–34	Sm.	–	–	–	–	–	–	–	–	–	–	–
	Total	624	94	4	0	90	10	7	26	7	261	219
35–69	Sm.	1457	542	418	29	95	257	19	404	–	235	–
	Total	6597	2876	504	53	2319	353	72	1638	140	913	605
		(22%)	(19%)	(83%)	(55%)	(4%)	(73%)	(26%)	(25%)		(26%)	
70+	Sm.	1721	411	282	42	87	387	54	691	–	178	–
	Total	20529	3982	373	99	3510	617	979	11304	81	2726	840
		(8%)	(10%)	(76%)	(42%)	(2%)	(63%)	(6%)	(6%)		(7%)	
Any age	Sm.	3178	953	700	71	182	644	73	1095	–	413	–
	Total	27750	6952	881	152	5919	980	1058	12968	228	3900	1664
		(11%)	(14%)	(79%)	(47%)	(3%)	(66%)	(7%)	(8%)		(11%)	
Males+Females												
0–34	Sm.	–	–	–	–	–	–	–	–	–	–	–
	Total	1929	207	5	0	202	18	21	64	26	652	941
35–69	Sm.	5104	2070	1469	179	422	670	44	1676	–	644	–
	Total	17181	6082	1630	273	4179	868	154	5801	462	2199	1615
		(30%)	(34%)	(90%)	(66%)	(10%)	(77%)	(29%)	(29%)		(29%)	
70+	Sm.	5964	2009	1333	144	532	1291	149	2055	–	460	–
	Total	38968	8227	1512	260	6455	1795	1710	20922	154	4710	1450
		(15%)	(24%)	(88%)	(55%)	(8%)	(72%)	(9%)	(10%)		(10%)	
Any age	Sm.	11068	4079	2802	323	954	1961	193	3731	–	1104	–
	Total	58078	14516	3147	533	10836	2681	1885	26787	642	7561	4006
		(19%)	(28%)	(89%)	(61%)	(9%)	(73%)	(10%)	(14%)		(15%)	

(To be conservative, no deaths before age 35, and none from liver cirrhosis or non–medical causes, were attributed to smoking.)

DENMARK: 1990

Smoking-attributed deaths (Sm.) and total deaths (Total)

		ALL CAUSES	ALL CANCER	Lung cancer	Upper aero-digestive ca.	Other cancer	COPD	Other respiratory	Vascular disease	Liver cirrhosis	Other medical	Non-medical
Males												
0–34	Sm.	–	–	–	–	–	–	–	–	–	–	–
	Total	1158	98	3	2	93	18	10	37	12	444	539
35–69	Sm.	3315	1435	957	173	305	357	26	1021	–	476	–
	Total	10283	3192	1030	267	1895	455	87	3598	396	1615	940
		(32%)	(45%)	(93%)	(65%)	(16%)	(78%)	(30%)	(28%)		(29%)	
70+	Sm.	4306	1636	1056	125	455	960	74	1308	–	328	–
	Total	19503	4524	1147	199	3178	1273	636	9826	78	2454	712
		(22%)	(36%)	(92%)	(63%)	(14%)	(75%)	(12%)	(13%)		(13%)	
Any age	Sm.	7621	3071	2013	298	760	1317	100	2329	–	804	–
	Total	30944	7814	2180	468	5166	1746	733	13461	486	4513	2191
		(25%)	(39%)	(92%)	(64%)	(15%)	(75%)	(14%)	(17%)		(18%)	
Females												
0–34	Sm.	–	–	–	–	–	–	–	–	–	–	–
	Total	569	75	2	0	73	4	5	31	4	284	166
35–69	Sm.	1823	687	527	45	115	339	17	476	–	304	–
	Total	6767	2999	614	73	2312	437	56	1609	156	1014	496
		(27%)	(23%)	(86%)	(62%)	(5%)	(78%)	(30%)	(30%)		(30%)	
70+	Sm.	2561	592	410	52	130	546	73	1044	–	306	–
	Total	22309	4137	502	98	3537	760	889	12095	66	3427	935
		(11%)	(14%)	(82%)	(53%)	(4%)	(72%)	(8%)	(9%)		(9%)	
Any age	Sm.	4384	1279	937	97	245	885	90	1520	–	610	–
	Total	29645	7211	1118	171	5922	1201	950	13735	226	4725	1597
		(15%)	(18%)	(84%)	(57%)	(4%)	(74%)	(9%)	(11%)		(13%)	
Males+Females												
0–34	Sm.	–	–	–	–	–	–	–	–	–	–	–
	Total	1727	173	5	2	166	22	15	68	16	728	705
35–69	Sm.	5138	2122	1484	218	420	696	43	1497	–	780	–
	Total	17050	6191	1644	340	4207	892	143	5207	552	2629	1436
		(30%)	(34%)	(90%)	(64%)	(10%)	(78%)	(30%)	(29%)		(30%)	
70+	Sm.	6867	2228	1466	177	585	1506	147	2352	–	634	–
	Total	41812	8661	1649	297	6715	2033	1525	21921	144	5881	1647
		(16%)	(26%)	(89%)	(60%)	(9%)	(74%)	(10%)	(11%)		(11%)	
Any age	Sm.	12005	4350	2950	395	1005	2202	190	3849	–	1414	–
	Total	60589	15025	3298	639	11088	2947	1683	27196	712	9238	3788
		(20%)	(29%)	(89%)	(62%)	(9%)	(75%)	(11%)	(14%)		(15%)	

DENMARK: 1995

Smoking-attributed deaths (Sm.) and total deaths (Total)

		ALL CAUSES	ALL CANCER	Lung cancer	Upper aero-digestive ca.	Other cancer	COPD	Other respiratory	Vascular disease	Liver cirrhosis	Other medical	Non-medical
Males												
0–34	Sm.	–	–	–	–	–	–	–	–	–	–	–
	Total	1047	85	2	3	80	24	9	36	14	478	401
35–69	Sm.	3067	1367	884	199	284	320	20	828	–	532	–
	Total	10142	3201	960	325	1916	412	81	3129	481	1985	853
		(30%)	(43%)	(92%)	(61%)	(15%)	(78%)	(25%)	(26%)		(27%)	
70+	Sm.	4246	1616	1013	148	455	981	58	1221	–	370	–
	Total	19955	4664	1106	242	3316	1319	535	9662	82	2910	783
		(21%)	(35%)	(92%)	(61%)	(14%)	(74%)	(11%)	(13%)		(13%)	
Any age	Sm.	7313	2983	1897	347	739	1301	78	2049	–	902	–
	Total	31144	7950	2068	570	5312	1755	625	12827	577	5373	2037
		(23%)	(38%)	(92%)	(61%)	(14%)	(74%)	(12%)	(16%)		(17%)	
Females												
0–34	Sm.	–	–	–	–	–	–	–	–	–	–	–
	Total	508	58	2	0	56	3	3	34	4	284	122
35–69	Sm.	2155	832	635	64	133	437	16	504	–	366	–
	Total	6884	3125	724	98	2303	540	48	1493	176	1089	413
		(31%)	(27%)	(88%)	(65%)	(6%)	(81%)	(33%)	(34%)		(34%)	
70+	Sm.	3423	819	587	62	170	702	80	1357	–	465	–
	Total	22637	4173	680	103	3390	903	731	11857	54	3954	965
		(15%)	(20%)	(86%)	(60%)	(5%)	(78%)	(11%)	(11%)		(12%)	
Any age	Sm.	5578	1651	1222	126	303	1139	96	1861	–	831	–
	Total	30029	7356	1406	201	5749	1446	782	13384	234	5327	1500
		(19%)	(22%)	(87%)	(63%)	(5%)	(79%)	(12%)	(14%)		(16%)	
Males+Females												
0–34	Sm.	–	–	–	–	–	–	–	–	–	–	–
	Total	1555	143	4	3	136	27	12	70	18	762	523
35–69	Sm.	5222	2199	1519	263	417	757	36	1332	–	898	–
	Total	17026	6326	1684	423	4219	952	129	4622	657	3074	1266
		(31%)	(35%)	(90%)	(62%)	(10%)	(80%)	(28%)	(29%)		(29%)	
70+	Sm.	7669	2435	1600	210	625	1683	138	2578	–	835	–
	Total	42592	8837	1786	345	6706	2222	1266	21519	136	6864	1748
		(18%)	(28%)	(90%)	(61%)	(9%)	(76%)	(11%)	(12%)		(12%)	
Any age	Sm.	12891	4634	3119	473	1042	2440	174	3910	–	1733	–
	Total	61173	15306	3474	771	11061	3201	1407	26211	811	10700	3537
		(21%)	(30%)	(90%)	(61%)	(9%)	(76%)	(12%)	(15%)		(16%)	

(To be conservative, no deaths before age 35, and none from liver cirrhosis or non-medical causes, were attributed to smoking.)

¶ESTONIA: 1990

		No. of deaths			Standardised rates (Defined on p.328)			Annual death rates / 100, 000						
		All ages	0–34	35–69	All ages	0–34	35–69	0–4	5–9	10–14	15–19	20–24	25–29	30–34
ALL CAUSES	M	9424	930	4888	1611.3	223.7	2019.9	363.5	70.2	66.8	172.2	257.7	284.5	350.9
	F	10106	354	2662	855.3	88.2	798.1	269.0	38.1	27.5	62.7	71.6	65.3	83.5
Tuberculosis	M	73	10	52	11.5	2.4	20.4	–	–	–	–	1.8	5.0	9.9
	F	13	1	9	1.3	0.2	2.6	–	–	–	–	–	–	1.6
Other infective	M	26	16	9	3.6	3.7	3.4	22.6	–	1.8	–	–	1.7	–
and parasitic	F	16	6	5	1.9	1.5	1.4	8.5	–	–	–	2.0	–	–
ALL CANCER	M	1682	32	1153	286.4	7.7	493.2	4.8	5.0	8.8	8.7	3.6	5.0	18.1
	F	1466	31	823	143.4	7.8	242.3	6.8	3.5	7.3	7.6	8.0	6.9	14.7
Mouth and	M	68	–	57	11.0	–	21.5	–	–	–	–	–	–	–
pharynx cancer	F	14	–	6	1.3	–	1.7	–	–	–	–	–	–	–
Oesophagus cancer	M	46	–	39	7.7	–	16.9	–	–	–	–	–	–	–
	F	13	1	6	1.3	0.2	1.8	–	–	–	–	–	–	1.6
Stomach cancer	M	256	4	175	43.7	1.0	74.2	–	–	–	1.7	1.8	–	3.3
	F	223	1	116	21.1	0.2	34.6	–	–	–	–	–	1.7	–
Colorectal cancer	M	136	1	77	24.1	0.2	32.9	–	–	–	–	–	–	1.6
	F	201	–	89	18.1	–	27.1	–	–	–	–	–	–	–
Liver cancer	M	...	...	...	...	...	...	...	...	...	...	...	...	...
	F	...	...	...	...	...	...	...	...	...	...	...	...	...
Pancreas cancer	M	...	...	...	...	...	...	...	...	...	...	...	...	...
	F	...	...	...	...	...	...	...	...	...	...	...	...	...
Larynx cancer	M	35	–	31	5.6	–	12.7	–	–	–	–	–	–	–
	F	2	–	2	0.2	–	0.6	–	–	–	–	–	–	–
Lung cancer	M	551	1	416	93.0	0.2	176.6	–	–	–	–	–	–	1.6
	F	104	–	61	10.1	–	18.4	–	–	–	–	–	–	–
Malignant melanoma	M	...	...	...	...	...	...	...	...	...	...	...	...	...
	F	...	...	...	...	...	...	...	...	...	...	...	...	...
Female breast cancer	F	218	4	152	22.7	0.9	43.7	–	–	–	–	–	–	6.5
Cervix cancer	F	69	2	42	7.1	0.5	12.0	–	–	–	–	–	1.7	1.6
Other uterine cancer	F	69	1	35	6.5	0.2	10.3	–	–	–	–	–	–	1.6
Ovarian cancer	F	...	...	...	...	...	...	...	...	...	...	...	...	...
Prostate cancer	M	103	–	43	19.1	–	21.6	–	–	–	–	–	–	–
Bladder cancer	M	...	...	...	...	...	...	...	...	...	...	...	...	...
	F	...	...	...	...	...	...	...	...	...	...	...	...	...
Other and ill–defined	M	398	17	263	67.5	4.1	114.5	3.2	1.7	7.0	5.2	–	3.3	8.2
cancer sites	F	470	14	268	46.5	3.6	78.8	3.4	1.7	5.5	5.7	4.0	3.4	1.6
Hodgkin's disease	M	...	...	...	...	...	...	...	...	...	...	...	...	...
	F	...	...	...	...	...	...	...	...	...	...	...	...	...
Myeloma and all	M	39	3	23	6.7	0.7	9.7	–	–	–	–	1.8	–	3.3
lymphomas	F	35	3	22	3.7	0.8	6.2	–	1.7	–	–	4.0	–	–
Leukaemia	M	50	6	29	8.2	1.4	12.6	1.6	3.3	1.8	1.7	–	1.7	–
	F	48	5	24	4.8	1.3	7.2	3.4	–	1.8	1.9	–	–	1.6
ALL VASCULAR	M	4917	40	2256	898.0	9.6	984.7	1.6	1.7	–	1.7	12.7	11.6	37.9
DISEASE	F	6903	14	1188	540.6	3.5	365.9	6.8	–	–	–	6.0	1.7	9.8
Rheumatic heart	M	48	2	42	7.4	0.5	16.2	–	–	–	–	–	1.7	1.6
disease and fever	F	58	–	45	6.0	–	13.3	–	–	–	–	–	–	–
Hypertensive disease	M	62	–	53	9.9	–	20.7	–	–	–	–	–	–	–
	F	66	1	25	5.9	0.2	7.7	–	–	–	–	–	–	1.6
Ischaemic heart	M	3199	17	1422	586.6	4.1	621.8	–	–	–	–	3.6	8.3	16.5
disease	F	4176	2	614	321.6	0.5	189.8	–	–	–	–	–	–	3.3
Pulmonary embolism	M	...	...	...	...	...	...	...	...	...	...	...	...	...
and other venous	F	...	...	...	...	...	...	...	...	...	...	...	...	...
Cerebrovascular	M	1313	9	535	245.2	2.2	242.6	1.6	1.7	–	–	3.6	1.7	6.6
disease	F	2381	2	417	186.9	0.5	129.0	–	–	–	–	–	1.7	1.6
Other vascular	M	295	12	204	48.8	2.9	83.4	–	–	–	1.7	5.4	–	13.2
disease, incl. venous	F	222	9	87	20.1	2.3	26.2	6.8	–	–	–	6.0	–	3.3
Chronic obstructive	M	225	1	133	40.1	0.2	60.5	–	–	–	1.7	–	–	–
pulmonary disease	F	125	2	62	11.8	0.5	18.6	–	–	–	–	2.0	1.7	–
Other respiratory	M	93	23	50	14.5	5.3	19.5	30.7	3.3	–	–	–	3.3	–
disease	F	45	19	12	4.9	4.6	3.7	25.4	–	1.8	1.9	–	–	3.3
Peptic ulcer	M	48	–	29	8.3	–	11.0	–	–	–	–	–	–	–
	F	27	–	12	2.3	–	3.6	–	–	–	–	–	–	–
Liver cirrhosis and	M	70	4	54	10.9	0.9	20.4	1.6	–	–	–	–	3.3	1.6
other liver disease	F	37	2	23	4.0	0.5	6.7	–	1.7	–	–	–	–	1.6
Renal disease	M	87	5	49	15.0	1.2	20.9	3.2	–	–	–	3.6	1.7	–
	F	130	3	69	12.2	0.8	20.4	–	–	–	1.9	2.0	–	1.6
Pregnancy and birth	F	7	4	3	0.9	1.0	0.8	–	–	–	–	2.0	1.7	3.3
Congenital and	M	137	132	5	17.7	30.6	1.5	193.9	8.4	3.5	3.5	1.8	1.7	1.6
perinatal causes	F	106	100	6	14.1	24.4	1.7	143.8	8.7	5.5	7.6	2.0	–	3.3
Ill–defined causes	M	132	7	30	25.3	1.7	11.2	3.2	–	–	–	1.8	3.3	3.3
	F	302	7	6	20.8	1.8	1.9	6.8	1.7	–	1.9	2.0	–	–
Other medical causes	M	382	54	232	61.9	12.9	91.6	30.7	–	1.8	10.4	9.1	13.3	24.7
	F	427	37	215	42.8	9.3	63.9	22.0	3.5	1.8	11.4	8.0	8.6	9.8
ALL NON–	M	1552	606	836	218.2	147.4	281.5	71.1	51.8	51.0	146.1	223.2	234.6	253.7
MEDICAL CAUSES	F	502	128	229	54.4	32.3	64.5	49.1	19.1	11.0	30.4	37.8	44.7	34.4
Motor vehicle	M	399	203	174	54.5	49.7	59.5	6.5	26.8	17.6	60.9	87.1	71.5	77.4
traffic accidents	F	127	49	52	14.4	12.7	14.6	6.8	6.9	7.3	15.2	23.9	17.2	11.5
Fire	M	67	25	29	10.0	5.9	10.3	17.8	5.0	1.8	3.5	1.8	3.3	8.2
	F	38	11	12	3.8	2.7	3.7	13.5	1.7	–	–	–	3.4	–
Suicide	M	307	94	187	44.0	22.8	63.4	–	–	5.3	20.9	30.9	54.9	47.8
	F	118	18	65	12.9	4.6	18.4	–	–	–	3.8	8.0	12.0	8.2
Homicide	M	138	56	76	19.0	13.7	24.5	1.6	1.7	1.8	12.2	25.4	34.9	18.1
	F	35	8	21	4.0	2.0	5.8	–	–	1.8	3.8	2.0	1.7	4.9
POPULATION (thousands):	M=males				739.1	412.0	293.2	61.9	59.8	56.9	57.5	55.1	60.1	60.7
	F=females				836.4	393.6	357.4	59.1	57.7	54.6	52.6	50.3	58.2	61.1

ESTONIA: 1990

9th ICD categories

Annual death rates / 100, 000

35–39	40–44	45–49	50–54	55–59	60–64	65–69	70–74	75–79	80+/NK	Sex	Cause	ICD
472.8	736.2	1069.4	1490.5	2206.4	3367.5	4796.2	6859.4	9111.1	17680.9	M	**ALL CAUSES**	001–999
154.8	211.4	350.2	500.9	739.6	1327.5	2302.2	3721.4	5941.4	14543.0	F		
5.3	14.3	6.9	12.7	34.4	31.3	37.9	62.5	17.1	10.6	M	**Tuberculosis**	010–018, 137
3.4	1.9	–	–	2.0	3.9	7.2	–	6.9	3.3	F		
1.8	4.1	2.3	2.1	–	8.5	4.7	–	8.5	–	M	**Other infective**	Rest of 001–139
–	–	2.1	5.5	–	–	2.4	7.6	3.4	6.6	F	**and parasitic**	
24.6	83.8	217.6	353.1	609.3	945.9	1218.0	1554.7	1547.0	1244.7	M	**ALL CANCER**	140–208
62.9	81.9	128.7	182.8	230.8	447.7	561.2	610.7	817.2	711.9	F		
1.8	8.2	13.9	35.9	22.1	39.9	28.4	46.9	25.6	21.3	M	**Mouth and**	140–149
1.7	–	–	1.8	–	5.8	2.4	11.5	3.4	13.2	F	**pharynx cancer**	
–	–	13.9	8.5	22.1	31.3	42.7	23.4	8.5	31.9	M	**Oesophagus cancer**	150
–	–	–	–	2.0	5.8	4.8	11.5	3.4	6.6	F		
3.5	18.4	30.1	57.1	115.5	105.4	189.6	203.1	230.8	255.3	M	**Stomach cancer**	151
6.8	9.5	14.8	18.3	45.4	56.2	91.1	91.6	165.5	112.6	F		
1.8	6.1	9.3	19.0	31.9	91.2	71.1	171.9	145.3	202.1	M	**Colorectal cancer**	153, 154
3.4	7.6	6.3	20.1	17.8	40.7	93.5	87.8	175.9	125.8	F		
...	...	...	...	...	...	...	...	...	...	M	**Liver cancer**	Not given separately
...	...	...	...	...	...	...	...	...	...	F		
...	...	...	...	...	...	...	...	...	...	M	**Pancreas cancer**	Not given separately
...	...	...	...	...	...	...	...	...	...	F		
–	6.1	4.6	19.0	4.9	25.6	28.4	15.6	17.1	–	M	**Larynx cancer**	161
–	–	–	–	2.0	1.9	–	–	–	–	F		
3.5	22.5	74.1	129.0	255.5	339.0	412.3	515.6	384.6	244.7	M	**Lung cancer**	162
1.7	1.9	2.1	11.0	21.7	32.9	57.6	64.9	48.3	39.7	F		
...	...	...	...	...	...	...	...	...	...	M	**Malignant melanoma**	Not given separately
...	...	...	...	...	...	...	...	...	...	F		
11.9	19.0	44.3	42.0	53.3	75.6	60.0	38.2	79.3	96.0	F	**Female breast cancer**	174
11.9	7.6	6.3	7.3	11.8	17.4	21.6	34.4	27.6	26.5	F	**Cervix cancer**	180
6.8	3.8	8.4	–	7.9	23.3	21.6	26.7	31.0	56.3	F	**Other uterine cancer**	179, 182
...	...	...	...	...	...	...	...	...	...	F	**Ovarian cancer**	Not given separately
–	–	–	–	22.1	48.4	80.6	132.8	213.7	191.5	M	**Prostate cancer**	185
...	...	...	...	...	...	...	...	...	...	M	**Bladder cancer**	Not given separately
...	...	...	...	...	...	...	...	...	...	F		
10.5	20.4	64.8	65.5	113.0	219.4	308.1	367.2	418.8	234.0	M	**Other and ill-defined**	Rest of 140–208,
13.6	24.8	42.2	69.5	63.1	158.9	179.9	209.9	248.3	202.0	F	**cancer sites**	incl. 155, 157, 172, 183, 188
...	...	...	...	...	...	...	...	...	...	M	**Hodgkin's disease**	Not given separately
...	...	...	...	...	...	...	...	...	...	F		
1.8	–	2.3	10.6	12.3	17.1	23.7	54.7	34.2	21.3	M	**Myeloma and all**	200–203,
3.4	5.7	2.1	7.3	3.9	13.6	7.2	7.6	17.2	9.9	F	**lymphomas**	incl. 201
1.8	2.0	4.6	8.5	9.8	28.5	33.2	23.4	68.4	42.6	M	**Leukaemia**	204–208
1.7	1.9	2.1	5.5	2.0	15.5	21.6	26.7	17.2	23.2	F		
117.8	216.8	405.1	634.2	1017.2	1743.6	2758.3	4367.2	6376.1	14000.0	M	**ALL VASCULAR**	390–459
18.7	40.0	103.4	148.1	276.1	629.8	1345.3	2694.7	4496.6	12221.9	F	**DISEASE**	
5.3	6.1	6.9	16.9	29.5	19.9	28.4	15.6	17.1	–	M	**Rheumatic heart**	390–398
–	7.6	4.2	7.3	13.8	29.1	31.2	19.1	24.1	3.3	F	**disease and fever**	
5.3	4.1	11.6	27.5	12.3	51.3	33.2	31.3	17.1	31.9	M	**Hypertensive disease**	401–405
–	1.9	10.5	5.5	3.9	7.8	24.0	19.1	48.3	69.5	F		
73.8	147.2	231.5	401.7	670.8	1059.8	1767.8	2632.8	4265.0	9829.8	M	**Ischaemic heart**	410–414
10.2	13.3	38.0	78.6	149.9	312.0	726.6	1587.8	2644.8	7870.9	F	**disease**	
...	...	...	...	...	...	...	...	...	...	M	**Pulmonary embolism**	Not given
...	...	...	...	...	...	...	...	...	...	F	**and other venous**	separately
8.8	34.8	90.3	135.3	226.0	458.7	744.1	1531.3	1812.0	3840.4	M	**Cerebrovascular**	430–438
6.8	11.4	31.6	34.7	84.8	244.2	489.2	1000.0	1682.8	4013.2	F	**disease**	
24.6	24.5	64.8	52.9	78.6	153.8	184.8	156.3	265.0	297.9	M	**Other vascular**	Rest of 390–459,
1.7	5.7	19.0	21.9	23.7	36.8	74.3	68.7	96.6	264.9	F	**disease, incl. venous**	incl. 415, 451–3
–	6.1	18.5	40.2	51.6	122.5	184.8	265.6	265.0	276.6	M	**Chronic obstructive**	490–496
–	5.7	12.7	12.8	19.7	29.1	50.4	45.8	89.7	76.2	F	**pulmonary disease**	
8.8	8.2	16.2	12.7	24.6	28.5	37.9	31.3	76.9	74.5	M	**Other respiratory**	Rest of 460–519
–	–	–	3.7	2.0	5.8	14.4	15.3	10.3	23.2	F	**disease**	
5.3	6.1	6.9	12.7	7.4	19.9	19.0	54.7	59.8	53.2	M	**Peptic ulcer**	531–533
–	–	2.1	3.7	5.9	3.9	9.6	–	20.7	29.8	F		
5.3	6.1	13.9	21.1	24.6	48.4	23.7	15.6	51.3	42.6	M	**Liver cirrhosis and**	570–573, 576,
1.7	–	8.4	7.3	3.9	13.6	12.0	22.9	20.7	–	F	**other liver disease**	575.2–579.9
5.3	2.0	13.9	16.9	19.7	31.3	56.9	70.3	102.6	127.7	M	**Renal disease**	580–590
1.7	5.7	–	20.1	27.6	34.9	52.8	34.4	82.8	82.8	F		
3.4	1.9	–	–	–	–	–	–	–	–	F	**Pregnancy and birth**	630–676
1.8	2.0	–	4.2	2.5	–	–	–	–	–	M	**Congenital and**	740–779
–	3.8	–	–	5.9	–	2.4	–	–	–	F	**perinatal causes**	
5.3	6.1	4.6	14.8	17.2	11.4	19.0	7.8	68.4	914.9	M	**Ill-defined causes**	780–799
1.7	–	2.1	–	2.0	–	7.2	3.8	44.8	910.6	F		
26.4	61.3	62.5	74.0	93.4	133.9	189.6	203.1	256.4	425.5	M	**Other medical causes**	Rest of 001–799
13.6	30.5	33.8	42.0	82.8	79.5	165.5	183.2	203.4	225.2	F		
265.4	319.0	300.9	291.8	304.7	242.2	246.4	226.6	282.1	510.6	M	**ALL NON-**	E800–E999
47.6	40.0	57.0	75.0	80.9	79.5	71.9	103.1	144.8	251.7	F	**MEDICAL CAUSES**	
58.0	61.3	62.5	55.0	73.7	39.9	66.4	23.4	68.4	117.0	M	**Motor vehicle**	E810–E819
15.3	5.7	6.3	18.3	21.7	15.5	19.2	26.7	17.2	46.4	F	**traffic accidents**	
7.0	8.2	4.6	14.8	4.9	22.8	9.5	23.4	25.6	74.5	M	**Fire**	E890–E899
1.7	–	–	3.7	–	5.8	14.4	7.6	17.2	26.5	F		
59.8	75.7	69.4	52.9	63.9	65.5	56.9	70.3	59.8	106.4	M	**Suicide**	E950–E959
8.5	11.4	23.2	27.4	17.8	21.3	19.2	38.2	34.5	49.7	F		
38.7	36.8	30.1	16.9	19.7	5.7	23.7	23.4	8.5	21.3	M	**Homicide**	E960–E969
5.1	7.6	6.3	9.1	3.9	5.8	2.4	3.8	3.4	13.2	F		
56.9	48.9	43.2	47.3	40.7	35.1	21.1	12.8	11.7	9.4	M	**POPULATION (thousands)**	
58.8	52.5	47.4	54.7	50.7	51.6	41.7	26.2	29.0	30.2	F		

ESTONIA: Males

	All ages	0–34	35–69	35–39	40–44	45–49	50–54	55–59	60–64	65–69	70–74	75–79	80+/NK
POPULATION (1000s)													
1985–90	720.5	405.6	279.9	54.1	43.7	48.1	44.5	41.4	29.8	18.3	14.8	11.4	8.8
1985	702.7	399.0	267.5	49.2	44.0	49.6	43.9	39.4	25.0	16.4	17.0	11.1	8.1
1990	**739.1**	**412.0**	**293.2**	**56.9**	**48.9**	**43.2**	**47.3**	**40.7**	**35.1**	**21.1**	**12.8**	**11.7**	**9.4**
1995 projected	*743.0*	*400.0*	*308.0*	*59.0*	*55.0*	*47.0*	*40.0*	*43.0*	*35.0*	*29.0*	*16.0*	*9.0*	*10.0*
NUMBER OF DEATHS													
All causes													
1985–90	8751	844	4272	236	280	467	622	885	951	831	962	1098	1575
1985	9098	901	4286	243	324	550	650	911	853	755	1180	1184	1547
1990	**9424**	**930**	**4888**	**269**	**360**	**462**	**705**	**898**	**1182**	**1012**	**878**	**1066**	**1662**
1995 projected	*9572*	*913*	*5246*	*267*	*395*	*496*	*580*	*930*	*1182*	*1396*	*1026*	*758*	*1629*
Lung cancer													
1985–90	527	1	399	4	7	32	52	109	116	79	57	47	23
1985	478	1	335	6	8	29	50	104	82	56	66	48	28
1990	**551**	**1**	**416**	**2**	**11**	**32**	**61**	**104**	**119**	**87**	**66**	**45**	**23**
1995 projected	*634*	*1*	*488*	*2*	*14*	*40*	*53*	*111*	*127*	*141*	*92*	*33*	*20*
ANNUAL DEATH RATE / 100,000 (*The rates for the age groups 0–34 and 35–69 are the means of seven five-yearly rates, but the all-ages rates are standardised to the conventional "European" age distribution)													
All causes													
1985–90	1561.0*	205.3*	1902.2*	436.2	640.7	970.9	1397.8	2137.7	3191.3	4541.0	6500.0	9631.6	17897.7
1985	1677.7*	222.0*	2021.1*	493.9	736.4	1108.9	1480.6	2312.2	3412.0	4603.7	6941.2	10666.7	19098.8
1990	**1611.3***	**223.7***	**2019.9***	**472.8**	**736.2**	**1069.4**	**1490.5**	**2206.4**	**3367.5**	**4796.2**	**6859.4**	**9111.1**	**17680.9**
1995 projected	*1551.2**	*231.1**	*2004.3**	*452.5*	*718.2*	*1055.3*	*1450.0*	*2162.8*	*3377.1*	*4813.8*	*6412.5*	*8422.2*	*16290.0*
All cancer													
1985–90	290.0*	10.1*	503.4*	38.8	82.4	193.3	337.1	632.9	966.4	1273.2	1391.9	1596.5	1420.5
1985	287.3*	11.3*	484.9*	36.6	102.3	197.6	334.9	634.5	924.0	1164.6	1411.8	1603.6	1469.1
1990	**286.4***	**7.7***	**493.2***	**24.6**	**83.8**	**217.6**	**353.1**	**609.3**	**945.9**	**1218.0**	**1554.7**	**1547.0**	**1244.7**
1995 projected	*286.0**	*5.7**	*503.8**	*18.6*	*83.6*	*221.3*	*352.5*	*607.0*	*957.1*	*1286.2*	*1600.0*	*1455.6*	*1150.0*
Lung cancer													
1985–90	92.1*	0.2*	184.4*	7.4	16.0	66.5	116.9	263.3	389.3	431.7	385.1	412.3	261.4
1985	87.4*	0.3*	162.3*	12.2	18.2	58.5	113.9	264.0	328.0	341.5	388.2	432.4	345.7
1990	**93.0***	**0.2***	**176.6***	**3.5**	**22.5**	**74.1**	**129.0**	**255.5**	**339.0**	**412.3**	**515.6**	**384.6**	**244.7**
1995 projected	*99.0**	*0.2**	*193.4**	*3.4*	*25.5*	*85.1*	*132.5*	*258.1*	*362.9*	*486.2*	*575.0*	*366.7*	*200.0*
Upper aerodigestive cancer (mouth, oesophagus, pharynx and larynx)													
1985–90	24.5*	–	50.2*	3.7	13.7	27.0	49.4	62.8	90.6	103.8	81.1	70.2	79.5
1985	23.8*	0.3*	48.9*	4.1	6.8	18.1	43.3	66.0	100.0	103.7	88.2	45.0	98.8
1990	**24.3***	**–**	**51.1***	**1.8**	**14.3**	**32.4**	**63.4**	**49.1**	**96.9**	**99.5**	**85.9**	**51.3**	**53.2**
1995 projected	*24.9**	*–*	*52.9**	*1.7*	*20.0*	*44.7*	*70.0*	*48.8*	*88.6*	*96.6*	*87.5*	*33.3*	*40.0*
Other cancer													
1985–90	173.4*	9.8*	268.9*	27.7	52.6	99.8	170.8	306.8	486.6	737.7	925.7	1114.0	1079.5
1985	176.1*	10.8*	273.8*	20.3	77.3	121.0	177.7	304.6	496.0	719.5	935.3	1126.1	1024.7
1990	**169.2***	**7.5***	**265.6***	**19.3**	**47.0**	**111.1**	**160.7**	**304.7**	**510.0**	**706.2**	**953.1**	**1111.1**	**946.8**
1995 projected	*162.1**	*5.4**	*257.5**	*13.6*	*38.2*	*91.5*	*150.0*	*300.0*	*505.7*	*703.4*	*937.5*	*1055.6*	*910.0*
Chronic obstructive pulmonary disease (COPD)													
1985–90	41.7*	1.2*	60.4*	3.7	9.2	20.8	42.7	65.2	117.4	163.9	216.2	271.9	375.0
1985	53.2*	1.2*	73.0*	6.1	11.4	28.2	63.8	78.7	140.0	182.9	282.4	414.4	456.8
1990	**40.1***	**0.2***	**60.5***	**–**	**6.1**	**18.5**	**40.2**	**51.6**	**122.5**	**184.8**	**265.6**	**265.0**	**276.6**
1995 projected	*31.8**	*0.3**	*52.1**	*–*	*3.6*	*12.8*	*27.5*	*39.5*	*108.6*	*172.4*	*212.5*	*188.9*	*190.0*
Other respiratory disease													
1985–90	14.1*	7.3*	17.1*	5.5	6.9	16.6	15.7	24.2	23.5	27.3	33.8	43.9	68.2
1985	19.1*	9.2*	26.1*	4.1	18.2	28.2	36.4	45.7	32.0	18.3	23.5	27.0	86.4
1990	**14.5***	**5.3***	**19.5***	**8.8**	**8.2**	**16.2**	**12.7**	**24.6**	**28.5**	**37.9**	**31.3**	**76.9**	**74.5**
1995 projected	*13.7**	*3.4**	*17.2**	*6.8*	*5.5*	*10.6*	*7.5*	*16.3*	*25.7*	*48.3*	*43.8*	*111.1*	*100.0*
Vascular disease													
1985–90	894.2*	12.0*	917.1*	107.2	203.7	365.9	600.0	963.8	1610.7	2568.3	4243.2	6868.4	14659.1
1985	971.0*	14.7*	977.8*	134.1	202.3	358.9	619.6	1007.6	1772.0	2750.0	4594.1	7657.7	16086.4
1990	**898.0***	**9.6***	**984.7***	**117.8**	**216.8**	**405.1**	**634.2**	**1017.2**	**1743.6**	**2758.3**	**4367.2**	**6376.1**	**14000.0**
1995 projected	*822.4**	*6.7**	*968.1**	*108.5*	*227.3*	*419.1*	*640.0*	*1004.7*	*1728.6*	*2648.3*	*3893.8*	*5588.9*	*12010.0*
Liver cirrhosis and other liver disease													
1985–90	11.7*	1.0*	22.9*	3.7	6.9	14.6	22.5	29.0	40.3	43.7	33.8	35.1	34.1
1985	18.1*	1.7*	36.2*	2.0	13.6	22.2	29.6	60.9	52.0	73.2	58.8	45.0	37.0
1990	**10.9***	**0.9***	**20.4***	**5.3**	**6.1**	**13.9**	**21.1**	**24.6**	**48.4**	**23.7**	**15.6**	**51.3**	**42.6**
1995 projected	*8.0**	*0.5**	*14.0**	*3.4*	*3.6*	*8.5*	*15.0*	*16.3*	*34.3*	*17.2*	*12.5*	*44.4*	*50.0*
Other medical causes													
1985–90	128.0*	62.4*	138.6*	51.8	70.9	91.5	128.1	159.4	211.4	256.8	364.9	535.1	920.5
1985	138.3*	76.0*	157.5*	73.2	70.5	153.2	132.1	185.3	244.0	243.9	335.3	594.6	642.0
1990	**143.2***	**52.5***	**160.0***	**51.0**	**96.1**	**97.2**	**137.4**	**174.4**	**236.5**	**327.0**	**398.4**	**512.8**	**1531.9**
1995 projected	*151.9**	*39.6**	*161.3**	*45.8*	*78.2*	*87.2*	*117.5*	*167.4*	*257.1*	*375.9*	*418.8*	*688.9*	*2160.0*
All non-medical causes													
1985–90	181.3*	111.3*	242.7*	225.5	260.9	268.2	251.7	263.3	221.5	207.7	216.2	280.7	420.5
1985	190.7*	107.9*	265.6*	237.8	318.2	320.6	264.2	299.5	248.0	170.7	235.3	324.3	321.0
1990	**218.2***	**147.4***	**281.5***	**265.4**	**319.0**	**300.9**	**291.8**	**304.7**	**242.2**	**246.4**	**226.6**	**282.1**	**510.6**
1995 projected	*237.4**	*175.0**	*287.8**	*269.5*	*316.4*	*295.7*	*290.0*	*311.6*	*265.7*	*265.5*	*231.3*	*344.4*	*630.0*

ESTONIA: Females

	All ages	0–34	35–69	35–39	40–44	45–49	50–54	55–59	60–64	65–69	70–74	75–79	80+/NK
POPULATION (1000s)													
1985–90	825.1	391.9	345.8	56.7	47.2	53.4	52.0	52.9	49.1	34.5	30.7	28.3	28.4
1985	810.4	386.8	334.0	52.2	47.6	55.3	51.7	53.2	44.6	29.4	35.6	27.1	26.9
1990	**836.4**	**393.6**	**357.4**	**58.8**	**52.5**	**47.4**	**54.7**	**50.7**	**51.6**	**41.7**	**26.2**	**29.0**	**30.2**
1995 projected	*829.0*	*379.0*	*362.0*	*60.0*	*58.0*	*51.0*	*46.0*	*52.0*	*48.0*	*47.0*	*36.0*	*20.0*	*32.0*
NUMBER OF DEATHS													
All causes													
1985–90	9978	384	2444	75	101	178	263	410	652	765	1097	1781	4272
1985	10245	373	2403	76	103	225	294	418	667	620	1249	1919	4301
1990	**10106**	**354**	**2662**	**91**	**111**	**166**	**274**	**375**	**685**	**960**	**975**	**1723**	**4392**
1995 projected	*9468*	*318*	*2669*	*88*	*114*	*159*	*208*	*347*	*635*	*1118*	*1262*	*1101*	*4118*
Lung cancer													
1985–90	104	–	62	1	1	2	7	12	20	19	16	15	11
1985	83	–	46	–	2	5	2	9	16	12	16	15	6
1990	**104**	–	**61**	**1**	**1**	**1**	**6**	**11**	**17**	**24**	**17**	**14**	**12**
1995 projected	*129*	–	*75*	*1*	*1*	*1*	*6*	*13*	*19*	*34*	*28*	*11*	*15*
ANNUAL DEATH RATE / 100,000 (*The rates for the age groups 0–34 and 35–69 are the means of seven five-yearly rates, but the all-ages rates are standardised to the conventional "European" age distribution)													
All causes													
1985–90	868.5*	95.6*	786.5*	132.3	214.0	333.3	505.8	775.0	1327.9	2217.4	3573.3	6293.3	15042.3
1985	915.8*	94.7*	818.2*	145.6	216.4	406.9	568.7	785.7	1495.5	2108.8	3508.4	7081.2	15988.8
1990	**855.3***	**88.2***	**798.1***	**154.8**	**211.4**	**350.2**	**500.9**	**739.6**	**1327.5**	**2302.2**	**3721.4**	**5941.4**	**14543.0**
1995 projected	*795.9**	*85.4**	*782.3**	*146.7*	*196.6*	*311.8*	*452.2*	*667.3*	*1322.9*	*2378.7*	*3505.6*	*5505.0*	*12868.8*
All cancer													
1985–90	144.1*	10.2*	239.5*	51.1	80.5	121.7	186.5	268.4	411.4	556.5	635.2	791.5	721.8
1985	143.8*	11.4*	237.5*	42.1	90.3	135.6	183.8	261.3	466.4	483.0	581.5	815.5	724.9
1990	**143.4***	**7.8***	**242.3***	**62.9**	**81.9**	**128.7**	**182.8**	**230.8**	**447.7**	**561.2**	**610.7**	**817.2**	**711.9**
1995 projected	*142.9**	*7.3**	*241.4**	*61.7*	*82.8*	*123.5*	*169.6*	*217.3*	*452.1*	*583.0*	*641.7*	*810.0*	*709.4*
Lung cancer													
1985–90	10.5*	–	19.9*	1.8	2.1	3.7	13.5	22.7	40.7	55.1	52.1	53.0	38.7
1985	8.5*	–	15.8*	–	4.2	9.0	3.9	16.9	35.9	40.8	44.9	55.4	22.3
1990	**10.1***	–	**18.4***	**1.7**	**1.9**	**2.1**	**11.0**	**21.7**	**32.9**	**57.6**	**64.9**	**48.3**	**39.7**
1995 projected	*12.0**	–	*22.2**	*1.7*	*1.7*	*2.0*	*13.0*	*25.0*	*39.6*	*72.3*	*77.8*	*55.0*	*46.9*
Upper aerodigestive cancer (mouth, oesophagus, pharynx and larynx)													
1985–90	3.0*	–	4.9*	1.8	2.1	1.9	3.8	5.7	10.2	8.7	13.0	17.7	17.6
1985	3.2*	–	6.1*	1.9	2.1	–	3.9	5.6	15.7	13.6	8.4	18.5	18.6
1990	**2.8***	**0.2***	**4.0***	**1.7**	–	–	**1.8**	**3.9**	**13.6**	**7.2**	**22.9**	**6.9**	**19.9**
1995 projected	*2.5**	*0.3**	*3.8**	*1.7*	–	–	*2.2*	*3.8*	*10.4*	*8.5*	*19.4*	*5.0*	*15.6*
Other cancer													
1985–90	130.7*	10.2*	214.6*	47.6	76.3	116.1	169.2	240.1	360.5	492.8	570.0	720.8	665.5
1985	132.0*	11.4*	215.6*	40.2	84.0	126.6	176.0	238.7	414.8	428.6	528.1	741.7	684.0
1990	**130.5***	**7.6***	**219.8***	**59.5**	**80.0**	**126.6**	**170.0**	**205.1**	**401.2**	**496.4**	**522.9**	**762.1**	**652.3**
1995 projected	*128.4**	*7.1**	*215.4**	*58.3*	*81.0*	*121.6*	*154.3*	*188.5*	*402.1*	*502.1*	*544.4*	*750.0*	*646.9*
Chronic obstructive pulmonary disease (COPD)													
1985–90	12.6*	0.7*	17.4*	1.8	4.2	11.2	13.5	18.9	28.5	43.5	61.9	88.3	109.2
1985	14.1*	0.5*	19.2*	–	4.2	7.2	19.3	18.8	33.6	51.0	67.4	99.6	141.3
1990	**11.8***	**0.5***	**18.6***	–	**5.7**	**12.7**	**12.8**	**19.7**	**29.1**	**50.4**	**45.8**	**89.7**	**76.2**
1995 projected	*10.0**	*0.3**	*16.6**	–	*6.9*	*11.8*	*13.0*	*17.3*	*27.1*	*40.4*	*38.9*	*65.0*	*56.3*
Other respiratory disease													
1985–90	5.5*	4.7*	4.0*	1.8	2.1	3.7	3.8	3.8	4.1	8.7	13.0	21.2	28.2
1985	5.8*	3.8*	4.4*	1.9	–	9.0	3.9	3.8	2.2	10.2	8.4	48.0	37.2
1990	**4.9***	**4.6***	**3.7***	–	–	–	**3.7**	**2.0**	**5.8**	**14.4**	**15.3**	**10.3**	**23.2**
1995 projected	*5.5**	*6.0**	*4.5**	–	–	–	*2.2*	*1.9*	*8.3*	*19.1*	*11.1*	*5.0*	*15.6*
Vascular disease													
1985–90	571.0*	3.7*	373.0*	15.9	42.4	84.3	155.8	302.5	674.1	1336.2	2550.5	4932.9	13390.8
1985	619.3*	3.9*	400.1*	17.2	35.7	117.5	181.8	285.7	778.0	1384.4	2564.6	5693.7	14524.2
1990	**540.6***	**3.5***	**365.9***	**18.7**	**40.0**	**103.4**	**148.1**	**276.1**	**629.8**	**1345.3**	**2694.7**	**4496.6**	**12221.9**
1995 projected	*468.0**	*2.9**	*339.5**	*20.0*	*36.2*	*88.2*	*132.6*	*230.8*	*568.8*	*1300.0*	*2372.2*	*3975.0*	*10106.3*
Liver cirrhosis and other liver disease													
1985–90	4.3*	0.2*	8.3*	1.8	2.1	7.5	5.8	9.5	14.3	17.4	16.3	14.1	14.1
1985	6.3*	0.8*	12.3*	5.7	2.1	18.1	7.7	13.2	15.7	23.8	16.9	18.5	7.4
1990	**4.0***	**0.5***	**6.7***	**1.7**	–	**8.4**	**7.3**	**3.9**	**13.6**	**12.0**	**22.9**	**20.7**	–
1995 projected	*3.2**	*0.5**	*5.0**	*1.7*	–	*5.9*	*4.3*	*1.9*	*10.4*	*10.6*	*22.2*	*20.0*	–
Other medical causes													
1985–90	79.6*	47.7*	84.1*	22.9	31.8	44.9	73.1	98.3	132.4	185.5	202.0	289.8	500.0
1985	73.7*	48.1*	83.4*	36.4	33.6	47.0	90.9	116.5	143.5	115.6	179.8	203.0	260.2
1990	**96.3***	**39.0***	**96.3***	**23.8**	**43.8**	**40.1**	**71.3**	**126.2**	**122.1**	**247.0**	**229.0**	**362.1**	**1258.3**
1995 projected	*111.5**	*31.7**	*108.6**	*20.0*	*37.9*	*35.3*	*65.2*	*113.5*	*158.3*	*329.8*	*322.2*	*510.0*	*1781.3*
All non-medical causes													
1985–90	51.3*	28.3*	60.2*	37.0	50.8	59.9	67.3	73.7	63.1	69.6	94.5	155.5	278.2
1985	52.8*	26.2*	61.4*	42.1	50.4	72.3	81.2	86.5	56.1	40.8	89.9	203.0	293.7
1990	**54.4***	**32.3***	**64.5***	**47.6**	**40.0**	**57.0**	**75.0**	**80.9**	**79.5**	**71.9**	**103.1**	**144.8**	**251.7**
1995 projected	*54.8**	*36.8**	*66.7**	*43.3*	*32.8*	*47.1*	*65.2*	*84.6*	*97.9*	*95.7*	*97.2*	*120.0*	*200.0*

ESTONIA: 1985–1990

Smoking-attributed deaths (Sm.) and total deaths (Total)

		ALL CAUSES	ALL CANCER	Lung cancer	Upper aero-digestive ca.	Other cancer	COPD	Other respiratory	Vascular disease	Cirrhosis/ other liver	Other medical	Non-medical
Males												
0–34	Sm.	–	–	–	–	–	–	–	–	–	–	–
	Total	844	41	1	0	40	5	31	49	4	262	452
35–69	Sm.	1702	607	381	88	138	108	18	818	–	151	–
	Total	4272	1083	399	115	569	127	43	1939	54	336	690
		(40%)	(56%)	(95%)	(77%)	(24%)	(85%)	(42%)	(42%)		(45%)	
70+	Sm.	535	169	114	15	40	67	1	277	–	21	–
	Total	3635	513	127	27	359	96	16	2701	12	196	101
		(15%)	(33%)	(90%)	(56%)	(11%)	(70%)	(6%)	(10%)		(11%)	
Any age	Sm.	2237	776	495	103	178	175	19	1095	–	172	–
	Total	8751	1637	527	142	968	228	90	4689	70	794	1243
		(26%)	(47%)	(94%)	(73%)	(18%)	(77%)	(21%)	(23%)		(22%)	
Females												
0–34	Sm.	–	–	–	–	–	–	–	–	–	–	–
	Total	384	41	0	0	41	3	19	15	1	193	112
35–69	Sm.	174	42	32	3	7	22	0	90	–	20	–
	Total	2444	765	62	16	687	55	13	1107	27	271	206
		(7%)	(5%)	(52%)	(19%)	(1%)	(40%)	(0%)	(8%)		(7%)	
70+	Sm.	124	21	16	2	3	19	0	79	–	5	–
	Total	7150	624	42	14	568	75	18	5982	13	286	152
		(2%)	(3%)	(38%)	(14%)	(1%)	(25%)	(0%)	(1%)		(2%)	
Any age	Sm.	298	63	48	5	10	41	0	169	–	25	–
	Total	9978	1430	104	30	1296	133	50	7104	41	750	470
		(3%)	(4%)	(46%)	(17%)	(1%)	(31%)	(0%)	(2%)		(3%)	
Males+Females												
0–34	Sm.	–	–	–	–	–	–	–	–	–	–	–
	Total	1228	82	1	0	81	8	50	64	5	455	564
35–69	Sm.	1876	649	413	91	145	130	18	908	–	171	–
	Total	6716	1848	461	131	1256	182	56	3046	81	607	896
		(28%)	(35%)	(90%)	(69%)	(12%)	(71%)	(32%)	(30%)		(28%)	
70+	Sm.	659	190	130	17	43	86	1	356	–	26	–
	Total	10785	1137	169	41	927	171	34	8683	25	482	253
		(6%)	(17%)	(77%)	(41%)	(5%)	(50%)	(3%)	(4%)		(5%)	
Any age	Sm.	2535	839	543	108	188	216	19	1264	–	197	–
	Total	18729	3067	631	172	2264	361	140	11793	111	1544	1713
		(14%)	(27%)	(86%)	(63%)	(8%)	(60%)	(14%)	(11%)		(13%)	

ESTONIA: 1985

Smoking-attributed deaths (Sm.) and total deaths (Total)

		ALL CAUSES	ALL CANCER	Lung cancer	Upper aero-digestive ca.	Other cancer	COPD	Other respiratory	Vascular disease	Cirrhosis/ other liver	Other medical	Non-medical
Males												
0–34	Sm.	–	–	–	–	–	–	–	–	–	–	–
	Total	901	45	1	1	43	5	38	59	7	312	435
35–69	Sm.	1604	518	320	76	122	123	33	763	–	167	–
	Total	4286	980	335	101	544	146	69	1896	80	375	740
		(37%)	(53%)	(96%)	(75%)	(22%)	(84%)	(48%)	(40%)		(45%)	
70+	Sm.	620	186	127	17	42	93	2	319	–	20	–
	Total	3911	537	142	28	367	131	14	2934	18	175	102
		(16%)	(35%)	(89%)	(61%)	(11%)	(71%)	(14%)	(11%)		(11%)	
Any age	Sm.	2224	704	447	93	164	216	35	1082	–	187	–
	Total	9098	1562	478	130	954	282	121	4889	105	862	1277
		(24%)	(45%)	(94%)	(72%)	(17%)	(77%)	(29%)	(22%)		(22%)	
Females												
0–34	Sm.	–	–	–	–	–	–	–	–	–	–	–
	Total	373	45	0	0	45	2	15	16	3	190	102
35–69	Sm.	107	23	17	3	3	15	0	58	–	11	–
	Total	2403	724	46	18	660	56	14	1091	39	268	211
		(4%)	(3%)	(37%)	(17%)	(0%)	(27%)	(0%)	(5%)		(4%)	
70+	Sm.	128	18	13	2	3	23	0	84	–	3	–
	Total	7469	623	37	13	573	89	26	6363	13	189	166
		(2%)	(3%)	(35%)	(15%)	(1%)	(26%)	(0%)	(1%)		(2%)	
Any age	Sm.	235	41	30	5	6	38	0	142	–	14	–
	Total	10245	1392	83	31	1278	147	55	7470	55	647	479
		(2%)	(3%)	(36%)	(16%)	(0%)	(26%)	(0%)	(2%)		(2%)	
Males+Females												
0–34	Sm.	–	–	–	–	–	–	–	–	–	–	–
	Total	1274	90	1	1	88	7	53	75	10	502	537
35–69	Sm.	1711	541	337	79	125	138	33	821	–	178	–
	Total	6689	1704	381	119	1204	202	83	2987	119	643	951
		(26%)	(32%)	(88%)	(66%)	(10%)	(68%)	(40%)	(27%)		(28%)	
70+	Sm.	748	204	140	19	45	116	2	403	–	23	–
	Total	11380	1160	179	41	940	220	40	9297	31	364	268
		(7%)	(18%)	(78%)	(46%)	(5%)	(53%)	(5%)	(4%)		(6%)	
Any age	Sm.	2459	745	477	98	170	254	35	1224	–	201	–
	Total	19343	2954	561	161	2232	429	176	12359	160	1509	1756
		(13%)	(25%)	(85%)	(61%)	(8%)	(59%)	(20%)	(10%)		(13%)	

(To be conservative, no deaths before age 35, and none from liver cirrhosis or non-medical causes, were attributed to smoking.)

ESTONIA: 1990

Smoking-attributed deaths (Sm.) and total deaths (Total)

			ALL CAUSES	ALL CANCER	Lung cancer	Upper aero-digestive ca.	Other cancer	COPD	Other respiratory	Vascular disease	Cirrhosis/ other liver	Other medical	Non-medical
Males													
	0–34	Sm.	–	–	–	–	–	–	–	–	–	–	–
		Total	930	32	1	0	31	1	23	40	4	224	606
	35–69	Sm.	1876	638	398	97	143	113	23	923	–	179	–
		Total	4888	1153	416	127	610	133	50	2256	54	406	836
			(38%)	(55%)	(96%)	(76%)	(23%)	(85%)	(46%)	(41%)		(44%)	
	70+	Sm.	548	174	120	13	41	65	3	279	–	27	–
		Total	3606	497	134	22	341	91	20	2621	12	255	110
			(15%)	(35%)	(90%)	(59%)	(12%)	(71%)	(15%)	(11%)		(11%)	
	Any age	Sm.	2424	812	518	110	184	178	26	1202	–	206	–
		Total	9424	1682	551	149	982	225	93	4917	70	885	1552
			(26%)	(48%)	(94%)	(74%)	(19%)	(79%)	(28%)	(24%)		(23%)	
Females													
	0–34	Sm.	–	–	–	–	–	–	–	–	–	–	–
		Total	354	31	0	1	30	2	19	14	2	158	128
	35–69	Sm.	165	37	29	3	5	22	1	86	–	19	–
		Total	2662	823	61	14	748	62	12	1188	23	325	229
			(6%)	(4%)	(48%)	(21%)	(1%)	(35%)	(8%)	(7%)		(6%)	
	70+	Sm.	117	22	17	2	3	13	0	75	–	7	–
		Total	7090	612	43	14	555	61	14	5701	12	545	145
			(2%)	(4%)	(40%)	(14%)	(1%)	(21%)	(0%)	(1%)		(1%)	
	Any age	Sm.	282	59	46	5	8	35	1	161	–	26	–
		Total	10106	1466	104	29	1333	125	45	6903	37	1028	502
			(3%)	(4%)	(44%)	(17%)	(1%)	(28%)	(2%)	(2%)		(3%)	
Males+Females													
	0–34	Sm.	–	–	–	–	–	–	–	–	–	–	–
		Total	1284	63	1	1	61	3	42	54	6	382	734
	35–69	Sm.	2041	675	427	100	148	135	24	1009	–	198	–
		Total	7550	1976	477	141	1358	195	62	3444	77	731	1065
			(27%)	(34%)	(90%)	(71%)	(11%)	(69%)	(39%)	(29%)		(27%)	
	70+	Sm.	665	196	137	15	44	78	3	354	–	34	–
		Total	10696	1109	177	36	896	152	34	8322	24	800	255
			(6%)	(18%)	(77%)	(42%)	(5%)	(51%)	(9%)	(4%)		(4%)	
	Any age	Sm.	2706	871	564	115	192	213	27	1363	–	232	–
		Total	19530	3148	655	178	2315	350	138	11820	107	1913	2054
			(14%)	(28%)	(86%)	(65%)	(8%)	(61%)	(20%)	(12%)		(12%)	

ESTONIA: 1995

Smoking-attributed deaths (Sm.) and total deaths (Total)

			ALL CAUSES	ALL CANCER	Lung cancer	Upper aero-digestive ca.	Other cancer	COPD	Other respiratory	Vascular disease	Cirrhosis/ other liver	Other medical	Non-medical
Males													
	0–34	Sm.	–	–	–	–	–	–	–	–	–	–	–
		Total	913	23	1	0	22	1	13	27	2	154	693
	35–69	Sm.	2070	733	467	109	157	107	20	1024	–	186	–
		Total	5246	1271	488	141	642	124	45	2447	38	429	892
			(39%)	(58%)	(96%)	(77%)	(24%)	(86%)	(44%)	(42%)		(43%)	
	70+	Sm.	554	189	132	12	45	50	4	274	–	37	–
		Total	3413	502	145	21	336	70	27	2327	11	345	131
			(16%)	(38%)	(91%)	(57%)	(13%)	(71%)	(15%)	(12%)		(11%)	
	Any age	Sm.	2624	922	599	121	202	157	24	1298	–	223	–
		Total	9572	1796	634	162	1000	195	85	4801	51	928	1716
			(27%)	(51%)	(94%)	(75%)	(20%)	(81%)	(28%)	(27%)		(24%)	
Females													
	0–34	Sm.	–	–	–	–	–	–	–	–	–	–	–
		Total	318	28	0	1	27	1	22	11	2	117	137
	35–69	Sm.	225	52	42	2	8	24	1	114	–	34	–
		Total	2669	830	75	13	742	57	15	1143	17	372	235
			(8%)	(6%)	(56%)	(15%)	(1%)	(42%)	(7%)	(10%)		(9%)	
	70+	Sm.	171	34	27	2	5	15	0	106	–	16	–
		Total	6481	620	54	13	553	45	10	4883	12	788	123
			(3%)	(5%)	(50%)	(15%)	(1%)	(33%)	(0%)	(2%)		(2%)	
	Any age	Sm.	396	86	69	4	13	39	1	220	–	50	–
		Total	9468	1478	129	27	1322	103	47	6037	31	1277	495
			(4%)	(6%)	(53%)	(15%)	(1%)	(38%)	(2%)	(4%)		(4%)	
Males+Females													
	0–34	Sm.	–	–	–	–	–	–	–	–	–	–	–
		Total	1231	51	1	1	49	2	35	38	4	271	830
	35–69	Sm.	2295	785	509	111	165	131	21	1138	–	220	–
		Total	7915	2101	563	154	1384	181	60	3590	55	801	1127
			(29%)	(37%)	(90%)	(72%)	(12%)	(72%)	(35%)	(32%)		(27%)	
	70+	Sm.	725	223	159	14	50	65	4	380	–	53	–
		Total	9894	1122	199	34	889	115	37	7210	23	1133	254
			(7%)	(20%)	(80%)	(41%)	(6%)	(57%)	(11%)	(5%)		(5%)	
	Any age	Sm.	3020	1008	668	125	215	196	25	1518	–	273	–
		Total	19040	3274	763	189	2322	298	132	10838	82	2205	2211
			(16%)	(31%)	(88%)	(66%)	(9%)	(66%)	(19%)	(14%)		(12%)	

(To be conservative, no deaths before age 35, and none from liver cirrhosis or non-medical causes, were attributed to smoking.)

FINLAND: 1990

		No. of deaths			Standardised rates (Defined on p.334)			Annual death rates / 100, 000						
		All ages	0–34	35–69	All ages	0–34	35–69	0–4	5–9	10–14	15–19	20–24	25–29	30–34
ALL CAUSES	M	25034	1434	10671	1150.6	114.9	1264.5	142.9	23.3	25.9	104.1	161.7	143.7	203.0
	F	25053	613	4886	624.6	53.2	499.2	136.1	18.2	12.6	48.7	53.2	39.6	64.3
Tuberculosis	M	89	–	42	4.1	–	5.0	–	–	–	–	–	–	–
	F	90	–	25	2.3	–	2.6	–	–	–	–	–	–	–
Other infective and parasitic	M	109	20	38	4.9	1.6	3.7	4.4	–	0.6	1.3	1.1	0.5	3.6
	F	147	8	38	4.0	0.7	3.9	3.3	0.6	–	0.7	–	–	0.5
ALL CANCER	M	5043	64	2317	233.8	5.0	294.9	4.4	1.2	3.0	1.3	5.6	8.3	11.2
	F	4766	76	1833	136.2	6.3	187.4	3.9	4.4	2.5	5.4	5.8	7.6	14.4
Mouth and pharynx cancer	M	69	2	41	3.2	0.1	5.0	–	–	–	–	–	0.5	0.5
	F	36	1	9	0.9	0.1	0.9	–	–	–	–	–	–	0.5
Oesophagus cancer	M	91	1	50	4.3	0.1	6.3	–	–	–	–	–	–	0.5
	F	84	–	20	2.1	–	2.1	–	–	–	–	–	–	–
Stomach cancer	M	422	3	195	19.5	0.2	25.4	–	–	–	–	0.6	–	1.0
	F	372	5	112	10.0	0.4	11.5	–	–	–	–	0.6	–	2.1
Colorectal cancer	M	402	3	171	18.8	0.2	21.2	–	–	–	–	0.6	0.5	0.5
	F	515	–	138	13.2	–	14.3	–	–	–	–	–	–	–
Liver cancer	M	111	2	53	5.1	0.2	7.2	–	–	–	–	0.6	0.5	–
	F	130	–	49	3.7	–	5.0	–	–	–	–	–	–	–
Pancreas cancer	M	278	1	141	12.8	0.1	17.4	–	–	–	–	–	–	0.5
	F	409	3	125	11.1	0.2	13.1	–	–	–	–	–	0.5	1.1
Larynx cancer	M	40	–	19	1.9	–	2.3	–	–	–	–	–	–	–
	F	5	–	2	0.1	–	0.2	–	–	–	–	–	–	–
Lung cancer	M	1599	1	825	73.7	0.1	108.0	–	–	–	–	–	–	0.5
	F	346	4	152	10.1	0.3	16.0	–	–	–	0.7	1.2	0.5	–
Malignant melanoma	M	64	3	41	2.9	0.2	4.4	0.6	–	–	–	–	0.5	0.5
	F	53	1	25	1.7	0.1	2.6	–	–	–	–	–	–	0.5
Female breast cancer	F	747	8	434	24.3	0.6	43.0	–	–	–	–	–	1.1	3.2
Cervix cancer	F	76	1	25	2.0	0.1	2.6	–	–	–	–	–	0.5	–
Other uterine cancer	F	145	1	48	3.9	0.1	5.1	–	–	–	–	–	–	0.5
Ovarian cancer	F	313	3	164	9.7	0.2	16.9	–	–	0.6	–	–	0.5	0.5
Prostate cancer	M	635	–	135	30.3	–	18.7	–	–	–	–	–	–	–
Bladder cancer	M	140	–	37	6.7	–	5.1	–	–	–	–	–	–	–
	F	68	–	13	1.6	–	1.4	–	–	–	–	–	–	–
Other and ill-defined cancer sites	M	758	29	418	34.7	2.3	50.9	1.9	0.6	3.0	0.6	1.7	4.7	3.6
	F	978	34	348	27.8	2.9	35.5	2.6	2.5	1.9	2.7	3.5	2.7	4.3
Hodgkin's disease	M	27	4	15	1.2	0.3	1.6	–	–	–	–	0.6	0.5	1.0
	F	16	–	7	0.5	–	0.6	–	–	–	–	–	–	–
Myeloma and non-Hodgkin lymphomas	M	249	5	113	11.5	0.4	13.8	0.6	–	–	–	1.1	–	1.0
	F	345	2	125	9.6	0.2	12.8	0.7	–	–	–	–	–	0.5
Leukaemia	M	158	10	63	7.3	0.8	7.6	1.3	0.6	–	0.6	0.6	1.0	1.5
	F	128	13	37	3.8	1.1	3.7	0.7	1.9	–	2.0	0.6	1.6	1.1
ALL VASCULAR DISEASE	M	11663	67	4743	545.3	5.1	592.6	1.3	1.8	1.2	3.2	2.8	4.7	20.8
	F	12926	28	1701	299.2	2.3	178.8	2.6	1.3	0.6	1.4	2.9	2.7	4.8
Rheumatic heart disease and fever	M	22	1	13	1.0	0.1	1.7	–	–	–	–	–	–	0.5
	F	57	–	15	1.5	–	1.6	–	–	–	–	–	–	–
Hypertensive disease	M	147	–	53	6.9	–	6.5	–	–	–	–	–	–	–
	F	271	–	35	6.2	–	3.8	–	–	–	–	–	–	–
Ischaemic heart disease	M	7520	13	3287	351.3	1.0	416.7	–	–	–	–	0.6	–	6.1
	F	6563	3	918	153.1	0.2	97.9	–	–	–	–	–	0.5	1.1
Pulmonary embolism and other venous	M	...	...	...	...	...	...	...	...	...	...	...	...	...
	F	...	...	...	...	...	...	...	...	...	...	...	...	...
Cerebrovascular disease	M	2288	25	746	107.2	1.9	90.9	–	–	0.6	1.3	0.6	2.6	8.1
	F	3722	11	460	85.7	0.9	47.7	–	0.6	0.6	1.4	1.8	2.2	–
Other vascular disease, incl. venous	M	1686	28	644	78.9	2.2	76.7	1.3	1.8	0.6	1.9	1.7	2.1	6.1
	F	2313	14	273	52.7	1.2	27.9	2.6	0.6	–	–	1.2	–	3.7
Chronic obstructive pulmonary disease	M	748	2	208	35.5	0.2	28.1	–	0.6	–	–	0.6	–	–
	F	205	–	65	5.4	–	6.8	–	–	–	–	–	–	–
Other respiratory disease	M	1247	20	233	60.1	1.6	28.9	4.4	–	–	–	0.6	2.1	4.1
	F	1546	8	125	33.8	0.7	12.9	2.6	1.3	–	–	–	0.5	0.5
Peptic ulcer	M	145	1	75	6.7	0.1	8.8	0.6	–	–	–	–	–	–
	F	178	–	21	4.1	–	2.2	–	–	–	–	–	–	–
Liver cirrhosis	M	373	12	332	16.1	0.9	33.8	–	–	–	–	–	1.0	5.1
	F	160	6	100	5.4	0.5	9.5	–	–	–	–	1.2	0.5	1.6
Renal disease	M	117	2	34	5.5	0.2	4.1	–	–	–	–	0.6	–	0.5
	F	254	2	23	5.6	0.2	2.5	1.3	–	–	–	–	–	–
Pregnancy and birth	F	4	2	2	0.2	0.2	0.2	–	–	–	0.7	–	–	0.5
Congenital and perinatal causes	M	205	179	19	9.8	15.9	1.7	93.8	5.4	3.0	2.6	4.5	1.0	1.0
	F	199	164	22	9.5	15.2	2.0	93.4	2.5	1.9	3.4	2.3	1.6	1.6
Ill-defined causes	M	131	42	63	5.8	3.5	6.6	13.8	–	0.6	–	2.8	2.1	5.1
	F	122	32	18	3.7	2.9	1.5	15.1	–	–	0.7	1.2	2.2	1.1
Other medical causes	M	1738	80	595	80.7	6.3	67.4	7.6	3.0	1.2	3.2	8.5	7.3	13.7
	F	3147	49	415	73.7	4.2	42.5	5.3	1.9	3.8	3.4	5.8	3.8	5.3
ALL NON-MEDICAL CAUSES	M	3426	945	1972	142.4	74.6	188.8	12.6	11.4	16.2	92.5	134.6	116.7	138.1
	F	1309	238	498	41.4	20.0	46.3	8.5	6.3	3.8	33.2	33.9	20.6	34.0
Motor vehicle traffic accidents	M	429	201	159	18.1	16.5	16.8	3.8	5.4	6.6	32.3	37.2	15.6	14.7
	F	199	87	65	7.4	7.6	6.2	1.3	5.0	3.8	21.0	11.1	7.6	3.7
Fire	M	67	16	40	2.7	1.3	3.6	0.6	0.6	0.6	1.3	2.3	1.6	2.0
	F	25	5	6	0.7	0.4	0.5	0.7	0.6	–	–	0.6	–	1.1
Suicide	M	1193	423	670	47.8	33.0	61.8	–	–	2.4	40.1	60.3	65.4	62.9
	F	319	83	199	11.9	6.7	18.0	–	–	–	5.4	15.8	8.1	17.5
Homicide	M	120	36	77	4.8	2.8	6.8	1.9	–	0.6	2.6	4.5	6.2	4.1
	F	40	18	22	1.6	1.5	2.0	0.7	–	–	3.4	2.3	1.1	3.2
POPULATION (thousands):	M=males				2419.3	1214.2	1059.2	158.9	167.2	166.2	154.6	177.5	192.8	197.0
	F=females				2566.8	1162.3	1104.8	152.1	159.7	159.1	147.8	171.0	184.5	188.1

FINLAND: 1990

Annual death rates / 100, 000

9th ICD categories

35–39	40–44	45–49	50–54	55–59	60–64	65–69	70–74	75–79	80+/NK			
286.8	407.7	564.6	850.0	1318.2	2123.3	3301.0	5170.5	8109.0	15532.3	M	ALL CAUSES	001–999
78.8	158.1	217.8	339.3	460.9	794.2	1445.0	2667.6	4653.1	12163.4	F		
0.5	1.8	1.9	5.8	4.9	7.7	12.1	21.5	44.9	33.6	M	Tuberculosis	010–018, 137
–	–	1.3	1.4	–	7.3	8.4	8.6	11.8	44.0	F		
3.4	4.0	3.2	0.7	4.1	5.1	5.5	23.2	15.0	77.5	M	Other infective	Rest of 001–139
–	1.9	1.3	3.6	6.1	5.8	8.4	12.5	19.3	68.5	F	and parasitic	
16.3	41.4	81.1	153.7	293.0	569.3	909.6	1365.9	1797.0	2573.6	M	ALL CANCER	140–208
24.1	55.2	94.3	150.6	202.9	313.1	471.8	650.3	880.1	1328.8	F		
–	0.4	2.5	5.8	4.9	9.4	12.1	13.2	10.7	33.6	M	Mouth and	140–149
–	0.5	0.7	1.4	–	1.5	2.3	1.9	8.6	15.7	F	pharynx cancer	
0.5	–	1.9	3.6	9.7	12.0	16.5	29.8	15.0	38.8	M	Oesophagus cancer	150
–	–	0.7	1.4	0.8	3.6	8.4	12.5	22.5	29.4	F		
0.5	4.4	4.4	9.5	26.0	42.8	90.4	104.3	153.8	230.0	M	Stomach cancer	151
1.5	1.9	6.5	7.2	8.4	27.0	28.2	49.0	76.0	130.1	F		
1.4	3.1	8.9	8.7	26.8	45.4	54.0	92.7	147.4	266.1	M	Colorectal cancer	153, 154
1.0	3.3	4.6	6.5	12.3	27.0	45.8	68.2	106.0	202.5	F		
0.5	0.4	1.9	2.2	1.6	12.8	30.9	24.8	44.9	51.7	M	Liver cancer	155.0
–	1.9	3.3	2.9	5.4	9.5	12.2	25.0	27.8	28.4	F		
1.4	3.1	5.7	11.7	20.3	32.5	47.4	71.2	106.8	111.1	M	Pancreas cancer	157
0.5	1.9	2.6	12.9	13.8	21.9	38.2	62.4	95.3	124.3	F		
–	–	0.6	2.2	5.7	3.4	4.4	14.9	15.0	12.9	M	Larynx cancer	161
–	–	–	–	–	–	1.5	1.9	1.1	–	F		
1.0	9.3	25.3	43.7	88.5	228.6	359.4	496.7	568.4	534.9	M	Lung cancer	162
0.5	2.8	2.0	12.9	13.8	24.8	55.0	55.7	70.7	64.6	F		
–	2.7	5.7	3.6	8.9	5.1	4.4	6.6	15.0	23.3	M	Malignant melanoma	172
–	0.9	0.7	4.3	4.6	2.2	5.3	6.7	6.4	13.7	F		
10.5	20.6	37.1	46.6	53.6	58.4	74.0	76.8	110.3	119.4	F	Female breast cancer	174
1.0	–	2.0	0.7	1.5	5.8	6.9	8.6	13.9	27.4	F	Cervix cancer	180
–	–	0.7	2.9	7.7	8.0	16.8	20.2	32.1	44.0	F	Other uterine cancer	179, 182
–	4.7	9.1	12.2	22.2	31.4	38.9	43.2	40.7	61.6	F	Ovarian cancer	183
–	0.4	0.6	2.2	15.4	34.2	78.3	195.4	305.6	617.6	M	Prostate cancer	185
–	0.4	–	1.5	1.6	12.0	19.8	33.1	59.8	142.1	M	Bladder cancer	188
–	0.5	–	–	3.1	2.2	3.8	3.8	20.3	31.3	F		
7.2	10.2	15.2	43.0	59.3	89.9	131.2	165.6	205.1	297.2	M	Other and ill-defined	Rest of 140–208
7.0	10.8	14.3	25.8	40.6	61.3	88.5	136.4	162.7	295.5	F	cancer sites	
1.0	0.4	1.3	0.7	4.1	2.6	1.1	3.3	6.4	7.8	M	Hodgkin's disease	201
1.0	0.5	0.7	0.7	–	–	1.5	1.9	3.2	3.9	F		
2.4	4.0	3.2	9.5	13.8	24.0	39.7	69.5	79.1	134.4	M	Myeloma and non-	200, 202–203
1.0	3.7	5.2	8.6	10.0	25.5	35.9	56.7	66.4	94.9	F	Hodgkin lymphomas	
0.5	2.2	3.8	5.8	6.5	14.6	19.8	44.7	64.1	72.4	M	Leukaemia	204–208
–	1.4	4.6	3.6	5.4	2.9	8.4	19.2	16.1	42.1	F		
49.4	103.6	186.9	363.4	636.4	1079.6	1728.8	2620.9	4480.8	8199.0	M	ALL VASCULAR	390–459
12.6	24.3	38.4	78.2	142.4	294.2	661.8	1438.0	2672.4	7048.9	F	DISEASE	
–	–	0.6	1.5	–	3.4	6.6	1.7	6.4	10.3	M	Rheumatic heart	390–398
–	–	0.7	–	–	3.6	6.9	14.4	12.8	14.7	F	disease and fever	
1.0	2.7	0.6	5.1	5.7	9.4	20.9	41.4	53.4	113.7	M	Hypertensive disease	401–405
–	–	0.7	0.7	2.3	6.6	16.0	34.6	38.5	160.5	F		
21.6	52.0	114.1	252.0	448.9	789.4	1239.3	1786.4	2829.1	4695.1	M	Ischaemic heart	410–414
1.0	5.6	13.7	29.4	78.1	158.4	399.2	828.0	1458.2	3344.4	F	disease	
...	...	...	...	...	...	...	...	...	...	M	Pulmonary embolism	Not given
...	...	...	...	...	...	...	...	...	...	F	and other venous	separately
12.9	26.7	39.9	45.9	93.3	149.8	267.9	496.7	989.3	1948.3	M	Cerebrovascular	430–438
6.5	9.8	13.7	28.7	42.1	79.6	153.4	370.8	769.8	2099.8	F	disease	
13.9	22.2	31.7	59.0	88.5	127.6	194.0	294.7	602.6	1431.5	M	Other vascular	Rest of 390–459,
5.0	8.9	9.8	19.4	19.9	46.0	86.3	190.2	392.9	1429.5	F	disease, incl. venous	incl. 415, 451–3
–	1.3	5.1	8.7	16.2	56.5	109.2	238.4	318.4	633.1	M	Chronic obstructive	490–496
–	0.9	2.0	3.6	6.9	13.9	20.6	23.1	33.2	83.2	F	pulmonary disease	
5.3	5.3	10.1	18.2	26.8	46.2	90.4	233.4	489.3	1612.4	M	Other respiratory	Rest of 460–519
3.5	2.3	5.9	8.6	11.5	10.2	48.1	91.3	228.1	1081.2	F	disease	
1.4	4.0	2.5	5.1	13.0	13.7	22.1	44.7	32.1	69.8	M	Peptic ulcer	531–533
–	–	2.0	2.2	–	7.3	3.8	20.2	34.3	101.8	F		
12.5	24.5	34.9	37.9	53.6	42.8	30.9	21.5	23.5	12.9	M	Liver cirrhosis	571
3.0	7.5	10.4	12.2	8.4	14.6	10.7	15.4	19.3	19.6	F		
1.4	0.4	2.5	1.5	1.6	9.4	12.1	34.8	51.3	93.0	M	Renal disease	580–590
–	–	–	0.7	1.5	5.1	9.9	17.3	51.4	159.5	F		
–	0.5	0.7	–	–	–	–	–	–	–	F	Pregnancy and birth	630–676
2.4	2.7	1.3	–	0.8	2.6	2.2	6.6	2.1	5.2	M	Congenital and	740–779
1.5	2.8	0.7	1.4	2.3	2.9	2.3	1.9	7.5	3.9	F	perinatal causes	
4.8	3.6	2.5	10.2	4.9	11.1	8.8	5.0	8.5	49.1	M	Ill-defined causes	780–799
–	4.2	0.7	1.4	1.5	0.7	2.3	1.9	7.5	61.6	F		
29.3	31.1	39.9	45.2	56.8	94.2	175.3	337.7	547.0	1558.1	M	Other medical causes	Rest of 001–799
9.0	11.7	15.0	33.0	30.6	60.6	137.4	303.6	571.7	1793.5	F		
160.2	184.1	192.6	199.6	206.2	184.9	194.0	216.9	299.1	615.0	M	ALL NON-	E800–E999
25.1	46.8	45.5	42.3	46.7	58.4	59.5	83.6	116.7	368.9	F	MEDICAL CAUSES	
8.2	12.0	12.7	15.3	22.7	13.7	33.1	44.7	57.7	38.8	M	Motor vehicle	E810–E819
3.5	4.2	5.2	5.0	9.2	6.6	9.9	16.3	11.8	18.6	F	traffic accidents	
4.3	4.4	2.5	3.6	4.9	3.4	2.2	5.0	10.7	7.8	M	Fire	E890–E899
0.5	0.9	0.7	–	0.8	0.7	–	2.9	3.2	7.8	F		
64.3	71.6	68.4	58.3	56.0	56.5	57.3	38.1	87.6	93.0	M	Suicide	E950–E959
12.0	22.9	19.5	15.1	17.6	21.9	16.8	16.3	11.8	8.8	F		
7.7	8.4	10.8	7.3	4.1	6.0	3.3	6.6	4.3	2.6	M	Homicide	E960–E969
2.0	2.3	2.0	1.4	0.8	2.9	2.3	–	–	–	F		
208.5	224.9	157.8	137.3	123.2	116.8	90.7	60.4	46.8	38.7	M	POPULATION (thousands)	
199.2	213.8	153.8	139.4	130.6	137.0	131.0	104.1	93.4	102.2	F		

FINLAND: Males

	All ages	0–34	35–69	35–39	40–44	45–49	50–54	55–59	60–64	65–69	70–74	75–79	80+/NK
POPULATION (1000s)													
1955	2031.0	1284.4	685.4	119.1	132.9	130.1	107.8	84.9	63.1	47.5	31.5	18.3	11.4
1965	2203.8	1348.3	780.0	150.8	134.9	111.6	121.2	113.3	87.1	61.1	38.7	22.7	14.1
1975	2278.1	1346.2	829.7	147.6	138.5	142.1	123.3	97.3	98.4	82.5	53.8	30.0	18.4
1985	2373.5	1265.6	967.5	227.7	161.1	142.0	130.0	127.6	104.2	74.9	65.6	44.4	30.4
1990	**2419.3**	**1214.2**	**1059.2**	**208.5**	**224.9**	**157.8**	**137.3**	**123.2**	**116.8**	**90.7**	**60.4**	**46.8**	**38.7**
1995 projected	*2446.5*	*1172.8*	*1118.0*	*193.8*	*204.9*	*220.6*	*153.7*	*130.6*	*112.8*	*101.6*	*72.6*	*42.2*	*40.9*
NUMBER OF DEATHS													
All causes													
1955	20439	3488	10206	451	736	1101	1483	1881	2143	2411	2291	2149	2305
1965	23261	2403	12404	593	773	966	1732	2485	2853	3002	2956	2498	3000
1975	23916	2048	12206	459	695	1114	1534	1761	2933	3710	3499	2954	3209
1985	24985	1378	10590	569	591	843	1255	1953	2616	2763	3865	4013	5139
1990	**25034**	**1434**	**10671**	**598**	**917**	**891**	**1167**	**1624**	**2480**	**2994**	**3123**	**3795**	**6011**
1995 projected	*24166*	*1542*	*10336*	*628*	*868*	*1179*	*1156*	*1476*	*2090*	*2939*	*3343*	*3082*	*5863*
Lung cancer													
1955	852	3	674	8	22	50	105	155	171	163	95	60	20
1965	1369	2	1019	12	18	48	137	241	278	285	205	102	41
1975	1564	1	1009	–	15	49	104	165	299	377	317	162	75
1985	1758	2	937	4	11	30	84	205	319	284	348	287	184
1990	**1599**	**1**	**825**	**2**	**21**	**40**	**60**	**109**	**267**	**326**	**300**	**266**	**207**
1995 projected	*1448*	*1*	*713*	*2*	*22*	*45*	*45*	*77*	*201*	*321*	*325*	*216*	*193*
ANNUAL DEATH RATE / 100,000 (*The rates for the age groups 0–34 and 35–69 are the means of seven five-yearly rates, but the all-ages rates are standardised to the conventional "European" age distribution)													
All causes													
1955	1719.0*	258.2*	1977.4*	378.7	553.8	846.3	1375.7	2215.5	3396.2	5075.8	7273.0	11743.2	20219.3
1965	1691.1*	186.2*	1949.0*	393.2	573.0	865.6	1429.0	2193.3	3275.5	4913.3	7638.2	11004.4	21276.6
1975	1456.5*	155.4*	1732.6*	311.0	501.8	784.0	1244.1	1809.9	2980.7	4497.0	6503.7	9846.7	17440.2
1985	1265.8*	104.8*	1415.1*	249.9	366.9	593.7	965.4	1530.6	2510.6	3688.9	5891.8	9038.3	16904.6
1990	**1150.6***	**114.9***	**1264.5***	**286.8**	**407.7**	**564.6**	**850.0**	**1318.2**	**2123.3**	**3301.0**	**5170.5**	**8109.0**	**15532.3**
1995 projected	*1053.7**	*128.5**	*1130.0**	*324.0*	*423.6*	*534.5*	*752.1*	*1130.2*	*1852.8*	*2892.7*	*4604.7*	*7303.3*	*14335.0*
All cancer													
1955	275.9*	12.6*	446.3*	41.1	72.2	128.4	302.4	524.1	881.1	1174.7	1368.3	1923.5	1473.7
1965	277.4*	12.1*	413.9*	41.8	64.5	123.7	264.0	479.3	732.5	1191.5	1571.1	1713.7	2120.6
1975	270.5*	10.8*	373.9*	24.4	46.2	115.4	227.1	392.6	695.1	1116.4	1490.7	1906.7	2516.3
1985	256.0*	8.0*	333.2*	21.5	52.1	91.5	192.3	348.7	666.0	959.9	1358.2	1900.9	2779.6
1990	**233.8***	**5.0***	**294.9***	**16.3**	**41.4**	**81.1**	**153.7**	**293.0**	**569.3**	**909.6**	**1365.9**	**1797.0**	**2573.6**
1995 projected	*213.4**	*3.7**	*263.5**	*12.4*	*34.2*	*63.5*	*130.1*	*247.3*	*500.9*	*856.3*	*1298.9*	*1654.0*	*2425.4*
Lung cancer													
1955	68.6*	0.3*	136.5*	6.7	16.6	38.4	97.4	182.6	271.0	343.2	301.6	327.9	175.4
1965	90.6*	0.2*	168.0*	8.0	13.3	43.0	113.0	212.7	319.2	466.4	529.7	449.3	290.8
1975	89.4*	0.1*	151.4*	–	10.8	34.5	84.3	169.6	303.9	457.0	589.2	540.0	407.6
1985	87.7*	0.1*	134.3*	1.8	6.8	21.1	64.6	160.7	306.1	379.2	530.5	646.4	605.3
1990	**73.7***	**0.1***	**108.0***	**1.0**	**9.3**	**25.3**	**43.7**	**88.5**	**228.6**	**359.4**	**496.7**	**568.4**	**534.9**
1995 projected	*62.5**	*0.1**	*87.8**	*1.0*	*10.7*	*20.4*	*29.3*	*59.0*	*178.2*	*315.9*	*447.7*	*511.8*	*471.9*
Upper aerodigestive cancer (mouth, oesophagus, pharynx and larynx)													
1955	24.5*	0.5*	36.1*	2.5	5.3	6.9	13.9	40.0	61.8	122.1	127.0	174.9	228.1
1965	17.3*	0.1*	24.4*	3.3	5.2	9.0	14.9	25.6	50.5	62.2	93.0	110.1	170.2
1975	12.5*	0.2*	17.2*	–	2.2	8.4	11.4	16.4	41.7	40.0	66.9	100.0	108.7
1985	10.1*	0.1*	14.5*	–	3.1	4.9	8.5	14.9	29.8	40.1	38.1	78.8	108.6
1990	**9.4***	**0.2***	**13.7***	**0.5**	**0.4**	**5.1**	**11.7**	**20.3**	**24.8**	**33.1**	**57.9**	**40.6**	**85.3**
1995 projected	*8.6**	*0.3**	*14.1**	*0.5*	*0.5*	*5.0*	*14.3*	*20.7*	*22.2*	*35.4*	*48.2*	*30.8*	*61.1*
Other cancer													
1955	182.8*	11.8*	273.7*	31.9	50.4	83.0	191.1	301.5	548.3	709.5	939.7	1420.8	1070.2
1965	169.6*	11.7*	221.6*	30.5	46.0	71.7	136.1	241.0	362.8	662.8	948.3	1154.2	1659.6
1975	168.6*	10.5*	205.3*	24.4	33.2	72.5	131.4	206.6	349.6	619.4	834.6	1266.7	2000.0
1985	158.2*	7.8*	184.4*	19.8	42.2	65.5	119.2	173.2	330.1	540.7	789.6	1175.7	2065.8
1990	**150.7***	**4.7***	**173.2***	**14.9**	**31.6**	**50.7**	**98.3**	**184.3**	**315.9**	**517.1**	**811.3**	**1188.0**	**1953.5**
1995 projected	*142.2**	*3.4**	*161.6**	*10.8*	*22.9*	*38.1*	*86.5*	*167.7*	*300.5*	*504.9*	*803.0*	*1111.4*	*1892.4*
Chronic obstructive pulmonary disease (COPD)													
1955	29.7*	1.2*	35.2*	–	2.3	7.7	18.6	42.4	61.8	113.7	193.7	229.5	324.6
1965	63.3*	1.1*	64.9*	4.6	5.9	15.2	28.1	70.6	144.7	184.9	315.2	497.8	1035.5
1975	60.8*	0.9*	61.1*	0.7	5.1	7.0	26.8	55.5	115.9	217.0	355.0	576.7	880.4
1985	50.6*	0.4*	42.7*	0.4	2.5	2.8	13.1	37.6	96.9	145.5	282.0	547.3	835.5
1990	**35.5***	**0.2***	**28.1***	**–**	**1.3**	**5.1**	**8.7**	**16.2**	**56.5**	**109.2**	**238.4**	**318.4**	**633.1**
1995 projected	*25.5**	*0.2**	*20.5**	*–*	*1.5*	*4.1*	*5.9*	*10.7*	*39.0*	*82.7*	*166.7*	*239.3*	*447.4*
Other respiratory disease													
1955	100.3*	23.0*	59.5*	9.2	14.3	16.1	22.3	60.1	96.7	197.9	400.0	847.0	1903.5
1965	85.3*	7.0*	39.4*	6.0	5.9	11.6	27.2	28.2	57.4	139.1	333.3	718.1	2177.3
1975	72.5*	2.8*	37.7*	2.7	7.2	15.5	19.5	26.7	60.0	132.1	262.1	576.7	1929.3
1985	64.0*	1.3*	25.7*	3.5	4.3	8.5	15.4	18.0	48.9	81.4	207.3	542.8	1865.1
1990	**60.1***	**1.6***	**28.9***	**5.3**	**5.3**	**10.1**	**18.2**	**26.8**	**46.2**	**90.4**	**233.4**	**489.3**	**1612.4**
1995 projected	*56.5**	*2.1**	*31.9**	*7.2*	*6.3*	*11.3*	*22.8*	*28.3*	*49.6*	*97.4*	*224.5*	*457.3*	*1405.9*
Vascular disease													
1955	819.7*	14.1*	947.1*	87.3	186.6	339.0	568.6	1035.3	1710.0	2703.2	4155.6	6623.0	10859.6
1965	890.5*	11.6*	1027.9*	114.1	235.7	435.5	763.2	1165.9	1796.8	2684.1	4333.3	6572.7	12390.1
1975	758.9*	7.1*	923.6*	77.9	182.7	374.4	661.8	991.8	1666.7	2510.3	3630.1	5640.0	9983.7
1985	651.9*	6.5*	737.6*	49.2	111.7	236.6	473.8	813.5	1360.8	2117.5	3372.0	5054.1	9194.1
1990	**545.3***	**5.1***	**592.6***	**49.4**	**103.6**	**186.9**	**363.4**	**636.4**	**1079.6**	**1728.8**	**2620.9**	**4480.8**	**8199.0**
1995 projected	*451.7**	*4.3**	*458.1**	*45.4*	*84.9*	*140.5*	*267.4*	*474.0*	*844.9*	*1349.4*	*2162.5*	*3824.6*	*7293.4*
Liver cirrhosis													
1955	6.2*	0.2*	13.3*	1.7	0.8	5.4	12.1	21.2	20.6	31.6	15.9	27.3	8.8
1965	5.8*	0.5*	8.9*	5.3	3.0	5.4	9.1	10.6	17.2	11.5	25.8	17.6	42.6
1975	11.8*	1.3*	21.3*	8.1	17.3	22.5	25.1	24.7	21.3	30.3	22.3	26.7	54.3
1985	11.3*	0.8*	23.5*	8.8	11.8	26.8	26.2	32.1	26.9	32.0	16.8	18.0	19.7
1990	**16.1***	**0.9***	**33.8***	**12.5**	**24.5**	**34.9**	**37.9**	**53.6**	**42.8**	**30.9**	**21.5**	**23.5**	**12.9**
1995 projected	*21.1**	*1.1**	*45.2**	*17.0*	*33.2*	*46.7*	*50.7*	*72.0*	*58.5*	*38.4*	*23.4*	*26.1*	*12.2*
Other medical causes													
1955	359.6*	128.0*	314.6*	104.1	137.7	185.2	271.8	374.6	454.8	673.7	955.6	1836.1	5210.5
1965	222.3*	74.5*	207.4*	54.4	79.3	96.8	153.5	232.1	324.9	510.6	816.5	1141.0	2851.1
1975	136.4*	49.3*	124.5*	40.7	62.1	61.9	99.8	131.6	194.1	281.2	470.3	823.3	1592.4
1985	111.4*	27.1*	94.8*	32.5	48.4	59.9	71.5	104.2	133.4	213.6	431.4	700.5	1677.6
1990	**117.5***	**27.6***	**97.3***	**43.2**	**47.6**	**53.9**	**68.5**	**86.0**	**143.8**	**238.1**	**473.5**	**700.9**	**1886.3**
1995 projected	*122.3**	*27.8**	*97.5**	*48.0*	*46.9*	*48.1*	*57.3*	*78.9*	*145.4*	*257.9*	*490.4*	*774.9*	*2053.8*
All non-medical causes													
1955	127.5*	79.3*	161.4*	135.2	140.0	164.5	180.0	157.8	171.2	181.1	184.1	256.8	438.6
1965	146.4*	79.4*	186.8*	167.1	178.7	177.4	184.0	206.5	202.1	191.5	242.9	343.6	659.6
1975	145.5*	83.2*	190.5*	156.5	181.2	187.2	184.1	187.1	227.6	209.7	273.2	296.7	483.7
1985	120.5*	60.8*	157.6*	133.9	135.9	167.6	173.1	176.3	177.5	138.9	224.1	274.8	532.9
1990	**142.4***	**74.6***	**188.8***	**160.2**	**184.1**	**192.6**	**199.6**	**206.2**	**184.9**	**194.0**	**216.9**	**299.1**	**615.0**
1995 projected	*163.2**	*89.3**	*213.3**	*194.0*	*216.7*	*220.3*	*218.0*	*219.0*	*214.5*	*210.6*	*238.3*	*327.0*	*696.8*

FINLAND: Females

	All ages	0–34	35–69	35–39	40–44	45–49	50–54	55–59	60–64	65–69	70–74	75–79	80+/NK
POPULATION (1000s)													
1955	2203.8	1262.9	829.9	139.4	151.0	147.8	125.8	107.9	85.5	72.5	53.3	34.0	23.7
1965	2359.9	1295.2	926.3	151.0	152.7	134.1	144.3	138.5	114.2	91.5	64.2	43.2	31.0
1975	2433.5	1284.1	955.5	143.8	136.5	146.7	146.9	127.1	133.0	121.5	90.4	59.7	43.8
1985	2528.7	1208.3	1038.7	214.5	154.9	141.2	133.2	141.4	138.4	115.1	112.1	88.8	80.8
1990	**2566.8**	**1162.3**	**1104.8**	**199.2**	**213.8**	**153.8**	**139.4**	**130.6**	**137.0**	**131.0**	**104.1**	**93.4**	**102.2**
1995 projected	*2584.1*	*1127.2*	*1142.1*	*187.2*	*197.9*	*212.2*	*152.1*	*136.9*	*126.3*	*129.5*	*118.6*	*86.1*	*110.1*
NUMBER OF DEATHS													
All causes													
1955	19134	2195	6612	302	421	582	787	1041	1363	2116	2696	3162	4469
1965	21212	1261	6994	190	353	460	747	1149	1618	2477	3085	3925	5947
1975	19937	829	6090	160	239	396	638	882	1447	2328	3109	3783	6126
1985	23360	555	4860	184	202	287	420	748	1204	1815	3157	4573	10215
1990	**25053**	**613**	**4886**	**157**	**338**	**335**	**473**	**602**	**1088**	**1893**	**2777**	**4346**	**12431**
1995 projected	*24985*	*686*	*4756*	*162*	*339*	*510*	*503*	*588*	*910*	*1744*	*2906*	*3689*	*12948*
Lung cancer													
1955	114	1	73	1	5	6	14	13	22	12	12	19	9
1965	120	–	78	1	3	5	9	19	18	23	12	19	11
1975	165	1	89	2	3	6	7	20	24	27	26	25	24
1985	320	–	153	4	3	5	15	27	41	58	62	48	57
1990	**346**	**4**	**152**	**1**	**6**	**3**	**18**	**18**	**34**	**72**	**58**	**66**	**66**
1995 projected	*353*	–	*139*	*1*	*4*	*4*	*16*	*16*	*29*	*69*	*74*	*63*	*77*
ANNUAL DEATH RATE / 100,000 (*The rates for the age groups 0–34 and 35–69 are the means of seven five-yearly rates, but the all-ages rates are standardised to the conventional "European" age distribution)													
All causes													
1955	1160.0*	160.4*	998.9*	216.6	278.8	393.8	625.6	964.8	1594.2	2918.6	5058.2	9300.0	18856.5
1965	1075.5*	98.5*	881.6*	125.8	231.2	343.0	517.7	829.6	1416.8	2707.1	4805.3	9085.6	19183.9
1975	788.2*	70.0*	669.8*	111.3	175.1	269.9	434.3	693.9	1088.0	1916.0	3439.2	6336.7	13986.3
1985	653.9*	45.9*	530.1*	85.8	130.4	203.3	315.3	529.0	869.9	1576.9	2816.2	5149.8	12642.3
1990	**624.6***	**53.2***	**499.2***	**78.8**	**158.1**	**217.8**	**339.3**	**460.9**	**794.2**	**1445.0**	**2667.6**	**4653.1**	**12163.4**
1995 projected	*599.8**	*61.9**	*475.1**	*86.5*	*171.3*	*240.3*	*330.7*	*429.5*	*720.5*	*1346.7*	*2450.3*	*4284.6*	*11760.2*
All cancer													
1955	166.8*	9.3*	238.3*	51.6	76.2	113.7	203.5	270.6	380.1	572.4	810.5	1135.3	1291.1
1965	156.1*	9.7*	212.8*	35.1	74.7	118.6	176.0	236.8	315.2	533.3	749.2	1034.7	1422.6
1975	143.7*	8.2*	196.5*	27.8	51.3	99.5	159.3	249.4	313.5	474.9	647.1	943.0	1404.1
1985	136.7*	4.7*	183.2*	25.2	47.1	80.7	136.6	203.7	324.4	464.8	646.7	973.0	1409.7
1990	**136.2***	**6.3***	**187.4***	**24.1**	**55.2**	**94.3**	**150.6**	**202.9**	**313.1**	**471.8**	**650.3**	**880.1**	**1328.8**
1995 projected	*134.0**	*7.3**	*188.8**	*26.7*	*61.6*	*105.1*	*157.1*	*201.6*	*307.2*	*462.5*	*618.0*	*833.9*	*1234.3*
Lung cancer													
1955	6.6*	0.1*	10.5*	0.7	3.3	4.1	11.1	12.0	25.7	16.6	22.5	55.9	38.0
1965	5.6*	–	9.6*	0.7	2.0	3.7	6.2	13.7	15.8	25.1	18.7	44.0	35.5
1975	6.4*	0.1*	9.8*	1.4	2.2	4.1	4.8	15.7	18.0	22.2	28.8	41.9	54.8
1985	10.1*	–	16.8*	1.9	1.9	3.5	11.3	19.1	29.6	50.4	55.3	54.1	70.5
1990	**10.1***	**0.3***	**16.0***	**0.5**	**2.8**	**2.0**	**12.9**	**13.8**	**24.8**	**55.0**	**55.7**	**70.7**	**64.6**
1995 projected	*9.8**	–	*14.7**	*0.5*	*2.0*	*1.9*	*10.5*	*11.7*	*23.0*	*53.3*	*62.4*	*73.2*	*69.9*
Upper aerodigestive cancer (mouth, oesophagus, pharynx and larynx)													
1955	12.5*	0.3*	16.6*	0.7	4.0	4.7	9.5	14.8	32.7	49.7	78.8	88.2	122.4
1965	9.0*	–	10.2*	–	3.9	1.5	5.5	9.4	15.8	35.0	43.6	85.6	122.6
1975	6.9*	0.1*	7.2*	0.7	0.7	2.7	4.1	7.9	14.3	19.8	39.8	60.3	95.9
1985	5.2*	–	5.9*	0.9	0.6	0.7	1.5	11.3	11.6	14.8	29.4	40.5	68.1
1990	**3.2***	**0.1***	**3.2***	–	**0.5**	**1.3**	**2.9**	**0.8**	**5.1**	**12.2**	**16.3**	**32.1**	**45.0**
1995 projected	*2.3**	*0.1**	*2.4**	–	*0.5*	*1.9*	*2.0*	*0.7*	*3.2*	*8.5*	*11.8*	*22.1*	*31.8*
Other cancer													
1955	147.6*	8.9*	211.2*	50.2	68.9	104.9	182.8	243.7	321.6	506.2	709.2	991.2	1130.8
1965	141.4*	9.7*	193.1*	34.4	68.8	113.3	164.2	213.7	283.7	473.2	686.9	905.1	1264.5
1975	130.4*	8.0*	179.6*	25.7	48.4	92.7	150.4	225.8	281.2	432.9	578.5	840.9	1253.4
1985	121.4*	4.7*	160.5*	22.4	44.5	76.5	123.9	173.3	283.2	399.7	562.0	878.4	1271.0
1990	**122.9***	**5.9***	**168.2***	**23.6**	**51.9**	**91.0**	**134.9**	**188.4**	**283.2**	**404.6**	**578.3**	**777.3**	**1219.2**
1995 projected	*122.0**	*7.2**	*171.8**	*26.2*	*59.1*	*101.3*	*144.6*	*189.2*	*281.1*	*400.8*	*543.8*	*738.7*	*1132.6*
Chronic obstructive pulmonary disease (COPD)													
1955	5.3*	0.7*	3.9*	0.7	1.3	0.7	–	2.8	9.4	12.4	26.3	29.4	109.7
1965	11.1*	0.6*	7.9*	0.7	2.6	3.7	4.2	8.7	15.8	19.7	28.0	106.5	248.4
1975	10.8*	0.8*	11.6*	–	2.2	4.8	15.7	13.4	19.5	25.5	50.9	70.4	153.0
1985	9.6*	0.5*	11.3*	1.4	1.9	3.5	6.8	12.0	27.5	26.1	41.9	76.6	122.5
1990	**5.4***	–	**6.8***	–	**0.9**	**2.0**	**3.6**	**6.9**	**13.9**	**20.6**	**23.1**	**33.2**	**83.2**
1995 projected	*3.7**	–	*4.6**	–	*0.5*	*1.4*	*2.6*	*4.4*	*9.5*	*13.9*	*16.0*	*23.2*	*58.1*
Other respiratory disease													
1955	85.7*	20.6*	39.9*	10.0	10.6	10.1	15.1	29.7	48.0	155.9	335.8	738.2	1797.5
1965	67.1*	5.5*	28.4*	2.6	3.3	6.0	6.2	16.6	44.7	119.1	236.8	594.9	1796.8
1975	47.3*	3.0*	15.0*	2.1	5.9	2.0	8.8	11.8	23.3	51.0	143.8	438.9	1369.9
1985	35.4*	1.0*	9.3*	1.9	1.3	2.1	4.5	7.8	8.7	39.1	87.4	266.9	1188.1
1990	**33.8***	**0.7***	**12.9***	**3.5**	**2.3**	**5.9**	**8.6**	**11.5**	**10.2**	**48.1**	**91.3**	**228.1**	**1081.2**
1995 projected	*31.8**	*0.6**	*15.3**	*4.8*	*3.0*	*8.0*	*11.8*	*15.3*	*12.7*	*51.7*	*83.5*	*200.9*	*973.7*
Vascular disease													
1955	604.7*	9.6*	512.5*	48.1	78.8	140.7	251.2	451.3	878.4	1739.3	3219.5	5885.3	10438.8
1965	616.0*	6.2*	446.2*	28.5	64.2	123.0	207.9	367.5	756.6	1576.0	2987.5	5923.6	12616.1
1975	432.7*	3.1*	310.8*	21.6	51.3	80.4	157.9	267.5	539.8	1056.8	2091.8	3978.2	9086.8
1985	342.8*	2.4*	217.9*	14.0	29.7	46.0	87.1	183.9	368.5	795.8	1672.6	3100.2	7787.1
1990	**299.2***	**2.3***	**178.8***	**12.6**	**24.3**	**38.4**	**78.2**	**142.4**	**294.2**	**661.8**	**1438.0**	**2672.4**	**7048.9**
1995 projected	*257.2**	*2.5**	*144.5**	*9.6*	*20.2*	*32.5*	*61.8*	*110.3*	*232.8*	*544.4*	*1210.8*	*2250.9*	*6295.2*
Liver cirrhosis													
1955	3.5*	0.1*	5.1*	0.7	2.6	3.4	4.0	4.6	8.2	12.4	11.3	32.4	25.3
1965	3.2*	0.5*	3.6*	0.7	3.9	3.0	1.4	0.7	7.9	7.7	23.4	27.8	16.1
1975	3.2*	0.6*	4.9*	0.7	2.9	2.0	4.8	7.9	8.3	7.4	8.8	16.8	18.3
1985	4.2*	0.5*	7.5*	1.4	3.2	5.0	8.3	9.2	10.8	14.8	12.5	16.9	17.3
1990	**5.4***	**0.5***	**9.5***	**3.0**	**7.5**	**10.4**	**12.2**	**8.4**	**14.6**	**10.7**	**15.4**	**19.3**	**19.6**
1995 projected	*6.4**	*0.3**	*11.5**	*4.3*	*10.6*	*14.6*	*16.4*	*10.2*	*13.5*	*10.8*	*15.2*	*22.1*	*21.8*
Other medical causes													
1955	251.5*	100.4*	164.5*	80.3	84.1	96.8	114.5	167.7	240.9	366.9	568.5	1297.1	4590.7
1965	176.0*	55.4*	143.5*	37.1	53.0	61.1	81.1	151.6	229.4	391.3	685.4	1182.9	2464.5
1975	108.8*	33.7*	84.7*	17.4	27.8	40.9	42.9	94.4	132.3	237.0	410.4	772.2	1595.9
1985	89.2*	22.6*	60.6*	12.6	17.4	30.5	27.0	54.5	91.8	190.3	300.6	591.2	1726.5
1990	**103.0***	**23.4***	**57.3***	**10.5**	**21.0**	**21.5**	**43.8**	**42.1**	**89.8**	**172.5**	**366.0**	**703.4**	**2232.9**
1995 projected	*119.1**	*24.6**	*56.5**	*10.7*	*18.2*	*24.0*	*40.8*	*40.9*	*79.2*	*181.5*	*412.3*	*829.3*	*2830.2*
All non-medical causes													
1955	42.7*	19.8*	34.7*	25.1	25.2	28.4	37.4	38.0	29.2	59.3	86.3	182.4	603.4
1965	46.0*	20.8*	39.2*	21.2	29.5	27.6	40.9	47.7	47.3	60.1	95.0	215.3	619.4
1975	41.7*	20.5*	46.4*	41.7	33.7	40.2	44.9	49.6	51.1	63.4	86.3	117.3	358.4
1985	36.0*	14.3*	40.3*	29.4	29.7	35.4	45.0	58.0	38.3	46.0	54.4	125.0	391.1
1990	**41.4***	**20.0***	**46.3***	**25.1**	**46.8**	**45.5**	**42.3**	**46.7**	**58.4**	**59.5**	**83.6**	**116.7**	**368.9**
1995 projected	*47.5**	*26.6**	*53.8**	*30.4*	*57.1*	*54.7*	*40.1*	*46.7*	*65.7*	*81.9*	*94.4*	*124.3*	*347.0*

FINLAND: 1975

Smoking-attributed deaths (Sm.) and total deaths (Total)

		ALL CAUSES	ALL CANCER	Lung cancer	Upper aero-digestive ca.	Other cancer	COPD	Other respiratory	Vascular disease	Liver cirrhosis	Other medical	Non-medical
Males												
0-34	Sm.	–	–	–	–	–	–	–	–	–	–	–
	Total	2048	145	1	3	141	11	34	98	18	576	1166
35-69	Sm.	4224	1311	952	84	275	327	85	2183	–	318	–
	Total	12206	2531	1009	119	1403	398	254	6392	169	908	1554
		(35%)	(52%)	(94%)	(71%)	(20%)	(82%)	(33%)	(34%)		(35%)	
70+	Sm.	2215	750	513	55	182	401	91	854	–	119	–
	Total	9662	1837	554	86	1197	526	669	5482	30	793	325
		(23%)	(41%)	(93%)	(64%)	(15%)	(76%)	(14%)	(16%)		(15%)	
Any age	Sm.	6439	2061	1465	139	457	728	176	3037	–	437	–
	Total	23916	4513	1564	208	2741	935	957	11972	217	2277	3045
		(27%)	(46%)	(94%)	(67%)	(17%)	(78%)	(18%)	(25%)		(19%)	
Females												
0-34	Sm.	–	–	–	–	–	–	–	–	–	–	–
	Total	829	104	1	1	102	10	35	39	8	371	262
35-69	Sm.	41	9	7	1	1	6	0	21	–	5	–
	Total	6090	1801	89	65	1647	107	135	2793	45	770	439
		(1%)	(0%)	(8%)	(2%)	(0%)	(6%)	(0%)	(1%)		(1%)	
70+	Sm.	60	15	9	4	2	11	3	26	–	5	–
	Total	13018	1763	75	114	1574	155	992	8246	26	1531	305
		(0%)	(1%)	(12%)	(4%)	(0%)	(7%)	(0%)	(0%)		(0%)	
Any age	Sm.	101	24	16	5	3	17	3	47	–	10	–
	Total	19937	3668	165	180	3323	272	1162	11078	79	2672	1006
		(1%)	(1%)	(10%)	(3%)	(0%)	(6%)	(0%)	(0%)		(0%)	
Males+Females												
0-34	Sm.	–	–	–	–	–	–	–	–	–	–	–
	Total	2877	249	2	4	243	21	69	137	26	947	1428
35-69	Sm.	4265	1320	959	85	276	333	85	2204	–	323	–
	Total	18296	4332	1098	184	3050	505	389	9185	214	1678	1993
		(23%)	(30%)	(87%)	(46%)	(9%)	(66%)	(22%)	(24%)		(19%)	
70+	Sm.	2275	765	522	59	184	412	94	880	–	124	–
	Total	22680	3600	629	200	2771	681	1661	13728	56	2324	630
		(10%)	(21%)	(83%)	(30%)	(7%)	(60%)	(6%)	(6%)		(5%)	
Any age	Sm.	6540	2085	1481	144	460	745	179	3084	–	447	–
	Total	43853	8181	1729	388	6064	1207	2119	23050	296	4949	4051
		(15%)	(25%)	(86%)	(37%)	(8%)	(62%)	(8%)	(13%)		(9%)	

FINLAND: 1985

Smoking-attributed deaths (Sm.) and total deaths (Total)

		ALL CAUSES	ALL CANCER	Lung cancer	Upper aero-digestive ca.	Other cancer	COPD	Other respiratory	Vascular disease	Liver cirrhosis	Other medical	Non-medical
Males												
0-34	Sm.	–	–	–	–	–	–	–	–	–	–	–
	Total	1378	104	2	1	101	5	17	90	11	330	821
35-69	Sm.	3370	1178	877	69	232	229	57	1662	–	244	–
	Total	10590	2371	937	103	1331	284	182	5286	204	762	1501
		(32%)	(50%)	(94%)	(67%)	(17%)	(81%)	(31%)	(31%)		(32%)	
70+	Sm.	3055	1088	760	62	266	531	133	1135	–	168	–
	Total	13017	2580	819	93	1668	682	944	7251	25	1104	431
		(23%)	(42%)	(93%)	(67%)	(16%)	(78%)	(14%)	(16%)		(15%)	
Any age	Sm.	6425	2266	1637	131	498	760	190	2797	–	412	–
	Total	24985	5055	1758	197	3100	971	1143	12627	240	2196	2753
		(26%)	(45%)	(93%)	(66%)	(16%)	(78%)	(17%)	(22%)		(19%)	
Females												
0-34	Sm.	–	–	–	–	–	–	–	–	–	–	–
	Total	555	60	0	0	60	6	11	31	7	259	181
35-69	Sm.	272	88	69	9	10	34	4	116	–	30	–
	Total	4860	1695	153	55	1487	105	83	1943	71	556	407
		(6%)	(5%)	(45%)	(16%)	(1%)	(32%)	(5%)	(6%)		(5%)	
70+	Sm.	381	101	69	17	15	57	16	173	–	34	–
	Total	17945	2728	167	124	2437	214	1295	10920	43	2257	488
		(2%)	(4%)	(41%)	(14%)	(1%)	(27%)	(1%)	(2%)		(2%)	
Any age	Sm.	653	189	138	26	25	91	20	289	–	64	–
	Total	23360	4483	320	179	3984	325	1389	12894	121	3072	1076
		(3%)	(4%)	(43%)	(15%)	(1%)	(28%)	(1%)	(2%)		(2%)	
Males+Females												
0-34	Sm.	–	–	–	–	–	–	–	–	–	–	–
	Total	1933	164	2	1	161	11	28	121	18	589	1002
35-69	Sm.	3642	1266	946	78	242	263	61	1778	–	274	–
	Total	15450	4066	1090	158	2818	389	265	7229	275	1318	1908
		(24%)	(31%)	(87%)	(49%)	(9%)	(68%)	(23%)	(25%)		(21%)	
70+	Sm.	3436	1189	829	79	281	588	149	1308	–	202	–
	Total	30962	5308	986	217	4105	896	2239	18171	68	3361	919
		(11%)	(22%)	(84%)	(36%)	(7%)	(66%)	(7%)	(7%)		(6%)	
Any age	Sm.	7078	2455	1775	157	523	851	210	3086	–	476	–
	Total	48345	9538	2078	376	7084	1296	2532	25521	361	5268	3829
		(15%)	(26%)	(85%)	(42%)	(7%)	(66%)	(8%)	(12%)		(9%)	

(To be conservative, no deaths before age 35, and none from liver cirrhosis or non-medical causes, were attributed to smoking.)

FINLAND: 1990

Smoking–attributed deaths (Sm.) and total deaths (Total)

		ALL CAUSES	ALL CANCER	Lung cancer	Upper aero-digestive ca.	Other cancer	COPD	Other respiratory	Vascular disease	Liver cirrhosis	Other medical	Non-medical
Males												
0–34	Sm.	–	–	–	–	–	–	–	–	–	–	–
	Total	1434	64	1	3	60	2	20	67	12	324	945
35–69	Sm.	2637	1018	757	66	195	158	59	1189	–	213	–
	Total	10671	2317	825	110	1382	208	233	4743	332	866	1972
		(25%)	(44%)	(92%)	(60%)	(14%)	(76%)	(25%)	(25%)		(25%)	
70+	Sm.	2669	1026	711	55	260	408	126	929	–	180	–
	Total	12929	2662	773	87	1802	538	994	6853	29	1344	509
		(21%)	(39%)	(92%)	(63%)	(14%)	(76%)	(13%)	(14%)		(13%)	
Any age	Sm.	5306	2044	1468	121	455	566	185	2118	–	393	–
	Total	25034	5043	1599	200	3244	748	1247	11663	373	2534	3426
		(21%)	(41%)	(92%)	(61%)	(14%)	(76%)	(15%)	(18%)		(16%)	
Females												
0–34	Sm.	–	–	–	–	–	–	–	–	–	–	–
	Total	613	76	4	1	71	0	8	28	6	257	238
35–69	Sm.	227	76	63	5	8	19	6	97	–	29	–
	Total	4886	1833	152	31	1650	65	125	1701	100	564	498
		(5%)	(4%)	(41%)	(16%)	(0%)	(29%)	(5%)	(6%)		(5%)	
70+	Sm.	544	139	97	20	22	51	30	251	–	73	–
	Total	19554	2857	190	93	2574	140	1413	11197	54	3320	573
		(3%)	(5%)	(51%)	(22%)	(1%)	(36%)	(2%)	(2%)		(2%)	
Any age	Sm.	771	215	160	25	30	70	36	348	–	102	–
	Total	25053	4766	346	125	4295	205	1546	12926	160	4141	1309
		(3%)	(5%)	(46%)	(20%)	(1%)	(34%)	(2%)	(3%)		(2%)	
Males+Females												
0–34	Sm.	–	–	–	–	–	–	–	–	–	–	–
	Total	2047	140	5	4	131	2	28	95	18	581	1183
35–69	Sm.	2864	1094	820	71	203	177	65	1286	–	242	–
	Total	15557	4150	977	141	3032	273	358	6444	432	1430	2470
		(18%)	(26%)	(84%)	(50%)	(7%)	(65%)	(18%)	(20%)		(17%)	
70+	Sm.	3213	1165	808	75	282	459	156	1180	–	253	–
	Total	32483	5519	963	180	4376	678	2407	18050	83	4664	1082
		(10%)	(21%)	(84%)	(42%)	(6%)	(68%)	(6%)	(7%)		(5%)	
Any age	Sm.	6077	2259	1628	146	485	636	221	2466	–	495	–
	Total	50087	9809	1945	325	7539	953	2793	24589	533	6675	4735
		(12%)	(23%)	(84%)	(45%)	(6%)	(67%)	(8%)	(10%)		(7%)	

FINLAND: 1995

Smoking–attributed deaths (Sm.) and total deaths (Total)

		ALL CAUSES	ALL CANCER	Lung cancer	Upper aero-digestive ca.	Other cancer	COPD	Other respiratory	Vascular disease	Liver cirrhosis	Other medical	Non-medical
Males												
0–34	Sm.	–	–	–	–	–	–	–	–	–	–	–
	Total	1542	46	1	4	41	2	25	55	15	314	1085
35–69	Sm.	1994	855	637	63	155	117	55	790	–	177	–
	Total	10336	2192	713	123	1356	163	279	3926	481	912	2383
		(19%)	(39%)	(89%)	(51%)	(11%)	(72%)	(20%)	(20%)		(19%)	
70+	Sm.	2323	954	669	45	240	298	110	773	–	188	–
	Total	12288	2633	734	73	1826	405	931	6167	33	1523	596
		(19%)	(36%)	(91%)	(62%)	(13%)	(74%)	(12%)	(13%)		(12%)	
Any age	Sm.	4317	1809	1306	108	395	415	165	1563	–	365	–
	Total	24166	4871	1448	200	3223	570	1235	10148	529	2749	4064
		(18%)	(37%)	(90%)	(54%)	(12%)	(73%)	(13%)	(15%)		(13%)	
Females												
0–34	Sm.	–	–	–	–	–	–	–	–	–	–	–
	Total	686	85	0	1	84	0	6	28	4	258	305
35–69	Sm.	167	60	49	3	8	11	6	67	–	23	–
	Total	4756	1897	139	24	1734	44	154	1371	130	560	600
		(4%)	(3%)	(35%)	(13%)	(0%)	(25%)	(4%)	(5%)		(4%)	
70+	Sm.	591	155	115	16	24	40	31	260	–	105	–
	Total	19543	2810	214	68	2528	103	1344	10305	61	4319	601
		(3%)	(6%)	(54%)	(24%)	(1%)	(39%)	(2%)	(3%)		(2%)	
Any age	Sm.	758	215	164	19	32	51	37	327	–	128	–
	Total	24985	4792	353	93	4346	147	1504	11704	195	5137	1506
		(3%)	(4%)	(46%)	(20%)	(1%)	(35%)	(2%)	(3%)		(2%)	
Males+Females												
0–34	Sm.	–	–	–	–	–	–	–	–	–	–	–
	Total	2228	131	1	5	125	2	31	83	19	572	1390
35–69	Sm.	2161	915	686	66	163	128	61	857	–	200	–
	Total	15092	4089	852	147	3090	207	433	5297	611	1472	2983
		(14%)	(22%)	(81%)	(45%)	(5%)	(62%)	(14%)	(16%)		(14%)	
70+	Sm.	2914	1109	784	61	264	338	141	1033	–	293	–
	Total	31831	5443	948	141	4354	508	2275	16472	94	5842	1197
		(9%)	(20%)	(83%)	(43%)	(6%)	(67%)	(6%)	(6%)		(5%)	
Any age	Sm.	5075	2024	1470	127	427	466	202	1890	–	493	–
	Total	49151	9663	1801	293	7569	717	2739	21852	724	7886	5570
		(10%)	(21%)	(82%)	(43%)	(6%)	(65%)	(7%)	(9%)		(6%)	

(To be conservative, no deaths before age 35, and none from liver cirrhosis or non-medical causes, were attributed to smoking.)

FRANCE: 1990

		No. of deaths			Standardised rates (Defined on p.340)			Annual death rates / 100, 000						
		All ages	0–34	35–69	All ages	0–34	35–69	0–4	5–9	10–14	15–19	20–24	25–29	30–34
ALL CAUSES	M	272664	17184	100533	922.7	117.9	1013.9	205.8	20.5	22.0	78.9	150.9	162.6	184.9
	F	253537	7516	43166	486.5	54.0	395.7	150.3	16.3	15.8	32.9	42.7	54.1	66.1
Tuberculosis	M	833	18	282	2.8	0.1	2.9	–	–	–	0.1	0.1	0.2	0.4
	F	556	9	88	1.1	0.1	0.8	0.1	–	–	–	0.0	0.2	0.1
Other infective	M	2576	138	732	8.5	1.0	7.4	3.6	0.1	0.2	0.3	0.6	0.9	1.1
and parasitic	F	2924	97	393	5.4	0.7	3.6	2.7	0.5	0.2	0.4	0.2	0.3	0.7
ALL CANCER	M	84202	989	41721	296.2	6.8	430.8	4.8	4.3	3.4	4.7	6.7	8.9	14.8
	F	53746	775	19547	128.9	5.4	180.2	3.4	2.5	3.4	3.7	4.3	7.1	13.3
Mouth and	M	4865	28	3619	18.6	0.2	36.1	–	–	0.1	0.1	0.2	0.1	0.9
pharynx cancer	F	672	9	347	1.9	0.1	3.2	–	–	–	0.1	0.0	0.1	0.2
Oesophagus cancer	M	4311	3	2910	16.0	0.0	29.8	–	–	–	–	–	0.0	0.1
	F	705	1	268	1.7	0.0	2.5	–	–	–	–	–	–	0.0
Stomach cancer	M	3962	6	1536	13.5	0.0	16.0	–	–	–	–	–	0.0	0.2
	F	2836	16	547	5.6	0.1	5.1	–	–	–	–	0.0	0.2	0.5
Colorectal cancer	M	7886	24	2999	26.7	0.2	31.6	0.1	–	–	0.1	0.1	0.2	0.6
	F	7599	26	1992	16.1	0.2	18.6	–	–	–	–	0.1	0.3	0.8
Liver cancer	M	2479	18	1505	9.0	0.1	15.9	0.2	–	0.1	–	0.2	0.1	0.2
	F	515	4	211	1.3	0.0	2.0	0.1	–	–	0.0	–	–	0.0
Pancreas cancer	M	3090	11	1523	10.9	0.1	15.9	–	–	–	–	–	0.1	0.4
	F	2647	10	763	5.8	0.1	7.1	–	0.1	–	–	0.1	0.1	0.2
Larynx cancer	M	2880	2	1990	10.8	0.0	20.3	–	–	–	–	–	–	0.1
	F	155	–	88	0.5	–	0.8	–	–	–	–	–	–	–
Lung cancer	M	18805	58	11185	68.0	0.4	115.7	0.2	0.1	–	0.1	–	0.3	2.1
	F	2812	19	1335	7.4	0.1	12.4	–	–	–	–	0.1	0.1	0.7
Malignant melanoma	M	502	24	295	1.8	0.2	2.9	–	–	–	0.0	0.1	0.4	0.6
	F	501	31	249	1.4	0.2	2.2	–	–	–	0.0	0.2	0.6	0.7
Female breast cancer	F	10173	79	5322	28.1	0.5	48.8	–	–	–	0.0	0.0	0.7	2.9
Cervix cancer	F	791	26	454	2.3	0.2	4.0	–	–	–	–	0.0	0.3	0.9
Other uterine cancer	F	2348	8	895	5.8	0.1	8.3	–	–	–	–	0.0	0.0	0.3
Ovarian cancer	F	3129	38	1474	8.3	0.3	13.7	–	–	–	0.2	0.2	0.3	1.0
Prostate cancer	M	9211	5	1587	29.2	0.0	17.5	–	–	–	–	0.1	0.1	0.0
Bladder cancer	M	3170	1	1126	10.7	0.0	11.9	–	–	–	–	–	–	0.0
	F	1105	4	169	2.1	0.0	1.6	–	–	–	0.0	–	0.1	0.0
Other and ill-defined	M	17811	446	9324	63.2	3.1	95.6	2.3	2.4	1.7	2.4	3.0	4.0	5.8
cancer sites	F	13003	281	4030	29.7	2.0	37.2	1.9	1.2	1.7	1.7	1.9	2.5	3.1
Hodgkin's disease	M	228	29	131	0.8	0.2	1.2	–	–	0.1	0.0	0.3	0.4	0.5
	F	109	17	37	0.3	0.1	0.3	–	–	–	0.1	0.2	0.2	0.3
Myeloma and non-	M	2487	80	1081	8.6	0.5	11.1	0.2	0.1	0.3	0.4	0.6	1.0	1.2
Hodgkin lymphomas	F	2414	51	733	5.6	0.4	6.8	0.1	0.3	0.2	0.4	0.2	0.7	0.6
Leukaemia	M	2515	254	910	8.6	1.8	9.2	1.9	1.7	1.2	1.5	2.0	2.1	2.0
	F	2232	155	633	5.2	1.1	5.8	1.2	0.9	1.5	1.1	1.0	0.9	1.2
ALL VASCULAR	M	79357	648	21803	258.5	4.4	226.5	3.6	0.8	0.8	1.9	4.3	7.1	12.4
DISEASE	F	95187	352	8027	156.4	2.4	74.8	3.1	0.3	0.7	2.2	1.7	3.6	5.5
Rheumatic heart	M	381	14	129	1.3	0.1	1.3	0.1	0.1	–	0.1	0.1	0.2	0.2
disease and fever	F	779	13	204	1.7	0.1	1.9	–	0.1	–	0.0	0.0	0.2	0.2
Hypertensive disease	M	2295	13	596	7.4	0.1	6.3	–	–	0.1	–	0.1	0.2	0.3
	F	3898	5	394	6.5	0.0	3.7	–	–	–	–	–	0.0	0.2
Ischaemic heart	M	26724	118	9713	89.9	0.8	100.9	0.1	–	0.1	0.1	0.4	0.9	3.9
disease	F	22564	22	2317	39.0	0.1	21.7	–	–	–	–	0.1	0.2	0.7
Pulmonary embolism	M	1909	20	563	6.3	0.1	5.8	–	–	–	0.0	0.1	0.1	0.6
and other venous	F	3299	21	456	5.9	0.1	4.2	–	–	0.1	0.1	–	0.3	0.5
Cerebrovascular	M	19718	173	4269	63.0	1.2	44.3	0.8	0.2	0.2	0.6	0.9	2.2	3.3
disease	F	28810	114	2360	47.2	0.8	21.9	0.3	0.1	0.3	0.6	0.8	1.3	2.2
Other vascular	M	28330	310	6533	90.6	2.1	67.9	2.6	0.6	0.6	1.0	2.6	3.4	4.0
disease	F	35837	177	2296	56.0	1.3	21.4	2.8	0.1	0.4	1.5	0.9	1.5	1.7
Chronic obstructive	M	8839	92	1920	28.3	0.6	20.5	0.7	0.1	0.7	0.9	0.7	0.6	0.7
pulmonary disease	F	6050	60	707	10.6	0.4	6.6	0.4	0.2	0.1	0.6	0.7	0.4	0.6
Other respiratory	M	10961	200	1969	34.4	1.4	20.5	4.3	0.3	0.3	0.9	1.0	1.0	2.0
disease	F	12236	136	634	18.7	1.0	5.8	3.1	0.4	0.5	0.5	0.8	0.6	0.9
Peptic ulcer	M	1032	5	343	3.4	0.0	3.5	–	–	–	–	–	0.0	0.2
	F	911	2	87	1.5	0.0	0.8	0.1	–	0.1	–	–	–	–
Liver cirrhosis	M	6931	113	5200	26.0	0.8	51.4	0.1	–	–	0.0	0.1	1.1	3.9
	F	3121	44	2236	10.2	0.3	20.3	–	0.1	0.1	–	0.1	0.4	1.4
Renal disease	M	2405	26	442	7.5	0.2	4.6	0.4	–	0.1	–	0.2	0.4	0.1
	F	2555	17	239	4.3	0.1	2.2	0.3	–	0.1	0.1	0.0	0.1	0.2
Pregnancy and birth	F	79	53	26	0.3	0.4	0.2	–	–	–	0.0	0.3	0.8	1.3
Congenital and	M	1804	1654	113	7.3	12.2	1.0	78.9	1.2	0.9	1.1	1.2	1.1	0.7
perinatal causes	F	1442	1286	97	5.9	9.9	0.8	63.7	1.4	1.1	0.9	0.6	0.9	0.6
Ill-defined causes	M	14020	2496	4007	47.3	17.6	38.5	69.9	1.0	1.0	4.6	11.9	16.9	18.0
	F	17448	1235	1496	30.9	9.2	13.4	45.9	0.9	0.4	1.5	4.7	5.0	5.9
Other medical causes	M	30665	2163	9704	101.6	14.8	94.5	15.3	3.5	3.9	5.2	11.1	27.1	37.1
	F	38067	936	4923	68.5	6.7	45.0	12.0	3.7	2.8	2.6	4.4	9.9	11.2
ALL NON-	M	29039	8642	12297	100.8	58.1	111.8	24.2	9.2	10.8	59.0	113.0	97.3	93.3
MEDICAL CAUSES	F	19215	2514	4666	43.8	17.5	41.1	15.5	6.4	6.3	20.4	24.8	24.8	24.4
Motor vehicle	M	7316	4063	2515	25.4	27.2	22.0	4.9	4.4	5.6	35.6	67.7	43.6	28.6
traffic accidents	F	2690	1123	1020	8.7	7.8	8.8	3.7	3.3	3.5	12.3	13.7	11.0	7.1
Fire	M	328	90	154	1.2	0.6	1.4	1.1	0.3	0.5	0.5	0.5	0.9	0.6
	F	251	55	69	0.7	0.4	0.6	1.1	0.3	0.2	0.2	0.1	0.5	0.5
Suicide	M	8178	1935	4456	29.0	12.9	39.8	–	–	0.7	8.0	20.1	26.1	35.2
	F	3225	581	1801	10.2	3.9	15.7	–	–	0.3	3.3	5.5	7.6	10.6
Homicide	M	389	162	204	1.4	1.1	1.7	0.7	0.2	0.2	0.6	1.2	1.9	2.8
	F	225	91	99	0.8	0.6	0.8	0.8	0.4	0.4	0.4	1.0	0.9	0.6
POPULATION (thousands):	M=males				27623	14248	11334	1934	1771	1934	2156	2163	2155	2135
	F=females				29112	13867	11758	1848	1690	1845	2060	2115	2158	2150

FRANCE: 1990
9th ICD categories

Annual death rates / 100, 000

35–39	40–44	45–49	50–54	55–59	60–64	65–69	70–74	75–79	80+/NK			
239.6	327.6	487.3	746.8	1152.2	1721.4	2422.7	3536.1	5895.7	13034.4	M	**ALL CAUSES**	001–999
98.1	134.6	207.3	303.0	440.2	635.9	950.9	1593.4	3099.6	10022.7	F		
0.5	0.9	1.1	2.0	3.1	4.9	7.7	14.1	23.2	40.3	M	**Tuberculosis**	010–018, 137
0.3	0.3	0.4	0.3	0.8	1.6	2.0	6.0	9.6	19.6	F		
1.8	2.8	3.7	4.8	7.4	11.8	19.3	36.5	58.0	152.2	M	**Other infective**	Rest of 001–139
0.7	1.3	1.7	2.3	4.2	5.6	9.5	17.2	36.8	121.6	F	**and parasitic**	
36.3	82.9	177.4	315.8	539.7	804.7	1059.1	1377.3	1912.5	2771.7	M	**ALL CANCER**	140–208
31.2	54.8	93.0	148.4	219.1	305.4	409.8	552.3	794.4	1299.9	F		
3.7	11.4	26.3	38.4	56.7	62.1	53.7	63.4	62.5	53.5	M	**Mouth and**	140–149
0.6	1.3	2.2	3.4	4.6	5.1	5.0	6.1	7.5	11.8	F	**pharynx cancer**	
1.5	5.2	13.0	27.0	46.0	56.5	59.7	64.3	67.1	73.8	M	**Oesophagus cancer**	150
0.2	0.5	1.5	2.1	3.2	4.6	5.3	6.1	10.9	17.2	F		
1.1	3.1	5.7	9.9	17.8	30.5	43.9	71.5	108.9	172.6	M	**Stomach cancer**	151
0.8	1.3	2.2	2.9	6.3	8.7	13.2	27.1	45.7	99.8	F		
1.9	4.3	8.1	16.4	34.2	59.6	97.1	137.0	217.9	354.0	M	**Colorectal cancer**	153, 154
1.8	3.1	6.2	12.1	20.4	34.9	51.5	74.5	120.2	235.3	F		
0.7	1.2	3.1	7.8	18.2	35.9	44.5	53.8	49.0	38.2	M	**Liver cancer**	155.0
0.1	0.3	0.4	1.0	2.0	3.7	6.2	8.3	8.7	8.7	F		
1.2	2.5	5.3	10.6	19.7	29.0	42.9	57.1	73.2	97.4	M	**Pancreas cancer**	157
0.5	1.2	2.6	3.6	7.8	12.9	21.3	27.6	46.1	73.8	F		
0.9	3.9	9.8	20.4	31.6	35.5	40.3	42.9	41.3	46.1	M	**Larynx cancer**	161
0.0	0.2	0.7	1.2	1.4	1.1	1.1	1.2	2.6	1.9	F		
7.9	21.6	49.5	83.3	143.8	219.8	283.9	324.4	393.6	393.5	M	**Lung cancer**	162
1.3	3.5	5.3	9.8	14.2	24.0	28.4	32.7	41.1	47.6	F		
1.2	1.2	1.6	2.6	2.9	4.9	5.9	6.5	9.8	10.6	M	**Malignant melanoma**	172
0.9	1.3	2.1	2.5	3.0	2.4	3.4	3.7	5.2	8.6	F		
9.8	19.8	31.7	51.7	65.3	75.1	88.1	97.3	118.7	171.6	F	**Female breast cancer**	174
2.3	2.6	3.3	3.8	4.7	5.4	6.0	7.1	8.7	10.1	F	**Cervix cancer**	180
1.2	2.2	3.5	5.7	10.8	14.1	20.3	30.6	37.3	50.4	F	**Other uterine cancer**	179, 182
1.6	3.8	6.4	12.2	17.5	23.5	30.6	36.8	46.1	52.1	F	**Ovarian cancer**	183
0.1	0.2	0.7	3.6	11.0	33.9	72.8	146.2	297.6	660.4	M	**Prostate cancer**	185
0.1	0.9	3.5	6.5	14.0	24.6	34.0	57.5	94.7	145.8	M	**Bladder cancer**	188
0.1	0.1	0.5	0.8	1.5	2.6	5.5	9.3	20.6	40.8	F		
10.8	20.6	41.5	73.7	121.8	177.3	223.9	273.6	374.2	527.4	M	**Other and ill-defined**	Rest of 140–208
6.5	9.5	17.8	26.0	42.8	66.0	92.1	134.0	195.6	350.7	F	**cancer sites**	
1.2	0.8	0.8	1.6	1.0	1.2	1.8	1.9	3.4	4.6	M	**Hodgkin's disease**	201
0.3	0.4	0.3	0.2	0.3	0.3	0.4	1.0	2.2	1.5	F		
1.7	2.8	5.1	8.4	11.1	19.1	29.4	41.5	63.1	89.2	M	**Myeloma and non-**	200, 202–203
1.2	1.3	3.0	4.6	7.4	11.5	18.6	27.1	46.2	58.4	F	**Hodgkin lymphomas**	
2.1	3.2	3.5	5.9	9.9	14.7	25.4	35.9	56.1	104.6	M	**Leukaemia**	204–208
1.9	2.3	3.3	4.9	5.7	9.7	12.6	21.8	31.1	59.4	F		
29.3	50.3	75.4	135.4	225.8	402.8	666.5	1090.3	2100.0	5046.6	M	**ALL VASCULAR**	390–459
8.7	12.7	23.1	36.9	69.6	125.5	247.2	520.6	1236.0	4440.9	F	**DISEASE**	
0.5	0.5	0.5	1.2	1.2	2.0	3.1	6.6	12.3	15.9	M	**Rheumatic heart**	390–398
0.3	0.4	0.8	0.9	2.1	3.5	5.2	11.0	13.9	20.6	F	**disease and fever**	
0.3	0.8	1.5	4.1	6.4	11.7	19.5	30.7	57.0	155.8	M	**Hypertensive disease**	401–405
0.2	0.4	0.8	1.7	3.6	5.9	13.2	22.3	50.6	177.8	F		
10.9	22.9	34.8	62.3	100.9	182.4	292.4	434.9	720.4	1302.5	M	**Ischaemic heart**	410–414
0.9	2.6	4.2	9.4	18.6	37.3	79.3	172.6	370.5	951.4	F	**disease**	
1.2	1.7	1.7	3.7	4.8	10.9	16.4	30.1	50.8	111.3	M	**Pulmonary embolism**	415.1, 451–453
0.8	1.3	1.6	1.7	4.3	6.7	12.8	24.6	46.5	135.9	F	**and other venous**	
6.2	10.0	16.1	26.6	43.0	77.2	131.1	247.6	540.5	1419.2	M	**Cerebrovascular**	430–438
3.5	4.4	8.4	12.1	20.9	35.9	68.2	147.8	379.2	1350.4	F	**disease**	
10.1	14.6	20.9	37.6	69.5	118.6	204.0	340.2	719.0	2041.8	M	**Other vascular**	Rest of 390–459
3.0	3.6	7.3	11.0	20.1	36.2	68.5	142.4	375.3	1804.9	F	**disease**	
1.3	2.0	3.5	8.7	18.6	38.9	70.6	121.5	248.2	617.9	M	**Chronic obstructive**	490–496
0.8	1.2	1.6	3.5	6.7	11.3	21.1	40.4	80.2	262.0	F	**pulmonary disease**	
3.3	4.7	6.9	11.3	20.4	32.9	63.8	115.0	250.6	898.7	M	**Other respiratory**	Rest of 460–519
1.2	2.0	1.9	4.2	5.8	8.9	16.8	39.2	106.5	640.5	F	**disease**	
0.6	1.1	1.7	1.7	3.8	6.4	9.4	12.8	26.3	60.0	M	**Peptic ulcer**	531–533
0.2	0.3	0.2	0.7	0.5	1.6	2.1	7.0	9.5	42.3	F		
11.4	20.1	29.6	48.0	74.5	87.1	89.2	86.9	87.4	64.5	M	**Liver cirrhosis**	571
5.4	11.3	17.9	24.0	26.5	29.4	27.3	29.9	24.2	20.8	F		
1.0	0.8	1.5	2.5	4.3	9.0	13.0	24.3	58.5	196.0	M	**Renal disease**	580–590
0.4	0.5	0.3	1.1	2.8	3.5	7.0	14.7	29.7	119.1	F		
0.9	0.2	0.1	–	–	–	–	–	–	–	F	**Pregnancy and birth**	630–676
0.8	0.8	1.2	1.0	0.8	1.4	1.1	1.5	1.7	2.3	M	**Congenital and**	740–779
0.6	0.7	0.5	0.7	1.1	1.0	1.1	1.6	1.4	2.0	F	**perinatal causes**	
18.2	22.2	26.8	34.1	40.3	56.6	71.0	115.3	197.0	767.9	M	**Ill-defined causes**	780–799
7.5	6.4	9.6	10.4	12.5	18.7	28.6	55.8	128.6	824.2	F		
42.7	47.4	54.5	69.4	102.4	140.0	205.3	356.9	649.3	1711.0	M	**Other medical causes**	Rest of 001–799
13.6	13.8	20.0	28.8	47.1	73.7	118.3	219.4	478.1	1619.8	F		
92.5	91.5	104.0	112.1	111.2	124.9	146.7	183.9	283.2	705.2	M	**ALL NON-**	E800–E999
26.8	28.9	36.9	41.7	43.6	49.7	60.0	89.3	164.7	610.1	F	**MEDICAL CAUSES**	
23.4	23.1	23.2	22.6	20.2	20.4	21.3	27.9	38.7	41.7	M	**Motor vehicle**	E810–E819
7.5	7.4	8.9	9.0	7.9	10.3	10.7	14.3	15.9	16.4	F	**traffic accidents**	
1.3	1.0	1.2	1.6	2.0	1.4	1.3	2.2	2.6	7.3	M	**Fire**	E890–E899
0.6	0.4	0.5	0.7	1.0	0.4	0.7	0.9	2.4	6.1	F		
38.3	36.0	39.9	42.3	37.9	38.8	45.1	50.9	77.9	131.6	M	**Suicide**	E950–E959
11.3	12.3	14.4	18.5	18.8	17.5	17.4	20.2	26.0	25.3	F		
2.4	2.4	1.9	2.1	1.4	0.9	0.7	0.6	1.1	1.7	M	**Homicide**	E960–E969
1.1	0.7	1.2	1.0	0.5	1.0	0.5	0.7	1.1	1.1	F		
2135	2205	1498	1430	1464	1385	1218	680	651	710	M	**POPULATION (thousands)**	
2133	2152	1457	1437	1541	1548	1491	903	1018	1566	F		

FRANCE: Males

	All ages	0–34	35–69	35–39	40–44	45–49	50–54	55–59	60–64	65–69	70–74	75–79	80+/NK
POPULATION (1000s)													
1955	20971	11712	8058	984	1422	1492	1439	1165	837	719	554	385	262
1965	23737	13227	9215	1704	1668	984	1369	1361	1223	907	580	397	318
1975	25819	14393	9627	1560	1658	1659	1563	969	1136	1081	865	540	394
1985	26900	14366	10441	2225	1540	1488	1546	1492	1358	792	830	663	600
1990	27623	14248	11334	2135	2205	1498	1430	1464	1385	1218	680	651	710
1995 projected	27924	14127	11690	2077	2107	2101	1443	1378	1364	1221	1015	459	633
NUMBER OF DEATHS													
All causes													
1955	266657	31102	109153	3248	6301	11113	17140	21425	22090	27836	34487	38330	53585
1965	278760	22731	124181	4990	7090	6809	13977	22860	32006	36449	34057	36745	61046
1975	291122	20909	114790	3899	6993	11179	15792	13863	25542	37522	46109	44964	64350
1985	286892	17840	99715	4929	5136	8172	13773	20309	25946	21450	35865	46380	87092
1990	272664	17184	100533	5114	7225	7299	10677	16863	23842	29513	24049	38393	92505
1995 projected	232709	16605	89968	5176	6594	9014	9181	13809	20799	25395	30320	22836	72980
Lung cancer													
1955	4294	31	3185	34	120	275	578	787	720	671	539	372	167
1965	8363	49	5993	79	172	245	739	1236	1795	1727	1102	746	473
1975	12555	47	7623	78	276	615	1042	1026	1998	2588	2432	1563	890
1985	17042	56	9365	132	305	637	1311	2209	2689	2082	2848	2548	2225
1990	18805	58	11185	168	477	741	1191	2105	3044	3459	2206	2563	2793
1995 projected	19353	68	11610	183	517	1071	1190	2019	3129	3501	3272	1806	2597
ANNUAL DEATH RATE / 100,000 (*The rates for the age groups 0–34 and 35–69 are the means of seven five-yearly rates, but the all-ages rates are standardised to the conventional "European" age distribution)													
All causes													
1955	1511.1*	243.6*	1580.0*	330.1	443.0	744.6	1190.9	1839.8	2640.8	3870.4	6227.3	9958.4	20475.7
1965	1396.0*	170.3*	1535.3*	292.9	425.0	692.2	1021.3	1680.1	2617.6	4017.7	5873.9	9246.4	19190.8
1975	1229.6*	145.2*	1358.0*	249.9	421.7	673.9	1010.2	1431.1	2247.6	3471.4	5328.1	8322.0	16336.6
1985	1047.6*	122.9*	1139.4*	221.5	333.4	549.2	891.1	1361.0	1910.9	2708.7	4322.6	6994.4	14512.9
1990	922.7*	117.9*	1013.9*	239.6	327.6	487.3	746.8	1152.2	1721.4	2422.7	3536.1	5895.7	13034.4
1995 projected	811.4*	115.0*	890.7*	249.2	313.0	429.1	636.2	1002.0	1524.4	2080.7	2988.7	4974.1	11529.2
All cancer													
1955	222.4*	9.5*	321.5*	26.9	49.9	112.5	233.4	408.1	598.9	820.5	1149.2	1484.8	1832.3
1965	265.4*	9.9*	389.3*	33.0	67.6	131.5	254.7	453.3	715.1	1069.9	1333.2	1729.7	2305.9
1975	284.9*	9.4*	414.6*	34.6	91.4	183.7	310.2	470.4	751.8	1060.2	1431.4	1903.6	2378.8
1985	302.4*	8.2*	436.2*	35.0	86.3	183.1	354.2	566.7	776.0	1052.5	1466.6	1961.8	2705.7
1990	296.2*	6.8*	430.8*	36.3	82.9	177.4	315.8	539.7	804.7	1059.1	1377.3	1912.5	2771.7
1995 projected	286.8*	5.8*	415.7*	34.1	80.4	163.2	292.9	519.7	795.0	1024.6	1314.8	1839.5	2788.2
Lung cancer													
1955	23.3*	0.3*	45.3*	3.5	8.4	18.4	40.2	67.6	86.1	93.3	97.3	96.6	63.8
1965	39.6*	0.4*	74.6*	4.6	10.3	24.9	54.0	90.8	146.8	190.4	190.1	187.7	148.7
1975	52.4*	0.3*	92.4*	5.0	16.6	37.1	66.7	105.9	175.8	239.4	281.0	289.3	225.9
1985	65.6*	0.4*	108.9*	5.9	19.8	42.8	84.8	148.0	198.0	262.9	343.3	384.3	370.8
1990	68.0*	0.4*	115.7*	7.9	21.6	49.5	83.3	143.8	219.8	283.9	324.4	393.6	393.5
1995 projected	69.4*	0.5*	118.5*	8.8	24.5	51.0	82.5	146.5	229.3	286.8	322.5	393.4	410.3
Upper aerodigestive cancer (mouth, oesophagus, pharynx and larynx)													
1955	37.3*	0.2*	67.3*	1.1	7.9	26.4	60.3	104.4	129.1	141.7	167.4	173.3	180.7
1965	50.3*	0.2*	95.6*	5.0	15.3	38.4	74.9	129.6	175.3	230.6	208.2	218.2	225.4
1975	58.1*	0.3*	107.2*	6.9	31.4	69.3	102.5	139.6	181.6	218.9	239.2	257.1	236.6
1985	52.6*	0.3*	100.6*	6.0	23.6	57.3	115.9	154.1	168.7	178.8	183.1	200.6	193.8
1990	45.3*	0.2*	86.2*	6.2	20.5	49.1	85.8	134.3	154.1	153.7	170.6	170.9	173.5
1995 projected	38.6*	0.2*	73.2*	5.5	17.7	38.1	69.6	112.5	133.2	135.9	147.6	150.1	151.5
Other cancer													
1955	161.9*	9.1*	208.8*	22.4	33.5	67.7	132.9	236.1	383.7	585.5	884.4	1214.9	1587.7
1965	175.5*	9.2*	219.2*	23.4	42.0	68.2	125.8	232.8	393.0	648.9	935.0	1323.9	1931.8
1975	174.3*	8.7*	215.1*	22.7	43.3	77.3	141.1	224.9	394.3	601.9	911.1	1357.2	1916.2
1985	184.3*	7.6*	226.7*	23.0	42.9	83.0	153.4	264.5	409.3	610.8	940.2	1377.0	2141.1
1990	182.9*	6.2*	228.9*	22.2	40.7	78.9	146.7	261.6	430.8	621.5	882.4	1348.0	2204.7
1995 projected	178.8*	5.2*	224.0*	19.8	38.2	74.1	140.8	260.6	432.4	601.8	844.8	1296.0	2226.4
Chronic obstructive pulmonary disease (COPD)													
1955	39.7*	3.2*	48.2*	4.9	10.4	20.4	32.2	57.9	82.7	129.3	186.2	275.7	470.0
1965	45.1*	2.0*	45.9*	4.3	7.5	16.2	25.1	47.4	80.6	140.1	222.5	361.6	695.7
1975	55.9*	1.7*	50.5*	4.3	6.9	16.2	31.7	51.7	84.7	157.7	280.2	474.6	964.2
1985	32.7*	0.7*	24.7*	1.7	3.4	6.1	11.8	26.9	45.7	77.0	158.9	284.0	666.2
1990	28.3*	0.6*	20.5*	1.3	2.0	3.5	8.7	18.6	38.9	70.6	121.5	248.2	617.9
1995 projected	24.3*	0.7*	16.4*	0.9	1.4	2.4	6.1	14.3	32.7	56.9	101.1	207.4	563.2
Other respiratory disease													
1955	72.1*	17.0*	40.0*	6.4	7.2	13.7	26.0	39.6	65.4	121.7	251.4	524.0	1522.0
1965	53.2*	5.0*	26.3*	3.0	5.0	8.8	12.6	23.7	45.6	85.5	186.4	409.2	1374.7
1975	29.2*	2.1*	17.2*	2.8	4.2	7.5	11.1	14.3	26.9	53.5	107.9	227.3	709.8
1985	36.8*	1.6*	23.4*	3.6	4.6	6.7	14.7	25.6	39.1	69.3	135.0	284.7	893.9
1990	34.4*	1.4*	20.5*	3.3	4.7	6.9	11.3	20.4	32.9	63.8	115.0	250.6	898.7
1995 projected	31.7*	1.2*	17.4*	3.2	4.7	6.0	9.2	16.3	28.1	54.4	99.3	219.3	876.5
Vascular disease													
1955	489.3*	10.6*	475.2*	43.4	67.4	141.3	274.0	507.0	851.6	1441.6	2554.0	4219.5	7774.9
1965	454.9*	7.1*	431.6*	39.0	73.1	139.1	233.1	425.2	771.7	1339.7	2256.0	3798.4	7808.6
1975	431.5*	6.2*	393.6*	35.3	73.4	135.5	244.5	375.7	681.3	1209.4	2126.9	3665.4	7605.2
1985	332.0*	5.4*	293.0*	30.0	57.1	101.3	179.9	319.0	533.4	830.7	1519.5	2756.6	6189.3
1990	258.5*	4.4*	226.5*	29.3	50.3	75.4	135.4	225.8	402.8	666.5	1090.3	2100.0	5046.6
1995 projected	198.3*	3.7*	168.4*	25.5	40.8	57.3	97.2	164.1	304.2	489.7	809.4	1570.5	4031.6
Liver cirrhosis													
1955	43.8*	0.8*	93.1*	11.3	26.0	54.4	95.0	131.1	162.1	171.4	150.6	92.8	54.3
1965	54.2*	1.3*	109.8*	18.9	34.8	57.5	90.2	142.6	195.3	229.1	211.3	176.9	104.4
1975	53.3*	1.2*	106.4*	16.2	42.1	67.5	98.6	129.9	175.2	215.7	198.2	179.3	113.0
1985	35.1*	0.8*	69.8*	12.4	22.0	41.7	70.8	98.5	117.8	125.3	122.1	117.2	80.3
1990	26.0*	0.8*	51.4*	11.4	20.1	29.6	48.0	74.5	87.1	89.2	86.9	87.4	64.5
1995 projected	19.0*	0.7*	37.2*	10.3	15.9	21.1	34.1	53.5	62.8	63.1	61.7	64.5	49.8
Other medical causes													
1955	524.5*	143.6*	446.5*	123.5	166.9	259.1	365.2	514.2	703.5	993.3	1695.2	3055.9	8238.4
1965	398.4*	81.3*	375.6*	86.1	121.5	194.1	255.8	402.5	618.7	950.3	1427.6	2441.9	6184.8
1975	256.7*	57.0*	241.9*	58.2	92.1	140.0	182.2	248.2	377.6	594.8	938.2	1536.7	3830.2
1985	200.0*	44.3*	173.1*	47.2	63.6	95.2	140.3	195.9	270.3	399.3	701.5	1265.0	3227.1
1990	178.5*	45.8*	152.4*	65.6	76.0	90.5	115.5	162.1	230.1	326.8	561.2	1014.0	2929.7
1995 projected	159.2*	48.6*	133.6*	87.4	84.4	83.9	97.2	133.2	187.6	261.5	443.6	831.0	2572.0
All non-medical causes													
1955	119.3*	58.9*	155.5*	113.7	115.2	143.3	165.1	182.0	176.4	192.6	240.9	305.8	583.9
1965	124.7*	63.7*	156.9*	108.6	115.6	145.0	149.8	185.5	190.6	203.2	237.0	328.6	716.8
1975	118.1*	67.6*	133.8*	98.5	111.6	123.6	131.9	140.9	150.1	180.1	245.3	335.2	735.5
1985	108.6*	61.9*	119.2*	91.6	96.3	115.1	119.4	128.4	128.7	154.6	219.2	325.1	750.4
1990	100.8*	58.1*	111.8*	92.5	91.5	104.0	112.1	111.2	124.9	146.7	183.9	283.2	705.2
1995 projected	92.1*	54.3*	101.9*	87.8	85.6	95.1	99.7	100.9	114.0	130.5	158.8	242.0	648.0

FRANCE: Females

	All ages	0–34	35–69	35–39	40–44	45–49	50–54	55–59	60–64	65–69	70–74	75–79	80+/NK
POPULATION (1000s)													
1955	22457	11350	9081	981	1439	1517	1486	1368	1218	1073	885	629	512
1965	25021	12643	9911	1658	1677	1012	1446	1476	1406	1236	998	749	721
1975	26886	13699	10053	1469	1609	1648	1633	1038	1313	1343	1202	922	1011
1985	28270	13928	10752	2152	1480	1456	1565	1583	1553	964	1156	1075	1360
1990	29112	13867	11758	2133	2152	1457	1437	1541	1548	1491	903	1018	1566
1995 projected	29215	13579	12085	2090	2107	2065	1428	1425	1504	1468	1383	722	1446
NUMBER OF DEATHS													
All causes													
1955	256051	21135	74269	2040	3870	6340	9171	12250	16751	23847	34005	43579	83063
1965	261581	13668	65888	2522	3596	3661	6858	10743	15712	22796	32342	43091	106592
1975	269251	11197	55243	1740	3045	4803	7048	6385	12005	20217	31436	44448	126927
1985	265604	8691	42744	2241	2120	3260	5464	7824	11208	10627	22909	39659	151601
1990	253537	7516	43166	2092	2896	3019	4354	6783	9843	14179	14385	31554	156916
1995 projected	210135	6393	37808	1911	2646	3851	3852	5528	8358	11662	18355	18659	128920
Lung cancer													
1955	1222	25	711	12	28	60	94	135	179	203	218	167	101
1965	1593	16	804	20	31	37	96	157	190	273	269	237	267
1975	1767	7	767	12	23	81	116	80	196	259	310	300	383
1985	2359	14	943	23	25	57	128	221	257	232	365	421	616
1990	2812	19	1335	27	76	77	141	219	371	424	295	418	745
1995 projected	3129	24	1598	37	104	145	155	247	431	479	475	310	722
ANNUAL DEATH RATE / 100,000 (*The rates for the age groups 0–34 and 35–69 are the means of seven five-yearly rates, but the all-ages rates are standardised to the conventional "European" age distribution)													
All causes													
1955	985.3*	167.9*	858.1*	207.9	268.9	417.9	617.3	895.7	1375.5	2223.1	3844.5	6925.0	16220.1
1965	820.4*	104.0*	699.0*	152.1	214.4	361.7	474.4	727.8	1117.7	1845.1	3242.0	5753.9	14788.0
1975	683.9*	81.9*	580.9*	118.5	189.2	291.5	431.6	615.1	914.3	1505.9	2616.4	4818.7	12559.6
1985	556.0*	62.8*	448.5*	104.2	143.3	224.0	349.1	494.3	721.5	1103.0	1981.7	3690.6	11147.1
1990	486.5*	54.0*	395.7*	98.1	134.6	207.3	303.0	440.2	635.9	950.9	1593.4	3099.6	10022.7
1995 projected	424.0*	46.9*	344.5*	91.5	125.6	186.5	269.8	387.9	555.8	794.5	1327.4	2583.6	8914.4
All cancer													
1955	155.8*	8.8*	220.9*	42.3	73.4	120.8	181.4	259.4	362.7	506.1	730.4	1001.4	1312.8
1965	152.3*	8.3*	213.3*	35.9	66.5	124.2	175.1	259.1	346.2	486.2	683.2	939.6	1424.1
1975	142.4*	7.3*	201.8*	30.4	60.0	108.9	174.6	244.7	343.8	450.4	628.9	861.9	1330.3
1985	132.0*	6.8*	183.8*	31.0	52.0	94.1	156.2	225.6	311.3	416.5	584.3	800.4	1301.1
1990	128.9*	5.4*	180.2*	31.2	54.8	93.0	148.4	219.1	305.4	409.8	552.3	794.4	1299.9
1995 projected	124.2*	4.4*	172.8*	30.6	55.1	90.2	141.7	210.1	295.2	386.7	526.0	761.8	1295.2
Lung cancer													
1955	4.8*	0.2*	8.1*	1.2	1.9	4.0	6.3	9.9	14.7	18.9	24.6	26.5	19.7
1965	5.4*	0.1*	8.5*	1.2	1.8	3.7	6.6	10.6	13.5	22.1	27.0	31.6	37.0
1975	5.2*	0.1*	8.0*	0.8	1.4	4.9	7.1	7.7	14.9	19.3	25.8	32.5	37.9
1985	6.4*	0.1*	9.9*	1.1	1.7	3.9	8.2	14.0	16.5	24.1	31.6	39.2	45.3
1990	7.4*	0.1*	12.4*	1.3	3.5	5.3	9.8	14.2	24.0	28.4	32.7	41.1	47.6
1995 projected	8.5*	0.2*	14.7*	1.8	4.9	7.0	10.9	17.3	28.7	32.6	34.4	42.9	49.9
Upper aerodigestive cancer (mouth, oesophagus, pharynx and larynx)													
1955	3.4*	0.1*	4.0*	0.5	1.2	1.8	2.5	4.3	6.8	10.9	17.3	26.9	44.3
1965	3.6*	0.1*	4.3*	0.8	1.1	2.1	3.5	4.6	6.5	11.5	15.1	25.5	49.9
1975	3.9*	0.1*	5.6*	0.5	1.6	3.3	4.8	9.1	9.6	10.2	15.3	22.3	41.4
1985	3.8*	0.1*	6.1*	0.7	1.3	4.0	6.2	10.0	10.3	10.5	12.9	17.4	33.2
1990	4.0*	0.1*	6.5*	0.8	2.0	4.4	6.7	9.3	10.8	11.5	13.4	20.9	31.0
1995 projected	4.2*	0.1*	6.7*	1.1	2.4	4.9	6.7	9.3	10.8	11.9	14.7	21.3	31.8
Other cancer													
1955	147.6*	8.5*	208.7*	40.6	70.3	115.0	172.6	245.2	341.2	476.3	688.4	948.0	1248.8
1965	143.3*	8.0*	200.5*	34.0	63.6	118.5	165.0	243.9	326.2	452.6	641.1	882.5	1337.1
1975	133.3*	7.2*	188.2*	29.1	57.0	100.6	162.7	227.9	319.3	420.9	587.8	807.0	1251.0
1985	121.9*	6.6*	167.8*	29.2	49.1	86.2	141.8	201.7	284.4	381.9	539.9	743.8	1222.6
1990	117.5*	5.2*	161.4*	29.1	49.3	83.3	131.9	195.6	270.7	369.9	506.2	732.4	1221.3
1995 projected	111.6*	4.2*	151.3*	27.7	47.8	78.3	124.2	183.5	255.7	342.2	476.9	697.6	1213.5
Chronic obstructive pulmonary disease (COPD)													
1955	19.5*	2.7*	15.7*	1.7	3.3	4.8	7.4	14.4	28.6	49.9	89.5	161.1	332.9
1965	20.3*	1.5*	12.2*	1.9	1.4	3.1	5.5	10.6	21.3	41.7	82.8	165.6	477.9
1975	20.2*	1.3*	12.9*	2.2	4.3	5.3	8.2	11.8	22.1	36.1	82.6	155.7	465.0
1985	10.8*	0.6*	8.2*	1.6	1.1	4.2	6.3	8.6	14.1	21.5	44.6	75.7	230.4
1990	10.6*	0.4*	6.6*	0.8	1.2	1.6	3.5	6.7	11.3	21.1	40.4	80.2	262.0
1995 projected	10.6*	0.3*	5.5*	0.5	0.8	1.1	2.5	4.9	9.8	18.7	39.4	77.8	293.0
Other respiratory disease													
1955	51.4*	14.6*	19.4*	2.3	3.8	4.7	9.4	16.5	32.8	66.3	153.1	375.7	1227.7
1965	34.9*	3.8*	12.0*	2.1	2.6	3.8	5.9	8.2	18.4	43.3	97.8	262.4	1027.6
1975	17.6*	1.5*	6.4*	1.2	2.0	2.5	4.0	6.0	8.6	20.8	50.9	129.0	521.6
1985	19.1*	1.1*	7.0*	1.4	1.1	2.9	5.2	5.4	11.0	21.6	41.9	114.3	623.8
1990	18.7*	1.0*	5.8*	1.2	2.0	1.9	4.2	5.8	8.9	16.8	39.2	106.5	640.5
1995 projected	18.3*	0.9*	5.0*	1.2	1.9	1.6	3.6	5.1	7.2	14.3	35.0	97.6	648.3
Vascular disease													
1955	335.7*	8.7*	274.3*	33.4	45.6	88.2	153.4	262.4	468.2	868.9	1649.7	3082.9	6191.8
1965	287.1*	5.0*	200.3*	18.9	32.7	59.1	95.2	181.2	340.2	674.7	1350.4	2555.6	6183.5
1975	260.3*	3.8*	156.2*	13.5	25.1	45.3	78.6	130.1	256.4	544.5	1127.6	2354.5	6181.8
1985	199.3*	3.1*	98.3*	10.1	16.0	27.3	50.2	86.8	170.3	327.8	767.1	1649.8	5382.6
1990	156.4*	2.4*	74.8*	8.7	12.7	23.1	36.9	69.6	125.5	247.2	520.6	1236.0	4440.9
1995 projected	121.1*	2.0*	54.1*	6.9	10.5	17.7	28.7	51.7	93.1	170.1	370.8	911.0	3584.9
Liver cirrhosis													
1955	21.2*	1.0*	44.9*	15.0	21.1	39.1	55.3	63.1	65.5	55.4	41.7	30.8	19.3
1965	20.5*	1.2*	41.3*	16.2	22.0	35.9	43.4	50.1	62.0	59.7	56.1	43.7	30.7
1975	19.6*	1.4*	38.8*	13.9	26.9	37.4	41.3	48.5	49.2	54.7	53.8	42.2	26.8
1985	12.7*	0.6*	25.5*	8.3	11.8	19.6	33.0	36.6	35.6	33.9	31.5	29.8	22.8
1990	10.2*	0.3*	20.3*	5.4	11.3	17.9	24.0	26.5	29.4	27.3	29.9	24.2	20.8
1995 projected	8.1*	0.2*	16.0*	4.3	9.8	14.6	18.1	19.8	22.6	22.8	24.9	21.3	17.8
Other medical causes													
1955	358.7*	115.7*	239.8*	90.5	97.2	126.6	165.5	232.7	362.5	603.8	1079.5	2089.0	6601.8
1965	254.3*	63.1*	176.4*	49.9	61.0	99.4	112.7	171.1	275.2	465.6	851.8	1573.1	4893.7
1975	170.4*	42.8*	121.4*	31.9	42.5	60.9	86.4	123.7	177.9	326.5	561.0	1053.9	3222.4
1985	132.8*	30.6*	79.7*	21.3	25.5	38.2	58.0	82.3	124.8	207.9	403.8	833.1	2902.5
1990	117.9*	27.0*	66.9*	24.1	23.6	32.9	44.3	68.9	105.6	168.7	321.7	693.7	2748.6
1995 projected	103.3*	23.9*	54.9*	25.1	22.0	26.8	35.7	56.1	85.7	132.9	257.2	576.7	2532.8
All non-medical causes													
1955	43.0*	16.4*	43.0*	22.6	24.5	33.7	45.0	47.2	55.3	72.7	100.6	184.0	533.7
1965	51.0*	21.1*	43.4*	27.2	28.2	36.4	36.5	47.4	54.3	73.9	119.7	213.9	750.4
1975	53.3*	23.7*	43.3*	25.2	28.5	31.2	38.6	50.3	56.3	72.9	111.6	221.6	811.7
1985	49.3*	19.9*	45.9*	30.4	35.6	37.6	40.3	49.0	54.5	73.8	108.5	187.5	684.0
1990	43.8*	17.5*	41.1*	26.8	28.9	36.9	41.7	43.6	49.7	60.0	89.3	164.7	610.1
1995 projected	38.4*	15.1*	36.3*	22.9	25.5	34.4	39.5	40.3	42.2	49.1	74.0	137.4	542.5

FRANCE: 1975

Smoking-attributed deaths (Sm.) and total deaths (Total)

Age		ALL CAUSES	ALL CANCER	Lung cancer	Upper aero-digestive ca.	Other cancer	COPD	Other respiratory	Vascular disease	Liver cirrhosis	Other medical	Non-medical
Males												
0–34	Sm.	–	–	–	–	–	–	–	–	–	–	–
	Total	20909	1315	47	41	1227	244	296	859	157	8274	9764
35–69	Sm.	30713	14608	6915	5446	2247	2991	341	7574	–	5199	–
	Total	114790	34512	7623	9163	17726	4115	1435	32291	9191	20729	12517
		(27%)	(42%)	(91%)	(59%)	(13%)	(73%)	(24%)	(23%)		(25%)	
70+	Sm.	21141	7984	4171	2036	1777	5311	347	5147	–	2352	–
	Total	155423	32042	4885	4391	22766	8787	4958	68167	3129	31509	6831
		(14%)	(25%)	(85%)	(46%)	(8%)	(60%)	(7%)	(8%)		(7%)	
Any age	Sm.	51854	22592	11086	7482	4024	8302	688	12721	–	7551	–
	Total	291122	67869	12555	13595	41719	13146	6689	101317	12477	60512	29112
		(18%)	(33%)	(88%)	(55%)	(10%)	(63%)	(10%)	(13%)		(12%)	
Females												
0–34	Sm.	–	–	–	–	–	–	–	–	–	–	–
	Total	11197	950	7	9	934	175	208	505	161	5945	3253
35–69	Sm.	0	0	0	0	0	0	0	0	–	0	–
	Total	55243	19158	767	522	17869	1221	611	14660	3810	11571	4212
		(0%)	(0%)	(0%)	(0%)	(0%)	(0%)	(0%)	(0%)		(0%)	
70+	Sm.	0	0	0	0	0	0	0	0	–	0	–
	Total	202811	28950	993	808	27149	7127	7073	97739	1306	49028	11588
		(0%)	(0%)	(0%)	(0%)	(0%)	(0%)	(0%)	(0%)		(0%)	
Any age	Sm.	0	0	0	0	0	0	0	0	–	0	–
	Total	269251	49058	1767	1339	45952	8523	7892	112904	5277	66544	19053
		(0%)	(0%)	(0%)	(0%)	(0%)	(0%)	(0%)	(0%)		(0%)	
Males+Females												
0–34	Sm.	–	–	–	–	–	–	–	–	–	–	–
	Total	32106	2265	54	50	2161	419	504	1364	318	14219	13017
35–69	Sm.	30713	14608	6915	5446	2247	2991	341	7574	–	5199	–
	Total	170033	53670	8390	9685	35595	5336	2046	46951	13001	32300	16729
		(18%)	(27%)	(82%)	(56%)	(6%)	(56%)	(17%)	(16%)		(16%)	
70+	Sm.	21141	7984	4171	2036	1777	5311	347	5147	–	2352	–
	Total	358234	60992	5878	5199	49915	15914	12031	165906	4435	80537	18419
		(6%)	(13%)	(71%)	(39%)	(4%)	(33%)	(3%)	(3%)		(3%)	
Any age	Sm.	51854	22592	11086	7482	4024	8302	688	12721	–	7551	–
	Total	560373	116927	14322	14934	87671	21669	14581	214221	17754	127056	48165
		(9%)	(19%)	(77%)	(50%)	(5%)	(38%)	(5%)	(6%)		(6%)	

FRANCE: 1985

Smoking-attributed deaths (Sm.) and total deaths (Total)

Age		ALL CAUSES	ALL CANCER	Lung cancer	Upper aero-digestive ca.	Other cancer	COPD	Other respiratory	Vascular disease	Liver cirrhosis	Other medical	Non-medical
Males												
0–34	Sm.	–	–	–	–	–	–	–	–	–	–	–
	Total	17840	1199	56	41	1102	102	224	802	118	6214	9181
35–69	Sm.	31436	17544	8652	5954	2938	1525	560	7057	–	4750	–
	Total	99715	37633	9365	9148	19120	1996	1939	24415	6393	15370	11969
		(32%)	(47%)	(92%)	(65%)	(15%)	(76%)	(29%)	(29%)		(31%)	
70+	Sm.	26532	11814	6728	2119	2967	4815	725	6166	–	3012	–
	Total	169337	41414	7621	4012	29781	7199	8372	68028	2272	33574	8478
		(16%)	(29%)	(88%)	(53%)	(10%)	(67%)	(9%)	(9%)		(9%)	
Any age	Sm.	57968	29358	15380	8073	5905	6340	1285	13223	–	7762	–
	Total	286892	80246	17042	13201	50003	9297	10535	93245	8783	55158	29628
		(20%)	(37%)	(90%)	(61%)	(12%)	(68%)	(12%)	(14%)		(14%)	
Females												
0–34	Sm.	–	–	–	–	–	–	–	–	–	–	–
	Total	8691	974	14	15	945	92	147	447	89	4089	2853
35–69	Sm.	304	122	92	15	15	48	5	71	–	58	–
	Total	42744	17672	943	609	16120	772	636	8814	2614	7543	4693
		(1%)	(1%)	(10%)	(2%)	(0%)	(6%)	(1%)	(1%)		(1%)	
70+	Sm.	810	193	141	22	30	248	20	229	–	120	–
	Total	214169	33051	1402	787	30862	4462	10195	99800	994	53095	12572
		(0%)	(1%)	(10%)	(3%)	(0%)	(6%)	(0%)	(0%)		(0%)	
Any age	Sm.	1114	315	233	37	45	296	25	300	–	178	–
	Total	265604	51697	2359	1411	47927	5326	10978	109061	3697	64727	20118
		(0%)	(1%)	(10%)	(3%)	(0%)	(6%)	(0%)	(0%)		(0%)	
Males+Females												
0–34	Sm.	–	–	–	–	–	–	–	–	–	–	–
	Total	26531	2173	70	56	2047	194	371	1249	207	10303	12034
35–69	Sm.	31740	17666	8744	5969	2953	1573	565	7128	–	4808	–
	Total	142459	55305	10308	9757	35240	2768	2575	33229	9007	22913	16662
		(22%)	(32%)	(85%)	(61%)	(8%)	(57%)	(22%)	(21%)		(21%)	
70+	Sm.	27342	12007	6869	2141	2997	5063	745	6395	–	3132	–
	Total	383506	74465	9023	4799	60643	11661	18567	167828	3266	86669	21050
		(7%)	(16%)	(76%)	(45%)	(5%)	(43%)	(4%)	(4%)		(4%)	
Any age	Sm.	59082	29673	15613	8110	5950	6636	1310	13523	–	7940	–
	Total	552496	131943	19401	14612	97930	14623	21513	202306	12480	119885	49746
		(11%)	(22%)	(80%)	(56%)	(6%)	(45%)	(6%)	(7%)		(7%)	

(To be conservative, no deaths before age 35, and none from liver cirrhosis or non-medical causes, were attributed to smoking.)

FRANCE: 1990

Smoking–attributed deaths (Sm.) and total deaths (Total)

		ALL CAUSES	ALL CANCER	Lung cancer	Upper aero–digestive ca.	Other cancer	COPD	Other respiratory	Vascular disease	Liver cirrhosis	Other medical	Non–medical
Males												
0–34	Sm.	–	–	–	–	–	–	–	–	–	–	–
	Total	17184	989	58	33	898	92	200	648	113	6500	8642
35–69	Sm.	32637	19452	10362	5608	3482	1479	561	6240	–	4905	–
	Total	100533	41721	11185	8519	22017	1920	1969	21803	5200	15623	12297
		(32%)	(47%)	(93%)	(66%)	(16%)	(77%)	(28%)	(29%)		(31%)	
70+	Sm.	24500	11530	6667	1841	3022	4576	741	4953	–	2700	–
	Total	154947	41492	7562	3504	30426	6827	8792	56906	1618	31212	8100
		(16%)	(28%)	(88%)	(53%)	(10%)	(67%)	(8%)	(9%)		(9%)	
Any age	Sm.	57137	30982	17029	7449	6504	6055	1302	11193	–	7605	–
	Total	272664	84202	18805	12056	53341	8839	10961	79357	6931	53335	29039
		(21%)	(37%)	(91%)	(62%)	(12%)	(69%)	(12%)	(14%)		(14%)	
Females												
0–34	Sm.	–	–	–	–	–	–	–	–	–	–	–
	Total	7516	775	19	10	746	60	136	352	44	3635	2514
35–69	Sm.	1028	486	368	61	57	124	17	210	–	191	–
	Total	43166	19547	1335	703	17509	707	634	8027	2236	7349	4666
		(2%)	(2%)	(28%)	(9%)	(0%)	(18%)	(3%)	(3%)		(3%)	
70+	Sm.	1192	278	202	33	43	430	35	279	–	170	–
	Total	202855	33424	1458	819	31147	5283	11466	86808	841	52998	12035
		(1%)	(1%)	(14%)	(4%)	(0%)	(8%)	(0%)	(0%)		(0%)	
Any age	Sm.	2220	764	570	94	100	554	52	489	–	361	–
	Total	253537	53746	2812	1532	49402	6050	12236	95187	3121	63982	19215
		(1%)	(1%)	(20%)	(6%)	(0%)	(9%)	(0%)	(1%)		(1%)	
Males+Females												
0–34	Sm.	–	–	–	–	–	–	–	–	–	–	–
	Total	24700	1764	77	43	1644	152	336	1000	157	10135	11156
35–69	Sm.	33665	19938	10730	5669	3539	1603	578	6450	–	5096	–
	Total	143699	61268	12520	9222	39526	2627	2603	29830	7436	22972	16963
		(23%)	(33%)	(86%)	(61%)	(9%)	(61%)	(22%)	(22%)		(22%)	
70+	Sm.	25692	11808	6869	1874	3065	5006	776	5232	–	2870	–
	Total	357802	74916	9020	4323	61573	12110	20258	143714	2459	84210	20135
		(7%)	(16%)	(76%)	(43%)	(5%)	(41%)	(4%)	(4%)		(3%)	
Any age	Sm.	59357	31746	17599	7543	6604	6609	1354	11682	–	7966	–
	Total	526201	137948	21617	13588	102743	14889	23197	174544	10052	117317	48254
		(11%)	(23%)	(81%)	(56%)	(6%)	(44%)	(6%)	(7%)		(7%)	

FRANCE: 1995

Smoking–attributed deaths (Sm.) and total deaths (Total)

		ALL CAUSES	ALL CANCER	Lung cancer	Upper aero–digestive ca.	Other cancer	COPD	Other respiratory	Vascular disease	Liver cirrhosis	Other medical	Non–medical
Males												
0–34	Sm.	–	–	–	–	–	–	–	–	–	–	–
	Total	16605	842	68	31	743	91	173	541	105	6933	7920
35–69	Sm.	30333	19143	10778	4859	3506	1178	493	4805	–	4714	–
	Total	89968	40570	11610	7319	21641	1524	1696	16384	3847	14346	11601
		(34%)	(47%)	(93%)	(66%)	(16%)	(77%)	(29%)	(29%)		(33%)	
70+	Sm.	21636	11287	6773	1658	2856	3719	659	3748	–	2223	–
	Total	126136	39433	7675	3145	28613	5543	7562	40941	1237	24596	6824
		(17%)	(29%)	(88%)	(53%)	(10%)	(67%)	(9%)	(9%)		(9%)	
Any age	Sm.	51969	30430	17551	6517	6362	4897	1152	8553	–	6937	–
	Total	232709	80845	19353	10495	50997	7158	9431	57866	5189	45875	26345
		(22%)	(38%)	(91%)	(62%)	(12%)	(68%)	(12%)	(15%)		(15%)	
Females												
0–34	Sm.	–	–	–	–	–	–	–	–	–	–	–
	Total	6393	624	24	9	591	43	121	279	32	3205	2089
35–69	Sm.	1511	823	626	106	91	152	24	247	–	265	–
	Total	37808	18795	1598	741	16456	578	541	5774	1811	6091	4218
		(4%)	(4%)	(39%)	(14%)	(1%)	(26%)	(4%)	(4%)		(4%)	
70+	Sm.	1484	374	275	44	55	576	45	288	–	201	–
	Total	165934	31506	1507	817	29182	5344	10565	63552	756	44351	9860
		(1%)	(1%)	(18%)	(5%)	(0%)	(11%)	(0%)	(0%)		(0%)	
Any age	Sm.	2995	1197	901	150	146	728	69	535	–	466	–
	Total	210135	50925	3129	1567	46229	5965	11227	69605	2599	53647	16167
		(1%)	(2%)	(29%)	(10%)	(0%)	(12%)	(1%)	(1%)		(1%)	
Males+Females												
0–34	Sm.	–	–	–	–	–	–	–	–	–	–	–
	Total	22998	1466	92	40	1334	134	294	820	137	10138	10009
35–69	Sm.	31844	19966	11404	4965	3597	1330	517	5052	–	4979	–
	Total	127776	59365	13208	8060	38097	2102	2237	22158	5658	20437	15819
		(25%)	(34%)	(86%)	(62%)	(9%)	(63%)	(23%)	(23%)		(24%)	
70+	Sm.	23120	11661	7048	1702	2911	4295	704	4036	–	2424	–
	Total	292070	70939	9182	3962	57795	10887	18127	104493	1993	68947	16684
		(8%)	(16%)	(77%)	(43%)	(5%)	(39%)	(4%)	(4%)		(4%)	
Any age	Sm.	54964	31627	18452	6667	6508	5625	1221	9088	–	7403	–
	Total	442844	131770	22482	12062	97226	13123	20658	127471	7788	99522	42512
		(12%)	(24%)	(82%)	(55%)	(7%)	(43%)	(6%)	(7%)		(7%)	

(To be conservative, no deaths before age 35, and none from liver cirrhosis or non–medical causes, were attributed to smoking.)

¶GEORGIA: 1990

		No. of deaths			Standardised rates (Defined on p.346)			Annual death rates / 100, 000						
		All ages	0–34	35–69	All ages	0–34	35–69	0–4	5–9	10–14	15–19	20–24	25–29	30–34
ALL CAUSES	M	22977	2649	11778	1224.9	171.6	1459.4	448.8	36.4	48.9	82.7	141.2	189.2	254.2
	F	22968	1438	6976	745.9	93.1	691.3	355.6	30.0	19.9	35.6	59.6	66.0	85.3
Tuberculosis	M	326	60	241	14.8	4.1	26.3	0.4	–	–	–	3.0	8.0	17.2
	F	61	9	44	2.2	0.6	4.0	–	–	–	–	0.5	1.7	1.8
Other infective	M	159	122	30	5.9	7.5	3.3	42.2	1.3	0.9	1.9	1.0	3.6	2.0
and parasitic	F	140	103	18	4.9	6.6	1.7	38.6	1.4	0.9	–	2.0	1.7	1.8
ALL CANCER	M	2903	134	2065	148.5	8.9	255.5	5.1	5.7	5.0	7.0	10.9	14.2	14.2
	F	2556	111	1655	89.4	7.3	157.3	3.1	3.6	3.8	6.0	4.0	7.9	22.3
Mouth and	M	99	2	75	5.1	0.1	8.7	–	–	–	0.5	0.5	–	–
pharynx cancer	F	26	–	14	0.9	–	1.2	–	–	–	–	–	–	–
Oesophagus cancer	M	55	3	38	2.7	0.2	4.2	–	–	–	0.5	–	0.4	0.5
	F	24	1	10	0.8	0.1	1.0	–	–	–	0.5	–	–	–
Stomach cancer	M	424	6	307	22.2	0.4	38.9	0.4	–	–	–	1.0	–	1.5
	F	289	6	170	9.9	0.4	16.4	–	–	–	0.5	0.5	0.4	1.4
Colorectal cancer	M	215	7	150	11.2	0.5	18.6	–	–	–	–	0.5	1.8	1.0
	F	226	3	125	7.7	0.2	12.1	–	–	–	–	–	0.4	0.9
Liver cancer	M	...	...	...	...	...	...	...	...	...	...	...	...	...
	F	...	...	...	...	...	...	...	...	...	...	...	...	...
Pancreas cancer	M	...	...	...	...	...	...	...	...	...	...	...	...	...
	F	...	...	...	...	...	...	...	...	...	...	...	...	...
Larynx cancer	M	157	–	127	8.0	–	15.8	–	–	–	–	–	–	–
	F	12	–	5	0.4	–	0.5	–	–	–	–	–	–	–
Lung cancer	M	830	6	634	42.5	0.4	79.1	–	–	–	–	0.5	0.4	2.0
	F	178	6	115	6.1	0.4	11.0	–	–	–	–	–	1.2	1.4
Malignant melanoma	M	...	...	...	...	...	...	...	...	...	...	...	...	...
	F	...	...	...	...	...	...	...	...	...	...	...	...	...
Female breast cancer	F	581	16	426	21.0	1.0	39.7	–	–	–	–	0.5	0.4	6.4
Cervix cancer	F	183	8	125	6.6	0.5	11.6	–	–	–	–	–	0.4	3.2
Other uterine cancer	F	158	4	106	5.5	0.2	10.3	–	–	–	–	–	0.8	0.9
Ovarian cancer	F	...	...	...	...	...	...	...	...	...	...	...	...	...
Prostate cancer	M	123	–	52	7.6	–	8.1	–	–	–	–	–	–	–
Bladder cancer	M	...	...	...	...	...	...	...	...	...	...	...	...	...
	F	...	...	...	...	...	...	...	...	...	...	...	...	...
Other and ill-defined	M	787	46	562	39.5	3.1	67.1	1.3	–	1.4	3.3	3.0	7.6	4.9
cancer sites	F	717	26	463	24.8	1.7	44.3	0.9	0.5	–	2.0	1.0	2.5	5.0
Hodgkin's disease	M	...	...	...	...	...	...	...	...	...	...	...	...	...
	F	...	...	...	...	...	...	...	...	...	...	...	...	...
Myeloma and all	M	127	34	79	5.8	2.2	9.5	2.1	1.3	1.4	1.4	3.5	3.6	2.5
lymphomas	F	87	16	54	3.0	1.1	5.2	0.9	0.9	0.9	0.5	1.5	1.2	1.4
Leukaemia	M	86	30	41	4.1	2.0	5.5	1.3	4.4	2.3	1.4	2.0	0.4	2.0
	F	75	25	42	2.6	1.7	3.8	1.3	2.3	2.8	2.5	0.5	0.4	1.8
ALL VASCULAR	M	13229	204	6261	765.2	14.0	809.2	1.3	2.2	0.9	7.0	13.9	16.0	56.4
DISEASE	F	16486	128	3917	522.9	8.4	399.1	5.8	1.8	0.9	6.0	13.9	12.5	17.8
Rheumatic heart	M	71	9	55	3.3	0.6	5.9	–	0.4	–	0.9	1.0	0.4	1.5
disease and fever	F	105	9	77	3.9	0.6	7.0	–	–	–	0.5	1.0	0.4	2.3
Hypertensive disease	M	15	1	4	0.9	0.1	0.5	–	–		–	0.5	–	–
	F	40	–	13	1.3	–	1.3	–	–	–	–	–	–	–
Ischaemic heart	M	8294	89	3998	478.4	6.2	510.9	–	–	–	2.8	5.4	4.0	30.9
disease	F	9624	42	2082	303.6	2.8	212.9	–	–	–	1.5	5.5	4.2	8.2
Pulmonary embolism	M	...	...	...	...	...	...	...	...	...	...	...	...	...
and other venous	F	...	...	...	...	...	...	...	...	...	...	...	...	...
Cerebrovascular	M	4430	70	1966	260.6	4.8	263.3	0.4	0.9	0.5	1.4	4.0	7.6	18.6
disease	F	6375	57	1620	202.9	3.7	165.6	3.6	1.8	0.9	3.0	5.5	6.6	4.6
Other vascular	M	419	35	238	22.1	2.3	28.6	0.9	0.9	0.5	1.9	3.0	4.0	5.4
disease, incl. venous	F	342	20	125	11.3	1.3	12.4	2.2	–	–	1.0	2.0	1.2	2.7
Chronic obstructive	M	637	18	311	36.3	1.2	39.3	2.1	–	–	–	1.0	1.3	3.9
pulmonary disease	F	573	18	154	18.4	1.1	15.2	0.9	–	–	–	1.5	2.9	2.7
Other respiratory	M	623	458	98	24.4	28.4	11.4	155.2	7.9	11.9	4.7	7.9	7.1	3.9
disease	F	515	381	50	17.7	24.6	4.7	137.2	11.4	6.6	5.0	5.0	4.2	2.7
Peptic ulcer	M	111	9	69	5.7	0.6	8.0	0.4	0.4	–	–	0.5	1.8	1.0
	F	59	1	28	2.0	0.1	2.8	–	–	–	–	–	–	0.5
Liver cirrhosis and	M	846	29	661	42.6	1.9	79.5	1.3	0.4	0.5	–	–	3.1	8.3
other liver disease	F	386	6	223	13.1	0.4	21.8	–	–	–	–	1.5	0.4	0.9
Renal disease	M	213	24	141	10.5	1.6	16.1	0.4	0.4	1.8	1.9	2.5	1.8	2.5
	F	182	23	101	6.2	1.5	9.5	0.4	0.5	–	1.0	3.5	2.5	2.7
Pregnancy and birth	F	19	14	5	0.6	0.9	0.4	–	–	–	0.5	1.0	3.3	1.4
Congenital and	M	424	424	–	14.5	25.8	–	180.3	–	–	–	–	–	0.5
perinatal causes	F	272	272	–	9.8	17.4	–	122.0	–	–	–	–	–	–
Ill-defined causes	M	393	69	236	19.4	4.5	26.5	10.7	1.3	0.9	1.4	3.0	3.6	10.8
	F	298	42	91	9.7	2.7	8.6	9.0	–	–	0.5	2.5	3.3	3.6
Other medical causes	M	780	125	457	39.4	8.1	57.6	14.9	3.1	5.0	6.5	4.5	10.7	12.3
	F	717	89	360	24.2	5.8	36.0	7.6	3.6	2.4	4.5	7.9	7.5	7.3
ALL NON-	M	2333	973	1208	97.7	65.0	126.7	34.5	13.6	21.9	52.4	93.1	118.2	121.2
MEDICAL CAUSES	F	704	241	330	24.8	15.7	30.3	30.9	7.7	5.2	12.0	16.4	18.3	19.6
Motor vehicle	M	575	248	288	24.1	16.6	29.6	3.8	1.3	6.4	11.2	24.8	35.1	33.9
traffic accidents	F	154	58	70	5.4	3.8	6.4	2.7	1.8	0.9	3.5	6.0	5.0	6.8
Fire	M	102	39	51	4.5	2.5	5.5	8.5	0.9	0.9	2.3	3.0	1.3	0.5
	F	77	27	27	2.7	1.7	2.5	6.3	2.7	0.5	0.5	0.5	0.8	0.9
Suicide	M	140	46	75	6.2	3.1	8.2	–	–	–	6.5	4.5	6.7	3.9
	F	56	8	36	2.0	0.5	3.2	–	–	–	0.5	1.5	1.2	0.5
Homicide	M	117	58	55	4.8	3.9	5.9	–	–	0.9	3.3	4.0	8.4	10.8
	F	34	8	24	1.2	0.5	2.2	0.4	–	0.5	–	–	1.7	0.9
POPULATION (thousands):	**M=males**				2571.1	1526.0	946.0	234.6	228.0	218.7	213.9	201.9	225.1	203.8
	F=females				2842.4	1514.8	1110.0	223.0	219.9	210.7	199.7	201.4	240.8	219.3

GEORGIA: 1990

Annual death rates / 100, 000 — 9th ICD categories

Cause	ICD	Sex	35–39	40–44	45–49	50–54	55–59	60–64	65–69	70–74	75–79	80+/NK
ALL CAUSES	001–999	M	336.7	511.5	729.5	1073.4	1597.4	2367.6	3599.7	5171.7	7366.1	14503.5
		F	110.9	180.4	239.3	462.3	657.8	1190.1	1998.2	3214.8	5400.8	12189.8
Tuberculosis	010–018, 137	M	18.5	20.2	31.5	24.6	30.9	27.9	30.4	13.6	20.8	45.1
		F	1.6	4.0	1.4	5.3	7.0	4.2	4.5	2.5	2.8	6.0
Other infective and parasitic	Rest of 001–139	M	1.1	2.2	2.5	4.1	1.5	7.4	4.6	2.7	11.9	6.9
		F	1.6	0.7	0.7	1.6	2.5	1.2	3.6	7.5	7.0	12.0
ALL CANCER	140–208	M	30.8	66.3	100.4	198.9	311.5	461.0	619.5	757.5	735.1	621.5
		F	36.4	72.7	77.4	155.0	167.6	260.2	331.6	381.9	362.9	340.8
Mouth and pharynx cancer	140–149	M	1.1	5.8	5.8	9.4	11.8	11.8	15.2	27.2	11.9	27.8
		F	0.5	–	–	0.5	4.4	2.4	0.9	5.0	5.6	6.0
Oesophagus cancer	150	M	0.6	1.4	–	6.5	3.7	11.0	6.1	16.3	17.9	6.9
		F	–	–	–	0.5	0.6	2.4	3.6	5.0	5.6	7.5
Stomach cancer	151	M	3.4	10.1	17.4	23.5	47.8	69.9	100.5	114.4	133.9	83.3
		F	3.1	5.9	6.4	12.7	16.4	30.9	39.2	49.0	49.2	58.3
Colorectal cancer	153, 154	M	1.7	7.9	7.5	12.3	23.5	33.1	44.1	54.5	68.5	52.1
		F	1.6	4.6	3.6	11.7	10.8	22.0	30.3	41.5	56.3	37.4
Liver cancer	Not given separately	M	...	...	...	...	...	...	...	...	...	...
		F	...	...	...	...	...	...	...	...	...	...
Pancreas cancer	Not given separately	M	...	...	...	...	...	...	...	...	...	...
		F	...	...	...	...	...	...	...	...	...	...
Larynx cancer	161	M	0.6	1.4	10.8	12.3	18.4	29.4	38.1	24.5	26.8	41.7
		F	–	0.7	–	0.5	0.6	0.6	0.9	2.5	2.8	4.5
Lung cancer	162	M	8.4	12.2	25.7	56.3	108.7	145.6	196.3	218.0	211.3	135.4
		F	–	2.0	5.0	10.6	13.3	21.4	25.0	28.9	28.1	20.9
Malignant melanoma	Not given separately	M	...	...	...	...	...	...	...	...	...	...
		F	...	...	...	...	...	...	...	...	...	...
Female breast cancer	174	F	15.6	28.4	23.6	50.4	40.5	48.7	70.4	74.1	56.3	59.8
Cervix cancer	180	F	3.6	9.9	7.9	12.7	10.1	19.0	17.8	32.7	18.3	16.4
Other uterine cancer	179, 182	F	1.0	4.0	6.4	8.5	8.2	18.4	25.8	25.1	26.7	13.5
Ovarian cancer	Not given separately	F	...	...	...	...	...	...	...	...	...	...
Prostate cancer	185	M	–	0.7	–	2.3	5.9	11.0	36.5	76.3	77.4	59.0
Bladder cancer	Not given separately	M	...	...	...	...	...	...	...	...	...	...
		F	...	...	...	...	...	...	...	...	...	...
Other and ill-defined cancer sites	Rest of 140–208, incl. 155, 157, 172, 183, 188	M	14.0	20.9	29.0	62.2	75.7	125.0	143.1	171.7	178.6	194.4
		F	7.3	12.6	20.8	39.8	54.4	76.6	98.9	101.8	106.9	106.1
Hodgkin's disease	Not given separately	M	...	...	...	...	...	...	...	...	...	...
		F	...	...	...	...	...	...	...	...	...	...
Myeloma and all lymphomas	200–203, incl. 201	M	1.1	4.3	3.3	8.8	10.3	17.6	21.3	30.0	6.0	3.5
		F	1.6	3.3	2.1	3.7	1.9	10.7	13.4	8.8	4.2	10.5
Leukaemia	204–208	M	–	1.4	0.8	5.3	5.9	6.6	18.3	24.5	3.0	17.4
		F	2.1	1.3	1.4	3.2	6.3	7.1	5.3	7.5	2.8	–
ALL VASCULAR DISEASE	390–459	M	103.1	188.0	308.7	522.9	850.8	1380.1	2310.5	3629.4	5636.9	12284.7
		F	28.6	50.2	102.4	204.4	344.7	708.9	1354.7	2441.0	4488.0	10922.3
Rheumatic heart disease and fever	390–398	M	1.7	5.0	4.1	8.2	7.3	8.8	6.1	8.2	6.0	6.9
		F	2.1	3.3	8.6	9.6	10.1	8.9	6.2	8.8	4.2	13.5
Hypertensive disease	401–405	M	–	–	–	0.6	0.7	0.7	1.5	8.2	11.9	10.4
		F	–	–	0.7	1.1	0.6	3.0	3.6	2.5	12.7	23.9
Ischaemic heart disease	410–414	M	75.6	116.0	205.8	352.7	570.9	845.6	1409.4	2098.1	3488.1	7864.6
		F	14.1	25.8	48.0	100.3	182.8	383.2	736.2	1378.1	2609.0	6798.2
Pulmonary embolism and other venous	Not given separately	M	...	...	...	...	...	...	...	...	...	...
		F	...	...	...	...	...	...	...	...	...	...
Cerebrovascular disease	430–438	M	19.6	54.8	81.3	140.3	237.3	475.7	834.1	1438.7	1985.1	4163.2
		F	8.3	15.2	40.1	83.9	141.7	297.7	572.2	1013.8	1791.8	3911.8
Other vascular disease, incl. venous	Rest of 390–459, incl. 415, 451–3	M	6.2	12.2	17.4	21.1	34.5	49.3	59.4	76.3	145.8	239.6
		F	4.2	5.9	5.0	9.6	9.5	16.0	36.5	37.7	70.3	174.9
Chronic obstructive pulmonary disease	490–496	M	1.7	7.9	19.9	32.3	45.6	65.4	102.0	174.4	282.7	517.4
		F	2.6	4.6	1.4	8.5	22.8	24.4	41.9	85.4	144.9	343.8
Other respiratory disease	Rest of 460–519	M	3.4	5.0	7.5	6.5	18.4	20.6	18.3	24.5	65.5	125.0
		F	2.6	3.3	1.4	2.1	5.7	8.9	8.9	8.8	38.0	74.7
Peptic ulcer	531–533	M	2.8	5.0	4.1	7.6	9.6	11.8	15.2	30.0	35.7	34.7
		F	1.0	–	–	1.6	1.9	5.9	8.9	15.1	15.5	10.5
Liver cirrhosis and other liver disease	570–573, 576, 575.2–579.9	M	17.9	35.3	58.1	69.8	78.6	126.5	170.5	158.0	148.8	166.7
		F	2.1	2.6	6.4	19.1	24.0	38.6	59.7	64.1	74.5	79.2
Renal disease	580–590	M	6.2	7.2	8.3	14.7	22.0	27.2	27.4	32.7	29.8	90.3
		F	1.6	4.0	3.6	11.1	12.0	14.9	19.6	20.1	32.3	28.4
Pregnancy and birth	630–676	F	2.1	–	–	–	–	0.6	–	–	–	–
Congenital and perinatal causes	740–779	M	–	–	–	–	–	–	–	–	–	–
		F	–	–	–	–	–	–	–	–	–	–
Ill-defined causes	780–799	M	11.8	15.9	29.0	28.2	30.1	32.4	38.1	46.3	38.7	201.4
		F	3.1	4.6	5.0	6.4	7.6	16.6	16.9	21.4	39.4	179.4
Other medical causes	Rest of 001–799	M	11.8	23.8	31.5	37.6	67.6	81.6	149.2	163.5	190.5	256.9
		F	5.2	8.6	13.6	18.0	32.3	67.1	107.0	114.3	147.7	107.6
ALL NON-MEDICAL CAUSES	E800–E999	M	127.7	134.7	127.8	126.2	130.8	125.7	114.2	139.0	169.6	152.8
		F	22.4	25.1	25.8	29.2	29.7	38.6	41.0	52.8	47.8	85.2
Motor vehicle traffic accidents	E810–E819	M	29.7	39.6	33.2	33.5	27.9	23.5	19.8	35.4	44.6	38.2
		F	7.8	4.6	3.6	5.3	7.0	6.5	9.8	12.6	11.3	12.0
Fire	E890–E899	M	4.5	4.3	9.1	2.9	3.7	9.6	4.6	10.9	11.9	13.9
		F	1.0	3.3	3.6	1.6	1.9	3.6	2.7	2.5	12.7	17.9
Suicide	E950–E959	M	3.9	9.4	5.0	10.6	6.6	11.0	10.7	13.6	17.9	27.8
		F	1.0	0.7	5.0	6.4	3.8	3.6	1.8	5.0	4.2	7.5
Homicide	E960–E969	M	7.8	7.9	6.6	4.1	3.7	3.7	7.6	5.4	3.0	3.5
		F	1.6	2.6	1.4	1.6	1.9	3.6	2.7	1.3	–	1.5
POPULATION (thousands)		M	178.5	138.8	120.5	170.4	136.1	136.0	65.7	36.7	33.6	28.8
		F	192.1	151.3	139.6	188.4	158.1	168.3	112.2	79.6	71.1	66.9

GEORGIA: Males

	All ages	0–34	35–69	35–39	40–44	45–49	50–54	55–59	60–64	65–69	70–74	75–79	80+/NK
POPULATION (1000s)													
1985–90	2524.4	1518.2	904.2	163.6	117.6	159.7	155.8	147.1	107.2	53.2	42.1	32.3	27.6
1985	2468.2	1499.5	862.7	140.9	122.8	179.4	146.3	150.2	76.8	46.3	47.6	31.3	27.1
1990	**2571.1**	**1526.0**	**946.0**	**178.5**	**138.8**	**120.5**	**170.4**	**136.1**	**136.0**	**65.7**	**36.7**	**33.6**	**28.8**
1995 projected	*2599.4*	*1542.8*	*956.4*	*180.5*	*140.3*	*121.8*	*172.3*	*137.6*	*137.5*	*66.4*	*37.1*	*34.0*	*29.1*
NUMBER OF DEATHS													
All causes													
1985–90	23194	2958	10921	544	574	1098	1678	2324	2737	1966	2277	2651	4387
1985	22915	3084	10048	456	574	1240	1551	2533	1980	1714	2633	2644	4506
1990	**22977**	**2649**	**11778**	**601**	**710**	**879**	**1829**	**2174**	**3220**	**2365**	**1898**	**2475**	**4177**
1995 projected	*21735*	*2413*	*11594*	*649*	*764*	*926*	*1830*	*2079*	*3092*	*2254*	*1750*	*2273*	*3705*
Lung cancer													
1985–90	816	7	634	9	19	52	100	165	182	107	88	56	31
1985	768	11	584	9	19	71	83	175	132	95	93	50	30
1990	**830**	**6**	**634**	**15**	**17**	**31**	**96**	**148**	**198**	**129**	**80**	**71**	**39**
1995 projected	*810*	*6*	*576*	*13*	*12*	*26*	*86*	*132*	*181*	*126*	*89*	*89*	*50*
ANNUAL DEATH RATE / 100,000 (*The rates for the age groups 0–34 and 35–69 are the means of seven five-yearly rates, but the all-ages rates are standardised to the conventional "European" age distribution)													
All causes													
1985–90	1295.3*	190.8*	1487.7*	332.5	488.1	687.5	1077.0	1579.9	2553.2	3695.5	5408.6	8207.4	15894.9
1985	1330.1*	203.2*	1501.3*	323.6	467.4	691.2	1060.2	1686.4	2578.1	3701.9	5531.5	8447.3	16627.3
1990	**1224.9***	**171.6***	**1459.4***	**336.7**	**511.5**	**729.5**	**1073.4**	**1597.4**	**2367.6**	**3599.7**	**5171.7**	**7366.1**	**14503.5**
1995 projected	*1139.3**	*156.1**	*1411.5**	*359.6*	*544.5*	*760.3*	*1062.1*	*1510.9*	*2248.7*	*3394.6*	*4717.0*	*6685.3*	*12732.0*
All cancer													
1985–90	151.5*	9.2*	265.4*	34.2	62.9	110.2	198.3	314.1	495.3	642.9	719.7	752.3	630.4
1985	150.1*	9.6*	260.4*	34.8	57.0	110.4	189.3	344.2	487.0	600.4	708.0	738.0	642.1
1990	**148.5***	**8.9***	**255.5***	**30.8**	**66.3**	**100.4**	**198.9**	**311.5**	**461.0**	**619.5**	**757.5**	**735.1**	**621.5**
1995 projected	*146.5**	*7.8**	*249.9**	*28.8*	*64.9*	*103.4*	*187.5*	*291.4*	*445.1*	*628.0*	*773.6*	*764.7*	*615.1*
Lung cancer													
1985–90	43.8*	0.5*	85.9*	5.5	16.2	32.6	64.2	112.2	169.8	201.1	209.0	173.4	112.3
1985	43.7*	0.8*	87.4*	6.4	15.5	39.6	56.7	116.5	171.9	205.2	195.4	159.7	110.7
1990	**42.5***	**0.4***	**79.1***	**8.4**	**12.2**	**25.7**	**56.3**	**108.7**	**145.6**	**196.3**	**218.0**	**211.3**	**135.4**
1995 projected	*42.1**	*0.4**	*72.0**	*7.2*	*8.6*	*21.3*	*49.9*	*95.9*	*131.6*	*189.8*	*239.9*	*261.8*	*171.8*
Upper aerodigestive cancer (mouth, oesophagus, pharynx and larynx)													
1985–90	16.2*	0.3*	29.4*	2.4	6.8	15.7	24.4	34.0	58.8	63.9	68.9	71.2	79.7
1985	15.8*	–	28.2*	4.3	3.3	12.3	23.2	37.3	67.7	49.7	73.5	79.9	70.1
1990	**15.8***	**0.3***	**28.7***	**2.2**	**8.6**	**16.6**	**28.2**	**33.8**	**52.2**	**59.4**	**68.1**	**56.5**	**76.4**
1995 projected	*15.5**	*0.1**	*28.7**	*2.8*	*11.4*	*22.2*	*30.2*	*29.8*	*48.7*	*55.7*	*62.0*	*55.9*	*68.7*
Other cancer													
1985–90	91.6*	8.5*	150.1*	26.3	40.0	62.0	109.8	167.9	266.8	377.8	441.8	507.7	438.4
1985	90.5*	8.8*	144.8*	24.1	38.3	58.5	109.4	190.4	247.4	345.6	439.1	498.4	461.3
1990	**90.2***	**8.1***	**147.7***	**20.2**	**45.4**	**58.1**	**114.4**	**169.0**	**263.2**	**363.8**	**471.4**	**467.3**	**409.7**
1995 projected	*88.9**	*7.4**	*149.1**	*18.8*	*44.9*	*59.9*	*107.4*	*165.7*	*264.7*	*382.5*	*471.7*	*447.1*	*374.6*
Chronic obstructive pulmonary disease (COPD)													
1985–90	43.6*	0.8*	46.8*	4.3	8.5	13.8	30.8	48.3	84.9	137.2	213.8	337.5	666.7
1985	46.1*	1.2*	44.4*	6.4	9.0	12.3	27.3	47.9	84.6	123.1	212.2	361.0	800.7
1990	**36.3***	**1.2***	**39.3***	**1.7**	**7.9**	**19.9**	**32.3**	**45.6**	**65.4**	**102.0**	**174.4**	**282.7**	**517.4**
1995 projected	*29.2**	*1.1**	*35.0**	*1.1*	*7.8*	*23.8*	*35.4*	*40.0*	*53.8*	*82.8*	*137.5*	*202.9*	*364.3*
Other respiratory disease													
1985–90	34.9*	40.6*	15.5*	6.1	6.0	7.5	12.2	19.7	25.2	32.0	54.6	89.8	155.8
1985	41.2*	46.8*	17.8*	7.8	9.0	7.2	16.4	26.6	27.3	30.2	60.9	134.2	191.9
1990	**24.4***	**28.4***	**11.4***	**3.4**	**5.0**	**7.5**	**6.5**	**18.4**	**20.6**	**18.3**	**24.5**	**65.5**	**125.0**
1995 projected	*17.8**	*21.6**	*7.9**	*2.2*	*3.6*	*4.9*	*4.6*	*13.1*	*14.5*	*12.0*	*16.2*	*44.1*	*85.9*
Vascular disease													
1985–90	816.3*	14.5*	827.0*	102.7	182.0	304.3	522.5	846.4	1481.3	2349.6	3817.1	6328.2	13572.5
1985	847.2*	15.3*	855.0*	100.8	179.2	314.9	515.4	908.8	1516.9	2449.2	3979.0	6559.1	14155.0
1990	**765.2***	**14.0***	**809.2***	**103.1**	**188.0**	**308.7**	**522.9**	**850.8**	**1380.1**	**2310.5**	**3629.4**	**5636.9**	**12284.7**
1995 projected	*683.6**	*11.6**	*749.4**	*100.8*	*182.5*	*303.8*	*497.4*	*783.4*	*1272.7*	*2105.4*	*3186.0*	*4950.0*	*10628.9*
Liver cirrhosis and other liver disease													
1985–90	42.5*	1.9*	77.8*	14.1	26.4	44.5	71.2	90.4	143.7	154.1	173.4	176.5	155.8
1985	45.9*	2.1*	83.8*	14.9	27.7	47.9	77.2	108.5	158.9	151.2	182.8	182.1	173.4
1990	**42.6***	**1.9***	**79.5***	**17.9**	**35.3**	**58.1**	**69.8**	**78.6**	**126.5**	**170.5**	**158.0**	**148.8**	**166.7**
1995 projected	*39.4**	*2.1**	*73.4**	*21.1*	*42.1*	*60.8*	*60.9*	*61.8*	*112.0*	*155.1*	*142.9*	*129.4*	*151.2*
Other medical causes													
1985–90	116.3*	62.9*	138.1*	56.8	77.4	96.4	119.4	144.8	207.1	265.0	313.5	383.9	550.7
1985	123.9*	73.4*	146.2*	61.0	92.8	109.3	134.7	146.5	226.6	252.7	289.9	348.2	538.7
1990	**110.3***	**52.3***	**137.8***	**52.1**	**74.2**	**107.1**	**116.8**	**161.6**	**188.2**	**264.8**	**288.8**	**327.4**	**635.4**
1995 projected	*99.3**	*37.1**	*127.3**	*40.4*	*63.4*	*92.0*	*113.2*	*146.1*	*183.3*	*253.0*	*280.3*	*376.5*	*687.3*
All non-medical causes													
1985–90	90.3*	60.9*	117.0*	114.3	125.0	110.8	122.6	116.2	115.7	114.7	116.4	139.3	163.0
1985	75.8*	54.8*	93.6*	97.9	92.8	89.2	99.8	103.9	76.8	95.0	98.7	124.6	125.5
1990	**97.7***	**65.0***	**126.7***	**127.7**	**134.7**	**127.8**	**126.2**	**130.8**	**125.7**	**114.2**	**139.0**	**169.6**	**152.8**
1995 projected	*123.5**	*74.8**	*168.7**	*165.1*	*180.3*	*171.6*	*163.1*	*175.1*	*167.3*	*158.1*	*180.6*	*217.6*	*199.3*

GEORGIA: Females

	All ages	0–34	35–69	35–39	40–44	45–49	50–54	55–59	60–64	65–69	70–74	75–79	80+/NK
POPULATION (1000s)													
1985–90	2807.4	1513.5	1078.0	177.2	131.0	180.2	171.4	169.7	148.5	100.0	85.9	66.0	64.0
1985	2761.7	1500.1	1045.7	153.4	142.2	195.8	161.4	174.2	126.4	92.3	92.1	62.4	61.4
1990	**2842.4**	**1514.8**	**1110.0**	**192.1**	**151.3**	**139.6**	**188.4**	**158.1**	**168.3**	**112.2**	**79.6**	**71.1**	**66.9**
1995 projected	*2873.5*	*1531.4*	*1122.1*	*194.2*	*153.0*	*141.1*	*190.5*	*159.8*	*170.1*	*113.4*	*80.5*	*71.9*	*67.6*
NUMBER OF DEATHS													
All causes													
1985–90	23405	1740	6702	214	227	480	779	1194	1836	1972	2862	3751	8350
1985	23238	1868	6392	214	208	564	708	1305	1593	1800	3097	3606	8275
1990	**22968**	**1438**	**6976**	**213**	**273**	**334**	**871**	**1040**	**2003**	**2242**	**2559**	**3840**	**8155**
1995 projected	*21793*	*1273*	*6798*	*225*	*255*	*341*	*810*	*992*	*1967*	*2208*	*2477*	*3668*	*7577*
Lung cancer													
1985–90	183	4	113	5	3	10	15	25	29	26	24	24	18
1985	191	6	124	3	4	13	14	32	21	37	28	14	19
1990	**178**	**6**	**115**	–	**3**	**7**	**20**	**21**	**36**	**28**	**23**	**20**	**14**
1995 projected	*156*	*5*	*99*	–	*2*	*7*	*17*	*21*	*28*	*24*	*20*	*19*	*13*
ANNUAL DEATH RATE / 100,000 (*The rates for the age groups 0–34 and 35–69 are the means of seven five-yearly rates, but the all-ages rates are standardised to the conventional "European" age distribution)													
All causes													
1985–90	788.3*	111.9*	703.8*	120.8	173.3	266.4	454.5	703.6	1236.4	1972.0	3331.8	5683.3	13046.9
1985	808.7*	122.1*	710.3*	139.5	146.3	288.0	438.7	749.1	1260.3	1950.2	3362.6	5778.8	13477.2
1990	**745.9***	**93.1***	**691.3***	**110.9**	**180.4**	**239.3**	**462.3**	**657.8**	**1190.1**	**1998.2**	**3214.8**	**5400.8**	**12189.8**
1995 projected	*700.5**	*81.9**	*667.7**	*115.9*	*166.7*	*241.7*	*425.2*	*620.8*	*1156.4*	*1947.1*	*3077.0*	*5101.5*	*11208.6*
All cancer													
1985–90	92.1*	7.9*	161.2*	37.2	63.4	96.6	145.3	196.2	260.6	329.0	374.9	392.4	359.4
1985	91.3*	6.5*	157.1*	49.5	54.1	106.2	136.3	206.1	250.8	296.9	393.1	381.4	381.1
1990	**89.4***	**7.3***	**157.3***	**36.4**	**72.7**	**77.4**	**155.0**	**167.6**	**260.2**	**331.6**	**381.9**	**362.9**	**340.8**
1995 projected	*86.0**	*6.8**	*153.3**	*38.6*	*63.4*	*78.0*	*136.5*	*160.8*	*257.5*	*338.6*	*378.9*	*338.0*	*316.6*
Lung cancer													
1985–90	6.5*	0.3*	11.4*	2.8	2.3	5.5	8.8	14.7	19.5	26.0	27.9	36.4	28.1
1985	7.1*	0.4*	13.6*	2.0	2.8	6.6	8.7	18.4	16.6	40.1	30.4	22.4	30.9
1990	**6.1***	**0.4***	**11.0***	–	**2.0**	**5.0**	**10.6**	**13.3**	**21.4**	**25.0**	**28.9**	**28.1**	**20.9**
1995 projected	*5.3**	*0.3**	*9.4**	–	*1.3*	*5.0*	*8.9*	*13.1*	*16.5*	*21.2*	*24.8*	*26.4*	*19.2*
Upper aerodigestive cancer (mouth, oesophagus, pharynx and larynx)													
1985–90	2.3*	0.1*	3.3*	0.6	0.8	1.1	2.9	4.1	5.4	8.0	12.8	15.2	18.8
1985	2.5*	0.1*	3.5*	–	0.7	1.0	3.7	4.6	4.7	9.8	17.4	14.4	16.3
1990	**2.1***	**0.1***	**2.7***	**0.5**	**0.7**	–	**1.6**	**5.7**	**5.3**	**5.3**	**12.6**	**14.1**	**17.9**
1995 projected	*1.9**	*0.1**	*2.3**	*0.5*	*0.7*	–	*1.0*	*5.6*	*4.7*	*3.5*	*9.9*	*13.9*	*19.2*
Other cancer													
1985–90	83.3*	7.5*	146.5*	33.9	60.3	89.9	133.6	177.4	235.7	295.0	334.1	340.9	312.5
1985	81.7*	6.1*	140.0*	47.6	50.6	98.6	123.9	183.1	229.4	247.0	345.3	344.6	333.9
1990	**81.2***	**6.8***	**143.5***	**35.9**	**70.1**	**72.3**	**142.8**	**148.6**	**233.5**	**301.2**	**340.5**	**320.7**	**301.9**
1995 projected	*78.9**	*6.5**	*141.6**	*38.1*	*61.4*	*73.0*	*126.5*	*142.1*	*236.3*	*313.9*	*344.1*	*297.6*	*278.1*
Chronic obstructive pulmonary disease (COPD)													
1985–90	20.1*	0.9*	15.9*	2.8	3.1	5.5	9.9	15.9	28.3	46.0	88.5	151.5	414.1
1985	22.1*	0.9*	15.5*	2.6	2.8	7.7	7.4	13.2	28.5	46.6	102.1	157.1	495.1
1990	**18.4***	**1.1***	**15.2***	**2.6**	**4.6**	**1.4**	**8.5**	**22.8**	**24.4**	**41.9**	**85.4**	**144.9**	**343.8**
1995 projected	*15.7**	*1.5**	*14.6**	*3.6*	*3.3*	*1.4*	*9.4*	*25.0*	*24.1*	*35.3*	*74.5*	*111.3*	*257.4*
Other respiratory disease													
1985–90	25.7*	34.8*	6.8*	2.3	3.1	2.8	4.7	7.1	13.5	14.0	27.9	48.5	104.7
1985	30.8*	40.1*	7.8*	2.0	2.1	4.1	6.2	11.5	19.0	9.8	33.7	67.3	158.0
1990	**17.7***	**24.6***	**4.7***	**2.6**	**3.3**	**1.4**	**2.1**	**5.7**	**8.9**	**8.9**	**8.8**	**38.0**	**74.7**
1995 projected	*13.5**	*19.2**	*3.5**	*3.6*	*2.6*	*0.7*	*1.6*	*3.8*	*5.9*	*6.2*	*6.2*	*26.4*	*53.3*
Vascular disease													
1985–90	550.8*	7.6*	409.4*	31.0	51.9	100.4	206.0	365.9	756.2	1354.0	2561.1	4731.8	11718.8
1985	567.7*	8.1*	426.4*	46.9	38.7	108.3	208.2	389.8	800.6	1392.2	2590.7	4879.8	12058.6
1990	**522.9***	**8.4***	**399.1***	**28.6**	**50.2**	**102.4**	**204.4**	**344.7**	**708.9**	**1354.7**	**2441.0**	**4488.0**	**10922.3**
1995 projected	*478.7**	*8.0**	*364.4**	*24.2*	*45.1*	*99.9*	*186.4*	*302.9*	*645.5*	*1246.9*	*2246.0*	*4166.9*	*9936.4*
Liver cirrhosis and other liver disease													
1985–90	14.5*	0.6*	23.1*	3.4	4.6	9.4	17.5	28.3	43.8	55.0	68.7	77.3	101.6
1985	16.6*	0.8*	27.9*	2.0	4.9	11.7	16.7	38.5	58.5	62.8	68.4	84.9	110.7
1990	**13.1***	**0.4***	**21.8***	**2.1**	**2.6**	**6.4**	**19.1**	**24.0**	**38.6**	**59.7**	**64.1**	**74.5**	**79.2**
1995 projected	*10.5**	*0.3**	*16.9**	*1.5*	*2.0*	*5.0*	*14.2*	*16.9*	*28.8*	*50.3*	*58.4*	*66.8*	*62.1*
Other medical causes													
1985–90	60.2*	43.6*	58.5*	22.6	24.4	28.9	43.8	60.1	97.0	133.0	161.8	209.1	265.6
1985	58.5*	49.7*	51.6*	23.5	27.4	29.6	43.4	59.7	73.6	104.0	132.5	166.7	197.1
1990	**59.6***	**35.6***	**62.9***	**16.1**	**21.8**	**24.4**	**44.1**	**63.3**	**110.5**	**160.4**	**180.9**	**244.7**	**343.8**
1995 projected	*67.2**	*28.8**	*77.8**	*13.9*	*16.3*	*21.3*	*43.0*	*76.3*	*152.3*	*221.3*	*252.2*	*342.1*	*486.7*
All non-medical causes													
1985–90	25.0*	16.5*	28.9*	21.4	22.9	22.8	27.4	30.1	37.0	41.0	48.9	72.7	82.8
1985	21.7*	16.0*	24.0*	13.0	16.2	20.4	20.4	30.4	29.3	37.9	42.3	41.7	76.5
1990	**24.8***	**15.7***	**30.3***	**22.4**	**25.1**	**25.8**	**29.2**	**29.7**	**38.6**	**41.0**	**52.8**	**47.8**	**85.2**
1995 projected	*28.9**	*17.2**	*37.1**	*30.4*	*34.0*	*35.4*	*34.1*	*35.0*	*42.3*	*48.5*	*60.9*	*50.1*	*96.2*

GEORGIA: 1985–1990

Smoking-attributed deaths (Sm.) and total deaths (Total)

		ALL CAUSES	ALL CANCER	Lung cancer	Upper aero-digestive ca.	Other cancer	COPD	Other respiratory	Vascular disease	Cirrhosis/ other liver	Other medical	Non-medical
Males												
0–34	Sm.	–	–	–	–	–	–	–	–	–	–	–
	Total	2958	137	7	4	126	12	662	208	27	1004	908
35–69	Sm.	2848	840	572	131	137	233	32	1444	–	299	–
	Total	10921	1950	634	222	1094	322	121	5765	605	1100	1058
		(26%)	(43%)	(90%)	(59%)	(13%)	(72%)	(26%)	(25%)		(27%)	
70+	Sm.	721	186	137	26	23	177	5	332	–	21	–
	Total	9315	720	175	74	471	383	95	7397	173	408	139
		(8%)	(26%)	(78%)	(35%)	(5%)	(46%)	(5%)	(4%)		(5%)	
Any age	Sm.	3569	1026	709	157	160	410	37	1776	–	320	–
	Total	23194	2807	816	300	1691	717	878	13370	805	2512	2105
		(15%)	(37%)	(87%)	(52%)	(9%)	(57%)	(4%)	(13%)		(13%)	
Females												
0–34	Sm.	–	–	–	–	–	–	–	–	–	–	–
	Total	1740	119	4	2	113	14	547	116	9	682	253
35–69	Sm.	138	32	26	2	4	21	0	73	–	12	–
	Total	6702	1621	113	32	1476	151	67	3755	227	578	303
		(2%)	(2%)	(23%)	(6%)	(0%)	(14%)	(0%)	(2%)		(2%)	
70+	Sm.	10	1	1	0	0	4	0	5	–	0	–
	Total	14963	811	66	33	712	441	123	12823	175	447	143
		(0%)	(0%)	(2%)	(0%)	(0%)	(1%)	(0%)	(0%)		(0%)	
Any age	Sm.	148	33	27	2	4	25	0	78	–	12	–
	Total	23405	2551	183	67	2301	606	737	16694	411	1707	699
		(1%)	(1%)	(15%)	(3%)	(0%)	(4%)	(0%)	(0%)		(1%)	
Males+Females												
0–34	Sm.	–	–	–	–	–	–	–	–	–	–	–
	Total	4698	256	11	6	239	26	1209	324	36	1686	1161
35–69	Sm.	2986	872	598	133	141	254	32	1517	–	311	–
	Total	17623	3571	747	254	2570	473	188	9520	832	1678	1361
		(17%)	(24%)	(80%)	(52%)	(5%)	(54%)	(17%)	(16%)		(19%)	
70+	Sm.	731	187	138	26	23	181	5	337	–	21	–
	Total	24278	1531	241	107	1183	824	218	20220	348	855	282
		(3%)	(12%)	(57%)	(24%)	(2%)	(22%)	(2%)	(2%)		(2%)	
Any age	Sm.	3717	1059	736	159	164	435	37	1854	–	332	–
	Total	46599	5358	999	367	3992	1323	1615	30064	1216	4219	2804
		(8%)	(20%)	(74%)	(43%)	(4%)	(33%)	(2%)	(6%)		(8%)	

GEORGIA: 1985

Smoking-attributed deaths (Sm.) and total deaths (Total)

		ALL CAUSES	ALL CANCER	Lung cancer	Upper aero-digestive ca.	Other cancer	COPD	Other respiratory	Vascular disease	Cirrhosis/ other liver	Other medical	Non-medical
Males												
0–34	Sm.	–	–	–	–	–	–	–	–	–	–	–
	Total	3084	140	11	0	129	17	748	209	29	1137	804
35–69	Sm.	2718	774	530	117	127	201	38	1392	–	313	–
	Total	10048	1763	584	197	982	276	134	5345	609	1104	817
		(27%)	(44%)	(91%)	(59%)	(13%)	(73%)	(28%)	(26%)		(28%)	
70+	Sm.	729	183	133	26	24	190	6	331	–	19	–
	Total	9783	742	173	79	490	431	123	7783	191	393	120
		(7%)	(25%)	(77%)	(33%)	(5%)	(44%)	(5%)	(4%)		(5%)	
Any age	Sm.	3447	957	663	143	151	391	44	1723	–	332	–
	Total	22915	2645	768	276	1601	724	1005	13337	829	2634	1741
		(15%)	(36%)	(86%)	(52%)	(9%)	(54%)	(4%)	(13%)		(13%)	
Females												
0–34	Sm.	–	–	–	–	–	–	–	–	–	–	–
	Total	1868	96	6	1	89	13	620	119	12	765	243
35–69	Sm.	211	48	39	4	5	28	1	118	–	16	–
	Total	6392	1531	124	32	1375	137	77	3651	259	496	241
		(3%)	(3%)	(31%)	(13%)	(0%)	(20%)	(1%)	(3%)		(3%)	
70+	Sm.	22	3	3	0	0	6	0	12	–	1	–
	Total	14978	834	61	35	738	496	170	12835	184	347	112
		(0%)	(0%)	(5%)	(0%)	(0%)	(1%)	(0%)	(0%)		(0%)	
Any age	Sm.	233	51	42	4	5	34	1	130	–	17	–
	Total	23238	2461	191	68	2202	646	867	16605	455	1608	596
		(1%)	(2%)	(22%)	(6%)	(0%)	(5%)	(0%)	(1%)		(1%)	
Males+Females												
0–34	Sm.	–	–	–	–	–	–	–	–	–	–	–
	Total	4952	236	17	1	218	30	1368	328	41	1902	1047
35–69	Sm.	2929	822	569	121	132	229	39	1510	–	329	–
	Total	16440	3294	708	229	2357	413	211	8996	868	1600	1058
		(18%)	(25%)	(80%)	(53%)	(6%)	(55%)	(18%)	(17%)		(21%)	
70+	Sm.	751	186	136	26	24	196	6	343	–	20	–
	Total	24761	1576	234	114	1228	927	293	20618	375	740	232
		(3%)	(12%)	(58%)	(23%)	(2%)	(21%)	(2%)	(2%)		(3%)	
Any age	Sm.	3680	1008	705	147	156	425	45	1853	–	349	–
	Total	46153	5106	959	344	3803	1370	1872	29942	1284	4242	2337
		(8%)	(20%)	(74%)	(43%)	(4%)	(31%)	(2%)	(6%)		(8%)	

(To be conservative, no deaths before age 35, and none from liver cirrhosis or non-medical causes, were attributed to smoking.)

GEORGIA: 1990

Smoking–attributed deaths (Sm.) and total deaths (Total)

		ALL CAUSES	ALL CANCER	Lung cancer	Upper aero–digestive ca.	Other cancer	COPD	Other respiratory	Vascular disease	Cirrhosis/ other liver	Other medical	Non–medical
Males												
0–34	Sm.	–	–	–	–	–	–	–	–	–	–	–
	Total	2649	134	6	5	123	18	458	204	29	833	973
35–69	Sm.	2782	839	568	135	136	218	24	1410	–	291	–
	Total	11778	2065	634	240	1191	311	98	6261	661	1174	1208
		(24%)	(41%)	(90%)	(56%)	(11%)	(70%)	(24%)	(23%)		(25%)	
70+	Sm.	735	205	153	26	26	158	4	347	–	21	–
	Total	8550	704	190	66	448	308	67	6764	156	399	152
		(9%)	(29%)	(81%)	(39%)	(6%)	(51%)	(6%)	(5%)		(5%)	
Any age	Sm.	3517	1044	721	161	162	376	28	1757	–	312	–
	Total	22977	2903	830	311	1762	637	623	13229	846	2406	2333
		(15%)	(36%)	(87%)	(52%)	(9%)	(59%)	(4%)	(13%)		(13%)	
Females												
0–34	Sm.	–	–	–	–	–	–	–	–	–	–	–
	Total	1438	111	6	1	104	18	381	128	6	553	241
35–69	Sm.	123	25	22	1	2	18	0	70	–	10	–
	Total	6976	1655	115	29	1511	154	50	3917	223	647	330
		(2%)	(2%)	(19%)	(3%)	(0%)	(12%)	(0%)	(2%)		(2%)	
70+	Sm.	8	1	1	0	0	2	0	5	–	0	–
	Total	14554	790	57	32	701	401	84	12441	157	548	133
		(0%)	(0%)	(2%)	(0%)	(0%)	(0%)	(0%)	(0%)		(0%)	
Any age	Sm.	131	26	23	1	2	20	0	75	–	10	–
	Total	22968	2556	178	62	2316	573	515	16486	386	1748	704
		(1%)	(1%)	(13%)	(2%)	(0%)	(3%)	(0%)	(0%)		(1%)	
Males+Females												
0–34	Sm.	–	–	–	–	–	–	–	–	–	–	–
	Total	4087	245	12	6	227	36	839	332	35	1386	1214
35–69	Sm.	2905	864	590	136	138	236	24	1480	–	301	–
	Total	18754	3720	749	269	2702	465	148	10178	884	1821	1538
		(15%)	(23%)	(79%)	(51%)	(5%)	(51%)	(16%)	(15%)		(17%)	
70+	Sm.	743	206	154	26	26	160	4	352	–	21	–
	Total	23104	1494	247	98	1149	709	151	19205	313	947	285
		(3%)	(14%)	(62%)	(27%)	(2%)	(23%)	(3%)	(2%)		(2%)	
Any age	Sm.	3648	1070	744	162	164	396	28	1832	–	322	–
	Total	45945	5459	1008	373	4078	1210	1138	29715	1232	4154	3037
		(8%)	(20%)	(74%)	(43%)	(4%)	(33%)	(2%)	(6%)		(8%)	

GEORGIA: 1995

Smoking–attributed deaths (Sm.) and total deaths (Total)

		ALL CAUSES	ALL CANCER	Lung cancer	Upper aero–digestive ca.	Other cancer	COPD	Other respiratory	Vascular disease	Cirrhosis/ other liver	Other medical	Non–medical
Males												
0–34	Sm.	–	–	–	–	–	–	–	–	–	–	–
	Total	2413	119	6	1	112	17	351	170	31	597	1128
35–69	Sm.	2414	760	509	130	121	195	15	1204	–	240	–
	Total	11594	2022	576	245	1201	287	69	5891	618	1090	1617
		(21%)	(38%)	(88%)	(53%)	(10%)	(68%)	(22%)	(20%)		(22%)	
70+	Sm.	775	246	190	26	30	129	3	370	–	27	–
	Total	7728	726	228	62	436	226	46	5958	141	432	199
		(10%)	(34%)	(83%)	(42%)	(7%)	(57%)	(7%)	(6%)		(6%)	
Any age	Sm.	3189	1006	699	156	151	324	18	1574	–	267	–
	Total	21735	2867	810	308	1749	530	466	12019	790	2119	2944
		(15%)	(35%)	(86%)	(51%)	(9%)	(61%)	(4%)	(13%)		(13%)	
Females												
0–34	Sm.	–	–	–	–	–	–	–	–	–	–	–
	Total	1273	105	5	1	99	23	300	122	4	453	266
35–69	Sm.	32	6	6	0	0	5	0	17	–	4	–
	Total	6798	1621	99	25	1497	153	38	3608	173	796	409
		(0%)	(0%)	(6%)	(0%)	(0%)	(3%)	(0%)	(0%)		(1%)	
70+	Sm.	0	0	0	0	0	0	0	0	–	0	–
	Total	13722	762	52	31	679	314	60	11521	137	778	150
		(0%)	(0%)	(0%)	(0%)	(0%)	(0%)	(0%)	(0%)		(0%)	
Any age	Sm.	32	6	6	0	0	5	0	17	–	4	–
	Total	21793	2488	156	57	2275	490	398	15251	314	2027	825
		(0%)	(0%)	(4%)	(0%)	(0%)	(1%)	(0%)	(0%)		(0%)	
Males+Females												
0–34	Sm.	–	–	–	–	–	–	–	–	–	–	–
	Total	3686	224	11	2	211	40	651	292	35	1050	1394
35–69	Sm.	2446	766	515	130	121	200	15	1221	–	244	–
	Total	18392	3643	675	270	2698	440	107	9499	791	1886	2026
		(13%)	(21%)	(76%)	(48%)	(4%)	(45%)	(14%)	(13%)		(13%)	
70+	Sm.	775	246	190	26	30	129	3	370	–	27	–
	Total	21450	1488	280	93	1115	540	106	17479	278	1210	349
		(4%)	(17%)	(68%)	(28%)	(3%)	(24%)	(3%)	(2%)		(2%)	
Any age	Sm.	3221	1012	705	156	151	329	18	1591	–	271	–
	Total	43528	5355	966	365	4024	1020	864	27270	1104	4146	3769
		(7%)	(19%)	(73%)	(43%)	(4%)	(32%)	(2%)	(6%)		(7%)	

(To be conservative, no deaths before age 35, and none from liver cirrhosis or non–medical causes, were attributed to smoking.)

¶Former GERMAN DEMOCRATIC REPUBLIC: 1990

		No. of deaths			Standardised rates (Defined on p.352)			Annual death rates / 100, 000						
		All ages	0–34	35–69	All ages	0–34	35–69	0–4	5–9	10–14	15–19	20–24	25–29	30–34
ALL CAUSES	M	94654	5216	39095	1317.5	129.7	1452.0	199.5	34.2	42.7	122.0	149.3	148.9	211.0
	F	113456	2336	23966	787.0	62.2	704.5	149.3	28.1	27.3	47.2	47.2	56.3	79.8
Tuberculosis	M	173	3	100	2.4	0.1	4.0	–	–	–	–	–	0.1	0.3
	F	104	3	37	0.8	0.1	1.1	–	–	–	–	–	0.5	–
Other infective and parasitic	M	140	29	66	2.0	0.8	2.2	3.3	0.4	–	0.4	0.7	0.3	0.3
	F	191	34	69	1.8	1.0	1.9	4.7	0.4	0.2	0.7	–	0.5	0.3
ALL CANCER	M	16668	316	9325	237.1	7.5	353.8	4.5	3.0	3.4	4.1	9.3	12.9	15.6
	F	16928	268	7482	142.0	6.7	217.4	4.1	2.2	1.8	4.7	5.4	10.0	18.4
Mouth and pharynx cancer	M	497	4	389	6.6	0.1	12.4	–	–	–	0.2	–	–	0.5
	F	138	2	59	1.1	0.0	1.7	–	–	–	–	–	0.2	0.2
Oesophagus cancer	M	412	–	293	5.7	–	10.2	–	–	–	–	–	–	–
	F	94	–	27	0.7	–	0.8	–	–	–	–	–	–	–
Stomach cancer	M	1754	11	856	25.1	0.2	33.4	–	–	–	–	–	0.1	1.6
	F	1602	11	512	12.2	0.3	15.1	–	–	–	0.2	0.2	0.8	0.7
Colorectal cancer	M	1961	8	970	28.2	0.2	37.8	–	–	–	–	–	0.4	0.8
	F	2781	11	929	21.3	0.3	27.4	–	–	–	–	0.4	0.6	0.8
Liver cancer	M	66	–	40	1.0	–	1.7	–	–	–	–	–	–	–
	F	44	–	26	0.4	–	0.8	–	–	–	–	–	–	–
Pancreas cancer	M	679	4	403	9.7	0.1	15.1	–	–	0.2	–	–	–	0.5
	F	821	1	295	6.4	0.0	8.7	–	–	–	–	–	–	0.2
Larynx cancer	M	228	–	160	3.1	–	5.5	–	–	–	–	–	–	–
	F	21	–	9	0.2	–	0.3	–	–	–	–	–	–	–
Lung cancer	M	4907	9	3150	70.5	0.2	120.9	–	–	–	–	0.2	–	1.3
	F	1011	6	521	8.9	0.1	15.2	–	–	–	–	0.5	0.2	0.3
Malignant melanoma	M	135	8	95	1.8	0.2	3.2	–	–	–	–	0.2	0.6	0.5
	F	153	3	81	1.4	0.1	2.2	–	–	–	–	0.2	–	0.3
Female breast cancer	F	2653	37	1495	24.5	0.9	42.6	–	–	–	–	0.2	0.3	5.6
Cervix cancer	F	739	42	426	7.1	1.0	12.1	0.2	–	–	–	–	2.8	3.8
Other uterine cancer	F	638	1	272	5.2	0.0	8.0	–	–	–	–	–	0.2	–
Ovarian cancer	F	1104	14	651	10.1	0.3	18.8	–	–	–	–	0.4	0.5	1.5
Prostate cancer	M	1206	1	270	17.4	0.0	12.7	–	–	–	–	–	–	0.2
Bladder cancer	M	747	1	304	10.7	0.0	12.8	–	–	–	–	–	0.1	–
	F	325	–	89	2.3	–	2.7	–	–	–	–	–	–	–
Other and ill-defined cancer sites	M	2998	170	1791	42.0	4.0	65.3	2.9	2.1	1.9	1.5	5.1	8.5	6.2
	F	3718	72	1597	30.9	1.9	46.5	2.3	1.1	1.2	2.0	1.8	2.8	2.0
Hodgkin's disease	M	97	14	61	1.3	0.3	2.0	–	–	–	0.2	0.9	0.9	0.3
	F	82	10	33	0.7	0.2	0.9	–	–	–	–	0.4	0.8	0.5
Myeloma and non-Hodgkin lymphomas	M	423	20	261	6.0	0.5	9.9	0.4	–	0.4	0.4	0.7	0.6	1.0
	F	464	16	218	4.0	0.4	6.4	0.6	0.2	–	0.9	0.5	0.3	0.5
Leukaemia	M	558	66	282	7.8	1.6	10.8	1.2	0.9	0.9	1.7	2.3	1.6	2.9
	F	540	42	242	4.8	1.1	7.0	1.0	0.9	0.6	1.6	0.9	0.8	2.0
ALL VASCULAR DISEASE	M	46980	392	14881	657.9	9.3	590.9	6.8	2.3	3.7	3.8	7.2	12.8	28.2
	F	69125	176	8784	430.3	4.5	263.8	4.1	1.3	4.5	2.9	4.0	4.6	10.1
Rheumatic heart disease and fever	M	192	9	143	2.7	0.2	5.2	–	–	–	0.2	–	0.3	1.0
	F	336	1	182	3.0	0.0	5.4	–	0.2	–	–	–	–	–
Hypertensive disease	M	4162	17	1712	59.3	0.4	67.3	0.2	–	–	–	0.3	0.3	1.9
	F	7931	9	1431	52.4	0.2	42.9	–	0.2	–	–	–	0.3	1.0
Ischaemic heart disease	M	17321	97	7062	245.4	2.2	277.8	–	–	–	0.2	0.7	3.5	10.8
	F	18077	14	2793	116.1	0.3	84.2	–	–	–	–	–	0.6	1.7
Pulmonary embolism and other venous	M	782	19	421	11.2	0.4	16.0	0.4	–	–	–	0.2	0.6	1.9
	F	1111	17	414	8.9	0.4	12.2	0.2	–	0.2	0.7	0.7	0.3	1.0
Cerebrovascular disease	M	7384	48	1577	102.6	1.1	65.2	0.4	0.4	0.2	0.2	1.6	2.2	2.9
	F	14043	27	1471	85.7	0.7	44.2	–	–	0.2	0.4	0.9	1.1	2.0
Other vascular disease	M	17139	202	3966	236.7	4.9	159.3	5.8	2.0	3.5	3.2	4.4	5.9	9.8
	F	27627	108	2493	164.2	2.8	74.9	3.9	0.9	4.1	1.8	2.4	2.3	4.5
Chronic obstructive pulmonary disease	M	3406	14	1156	48.7	0.4	48.6	0.2	0.2	0.2	0.6	0.3	0.3	0.6
	F	1529	11	417	10.9	0.3	12.4	0.4	–	0.4	–	0.4	–	0.8
Other respiratory disease	M	3380	120	1047	46.7	3.0	40.0	7.6	0.5	0.7	2.3	2.6	2.3	5.1
	F	3846	81	546	24.8	2.2	16.2	8.8	0.6	0.6	0.2	0.7	2.2	2.2
Peptic ulcer	M	645	16	334	9.0	0.4	11.8	–	–	–	–	0.3	1.2	1.0
	F	549	2	135	3.8	0.0	4.0	–	–	–	–	–	–	0.3
Liver cirrhosis	M	2606	131	2135	34.9	2.9	68.9	–	–	–	0.2	0.9	4.3	15.2
	F	1197	47	841	12.2	1.1	23.9	0.4	–	0.2	0.2	–	1.8	5.1
Renal disease	M	882	34	370	12.3	0.8	13.9	0.6	–	–	0.2	0.9	1.6	2.2
	F	1113	17	393	8.8	0.4	11.6	0.2	0.2	0.2	–	0.4	0.9	1.0
Pregnancy and birth	F	29	27	2	0.3	0.7	0.1	–	–	–	0.2	1.8	1.4	1.2
Congenital and perinatal causes	M	727	666	54	11.0	18.4	1.7	118.6	2.7	1.7	1.9	1.0	1.2	1.6
	F	545	481	47	8.4	14.0	1.4	91.4	2.1	1.8	0.9	0.4	0.9	0.5
Ill-defined causes	M	3231	493	1618	43.7	12.1	55.1	10.3	6.8	12.9	8.5	13.5	15.3	17.8
	F	3119	219	783	23.7	5.8	22.6	6.4	6.0	9.8	3.8	6.0	4.2	4.8
Other medical causes	M	7759	514	3977	107.1	12.4	138.6	18.1	3.6	4.1	6.0	7.7	15.1	32.4
	F	9895	245	2855	74.4	6.4	83.6	11.3	3.2	3.1	3.8	5.8	7.2	10.1
ALL NON-MEDICAL CAUSES	M	8057	2488	4032	104.9	61.6	122.4	29.6	14.8	16.0	93.8	104.9	81.6	90.8
	F	5286	725	1575	44.8	19.1	44.4	17.4	12.2	4.7	29.7	22.4	22.1	25.0
Motor vehicle traffic accidents	M	2197	1183	813	28.2	30.0	24.1	6.2	7.3	8.0	64.5	61.5	34.5	28.2
	F	946	347	336	10.2	9.4	9.4	4.3	6.9	3.1	22.7	11.0	8.9	8.8
Fire	M	138	42	70	1.8	1.1	2.2	1.4	0.7	0.2	1.1	2.1	1.2	0.8
	F	83	14	30	0.8	0.4	0.9	1.0	0.6	0.2	0.2	–	0.3	0.3
Suicide	M	2681	469	1627	34.9	10.9	49.5	–	0.4	1.3	7.0	15.7	20.8	30.9
	F	1248	126	621	11.8	3.0	17.5	–	0.7	0.4	1.3	5.1	7.1	6.6
Homicide	M	96	31	60	1.2	0.8	1.7	1.0	0.4	–	1.3	0.9	1.2	0.8
	F	68	25	31	0.8	0.7	0.9	1.6	0.6	–	0.7	0.7	0.3	0.8
POPULATION (thousands):	M=males				7693.7	3964.0	3281.8	513.7	562.2	536.0	468.2	572.1	681.6	630.2
	F=females				8417.2	3782.6	3596.9	487.7	534.7	508.6	444.5	553.1	650.3	603.7

Former GERMAN DEMOCRATIC REPUBLIC: 1990

Annual death rates / 100, 000 — 9th ICD categories

35–39	40–44	45–49	50–54	55–59	60–64	65–69	70–74	75–79	80+/NK			
300.5	393.8	684.9	1014.4	1621.3	2331.0	3818.0	5482.5	9684.3	17987.7	M	ALL CAUSES	001–999
121.8	172.6	293.5	434.1	721.5	1186.6	2001.1	3185.2	6249.3	14016.0	F		
0.6	0.2	1.2	1.6	3.8	8.8	11.3	10.0	17.0	19.4	M	Tuberculosis	010–018, 137
0.2	–	0.2	1.0	0.8	2.3	3.1	3.5	5.1	9.0	F		
0.6	1.1	1.7	2.5	2.6	2.9	4.0	10.0	8.5	11.6	M	Other infective	Rest of 001–139
0.7	0.2	1.5	2.2	2.0	3.6	3.3	4.5	7.4	12.2	F	and parasitic	
29.1	52.2	135.8	239.8	432.2	629.9	957.5	1214.1	1665.4	1794.6	M	ALL CANCER	140–208
37.5	52.7	105.1	168.5	262.9	370.2	525.0	629.6	893.3	1059.0	F		
1.3	3.8	13.1	18.0	16.2	19.3	15.4	12.8	25.5	30.4	M	Mouth and	140–149
0.2	0.5	1.5	1.1	2.8	2.7	3.1	2.4	6.5	11.7	F	pharynx cancer	
0.3	1.8	7.5	10.3	14.7	17.4	19.0	20.7	23.5	34.9	M	Oesophagus cancer	150
0.2	0.2	0.2	0.2	1.4	1.1	2.4	3.5	6.5	8.5	F		
3.1	3.6	9.3	21.3	40.3	53.0	103.6	139.9	197.4	251.3	M	Stomach cancer	151
2.3	3.2	7.4	8.2	12.4	27.4	44.8	65.7	107.0	128.7	F		
2.3	6.8	12.8	23.0	42.2	65.8	111.7	159.9	219.6	273.3	M	Colorectal cancer	153, 154
2.0	4.6	9.3	17.5	26.4	47.2	84.9	115.7	177.9	221.2	F		
–	0.5	0.4	0.7	1.1	2.7	6.9	5.0	7.8	4.5	M	Liver cancer	155.0
0.2	0.7	0.4	–	1.0	1.5	1.8	0.7	2.8	1.5	F		
1.4	3.4	7.7	10.2	18.8	24.1	40.0	48.5	69.3	63.3	M	Pancreas cancer	157
1.2	0.9	3.4	4.8	9.3	15.0	26.3	36.3	51.2	60.2	F		
0.5	1.1	4.3	4.8	7.7	11.2	9.3	7.9	13.1	23.9	M	Larynx cancer	161
–	–	–	0.2	0.8	0.6	0.2	1.7	0.6	1.2	F		
3.5	10.8	36.7	73.5	160.3	239.5	321.6	384.0	449.7	337.2	M	Lung cancer	162
1.3	2.5	7.1	11.1	21.5	25.3	37.5	40.9	52.4	45.7	F		
1.0	0.9	1.7	3.0	5.8	4.8	5.3	5.0	8.5	7.8	M	Malignant melanoma	172
2.3	0.9	2.3	2.2	2.4	2.5	2.9	3.5	6.0	9.5	F		
9.5	16.6	31.1	43.8	59.5	66.2	71.3	88.4	99.9	129.2	F	Female breast cancer	174
6.7	5.5	7.6	10.9	16.1	17.7	20.1	22.7	26.5	28.2	F	Cervix cancer	180
1.2	0.7	1.5	4.0	10.0	15.8	23.2	26.2	33.6	43.0	F	Other uterine cancer	179, 182
1.0	4.6	8.0	18.3	24.6	32.3	43.0	34.6	45.0	45.5	F	Ovarian cancer	183
–	0.5	0.6	2.1	6.6	20.6	58.3	110.6	214.4	292.0	M	Prostate cancer	185
–	0.5	1.9	5.2	13.4	21.4	47.3	57.1	115.0	120.2	M	Bladder cancer	188
–	–	0.6	1.0	2.2	4.8	10.1	11.2	22.2	31.5	F		
10.0	13.3	29.4	50.7	85.1	115.1	153.7	197.0	227.5	266.8	M	Other and ill-defined	Rest of 140–208
6.5	7.4	20.8	34.1	57.5	82.6	116.9	135.6	200.1	239.4	F	cancer sites	
1.3	0.9	1.9	1.6	2.1	2.4	4.0	4.3	5.2	5.2	M	Hodgkin's disease	201
0.3	0.5	0.2	1.3	0.6	1.1	2.6	3.5	4.6	3.2	F		
1.9	1.8	3.3	7.9	9.0	16.9	28.7	26.4	35.9	32.3	M	Myeloma and non-	200, 202–203
0.2	0.7	1.0	4.8	7.7	13.5	17.0	18.5	25.6	21.7	F	Hodgkin lymphomas	
2.6	2.5	5.2	7.5	9.0	15.8	32.8	35.0	52.9	51.7	M	Leukaemia	204–208
2.3	3.0	2.7	5.0	6.5	12.9	17.0	18.5	25.0	28.7	F		
57.1	89.0	181.8	316.7	606.8	1013.9	1871.0	2960.7	5773.2	12096.9	M	ALL VASCULAR	390–459
19.4	35.4	61.1	99.6	216.0	458.1	957.2	1799.8	4036.1	10205.2	F	DISEASE	
0.2	0.5	1.9	3.4	8.1	12.3	10.1	10.7	9.8	6.5	M	Rheumatic heart	390–398
0.2	1.2	1.1	2.7	6.1	10.8	15.9	15.4	13.7	15.2	F	disease and fever	
4.7	8.8	21.3	39.5	69.7	124.2	203.1	319.8	517.0	771.3	M	Hypertensive disease	401–405
1.5	5.3	8.8	19.4	37.4	70.2	157.7	262.4	513.1	984.0	F		
25.3	42.2	84.6	151.5	310.2	483.5	847.1	1233.4	2058.8	3413.4	M	Ischaemic heart	410–414
3.8	7.4	15.8	27.3	67.9	155.2	312.2	558.4	1137.2	2418.4	F	disease	
2.1	4.5	6.2	10.3	15.6	30.0	43.7	62.1	74.5	91.1	M	Pulmonary embolism	415.1, 451–453
1.0	4.6	7.4	8.0	11.4	19.4	33.3	41.6	64.3	83.7	F	and other venous	
4.5	7.5	19.5	29.2	58.2	102.8	234.6	434.7	1014.4	2324.3	M	Cerebrovascular	430–438
5.5	7.2	11.1	14.5	32.3	75.7	163.5	363.0	844.3	2134.2	F	disease	
20.4	25.5	48.3	82.7	145.0	261.2	532.4	900.1	2098.7	5490.3	M	Other vascular	Rest of 390–459
7.4	9.7	16.8	27.6	61.0	126.9	274.7	559.0	1463.6	4569.6	F	disease	
2.3	3.8	7.5	16.7	47.8	88.3	173.9	263.4	451.6	759.7	M	Chronic obstructive	490–496
1.2	0.7	3.1	5.6	12.6	24.0	39.7	48.9	83.4	167.0	F	pulmonary disease	
6.8	8.6	16.2	22.8	45.6	67.2	112.9	174.9	389.5	886.3	M	Other respiratory	Rest of 460–519
3.0	3.9	5.5	7.5	12.4	27.8	53.4	90.5	195.5	568.1	F	disease	
2.7	5.2	5.8	9.0	16.4	19.3	24.3	40.0	54.2	100.8	M	Peptic ulcer	531–533
0.2	0.2	1.7	2.4	6.1	5.9	11.3	13.6	31.0	66.0	F		
27.2	35.0	58.0	78.4	92.3	99.8	91.8	75.7	75.2	76.9	M	Liver cirrhosis	571
8.4	12.5	18.5	22.6	35.8	35.0	34.6	24.8	30.4	32.7	F		
2.4	4.7	4.8	10.8	14.9	19.8	40.0	49.3	92.8	172.5	M	Renal disease	580–590
1.5	1.4	4.2	6.1	14.4	23.0	30.4	46.1	73.1	78.5	F		
0.2	0.2	–	–	–	–	–	–	–	–	F	Pregnancy and birth	630–676
1.3	1.4	1.5	1.1	1.5	4.0	1.2	1.4	2.6	0.6	M	Congenital and	740–779
0.3	1.6	1.1	1.1	1.0	2.5	1.8	1.4	1.7	1.7	F	perinatal causes	
23.8	26.4	40.6	52.3	59.9	72.5	110.0	121.3	207.8	408.3	M	Ill-defined causes	780–799
6.9	9.9	13.7	18.1	23.6	33.5	52.7	78.6	140.9	349.2	F		
47.3	61.9	95.8	121.2	152.5	192.9	298.5	407.6	668.0	1082.0	M	Other medical causes	Rest of 001–799
18.7	24.7	33.8	54.1	87.0	143.4	223.7	340.0	557.2	965.8	F		
99.2	104.3	134.1	141.4	145.0	111.6	121.4	154.2	278.4	578.2	M	ALL NON-	E800–E999
23.8	29.1	43.9	45.1	46.9	57.1	64.9	103.8	194.1	501.6	F	MEDICAL CAUSES	
24.9	21.9	22.6	28.0	29.0	26.0	16.2	27.1	43.8	62.0	M	Motor vehicle	E810–E819
7.7	8.3	8.4	9.8	8.3	11.2	12.1	12.6	25.3	34.5	F	traffic accidents	
1.8	2.5	1.7	1.8	3.0	1.9	2.8	2.1	3.9	11.0	M	Fire	E890–E899
0.5	0.7	1.1	0.6	0.6	1.1	1.3	2.8	3.1	5.0	F		
35.5	40.2	52.0	61.2	64.6	42.0	51.0	62.1	117.6	205.4	M	Suicide	E950–E959
7.5	10.9	18.3	19.0	19.1	21.3	26.5	31.8	46.1	62.0	F		
1.9	2.5	2.5	2.1	1.3	1.1	0.4	0.7	1.3	1.3	M	Homicide	E960–E969
1.2	0.9	1.0	0.6	1.8	–	0.4	1.7	0.6	1.2	F		
621.7	442.9	517.6	609.7	469.0	373.7	247.2	140.1	153.0	154.8	M	**POPULATION (thousands)**	
597.6	432.8	524.1	622.6	492.2	474.3	453.3	286.2	351.4	400.1	F		

Former GERMAN DEMOCRATIC REPUBLIC: Males

	All ages	0–34	35–69	35–39	40–44	45–49	50–54	55–59	60–64	65–69	70–74	75–79	80+/NK
POPULATION (1000s)													
1955	8018.0	4214.5	3253.5	277.9	465.4	578.7	625.2	524.1	417.6	364.6	267.1	179.0	103.9
1965	7762.1	4341.2	2849.1	458.0	357.9	241.0	406.3	495.1	508.5	382.3	260.2	178.8	132.8
1975	7823.1	4269.7	2920.3	659.3	528.2	444.6	339.7	221.2	349.5	377.8	320.4	184.9	127.8
1985	7870.2	4302.3	2998.1	447.8	562.8	629.5	493.4	402.1	290.5	172.0	229.1	190.6	150.1
1990	**7693.7**	**3964.0**	**3281.8**	**621.7**	**442.9**	**517.6**	**609.7**	**469.0**	**373.7**	**247.2**	**140.1**	**153.0**	**154.8**
1995 projected	*7830.7*	*3906.8*	*3499.2*	*635.6*	*620.1*	*422.6*	*522.5*	*565.3*	*418.9*	*314.2*	*197.1*	*90.5*	*137.1*
NUMBER OF DEATHS													
All causes													
1955	104841	13754	41301	626	1670	3119	5581	7719	9540	13046	15213	16560	18013
1965	111130	8949	42007	996	1156	1187	3411	7204	12574	15479	16341	17794	26039
1975	110117	5944	35754	1428	1941	2427	2984	3114	8422	15438	22033	20164	26222
1985	99370	5477	29826	952	1922	3510	4613	5822	6718	6289	14405	19968	29694
1990	**94654**	**5216**	**39095**	**1868**	**1744**	**3545**	**6185**	**7604**	**8711**	**9438**	**7681**	**14817**	**27845**
1995 projected	*92545*	*5723*	*46018*	*2394*	*3029*	*3301*	*5987*	*9694*	*10231*	*11382*	*10045*	*7940*	*22819*
Lung cancer													
1955	...	...	...	...	...	...	...	...	...	...	...	...	...
1965	...	...	...	...	...	...	...	...	...	...	...	...	...
1975	5850	10	3125	42	84	187	281	300	869	1362	1507	844	364
1985	5215	10	2730	12	100	259	471	676	662	550	974	898	603
1990	**4907**	**9**	**3150**	**22**	**48**	**190**	**448**	**752**	**895**	**795**	**538**	**688**	**522**
1995 projected	*4930*	*12*	*3419*	*17*	*59*	*125*	*350*	*880*	*1012*	*976*	*714*	*368*	*417*
ANNUAL DEATH RATE / 100,000 (*The rates for the age groups 0–34 and 35–69 are the means of seven five-yearly rates, but the all-ages rates are standardised to the conventional "European" age distribution)													
All causes													
1955	1348.5*	297.7*	1335.9*	225.3	358.8	539.0	892.7	1472.8	2284.5	3578.2	5695.6	9251.4	17336.9
1965	1385.1*	193.6*	1407.0*	217.5	323.0	492.5	839.5	1455.1	2472.8	4048.9	6280.2	9951.9	19607.7
1975	1420.5*	148.6*	1416.0*	216.6	367.5	545.9	878.4	1407.8	2409.7	4086.3	6876.7	10905.4	20518.0
1985	1349.1*	123.6*	1351.9*	212.6	341.5	557.6	934.9	1447.9	2312.6	3656.4	6287.6	10476.4	19782.8
1990	**1317.5***	**129.7***	**1452.0***	**300.5**	**393.8**	**684.9**	**1014.4**	**1621.3**	**2331.0**	**3818.0**	**5482.5**	**9684.3**	**17987.7**
1995 projected	*1297.6**	*141.8**	*1510.3**	*376.7*	*488.5*	*781.1*	*1145.8*	*1714.8*	*2442.3*	*3622.5*	*5096.4*	*8773.5*	*16644.1*
All cancer													
1955	...	...	...	...	...	...	...	...	...	...	...	...	...
1965	...	...	...	...	...	...	...	...	...	...	...	...	...
1975	237.4*	11.7*	356.3*	34.4	71.8	132.5	229.3	384.3	670.7	971.1	1375.5	1591.7	1512.5
1985	244.2*	9.8*	356.1*	28.4	72.9	138.7	265.7	433.2	631.0	922.7	1342.2	1671.6	1786.8
1990	**237.1***	**7.5***	**353.8***	**29.1**	**52.2**	**135.8**	**239.8**	**432.2**	**629.9**	**957.5**	**1214.1**	**1665.4**	**1794.6**
1995 projected	*232.0**	*6.1**	*348.2**	*25.2*	*50.6*	*129.0*	*240.2*	*428.1*	*643.1*	*921.1*	*1175.0*	*1585.6*	*1811.1*
Lung cancer													
1955	...	...	...	...	...	...	...	...	...	...	...	...	...
1965	...	...	...	...	...	...	...	...	...	...	...	...	...
1975	74.3*	0.3*	127.4*	6.4	15.9	42.1	82.7	135.6	248.6	360.5	470.3	456.5	284.8
1985	75.6*	0.2*	124.7*	2.7	17.8	41.1	95.5	168.1	227.9	319.8	425.1	471.1	401.7
1990	**70.5***	**0.2***	**120.9***	**3.5**	**10.8**	**36.7**	**73.5**	**160.3**	**239.5**	**321.6**	**384.0**	**449.7**	**337.2**
1995 projected	*66.7**	*0.3**	*116.7**	*2.7*	*9.5*	*29.6*	*67.0*	*155.7*	*241.6*	*310.6*	*362.3*	*406.6*	*304.2*
Upper aerodigestive cancer (mouth, oesophagus, pharynx and larynx)													
1955	...	...	...	...	...	...	...	...	...	...	...	...	...
1965	...	...	...	...	...	...	...	...	...	...	...	...	...
1975	10.6*	0.1*	17.1*	1.2	5.1	10.6	12.7	19.0	26.9	44.2	55.9	66.0	61.8
1985	14.0*	0.2*	23.5*	0.9	6.0	17.6	30.4	37.1	30.6	41.9	58.9	64.0	78.6
1990	**15.5***	**0.1***	**28.2***	**2.1**	**6.8**	**24.9**	**33.1**	**38.6**	**47.9**	**43.7**	**41.4**	**62.1**	**89.1**
1995 projected	*17.4**	*0.1**	*32.9**	*2.8*	*9.8*	*30.8*	*38.7*	*47.4*	*57.1*	*43.9*	*36.5*	*57.5*	*94.1*
Other cancer													
1955	...	...	...	...	...	...	...	...	...	...	...	...	...
1965	...	...	...	...	...	...	...	...	...	...	...	...	...
1975	152.4*	11.3*	211.8*	26.8	50.7	79.8	133.9	229.7	395.1	566.4	849.3	1069.2	1165.9
1985	154.6*	9.5*	207.9*	24.8	49.0	79.9	139.8	228.1	372.5	561.0	858.1	1136.4	1306.5
1990	**151.1***	**7.2***	**204.8***	**23.5**	**34.5**	**74.2**	**133.2**	**233.3**	**342.5**	**592.2**	**788.7**	**1153.6**	**1368.2**
1995 projected	*148.0**	*5.7**	*198.6**	*19.7*	*31.3*	*68.6*	*134.5*	*225.0*	*344.5*	*566.5*	*776.3*	*1121.5*	*1412.8*
Chronic obstructive pulmonary disease (COPD)													
1955	...	...	...	...	...	...	...	...	...	...	...	...	...
1965	...	...	...	...	...	...	...	...	...	...	...	...	...
1975	104.3*	0.6*	104.2*	2.7	7.8	23.2	46.8	82.3	182.5	383.8	683.5	1026.5	1397.5
1985	69.8*	0.5*	59.7*	0.7	4.8	9.5	23.3	51.0	123.2	205.2	433.9	707.8	1114.6
1990	**48.7***	**0.4***	**48.6***	**2.3**	**3.8**	**7.5**	**16.7**	**47.8**	**88.3**	**173.9**	**263.4**	**451.6**	**759.7**
1995 projected	*35.4**	*0.3**	*36.9**	*2.7*	*3.7*	*5.7*	*14.7*	*37.1*	*72.1*	*122.2*	*184.7*	*316.0*	*537.6*
Other respiratory disease													
1955	...	...	...	...	...	...	...	...	...	...	...	...	...
1965	...	...	...	...	...	...	...	...	...	...	...	...	...
1975	35.5*	5.8*	28.0*	4.6	10.4	9.9	16.2	27.1	44.1	83.6	144.5	292.6	605.6
1985	41.1*	3.7*	34.6*	6.5	8.2	12.9	21.3	40.5	59.6	93.0	165.9	339.5	742.2
1990	**46.7***	**3.0***	**40.0***	**6.8**	**8.6**	**16.2**	**22.8**	**45.6**	**67.2**	**112.9**	**174.9**	**389.5**	**886.3**
1995 projected	*53.3**	*2.7**	*45.5**	*7.9*	*10.3*	*18.7*	*26.6*	*51.3*	*78.5*	*125.1*	*196.3*	*430.9*	*1046.0*
Vascular disease													
1955	...	...	...	...	...	...	...	...	...	...	...	...	...
1965	...	...	...	...	...	...	...	...	...	...	...	...	...
1975	723.5*	4.8*	594.7*	35.2	89.9	175.9	335.3	553.3	1022.6	1950.5	3647.9	6407.8	13829.4
1985	709.2*	6.2*	582.0*	30.1	72.1	153.9	320.2	567.3	1070.9	1859.3	3439.5	6314.8	13716.2
1990	**657.9***	**9.3***	**590.9***	**57.1**	**89.0**	**181.8**	**316.7**	**606.8**	**1013.9**	**1871.0**	**2960.7**	**5773.2**	**12096.9**
1995 projected	*612.4**	*12.9**	*582.3**	*85.4*	*120.0*	*201.1*	*344.9*	*604.8*	*1012.7*	*1707.5*	*2682.9*	*5090.6*	*10793.6*
Liver cirrhosis													
1955	...	...	...	...	...	...	...	...	...	...	...	...	...
1965	...	...	...	...	...	...	...	...	...	...	...	...	...
1975	16.9*	0.8*	31.1*	5.6	12.7	16.4	20.6	38.4	51.5	72.3	63.4	76.3	75.1
1985	23.3*	1.2*	44.4*	10.3	20.4	32.6	47.6	54.5	66.1	79.7	70.3	87.6	68.6
1990	**34.9***	**2.9***	**68.9***	**27.2**	**35.0**	**58.0**	**78.4**	**92.3**	**99.8**	**91.8**	**75.7**	**75.2**	**76.9**
1995 projected	*47.2**	*4.4**	*96.7**	*40.6*	*52.2*	*84.2*	*113.7*	*131.6*	*141.3*	*113.0*	*76.6*	*71.8*	*74.4*
Other medical causes													
1955	...	...	...	...	...	...	...	...	...	...	...	...	...
1965	...	...	...	...	...	...	...	...	...	...	...	...	...
1975	195.1*	61.4*	182.4*	36.6	65.5	89.1	122.5	198.9	301.9	462.7	744.4	1181.2	2413.9
1985	212.4*	68.4*	225.8*	94.2	115.1	157.3	204.1	249.9	311.2	448.8	763.4	1237.1	2031.3
1990	**187.4***	**44.9***	**227.3***	**78.8**	**100.9**	**151.5**	**198.6**	**251.6**	**320.3**	**489.5**	**639.5**	**1051.0**	**1795.2**
1995 projected	*168.8**	*31.4**	*223.7**	*66.6*	*96.1*	*147.4*	*200.6*	*255.3*	*336.8*	*463.1*	*564.7*	*889.5*	*1563.8*
All non-medical causes													
1955	...	...	...	...	...	...	...	...	...	...	...	...	...
1965	...	...	...	...	...	...	...	...	...	...	...	...	...
1975	107.9*	63.5*	119.4*	97.5	109.4	99.0	107.7	123.4	136.5	162.3	217.5	329.4	683.9
1985	49.0*	33.7*	49.4*	42.4	48.0	52.7	52.7	51.5	50.6	47.7	72.5	118.0	323.1
1990	**104.9***	**61.6***	**122.4***	**99.2**	**104.3**	**134.1**	**141.4**	**145.0**	**111.6**	**121.4**	**154.2**	**278.4**	**578.2**
1995 projected	*148.5**	*84.1**	*177.0**	*148.4*	*155.5*	*195.0*	*205.2*	*206.6*	*157.8*	*170.6*	*216.1*	*389.0*	*817.7*

Former GERMAN DEMOCRATIC REPUBLIC: Females

	All ages	0–34	35–69	35–39	40–44	45–49	50–54	55–59	60–64	65–69	70–74	75–79	80+/NK
POPULATION (1000s)													
1955	9926.0	4504.4	4654.5	455.9	736.0	817.7	781.9	720.5	622.2	520.3	368.7	245.0	153.4
1965	9257.5	4196.0	4102.3	540.7	571.2	394.4	648.7	713.6	662.5	571.2	441.4	298.6	219.2
1975	9027.2	4089.4	3809.6	651.1	524.2	529.3	550.3	372.2	584.8	597.7	496.4	351.0	280.8
1985	8774.0	4107.5	3470.0	439.6	566.0	635.1	506.1	501.7	502.9	318.6	455.0	389.9	351.6
1990	8417.2	3782.6	3596.9	597.6	432.8	524.1	622.6	492.2	474.3	453.3	286.2	351.4	400.1
1995 projected	8388.0	3727.9	3669.0	612.4	603.4	420.8	539.2	596.3	460.9	436.0	401.5	213.7	375.9
NUMBER OF DEATHS													
All causes													
1955	109222	10524	38375	902	2155	3127	4521	6186	8803	12681	16331	19872	24120
1965	119128	5701	34776	842	1376	1379	3416	5763	8772	13228	18634	23116	36901
1975	130272	3216	30247	816	1055	1641	2777	2870	7610	13478	20841	27161	48807
1985	125983	2759	21924	508	998	1768	2353	3592	6303	6402	17199	26888	57213
1990	113456	2336	23966	728	747	1538	2703	3551	5628	9071	9116	21960	56078
1995 projected	94670	2191	22781	767	1075	1208	2325	4138	5373	7895	11529	11538	46631
Lung cancer													
1955	...	...	...	...	...	...	...	...	...	...	...	...	...
1965	...	...	...	...	...	...	...	...	...	...	...	...	...
1975	817	1	429	6	17	24	46	42	134	160	167	139	81
1985	959	7	437	7	18	32	62	99	122	97	201	171	143
1990	1011	6	521	8	11	37	69	106	120	170	117	184	183
1995 projected	1056	6	549	7	17	29	64	131	131	170	179	122	200
ANNUAL DEATH RATE / 100,000 (*The rates for the age groups 0–34 and 35–69 are the means of seven five-yearly rates, but the all-ages rates are standardised to the conventional "European" age distribution)													
All causes													
1955	1051.8*	225.3*	880.3*	197.9	292.8	382.4	578.2	858.6	1414.8	2437.2	4429.3	8111.0	15723.6
1965	981.3*	125.9*	817.2*	155.7	240.9	349.6	526.6	807.6	1324.1	2315.8	4221.6	7741.5	16834.4
1975	955.1*	86.4*	781.2*	125.3	201.3	310.0	504.6	771.1	1301.3	2255.0	4198.4	7738.2	17381.4
1985	869.8*	66.4*	716.3*	115.6	176.3	278.4	464.9	716.0	1253.3	2009.4	3780.0	6896.1	16272.2
1990	787.0*	62.2*	704.5*	121.8	172.6	293.5	434.1	721.5	1186.6	2001.1	3185.2	6249.3	14016.0
1995 projected	715.9*	58.5*	670.3*	125.2	178.2	287.1	431.2	693.9	1165.8	1810.8	2871.5	5399.2	12405.2
All cancer													
1955	...	...	...	...	...	...	...	...	...	...	...	...	...
1965	...	...	...	...	...	...	...	...	...	...	...	...	...
1975	152.1*	9.2*	238.0*	40.4	84.3	128.1	211.5	284.5	401.2	516.0	690.4	882.3	945.5
1985	148.6*	7.9*	223.6*	44.1	69.1	108.6	176.6	267.9	402.9	495.6	724.8	907.7	1042.4
1990	142.0*	6.7*	217.4*	37.5	52.7	105.1	168.5	262.9	370.2	525.0	629.6	893.3	1059.0
1995 projected	135.2*	5.7*	205.5*	31.4	46.4	94.8	163.2	247.0	365.6	490.4	599.8	849.3	1060.4
Lung cancer													
1955	...	...	...	...	...	...	...	...	...	...	...	...	...
1965	...	...	...	...	...	...	...	...	...	...	...	...	...
1975	6.5*	0.0*	11.1*	0.9	3.2	4.5	8.4	11.3	22.9	26.8	33.6	39.6	28.8
1985	8.3*	0.2*	13.8*	1.6	3.2	5.0	12.3	19.7	24.3	30.4	44.2	43.9	40.7
1990	8.9*	0.1*	15.2*	1.3	2.5	7.1	11.1	21.5	25.3	37.5	40.9	52.4	45.7
1995 projected	9.5*	0.2*	16.0*	1.1	2.8	6.9	11.9	22.0	28.4	39.0	44.6	57.1	53.2
Upper aerodigestive cancer (mouth, oesophagus, pharynx and larynx)													
1955	...	...	...	...	...	...	...	...	...	...	...	...	...
1965	...	...	...	...	...	...	...	...	...	...	...	...	...
1975	1.8*	0.1*	2.3*	0.2	1.1	1.1	1.8	3.2	2.9	5.7	10.7	12.5	18.9
1985	2.4*	0.1*	3.6*	0.5	0.7	1.3	3.0	6.2	6.4	7.5	9.2	11.3	21.3
1990	2.0*	0.0*	2.8*	0.3	0.7	1.7	1.4	5.1	4.4	5.7	7.7	13.7	21.5
1995 projected	1.8*	0.0*	2.1*	0.3	0.8	1.4	1.1	3.5	3.3	4.4	7.2	14.0	23.1
Other cancer													
1955	...	...	...	...	...	...	...	...	...	...	...	...	...
1965	...	...	...	...	...	...	...	...	...	...	...	...	...
1975	143.8*	9.1*	224.6*	39.3	79.9	122.4	201.3	270.0	375.3	483.5	646.1	830.2	897.8
1985	138.0*	7.6*	206.1*	42.1	65.2	102.3	161.4	242.0	372.2	457.6	671.4	852.5	980.4
1990	131.1*	6.5*	199.5*	35.8	49.4	96.4	156.0	236.3	340.5	481.8	581.1	827.3	991.8
1995 projected	123.9*	5.5*	187.4*	29.9	42.8	86.5	150.2	221.5	333.9	447.0	547.9	778.2	984.0
Chronic obstructive pulmonary disease (COPD)													
1955	...	...	...	...	...	...	...	...	...	...	...	...	...
1965	...	...	...	...	...	...	...	...	...	...	...	...	...
1975	25.3*	0.6*	19.7*	1.7	2.3	5.9	11.1	20.2	31.8	65.1	129.7	235.0	477.9
1985	15.4*	0.4*	15.1*	2.0	2.1	4.9	6.7	16.1	27.8	45.8	71.0	124.1	266.5
1990	10.9*	0.3*	12.4*	1.2	0.7	3.1	5.6	12.6	24.0	39.7	48.9	83.4	167.0
1995 projected	8.1*	0.2*	9.9*	0.8	0.5	2.1	4.3	10.4	20.2	30.7	34.6	58.0	118.1
Other respiratory disease													
1955	...	...	...	...	...	...	...	...	...	...	...	...	...
1965	...	...	...	...	...	...	...	...	...	...	...	...	...
1975	22.9*	3.9*	16.7*	3.1	4.0	7.6	10.2	16.4	27.4	48.7	91.3	183.5	416.0
1985	23.9*	2.6*	14.4*	2.7	3.7	6.5	10.1	12.2	22.1	43.6	81.3	183.4	561.4
1990	24.8*	2.2*	16.2*	3.0	3.9	5.5	7.5	12.4	27.8	53.4	90.5	195.5	568.1
1995 projected	25.8*	2.0*	18.0*	2.9	3.8	4.5	6.7	13.2	33.2	61.9	98.4	198.4	582.3
Vascular disease													
1955	...	...	...	...	...	...	...	...	...	...	...	...	...
1965	...	...	...	...	...	...	...	...	...	...	...	...	...
1975	542.6*	3.7*	303.7*	17.2	28.4	57.1	116.1	225.4	515.0	1166.8	2506.2	5237.0	12976.5
1985	504.0*	4.2*	274.8*	16.6	28.3	53.2	113.2	213.7	493.1	1005.3	2233.6	4648.6	12470.1
1990	430.3*	4.5*	263.8*	19.4	35.4	61.1	99.6	216.0	458.1	957.2	1799.8	4036.1	10205.2
1995 projected	365.6*	4.9*	239.6*	23.4	41.6	60.1	98.3	202.2	433.3	818.3	1532.5	3263.0	8489.5
Liver cirrhosis													
1955	...	...	...	...	...	...	...	...	...	...	...	...	...
1965	...	...	...	...	...	...	...	...	...	...	...	...	...
1975	6.7*	0.3*	9.8*	1.8	3.1	5.3	10.2	7.8	17.1	23.4	34.0	42.5	48.4
1985	9.0*	0.3*	16.2*	2.3	6.2	11.5	17.8	21.9	28.6	25.1	30.5	39.8	39.8
1990	12.2*	1.1*	23.9*	8.4	12.5	18.5	22.6	35.8	35.0	34.6	24.8	30.4	32.7
1995 projected	15.4*	1.5*	31.8*	12.1	17.6	25.7	31.9	48.5	48.4	38.5	23.2	23.4	25.8
Other medical causes													
1955	...	...	...	...	...	...	...	...	...	...	...	...	...
1965	...	...	...	...	...	...	...	...	...	...	...	...	...
1975	148.9*	49.0*	139.7*	31.2	43.9	69.5	94.9	156.6	232.2	349.7	584.2	876.1	1779.6
1985	145.0*	41.1*	153.6*	37.8	55.3	80.8	124.3	165.8	255.5	355.9	578.5	861.5	1538.7
1990	122.1*	28.3*	126.3*	28.6	38.4	56.3	85.1	134.9	214.2	326.3	487.8	816.4	1482.4
1995 projected	104.2*	20.0*	103.0*	20.6	27.2	39.0	63.2	106.7	184.9	279.8	437.9	736.5	1419.8
All non-medical causes													
1955	...	...	...	...	...	...	...	...	...	...	...	...	...
1965	...	...	...	...	...	...	...	...	...	...	...	...	...
1975	56.7*	19.7*	53.5*	29.9	35.3	36.7	50.7	60.2	76.6	85.3	162.6	281.8	737.5
1985	22.3*	10.0*	18.6*	10.0	11.7	12.9	16.2	18.3	23.3	38.0	60.2	131.1	353.2
1990	44.8*	19.1*	44.4*	23.8	29.1	43.9	45.1	46.9	57.1	64.9	103.8	194.1	501.6
1995 projected	61.6*	24.3*	62.4*	34.1	41.1	60.8	63.6	65.9	80.3	91.1	145.2	270.5	709.2

Former GERMAN DEMOCRATIC REPUBLIC: 1975

Smoking-attributed deaths (Sm.) and total deaths (Total)

		ALL CAUSES	ALL CANCER	Lung cancer	Upper aero-digestive ca.	Other cancer	COPD	Other respiratory	Vascular disease	Liver cirrhosis	Other medical	Non-medical
Males												
0–34	Sm.	–	–	–	–	–	–	–	–	–	–	–
	Total	5944	489	10	5	474	23	223	197	31	2290	2691
35–69	Sm.	12025	4101	2915	287	899	2052	212	4253	–	1407	–
	Total	35754	8837	3125	428	5284	2591	714	14795	785	4642	3390
		(34%)	(46%)	(93%)	(67%)	(17%)	(79%)	(30%)	(29%)		(30%)	
70+	Sm.	13991	3496	2471	226	799	4267	213	5052	–	963	–
	Total	68419	9283	2715	380	6188	5874	1778	41210	440	7654	2180
		(20%)	(38%)	(91%)	(59%)	(13%)	(73%)	(12%)	(12%)		(13%)	
Any age	Sm.	26016	7597	5386	513	1698	6319	425	9305	–	2370	–
	Total	110117	18609	5850	813	11946	8488	2715	56202	1256	14586	8261
		(24%)	(41%)	(92%)	(63%)	(14%)	(74%)	(16%)	(17%)		(16%)	
Females												
0–34	Sm.	–	–	–	–	–	–	–	–	–	–	–
	Total	3216	366	1	3	362	25	144	144	12	1742	783
35–69	Sm.	552	109	87	4	18	99	11	238	–	95	–
	Total	30247	9036	429	86	8521	765	649	12027	381	5354	2035
		(2%)	(1%)	(20%)	(5%)	(0%)	(13%)	(2%)	(2%)		(2%)	
70+	Sm.	570	73	54	6	13	203	8	240	–	46	–
	Total	96809	9179	387	150	8642	2811	2265	67261	454	10972	3867
		(1%)	(1%)	(14%)	(4%)	(0%)	(7%)	(0%)	(0%)		(0%)	
Any age	Sm.	1122	182	141	10	31	302	19	478	–	141	–
	Total	130272	18581	817	239	17525	3601	3058	79432	847	18068	6685
		(1%)	(1%)	(17%)	(4%)	(0%)	(8%)	(1%)	(1%)		(1%)	
Males+Females												
0–34	Sm.	–	–	–	–	–	–	–	–	–	–	–
	Total	9160	855	11	8	836	48	367	341	43	4032	3474
35–69	Sm.	12577	4210	3002	291	917	2151	223	4491	–	1502	–
	Total	66001	17873	3554	514	13805	3356	1363	26822	1166	9996	5425
		(19%)	(24%)	(84%)	(57%)	(7%)	(64%)	(16%)	(17%)		(15%)	
70+	Sm.	14561	3569	2525	232	812	4470	221	5292	–	1009	–
	Total	165228	18462	3102	530	14830	8685	4043	108471	894	18626	6047
		(9%)	(19%)	(81%)	(44%)	(5%)	(51%)	(5%)	(5%)		(5%)	
Any age	Sm.	27138	7779	5527	523	1729	6621	444	9783	–	2511	–
	Total	240389	37190	6667	1052	29471	12089	5773	135634	2103	32654	14946
		(11%)	(21%)	(83%)	(50%)	(6%)	(55%)	(8%)	(7%)		(8%)	

Former GERMAN DEMOCRATIC REPUBLIC: 1985

Smoking-attributed deaths (Sm.) and total deaths (Total)

		ALL CAUSES	ALL CANCER	Lung cancer	Upper aero-digestive ca.	Other cancer	COPD	Other respiratory	Vascular disease	Liver cirrhosis	Other medical	Non-medical
Males												
0–34	Sm.	–	–	–	–	–	–	–	–	–	–	–
	Total	5477	441	10	7	424	24	159	282	55	2986	1530
35–69	Sm.	10663	3755	2549	417	789	884	252	3721	–	2051	–
	Total	29826	7883	2730	609	4544	1121	757	11680	1149	5748	1488
		(36%)	(48%)	(93%)	(68%)	(17%)	(79%)	(33%)	(32%)		(36%)	
70+	Sm.	11687	3206	2239	218	749	2888	236	4525	–	832	–
	Total	64067	8943	2475	375	6093	4016	2141	40504	431	7156	876
		(18%)	(36%)	(90%)	(58%)	(12%)	(72%)	(11%)	(11%)		(12%)	
Any age	Sm.	22350	6961	4788	635	1538	3772	488	8246	–	2883	–
	Total	99370	17267	5215	991	11061	5161	3057	52466	1635	15890	3894
		(22%)	(40%)	(92%)	(64%)	(14%)	(73%)	(16%)	(16%)		(18%)	
Females												
0–34	Sm.	–	–	–	–	–	–	–	–	–	–	–
	Total	2759	333	7	5	321	15	105	182	12	1691	421
35–69	Sm.	804	203	158	14	31	106	18	286	–	191	–
	Total	21924	7118	437	116	6565	453	436	7899	542	4872	604
		(4%)	(3%)	(36%)	(12%)	(0%)	(23%)	(4%)	(4%)		(4%)	
70+	Sm.	1108	179	136	13	30	252	22	546	–	109	–
	Total	101300	10502	515	161	9826	1744	3059	72133	434	11401	2027
		(1%)	(2%)	(26%)	(8%)	(0%)	(14%)	(1%)	(1%)		(1%)	
Any age	Sm.	1912	382	294	27	61	358	40	832	–	300	–
	Total	125983	17953	959	282	16712	2212	3600	80214	988	17964	3052
		(2%)	(2%)	(31%)	(10%)	(0%)	(16%)	(1%)	(1%)		(2%)	
Males+Females												
0–34	Sm.	–	–	–	–	–	–	–	–	–	–	–
	Total	8236	774	17	12	745	39	264	464	67	4677	1951
35–69	Sm.	11467	3958	2707	431	820	990	270	4007	–	2242	–
	Total	51750	15001	3167	725	11109	1574	1193	19579	1691	10620	2092
		(22%)	(26%)	(85%)	(59%)	(7%)	(63%)	(23%)	(20%)		(21%)	
70+	Sm.	12795	3385	2375	231	779	3140	258	5071	–	941	–
	Total	165367	19445	2990	536	15919	5760	5200	112637	865	18557	2903
		(8%)	(17%)	(79%)	(43%)	(5%)	(55%)	(5%)	(5%)		(5%)	
Any age	Sm.	24262	7343	5082	662	1599	4130	528	9078	–	3183	–
	Total	225353	35220	6174	1273	27773	7373	6657	132680	2623	33854	6946
		(11%)	(21%)	(82%)	(52%)	(6%)	(56%)	(8%)	(7%)		(9%)	

(To be conservative, no deaths before age 35, and none from liver cirrhosis or non-medical causes, were attributed to smoking.)

Former GERMAN DEMOCRATIC REPUBLIC: 1990

Smoking–attributed deaths (Sm.) and total deaths (Total)

		ALL CAUSES	ALL CANCER	Lung cancer	Upper aero–digestive ca.	Other cancer	COPD	Other respiratory	Vascular disease	Liver cirrhosis	Other medical	Non–medical
Males												
0–34	Sm.	–	–	–	–	–	–	–	–	–	–	–
	Total	5216	316	9	4	303	14	120	392	131	1755	2488
35–69	Sm.	12190	4357	2928	557	872	905	324	4485	–	2119	–
	Total	39095	9325	3150	842	5333	1156	1047	14881	2135	6519	4032
		(31%)	(47%)	(93%)	(66%)	(16%)	(78%)	(31%)	(30%)		(33%)	
70+	Sm.	7813	2302	1569	164	569	1575	218	3173	–	545	–
	Total	50343	7027	1748	291	4988	2236	2213	31707	340	5283	1537
		(16%)	(33%)	(90%)	(56%)	(11%)	(70%)	(10%)	(10%)		(10%)	
Any age	Sm.	20003	6659	4497	721	1441	2480	542	7658	–	2664	–
	Total	94654	16668	4907	1137	10624	3406	3380	46980	2606	13557	8057
		(21%)	(40%)	(92%)	(63%)	(14%)	(73%)	(16%)	(16%)		(20%)	
Females												
0–34	Sm.	–	–	–	–	–	–	–	–	–	–	–
	Total	2336	268	6	2	260	11	81	176	47	1028	725
35–69	Sm.	1008	265	212	13	40	119	24	400	–	200	–
	Total	23966	7482	521	95	6866	417	546	8784	841	4321	1575
		(4%)	(4%)	(41%)	(14%)	(1%)	(29%)	(4%)	(5%)		(5%)	
70+	Sm.	1212	212	159	18	35	239	33	617	–	111	–
	Total	87154	9178	484	156	8538	1101	3219	60165	309	10196	2986
		(1%)	(2%)	(33%)	(12%)	(0%)	(22%)	(1%)	(1%)		(1%)	
Any age	Sm.	2220	477	371	31	75	358	57	1017	–	311	–
	Total	113456	16928	1011	253	15664	1529	3846	69125	1197	15545	5286
		(2%)	(3%)	(37%)	(12%)	(0%)	(23%)	(1%)	(1%)		(2%)	
Males+Females												
0–34	Sm.	–	–	–	–	–	–	–	–	–	–	–
	Total	7552	584	15	6	563	25	201	568	178	2783	3213
35–69	Sm.	13198	4622	3140	570	912	1024	348	4885	–	2319	–
	Total	63061	16807	3671	937	12199	1573	1593	23665	2976	10840	5607
		(21%)	(28%)	(86%)	(61%)	(7%)	(65%)	(22%)	(21%)		(21%)	
70+	Sm.	9025	2514	1728	182	604	1814	251	3790	–	656	–
	Total	137497	16205	2232	447	13526	3337	5432	91872	649	15479	4523
		(7%)	(16%)	(77%)	(41%)	(4%)	(54%)	(5%)	(4%)		(4%)	
Any age	Sm.	22223	7136	4868	752	1516	2838	599	8675	–	2975	–
	Total	208110	33596	5918	1390	26288	4935	7226	116105	3803	29102	13343
		(11%)	(21%)	(82%)	(54%)	(6%)	(58%)	(8%)	(7%)		(10%)	

¶The acceding part of GERMANY: 1995

Smoking–attributed deaths (Sm.) and total deaths (Total)

		ALL CAUSES	ALL CANCER	Lung cancer	Upper aero–digestive ca.	Other cancer	COPD	Other respiratory	Vascular disease	Liver cirrhosis	Other medical	Non–medical
Males												
0–34	Sm.	–	–	–	–	–	–	–	–	–	–	–
	Total	5723	256	12	5	239	14	110	559	207	1198	3379
35–69	Sm.	13058	4764	3167	685	912	804	395	4939	–	2156	–
	Total	46018	10282	3419	1056	5807	1037	1344	16965	3223	6999	6168
		(28%)	(46%)	(93%)	(65%)	(16%)	(78%)	(29%)	(29%)		(31%)	
70+	Sm.	5950	1950	1336	136	478	950	210	2422	–	418	–
	Total	40804	6234	1499	253	4482	1387	2211	24693	318	4062	1899
		(15%)	(31%)	(89%)	(54%)	(11%)	(68%)	(9%)	(10%)		(10%)	
Any age	Sm.	19008	6714	4503	821	1390	1754	605	7361	–	2574	–
	Total	92545	16772	4930	1314	10528	2438	3665	42217	3748	12259	11446
		(21%)	(40%)	(91%)	(62%)	(13%)	(72%)	(17%)	(17%)		(21%)	
Females												
0–34	Sm.	–	–	–	–	–	–	–	–	–	–	–
	Total	2191	233	6	2	225	8	70	193	66	698	923
35–69	Sm.	1017	292	238	12	42	102	31	410	–	182	–
	Total	22781	7047	549	74	6424	329	598	7948	1140	3503	2216
		(4%)	(4%)	(43%)	(16%)	(1%)	(31%)	(5%)	(5%)		(5%)	
70+	Sm.	1240	255	194	20	41	187	42	626	–	130	–
	Total	69698	8209	501	146	7562	707	3008	45038	240	8669	3827
		(2%)	(3%)	(39%)	(14%)	(1%)	(26%)	(1%)	(1%)		(1%)	
Any age	Sm.	2257	547	432	32	83	289	73	1036	–	312	–
	Total	94670	15489	1056	222	14211	1044	3676	53179	1446	12870	6966
		(2%)	(4%)	(41%)	(14%)	(1%)	(28%)	(2%)	(2%)		(2%)	
Males+Females												
0–34	Sm.	–	–	–	–	–	–	–	–	–	–	–
	Total	7914	489	18	7	464	22	180	752	273	1896	4302
35–69	Sm.	14075	5056	3405	697	954	906	426	5349	–	2338	–
	Total	68799	17329	3968	1130	12231	1366	1942	24913	4363	10502	8384
		(20%)	(29%)	(86%)	(62%)	(8%)	(66%)	(22%)	(21%)		(22%)	
70+	Sm.	7190	2205	1530	156	519	1137	252	3048	–	548	–
	Total	110502	14443	2000	399	12044	2094	5219	69731	558	12731	5726
		(7%)	(15%)	(77%)	(39%)	(4%)	(54%)	(5%)	(4%)		(4%)	
Any age	Sm.	21265	7261	4935	853	1473	2043	678	8397	–	2886	–
	Total	187215	32261	5986	1536	24739	3482	7341	95396	5194	25129	18412
		(11%)	(23%)	(82%)	(56%)	(6%)	(59%)	(9%)	(9%)		(11%)	

(To be conservative, no deaths before age 35, and none from liver cirrhosis or non-medical causes, were attributed to smoking.)

¶FEDERAL REPUBLIC OF GERMANY (within its territorial boundaries up to 3.10.90): 1990

		No. of deaths			Standardised rates (Defined on p.358)			Annual death rates / 100, 000						
		All ages	0–34	35–69	All ages	0–34	35–69	0–4	5–9	10–14	15–19	20–24	25–29	30–34
ALL CAUSES	M	330439	14531	122878	1038.4	92.9	1072.5	202.7	20.9	18.0	71.6	101.3	104.9	130.7
	F	382896	7000	70504	615.1	50.3	514.9	156.0	16.7	12.8	28.7	39.1	40.4	58.2
Tuberculosis	M	731	13	355	2.3	0.1	3.0	–	–	–	0.1	0.0	0.1	0.3
	F	350	6	99	0.6	0.0	0.7	–	–	0.1	0.1	0.0	–	0.1
Other infective	M	1838	153	701	5.9	1.1	6.1	4.1	0.4	0.4	0.8	0.6	0.6	0.8
and parasitic	F	2486	102	473	4.2	0.8	3.5	2.9	0.7	0.1	0.6	0.2	0.3	0.7
ALL CANCER	M	86251	1083	40764	273.7	6.6	357.9	4.0	3.7	2.7	5.6	7.0	8.8	14.5
	F	85301	874	31228	163.3	5.6	227.6	3.5	3.0	2.4	3.2	3.6	7.1	16.6
Mouth and	M	2911	17	2350	9.2	0.1	18.3	0.1	–	0.1	0.1	0.1	0.1	0.4
pharynx cancer	F	695	4	401	1.6	0.0	2.9	–	–	–	0.1	0.0	0.1	–
Oesophagus cancer	M	2298	3	1644	7.3	0.0	13.4	–	–	–	–	–	–	0.1
	F	651	1	251	1.3	0.0	1.8	–	–	–	–	–	–	0.0
Stomach cancer	M	7065	33	2923	22.3	0.2	26.1	–	–	0.1	0.1	0.1	0.2	0.9
	F	6864	47	1816	11.8	0.3	13.3	0.1	–	–	–	0.2	0.4	1.2
Colorectal cancer	M	10597	41	4384	33.4	0.2	39.3	–	–	–	0.1	0.1	0.4	1.1
	F	13843	34	3708	23.8	0.2	27.2	–	–	–	–	–	0.3	1.1
Liver cancer	M	1159	9	626	3.7	0.1	5.7	0.1	–	–	0.1	0.0	0.1	0.0
	F	687	5	244	1.3	0.0	1.8	0.1	–	–	0.1	–	0.1	0.0
Pancreas cancer	M	3972	10	2045	12.8	0.1	18.0	–	–	–	–	0.0	0.2	0.2
	F	4509	6	1395	8.1	0.0	10.3	–	–	–	–	–	0.0	0.2
Larynx cancer	M	1299	4	857	4.1	0.0	6.9	–	–	–	–	–	0.1	0.1
	F	137	1	70	0.3	0.0	0.5	–	–	–	–	–	–	0.0
Lung cancer	M	22516	42	12944	72.3	0.2	115.1	–	–	–	0.1	0.3	0.2	1.1
	F	5784	18	2713	12.1	0.1	19.9	0.1	–	–	–	0.1	0.1	0.5
Malignant melanoma	M	823	42	520	2.6	0.2	4.2	–	–	–	0.2	0.3	0.4	0.8
	F	809	31	374	1.8	0.2	2.7	–	–	–	–	0.2	0.3	0.7
Female breast cancer	F	14891	137	7834	32.7	0.8	56.5	–	–	–	–	0.1	0.9	4.7
Cervix cancer	F	1850	54	1036	4.3	0.3	7.5	–	–	–	–	0.1	0.4	1.7
Other uterine cancer	F	2503	6	840	4.6	0.0	6.2	–	–	0.1	–	–	–	0.2
Ovarian cancer	F	5222	41	2535	11.1	0.2	18.5	–	–	0.1	0.1	0.2	0.4	0.9
Prostate cancer	M	9290	9	1660	28.9	0.0	16.6	0.1	–	–	–	–	0.2	0.1
Bladder cancer	M	3504	5	999	11.0	0.0	9.5	–	0.1	–	–	0.0	0.0	0.1
	F	1717	2	323	2.7	0.0	2.4	–	–	–	–	–	0.0	0.0
Other and ill-defined	M	14949	528	7138	47.5	3.3	61.6	2.6	2.5	1.4	2.8	3.8	4.2	5.8
cancer sites	F	18954	279	5665	34.1	2.0	41.5	2.3	2.2	1.4	1.5	1.2	2.2	3.0
Hodgkin's disease	M	328	56	169	1.0	0.3	1.4	–	–	–	0.2	0.4	0.6	1.1
	F	328	37	127	0.7	0.2	0.9	–	–	0.1	0.1	0.3	0.3	0.8
Myeloma and non-	M	2847	78	1418	9.0	0.5	12.4	–	0.1	0.3	0.3	0.6	0.6	1.2
Hodgkin lymphomas	F	3185	31	1077	6.0	0.2	7.9	0.1	0.1	–	0.1	0.2	0.3	0.6
Leukaemia	M	2693	206	1087	8.5	1.3	9.5	1.2	1.1	0.9	1.8	1.3	1.6	1.5
	F	2672	140	819	5.1	1.0	5.9	1.0	0.7	0.7	1.4	1.0	1.2	0.9
ALL VASCULAR	M	145861	771	44296	454.8	4.6	403.2	2.9	0.7	1.1	3.1	3.7	5.8	14.5
DISEASE	F	201026	458	20259	283.5	2.9	149.4	2.8	0.8	0.8	2.4	3.3	4.3	6.2
Rheumatic heart	M	533	11	272	1.7	0.1	2.5	0.1	–	–	0.1	0.1	0.1	0.2
disease and fever	F	1498	6	409	2.6	0.0	3.0	0.1	–	–	–	0.0	0.1	0.0
Hypertensive disease	M	2675	15	777	8.3	0.1	7.0	0.1	–	–	0.1	–	0.1	0.3
	F	6228	10	647	8.7	0.1	4.8	0.1	–	–	0.1	0.1	0.1	0.1
Ischaemic heart	M	68442	171	25252	215.7	0.9	230.4	–	–	–	0.2	0.5	1.4	4.6
disease	F	68671	40	8641	100.5	0.2	64.0	–	–	–	–	0.3	0.6	0.7
Pulmonary embolism	M	2900	44	1123	9.2	0.2	10.0	–	–	–	0.1	0.3	0.5	0.8
and other venous	F	4805	67	1080	8.1	0.4	7.9	–	–	0.1	0.5	0.7	0.4	1.2
Cerebrovascular	M	30454	125	6434	93.9	0.8	59.9	0.3	0.2	0.4	0.5	0.8	0.9	2.1
disease	F	53788	114	4435	74.3	0.7	32.6	0.4	0.3	0.1	0.5	0.7	1.3	1.7
Other vascular	M	40857	405	10438	126.0	2.5	93.5	2.5	0.5	0.6	2.2	2.1	2.9	6.5
disease	F	66036	221	5047	89.3	1.5	37.1	2.3	0.5	0.7	1.4	1.4	1.8	2.4
Chronic obstructive	M	15714	110	4103	49.2	0.7	39.3	0.5	0.1	0.4	0.6	0.7	1.2	1.1
pulmonary disease	F	8896	87	1668	14.3	0.6	12.3	0.6	0.2	0.1	0.4	0.9	0.8	0.9
Other respiratory	M	9060	180	1635	27.8	1.3	15.0	4.7	0.5	0.3	0.5	0.4	1.0	1.3
disease	F	11830	139	868	16.2	1.1	6.4	3.8	0.8	0.3	0.6	0.4	0.9	0.6
Peptic ulcer	M	1444	12	454	4.5	0.1	4.0	–	–	–	0.1	0.0	0.1	0.3
	F	1644	4	228	2.4	0.0	1.7	–	–	–	–	–	0.1	0.1
Liver cirrhosis	M	9045	217	6663	28.7	1.2	53.5	0.1	–	0.2	0.1	0.3	1.8	6.0
	F	5265	109	3007	12.1	0.6	21.6	0.1	–	–	0.1	0.0	1.0	3.3
Renal disease	M	2707	30	755	8.4	0.2	6.7	0.1	–	–	0.1	0.2	0.3	0.5
	F	3621	21	609	5.6	0.1	4.5	0.2	0.1	0.1	0.2	0.2	0.1	0.2
Pregnancy and birth	F	53	41	12	0.2	0.2	0.1	–	–	–	0.1	0.3	0.6	0.7
Congenital and	M	2193	2021	134	9.6	16.4	1.0	107.6	1.8	1.5	1.5	1.0	0.8	0.4
perinatal causes	F	1697	1527	102	7.6	13.0	0.7	84.8	1.9	1.3	1.0	0.8	0.8	0.6
Ill-defined causes	M	9739	1459	4104	31.5	10.4	32.9	49.7	1.2	0.4	2.0	4.9	5.6	9.2
	F	11531	809	1738	19.6	6.4	12.5	35.8	0.8	0.2	0.8	2.0	2.5	2.9
Other medical causes	M	26410	2014	10498	82.3	11.9	86.9	10.4	3.1	3.1	5.8	12.9	19.4	28.5
	F	36022	867	6769	58.7	5.8	49.5	9.4	2.3	2.6	2.9	7.1	6.9	9.1
ALL NON-	M	19446	6468	8416	59.7	38.5	63.0	18.6	9.3	7.8	51.4	69.5	59.3	53.2
MEDICAL CAUSES	F	13174	1956	3444	26.6	13.0	24.5	12.1	6.2	4.8	16.3	20.2	15.0	16.2
Motor vehicle	M	5272	3006	1669	16.0	17.9	12.4	4.1	4.2	3.0	32.5	39.3	25.8	16.6
traffic accidents	F	2163	850	666	5.8	5.7	4.7	3.1	2.9	2.5	10.6	11.0	5.5	4.3
Fire	M	321	118	144	1.1	0.8	1.1	2.3	0.8	0.1	0.4	0.6	0.5	1.0
	F	245	52	63	0.5	0.4	0.5	1.1	0.5	–	0.2	0.4	0.1	0.4
Suicide	M	6853	1841	3699	20.9	10.3	27.5	–	–	0.8	9.6	18.6	19.8	23.0
	F	3142	545	1603	7.8	3.2	11.4	–	0.1	0.1	2.4	5.9	6.3	7.5
Homicide	M	369	147	206	1.2	0.9	1.5	0.9	0.4	0.1	0.9	1.3	1.2	1.5
	F	267	120	102	0.8	0.8	0.7	1.4	0.5	0.3	1.2	0.7	0.7	1.1
POPULATION (thousands):	M=males				30583	14874	13619	1748	1627	1565	1826	2700	2887	2523
	F=females				32671	14046	14184	1657	1543	1481	1730	2561	2701	2373

FEDERAL REPUBLIC OF GERMANY (within its territorial boundaries up to 3.10.90): 1990

Annual death rates / 100, 000 9th ICD categories

35–39	40–44	45–49	50–54	55–59	60–64	65–69	70–74	75–79	80+/NK			
175.4	257.4	431.5	688.8	1158.4	1861.0	2934.7	4594.6	7650.7	15569.0	M	ALL CAUSES	001–999
98.5	146.8	231.6	327.3	528.8	851.2	1420.0	2386.2	4473.7	12024.9	F		
0.8	1.2	1.6	2.3	2.7	4.8	7.9	13.7	15.5	23.1	M	Tuberculosis	010–018, 137
0.1	0.2	0.4	0.2	1.0	0.9	2.2	2.5	5.1	7.9	F		
1.6	1.4	2.9	3.6	6.3	10.7	16.1	24.6	39.1	78.1	M	Other infective	Rest of 001–139
0.8	1.3	1.3	1.7	3.2	7.0	9.2	17.1	28.2	73.5	F	and parasitic	
28.2	61.7	133.7	236.5	410.2	655.5	979.4	1396.8	1990.9	2994.9	M	ALL CANCER	140–208
38.5	68.7	116.0	168.8	263.3	383.9	553.7	740.6	1025.1	1661.5	F		
2.9	7.8	15.3	22.6	26.4	25.5	27.6	25.0	23.7	29.5	M	Mouth and	140–149
0.5	1.0	3.0	3.0	3.3	4.5	4.8	4.4	4.6	9.7	F	pharynx cancer	
0.8	3.4	8.7	13.2	18.5	25.5	23.8	27.1	30.7	35.7	M	Oesophagus cancer	150
0.2	0.5	1.0	2.0	2.1	3.8	3.2	5.6	7.5	12.6	F		
2.5	4.7	7.7	15.7	27.6	46.8	77.8	113.1	183.0	294.6	M	Stomach cancer	151
2.1	3.8	5.5	8.8	15.3	20.5	36.9	52.7	87.1	175.8	F		
1.8	3.8	11.2	24.6	43.6	73.2	116.6	168.0	269.3	450.4	M	Colorectal cancer	153, 154
2.3	4.0	10.8	17.0	30.0	49.2	77.1	116.4	187.8	338.0	F		
0.3	0.4	1.6	3.2	5.5	11.1	17.6	21.8	27.3	26.0	M	Liver cancer	155.0
0.4	0.2	0.9	0.8	1.2	3.5	5.6	7.1	9.9	11.7	F		
1.0	2.7	6.8	12.4	20.5	32.0	50.6	76.5	89.0	109.8	M	Pancreas cancer	157
0.5	1.3	3.0	6.1	10.3	18.8	31.7	45.0	65.9	90.7	F		
0.4	2.4	5.0	7.4	9.2	12.0	11.7	16.5	20.4	26.0	M	Larynx cancer	161
0.0	0.2	0.5	0.5	0.5	0.8	1.0	0.8	1.4	2.0	F		
4.5	13.1	36.3	67.0	139.8	227.2	317.6	396.2	472.6	497.9	M	Lung cancer	162
1.9	5.7	9.6	13.3	22.6	36.0	49.9	65.3	65.0	74.3	F		
1.4	2.4	2.5	3.8	4.3	6.3	9.0	10.7	12.2	14.5	M	Malignant melanoma	172
1.3	1.4	1.9	2.6	3.0	4.3	4.3	7.3	7.8	11.4	F		
13.8	26.0	38.4	55.8	72.5	85.2	103.7	113.8	138.7	199.5	F	Female breast cancer	174
4.0	6.1	6.1	5.1	7.8	10.2	13.0	12.9	17.8	19.4	F	Cervix cancer	180
0.9	1.0	1.6	2.8	6.3	12.1	18.8	26.5	32.1	49.2	F	Other uterine cancer	179, 182
1.4	4.1	9.1	15.2	23.6	34.4	41.7	52.7	55.6	67.7	F	Ovarian cancer	183
0.1	0.1	1.0	3.5	10.4	30.5	70.7	158.0	310.6	628.9	M	Prostate cancer	185
0.1	0.7	1.5	3.4	7.7	18.0	35.4	58.5	105.1	196.2	M	Bladder cancer	188
0.2	0.3	0.4	0.9	2.1	4.9	7.9	15.5	24.8	47.9	F		
7.8	13.9	26.0	44.8	72.3	107.7	158.4	234.4	309.9	503.7	M	Other and ill-defined	Rest of 140–208
6.0	9.6	17.6	25.4	46.5	71.9	113.6	152.2	236.3	438.6	F	cancer sites	
1.0	0.9	0.7	1.0	1.4	1.7	3.0	4.1	4.7	6.0	M	Hodgkin's disease	201
0.6	0.6	0.4	0.5	1.1	1.3	2.0	2.7	3.4	4.6	F		
1.5	3.2	4.9	8.0	12.9	22.7	33.6	46.3	68.9	78.4	M	Myeloma and non–	200, 202–203
0.7	1.3	3.1	4.8	9.2	13.7	22.4	35.6	45.6	55.5	F	Hodgkin lymphomas	
2.1	2.1	4.3	6.0	10.1	15.2	26.2	40.6	63.4	97.2	M	Leukaemia	204–208
1.8	1.7	3.1	4.4	5.7	8.9	16.0	23.9	33.6	53.0	F		
27.3	60.5	112.1	202.6	404.2	743.0	1272.4	2139.7	3858.1	8535.1	M	ALL VASCULAR	390–459
14.9	21.5	35.0	60.6	125.5	256.0	532.4	1088.3	2410.1	7517.6	F	DISEASE	
0.2	0.2	0.6	1.1	2.8	4.7	7.7	10.9	11.0	14.1	M	Rheumatic heart	390–398
–	0.4	0.7	1.7	2.6	6.4	9.3	15.4	23.3	31.6	F	disease and fever	
0.5	1.0	2.0	3.4	8.2	12.8	21.0	36.0	66.5	169.3	M	Hypertensive disease	401–405
0.1	0.6	0.8	2.3	4.2	7.9	17.5	31.6	69.1	238.3	F		
10.8	30.6	61.1	113.9	235.1	436.1	725.1	1139.0	1866.0	3182.7	M	Ischaemic heart	410–414
2.8	5.4	11.3	20.8	51.4	114.7	241.7	466.5	952.9	2301.0	F	disease	
1.2	2.5	2.9	5.2	11.1	19.4	27.3	54.1	75.9	119.2	M	Pulmonary embolism	415.1, 451–453
1.5	2.0	2.4	4.4	8.5	13.6	23.2	39.9	67.5	124.4	F	and other venous	
4.6	8.0	15.6	24.8	54.4	103.0	208.7	407.1	882.6	2157.7	M	Cerebrovascular	430–438
4.9	7.4	9.9	14.3	26.6	50.2	114.7	266.7	668.5	2065.3	F	disease	
9.9	18.3	29.8	54.1	92.5	167.1	282.6	492.6	956.2	2892.1	M	Other vascular	Rest of 390–459
5.4	5.8	10.0	17.2	32.2	63.2	126.0	268.2	628.9	2757.0	F	disease	
1.4	2.0	5.6	12.9	32.4	73.9	147.2	268.0	461.7	927.2	M	Chronic obstructive	490–496
1.2	1.6	4.4	5.7	10.8	22.7	39.5	73.8	113.6	261.0	F	pulmonary disease	
2.2	3.0	4.7	7.2	12.3	24.1	51.5	99.3	226.1	722.8	M	Other respiratory	Rest of 460–519
1.1	1.7	2.1	3.2	5.8	11.3	19.5	42.4	114.0	493.1	F	disease	
0.5	0.5	1.5	2.6	4.6	6.6	11.7	16.5	35.7	89.0	M	Peptic ulcer	531–533
0.3	0.4	0.8	0.9	1.6	1.9	5.7	9.7	20.1	57.0	F		
13.3	22.4	35.1	53.5	69.8	84.1	96.2	93.8	102.1	115.0	M	Liver cirrhosis	571
6.9	12.1	17.7	20.8	25.2	31.4	37.1	39.6	46.1	56.4	F		
0.4	1.2	1.7	4.5	8.1	11.8	19.2	35.9	67.9	173.7	M	Renal disease	580–590
0.5	0.5	1.2	2.4	4.0	8.3	14.5	23.9	46.4	115.2	F		
0.4	0.2	–	–	–	–	–	–	–	–	F	Pregnancy and birth	630–676
0.9	0.7	0.8	1.2	1.1	1.1	1.1	0.6	2.5	2.3	M	Congenital and	740–779
0.7	0.5	0.8	1.1	0.5	0.6	0.8	1.0	1.7	1.8	F	perinatal causes	
12.3	15.4	22.3	30.7	41.2	47.2	61.2	84.9	119.1	401.0	M	Ill-defined causes	780–799
5.1	5.6	9.1	10.0	11.5	19.3	26.9	47.8	81.4	411.8	F		
34.4	38.4	50.4	66.6	94.8	127.4	196.0	318.9	563.6	1119.2	M	Other medical causes	Rest of 001–799
11.4	16.1	21.5	28.1	50.0	79.9	139.4	241.7	480.8	1049.0	F		
52.0	48.8	59.1	64.7	70.8	71.0	74.8	102.1	168.5	387.7	M	ALL NON–	E800–E999
16.6	16.5	21.4	23.7	26.2	27.9	39.2	57.7	101.1	319.0	F	MEDICAL CAUSES	
13.8	10.1	11.8	11.9	12.5	12.4	13.9	19.0	28.9	37.7	M	Motor vehicle	E810–E819
4.4	3.2	4.3	4.5	4.9	5.2	6.5	11.6	15.0	16.2	F	traffic accidents	
0.7	1.0	1.1	1.2	1.0	1.0	1.5	0.7	2.7	5.0	M	Fire	E890–E899
0.2	0.4	0.3	0.3	0.7	0.3	1.0	0.7	2.9	4.5	F		
22.5	21.9	27.8	28.4	32.2	29.7	29.8	43.4	54.7	90.9	M	Suicide	E950–E959
7.2	8.1	11.1	11.7	12.5	13.1	15.9	19.0	22.2	24.9	F		
1.8	1.7	1.5	1.6	1.6	1.2	0.8	1.0	0.3	1.0	M	Homicide	E960–E969
0.9	1.1	0.7	0.6	0.9	0.3	0.5	0.7	0.8	1.4	F		
2233	2054	2205	2443	1834	1633	1216	680	729	681	M	POPULATION (thousands)	
2166	1959	2090	2352	1829	1851	1939	1214	1479	1749	F		

FEDERAL REPUBLIC OF GERMANY (within its territorial boundaries up to 3.10.90): Males

	All ages	0–34	35–69	35–39	40–44	45–49	50–54	55–59	60–64	65–69	70–74	75–79	80+/NK
POPULATION (1000s)													
1955	23539	12941	9269	1056	1581	1746	1726	1345	994	822	635	431	262
1965	28977	16005	11286	2038	1716	1159	1703	1813	1671	1187	774	514	399
1975	29499	15637	11846	2593	2030	1909	1564	1016	1403	1332	1043	574	399
1985	29181	14562	12323	1992	2147	2430	1871	1724	1347	811	982	733	582
1990	**30583**	**14874**	**13619**	**2233**	**2054**	**2205**	**2443**	**1834**	**1633**	**1216**	**680**	**729**	**681**
1995 projected	*29630*	*13511*	*13991*	*2448*	*2177*	*1961*	*2066*	*2265*	*1661*	*1414*	*977*	*481*	*670*
NUMBER OF DEATHS													
All causes													
1955	279500	36668	111448	2526	5543	10037	16759	21478	24337	30768	38247	43056	50081
1965	365756	33120	158819	4741	6084	6233	16083	29292	45294	51092	49896	50539	73382
1975	371074	23893	144267	6110	7830	11305	14754	14775	34317	55176	69279	59078	74557
1985	334382	14543	111580	3453	6297	11689	15088	22032	27339	25682	51874	63524	92861
1990	**330439**	**14531**	**122878**	**3917**	**5287**	**9516**	**16828**	**21243**	**30389**	**35698**	**31239**	**55766**	**106025**
1995 projected	*302683*	*12561*	*118450*	*4082*	*5112*	*7375*	*12639*	*23646*	*28424*	*37172*	*39826*	*33138*	*98708*
Lung cancer													
1955	7925	52	6132	29	133	423	1061	1581	1594	1311	992	525	224
1965	16995	75	11935	78	184	297	979	2448	3952	3997	2698	1472	815
1975	20035	42	10774	121	263	626	1022	1204	3071	4467	4818	2917	1484
1985	21707	45	10592	96	332	750	1441	2461	2954	2558	4228	3871	2971
1990	**22516**	**42**	**12944**	**101**	**270**	**801**	**1636**	**2563**	**3710**	**3863**	**2694**	**3445**	**3391**
1995 projected	*22312*	*36*	*13510*	*92*	*296*	*657*	*1305*	*3064*	*3765*	*4331*	*3574*	*2073*	*3119*
ANNUAL DEATH RATE / 100,000 (*The rates for the age groups 0–34 and 35–69 are the means of seven five-yearly rates, but the all-ages rates are standardised to the conventional "European" age distribution)													
All causes													
1955	1429.4*	282.3*	1418.0*	239.2	350.7	575.0	970.9	1597.4	2447.7	3744.9	6026.0	9982.8	19093.0
1965	1409.5*	194.1*	1528.6*	232.7	354.6	537.9	944.6	1616.0	2710.3	4304.3	6449.0	9828.7	18414.6
1975	1391.5*	167.1*	1457.2*	235.7	385.8	592.3	943.4	1454.2	2446.3	4142.7	6640.4	10297.7	18676.6
1985	1130.0*	99.8*	1175.4*	173.4	293.2	481.0	806.3	1278.0	2030.1	3165.5	5284.6	8666.3	15963.7
1990	**1038.4***	**92.9***	**1072.5***	**175.4**	**257.4**	**431.5**	**688.8**	**1158.4**	**1861.0**	**2934.7**	**4594.6**	**7650.7**	**15569.0**
1995 projected	*949.8**	*87.0**	*967.8**	*166.7*	*234.8*	*376.1*	*611.8*	*1044.0*	*1711.7*	*2629.4*	*4074.7*	*6896.6*	*14728.1*
All cancer													
1955	227.5*	10.4*	323.8*	28.0	52.1	111.9	220.8	387.6	601.2	865.0	1227.8	1591.2	1841.0
1965	262.8*	12.0*	367.8*	31.0	59.9	106.2	206.2	404.7	694.3	1072.5	1461.9	1826.5	2317.7
1975	278.4*	9.7*	364.2*	29.7	61.2	122.1	219.0	383.7	665.7	1067.6	1601.1	2170.6	2645.5
1985	276.4*	7.6*	358.5*	29.9	70.0	126.5	244.8	409.7	650.1	978.3	1445.7	2069.8	2933.1
1990	**273.7***	**6.6***	**357.9***	**28.2**	**61.7**	**133.7**	**236.5**	**410.2**	**655.5**	**979.4**	**1396.8**	**1990.9**	**2994.9**
1995 projected	*267.9**	*5.6**	*351.8**	*24.2*	*59.9*	*128.8*	*232.5*	*405.2*	*654.2*	*957.8*	*1345.7*	*1914.3*	*2996.1*
Lung cancer													
1955	37.3*	0.4*	76.3*	2.7	8.4	24.2	61.5	117.6	160.3	159.6	156.3	121.7	85.4
1965	60.7*	0.5*	115.1*	3.8	10.7	25.6	57.5	135.1	236.5	336.7	348.7	286.3	204.5
1975	71.2*	0.3*	112.7*	4.7	13.0	32.8	65.3	118.5	218.9	335.4	461.8	508.5	371.7
1985	75.0*	0.3*	115.1*	4.8	15.5	30.9	77.0	142.7	219.4	315.3	430.7	528.1	510.7
1990	**72.3***	**0.2***	**115.1***	**4.5**	**13.1**	**36.3**	**67.0**	**139.8**	**227.2**	**317.6**	**396.2**	**472.6**	**497.9**
1995 projected	*68.7**	*0.2**	*111.8**	*3.8*	*13.6*	*33.5*	*63.2*	*135.3*	*226.7*	*306.4*	*365.7*	*431.4*	*465.4*
Upper aerodigestive cancer (mouth, oesophagus, pharynx and larynx)													
1955	11.5*	0.1*	14.4*	0.8	1.3	4.1	8.9	17.0	27.6	41.3	61.3	101.3	124.3
1965	11.8*	0.1*	15.2*	0.8	1.9	3.3	7.8	16.9	30.5	45.3	64.6	84.4	142.0
1975	13.1*	0.1*	19.3*	1.7	4.8	9.2	14.5	21.9	33.4	49.6	70.0	87.3	105.5
1985	18.4*	0.2*	32.3*	3.7	15.1	24.3	37.5	43.0	47.1	55.1	64.9	76.7	100.1
1990	**20.7***	**0.1***	**38.6***	**4.0**	**13.6**	**29.0**	**43.1**	**54.2**	**63.0**	**63.1**	**68.5**	**74.9**	**91.2**
1995 projected	*23.1**	*0.1**	*45.2**	*3.5*	*14.4*	*31.6*	*50.6*	*66.7*	*77.2*	*72.6*	*71.3*	*69.9*	*85.6*
Other cancer													
1955	178.7*	9.8*	233.1*	24.5	42.4	83.6	150.4	253.0	413.4	664.2	1010.2	1368.2	1631.3
1965	190.3*	11.4*	237.5*	26.4	47.3	77.2	140.8	252.7	427.4	690.5	1048.6	1455.9	1971.1
1975	194.2*	9.3*	232.2*	23.3	43.5	80.1	139.2	243.2	413.3	682.7	1069.3	1574.9	2168.3
1985	183.1*	7.1*	211.2*	21.4	39.4	71.4	130.3	224.0	383.7	607.9	950.1	1465.1	2322.3
1990	**180.7***	**6.2***	**204.3***	**19.6**	**35.0**	**68.4**	**126.4**	**216.3**	**365.3**	**598.8**	**932.0**	**1443.4**	**2405.7**
1995 projected	*176.1**	*5.3**	*194.8**	*17.0*	*31.9*	*63.7*	*118.8*	*203.2*	*350.3*	*578.8*	*908.7*	*1412.9*	*2445.1*
Chronic obstructive pulmonary disease (COPD)													
1955	43.3*	1.3*	52.5*	1.2	3.2	13.2	40.8	70.1	98.2	140.9	177.1	301.0	623.3
1965	53.0*	0.9*	64.5*	1.4	2.9	7.6	20.0	59.4	137.1	223.3	292.1	405.3	703.4
1975	70.2*	1.0*	65.5*	2.1	5.6	11.9	23.0	53.5	113.7	248.6	462.8	717.4	981.5
1985	53.5*	0.8*	44.7*	1.7	2.7	7.1	17.5	40.2	83.9	159.5	295.9	525.2	937.8
1990	**49.2***	**0.7***	**39.3***	**1.4**	**2.0**	**5.6**	**12.9**	**32.4**	**73.9**	**147.2**	**268.0**	**461.7**	**927.2**
1995 projected	*44.7**	*0.6**	*34.4**	*1.1*	*1.6*	*4.1*	*9.8*	*26.7*	*65.2*	*132.1*	*237.5*	*417.5*	*880.2*
Other respiratory disease													
1955	75.3*	22.4*	44.0*	5.2	7.7	12.7	24.1	45.9	74.7	137.9	275.7	573.6	1388.5
1965	47.7*	7.4*	30.2*	3.5	4.8	8.0	13.7	27.6	52.4	101.6	193.4	378.3	990.5
1975	42.5*	5.1*	26.4*	3.9	5.7	7.6	15.8	22.6	41.6	87.7	172.3	360.8	905.1
1985	31.3*	1.7*	15.6*	2.3	3.0	5.4	7.7	14.3	27.0	49.4	124.8	279.7	778.6
1990	**27.8***	**1.3***	**15.0***	**2.2**	**3.0**	**4.7**	**7.2**	**12.3**	**24.1**	**51.5**	**99.3**	**226.1**	**722.8**
1995 projected	*24.2**	*1.0**	*13.3**	*2.0*	*2.8*	*4.3*	*6.2*	*10.7*	*23.0*	*44.2*	*81.6*	*182.9*	*648.2*
Vascular disease													
1955	542.2*	8.2*	524.1*	36.9	67.8	140.7	280.9	545.7	965.8	1631.0	2879.0	4945.7	8488.4
1965	589.9*	6.2*	612.0*	44.8	94.6	173.4	338.7	612.5	1112.0	1908.1	3060.6	4977.8	9060.5
1975	610.1*	5.6*	578.8*	36.9	88.6	178.1	336.0	553.5	1023.4	1835.5	3114.3	5157.7	10407.8
1985	530.7*	4.7*	490.5*	34.5	69.9	142.2	286.6	521.5	897.1	1481.8	2671.4	4621.1	9153.3
1990	**454.8***	**4.6***	**403.2***	**27.3**	**60.5**	**112.1**	**202.6**	**404.2**	**743.0**	**1272.4**	**2139.7**	**3858.1**	**8535.1**
1995 projected	*385.7**	*4.2**	*323.4**	*22.4*	*48.0*	*82.4*	*149.1*	*313.4*	*612.1*	*1036.2*	*1757.0*	*3267.6*	*7679.6*
Liver cirrhosis													
1955	19.5*	0.5*	33.6*	4.4	8.7	14.8	27.7	44.1	58.2	77.0	102.3	98.5	85.4
1965	33.1*	0.8*	56.7*	7.4	14.3	26.0	43.3	71.3	102.5	131.8	151.6	178.9	174.2
1975	42.6*	2.5*	77.1*	20.7	39.2	55.2	70.0	86.6	117.6	150.2	160.7	166.8	157.1
1985	32.3*	1.6*	59.6*	14.4	27.5	43.3	60.8	71.7	92.2	107.6	115.4	126.5	106.2
1990	**28.7***	**1.2***	**53.5***	**13.3**	**22.4**	**35.1**	**53.5**	**69.8**	**84.1**	**96.2**	**93.8**	**102.1**	**115.0**
1995 projected	*25.0**	*1.0**	*46.7**	*10.7*	*18.3*	*29.0*	*46.9*	*63.1*	*76.5*	*82.8*	*77.8*	*91.4*	*107.1*
Other medical causes													
1955	402.6*	159.5*	312.3*	68.9	105.6	162.4	245.8	364.8	501.1	737.7	1150.1	2159.5	6019.8
1965	311.3*	97.9*	275.6*	57.3	89.0	121.4	196.3	297.3	460.0	707.8	1075.7	1741.7	4456.0
1975	245.4*	71.9*	237.5*	57.2	87.6	117.5	177.4	246.5	366.6	610.1	948.7	1470.3	3008.8
1985	136.3*	38.9*	131.4*	34.8	53.2	77.5	108.1	145.2	202.7	298.3	501.4	852.5	1664.6
1990	**144.5***	**40.1***	**140.5***	**51.0**	**58.8**	**81.2**	**111.5**	**158.7**	**209.4**	**313.2**	**494.9**	**843.3**	**1886.5**
1995 projected	*151.4**	*41.9**	*146.5**	*64.2*	*66.5*	*83.6*	*115.2*	*163.5*	*218.1*	*314.7*	*490.3*	*872.0*	*2046.1*
All non-medical causes													
1955	118.9*	80.0*	127.6*	94.6	105.5	119.2	130.8	139.1	148.4	155.3	214.0	313.2	646.6
1965	111.8*	69.0*	121.8*	87.4	89.0	95.4	126.4	143.2	152.1	159.2	213.6	320.1	712.4
1975	102.4*	71.3*	107.7*	85.1	97.9	99.9	102.2	107.8	117.8	143.0	180.4	254.0	570.9
1985	69.4*	44.6*	75.1*	55.8	66.9	79.0	80.8	75.3	77.0	90.6	130.0	191.4	390.1
1990	**59.7***	**38.5***	**63.0***	**52.0**	**48.8**	**59.1**	**64.7**	**70.8**	**71.0**	**74.8**	**102.1**	**168.5**	**387.7**
1995 projected	*50.8**	*32.8**	*51.7**	*42.1*	*37.9*	*44.0*	*52.1*	*61.5*	*62.6*	*61.7*	*84.8*	*150.9*	*370.8*

FEDERAL REPUBLIC OF GERMANY (within its territorial boundaries up to 3.10.90): Females

	All ages	0–34	35–69	35–39	40–44	45–49	50–54	55–59	60–64	65–69	70–74	75–79	80+/NK
POPULATION (1000s)													
1955	26474	13071	11695	1430	2067	2118	1913	1675	1385	1108	820	543	345
1965	32235	14951	14435	2051	2295	1598	2310	2353	2080	1749	1323	868	658
1975	32330	14820	13906	2385	1893	1967	2154	1461	2061	1985	1592	1104	907
1985	31843	13831	13398	1898	2063	2347	1844	1890	2026	1330	1748	1454	1412
1990	32671	14046	14184	2166	1959	2090	2352	1829	1851	1939	1214	1479	1749
1995 projected	31481	12833	14101	2292	2107	1894	2037	2283	1756	1734	1743	1015	1789
NUMBER OF DEATHS													
All causes													
1955	261824	24994	90527	2676	5215	8084	10984	14664	20136	28768	39552	46878	59873
1965	351477	19985	113583	3056	5292	5474	12385	18823	28350	40203	53985	62286	101638
1975	378186	12890	98369	3019	3830	6300	10859	10575	23839	39947	58104	73657	135166
1985	369914	7483	67571	1862	3196	5604	6936	11112	18883	19978	47053	71833	175974
1990	382896	7000	70504	2133	2875	4841	7698	9670	15753	27534	28956	66144	210292
1995 projected	351316	5775	62297	2162	3000	4021	6027	10867	13852	22368	37694	41118	204432
Lung cancer													
1955	1575	44	1032	15	55	117	134	217	216	278	239	188	72
1965	3003	42	1751	34	67	81	216	311	491	551	562	403	245
1975	3282	17	1633	27	44	92	193	208	482	587	608	541	483
1985	4560	23	1949	32	67	138	199	387	573	553	881	783	924
1990	5784	18	2713	41	111	201	312	413	667	968	793	961	1299
1995 projected	6953	16	3236	61	167	252	325	613	749	1069	1383	766	1552
ANNUAL DEATH RATE / 100,000	(*The rates for the age groups 0–34 and 35–69 are the means of seven five-yearly rates, but the all-ages rates are standardised to the conventional "European" age distribution)												
All causes													
1955	1096.2*	195.2*	903.1*	187.1	252.3	381.7	574.2	875.5	1454.1	2596.9	4822.8	8636.3	17369.6
1965	936.1*	122.2*	817.2*	149.0	230.6	342.5	536.1	800.1	1363.0	2298.9	4081.4	7172.5	15451.2
1975	854.9*	97.8*	720.8*	126.6	202.4	320.3	504.1	723.6	1156.8	2012.0	3649.5	6669.4	14900.9
1985	661.9*	58.3*	555.7*	98.1	154.9	238.8	376.2	588.1	932.0	1501.8	2692.1	4941.1	12459.2
1990	615.1*	50.3*	514.9*	98.5	146.8	231.6	327.3	528.8	851.2	1420.0	2386.2	4473.7	12024.9
1995 projected	569.1*	44.1*	471.4*	94.3	142.4	212.3	295.9	476.1	788.7	1290.2	2162.8	4049.4	11428.4
All cancer													
1955	187.9*	10.8*	268.1*	54.7	94.1	148.5	215.0	304.2	432.6	627.8	903.7	1239.9	1488.8
1965	189.9*	10.5*	268.5*	49.0	94.1	140.2	228.0	305.0	442.1	621.3	889.2	1202.2	1646.5
1975	178.9*	8.1*	250.5*	38.6	75.1	131.6	217.0	297.8	415.7	577.7	814.8	1153.0	1661.3
1985	165.8*	6.6*	228.7*	37.0	71.4	111.2	178.8	277.3	392.9	532.1	755.8	1056.9	1665.5
1990	163.3*	5.6*	227.6*	38.5	68.7	116.0	168.8	263.3	383.9	553.7	740.6	1025.1	1661.5
1995 projected	159.5*	5.0*	222.6*	37.3	69.3	113.1	161.8	251.0	379.6	545.8	724.5	993.4	1640.0
Lung cancer													
1955	5.8*	0.3*	10.0*	1.0	2.7	5.5	7.0	13.0	15.6	25.1	29.1	34.6	20.9
1965	7.7*	0.3*	12.5*	1.7	2.9	5.1	9.3	13.2	23.6	31.5	42.5	46.4	37.2
1975	7.6*	0.1*	12.0*	1.1	2.3	4.7	9.0	14.2	23.4	29.6	38.2	49.0	53.2
1985	9.8*	0.2*	16.0*	1.7	3.2	5.9	10.8	20.5	28.3	41.6	50.4	53.9	65.4
1990	12.1*	0.1*	19.9*	1.9	5.7	9.6	13.3	22.6	36.0	49.9	65.3	65.0	74.3
1995 projected	14.7*	0.1*	24.4*	2.7	7.9	13.3	16.0	26.9	42.6	61.7	79.4	75.4	86.8
Upper aerodigestive cancer (mouth, oesophagus, pharynx and larynx)													
1955	3.1*	0.0*	2.8*	0.7	0.3	1.1	1.5	3.1	5.1	8.0	16.9	30.6	45.3
1965	2.8*	0.1*	2.6*	0.3	0.5	1.0	1.7	2.3	4.7	7.4	14.3	27.1	43.8
1975	2.4*	0.1*	2.7*	0.3	0.8	2.0	2.6	2.4	4.2	6.7	9.7	17.9	37.2
1985	2.7*	0.1*	4.0*	0.3	1.0	2.8	3.3	5.0	7.3	8.5	9.3	14.2	26.3
1990	3.1*	0.0*	5.2*	0.7	1.6	4.5	5.4	6.0	9.1	9.0	10.8	13.5	24.2
1995 projected	3.7*	0.0*	6.5*	1.0	2.3	6.2	7.6	7.8	10.5	10.2	11.0	13.7	22.5
Other cancer													
1955	179.0*	10.5*	255.3*	52.9	91.1	141.9	206.5	288.1	412.0	594.7	857.6	1174.6	1422.7
1965	179.5*	10.1*	253.5*	47.0	90.6	134.2	216.9	289.4	413.8	582.5	832.5	1128.7	1565.5
1975	168.8*	7.9*	235.7*	37.2	72.0	124.9	205.4	281.2	388.1	541.5	766.9	1086.1	1570.9
1985	153.4*	6.3*	208.7*	35.0	67.2	102.5	164.7	251.9	357.3	482.1	696.0	988.8	1573.7
1990	148.1*	5.5*	202.5*	35.9	61.4	101.9	150.0	234.8	338.7	494.8	664.4	946.6	1563.0
1995 projected	141.1*	4.9*	191.6*	33.7	59.1	93.6	138.3	216.3	326.4	473.9	634.2	904.3	1530.7
Chronic obstructive pulmonary disease (COPD)													
1955	16.7*	0.9*	8.8*	1.0	1.4	2.0	3.7	7.9	14.3	30.9	71.7	155.7	396.0
1965	13.8*	0.5*	8.9*	0.6	1.1	2.3	3.6	6.1	16.0	32.7	59.0	125.2	313.2
1975	17.0*	0.9*	14.2*	2.7	3.3	5.7	8.4	11.6	23.8	43.9	82.8	142.9	307.7
1985	14.3*	0.8*	13.3*	1.9	2.9	4.8	7.9	13.5	22.3	39.6	67.6	104.1	255.6
1990	14.3*	0.6*	12.3*	1.2	1.6	4.4	5.7	10.8	22.7	39.5	73.8	113.6	261.0
1995 projected	14.3*	0.5*	11.7*	0.9	1.2	3.2	4.5	9.6	21.7	40.7	77.9	114.6	271.9
Other respiratory disease													
1955	61.7*	19.9*	29.3*	5.4	7.1	8.4	12.6	23.2	48.0	100.2	246.4	506.4	1153.5
1965	32.8*	5.9*	16.4*	2.2	3.6	5.0	8.4	13.9	27.6	53.9	125.3	273.1	734.1
1975	27.3*	4.3*	13.0*	2.6	2.5	4.7	7.2	11.2	21.6	40.8	96.4	222.8	655.2
1985	17.4*	1.2*	6.6*	1.2	1.2	2.5	3.4	5.7	10.1	22.4	52.4	134.3	511.9
1990	16.2*	1.1*	6.4*	1.1	1.7	2.1	3.2	5.8	11.3	19.5	42.4	114.0	493.1
1995 projected	14.8*	0.9*	5.9*	1.1	1.7	2.0	3.0	6.0	10.6	16.6	35.0	96.7	463.3
Vascular disease													
1955	454.1*	7.2*	346.1*	25.9	41.3	79.6	151.2	287.5	589.8	1247.1	2557.4	4644.1	8176.4
1965	410.5*	3.8*	293.4*	20.3	36.8	66.1	127.6	245.2	516.6	1041.5	2108.6	3999.3	8282.2
1975	394.2*	3.4*	237.7*	17.4	32.8	64.0	105.6	187.4	397.4	859.1	1817.2	3736.5	9120.5
1985	322.7*	2.8*	180.8*	13.1	23.7	42.3	81.9	161.0	314.4	629.4	1360.9	2864.4	8067.3
1990	283.5*	2.9*	149.4*	14.9	21.5	35.0	60.6	125.5	256.0	532.4	1088.3	2410.1	7517.6
1995 projected	246.1*	3.2*	119.9*	14.0	19.3	27.2	46.2	98.1	208.5	425.7	887.5	2022.7	6827.3
Liver cirrhosis													
1955	8.1*	0.3*	12.2*	1.2	3.0	5.3	8.8	14.9	19.9	32.1	46.6	51.8	54.5
1965	13.7*	0.4*	19.8*	2.0	5.1	9.6	12.6	21.5	36.0	51.4	74.0	92.5	113.3
1975	14.2*	0.9*	22.6*	7.1	12.5	16.8	22.8	28.1	30.4	40.4	54.1	74.6	81.2
1985	12.3*	0.7*	21.4*	8.2	10.9	16.5	21.3	26.7	32.1	34.2	42.3	51.5	57.1
1990	12.1*	0.6*	21.6*	6.9	12.1	17.7	20.8	25.2	31.4	37.1	39.6	46.1	56.4
1995 projected	11.8*	0.6*	21.3*	6.8	12.3	18.0	20.2	24.1	31.2	36.3	37.4	42.5	53.2
Other medical causes													
1955	316.8*	134.9*	197.9*	75.7	80.0	106.1	143.3	193.8	300.0	486.7	865.3	1766.8	5385.6
1965	220.1*	80.2*	165.8*	51.5	63.2	83.9	113.6	163.7	266.5	418.3	682.0	1204.4	3508.1
1975	172.6*	55.0*	139.9*	30.6	46.1	63.7	97.3	140.4	217.8	383.5	672.2	1131.8	2430.4
1985	97.5*	30.5*	74.4*	18.0	23.3	35.1	51.9	72.7	123.2	196.6	342.7	617.7	1551.5
1990	99.0*	26.5*	73.1*	19.4	24.7	35.1	44.4	72.0	117.9	198.6	343.7	663.6	1716.3
1995 projected	100.4*	23.2*	70.8*	20.3	25.3	32.5	41.4	67.1	114.9	194.3	351.8	691.6	1883.0
All non-medical causes													
1955	50.9*	21.2*	40.8*	23.2	25.4	31.9	39.7	44.0	49.4	72.0	131.8	271.7	714.8
1965	55.2*	20.9*	44.3*	23.4	26.8	35.4	42.2	44.8	58.1	79.7	143.1	275.8	853.9
1975	50.7*	25.2*	43.0*	27.5	29.9	33.8	45.7	47.2	50.2	66.7	112.1	207.7	644.6
1985	31.8*	15.8*	30.5*	18.7	21.6	26.5	31.1	31.2	37.1	47.4	70.5	112.2	350.3
1990	26.6*	13.0*	24.5*	16.6	16.5	21.4	23.7	26.2	27.9	39.2	57.7	101.1	319.0
1995 projected	22.2*	10.6*	19.4*	13.9	13.3	16.3	18.7	20.2	22.2	31.0	48.8	87.9	289.8

FEDERAL REPUBLIC OF GERMANY (within its territorial boundaries up to 3.10.90): 1975

Smoking-attributed deaths (Sm.) and total deaths (Total)

		ALL CAUSES	ALL CANCER	Lung cancer	Upper aero-digestive ca.	Other cancer	COPD	Other respiratory	Vascular disease	Liver cirrhosis	Other medical	Non-medical
Males												
0-34	Sm.	–	–	–	–	–	–	–	–	–	–	–
	Total	23893	1508	42	20	1446	152	677	866	389	9383	10918
35-69	Sm.	41574	14576	9947	1208	3421	4788	690	14860	–	6660	–
	Total	144267	35226	10774	1897	22555	6204	2589	55835	8011	24050	12352
		(29%)	(41%)	(92%)	(64%)	(15%)	(77%)	(27%)	(27%)		(28%)	
70+	Sm.	41447	13283	8422	1003	3858	9517	934	13672	–	4041	–
	Total	202914	39718	9219	1652	28847	12862	7481	103630	3261	30344	5618
		(20%)	(33%)	(91%)	(61%)	(13%)	(74%)	(12%)	(13%)		(13%)	
Any age	Sm.	83021	27859	18369	2211	7279	14305	1624	28532	–	10701	–
	Total	371074	76452	20035	3569	52848	19218	10747	160331	11661	63777	28888
		(22%)	(36%)	(92%)	(62%)	(14%)	(74%)	(15%)	(18%)		(17%)	
Females												
0-34	Sm.	–	–	–	–	–	–	–	–	–	–	–
	Total	12890	1180	17	9	1154	128	543	493	130	6803	3613
35-69	Sm.	2192	544	420	31	93	328	43	825	–	452	–
	Total	98369	33994	1633	373	31988	1950	1778	32552	3067	19108	5920
		(2%)	(2%)	(26%)	(8%)	(0%)	(17%)	(2%)	(3%)		(2%)	
70+	Sm.	3619	652	459	64	129	1034	88	1407	–	438	–
	Total	266927	40776	1632	689	38455	5687	9939	152929	2422	45248	9926
		(1%)	(2%)	(28%)	(9%)	(0%)	(18%)	(1%)	(1%)		(1%)	
Any age	Sm.	5811	1196	879	95	222	1362	131	2232	–	890	–
	Total	378186	75950	3282	1071	71597	7765	12260	185974	5619	71159	19459
		(2%)	(2%)	(27%)	(9%)	(0%)	(18%)	(1%)	(1%)		(1%)	
Males+Females												
0-34	Sm.	–	–	–	–	–	–	–	–	–	–	–
	Total	36783	2688	59	29	2600	280	1220	1359	519	16186	14531
35-69	Sm.	43766	15120	10367	1239	3514	5116	733	15685	–	7112	–
	Total	242636	69220	12407	2270	54543	8154	4367	88387	11078	43158	18272
		(18%)	(22%)	(84%)	(55%)	(6%)	(63%)	(17%)	(18%)		(16%)	
70+	Sm.	45066	13935	8881	1067	3987	10551	1022	15079	–	4479	–
	Total	469841	80494	10851	2341	67302	18549	17420	256559	5683	75592	15544
		(10%)	(17%)	(82%)	(46%)	(6%)	(57%)	(6%)	(6%)		(6%)	
Any age	Sm.	88832	29055	19248	2306	7501	15667	1755	30764	–	11591	–
	Total	749260	152402	23317	4640	124445	26983	23007	346305	17280	134936	48347
		(12%)	(19%)	(83%)	(50%)	(6%)	(58%)	(8%)	(9%)		(9%)	

FEDERAL REPUBLIC OF GERMANY (within its territorial boundaries up to 3.10.90): 1985

Smoking-attributed deaths (Sm.) and total deaths (Total)

		ALL CAUSES	ALL CANCER	Lung cancer	Upper aero-digestive ca.	Other cancer	COPD	Other respiratory	Vascular disease	Liver cirrhosis	Other medical	Non-medical
Males												
0-34	Sm.	–	–	–	–	–	–	–	–	–	–	–
	Total	14543	1192	45	36	1111	126	214	737	254	4726	7294
35-69	Sm.	35500	15110	9803	2276	3031	2871	408	12936	–	4175	–
	Total	111580	33511	10592	3513	19406	3709	1398	44100	6418	13394	9050
		(32%)	(45%)	(93%)	(65%)	(16%)	(77%)	(29%)	(29%)		(31%)	
70+	Sm.	42198	15606	10090	1075	4441	9013	920	14063	–	2596	–
	Total	208259	46425	11070	1781	33574	12210	7804	113340	2678	20854	4948
		(20%)	(34%)	(91%)	(60%)	(13%)	(74%)	(12%)	(12%)		(12%)	
Any age	Sm.	77698	30716	19893	3351	7472	11884	1328	26999	–	6771	–
	Total	334382	81128	21707	5330	54091	16045	9416	158177	9350	38974	21292
		(23%)	(38%)	(92%)	(63%)	(14%)	(74%)	(14%)	(17%)		(17%)	
Females												
0-34	Sm.	–	–	–	–	–	–	–	–	–	–	–
	Total	7483	941	23	13	905	128	138	419	99	3448	2310
35-69	Sm.	3180	1088	838	82	168	485	41	1102	–	464	–
	Total	67571	28359	1949	507	25903	1587	778	21023	2770	9086	3968
		(5%)	(4%)	(43%)	(16%)	(1%)	(31%)	(5%)	(5%)		(5%)	
70+	Sm.	5988	1347	994	99	254	1577	126	2413	–	525	–
	Total	294860	52097	2588	742	48767	6306	10098	179371	2294	36883	7811
		(2%)	(3%)	(38%)	(13%)	(1%)	(25%)	(1%)	(1%)		(1%)	
Any age	Sm.	9168	2435	1832	181	422	2062	167	3515	–	989	–
	Total	369914	81397	4560	1262	75575	8021	11014	200813	5163	49417	14089
		(2%)	(3%)	(40%)	(14%)	(1%)	(26%)	(2%)	(2%)		(2%)	
Males+Females												
0-34	Sm.	–	–	–	–	–	–	–	–	–	–	–
	Total	22026	2133	68	49	2016	254	352	1156	353	8174	9604
35-69	Sm.	38680	16198	10641	2358	3199	3356	449	14038	–	4639	–
	Total	179151	61870	12541	4020	45309	5296	2176	65123	9188	22480	13018
		(22%)	(26%)	(85%)	(59%)	(7%)	(63%)	(21%)	(22%)		(21%)	
70+	Sm.	48186	16953	11084	1174	4695	10590	1046	16476	–	3121	–
	Total	503119	98522	13658	2523	82341	18516	17902	292711	4972	57737	12759
		(10%)	(17%)	(81%)	(47%)	(6%)	(57%)	(6%)	(6%)		(5%)	
Any age	Sm.	86866	33151	21725	3532	7894	13946	1495	30514	–	7760	–
	Total	704296	162525	26267	6592	129666	24066	20430	358990	14513	88391	35381
		(12%)	(20%)	(83%)	(54%)	(6%)	(58%)	(7%)	(8%)		(9%)	

(To be conservative, no deaths before age 35, and none from liver cirrhosis or non-medical causes, were attributed to smoking.)

FEDERAL REPUBLIC OF GERMANY (within its territorial boundaries up to 3.10.90): 1990

Smoking–attributed deaths (Sm.) and total deaths (Total)

		ALL CAUSES	ALL CANCER	Lung cancer	Upper aero–digestive ca.	Other cancer	COPD	Other respiratory	Vascular disease	Liver cirrhosis	Other medical	Non–medical
Males												
0–34	Sm.	–	–	–	–	–	–	–	–	–	–	–
	Total	14531	1083	42	24	1017	110	180	771	217	5702	6468
35–69	Sm.	39909	18659	11974	3123	3562	3173	457	12482	–	5138	–
	Total	122878	40764	12944	4851	22969	4103	1635	44296	6663	17001	8416
		(32%)	(46%)	(93%)	(64%)	(16%)	(77%)	(28%)	(28%)		(30%)	
70+	Sm.	35472	13490	8591	940	3959	8214	736	10657	–	2375	–
	Total	193030	44404	9530	1633	33241	11501	7245	100794	2165	22359	4562
		(18%)	(30%)	(90%)	(58%)	(12%)	(71%)	(10%)	(11%)		(11%)	
Any age	Sm.	75381	32149	20565	4063	7521	11387	1193	23139	–	7513	–
	Total	330439	86251	22516	6508	57227	15714	9060	145861	9045	45062	19446
		(23%)	(37%)	(91%)	(62%)	(13%)	(72%)	(13%)	(16%)		(17%)	
Females												
0–34	Sm.	–	–	–	–	–	–	–	–	–	–	–
	Total	7000	874	18	6	850	87	139	458	109	3377	1956
35–69	Sm.	4992	1918	1470	168	280	678	67	1558	–	771	–
	Total	70504	31228	2713	722	27793	1668	868	20259	3007	10030	3444
		(7%)	(6%)	(54%)	(23%)	(1%)	(41%)	(8%)	(8%)		(8%)	
70+	Sm.	9041	2047	1502	147	398	2451	196	3462	–	885	–
	Total	305392	53199	3053	755	49391	7141	10823	180309	2149	43997	7774
		(3%)	(4%)	(49%)	(19%)	(1%)	(34%)	(2%)	(2%)		(2%)	
Any age	Sm.	14033	3965	2972	315	678	3129	263	5020	–	1656	–
	Total	382896	85301	5784	1483	78034	8896	11830	201026	5265	57404	13174
		(4%)	(5%)	(51%)	(21%)	(1%)	(35%)	(2%)	(2%)		(3%)	
Males+Females												
0–34	Sm.	–	–	–	–	–	–	–	–	–	–	–
	Total	21531	1957	60	30	1867	197	319	1229	326	9079	8424
35–69	Sm.	44901	20577	13444	3291	3842	3851	524	14040	–	5909	–
	Total	193382	71992	15657	5573	50762	5771	2503	64555	9670	27031	11860
		(23%)	(29%)	(86%)	(59%)	(8%)	(67%)	(21%)	(22%)		(22%)	
70+	Sm.	44513	15537	10093	1087	4357	10665	932	14119	–	3260	–
	Total	498422	97603	12583	2388	82632	18642	18068	281103	4314	66356	12336
		(9%)	(16%)	(80%)	(46%)	(5%)	(57%)	(5%)	(5%)		(5%)	
Any age	Sm.	89414	36114	23537	4378	8199	14516	1456	28159	–	9169	–
	Total	713335	171552	28300	7991	135261	24610	20890	346887	14310	102466	32620
		(13%)	(21%)	(83%)	(55%)	(6%)	(59%)	(7%)	(8%)		(9%)	

¶GERMANY, the 11 old Länder: 1995

Smoking–attributed deaths (Sm.) and total deaths (Total)

		ALL CAUSES	ALL CANCER	Lung cancer	Upper aero–digestive ca.	Other cancer	COPD	Other respiratory	Vascular disease	Liver cirrhosis	Other medical	Non–medical
Males												
0–34	Sm.	–	–	–	–	–	–	–	–	–	–	–
	Total	12561	855	36	20	799	83	143	662	178	5839	4801
35–69	Sm.	39030	19728	12464	3738	3526	2993	426	10370	–	5513	–
	Total	118450	42807	13510	5883	23414	3899	1571	38200	6065	18811	7097
		(33%)	(46%)	(92%)	(64%)	(15%)	(77%)	(27%)	(27%)		(29%)	
70+	Sm.	30830	12264	7837	894	3533	7111	578	8561	–	2316	–
	Total	171672	42431	8766	1607	32058	10226	6021	84343	1917	22695	4039
		(18%)	(29%)	(89%)	(56%)	(11%)	(70%)	(10%)	(10%)		(10%)	
Any age	Sm.	69860	31992	20301	4632	7059	10104	1004	18931	–	7829	–
	Total	302683	86093	22312	7510	56271	14208	7735	123205	8160	47345	15937
		(23%)	(37%)	(91%)	(62%)	(13%)	(71%)	(13%)	(15%)		(17%)	
Females												
0–34	Sm.	–	–	–	–	–	–	–	–	–	–	–
	Total	5775	770	16	5	749	64	117	453	101	2846	1424
35–69	Sm.	6102	2660	2028	266	366	739	83	1624	–	996	–
	Total	62297	29609	3236	880	25493	1504	772	15464	2894	9376	2678
		(10%)	(9%)	(63%)	(30%)	(1%)	(49%)	(11%)	(11%)		(11%)	
70+	Sm.	11923	2884	2154	188	542	3118	249	4310	–	1362	–
	Total	283244	52050	3701	734	47615	7384	9880	158131	2035	46837	6927
		(4%)	(6%)	(58%)	(26%)	(1%)	(42%)	(3%)	(3%)		(3%)	
Any age	Sm.	18025	5544	4182	454	908	3857	332	5934	–	2358	–
	Total	351316	82429	6953	1619	73857	8952	10769	174048	5030	59059	11029
		(5%)	(7%)	(60%)	(28%)	(1%)	(43%)	(3%)	(3%)		(4%)	
Males+Females												
0–34	Sm.	–	–	–	–	–	–	–	–	–	–	–
	Total	18336	1625	52	25	1548	147	260	1115	279	8685	6225
35–69	Sm.	45132	22388	14492	4004	3892	3732	509	11994	–	6509	–
	Total	180747	72416	16746	6763	48907	5403	2343	53664	8959	28187	9775
		(25%)	(31%)	(87%)	(59%)	(8%)	(69%)	(22%)	(22%)		(23%)	
70+	Sm.	42753	15148	9991	1082	4075	10229	827	12871	–	3678	–
	Total	454916	94481	12467	2341	79673	17610	15901	242474	3952	69532	10966
		(9%)	(16%)	(80%)	(46%)	(5%)	(58%)	(5%)	(5%)		(5%)	
Any age	Sm.	87885	37536	24483	5086	7967	13961	1336	24865	–	10187	–
	Total	653999	168522	29265	9129	130128	23160	18504	297253	13190	106404	26966
		(13%)	(22%)	(84%)	(56%)	(6%)	(60%)	(7%)	(8%)		(10%)	

(To be conservative, no deaths before age 35, and none from liver cirrhosis or non–medical causes, were attributed to smoking.)

¶GERMANY: 1990

		No. of deaths			Standardised rates (Defined on p.364)			Annual death rates / 100, 000						
		All ages	0–34	35–69	All ages	0–34	35–69	0–4	5–9	10–14	15–19	20–24	25–29	30–34
ALL CAUSES	M	425093	19747	161973	1090.2	100.3	1143.3	202.0	24.3	24.3	81.9	109.7	113.3	146.7
	F	496352	9336	94470	648.6	52.8	552.6	154.5	19.6	16.5	32.5	40.5	43.4	62.6
Tuberculosis	M	904	16	455	2.4	0.1	3.2	–	–	–	0.0	0.0	0.1	0.3
	F	454	9	136	0.7	0.0	0.8	–	–	0.1	0.0	0.0	0.1	0.1
Other infective and parasitic	M	1978	182	767	5.2	1.0	5.4	3.9	0.4	0.3	0.7	0.6	0.5	0.7
	F	2677	136	542	3.8	0.8	3.2	3.3	0.6	0.2	0.6	0.2	0.3	0.6
ALL CANCER	M	102919	1399	50089	267.1	6.8	357.3	4.1	3.6	2.9	5.3	7.4	9.6	14.7
	F	102229	1142	38710	159.3	5.8	225.6	3.6	2.8	2.2	3.5	3.9	7.7	17.0
Mouth and pharynx cancer	M	3408	21	2739	8.7	0.1	17.2	0.0	–	0.0	0.1	0.1	0.1	0.4
	F	833	6	460	1.5	0.0	2.6	–	–	–	0.0	0.0	0.1	0.0
Oesophagus cancer	M	2710	3	1937	7.0	0.0	12.8	–	–	–	–	–	–	0.1
	F	745	1	278	1.2	0.0	1.6	–	–	–	–	–	–	0.0
Stomach cancer	M	8819	44	3779	22.8	0.2	27.5	–	–	0.0	0.0	0.1	0.2	1.0
	F	8466	58	2328	11.9	0.3	13.6	0.0	–	–	0.0	0.2	0.5	1.1
Colorectal cancer	M	12558	49	5354	32.4	0.2	39.0	–	–	–	0.0	0.1	0.4	1.0
	F	16624	45	4637	23.4	0.2	27.2	–	–	–	–	0.1	0.4	1.0
Liver cancer	M	1225	9	666	3.2	0.0	5.0	0.0	–	–	0.1	0.0	0.1	0.0
	F	731	5	270	1.1	0.0	1.6	0.0	–	–	0.0	–	0.1	0.0
Pancreas cancer	M	4651	14	2448	12.2	0.1	17.5	–	–	0.0	–	0.0	0.1	0.2
	F	5330	7	1690	7.8	0.0	9.9	–	–	–	–	–	0.0	0.2
Larynx cancer	M	1527	4	1017	3.9	0.0	6.6	–	–	–	–	–	0.1	0.1
	F	158	1	79	0.3	0.0	0.5	–	–	–	–	–	–	0.0
Lung cancer	M	27423	51	16094	72.0	0.2	116.2	–	–	–	0.0	0.2	0.1	1.2
	F	6795	24	3234	11.5	0.1	18.9	0.0	–	–	–	0.2	0.1	0.4
Malignant melanoma	M	958	50	615	2.5	0.2	4.1	–	–	–	0.1	0.3	0.4	0.7
	F	962	34	455	1.7	0.2	2.6	–	–	–	–	0.2	0.3	0.6
Female breast cancer	F	17544	174	9329	31.1	0.8	53.7	–	–	–	–	0.1	0.7	4.9
Cervix cancer	F	2589	96	1462	4.8	0.4	8.4	0.0	–	–	–	0.1	0.9	2.1
Other uterine cancer	F	3141	7	1112	4.7	0.0	6.6	–	–	0.1	–	–	0.0	0.2
Ovarian cancer	F	6326	55	3186	10.9	0.3	18.6	–	–	0.1	0.0	0.2	0.4	1.0
Prostate cancer	M	10496	10	1930	26.8	0.0	15.9	0.0	–	–	–	–	0.2	0.1
Bladder cancer	M	4251	6	1303	10.9	0.0	10.1	–	0.0	–	–	0.0	0.1	0.1
	F	2042	2	412	2.7	0.0	2.4	–	–	–	–	–	0.0	0.0
Other and ill-defined cancer sites	M	17947	698	8929	46.5	3.4	62.3	2.7	2.4	1.5	2.5	4.0	5.0	5.9
	F	22672	351	7262	33.5	1.9	42.6	2.3	1.9	1.3	1.6	1.3	2.3	2.8
Hodgkin's disease	M	425	70	230	1.1	0.3	1.5	–	–	–	0.2	0.5	0.6	0.9
	F	410	47	160	0.7	0.2	0.9	–	–	0.1	0.0	0.3	0.4	0.7
Myeloma and non-Hodgkin lymphomas	M	3270	98	1679	8.5	0.5	11.9	0.1	0.1	0.3	0.3	0.6	0.6	1.2
	F	3649	47	1295	5.6	0.2	7.6	0.2	0.1	–	0.3	0.3	0.3	0.6
Leukaemia	M	3251	272	1369	8.4	1.4	9.7	1.2	1.1	0.9	1.8	1.5	1.6	1.8
	F	3212	182	1061	5.1	1.0	6.2	1.0	0.8	0.7	1.4	1.0	1.1	1.1
ALL VASCULAR DISEASE	M	192841	1163	59177	491.7	5.5	437.5	3.8	1.1	1.8	3.3	4.3	7.1	17.3
	F	270151	634	29043	311.7	3.3	172.0	3.1	0.9	1.8	2.5	3.4	4.4	7.0
Rheumatic heart disease and fever	M	725	20	415	1.9	0.1	3.0	0.0	–	–	0.1	0.1	0.1	0.3
	F	1834	7	591	2.7	0.0	3.5	0.0	0.0	–	–	0.0	0.1	0.0
Hypertensive disease	M	6837	32	2489	17.5	0.2	18.0	0.1	–	–	0.1	0.1	0.2	0.6
	F	14159	19	2078	17.1	0.1	12.3	0.0	0.0	–	0.0	0.1	0.1	0.3
Ischaemic heart disease	M	85763	268	32314	221.2	1.2	239.2	–	–	–	0.2	0.5	1.8	5.8
	F	86748	54	11434	103.5	0.2	68.0	–	–	–	–	0.3	0.6	0.9
Pulmonary embolism and other venous	M	3682	63	1544	9.6	0.3	11.1	0.1	–	–	0.1	0.2	0.5	1.0
	F	5916	84	1494	8.2	0.4	8.8	0.0	–	0.1	0.5	0.7	0.4	1.2
Cerebrovascular disease	M	37838	173	8011	95.4	0.8	60.8	0.3	0.3	0.4	0.4	0.9	1.1	2.3
	F	67831	141	5906	76.5	0.7	34.9	0.3	0.2	0.1	0.5	0.7	1.3	1.8
Other vascular disease	M	57996	607	14404	146.1	3.0	105.4	3.2	0.9	1.4	2.4	2.5	3.4	7.2
	F	93663	329	7540	103.6	1.8	44.5	2.7	0.6	1.6	1.5	1.6	1.9	2.8
Chronic obstructive pulmonary disease	M	19120	124	5259	49.1	0.6	41.1	0.4	0.1	0.3	0.6	0.7	1.0	1.0
	F	10425	98	2085	13.6	0.5	12.3	0.6	0.1	0.2	0.3	0.8	0.7	0.9
Other respiratory disease	M	12440	300	2682	31.3	1.6	19.6	5.4	0.5	0.4	0.9	0.8	1.3	2.1
	F	15676	220	1414	17.9	1.3	8.3	4.9	0.7	0.4	0.6	0.4	1.2	0.9
Peptic ulcer	M	2089	28	788	5.3	0.1	5.5	–	–	–	0.0	0.1	0.3	0.4
	F	2193	6	363	2.7	0.0	2.1	–	–	–	–	–	0.1	0.1
Liver cirrhosis	M	11651	348	8798	29.9	1.5	56.5	0.0	–	0.1	0.1	0.4	2.3	7.8
	F	6462	156	3848	12.2	0.7	22.1	0.2	–	0.1	0.1	0.0	1.2	3.7
Renal disease	M	3589	64	1125	9.1	0.3	8.0	0.2	–	–	0.1	0.3	0.5	0.9
	F	4734	38	1002	6.2	0.2	5.9	0.2	0.1	0.1	0.1	0.2	0.3	0.4
Pregnancy and birth	F	82	68	14	0.2	0.3	0.1	–	–	–	0.1	0.5	0.7	0.8
Congenital and perinatal causes	M	2920	2687	188	9.9	16.8	1.1	110.1	2.0	1.5	1.6	1.0	0.8	0.7
	F	2242	2008	149	7.8	13.3	0.8	86.3	1.9	1.4	1.0	0.7	0.8	0.6
Ill-defined causes	M	12970	1952	5722	33.7	10.7	37.1	40.7	2.6	3.6	3.3	6.4	7.5	10.9
	F	14650	1028	2521	20.4	6.3	14.5	29.1	2.1	2.7	1.4	2.7	2.8	3.3
Other medical causes	M	34169	2528	14475	87.0	12.1	96.5	12.2	3.2	3.4	5.8	12.0	18.6	29.3
	F	45917	1112	9624	61.9	5.9	56.3	9.8	2.6	2.8	3.1	6.9	7.0	9.3
ALL NON-MEDICAL CAUSES	M	27503	8956	12448	68.5	43.1	74.5	21.1	10.7	9.9	60.1	75.7	63.6	60.7
	F	18460	2681	5019	30.2	14.3	28.5	13.3	7.7	4.8	19.0	20.6	16.4	18.0
Motor vehicle traffic accidents	M	7469	4189	2482	18.4	20.4	14.6	4.6	5.0	4.3	39.1	43.2	27.5	18.9
	F	3109	1197	1002	6.7	6.5	5.7	3.4	3.9	2.7	13.1	11.0	6.1	5.2
Fire	M	459	160	214	1.2	0.9	1.3	2.1	0.8	0.1	0.6	0.9	0.6	0.9
	F	328	66	93	0.6	0.4	0.5	1.1	0.5	0.1	0.2	0.3	0.1	0.4
Suicide	M	9534	2310	5326	23.6	10.4	31.7	–	0.1	1.0	9.1	18.1	20.0	24.6
	F	4390	671	2224	8.6	3.2	12.6	–	0.2	0.2	2.2	5.8	6.4	7.3
Homicide	M	465	178	266	1.2	0.9	1.5	0.9	0.4	0.0	1.0	1.2	1.2	1.4
	F	335	145	133	0.8	0.8	0.7	1.4	0.5	0.2	1.1	0.7	0.7	1.1
POPULATION (thousands):	**M=males**				38276	18838	16900	2261	2189	2101	2294	3272	3568	3153
	F=females				41088	17829	17781	2144	2078	1990	2174	3114	3352	2976

GERMANY: 1990
9th ICD categories

Annual death rates / 100, 000

35–39	40–44	45–49	50–54	55–59	60–64	65–69	70–74	75–79	80+/NK			
202.6	281.6	479.7	753.8	1252.6	1948.6	3083.9	4746.3	8003.5	16017.0	M	ALL CAUSES	001–999
103.5	151.5	244.0	349.7	569.7	919.7	1530.1	2538.6	4814.7	12395.6	F		
0.7	1.0	1.5	2.1	2.9	5.5	8.5	13.0	15.8	22.4	M	Tuberculosis	010–018, 137
0.1	0.2	0.4	0.4	1.0	1.2	2.3	2.7	5.1	8.1	F		
1.4	1.4	2.7	3.4	5.5	9.2	14.1	22.1	33.8	65.8	M	Other infective	Rest of 001–139
0.8	1.1	1.3	1.8	2.9	6.3	8.1	14.7	24.2	62.1	F	and parasitic	
28.4	60.0	134.1	237.2	414.7	650.7	975.7	1365.6	1934.5	2772.6	M	ALL CANCER	140–208
38.3	65.8	113.8	168.7	263.2	381.1	548.3	719.4	999.8	1549.3	F		
2.5	7.1	14.9	21.7	24.4	24.3	25.6	22.9	24.0	29.7	M	Mouth and	140–149
0.4	0.9	2.7	2.6	3.2	4.2	4.5	4.0	5.0	10.1	F	pharynx cancer	
0.7	3.1	8.4	12.6	17.8	24.0	23.0	26.0	29.5	35.5	M	Oesophagus cancer	150
0.2	0.4	0.8	1.6	2.0	3.2	3.1	5.2	7.3	11.8	F		
2.6	4.5	8.0	16.8	30.2	48.0	82.1	117.7	185.5	286.6	M	Stomach cancer	151
2.2	3.7	5.9	8.6	14.7	21.9	38.4	55.1	90.9	167.0	F		
1.9	4.4	11.5	24.3	43.3	71.9	115.7	166.6	260.7	417.6	M	Colorectal cancer	153, 154
2.2	4.1	10.5	17.1	29.3	48.8	78.6	116.3	185.9	316.3	F		
0.2	0.4	1.4	2.7	4.6	9.6	15.8	18.9	23.9	22.0	M	Liver cancer	155.0
0.3	0.3	0.8	0.6	1.2	3.1	4.8	5.9	8.6	9.8	F		
1.1	2.8	7.0	12.0	20.1	30.5	48.8	71.7	85.6	101.2	M	Pancreas cancer	157
0.7	1.2	3.1	5.8	10.1	18.0	30.7	43.3	63.1	85.1	F		
0.4	2.2	4.9	6.8	8.9	11.9	11.3	15.0	19.2	25.6	M	Larynx cancer	161
0.0	0.1	0.4	0.4	0.6	0.8	0.9	1.0	1.3	1.9	F		
4.3	12.7	36.4	68.3	143.9	229.5	318.3	394.1	468.6	468.2	M	Lung cancer	162
1.8	5.1	9.1	12.8	22.4	33.9	47.6	60.7	62.6	69.0	F		
1.3	2.1	2.4	3.6	4.6	6.0	8.4	9.8	11.6	13.3	M	Malignant melanoma	172
1.6	1.3	2.0	2.5	2.9	3.9	4.1	6.6	7.5	11.0	F		
12.8	24.3	36.9	53.3	69.8	81.3	97.5	109.0	131.3	186.4	F	Female breast cancer	174
4.6	6.0	6.4	6.3	9.6	11.7	14.3	14.8	19.5	21.1	F	Cervix cancer	180
0.9	1.0	1.6	3.0	7.1	12.8	19.6	26.5	32.4	48.0	F	Other uterine cancer	179, 182
1.3	4.2	8.9	15.8	23.8	33.9	42.0	49.3	53.6	63.6	F	Ovarian cancer	183
0.1	0.2	0.9	3.2	9.6	28.7	68.6	149.9	293.9	566.5	M	Prostate cancer	185
0.1	0.7	1.6	3.8	8.9	18.6	37.4	58.3	106.8	182.1	M	Bladder cancer	188
0.1	0.3	0.4	0.9	2.1	4.9	8.4	14.7	24.3	44.9	F		
8.3	13.8	26.7	46.0	74.9	109.1	157.6	228.0	295.6	459.8	M	Other and ill-defined	Rest of 140–208
6.1	9.2	18.2	27.2	48.9	74.1	114.2	149.0	229.3	401.5	F	cancer sites	
1.1	0.9	1.0	1.1	1.5	1.8	3.1	4.1	4.8	5.9	M	Hodgkin's disease	201
0.5	0.5	0.4	0.6	1.0	1.2	2.1	2.9	3.7	4.3	F		
1.6	3.0	4.6	8.0	12.1	21.6	32.8	42.9	63.2	69.9	M	Myeloma and non-	200, 202–203
0.6	1.2	2.7	4.8	8.9	13.6	21.4	32.3	41.8	49.2	F	Hodgkin lymphomas	
2.2	2.2	4.5	6.3	9.9	15.3	27.3	39.6	61.6	88.8	M	Leukaemia	204–208
1.9	1.9	3.0	4.5	5.9	9.7	16.2	22.9	32.0	48.4	F		
33.8	65.6	125.3	225.4	445.4	793.5	1373.5	2280.0	4190.4	9194.8	M	ALL VASCULAR	390–459
15.9	24.0	40.2	68.8	144.7	297.3	612.9	1224.1	2722.4	8018.0	F	DISEASE	
0.2	0.2	0.9	1.6	3.9	6.1	8.1	10.9	10.8	12.7	M	Rheumatic heart	390–398
0.0	0.5	0.8	1.9	3.4	7.3	10.6	15.4	21.4	28.5	F	disease and fever	
1.4	2.4	5.7	10.6	20.8	33.5	51.8	84.5	144.7	280.8	M	Hypertensive disease	401–405
0.4	1.5	2.4	5.9	11.2	20.6	44.1	75.6	154.3	377.1	F		
14.0	32.6	65.6	121.4	250.4	444.9	745.7	1155.1	1899.4	3225.4	M	Ischaemic heart	410–414
3.0	5.7	12.2	22.2	54.9	123.0	255.1	484.0	988.3	2322.9	F	disease	
1.4	2.9	3.5	6.3	12.0	21.3	30.1	55.5	75.6	114.0	M	Pulmonary embolism	415.1, 451–453
1.4	2.5	3.4	5.1	9.1	14.8	25.1	40.2	66.9	116.9	F	and other venous	
4.6	7.9	16.3	25.6	55.2	103.0	213.1	411.8	905.4	2188.6	M	Cerebrovascular	430–438
5.1	7.3	10.1	14.4	27.8	55.4	123.9	285.1	702.3	2078.1	F	disease	
12.2	19.5	33.3	59.8	103.2	184.6	324.7	562.2	1154.4	3373.3	M	Other vascular	Rest of 390–459
5.9	6.5	11.3	19.4	38.3	76.2	154.2	323.7	789.2	3094.5	F	disease	
1.6	2.4	6.0	13.7	35.5	76.6	151.7	267.2	459.9	896.1	M	Chronic obstructive	490–496
1.2	1.4	4.1	5.7	11.2	23.0	39.5	69.1	107.8	243.5	F	pulmonary disease	
3.2	4.0	6.9	10.3	19.1	32.1	61.8	112.2	254.5	753.1	M	Other respiratory	Rest of 460–519
1.5	2.1	2.8	4.1	7.2	14.7	26.0	51.5	129.6	507.1	F	disease	
1.0	1.3	2.3	3.9	7.0	9.0	13.8	20.5	38.9	91.2	M	Peptic ulcer	531–533
0.3	0.3	1.0	1.2	2.6	2.8	6.7	10.5	22.2	58.7	F		
16.4	24.7	39.5	58.4	74.4	87.0	95.4	90.7	97.4	107.9	M	Liver cirrhosis	571
7.2	12.2	17.8	21.2	27.4	32.2	36.6	36.8	43.1	52.0	F		
0.9	1.8	2.3	5.7	9.5	13.3	22.8	38.2	72.2	173.5	M	Renal disease	580–590
0.7	0.6	1.8	3.2	6.2	11.3	17.5	28.1	51.5	108.4	F		
0.4	0.2	–	–	–	–	–	–	–	–	F	Pregnancy and birth	630–676
1.0	0.8	0.9	1.2	1.2	1.6	1.1	0.7	2.5	2.0	M	Congenital and	740–779
0.6	0.7	0.8	1.1	0.6	1.0	1.0	1.1	1.7	1.8	F	perinatal causes	
14.8	17.4	25.8	35.0	45.0	51.9	69.5	91.1	134.5	402.4	M	Ill-defined causes	780–799
5.5	6.4	10.1	11.7	14.1	22.2	31.8	53.7	92.8	400.1	F		
37.2	42.5	59.1	77.5	106.5	139.6	213.3	334.0	581.7	1112.3	M	Other medical causes	Rest of 001–799
13.0	17.6	23.9	33.6	57.9	92.9	155.3	260.5	495.4	1033.5	F		
62.3	58.7	73.3	80.0	85.9	78.6	82.7	111.0	187.5	422.9	M	ALL NON-	E800–E999
18.1	18.8	25.9	28.2	30.6	33.9	44.1	66.5	119.0	353.0	F	MEDICAL CAUSES	
16.2	12.2	13.9	15.1	15.9	14.9	14.3	20.4	31.5	42.2	M	Motor vehicle	E810–E819
5.1	4.1	5.1	5.6	5.6	6.4	7.6	11.8	17.0	19.6	F	traffic accidents	
0.9	1.3	1.2	1.3	1.4	1.1	1.7	1.0	2.9	6.1	M	Fire	E890–E899
0.3	0.4	0.5	0.4	0.6	0.5	1.1	1.1	3.0	4.6	F		
25.3	25.2	32.4	35.0	38.8	32.0	33.3	46.6	65.7	112.1	M	Suicide	E950–E959
7.3	8.6	12.5	13.2	13.9	14.8	17.9	21.4	26.8	31.8	F		
1.9	1.8	1.7	1.7	1.5	1.1	0.8	1.0	0.5	1.1	M	Homicide	E960–E969
1.0	1.1	0.8	0.6	1.1	0.2	0.5	0.9	0.8	1.3	F		
2855	2497	2723	3053	2303	2007	1464	820	882	836	M	**POPULATION (thousands)**	
2763	2391	2614	2975	2321	2325	2392	1500	1830	2149	F		

GERMANY: Males

	All ages	0–34	35–69	35–39	40–44	45–49	50–54	55–59	60–64	65–69	70–74	75–79	80+/NK
POPULATION (1000s)													
1955	31557	17156	12522	1334	2046	2324	2351	1869	1412	1186	902	610	366
1965	36739	20346	14135	2496	2074	1400	2109	2308	2180	1569	1034	693	531
1975	37322	19907	14766	3252	2558	2353	1904	1237	1752	1710	1364	759	527
1985	37051	18864	15321	2440	2710	3060	2365	2126	1637	983	1211	924	732
1990	**38276**	**18838**	**16900**	**2855**	**2497**	**2723**	**3053**	**2303**	**2007**	**1464**	**820**	**882**	**836**
1995 projected	*37461*	*17418*	*17490*	*3084*	*2797*	*2384*	*2588*	*2830*	*2080*	*1728*	*1175*	*571*	*807*
NUMBER OF DEATHS													
All causes													
1955	384341	50422	152749	3152	7213	13156	22340	29197	33877	43814	53460	59616	68094
1965	476886	42069	200826	5737	7240	7420	19494	36496	57868	66571	66237	68333	99421
1975	481191	29837	180021	7538	9771	13732	17738	17889	42739	70614	91312	79242	100779
1985	433752	20020	141406	4405	8219	15199	19701	27854	34057	31971	66279	83492	122555
1990	**425093**	**19747**	**161973**	**5785**	**7031**	**13061**	**23013**	**28847**	**39100**	**45136**	**38920**	**70583**	**133870**
1995 projected	*392243*	*17867*	*162852*	*6365*	*7742*	*10607*	*18374*	*33198*	*38346*	*48220*	*49683*	*41010*	*120831*
Lung cancer													
1955	10898	65	8412	36	173	554	1414	2149	2219	1867	1387	727	307
1965	21930	94	15161	94	219	354	1187	3050	5049	5208	3582	1990	1103
1975	25885	52	13899	163	347	813	1303	1504	3940	5829	6325	3761	1848
1985	26922	55	13322	108	432	1009	1912	3137	3616	3108	5202	4769	3574
1990	**27423**	**51**	**16094**	**123**	**318**	**991**	**2084**	**3315**	**4605**	**4658**	**3232**	**4133**	**3913**
1995 projected	*27223*	*46*	*16905*	*111*	*355*	*774*	*1645*	*3934*	*4771*	*5315*	*4299*	*2449*	*3524*
ANNUAL DEATH RATE / 100,000 (*The rates for the age groups 0–34 and 35–69 are the means of seven five-yearly rates, but the all-ages rates are standardised to the conventional "European" age distribution)													
All causes													
1955	1406.4*	287.1*	1394.3*	236.3	352.5	566.0	950.1	1562.4	2399.4	3693.6	5928.1	9768.3	18594.8
1965	1404.9*	194.1*	1501.7*	229.9	349.1	530.1	924.4	1581.5	2654.9	4242.1	6406.5	9860.5	18712.8
1975	1399.6*	163.0*	1449.2*	231.8	382.0	583.5	931.8	1445.9	2439.0	4130.2	6695.9	10445.8	19123.1
1985	1173.7*	105.4*	1207.9*	180.6	303.3	496.8	833.2	1310.1	2080.2	3251.4	5474.4	9039.8	16747.1
1990	**1090.2***	**100.3***	**1143.3***	**202.6**	**281.6**	**479.7**	**753.8**	**1252.6**	**1948.6**	**3083.9**	**4746.3**	**8003.5**	**16017.0**
1995 projected	*1007.8**	*96.7**	*1063.7**	*206.4*	*276.8*	*445.0*	*709.9*	*1173.0*	*1844.0*	*2790.7*	*4230.1*	*7182.1*	*14967.3*
All cancer													
1955	223.3*	10.3*	318.3*	27.7	52.4	110.2	216.1	379.1	589.3	853.2	1207.9	1557.1	1800.9
1965	261.1*	12.0*	361.3*	30.6	59.0	104.6	201.7	396.0	680.1	1057.0	1452.4	1832.5	2354.4
1975	268.4*	10.2*	362.3*	30.7	63.4	124.1	220.8	383.8	666.7	1046.3	1548.1	2029.5	2370.8
1985	269.9*	8.1*	358.3*	29.6	70.6	129.0	249.2	414.2	646.7	968.6	1426.1	1987.7	2698.0
1990	**267.1***	**6.8***	**357.3***	**28.4**	**60.0**	**134.1**	**237.2**	**414.7**	**650.7**	**975.7**	**1365.6**	**1934.5**	**2772.6**
1995 projected	*262.2**	*5.7**	*351.1**	*24.7*	*58.2*	*128.4*	*232.9*	*408.6*	*651.7*	*953.5*	*1322.4*	*1871.5*	*2797.7*
Lung cancer													
1955	36.6*	0.4*	75.0*	2.7	8.5	23.8	60.1	115.0	157.2	157.4	153.8	119.1	83.8
1965	60.0*	0.5*	113.1*	3.8	10.6	25.3	56.3	132.2	231.6	331.9	346.5	287.2	207.6
1975	71.7*	0.3*	115.6*	5.0	13.6	34.5	68.4	121.6	224.8	340.9	463.8	495.8	350.7
1985	75.0*	0.3*	117.0*	4.4	15.9	33.0	80.9	147.5	220.9	316.1	429.7	516.3	488.4
1990	**72.0***	**0.2***	**116.2***	**4.3**	**12.7**	**36.4**	**68.3**	**143.9**	**229.5**	**318.3**	**394.1**	**468.6**	**468.2**
1995 projected	*68.4**	*0.2**	*112.6**	*3.6*	*12.7*	*32.5*	*63.6*	*139.0*	*229.4*	*307.6*	*366.0*	*428.9*	*436.5*
Upper aerodigestive cancer (mouth, oesophagus, pharynx and larynx)													
1955	11.3*	0.1*	14.2*	0.7	1.3	4.0	8.7	16.6	27.0	40.7	60.3	99.1	121.5
1965	11.8*	0.1*	14.9*	0.8	1.9	3.2	7.6	16.6	29.8	44.7	64.2	84.7	144.2
1975	12.5*	0.1*	18.9*	1.6	4.9	9.5	14.1	21.4	32.1	48.4	66.7	82.1	94.9
1985	17.5*	0.2*	30.6*	3.2	13.2	22.9	36.0	41.9	44.2	52.8	63.8	74.1	95.7
1990	**19.7***	**0.1***	**36.6***	**3.6**	**12.4**	**28.2**	**41.1**	**51.0**	**60.2**	**59.8**	**63.9**	**72.7**	**90.8**
1995 projected	*22.0**	*0.1**	*42.9**	*3.4*	*13.8*	*31.5*	*48.1*	*62.5*	*73.3*	*67.8*	*65.3*	*68.3*	*87.5*
Other cancer													
1955	175.5*	9.8*	229.2*	24.2	42.7	82.3	147.2	247.5	405.2	655.1	993.8	1338.8	1595.6
1965	189.3*	11.4*	233.3*	26.0	46.5	76.1	137.8	247.3	418.6	680.5	1041.7	1460.6	2002.6
1975	184.2*	9.8*	227.8*	24.0	45.0	80.1	138.3	240.8	409.7	657.0	1017.6	1451.6	1925.2
1985	177.4*	7.6*	210.7*	22.0	41.4	73.1	132.3	224.8	381.7	599.7	932.7	1397.2	2114.0
1990	**175.4***	**6.4***	**204.4***	**20.5**	**34.9**	**69.5**	**127.8**	**219.7**	**361.1**	**597.7**	**907.6**	**1393.1**	**2213.6**
1995 projected	*171.8**	*5.3**	*195.6**	*17.8*	*31.7*	*64.4*	*121.2*	*207.0*	*349.0*	*578.1*	*891.1*	*1374.3*	*2273.8*
Chronic obstructive pulmonary disease (COPD)													
1955	42.5*	1.4*	51.6*	1.2	3.2	13.0	40.0	68.6	96.3	139.0	174.2	294.4	607.0
1965	52.8*	0.9*	63.4*	1.4	2.8	7.5	19.6	58.2	134.3	220.0	290.2	406.6	714.9
1975	77.9*	0.9*	73.4*	2.2	6.0	14.0	27.3	58.7	127.4	278.5	514.6	792.8	1082.4
1985	56.7*	0.7*	47.4*	1.5	3.1	7.6	18.7	42.2	90.9	167.5	322.0	562.9	974.0
1990	**49.1***	**0.6***	**41.1***	**1.6**	**2.4**	**6.0**	**13.7**	**35.5**	**76.6**	**151.7**	**267.2**	**459.9**	**896.1**
1995 projected	*41.9**	*0.5**	*34.6**	*1.4*	*1.9*	*4.4*	*10.7*	*28.9*	*66.5*	*128.4*	*221.5*	*387.4*	*790.7*
Other respiratory disease													
1955	74.4*	23.2*	43.3*	5.2	7.8	12.5	23.6	44.9	73.2	136.0	271.2	561.4	1351.4
1965	47.8*	7.5*	29.7*	3.5	4.7	7.9	13.5	27.0	51.3	100.1	192.1	379.5	1006.8
1975	40.8*	5.3*	26.7*	4.0	6.6	8.0	15.9	23.4	42.1	86.8	165.8	344.2	832.4
1985	33.2*	2.2*	19.1*	3.1	4.1	6.9	10.5	19.3	32.8	57.1	132.6	292.0	771.1
1990	**31.3***	**1.6***	**19.6***	**3.2**	**4.0**	**6.9**	**10.3**	**19.1**	**32.1**	**61.8**	**112.2**	**254.5**	**753.1**
1995 projected	*29.0**	*1.3**	*18.8**	*3.2*	*4.0*	*6.7*	*10.0*	*18.4*	*32.9*	*56.8*	*99.0*	*220.5*	*713.6*
Vascular disease													
1955	531.2*	8.1*	515.3*	36.5	68.2	138.5	274.9	533.7	946.7	1608.7	2832.2	4839.4	8276.6
1965	588.7*	6.2*	601.3*	44.3	93.2	170.9	331.5	599.5	1089.2	1880.5	3040.4	4993.8	9207.6
1975	637.4*	5.4*	582.4*	36.6	88.9	177.7	335.8	553.5	1023.2	1860.9	3239.7	5462.4	11237.6
1985	566.3*	5.0*	506.9*	33.7	70.4	144.6	293.6	530.1	927.9	1547.8	2816.7	4970.7	10089.2
1990	**491.7***	**5.5***	**437.5***	**33.8**	**65.6**	**125.3**	**225.4**	**445.4**	**793.5**	**1373.5**	**2280.0**	**4190.4**	**9194.8**
1995 projected	*422.5**	*5.9**	*366.7**	*32.6*	*58.8*	*101.1*	*181.4*	*365.8*	*682.3*	*1144.8*	*1901.4*	*3553.9*	*8172.3*
Liver cirrhosis													
1955	19.2*	0.5*	33.0*	4.3	8.8	14.5	27.1	43.1	57.1	76.0	100.6	96.3	83.6
1965	32.7*	0.8*	55.6*	7.3	14.1	25.6	42.3	69.8	100.4	129.9	150.6	179.5	176.9
1975	37.3*	2.1*	68.0*	17.7	33.7	47.9	61.2	78.0	104.4	132.9	137.9	144.7	137.2
1985	30.6*	1.5*	56.8*	13.6	26.0	41.1	58.1	68.4	87.6	102.7	106.9	118.4	98.5
1990	**29.9***	**1.5***	**56.5***	**16.4**	**24.7**	**39.5**	**58.4**	**74.4**	**87.0**	**95.4**	**90.7**	**97.4**	**107.9**
1995 projected	*28.9**	*1.7**	*55.1**	*16.8*	*24.5*	*38.1*	*58.8*	*75.0*	*85.5*	*87.0*	*77.8*	*88.6*	*102.1*
Other medical causes													
1955	398.8*	164.9*	307.2*	68.0	106.2	159.9	240.5	356.8	491.2	727.6	1131.5	2113.1	5847.1
1965	310.8*	97.8*	270.7*	56.6	87.7	119.7	192.1	290.9	450.6	697.5	1068.7	1747.3	4528.7
1975	234.2*	69.6*	226.4*	53.0	83.0	112.1	167.6	238.0	353.6	577.5	900.7	1399.8	2864.5
1985	151.6*	45.5*	149.3*	45.7	66.0	93.9	128.1	165.0	222.0	324.6	551.0	931.9	1739.8
1990	**152.5***	**41.1***	**156.8***	**57.1**	**66.3**	**94.6**	**128.9**	**177.6**	**230.1**	**343.0**	**519.6**	**879.4**	**1869.6**
1995 projected	*151.8**	*37.5**	*159.6**	*62.1*	*69.8*	*93.8*	*130.7*	*181.7*	*240.2*	*338.7*	*497.1*	*862.9*	*1923.7*
All non-medical causes													
1955	116.9*	78.7*	125.7*	93.5	106.1	117.4	127.9	136.1	145.5	153.2	210.5	306.6	628.1
1965	111.0*	68.9*	119.7*	86.3	87.6	93.9	123.7	140.1	149.0	156.9	212.2	321.2	723.5
1975	103.6*	69.5*	110.0*	87.6	100.3	99.7	103.2	110.6	121.6	147.2	189.1	272.3	598.3
1985	65.3*	42.3*	70.2*	53.4	62.9	73.6	74.9	70.8	72.3	83.1	119.1	176.3	376.3
1990	**68.5***	**43.1***	**74.5***	**62.3**	**58.7**	**73.3**	**80.0**	**85.9**	**78.6**	**82.7**	**111.0**	**187.5**	**422.9**
1995 projected	*71.4**	*44.1**	*77.7**	*65.6*	*59.6*	*72.5*	*85.4*	*94.7*	*85.0*	*81.3*	*110.9*	*197.4*	*467.2*

GERMANY: Females

	All ages	0–34	35–69	35–39	40–44	45–49	50–54	55–59	60–64	65–69	70–74	75–79	80+/NK
POPULATION (1000s)													
1955	36400	17576	16350	1886	2803	2935	2695	2395	2007	1628	1189	788	498
1965	41493	19147	18538	2592	2866	1993	2959	3066	2743	2320	1764	1167	877
1975	41357	18910	17716	3036	2417	2496	2705	1834	2646	2583	2089	1455	1188
1985	40617	17939	16868	2338	2629	2982	2350	2391	2529	1649	2203	1844	1764
1990	41088	17829	17781	2763	2391	2614	2975	2321	2325	2392	1500	1830	2149
1995 projected	39869	16561	17770	2904	2710	2314	2576	2879	2217	2170	2144	1229	2165
NUMBER OF DEATHS													
All causes													
1955	371046	35518	128902	3578	7370	11211	15505	20850	28939	41449	55883	66750	83993
1965	470605	25686	148359	3898	6668	6853	15801	24586	37122	53431	72619	85402	138539
1975	508458	16106	128616	3835	4885	7941	13636	13445	31449	53425	78945	100818	183973
1985	495897	10242	89495	2370	4194	7372	9289	14704	25186	26380	64252	98721	233187
1990	496352	9336	94470	2861	3622	6379	10401	13221	21381	36605	38072	88104	266370
1995 projected	443517	7854	84789	2923	4032	5249	8333	15033	19176	30043	48990	52672	249212
Lung cancer													
1955	2236	60	1469	20	78	162	189	309	310	401	338	268	101
1965	3982	54	2285	43	84	101	276	406	643	732	756	553	334
1975	4099	18	2062	33	61	116	239	250	616	747	775	680	564
1985	5519	30	2386	39	85	170	261	486	695	650	1082	954	1067
1990	6795	24	3234	49	122	238	381	519	787	1138	910	1145	1482
1995 projected	8025	20	3805	68	194	279	388	746	884	1246	1561	889	1750
ANNUAL DEATH RATE / 100,000 (*The rates for the age groups 0–34 and 35–69 are the means of seven five-yearly rates, but the all-ages rates are standardised to the conventional "European" age distribution)													
All causes													
1955	1081.6*	203.2*	895.4*	189.7	262.9	381.9	575.3	870.4	1441.9	2545.9	4700.8	8473.0	16862.7
1965	947.3*	123.0*	817.1*	150.4	232.7	343.9	534.0	801.8	1353.6	2303.1	4116.5	7318.1	15796.9
1975	878.6*	95.2*	734.4*	126.3	202.1	318.1	504.2	733.3	1188.8	2068.3	3780.0	6927.2	15487.2
1985	704.3*	60.2*	587.7*	101.4	159.5	247.2	395.3	614.9	995.9	1599.9	2916.8	5354.5	13219.2
1990	648.6*	52.8*	552.6*	103.5	151.5	244.0	349.7	569.7	919.7	1530.1	2538.6	4814.7	12395.6
1995 projected	594.6*	46.7*	510.2*	100.6	148.8	226.8	323.5	522.2	864.9	1384.7	2284.7	4285.4	11512.5
All cancer													
1955	185.8*	11.3*	266.3*	55.4	98.1	148.5	215.4	302.5	429.0	615.5	880.8	1216.4	1447.7
1965	191.5*	10.7*	268.5*	49.5	94.9	140.8	227.1	305.6	439.1	622.5	896.8	1226.6	1683.8
1975	172.6*	8.3*	247.7*	39.0	77.1	130.8	215.9	295.1	412.5	563.4	785.2	1087.7	1492.1
1985	162.4*	6.9*	227.6*	38.3	70.9	110.6	178.3	275.3	394.9	525.1	749.4	1025.3	1541.3
1990	159.3*	5.8*	225.6*	38.3	65.8	113.8	168.7	263.2	381.1	548.3	719.4	999.8	1549.3
1995 projected	155.3*	5.1*	219.6*	36.0	65.1	110.0	161.7	250.7	377.7	536.3	703.0	969.9	1539.0
Lung cancer													
1955	5.8*	0.3*	9.9*	1.1	2.8	5.5	7.0	12.9	15.4	24.6	28.4	34.0	20.3
1965	7.7*	0.3*	12.5*	1.7	2.9	5.1	9.3	13.2	23.4	31.6	42.9	47.4	38.1
1975	7.4*	0.1*	11.8*	1.1	2.5	4.6	8.8	13.6	23.3	28.9	37.1	46.7	47.5
1985	9.5*	0.2*	15.6*	1.7	3.2	5.7	11.1	20.3	27.5	39.4	49.1	51.7	60.5
1990	11.5*	0.1*	18.9*	1.8	5.1	9.1	12.8	22.4	33.9	47.6	60.7	62.6	69.0
1995 projected	13.7*	0.1*	22.8*	2.3	7.2	12.1	15.1	25.9	39.9	57.4	72.8	72.3	80.8
Upper aerodigestive cancer (mouth, oesophagus, pharynx and larynx)													
1955	3.0*	0.0*	2.8*	0.7	0.4	1.1	1.5	3.1	5.0	7.9	16.5	30.0	44.0
1965	2.8*	0.1*	2.6*	0.3	0.5	1.0	1.7	2.3	4.7	7.4	14.4	27.6	44.7
1975	2.3*	0.1*	2.6*	0.3	0.9	1.8	2.4	2.6	3.9	6.5	9.9	16.6	32.8
1985	2.6*	0.1*	3.9*	0.3	0.9	2.5	3.2	5.2	7.1	8.3	9.3	13.6	25.3
1990	2.9*	0.0*	4.7*	0.6	1.5	3.9	4.6	5.8	8.2	8.4	10.2	13.6	23.7
1995 projected	3.3*	0.0*	5.6*	0.9	2.1	5.5	5.9	6.8	8.8	9.0	10.4	13.8	22.7
Other cancer													
1955	177.0*	10.9*	253.6*	53.7	94.9	141.9	206.9	286.5	408.5	583.0	835.9	1152.4	1383.5
1965	181.0*	10.3*	253.5*	47.5	91.4	134.7	216.1	290.0	410.9	583.5	839.6	1151.7	1601.0
1975	162.9*	8.2*	233.2*	37.6	73.7	124.4	204.6	278.9	385.3	528.0	738.2	1024.4	1411.8
1985	150.3*	6.6*	208.1*	36.3	66.8	102.4	164.0	249.8	360.3	477.3	690.9	960.0	1455.4
1990	144.9*	5.7*	202.0*	35.9	59.2	100.8	151.3	235.1	339.1	492.3	648.5	923.7	1456.6
1995 projected	138.3*	5.0*	191.2*	32.8	55.9	92.5	140.7	217.9	329.1	469.9	619.8	883.7	1435.4
Chronic obstructive pulmonary disease (COPD)													
1955	16.3*	0.9*	8.7*	1.1	1.5	2.0	3.7	7.9	14.2	30.3	69.9	152.7	384.5
1965	14.0*	0.5*	8.9*	0.6	1.1	2.3	3.6	6.1	15.9	32.8	59.6	127.7	320.2
1975	18.9*	0.8*	15.4*	2.5	3.1	5.7	8.9	13.3	25.6	48.8	93.9	165.1	347.9
1985	14.6*	0.7*	13.6*	2.0	2.7	4.8	7.6	14.1	23.4	40.8	68.3	108.4	257.8
1990	13.6*	0.5*	12.3*	1.2	1.4	4.1	5.7	11.2	23.0	39.5	69.1	107.8	243.5
1995 projected	12.8*	0.4*	11.3*	0.9	1.0	3.0	4.5	9.8	21.5	38.7	67.7	99.6	233.7
Other respiratory disease													
1955	61.0*	20.8*	29.0*	5.5	7.4	8.3	12.6	23.0	47.6	98.2	240.2	496.8	1119.7
1965	33.3*	5.9*	16.4*	2.2	3.6	5.0	8.3	13.9	27.5	54.0	126.4	278.7	750.5
1975	26.2*	4.2*	13.8*	2.7	2.9	5.3	7.8	12.2	22.9	42.6	95.2	213.3	598.6
1985	18.8*	1.5*	8.2*	1.5	1.7	3.3	4.9	7.0	12.5	26.5	58.4	144.7	521.8
1990	17.9*	1.3*	8.3*	1.5	2.1	2.8	4.1	7.2	14.7	26.0	51.5	129.6	507.1
1995 projected	16.8*	1.1*	8.1*	1.5	2.0	2.5	3.7	7.6	15.1	24.2	45.8	114.8	484.5
Vascular disease													
1955	444.7*	7.4*	342.0*	26.2	43.0	79.6	151.5	285.8	584.9	1222.6	2492.6	4556.2	7942.0
1965	416.4*	3.9*	293.3*	20.5	37.2	66.3	127.1	245.7	513.0	1043.4	2126.8	4080.5	8468.1
1975	429.2*	3.5*	252.6*	17.3	31.9	62.5	107.7	195.1	423.4	930.3	1980.9	4098.4	10032.0
1985	359.4*	3.1*	199.4*	13.8	24.6	44.6	88.6	172.0	349.9	702.0	1541.1	3241.7	8944.9
1990	311.7*	3.3*	172.0*	15.9	24.0	40.2	68.8	144.7	297.3	612.9	1224.1	2722.4	8018.0
1995 projected	266.9*	3.6*	142.7*	15.7	23.0	33.3	56.3	119.7	253.5	497.3	1002.5	2246.2	7066.5
Liver cirrhosis													
1955	8.0*	0.3*	12.1*	1.2	3.1	5.3	8.8	14.8	19.8	31.5	45.4	50.8	53.0
1965	13.9*	0.4*	19.7*	2.0	5.2	9.7	12.5	21.5	35.8	51.5	74.7	94.3	115.8
1975	12.5*	0.8*	19.8*	6.0	10.5	14.4	20.2	23.9	27.4	36.5	49.3	66.9	73.5
1985	11.6*	0.6*	20.4*	7.1	9.9	15.4	20.6	25.7	31.4	32.4	39.9	49.0	53.7
1990	12.2*	0.7*	22.1*	7.2	12.2	17.8	21.2	27.4	32.2	36.6	36.8	43.1	52.0
1995 projected	12.6*	0.8*	23.3*	8.3	13.8	19.5	22.5	28.2	34.2	36.8	34.8	39.1	48.2
Other medical causes													
1955	314.9*	140.3*	196.7*	76.8	83.4	106.1	143.6	192.7	297.5	477.2	843.4	1733.3	5222.6
1965	222.3*	80.3*	165.9*	52.0	63.8	84.3	113.2	164.0	264.6	419.1	687.9	1228.9	3585.6
1975	167.0*	53.6*	139.8*	30.8	45.6	64.9	96.8	143.7	221.0	375.7	651.3	1070.2	2276.5
1985	107.4*	32.8*	90.5*	21.7	30.2	44.8	67.5	92.2	149.5	227.4	391.4	669.3	1549.0
1990	103.7*	26.9*	83.8*	21.4	27.1	39.4	53.0	85.3	137.6	222.8	371.2	693.0	1672.7
1995 projected	100.2*	21.9*	76.5*	19.6	24.4	32.4	45.3	75.3	129.3	209.1	365.4	696.3	1783.9
All non-medical causes													
1955	50.7*	22.1*	40.7*	23.5	26.5	31.9	39.7	43.8	49.0	70.6	128.5	266.7	693.2
1965	55.9*	21.3*	44.4*	23.6	27.0	35.6	42.1	44.9	57.7	79.8	144.4	281.4	872.9
1975	52.1*	24.0*	45.3*	28.1	31.1	34.4	46.7	49.8	56.0	71.0	124.1	225.6	666.6
1985	30.1*	14.6*	28.1*	17.1	19.5	23.6	27.9	28.5	34.3	45.5	68.4	116.2	350.9
1990	30.2*	14.3*	28.5*	18.1	18.8	25.9	28.2	30.6	33.9	44.1	66.5	119.0	353.0
1995 projected	30.2*	13.8*	28.7*	18.8	19.4	26.1	29.4	30.9	33.6	42.3	65.3	119.6	356.8

GERMANY: 1975

Smoking–attributed deaths (Sm.) and total deaths (Total)

		ALL CAUSES	ALL CANCER	Lung cancer	Upper aero–digestive ca.	Other cancer	COPD	Other respiratory	Vascular disease	Liver cirrhosis	Other medical	Non–medical
Males												
0–34	Sm.	–	–	–	–	–	–	–	–	–	–	–
	Total	29837	1997	52	25	1920	175	900	1063	420	11673	13609
35–69	Sm.	53639	18682	12861	1495	4326	6828	899	19121	–	8109	–
	Total	180021	44063	13899	2325	27839	8795	3303	70630	8796	28692	15742
		(30%)	(42%)	(93%)	(64%)	(16%)	(78%)	(27%)	(27%)		(28%)	
70+	Sm.	55475	16757	10893	1226	4638	13806	1143	18773	–	4996	–
	Total	271333	49001	11934	2032	35035	18736	9259	144840	3701	37998	7798
		(20%)	(34%)	(91%)	(60%)	(13%)	(74%)	(12%)	(13%)		(13%)	
Any age	Sm.	109114	35439	23754	2721	8964	20634	2042	37894	–	13105	–
	Total	481191	95061	25885	4382	64794	27706	13462	216533	12917	78363	37149
		(23%)	(37%)	(92%)	(62%)	(14%)	(74%)	(15%)	(18%)		(17%)	
Females												
0–34	Sm.	–	–	–	–	–	–	–	–	–	–	–
	Total	16106	1546	18	12	1516	153	687	637	142	8545	4396
35–69	Sm.	2768	655	508	35	112	435	57	1075	–	546	–
	Total	128616	43030	2062	459	40509	2715	2427	44579	3448	24462	7955
		(2%)	(2%)	(25%)	(8%)	(0%)	(16%)	(2%)	(2%)		(2%)	
70+	Sm.	4342	706	506	65	135	1344	93	1729	–	470	–
	Total	363736	49955	2019	839	47097	8498	12204	220190	2876	56220	13793
		(1%)	(1%)	(25%)	(8%)	(0%)	(16%)	(1%)	(1%)		(1%)	
Any age	Sm.	7110	1361	1014	100	247	1779	150	2804	–	1016	–
	Total	508458	94531	4099	1310	89122	11366	15318	265406	6466	89227	26144
		(1%)	(1%)	(25%)	(8%)	(0%)	(16%)	(1%)	(1%)		(1%)	
Males+Females												
0–34	Sm.	–	–	–	–	–	–	–	–	–	–	–
	Total	45943	3543	70	37	3436	328	1587	1700	562	20218	18005
35–69	Sm.	56407	19337	13369	1530	4438	7263	956	20196	–	8655	–
	Total	308637	87093	15961	2784	68348	11510	5730	115209	12244	53154	23697
		(18%)	(22%)	(84%)	(55%)	(6%)	(63%)	(17%)	(18%)		(16%)	
70+	Sm.	59817	17463	11399	1291	4773	15150	1236	20502	–	5466	–
	Total	635069	98956	13953	2871	82132	27234	21463	365030	6577	94218	21591
		(9%)	(18%)	(82%)	(45%)	(6%)	(56%)	(6%)	(6%)		(6%)	
Any age	Sm.	116224	36800	24768	2821	9211	22413	2192	40698	–	14121	–
	Total	989649	189592	29984	5692	153916	39072	28780	481939	19383	167590	63293
		(12%)	(19%)	(83%)	(50%)	(6%)	(57%)	(8%)	(8%)		(8%)	

GERMANY: 1985

Smoking–attributed deaths (Sm.) and total deaths (Total)

		ALL CAUSES	ALL CANCER	Lung cancer	Upper aero–digestive ca.	Other cancer	COPD	Other respiratory	Vascular disease	Liver cirrhosis	Other medical	Non–medical
Males												
0–34	Sm.	–	–	–	–	–	–	–	–	–	–	–
	Total	20020	1633	55	43	1535	150	373	1019	309	7712	8824
35–69	Sm.	46084	18871	12353	2700	3818	3753	651	16654	–	6155	–
	Total	141406	41394	13322	4122	23950	4830	2155	55780	7567	19142	10538
		(33%)	(46%)	(93%)	(66%)	(16%)	(78%)	(30%)	(30%)		(32%)	
70+	Sm.	53985	18790	12329	1293	5168	11918	1157	18680	–	3440	–
	Total	272326	55368	13545	2156	39667	16226	9945	153844	3109	28010	5824
		(20%)	(34%)	(91%)	(60%)	(13%)	(73%)	(12%)	(12%)		(12%)	
Any age	Sm.	100069	37661	24682	3993	8986	15671	1808	35334	–	9595	–
	Total	433752	98395	26922	6321	65152	21206	12473	210643	10985	54864	25186
		(23%)	(38%)	(92%)	(63%)	(14%)	(74%)	(14%)	(17%)		(17%)	
Females												
0–34	Sm.	–	–	–	–	–	–	–	–	–	–	–
	Total	10242	1274	30	18	1226	143	243	601	111	5139	2731
35–69	Sm.	4057	1293	996	97	200	600	59	1428	–	677	–
	Total	89495	35477	2386	623	32468	2040	1214	28922	3312	13958	4572
		(5%)	(4%)	(42%)	(16%)	(1%)	(29%)	(5%)	(5%)		(5%)	
70+	Sm.	7237	1512	1123	110	279	1851	150	3080	–	644	–
	Total	396160	62599	3103	903	58593	8050	13157	251504	2728	48284	9838
		(2%)	(2%)	(36%)	(12%)	(0%)	(23%)	(1%)	(1%)		(1%)	
Any age	Sm.	11294	2805	2119	207	479	2451	209	4508	–	1321	–
	Total	495897	99350	5519	1544	92287	10233	14614	281027	6151	67381	17141
		(2%)	(3%)	(38%)	(13%)	(1%)	(24%)	(1%)	(2%)		(2%)	
Males+Females												
0–34	Sm.	–	–	–	–	–	–	–	–	–	–	–
	Total	30262	2907	85	61	2761	293	616	1620	420	12851	11555
35–69	Sm.	50141	20164	13349	2797	4018	4353	710	18082	–	6832	–
	Total	230901	76871	15708	4745	56418	6870	3369	84702	10879	33100	15110
		(22%)	(26%)	(85%)	(59%)	(7%)	(63%)	(21%)	(21%)		(21%)	
70+	Sm.	61222	20302	13452	1403	5447	13769	1307	21760	–	4084	–
	Total	668486	117967	16648	3059	98260	24276	23102	405348	5837	76294	15662
		(9%)	(17%)	(81%)	(46%)	(6%)	(57%)	(6%)	(5%)		(5%)	
Any age	Sm.	111363	40466	26801	4200	9465	18122	2017	39842	–	10916	–
	Total	929649	197745	32441	7865	157439	31439	27087	491670	17136	122245	42327
		(12%)	(20%)	(83%)	(53%)	(6%)	(58%)	(7%)	(8%)		(9%)	

(To be conservative, no deaths before age 35, and none from liver cirrhosis or non–medical causes, were attributed to smoking.)

GERMANY: 1990

Smoking–attributed deaths (Sm.) and total deaths (Total)

		ALL CAUSES	ALL CANCER	Lung cancer	Upper aero–digestive ca.	Other cancer	COPD	Other respiratory	Vascular disease	Liver cirrhosis	Other medical	Non–medical
Males												
0–34	Sm.	–	–	–	–	–	–	–	–	–	–	–
	Total	19747	1399	51	28	1320	124	300	1163	348	7457	8956
35–69	Sm.	52014	23021	14902	3686	4433	4077	773	16919	–	7224	–
	Total	161973	50089	16094	5693	28302	5259	2682	59177	8798	23520	12448
		(32%)	(46%)	(93%)	(65%)	(16%)	(78%)	(29%)	(29%)		(31%)	
70+	Sm.	43320	15783	10159	1103	4521	9787	957	13870	–	2923	–
	Total	243373	51431	11278	1924	38229	13737	9458	132501	2505	27642	6099
		(18%)	(31%)	(90%)	(57%)	(12%)	(71%)	(10%)	(10%)		(11%)	
Any age	Sm.	95334	38804	25061	4789	8954	13864	1730	30789	–	10147	–
	Total	425093	102919	27423	7645	67851	19120	12440	192841	11651	58619	27503
		(22%)	(38%)	(91%)	(63%)	(13%)	(73%)	(14%)	(16%)		(17%)	
Females												
0–34	Sm.	–	–	–	–	–	–	–	–	–	–	–
	Total	9336	1142	24	8	1110	98	220	634	156	4405	2681
35–69	Sm.	6169	2183	1684	178	321	803	100	2062	–	1021	–
	Total	94470	38710	3234	817	34659	2085	1414	29043	3848	14351	5019
		(7%)	(6%)	(52%)	(22%)	(1%)	(39%)	(7%)	(7%)		(7%)	
70+	Sm.	10374	2243	1654	165	424	2661	236	4230	–	1004	–
	Total	392546	62377	3537	911	57929	8242	14042	240474	2458	54193	10760
		(3%)	(4%)	(47%)	(18%)	(1%)	(32%)	(2%)	(2%)		(2%)	
Any age	Sm.	16543	4426	3338	343	745	3464	336	6292	–	2025	–
	Total	496352	102229	6795	1736	93698	10425	15676	270151	6462	72949	18460
		(3%)	(4%)	(49%)	(20%)	(1%)	(33%)	(2%)	(2%)		(3%)	
Males+Females												
0–34	Sm.	–	–	–	–	–	–	–	–	–	–	–
	Total	29083	2541	75	36	2430	222	520	1797	504	11862	11637
35–69	Sm.	58183	25204	16586	3864	4754	4880	873	18981	–	8245	–
	Total	256443	88799	19328	6510	62961	7344	4096	88220	12646	37871	17467
		(23%)	(28%)	(86%)	(59%)	(8%)	(66%)	(21%)	(22%)		(22%)	
70+	Sm.	53694	18026	11813	1268	4945	12448	1193	18100	–	3927	–
	Total	635919	113808	14815	2835	96158	21979	23500	372975	4963	81835	16859
		(8%)	(16%)	(80%)	(45%)	(5%)	(57%)	(5%)	(5%)		(5%)	
Any age	Sm.	111877	43230	28399	5132	9699	17328	2066	37081	–	12172	–
	Total	921445	205148	34218	9381	161549	29545	28116	462992	18113	131568	45963
		(12%)	(21%)	(83%)	(55%)	(6%)	(59%)	(7%)	(8%)		(9%)	

GERMANY: 1995

Smoking–attributed deaths (Sm.) and total deaths (Total)

		ALL CAUSES	ALL CANCER	Lung cancer	Upper aero–digestive ca.	Other cancer	COPD	Other respiratory	Vascular disease	Liver cirrhosis	Other medical	Non–medical
Males												
0–34	Sm.	–	–	–	–	–	–	–	–	–	–	–
	Total	17867	1105	46	25	1034	99	245	1197	392	6609	8220
35–69	Sm.	51440	24463	15606	4429	4428	3766	784	14898	–	7529	–
	Total	162852	53071	16905	6951	29215	4898	2813	54076	9036	25476	13482
		(32%)	(46%)	(92%)	(64%)	(15%)	(77%)	(28%)	(28%)		(30%)	
70+	Sm.	36502	14242	9180	1033	4029	7775	789	11000	–	2696	–
	Total	211524	48804	10272	1863	36669	11196	8183	108600	2244	26295	6202
		(17%)	(29%)	(89%)	(55%)	(11%)	(69%)	(10%)	(10%)		(10%)	
Any age	Sm.	87942	38705	24786	5462	8457	11541	1573	25898	–	10225	–
	Total	392243	102980	27223	8839	66918	16193	11241	163873	11672	58380	27904
		(22%)	(38%)	(91%)	(62%)	(13%)	(71%)	(14%)	(16%)		(18%)	
Females												
0–34	Sm.	–	–	–	–	–	–	–	–	–	–	–
	Total	7854	994	20	7	967	73	181	640	179	3404	2383
35–69	Sm.	7380	2964	2288	265	411	852	127	2211	–	1226	–
	Total	84789	36747	3805	946	31996	1834	1328	23157	4018	12718	4987
		(9%)	(8%)	(60%)	(28%)	(1%)	(46%)	(10%)	(10%)		(10%)	
70+	Sm.	13119	3124	2341	210	573	3099	307	5104	–	1485	–
	Total	350874	60309	4200	884	55225	7735	12882	202073	2270	55011	10594
		(4%)	(5%)	(56%)	(24%)	(1%)	(40%)	(2%)	(3%)		(3%)	
Any age	Sm.	20499	6088	4629	475	984	3951	434	7315	–	2711	–
	Total	443517	98050	8025	1837	88188	9642	14391	225870	6467	71133	17964
		(5%)	(6%)	(58%)	(26%)	(1%)	(41%)	(3%)	(3%)		(4%)	
Males+Females												
0–34	Sm.	–	–	–	–	–	–	–	–	–	–	–
	Total	25721	2099	66	32	2001	172	426	1837	571	10013	10603
35–69	Sm.	58820	27427	17894	4694	4839	4618	911	17109	–	8755	–
	Total	247641	89818	20710	7897	61211	6732	4141	77233	13054	38194	18469
		(24%)	(31%)	(86%)	(59%)	(8%)	(69%)	(22%)	(22%)		(23%)	
70+	Sm.	49621	17366	11521	1243	4602	10874	1096	16104	–	4181	–
	Total	562398	109113	14472	2747	91894	18931	21065	310673	4514	81306	16796
		(9%)	(16%)	(80%)	(45%)	(5%)	(57%)	(5%)	(5%)		(5%)	
Any age	Sm.	108441	44793	29415	5937	9441	15492	2007	33213	–	12936	–
	Total	835760	201030	35248	10676	155106	25835	25632	389743	18139	129513	45868
		(13%)	(22%)	(83%)	(56%)	(6%)	(60%)	(8%)	(9%)		(10%)	

(To be conservative, no deaths before age 35, and none from liver cirrhosis or non–medical causes, were attributed to smoking.)

GREECE: 1990

		No. of deaths			Standardised rates (Defined on p.370)			Annual death rates / 100, 000						
		All ages	0–34	35–69	All ages	0–34	35–69	0–4	5–9	10–14	15–19	20–24	25–29	30–34
ALL CAUSES	M	49433	2349	15547	865.5	97.8	846.3	216.3	25.2	25.9	81.2	125.9	98.1	111.8
	F	44719	1251	8236	577.4	58.4	409.0	205.3	18.2	14.4	29.3	39.6	49.2	53.0
Tuberculosis	M	110	3	39	2.0	0.1	2.1	–	–	–	–	–	0.5	0.3
	F	48	1	11	0.6	0.0	0.6	–	–	–	–	–	–	0.3
Other infective	M	226	5	57	3.8	0.2	3.1	–	0.6	–	0.3	0.2	–	0.3
and parasitic	F	220	7	47	2.8	0.3	2.4	–	–	–	0.6	0.3	0.8	0.3
ALL CANCER	M	12032	180	5475	216.1	7.1	299.8	3.6	4.7	4.0	8.0	7.7	7.9	13.9
	F	7400	163	3379	110.6	6.8	162.7	5.8	3.4	3.5	4.1	4.3	9.0	17.7
Mouth and	M	114	1	65	2.1	0.0	3.5	–	–	–	–	–	–	0.3
pharynx cancer	F	62	–	18	0.8	–	0.9	–	–	–	–	–	–	–
Oesophagus cancer	M	132	–	66	2.4	–	3.7	–	–	–	–	–	–	–
	F	50	–	15	0.7	–	0.7	–	–	–	–	–	–	–
Stomach cancer	M	816	10	395	14.7	0.4	21.2	–	–	–	–	0.2	1.1	1.4
	F	531	7	190	7.5	0.3	9.3	–	–	–	–	–	0.3	1.7
Colorectal cancer	M	624	4	232	11.0	0.2	12.7	–	–	–	0.3	–	0.3	0.6
	F	619	3	204	8.5	0.1	9.8	–	–	–	0.3	–	–	0.6
Liver cancer	M	32	–	20	0.6	–	1.1	–	–	–	–	–	–	–
	F	7	–	4	0.1	–	0.2	–	–	–	–	–	–	–
Pancreas cancer	M	493	4	225	8.9	0.2	12.4	–	0.3	–	–	0.2	–	0.6
	F	343	2	130	4.8	0.1	6.5	0.4	–	–	–	–	–	0.3
Larynx cancer	M	323	1	140	5.8	0.0	7.9	–	–	–	–	–	–	0.3
	F	28	–	10	0.4	–	0.5	–	–	–	–	–	–	–
Lung cancer	M	4034	18	2168	73.8	0.7	118.9	0.4	–	0.3	–	0.5	1.1	2.8
	F	714	7	336	10.6	0.3	16.1	–	–	–	0.3	–	0.6	1.1
Malignant melanoma	M	34	2	22	0.7	0.1	1.1	–	–	–	–	–	0.3	0.3
	F	32	2	21	0.5	0.1	1.0	–	–	–	–	–	0.3	0.3
Female breast cancer	F	1272	18	824	20.9	0.7	38.6	–	–	–	0.3	–	2.0	2.8
Cervix cancer	F	113	5	67	1.9	0.2	3.2	–	–	–	–	–	0.3	1.1
Other uterine cancer	F	251	7	116	3.8	0.3	5.6	–	–	–	–	0.3	0.3	1.4
Ovarian cancer	F	260	7	169	4.3	0.3	7.9	–	–	–	–	–	0.3	1.7
Prostate cancer	M	831	1	131	13.8	0.0	7.8	–	–	–	0.3	–	–	–
Bladder cancer	M	659	1	202	11.4	0.0	11.7	–	–	–	–	0.2	–	–
	F	136	–	33	1.8	–	1.7	–	–	–	–	–	–	–
Other and ill–defined	M	3182	82	1485	57.5	3.3	80.1	3.3	2.6	2.2	3.6	3.7	2.4	5.4
cancer sites	F	2479	67	1025	36.3	2.8	50.2	2.7	2.2	0.9	1.8	3.2	3.1	5.9
Hodgkin's disease	M	96	6	57	1.8	0.2	3.0	–	–	–	0.3	0.2	0.5	0.6
	F	53	3	24	0.8	0.1	1.2	–	–	–	–	0.3	0.6	–
Myeloma and non–	M	226	8	110	4.1	0.3	5.8	–	–	0.3	1.1	0.5	–	0.3
Hodgkin lymphomas	F	185	5	80	2.7	0.2	4.0	0.4	–	0.3	0.6	0.3	–	–
Leukaemia	M	436	42	157	7.7	1.6	8.7	–	1.8	1.3	2.5	2.0	2.4	1.4
	F	265	30	113	4.1	1.3	5.5	2.3	1.3	2.3	0.9	0.3	1.4	0.8
ALL VASCULAR	M	23580	175	6454	401.9	6.8	355.3	0.7	0.6	1.3	2.2	8.7	12.4	21.5
DISEASE	F	25499	107	3053	307.5	4.3	157.0	0.8	0.9	1.7	2.3	4.5	8.2	11.8
Rheumatic heart	M	8	–	4	0.1	–	0.2	–	–	–	–	–	–	–
disease and fever	F	23	2	10	0.4	0.1	0.5	–	–	–	0.3	0.3	–	–
Hypertensive disease	M	446	3	83	7.4	0.1	4.7	–	–	–	–	–	0.3	0.6
	F	578	4	54	6.9	0.2	2.8	–	–	–	–	–	0.8	0.3
Ischaemic heart	M	7581	52	3385	135.5	2.0	182.7	–	–	–	–	1.5	2.4	10.5
disease	F	4528	12	931	57.9	0.5	47.7	–	–	–	–	0.5	1.7	1.1
Pulmonary embolism	M	319	13	124	5.6	0.5	6.4	–	0.3	–	–	0.7	0.8	1.7
and other venous	F	419	7	123	5.7	0.3	6.1	–	–	–	–	0.5	0.6	0.8
Cerebrovascular	M	7518	44	1300	124.5	1.7	74.2	0.4	0.3	1.3	1.1	1.7	4.2	2.8
disease	F	10754	42	997	127.6	1.7	51.6	0.8	0.9	1.4	1.5	1.6	2.2	3.6
Other vascular	M	7708	63	1558	128.7	2.4	87.0	0.4	–	–	1.1	4.7	4.7	5.9
disease	F	9197	40	938	108.9	1.6	48.4	–	–	0.3	0.6	1.6	2.8	5.9
Chronic obstructive	M	531	1	118	8.9	0.0	6.8	–	–	–	–	0.2	–	–
pulmonary disease	F	259	1	41	3.2	0.0	2.1	–	–	–	–	0.3	–	–
Other respiratory	M	2245	57	488	37.9	2.2	27.0	1.5	0.6	0.8	0.6	5.0	3.4	3.7
disease	F	2136	29	293	26.5	1.3	14.7	3.9	0.6	–	0.6	1.3	1.7	1.1
Peptic ulcer	M	76	5	25	1.3	0.2	1.3	–	–	–	–	0.2	0.3	0.8
	F	48	1	8	0.6	0.0	0.4	–	–	–	–	–	0.3	–
Liver cirrhosis	M	676	8	386	12.6	0.3	20.8	0.4	–	–	–	–	0.8	1.1
	F	283	8	97	4.0	0.3	4.9	–	–	–	0.3	0.3	1.1	0.6
Renal disease	M	966	21	210	16.3	0.8	11.5	0.4	0.3	–	0.6	1.7	1.3	1.4
	F	852	9	145	10.7	0.4	7.3	0.4	–	–	0.6	–	0.6	1.1
Pregnancy and birth	F	1	1	–	0.0	0.0	–	–	–	–	–	0.3	–	–
Congenital and	M	551	550	1	15.6	28.0	0.1	183.3	3.2	3.8	5.2	0.2	–	–
perinatal causes	F	490	487	2	14.8	26.5	0.1	177.4	2.2	2.9	2.3	0.3	0.3	0.3
Ill–defined causes	M	3675	61	562	60.8	2.5	31.5	4.4	1.5	0.5	1.9	3.2	2.9	3.1
	F	4205	35	358	49.1	1.5	18.1	2.3	0.9	0.9	0.6	1.1	2.5	2.2
Other medical causes	M	1712	102	472	29.9	4.1	25.2	4.0	1.2	1.9	5.2	3.7	4.5	8.2
	F	1897	71	364	24.6	2.9	18.2	1.9	1.3	1.7	2.3	4.5	3.9	4.8
ALL NON–	M	3053	1181	1260	58.5	45.4	61.9	18.1	12.6	13.5	57.3	94.9	64.2	57.5
MEDICAL CAUSES	F	1381	331	438	22.2	13.8	20.5	12.8	8.8	3.8	15.5	22.5	20.8	12.9
Motor vehicle	M	1686	790	662	32.3	30.1	32.3	5.8	8.5	9.2	45.4	70.1	39.5	32.0
traffic accidents	F	561	212	217	9.9	8.6	10.0	1.9	5.3	3.2	11.7	18.2	12.1	7.8
Fire	M	65	11	26	1.2	0.4	1.4	–	0.3	0.3	0.3	0.5	1.1	0.6
	F	78	2	17	1.1	0.1	0.8	–	–	–	–	–	0.6	–
Suicide	M	271	89	125	5.1	3.4	6.1	–	–	0.8	2.2	7.9	6.3	6.2
	F	78	19	48	1.4	0.8	2.3	–	–	–	0.6	1.6	1.4	1.7
Homicide	M	73	36	33	1.4	1.4	1.5	–	–	0.3	1.9	1.2	3.2	3.1
	F	34	14	14	0.6	0.6	0.6	–	–	–	0.6	0.8	2.0	0.6
POPULATION (thousands):	M=males				4968.3	2488.0	2065.6	275.5	341.5	370.6	363.3	403.6	380.2	353.3
	F=females				5120.6	2352.3	2203.6	258.7	319.3	346.1	341.5	374.1	355.8	356.8

GREECE: 1990

Annual death rates / 100, 000

9th ICD categories

35–39	40–44	45–49	50–54	55–59	60–64	65–69	70–74	75–79	80+/NK			
143.7	226.2	311.7	534.4	875.2	1482.4	2350.4	3858.1	6165.2	13530.0	M	ALL CAUSES	001–999
65.9	102.7	168.0	234.2	382.1	675.5	1234.9	2354.1	4291.9	12209.4	F		
0.3	0.9	1.5	1.3	2.2	3.5	4.9	12.6	19.2	17.9	M	Tuberculosis	010–018, 137
0.3	–	0.3	–	0.3	0.9	2.1	1.5	7.7	10.2	F		
1.2	1.2	0.7	2.6	1.6	4.9	9.9	15.9	36.1	70.9	M	Other infective	Rest of 001–139
–	0.3	1.4	1.5	1.7	4.4	7.3	9.7	20.3	58.9	F	and parasitic	
28.1	54.1	101.2	190.5	318.9	559.4	846.0	1205.6	1551.6	1913.5	M	ALL CANCER	140–208
29.0	50.8	94.2	133.4	183.9	262.0	385.3	496.9	673.1	888.1	F		
0.3	0.9	1.1	2.9	3.2	7.0	9.4	7.3	10.3	17.9	M	Mouth and	140–149
–	–	0.3	–	1.1	2.2	2.6	4.6	4.9	13.9	F	pharynx cancer	
0.3	0.6	0.4	1.6	4.1	7.0	11.8	10.6	14.7	23.4	M	Oesophagus cancer	150
–	0.3	–	0.6	1.7	1.3	0.9	3.1	6.0	9.6	F		
2.0	4.5	7.6	17.1	20.8	44.3	52.3	68.3	109.1	124.7	M	Stomach cancer	151
0.9	3.0	4.8	7.6	9.1	13.8	26.1	34.8	66.3	77.7	F		
1.2	1.2	2.2	9.0	16.1	22.3	37.0	69.0	91.4	124.7	M	Colorectal cancer	153, 154
0.6	1.8	5.1	8.2	12.5	17.6	22.6	44.5	63.0	112.5	F		
–	–	0.4	1.3	1.6	1.7	2.5	3.3	2.9	2.3	M	Liver cancer	155.0
–	–	–	–	0.6	0.3	0.4	0.5	1.1	–	F		
0.9	0.9	4.7	10.0	13.9	19.5	37.0	46.4	66.4	81.1	M	Pancreas cancer	157
–	0.3	0.7	5.6	7.4	10.1	21.4	25.1	39.4	48.2	F		
–	0.9	2.5	4.5	7.6	13.6	26.2	37.8	51.6	42.9	M	Larynx cancer	161
–	–	0.3	0.3	0.6	0.6	1.7	1.5	2.2	5.9	F		
6.7	21.0	41.2	72.3	129.8	224.1	337.1	429.0	472.7	436.5	M	Lung cancer	162
2.1	4.8	8.9	13.2	19.9	27.3	36.3	49.1	68.5	80.3	F		
–	1.2	0.4	1.6	0.9	1.4	2.5	2.0	2.2	3.1	M	Malignant melanoma	172
0.3	0.9	0.7	0.6	0.3	2.2	2.1	0.5	2.7	1.6	F		
11.2	18.2	31.8	41.3	46.7	52.8	68.3	63.5	73.9	91.6	F	Female breast cancer	174
0.6	1.8	3.1	3.8	2.8	4.1	6.0	7.2	6.6	8.0	F	Cervix cancer	180
3.0	1.2	3.4	3.2	6.3	8.2	14.1	15.4	17.5	35.4	F	Other uterine cancer	179, 182
1.5	3.6	4.4	7.0	10.8	14.5	13.2	17.9	13.1	13.4	F	Ovarian cancer	183
–	0.3	1.1	1.9	6.3	11.9	33.1	86.9	141.6	293.1	M	Prostate cancer	185
–	0.9	1.8	3.6	10.7	20.9	43.9	75.6	104.7	155.9	M	Bladder cancer	188
0.3	–	1.4	–	1.1	4.1	4.7	12.3	20.3	22.5	F		
11.7	15.3	31.7	53.0	87.6	156.8	204.8	315.0	389.4	477.0	M	Other and ill-defined	Rest of 140–208
6.6	12.2	25.9	33.4	51.5	86.4	135.0	182.2	241.5	316.0	F	cancer sites	
2.0	1.2	1.5	2.3	3.2	3.5	7.4	6.0	12.5	5.5	M	Hodgkin's disease	201
–	1.2	0.7	0.9	0.9	1.3	3.4	4.6	3.8	5.4	F		
1.2	2.7	1.8	3.9	6.3	11.5	13.3	17.9	24.3	37.4	M	Myeloma and non–	200, 202–203
–	0.3	1.7	2.6	5.4	5.7	12.0	15.4	20.3	17.7	F	Hodgkin lymphomas	
1.8	2.4	2.9	5.5	6.9	13.9	27.6	30.5	57.5	88.1	M	Leukaemia	204–208
1.8	1.2	1.0	5.0	5.1	9.7	14.5	14.8	21.9	28.4	F		
41.9	77.5	115.1	208.3	368.1	626.4	1049.9	1767.9	3131.3	7824.6	M	ALL VASCULAR	390–459
12.4	23.3	31.8	54.8	126.1	260.1	590.8	1340.3	2624.3	7995.7	F	DISEASE	
–	–	0.4	–	–	0.3	1.0	0.7	–	2.3	M	Rheumatic heart	390–398
0.9	–	0.7	–	0.3	0.3	1.3	2.6	1.1	2.1	F	disease and fever	
–	0.3	1.8	1.6	4.1	9.1	16.3	27.9	66.4	177.7	M	Hypertensive disease	401–405
0.6	–	0.3	1.8	2.3	4.1	10.3	35.8	56.4	185.9	F		
22.8	49.0	68.1	120.4	210.8	330.8	476.8	685.7	908.6	1463.8	M	Ischaemic heart	410–414
2.1	4.5	9.9	17.0	43.6	80.7	176.0	331.6	532.3	1052.5	F	disease	
1.8	2.4	3.3	5.2	7.2	12.9	12.3	17.2	38.3	81.1	M	Pulmonary embolism	415.1, 451–453
0.6	2.7	2.4	5.0	4.3	8.8	19.2	25.1	37.8	91.6	F	and other venous	
5.3	12.9	14.6	37.5	62.1	120.3	267.0	515.9	1126.8	3014.8	M	Cerebrovascular	430–438
3.6	6.9	9.2	15.5	39.3	86.7	199.9	555.8	1186.7	3461.2	F	disease	
12.0	12.9	26.9	43.6	83.8	153.0	276.4	520.6	991.2	3085.0	M	Other vascular	Rest of 390–459
4.5	9.3	9.2	15.5	36.4	79.5	184.1	389.5	810.0	3202.5	F	disease	
0.3	0.9	1.8	1.6	4.1	14.6	24.2	42.4	92.9	173.0	M	Chronic obstructive	490–496
0.3	0.6	0.3	0.3	1.7	3.8	7.7	13.3	24.1	78.7	F	pulmonary disease	
5.6	4.8	9.5	10.3	26.5	50.9	81.4	179.7	314.9	781.0	M	Other respiratory	Rest of 460–519
1.2	4.5	6.8	6.7	14.2	21.0	48.7	119.2	205.4	646.0	F	disease	
0.3	0.3	0.7	1.0	1.9	1.7	3.5	5.3	8.8	20.3	M	Peptic ulcer	531–533
–	0.3	–	0.3	–	0.3	2.1	3.6	3.3	13.9	F		
3.2	7.5	6.6	18.7	20.8	34.2	54.3	63.7	60.5	81.1	M	Liver cirrhosis	571
0.6	0.6	2.0	2.6	2.8	10.1	15.4	28.1	27.9	38.6	F		
1.5	2.7	4.0	5.8	13.6	20.6	32.1	80.2	149.0	321.1	M	Renal disease	580–590
0.6	1.2	2.0	2.1	5.7	15.4	24.3	57.3	95.8	220.1	F		
–	–	–	–	–	–	–	–	–	–	F	Pregnancy and birth	630–676
–	–	0.4	–	–	–	–	–	–	–	M	Congenital and	740–779
0.3	–	–	–	–	0.3	–	–	–	0.5	F	perinatal causes	
3.8	7.5	4.7	16.5	26.8	57.5	103.7	238.7	465.3	1606.4	M	Ill-defined causes	780–799
3.6	3.3	5.8	6.4	12.8	34.6	60.2	127.9	328.6	1586.5	F		
7.3	12.6	12.0	16.5	22.1	42.9	63.2	143.2	219.0	487.1	M	Other medical causes	Rest of 001–799
3.0	5.1	7.9	7.3	14.2	33.9	56.0	102.9	207.0	473.0	F		
50.4	56.2	53.5	61.3	68.7	65.9	77.5	102.8	116.5	233.0	M	ALL NON–	E800–E999
14.5	12.8	15.4	18.8	18.5	28.6	35.0	53.2	74.5	199.3	F	MEDICAL CAUSES	
24.3	30.3	29.1	31.6	38.4	38.3	33.6	49.1	47.9	74.0	M	Motor vehicle	E810–E819
7.3	6.6	7.9	10.6	11.4	12.9	13.2	15.9	23.5	31.1	F	traffic accidents	
0.6	1.2	1.1	1.0	0.9	1.7	3.0	2.0	5.9	13.3	M	Fire	E890–E899
0.3	0.9	0.7	0.9	1.1	–	1.7	5.6	5.5	20.4	F		
5.0	6.0	4.0	6.5	7.2	7.0	6.9	7.3	13.3	21.8	M	Suicide	E950–E959
0.9	0.9	3.1	2.9	0.9	3.5	3.8	1.0	2.2	2.7	F		
2.3	1.8	1.1	2.3	1.3	1.7	–	–	–	3.1	M	Homicide	E960–E969
1.2	0.9	–	0.3	0.3	0.9	0.9	1.0	0.5	1.6	F		
341.6	332.9	274.6	309.7	317.3	286.9	202.6	150.8	135.6	128.3	M	**POPULATION (thousands)**	
331.0	334.9	292.9	341.2	351.2	318.3	234.1	195.4	182.6	186.7	F		

GREECE: Males

	All ages	0–34	35–69	35–39	40–44	45–49	50–54	55–59	60–64	65–69	70–74	75–79	80+/NK
POPULATION (1000s)													
1955	3888.6	2449.9	1274.5	233.4	240.3	232.0	199.5	154.3	119.3	95.7	74.7	50.2	39.3
1965	4157.3	2427.5	1525.1	315.5	237.1	206.7	237.9	215.9	181.3	130.7	86.0	63.0	55.7
1975	4431.5	2361.1	1767.7	291.2	317.8	308.3	240.8	200.8	219.4	189.4	142.1	85.4	75.2
1985	4886.9	2530.4	1950.4	331.8	275.8	314.3	327.0	303.4	222.6	175.5	172.8	124.3	109.0
1990	**4968.3**	**2488.0**	**2065.6**	**341.6**	**332.9**	**274.6**	**309.7**	**317.3**	**286.9**	**202.6**	**150.8**	**135.6**	**128.3**
1995 projected	*4993.6*	*2459.7*	*2104.9*	*334.2*	*326.4*	*326.4*	*262.2*	*308.4*	*297.4*	*249.9*	*164.3*	*134.4*	*130.3*
NUMBER OF DEATHS													
All causes													
1955	27728	6714	9584	488	689	970	1330	1647	2005	2455	2951	3166	5313
1965	34441	5076	12787	537	608	816	1565	2386	3161	3714	3807	4319	8452
1975	41361	3773	14596	432	690	1113	1423	2155	3625	5158	6058	6046	10888
1985	48452	2899	14934	470	562	1141	1818	2971	3580	4392	7144	8442	15033
1990	**49433**	**2349**	**15547**	**491**	**753**	**856**	**1655**	**2777**	**4253**	**4762**	**5818**	**8360**	**17359**
1995 projected	*48379*	*2081*	*15501*	*506*	*710*	*973*	*1271*	*2485*	*4078*	*5478*	*5840*	*7731*	*17226*
Lung cancer													
1955 estimated	*909*	*7*	*636*	*18*	*22*	*59*	*58*	*121*	*153*	*205*	*142*	*70*	*54*
1965	1462	9	988	17	23	57	101	195	278	317	217	144	104
1975	2434	14	1415	11	32	92	149	209	403	519	475	319	211
1985	3683	15	1918	24	32	112	236	407	533	574	736	563	451
1990	**4034**	**18**	**2168**	**23**	**70**	**113**	**224**	**412**	**643**	**683**	**647**	**641**	**560**
1995 projected	*4271*	*18*	*2299*	*32*	*86*	*150*	*189*	*377*	*644*	*821*	*706*	*651*	*597*
ANNUAL DEATH RATE / 100,000 (*The rates for the age groups 0–34 and 35–69 are the means of seven five-yearly rates, but the all-ages rates are standardised to the conventional "European" age distribution)													
All causes													
1955	1017.8*	264.5*	984.8*	209.1	286.7	418.1	666.7	1067.4	1680.6	2565.3	3950.5	6306.8	13519.1
1965	1050.9*	200.5*	1024.2*	170.2	256.4	394.8	657.8	1105.1	1743.5	2841.6	4426.7	6855.6	15174.1
1975	991.1*	158.8*	966.6*	148.4	217.1	361.0	590.9	1073.2	1652.2	2723.3	4263.2	7079.6	14478.7
1985	924.0*	117.0*	907.8*	141.7	203.8	363.0	556.0	979.2	1608.3	2502.6	4134.3	6791.6	13791.7
1990	**865.5***	**97.8***	**846.3***	**143.7**	**226.2**	**311.7**	**534.4**	**875.2**	**1482.4**	**2350.4**	**3858.1**	**6165.2**	**13530.0**
1995 projected	*814.1**	*84.3**	*788.7**	*151.4*	*217.5*	*298.1*	*484.7*	*805.8*	*1371.2*	*2192.1*	*3554.5*	*5752.2*	*13220.3*
All cancer													
1955 estimated	*158.8**	*10.0**	*251.4**	*33.8*	*51.6*	*88.4*	*168.4*	*291.6*	*489.5*	*636.4*	*788.5*	*882.5*	*1056.0*
1965	176.4*	10.6*	272.1*	31.1	50.2	95.8	177.0	315.0	505.2	730.7	911.6	1092.1	1186.7
1975	200.5*	12.6*	298.5*	29.2	50.0	104.4	193.9	341.6	530.5	839.5	1061.9	1378.2	1389.6
1985	215.2*	8.4*	305.6*	29.2	45.3	107.2	185.9	340.8	604.2	826.2	1219.9	1501.2	1745.0
1990	**216.1***	**7.1***	**299.8***	**28.1**	**54.1**	**101.2**	**190.5**	**318.9**	**559.4**	**846.0**	**1205.6**	**1551.6**	**1913.5**
1995 projected	*214.5**	*6.4**	*288.0**	*29.3*	*56.1*	*103.9*	*181.9*	*297.0*	*533.6*	*814.3*	*1194.2*	*1578.1*	*2045.3*
Lung cancer													
1955 estimated	*36.1**	*0.3**	*70.3**	*7.7*	*9.2*	*25.4*	*29.1*	*78.4*	*128.2*	*214.2*	*190.1*	*139.4*	*137.4*
1965	44.8*	0.4*	81.6*	5.4	9.7	27.6	42.5	90.3	153.3	242.5	252.3	228.6	186.7
1975	57.2*	0.7*	95.3*	3.8	10.1	29.8	61.9	104.1	183.7	274.0	334.3	373.5	280.6
1985	72.4*	0.6*	118.2*	7.2	11.6	35.6	72.2	134.1	239.4	327.1	425.9	452.9	413.8
1990	**73.8***	**0.7***	**118.9***	**6.7**	**21.0**	**41.2**	**72.3**	**129.8**	**224.1**	**337.1**	**429.0**	**472.7**	**436.5**
1995 projected	*74.2**	*0.7**	*117.3**	*9.6*	*26.3*	*46.0*	*72.1*	*122.2*	*216.5*	*328.5*	*429.7*	*484.4*	*458.2*
Upper aerodigestive cancer (mouth, oesophagus, pharynx and larynx)													
1955 estimated	*10.6**	*0.3**	*18.8**	*2.1*	*7.5*	*6.9*	*20.6*	*14.3*	*50.3*	*30.3*	*34.8*	*57.8*	*53.4*
1965	10.0*	0.4*	16.9*	1.3	3.8	5.3	13.5	18.1	36.4	39.8	46.5	63.5	52.1
1975	10.3*	0.1*	16.7*	0.7	1.6	4.2	8.7	22.9	26.4	52.3	61.2	70.3	59.8
1985	11.0*	0.3*	16.9*	0.9	2.9	5.7	10.4	20.4	27.4	50.7	57.9	69.2	83.5
1990	**10.2***	**0.1***	**15.1***	**0.6**	**2.4**	**4.0**	**9.0**	**14.8**	**27.5**	**47.4**	**55.7**	**76.7**	**84.2**
1995 projected	*9.7**	*0.0**	*13.5**	*0.3*	*1.8*	*3.4*	*6.9*	*13.0*	*24.5*	*44.4*	*54.8*	*78.9*	*89.0*
Other cancer													
1955 estimated	*112.2**	*9.4**	*162.2**	*24.0*	*35.0*	*56.0*	*118.8*	*199.0*	*311.0*	*391.8*	*563.6*	*685.3*	*865.1*
1965	121.5*	9.9*	173.6*	24.4	36.7	62.9	121.1	206.6	315.5	448.4	612.8	800.0	947.9
1975	132.9*	11.8*	186.4*	24.7	38.4	70.4	123.3	214.6	320.4	513.2	666.4	934.4	1049.2
1985	131.8*	7.5*	170.5*	21.1	30.8	65.9	103.4	186.2	337.4	448.4	736.1	979.1	1247.7
1990	**132.1***	**6.3***	**165.7***	**20.8**	**30.6**	**56.1**	**109.1**	**174.3**	**307.8**	**461.5**	**720.8**	**1002.2**	**1392.8**
1995 projected	*130.7**	*5.7**	*157.2**	*19.4*	*27.9*	*54.5*	*103.0*	*161.8*	*292.5*	*441.4*	*709.7*	*1014.9*	*1498.1*
Chronic obstructive pulmonary disease (COPD)													
1955 estimated	*12.2**	*1.7**	*11.3**	*2.1*	*7.9*	*3.0*	*7.0*	*12.3*	*15.1*	*31.3*	*66.9*	*89.6*	*167.9*
1965	28.4*	1.3*	25.3*	1.9	5.5	5.3	12.6	25.5	39.7	86.5	161.6	223.8	481.1
1975	57.6*	1.4*	45.2*	1.7	3.1	7.8	17.0	42.8	78.4	165.8	289.2	543.3	1105.1
1985	20.7*	0.1*	13.6*	0.9	0.7	1.9	3.7	9.9	24.3	53.6	118.6	204.3	429.4
1990	**8.9***	**0.0***	**6.8***	**0.3**	**0.9**	**1.8**	**1.6**	**4.1**	**14.6**	**24.2**	**42.4**	**92.9**	**173.0**
1995 projected	*6.2**	*0.0**	*4.7**	*0.3*	*0.6*	*1.2*	*1.1*	*2.9*	*10.1*	*16.8*	*29.2*	*64.0*	*122.8*
Other respiratory disease													
1955 estimated	*45.6**	*43.8**	*16.3**	*4.3*	*2.9*	*6.0*	*4.0*	*16.2*	*29.3*	*51.2*	*79.0*	*143.4*	*514.0*
1965	45.9*	22.9*	21.4*	2.2	3.8	6.8	6.7	19.5	37.0	74.2	125.6	247.6	854.6
1975	45.9*	11.1*	21.5*	1.0	4.1	6.2	8.7	18.9	36.0	75.5	147.8	345.4	1053.2
1985	34.4*	2.7*	22.6*	3.3	4.0	9.2	11.0	20.1	43.1	67.2	136.6	285.6	759.6
1990	**37.9***	**2.2***	**27.0***	**5.6**	**4.8**	**9.5**	**10.3**	**26.5**	**50.9**	**81.4**	**179.7**	**314.9**	**781.0**
1995 projected	*42.0**	*2.8**	*32.4**	*7.8*	*5.8*	*9.5*	*11.8*	*30.8*	*60.5*	*100.4*	*206.3*	*337.8*	*818.9*
Vascular disease													
1955 estimated	*205.2**	*8.6**	*196.8**	*25.3*	*25.0*	*51.3*	*125.8*	*210.6*	*360.4*	*578.9*	*1096.4*	*1683.3*	*3229.0*
1965	309.6*	7.3*	300.0*	28.2	43.0	84.7	176.1	315.4	541.6	911.2	1588.4	2488.9	5140.0
1975	355.2*	6.1*	343.6*	29.2	59.8	111.6	187.7	385.0	621.7	1010.6	1715.7	2963.7	5984.0
1985	405.7*	6.8*	367.1*	37.7	69.6	130.8	216.5	398.5	633.0	1083.8	1860.5	3366.9	7420.2
1990	**401.9***	**6.8***	**355.3***	**41.9**	**77.5**	**115.1**	**208.3**	**368.1**	**626.4**	**1049.9**	**1767.9**	**3131.3**	**7824.6**
1995 projected	*389.9**	*6.8**	*336.2**	*46.7*	*75.7*	*109.7*	*191.1*	*349.2*	*593.1*	*987.6*	*1625.1*	*2957.6*	*7948.6*
Liver cirrhosis													
1955 estimated	*29.3**	*1.3**	*50.5**	*5.6*	*12.1*	*35.3*	*41.6*	*86.2*	*82.1*	*90.9*	*133.9*	*107.6*	*150.1*
1965	27.5*	1.4*	46.2*	4.1	10.5	27.1	38.7	64.8	82.2	95.6	131.4	120.6	150.8
1975	19.8*	0.6*	32.6*	2.7	7.6	16.5	27.4	39.8	62.9	71.3	95.7	108.9	114.4
1985	15.3*	0.4*	25.2*	2.4	5.4	15.0	19.0	37.2	49.9	47.9	70.6	85.3	88.1
1990	**12.6***	**0.3***	**20.8***	**3.2**	**7.5**	**6.6**	**18.7**	**20.8**	**34.2**	**54.3**	**63.7**	**60.5**	**81.1**
1995 projected	*10.2**	*0.3**	*16.9**	*4.2*	*5.5*	*5.5*	*13.0*	*14.6*	*27.2*	*48.0*	*54.2*	*45.4*	*66.8*
Other medical causes													
1955 estimated	*513.4**	*155.9**	*412.9**	*105.0*	*141.1*	*197.0*	*282.7*	*388.9*	*647.1*	*1128.5*	*1653.3*	*3268.9*	*8109.4*
1965	401.6*	115.1*	299.0*	56.7	86.9	123.4	196.3	298.3	468.3	863.0	1373.3	2503.2	6958.7
1975	249.2*	83.8*	161.8*	25.4	36.5	56.8	103.8	186.3	258.4	465.2	850.1	1543.3	4425.5
1985	166.1*	49.1*	103.9*	16.6	20.7	30.2	54.4	100.9	179.2	325.4	614.0	1173.8	3038.5
1990	**129.6***	**35.9***	**74.8***	**14.3**	**25.2**	**24.0**	**43.6**	**68.1**	**131.1**	**217.2**	**496.0**	**897.5**	**2523.8**
1995 projected	*100.4**	*26.7**	*55.8**	*15.0*	*23.6*	*21.1*	*31.7*	*48.6*	*90.8*	*160.1*	*368.8*	*683.8*	*2049.9*
All non-medical causes													
1955 estimated	*53.2**	*43.2**	*45.7**	*33.0*	*46.2*	*37.1*	*37.1*	*61.6*	*57.0*	*48.1*	*132.5*	*131.5*	*292.6*
1965	61.6*	42.0*	60.2*	46.0	56.5	51.8	50.4	66.7	69.5	80.3	134.9	179.4	402.2
1975	63.0*	43.3*	63.4*	59.1	56.0	57.7	52.3	58.8	64.3	95.6	102.7	196.7	406.9
1985	66.7*	49.5*	69.8*	51.5	58.0	68.7	65.4	71.9	74.6	98.6	114.0	174.6	311.0
1990	**58.5***	**45.4***	**61.9***	**50.4**	**56.2**	**53.5**	**61.3**	**68.7**	**65.9**	**77.5**	**102.8**	**116.5**	**233.0**
1995 projected	*50.8**	*41.2**	*54.7**	*48.2*	*50.2*	*47.2*	*54.2*	*62.6*	*55.8*	*64.8*	*76.7*	*85.6*	*168.1*

GREECE: Females

	All ages	0–34	35–69	35–39	40–44	45–49	50–54	55–59	60–64	65–69	70–74	75–79	80+/NK
POPULATION (1000s)													
1955	4077.0	2440.7	1424.3	259.4	262.2	245.2	212.5	174.7	147.1	123.2	96.1	63.8	52.1
1965	4392.9	2430.7	1685.1	349.4	263.4	230.7	258.2	225.3	198.3	159.8	114.2	85.5	77.4
1975	4614.9	2276.2	1936.4	324.7	338.2	328.3	258.8	228.5	245.7	212.2	173.4	115.5	113.4
1985	5047.4	2402.5	2112.1	334.6	293.4	343.1	355.8	326.5	244.9	213.8	214.9	157.7	160.2
1990	**5120.6**	**2352.3**	**2203.6**	**331.0**	**334.9**	**292.9**	**341.2**	**351.2**	**318.3**	**234.1**	**195.4**	**182.6**	**186.7**
1995 projected	*5130.3*	*2297.2*	*2261.1*	*344.1*	*326.5*	*331.4*	*289.3*	*341.7*	*338.9*	*289.2*	*202.2*	*183.1*	*186.7*
NUMBER OF DEATHS													
All causes													
1955	27059	5821	7810	450	572	750	956	1187	1642	2253	2903	3332	7193
1965	32828	3804	9087	441	459	579	995	1421	2132	3060	3771	5035	11131
1975	38716	2453	9374	283	425	727	858	1223	2361	3497	5149	6691	15049
1985	44434	1467	8784	242	305	630	1001	1556	1905	3145	5695	7978	20510
1990	**44719**	**1251**	**8236**	**218**	**344**	**492**	**799**	**1342**	**2150**	**2891**	**4600**	**7837**	**22795**
1995 projected	*41649*	*1192*	*7726*	*219*	*313*	*495*	*564*	*1100*	*1927*	*3108*	*4088*	*7236*	*21407*
Lung cancer													
1955 estimated	*273*	*18*	*199*	*17*	*8*	*32*	*25*	*49*	*35*	*33*	*24*	*14*	*18*
1965	344	12	232	14	10	23	32	48	53	52	39	29	32
1975	488	4	279	8	17	25	34	37	73	85	81	59	65
1985	632	4	320	9	12	28	30	75	74	92	93	88	127
1990	**714**	**7**	**336**	**7**	**16**	**26**	**45**	**70**	**87**	**85**	**96**	**125**	**150**
1995 projected	*743*	*7*	*336*	*8*	*16*	*37*	*38*	*64*	*77*	*96*	*102*	*133*	*165*
ANNUAL DEATH RATE / 100,000 (*The rates for the age groups 0–34 and 35–69 are the means of seven five-yearly rates, but the all-ages rates are standardised to the conventional "European" age distribution)													
All causes													
1955	850.2*	239.3*	681.7*	173.5	218.2	305.9	449.9	679.5	1116.2	1828.7	3020.8	5222.6	13806.1
1965	820.9*	153.3*	651.1*	126.2	174.3	251.0	385.4	630.7	1075.1	1914.9	3302.1	5888.9	14381.1
1975	727.4*	107.0*	558.6*	87.2	125.7	221.4	331.5	535.2	960.9	1648.0	2969.4	5793.1	13270.7
1985	641.4*	63.3*	481.0*	72.3	104.0	183.6	281.3	476.6	777.9	1471.0	2650.1	5059.0	12802.7
1990	**577.4***	**58.4***	**409.0***	**65.9**	**102.7**	**168.0**	**234.2**	**382.1**	**675.5**	**1234.9**	**2354.1**	**4291.9**	**12209.4**
1995 projected	*523.2**	*54.0**	*352.7**	*63.6*	*95.9*	*149.4*	*195.0*	*321.9*	*568.6*	*1074.7*	*2021.8*	*3951.9*	*11466.0*
All cancer													
1955 estimated	*108.6**	*8.0**	*185.2**	*49.3*	*66.4*	*104.0*	*151.5*	*205.5*	*248.8*	*470.8*	*374.6*	*525.1*	*656.4*
1965	108.4*	8.5*	175.8*	40.1	63.0	101.4	149.1	199.7	270.8	406.1	424.7	570.8	670.5
1975	111.6*	10.0*	169.5*	33.0	61.2	99.9	147.2	196.1	295.1	354.4	485.6	626.8	744.3
1985	115.9*	6.9*	174.9*	33.5	60.0	95.6	135.5	208.6	291.5	399.9	530.5	676.0	860.8
1990	**110.6***	**6.8***	**162.7***	**29.0**	**50.8**	**94.2**	**133.4**	**183.9**	**262.0**	**385.3**	**496.9**	**673.1**	**888.1**
1995 projected	*102.8**	*6.7**	*144.5**	*26.2*	*46.2*	*88.7*	*116.8*	*160.4*	*231.3*	*342.0*	*457.5*	*664.7*	*906.8*
Lung cancer													
1955 estimated	*8.6**	*0.8**	*16.1**	*6.6*	*3.1*	*13.1*	*11.8*	*28.0*	*23.8*	*26.8*	*25.0*	*21.9*	*34.5*
1965	8.8*	0.5*	15.8*	4.0	3.8	10.0	12.4	21.3	26.7	32.5	34.2	33.9	41.3
1975	9.7*	0.2*	16.3*	2.5	5.0	7.6	13.1	16.2	29.7	40.1	46.7	51.1	57.3
1985	10.3*	0.2*	17.1*	2.7	4.1	8.2	8.4	23.0	30.2	43.0	43.3	55.8	79.3
1990	**10.6***	**0.3***	**16.1***	**2.1**	**4.8**	**8.9**	**13.2**	**19.9**	**27.3**	**36.3**	**49.1**	**68.5**	**80.3**
1995 projected	*10.7**	*0.3**	*15.2**	*2.3*	*4.9*	*11.2*	*13.1*	*18.7*	*22.7*	*33.2*	*50.4*	*72.6*	*88.4*
Upper aerodigestive cancer (mouth, oesophagus, pharynx and larynx)													
1955 estimated	*2.1**	*0.1**	*4.3**	–	*3.8*	*6.1*	*3.3*	*6.3*	*4.8*	*5.7*	*3.1*	*7.8*	*3.8*
1965	2.0*	0.1*	3.5*	0.3	1.9	3.0	3.1	4.9	5.5	5.6	5.3	11.7	7.8
1975	2.7*	0.3*	3.1*	0.6	0.9	0.3	3.1	3.9	6.9	5.7	10.4	18.2	37.9
1985	1.8*	0.2*	2.4*	0.3	1.4	0.6	0.8	1.5	4.5	8.0	7.9	11.4	18.1
1990	**1.9***	–	**2.1***	–	**0.3**	**0.7**	**0.9**	**3.4**	**4.1**	**5.1**	**9.2**	**13.1**	**29.5**
1995 projected	*2.2**	–	*2.0**	–	*0.3*	*0.6*	*1.0*	*4.1*	*3.5*	*4.5*	*8.9*	*18.0*	*41.8*
Other cancer													
1955 estimated	*97.8**	*7.1**	*164.8**	*42.8*	*59.5*	*84.8*	*136.5*	*171.2*	*220.3*	*438.3*	*346.5*	*495.3*	*618.0*
1965	97.6*	7.9*	156.5*	35.8	57.3	88.4	133.6	173.5	238.5	368.0	385.3	525.1	621.4
1975	99.2*	9.5*	150.2*	29.9	55.3	92.0	131.0	175.9	258.4	308.7	428.5	557.6	649.0
1985	103.8*	6.6*	155.4*	30.5	54.5	86.9	126.2	184.1	256.8	348.9	479.3	608.8	763.4
1990	**98.1***	**6.5***	**144.5***	**26.9**	**45.7**	**84.7**	**119.3**	**160.6**	**230.6**	**343.9**	**438.6**	**591.5**	**778.3**
1995 projected	*89.9**	*6.4**	*127.3**	*23.8*	*41.0*	*76.9*	*102.7*	*137.5*	*205.1*	*304.3*	*398.1*	*574.0*	*776.6*
Chronic obstructive pulmonary disease (COPD)													
1955 estimated	*8.9**	*2.7**	*8.5**	*4.6*	*3.1*	*2.4*	*6.6*	*6.9*	*10.2*	*26.0*	*32.3*	*53.3*	*117.1*
1965	17.3*	1.6*	14.6*	2.6	2.3	3.0	7.0	12.0	22.7	52.6	84.9	133.3	311.4
1975	33.6*	1.1*	21.4*	0.9	1.5	4.0	6.6	17.1	41.9	78.2	168.4	316.0	727.5
1985	8.1*	0.2*	4.0*	0.3	0.7	1.7	2.0	3.7	5.3	14.5	32.1	78.0	206.6
1990	**3.2***	**0.0***	**2.1***	**0.3**	**0.6**	**0.3**	**0.3**	**1.7**	**3.8**	**7.7**	**13.3**	**24.1**	**78.7**
1995 projected	*2.2**	*0.0**	*1.5**	*0.3*	*0.3*	*0.3*	*0.3*	*1.2*	*2.7*	*5.2*	*8.9*	*16.4*	*55.7*
Other respiratory disease													
1955 estimated	*45.6**	*42.2**	*12.8**	*4.6*	*0.8*	*1.6*	*2.8*	*26.9*	*17.7*	*34.9*	*117.6*	*169.3*	*535.5*
1965	41.9*	21.1*	14.8*	2.9	1.1	3.0	5.0	17.8	22.2	51.3	132.2	245.6	812.7
1975	39.5*	9.9*	15.2*	1.5	1.8	6.4	7.7	9.6	24.0	55.6	111.9	284.8	986.8
1985	26.9*	2.3*	13.1*	1.2	2.4	5.0	12.1	11.0	19.2	41.2	96.3	220.7	680.4
1990	**26.5***	**1.3***	**14.7***	**1.2**	**4.5**	**6.8**	**6.7**	**14.2**	**21.0**	**48.7**	**119.2**	**205.4**	**646.0**
1995 projected	*26.0**	*1.1**	*16.1**	*1.5*	*6.1*	*6.3*	*6.2*	*13.5*	*23.6*	*55.7*	*118.2*	*202.6*	*610.1*
Vascular disease													
1955 estimated	*222.6**	*15.5**	*194.4**	*16.6*	*24.0*	*77.9*	*94.6*	*173.4*	*382.7*	*591.7*	*1130.1*	*1866.8*	*3775.4*
1965	281.5*	8.2*	217.4*	16.9	28.1	63.7	93.7	190.0	390.8	738.4	1441.3	2566.1	5413.4
1975	291.0*	4.9*	196.6*	15.1	27.8	51.5	84.2	172.0	341.5	684.3	1384.1	2826.8	6161.4
1985	317.3*	3.6*	176.0*	15.5	19.8	39.1	67.2	139.4	287.1	663.7	1368.5	2909.3	7857.7
1990	**307.5***	**4.3***	**157.0***	**12.4**	**23.3**	**31.8**	**54.8**	**126.1**	**260.1**	**590.8**	**1340.3**	**2624.3**	**7995.7**
1995 projected	*292.0**	*4.5**	*137.8**	*13.1*	*20.8*	*27.2*	*44.6*	*107.4*	*222.8*	*529.0*	*1173.1*	*2535.8*	*7887.5*
Liver cirrhosis													
1955 estimated	*13.7**	*1.1**	*21.2**	*1.5*	*10.7*	*4.1*	*19.8*	*20.6*	*41.5*	*50.3*	*67.6*	*50.2*	*109.4*
1965	11.2*	0.7*	16.5*	1.4	6.5	3.9	10.8	17.8	32.3	42.6	54.3	59.6	103.4
1975	7.5*	0.4*	10.2*	1.2	0.3	3.7	5.4	12.7	21.6	26.9	32.9	56.3	78.5
1985	5.1*	0.1*	7.0*	0.6	0.7	2.0	4.8	8.9	15.5	16.4	27.0	38.7	47.4
1990	**4.0***	**0.3***	**4.9***	**0.6**	**0.6**	**2.0**	**2.6**	**2.8**	**10.1**	**15.4**	**28.1**	**27.9**	**38.6**
1995 projected	*3.3**	*0.4**	*3.8**	*0.6*	*0.6*	*1.5*	*1.7*	*2.0*	*6.8*	*13.1*	*23.2*	*24.0*	*30.0*
Other medical causes													
1955 estimated	*424.2**	*155.8**	*240.9**	*89.1*	*96.5*	*108.9*	*161.4*	*223.2*	*388.2*	*619.3*	*1194.6*	*2388.7*	*8332.1*
1965	331.2*	101.3*	188.3*	50.9	57.3	64.6	101.9	167.8	303.6	572.0	1065.7	2129.8	6695.1
1975	213.9*	67.3*	119.6*	20.6	20.4	37.8	58.3	104.2	203.1	392.6	715.7	1522.1	4169.3
1985	141.8*	36.3*	81.0*	8.1	9.2	22.4	36.3	77.8	127.8	285.3	537.5	1026.0	2870.8
1990	**103.3***	**31.7***	**47.1***	**7.9**	**10.2**	**17.4**	**17.6**	**34.7**	**89.9**	**152.1**	**303.0**	**662.7**	**2363.1**
1995 projected	*78.2**	*27.1**	*32.5**	*8.4*	*8.9*	*12.1*	*11.8*	*23.4*	*60.8*	*102.0*	*203.3*	*457.1*	*1835.0*
All non-medical causes													
1955 estimated	*26.6**	*14.0**	*18.6**	*7.7*	*16.8*	*6.9*	*13.2*	*22.9*	*27.2*	*35.7*	*104.1*	*169.3*	*280.2*
1965	29.4*	11.9*	23.8*	11.4	15.9	11.3	17.8	25.7	32.8	51.9	98.9	183.6	374.7
1975	30.3*	13.3*	25.9*	14.8	12.7	18.3	22.0	23.6	33.8	56.1	70.9	160.2	403.0
1985	26.3*	13.9*	24.9*	13.2	11.2	17.8	23.6	27.3	31.4	50.0	58.2	110.3	279.0
1990	**22.2***	**13.8***	**20.5***	**14.5**	**12.8**	**15.4**	**18.8**	**18.5**	**28.6**	**35.0**	**53.2**	**74.5**	**199.3**
1995 projected	*18.7**	*14.2**	*16.5**	*13.7*	*12.9*	*13.3*	*13.5*	*14.0*	*20.7*	*27.7*	*37.6*	*51.3*	*140.9*

GREECE: 1975

Smoking–attributed deaths (Sm.) and total deaths (Total)

		ALL CAUSES	ALL CANCER	Lung cancer	Upper aero–digestive ca.	Other cancer	COPD	Other respiratory	Vascular disease	Liver cirrhosis	Other medical	Non–medical
Males												
0–34	Sm.	–	–	–	–	–	–	–	–	–	–	–
	Total	3773	285	14	2	269	32	275	130	12	2058	981
35–69	Sm.	4160	1795	1286	146	363	479	74	1223	–	589	–
	Total	14596	4473	1415	244	2814	652	316	5122	502	2437	1094
		(29%)	(40%)	(91%)	(60%)	(13%)	(73%)	(23%)	(24%)		(24%)	
70+	Sm.	3892	1236	886	101	249	1133	112	886	–	525	–
	Total	22992	3731	1005	192	2534	1706	1297	9469	315	5854	620
		(17%)	(33%)	(88%)	(53%)	(10%)	(66%)	(9%)	(9%)		(9%)	
Any age	Sm.	8052	3031	2172	247	612	1612	186	2109	–	1114	–
	Total	41361	8489	2434	438	5617	2390	1888	14721	829	10349	2695
		(19%)	(36%)	(89%)	(56%)	(11%)	(67%)	(10%)	(14%)		(11%)	
Females												
0–34	Sm.	–	–	–	–	–	–	–	–	–	–	–
	Total	2453	219	4	6	209	25	231	108	8	1561	301
35–69	Sm.	556	149	124	7	18	112	13	175	–	107	–
	Total	9374	2948	279	52	2617	346	251	3214	170	1981	464
		(6%)	(5%)	(44%)	(13%)	(1%)	(32%)	(5%)	(5%)		(5%)	
70+	Sm.	690	91	72	10	9	327	19	160	–	93	–
	Total	26889	2410	205	82	2123	1482	1642	12652	211	7727	765
		(3%)	(4%)	(35%)	(12%)	(0%)	(22%)	(1%)	(1%)		(1%)	
Any age	Sm.	1246	240	196	17	27	439	32	335	–	200	–
	Total	38716	5577	488	140	4949	1853	2124	15974	389	11269	1530
		(3%)	(4%)	(40%)	(12%)	(1%)	(24%)	(2%)	(2%)		(2%)	
Males+Females												
0–34	Sm.	–	–	–	–	–	–	–	–	–	–	–
	Total	6226	504	18	8	478	57	506	238	20	3619	1282
35–69	Sm.	4716	1944	1410	153	381	591	87	1398	–	696	–
	Total	23970	7421	1694	296	5431	998	567	8336	672	4418	1558
		(20%)	(26%)	(83%)	(52%)	(7%)	(59%)	(15%)	(17%)		(16%)	
70+	Sm.	4582	1327	958	111	258	1460	131	1046	–	618	–
	Total	49881	6141	1210	274	4657	3188	2939	22121	526	13581	1385
		(9%)	(22%)	(79%)	(41%)	(6%)	(46%)	(4%)	(5%)		(5%)	
Any age	Sm.	9298	3271	2368	264	639	2051	218	2444	–	1314	–
	Total	80077	14066	2922	578	10566	4243	4012	30695	1218	21618	4225
		(12%)	(23%)	(81%)	(46%)	(6%)	(48%)	(5%)	(8%)		(6%)	

GREECE: 1985

Smoking–attributed deaths (Sm.) and total deaths (Total)

		ALL CAUSES	ALL CANCER	Lung cancer	Upper aero–digestive ca.	Other cancer	COPD	Other respiratory	Vascular disease	Liver cirrhosis	Other medical	Non–medical
Males												
0–34	Sm.	–	–	–	–	–	–	–	–	–	–	–
	Total	2899	209	15	8	186	3	66	169	9	1186	1257
35–69	Sm.	4887	2402	1778	178	446	157	105	1742	–	481	–
	Total	14934	4996	1918	275	2803	201	362	5956	440	1661	1318
		(33%)	(48%)	(93%)	(65%)	(16%)	(78%)	(29%)	(29%)		(29%)	
70+	Sm.	5348	2203	1580	160	463	660	151	1706	–	628	–
	Total	30619	5876	1750	277	3849	927	1419	15488	324	5832	753
		(17%)	(37%)	(90%)	(58%)	(12%)	(71%)	(11%)	(11%)		(11%)	
Any age	Sm.	10235	4605	3358	338	909	817	256	3448	–	1109	–
	Total	48452	11081	3683	560	6838	1131	1847	21613	773	8679	3328
		(21%)	(42%)	(91%)	(60%)	(13%)	(72%)	(14%)	(16%)		(13%)	
Females												
0–34	Sm.	–	–	–	–	–	–	–	–	–	–	–
	Total	1467	166	4	4	158	4	54	87	2	821	333
35–69	Sm.	482	180	150	8	22	25	13	180	–	84	–
	Total	8784	3348	320	43	2985	72	242	3060	130	1437	495
		(5%)	(5%)	(47%)	(19%)	(1%)	(35%)	(5%)	(6%)		(6%)	
70+	Sm.	652	137	114	7	16	131	21	265	–	98	–
	Total	34183	3585	308	64	3213	523	1645	20117	195	7372	746
		(2%)	(4%)	(37%)	(11%)	(0%)	(25%)	(1%)	(1%)		(1%)	
Any age	Sm.	1134	317	264	15	38	156	34	445	–	182	–
	Total	44434	7099	632	111	6356	599	1941	23264	327	9630	1574
		(3%)	(4%)	(42%)	(14%)	(1%)	(26%)	(2%)	(2%)		(2%)	
Males+Females												
0–34	Sm.	–	–	–	–	–	–	–	–	–	–	–
	Total	4366	375	19	12	344	7	120	256	11	2007	1590
35–69	Sm.	5369	2582	1928	186	468	182	118	1922	–	565	–
	Total	23718	8344	2238	318	5788	273	604	9016	570	3098	1813
		(23%)	(31%)	(86%)	(58%)	(8%)	(67%)	(20%)	(21%)		(18%)	
70+	Sm.	6000	2340	1694	167	479	791	172	1971	–	726	–
	Total	64802	9461	2058	341	7062	1450	3064	35605	519	13204	1499
		(9%)	(25%)	(82%)	(49%)	(7%)	(55%)	(6%)	(6%)		(5%)	
Any age	Sm.	11369	4922	3622	353	947	973	290	3893	–	1291	–
	Total	92886	18180	4315	671	13194	1730	3788	44877	1100	18309	4902
		(12%)	(27%)	(84%)	(53%)	(7%)	(56%)	(8%)	(9%)		(7%)	

(To be conservative, no deaths before age 35, and none from liver cirrhosis or non-medical causes, were attributed to smoking.)

GREECE: 1990

Smoking–attributed deaths (Sm.) and total deaths (Total)

		ALL CAUSES	ALL CANCER	Lung cancer	Upper aero–digestive ca.	Other cancer	COPD	Other respiratory	Vascular disease	Liver cirrhosis	Other medical	Non–medical
Males												
0–34	Sm.	–	–	–	–	–	–	–	–	–	–	–
	Total	2349	180	18	2	160	1	57	175	8	747	1181
35–69	Sm.	5180	2673	2011	177	485	92	141	1876	–	398	–
	Total	15547	5475	2168	271	3036	118	488	6454	386	1366	1260
		(33%)	(49%)	(93%)	(65%)	(16%)	(78%)	(29%)	(29%)		(29%)	
70+	Sm.	5248	2362	1672	172	518	296	186	1844	–	560	–
	Total	31537	6377	1848	296	4233	412	1700	16951	282	5203	612
		(17%)	(37%)	(90%)	(58%)	(12%)	(72%)	(11%)	(11%)		(11%)	
Any age	Sm.	10428	5035	3683	349	1003	388	327	3720	–	958	–
	Total	49433	12032	4034	569	7429	531	2245	23580	676	7316	3053
		(21%)	(42%)	(91%)	(61%)	(14%)	(73%)	(15%)	(16%)		(13%)	
Females												
0–34	Sm.	–	–	–	–	–	–	–	–	–	–	–
	Total	1251	163	7	0	156	1	29	107	8	612	331
35–69	Sm.	409	177	150	7	20	12	15	156	–	49	–
	Total	8236	3379	336	43	3000	41	293	3053	97	935	438
		(5%)	(5%)	(45%)	(16%)	(1%)	(29%)	(5%)	(5%)		(5%)	
70+	Sm.	903	223	177	19	27	76	37	445	–	122	–
	Total	35232	3858	371	97	3390	217	1814	22339	178	6214	612
		(3%)	(6%)	(48%)	(20%)	(1%)	(35%)	(2%)	(2%)		(2%)	
Any age	Sm.	1312	400	327	26	47	88	52	601	–	171	–
	Total	44719	7400	714	140	6546	259	2136	25499	283	7761	1381
		(3%)	(5%)	(46%)	(19%)	(1%)	(34%)	(2%)	(2%)		(2%)	
Males+Females												
0–34	Sm.	–	–	–	–	–	–	–	–	–	–	–
	Total	3600	343	25	2	316	2	86	282	16	1359	1512
35–69	Sm.	5589	2850	2161	184	505	104	156	2032	–	447	–
	Total	23783	8854	2504	314	6036	159	781	9507	483	2301	1698
		(23%)	(32%)	(86%)	(59%)	(8%)	(65%)	(20%)	(21%)		(19%)	
70+	Sm.	6151	2585	1849	191	545	372	223	2289	–	682	–
	Total	66769	10235	2219	393	7623	629	3514	39290	460	11417	1224
		(9%)	(25%)	(83%)	(49%)	(7%)	(59%)	(6%)	(6%)		(6%)	
Any age	Sm.	11740	5435	4010	375	1050	476	379	4321	–	1129	–
	Total	94152	19432	4748	709	13975	790	4381	49079	959	15077	4434
		(12%)	(28%)	(84%)	(53%)	(8%)	(60%)	(9%)	(9%)		(7%)	

GREECE: 1995

Smoking–attributed deaths (Sm.) and total deaths (Total)

		ALL CAUSES	ALL CANCER	Lung cancer	Upper aero–digestive ca.	Other cancer	COPD	Other respiratory	Vascular disease	Liver cirrhosis	Other medical	Non–medical
Males												
0–34	Sm.	–	–	–	–	–	–	–	–	–	–	–
	Total	2081	164	18	1	145	1	73	179	9	592	1063
35–69	Sm.	5212	2786	2130	170	486	70	176	1863	–	317	–
	Total	15501	5635	2299	260	3076	91	633	6571	330	1099	1142
		(34%)	(49%)	(93%)	(65%)	(16%)	(77%)	(28%)	(28%)		(29%)	
70+	Sm.	5277	2512	1771	183	558	213	210	1882	–	460	–
	Total	30797	6748	1954	312	4482	294	1860	17002	237	4196	460
		(17%)	(37%)	(91%)	(59%)	(12%)	(72%)	(11%)	(11%)		(11%)	
Any age	Sm.	10489	5298	3901	353	1044	283	386	3745	–	777	–
	Total	48379	12547	4271	573	7703	386	2566	23752	576	5887	2665
		(22%)	(42%)	(91%)	(62%)	(14%)	(73%)	(15%)	(16%)		(13%)	
Females												
0–34	Sm.	–	–	–	–	–	–	–	–	–	–	–
	Total	1192	155	7	0	148	1	25	111	10	551	339
35–69	Sm.	340	164	140	7	17	6	14	125	–	31	–
	Total	7726	3194	336	45	2813	32	351	2984	82	713	370
		(4%)	(5%)	(42%)	(16%)	(1%)	(19%)	(4%)	(4%)		(4%)	
70+	Sm.	933	257	201	27	29	56	40	478	–	102	–
	Total	32731	3835	400	129	3306	152	1749	21741	147	4674	433
		(3%)	(7%)	(50%)	(21%)	(1%)	(37%)	(2%)	(2%)		(2%)	
Any age	Sm.	1273	421	341	34	46	62	54	603	–	133	–
	Total	41649	7184	743	174	6267	185	2125	24836	239	5938	1142
		(3%)	(6%)	(46%)	(20%)	(1%)	(34%)	(3%)	(2%)		(2%)	
Males+Females												
0–34	Sm.	–	–	–	–	–	–	–	–	–	–	–
	Total	3273	319	25	1	293	2	98	290	19	1143	1402
35–69	Sm.	5552	2950	2270	177	503	76	190	1988	–	348	–
	Total	23227	8829	2635	305	5889	123	984	9555	412	1812	1512
		(24%)	(33%)	(86%)	(58%)	(9%)	(62%)	(19%)	(21%)		(19%)	
70+	Sm.	6210	2769	1972	210	587	269	250	2360	–	562	–
	Total	63528	10583	2354	441	7788	446	3609	38743	384	8870	893
		(10%)	(26%)	(84%)	(48%)	(8%)	(60%)	(7%)	(6%)		(6%)	
Any age	Sm.	11762	5719	4242	387	1090	345	440	4348	–	910	–
	Total	90028	19731	5014	747	13970	571	4691	48588	815	11825	3807
		(13%)	(29%)	(85%)	(52%)	(8%)	(60%)	(9%)	(9%)		(8%)	

(To be conservative, no deaths before age 35, and none from liver cirrhosis or non–medical causes, were attributed to smoking.)

HUNGARY: 1990

		No. of deaths			Standardised rates (Defined on p.376)			Annual death rates / 100, 000						
		All ages	0–34	35–69	All ages	0–34	35–69	0–4	5–9	10–14	15–19	20–24	25–29	30–34
ALL CAUSES	M	76936	4243	38981	1630.9	175.1	2075.5	379.7	31.1	33.0	101.2	155.1	203.2	322.8
	F	68724	2115	20607	925.8	92.1	905.8	303.5	27.5	20.6	44.2	56.7	65.6	126.2
Tuberculosis	M	514	12	325	10.8	0.5	17.2	–	–	–	–	–	0.3	2.9
	F	185	5	81	2.6	0.2	3.5	–	–	–	0.3	–	–	1.1
Other infective	M	126	30	59	2.7	1.3	3.1	6.7	–	0.2	0.2	0.3	0.6	1.1
and parasitic	F	131	23	43	2.0	1.0	1.9	5.3	0.3	0.2	0.5	0.3	–	0.5
ALL CANCER	M	17497	282	10444	368.6	11.3	567.9	5.7	5.4	4.7	5.7	13.3	15.4	28.7
	F	13374	257	6360	193.4	10.4	278.9	4.7	4.7	4.9	7.0	9.5	11.9	30.3
Mouth and	M	945	15	754	20.0	0.6	38.2	–	–	–	0.5	0.6	0.3	2.7
pharynx cancer	F	175	5	96	2.7	0.2	4.1	0.3	–	–	0.3	0.6	0.3	–
Oesophagus cancer	M	519	–	418	11.0	–	21.9	–	–	–	–	–	–	–
	F	67	–	38	1.0	–	1.6	–	–	–	–	–	–	–
Stomach cancer	M	1760	4	920	37.1	0.2	51.6	–	–	–	–	–	0.6	0.5
	F	1135	11	388	15.4	0.5	17.1	–	–	–	–	0.3	1.0	1.9
Colorectal cancer	M	2146	17	1077	45.1	0.7	60.1	0.3	–	–	–	0.3	1.9	2.4
	F	2090	12	813	28.4	0.5	36.1	–	–	–	–	0.6	–	2.7
Liver cancer	M	571	6	325	11.9	0.2	18.2	–	–	–	0.5	0.3	–	0.8
	F	409	3	178	5.7	0.1	7.9	–	–	0.2	–	–	–	0.5
Pancreas cancer	M	780	7	475	16.4	0.3	25.8	–	–	–	–	–	–	1.9
	F	680	3	280	9.4	0.1	12.4	–	–	–	–	0.3	–	0.5
Larynx cancer	M	558	2	426	11.8	0.1	22.4	–	–	–	–	–	–	0.5
	F	49	2	31	0.8	0.1	1.4	–	–	–	–	–	–	0.5
Lung cancer	M	5416	22	3804	114.0	0.9	207.0	–	–	–	–	0.6	1.3	4.3
	F	1492	13	825	22.4	0.5	36.1	–	–	–	–	0.6	1.0	2.1
Malignant melanoma	M	165	5	122	3.4	0.2	6.3	–	–	–	–	–	0.3	1.1
	F	130	6	74	2.0	0.3	3.2	–	–	–	–	0.6	0.7	0.5
Female breast cancer	F	2097	21	1248	32.1	0.8	54.2	–	–	–	–	0.3	0.7	4.8
Cervix cancer	F	602	30	381	9.6	1.2	16.2	–	–	–	–	–	1.3	7.0
Other uterine cancer	F	489	5	213	6.9	0.2	9.4	–	–	–	–	0.3	–	1.1
Ovarian cancer	F	652	14	372	10.0	0.6	16.3	–	–	–	0.5	0.9	1.0	1.6
Prostate cancer	M	1237	3	289	26.4	0.1	17.3	0.3	–	–	–	–	0.3	0.3
Bladder cancer	M	548	–	223	11.7	–	12.7	–	–	–	–	–	–	–
	F	204	–	74	2.8	–	3.3	–	–	–	–	–	–	–
Other and ill-defined	M	1910	116	1120	40.1	4.7	59.7	3.8	2.1	2.1	3.2	6.0	8.0	7.7
cancer sites	F	2297	63	1000	32.6	2.6	44.1	3.0	2.5	2.2	2.1	2.4	3.6	2.7
Hodgkin's disease	M	77	15	47	1.6	0.6	2.3	–	–	0.2	0.2	1.1	0.3	2.1
	F	64	14	27	1.0	0.6	1.2	–	–	0.2	0.8	0.3	1.0	1.6
Myeloma and non-	M	359	19	198	7.6	0.7	10.9	0.3	0.9	0.9	0.2	1.1	0.6	1.1
Hodgkin lymphomas	F	320	12	144	4.6	0.5	6.4	0.3	–	0.5	–	1.5	–	1.1
Leukaemia	M	506	51	246	10.5	2.0	13.3	1.0	2.4	1.4	1.0	3.4	1.6	3.5
	F	422	43	178	6.3	1.7	7.8	1.0	2.2	1.7	3.4	0.9	1.3	1.6
ALL VASCULAR	M	36435	375	15957	777.4	14.8	874.5	1.6	0.6	2.1	6.2	6.2	24.4	62.7
DISEASE	F	39934	150	8630	501.6	6.0	384.4	2.3	1.3	0.5	3.1	3.9	5.9	25.2
Rheumatic heart	M	342	2	222	7.3	0.1	11.7	–	–	–	–	–	0.3	0.3
disease and fever	F	560	7	298	8.2	0.3	13.2	–	–	–	–	0.3	–	1.6
Hypertensive disease	M	2027	5	846	43.4	0.2	47.6	–	–	–	–	0.3	0.3	0.8
	F	3746	9	726	46.5	0.4	32.6	–	–	–	–	0.3	0.3	1.9
Ischaemic heart	M	15316	169	7917	325.0	6.7	430.2	–	–	0.2	0.7	2.3	11.9	31.9
disease	F	12875	29	3333	165.0	1.2	148.5	–	–	–	0.3	–	1.6	6.2
Pulmonary embolism	M	911	18	378	19.2	0.7	20.9	–	–	–	0.2	–	1.9	2.9
and other venous	F	1310	8	337	16.7	0.3	15.1	–	–	–	–	0.6	0.3	1.3
Cerebrovascular	M	9616	78	3938	204.7	3.1	218.7	0.6	–	0.7	2.5	1.4	4.5	11.7
disease	F	11731	46	2626	148.3	1.8	116.9	0.7	0.3	0.2	0.5	0.6	1.6	8.8
Other vascular	M	8223	103	2656	177.9	4.0	145.5	1.0	0.6	1.2	2.7	2.3	5.5	15.1
disease	F	9712	51	1310	117.0	2.1	58.2	1.7	0.9	0.2	2.3	2.1	2.0	5.4
Chronic obstructive	M	3181	23	1215	68.3	0.9	67.9	1.9	–	0.7	0.2	0.3	1.0	2.4
pulmonary disease	F	1896	19	477	24.6	0.8	21.1	0.3	0.3	–	0.3	1.2	1.0	2.4
Other respiratory	M	898	132	377	19.4	5.7	19.6	26.3	–	1.6	2.0	1.7	2.9	5.0
disease	F	669	87	175	9.9	3.9	7.4	15.6	0.6	0.2	1.8	2.4	3.3	3.2
Peptic ulcer	M	569	17	326	12.1	0.7	17.2	0.6	–	–	–	–	1.3	2.9
	F	434	2	137	5.7	0.1	6.0	–	–	–	–	0.3	–	0.3
Liver cirrhosis	M	3726	173	3051	77.0	6.8	152.3	–	–	–	–	1.1	8.7	37.7
	F	1721	60	1366	29.3	2.4	58.4	–	–	–	–	–	4.3	12.6
Renal disease	M	476	19	191	10.2	0.8	10.3	1.0	–	0.2	–	1.4	1.3	1.6
	F	545	13	189	7.4	0.5	8.4	1.3	–	0.2	–	0.9	–	1.3
Pregnancy and birth	F	26	20	6	0.5	0.8	0.2	–	–	–	0.3	1.8	1.0	2.7
Congenital and	M	973	933	30	24.1	41.9	1.4	275.9	4.8	1.6	3.5	4.0	2.3	1.6
perinatal causes	F	779	743	30	20.1	35.0	1.3	233.7	3.5	1.7	1.6	2.4	1.0	1.3
Ill-defined causes	M	87	28	22	2.0	1.3	1.1	8.3	–	–	–	0.3	–	0.3
	F	86	16	5	1.2	0.8	0.2	5.0	–	–	–	0.3	–	–
Other medical causes	M	3995	343	2270	84.2	14.1	117.6	26.0	7.3	3.5	7.9	8.8	17.7	27.6
	F	4128	232	1573	58.6	9.9	68.8	19.6	6.0	3.2	6.2	8.9	10.2	15.0
ALL NON-	M	8459	1876	4714	174.2	75.1	225.5	25.7	13.0	18.3	75.5	117.6	127.3	148.2
MEDICAL CAUSES	F	4816	488	1535	68.8	20.2	65.2	15.6	10.7	9.6	23.1	24.9	27.0	30.3
Motor vehicle	M	1929	745	954	38.8	29.6	44.9	4.8	7.0	4.7	45.7	62.8	43.1	39.1
traffic accidents	F	680	200	303	11.6	8.2	12.8	3.0	8.8	3.7	13.0	11.3	9.6	8.3
Fire	M	172	23	104	3.6	1.0	5.2	1.6	–	0.2	–	0.9	1.9	2.1
	F	82	6	29	1.2	0.3	1.3	0.7	0.3	–	0.3	0.3	–	0.3
Suicide	M	2980	556	1916	60.9	22.3	90.0	–	0.3	4.2	12.6	28.7	47.6	63.0
	F	1153	145	658	18.8	5.9	27.7	–	–	1.5	6.8	9.8	10.2	13.1
Homicide	M	211	58	131	4.3	2.4	5.9	2.5	1.2	0.2	1.0	2.3	3.9	5.6
	F	111	38	56	2.0	1.6	2.3	2.3	0.6	0.5	0.8	1.5	2.6	2.9
POPULATION (thousands):	**M=males**				4978.6	2517.9	2152.0	315.0	330.9	427.2	405.2	352.1	311.1	376.4
	F=females				5386.3	2421.8	2420.1	300.8	316.4	406.8	384.5	336.7	303.5	373.1

HUNGARY: 1990
9th ICD categories

Annual death rates / 100, 000

35–39	40–44	45–49	50–54	55–59	60–64	65–69	70–74	75–79	80+/NK			
489.9	710.2	1151.4	1673.7	2459.0	3415.4	4628.8	6327.4	10045.3	18266.4	M	**ALL CAUSES**	001–999
194.5	303.3	445.5	651.0	960.5	1461.8	2324.0	3735.7	6654.7	14859.5	F		
3.7	5.5	11.0	16.1	20.3	28.6	35.2	34.7	60.4	83.6	M	**Tuberculosis**	010–018, 137
1.2	0.3	2.6	2.2	5.9	4.0	8.7	8.2	21.3	24.4	F		
1.4	0.8	1.8	2.1	2.9	5.0	7.7	8.0	8.9	21.5	M	**Other infective**	Rest of 001–139
0.5	0.5	0.9	1.9	2.8	3.4	3.2	2.9	10.4	22.2	F	**and parasitic**	
62.3	141.2	274.0	449.9	716.6	1001.9	1329.3	1687.7	2209.6	2850.7	M	**ALL CANCER**	140–208
56.5	91.1	160.0	225.5	337.8	465.5	616.0	858.8	1187.7	1662.4	F		
5.6	23.1	38.6	46.2	53.0	55.6	45.6	46.3	48.8	82.4	M	**Mouth and**	140–149
1.4	2.7	3.2	4.4	6.5	4.6	6.2	7.0	12.4	21.1	F	**pharynx cancer**	
2.1	6.9	15.6	26.1	38.1	30.9	33.8	32.0	32.9	33.5	M	**Oesophagus cancer**	150
0.2	1.4	1.2	1.6	0.9	3.4	2.9	4.7	4.7	6.7	F		
2.3	7.4	22.4	26.9	55.5	95.1	151.6	208.2	271.8	353.6	M	**Stomach cancer**	151
2.3	4.9	8.1	13.7	19.1	27.7	44.1	78.2	128.0	197.1	F		
5.6	9.1	23.6	33.3	60.6	116.7	171.9	242.9	357.9	449.2	M	**Colorectal cancer**	153, 154
3.7	6.8	11.0	24.9	36.7	68.4	101.4	135.4	215.7	342.6	F		
1.9	2.5	7.0	9.3	19.6	32.1	55.0	68.5	84.4	81.2	M	**Liver cancer**	155.0
1.9	1.6	2.3	6.5	7.4	14.8	20.4	27.4	47.2	50.0	F		
3.0	7.2	12.0	18.6	30.1	50.2	59.5	79.2	89.7	129.0	M	**Pancreas cancer**	157
1.6	1.4	3.8	6.5	15.7	23.1	35.0	51.3	69.5	97.2	F		
3.0	7.4	15.9	24.4	29.8	38.6	37.9	44.5	42.6	38.2	M	**Larynx cancer**	161
0.2	0.5	0.3	2.2	2.2	2.8	1.3	1.2	2.1	5.6	F		
15.7	46.0	90.1	180.5	295.0	370.2	451.5	487.5	510.7	557.9	M	**Lung cancer**	162
7.9	11.1	21.5	33.0	46.0	62.5	70.6	110.9	106.3	143.8	F		
2.8	1.9	3.7	5.0	9.1	11.2	10.4	9.8	13.3	14.3	M	**Malignant melanoma**	172
1.2	0.5	2.9	4.4	4.0	4.6	4.9	5.3	9.3	12.8	F		
12.8	25.5	40.7	54.7	69.5	84.1	92.4	110.3	129.6	216.0	F	**Female breast cancer**	174
9.3	10.8	17.1	14.9	16.1	18.8	26.2	26.8	36.8	41.1	F	**Cervix cancer**	180
1.4	0.8	4.6	3.7	13.9	19.7	21.7	37.9	50.8	60.0	F	**Other uterine cancer**	179, 182
2.3	8.7	9.9	16.2	21.0	23.4	32.4	46.7	51.3	48.3	F	**Ovarian cancer**	183
–	0.3	1.2	3.6	12.0	26.7	77.6	139.7	319.7	511.4	M	**Prostate cancer**	185
0.2	0.8	1.5	6.4	16.7	25.9	37.4	72.1	98.6	158.9	M	**Bladder cancer**	188
–	0.3	0.9	0.9	2.8	8.0	10.4	21.6	18.1	32.2	F		
15.5	18.4	31.0	52.7	64.9	103.9	131.3	164.6	210.5	301.1	M	**Other and ill-defined**	Rest of 140–208
7.2	9.8	25.3	29.2	56.2	74.9	106.0	139.4	229.1	307.1	F	**cancer sites**	
1.4	1.9	1.2	1.4	4.4	2.3	3.6	4.4	6.2	3.6	M	**Hodgkin's disease**	201
0.7	0.8	0.6	1.6	0.6	1.2	2.6	2.3	5.2	5.0	F		
0.9	2.5	3.4	8.6	15.6	18.5	26.6	39.1	41.7	60.9	M	**Myeloma and non–**	200, 202–203
0.7	1.6	1.2	3.7	8.6	10.8	18.1	23.3	33.7	32.8	F	**Hodgkin lymphomas**	
2.1	5.8	6.7	6.8	12.3	24.0	35.6	48.9	80.8	75.3	M	**Leukaemia**	204–208
1.4	1.9	5.5	3.4	10.5	12.6	19.4	29.2	37.8	43.3	F		
115.7	196.2	373.3	608.2	1032.7	1545.2	2250.3	3326.5	5853.5	11676.2	M	**ALL VASCULAR**	390–459
42.0	76.2	116.8	210.0	360.0	657.7	1228.5	2184.4	4278.4	10636.9	F	**DISEASE**	
2.3	5.0	7.7	11.8	16.0	14.7	24.4	36.5	34.6	45.4	M	**Rheumatic heart**	390–398
2.6	2.2	3.8	9.3	18.2	25.9	30.1	39.1	47.7	53.3	F	**disease and fever**	
2.1	5.0	14.1	35.5	52.6	87.7	136.2	193.1	342.8	684.6	M	**Hypertensive disease**	401–405
1.2	3.3	8.4	16.5	27.5	57.9	113.4	215.3	424.6	1012.2	F		
62.8	105.4	200.1	319.1	538.5	755.0	1030.2	1447.5	2175.8	3767.0	M	**Ischaemic heart**	410–414
14.9	26.8	47.3	79.3	137.7	267.7	465.7	788.8	1383.6	3049.4	F	**disease**	
2.6	4.7	8.9	10.0	23.2	39.0	57.7	79.2	173.2	276.0	M	**Pulmonary embolism**	415.1, 451–453
1.4	3.5	2.9	9.0	11.1	23.1	54.4	77.0	155.5	295.9	F	**and other venous**	
23.9	42.7	79.7	130.7	242.0	392.2	619.8	950.2	1717.6	3103.9	M	**Cerebrovascular**	430–438
12.8	25.8	39.8	64.7	111.1	190.1	373.9	693.1	1359.8	2913.9	F	**disease**	
22.0	33.6	62.8	101.0	160.4	256.6	382.0	620.1	1409.4	3799.3	M	**Other vascular**	Rest of 390–459
9.1	14.6	14.5	31.1	54.3	93.0	190.9	371.1	907.2	3312.0	F	**disease**	
4.4	12.7	21.1	47.3	75.1	119.8	194.9	325.6	568.4	1119.5	M	**Chronic obstructive**	490–496
3.3	4.3	7.3	20.2	23.5	35.4	53.8	102.7	169.5	498.1	F	**pulmonary disease**	
7.5	9.9	8.9	16.5	25.4	31.3	37.4	51.6	103.9	255.7	M	**Other respiratory**	Rest of 460–519
4.0	6.0	5.2	8.1	9.3	10.5	9.1	26.8	51.3	145.5	F	**disease**	
3.7	7.4	12.0	15.0	16.7	28.2	37.4	47.2	60.4	125.4	M	**Peptic ulcer**	531–533
1.6	1.9	3.5	4.0	4.6	9.6	16.9	22.2	44.1	95.5	F		
69.8	88.6	130.2	164.0	201.4	215.6	196.2	167.3	174.1	141.0	M	**Liver cirrhosis**	571
24.7	42.6	48.5	74.0	75.9	72.4	70.3	59.5	61.2	41.6	F		
2.3	4.1	4.0	8.6	9.1	17.0	27.1	45.4	77.3	152.9	M	**Renal disease**	580–590
1.2	1.9	3.5	5.9	8.6	13.2	24.3	36.2	51.3	101.1	F		
1.4	–	–	–	–	–	–	–	–	–	F	**Pregnancy and birth**	630–676
1.9	0.8	0.6	2.9	1.1	1.2	1.4	0.9	2.7	7.2	M	**Congenital and**	740–779
0.7	1.1	1.2	1.6	0.9	2.5	1.0	1.8	1.0	0.6	F	**perinatal causes**	
0.9	0.6	0.6	1.8	0.7	0.8	2.3	2.7	4.4	34.6	M	**Ill–defined causes**	780–799
–	0.3	–	–	–	0.3	1.0	1.2	2.1	32.8	F		
43.8	58.1	75.1	108.5	127.7	170.8	239.1	302.5	393.4	715.7	M	**Other medical causes**	Rest of 001–799
20.3	28.2	32.8	40.4	66.4	113.4	180.2	268.4	411.1	594.1	F		
172.4	184.4	238.7	232.8	229.3	250.0	270.6	327.4	528.4	1082.4	M	**ALL NON–**	E800–E999
37.1	49.1	63.3	57.2	64.8	73.9	111.1	162.8	365.5	1004.4	F	**MEDICAL CAUSES**	
40.7	41.0	46.0	45.8	47.2	42.9	50.5	49.8	72.8	109.9	M	**Motor vehicle**	E810–E819
8.2	11.1	13.9	11.2	11.1	13.6	20.4	27.4	37.3	32.2	F	**traffic accidents**	
2.6	3.6	2.8	6.8	6.9	6.2	7.7	8.0	16.0	21.5	M	**Fire**	E890–E899
–	0.8	0.6	1.2	1.9	1.8	2.6	4.1	8.3	13.3	F		
76.3	83.1	103.9	94.6	84.2	96.6	91.6	108.5	159.0	247.3	M	**Suicide**	E950–E959
18.0	23.0	33.4	26.1	27.8	29.9	35.6	39.7	64.3	87.7	F		
7.5	5.8	8.0	5.7	5.4	4.3	4.5	4.4	4.4	14.3	M	**Homicide**	E960–E969
2.6	3.3	2.6	3.1	1.9	1.2	1.3	1.8	5.2	2.2	F		
427.0	363.4	326.3	279.2	275.6	258.8	221.7	112.4	112.6	83.7	M	**POPULATION (thousands)**	
428.3	368.9	344.3	321.5	323.9	324.6	308.6	171.4	192.9	180.1	F		

HUNGARY: Males

	All ages	0–34	35–69	35–39	40–44	45–49	50–54	55–59	60–64	65–69	70–74	75–79	80+/NK
POPULATION (1000s)													
1955	4752.2	2787.6	1759.9	230.9	338.8	328.3	295.2	247.8	178.5	140.4	104.7	61.6	38.4
1965	4903.4	2668.7	1989.4	362.7	355.6	218.8	315.5	295.8	250.0	191.0	119.0	74.1	52.2
1975	5113.0	2749.9	2042.7	325.0	338.5	347.6	334.3	199.2	270.5	227.6	162.7	97.6	60.1
1985	5143.7	2720.9	2060.8	384.0	347.4	302.6	306.7	299.9	271.7	148.5	172.3	112.4	77.3
1990	**4978.6**	**2517.9**	**2152.0**	**427.0**	**363.4**	**326.3**	**279.2**	**275.6**	**258.8**	**221.7**	**112.4**	**112.6**	**83.7**
1995 projected	*5063.5*	*2480.0*	*2247.5*	*390.0*	*437.7*	*363.6*	*318.4*	*264.2*	*250.4*	*223.2*	*174.4*	*74.6*	*87.0*
NUMBER OF DEATHS													
All causes													
1955	49780	11286	19576	558	1185	1926	2717	3720	4224	5246	6084	5859	6975
1965	55483	5829	23910	946	1259	1103	2728	4314	6099	7461	7745	7684	10315
1975	68229	6704	28577	958	1622	2604	3649	3071	7213	9460	11005	10334	11609
1985	78034	4828	34405	1682	2416	3295	4773	6933	8789	6517	12133	11899	14769
1990	**76936**	**4243**	**38981**	**2092**	**2581**	**3757**	**4673**	**6777**	**8839**	**10262**	**7112**	**11311**	**15289**
1995 projected	*78403*	*4174*	*41525*	*2052*	*3290*	*4430*	*5680*	*6906*	*9042*	*10125*	*10525*	*7022*	*15157*
Lung cancer													
1955	1089	10	878	9	28	78	138	204	239	182	132	51	18
1965	2290	19	1641	21	38	41	165	342	462	572	358	182	90
1975	3414	16	1976	26	59	137	243	232	549	730	754	483	185
1985	4721	26	2891	53	113	255	426	681	852	511	803	603	398
1990	**5416**	**22**	**3804**	**67**	**167**	**294**	**504**	**813**	**958**	**1001**	**548**	**575**	**467**
1995 projected	*6514*	*22*	*4706*	*79*	*230*	*400*	*713*	*959*	*1161*	*1164*	*908*	*385*	*493*
ANNUAL DEATH RATE / 100,000													
All causes													
1955	1425.9*	360.1*	1386.1*	241.7	349.8	586.7	920.4	1501.2	2366.4	3736.5	5810.9	9511.4	18164.1
1965	1430.3*	240.2*	1398.3*	260.8	354.0	504.1	864.7	1458.4	2439.6	3906.3	6508.4	10369.8	19760.5
1975	1502.1*	237.5*	1568.5*	294.8	479.2	749.1	1091.5	1541.7	2666.5	4156.4	6764.0	10588.1	19316.1
1985	1640.4*	183.4*	1959.1*	438.0	695.5	1088.9	1556.2	2311.8	3234.8	4388.6	7041.8	10586.3	19106.1
1990	**1630.9***	**175.1***	**2075.5***	**489.9**	**710.2**	**1151.4**	**1673.7**	**2459.0**	**3415.4**	**4628.8**	**6327.4**	**10045.3**	**18266.4**
1995 projected	*1622.7**	*170.5**	*2148.8**	*526.2*	*751.7*	*1218.4*	*1783.9*	*2613.9*	*3611.0*	*4536.3*	*6035.0*	*9412.9*	*17421.8*
All cancer													
1955	189.4*	9.1*	306.4*	26.9	54.6	107.2	208.0	358.4	572.5	817.0	1025.8	1110.4	1065.1
1965	242.1*	10.9*	354.8*	40.5	55.7	109.7	213.6	394.2	637.6	1031.9	1338.7	1685.6	1829.5
1975	290.8*	13.2*	400.8*	43.7	75.9	158.5	267.4	419.7	727.9	1112.5	1627.5	2146.5	2412.6
1985	329.4*	12.2*	480.5*	48.4	108.8	233.0	368.4	596.2	863.5	1145.5	1635.5	2094.3	2728.3
1990	**368.6***	**11.3***	**567.9***	**62.3**	**141.2**	**274.0**	**449.9**	**716.6**	**1001.9**	**1329.3**	**1687.7**	**2209.6**	**2850.7**
1995 projected	*410.5**	*11.1**	*656.2**	*75.4*	*170.0*	*329.2*	*538.9*	*850.9*	*1171.7*	*1457.0*	*1794.7*	*2276.1*	*2992.0*
Lung cancer													
1955	29.2*	0.4*	61.2*	3.9	8.3	23.8	46.7	82.3	133.9	129.6	126.1	82.8	46.9
1965	52.1*	0.8*	98.2*	5.8	10.7	18.7	52.3	115.6	184.8	299.5	300.8	245.6	172.4
1975	69.8*	0.6*	111.1*	8.0	17.4	39.4	72.7	116.5	203.0	320.7	463.4	494.9	307.8
1985	97.4*	0.9*	164.9*	13.8	32.5	84.3	138.9	227.1	313.6	344.1	466.0	536.5	514.9
1990	**114.0***	**0.9***	**207.0***	**15.7**	**46.0**	**90.1**	**180.5**	**295.0**	**370.2**	**451.5**	**487.5**	**510.7**	**557.9**
1995 projected	*132.0**	*0.9**	*250.7**	*20.3*	*52.5*	*110.0*	*223.9*	*363.0*	*463.7*	*521.5*	*520.6*	*516.1*	*566.7*
Upper aerodigestive cancer (mouth, oesophagus, pharynx and larynx)													
1955	16.3*	0.2*	25.4*	1.3	4.7	8.2	17.3	35.1	40.9	70.5	78.3	107.1	125.0
1965	16.2*	0.3*	22.8*	0.6	2.5	9.1	15.2	28.7	45.2	58.1	70.6	114.7	170.5
1975	21.1*	0.2*	33.0*	1.8	5.6	23.0	35.6	37.1	54.7	72.9	91.0	124.0	164.7
1985	33.4*	0.5*	60.4*	6.8	25.0	47.3	63.6	80.7	106.0	93.6	124.2	121.0	159.1
1990	**42.8***	**0.7***	**82.6***	**10.8**	**37.4**	**70.2**	**96.7**	**120.8**	**125.2**	**117.3**	**122.8**	**124.3**	**154.1**
1995 projected	*53.8**	*0.9**	*107.9**	*14.9*	*52.1*	*97.9*	*135.1*	*163.5*	*160.9*	*131.3*	*130.7*	*115.3*	*152.9*
Other cancer													
1955	144.0*	8.6*	219.7*	21.7	41.6	75.2	144.0	240.9	397.8	616.8	821.4	920.5	893.2
1965	173.9*	9.8*	233.8*	34.2	42.5	81.8	146.1	249.8	407.6	674.3	967.2	1325.2	1486.6
1975	199.9*	12.4*	256.7*	33.8	52.9	96.1	159.1	266.1	470.2	718.8	1073.1	1527.7	1940.1
1985	198.6*	10.8*	255.2*	27.9	51.2	101.5	166.0	288.4	443.9	707.7	1045.3	1436.8	2054.3
1990	**211.8***	**9.8***	**278.3***	**35.8**	**57.8**	**113.7**	**172.6**	**300.8**	**506.6**	**760.5**	**1077.4**	**1574.6**	**2138.6**
1995 projected	*224.7**	*9.2**	*297.5**	*40.3*	*65.3*	*121.3*	*180.0*	*324.4*	*547.1*	*804.2*	*1143.3*	*1644.8*	*2272.4*
Chronic obstructive pulmonary disease (COPD)													
1955	33.2*	0.7*	39.5*	2.6	3.5	11.3	23.0	44.0	75.6	116.1	158.5	305.2	401.0
1965	40.8*	0.6*	48.9*	2.2	3.7	9.1	24.1	55.1	104.4	143.5	246.2	322.5	484.7
1975	60.1*	1.6*	60.3*	3.1	11.8	12.9	34.4	55.2	107.2	197.7	351.0	521.5	868.6
1985	78.8*	1.1*	71.1*	5.5	14.7	23.5	48.3	82.7	134.7	188.6	399.9	706.4	1320.8
1990	**68.3***	**0.9***	**67.9***	**4.4**	**12.7**	**21.1**	**47.3**	**75.1**	**119.8**	**194.9**	**325.6**	**568.4**	**1119.5**
1995 projected	*58.1**	*0.6**	*61.6**	*4.1*	*11.0*	*19.5*	*43.3*	*67.8*	*114.2*	*171.1*	*271.8*	*445.0*	*931.0*
Other respiratory disease													
1955	103.0*	62.8*	68.4*	9.5	13.3	23.8	37.6	79.1	112.0	203.7	337.2	514.6	1169.3
1965	44.8*	20.1*	27.3*	4.7	8.4	11.0	18.7	31.4	42.4	74.3	147.1	279.4	687.7
1975	36.6*	14.0*	25.4*	6.2	8.6	13.2	19.7	17.1	40.3	72.5	135.8	251.0	529.1
1985	21.9*	8.2*	21.7*	10.4	12.1	18.5	20.5	26.0	33.5	31.0	74.9	108.5	214.7
1990	**19.4***	**5.7***	**19.6***	**7.5**	**9.9**	**8.9**	**16.5**	**25.4**	**31.3**	**37.4**	**51.6**	**103.9**	**255.7**
1995 projected	*17.9**	*4.0**	*17.0**	*5.6*	*6.9*	*6.3*	*12.6*	*23.1*	*32.3*	*32.3*	*45.9*	*111.3*	*283.9*
Vascular disease													
1955	513.7*	13.5*	538.3*	44.6	85.0	164.8	306.6	557.7	959.7	1649.6	2785.1	4500.0	7200.5
1965	724.4*	11.7*	594.8*	54.0	98.7	159.0	310.0	558.8	1082.0	1901.0	3626.1	6489.9	13643.7
1975	742.2*	11.0*	692.8*	75.7	149.8	273.3	405.9	655.6	1228.5	2060.6	3620.2	6131.1	12955.1
1985	820.6*	14.1*	878.8*	116.7	213.3	375.4	620.1	1032.0	1537.0	2257.2	3886.8	6217.1	12543.3
1990	**777.4***	**14.8***	**874.5***	**115.7**	**196.2**	**373.3**	**608.2**	**1032.7**	**1545.2**	**2250.3**	**3326.5**	**5853.5**	**11676.2**
1995 projected	*732.3**	*15.4**	*839.3**	*111.0*	*187.6*	*358.9*	*596.7*	*1019.7*	*1533.5*	*2067.7*	*3051.6*	*5343.2*	*10900.0*
Liver cirrhosis													
1955	10.3*	0.6*	19.4*	3.9	6.5	11.0	16.3	24.6	25.8	47.7	44.9	27.6	41.7
1965	14.7*	0.2*	25.0*	2.5	8.7	17.8	22.5	30.8	45.2	47.6	89.9	51.3	63.2
1975	26.7*	1.5*	49.7*	9.8	19.2	34.2	43.7	62.2	89.5	89.2	91.6	92.2	106.5
1985	66.2*	4.6*	133.9*	46.1	73.7	105.4	133.0	174.1	204.3	200.7	169.5	153.9	100.9
1990	**77.0***	**6.8***	**152.3***	**69.8**	**88.6**	**130.2**	**164.0**	**201.4**	**215.6**	**196.2**	**167.3**	**174.1**	**141.0**
1995 projected	*89.1**	*9.5**	*172.6**	*95.1*	*111.7*	*157.9*	*194.7*	*226.3*	*226.4*	*196.2*	*170.3*	*201.1*	*173.6*
Other medical causes													
1955	484.0*	211.3*	311.6*	85.8	108.6	177.9	232.0	324.9	501.4	750.7	1299.9	2785.7	7830.7
1965	254.5*	136.7*	223.1*	48.5	72.0	90.0	152.8	253.9	393.6	550.8	851.3	1215.9	2348.7
1975	199.1*	132.9*	150.5*	30.2	54.4	84.0	112.2	142.6	256.6	373.9	622.0	958.0	1592.3
1985	151.3*	72.4*	150.9*	39.8	70.2	103.4	132.4	170.7	224.9	314.5	488.1	756.2	1179.8
1990	**146.0***	**60.6***	**167.9***	**57.8**	**77.3**	**105.1**	**155.1**	**178.5**	**251.5**	**350.0**	**441.3**	**607.5**	**1141.0**
1995 projected	*140.5**	*51.3**	*179.5**	*69.7*	*85.7*	*114.4*	*165.2*	*195.7*	*274.0*	*352.2*	*392.8*	*530.8*	*1029.9*
All non-medical causes													
1955	92.3*	62.1*	102.6*	68.4	78.2	90.8	96.9	112.6	119.3	151.7	159.5	267.9	455.7
1965	108.9*	60.0*	124.5*	108.4	106.9	107.4	123.0	134.2	134.4	157.1	209.2	325.2	703.1
1975	146.4*	63.3*	189.0*	126.2	159.5	172.9	208.2	189.3	216.6	250.0	315.9	487.7	851.9
1985	172.2*	70.7*	222.2*	171.1	202.6	229.7	233.5	230.1	237.0	251.2	387.1	549.8	1018.1
1990	**174.2***	**75.1***	**225.5***	**172.4**	**184.4**	**238.7**	**232.8**	**229.3**	**250.0**	**270.6**	**327.4**	**528.4**	**1082.4**
1995 projected	*174.1**	*78.7**	*222.5**	*165.1*	*178.9*	*232.1*	*232.4*	*230.5*	*258.8*	*259.9*	*307.9*	*505.4*	*1111.5*

(*The rates for the age groups 0–34 and 35–69 are the means of seven five-yearly rates, but the all-ages rates are standardised to the conventional "European" age distribution)

HUNGARY: Females

	All ages	0–34	35–69	35–39	40–44	45–49	50–54	55–59	60–64	65–69	70–74	75–79	80+/NK
POPULATION (1000s)													
1955	5072.7	2777.1	2018.8	259.8	376.9	357.8	318.0	288.8	230.8	186.7	140.8	82.8	53.2
1965	5244.5	2630.2	2245.6	382.0	392.1	248.6	357.6	334.3	286.9	244.1	173.3	112.7	82.7
1975	5427.6	2634.2	2298.2	345.2	355.8	371.6	376.9	233.7	326.4	288.6	222.2	155.6	117.4
1985	5505.0	2596.9	2304.2	380.2	355.4	334.3	340.9	347.9	343.4	202.1	254.6	187.7	161.6
1990	**5386.3**	**2421.8**	**2420.1**	**428.3**	**368.9**	**344.3**	**321.5**	**323.9**	**324.6**	**308.6**	**171.4**	**192.9**	**180.1**
1995 projected	*5445.5*	*2358.5*	*2458.2*	*380.2*	*434.7*	*370.0*	*340.9*	*313.7*	*306.8*	*311.9*	*305.4*	*139.5*	*183.9*
NUMBER OF DEATHS													
All causes													
1955	48068	8174	17252	530	1077	1446	2027	2928	3971	5273	6858	6968	8816
1965	52636	3777	17444	583	916	879	1870	2907	4089	6200	7882	9261	14272
1975	62873	4133	18500	480	854	1464	2245	2014	4565	6878	9440	11844	18956
1985	69580	2536	18724	708	1020	1476	2265	3455	5080	4720	10364	13174	24782
1990	**68724**	**2115**	**20607**	**833**	**1119**	**1534**	**2093**	**3111**	**4745**	**7172**	**6403**	**12837**	**26762**
1995 projected	*68015*	*1900*	*20263*	*779*	*1359*	*1656*	*2173*	*2955*	*4428*	*6913*	*10806*	*8754*	*26292*
Lung cancer													
1955	341	12	238	5	12	17	42	52	57	53	46	34	11
1965	573	9	336	11	16	19	40	56	94	100	104	68	56
1975	755	8	371	10	23	30	56	47	98	107	144	137	95
1985	1115	10	586	12	33	59	75	124	152	131	177	188	154
1990	**1492**	**13**	**825**	**34**	**41**	**74**	**106**	**149**	**203**	**218**	**190**	**205**	**259**
1995 projected	*2047*	*17*	*1085*	*42*	*63*	*104*	*146*	*197*	*235*	*298*	*412*	*194*	*339*
ANNUAL DEATH RATE / 100,000 (*The rates for the age groups 0–34 and 35–69 are the means of seven five-yearly rates, but the all-ages rates are standardised to the conventional "European" age distribution)													
All causes													
1955	1156.3*	265.7*	1012.9*	204.0	285.8	404.1	637.4	1013.9	1720.5	2824.3	4870.7	8415.5	16571.4
1965	1047.1*	162.7*	871.1*	152.6	233.6	353.6	522.9	869.6	1425.2	2539.9	4548.2	8217.4	17257.6
1975	998.4*	153.7*	858.9*	139.0	240.0	394.0	595.6	861.8	1398.6	2383.2	4248.4	7611.8	16146.5
1985	961.2*	102.9*	912.4*	186.2	287.0	441.5	664.4	993.1	1479.3	2335.5	4070.7	7018.6	15335.4
1990	**925.8***	**92.1***	**905.8***	**194.5**	**303.3**	**445.5**	**651.0**	**960.5**	**1461.8**	**2324.0**	**3735.7**	**6654.7**	**14859.5**
1995 projected	*890.2**	*83.3**	*886.3**	*204.9*	*312.6*	*447.6*	*637.4*	*942.0*	*1443.3*	*2216.4*	*3538.3*	*6275.3*	*14296.9*
All cancer													
1955	162.5*	9.4*	264.5*	50.8	92.6	133.3	200.6	321.7	468.8	583.8	781.3	880.4	864.7
1965	176.0*	9.4*	255.6*	49.5	90.8	144.4	192.4	283.3	414.8	614.1	871.3	1110.9	1362.8
1975	188.4*	10.5*	267.9*	44.0	95.0	151.5	231.1	307.2	427.7	618.5	846.5	1207.6	1631.2
1985	184.7*	9.8*	267.4*	53.7	85.3	154.1	228.8	315.9	428.7	605.6	817.0	1143.8	1562.5
1990	**193.4***	**10.4***	**278.9***	**56.5**	**91.1**	**160.0**	**225.5**	**337.8**	**465.5**	**616.0**	**858.8**	**1187.7**	**1662.4**
1995 projected	*201.4**	*10.8**	*290.4**	*60.0*	*94.3*	*161.1*	*230.9*	*355.1*	*487.9*	*643.8*	*890.6*	*1228.0*	*1757.5*
Lung cancer													
1955	7.5*	0.4*	13.5*	1.9	3.2	4.8	13.2	18.0	24.7	28.4	32.7	41.1	20.7
1965	10.6*	0.4*	16.6*	2.9	4.1	7.6	11.2	16.8	32.8	41.0	60.0	60.3	67.7
1975	11.9*	0.3*	17.1*	2.9	6.5	8.1	14.9	20.1	30.0	37.1	64.8	88.0	80.9
1985	16.8*	0.3*	28.1*	3.2	9.3	17.6	22.0	35.6	44.3	64.8	69.5	100.2	95.3
1990	**22.4***	**0.5***	**36.1***	**7.9**	**11.1**	**21.5**	**33.0**	**46.0**	**62.5**	**70.6**	**110.9**	**106.3**	**143.8**
1995 projected	*29.0**	*0.7**	*47.3**	*11.0*	*14.5*	*28.1*	*42.8*	*62.8*	*76.6*	*95.5*	*134.9*	*139.1*	*184.3*
Upper aerodigestive cancer (mouth, oesophagus, pharynx and larynx)													
1955	3.7*	0.1*	4.1*	1.2	1.6	2.2	2.2	4.5	8.7	8.6	17.0	25.4	50.8
1965	3.0*	0.1*	3.4*	0.5	0.8	1.6	2.5	1.8	6.6	10.2	10.4	18.6	53.2
1975	2.5*	0.1*	3.2*	0.6	1.1	1.6	3.4	2.1	4.0	9.4	9.0	21.9	29.0
1985	3.7*	0.1*	5.2*	1.3	3.1	4.2	6.2	6.6	6.4	8.4	14.9	19.2	38.4
1990	**4.5***	**0.3***	**7.1***	**1.9**	**4.6**	**4.6**	**8.1**	**9.6**	**10.8**	**10.4**	**12.8**	**19.2**	**33.3**
1995 projected	*5.2**	*0.2**	*9.3**	*2.6*	*5.8*	*5.9*	*10.3*	*13.4*	*15.0*	*11.9*	*12.8*	*17.9*	*30.5*
Other cancer													
1955	151.4*	8.8*	246.9*	47.7	87.8	126.3	185.2	299.2	435.4	546.9	731.5	814.0	793.2
1965	162.4*	9.0*	235.6*	46.1	85.9	135.2	178.7	264.7	375.4	562.9	800.9	1031.9	1241.8
1975	174.0*	10.0*	247.6*	40.6	87.4	141.8	212.8	285.0	393.7	572.1	772.7	1097.7	1521.3
1985	164.2*	9.4*	234.1*	49.2	72.9	132.2	200.6	273.6	378.0	532.4	732.5	1024.5	1428.8
1990	**166.5***	**9.6***	**235.7***	**46.7**	**75.4**	**133.9**	**184.4**	**282.2**	**392.2**	**535.0**	**735.1**	**1062.2**	**1485.3**
1995 projected	*167.2**	*9.8**	*233.8**	*46.3*	*74.1*	*127.0*	*177.8*	*278.9*	*396.3*	*536.4*	*743.0*	*1071.0*	*1542.7*
Chronic obstructive pulmonary disease (COPD)													
1955	14.5*	0.4*	12.0*	0.8	0.5	1.1	4.4	10.0	20.8	46.6	89.5	140.1	240.6
1965	16.0*	0.4*	12.4*	0.5	1.5	3.2	7.6	9.0	22.7	42.2	85.4	157.1	295.0
1975	20.7*	0.6*	17.2*	2.0	1.4	9.7	7.7	15.4	31.9	52.0	107.6	162.6	392.7
1985	27.4*	0.8*	20.7*	3.2	7.0	8.1	18.2	27.6	31.5	49.5	122.5	213.1	567.5
1990	**24.6***	**0.8***	**21.1***	**3.3**	**4.3**	**7.3**	**20.2**	**23.5**	**35.4**	**53.8**	**102.7**	**169.5**	**498.1**
1995 projected	*21.9**	*0.9**	*20.3**	*2.9*	*3.5*	*6.8*	*18.5*	*23.6*	*36.5*	*50.3*	*86.1*	*145.5*	*426.3*
Other respiratory disease													
1955	77.6*	50.0*	44.0*	6.5	12.2	12.3	25.8	39.5	72.8	138.7	237.9	462.6	902.3
1965	30.9*	16.0*	13.4*	2.6	3.8	3.6	5.3	13.2	20.9	44.7	90.6	196.1	536.9
1975	24.5*	10.5*	13.7*	3.2	4.8	4.6	7.2	13.7	23.9	38.5	74.7	173.5	400.3
1985	11.3*	6.0*	8.0*	4.2	3.4	6.0	5.0	8.9	11.9	16.3	32.6	59.1	139.9
1990	**9.9***	**3.9***	**7.4***	**4.0**	**6.0**	**5.2**	**8.1**	**9.3**	**10.5**	**9.1**	**26.8**	**51.3**	**145.5**
1995 projected	*9.3**	*3.2**	*7.4**	*5.0*	*6.4*	*6.8*	*8.8*	*9.9*	*8.1*	*6.7*	*21.6*	*45.9*	*144.1*
Vascular disease													
1955	475.2*	12.0*	452.0*	43.5	67.9	129.4	242.5	405.8	807.2	1467.6	2587.4	4438.4	7282.0
1965	594.8*	8.6*	405.5*	32.2	62.5	99.0	182.9	367.0	688.0	1406.8	2847.1	5669.0	12633.6
1975	547.3*	6.4*	380.9*	34.2	57.3	117.1	203.8	335.0	638.8	1280.0	2589.6	5073.3	11647.4
1985	535.2*	5.5*	410.0*	45.2	84.4	139.1	227.3	393.5	702.1	1278.1	2465.4	4656.9	11037.1
1990	**501.6***	**6.0***	**384.4***	**42.0**	**76.2**	**116.8**	**210.0**	**360.0**	**657.7**	**1228.5**	**2184.4**	**4278.4**	**10636.9**
1995 projected	*466.0**	*6.0**	*350.1**	*40.8*	*64.9*	*101.9*	*184.8*	*327.7*	*615.7*	*1114.8*	*1984.0*	*3941.9*	*10111.5*
Liver cirrhosis													
1955	5.8*	0.4*	10.0*	2.3	3.7	5.0	8.5	11.8	16.0	22.5	22.0	29.0	26.3
1965	7.0*	0.2*	11.1*	1.3	2.0	4.0	8.4	16.5	18.1	27.0	38.7	44.4	37.5
1975	10.7*	0.6*	18.3*	2.9	5.9	12.1	22.0	23.5	29.4	32.2	39.2	46.3	57.9
1985	22.7*	2.1*	43.5*	13.4	24.5	38.6	51.0	64.1	62.3	50.5	58.9	49.0	53.2
1990	**29.3***	**2.4***	**58.4***	**24.7**	**42.6**	**48.5**	**74.0**	**75.9**	**72.4**	**70.3**	**59.5**	**61.2**	**41.6**
1995 projected	*36.9**	*3.3**	*73.9**	*34.7*	*58.7*	*67.0*	*93.0*	*93.4*	*88.7*	*82.1*	*71.1*	*63.8*	*41.9*
Other medical causes													
1955	382.5*	175.6*	193.8*	76.2	84.6	93.9	126.1	186.6	296.4	492.8	1061.1	2309.2	6817.7
1965	173.0*	110.9*	131.0*	42.1	47.9	59.9	92.6	139.1	210.2	325.3	480.1	779.1	1659.0
1975	145.7*	108.5*	102.1*	24.9	35.1	52.5	75.1	101.4	172.5	253.3	430.2	618.9	1128.6
1985	110.2*	59.4*	98.6*	26.6	34.9	47.0	72.2	111.5	163.4	234.5	391.6	543.4	906.6
1990	**98.2***	**48.3***	**90.3***	**26.9**	**34.2**	**44.4**	**56.0**	**89.2**	**146.3**	**235.3**	**340.7**	**541.2**	**870.6**
1995 projected	*87.1**	*38.5**	*80.2**	*26.0*	*32.4*	*37.8*	*44.9*	*73.6*	*133.6*	*213.2*	*322.9*	*504.7*	*847.7*
All non-medical causes													
1955	38.3*	17.9*	36.6*	23.9	24.1	29.1	29.6	38.4	38.6	72.3	91.6	155.8	438.0
1965	49.4*	17.2*	42.1*	24.3	25.0	39.4	33.8	41.6	50.5	79.9	135.0	260.9	732.8
1975	61.0*	16.6*	58.9*	27.8	40.5	46.6	48.8	65.5	74.4	108.8	160.7	329.7	888.4
1985	69.7*	19.3*	64.3*	40.0	47.6	48.8	61.9	71.6	79.5	100.9	182.6	353.2	1068.7
1990	**68.8***	**20.2***	**65.2***	**37.1**	**49.1**	**63.3**	**57.2**	**64.8**	**73.9**	**111.1**	**162.8**	**365.5**	**1004.4**
1995 projected	*67.6**	*20.7**	*63.9**	*35.5*	*52.4*	*66.2*	*56.6*	*58.7*	*72.7*	*105.5*	*162.1*	*345.5*	*967.9*

HUNGARY: 1975

Smoking-attributed deaths (Sm.) and total deaths (Total)

		ALL CAUSES	ALL CANCER	Lung cancer	Upper aero-digestive ca.	Other cancer	COPD	Other respiratory	Vascular disease	Liver cirrhosis	Other medical	Non-medical
Males												
0–34	Sm.	–	–	–	–	–	–	–	–	–	–	–
	Total	6704	364	16	6	342	45	396	300	40	3767	1792
35–69	Sm.	7970	2900	1822	389	689	812	129	3350	–	779	–
	Total	28577	7181	1976	612	4593	1060	469	12379	931	2778	3779
		(28%)	(40%)	(92%)	(64%)	(15%)	(77%)	(28%)	(27%)		(28%)	
70+	Sm.	6300	2099	1297	220	582	1179	100	2534	–	388	–
	Total	32948	6193	1422	368	4403	1602	784	19660	303	2904	1502
		(19%)	(34%)	(91%)	(60%)	(13%)	(74%)	(13%)	(13%)		(13%)	
Any age	Sm.	14270	4999	3119	609	1271	1991	229	5884	–	1167	–
	Total	68229	13738	3414	986	9338	2707	1649	32339	1274	9449	7073
		(21%)	(36%)	(91%)	(62%)	(14%)	(74%)	(14%)	(18%)		(12%)	
Females												
0–34	Sm.	–	–	–	–	–	–	–	–	–	–	–
	Total	4133	278	8	3	267	16	283	171	17	2918	450
35–69	Sm.	971	231	176	13	42	123	17	464	–	136	–
	Total	18500	5823	371	70	5382	367	293	8087	403	2220	1307
		(5%)	(4%)	(47%)	(19%)	(1%)	(34%)	(6%)	(6%)		(6%)	
70+	Sm.	1848	315	225	25	65	439	30	944	–	120	–
	Total	40240	5675	376	88	5211	953	906	27322	227	3244	1913
		(5%)	(6%)	(60%)	(28%)	(1%)	(46%)	(3%)	(3%)		(4%)	
Any age	Sm.	2819	546	401	38	107	562	47	1408	–	256	–
	Total	62873	11776	755	161	10860	1336	1482	35580	647	8382	3670
		(4%)	(5%)	(53%)	(24%)	(1%)	(42%)	(3%)	(4%)		(3%)	
Males+Females												
0–34	Sm.	–	–	–	–	–	–	–	–	–	–	–
	Total	10837	642	24	9	609	61	679	471	57	6685	2242
35–69	Sm.	8941	3131	1998	402	731	935	146	3814	–	915	–
	Total	47077	13004	2347	682	9975	1427	762	20466	1334	4998	5086
		(19%)	(24%)	(85%)	(59%)	(7%)	(66%)	(19%)	(19%)		(18%)	
70+	Sm.	8148	2414	1522	245	647	1618	130	3478	–	508	–
	Total	73188	11868	1798	456	9614	2555	1690	46982	530	6148	3415
		(11%)	(20%)	(85%)	(54%)	(7%)	(63%)	(8%)	(7%)		(8%)	
Any age	Sm.	17089	5545	3520	647	1378	2553	276	7292	–	1423	–
	Total	131102	25514	4169	1147	20198	4043	3131	67919	1921	17831	10743
		(13%)	(22%)	(84%)	(56%)	(7%)	(63%)	(9%)	(11%)		(8%)	

HUNGARY: 1985

Smoking-attributed deaths (Sm.) and total deaths (Total)

		ALL CAUSES	ALL CANCER	Lung cancer	Upper aero-digestive ca.	Other cancer	COPD	Other respiratory	Vascular disease	Liver cirrhosis	Other medical	Non-medical
Males												
0–34	Sm.	–	–	–	–	–	–	–	–	–	–	–
	Total	4828	342	26	15	301	29	204	413	140	1759	1941
35–69	Sm.	12902	4551	2751	844	956	995	187	6009	–	1160	–
	Total	34405	8234	2891	1120	4223	1185	416	14850	2535	2706	4479
		(38%)	(55%)	(95%)	(75%)	(23%)	(84%)	(45%)	(40%)		(43%)	
70+	Sm.	8035	2632	1652	291	689	1866	57	3123	–	357	–
	Total	38801	7281	1804	473	5004	2504	417	23381	543	2603	2072
		(21%)	(36%)	(92%)	(62%)	(14%)	(75%)	(14%)	(13%)		(14%)	
Any age	Sm.	20937	7183	4403	1135	1645	2861	244	9132	–	1517	–
	Total	78034	15857	4721	1608	9528	3718	1037	38644	3218	7068	8492
		(27%)	(45%)	(93%)	(71%)	(17%)	(77%)	(24%)	(24%)		(21%)	
Females												
0–34	Sm.	–	–	–	–	–	–	–	–	–	–	–
	Total	2536	272	10	2	260	20	141	152	61	1383	507
35–69	Sm.	2117	533	401	41	91	238	24	1044	–	278	–
	Total	18724	5597	586	113	4898	430	170	8075	980	2051	1421
		(11%)	(10%)	(68%)	(36%)	(2%)	(55%)	(14%)	(13%)		(14%)	
70+	Sm.	2797	468	332	43	93	832	17	1330	–	150	–
	Total	48320	6752	519	136	6097	1629	420	32854	328	3482	2855
		(6%)	(7%)	(64%)	(32%)	(2%)	(51%)	(4%)	(4%)		(4%)	
Any age	Sm.	4914	1001	733	84	184	1070	41	2374	–	428	–
	Total	69580	12621	1115	251	11255	2079	731	41081	1369	6916	4783
		(7%)	(8%)	(66%)	(33%)	(2%)	(51%)	(6%)	(6%)		(6%)	
Males+Females												
0–34	Sm.	–	–	–	–	–	–	–	–	–	–	–
	Total	7364	614	36	17	561	49	345	565	201	3142	2448
35–69	Sm.	15019	5084	3152	885	1047	1233	211	7053	–	1438	–
	Total	53129	13831	3477	1233	9121	1615	586	22925	3515	4757	5900
		(28%)	(37%)	(91%)	(72%)	(11%)	(76%)	(36%)	(31%)		(30%)	
70+	Sm.	10832	3100	1984	334	782	2698	74	4453	–	507	–
	Total	87121	14033	2323	609	11101	4133	837	56235	871	6085	4927
		(12%)	(22%)	(85%)	(55%)	(7%)	(65%)	(9%)	(8%)		(8%)	
Any age	Sm.	25851	8184	5136	1219	1829	3931	285	11506	–	1945	–
	Total	147614	28478	5836	1859	20783	5797	1768	79725	4587	13984	13275
		(18%)	(29%)	(88%)	(66%)	(9%)	(68%)	(16%)	(14%)		(14%)	

(To be conservative, no deaths before age 35, and none from liver cirrhosis or non-medical causes, were attributed to smoking.)

HUNGARY: 1990

Smoking–attributed deaths (Sm.) and total deaths (Total)

		ALL CAUSES	ALL CANCER	Lung cancer	Upper aero-digestive ca.	Other cancer	COPD	Other respiratory	Vascular disease	Liver cirrhosis	Other medical	Non-medical
Males												
0–34	Sm.	–	–	–	–	–	–	–	–	–	–	–
	Total	4243	282	22	17	243	23	132	375	173	1382	1876
35–69	Sm.	15985	6237	3651	1268	1318	1048	178	7012	–	1510	–
	Total	38981	10444	3804	1598	5042	1215	377	15957	3051	3223	4714
		(41%)	(60%)	(96%)	(79%)	(26%)	(86%)	(47%)	(44%)		(47%)	
70+	Sm.	6524	2336	1451	248	637	1430	45	2443	–	270	–
	Total	33712	6771	1590	407	4774	1943	389	20103	502	2135	1869
		(19%)	(35%)	(91%)	(61%)	(13%)	(74%)	(12%)	(12%)		(13%)	
Any age	Sm.	22509	8573	5102	1516	1955	2478	223	9455	–	1780	–
	Total	76936	17497	5416	2022	10059	3181	898	36435	3726	6740	8459
		(29%)	(49%)	(94%)	(75%)	(19%)	(78%)	(25%)	(26%)		(26%)	
Females												
0–34	Sm.	–	–	–	–	–	–	–	–	–	–	–
	Total	2115	257	13	7	237	19	87	150	60	1054	488
35–69	Sm.	2955	832	619	74	139	297	35	1428	–	363	–
	Total	20607	6360	825	165	5370	477	175	8630	1366	2064	1535
		(14%)	(13%)	(75%)	(45%)	(3%)	(62%)	(20%)	(17%)		(18%)	
70+	Sm.	3069	615	455	44	116	776	19	1490	–	169	–
	Total	46002	6757	654	119	5984	1400	407	31154	295	3196	2793
		(7%)	(9%)	(70%)	(37%)	(2%)	(55%)	(5%)	(5%)		(5%)	
Any age	Sm.	6024	1447	1074	118	255	1073	54	2918	–	532	–
	Total	68724	13374	1492	291	11591	1896	669	39934	1721	6314	4816
		(9%)	(11%)	(72%)	(41%)	(2%)	(57%)	(8%)	(7%)		(8%)	
Males+Females												
0–34	Sm.	–	–	–	–	–	–	–	–	–	–	–
	Total	6358	539	35	24	480	42	219	525	233	2436	2364
35–69	Sm.	18940	7069	4270	1342	1457	1345	213	8440	–	1873	–
	Total	59588	16804	4629	1763	10412	1692	552	24587	4417	5287	6249
		(32%)	(42%)	(92%)	(76%)	(14%)	(79%)	(39%)	(34%)		(35%)	
70+	Sm.	9593	2951	1906	292	753	2206	64	3933	–	439	–
	Total	79714	13528	2244	526	10758	3343	796	51257	797	5331	4662
		(12%)	(22%)	(85%)	(56%)	(7%)	(66%)	(8%)	(8%)		(8%)	
Any age	Sm.	28533	10020	6176	1634	2210	3551	277	12373	–	2312	–
	Total	145660	30871	6908	2313	21650	5077	1567	76369	5447	13054	13275
		(20%)	(32%)	(89%)	(71%)	(10%)	(70%)	(18%)	(16%)		(18%)	

HUNGARY: 1995

Smoking–attributed deaths (Sm.) and total deaths (Total)

		ALL CAUSES	ALL CANCER	Lung cancer	Upper aero-digestive ca.	Other cancer	COPD	Other respiratory	Vascular disease	Liver cirrhosis	Other medical	Non-medical
Males												
0–34	Sm.	–	–	–	–	–	–	–	–	–	–	–
	Total	4174	273	22	23	228	14	93	373	221	1176	2024
35–69	Sm.	18750	8034	4551	1822	1661	991	169	7679	–	1877	–
	Total	41525	12385	4706	2200	5479	1120	329	15608	3657	3578	4848
		(45%)	(65%)	(97%)	(83%)	(30%)	(88%)	(51%)	(49%)		(52%)	
70+	Sm.	6752	2654	1640	280	734	1205	53	2556	–	284	–
	Total	32704	7431	1786	447	5198	1616	410	18791	598	1977	1881
		(21%)	(36%)	(92%)	(63%)	(14%)	(75%)	(13%)	(14%)		(14%)	
Any age	Sm.	25502	10688	6191	2102	2395	2196	222	10235	–	2161	–
	Total	78403	20089	6514	2670	10905	2750	832	34772	4476	6731	8753
		(33%)	(53%)	(95%)	(79%)	(22%)	(80%)	(27%)	(29%)		(32%)	
Females												
0–34	Sm.	–	–	–	–	–	–	–	–	–	–	–
	Total	1900	254	17	5	232	20	73	136	73	842	502
35–69	Sm.	3684	1190	878	119	193	319	47	1707	–	421	–
	Total	20263	6640	1085	217	5338	457	179	7838	1773	1839	1537
		(18%)	(18%)	(81%)	(55%)	(4%)	(70%)	(26%)	(22%)		(23%)	
70+	Sm.	4297	970	729	56	185	809	28	2220	–	270	–
	Total	45852	7665	945	120	6600	1250	395	30153	383	3249	2757
		(9%)	(13%)	(77%)	(47%)	(3%)	(65%)	(7%)	(7%)		(8%)	
Any age	Sm.	7981	2160	1607	175	378	1128	75	3927	–	691	–
	Total	68015	14559	2047	342	12170	1727	647	38127	2229	5930	4796
		(12%)	(15%)	(79%)	(51%)	(3%)	(65%)	(12%)	(10%)		(12%)	
Males+Females												
0–34	Sm.	–	–	–	–	–	–	–	–	–	–	–
	Total	6074	527	39	28	460	34	166	509	294	2018	2526
35–69	Sm.	22434	9224	5429	1941	1854	1310	216	9386	–	2298	–
	Total	61788	19025	5791	2417	10817	1577	508	23446	5430	5417	6385
		(36%)	(48%)	(94%)	(80%)	(17%)	(83%)	(43%)	(40%)		(42%)	
70+	Sm.	11049	3624	2369	336	919	2014	81	4776	–	554	–
	Total	78556	15096	2731	567	11798	2866	805	48944	981	5226	4638
		(14%)	(24%)	(87%)	(59%)	(8%)	(70%)	(10%)	(10%)		(11%)	
Any age	Sm.	33483	12848	7798	2277	2773	3324	297	14162	–	2852	–
	Total	146418	34648	8561	3012	23075	4477	1479	72899	6705	12661	13549
		(23%)	(37%)	(91%)	(76%)	(12%)	(74%)	(20%)	(19%)		(23%)	

(To be conservative, no deaths before age 35, and none from liver cirrhosis or non-medical causes, were attributed to smoking.)

IRELAND: 1990

		No. of deaths			Standardised rates (Defined on p.382)			Annual death rates / 100, 000						
		All ages	0–34	35–69	All ages	0–34	35–69	0–4	5–9	10–14	15–19	20–24	25–29	30–34
ALL CAUSES	M	16828	883	5475	1152.9	91.2	1148.9	213.6	20.1	20.1	62.7	106.9	115.4	99.5
	F	14542	498	3245	710.0	52.7	630.6	159.7	13.7	15.3	34.9	37.6	54.7	52.7
Tuberculosis	M	38	2	14	2.6	0.2	2.9	–	–	–	–	–	–	1.6
	F	30	–	10	1.6	–	2.1	–	–	–	–	–	–	–
Other infective	M	65	22	15	4.1	2.3	3.0	4.9	1.2	0.6	1.7	0.7	4.3	2.5
and parasitic	F	57	6	15	3.0	0.6	3.0	2.2	0.6	–	0.6	–	0.9	–
ALL CANCER	M	3854	62	1601	265.7	6.4	338.0	5.6	2.3	2.3	5.8	8.1	3.5	17.3
	F	3261	65	1374	181.0	7.1	264.0	2.2	3.1	4.7	1.8	8.8	6.8	22.2
Mouth and	M	82	1	38	5.7	0.1	7.9	–	–	–	–	0.7	–	–
pharynx cancer	F	23	–	6	1.1	–	1.2	–	–	–	–	–	–	–
Oesophagus cancer	M	162	2	83	11.5	0.2	17.5	–	–	–	–	–	–	1.6
	F	124	1	35	6.2	0.1	7.0	–	–	–	–	–	–	0.8
Stomach cancer	M	264	1	97	18.3	0.1	20.8	–	–	–	–	–	–	0.8
	F	182	–	55	9.2	–	10.8	–	–	–	–	–	–	–
Colorectal cancer	M	471	–	201	33.0	–	42.2	–	–	–	–	–	–	–
	F	398	2	141	21.0	0.2	27.4	–	–	–	–	–	–	1.6
Liver cancer	M	10	–	6	0.7	–	1.3	–	–	–	–	–	–	–
	F	2	–	–	0.1	–	–	–	–	–	–	–	–	–
Pancreas cancer	M	188	–	94	13.2	–	19.5	–	–	–	–	–	–	–
	F	183	–	67	9.6	–	13.1	–	–	–	–	–	–	–
Larynx cancer	M	51	–	26	3.7	–	5.4	–	–	–	–	–	–	–
	F	9	–	5	0.5	–	0.9	–	–	–	–	–	–	–
Lung cancer	M	1044	1	490	71.7	0.1	105.6	–	–	–	–	–	–	0.8
	F	485	1	217	27.5	0.1	43.0	–	–	–	0.6	–	–	–
Malignant melanoma	M	20	–	12	1.4	–	2.6	–	–	–	–	–	–	–
	F	26	4	13	1.5	0.5	2.4	–	–	–	–	1.6	–	1.6
Female breast cancer	F	603	7	331	36.4	0.8	61.4	–	–	–	–	–	1.7	4.1
Cervix cancer	F	65	5	39	4.1	0.6	6.9	–	–	–	–	–	–	4.1
Other uterine cancer	F	79	–	32	4.4	–	6.3	–	–	–	–	–	–	–
Ovarian cancer	F	196	2	113	12.1	0.2	21.6	–	–	–	–	–	1.7	–
Prostate cancer	M	465	–	87	31.5	–	19.5	–	–	–	–	–	–	–
Bladder cancer	M	115	–	37	7.9	–	8.4	–	–	–	–	–	–	–
	F	40	–	14	2.1	–	2.8	–	–	–	–	–	–	–
Other and ill-defined	M	627	31	274	43.1	3.1	55.6	3.5	1.7	1.7	3.5	2.2	1.7	7.4
cancer sites	F	601	25	208	32.0	2.6	40.2	1.5	2.5	2.9	1.2	4.0	1.7	4.1
Hodgkin's disease	M	20	5	11	1.3	0.5	1.9	–	–	–	–	2.9	0.9	–
	F	5	3	1	0.3	0.3	0.2	–	–	0.6	–	–	–	1.6
Myeloma and non-	M	196	6	98	13.3	0.6	20.8	–	0.6	–	1.7	–	0.9	0.8
Hodgkin lymphomas	F	139	3	69	8.0	0.3	13.6	–	–	–	–	0.8	–	1.6
Leukaemia	M	139	15	47	9.5	1.6	9.1	2.1	–	0.6	0.6	2.2	–	5.8
	F	101	12	28	5.1	1.3	5.2	0.7	0.6	1.2	–	2.4	1.7	2.5
ALL VASCULAR	M	7642	42	2571	529.6	4.6	550.6	2.8	1.2	1.2	2.3	3.7	6.1	14.8
DISEASE	F	6669	33	1088	308.7	3.8	216.4	2.2	–	0.6	1.2	3.2	10.3	9.1
Rheumatic heart	M	27	–	16	1.9	–	3.5	–	–	–	–	–	–	–
disease and fever	F	77	1	33	4.3	0.1	6.5	–	–	–	–	–	0.9	–
Hypertensive disease	M	99	–	28	6.9	–	6.1	–	–	–	–	–	–	–
	F	126	–	13	5.6	–	2.6	–	–	–	–	–	–	–
Ischaemic heart	M	4793	10	1913	332.0	1.2	409.3	–	–	–	–	0.7	1.7	5.8
disease	F	3246	5	644	153.2	0.6	129.6	–	–	–	–	–	–	4.1
Pulmonary embolism	M	104	–	37	7.1	–	7.9	–	–	–	–	–	–	–
and other venous	F	103	1	28	5.1	0.1	5.5	–	–	–	–	–	0.9	–
Cerebrovascular	M	1274	12	279	88.0	1.3	59.5	1.4	–	0.6	1.2	–	1.7	4.1
disease	F	1697	15	219	77.1	1.7	42.9	–	–	–	1.2	1.6	5.1	4.1
Other vascular	M	1345	20	298	93.6	2.1	64.4	1.4	1.2	0.6	1.2	2.9	2.6	4.9
disease	F	1420	11	151	63.3	1.2	29.3	2.2	–	0.6	–	1.6	3.4	0.8
Chronic obstructive	M	1270	11	277	86.3	1.1	61.0	0.7	–	1.2	1.7	0.7	0.9	2.5
pulmonary disease	F	711	10	168	34.5	1.1	33.6	–	–	1.2	1.2	–	3.4	1.6
Other respiratory	M	1136	21	153	79.4	2.2	33.2	9.1	–	–	–	1.5	2.6	2.5
disease	F	1344	16	105	58.8	1.7	20.5	5.9	0.6	–	1.8	0.8	1.7	0.8
Peptic ulcer	M	112	–	23	7.7	–	5.0	–	–	–	–	–	–	–
	F	93	–	9	4.1	–	1.8	–	–	–	–	–	–	–
Liver cirrhosis	M	45	–	35	3.2	–	6.5	–	–	–	–	–	–	–
	F	37	–	16	2.1	–	3.0	–	–	–	–	–	–	–
Renal disease	M	223	3	46	15.6	0.3	9.6	1.4	–	0.6	–	–	–	–
	F	206	3	33	9.7	0.3	6.5	1.5	–	–	–	–	0.9	–
Pregnancy and birth	F	2	2	–	0.1	0.2	–	–	–	–	–	–	–	1.6
Congenital and	M	188	179	9	10.6	17.9	1.6	116.9	1.7	–	2.3	1.5	2.6	–
perinatal causes	F	177	158	16	10.4	16.5	2.7	102.3	3.1	1.2	2.4	2.4	3.4	0.8
Ill-defined causes	M	123	65	10	7.8	6.5	2.0	45.5	–	–	–	–	–	–
	F	110	37	6	5.4	3.9	1.2	26.5	–	–	–	0.8	–	–
Other medical causes	M	1142	67	311	78.0	6.7	64.6	12.6	4.6	1.7	6.9	4.4	8.7	8.2
	F	1366	36	265	65.2	3.7	51.5	9.6	1.2	1.8	3.6	3.2	4.3	2.5
ALL NON-	M	990	409	410	62.3	43.0	70.9	14.0	9.2	12.7	42.0	86.3	86.7	50.2
MEDICAL CAUSES	F	479	132	140	25.5	13.7	24.3	7.4	5.0	5.9	22.2	18.4	23.1	14.0
Motor vehicle	M	335	181	111	20.0	18.7	19.4	4.9	5.2	5.8	20.7	43.5	32.1	18.9
traffic accidents	F	121	64	31	6.6	6.4	5.5	2.2	3.1	4.1	13.8	8.8	6.8	5.8
Fire	M	34	9	13	2.2	0.9	2.5	2.1	1.2	–	0.6	0.7	1.7	–
	F	22	4	5	1.1	0.4	0.8	2.2	–	–	–	–	0.9	–
Suicide	M	251	99	130	16.2	10.8	21.8	–	–	2.3	10.4	19.2	29.5	14.0
	F	83	32	47	5.3	3.7	7.9	–	–	–	2.4	6.4	11.1	5.8
Homicide	M	19	10	8	1.2	1.1	1.5	0.7	–	–	0.6	0.7	4.3	1.6
	F	3	1	2	0.2	0.1	0.3	–	–	–	0.6	–	–	–
POPULATION (thousands):	M=males				1748.6	1036.9	600.8	142.8	173.9	173.9	173.8	135.6	115.3	121.6
	F=females				1754.1	995.9	600.1	135.9	160.6	169.7	166.3	125.0	117.0	121.4

IRELAND: 1990

Annual death rates / 100, 000

9th ICD categories

35–39	40–44	45–49	50–54	55–59	60–64	65–69	70–74	75–79	80+/NK			
123.2	223.0	360.5	580.0	1189.9	2105.5	3459.9	5292.6	8886.4	18220.9	M	ALL CAUSES	001–999
89.8	119.7	246.9	384.5	673.0	1081.1	1819.5	2928.6	5184.4	13250.5	F		
–	0.9	–	2.5	2.9	9.2	5.0	16.0	14.2	34.9	M	Tuberculosis	010–018, 137
–	–	–	–	4.4	2.8	7.2	8.3	8.2	22.4	F		
–	2.6	–	1.2	1.4	7.6	8.4	14.0	22.7	50.4	M	Other infective	Rest of 001–139
–	–	–	3.9	5.8	4.3	7.2	15.0	18.4	36.7	F	and parasitic	
27.8	51.0	89.3	192.1	387.1	625.4	993.3	1434.9	1960.2	3042.6	M	ALL CANCER	140–208
38.4	61.7	139.8	211.6	315.4	479.4	601.7	833.9	1163.9	1531.6	F		
–	0.9	4.4	8.6	8.6	10.7	21.7	40.1	31.3	46.5	M	Mouth and	140–149
–	0.9	–	–	–	1.4	5.7	15.0	6.1	10.2	F	pharynx cancer	
–	2.6	5.5	14.8	21.6	26.0	51.8	40.1	68.2	127.9	M	Oesophagus cancer	150
–	–	2.3	2.6	4.4	19.9	20.1	29.9	65.6	77.4	F		
1.7	3.5	3.3	7.4	24.5	39.8	65.2	134.3	90.9	259.7	M	Stomach cancer	151
0.9	1.8	3.4	6.5	8.7	19.9	34.4	36.5	79.9	134.4	F		
4.2	6.9	9.9	19.7	61.9	82.6	110.4	148.3	247.2	422.5	M	Colorectal cancer	153, 154
2.6	4.5	15.8	16.8	34.9	49.8	67.3	76.4	172.1	254.6	F		
–	–	–	1.2	1.4	1.5	5.0	2.0	8.5	–	M	Liver cancer	155.0
–	–	–	–	–	–	–	–	4.1	–	F		
3.4	1.7	6.6	16.0	14.4	47.4	46.8	60.1	85.2	131.8	M	Pancreas cancer	157
1.7	1.8	5.6	5.2	11.6	24.2	41.5	54.8	63.5	105.9	F		
–	–	3.3	4.9	10.1	7.6	11.7	18.0	14.2	42.6	M	Larynx cancer	161
–	–	2.3	–	1.5	1.4	1.4	1.7	2.0	4.1	F		
2.5	10.4	19.8	55.4	116.5	200.3	334.4	408.8	582.4	558.1	M	Lung cancer	162
1.7	3.6	13.5	29.7	56.7	95.3	100.3	169.4	215.2	122.2	F		
0.8	–	1.1	–	2.9	3.1	10.0	10.0	2.8	7.8	M	Malignant melanoma	172
0.9	0.9	2.3	1.3	1.5	2.8	7.2	–	10.2	8.1	F		
15.7	22.7	53.0	64.5	79.9	93.9	100.3	131.2	139.3	240.3	F	Female breast cancer	174
3.5	6.3	3.4	9.0	8.7	11.4	5.7	13.3	10.2	16.3	F	Cervix cancer	180
–	0.9	–	9.0	7.3	11.4	15.8	23.3	26.6	40.7	F	Other uterine cancer	179, 182
1.7	3.6	16.9	25.8	29.1	31.3	43.0	48.2	53.3	53.0	F	Ovarian cancer	183
–	–	1.1	2.5	21.6	42.8	68.6	206.4	335.2	608.5	M	Prostate cancer	185
–	–	–	1.2	8.6	16.8	31.8	34.1	71.0	139.5	M	Bladder cancer	188
–	–	2.3	–	2.9	7.1	7.2	6.6	22.5	22.4	F		
10.1	13.8	23.2	40.6	66.2	96.3	138.8	218.4	275.6	449.6	M	Other and ill-defined	Rest of 140–208
5.2	11.8	13.5	28.4	49.4	82.5	90.3	157.8	217.2	340.1	F	cancer sites	
–	2.6	1.1	3.7	1.4	3.1	1.7	4.0	2.8	3.9	M	Hodgkin's disease	201
–	–	–	–	–	1.4	–	–	–	2.0	F		
1.7	5.2	4.4	8.6	17.3	36.7	71.9	76.2	79.5	100.8	M	Myeloma and non-	200, 202–203
2.6	0.9	2.3	10.3	17.4	19.9	41.5	48.2	32.8	44.8	F	Hodgkin lymphomas	
3.4	3.5	5.5	7.4	10.1	10.7	23.4	34.1	65.3	143.4	M	Leukaemia	204–208
1.7	1.8	3.4	2.6	1.5	5.7	20.1	21.6	43.0	55.0	F		
27.0	70.0	148.8	250.0	542.4	1055.0	1760.9	2563.1	4207.4	8794.6	M	ALL VASCULAR	390–459
17.4	18.1	50.7	78.7	200.6	374.1	775.1	1317.3	2592.2	7107.9	F	DISEASE	
–	–	–	2.5	2.9	12.2	6.7	12.0	5.7	11.6	M	Rheumatic heart	390–398
–	0.9	4.5	1.3	13.1	10.0	15.8	26.6	26.6	28.5	F	disease and fever	
–	0.9	1.1	2.5	2.9	16.8	18.4	34.1	45.5	147.3	M	Hypertensive disease	401–405
–	–	–	2.6	2.9	1.4	11.5	21.6	43.0	160.9	F		
17.7	51.9	109.2	186.0	433.1	799.7	1267.6	1663.3	2579.5	4387.6	M	Ischaemic heart	410–414
4.4	5.4	16.9	45.2	109.0	250.4	475.6	697.7	1379.1	3063.1	F	disease	
–	0.9	5.5	1.2	7.2	15.3	25.1	44.1	56.8	96.9	M	Pulmonary embolism	415.1, 451–453
1.7	–	2.3	1.3	7.3	10.0	15.8	21.6	59.4	65.2	F	and other venous	
3.4	10.4	15.4	30.8	47.5	113.1	195.7	432.9	769.9	1922.5	M	Cerebrovascular	430–438
6.1	8.2	11.3	14.2	40.7	71.1	149.0	335.5	641.4	1930.8	F	disease	
5.9	6.1	17.6	27.1	48.9	97.9	247.5	376.8	750.0	2228.7	M	Other vascular	Rest of 390–459
5.2	3.6	15.8	14.2	27.6	31.3	107.4	214.3	442.6	1859.5	F	disease	
3.4	5.2	8.8	9.9	54.7	116.2	229.1	412.8	948.9	1713.2	M	Chronic obstructive	490–496
3.5	1.8	3.4	12.9	33.4	56.9	123.2	179.4	272.5	594.7	F	pulmonary disease	
–	6.9	8.8	8.6	27.3	53.5	127.1	264.5	715.9	2240.3	M	Other respiratory	Rest of 460–519
1.7	5.4	5.6	10.3	18.9	24.2	77.4	174.4	387.3	1892.1	F	disease	
–	–	2.2	1.2	7.2	9.2	15.1	40.1	82.4	155.0	M	Peptic ulcer	531–533
–	–	–	–	–	2.8	10.0	16.6	41.0	110.0	F		
0.8	6.1	5.5	4.9	5.8	9.2	13.4	8.0	14.2	3.9	M	Liver cirrhosis	571
0.9	1.8	–	1.3	8.7	5.7	2.9	8.3	12.3	20.4	F		
–	4.3	3.3	1.2	10.1	19.9	28.4	52.1	136.4	387.6	M	Renal disease	580–590
0.9	–	2.3	6.5	7.3	8.5	20.1	43.2	71.7	222.0	F		
–	–	–	–	–	–	–	–	–	–	F	Pregnancy and birth	630–676
0.8	–	5.5	–	1.4	1.5	1.7	–	–	–	M	Congenital and	740–779
2.6	0.9	3.4	5.2	1.5	1.4	4.3	1.7	2.0	2.0	F	perinatal causes	
–	1.7	1.1	–	1.4	4.6	5.0	8.0	31.3	127.9	M	Ill-defined causes	780–799
–	–	1.1	1.3	2.9	1.4	1.4	8.3	14.3	112.0	F		
13.5	12.1	17.6	39.4	57.6	117.7	194.0	376.8	590.9	1426.4	M	Other medical causes	Rest of 001–799
7.0	10.9	16.9	32.3	49.4	95.3	149.0	260.8	508.2	1344.2	F		
49.8	62.2	69.5	69.0	90.6	76.5	78.6	102.2	161.9	244.2	M	ALL NON-	E800–E999
17.4	19.0	23.7	20.6	24.7	24.2	40.1	61.5	92.2	254.6	F	MEDICAL CAUSES	
16.0	13.0	17.6	18.5	28.8	19.9	21.7	28.1	56.8	34.9	M	Motor vehicle	E810–E819
3.5	2.7	4.5	6.5	7.3	5.7	8.6	16.6	18.4	14.3	F	traffic accidents	
0.8	0.9	4.4	1.2	–	1.5	8.4	8.0	11.4	15.5	M	Fire	E890–E899
1.7	0.9	–	–	–	1.4	1.4	10.0	4.1	10.2	F		
16.9	21.6	24.3	22.2	30.2	26.0	11.7	26.1	17.0	11.6	M	Suicide	E950–E959
7.0	7.3	9.0	6.5	5.8	10.0	10.0	3.3	2.0	2.0	F		
0.8	0.9	1.1	1.2	1.4	1.5	3.3	2.0	–	–	M	Homicide	E960–E969
–	0.9	1.1	–	–	–	–	–	–	–	F		
118.5	115.7	90.7	81.2	69.5	65.4	59.8	49.9	35.2	25.8	M	**POPULATION (thousands)**	
114.7	110.3	88.7	77.5	68.8	70.3	69.8	60.2	48.8	49.1	F		

IRELAND: Males

	All ages	0–34	35–69	35–39	40–44	45–49	50–54	55–59	60–64	65–69	70–74	75–79	80+/NK
POPULATION (1000s)													
1955	1479.1	837.6	540.9	92.1	94.5	87.9	77.6	74.8	58.8	55.2	46.2	32.3	22.1
1965	1445.8	830.2	519.9	77.8	82.0	84.9	84.0	74.5	62.3	54.4	42.7	29.0	24.0
1975	1568.2	957.8	514.0	78.6	75.7	77.0	78.1	76.1	70.3	58.2	43.9	29.6	22.9
1985	1771.0	1095.9	568.5	113.6	95.9	82.2	75.6	71.5	67.7	62.0	50.6	32.0	24.0
1990	1748.6	1036.9	600.8	118.5	115.7	90.7	81.2	69.5	65.4	59.8	49.9	35.2	25.8
1995 projected	1956.7	1194.7	652.8	131.8	121.8	109.1	90.2	75.6	66.2	58.1	47.2	34.4	27.6
NUMBER OF DEATHS													
All causes													
1955	19773	2209	6623	217	324	479	811	1125	1570	2097	3024	3220	4697
1965	17965	1533	6510	163	301	401	774	1125	1626	2120	2633	2642	4647
1975	18077	1450	6779	150	231	417	759	1103	1775	2344	2786	2749	4313
1985	18201	1048	6228	160	216	345	548	1006	1651	2302	3215	3106	4604
1990	16828	883	5475	146	258	327	471	827	1377	2069	2641	3128	4701
1995 projected	15764	1026	4922	148	244	333	439	765	1246	1747	2228	2822	4766
Lung cancer													
1955	338	3	271	4	11	35	40	75	58	48	29	24	11
1965	570	–	418	2	12	14	53	87	129	121	92	39	21
1975	891	–	555	6	7	26	66	84	164	202	176	111	49
1985	1112	2	588	3	6	25	53	91	171	239	222	173	127
1990	1044	1	490	3	12	18	45	81	131	200	204	205	144
1995 projected	975	1	425	5	10	16	41	72	112	169	185	200	164
ANNUAL DEATH RATE / 100,000	(*The rates for the age groups 0–34 and 35–69 are the means of seven five-yearly rates, but the all-ages rates are standardised to the conventional "European" age distribution)												
All causes													
1955	1474.2*	236.9*	1448.8*	235.6	342.9	544.9	1045.1	1504.0	2670.1	3798.9	6545.5	9969.0	21253.4
1965	1356.4*	164.3*	1426.8*	209.5	367.1	472.3	921.4	1510.1	2610.0	3897.1	6166.3	9110.3	19362.5
1975	1343.2*	144.4*	1430.2*	190.8	305.2	541.6	971.8	1449.4	2524.9	4027.5	6346.2	9287.2	18834.1
1985	1279.4*	98.4*	1295.6*	140.8	225.2	419.7	724.9	1407.0	2438.7	3712.9	6353.8	9706.3	19183.3
1990	1152.9*	91.2*	1148.9*	123.2	223.0	360.5	580.0	1189.9	2105.5	3459.9	5292.6	8886.4	18220.9
1995 projected	1047.8*	86.3*	1000.8*	112.3	200.3	305.2	486.7	1011.9	1882.2	3006.9	4720.3	8203.5	17268.1
All cancer													
1955	196.3*	11.6*	284.3*	26.1	59.3	120.6	220.4	342.2	551.0	670.3	1095.2	1176.5	1470.6
1965	208.8*	12.3*	305.0*	27.0	79.3	83.6	217.9	330.2	571.4	825.4	1138.2	1382.8	1545.8
1975	246.4*	11.1*	352.0*	34.4	62.1	118.2	248.4	352.2	633.0	1015.5	1321.2	1530.4	2240.2
1985	262.5*	7.7*	360.1*	27.3	50.1	125.3	206.3	432.2	680.9	998.4	1419.0	1865.6	2512.5
1990	265.7*	6.4*	338.0*	27.8	51.0	89.3	192.1	387.1	625.4	993.3	1434.9	1960.2	3042.6
1995 projected	269.7*	5.8*	318.0*	27.3	40.2	75.2	165.2	350.5	595.2	972.5	1457.6	2098.8	3492.8
Lung cancer													
1955	26.5*	0.5*	56.2*	4.3	11.6	39.8	51.5	100.3	98.6	87.0	62.8	74.3	49.8
1965	43.9*	–	91.9*	2.6	14.6	16.5	63.1	116.8	207.1	222.4	215.5	134.5	87.5
1975	65.4*	–	118.0*	7.6	9.2	33.8	84.5	110.4	233.3	347.1	400.9	375.0	214.0
1985	78.0*	0.2*	125.0*	2.6	6.3	30.4	70.1	127.3	252.6	385.5	438.7	540.6	529.2
1990	71.7*	0.1*	105.6*	2.5	10.4	19.8	55.4	116.5	200.3	334.4	408.8	582.4	558.1
1995 projected	66.2*	0.1*	89.6*	3.8	8.2	14.7	45.5	95.2	169.2	290.9	391.9	581.4	594.2
Upper aerodigestive cancer (mouth, oesophagus, pharynx and larynx)													
1955	23.3*	0.3*	25.5*	–	6.3	5.7	14.2	22.7	64.6	65.2	171.0	179.6	271.5
1965	17.4*	–	21.2*	2.6	3.7	7.1	10.7	9.4	41.7	73.5	114.8	165.5	170.8
1975	18.9*	0.2*	21.5*	5.1	4.0	6.5	19.2	21.0	39.8	55.0	113.9	125.0	253.3
1985	20.3*	0.1*	31.3*	0.9	4.2	14.6	15.9	44.8	70.9	67.7	110.7	90.6	183.3
1990	20.9*	0.3*	30.7*	–	3.5	13.2	28.3	40.3	44.3	85.3	98.2	113.6	217.1
1995 projected	21.7*	0.5*	28.8*	–	2.5	16.5	29.9	34.4	40.8	77.5	108.1	122.1	260.9
Other cancer													
1955	146.5*	10.9*	202.5*	21.7	41.3	75.1	154.6	219.3	387.8	518.1	861.5	922.6	1149.3
1965	147.4*	12.3*	191.9*	21.9	61.0	60.1	144.0	204.0	322.6	529.4	808.0	1082.8	1287.5
1975	162.0*	10.9*	212.5*	21.6	48.9	77.9	144.7	220.8	359.9	613.4	806.4	1030.4	1772.9
1985	164.2*	7.4*	203.8*	23.8	39.6	80.3	120.4	260.1	357.5	545.2	869.6	1234.4	1800.0
1990	173.1*	5.9*	201.7*	25.3	37.2	56.2	108.4	230.2	380.7	573.6	927.9	1264.2	2267.4
1995 projected	181.8*	5.3*	199.6*	23.5	29.6	44.0	89.8	220.9	385.2	604.1	957.6	1395.3	2637.7
Chronic obstructive pulmonary disease (COPD)													
1955	59.9*	2.7*	67.2*	6.5	14.8	15.9	58.0	49.5	141.2	184.8	307.4	365.3	891.4
1965	84.6*	1.2*	114.0*	6.4	7.3	29.4	54.8	108.7	242.4	349.3	442.6	620.7	941.7
1975	90.4*	5.1*	93.9*	3.8	7.9	24.7	42.3	105.1	145.1	328.2	480.6	723.0	1323.1
1985	93.7*	0.9*	78.9*	2.6	7.3	7.3	31.7	55.9	165.4	282.3	592.9	934.4	1520.8
1990	86.3*	1.1*	61.0*	3.4	5.2	8.8	9.9	54.7	116.2	229.1	412.8	948.9	1713.2
1995 projected	82.4*	1.3*	45.3*	3.0	4.9	5.5	7.8	38.4	92.1	165.2	358.1	941.9	1858.7
Other respiratory disease													
1955	63.0*	21.8*	51.3*	10.9	8.5	26.2	29.6	61.5	90.1	132.2	244.6	328.2	918.6
1965	64.0*	12.7*	54.7*	6.4	19.5	18.8	29.8	41.6	99.5	167.3	285.7	406.9	1054.2
1975	82.7*	11.2*	60.3*	11.5	6.6	11.7	30.7	57.8	108.1	195.9	350.8	621.6	1637.6
1985	92.0*	2.1*	39.4*	0.9	8.3	10.9	17.2	35.0	65.0	138.7	355.7	728.1	2608.3
1990	79.4*	2.2*	33.2*	–	6.9	8.8	8.6	27.3	53.5	127.1	264.5	715.9	2240.3
1995 projected	69.0*	2.9*	26.3*	–	4.9	5.5	5.5	21.2	46.8	99.8	237.3	598.8	1981.9
Vascular disease													
1955	690.3*	14.5*	683.2*	47.8	89.9	198.0	416.2	644.4	1297.6	2088.8	3725.1	5919.5	10660.6
1965	701.9*	10.4*	704.5*	68.1	141.5	215.5	441.7	753.0	1311.4	2000.0	3449.6	5393.1	11700.0
1975	698.3*	6.8*	723.3*	56.0	126.8	261.0	499.4	735.9	1308.7	2075.6	3473.8	5307.4	11296.9
1985	632.8*	5.5*	644.5*	41.4	87.6	176.4	347.9	696.5	1273.3	1888.7	3334.0	5006.3	10162.5
1990	529.6*	4.6*	550.6*	27.0	70.0	148.8	250.0	542.4	1055.0	1760.9	2563.1	4207.4	8794.6
1995 projected	441.3*	3.1*	450.0*	19.7	54.2	107.2	186.3	424.6	912.4	1445.8	2114.4	3552.3	7532.6
Liver cirrhosis													
1955	2.9*	–	6.2*	–	2.1	2.3	7.7	12.0	13.6	5.4	2.2	15.5	4.5
1965	4.6*	0.1*	8.6*	2.6	1.2	4.7	4.8	16.1	16.1	14.7	21.1	17.2	12.5
1975	3.7*	–	8.2*	2.5	2.6	1.3	3.8	9.2	22.8	15.5	6.8	20.3	4.4
1985	3.7*	0.1*	8.1*	1.8	2.1	4.9	6.6	7.0	14.8	19.4	7.9	12.5	8.3
1990	3.2*	–	6.5*	0.8	6.1	5.5	4.9	5.8	9.2	13.4	8.0	14.2	3.9
1995 projected	2.9*	–	5.8*	1.5	8.2	6.4	4.4	4.0	6.0	10.3	6.4	11.6	3.6
Other medical causes													
1955	412.0*	151.7*	300.4*	107.5	122.8	142.2	260.3	327.5	510.2	632.2	1069.3	2049.5	7095.0
1965	240.8*	93.9*	180.2*	55.3	80.5	80.1	107.1	208.1	298.6	432.0	747.1	1162.1	3820.8
1975	148.3*	59.0*	113.6*	22.9	33.0	57.1	73.0	95.9	200.6	312.7	564.9	922.3	1969.4
1985	131.7*	36.6*	97.4*	21.1	21.9	37.7	63.5	109.1	149.2	279.0	525.7	1000.0	2041.7
1990	126.3*	33.9*	88.7*	14.3	21.6	29.8	45.6	82.0	169.7	257.5	507.0	877.8	2182.2
1995 projected	120.3*	31.7*	80.9*	10.6	16.4	22.0	33.3	74.1	160.1	249.6	455.5	860.5	2195.7
All non-medical causes													
1955	49.9*	34.6*	56.2*	36.9	45.5	39.8	52.8	66.8	66.3	85.1	101.7	114.6	212.7
1965	51.8*	33.7*	59.8*	43.7	37.8	40.0	65.5	52.3	70.6	108.5	82.0	127.6	287.5
1975	73.4*	51.2*	78.8*	59.8	66.1	67.5	74.3	93.3	106.7	84.2	148.1	162.2	362.4
1985	63.0*	45.5*	67.2*	45.8	48.0	57.2	51.6	71.3	90.1	106.5	118.6	159.4	329.2
1990	62.3*	43.0*	70.9*	49.8	62.2	69.5	69.0	90.6	76.5	78.6	102.2	161.9	244.2
1995 projected	62.3*	41.5*	74.5*	50.1	71.4	83.4	84.3	99.2	69.5	63.7	91.1	139.5	202.9

IRELAND: Females

	All ages	0–34	35–69	35–39	40–44	45–49	50–54	55–59	60–64	65–69	70–74	75–79	80+/NK
POPULATION (1000s)													
1955	1442.3	807.5	526.7	94.1	90.0	82.9	73.3	73.0	59.6	53.8	48.5	33.6	26.0
1965	1430.0	798.7	517.4	79.4	83.2	83.5	79.7	70.5	63.2	57.9	48.1	34.0	31.8
1975	1558.8	917.8	515.9	76.5	74.6	77.6	79.6	76.3	70.7	60.6	51.4	39.8	33.9
1985	1769.0	1055.7	568.1	110.0	91.6	78.4	73.2	73.0	72.9	69.0	59.3	42.3	43.6
1990	1754.1	995.9	600.1	114.7	110.3	88.7	77.5	68.8	70.3	69.8	60.2	48.8	49.1
1995 projected	1942.9	1136.1	650.5	128.8	119.3	105.7	87.4	74.6	68.7	66.0	59.3	48.1	48.9
NUMBER OF DEATHS													
All causes													
1955	16988	1702	4869	200	287	394	594	749	1164	1481	2664	2910	4843
1965	15057	1087	4106	114	203	349	504	613	967	1356	2112	2476	5276
1975	15096	875	4037	94	142	280	467	672	987	1395	2056	2586	5542
1985	15012	562	3589	92	140	184	316	545	947	1365	2094	2410	6357
1990	14542	498	3245	103	132	219	298	463	760	1270	1763	2530	6506
1995 projected	13274	615	2912	101	139	238	312	434	659	1029	1539	2221	5987
Lung cancer													
1955	97	–	78	3	4	4	14	19	17	17	10	8	1
1965	146	1	95	4	4	9	14	16	22	26	30	11	9
1975	300	1	184	1	4	13	29	41	45	51	46	35	34
1985	430	4	208	–	3	6	20	30	75	74	96	75	47
1990	485	1	217	2	4	12	23	39	67	70	102	105	60
1995 projected	524	1	230	2	6	17	33	44	64	64	107	115	71
ANNUAL DEATH RATE / 100,000 (*The rates for the age groups 0–34 and 35–69 are the means of seven five-yearly rates, but the all-ages rates are standardised to the conventional "European" age distribution)													
All causes													
1955	1208.0*	190.5*	1078.4*	212.5	318.9	475.3	810.4	1026.0	1953.0	2752.8	5492.8	8660.7	18626.9
1965	995.2*	118.0*	882.8*	143.6	244.0	418.0	632.4	869.5	1530.1	2342.0	4390.9	7282.4	16591.2
1975	926.6*	87.8*	834.2*	122.9	190.3	360.8	586.7	880.7	1396.0	2302.0	4000.0	6497.5	16348.1
1985	791.5*	53.2*	703.8*	83.6	152.8	234.7	431.7	746.6	1299.0	1978.3	3531.2	5697.4	14580.3
1990	710.0*	52.7*	630.6*	89.8	119.7	246.9	384.5	673.0	1081.1	1819.5	2928.6	5184.4	13250.5
1995 projected	642.7*	54.4*	553.9*	78.4	116.5	225.2	357.0	581.8	959.2	1559.1	2595.3	4617.5	12243.4
All cancer													
1955	156.3*	9.2*	249.2*	32.9	100.0	137.5	237.4	284.9	429.5	522.3	758.8	791.7	903.8
1965	160.3*	10.2*	242.9*	49.1	88.9	167.7	229.6	262.4	403.5	499.1	738.0	850.0	1135.2
1975	190.2*	7.3*	294.2*	51.0	73.7	179.1	263.8	355.2	479.5	656.8	778.2	1060.3	1533.9
1985	176.6*	6.7*	266.8*	38.2	81.9	132.7	218.6	323.3	504.8	568.1	828.0	1016.5	1385.3
1990	181.0*	7.1*	264.0*	38.4	61.7	139.8	211.6	315.4	479.4	601.7	833.9	1163.9	1531.6
1995 projected	184.0*	7.9*	255.8*	32.6	57.0	129.6	203.7	300.3	468.7	598.5	878.6	1222.5	1717.8
Lung cancer													
1955	7.6*	–	16.8*	3.2	4.4	4.8	19.1	26.0	28.5	31.6	20.6	23.8	3.8
1965	10.8*	0.2*	20.1*	5.0	4.8	10.8	17.6	22.7	34.8	44.9	62.4	32.4	28.3
1975	20.5*	0.2*	37.3*	1.3	5.4	16.8	36.4	53.7	63.6	84.2	89.5	87.9	100.3
1985	25.3*	0.4*	41.4*	–	3.3	7.7	27.3	41.1	102.9	107.2	161.9	177.3	107.8
1990	27.5*	0.1*	43.0*	1.7	3.6	13.5	29.7	56.7	95.3	100.3	169.4	215.2	122.2
1995 projected	29.4*	0.1*	44.2*	1.6	5.0	16.1	37.8	59.0	93.2	97.0	180.4	239.1	145.2
Upper aerodigestive cancer (mouth, oesophagus, pharynx and larynx)													
1955	10.6*	0.2*	16.0*	1.1	5.6	6.0	20.5	15.1	30.2	33.5	57.7	71.4	65.4
1965	9.1*	0.5*	12.6*	2.5	3.6	8.4	15.1	8.5	22.2	27.6	37.4	50.0	97.5
1975	10.3*	0.2*	14.1*	1.3	2.7	5.2	12.6	21.0	19.8	36.3	42.8	75.4	112.1
1985	8.7*	0.1*	12.4*	1.8	2.2	1.3	5.5	11.0	30.2	34.8	43.8	37.8	112.4
1990	7.9*	0.1*	9.1*	–	0.9	4.5	2.6	5.8	22.8	27.2	46.5	73.8	91.6
1995 projected	7.9*	0.1*	7.3*	–	0.8	3.8	2.3	4.0	16.0	24.2	57.3	83.2	100.2
Other cancer													
1955	138.0*	9.0*	216.4*	28.7	90.0	126.7	197.8	243.8	370.8	457.2	680.4	696.4	834.6
1965	140.4*	9.5*	210.3*	41.6	80.5	148.5	197.0	231.2	346.5	426.6	638.3	767.6	1009.4
1975	159.3*	7.0*	242.7*	48.4	65.7	157.2	214.8	280.5	396.0	536.3	645.9	897.0	1321.5
1985	142.5*	6.2*	213.1*	36.4	76.4	123.7	185.8	271.2	371.7	426.1	622.3	801.4	1165.1
1990	145.6*	6.9*	211.9*	36.6	57.1	121.8	179.4	252.9	361.3	474.2	617.9	875.0	1317.7
1995 projected	146.7*	7.7*	204.2*	31.1	51.1	109.7	163.6	237.3	359.5	477.3	640.8	900.2	1472.4
Chronic obstructive pulmonary disease (COPD)													
1955	36.3*	2.1*	26.6*	6.4	6.7	10.9	12.3	20.5	55.4	74.3	216.5	342.3	615.4
1965	42.7*	1.4*	40.3*	1.3	9.6	19.2	21.3	51.1	72.8	107.1	222.5	320.6	713.8
1975	38.0*	2.8*	37.5*	–	8.0	16.8	27.6	38.0	65.1	107.3	163.4	266.3	637.2
1985	39.2*	0.3*	40.2*	–	3.3	6.4	21.9	47.9	70.0	131.9	256.3	309.7	566.5
1990	34.5*	1.1*	33.6*	3.5	1.8	3.4	12.9	33.4	56.9	123.2	179.4	272.5	594.7
1995 projected	30.6*	1.3*	26.4*	4.7	1.7	1.9	9.2	24.1	48.0	95.5	145.0	249.5	589.0
Other respiratory disease													
1955	58.1*	16.5*	39.4*	9.6	7.8	19.3	20.5	32.9	70.5	115.2	249.5	482.1	896.2
1965	48.3*	9.9*	30.5*	3.8	6.0	16.8	18.8	31.2	49.1	88.1	237.0	352.9	886.8
1975	67.2*	8.0*	35.4*	5.2	8.0	10.3	17.6	31.5	56.6	118.8	254.9	507.5	1637.2
1985	63.2*	1.0*	25.6*	2.7	2.2	3.8	15.0	24.7	42.5	88.4	210.8	437.4	1942.7
1990	58.8*	1.7*	20.5*	1.7	5.4	5.6	10.3	18.9	24.2	77.4	174.4	387.3	1892.1
1995 projected	54.5*	2.2*	16.9*	2.3	7.5	5.7	8.0	13.4	18.9	62.1	148.4	334.7	1816.0
Vascular disease													
1955	581.2*	14.8*	515.4*	60.6	86.7	152.0	326.1	460.3	1003.4	1518.6	3208.2	5080.4	9684.6
1965	517.2*	9.6*	410.0*	35.3	66.1	129.3	245.9	373.0	723.1	1297.1	2548.9	4605.9	10003.1
1975	465.6*	3.7*	336.2*	18.3	49.6	92.8	184.7	329.0	598.3	1080.9	2231.5	3768.8	10221.2
1985	386.9*	3.8*	265.7*	13.6	26.2	48.5	110.7	239.7	517.1	904.3	1809.4	3144.2	8876.1
1990	308.7*	3.8*	216.4*	17.4	18.1	50.7	78.7	200.6	374.1	775.1	1317.3	2592.2	7107.9
1995 projected	244.5*	4.2*	165.6*	14.0	17.6	38.8	62.9	147.5	296.9	581.8	1028.7	2018.7	5742.3
Liver cirrhosis													
1955	2.3*	0.5*	4.4*	1.1	1.1	1.2	2.7	6.8	8.4	9.3	–	11.9	11.5
1965	2.3*	–	4.7*	1.3	2.4	1.2	7.5	8.5	3.2	8.6	4.2	5.9	9.4
1975	3.0*	0.4*	4.8*	1.3	2.7	3.9	2.5	5.2	11.3	6.6	5.8	12.6	23.6
1985	2.7*	0.1*	5.7*	–	5.5	3.8	2.7	13.7	6.9	7.2	1.7	14.2	2.3
1990	2.1*	–	3.0*	0.9	1.8	–	1.3	8.7	5.7	2.9	8.3	12.3	20.4
1995 projected	2.0*	–	2.2*	0.8	0.8	–	1.1	5.4	4.4	3.0	8.4	16.6	28.6
Other medical causes													
1955	349.0*	136.0*	229.2*	94.6	112.2	147.2	197.8	201.4	365.8	485.1	981.4	1800.6	6115.4
1965	198.7*	77.6*	132.8*	45.3	67.3	68.3	86.6	122.0	250.0	290.2	573.8	1023.5	3430.8
1975	124.0*	51.8*	93.4*	24.8	25.5	36.1	61.6	89.1	151.3	265.7	447.5	653.3	1769.9
1985	96.8*	29.3*	74.0*	11.8	15.3	21.7	38.3	69.9	124.8	236.2	367.6	678.5	1513.8
1990	99.4*	25.3*	68.9*	10.5	11.8	23.7	49.0	71.2	116.6	199.1	353.8	663.9	1849.3
1995 projected	101.6*	22.1*	64.3*	7.8	10.9	25.5	52.6	71.0	101.9	180.3	327.2	698.5	2122.7
All non-medical causes													
1955	24.8*	11.4*	14.3*	7.4	4.4	7.2	13.6	19.2	20.1	27.9	78.4	151.8	400.0
1965	25.8*	9.3*	21.6*	7.6	3.6	15.6	22.6	21.3	28.5	51.8	66.5	123.5	411.9
1975	38.6*	13.8*	32.6*	22.2	22.8	21.9	28.9	32.8	33.9	66.0	118.7	228.6	525.1
1985	26.0*	12.0*	25.8*	17.3	18.6	17.9	24.6	27.4	32.9	42.0	57.3	96.9	293.6
1990	25.5*	13.7*	24.3*	17.4	19.0	23.7	20.6	24.7	24.2	40.1	61.5	92.2	254.6
1995 projected	25.5*	16.7*	22.7*	16.3	21.0	23.7	19.5	20.1	20.4	37.9	59.0	76.9	227.0

IRELAND: 1975

Smoking-attributed deaths (Sm.) and total deaths (Total)

Age		ALL CAUSES	ALL CANCER	Lung cancer	Upper aero-digestive ca.	Other cancer	COPD	Other respiratory	Vascular disease	Liver cirrhosis	Other medical	Non-medical
Males												
0–34	Sm.	–	–	–	–	–	–	–	–	–	–	–
	Total	1450	93	0	1	92	60	124	52	0	672	449
35–69	Sm.	2276	738	515	66	157	337	79	968	–	154	–
	Total	6779	1663	555	103	1005	434	281	3419	40	540	402
		(34%)	(44%)	(93%)	(64%)	(16%)	(78%)	(28%)	(28%)		(29%)	
70+	Sm.	1729	490	300	78	112	494	69	578	–	98	–
	Total	9848	1546	336	145	1065	728	713	5683	10	972	196
		(18%)	(32%)	(89%)	(54%)	(11%)	(68%)	(10%)	(10%)		(10%)	
Any age	Sm.	4005	1228	815	144	269	831	148	1546	–	252	–
	Total	18077	3302	891	249	2162	1222	1118	9154	50	2184	1047
		(22%)	(37%)	(91%)	(58%)	(12%)	(68%)	(13%)	(17%)		(12%)	
Females												
0–34	Sm.	–	–	–	–	–	–	–	–	–	–	–
	Total	875	57	1	1	55	29	83	26	3	558	119
35–69	Sm.	712	202	140	31	31	117	29	283	–	81	–
	Total	4037	1451	184	69	1198	181	168	1599	24	451	163
		(18%)	(14%)	(76%)	(45%)	(3%)	(65%)	(17%)	(18%)		(18%)	
70+	Sm.	639	117	73	27	17	198	33	246	–	45	–
	Total	10184	1342	115	90	1137	406	888	6112	16	1090	330
		(6%)	(9%)	(63%)	(30%)	(1%)	(49%)	(4%)	(4%)		(4%)	
Any age	Sm.	1351	319	213	58	48	315	62	529	–	126	–
	Total	15096	2850	300	160	2390	616	1139	7737	43	2099	612
		(9%)	(11%)	(71%)	(36%)	(2%)	(51%)	(5%)	(7%)		(6%)	
Males+Females												
0–34	Sm.	–	–	–	–	–	–	–	–	–	–	–
	Total	2325	150	1	2	147	89	207	78	3	1230	568
35–69	Sm.	2988	940	655	97	188	454	108	1251	–	235	–
	Total	10816	3114	739	172	2203	615	449	5018	64	991	565
		(28%)	(30%)	(89%)	(56%)	(9%)	(74%)	(24%)	(25%)		(24%)	
70+	Sm.	2368	607	373	105	129	692	102	824	–	143	–
	Total	20032	2888	451	235	2202	1134	1601	11795	26	2062	526
		(12%)	(21%)	(83%)	(45%)	(6%)	(61%)	(6%)	(7%)		(7%)	
Any age	Sm.	5356	1547	1028	202	317	1146	210	2075	–	378	–
	Total	33173	6152	1191	409	4552	1838	2257	16891	93	4283	1659
		(16%)	(25%)	(86%)	(49%)	(7%)	(62%)	(9%)	(12%)		(9%)	

IRELAND: 1985

Smoking-attributed deaths (Sm.) and total deaths (Total)

Age		ALL CAUSES	ALL CANCER	Lung cancer	Upper aero-digestive ca.	Other cancer	COPD	Other respiratory	Vascular disease	Liver cirrhosis	Other medical	Non-medical
Males												
0–34	Sm.	–	–	–	–	–	–	–	–	–	–	–
	Total	1048	78	2	1	75	10	23	52	1	421	463
35–69	Sm.	2179	806	547	99	160	290	53	891	–	139	–
	Total	6228	1727	588	151	988	367	186	3070	40	476	362
		(35%)	(47%)	(93%)	(66%)	(16%)	(79%)	(28%)	(29%)		(29%)	
70+	Sm.	2464	728	477	79	172	716	127	756	–	137	–
	Total	10925	1918	522	129	1267	964	1039	5728	10	1076	190
		(23%)	(38%)	(91%)	(61%)	(14%)	(74%)	(12%)	(13%)		(13%)	
Any age	Sm.	4643	1534	1024	178	332	1006	180	1647	–	276	–
	Total	18201	3723	1112	281	2330	1341	1248	8850	51	1973	1015
		(26%)	(41%)	(92%)	(63%)	(14%)	(75%)	(14%)	(19%)		(14%)	
Females												
0–34	Sm.	–	–	–	–	–	–	–	–	–	–	–
	Total	562	64	4	1	59	3	11	35	1	325	123
35–69	Sm.	726	225	162	30	33	132	24	271	–	74	–
	Total	3589	1377	208	63	1106	201	129	1334	30	377	141
		(20%)	(16%)	(78%)	(48%)	(3%)	(66%)	(19%)	(20%)		(20%)	
70+	Sm.	1432	270	177	48	45	379	98	576	–	109	–
	Total	10861	1525	218	91	1216	530	1157	6273	8	1165	203
		(13%)	(18%)	(81%)	(53%)	(4%)	(72%)	(8%)	(9%)		(9%)	
Any age	Sm.	2158	495	339	78	78	511	122	847	–	183	–
	Total	15012	2966	430	155	2381	734	1297	7642	39	1867	467
		(14%)	(17%)	(79%)	(50%)	(3%)	(70%)	(9%)	(11%)		(10%)	
Males+Females												
0–34	Sm.	–	–	–	–	–	–	–	–	–	–	–
	Total	1610	142	6	2	134	13	34	87	2	746	586
35–69	Sm.	2905	1031	709	129	193	422	77	1162	–	213	–
	Total	9817	3104	796	214	2094	568	315	4404	70	853	503
		(30%)	(33%)	(89%)	(60%)	(9%)	(74%)	(24%)	(26%)		(25%)	
70+	Sm.	3896	998	654	127	217	1095	225	1332	–	246	–
	Total	21786	3443	740	220	2483	1494	2196	12001	18	2241	393
		(18%)	(29%)	(88%)	(58%)	(9%)	(73%)	(10%)	(11%)		(11%)	
Any age	Sm.	6801	2029	1363	256	410	1517	302	2494	–	459	–
	Total	33213	6689	1542	436	4711	2075	2545	16492	90	3840	1482
		(20%)	(30%)	(88%)	(59%)	(9%)	(73%)	(12%)	(15%)		(12%)	

(To be conservative, no deaths before age 35, and none from liver cirrhosis or non-medical causes, were attributed to smoking.)

IRELAND: 1990

Smoking-attributed deaths (Sm.) and total deaths (Total)

		ALL CAUSES	ALL CANCER	Lung cancer	Upper aero-digestive ca.	Other cancer	COPD	Other respiratory	Vascular disease	Liver cirrhosis	Other medical	Non-medical
Males												
0–34	Sm.	–	–	–	–	–	–	–	–	–	–	–
	Total	883	62	1	3	58	11	21	42	0	338	409
35–69	Sm.	1681	675	449	90	136	210	37	649	–	110	–
	Total	5475	1601	490	147	964	277	153	2571	35	428	410
		(31%)	(42%)	(92%)	(61%)	(14%)	(76%)	(24%)	(25%)		(26%)	
70+	Sm.	2469	804	507	89	208	738	120	661	–	146	–
	Total	10470	2191	553	145	1493	982	962	5029	10	1125	171
		(24%)	(37%)	(92%)	(61%)	(14%)	(75%)	(12%)	(13%)		(13%)	
Any age	Sm.	4150	1479	956	179	344	948	157	1310	–	256	–
	Total	16828	3854	1044	295	2515	1270	1136	7642	45	1891	990
		(25%)	(38%)	(92%)	(61%)	(14%)	(75%)	(14%)	(17%)		(14%)	
Females												
0–34	Sm.	–	–	–	–	–	–	–	–	–	–	–
	Total	498	65	1	1	63	10	16	33	0	242	132
35–69	Sm.	657	229	171	23	35	114	21	222	–	71	–
	Total	3245	1374	217	46	1111	168	105	1088	16	354	140
		(20%)	(17%)	(79%)	(50%)	(3%)	(68%)	(20%)	(20%)		(20%)	
70+	Sm.	1610	350	224	63	63	401	122	584	–	153	–
	Total	10799	1822	267	109	1446	533	1223	5548	21	1445	207
		(15%)	(19%)	(84%)	(58%)	(4%)	(75%)	(10%)	(11%)		(11%)	
Any age	Sm.	2267	579	395	86	98	515	143	806	–	224	–
	Total	14542	3261	485	156	2620	711	1344	6669	37	2041	479
		(16%)	(18%)	(81%)	(55%)	(4%)	(72%)	(11%)	(12%)		(11%)	
Males+Females												
0–34	Sm.	–	–	–	–	–	–	–	–	–	–	–
	Total	1381	127	2	4	121	21	37	75	0	580	541
35–69	Sm.	2338	904	620	113	171	324	58	871	–	181	–
	Total	8720	2975	707	193	2075	445	258	3659	51	782	550
		(27%)	(30%)	(88%)	(59%)	(8%)	(73%)	(22%)	(24%)		(23%)	
70+	Sm.	4079	1154	731	152	271	1139	242	1245	–	299	–
	Total	21269	4013	820	254	2939	1515	2185	10577	31	2570	378
		(19%)	(29%)	(89%)	(60%)	(9%)	(75%)	(11%)	(12%)		(12%)	
Any age	Sm.	6417	2058	1351	265	442	1463	300	2116	–	480	–
	Total	31370	7115	1529	451	5135	1981	2480	14311	82	3932	1469
		(20%)	(29%)	(88%)	(59%)	(9%)	(74%)	(12%)	(15%)		(12%)	

IRELAND: 1995

Smoking-attributed deaths (Sm.) and total deaths (Total)

		ALL CAUSES	ALL CANCER	Lung cancer	Upper aero-digestive ca.	Other cancer	COPD	Other respiratory	Vascular disease	Liver cirrhosis	Other medical	Non-medical
Males												
0–34	Sm.	–	–	–	–	–	–	–	–	–	–	–
	Total	1026	67	1	5	61	15	34	35	0	382	493
35–69	Sm.	1314	582	383	82	117	152	26	468	–	86	–
	Total	4922	1540	425	146	969	209	122	2142	36	395	478
		(27%)	(38%)	(90%)	(56%)	(12%)	(73%)	(21%)	(22%)		(22%)	
70+	Sm.	2387	832	503	101	228	756	106	552	–	141	–
	Total	9816	2374	549	165	1660	1006	865	4299	8	1117	147
		(24%)	(35%)	(92%)	(61%)	(14%)	(75%)	(12%)	(13%)		(13%)	
Any age	Sm.	3701	1414	886	183	345	908	132	1020	–	227	–
	Total	15764	3981	975	316	2690	1230	1021	6476	44	1894	1118
		(23%)	(36%)	(91%)	(58%)	(13%)	(74%)	(13%)	(16%)		(12%)	
Females												
0–34	Sm.	–	–	–	–	–	–	–	–	–	–	–
	Total	615	86	1	1	84	14	25	46	0	253	191
35–69	Sm.	586	235	182	17	36	88	18	173	–	72	–
	Total	2912	1366	230	37	1099	132	89	833	12	338	142
		(20%)	(17%)	(79%)	(46%)	(3%)	(67%)	(20%)	(21%)		(21%)	
70+	Sm.	1594	398	250	74	74	382	125	509	–	180	–
	Total	9747	1949	293	123	1533	494	1137	4389	27	1568	183
		(16%)	(20%)	(85%)	(60%)	(5%)	(77%)	(11%)	(12%)		(11%)	
Any age	Sm.	2180	633	432	91	110	470	143	682	–	252	–
	Total	13274	3401	524	161	2716	640	1251	5268	39	2159	516
		(16%)	(19%)	(82%)	(57%)	(4%)	(73%)	(11%)	(13%)		(12%)	
Males+Females												
0–34	Sm.	–	–	–	–	–	–	–	–	–	–	–
	Total	1641	153	2	6	145	29	59	81	0	635	684
35–69	Sm.	1900	817	565	99	153	240	44	641	–	158	–
	Total	7834	2906	655	183	2068	341	211	2975	48	733	620
		(24%)	(28%)	(86%)	(54%)	(7%)	(70%)	(21%)	(22%)		(22%)	
70+	Sm.	3981	1230	753	175	302	1138	231	1061	–	321	–
	Total	19563	4323	842	288	3193	1500	2002	8688	35	2685	330
		(20%)	(28%)	(89%)	(61%)	(9%)	(76%)	(12%)	(12%)		(12%)	
Any age	Sm.	5881	2047	1318	274	455	1378	275	1702	–	479	–
	Total	29038	7382	1499	477	5406	1870	2272	11744	83	4053	1634
		(20%)	(28%)	(88%)	(57%)	(8%)	(74%)	(12%)	(14%)		(12%)	

(To be conservative, no deaths before age 35, and none from liver cirrhosis or non-medical causes, were attributed to smoking.)

ITALY: 1990

		No. of deaths			Standardised rates (Defined on p.388)			Annual death rates / 100, 000						
		All ages	0–34	35–69	All ages	0–34	35–69	0–4	5–9	10–14	15–19	20–24	25–29	30–34
ALL CAUSES	M	282018	14281	102021	939.7	101.5	954.2	207.2	19.1	24.1	83.0	109.0	132.2	136.1
	F	261690	6015	53017	547.0	49.0	432.0	166.3	14.3	14.4	26.3	32.3	39.5	49.7
Tuberculosis	M	526	12	265	1.7	0.1	2.5	0.1	–	–	–	–	0.2	0.3
	F	259	8	77	0.6	0.1	0.6	0.1	–	–	–	0.0	0.1	0.1
Other infective and parasitic	M	616	103	234	2.1	0.8	2.1	1.9	0.1	0.2	0.4	0.5	1.1	1.1
	F	609	66	180	1.5	0.6	1.5	2.0	0.3	0.2	0.2	0.4	0.5	0.3
ALL CANCER	M	85244	1114	42879	284.9	7.6	403.1	3.4	5.1	5.3	7.3	7.6	9.7	14.6
	F	59792	918	24896	144.2	6.5	201.7	3.4	4.0	3.6	4.8	5.0	8.1	16.6
Mouth and pharynx cancer	M	2454	21	1671	8.4	0.1	15.2	–	–	–	0.1	0.2	0.2	0.4
	F	595	9	247	1.5	0.1	2.0	–	–	–	0.1	–	0.1	0.1
Oesophagus cancer	M	1801	5	1102	6.1	0.0	10.1	–	–	–	–	–	0.0	0.2
	F	457	1	153	1.0	0.0	1.2	–	–	–	–	0.0	–	–
Stomach cancer	M	8027	33	3465	26.6	0.2	32.6	–	–	–	–	0.1	0.3	1.1
	F	5757	37	1647	12.6	0.2	13.4	–	–	–	0.0	0.1	0.3	1.3
Colorectal cancer	M	7255	29	3090	24.1	0.2	29.1	–	–	–	0.0	0.1	0.3	0.9
	F	6902	30	2320	15.6	0.2	18.9	0.1	–	–	0.0	0.2	0.4	0.7
Liver cancer	M	3308	7	1972	11.1	0.1	18.7	0.1	0.1	0.1	–	0.0	0.0	0.1
	F	1518	10	548	3.5	0.1	4.5	–	0.1	0.1	0.0	0.1	0.0	0.2
Pancreas cancer	M	3368	15	1830	11.3	0.1	17.2	–	–	–	–	0.0	0.1	0.5
	F	3041	5	1088	6.9	0.0	8.9	–	–	–	–	0.0	0.1	0.1
Larynx cancer	M	2374	1	1389	8.0	0.0	13.0	–	–	–	0.0	–	–	–
	F	128	3	56	0.3	0.0	0.5	–	–	0.1	–	0.0	–	0.0
Lung cancer	M	25168	40	15105	84.4	0.3	142.8	0.1	–	–	0.0	0.2	0.4	1.2
	F	4431	20	2034	10.9	0.1	16.6	–	–	–	0.1	0.1	0.3	0.5
Malignant melanoma	M	615	29	382	2.1	0.2	3.4	–	–	–	–	0.2	0.5	0.7
	F	552	25	280	1.5	0.2	2.2	–	–	–	0.0	0.1	0.3	0.7
Female breast cancer	F	10924	119	6375	29.3	0.8	51.1	–	–	0.1	0.1	0.2	1.0	4.2
Cervix cancer	F	490	11	281	1.3	0.1	2.2	–	–	–	–	–	0.1	0.4
Other uterine cancer	F	2777	23	1259	6.8	0.2	10.2	–	–	–	–	0.0	0.2	0.9
Ovarian cancer	F	2611	42	1494	6.9	0.3	12.1	–	–	–	0.2	0.2	0.5	1.0
Prostate cancer	M	6152	1	1257	20.0	0.0	12.5	–	–	–	0.0	–	–	–
Bladder cancer	M	4285	2	1560	14.1	0.0	15.1	–	–	–	–	–	–	0.1
	F	1114	2	245	2.3	0.0	2.0	–	–	–	–	0.0	–	0.0
Other and ill-defined cancer sites	M	14704	456	7412	49.3	3.1	69.1	1.5	2.6	2.3	3.1	3.5	3.8	5.0
	F	13559	295	4951	31.7	2.2	40.3	2.0	2.0	1.8	2.0	1.7	2.2	3.5
Hodgkin's disease	M	339	63	186	1.2	0.4	1.7	–	0.1	0.1	0.2	0.6	0.8	1.0
	F	228	43	113	0.7	0.3	0.9	0.1	–	–	0.2	0.3	0.6	0.7
Myeloma and non-Hodgkin lymphomas	M	2742	123	1400	9.3	0.8	12.9	0.3	0.5	0.8	0.8	0.8	1.2	1.3
	F	2530	58	997	6.1	0.4	8.1	0.1	0.1	0.2	0.3	0.4	0.6	1.0
Leukaemia	M	2652	289	1058	8.9	2.0	9.8	1.4	1.7	2.1	2.9	2.0	1.9	2.1
	F	2178	185	808	5.4	1.4	6.5	1.1	1.9	1.4	1.6	1.3	1.2	1.2
ALL VASCULAR DISEASE	M	108580	741	30769	356.9	5.0	291.6	4.0	0.8	1.1	3.2	4.8	7.6	13.3
	F	126183	384	14060	238.1	2.8	115.8	4.1	0.7	1.8	2.0	2.4	3.2	5.4
Rheumatic heart disease and fever	M	616	18	346	2.1	0.1	3.2	–	–	–	0.0	0.2	0.2	0.3
	F	1271	21	552	3.1	0.1	4.5	–	0.1	0.1	0.1	0.1	0.3	0.3
Hypertensive disease	M	5451	7	1235	17.8	0.0	11.9	–	–	0.1	0.0	0.1	0.1	0.0
	F	9772	10	1096	18.4	0.1	9.1	0.1	0.1	–	0.0	–	0.2	0.1
Ischaemic heart disease	M	39920	165	16057	132.2	1.1	151.2	–	0.1	–	0.1	0.9	2.0	4.5
	F	31296	32	4697	61.2	0.2	38.8	–	–	0.1	0.1	0.3	0.2	0.7
Pulmonary embolism and other venous	M	905	13	337	3.0	0.1	3.2	–	–	0.1	0.0	0.1	0.2	0.1
	F	1295	15	293	2.7	0.1	2.4	0.1	–	–	0.0	0.2	0.2	0.2
Cerebrovascular disease	M	30766	175	6466	100.4	1.2	61.9	0.6	0.3	0.4	0.9	0.9	1.6	3.5
	F	41893	135	4292	78.8	1.0	35.3	0.9	0.3	0.8	0.9	0.6	1.2	2.0
Other vascular disease	M	30922	363	6328	101.5	2.5	60.1	3.4	0.4	0.6	2.0	2.6	3.6	4.8
	F	40656	171	3130	73.9	1.3	25.8	3.1	0.3	0.8	0.8	1.0	1.2	2.0
Chronic obstructive pulmonary disease	M	14015	56	2808	45.7	0.4	27.7	0.7	–	0.4	0.4	0.3	0.4	0.7
	F	6739	40	817	12.9	0.3	6.8	0.1	0.1	0.4	0.3	0.3	0.3	0.4
Other respiratory disease	M	7678	273	1548	25.4	2.2	14.8	8.0	0.3	0.5	1.1	1.4	1.9	1.9
	F	7188	154	645	13.6	1.4	5.3	6.4	0.3	0.3	0.5	0.3	1.0	0.8
Peptic ulcer	M	1338	11	403	4.4	0.1	3.9	–	–	–	0.0	0.1	0.1	0.2
	F	947	1	124	1.8	0.0	1.0	–	–	–	–	0.0	–	–
Liver cirrhosis	M	9761	165	6218	33.2	1.1	56.8	0.2	0.2	–	0.0	0.3	2.0	5.0
	F	5704	64	2672	14.1	0.4	21.7	0.1	–	0.1	0.0	0.3	0.7	1.8
Renal disease	M	2886	43	727	9.5	0.3	6.9	1.0	0.2	0.2	0.2	0.1	0.1	0.7
	F	2790	25	480	5.6	0.2	3.9	0.6	–	0.1	0.1	0.2	0.1	0.3
Pregnancy and birth	F	50	34	16	0.2	0.2	0.1	–	–	–	0.0	0.4	0.5	0.6
Congenital and perinatal causes	M	2683	2487	128	14.0	24.0	1.1	159.8	2.0	1.3	1.7	1.0	0.8	1.0
	F	2057	1869	113	11.2	19.1	0.9	127.8	1.4	0.9	1.3	0.7	0.9	0.7
Ill-defined causes	M	4878	485	963	16.4	3.4	8.7	6.7	0.3	0.4	1.9	4.4	5.6	4.5
	F	7284	181	386	13.2	1.5	3.1	5.2	0.4	0.2	0.5	1.3	1.2	1.4
Other medical causes	M	25512	2829	7882	84.2	18.6	73.3	12.8	3.1	3.5	8.3	19.4	43.8	39.5
	F	31202	940	6211	65.3	6.8	50.9	9.8	2.9	2.5	4.1	6.5	11.3	10.6
ALL NON-MEDICAL CAUSES	M	18301	5962	7197	61.3	38.1	61.7	8.5	6.9	11.3	58.6	69.3	58.9	53.3
	F	10886	1331	2340	24.8	9.2	18.7	6.7	4.2	4.5	12.5	14.5	11.7	10.7
Motor vehicle traffic accidents	M	7006	3203	2656	23.2	20.3	22.8	2.0	3.8	6.5	40.8	41.7	26.1	21.1
	F	2117	746	834	6.3	5.1	6.6	2.2	2.9	2.9	8.3	9.2	6.2	4.0
Fire	M	215	38	98	0.7	0.2	0.8	0.1	0.1	0.1	0.1	0.4	0.5	0.5
	F	145	16	52	0.4	0.1	0.4	0.2	0.2	–	0.0	0.2	0.1	0.1
Suicide	M	3181	729	1567	10.7	4.6	13.5	–	–	0.6	3.3	8.3	10.0	9.7
	F	1221	228	684	3.6	1.5	5.4	–	–	0.3	1.6	2.4	2.5	3.6
Homicide	M	1351	647	659	4.6	4.1	5.3	0.5	0.6	0.6	3.6	6.1	8.3	9.3
	F	176	78	72	0.6	0.5	0.6	0.3	0.2	0.1	0.5	0.7	0.9	1.1
POPULATION (thousands):	M=males				28021	14040	11914	1457	1563	1864	2258	2420	2395	2083
	F=females				29641	13499	12766	1373	1479	1767	2153	2337	2335	2057

ITALY: 1990

Annual death rates / 100, 000 — 9th ICD categories

35–39	40–44	45–49	50–54	55–59	60–64	65–69	70–74	75–79	80+/NK			
154.9	212.1	344.4	569.4	1019.8	1696.6	2682.4	4227.6	6884.8	14018.3	M	ALL CAUSES	001–999
73.2	114.1	180.1	276.3	452.0	722.2	1206.2	2119.5	3940.7	11122.3	F		
0.3	0.8	0.4	1.2	2.2	4.9	7.9	8.9	14.5	13.0	M	Tuberculosis	010–018, 137
0.2	0.0	0.3	0.2	0.8	0.9	2.1	3.1	4.8	7.2	F		
0.5	1.0	1.3	1.8	1.3	3.6	5.7	5.7	13.2	23.4	M	Other infective	Rest of 001–139
0.5	0.5	0.9	1.0	2.0	1.8	3.6	4.0	8.1	18.7	F	and parasitic	
28.6	62.6	134.5	239.6	466.0	765.4	1124.8	1564.6	1991.4	2528.6	M	ALL CANCER	140–208
35.0	63.0	101.9	159.0	237.4	341.3	474.3	652.0	928.1	1372.8	F		
1.4	4.0	9.0	12.9	21.7	27.7	29.5	34.3	33.2	44.5	M	Mouth and	140–149
0.3	0.4	1.3	2.3	2.6	3.1	3.8	6.4	8.8	14.3	F	pharynx cancer	
0.6	1.8	4.5	8.9	14.6	17.9	22.7	30.2	34.2	36.9	M	Oesophagus cancer	150
0.1	0.2	0.2	1.0	1.3	2.4	3.5	4.9	7.1	14.1	F		
3.2	6.0	11.5	18.6	34.6	62.2	91.8	143.6	216.8	314.2	M	Stomach cancer	151
2.6	4.0	5.9	8.5	14.2	20.3	38.4	60.8	101.9	187.6	F		
2.2	3.7	10.3	18.3	32.2	52.6	84.6	131.4	188.6	297.9	M	Colorectal cancer	153, 154
2.1	4.9	8.4	13.4	21.1	30.6	51.7	74.0	117.5	201.3	F		
0.5	1.4	3.8	10.7	22.0	39.5	52.8	65.5	65.8	61.1	M	Liver cancer	155.0
0.1	0.3	1.4	2.4	4.5	8.5	14.5	23.4	30.0	31.2	F		
1.0	2.9	6.0	11.1	20.5	31.1	47.4	62.7	76.2	84.2	M	Pancreas cancer	157
0.5	1.8	1.9	5.1	8.9	17.5	26.7	36.0	57.9	75.5	F		
0.3	2.0	4.9	8.5	17.6	24.2	33.2	41.8	51.5	50.0	M	Larynx cancer	161
–	0.2	0.2	0.5	0.4	0.8	1.0	1.3	1.9	2.8	F		
4.6	14.8	39.4	77.7	169.1	289.2	405.1	487.3	508.5	453.8	M	Lung cancer	162
1.9	3.7	6.9	10.6	18.6	32.2	42.0	59.1	72.8	77.6	F		
1.3	1.6	2.8	3.3	4.1	5.3	5.3	8.2	9.3	12.6	M	Malignant melanoma	172
1.3	1.4	1.9	2.2	2.5	2.7	3.6	5.6	5.9	10.0	F		
11.5	22.0	35.4	55.3	67.3	76.5	90.0	97.8	121.1	168.4	F	Female breast cancer	174
0.9	1.7	1.4	2.5	2.3	3.1	3.7	5.0	6.1	6.4	F	Cervix cancer	180
1.6	3.5	5.2	7.3	13.8	17.0	23.0	31.1	42.6	56.8	F	Other uterine cancer	179, 182
1.5	3.8	7.8	10.0	14.6	21.7	25.1	28.7	33.4	33.0	F	Ovarian cancer	183
–	0.1	1.1	2.6	9.6	21.5	52.5	118.1	223.0	398.4	M	Prostate cancer	185
0.2	0.7	1.9	6.9	13.8	30.0	52.2	89.3	125.5	191.1	M	Bladder cancer	188
0.1	0.2	0.4	0.5	2.7	4.0	6.1	11.0	22.2	41.1	F		
8.0	14.8	28.0	43.5	79.9	124.6	185.0	254.2	332.6	422.1	M	Other and ill-defined	Rest of 140–208
6.5	9.7	16.2	26.8	45.1	75.8	101.7	150.7	219.4	350.2	F	cancer sites	
0.6	1.3	1.2	1.4	1.5	2.1	3.5	4.2	3.7	5.3	M	Hodgkin's disease	201
0.8	0.6	1.0	0.6	0.6	1.2	1.5	2.2	2.1	2.1	F		
2.3	3.7	6.3	9.0	14.7	21.8	32.7	49.2	58.8	71.2	M	Myeloma and non–	200, 202–203
1.6	1.7	3.2	5.5	9.5	14.3	20.8	33.3	43.0	53.0	F	Hodgkin lymphomas	
2.4	3.9	3.7	6.0	10.3	15.6	26.6	44.5	63.7	85.2	M	Leukaemia	204–208
1.8	2.6	3.3	4.2	7.4	9.6	17.0	20.8	34.5	47.6	F		
26.9	51.2	86.3	157.4	289.8	525.9	903.7	1579.5	3001.4	7234.0	M	ALL VASCULAR	390–459
10.2	16.4	30.6	49.9	101.9	194.6	407.3	889.8	1933.9	6583.4	F	DISEASE	
0.7	0.9	1.1	2.2	3.1	5.9	8.5	10.9	12.7	13.1	M	Rheumatic heart	390–398
0.5	0.8	1.4	3.3	4.7	7.6	13.3	20.5	18.9	22.5	F	disease and fever	
0.3	1.5	2.1	5.8	11.2	21.1	41.3	83.4	163.0	399.7	M	Hypertensive disease	401–405
0.2	0.5	1.3	3.6	7.4	15.4	35.2	69.9	162.5	498.2	F		
12.8	27.8	47.6	89.1	162.4	279.9	439.0	667.4	1059.2	1837.6	M	Ischaemic heart	410–414
2.3	4.7	8.5	13.7	33.3	67.6	141.4	286.3	553.8	1416.8	F	disease	
0.4	0.5	0.9	1.2	3.0	6.5	9.9	15.1	27.5	40.4	M	Pulmonary embolism	415.1, 451–453
0.6	0.5	0.7	1.3	2.4	4.3	6.9	13.0	24.5	47.1	F	and other venous	
5.0	9.6	16.6	28.9	54.4	108.0	211.1	429.3	950.7	2330.3	M	Cerebrovascular	430–438
3.9	6.2	11.1	16.3	31.0	56.0	122.7	297.8	686.5	2172.8	F	disease	
7.7	10.9	18.0	30.1	55.8	104.5	194.0	373.5	788.2	2612.9	M	Other vascular	Rest of 390–459
2.7	3.6	7.7	11.7	23.1	43.7	87.9	202.4	487.6	2426.0	F	disease	
0.8	1.3	3.2	6.4	20.4	51.1	110.4	236.7	453.3	1013.6	M	Chronic obstructive	490–496
0.3	0.5	2.0	2.8	5.4	11.6	24.5	53.6	109.5	333.9	F	pulmonary disease	
1.9	2.4	4.6	6.6	12.6	25.8	49.6	103.8	198.1	605.9	M	Other respiratory	Rest of 460–519
0.9	1.5	1.7	2.7	4.7	9.4	16.0	36.1	87.0	410.4	F	disease	
0.5	0.6	1.2	1.8	3.4	5.9	13.5	21.4	40.4	78.4	M	Peptic ulcer	531–533
–	–	0.3	0.5	1.0	1.7	3.7	8.2	14.5	46.8	F		
10.3	15.2	28.3	46.8	71.8	98.5	126.9	140.4	172.1	181.2	M	Liver cirrhosis	571
3.8	5.1	8.6	15.3	24.4	37.8	57.2	76.1	88.2	97.4	F		
0.9	1.3	1.8	2.9	6.9	11.8	23.0	44.0	80.5	200.1	M	Renal disease	580–590
0.6	0.8	1.4	2.2	4.6	6.1	11.8	25.4	47.0	121.9	F		
0.4	0.4	–	–	–	–	–	–	–	–	F	Pregnancy and birth	630–676
0.8	1.1	0.9	1.1	1.2	0.9	1.7	2.6	3.3	4.2	M	Congenital and	740–779
0.8	0.8	0.7	1.1	0.7	1.1	1.0	1.6	1.9	3.1	F	perinatal causes	
4.6	4.3	4.2	5.7	9.7	12.7	19.7	31.3	58.9	460.0	M	Ill-defined causes	780–799
1.5	1.2	1.8	2.0	2.6	4.6	8.1	14.6	44.7	493.9	F		
26.6	20.5	26.0	41.3	67.3	120.5	211.1	360.3	654.4	1225.3	M	Other medical causes	Rest of 001–799
8.5	11.3	15.6	25.0	44.5	86.9	164.4	297.8	551.5	1204.4	F		
52.3	50.1	51.7	56.8	67.2	69.6	84.4	128.4	203.4	450.7	M	ALL NON–	E800–E999
10.6	12.4	14.1	14.8	22.1	24.4	32.2	57.2	121.6	428.4	F	MEDICAL CAUSES	
19.2	17.8	19.2	20.7	26.3	24.9	31.5	46.0	58.5	63.4	M	Motor vehicle	E810–E819
4.8	4.5	5.6	5.2	8.0	8.4	10.0	14.0	20.5	13.3	F	traffic accidents	
0.6	0.6	1.1	0.7	1.0	0.8	1.3	2.3	3.6	6.0	M	Fire	E890–E899
0.2	0.4	0.2	0.2	0.4	0.6	0.8	0.4	1.7	4.4	F		
10.1	10.5	10.6	12.3	14.6	16.6	20.1	29.3	43.8	58.1	M	Suicide	E950–E959
3.1	4.4	4.4	5.0	6.9	7.2	7.0	8.4	10.1	9.0	F		
9.6	7.6	5.9	4.4	4.2	2.8	2.6	2.2	2.3	2.0	M	Homicide	E960–E969
0.7	0.3	0.6	0.9	0.4	0.6	0.5	0.8	0.6	0.9	F		
1904	1987	1706	1785	1654	1548	1331	734	730	602	M	POPULATION (thousands)	
1911	2005	1750	1875	1795	1758	1674	1017	1131	1228	F		

ITALY: Males

	All ages	0–34	35–69	35–39	40–44	45–49	50–54	55–59	60–64	65–69	70–74	75–79	80+/NK
POPULATION (1000s)													
1955	23816	14187	8481	1251	1720	1568	1307	1060	856	719	549	358	240
1965	25428	14323	9781	1870	1797	1185	1597	1409	1102	821	588	406	329
1975	27305	14797	10835	1904	1811	1794	1691	1078	1391	1167	820	470	383
1985	27767	14400	11278	1995	1725	1825	1723	1653	1480	877	981	638	470
1990	**28021**	**14040**	**11914**	**1904**	**1987**	**1706**	**1785**	**1654**	**1548**	**1331**	**734**	**730**	**602**
1995 projected	*27776*	*13424*	*12091*	*2029*	*1878*	*1922*	*1690*	*1686*	*1536*	*1350*	*1084*	*527*	*651*
NUMBER OF DEATHS													
All causes													
1955	234315	44570	87750	2977	5993	9073	12249	15188	18833	23437	28647	32151	41197
1965	275437	35232	112685	4520	6350	6665	14381	21252	27683	31834	34245	36609	56666
1975	294941	21547	121072	3418	5651	9729	15037	15206	31043	40988	44500	42411	65411
1985	286799	13303	102579	2886	4094	7193	12399	20594	28981	26432	47288	50514	73115
1990	**282018**	**14281**	**102021**	**2949**	**4214**	**5875**	**10165**	**16869**	**26257**	**35692**	**31039**	**50259**	**84418**
1995 projected	*258274*	*15621*	*89151*	*3247*	*3651*	*5516*	*7885*	*14402*	*22621*	*31829*	*40127*	*32128*	*81247*
Lung cancer													
1955	3741	46	3139	41	183	384	638	772	639	482	297	187	72
1965	8810	72	7023	127	276	351	982	1581	2022	1684	997	474	244
1975	15957	74	10984	112	335	831	1567	1585	3083	3471	2725	1513	661
1985	23597	64	13874	124	303	796	1744	3170	4412	3325	4437	3264	1958
1990	**25168**	**40**	**15105**	**88**	**295**	**672**	**1387**	**2797**	**4476**	**5390**	**3578**	**3712**	**2733**
1995 projected	*25704*	*33*	*14464*	*74*	*238*	*598*	*1091*	*2535*	*4329*	*5599*	*5397*	*2750*	*3060*
ANNUAL DEATH RATE / 100,000 (*The rates for the age groups 0–34 and 35–69 are the means of seven five-yearly rates, but the all-ages rates are standardised to the conventional "European" age distribution)													
All causes													
1955	1318.9*	311.0*	1285.1*	237.9	348.5	578.7	936.9	1432.3	2200.6	3261.0	5215.2	8975.7	17151.1
1965	1336.0*	228.2*	1422.2*	241.7	353.4	562.6	900.3	1508.8	2511.8	3877.0	5822.0	9017.0	17202.8
1975	1232.7*	145.2*	1297.0*	179.5	312.1	542.4	889.1	1410.6	2232.5	3512.6	5425.5	9023.6	17092.0
1985	1062.9*	98.2*	1102.1*	144.7	237.4	394.1	719.6	1245.7	1957.8	3015.3	4818.4	7916.3	15569.6
1990	**939.7***	**101.5***	**954.2***	**154.9**	**212.1**	**344.4**	**569.4**	**1019.8**	**1696.6**	**2682.4**	**4227.6**	**6884.8**	**14018.3**
1995 projected	*834.1**	*107.9**	*827.5**	*160.0*	*194.5*	*286.9*	*466.7*	*854.1*	*1472.9*	*2357.5*	*3702.8*	*6097.6*	*12489.9*
All cancer													
1955	176.9*	10.6*	279.9*	30.1	60.0	121.5	219.1	358.1	498.7	671.6	878.6	1100.5	990.0
1965	223.6*	12.2*	354.8*	41.1	70.8	131.6	231.8	412.1	669.8	926.4	1128.7	1351.7	1401.6
1975	252.7*	11.1*	381.0*	35.6	73.8	151.9	280.8	443.1	694.0	987.9	1288.5	1694.5	1789.9
1985	286.9*	8.9*	414.8*	33.8	69.4	135.2	270.8	511.7	782.3	1100.2	1509.2	2006.7	2378.8
1990	**284.9***	**7.6***	**403.1***	**28.6**	**62.6**	**134.5**	**239.6**	**466.0**	**765.4**	**1124.8**	**1564.6**	**1991.4**	**2528.6**
1995 projected	*280.1**	*7.0**	*387.7**	*25.4*	*58.1*	*121.3*	*215.7*	*430.1*	*740.0*	*1123.6*	*1556.7*	*2027.1*	*2614.0*
Lung cancer													
1955	20.3*	0.3*	43.1*	3.3	10.6	24.5	48.8	72.8	74.7	67.1	54.1	52.2	30.0
1965	41.2*	0.5*	87.7*	6.8	15.4	29.6	61.5	112.2	183.5	205.1	169.5	116.7	74.1
1975	63.4*	0.6*	118.5*	5.9	18.5	46.3	92.7	147.0	221.7	297.5	332.2	321.9	172.7
1985	85.7*	0.5*	148.2*	6.2	17.6	43.6	101.2	191.7	298.0	379.3	452.1	511.5	417.0
1990	**84.4***	**0.3***	**142.8***	**4.6**	**14.8**	**39.4**	**77.7**	**169.1**	**289.2**	**405.1**	**487.3**	**508.5**	**453.8**
1995 projected	*82.4**	*0.2**	*137.0**	*3.6*	*12.7*	*31.1*	*64.6*	*150.3*	*281.9*	*414.7*	*498.0*	*521.9*	*470.4*
Upper aerodigestive cancer (mouth, oesophagus, pharynx and larynx)													
1955	18.8*	0.2*	30.2*	1.6	4.9	11.5	21.4	43.0	54.9	74.2	97.2	122.8	112.4
1965	23.1*	0.4*	37.7*	3.0	7.0	15.9	25.0	44.9	71.6	96.7	120.7	140.6	139.6
1975	25.1*	0.3*	41.3*	2.4	7.2	21.9	37.5	52.3	73.5	94.4	117.0	154.3	147.4
1985	25.9*	0.2*	44.3*	2.8	9.0	18.1	36.9	62.8	83.2	97.3	116.2	138.4	155.0
1990	**22.5***	**0.2***	**38.3***	**2.3**	**7.8**	**18.5**	**30.4**	**53.9**	**69.9**	**85.4**	**106.4**	**118.9**	**131.4**
1995 projected	*19.3**	*0.2**	*32.6**	*1.9*	*7.2*	*15.9*	*25.9*	*44.5*	*58.9*	*73.7*	*92.0*	*103.2*	*112.1*
Other cancer													
1955	137.8*	10.1*	206.6*	25.3	44.5	85.5	148.8	242.3	369.1	530.4	727.3	925.5	847.6
1965	159.3*	11.3*	229.4*	31.3	48.4	86.1	145.3	255.0	414.8	624.6	838.5	1094.3	1187.9
1975	164.2*	10.3*	221.2*	27.3	48.2	83.6	150.7	243.8	398.8	596.1	839.2	1218.3	1469.8
1985	175.2*	8.2*	222.2*	24.9	42.8	73.5	132.7	257.2	401.1	623.5	940.9	1356.8	1806.9
1990	**178.0***	**7.1***	**221.9***	**21.7**	**40.0**	**76.7**	**131.5**	**243.1**	**406.3**	**634.3**	**970.9**	**1364.0**	**1943.4**
1995 projected	*178.4**	*6.6**	*218.2**	*19.9*	*38.2*	*74.3*	*125.2*	*235.2*	*399.2*	*635.2*	*966.7*	*1402.0*	*2031.5*
Chronic obstructive pulmonary disease (COPD)													
1955	37.8*	2.8*	40.9*	2.5	5.7	14.4	32.0	52.0	75.8	103.8	152.6	266.9	577.4
1965	63.8*	1.2*	79.3*	3.3	8.0	15.4	33.1	78.5	162.6	254.0	356.5	491.1	774.1
1975	73.6*	0.9*	73.3*	2.4	5.6	14.4	33.6	67.3	129.3	260.8	434.8	734.3	1027.7
1985	52.0*	0.5*	36.2*	0.9	1.7	4.2	12.3	31.0	65.1	138.3	269.2	518.7	1068.4
1990	**45.7***	**0.4***	**27.7***	**0.8**	**1.3**	**3.2**	**6.4**	**20.4**	**51.1**	**110.4**	**236.7**	**453.3**	**1013.6**
1995 projected	*40.0**	*0.4**	*21.8**	*0.6*	*1.0*	*2.2*	*4.4*	*14.4*	*38.9*	*91.0*	*200.4*	*402.2*	*936.8*
Other respiratory disease													
1955	78.7*	39.3*	41.4*	5.7	9.3	16.8	29.8	42.5	67.8	117.9	222.1	516.8	1253.1
1965	58.5*	22.8*	32.2*	5.3	7.0	11.1	15.3	27.7	57.0	102.3	197.4	381.0	1049.2
1975	47.3*	9.6*	25.5*	2.7	5.1	8.1	12.1	24.1	40.4	85.9	172.9	367.7	1030.6
1985	34.2*	2.7*	23.7*	2.6	3.2	5.3	12.0	21.7	43.1	78.1	144.7	278.5	735.3
1990	**25.4***	**2.2***	**14.8***	**1.9**	**2.4**	**4.6**	**6.6**	**12.6**	**25.8**	**49.6**	**103.8**	**198.1**	**605.9**
1995 projected	*19.1**	*1.8**	*10.3**	*1.5*	*1.9*	*3.1*	*4.6*	*8.8*	*17.9*	*34.3*	*71.9*	*142.0*	*480.6*
Vascular disease													
1955	539.5*	12.7*	489.4*	44.4	71.9	142.2	266.1	484.3	887.5	1529.4	2774.8	5025.1	8909.7
1965	597.2*	9.8*	560.4*	53.3	97.2	170.7	294.9	535.2	1007.1	1764.6	3044.5	5162.3	10083.2
1975	549.3*	6.8*	491.2*	38.0	81.5	168.6	299.9	507.1	863.0	1480.4	2591.1	4758.1	9956.6
1985	439.2*	6.1*	372.1*	30.7	62.1	110.1	220.0	391.7	669.8	1120.2	2010.8	3753.0	8471.3
1990	**356.9***	**5.0***	**291.6***	**26.9**	**51.2**	**86.3**	**157.4**	**289.8**	**525.9**	**903.7**	**1579.5**	**3001.4**	**7234.0**
1995 projected	*286.7**	*4.4**	*223.2**	*22.5*	*40.5*	*63.1*	*113.7*	*215.7*	*406.6*	*700.2*	*1232.8*	*2416.2*	*6056.7*
Liver cirrhosis													
1955	26.0*	0.6*	51.2*	3.5	12.1	24.4	40.2	56.3	104.1	117.7	112.3	105.0	66.2
1965	41.1*	1.2*	77.2*	12.5	22.2	39.2	65.2	100.8	133.4	167.1	172.9	181.3	126.0
1975	52.8*	1.7*	97.0*	14.7	35.2	60.3	84.2	120.5	160.2	203.9	207.5	238.1	200.4
1985	45.6*	1.4*	79.8*	10.9	23.4	43.1	72.4	105.7	135.9	167.4	200.4	215.3	215.9
1990	**33.2***	**1.1***	**56.8***	**10.3**	**15.2**	**28.3**	**46.8**	**71.8**	**98.5**	**126.9**	**140.4**	**172.1**	**181.2**
1995 projected	*24.3**	*1.1**	*40.0**	*7.8*	*10.5*	*19.5*	*32.4*	*49.8*	*70.3*	*90.2*	*103.6*	*134.2*	*148.3*
Other medical causes													
1955	381.4*	194.4*	286.2*	89.4	115.7	170.8	247.6	336.9	452.1	590.6	932.6	1782.8	5077.4
1965	271.4*	134.2*	222.6*	61.8	81.4	117.6	167.5	248.1	361.0	520.9	754.3	1208.6	3356.7
1975	180.0*	71.0*	141.9*	29.1	49.2	67.2	98.0	154.5	233.7	361.7	565.6	977.7	2606.0
1985	139.7*	40.9*	105.8*	18.1	25.5	38.1	65.8	106.0	179.2	308.1	524.0	926.2	2262.4
1990	**132.3***	**47.2***	**98.6***	**34.1**	**29.4**	**35.8**	**55.8**	**92.0**	**160.3**	**282.6**	**474.1**	**865.2**	**2004.3**
1995 projected	*125.0**	*52.3**	*90.7**	*48.0*	*34.8*	*32.5*	*47.7*	*79.2*	*141.8*	*250.7*	*428.4*	*783.6*	*1803.7*
All non-medical causes													
1955	78.5*	50.7*	96.2*	62.3	73.9	88.5	102.1	102.3	114.6	130.0	142.2	178.7	277.3
1965	80.4*	46.8*	95.7*	64.4	66.8	77.1	92.5	106.4	121.0	141.6	167.6	240.9	412.0
1975	76.9*	44.0*	87.0*	57.0	61.7	71.9	80.4	93.9	112.0	132.0	165.2	253.4	480.8
1985	65.1*	37.7*	69.6*	47.6	52.1	58.1	66.3	77.8	82.5	103.0	160.1	217.8	437.6
1990	**61.3***	**38.1***	**61.7***	**52.3**	**50.1**	**51.7**	**56.8**	**67.2**	**69.6**	**84.4**	**128.4**	**203.4**	**450.7**
1995 projected	*58.9**	*41.0**	*53.8**	*54.2*	*47.7*	*45.2*	*48.2*	*56.2*	*57.4*	*67.5*	*108.9*	*192.3*	*449.8*

ITALY: Females

	All ages	0–34	35–69	35–39	40–44	45–49	50–54	55–59	60–64	65–69	70–74	75–79	80+/NK
POPULATION (1000s)													
1955	24817	13969	9409	1339	1794	1627	1394	1258	1079	918	682	436	321
1965	26560	13935	10722	1913	1917	1292	1710	1529	1276	1085	846	571	486
1975	28525	14264	11711	1941	1856	1858	1853	1218	1584	1402	1094	753	703
1985	29376	13932	12148	2008	1758	1891	1821	1804	1756	1110	1334	990	971
1990	**29641**	**13499**	**12766**	**1911**	**2005**	**1750**	**1875**	**1795**	**1758**	**1674**	**1017**	**1131**	**1228**
1995 projected	*29338*	*12859*	*12845*	*2012*	*1893*	*1957*	*1763*	*1823*	*1745*	*1652*	*1521*	*831*	*1282*
NUMBER OF DEATHS													
All causes													
1955	212374	33943	66828	2410	4387	5588	7499	10290	14863	21791	28898	33136	49569
1965	242571	24214	69889	2689	4038	4084	8360	11248	16150	23320	33495	41315	73658
1975	259405	13386	66251	1937	3050	4818	7846	7985	16375	24240	33736	45466	100566
1985	260637	6794	53185	1568	2178	3726	5840	9346	14739	15788	33277	46420	120961
1990	**261690**	**6015**	**53017**	**1399**	**2287**	**3152**	**5181**	**8111**	**12693**	**20194**	**21545**	**44565**	**136548**
1995 projected	*231846*	*5542*	*45663*	*1397*	*1990*	*3135*	*4272*	*7122*	*10793*	*16954*	*27218*	*28080*	*125343*
Lung cancer													
1955	1014	34	692	24	50	70	101	130	146	171	148	94	46
1965	1667	33	1016	26	52	71	141	201	229	296	270	211	137
1975	2480	33	1312	26	56	107	184	176	354	409	436	370	329
1985	3714	29	1714	43	50	111	181	353	530	446	690	670	611
1990	**4431**	**20**	**2034**	**37**	**74**	**121**	**198**	**334**	**566**	**704**	**601**	**823**	**953**
1995 projected	*4900*	*15*	*2111*	*41*	*80*	*151*	*186*	*342*	*568*	*743*	*961*	*666*	*1147*
ANNUAL DEATH RATE / 100,000 (*The rates for the age groups 0–34 and 35–69 are the means of seven five-yearly rates, but the all-ages rates are standardised to the conventional "European" age distribution)													
All causes													
1955	1024.0*	243.7*	839.4*	180.0	244.6	343.4	537.9	817.8	1377.0	2374.8	4237.9	7607.0	15446.9
1965	927.5*	160.5*	758.2*	140.6	210.6	316.2	488.9	735.8	1266.0	2149.1	3959.7	7230.5	15165.3
1975	775.6*	93.2*	623.6*	99.8	164.4	259.3	423.4	655.8	1034.0	1728.6	3084.0	6034.8	14309.3
1985	627.1*	55.3*	500.0*	78.1	123.9	197.0	320.6	518.0	839.4	1422.7	2494.7	4688.4	12452.2
1990	**547.0***	**49.0***	**432.0***	**73.2**	**114.1**	**180.1**	**276.3**	**452.0**	**722.2**	**1206.2**	**2119.5**	**3940.7**	**11122.3**
1995 projected	*475.3**	*43.7**	*373.2**	*69.5*	*105.1*	*160.2*	*242.3*	*390.7*	*618.4*	*1026.4*	*1789.6*	*3377.4*	*9774.1*
All cancer													
1955	139.0*	9.8*	214.3*	45.7	79.0	115.9	178.8	248.4	345.6	486.9	641.1	810.8	881.3
1965	149.1*	10.2*	221.2*	44.1	80.4	124.6	187.1	249.1	364.4	498.7	703.2	920.9	1043.6
1975	144.8*	9.4*	213.4*	38.6	70.9	116.0	184.4	255.2	354.8	474.3	625.7	908.4	1123.8
1985	146.8*	7.6*	207.8*	35.2	62.9	104.9	161.6	243.8	344.9	501.2	681.0	925.0	1335.6
1990	**144.2***	**6.5***	**201.7***	**35.0**	**63.0**	**101.9**	**159.0**	**237.4**	**341.3**	**474.3**	**652.0**	**928.1**	**1372.8**
1995 projected	*139.6**	*5.5**	*192.1**	*34.0*	*61.3*	*98.9*	*152.0*	*228.6*	*323.1*	*446.9*	*624.5*	*912.3*	*1397.5*
Lung cancer													
1955	4.7*	0.2*	8.4*	1.8	2.8	4.3	7.2	10.3	13.5	18.6	21.7	21.6	14.3
1965	6.4*	0.2*	10.9*	1.4	2.7	5.5	8.2	13.1	18.0	27.3	31.9	36.9	28.2
1975	7.8*	0.2*	12.3*	1.3	3.0	5.8	9.9	14.5	22.4	29.2	39.9	49.1	46.8
1985	10.0*	0.2*	15.8*	2.1	2.8	5.9	9.9	19.6	30.2	40.2	51.7	67.7	62.9
1990	**10.9***	**0.1***	**16.6***	**1.9**	**3.7**	**6.9**	**10.6**	**18.6**	**32.2**	**42.0**	**59.1**	**72.8**	**77.6**
1995 projected	*11.6**	*0.1**	*17.3**	*2.0*	*4.2*	*7.7*	*10.6*	*18.8*	*32.5*	*45.0*	*63.2*	*80.1*	*89.4*
Upper aerodigestive cancer (mouth, oesophagus, pharynx and larynx)													
1955	3.1*	0.2*	4.0*	0.7	1.1	1.9	2.7	4.7	7.0	9.7	16.7	22.0	32.1
1965	3.0*	0.2*	3.4*	0.7	0.9	1.2	2.9	4.3	6.0	8.0	17.9	23.5	31.1
1975	3.3*	0.1*	4.5*	0.6	1.2	1.9	3.9	5.2	7.7	11.2	15.1	23.5	31.4
1985	3.2*	0.1*	4.3*	0.7	1.1	2.2	3.5	5.8	6.2	10.7	14.1	21.9	33.5
1990	**2.8***	**0.1***	**3.7***	**0.4**	**0.9**	**1.7**	**3.9**	**4.3**	**6.3**	**8.3**	**12.6**	**17.8**	**31.1**
1995 projected	*2.4**	*0.1**	*3.2**	*0.3*	*0.7*	*1.6*	*3.3*	*4.0*	*5.2*	*7.1*	*10.2*	*15.5*	*27.5*
Other cancer													
1955	131.2*	9.4*	202.0*	43.2	75.1	109.7	168.9	233.3	325.0	458.6	602.7	767.2	834.8
1965	139.7*	9.8*	206.9*	42.0	76.7	117.8	176.0	231.6	340.5	463.4	653.4	860.5	984.4
1975	133.7*	9.1*	196.6*	36.7	66.7	108.3	170.6	235.5	324.7	433.9	570.8	835.8	1045.5
1985	133.7*	7.3*	187.6*	32.3	59.0	96.9	148.2	218.4	308.5	450.3	615.2	835.4	1239.2
1990	**130.5***	**6.3***	**181.4***	**32.7**	**58.4**	**93.3**	**144.5**	**214.5**	**302.7**	**423.9**	**580.3**	**837.6**	**1264.1**
1995 projected	*125.6**	*5.3**	*171.7**	*31.7*	*56.4*	*89.5*	*138.2*	*205.8*	*285.4*	*394.8*	*551.1*	*816.7*	*1280.6*
Chronic obstructive pulmonary disease (COPD)													
1955	23.4*	2.4*	15.7*	1.6	2.2	3.4	7.5	12.6	29.3	53.1	108.4	199.7	475.2
1965	27.1*	0.8*	20.6*	1.5	2.9	3.6	9.4	18.0	37.1	71.6	141.7	259.4	508.8
1975	23.6*	0.8*	16.7*	1.6	2.9	4.1	7.3	16.0	29.2	55.6	104.9	224.4	488.9
1985	14.2*	0.3*	8.4*	0.6	1.3	2.0	3.6	5.9	14.5	31.2	59.3	123.4	350.3
1990	**12.9***	**0.3***	**6.8***	**0.3**	**0.5**	**2.0**	**2.8**	**5.4**	**11.6**	**24.5**	**53.6**	**109.5**	**333.9**
1995 projected	*11.6**	*0.3**	*5.5**	*0.2*	*0.4*	*1.6*	*2.5*	*4.4*	*9.2*	*20.6*	*46.1*	*98.7*	*312.5*
Other respiratory disease													
1955	62.9*	36.3*	22.9*	4.6	5.5	7.5	11.5	18.1	38.1	75.2	180.7	409.6	1059.8
1965	45.0*	20.2*	16.1*	2.7	4.1	4.8	8.8	13.5	25.5	53.6	130.4	307.3	905.7
1975	32.2*	8.7*	12.7*	2.5	3.1	4.4	7.2	10.6	21.3	39.6	91.1	228.6	781.4
1985	18.0*	2.3*	7.9*	1.3	1.5	2.6	4.0	7.4	13.3	25.1	55.3	119.1	500.0
1990	**13.6***	**1.4***	**5.3***	**0.9**	**1.5**	**1.7**	**2.7**	**4.7**	**9.4**	**16.0**	**36.1**	**87.0**	**410.4**
1995 projected	*10.4**	*1.0**	*3.7**	*0.7*	*1.2*	*1.2*	*1.9*	*3.2*	*6.5*	*11.1*	*25.1*	*62.7*	*329.7*
Vascular disease													
1955	472.5*	13.7*	373.6*	38.7	61.6	102.6	182.1	318.3	636.4	1275.4	2507.0	4660.0	8422.2
1965	468.3*	8.3*	324.7*	30.1	50.2	91.2	158.3	277.3	558.0	1107.8	2318.6	4587.7	9547.9
1975	393.0*	4.4*	237.4*	18.5	33.2	63.6	118.8	213.0	403.7	811.0	1716.1	3676.5	9200.6
1985	294.3*	3.4*	155.3*	12.6	21.3	37.5	72.8	133.5	266.0	543.4	1153.8	2547.2	7694.6
1990	**238.1***	**2.8***	**115.8***	**10.2**	**16.4**	**30.6**	**49.9**	**101.9**	**194.6**	**407.3**	**889.8**	**1933.9**	**6583.4**
1995 projected	*190.0**	*2.4**	*85.4**	*7.8*	*12.9*	*22.2*	*36.5*	*73.1*	*142.2*	*303.0*	*663.9*	*1505.8*	*5475.1*
Liver cirrhosis													
1955	9.2*	0.3*	16.4*	2.2	3.2	8.0	14.0	23.9	30.7	32.7	38.4	48.0	35.2
1965	13.0*	0.3*	23.1*	3.8	6.9	10.8	19.6	29.1	42.4	49.1	59.3	60.9	56.6
1975	17.7*	0.7*	30.1*	5.9	10.1	16.5	26.1	40.8	48.2	62.7	74.5	91.2	90.6
1985	16.7*	0.6*	27.1*	4.7	7.2	12.6	19.5	33.3	47.6	64.5	79.2	103.0	97.3
1990	**14.1***	**0.4***	**21.7***	**3.8**	**5.1**	**8.6**	**15.3**	**24.4**	**37.8**	**57.2**	**76.1**	**88.2**	**97.4**
1995 projected	*11.9**	*0.3**	*17.5**	*2.8*	*3.6*	*6.2*	*11.0*	*18.4*	*30.4*	*50.1*	*67.1*	*83.4*	*90.3*
Other medical causes													
1955	295.2*	169.5*	175.1*	75.6	80.2	92.8	124.7	172.2	267.0	413.5	706.4	1385.0	4383.6
1965	196.7*	109.2*	128.4*	46.8	53.8	63.1	84.3	123.1	204.8	322.8	526.4	938.4	2724.9
1975	131.8*	57.0*	88.1*	19.5	29.2	37.4	55.0	93.1	143.0	239.4	395.6	729.4	2096.0
1985	109.4*	31.3*	70.1*	10.8	14.8	22.7	39.4	67.8	121.3	214.2	394.9	741.1	2040.8
1990	**99.3***	**28.4***	**62.1***	**12.5**	**15.1**	**21.1**	**31.9**	**56.2**	**103.1**	**194.7**	**354.6**	**672.4**	**1896.1**
1995 projected	*89.6**	*25.8**	*54.2**	*15.0*	*15.1*	*18.4*	*26.3*	*46.0*	*88.6*	*170.2*	*314.6*	*606.2*	*1750.7*
All non-medical causes													
1955	21.8*	11.7*	21.4*	11.6	12.9	13.3	19.4	24.3	30.0	38.0	55.9	93.9	189.5
1965	28.4*	11.5*	24.1*	11.6	12.3	18.1	21.5	25.8	33.9	45.4	80.0	155.9	377.8
1975	32.4*	12.0*	25.2*	13.1	14.9	17.2	24.6	27.0	33.7	46.0	76.2	176.3	527.9
1985	27.6*	9.9*	23.4*	12.8	14.9	14.8	19.7	26.4	32.0	43.2	71.3	129.6	433.7
1990	**24.8***	**9.2***	**18.7***	**10.6**	**12.4**	**14.1**	**14.8**	**22.1**	**24.4**	**32.2**	**57.2**	**121.6**	**428.4**
1995 projected	*22.1**	*8.3**	*14.8**	*8.9*	*10.7*	*11.6*	*12.1*	*17.0*	*18.5*	*24.5*	*48.4*	*108.4*	*418.3*

ITALY: 1975

Smoking-attributed deaths (Sm.) and total deaths (Total)

		ALL CAUSES	ALL CANCER	Lung cancer	Upper aero-digestive ca.	Other cancer	COPD	Other respiratory	Vascular disease	Liver cirrhosis	Other medical	Non-medical
Males												
0–34	Sm.	–	–	–	–	–	–	–	–	–	–	–
	Total	21547	1595	74	38	1483	134	1481	928	227	10872	6310
35–69	Sm.	38849	16085	10194	2564	3327	5067	654	12964	–	4079	–
	Total	121072	35444	10984	3891	20569	6541	2318	45037	9327	13444	8961
		(32%)	(45%)	(93%)	(66%)	(16%)	(77%)	(28%)	(29%)		(30%)	
70+	Sm.	23240	7045	4280	1120	1645	7014	571	6996	–	1614	–
	Total	152322	25382	4899	2249	18234	10950	7090	81719	3588	19207	4386
		(15%)	(28%)	(87%)	(50%)	(9%)	(64%)	(8%)	(9%)		(8%)	
Any age	Sm.	62089	23130	14474	3684	4972	12081	1225	19960	–	5693	–
	Total	294941	62421	15957	6178	40286	17625	10889	127684	13142	43523	19657
		(21%)	(37%)	(91%)	(60%)	(12%)	(69%)	(11%)	(16%)		(13%)	
Females												
0–34	Sm.	–	–	–	–	–	–	–	–	–	–	–
	Total	13386	1302	33	15	1254	119	1268	605	98	8303	1691
35–69	Sm.	1692	469	357	44	68	308	35	639	–	241	–
	Total	66251	23013	1312	482	21219	1735	1345	24720	3233	9390	2815
		(3%)	(2%)	(27%)	(9%)	(0%)	(18%)	(3%)	(3%)		(3%)	
70+	Sm.	2995	458	333	54	71	1173	73	1055	–	236	–
	Total	179768	21587	1135	563	19889	6274	8210	111133	2139	24553	5872
		(2%)	(2%)	(29%)	(10%)	(0%)	(19%)	(1%)	(1%)		(1%)	
Any age	Sm.	4687	927	690	98	139	1481	108	1694	–	477	–
	Total	259405	45902	2480	1060	42362	8128	10823	136458	5470	42246	10378
		(2%)	(2%)	(28%)	(9%)	(0%)	(18%)	(1%)	(1%)		(1%)	
Males+Females												
0–34	Sm.	–	–	–	–	–	–	–	–	–	–	–
	Total	34933	2897	107	53	2737	253	2749	1533	325	19175	8001
35–69	Sm.	40541	16554	10551	2608	3395	5375	689	13603	–	4320	–
	Total	187323	58457	12296	4373	41788	8276	3663	69757	12560	22834	11776
		(22%)	(28%)	(86%)	(60%)	(8%)	(65%)	(19%)	(20%)		(19%)	
70+	Sm.	26235	7503	4613	1174	1716	8187	644	8051	–	1850	–
	Total	332090	46969	6034	2812	38123	17224	15300	192852	5727	43760	10258
		(8%)	(16%)	(76%)	(42%)	(5%)	(48%)	(4%)	(4%)		(4%)	
Any age	Sm.	66776	24057	15164	3782	5111	13562	1333	21654	–	6170	–
	Total	554346	108323	18437	7238	82648	25753	21712	264142	18612	85769	30035
		(12%)	(22%)	(82%)	(52%)	(6%)	(53%)	(6%)	(8%)		(7%)	

ITALY: 1985

Smoking-attributed deaths (Sm.) and total deaths (Total)

		ALL CAUSES	ALL CANCER	Lung cancer	Upper aero-digestive ca.	Other cancer	COPD	Other respiratory	Vascular disease	Liver cirrhosis	Other medical	Non-medical
Males												
0–34	Sm.	–	–	–	–	–	–	–	–	–	–	–
	Total	13303	1271	64	26	1181	66	335	870	189	4853	5719
35–69	Sm.	38681	20215	13087	3062	4066	2471	720	11817	–	3458	–
	Total	102579	38691	13874	4299	20518	3023	2092	33694	7881	9737	7461
		(38%)	(52%)	(94%)	(71%)	(20%)	(82%)	(34%)	(35%)		(36%)	
70+	Sm.	35880	13969	8812	1663	3494	8066	810	10346	–	2689	–
	Total	170917	38787	9659	2751	26377	10969	6650	83463	4355	21677	5016
		(21%)	(36%)	(91%)	(60%)	(13%)	(74%)	(12%)	(12%)		(12%)	
Any age	Sm.	74561	34184	21899	4725	7560	10537	1530	22163	–	6147	–
	Total	286799	78749	23597	7076	48076	14058	9077	118027	12425	36267	18196
		(26%)	(43%)	(93%)	(67%)	(16%)	(75%)	(17%)	(19%)		(17%)	
Females												
0–34	Sm.	–	–	–	–	–	–	–	–	–	–	–
	Total	6794	1051	29	10	1012	35	266	476	79	3470	1417
35–69	Sm.	2419	928	727	72	129	259	42	815	–	375	–
	Total	53185	22754	1714	470	20570	844	821	15771	2967	7352	2676
		(5%)	(4%)	(42%)	(15%)	(1%)	(31%)	(5%)	(5%)		(5%)	
70+	Sm.	6344	1310	944	141	225	1880	134	2343	–	677	–
	Total	200658	31216	1971	730	28515	5416	6773	115355	3021	32430	6447
		(3%)	(4%)	(48%)	(19%)	(1%)	(35%)	(2%)	(2%)		(2%)	
Any age	Sm.	8763	2238	1671	213	354	2139	176	3158	–	1052	–
	Total	260637	55021	3714	1210	50097	6295	7860	131602	6067	43252	10540
		(3%)	(4%)	(45%)	(18%)	(1%)	(34%)	(2%)	(2%)		(2%)	
Males+Females												
0–34	Sm.	–	–	–	–	–	–	–	–	–	–	–
	Total	20097	2322	93	36	2193	101	601	1346	268	8323	7136
35–69	Sm.	41100	21143	13814	3134	4195	2730	762	12632	–	3833	–
	Total	155764	61445	15588	4769	41088	3867	2913	49465	10848	17089	10137
		(26%)	(34%)	(89%)	(66%)	(10%)	(71%)	(26%)	(26%)		(22%)	
70+	Sm.	42224	15279	9756	1804	3719	9946	944	12689	–	3366	–
	Total	371575	70003	11630	3481	54892	16385	13423	198818	7376	54107	11463
		(11%)	(22%)	(84%)	(52%)	(7%)	(61%)	(7%)	(6%)		(6%)	
Any age	Sm.	83324	36422	23570	4938	7914	12676	1706	25321	–	7199	–
	Total	547436	133770	27311	8286	98173	20353	16937	249629	18492	79519	28736
		(15%)	(27%)	(86%)	(60%)	(8%)	(62%)	(10%)	(10%)		(9%)	

(To be conservative, no deaths before age 35, and none from liver cirrhosis or non-medical causes, were attributed to smoking.)

ITALY: 1990

Smoking–attributed deaths (Sm.) and total deaths (Total)

		ALL CAUSES	ALL CANCER	Lung cancer	Upper aero–digestive ca.	Other cancer	COPD	Other respiratory	Vascular disease	Liver cirrhosis	Other medical	Non–medical
Males												
0–34	Sm.	–	–	–	–	–	–	–	–	–	–	–
	Total	14281	1114	40	27	1047	56	273	741	165	5970	5962
35–69	Sm.	37769	21510	14191	2888	4431	2284	496	9979	–	3500	–
	Total	102021	42879	15105	4162	23612	2808	1548	30769	6218	10602	7197
		(37%)	(50%)	(94%)	(69%)	(19%)	(81%)	(32%)	(32%)		(33%)	
70+	Sm.	34939	14449	9149	1480	3820	8188	674	9041	–	2587	–
	Total	165716	41251	10023	2440	28788	11151	5857	77070	3378	21867	5142
		(21%)	(35%)	(91%)	(61%)	(13%)	(73%)	(12%)	(12%)		(12%)	
Any age	Sm.	72708	35959	23340	4368	8251	10472	1170	19020	–	6087	–
	Total	282018	85244	25168	6629	53447	14015	7678	108580	9761	38439	18301
		(26%)	(42%)	(93%)	(66%)	(15%)	(75%)	(15%)	(18%)		(16%)	
Females												
0–34	Sm.	–	–	–	–	–	–	–	–	–	–	–
	Total	6015	918	20	13	885	40	154	384	64	3124	1331
35–69	Sm.	2669	1151	917	78	156	269	35	792	–	422	–
	Total	53017	24896	2034	456	22406	817	645	14060	2672	7587	2340
		(5%)	(5%)	(45%)	(17%)	(1%)	(33%)	(5%)	(6%)		(6%)	
70+	Sm.	7436	1693	1247	157	289	2263	141	2534	–	805	–
	Total	202658	33978	2377	711	30890	5882	6389	111739	2968	34487	7215
		(4%)	(5%)	(52%)	(22%)	(1%)	(38%)	(2%)	(2%)		(2%)	
Any age	Sm.	10105	2844	2164	235	445	2532	176	3326	–	1227	–
	Total	261690	59792	4431	1180	54181	6739	7188	126183	5704	45198	10886
		(4%)	(5%)	(49%)	(20%)	(1%)	(38%)	(2%)	(3%)		(3%)	
Males+Females												
0–34	Sm.	–	–	–	–	–	–	–	–	–	–	–
	Total	20296	2032	60	40	1932	96	427	1125	229	9094	7293
35–69	Sm.	40438	22661	15108	2966	4587	2553	531	10771	–	3922	–
	Total	155038	67775	17139	4618	46018	3625	2193	44829	8890	18189	9537
		(26%)	(33%)	(88%)	(64%)	(10%)	(70%)	(24%)	(24%)		(22%)	
70+	Sm.	42375	16142	10396	1637	4109	10451	815	11575	–	3392	–
	Total	368374	75229	12400	3151	59678	17033	12246	188809	6346	56354	12357
		(12%)	(21%)	(84%)	(52%)	(7%)	(61%)	(7%)	(6%)		(6%)	
Any age	Sm.	82813	38803	25504	4603	8696	13004	1346	22346	–	7314	–
	Total	543708	145036	29599	7809	107628	20754	14866	234763	15465	83637	29187
		(15%)	(27%)	(86%)	(59%)	(8%)	(63%)	(9%)	(10%)		(9%)	

ITALY: 1995

Smoking–attributed deaths (Sm.) and total deaths (Total)

		ALL CAUSES	ALL CANCER	Lung cancer	Upper aero–digestive ca.	Other cancer	COPD	Other respiratory	Vascular disease	Liver cirrhosis	Other medical	Non–medical
Males												
0–34	Sm.	–	–	–	–	–	–	–	–	–	–	–
	Total	15621	1018	33	28	957	51	248	667	170	7233	6234
35–69	Sm.	32765	20139	13543	2411	4185	1795	336	7354	–	3141	–
	Total	89151	41369	14464	3566	23339	2218	1089	23687	4412	9956	6420
		(37%)	(49%)	(94%)	(68%)	(18%)	(81%)	(31%)	(31%)		(32%)	
70+	Sm.	35130	15979	10276	1405	4298	7703	569	8247	–	2632	–
	Total	153502	44555	11207	2270	31078	10385	4653	65490	2795	20505	5119
		(23%)	(36%)	(92%)	(62%)	(14%)	(74%)	(12%)	(13%)		(13%)	
Any age	Sm.	67895	36118	23819	3816	8483	9498	905	15601	–	5773	–
	Total	258274	86942	25704	5864	55374	12654	5990	89844	7377	37694	17773
		(26%)	(42%)	(93%)	(65%)	(15%)	(75%)	(15%)	(17%)		(15%)	
Females												
0–34	Sm.	–	–	–	–	–	–	–	–	–	–	–
	Total	5542	776	15	13	748	42	119	317	54	3091	1143
35–69	Sm.	2515	1229	997	72	160	232	28	629	–	397	–
	Total	45663	23648	2111	390	21147	667	449	10298	2135	6606	1860
		(6%)	(5%)	(47%)	(18%)	(1%)	(35%)	(6%)	(6%)		(6%)	
70+	Sm.	8078	2083	1571	161	351	2361	137	2566	–	931	–
	Total	180641	35005	2774	637	31594	5529	5130	92830	2871	32275	7001
		(4%)	(6%)	(57%)	(25%)	(1%)	(43%)	(3%)	(3%)		(3%)	
Any age	Sm.	10593	3312	2568	233	511	2593	165	3195	–	1328	–
	Total	231846	59429	4900	1040	53489	6238	5698	103445	5060	41972	10004
		(5%)	(6%)	(52%)	(22%)	(1%)	(42%)	(3%)	(3%)		(3%)	
Males+Females												
0–34	Sm.	–	–	–	–	–	–	–	–	–	–	–
	Total	21163	1794	48	41	1705	93	367	984	224	10324	7377
35–69	Sm.	35280	21368	14540	2483	4345	2027	364	7983	–	3538	–
	Total	134814	65017	16575	3956	44486	2885	1538	33985	6547	16562	8280
		(26%)	(33%)	(88%)	(63%)	(10%)	(70%)	(24%)	(23%)		(21%)	
70+	Sm.	43208	18062	11847	1566	4649	10064	706	10813	–	3563	–
	Total	334143	79560	13981	2907	62672	15914	9783	158320	5666	52780	12120
		(13%)	(23%)	(85%)	(54%)	(7%)	(63%)	(7%)	(7%)		(7%)	
Any age	Sm.	78488	39430	26387	4049	8994	12091	1070	18796	–	7101	–
	Total	490120	146371	30604	6904	108863	18892	11688	193289	12437	79666	27777
		(16%)	(27%)	(86%)	(59%)	(8%)	(64%)	(9%)	(10%)		(9%)	

(To be conservative, no deaths before age 35, and none from liver cirrhosis or non–medical causes, were attributed to smoking.)

JAPAN: 1990

		No. of deaths			Standardised rates (Defined on p.394)			Annual death rates / 100, 000						
		All ages	0–34	35–69	All ages	0–34	35–69	0–4	5–9	10–14	15–19	20–24	25–29	30–34
ALL CAUSES	M	443718	18986	167928	787.3	67.6	752.6	136.6	22.2	17.4	62.7	78.1	72.3	83.9
	F	376587	10079	88120	454.3	38.8	353.0	109.5	14.7	11.6	23.6	31.0	34.5	46.4
Tuberculosis	M	3776	28	1515	6.7	0.1	7.3	–	0.0	–	–	0.2	0.1	0.4
	F	1369	11	507	1.7	0.0	2.1	–	–	–	0.0	0.0	0.1	0.2
Other infective	M	3389	303	1383	6.0	1.2	6.1	4.0	0.7	0.2	0.5	0.6	0.9	1.2
and parasitic	F	3472	235	883	4.4	0.9	3.5	3.5	0.5	0.5	0.4	0.5	0.6	0.6
ALL CANCER	M	130395	1771	66998	227.1	6.1	307.7	3.8	3.3	3.8	5.4	6.1	8.1	12.4
	F	87018	1563	38653	112.9	5.7	152.5	3.1	2.8	2.8	3.0	4.5	7.2	16.4
Mouth and	M	1866	28	1211	3.2	0.1	5.3	0.0	–	–	0.1	0.1	0.2	0.3
pharynx cancer	F	741	13	334	1.0	0.0	1.3	0.0	–	–	0.1	0.0	0.1	0.1
Oesophagus cancer	M	6004	5	3528	10.4	0.0	16.4	–	–	–	–	–	–	0.1
	F	1270	2	429	1.6	0.0	1.7	–	–	–	–	–	–	0.1
Stomach cancer	M	29909	174	15166	52.2	0.6	69.3	–	–	–	0.2	0.4	1.2	2.6
	F	17562	277	7466	22.6	1.0	29.2	–	–	–	0.0	0.6	1.9	4.7
Colorectal cancer	M	13360	101	7048	23.3	0.4	31.8	–	–	0.0	0.1	0.3	0.6	1.5
	F	11419	82	4925	14.7	0.3	19.6	–	–	–	–	0.4	0.3	1.4
Liver cancer	M	13394	39	9733	22.6	0.1	43.2	0.2	–	0.0	0.1	0.1	0.1	0.5
	F	4487	23	2058	5.8	0.1	8.7	0.1	0.0	0.0	–	0.1	0.1	0.2
Pancreas cancer	M	7317	14	3767	12.8	0.1	17.4	–	–	–	–	0.0	0.0	0.3
	F	6001	21	2180	7.5	0.1	9.0	–	–	–	0.0	0.0	0.1	0.4
Larynx cancer	M	770	2	365	1.4	0.0	1.8	–	–	0.0	–	–	–	0.0
	F	77	–	18	0.1	–	0.1	–	–	–	–	–	–	–
Lung cancer	M	26872	62	11840	47.4	0.2	57.5	–	–	–	0.0	0.1	0.4	1.0
	F	9614	37	3674	12.2	0.1	15.0	–	–	–	0.0	–	0.2	0.7
Malignant melanoma	M	191	8	103	0.3	0.0	0.4	0.0	–	–	0.0	–	0.0	0.1
	F	144	6	74	0.2	0.0	0.3	–	–	–	–	0.0	–	0.1
Female breast cancer	F	5848	131	4509	8.4	0.5	16.3	–	–	–	–	0.0	0.8	2.6
Cervix cancer	F	1875	40	1141	2.6	0.1	4.4	–	–	–	–	0.1	0.3	0.6
Other uterine cancer	F	2700	23	1244	3.5	0.1	4.9	–	–	–	–	0.1	0.1	0.3
Ovarian cancer	F	3330	83	2232	4.7	0.3	8.3	–	–	0.0	0.1	0.4	0.6	0.9
Prostate cancer	M	3460	10	662	6.3	0.0	3.4	–	–	–	0.0	0.0	0.1	0.1
Bladder cancer	M	2110	8	630	3.8	0.0	3.1	0.0	0.0	0.0	–	0.0	–	0.1
	F	938	2	181	1.1	0.0	0.8	–	0.0	–	–	–	–	0.0
Other and ill-defined	M	17658	554	9024	30.7	1.9	41.1	1.8	1.4	1.3	2.0	1.9	2.3	2.6
cancer sites	F	15504	356	5600	19.6	1.3	22.9	1.4	1.1	1.3	1.2	0.9	1.2	2.0
Hodgkin's disease	M	87	14	45	0.1	0.0	0.2	–	–	0.0	0.1	0.0	0.1	0.1
	F	42	2	20	0.1	0.0	0.1	–	–	–	–	–	0.0	0.0
Myeloma and non-	M	4172	182	2133	7.2	0.6	9.6	0.3	0.5	0.3	0.6	0.8	0.9	1.0
Hodgkin lymphomas	F	3058	95	1297	4.0	0.3	5.2	0.3	0.2	0.1	0.3	0.5	0.2	0.6
Leukaemia	M	3225	570	1743	5.4	1.9	7.2	1.4	1.4	2.0	2.2	2.3	2.1	2.2
	F	2408	370	1271	3.4	1.3	4.8	1.4	1.4	1.2	1.2	1.2	1.3	1.6
ALL VASCULAR	M	147230	1925	45734	264.1	6.8	207.0	6.3	1.2	1.9	3.6	7.1	10.2	17.4
DISEASE	F	157218	958	23805	180.4	3.6	98.1	6.1	1.0	1.3	2.3	3.0	4.4	6.9
Rheumatic heart	M	444	4	215	0.8	0.0	1.0	–	–	–	0.0	–	0.0	0.0
disease and fever	F	943	9	384	1.2	0.0	1.6	–	–	–	0.0	0.0	0.1	0.1
Hypertensive disease	M	3399	7	576	6.3	0.0	2.8	–	–	–	0.0	–	0.0	0.1
	F	5847	2	430	6.4	0.0	1.8	–	–	–	–	–	–	0.1
Ischaemic heart	M	27349	126	9289	48.9	0.4	43.4	–	0.1	0.0	0.1	0.6	0.5	1.7
disease	F	24088	44	3510	27.6	0.2	15.0	0.0	0.0	–	0.1	0.1	0.3	0.6
Pulmonary embolism	M	363	17	157	0.6	0.1	0.7	–	–	0.0	0.0	0.1	0.2	0.1
and other venous	F	456	9	178	0.6	0.0	0.7	–	–	–	0.0	0.1	0.0	0.1
Cerebrovascular	M	57627	360	17881	103.3	1.3	80.2	0.8	0.2	0.2	0.4	1.1	2.1	4.2
disease	F	64317	184	10695	74.1	0.7	43.5	0.6	0.1	0.2	0.3	0.7	1.0	1.8
Other vascular	M	58048	1411	17616	104.2	5.0	78.9	5.5	0.9	1.7	3.0	5.3	7.3	11.2
disease	F	61567	710	8608	70.5	2.7	35.4	5.4	0.9	1.0	1.9	2.1	3.0	4.2
Chronic obstructive	M	10791	280	1909	19.6	0.9	9.6	0.7	0.4	0.6	1.2	1.3	1.3	1.0
pulmonary disease	F	6060	143	1086	7.1	0.5	4.5	0.6	0.2	0.4	0.6	0.7	0.7	0.4
Other respiratory	M	47659	561	7988	87.5	2.1	39.9	7.4	1.4	0.5	1.0	1.3	1.5	1.9
disease	F	35549	386	3475	40.0	1.5	14.7	4.9	0.7	0.7	0.6	1.1	1.3	1.3
Peptic ulcer	M	1933	17	675	3.4	0.1	3.0	0.0	–	–	0.1	0.0	0.0	0.3
	F	1682	6	202	1.9	0.0	0.8	0.0	–	–	–	0.0	0.1	0.0
Liver cirrhosis	M	11516	76	8664	19.3	0.3	35.6	0.0	–	0.0	0.0	0.2	0.3	1.4
	F	5288	22	2465	6.9	0.1	10.0	–	–	0.1	0.0	0.0	0.2	0.3
Renal disease	M	8584	121	2328	15.5	0.5	11.0	1.4	0.0	0.1	0.2	0.3	0.4	0.8
	F	9467	99	1561	11.0	0.4	6.6	1.4	0.1	0.1	0.1	0.2	0.4	0.5
Pregnancy and birth	F	105	69	36	0.2	0.2	0.1	–	–	–	0.0	0.2	0.9	0.7
Congenital and	M	2933	2590	242	6.6	10.9	1.0	71.1	1.6	0.8	1.0	0.8	0.4	0.7
perinatal causes	F	2432	2088	216	5.6	9.3	0.8	60.6	1.2	1.0	0.9	0.5	0.3	0.4
Ill-defined causes	M	11895	417	1012	22.5	1.7	4.6	9.4	0.2	0.3	0.2	0.5	0.6	0.7
	F	19078	250	487	20.6	1.1	2.0	6.0	0.2	0.1	0.1	0.3	0.3	0.5
Other medical causes	M	26953	1366	10462	47.7	4.9	46.5	9.8	2.8	2.5	4.0	4.1	5.2	5.9
	F	28901	1003	6955	35.2	3.8	28.1	7.6	3.1	1.9	2.4	3.2	3.8	4.4
ALL NON-	M	36664	9531	19018	61.2	32.0	73.4	22.6	10.6	6.6	45.7	55.5	43.2	39.9
MEDICAL CAUSES	F	18948	3246	7789	26.4	11.7	29.0	15.6	4.8	2.8	13.2	16.8	14.6	13.8
Motor vehicle	M	10345	4611	4069	16.8	14.7	15.9	4.7	4.4	2.2	35.0	31.4	15.3	10.0
traffic accidents	F	4053	1142	1702	5.9	3.9	6.4	2.7	2.4	1.3	8.2	7.2	2.9	2.4
Fire	M	703	137	308	1.2	0.5	1.2	1.0	0.5	0.2	0.2	0.5	0.6	0.6
	F	505	86	156	0.7	0.3	0.6	1.0	0.4	0.2	0.2	0.2	0.1	0.3
Suicide	M	12316	2367	7821	20.3	8.1	29.2	–	–	0.7	4.8	14.2	17.5	19.5
	F	7772	1149	4121	11.0	4.0	15.0	–	–	0.4	2.8	6.9	9.1	8.8
Homicide	M	428	162	227	0.7	0.6	0.8	1.2	0.7	0.2	0.3	0.7	0.5	0.6
	F	316	122	139	0.5	0.5	0.5	1.5	0.4	0.2	0.2	0.4	0.4	0.2
POPULATION (thousands): M=males					60249	28959	27501	3318	3810	4358	5108	4438	4036	3892
F=females					62472	27822	28661	3152	3627	4138	4860	4284	3941	3821

JAPAN: 1990

Annual death rates / 100, 000

9th ICD categories

35–39	40–44	45–49	50–54	55–59	60–64	65–69	70–74	75–79	80+/NK			
121.1	183.2	317.9	505.2	870.7	1321.5	1948.8	3323.7	5793.6	13104.3	M	ALL CAUSES	001–999
69.8	104.9	166.2	247.6	371.7	570.8	939.7	1689.8	3201.7	9494.2	F		
0.5	1.0	2.2	3.9	6.8	12.2	24.3	38.4	58.3	90.6	M	Tuberculosis	010–018, 137
0.3	0.3	0.5	1.0	2.2	4.2	6.4	9.0	13.3	21.2	F		
1.1	1.8	3.1	4.3	6.8	10.1	15.6	23.9	42.4	79.5	M	Other infective	Rest of 001–139
0.7	1.2	1.7	2.5	3.8	5.3	9.5	16.8	30.6	74.0	F	and parasitic	
26.4	49.2	98.3	181.9	372.6	596.8	828.6	1200.1	1640.5	2250.9	M	ALL CANCER	140–208
32.0	49.7	80.4	118.5	175.7	248.5	362.9	527.1	741.2	1118.3	F		
0.5	1.2	2.7	4.1	6.9	9.5	12.5	15.4	15.0	20.0	M	Mouth and	140–149
0.2	0.5	0.7	1.0	1.3	2.3	3.1	4.1	5.1	10.9	F	pharynx cancer	
0.4	1.2	4.5	10.7	21.3	32.2	44.4	57.8	66.9	74.4	M	Oesophagus cancer	150
0.2	0.2	0.6	1.3	2.3	2.9	4.8	8.4	13.8	20.8	F		
7.0	12.1	24.6	44.3	79.1	131.8	186.4	273.5	385.5	550.1	M	Stomach cancer	151
8.7	12.8	15.8	23.0	30.0	45.2	68.6	98.1	150.0	254.5	F		
3.0	6.0	12.1	21.5	38.9	60.2	81.0	110.4	150.9	259.4	M	Colorectal cancer	153, 154
2.7	4.9	10.2	15.6	23.7	33.3	46.7	67.9	97.4	162.2	F		
2.0	5.6	12.2	27.4	74.5	89.7	90.6	93.2	95.6	99.2	M	Liver cancer	155.0
0.4	0.7	1.4	3.7	9.3	18.2	27.3	34.4	39.1	48.0	F		
1.3	2.8	6.3	11.0	18.5	33.0	49.0	71.5	99.5	119.0	M	Pancreas cancer	157
1.0	1.2	2.8	5.0	9.7	16.1	27.5	42.2	63.3	88.6	F		
0.0	0.1	0.3	0.8	2.3	3.2	5.5	8.2	9.4	15.6	M	Larynx cancer	161
–	–	–	0.1	0.1	0.1	0.2	0.7	1.1	1.2	F		
3.3	6.8	12.9	23.0	53.4	113.0	190.2	300.3	419.7	509.0	M	Lung cancer	162
2.0	3.1	5.7	10.4	15.7	25.3	42.7	69.3	99.6	132.0	F		
0.0	0.2	0.3	0.4	0.7	0.6	0.8	1.6	1.8	3.3	M	Malignant melanoma	172
0.1	0.2	0.2	0.1	0.3	0.5	0.6	0.6	0.6	2.1	F		
6.4	10.8	15.8	19.2	22.5	20.2	19.6	20.1	18.5	21.8	F	Female breast cancer	174
1.5	2.0	2.9	4.1	5.3	5.9	8.7	9.4	12.6	13.2	F	Cervix cancer	180
0.8	1.1	2.5	3.5	7.0	8.4	11.3	15.8	21.5	35.8	F	Other uterine cancer	179, 182
2.1	3.8	7.5	9.6	11.5	12.0	11.6	15.3	17.2	18.7	F	Ovarian cancer	183
0.0	0.1	0.1	0.6	2.4	7.6	13.4	35.2	65.4	140.7	M	Prostate cancer	185
–	0.3	0.7	1.2	3.1	6.1	10.3	20.6	34.9	70.9	M	Bladder cancer	188
0.0	0.1	0.2	0.3	0.5	1.5	2.9	5.3	10.8	22.9	F		
4.6	7.2	13.2	25.3	50.9	79.0	107.4	155.7	218.1	294.1	M	Other and ill-defined	Rest of 140–208
2.6	4.4	8.3	14.0	24.9	40.8	65.5	103.8	149.8	233.9	F	cancer sites	
0.1	0.1	0.1	0.1	0.2	0.4	0.3	0.6	0.7	1.0	M	Hodgkin's disease	201
0.1	–	–	0.0	0.2	0.1	0.2	0.3	0.4	0.3	F		
1.2	2.1	4.0	5.4	12.0	18.7	23.5	37.8	52.6	61.7	M	Myeloma and non–	200, 202–203
0.9	1.5	2.2	3.3	5.8	9.4	13.3	20.9	28.5	35.2	F	Hodgkin lymphomas	
3.1	3.5	4.3	6.0	8.3	11.9	13.2	18.2	24.5	32.4	M	Leukaemia	204–208
2.5	2.6	3.7	4.3	5.6	6.5	8.2	10.6	12.0	16.2	F		
28.7	48.3	87.9	140.6	226.1	353.3	564.0	1082.6	2145.2	5507.5	M	ALL VASCULAR	390–459
10.6	21.5	36.8	58.0	92.4	162.2	305.2	650.0	1450.5	4767.3	F	DISEASE	
0.2	0.2	0.3	0.5	1.3	1.8	2.6	4.4	5.8	8.4	M	Rheumatic heart	390–398
0.1	0.2	0.5	0.8	2.2	2.3	5.1	6.1	8.0	13.9	F	disease and fever	
0.2	0.3	0.9	1.4	2.6	4.9	9.0	19.4	48.6	186.5	M	Hypertensive disease	401–405
0.1	0.2	0.5	0.6	1.8	2.8	6.8	15.4	43.2	223.2	F		
3.0	6.5	14.9	24.7	45.5	81.3	128.1	240.8	415.7	889.2	M	Ischaemic heart	410–414
0.7	1.5	3.1	6.0	12.2	26.7	55.1	119.5	254.4	689.1	F	disease	
0.2	0.2	0.3	0.3	0.8	1.0	2.1	3.2	4.2	8.6	M	Pulmonary embolism	415.1, 451–453
0.1	0.3	0.3	0.3	0.8	1.3	1.8	2.5	4.1	7.1	F	and other venous	
9.8	19.6	35.6	58.6	91.1	136.8	210.1	425.9	865.0	2163.0	M	Cerebrovascular	430–438
4.0	10.9	19.4	29.9	43.1	70.2	127.3	270.6	603.3	1896.3	F	disease	
15.3	21.6	35.9	55.1	84.9	127.4	212.0	388.9	805.9	2251.8	M	Other vascular	Rest of 390–459
5.5	8.4	12.9	20.4	32.3	58.9	109.3	235.9	537.4	1937.6	F	disease	
1.0	1.4	2.1	2.9	6.2	16.7	37.0	94.7	200.3	456.7	M	Chronic obstructive	490–496
0.9	1.2	1.5	2.7	3.9	6.7	14.3	31.1	59.8	158.6	F	pulmonary disease	
2.4	4.0	8.0	14.6	33.3	68.9	148.1	360.5	813.9	2293.8	M	Other respiratory	Rest of 460–519
2.1	2.0	3.4	6.4	12.2	24.5	52.5	128.8	307.5	1209.3	F	disease	
0.4	0.7	1.5	2.1	3.5	5.3	7.5	14.3	28.3	65.6	M	Peptic ulcer	531–533
0.1	0.2	0.1	0.4	1.1	1.1	2.8	5.9	15.2	55.5	F		
4.7	11.1	23.2	37.0	58.2	59.7	55.4	60.4	71.0	95.3	M	Liver cirrhosis	571
0.9	1.6	3.3	6.6	12.7	19.4	25.5	38.3	48.1	55.5	F		
1.4	1.7	3.2	5.8	10.6	20.2	34.0	63.9	137.7	337.3	M	Renal disease	580–590
0.8	1.1	2.0	3.7	5.3	10.5	22.5	41.8	95.2	267.6	F		
0.5	0.2	0.0	–	–	–	–	–	–	–	F	Pregnancy and birth	630–676
0.8	0.6	0.7	0.8	1.0	1.3	1.6	2.0	2.8	3.5	M	Congenital and	740–779
0.6	0.4	0.4	0.6	1.0	1.2	1.6	1.6	2.5	2.5	F	perinatal causes	
0.9	1.3	1.9	2.7	4.9	6.8	13.8	34.8	108.4	832.8	M	Ill-defined causes	780–799
0.3	0.5	0.9	0.8	1.9	3.1	6.6	20.1	65.4	870.6	F		
8.3	12.5	20.3	32.9	54.6	78.7	118.2	207.2	350.7	743.6	M	Other medical causes	Rest of 001–799
6.3	7.8	11.6	17.9	27.6	46.3	79.4	143.8	258.7	677.8	F		
44.6	49.4	65.5	75.9	86.2	91.5	100.7	141.0	194.2	347.1	M	ALL NON–	E800–E999
13.6	17.4	23.5	28.5	31.8	37.8	50.4	75.4	113.9	216.1	F	MEDICAL CAUSES	
10.6	10.6	12.6	14.6	17.6	20.8	24.8	34.7	46.7	54.6	M	Motor vehicle	E810–E819
2.5	3.4	4.5	6.0	7.6	9.1	11.8	15.8	21.7	23.9	F	traffic accidents	
0.7	0.9	0.8	1.1	1.4	1.8	1.9	3.2	4.7	14.7	M	Fire	E890–E899
0.4	0.5	0.4	0.6	0.6	0.5	1.2	2.0	4.2	7.4	F		
20.4	22.4	30.4	33.8	33.8	31.1	32.7	42.1	50.5	83.9	M	Suicide	E950–E959
8.1	10.1	13.7	16.4	16.8	18.4	21.8	29.7	42.3	55.4	F		
0.6	0.9	1.2	0.9	0.9	0.4	0.5	0.9	0.8	1.4	M	Homicide	E960–E969
0.5	0.4	0.6	0.3	0.6	0.7	0.3	0.8	0.8	1.1	F		
4500	5333	4472	3991	3782	3234	2189	1557	1197	1036	M	**POPULATION (thousands)**	
4446	5284	4518	4078	3932	3501	2902	2253	1818	1918	F		

JAPAN: Males

	All ages	0–34	35–69	35–39	40–44	45–49	50–54	55–59	60–64	65–69	70–74	75–79	80+/NK
POPULATION (1000s)													
1955	43861	30289	12463	2320	2325	2136	1929	1608	1227	919	594	342	173
1965	48245	31094	15649	3748	2730	2225	2173	1931	1625	1219	789	452	261
1975	54760	32427	20080	4190	4109	3641	2615	2046	1910	1570	1133	686	433
1985	59044	30423	25344	5389	4494	4053	3898	3391	2349	1771	1486	997	794
1990	**60249**	**28959**	**27501**	**4500**	**5333**	**4472**	**3991**	**3782**	**3234**	**2189**	**1557**	**1197**	**1036**
1995 projected	*61932*	*29150*	*28578*	*3915*	*4505*	*5293*	*4407*	*3873*	*3609*	*2977*	*1894*	*1197*	*1113*
NUMBER OF DEATHS													
All causes													
1955	365246	102157	155838	8017	10847	15238	21269	27138	33421	39908	41481	35900	29870
1965	378716	56233	169254	9747	9827	12610	19393	28288	40357	49032	52399	48811	52019
1975	377827	38184	156049	8137	12971	16696	16991	22026	33116	46112	57697	56734	69163
1985	407769	22188	156625	7110	10234	15063	24347	30747	30884	38240	55100	65593	108263
1990	**443718**	**18986**	**167928**	**5449**	**9769**	**14218**	**20161**	**32925**	**42742**	**42664**	**51737**	**69320**	**135747**
1995 projected	*451047*	*17933*	*175039*	*4063*	*7020*	*13833*	*19818*	*31959*	*45084*	*53262*	*55962*	*62882*	*139231*
Lung cancer													
1955	1893	48	1373	18	47	105	195	249	362	397	306	124	42
1965	5404	80	3592	67	99	188	407	618	1078	1135	935	570	227
1975	10711	72	5851	78	201	416	541	903	1533	2179	2407	1635	746
1985	20837	61	9176	156	275	451	984	1818	2321	3171	4228	4018	3354
1990	**26872**	**62**	**11840**	**148**	**360**	**578**	**917**	**2018**	**3654**	**4165**	**4675**	**5022**	**5273**
1995 projected	*32410*	*78*	*14670*	*142*	*344*	*682*	*1001*	*2190*	*4336*	*5975*	*5862*	*5424*	*6376*
ANNUAL DEATH RATE / 100,000 (*The rates for the age groups 0–34 and 35–69 are the means of seven five-yearly rates, but the all-ages rates are standardised to the conventional "European" age distribution)													
All causes													
1955	1535.3*	335.9*	1626.1*	345.6	466.6	713.6	1102.5	1688.0	2724.2	4342.1	6985.7	10494.0	17236.0
1965	1430.3*	187.1*	1435.8*	260.1	360.0	566.8	892.5	1465.3	2483.4	4022.6	6641.2	10801.3	19945.9
1975	1078.3*	113.8*	1052.3*	194.2	315.7	458.6	649.7	1076.6	1734.0	2937.4	5091.1	8269.1	15969.3
1985	855.6*	75.8*	819.6*	131.9	227.7	371.7	624.6	906.7	1314.9	2159.4	3707.7	6581.0	13630.0
1990	**787.3***	**67.6***	**752.6***	**121.1**	**183.2**	**317.9**	**505.2**	**870.7**	**1321.5**	**1948.8**	**3323.7**	**5793.6**	**13104.3**
1995 projected	*726.2**	*60.6**	*690.6**	*103.8*	*155.8*	*261.4*	*449.7*	*825.2*	*1249.1*	*1789.2*	*2954.7*	*5254.6*	*12507.3*
All cancer													
1955	176.8*	7.5*	307.7*	33.5	65.2	126.5	218.7	351.7	570.2	787.7	974.1	910.6	669.4
1965	205.8*	9.7*	327.5*	35.4	60.3	119.7	219.6	366.3	606.8	884.8	1128.6	1316.9	1130.8
1975	209.2*	9.1*	305.2*	33.4	60.7	112.5	186.3	347.8	545.3	850.6	1218.6	1469.0	1453.5
1985	227.2*	7.0*	306.7*	28.9	54.2	103.2	213.5	363.9	546.7	836.9	1224.6	1730.8	2086.6
1990	**227.1***	**6.1***	**307.7***	**26.4**	**49.2**	**98.3**	**181.9**	**372.6**	**596.8**	**828.6**	**1200.1**	**1640.5**	**2250.9**
1995 projected	*224.2**	*5.5**	*305.5**	*23.7*	*45.9*	*87.0*	*174.0*	*379.2*	*606.9*	*821.5*	*1142.2*	*1606.8*	*2299.3*
Lung cancer													
1955	8.2*	0.2*	15.1*	0.8	2.0	4.9	10.1	15.5	29.5	43.2	51.5	36.2	24.2
1965	19.2*	0.3*	32.0*	1.8	3.6	8.5	18.7	32.0	66.3	93.1	118.5	126.1	87.0
1975	29.6*	0.2*	43.2*	1.9	4.9	11.4	20.7	44.1	80.3	138.8	212.4	238.3	172.2
1985	43.6*	0.2*	53.8*	2.9	6.1	11.1	25.2	53.6	98.8	179.1	284.5	403.1	422.3
1990	**47.4***	**0.2***	**57.5***	**3.3**	**6.8**	**12.9**	**23.0**	**53.4**	**113.0**	**190.2**	**300.3**	**419.7**	**509.0**
1995 projected	*50.6**	*0.3**	*60.6**	*3.6*	*7.6*	*12.9*	*22.7*	*56.5*	*120.1*	*200.7*	*309.5*	*453.2*	*572.8*
Upper aerodigestive cancer (mouth, oesophagus, pharynx and larynx)													
1955	14.0*	0.2*	23.5*	1.1	2.2	5.1	13.5	25.7	45.6	71.3	90.1	84.8	67.5
1965	14.9*	0.1*	23.2*	0.9	2.6	5.4	11.7	24.3	45.0	72.5	93.2	100.9	100.5
1975	15.5*	0.1*	23.1*	1.0	2.6	6.4	13.2	24.8	44.9	68.8	91.2	120.7	108.3
1985	14.9*	0.1*	22.3*	1.0	2.8	7.1	15.9	29.0	41.3	59.3	77.5	106.3	116.5
1990	**15.0***	**0.1***	**23.5***	**0.8**	**2.5**	**7.5**	**15.6**	**30.5**	**44.9**	**62.4**	**81.4**	**91.4**	**110.0**
1995 projected	*14.8**	*0.1**	*24.4**	*0.8*	*2.5*	*7.5*	*16.1*	*32.0*	*47.2*	*65.0*	*77.3*	*85.2*	*99.5*
Other cancer													
1955	154.5*	7.2*	269.0*	31.7	61.0	116.5	195.2	310.6	495.1	673.3	832.4	789.5	577.6
1965	171.7*	9.3*	272.3*	32.7	54.1	105.8	189.1	310.0	495.5	719.2	917.0	1089.8	943.3
1975	164.1*	8.7*	239.0*	30.6	53.2	94.7	152.4	278.9	420.2	642.9	914.9	1110.0	1172.9
1985	168.7*	6.7*	230.6*	25.1	45.3	85.0	172.4	281.2	406.6	598.6	862.6	1221.4	1547.9
1990	**164.8***	**5.8***	**226.7***	**22.2**	**40.0**	**77.9**	**143.3**	**288.7**	**438.9**	**575.9**	**818.4**	**1129.3**	**1631.8**
1995 projected	*158.7**	*5.1**	*220.4**	*19.3*	*35.8*	*66.7*	*135.2*	*290.6*	*439.6*	*555.8*	*755.4*	*1068.4*	*1627.0*
Chronic obstructive pulmonary disease (COPD)													
1955	20.6*	2.1*	14.5*	1.2	2.0	3.0	5.1	11.1	24.0	55.3	126.3	208.1	333.5
1965	18.1*	0.8*	12.0*	0.9	1.4	2.9	4.0	10.5	21.4	42.7	93.8	170.2	371.9
1975	31.9*	1.1*	22.0*	1.7	2.9	4.8	8.4	18.8	39.0	78.5	173.7	319.5	616.5
1985	23.0*	0.8*	12.8*	0.9	1.0	2.8	4.7	10.2	19.6	50.3	115.2	242.4	500.7
1990	**19.6***	**0.9***	**9.6***	**1.0**	**1.4**	**2.1**	**2.9**	**6.2**	**16.7**	**37.0**	**94.7**	**200.3**	**456.7**
1995 projected	*16.7**	*1.2**	*7.4**	*1.2*	*1.3*	*1.6*	*2.0*	*4.6*	*12.3*	*29.1*	*75.6*	*166.7*	*403.8*
Other respiratory disease													
1955	76.3*	32.5*	47.3*	7.8	8.7	15.1	24.6	41.1	79.2	154.7	310.5	573.2	1057.7
1965	89.2*	14.3*	48.0*	5.8	7.7	11.2	19.0	39.5	80.7	172.2	370.2	781.4	1919.1
1975	62.7*	5.9*	35.3*	4.3	6.1	8.7	15.3	27.2	56.5	128.9	289.5	560.1	1383.5
1985	72.1*	2.2*	35.7*	2.6	4.6	7.6	15.4	28.0	60.5	131.0	316.7	708.4	1760.5
1990	**87.5***	**2.1***	**39.9***	**2.4**	**4.0**	**8.0**	**14.6**	**33.3**	**68.9**	**148.1**	**360.5**	**813.9**	**2293.8**
1995 projected	*104.7**	*2.0**	*44.3**	*2.2*	*3.9*	*7.6*	*15.9*	*37.2*	*77.7*	*165.4*	*404.6*	*949.7*	*2887.0*
Vascular disease													
1955	486.4*	12.5*	596.2*	44.8	87.6	174.7	345.3	608.3	1084.4	1828.3	2943.8	4007.6	5110.2
1965	596.8*	9.6*	601.2*	46.9	83.6	161.7	309.1	578.1	1104.9	1923.9	3384.4	5445.0	8630.8
1975	472.4*	8.1*	396.8*	43.2	87.4	137.6	206.0	371.9	670.1	1261.1	2434.9	4307.0	8483.7
1985	316.2*	7.3*	245.3*	29.2	59.6	96.6	167.7	249.6	396.4	717.9	1400.2	2740.6	6376.9
1990	**264.1***	**6.8***	**207.0***	**28.7**	**48.3**	**87.9**	**140.6**	**226.1**	**353.3**	**564.0**	**1082.6**	**2145.2**	**5507.5**
1995 projected	*216.9**	*6.4**	*171.3**	*25.3*	*42.7*	*74.6*	*124.0*	*198.9*	*292.7*	*441.0*	*829.0*	*1676.8*	*4622.5*
Liver cirrhosis													
1955	20.0*	0.9*	30.9*	4.5	9.9	16.7	26.1	33.8	49.0	76.1	101.5	124.2	124.1
1965	22.5*	1.0*	34.3*	7.7	13.3	22.3	31.2	43.9	54.7	66.8	102.8	128.8	155.3
1975	27.6*	0.8*	47.6*	13.2	29.2	38.1	45.9	55.4	69.5	81.8	96.5	113.7	153.8
1985	23.2*	0.4*	41.4*	5.9	15.4	31.2	57.2	59.3	59.0	61.6	74.0	91.8	118.3
1990	**19.3***	**0.3***	**35.6***	**4.7**	**11.1**	**23.2**	**37.0**	**58.2**	**59.7**	**55.4**	**60.4**	**71.0**	**95.3**
1995 projected	*16.1**	*0.2**	*30.7**	*3.6*	*8.2*	*16.3*	*29.5*	*51.1*	*56.9*	*49.1*	*48.7*	*55.2*	*75.4*
Other medical causes													
1955	649.6*	195.9*	517.6*	172.5	209.9	277.6	373.0	518.7	782.2	1289.6	2344.6	4418.0	9624.9
1965	399.1*	89.0*	295.8*	83.0	107.0	147.4	201.2	305.0	464.7	762.3	1358.6	2697.3	7343.2
1975	194.0*	40.9*	151.4*	35.7	54.2	76.8	102.0	155.3	236.7	398.8	701.5	1263.4	3486.5
1985	123.2*	22.2*	88.8*	14.5	23.2	39.3	64.8	94.6	137.5	247.6	431.5	856.4	2440.8
1990	**108.5***	**19.3***	**79.5***	**13.4**	**19.7**	**32.9**	**52.4**	**88.1**	**134.6**	**215.0**	**384.4**	**728.5**	**2153.0**
1995 projected	*94.4**	*16.8**	*70.6**	*11.7*	*16.8*	*27.0*	*45.7*	*81.3*	*121.5*	*190.1*	*326.2*	*613.9*	*1881.6*
All non-medical causes													
1955	105.6*	84.5*	111.9*	81.3	83.3	100.1	109.7	123.3	135.1	150.4	184.9	252.3	316.2
1965	98.7*	62.6*	117.1*	80.5	86.7	101.6	108.5	122.1	150.1	169.9	202.8	261.8	394.9
1975	80.5*	48.0*	94.1*	62.7	75.2	80.0	85.6	100.2	116.9	137.9	176.4	236.4	391.8
1985	70.7*	36.0*	88.9*	49.8	69.9	90.9	101.4	101.1	95.3	114.1	145.5	210.5	346.1
1990	**61.2***	**32.0***	**73.4***	**44.6**	**49.4**	**65.5**	**75.9**	**86.2**	**91.5**	**100.7**	**141.0**	**194.2**	**347.1**
1995 projected	*53.2**	*28.6**	*60.9**	*36.0*	*37.1*	*47.3*	*58.7*	*73.0*	*81.1*	*93.0*	*128.4*	*185.5*	*337.7*

JAPAN: Females

	All ages	0–34	35–69	35–39	40–44	45–49	50–54	55–59	60–64	65–69	70–74	75–79	80+/NK
POPULATION (1000s)													
1955	45415	30259	13484	2796	2621	2232	1920	1598	1270	1048	799	534	339
1965	50030	30614	17299	3751	3232	2697	2485	2072	1719	1343	956	644	517
1975	56514	31484	21910	4188	4071	3683	3158	2578	2344	1889	1406	939	774
1985	61222	29381	26932	5288	4554	4140	3971	3574	3011	2394	2046	1438	1425
1990	62472	27822	28661	4446	5284	4518	4078	3932	3501	2902	2253	1818	1918
1995 projected	63972	27839	29319	3853	4464	5274	4499	4027	3843	3359	2699	1960	2155
NUMBER OF DEATHS													
All causes													
1955	328277	84426	114957	8435	9895	11717	14773	17855	22238	30044	38691	41438	48765
1965	321722	36885	111317	6352	7628	9932	13839	17653	23945	31968	40016	49023	84481
1975	324448	23687	101156	4673	6816	9306	12367	15294	22188	30512	43244	53135	103226
1985	344514	12425	90094	4017	5650	7644	11504	14828	19961	26490	40891	55657	145447
1990	376587	10079	88120	3102	5542	7510	10097	14616	19986	27267	38076	58203	182109
1995 projected	369982	9302	82654	2324	4149	7602	9842	13024	18900	26813	38127	53455	186444
Lung cancer													
1955	818	40	595	32	49	67	85	105	119	138	113	50	20
1965	2321	58	1513	67	87	105	231	293	356	374	343	269	138
1975	4048	55	2297	73	100	200	296	413	544	671	727	556	413
1985	7753	34	3312	95	149	220	373	587	844	1044	1352	1392	1663
1990	9614	37	3674	88	164	257	424	616	885	1240	1561	1811	2531
1995 projected	10913	48	3929	80	143	318	473	596	912	1407	1881	1972	3083
ANNUAL DEATH RATE / 100,000 (*The rates for the age groups 0–34 and 35–69 are the means of seven five-yearly rates, but the all-ages rates are standardised to the conventional "European" age distribution)													
All causes													
1955	1143.0*	280.6*	1101.3*	301.7	377.6	525.0	769.3	1117.5	1751.3	2866.8	4843.0	7765.7	14368.0
1965	980.2*	126.6*	850.7*	169.3	236.0	368.2	556.9	852.2	1392.6	2379.6	4187.5	7612.3	16331.1
1975	721.7*	72.0*	582.6*	111.6	167.4	252.7	391.6	593.3	946.4	1615.3	3075.9	5658.1	13329.8
1985	514.2*	44.5*	408.4*	76.0	124.1	184.6	289.7	414.9	663.0	1106.4	1998.4	3871.3	10209.0
1990	454.3*	38.8*	353.0*	69.8	104.9	166.2	247.6	371.7	570.8	939.7	1689.8	3201.7	9494.2
1995 projected	399.6*	33.9*	304.2*	60.3	92.9	144.1	218.8	323.4	491.9	798.2	1412.4	2727.0	8652.1
All cancer													
1955	130.8*	8.0*	229.6*	49.9	91.6	138.1	201.8	273.3	367.1	485.3	578.5	600.1	482.3
1965	136.0*	9.8*	219.7*	45.5	74.0	120.6	188.6	262.3	358.1	488.8	642.6	756.1	677.2
1975	126.5*	9.0*	190.4*	38.8	63.5	101.9	156.1	222.3	307.9	442.1	623.4	783.2	804.5
1985	118.8*	6.8*	164.4*	31.8	55.4	83.5	128.9	185.7	275.6	389.7	565.3	807.2	1041.1
1990	112.9*	5.7*	152.5*	32.0	49.7	80.4	118.5	175.7	248.5	362.9	527.1	741.2	1118.3
1995 projected	105.9*	4.9*	139.8*	29.5	47.0	74.2	110.6	160.1	227.1	330.3	479.8	704.7	1125.6
Lung cancer													
1955	2.9*	0.2*	5.7*	1.1	1.9	3.0	4.4	6.6	9.4	13.2	14.1	9.4	5.9
1965	6.8*	0.2*	11.5*	1.8	2.7	3.9	9.3	14.1	20.7	27.8	35.9	41.8	26.7
1975	8.8*	0.2*	13.4*	1.7	2.5	5.4	9.4	16.0	23.2	35.5	51.7	59.2	53.3
1985	11.8*	0.1*	15.4*	1.8	3.3	5.3	9.4	16.4	28.0	43.6	66.1	96.8	116.7
1990	12.2*	0.1*	15.0*	2.0	3.1	5.7	10.4	15.7	25.3	42.7	69.3	99.6	132.0
1995 projected	12.3*	0.2*	14.6*	2.1	3.2	6.0	10.5	14.8	23.7	41.9	69.7	100.6	143.1
Upper aerodigestive cancer (mouth, oesophagus, pharynx and larynx)													
1955	4.9*	0.1*	7.7*	0.9	2.1	2.9	5.1	8.6	13.6	20.5	26.9	33.9	30.3
1965	4.8*	0.1*	6.7*	0.6	0.8	1.9	4.3	8.7	11.6	18.5	30.0	36.6	36.3
1975	3.9*	0.1*	5.0*	0.5	1.0	1.6	3.5	5.5	9.6	13.5	20.6	30.0	40.5
1985	2.8*	0.0*	3.4*	0.2	0.7	1.3	2.0	3.9	5.5	10.6	14.1	23.4	35.0
1990	2.6*	0.1*	3.1*	0.4	0.7	1.3	2.4	3.7	5.3	8.1	13.2	19.9	32.9
1995 projected	2.4*	0.1*	2.9*	0.5	0.8	1.5	2.4	3.7	4.5	7.1	11.2	16.8	29.9
Other cancer													
1955	123.0*	7.8*	216.3*	47.9	87.7	132.2	192.3	258.1	344.1	451.6	537.5	556.8	446.1
1965	124.4*	9.5*	201.6*	43.1	70.4	114.8	175.0	239.4	325.8	442.4	576.7	677.6	614.2
1975	113.9*	8.7*	172.0*	36.6	60.1	94.9	143.1	200.7	275.1	393.0	551.1	694.0	710.6
1985	104.1*	6.6*	145.5*	29.7	51.4	76.9	117.4	165.4	242.1	335.5	485.2	687.0	889.4
1990	98.1*	5.5*	134.4*	29.6	45.9	73.4	105.7	156.3	217.9	312.0	444.6	621.7	953.4
1995 projected	91.2*	4.7*	122.3*	26.9	42.9	66.7	97.7	141.6	198.8	281.3	399.0	587.3	952.6
Chronic obstructive pulmonary disease (COPD)													
1955	11.6*	1.9*	7.8*	1.1	1.4	1.7	3.6	5.5	13.7	27.5	60.1	103.8	200.4
1965	9.2*	0.6*	5.5*	0.9	1.2	1.3	1.9	4.4	9.1	19.6	39.5	81.2	208.8
1975	14.4*	0.9*	9.6*	1.5	1.8	3.4	5.4	9.1	17.1	28.5	61.7	124.5	308.8
1985	8.5*	0.6*	5.7*	0.7	1.3	1.8	3.0	5.7	9.0	18.5	38.3	76.0	177.6
1990	7.1*	0.5*	4.5*	0.9	1.2	1.5	2.7	3.9	6.7	14.3	31.1	59.8	158.6
1995 projected	5.9*	0.5*	3.5*	0.8	1.1	1.3	2.0	2.9	5.0	11.2	24.2	48.9	136.7
Other respiratory disease													
1955	54.9*	32.1*	29.9*	8.2	8.9	9.9	16.0	26.3	46.9	92.8	177.2	334.3	734.5
1965	58.6*	13.0*	27.6*	4.8	6.8	8.7	13.6	23.4	45.3	90.6	202.5	453.9	1338.9
1975	39.8*	5.4*	18.4*	2.9	4.1	6.0	8.6	16.4	31.0	59.5	147.1	323.9	979.2
1985	35.3*	2.1*	14.4*	1.9	2.4	3.4	7.2	11.1	23.7	51.0	118.0	296.7	988.3
1990	40.0*	1.5*	14.7*	2.1	2.0	3.4	6.4	12.2	24.5	52.5	128.8	307.5	1209.3
1995 projected	44.9*	1.2*	15.1*	1.9	1.9	3.1	6.4	12.4	25.2	55.2	132.7	331.0	1427.4
Vascular disease													
1955	366.1*	14.6*	427.9*	47.4	78.8	152.8	272.4	434.5	736.6	1272.9	2137.3	3062.6	4054.8
1965	415.5*	7.6*	365.8*	28.8	54.2	109.9	189.4	336.5	636.2	1205.5	2242.6	4017.1	6857.7
1975	339.2*	4.8*	221.4*	20.5	37.7	64.2	117.0	199.7	378.5	732.1	1605.3	3228.9	7355.0
1985	219.2*	3.9*	127.1*	12.6	25.1	44.7	76.2	112.6	206.6	412.1	871.9	1908.3	5413.3
1990	180.4*	3.6*	98.1*	10.6	21.5	36.8	58.0	92.4	162.2	305.2	650.0	1450.5	4767.3
1995 projected	145.9*	3.2*	74.6*	9.0	17.9	29.1	46.1	72.4	122.7	225.0	480.8	1110.9	4048.6
Liver cirrhosis													
1955	11.5*	0.7*	17.4*	3.4	5.1	8.2	15.5	21.7	29.2	38.4	59.2	69.2	71.6
1965	9.9*	0.4*	13.9*	2.1	4.0	7.4	10.6	16.6	21.6	34.7	46.3	67.4	93.8
1975	9.2*	0.2*	13.5*	2.0	3.5	6.2	11.2	15.9	23.6	32.2	46.4	55.5	78.5
1985	7.9*	0.1*	11.9*	1.1	2.3	4.7	8.8	15.3	20.9	30.4	39.9	53.2	62.2
1990	6.9*	0.1*	10.0*	0.9	1.6	3.3	6.6	12.7	19.4	25.5	38.3	48.1	55.5
1995 projected	6.0*	0.1*	8.5*	0.7	1.1	2.4	5.2	10.8	16.6	22.8	34.0	43.0	49.8
Other medical causes													
1955	523.8*	187.2*	349.3*	166.7	166.3	187.0	229.2	317.4	503.9	874.7	1724.6	3449.2	8618.7
1965	311.4*	73.2*	179.2*	66.2	75.3	94.4	119.7	169.2	267.3	462.0	896.4	2071.0	6855.6
1975	157.3*	33.4*	94.5*	26.3	34.2	45.1	63.9	94.9	143.4	254.0	485.7	978.2	3516.9
1985	96.8*	19.0*	53.9*	11.0	15.7	21.5	34.0	53.8	88.6	152.4	290.0	608.8	2310.5
1990	80.6*	15.8*	44.1*	9.6	11.6	17.2	26.9	43.0	71.7	128.8	239.2	480.8	1969.1
1995 projected	66.0*	12.9*	35.5*	7.2	9.2	13.3	21.2	34.1	58.5	104.9	189.6	378.8	1652.5
All non-medical causes													
1955	44.3*	36.1*	39.5*	25.0	25.5	27.3	30.8	38.8	53.9	75.2	106.0	146.6	205.7
1965	39.5*	22.1*	39.1*	21.0	20.6	25.9	33.0	39.8	55.0	78.5	117.7	165.7	299.2
1975	35.3*	18.3*	34.9*	19.5	22.6	25.9	29.4	35.0	45.0	67.0	106.3	163.9	286.9
1985	27.6*	12.1*	31.0*	16.9	21.8	25.0	31.6	30.6	38.7	52.2	74.9	121.2	216.0
1990	26.4*	11.7*	29.0*	13.6	17.4	23.5	28.5	31.8	37.8	50.4	75.4	113.9	216.1
1995 projected	24.9*	11.1*	27.2*	11.1	14.7	20.6	27.2	30.7	37.0	48.9	71.4	109.7	211.5

JAPAN: 1975

Smoking-attributed deaths (Sm.) and total deaths (Total)

		ALL CAUSES	ALL CANCER	Lung cancer	Upper aero-digestive ca.	Other cancer	COPD	Other respiratory	Vascular disease	Liver cirrhosis	Other medical	Non-medical
Males												
0–34	Sm.	–	–	–	–	–	–	–	–	–	–	–
	Total	38184	2992	72	40	2880	351	2010	2699	271	14117	15744
35–69	Sm.	17842	7519	4604	1129	1786	1515	501	5863	–	2444	–
	Total	156049	43746	5851	3172	34723	2945	4806	56003	8087	23146	17316
		(11%)	(17%)	(79%)	(36%)	(5%)	(51%)	(10%)	(10%)		(11%)	
70+	Sm.	18240	6270	3913	924	1433	3712	761	5655	–	1842	–
	Total	183594	30184	4788	2331	23065	6830	13116	93888	2540	31718	5318
		(10%)	(21%)	(82%)	(40%)	(6%)	(54%)	(6%)	(6%)		(6%)	
Any age	Sm.	36082	13789	8517	2053	3219	5227	1262	11518	–	4286	–
	Total	377827	76922	10711	5543	60668	10126	19932	152590	10898	68981	38378
		(10%)	(18%)	(80%)	(37%)	(5%)	(52%)	(6%)	(8%)		(6%)	
Females												
0–34	Sm.	–	–	–	–	–	–	–	–	–	–	–
	Total	23687	2919	55	28	2836	284	1798	1578	70	11109	5929
35–69	Sm.	3106	934	721	94	119	344	100	1204	–	524	–
	Total	101156	34193	2297	851	31045	1610	3054	36298	2380	16778	6843
		(3%)	(3%)	(31%)	(11%)	(0%)	(21%)	(3%)	(3%)		(3%)	
70+	Sm.	5243	1012	738	144	130	1297	216	1987	–	731	–
	Total	199605	22349	1696	885	19768	4428	12693	109849	1781	43249	5256
		(3%)	(5%)	(44%)	(16%)	(1%)	(29%)	(2%)	(2%)		(2%)	
Any age	Sm.	8349	1946	1459	238	249	1641	316	3191	–	1255	–
	Total	324448	59461	4048	1764	53649	6322	17545	147725	4231	71136	18028
		(3%)	(3%)	(36%)	(13%)	(0%)	(26%)	(2%)	(2%)		(2%)	
Males+Females												
0–34	Sm.	–	–	–	–	–	–	–	–	–	–	–
	Total	61871	5911	127	68	5716	635	3808	4277	341	25226	21673
35–69	Sm.	20948	8453	5325	1223	1905	1859	601	7067	–	2968	–
	Total	257205	77939	8148	4023	65768	4555	7860	92301	10467	39924	24159
		(8%)	(11%)	(65%)	(30%)	(3%)	(41%)	(8%)	(8%)		(7%)	
70+	Sm.	23483	7282	4651	1068	1563	5009	977	7642	–	2573	–
	Total	383199	52533	6484	3216	42833	11258	25809	203737	4321	74967	10574
		(6%)	(14%)	(72%)	(33%)	(4%)	(44%)	(4%)	(4%)		(3%)	
Any age	Sm.	44431	15735	9976	2291	3468	6868	1578	14709	–	5541	–
	Total	702275	136383	14759	7307	114317	16448	37477	300315	15129	140117	56406
		(6%)	(12%)	(68%)	(31%)	(3%)	(42%)	(4%)	(5%)		(4%)	

JAPAN: 1985

Smoking-attributed deaths (Sm.) and total deaths (Total)

		ALL CAUSES	ALL CANCER	Lung cancer	Upper aero-digestive ca.	Other cancer	COPD	Other respiratory	Vascular disease	Liver cirrhosis	Other medical	Non-medical
Males												
0–34	Sm.	–	–	–	–	–	–	–	–	–	–	–
	Total	22188	2138	61	32	2045	231	623	2165	109	6170	10752
35–69	Sm.	22282	12015	7575	1652	2788	1207	788	6030	–	2242	–
	Total	156625	56498	9176	4087	43235	2087	5946	45191	8991	16765	21147
		(14%)	(21%)	(83%)	(40%)	(6%)	(58%)	(13%)	(13%)		(13%)	
70+	Sm.	35154	15446	10191	1621	3634	5428	2292	8925	–	3063	–
	Total	228956	52024	11600	3136	37288	8105	25751	98777	2954	34336	7009
		(15%)	(30%)	(88%)	(52%)	(10%)	(67%)	(9%)	(9%)		(9%)	
Any age	Sm.	57436	27461	17766	3273	6422	6635	3080	14955	–	5305	–
	Total	407769	110660	20837	7255	82568	10423	32320	146133	12054	57271	38908
		(14%)	(25%)	(85%)	(45%)	(8%)	(64%)	(10%)	(10%)		(9%)	
Females												
0–34	Sm.	–	–	–	–	–	–	–	–	–	–	–
	Total	12425	2010	34	14	1962	162	565	1129	39	5078	3442
35–69	Sm.	3804	1576	1291	108	177	335	141	1233	–	519	–
	Total	90094	37039	3312	730	32997	1212	2970	26794	2613	11775	7691
		(4%)	(4%)	(39%)	(15%)	(1%)	(28%)	(5%)	(5%)		(4%)	
70+	Sm.	12755	3557	2753	341	463	2186	753	4525	–	1734	–
	Total	241995	38005	4407	1122	32476	4406	20762	122398	2468	47603	6353
		(5%)	(9%)	(62%)	(30%)	(1%)	(50%)	(4%)	(4%)		(4%)	
Any age	Sm.	16559	5133	4044	449	640	2521	894	5758	–	2253	–
	Total	344514	77054	7753	1866	67435	5780	24297	150321	5120	64456	17486
		(5%)	(7%)	(52%)	(24%)	(1%)	(44%)	(4%)	(4%)		(3%)	
Males+Females												
0–34	Sm.	–	–	–	–	–	–	–	–	–	–	–
	Total	34613	4148	95	46	4007	393	1188	3294	148	11248	14194
35–69	Sm.	26086	13591	8866	1760	2965	1542	929	7263	–	2761	–
	Total	246719	93537	12488	4817	76232	3299	8916	71985	11604	28540	28838
		(11%)	(15%)	(71%)	(37%)	(4%)	(47%)	(10%)	(10%)		(10%)	
70+	Sm.	47909	19003	12944	1962	4097	7614	3045	13450	–	4797	–
	Total	470951	90029	16007	4258	69764	12511	46513	221175	5422	81939	13362
		(10%)	(21%)	(81%)	(46%)	(6%)	(61%)	(7%)	(6%)		(6%)	
Any age	Sm.	73995	32594	21810	3722	7062	9156	3974	20713	–	7558	–
	Total	752283	187714	28590	9121	150003	16203	56617	296454	17174	121727	56394
		(10%)	(17%)	(76%)	(41%)	(5%)	(57%)	(7%)	(7%)		(6%)	

(To be conservative, no deaths before age 35, and none from liver cirrhosis or non-medical causes, were attributed to smoking.)

JAPAN: 1990

Smoking–attributed deaths (Sm.) and total deaths (Total)

		ALL CAUSES	ALL CANCER	Lung cancer	Upper aero-digestive ca.	Other cancer	COPD	Other respiratory	Vascular disease	Liver cirrhosis	Other medical	Non-medical
Males												
0–34	Sm.	–	–	–	–	–	–	–	–	–	–	–
	Total	18986	1771	62	35	1674	280	561	1925	76	4842	9531
35–69	Sm.	26830	15657	9929	2177	3551	1149	1125	6425	–	2474	–
	Total	167928	66998	11840	5104	50054	1909	7988	45734	8664	17617	19018
		(16%)	(23%)	(84%)	(43%)	(7%)	(60%)	(14%)	(14%)		(14%)	
70+	Sm.	41512	19504	13236	1854	4414	5857	3558	9191	–	3402	–
	Total	256804	61626	14970	3501	43155	8602	39110	99571	2776	37004	8115
		(16%)	(32%)	(88%)	(53%)	(10%)	(68%)	(9%)	(9%)		(9%)	
Any age	Sm.	68342	35161	23165	4031	7965	7006	4683	15616	–	5876	–
	Total	443718	130395	26872	8640	94883	10791	47659	147230	11516	59463	36664
		(15%)	(27%)	(86%)	(47%)	(8%)	(65%)	(10%)	(11%)		(10%)	
Females												
0–34	Sm.	–	–	–	–	–	–	–	–	–	–	–
	Total	10079	1563	37	15	1511	143	386	958	22	3761	3246
35–69	Sm.	3629	1681	1398	107	176	291	158	1036	–	463	–
	Total	88120	38653	3674	781	34198	1086	3475	23805	2465	10847	7789
		(4%)	(4%)	(38%)	(14%)	(1%)	(27%)	(5%)	(4%)		(4%)	
70+	Sm.	15411	4786	3776	409	601	2466	1183	5019	–	1957	–
	Total	278388	46802	5903	1292	39607	4831	31688	132455	2801	51898	7913
		(6%)	(10%)	(64%)	(32%)	(2%)	(51%)	(4%)	(4%)		(4%)	
Any age	Sm.	19040	6467	5174	516	777	2757	1341	6055	–	2420	–
	Total	376587	87018	9614	2088	75316	6060	35549	157218	5288	66506	18948
		(5%)	(7%)	(54%)	(25%)	(1%)	(45%)	(4%)	(4%)		(4%)	
Males+Females												
0–34	Sm.	–	–	–	–	–	–	–	–	–	–	–
	Total	29065	3334	99	50	3185	423	947	2883	98	8603	12777
35–69	Sm.	30459	17338	11327	2284	3727	1440	1283	7461	–	2937	–
	Total	256048	105651	15514	5885	84252	2995	11463	69539	11129	28464	26807
		(12%)	(16%)	(73%)	(39%)	(4%)	(48%)	(11%)	(11%)		(10%)	
70+	Sm.	56923	24290	17012	2263	5015	8323	4741	14210	–	5359	–
	Total	535192	108428	20873	4793	82762	13433	70798	232026	5577	88902	16028
		(11%)	(22%)	(82%)	(47%)	(6%)	(62%)	(7%)	(6%)		(6%)	
Any age	Sm.	87382	41628	28339	4547	8742	9763	6024	21671	–	8296	–
	Total	820305	217413	36486	10728	170199	16851	83208	304448	16804	125969	55612
		(11%)	(19%)	(78%)	(42%)	(5%)	(58%)	(7%)	(7%)		(7%)	

JAPAN: 1995

Smoking–attributed deaths (Sm.) and total deaths (Total)

		ALL CAUSES	ALL CANCER	Lung cancer	Upper aero-digestive ca.	Other cancer	COPD	Other respiratory	Vascular disease	Liver cirrhosis	Other medical	Non-medical
Males												
0–34	Sm.	–	–	–	–	–	–	–	–	–	–	–
	Total	17933	1636	78	40	1518	367	556	1924	64	4520	8866
35–69	Sm.	31283	19508	12475	2745	4288	1101	1564	6468	–	2642	–
	Total	175039	76316	14670	6125	55521	1768	10530	43722	8165	17846	16692
		(18%)	(26%)	(85%)	(45%)	(8%)	(62%)	(15%)	(15%)		(15%)	
70+	Sm.	45162	22596	15731	1955	4910	5519	4993	8640	–	3414	–
	Total	258075	66459	17662	3591	45206	7922	51166	87225	2421	34472	8410
		(17%)	(34%)	(89%)	(54%)	(11%)	(70%)	(10%)	(10%)		(10%)	
Any age	Sm.	76445	42104	28206	4700	9198	6620	6557	15108	–	6056	–
	Total	451047	144411	32410	9756	102245	10057	62252	132871	10650	56838	33968
		(17%)	(29%)	(87%)	(48%)	(9%)	(66%)	(11%)	(11%)		(11%)	
Females												
0–34	Sm.	–	–	–	–	–	–	–	–	–	–	–
	Total	9302	1403	48	20	1335	151	324	898	17	3296	3213
35–69	Sm.	3336	1718	1450	103	165	239	171	819	–	389	–
	Total	82654	38392	3929	804	33659	926	3929	19943	2275	9491	7698
		(4%)	(4%)	(37%)	(13%)	(0%)	(26%)	(4%)	(4%)		(4%)	
70+	Sm.	15924	5524	4456	408	660	2344	1541	4671	–	1844	–
	Total	278026	51022	6936	1275	42811	4557	40830	121998	2833	48152	8634
		(6%)	(11%)	(64%)	(32%)	(2%)	(51%)	(4%)	(4%)		(4%)	
Any age	Sm.	19260	7242	5906	511	825	2583	1712	5490	–	2233	–
	Total	369982	90817	10913	2099	77805	5634	45083	142839	5125	60939	19545
		(5%)	(8%)	(54%)	(24%)	(1%)	(46%)	(4%)	(4%)		(4%)	
Males+Females												
0–34	Sm.	–	–	–	–	–	–	–	–	–	–	–
	Total	27235	3039	126	60	2853	518	880	2822	81	7816	12079
35–69	Sm.	34619	21226	13925	2848	4453	1340	1735	7287	–	3031	–
	Total	257693	114708	18599	6929	89180	2694	14459	63665	10440	27337	24390
		(13%)	(19%)	(75%)	(41%)	(5%)	(50%)	(12%)	(11%)		(11%)	
70+	Sm.	61086	28120	20187	2363	5570	7863	6534	13311	–	5258	–
	Total	536101	117481	24598	4866	88017	12479	91996	209223	5254	82624	17044
		(11%)	(24%)	(82%)	(49%)	(6%)	(63%)	(7%)	(6%)		(6%)	
Any age	Sm.	95705	49346	34112	5211	10023	9203	8269	20598	–	8289	–
	Total	821029	235228	43323	11855	180050	15691	107335	275710	15775	117777	53513
		(12%)	(21%)	(79%)	(44%)	(6%)	(59%)	(8%)	(7%)		(7%)	

(To be conservative, no deaths before age 35, and none from liver cirrhosis or non-medical causes, were attributed to smoking.)

¶KAZAKHSTAN: 1990

		No. of deaths			Standardised rates (Defined on p.400)			Annual death rates / 100, 000						
		All ages	0–34	35–69	All ages	0–34	35–69	0–4	5–9	10–14	15–19	20–24	25–29	30–34
ALL CAUSES	M	68134	15994	35124	1606.1	276.3	2014.8	740.5	81.5	70.7	131.6	226.1	299.7	384.1
	F	60653	8868	20091	884.6	150.0	893.5	579.7	46.3	33.2	71.1	100.5	97.7	121.6
Tuberculosis	M	1303	273	935	24.6	5.4	43.9	1.3	0.3	0.5	0.8	4.6	9.2	20.8
	F	391	109	215	5.5	2.1	8.2	1.5	0.4	0.1	1.1	3.0	4.6	4.1
Other infective	M	1151	1038	98	11.2	15.5	4.7	98.5	1.4	2.1	1.6	2.2	1.4	1.6
and parasitic	F	993	879	80	9.4	13.6	3.4	87.0	1.6	0.6	0.1	2.2	2.0	1.3
ALL CANCER	M	12678	618	9357	323.7	11.4	564.7	9.4	9.3	5.3	8.6	9.7	14.0	23.5
	F	9938	534	5896	156.4	10.2	256.9	6.9	4.8	4.6	7.0	8.9	14.7	24.6
Mouth and	M	410	20	329	9.7	0.4	18.9	0.5	0.1	0.1	0.5	–	0.3	1.0
pharynx cancer	F	143	5	78	2.3	0.1	3.6	0.1	–	0.1	0.1	0.2	0.1	–
Oesophagus cancer	M	1241	8	870	35.0	0.2	56.3	–	–	–	0.1	0.3	0.1	0.6
	F	1119	8	554	17.9	0.2	26.0	–	0.1	–	0.1	–	0.5	0.3
Stomach cancer	M	2130	43	1582	56.6	0.9	97.0	–	–	–	0.3	0.3	1.2	4.3
	F	1600	44	894	25.3	0.9	39.2	–	–	–	0.7	0.8	2.1	2.6
Colorectal cancer	M	648	28	426	17.9	0.6	27.8	–	0.1	–	0.1	0.4	1.2	2.0
	F	864	23	513	13.7	0.4	22.8	0.1	–	0.1	0.1	0.2	1.2	1.4
Liver cancer	M	...	...	...	...	...	...	...	...	...	...	...	...	...
	F	...	...	...	...	...	...	...	...	...	...	...	...	...
Pancreas cancer	M	...	...	...	...	...	...	...	...	...	...	...	...	...
	F	...	...	...	...	...	...	...	...	...	...	...	...	...
Larynx cancer	M	387	3	314	9.8	0.1	18.9	0.1	–	–	–	0.1	–	0.1
	F	57	–	41	0.9	–	1.7	–	–	–	–	–	–	–
Lung cancer	M	4024	37	3314	100.8	0.7	197.7	0.3	0.1	–	0.3	0.9	0.9	2.6
	F	857	19	550	13.9	0.4	25.1	–	–	–	–	0.6	0.8	1.3
Malignant melanoma	M	...	...	...	...	...	...	...	...	...	...	...	...	...
	F	...	...	...	...	...	...	...	...	...	...	...	...	...
Female breast cancer	F	1003	55	751	15.9	1.1	30.2	–	–	–	0.1	0.2	1.7	5.7
Cervix cancer	F	605	25	393	9.6	0.5	16.9	–	–	–	–	0.2	1.1	2.3
Other uterine cancer	F	471	7	296	7.5	0.1	12.9	–	–	0.1	–	–	0.3	0.6
Ovarian cancer	F	...	...	...	...	...	...	...	...	...	...	...	...	...
Prostate cancer	M	240	1	104	8.1	0.0	7.9	0.1	–	–	–	–	–	–
Bladder cancer	M	...	...	...	...	...	...	...	...	...	...	...	...	...
	F	...	...	...	...	...	...	...	...	...	...	...	...	...
Other and ill-defined	M	2991	273	2102	73.7	5.0	122.8	4.8	3.6	2.9	3.3	4.7	6.5	9.1
cancer sites	F	2790	219	1602	43.4	4.2	69.4	3.1	2.5	2.3	3.7	4.7	4.9	8.2
Hodgkin's disease	M	...	...	...	...	...	...	...	...	...	...	...	...	...
	F	...	...	...	...	...	...	...	...	...	...	...	...	...
Myeloma and all	M	308	69	194	6.6	1.3	10.7	0.7	0.8	0.7	1.7	1.5	1.7	1.9
lymphomas	F	212	50	120	3.1	0.9	5.0	1.4	0.2	0.8	0.8	1.3	1.1	1.0
Leukaemia	M	299	136	122	5.5	2.4	6.7	2.9	4.6	1.5	2.1	1.5	2.1	2.0
	F	217	79	104	2.9	1.4	4.1	2.2	2.0	1.3	1.3	0.9	0.9	1.3
ALL VASCULAR	M	25021	717	13622	758.1	14.1	838.8	2.9	1.6	1.4	7.5	11.1	23.2	50.9
DISEASE	F	32379	364	8693	494.5	7.2	407.2	3.2	0.7	1.3	4.6	9.1	12.2	19.2
Rheumatic heart	M	433	72	340	8.2	1.4	15.8	–	0.2	0.1	0.8	1.9	3.0	3.8
disease and fever	F	592	72	470	9.2	1.4	18.7	0.1	0.1	0.1	0.7	1.1	3.2	4.7
Hypertensive disease	M	656	16	428	18.7	0.3	27.1	–	–	–	0.3	–	1.1	0.9
	F	966	14	466	15.2	0.3	21.3	0.1	0.1	–	–	–	0.8	0.9
Ischaemic heart	M	13888	271	7873	416.9	5.4	474.8	–	–	0.4	1.3	1.9	7.6	26.6
disease	F	15478	76	3572	235.9	1.6	171.7	–	–	–	0.8	2.8	2.7	4.6
Pulmonary embolism	M	...	...	...	...	...	...	...	...	...	...	...	...	...
and other venous	F	...	...	...	...	...	...	...	...	...	...	...	...	...
Cerebrovascular	M	7408	160	3743	234.3	3.2	245.7	0.5	0.2	–	1.9	3.4	5.5	10.5
disease	F	11894	95	3471	182.7	1.9	162.6	0.8	0.2	0.5	0.8	3.6	2.3	5.0
Other vascular	M	2636	198	1238	79.9	3.8	75.4	2.4	1.1	0.9	3.2	3.8	5.9	9.0
disease, incl. venous	F	3449	107	714	51.6	2.0	32.8	2.1	0.2	0.6	2.3	1.6	3.3	4.1
Chronic obstructive	M	4053	116	2145	126.1	2.1	145.4	2.8	1.3	0.9	1.1	1.6	2.9	4.3
pulmonary disease	F	3210	129	1019	48.8	2.4	46.8	3.1	1.1	1.1	1.0	3.4	3.4	3.8
Other respiratory	M	2769	2273	345	32.4	33.8	19.4	218.8	5.6	3.1	2.4	1.9	2.2	2.6
disease	F	2235	1875	159	21.6	28.9	6.7	184.5	5.5	2.6	2.7	2.5	2.3	2.1
Peptic ulcer	M	293	18	217	7.1	0.3	12.1	0.1	0.2	–	–	0.3	0.8	1.0
	F	97	7	57	1.5	0.1	2.7	–	0.1	–	–	–	0.3	0.6
Liver cirrhosis and	M	1250	87	909	31.1	1.6	53.1	2.1	0.5	0.9	0.7	1.2	2.2	3.7
other liver disease	F	1143	59	626	17.9	1.1	27.4	1.2	0.5	0.8	0.4	1.7	1.2	2.1
Renal disease	M	701	126	390	17.1	2.4	22.1	1.1	0.6	0.6	1.1	3.4	3.8	6.4
	F	697	118	421	10.5	2.3	17.4	1.0	0.5	0.6	1.8	4.2	3.7	4.6
Pregnancy and birth	F	199	147	52	2.2	3.0	1.5	–	–	–	1.0	6.7	5.6	7.8
Congenital and	M	2802	2782	20	23.2	41.0	0.9	279.0	2.8	1.6	1.6	0.7	0.9	0.1
perinatal causes	F	1957	1942	13	16.8	29.6	0.5	199.3	2.2	1.9	1.5	0.9	0.8	0.7
Ill-defined causes	M	751	240	245	18.5	4.1	12.6	13.0	0.8	1.0	1.9	3.7	3.8	4.3
	F	953	152	115	13.3	2.6	5.2	10.5	0.5	0.4	1.4	2.0	1.7	1.4
Other medical causes	M	2136	703	1022	44.6	12.2	56.1	28.7	6.5	6.9	9.6	10.0	10.5	12.8
	F	2362	575	1099	33.9	10.3	47.1	22.3	6.5	5.8	8.7	9.7	9.1	10.0
ALL NON-	M	13226	7003	5819	188.3	132.4	241.0	82.8	50.6	46.6	94.8	175.6	224.6	252.1
MEDICAL CAUSES	F	4099	1978	1646	52.3	36.5	62.8	59.4	22.0	13.4	39.5	46.0	36.0	39.2
Motor vehicle	M	2868	1685	1108	39.0	32.5	45.4	7.1	13.2	10.6	21.0	47.8	59.7	68.4
traffic accidents	F	772	390	285	9.7	7.4	10.8	6.7	6.3	4.6	8.9	9.2	6.2	9.5
Fire	M	277	164	102	3.8	2.8	4.2	6.7	1.6	1.2	1.1	1.8	3.0	4.6
	F	158	95	41	1.9	1.6	1.7	5.6	1.4	0.6	0.7	0.8	1.1	1.0
Suicide	M	2398	1030	1246	37.9	20.3	52.4	–	0.1	6.4	20.9	32.3	40.0	42.5
	F	780	281	376	10.7	5.8	14.2	–	–	0.9	11.4	13.9	7.6	6.7
Homicide	M	1578	898	657	21.3	17.8	26.0	0.5	0.5	1.5	11.6	31.1	38.9	40.5
	F	392	171	190	5.2	3.4	6.7	1.0	0.7	0.6	3.8	5.2	6.6	5.8
POPULATION (thousands):	**M=males**				8057.4	5551.5	2336.2	974.7	877.2	813.7	747.0	678.1	759.1	701.7
	F=females				8561.0	5404.6	2715.4	943.2	855.5	798.9	710.5	638.6	754.7	703.2

KAZAKHSTAN: 1990

9th ICD categories

Annual death rates / 100, 000

35–39	40–44	45–49	50–54	55–59	60–64	65–69	70–74	75–79	80+/NK			
475.8	702.2	968.0	1573.8	2245.9	3435.5	4702.4	6463.6	9046.7	16674.9	M	**ALL CAUSES**	001–999
166.8	271.4	375.2	627.0	924.3	1491.9	2398.1	3651.9	5808.8	12640.2	F		
27.8	30.1	32.7	45.8	51.6	63.5	55.8	59.4	53.6	53.8	M	**Tuberculosis**	010–018, 137
7.1	5.2	6.6	8.2	7.7	11.2	11.3	13.1	13.3	19.7	F		
1.7	2.5	4.6	5.3	7.0	6.7	5.2	8.9	3.5	15.7	M	**Other infective**	Rest of 001–139
1.4	2.4	4.5	2.9	2.0	2.5	7.8	5.9	6.0	11.7	F	**and parasitic**	
46.8	100.6	203.0	447.7	713.0	1090.9	1350.8	1560.2	1707.6	1493.3	M	**ALL CANCER**	140–208
51.3	82.9	119.1	199.8	303.1	438.7	603.2	757.7	812.1	819.4	F		
2.6	4.7	9.9	16.9	23.3	33.7	41.0	26.7	50.2	31.4	M	**Mouth and**	140–149
0.3	1.4	0.6	2.3	4.7	4.7	11.3	9.8	10.6	21.1	F	**pharynx cancer**	
1.2	6.2	17.8	38.6	69.4	101.6	158.8	173.8	237.0	244.4	M	**Oesophagus cancer**	150
0.3	1.2	8.7	16.7	28.1	46.6	80.0	105.2	119.5	157.3	F		
8.9	19.2	27.4	69.4	128.8	183.0	242.6	291.2	288.9	318.4	M	**Stomach cancer**	151
7.8	12.6	18.0	28.9	43.9	67.7	95.2	129.3	164.0	158.0	F		
2.3	4.7	5.6	18.0	28.7	50.8	84.6	101.0	138.4	103.1	M	**Colorectal cancer**	153, 154
2.9	8.1	10.5	15.1	21.8	42.5	58.7	70.5	77.7	75.0	F		
...	...	...	...	...	...	...	...	...	...	M	**Liver cancer**	Not given separately
...	...	...	...	...	...	...	...	...	...	F		
...	...	...	...	...	...	...	...	...	...	M	**Pancreas cancer**	Not given separately
...	...	...	...	...	...	...	...	...	...	F		
1.0	2.7	5.6	15.7	26.8	37.3	42.8	32.7	46.7	47.1	M	**Larynx cancer**	161
0.3	0.2	0.6	2.1	3.7	2.2	3.0	3.9	2.0	5.1	F		
8.7	32.1	74.0	166.6	261.4	402.9	438.0	453.2	460.2	228.7	M	**Lung cancer**	162
2.4	4.5	8.4	14.4	32.8	46.3	66.5	75.8	71.0	47.3	F		
...	...	...	...	...	...	...	...	...	...	M	**Malignant melanoma**	Not given
...	...	...	...	...	...	...	...	...	...	F		separately
11.2	15.7	22.9	35.4	34.8	44.7	46.5	50.3	36.5	47.3	F	**Female breast cancer**	174
4.7	4.8	7.5	14.2	21.8	27.4	37.8	49.6	44.5	32.0	F	**Cervix cancer**	180
1.9	5.5	6.0	9.6	14.4	22.8	30.4	32.0	43.2	39.3	F	**Other uterine cancer**	179, 182
...	...	...	...	...	...	...	...	...	...	F	**Ovarian cancer**	Not given separately
0.2	–	0.7	2.1	6.2	16.7	29.7	52.0	90.0	107.6	M	**Prostate cancer**	185
...	...	...	...	...	...	...	...	...	...	M	**Bladder cancer**	Not given separately
...	...	...	...	...	...	...	...	...	...	F		
16.0	25.9	54.1	104.8	147.8	234.6	276.6	356.6	359.9	376.7	M	**Other and ill-defined**	Rest of 140–208,
15.1	23.1	31.3	53.1	86.1	120.6	156.9	209.7	226.4	223.6	F	**cancer sites**	incl. 155, 157, 172, 183, 188
...	...	...	...	...	...	...	...	...	...	M	**Hodgkin's disease**	Not given separately
...	...	...	...	...	...	...	...	...	...	F		
3.8	2.7	4.6	9.7	12.8	17.9	23.6	35.7	19.0	22.4	M	**Myeloma and all**	200–203,
1.7	4.0	2.4	4.0	6.7	6.6	9.6	11.8	9.3	7.3	F	**lymphomas**	incl. 201
2.1	2.2	3.3	5.8	7.8	12.3	13.1	37.1	17.3	13.5	M	**Leukaemia**	204–208
2.7	1.9	2.1	4.0	4.4	6.6	7.4	9.8	7.3	5.8	F		
102.4	215.4	355.9	570.1	878.2	1504.2	2245.2	3435.4	5408.3	11757.8	M	**ALL VASCULAR**	390–459
31.3	67.0	118.5	227.0	376.1	707.2	1323.3	2234.5	4053.8	10048.1	F	**DISEASE**	
8.9	9.2	16.2	19.2	17.8	21.0	18.3	14.9	8.7	13.5	M	**Rheumatic heart**	390–398
7.6	10.0	13.5	22.6	25.5	25.5	26.5	15.7	11.3	6.6	F	**disease and fever**	
2.3	6.0	11.6	17.4	27.9	48.4	75.9	93.6	112.5	188.3	M	**Hypertensive disease**	401–405
1.2	4.0	9.3	14.2	26.1	35.9	58.2	60.1	112.2	163.9	F		
62.8	136.2	219.5	350.3	501.6	830.5	1222.5	1809.8	2923.9	6358.7	M	**Ischaemic heart**	410–414
7.6	23.8	38.2	71.8	145.7	309.3	605.8	1089.5	2011.3	5195.2	F	**disease**	
...	...	...	...	...	...	...	...	...	...	M	**Pulmonary embolism**	Not given
...	...	...	...	...	...	...	...	...	...	F	**and other venous**	separately
15.5	39.1	78.2	131.4	256.0	478.4	721.6	1200.6	1827.0	3679.4	M	**Cerebrovascular**	430–438
10.8	22.3	47.8	95.2	152.4	282.7	527.2	869.4	1520.6	3428.3	F	**disease**	
13.0	24.9	30.4	51.8	74.9	125.8	206.8	316.5	536.3	1517.9	M	**Other vascular**	Rest of 390–459,
4.1	6.9	9.6	23.2	26.5	53.7	105.6	199.9	398.4	1254.2	F	**disease, incl. venous**	incl. 415, 451–3
7.6	17.9	30.7	74.0	148.6	281.1	458.1	711.7	953.3	1708.5	M	**Chronic obstructive**	490–496
4.9	8.3	12.3	27.6	40.5	91.6	142.1	249.5	395.8	789.5	F	**pulmonary disease**	
2.6	7.5	10.2	18.0	25.2	31.8	40.1	62.4	77.9	143.5	M	**Other respiratory**	Rest of 460–519
2.2	3.6	1.8	5.4	7.4	12.1	14.3	33.3	35.2	70.6	F	**disease**	
3.1	4.5	3.3	11.1	16.7	19.8	26.2	31.2	38.1	33.6	M	**Peptic ulcer**	531–533
–	0.5	0.3	1.3	4.4	4.9	7.4	3.3	9.3	10.2	F		
7.0	17.4	23.8	48.4	55.5	89.7	130.0	112.9	148.8	206.3	M	**Liver cirrhosis and**	570–573, 576,
3.4	6.7	14.4	23.6	32.8	47.7	63.0	81.0	104.2	128.9	F	**other liver disease**	575.2–579.9
4.7	8.5	10.9	23.4	19.0	32.6	55.8	72.8	114.2	157.0	M	**Renal disease**	580–590
4.9	7.8	11.4	18.8	19.4	27.1	32.2	35.3	30.5	42.2	F		
5.6	3.3	0.6	0.4	0.3	–	–	–	–	–	F	**Pregnancy and birth**	630–676
1.0	0.2	–	1.2	1.6	0.8	1.7	–	–	–	M	**Congenital and**	740–779
0.5	0.5	1.2	0.4	0.7	–	–	0.7		0.7	F	**perinatal causes**	
4.3	5.5	8.3	13.0	16.7	20.2	20.1	44.6	86.5	417.0	M	**Ill-defined causes**	780–799
0.7	2.4	2.7	4.0	6.0	5.8	14.8	22.9	82.3	383.8	F		
18.3	22.2	36.0	45.3	67.9	83.8	119.5	173.8	264.7	316.1	M	**Other medical causes**	Rest of 001–799
12.2	19.7	24.7	39.3	54.9	72.9	106.0	131.3	154.1	185.7	F		
248.4	269.9	248.6	270.5	245.2	210.4	193.7	190.2	190.3	372.2	M	**ALL NON-**	E800–E999
41.3	61.1	57.1	68.2	69.0	70.2	72.6	83.6	112.2	129.6	F	**MEDICAL CAUSES**	
54.9	50.3	41.9	47.2	46.9	36.5	40.1	40.1	41.5	53.8	M	**Motor vehicle**	E810–E819
8.1	8.1	9.0	12.6	12.1	13.2	12.6	19.6	25.2	21.1	F	**traffic accidents**	
3.0	4.5	4.3	6.7	3.9	4.8	2.6	4.5	6.9	9.0	M	**Fire**	E890–E899
0.8	1.0	2.1	1.0	2.7	1.1	3.5	2.0	4.6	8.7	F		
50.2	49.6	57.8	60.6	57.0	50.4	41.0	52.0	67.5	107.6	M	**Suicide**	E950–E959
8.3	12.6	11.4	17.8	14.4	20.3	14.8	24.2	33.2	26.2	F		
34.1	40.3	30.0	21.5	17.8	18.7	19.2	11.9	8.7	22.4	M	**Homicide**	E960–E969
7.1	12.4	5.7	6.3	5.0	5.5	5.2	9.1	2.7	9.5	F		
575.2	401.6	302.9	432.2	257.8	251.9	114.6	67.3	57.8	44.6	M	**POPULATION (thousands)**	
590.6	420.8	332.6	478.0	298.6	364.7	230.1	153.1	150.6	137.3	F		

KAZAKHSTAN: Males

	All ages	0–34	35–69	35–39	40–44	45–49	50–54	55–59	60–64	65–69	70–74	75–79	80+/NK
POPULATION (1000s)													
1985–90	7813.4	5471.9	2165.7	513.4	313.1	415.4	344.9	287.8	194.4	96.7	76.5	54.4	44.9
1985	7568.3	5372.4	2011.8	419.0	318.9	466.3	286.7	291.0	140.4	89.5	86.3	52.8	45.0
1990	**8057.4**	**5551.5**	**2336.2**	**575.2**	**401.6**	**302.9**	**432.2**	**257.8**	**251.9**	**114.6**	**67.3**	**57.8**	**44.6**
1995 projected	*8454.0*	*5824.8*	*2451.2*	*603.5*	*421.4*	*317.8*	*453.5*	*270.5*	*264.3*	*120.2*	*70.6*	*60.6*	*46.8*
NUMBER OF DEATHS													
All causes													
1985–90	65553	16684	31575	2413	2190	4054	5370	6379	6650	4519	4968	5147	7179
1985	67166	18062	31105	2419	2515	5184	4808	7018	4919	4242	5810	5211	6978
1990	**68134**	**15994**	**35124**	**2737**	**2820**	**2932**	**6802**	**5790**	**8654**	**5389**	**4350**	**5229**	**7437**
1995 projected	*66282*	*14035*	*34607*	*2516*	*2562*	*2790*	*6572*	*5804*	*8851*	*5512*	*4322*	*5371*	*7947*
Lung cancer													
1985–90	3470	31	2808	44	83	295	518	747	740	381	328	209	94
1985	2977	38	2352	30	110	330	410	708	459	305	348	156	83
1990	**4024**	**37**	**3314**	**50**	**129**	**224**	**720**	**674**	**1015**	**502**	**305**	**266**	**102**
1995 projected	*4891*	*36*	*3931*	*45*	*127*	*245*	*811*	*810*	*1265*	*628*	*409*	*364*	*151*
ANNUAL DEATH RATE / 100,000 (*The rates for the age groups 0–34 and 35–69 are the means of seven five–yearly rates, but the all–ages rates are standardised to the conventional "European" age distribution)													
All causes													
1985–90	1604.3*	288.5*	2001.8*	470.0	699.5	975.9	1557.0	2216.5	3420.8	4673.2	6494.1	9461.4	15988.9
1985	1678.4*	323.1*	2115.7*	577.3	788.6	1111.7	1677.0	2411.7	3503.6	4739.7	6732.3	9869.3	15506.7
1990	**1606.1***	**276.3***	**2014.8***	**475.8**	**702.2**	**968.0**	**1573.8**	**2245.9**	**3435.5**	**4702.4**	**6463.6**	**9046.7**	**16674.9**
1995 projected	*1535.4**	*235.4**	*1918.9**	*416.9*	*608.0*	*877.9*	*1449.2*	*2145.7*	*3348.8*	*4585.7*	*6121.8*	*8863.0*	*16980.8*
All cancer													
1985–90	316.4*	10.6*	555.0*	46.6	101.9	217.9	434.6	714.0	1066.9	1303.0	1520.3	1667.3	1389.8
1985	300.3*	11.0*	522.3*	53.2	116.7	232.3	420.0	700.7	965.8	1167.6	1456.5	1505.7	1322.2
1990	**323.7***	**11.4***	**564.7***	**46.8**	**100.6**	**203.0**	**447.7**	**713.0**	**1090.9**	**1350.8**	**1560.2**	**1707.6**	**1493.3**
1995 projected	*346.4**	*10.1**	*600.2**	*36.1*	*81.4*	*190.4*	*443.4*	*759.0*	*1199.8*	*1491.7*	*1733.7*	*1892.7*	*1685.9*
Lung cancer													
1985–90	93.4*	0.6*	184.4*	8.6	26.5	71.0	150.2	259.6	380.7	394.0	428.8	384.2	209.4
1985	84.6*	0.8*	166.6*	7.2	34.5	70.8	143.0	243.3	326.9	340.8	403.2	295.5	184.4
1990	**100.8***	**0.7***	**197.7***	**8.7**	**32.1**	**74.0**	**166.6**	**261.4**	**402.9**	**438.0**	**453.2**	**460.2**	**228.7**
1995 projected	*119.5**	*0.7**	*227.7**	*7.5*	*30.1*	*77.1*	*178.8*	*299.4*	*478.6*	*522.5*	*579.3*	*600.7*	*322.6*
Upper aerodigestive cancer (mouth, oesophagus, pharynx and larynx)													
1985–90	54.7*	0.5*	92.5*	4.5	15.0	36.8	72.5	120.6	172.8	225.4	244.4	314.3	347.4
1985	53.5*	0.5*	85.5*	5.3	14.4	42.0	62.8	122.3	173.8	177.7	243.3	361.7	344.4
1990	**54.6***	**0.6***	**94.0***	**4.9**	**13.7**	**33.3**	**71.3**	**119.5**	**172.7**	**242.6**	**233.3**	**333.9**	**322.9**
1995 projected	*54.7**	*0.6**	*98.1**	*4.0*	*10.7*	*31.5*	*68.8*	*119.0*	*191.4*	*261.2*	*238.0*	*305.3*	*299.1*
Other cancer													
1985–90	168.3*	9.5*	278.1*	33.5	60.4	110.0	211.9	333.9	513.4	683.6	847.1	968.8	833.0
1985	162.2*	9.7*	270.2*	40.8	67.7	119.5	214.2	335.1	465.1	649.2	810.0	848.5	793.3
1990	**168.4***	**10.1***	**273.0***	**33.2**	**54.8**	**95.7**	**209.9**	**332.0**	**515.3**	**670.2**	**873.7**	**913.5**	**941.7**
1995 projected	*172.2**	*8.8**	*274.4**	*24.7*	*40.6*	*81.8*	*195.8*	*340.5*	*529.7*	*708.0*	*916.4*	*986.8*	*1064.1*
Chronic obstructive pulmonary disease (COPD)													
1985–90	135.5*	2.9*	155.5*	10.5	22.0	39.0	87.9	161.6	296.3	471.6	745.1	1117.6	1741.6
1985	156.8*	3.7*	183.6*	16.0	30.4	53.8	120.3	195.2	321.9	547.5	881.8	1287.9	1875.6
1990	**126.1***	**2.1***	**145.4***	**7.6**	**17.9**	**30.7**	**74.0**	**148.6**	**281.1**	**458.1**	**711.7**	**953.3**	**1708.5**
1995 projected	*100.7**	*1.3**	*115.4**	*4.8*	*11.6*	*20.8*	*51.2*	*115.3*	*230.0*	*374.4*	*548.2*	*760.7*	*1438.0*
Other respiratory disease													
1985–90	45.2*	51.1*	24.0*	5.8	9.3	13.2	20.3	28.8	40.1	50.7	73.2	104.8	169.3
1985	59.9*	70.8*	32.8*	11.5	15.1	19.1	22.7	36.8	65.5	59.2	73.0	117.4	175.6
1990	**32.4***	**33.8***	**19.4***	**2.6**	**7.5**	**10.2**	**18.0**	**25.2**	**31.8**	**40.1**	**62.4**	**77.9**	**143.5**
1995 projected	*21.0**	*20.2**	*13.4**	*1.7*	*4.7*	*6.9*	*12.6*	*17.4*	*21.9*	*28.3*	*43.9*	*59.4*	*109.0*
Vascular disease													
1985–90	746.5*	13.8*	822.9*	103.4	215.6	339.0	565.1	831.8	1477.9	2227.5	3428.8	5614.0	11300.7
1985	766.7*	15.8*	859.6*	119.1	241.5	375.7	576.9	900.7	1552.7	2250.3	3560.8	5960.2	10962.2
1990	**758.1***	**14.1***	**838.8***	**102.4**	**215.4**	**355.9**	**570.1**	**878.2**	**1504.2**	**2245.2**	**3435.4**	**5408.3**	**11757.8**
1995 projected	*732.9**	*10.9**	*797.8**	*81.0*	*181.3*	*323.2*	*542.9*	*841.4*	*1452.5*	*2162.2*	*3185.6*	*5244.2*	*11927.4*
Liver cirrhosis and other liver disease													
1985–90	32.8*	1.7*	55.2*	8.0	18.8	30.3	47.8	65.7	93.6	122.0	134.6	165.4	187.1
1985	37.9*	2.4*	67.0*	13.6	23.8	39.2	56.5	86.9	108.3	140.8	139.0	185.6	160.0
1990	**31.1***	**1.6***	**53.1***	**7.0**	**17.4**	**23.8**	**48.4**	**55.5**	**89.7**	**130.0**	**112.9**	**148.8**	**206.3**
1995 projected	*25.6**	*1.1**	*41.5**	*4.5*	*11.4*	*17.0*	*33.5*	*41.8*	*72.3*	*109.8*	*93.5*	*143.6*	*211.5*
Other medical causes													
1985–90	159.0*	91.0*	172.6*	69.3	95.8	118.4	157.4	196.3	251.5	319.5	403.9	577.2	908.7
1985	178.7*	107.6*	209.6*	113.6	137.7	159.3	206.8	235.4	265.0	349.7	403.2	554.9	673.3
1990	**146.5***	**80.9***	**152.5***	**61.0**	**73.5**	**95.7**	**145.1**	**180.4**	**227.5**	**284.5**	**390.8**	**560.6**	**993.3**
1995 projected	*124.8**	*58.3**	*117.2**	*38.8*	*47.7*	*64.2*	*100.3*	*138.6*	*182.0*	*248.8*	*364.0*	*602.3*	*1256.4*
All non–medical causes													
1985–90	168.8*	117.4*	216.6*	226.3	236.0	218.1	243.8	218.2	194.4	178.9	188.2	215.1	291.8
1985	178.2*	111.7*	240.7*	250.4	223.6	232.3	273.8	256.0	224.4	224.6	217.8	257.6	337.8
1990	**188.3***	**132.4***	**241.0***	**248.4**	**269.9**	**248.6**	**270.5**	**245.2**	**210.4**	**193.7**	**190.2**	**190.3**	**372.2**
1995 projected	*184.1**	*133.5**	*233.4**	*250.0*	*269.8*	*255.5*	*265.3*	*232.2*	*190.3*	*170.5*	*153.0*	*160.1*	*352.6*

KAZAKHSTAN: Females

	All ages	0–34	35–69	35–39	40–44	45–49	50–54	55–59	60–64	65–69	70–74	75–79	80+/NK
POPULATION (1000s)													
1985–90	8348.0	5355.2	2551.8	529.6	330.4	450.9	377.7	353.5	315.6	194.1	173.7	137.8	129.5
1985	8127.8	5276.8	2406.6	432.7	342.9	497.0	310.8	387.4	256.4	179.4	194.7	128.3	121.4
1990	**8561.0**	**5404.6**	**2715.4**	**590.6**	**420.8**	**332.6**	**478.0**	**298.6**	**364.7**	**230.1**	**153.1**	**150.6**	**137.3**
1995 projected	*8982.2*	*5670.5*	*2849.0*	*619.7*	*441.5*	*349.0*	*501.5*	*313.3*	*382.6*	*241.4*	*160.6*	*158.0*	*144.1*
NUMBER OF DEATHS													
All causes													
1985–90	59606	9901	19016	936	907	1749	2477	3359	4857	4731	6423	8425	15841
1985	59620	10812	18870	937	968	2273	2214	4038	4135	4305	7322	7976	14640
1990	**60653**	**8868**	**20091**	**985**	**1142**	**1248**	**2997**	**2760**	**5441**	**5518**	**5591**	**8748**	**17355**
1995 projected	*60128*	*7513*	*19468*	*892*	*1019*	*1148*	*2738*	*2617*	*5437*	*5617*	*5618*	*9136*	*18393*
Lung cancer													
1985–90	772	20	476	14	16	36	61	95	141	113	118	99	59
1985	694	15	433	11	16	51	42	102	113	98	107	85	54
1990	**857**	**19**	**550**	**14**	**19**	**28**	**69**	**98**	**169**	**153**	**116**	**107**	**65**
1995 projected	*1039*	*22*	*654*	*14*	*17*	*28*	*80*	*114*	*206*	*195*	*146*	*144*	*73*
ANNUAL DEATH RATE / 100,000													
All causes													
1985–90	903.1*	167.2*	917.4*	176.7	274.5	387.9	655.8	950.2	1539.0	2437.4	3697.8	6113.9	12232.4
1985	935.0*	188.3*	960.5*	216.5	282.3	457.3	712.4	1042.3	1612.7	2399.7	3760.7	6216.7	12059.3
1990	**884.6***	**150.0***	**893.5***	**166.8**	**271.4**	**375.2**	**627.0**	**924.3**	**1491.9**	**2398.1**	**3651.9**	**5808.8**	**12640.2**
1995 projected	*842.5**	*124.2**	*833.3**	*143.9*	*230.8*	*328.9*	*546.0*	*835.3*	*1421.1*	*2326.8*	*3498.1*	*5782.3*	*12764.1*
All cancer													
1985–90	155.5*	10.2*	261.5*	47.8	79.3	122.6	213.4	310.9	454.7	601.8	718.5	812.0	737.5
1985	153.9*	9.9*	263.3*	47.8	69.1	134.8	207.5	332.7	467.6	583.6	667.7	776.3	729.0
1990	**156.4***	**10.2***	**256.9***	**51.3**	**82.9**	**119.1**	**199.8**	**303.1**	**438.7**	**603.2**	**757.7**	**812.1**	**819.4**
1995 projected	*158.8**	*10.3**	*253.0**	*53.9*	*81.8*	*115.2*	*182.9*	*282.5*	*426.3*	*628.8*	*805.7*	*901.3*	*887.6*
Lung cancer													
1985–90	13.0*	0.4*	23.1*	2.6	4.8	8.0	16.2	26.9	44.7	58.2	67.9	71.8	45.6
1985	12.2*	0.3*	22.3*	2.5	4.7	10.3	13.5	26.3	44.1	54.6	55.0	66.3	44.5
1990	**13.9***	**0.4***	**25.1***	**2.4**	**4.5**	**8.4**	**14.4**	**32.8**	**46.3**	**66.5**	**75.8**	**71.0**	**47.3**
1995 projected	*16.0**	*0.4**	*28.7**	*2.3*	*3.9*	*8.0*	*16.0*	*36.4*	*53.8*	*80.8*	*90.9*	*91.1*	*50.7*
Upper aerodigestive cancer (mouth, oesophagus, pharynx and larynx)													
1985–90	21.2*	0.3*	32.6*	1.5	3.9	10.6	22.5	37.3	59.9	92.2	116.9	131.3	164.5
1985	22.1*	0.2*	33.8*	1.6	3.8	11.1	27.0	44.7	65.1	83.1	108.4	139.5	179.6
1990	**21.1***	**0.2***	**31.3***	**1.0**	**2.9**	**9.9**	**21.1**	**36.5**	**53.5**	**94.3**	**118.9**	**132.1**	**183.5**
1995 projected	*20.2**	*0.2**	*29.4**	*0.6*	*2.3*	*8.0*	*17.1*	*29.4*	*51.0*	*97.3*	*122.7*	*132.9*	*181.8*
Other cancer													
1985–90	121.3*	9.5*	205.9*	43.6	70.5	104.0	174.7	246.7	350.1	451.3	533.7	608.9	527.4
1985	119.7*	9.3*	207.3*	43.7	60.7	113.5	167.0	261.7	358.4	445.9	504.4	570.5	504.9
1990	**121.5***	**9.6***	**200.5***	**47.9**	**75.6**	**100.7**	**164.2**	**233.8**	**338.9**	**442.4**	**563.0**	**608.9**	**588.5**
1995 projected	*122.6**	*9.7**	*194.9**	*51.0*	*75.7*	*99.1*	*149.8*	*216.7*	*321.5*	*450.7*	*592.2*	*677.2*	*655.1*
Chronic obstructive pulmonary disease (COPD)													
1985–90	52.4*	2.5*	51.5*	5.5	10.0	14.4	28.9	53.5	89.7	158.7	261.4	441.2	816.2
1985	61.2*	3.5*	60.3*	8.1	10.5	18.9	40.5	66.6	112.7	165.0	320.0	480.9	928.3
1990	**48.8***	**2.4***	**46.8***	**4.9**	**8.3**	**12.3**	**27.6**	**40.5**	**91.6**	**142.1**	**249.5**	**395.8**	**789.5**
1995 projected	*39.3**	*1.9**	*36.1**	*3.2*	*5.7*	*8.6*	*19.3*	*29.0*	*72.7*	*113.9*	*201.1*	*325.3*	*664.1*
Other respiratory disease													
1985–90	30.8*	43.3*	8.3*	2.3	3.6	4.0	6.1	8.2	13.9	20.1	32.8	48.6	82.6
1985	40.8*	58.8*	10.1*	2.1	5.2	5.2	6.4	9.6	19.5	22.9	40.1	51.4	101.3
1990	**21.6***	**28.9***	**6.7***	**2.2**	**3.6**	**1.8**	**5.4**	**7.4**	**12.1**	**14.3**	**33.3**	**35.2**	**70.6**
1995 projected	*13.8**	*17.9**	*4.7**	*1.5*	*2.5*	*1.1*	*3.8*	*5.1*	*8.6*	*10.4*	*23.7*	*24.7*	*50.0*
Vascular disease													
1985–90	502.4*	7.6*	415.4*	34.2	69.9	122.4	239.3	381.6	731.0	1329.2	2322.4	4322.9	9861.8
1985	512.7*	8.0*	431.7*	43.7	74.1	146.1	271.6	417.1	767.6	1301.6	2379.0	4456.0	9763.6
1990	**494.5***	**7.2***	**407.2***	**31.3**	**67.0**	**118.5**	**227.0**	**376.1**	**707.2**	**1323.3**	**2234.5**	**4053.8**	**10048.1**
1995 projected	*472.9**	*6.3**	*378.2**	*25.3*	*53.7*	*98.0*	*194.4*	*335.5*	*682.2*	*1258.1*	*2069.7*	*3892.4*	*9965.3*
Liver cirrhosis and other liver disease													
1985–90	18.2*	1.3*	28.0*	4.9	7.6	14.0	21.7	32.2	47.5	68.0	81.8	104.5	131.3
1985	18.9*	1.4*	31.0*	6.9	11.4	18.1	22.2	38.7	45.2	74.7	79.6	97.4	111.2
1990	**17.9***	**1.1***	**27.4***	**3.4**	**6.7**	**14.4**	**23.6**	**32.8**	**47.7**	**63.0**	**81.0**	**104.2**	**128.9**
1995 projected	*17.4**	*1.0**	*25.0**	*2.3*	*4.5*	*12.3*	*20.9*	*31.9*	*43.1*	*60.1*	*79.1*	*119.0*	*144.3*
Other medical causes													
1985–90	94.5*	69.5*	92.7*	42.1	50.5	55.7	79.2	98.7	134.3	188.6	196.9	274.3	471.0
1985	93.9*	74.1*	95.1*	54.1	53.7	68.8	82.4	99.1	128.7	178.9	188.0	244.7	290.8
1990	**93.0***	**63.7***	**85.8***	**32.3**	**41.8**	**52.0**	**75.3**	**95.4**	**124.5**	**179.5**	**212.3**	**295.5**	**654.0**
1995 projected	*90.0**	*48.4**	*79.5**	*21.8*	*29.2*	*42.4*	*66.4*	*90.0*	*121.8*	*185.2*	*236.0*	*412.7*	*924.4*
All non-medical causes													
1985–90	49.4*	32.9*	59.9*	40.0	53.6	54.8	67.2	65.1	67.8	71.1	84.1	110.3	132.0
1985	53.5*	32.7*	68.9*	53.8	58.3	65.4	81.7	78.5	71.4	73.0	86.3	109.9	135.1
1990	**52.3***	**36.5***	**62.8***	**41.3**	**61.1**	**57.1**	**68.2**	**69.0**	**70.2**	**72.6**	**83.6**	**112.2**	**129.6**
1995 projected	*50.3**	*38.5**	*56.7**	*36.0*	*53.5*	*51.3*	*58.2*	*61.3*	*66.4*	*70.4*	*82.8*	*107.0*	*128.4*

(*The rates for the age groups 0–34 and 35–69 are the means of seven five-yearly rates, but the all-ages rates are standardised to the conventional "European" age distribution)

KAZAKHSTAN: 1985–1990

Smoking–attributed deaths (Sm.) and total deaths (Total)

		ALL CAUSES	ALL CANCER	Lung cancer	Upper aero–digestive ca.	Other cancer	COPD	Other respiratory	Vascular disease	Cirrhosis/other liver	Other medical	Non–medical
Males												
0–34	Sm.	–	–	–	–	–	–	–	–	–	–	–
	Total	16684	559	31	23	505	158	3375	682	87	5685	6138
35–69	Sm.	13577	4804	2689	1056	1059	1785	184	5349	–	1455	–
	Total	31575	8351	2808	1374	4169	2085	394	11984	880	3054	4827
		(43%)	(58%)	(96%)	(77%)	(25%)	(86%)	(47%)	(45%)		(48%)	
70+	Sm.	3614	1022	565	282	175	1347	20	1112	–	113	–
	Total	17294	2694	631	514	1549	1960	189	10751	277	1031	392
		(21%)	(38%)	(90%)	(55%)	(11%)	(69%)	(11%)	(10%)		(11%)	
Any age	Sm.	17191	5826	3254	1338	1234	3132	204	6461	–	1568	–
	Total	65553	11604	3470	1911	6223	4203	3958	23417	1244	9770	11357
		(26%)	(50%)	(94%)	(70%)	(20%)	(75%)	(5%)	(28%)		(16%)	
Females												
0–34	Sm.	–	–	–	–	–	–	–	–	–	–	–
	Total	9901	521	20	14	487	132	2773	384	65	4225	1801
35–69	Sm.	2020	530	287	186	57	473	18	800	–	199	–
	Total	19016	5576	476	654	4446	1016	177	8104	592	2079	1472
		(11%)	(10%)	(60%)	(28%)	(1%)	(47%)	(10%)	(10%)		(10%)	
70+	Sm.	1823	319	152	141	26	837	6	619	–	42	–
	Total	30689	3322	276	597	2449	2119	231	22762	456	1330	469
		(6%)	(10%)	(55%)	(24%)	(1%)	(39%)	(3%)	(3%)		(3%)	
Any age	Sm.	3843	849	439	327	83	1310	24	1419	–	241	–
	Total	59606	9419	772	1265	7382	3267	3181	31250	1113	7634	3742
		(6%)	(9%)	(57%)	(26%)	(1%)	(40%)	(1%)	(5%)		(3%)	
Males+Females												
0–34	Sm.	–	–	–	–	–	–	–	–	–	–	–
	Total	26585	1080	51	37	992	290	6148	1066	152	9910	7939
35–69	Sm.	15597	5334	2976	1242	1116	2258	202	6149	–	1654	–
	Total	50591	13927	3284	2028	8615	3101	571	20088	1472	5133	6299
		(31%)	(38%)	(91%)	(61%)	(13%)	(73%)	(35%)	(31%)		(32%)	
70+	Sm.	5437	1341	717	423	201	2184	26	1731	–	155	–
	Total	47983	6016	907	1111	3998	4079	420	33513	733	2361	861
		(11%)	(22%)	(79%)	(38%)	(5%)	(54%)	(6%)	(5%)		(7%)	
Any age	Sm.	21034	6675	3693	1665	1317	4442	228	7880	–	1809	–
	Total	125159	21023	4242	3176	13605	7470	7139	54667	2357	17404	15099
		(17%)	(32%)	(87%)	(52%)	(10%)	(59%)	(3%)	(14%)		(10%)	

KAZAKHSTAN: 1985

Smoking–attributed deaths (Sm.) and total deaths (Total)

		ALL CAUSES	ALL CANCER	Lung cancer	Upper aero–digestive ca.	Other cancer	COPD	Other respiratory	Vascular disease	Cirrhosis/other liver	Other medical	Non–medical
Males												
0–34	Sm.	–	–	–	–	–	–	–	–	–	–	–
	Total	18062	557	38	25	494	195	4463	743	118	6291	5695
35–69	Sm.	12943	4068	2246	911	911	1919	229	5009	–	1718	–
	Total	31105	7322	2352	1203	3767	2270	502	11490	1009	3621	4891
		(42%)	(56%)	(95%)	(76%)	(24%)	(85%)	(46%)	(44%)		(47%)	
70+	Sm.	3531	943	517	277	149	1461	19	1011	–	97	–
	Total	17999	2647	587	556	1504	2285	204	11153	290	944	476
		(20%)	(36%)	(88%)	(50%)	(10%)	(64%)	(9%)	(9%)		(10%)	
Any age	Sm.	16474	5011	2763	1188	1060	3380	248	6020	–	1815	–
	Total	67166	10526	2977	1784	5765	4750	5169	23386	1417	10856	11062
		(25%)	(48%)	(93%)	(67%)	(18%)	(71%)	(5%)	(26%)		(17%)	
Females												
0–34	Sm.	–	–	–	–	–	–	–	–	–	–	–
	Total	10812	484	15	12	457	182	3616	393	68	4317	1752
35–69	Sm.	1940	482	254	177	51	512	19	740	–	187	–
	Total	18870	5294	433	648	4213	1134	201	7932	628	2051	1630
		(10%)	(9%)	(59%)	(27%)	(1%)	(45%)	(9%)	(9%)		(9%)	
70+	Sm.	1600	257	119	118	20	818	6	492	–	27	–
	Total	29938	3181	246	608	2327	2367	267	22202	415	1033	473
		(5%)	(8%)	(48%)	(19%)	(1%)	(35%)	(2%)	(2%)		(3%)	
Any age	Sm.	3540	739	373	295	71	1330	25	1232	–	214	–
	Total	59620	8959	694	1268	6997	3683	4084	30527	1111	7401	3855
		(6%)	(8%)	(54%)	(23%)	(1%)	(36%)	(1%)	(4%)		(3%)	
Males+Females												
0–34	Sm.	–	–	–	–	–	–	–	–	–	–	–
	Total	28874	1041	53	37	951	377	8079	1136	186	10608	7447
35–69	Sm.	14883	4550	2500	1088	962	2431	248	5749	–	1905	–
	Total	49975	12616	2785	1851	7980	3404	703	19422	1637	5672	6521
		(30%)	(36%)	(90%)	(59%)	(12%)	(71%)	(35%)	(30%)		(34%)	
70+	Sm.	5131	1200	636	395	169	2279	25	1503	–	124	–
	Total	47937	5828	833	1164	3831	4652	471	33355	705	1977	949
		(11%)	(21%)	(76%)	(34%)	(4%)	(49%)	(5%)	(5%)		(6%)	
Any age	Sm.	20014	5750	3136	1483	1131	4710	273	7252	–	2029	–
	Total	126786	19485	3671	3052	12762	8433	9253	53913	2528	18257	14917
		(16%)	(30%)	(85%)	(49%)	(9%)	(56%)	(3%)	(13%)		(11%)	

(To be conservative, no deaths before age 35, and none from liver cirrhosis or non–medical causes, were attributed to smoking.)

KAZAKHSTAN: 1990

Smoking–attributed deaths (Sm.) and total deaths (Total)

		ALL CAUSES	ALL CANCER	Lung cancer	Upper aero–digestive ca.	Other cancer	COPD	Other respiratory	Vascular disease	Cirrhosis/ other liver	Other medical	Non–medical
Males												
0–34	Sm.	–	–	–	–	–	–	–	–	–	–	–
	Total	15994	618	37	31	550	116	2273	717	87	5180	7003
35–69	Sm.	15180	5557	3181	1177	1199	1853	164	6189	–	1417	–
	Total	35124	9357	3314	1513	4530	2145	345	13622	909	2927	5819
		(43%)	(59%)	(96%)	(78%)	(26%)	(86%)	(48%)	(45%)		(48%)	
70+	Sm.	3739	1089	609	287	193	1289	18	1221	–	122	–
	Total	17016	2703	673	494	1536	1792	151	10682	254	1030	404
		(22%)	(40%)	(90%)	(58%)	(13%)	(72%)	(12%)	(11%)		(12%)	
Any age	Sm.	18919	6646	3790	1464	1392	3142	182	7410	–	1539	–
	Total	68134	12678	4024	2038	6616	4053	2769	25021	1250	9137	13226
		(28%)	(52%)	(94%)	(72%)	(21%)	(78%)	(7%)	(30%)		(17%)	
Females												
0–34	Sm.	–	–	–	–	–	–	–	–	–	–	–
	Total	8868	534	19	13	502	129	1875	364	59	3929	1978
35–69	Sm.	2336	625	348	209	68	512	18	962	–	219	–
	Total	20091	5896	550	673	4673	1019	159	8693	626	2052	1646
		(12%)	(11%)	(63%)	(31%)	(1%)	(50%)	(11%)	(11%)		(11%)	
70+	Sm.	1853	343	161	153	29	818	7	635	–	50	–
	Total	31694	3508	288	633	2587	2062	201	23322	458	1668	475
		(6%)	(10%)	(56%)	(24%)	(1%)	(40%)	(3%)	(3%)		(3%)	
Any age	Sm.	4189	968	509	362	97	1330	25	1597	–	269	–
	Total	60653	9938	857	1319	7762	3210	2235	32379	1143	7649	4099
		(7%)	(10%)	(59%)	(27%)	(1%)	(41%)	(1%)	(5%)		(4%)	
Males+Females												
0–34	Sm.	–	–	–	–	–	–	–	–	–	–	–
	Total	24862	1152	56	44	1052	245	4148	1081	146	9109	8981
35–69	Sm.	17516	6182	3529	1386	1267	2365	182	7151	–	1636	–
	Total	55215	15253	3864	2186	9203	3164	504	22315	1535	4979	7465
		(32%)	(41%)	(91%)	(63%)	(14%)	(75%)	(36%)	(32%)		(33%)	
70+	Sm.	5592	1432	770	440	222	2107	25	1856	–	172	–
	Total	48710	6211	961	1127	4123	3854	352	34004	712	2698	879
		(11%)	(23%)	(80%)	(39%)	(5%)	(55%)	(7%)	(5%)		(6%)	
Any age	Sm.	23108	7614	4299	1826	1489	4472	207	9007	–	1808	–
	Total	128787	22616	4881	3357	14378	7263	5004	57400	2393	16786	17325
		(18%)	(34%)	(88%)	(54%)	(10%)	(62%)	(4%)	(16%)		(11%)	

KAZAKHSTAN: 1995

Smoking–attributed deaths (Sm.) and total deaths (Total)

		ALL CAUSES	ALL CANCER	Lung cancer	Upper aero–digestive ca.	Other cancer	COPD	Other respiratory	Vascular disease	Cirrhosis/ other liver	Other medical	Non–medical
Males												
0–34	Sm.	–	–	–	–	–	–	–	–	–	–	–
	Total	14035	572	36	32	504	77	1424	581	62	3955	7364
35–69	Sm.	15753	6435	3792	1298	1345	1535	125	6520	–	1138	–
	Total	34607	10194	3931	1623	4640	1746	248	13456	717	2249	5997
		(46%)	(63%)	(96%)	(80%)	(29%)	(88%)	(50%)	(48%)		(51%)	
70+	Sm.	4401	1455	857	321	277	1174	17	1580	–	175	–
	Total	17640	3160	924	493	1743	1521	118	11009	252	1210	370
		(25%)	(46%)	(93%)	(65%)	(16%)	(77%)	(14%)	(14%)		(14%)	
Any age	Sm.	20154	7890	4649	1619	1622	2709	142	8100	–	1313	–
	Total	66282	13926	4891	2148	6887	3344	1790	25046	1031	7414	13731
		(30%)	(57%)	(95%)	(75%)	(24%)	(81%)	(8%)	(32%)		(18%)	
Females												
0–34	Sm.	–	–	–	–	–	–	–	–	–	–	–
	Total	7513	563	22	11	530	103	1209	332	54	3125	2127
35–69	Sm.	2584	758	443	232	83	451	14	1117	–	244	–
	Total	19468	6048	654	650	4744	816	117	8409	592	1940	1546
		(13%)	(13%)	(68%)	(36%)	(2%)	(55%)	(12%)	(13%)		(13%)	
70+	Sm.	2419	496	236	213	47	893	7	928	–	95	–
	Total	33147	3997	363	669	2965	1794	149	23834	523	2363	487
		(7%)	(12%)	(65%)	(32%)	(2%)	(50%)	(5%)	(4%)		(4%)	
Any age	Sm.	5003	1254	679	445	130	1344	21	2045	–	339	–
	Total	60128	10608	1039	1330	8239	2713	1475	32575	1169	7428	4160
		(8%)	(12%)	(65%)	(33%)	(2%)	(50%)	(1%)	(6%)		(5%)	
Males+Females												
0–34	Sm.	–	–	–	–	–	–	–	–	–	–	–
	Total	21548	1135	58	43	1034	180	2633	913	116	7080	9491
35–69	Sm.	18337	7193	4235	1530	1428	1986	139	7637	–	1382	–
	Total	54075	16242	4585	2273	9384	2562	365	21865	1309	4189	7543
		(34%)	(44%)	(92%)	(67%)	(15%)	(78%)	(38%)	(35%)		(33%)	
70+	Sm.	6820	1951	1093	534	324	2067	24	2508	–	270	–
	Total	50787	7157	1287	1162	4708	3315	267	34843	775	3573	857
		(13%)	(27%)	(85%)	(46%)	(7%)	(62%)	(9%)	(7%)		(8%)	
Any age	Sm.	25157	9144	5328	2064	1752	4053	163	10145	–	1652	–
	Total	126410	24534	5930	3478	15126	6057	3265	57621	2200	14842	17891
		(20%)	(37%)	(90%)	(59%)	(12%)	(67%)	(5%)	(18%)		(11%)	

(To be conservative, no deaths before age 35, and none from liver cirrhosis or non–medical causes, were attributed to smoking.)

¶KYRGYZSTAN: 1990

		No. of deaths			Standardised rates (Defined on p.406)			Annual death rates / 100, 000						
		All ages	0–34	35–69	All ages	0–34	35–69	0–4	5–9	10–14	15–19	20–24	25–29	30–34
ALL CAUSES	M	16338	5192	7092	1491.6	299.9	1752.4	961.4	73.2	78.3	106.1	201.1	290.1	389.2
	F	14242	3362	4235	875.7	183.5	849.7	761.7	53.9	35.4	65.1	91.1	117.7	159.8
Tuberculosis	M	209	37	154	18.4	3.0	33.3	0.6	–	–	1.4	1.6	5.3	11.7
	F	89	33	48	5.4	2.5	8.1	0.6	–	–	–	6.7	7.8	2.4
Other infective and parasitic	M	486	448	30	15.7	21.0	6.4	128.4	5.9	3.4	2.8	3.3	1.6	1.8
	F	433	407	18	13.1	20.4	3.4	110.6	7.2	1.7	2.4	7.8	6.8	6.7
ALL CANCER	M	1888	152	1365	198.7	10.9	348.6	5.7	2.2	7.7	11.3	13.0	12.3	24.0
	F	1446	99	854	104.2	7.5	169.6	2.6	1.1	3.0	4.3	3.9	13.1	24.2
Mouth and pharynx cancer	M	58	6	45	5.7	0.5	10.6	–	–	–	0.5	0.5	1.6	0.6
	F	13	2	5	0.9	0.2	1.1	–	–	–	–	0.6	0.5	–
Oesophagus cancer	M	118	1	87	13.4	0.1	22.0	–	–	–	–	0.5	–	–
	F	77	1	34	5.6	0.1	6.7	–	–	–	–	–	–	0.6
Stomach cancer	M	391	18	305	41.7	1.5	79.6	–	–	–	0.5	1.1	2.1	6.8
	F	254	15	155	18.4	1.2	31.2	–	–	–	–	0.6	2.1	6.1
Colorectal cancer	M	113	9	72	12.8	0.7	18.9	–	–	–	0.9	1.1	1.6	1.2
	F	129	5	67	9.2	0.4	13.0	–	–	–	–	–	1.6	1.2
Liver cancer	M	...	...	...	...	...	...	...	...	...	...	...	...	...
	F	...	...	...	...	...	...	...	...	...	...	...	...	...
Pancreas cancer	M	...	...	...	...	...	...	...	...	...	...	...	...	...
	F	...	...	...	...	...	...	...	...	...	...	...	...	...
Larynx cancer	M	58	1	50	6.1	0.1	13.5	–	–	–	0.5	–	–	–
	F	6	1	3	0.4	0.1	0.5	–	–	–	0.5	–	–	–
Lung cancer	M	467	2	375	50.9	0.2	95.1	–	–	–	–	–	–	1.2
	F	120	7	66	8.7	0.6	13.6	–	–	–	–	0.6	1.6	1.8
Malignant melanoma	M	...	...	...	...	...	...	...	...	...	...	...	...	...
	F	...	...	...	...	...	...	...	...	...	...	...	...	...
Female breast cancer	F	156	5	107	12.0	0.4	21.1	–	–	–	–	–	–	3.0
Cervix cancer	F	122	7	68	9.0	0.6	13.3	–	–	–	–	–	1.0	3.0
Other uterine cancer	F	52	–	35	4.0	–	7.4	–	–	–	–	–	–	–
Ovarian cancer	F	...	...	...	...	...	...	...	...	...	...	...	...	...
Prostate cancer	M	41	–	23	5.6	–	8.0	–	–	–	–	–	–	–
Bladder cancer	M	...	...	...	...	...	...	...	...	...	...	...	...	...
	F	...	...	...	...	...	...	...	...	...	...	...	...	...
Other and ill-defined cancer sites	M	508	56	344	53.0	4.0	86.7	1.6	0.4	3.0	5.6	3.8	5.3	8.6
	F	440	29	277	31.4	2.0	54.7	1.6	0.4	0.9	2.9	–	4.2	4.2
Hodgkin's disease	M	...	...	...	...	...	...	...	...	...	...	...	...	...
	F	...	...	...	...	...	...	...	...	...	...	...	...	...
Myeloma and all lymphomas	M	66	21	37	5.3	1.5	7.6	0.9	0.7	2.1	0.9	1.1	–	4.3
	F	30	7	15	1.9	0.6	3.2	–	–	0.4	–	0.6	1.0	1.8
Leukaemia	M	68	38	27	4.1	2.4	6.7	3.2	1.1	2.6	2.3	4.9	1.6	1.2
	F	47	20	22	2.7	1.4	4.0	1.0	0.8	1.7	1.0	1.7	1.0	2.4
ALL VASCULAR DISEASE	M	5250	174	2709	659.7	13.7	720.6	0.6	1.5	1.7	8.9	9.2	29.9	44.3
	F	6434	123	1963	452.1	9.5	409.2	2.3	0.8	2.6	2.9	11.2	18.8	27.8
Rheumatic heart disease and fever	M	112	38	71	8.3	2.9	15.0	–	0.7	0.4	3.8	2.2	7.5	5.5
	F	157	37	103	10.6	2.9	18.2	–	0.4	0.9	2.4	1.7	3.7	11.5
Hypertensive disease	M	224	7	147	26.0	0.5	39.4	–	–	0.9	0.9	–	–	1.8
	F	232	3	120	17.0	0.2	24.4	0.3	–	–	–	–	1.0	–
Ischaemic heart disease	M	2714	52	1344	350.2	4.3	358.3	–	–	–	0.9	1.1	7.5	20.9
	F	3005	17	795	210.8	1.3	171.3	0.3	–	–	–	2.8	2.6	3.6
Pulmonary embolism and other venous	M	...	...	...	...	...	...	...	...	...	...	...	...	...
	F	...	...	...	...	...	...	...	...	...	...	...	...	...
Cerebrovascular disease	M	1910	39	986	243.4	3.1	268.6	0.3	–	0.4	1.4	3.3	6.4	9.9
	F	2751	28	837	194.0	2.1	174.0	0.3	0.4	0.9	–	2.2	6.3	4.8
Other vascular disease, incl. venous	M	290	38	161	31.8	2.9	39.3	0.3	0.7	–	1.9	2.7	8.5	6.2
	F	289	38	108	19.7	2.9	21.3	1.3	–	0.9	0.5	4.5	5.2	7.9
Chronic obstructive pulmonary disease	M	1363	50	639	176.0	3.4	181.4	5.1	–	0.9	3.3	2.2	3.7	8.6
	F	1230	46	353	84.4	3.3	72.6	3.6	0.4	–	1.4	2.8	6.3	8.5
Other respiratory disease	M	1531	1438	56	48.1	66.2	13.5	433.4	11.1	5.5	3.8	3.3	2.1	4.3
	F	1280	1199	30	37.2	56.5	6.2	367.4	11.7	5.6	5.7	1.7	3.1	0.6
Peptic ulcer	M	62	6	45	6.1	0.5	9.9	–	–	0.4	0.5	0.5	–	1.8
	F	31	1	15	2.3	0.1	3.2	–	–	–	–	–	0.5	–
Liver cirrhosis and other liver disease	M	451	41	352	43.8	2.9	82.1	2.5	0.7	0.9	3.3	1.6	4.8	6.2
	F	381	42	223	26.4	3.0	42.6	2.6	0.4	0.4	2.4	4.5	4.2	6.7
Renal disease	M	198	55	108	17.7	4.0	25.0	2.2	1.1	1.3	1.9	4.3	8.0	9.2
	F	199	63	97	11.8	4.5	17.9	3.6	1.9	0.4	2.4	6.1	6.8	10.3
Pregnancy and birth	F	81	60	21	3.7	4.8	2.8	–	–	–	2.9	9.5	6.3	15.1
Congenital and perinatal causes	M	828	824	3	21.4	37.8	0.4	250.9	3.3	3.8	3.3	1.6	0.5	1.2
	F	523	513	9	14.2	24.2	1.5	159.9	1.9	0.4	2.4	1.1	3.1	0.6
Ill-defined causes	M	431	56	77	57.6	3.3	21.0	10.4	1.1	–	–	1.1	5.3	4.9
	F	640	50	45	41.4	2.7	9.6	11.0	1.1	–	2.4	–	1.6	3.0
Other medical causes	M	558	218	268	42.8	13.2	60.7	30.7	6.3	7.7	8.0	9.2	10.7	19.7
	F	508	188	230	30.2	11.5	44.1	25.9	6.0	5.6	7.7	7.8	14.7	12.7
ALL NON-MEDICAL CAUSES	M	3083	1693	1286	185.6	120.1	249.4	90.8	39.9	45.1	57.7	150.0	205.7	251.2
	F	967	538	329	49.1	32.9	58.9	71.7	21.5	15.6	28.2	27.9	24.6	41.2
Motor vehicle traffic accidents	M	811	486	304	46.5	36.4	58.7	7.0	12.6	13.6	16.0	53.3	74.3	78.2
	F	195	103	64	10.2	6.8	11.5	5.5	7.2	3.5	9.1	5.0	7.3	10.3
Fire	M	24	18	5	1.2	1.2	1.2	2.8	–	–	–	1.1	0.5	3.7
	F	15	11	1	0.6	0.6	0.2	1.9	1.5	0.4	–	–	–	–
Suicide	M	400	169	209	28.2	13.1	41.4	–	–	6.8	10.8	16.8	23.5	33.9
	F	147	58	69	8.8	4.4	12.7	–	–	1.7	7.2	8.9	4.7	8.5
Homicide	M	497	281	200	30.0	22.2	36.7	1.6	1.1	0.9	10.3	31.5	50.7	59.1
	F	115	46	62	7.1	3.4	10.7	1.6	0.8	2.2	1.9	2.8	4.2	10.3
POPULATION (thousands):	M=males				2118.0	1568.1	508.7	316.1	270.5	234.9	213.0	184.0	187.2	162.4
	F=females				2216.5	1549.4	573.2	308.4	265.2	231.5	209.0	179.0	191.1	165.2

KYRGYZSTAN: 1990

Annual death rates / 100, 000 — 9th ICD categories

35–39	40–44	45–49	50–54	55–59	60–64	65–69	70–74	75–79	80+/NK			
465.1	783.9	905.5	1402.6	1869.9	2754.8	4085.0	6379.1	8503.7	15564.5	M	ALL CAUSES	001–999
191.6	299.0	375.6	612.0	913.2	1395.5	2161.0	3483.3	5440.4	12519.5	F		
17.5	28.9	27.7	33.3	37.8	40.3	47.6	71.9	22.2	32.3	M	Tuberculosis	010–018, 137
7.8	4.8	3.3	16.4	13.2	3.8	7.6	15.2	6.6	3.2	F		
3.2	3.8	8.1	5.9	7.6	9.7	6.8	26.1	14.8	16.1	M	Other infective	Rest of 001–139
0.8	4.8	4.9	3.3	2.6	3.8	3.8	–	13.2	13.0	F	and parasitic	
32.5	86.7	141.7	313.5	405.4	633.9	826.5	1098.0	948.1	604.8	M	ALL CANCER	140–208
39.6	70.2	108.9	136.6	156.6	285.4	390.2	480.2	612.6	487.0	F		
1.6	3.8	6.5	9.5	16.6	19.4	17.0	32.7	7.4	8.1	M	Mouth and	140–149
0.8	–	1.6	–	1.3	–	3.8	9.1	6.6	3.2	F	pharynx cancer	
–	3.8	4.9	28.5	30.3	35.5	51.0	78.4	81.5	56.5	M	Oesophagus cancer	150
2.3	1.2	6.5	3.3	5.3	15.0	13.3	33.4	49.7	51.9	F		
8.7	30.2	39.1	55.8	78.7	140.3	204.1	189.5	163.0	137.1	M	Stomach cancer	151
7.8	12.1	16.3	18.6	31.6	52.6	79.5	91.2	82.8	94.2	F		
3.2	1.3	4.9	17.8	13.6	40.3	51.0	117.6	44.4	64.5	M	Colorectal cancer	153, 154
2.3	2.4	3.3	12.0	9.2	35.0	26.5	54.7	76.2	51.9	F		
...	...	...	...	...	...	...	...	...	...	M	Liver cancer	Not given separately
...	...	...	...	...	...	...	...	...	...	F		
...	...	...	...	...	...	...	...	...	...	M	Pancreas cancer	Not given separately
...	...	...	...	...	...	...	...	...	...	F		
0.8	2.5	3.3	8.3	19.7	22.6	37.4	19.6	7.4	24.2	M	Larynx cancer	161
0.8	–	–	1.1	–	–	1.9	–	6.6	–	F		
4.0	17.6	29.3	85.5	133.1	188.7	207.5	281.0	259.3	96.8	M	Lung cancer	162
4.7	3.6	11.4	12.0	5.3	16.3	41.7	42.6	59.6	48.7	F		
...	...	...	...	...	...	...	...	...	...	M	Malignant melanoma	Not given
...	...	...	...	...	...	...	...	...	...	F		separately
3.1	19.4	22.8	21.9	17.1	23.8	39.8	48.6	46.4	45.5	F	Female breast cancer	174
2.3	6.1	11.4	15.3	14.5	18.8	24.6	42.6	56.3	51.9	F	Cervix cancer	180
0.8	2.4	6.5	3.3	9.2	8.8	20.8	12.2	23.2	19.5	F	Other uterine cancer	179, 182
...	...	...	...	...	...	...	...	...	...	F	Ovarian cancer	Not given separately
–	–	–	2.4	3.0	12.9	37.4	58.8	44.4	24.2	M	Prostate cancer	185
...	...	...	...	...	...	...	...	...	...	M	Bladder cancer	Not given separately
...	...	...	...	...	...	...	...	...	...	F		
9.5	17.6	48.9	86.7	98.3	148.4	197.3	300.7	325.9	145.2	M	Other and ill-defined	Rest of 140–208,
13.2	19.4	24.4	44.8	53.9	100.1	126.9	136.8	185.4	107.1	F	cancer sites	incl. 155, 157, 172, 183, 188
...	...	...	...	...	...	...	...	...	...	M	Hodgkin's disease	Not given separately
...	...	...	...	...	...	...	...	...	...	F		
2.4	7.5	3.3	13.1	7.6	12.9	6.8	19.6	–	40.3	M	Myeloma and all	200–203,
0.8	–	–	1.1	2.6	6.3	11.4	6.1	13.2	6.5	F	lymphomas	incl. 201
2.4	2.5	1.6	5.9	4.5	12.9	17.0	–	14.8	8.1	M	Leukaemia	204–208
0.8	3.6	4.9	3.3	6.6	8.8	–	3.0	6.6	6.5	F		
78.6	194.7	304.6	515.4	748.9	1219.4	1983.0	3418.3	4925.9	9508.1	M	ALL VASCULAR	390–459
43.4	76.3	131.7	233.9	426.3	715.9	1236.7	2182.4	3596.0	8259.7	F	DISEASE	
4.0	18.8	16.3	16.6	16.6	19.4	13.6	6.5	7.4	8.1	M	Rheumatic heart	390–398
15.5	12.1	22.8	20.8	19.7	21.3	15.2	21.3	23.2	9.7	F	disease and fever	
2.4	7.5	17.9	21.4	40.8	83.9	102.0	104.6	125.9	298.4	M	Hypertensive disease	401–405
0.8	1.2	13.0	21.9	31.6	43.8	58.7	94.2	56.3	198.1	F		
48.4	89.2	140.1	263.7	370.7	582.3	1013.6	1941.2	2607.4	5395.2	M	Ischaemic heart	410–414
7.0	21.8	35.8	65.6	147.4	322.9	598.5	1045.6	1784.8	4253.2	F	disease	
...	...	...	...	...	...	...	...	...	...	M	Pulmonary embolism	Not given
...	...	...	...	...	...	...	...	...	...	F	and other venous	separately
15.9	57.8	97.7	178.1	285.9	475.8	768.7	1235.3	2037.0	3395.2	M	Cerebrovascular	430–438
13.2	33.9	53.7	109.3	194.7	301.6	511.4	914.9	1645.7	3532.5	F	disease	
7.9	21.4	32.6	35.6	34.8	58.1	85.0	130.7	148.1	411.3	M	Other vascular	Rest of 390–459,
7.0	7.3	6.5	16.4	32.9	26.3	53.0	106.4	86.1	266.2	F	disease, incl. venous	incl. 415, 451–3
9.5	38.9	60.3	90.3	163.4	332.3	574.8	915.0	1474.1	2701.6	M	Chronic obstructive	490–496
6.2	13.3	13.0	43.7	89.5	137.7	204.5	325.2	582.8	1779.2	F	pulmonary disease	
4.8	3.8	14.7	7.1	21.2	16.1	27.2	45.8	74.1	161.3	M	Other respiratory	Rest of 460–519
1.6	4.8	3.3	3.3	3.9	7.5	18.9	30.4	23.2	110.4	F	disease	
4.8	10.1	6.5	4.8	13.6	16.1	13.6	39.2	37.0	–	M	Peptic ulcer	531–533
–	–	1.6	2.2	5.3	3.8	9.5	18.2	16.6	13.0	F		
20.6	44.0	53.7	80.8	95.3	137.1	142.9	189.5	111.1	112.9	M	Liver cirrhosis and	570–573, 576,
9.3	12.1	16.3	47.0	68.4	71.3	73.9	94.2	99.3	178.6	F	other liver disease	575.2–579.9
9.5	16.3	16.3	15.4	34.8	38.7	44.2	65.4	74.1	121.0	M	Renal disease	580–590
13.2	7.3	6.5	13.1	17.1	33.8	34.1	18.2	33.1	74.7	F		
10.1	8.5	–	–	1.3	–	–	–	–	–	F	Pregnancy and birth	630–676
1.6	–	–	1.2	–	–	–	–	–	8.1	M	Congenital and	740–779
0.8	2.4	–	4.4	2.6	–	–	–	3.3	–	F	perinatal causes	
4.0	7.5	8.1	20.2	18.2	17.7	71.4	183.0	414.8	1725.8	M	Ill-defined causes	780–799
2.3	3.6	4.9	3.3	9.2	10.0	34.1	121.6	274.8	1370.1	F		
24.6	44.0	27.7	62.9	66.6	90.3	108.8	143.8	207.4	177.4	M	Other medical causes	Rest of 001–799
14.7	26.6	29.3	33.9	63.2	65.1	75.8	118.5	96.0	71.4	F		
254.0	305.3	236.2	251.8	257.2	203.2	238.1	183.0	200.0	395.2	M	ALL NON–	E800–E999
41.9	64.2	52.0	71.0	53.9	57.6	72.0	79.0	82.8	159.1	F	MEDICAL CAUSES	
73.8	80.4	37.5	51.1	53.0	37.1	78.2	19.6	37.0	104.8	M	Motor vehicle	E810–E819
8.5	8.5	9.8	15.3	11.8	11.3	15.2	21.3	16.6	51.9	F	traffic accidents	
0.8	1.3	–	–	1.5	1.6	3.4	6.5	–	–	M	Fire	E890–E899
–	1.2	–	–	–	–	–	6.1	–	3.2	F		
35.7	41.5	53.7	45.1	42.4	33.9	37.4	52.3	37.0	72.6	M	Suicide	E950–E959
8.5	8.5	13.0	10.9	14.5	16.3	17.0	15.2	16.6	32.5	F		
43.7	52.8	37.5	41.6	31.8	29.0	20.4	19.6	37.0	64.5	M	Homicide	E960–E969
10.1	19.4	11.4	12.0	10.5	3.8	7.6	12.2	6.6	3.2	F		
126.0	79.6	61.4	84.2	66.1	62.0	29.4	15.3	13.5	12.4	M	**POPULATION (thousands)**	
128.9	82.6	61.5	91.5	76.0	79.9	52.8	32.9	30.2	30.8	F		

KYRGYZSTAN: Males

	All ages	0–34	35–69	35–39	40–44	45–49	50–54	55–59	60–64	65–69	70–74	75–79	80+/NK
POPULATION (1000s)													
1985–90	2018.6	1500.0	474.8	108.9	62.9	82.5	76.9	71.2	48.5	23.9	17.4	13.2	13.2
1985	1921.0	1432.2	442.0	85.1	66.0	91.1	73.1	70.4	35.9	20.4	20.1	12.7	14.0
1990	**2118.0**	**1568.1**	**508.7**	**126.0**	**79.6**	**61.4**	**84.2**	**66.1**	**62.0**	**29.4**	**15.3**	**13.5**	**12.4**
1995 projected	*2293.2*	*1697.8*	*550.8*	*136.4*	*86.2*	*66.5*	*91.2*	*71.6*	*67.1*	*31.8*	*16.6*	*14.6*	*13.4*
NUMBER OF DEATHS													
All causes													
1985–90	16117	5794	6181	478	407	701	983	1275	1363	974	1029	1146	1967
1985	16686	6275	5993	431	394	851	1030	1351	1056	880	1251	1150	2017
1990	**16338**	**5192**	**7092**	**586**	**624**	**556**	**1181**	**1236**	**1708**	**1201**	**976**	**1148**	**1930**
1995 projected	*16949*	*4852*	*7662*	*746*	*715*	*633*	*1252*	*1287*	*1755*	*1274*	*1025*	*1311*	*2099*
Lung cancer													
1985–90	432	5	351	7	12	28	65	92	90	57	40	25	11
1985	378	4	306	10	9	34	56	104	51	42	41	20	7
1990	**467**	**2**	**375**	**5**	**14**	**18**	**72**	**88**	**117**	**61**	**43**	**35**	**12**
1995 projected	*553*	*1*	*419*	*4*	*12*	*20*	*70*	*101*	*133*	*79*	*60*	*54*	*19*
ANNUAL DEATH RATE / 100,000 (*The rates for the age groups 0–34 and 35–69 are the means of seven five-yearly rates, but the all-ages rates are standardised to the conventional "European" age distribution)													
All causes													
1985–90	1460.3*	330.7*	1698.6*	438.9	647.1	849.7	1278.3	1790.7	2810.3	4075.3	5913.8	8681.8	14901.5
1985	1530.4*	371.7*	1803.0*	506.5	597.0	934.1	1409.0	1919.0	2941.5	4313.7	6223.9	9055.1	14407.1
1990	**1491.6***	**299.9***	**1752.4***	**465.1**	**783.9**	**905.5**	**1402.6**	**1869.9**	**2754.8**	**4085.0**	**6379.1**	**8503.7**	**15564.5**
1995 projected	*1477.7**	*275.1**	*1731.5**	*546.9*	*829.5*	*951.9*	*1372.8*	*1797.5*	*2615.5*	*4006.3*	*6174.7*	*8979.5*	*15664.2*
All cancer													
1985–90	195.5*	9.6*	358.6*	40.4	84.3	152.7	283.5	443.8	635.1	870.3	948.3	931.8	560.6
1985	189.9*	8.1*	355.4*	50.5	65.2	153.7	276.3	491.5	607.2	843.1	890.5	826.8	542.9
1990	**198.7***	**10.9***	**348.6***	**32.5**	**86.7**	**141.7**	**313.5**	**405.4**	**633.9**	**826.5**	**1098.0**	**948.1**	**604.8**
1995 projected	*206.0**	*11.7**	*345.6**	*34.5*	*81.2*	*151.9*	*278.5*	*384.1*	*602.1*	*886.8*	*1216.9*	*1184.9*	*656.7*
Lung cancer													
1985–90	49.2*	0.5*	99.6*	6.4	19.1	33.9	84.5	129.2	185.6	238.5	229.9	189.4	83.3
1985	44.4*	0.4*	90.7*	11.8	13.6	37.3	76.6	147.7	142.1	205.9	204.0	157.5	50.0
1990	**50.9***	**0.2***	**95.1***	**4.0**	**17.6**	**29.3**	**85.5**	**133.1**	**188.7**	**207.5**	**281.0**	**259.3**	**96.8**
1995 projected	*58.1**	*0.1**	*101.6**	*2.9*	*13.9*	*30.1*	*76.8*	*141.1*	*198.2*	*248.4*	*361.4*	*369.9*	*141.8*
Upper aerodigestive cancer (mouth, oesophagus, pharynx and larynx)													
1985–90	24.7*	0.5*	46.1*	2.8	7.9	18.2	40.3	64.6	84.5	104.6	97.7	121.2	98.5
1985	24.2*	0.3*	48.8*	1.2	1.5	18.7	42.4	81.0	89.1	107.8	84.6	63.0	107.1
1990	**25.1***	**0.6***	**46.1***	**2.4**	**10.1**	**14.7**	**46.3**	**66.6**	**77.4**	**105.4**	**130.7**	**96.3**	**88.7**
1995 projected	*26.5**	*0.8**	*44.8**	*3.7*	*11.6*	*16.5*	*39.5*	*57.3*	*68.6*	*116.4*	*168.7*	*137.0*	*89.6*
Other cancer													
1985–90	121.6*	8.7*	212.8*	31.2	57.2	100.6	158.6	250.0	364.9	527.2	620.7	621.2	378.8
1985	121.3*	7.4*	215.8*	37.6	50.0	97.7	157.3	262.8	376.0	529.4	602.0	606.3	385.7
1990	**122.6***	**10.1***	**207.4***	**26.2**	**59.0**	**97.7**	**181.7**	**205.7**	**367.7**	**513.6**	**686.3**	**592.6**	**419.4**
1995 projected	*121.4**	*10.9**	*199.2**	*27.9*	*55.7*	*105.3*	*162.3*	*185.8*	*335.3*	*522.0*	*686.7*	*678.1*	*425.4*
Chronic obstructive pulmonary disease (COPD)													
1985–90	191.7*	3.4*	190.9*	11.9	33.4	52.1	106.6	189.6	348.5	594.1	1000.0	1628.8	3030.3
1985	236.0*	4.7*	249.2*	16.5	42.4	71.4	162.8	244.3	501.4	705.9	1273.6	1960.6	3385.7
1990	**176.0***	**3.4***	**181.4***	**9.5**	**38.9**	**60.3**	**90.3**	**163.4**	**332.3**	**574.8**	**915.0**	**1474.1**	**2701.6**
1995 projected	*131.8**	*2.7**	*128.8**	*7.3*	*31.3*	*40.6*	*60.3*	*110.3*	*239.9*	*411.9*	*668.7*	*1171.2*	*2104.5*
Other respiratory disease													
1985–90	67.3*	102.9*	13.3*	5.5	4.8	10.9	10.4	15.4	20.6	25.1	34.5	53.0	136.4
1985	89.4*	143.4*	13.6*	5.9	6.1	8.8	15.0	15.6	19.5	24.5	24.9	23.6	142.9
1990	**48.1***	**66.2***	**13.5***	**4.8**	**3.8**	**14.7**	**7.1**	**21.2**	**16.1**	**27.2**	**45.8**	**74.1**	**161.3**
1995 projected	*37.9**	*43.6**	*13.7**	*3.7*	*3.5*	*12.0*	*7.7*	*18.2*	*16.4*	*34.6*	*60.2*	*102.7*	*231.3*
Vascular disease													
1985–90	668.8*	13.0*	718.8*	90.0	182.8	289.7	475.9	693.8	1270.1	2029.3	3264.4	5242.4	10030.3
1985	676.5*	14.2*	736.9*	96.4	184.8	308.5	518.5	664.8	1273.0	2112.7	3393.0	5622.0	9485.7
1990	**659.7***	**13.7***	**720.6***	**78.6**	**194.7**	**304.6**	**515.4**	**748.9**	**1219.4**	**1983.0**	**3418.3**	**4925.9**	**9508.1**
1995 projected	*633.5**	*11.6**	*693.6**	*74.8*	*181.0*	*296.2*	*516.4*	*722.1*	*1168.4*	*1896.2*	*3090.4*	*5054.8*	*9082.1*
Liver cirrhosis and other liver disease													
1985–90	43.4*	3.2*	76.8*	18.4	33.4	48.5	74.1	91.3	134.0	138.1	155.2	189.4	174.2
1985	48.5*	3.4*	87.4*	23.5	33.3	61.5	87.6	119.3	139.3	147.1	154.2	173.2	214.3
1990	**43.8***	**2.9***	**82.1***	**20.6**	**44.0**	**53.7**	**80.8**	**95.3**	**137.1**	**142.9**	**189.5**	**111.1**	**112.9**
1995 projected	*39.9**	*2.6**	*76.4**	*20.5*	*41.8*	*51.1*	*65.8*	*82.4*	*125.2*	*147.8*	*174.7*	*102.7*	*82.1*
Other medical causes													
1985–90	149.7*	102.1*	151.8*	69.8	90.6	113.9	136.5	169.9	222.7	259.4	333.3	469.7	727.3
1985	160.8*	117.8*	182.1*	102.2	101.5	152.6	161.4	225.9	217.3	313.7	313.4	315.0	428.6
1990	**179.7***	**82.7***	**156.8***	**65.1**	**110.6**	**94.5**	**143.7**	**178.5**	**212.9**	**292.5**	**529.4**	**770.4**	**2080.6**
1995 projected	*188.2**	*56.5**	*143.9**	*52.8*	*80.0*	*76.7*	*105.3*	*150.8*	*189.3*	*352.2*	*728.9*	*1102.7*	*2947.8*
All non-medical causes													
1985–90	143.9*	96.5*	188.4*	202.9	217.8	181.8	191.2	186.8	179.4	159.0	178.2	166.7	242.4
1985	129.3*	80.0*	178.4*	211.5	163.6	177.8	187.4	157.7	183.8	166.7	174.1	133.9	207.1
1990	**185.6***	**120.1***	**249.4***	**254.0**	**305.3**	**236.2**	**251.8**	**257.2**	**203.2**	**238.1**	**183.0**	**200.0**	**395.2**
1995 projected	*240.4**	*146.3**	*329.5**	*353.4*	*410.7*	*323.3*	*338.8*	*329.6*	*274.2*	*276.7*	*234.9*	*260.3*	*559.7*

KYRGYZSTAN: Females

	All ages	0–34	35–69	35–39	40–44	45–49	50–54	55–59	60–64	65–69	70–74	75–79	80+/NK
POPULATION (1000s)													
1985–90	2124.8	1483.3	544.2	111.3	63.2	85.5	83.4	84.8	70.6	45.4	36.7	29.2	31.4
1985	2032.7	1416.0	516.5	86.8	65.2	95.9	80.8	86.4	61.1	40.3	41.2	27.7	31.3
1990	2216.5	1549.4	573.2	128.9	82.6	61.5	91.5	76.0	79.9	52.8	32.9	30.2	30.8
1995 projected	2399.9	1677.5	620.7	139.6	89.4	66.6	99.1	82.3	86.5	57.2	35.6	32.7	33.4
NUMBER OF DEATHS													
All causes													
1985–90	14852	4191	4066	226	192	339	527	763	1007	1012	1271	1663	3661
1985	15646	4790	3998	193	210	432	545	825	886	907	1458	1595	3805
1990	14242	3362	4235	247	247	231	560	694	1115	1141	1146	1643	3856
1995 projected	14248	2836	4334	250	233	222	554	713	1159	1203	1190	1820	4068
Lung cancer													
1985–90	94	3	58	2	2	4	8	12	14	16	15	10	8
1985	64	2	43	2	–	4	7	12	7	11	12	2	5
1990	120	7	66	6	3	7	11	4	13	22	14	18	15
1995 projected	171	10	89	9	4	10	12	4	17	33	21	28	23
ANNUAL DEATH RATE / 100,000 (*The rates for the age groups 0–34 and 35–69 are the means of seven five-yearly rates, but the all-ages rates are standardised to the conventional "European" age distribution)													
All causes													
1985–90	897.1*	231.0*	870.1*	203.1	303.8	396.5	631.9	899.8	1426.3	2229.1	3463.2	5695.2	11659.2
1985	951.6*	278.1*	903.6*	222.4	322.1	450.5	674.5	954.9	1450.1	2250.6	3538.8	5758.1	12156.5
1990	875.7*	183.5*	849.7*	191.6	299.0	375.6	612.0	913.2	1395.5	2161.0	3483.3	5440.4	12519.5
1995 projected	829.7*	148.6*	805.9*	179.1	260.6	333.3	559.0	866.3	1339.9	2103.1	3342.7	5565.7	12179.6
All cancer													
1985–90	104.6*	7.8*	182.3*	40.4	71.2	100.6	149.9	204.0	315.9	394.3	479.6	489.7	372.6
1985	104.0*	8.3*	182.5*	33.4	66.0	109.5	163.4	217.6	330.6	357.3	485.4	433.2	338.7
1990	104.2*	7.5*	169.6*	39.6	70.2	108.9	136.6	156.6	285.4	390.2	480.2	612.6	487.0
1995 projected	105.0*	6.7*	154.1*	40.8	63.8	97.6	109.0	122.7	260.1	384.6	533.7	755.4	649.7
Lung cancer													
1985–90	7.1*	0.2*	12.6*	1.8	3.2	4.7	9.6	14.2	19.8	35.2	40.9	34.2	25.5
1985	5.0*	0.2*	9.7*	2.3	–	4.2	8.7	13.9	11.5	27.3	29.1	7.2	16.0
1990	8.7*	0.6*	13.6*	4.7	3.6	11.4	12.0	5.3	16.3	41.7	42.6	59.6	48.7
1995 projected	11.5*	0.7*	17.2*	6.4	4.5	15.0	12.1	4.9	19.7	57.7	59.0	85.6	68.9
Upper aerodigestive cancer (mouth, oesophagus, pharynx and larynx)													
1985–90	6.4*	0.2*	9.9*	1.8	1.6	4.7	7.2	9.4	18.4	26.4	32.7	44.5	44.6
1985	6.4*	0.2*	9.1*	–	3.1	3.1	6.2	6.9	14.7	29.8	46.1	39.7	47.9
1990	6.9*	0.3*	8.3*	3.9	1.2	8.1	4.4	6.6	15.0	18.9	42.6	62.9	55.2
1995 projected	7.5*	0.4*	7.7*	5.0	1.1	9.0	5.0	6.1	11.6	15.7	44.9	73.4	74.9
Other cancer													
1985–90	91.1*	7.4*	159.8*	36.8	66.5	91.2	133.1	180.4	277.6	332.6	406.0	411.0	302.5
1985	92.6*	8.0*	163.7*	31.1	62.9	102.2	148.5	196.8	304.4	300.2	410.2	386.3	274.8
1990	88.6*	6.6*	147.8*	31.0	65.4	89.4	120.2	144.7	254.1	329.5	395.1	490.1	383.1
1995 projected	86.0*	5.6*	129.3*	29.4	58.2	73.6	91.8	111.8	228.9	311.2	429.8	596.3	506.0
Chronic obstructive pulmonary disease (COPD)													
1985–90	93.4*	3.4*	82.2*	9.9	17.4	24.6	51.6	84.9	140.2	246.7	384.2	715.8	1831.2
1985	110.1*	3.6*	97.3*	13.8	15.3	32.3	71.8	101.9	165.3	280.4	500.0	841.2	2079.9
1990	84.4*	3.3*	72.6*	6.2	13.3	13.0	43.7	89.5	137.7	204.5	325.2	582.8	1779.2
1995 projected	64.5*	2.7*	53.0*	4.3	8.9	9.0	30.3	69.3	107.5	141.6	224.7	437.3	1440.1
Other respiratory disease													
1985–90	54.7*	88.8*	5.8*	2.7	4.7	3.5	4.8	4.7	7.1	13.2	19.1	30.8	92.4
1985	76.6*	129.7*	5.8*	2.3	9.2	1.0	1.2	3.5	13.1	9.9	12.1	14.4	76.7
1990	37.2*	56.5*	6.2*	1.6	4.8	3.3	3.3	3.9	7.5	18.9	30.4	23.2	110.4
1995 projected	29.0*	38.8*	7.0*	0.7	3.4	3.0	4.0	3.6	8.1	26.2	42.1	33.6	155.7
Vascular disease													
1985–90	472.9*	9.6*	422.0*	50.3	85.4	149.7	260.2	412.7	722.4	1273.1	2234.3	3996.6	8560.5
1985	497.2*	11.3*	441.7*	64.5	101.2	185.6	274.8	438.7	726.7	1300.2	2254.9	4111.9	9162.9
1990	452.1*	9.5*	409.2*	43.4	76.3	131.7	233.9	426.3	715.9	1236.7	2182.4	3596.0	8259.7
1995 projected	411.2*	7.5*	375.5*	30.1	51.5	97.6	198.8	394.9	684.4	1171.3	1963.5	3492.4	7377.2
Liver cirrhosis and other liver disease													
1985–90	25.8*	2.6*	42.4*	9.0	14.2	21.1	38.4	51.9	65.2	96.9	84.5	119.9	178.3
1985	27.5*	2.7*	46.5*	13.8	18.4	20.9	42.1	49.8	63.8	116.6	82.5	119.1	191.7
1990	26.4*	3.0*	42.6*	9.3	12.1	16.3	47.0	68.4	71.3	73.9	94.2	99.3	178.6
1995 projected	25.4*	3.0*	42.0*	6.4	7.8	13.5	53.5	80.2	65.9	66.4	78.7	97.9	158.7
Other medical causes													
1985–90	101.1*	88.4*	83.8*	52.1	63.3	51.5	70.7	89.6	116.1	143.2	177.1	239.7	496.8
1985	95.0*	93.6*	82.5*	50.7	78.2	59.4	64.4	86.8	101.5	136.5	126.2	173.3	191.7
1990	122.2*	70.8*	90.6*	49.7	58.1	50.4	76.5	114.5	120.2	164.8	291.8	443.7	1545.5
1995 projected	137.6*	54.8*	104.3*	43.0	45.9	43.5	84.8	137.3	146.8	229.0	404.5	639.1	2185.6
All non-medical causes													
1985–90	44.5*	30.4*	51.6*	38.6	47.5	45.6	56.4	51.9	59.5	61.7	84.5	102.7	127.4
1985	41.1*	28.9*	47.4*	43.8	33.7	41.7	56.9	56.7	49.1	49.6	77.7	65.0	115.0
1990	49.1*	32.9*	58.9*	41.9	64.2	52.0	71.0	53.9	57.6	72.0	79.0	82.8	159.1
1995 projected	57.0*	35.1*	70.0*	53.7	79.4	69.1	78.7	58.3	67.1	83.9	95.5	110.1	212.6

KYRGYZSTAN: 1985–1990

Smoking–attributed deaths (Sm.) and total deaths (Total)

		ALL CAUSES	ALL CANCER	Lung cancer	Upper aero–digestive ca.	Other cancer	COPD	Other respiratory	Vascular disease	Cirrhosis/ other liver	Other medical	Non–medical
Males												
0–34	Sm.	–	–	–	–	–	–	–	–	–	–	–
	Total	5794	130	5	6	119	47	2138	155	42	1936	1346
35–69	Sm.	1896	535	321	104	110	455	16	693	–	197	–
	Total	6181	1273	351	166	756	605	53	2413	301	623	913
		(31%)	(42%)	(91%)	(63%)	(15%)	(75%)	(30%)	(29%)		(32%)	
70+	Sm.	623	92	61	17	14	388	1	130	–	12	–
	Total	4142	362	76	46	240	789	31	2584	75	216	85
		(15%)	(25%)	(80%)	(37%)	(6%)	(49%)	(3%)	(5%)		(6%)	
Any age	Sm.	2519	627	382	121	124	843	17	823	–	209	–
	Total	16117	1765	432	218	1115	1441	2222	5152	418	2775	2344
		(16%)	(36%)	(88%)	(56%)	(11%)	(59%)	(1%)	(16%)		(8%)	
Females												
0–34	Sm.	–	–	–	–	–	–	–	–	–	–	–
	Total	4191	101	3	2	96	48	1800	119	34	1599	490
35–69	Sm.	146	21	15	4	2	65	0	50	–	10	–
	Total	4066	876	58	46	772	369	28	1893	203	424	273
		(4%)	(2%)	(26%)	(9%)	(0%)	(18%)	(0%)	(3%)		(2%)	
70+	Sm.	58	7	5	1	1	32	0	18	–	1	–
	Total	6595	436	33	39	364	925	45	4675	122	291	101
		(1%)	(2%)	(15%)	(3%)	(0%)	(3%)	(0%)	(0%)		(0%)	
Any age	Sm.	204	28	20	5	3	97	0	68	–	11	–
	Total	14852	1413	94	87	1232	1342	1873	6687	359	2314	864
		(1%)	(2%)	(21%)	(6%)	(0%)	(7%)	(0%)	(1%)		(0%)	
Males+Females												
0–34	Sm.	–	–	–	–	–	–	–	–	–	–	–
	Total	9985	231	8	8	215	95	3938	274	76	3535	1836
35–69	Sm.	2042	556	336	108	112	520	16	743	–	207	–
	Total	10247	2149	409	212	1528	974	81	4306	504	1047	1186
		(20%)	(26%)	(82%)	(51%)	(7%)	(53%)	(20%)	(17%)		(20%)	
70+	Sm.	681	99	66	18	15	420	1	148	–	13	–
	Total	10737	798	109	85	604	1714	76	7259	197	507	186
		(6%)	(12%)	(61%)	(21%)	(2%)	(25%)	(1%)	(2%)		(3%)	
Any age	Sm.	2723	655	402	126	127	940	17	891	–	220	–
	Total	30969	3178	526	305	2347	2783	4095	11839	777	5089	3208
		(9%)	(21%)	(76%)	(41%)	(5%)	(34%)	(0%)	(8%)		(4%)	

KYRGYZSTAN: 1985

Smoking–attributed deaths (Sm.) and total deaths (Total)

		ALL CAUSES	ALL CANCER	Lung cancer	Upper aero–digestive ca.	Other cancer	COPD	Other respiratory	Vascular disease	Cirrhosis/ other liver	Other medical	Non–medical
Males												
0–34	Sm.	–	–	–	–	–	–	–	–	–	–	–
	Total	6275	104	4	4	96	59	2785	159	39	2042	1087
35–69	Sm.	1903	482	280	102	100	534	16	638	–	233	–
	Total	5993	1164	306	161	697	722	51	2220	326	712	798
		(32%)	(41%)	(92%)	(63%)	(14%)	(74%)	(31%)	(29%)		(33%)	
70+	Sm.	642	79	53	13	13	435	0	119	–	9	–
	Total	4418	360	68	40	252	979	28	2724	83	163	81
		(15%)	(22%)	(78%)	(33%)	(5%)	(44%)	(0%)	(4%)		(6%)	
Any age	Sm.	2545	561	333	115	113	969	16	757	–	242	–
	Total	16686	1628	378	205	1045	1760	2864	5103	448	2917	1966
		(15%)	(34%)	(88%)	(56%)	(11%)	(55%)	(1%)	(15%)		(8%)	
Females												
0–34	Sm.	–	–	–	–	–	–	–	–	–	–	–
	Total	4790	101	2	2	97	45	2433	129	31	1607	444
35–69	Sm.	21	2	2	0	0	12	0	6	–	1	–
	Total	3998	843	43	37	763	413	25	1869	207	396	245
		(1%)	(0%)	(5%)	(0%)	(0%)	(3%)	(0%)	(0%)		(0%)	
70+	Sm.	0	0	0	0	0	0	0	0	–	0	–
	Total	6858	426	19	45	362	1090	33	4936	127	160	86
		(0%)	(0%)	(0%)	(0%)	(0%)	(0%)	(0%)	(0%)		(0%)	
Any age	Sm.	21	2	2	0	0	12	0	6	–	1	–
	Total	15646	1370	64	84	1222	1548	2491	6934	365	2163	775
		(0%)	(0%)	(3%)	(0%)	(0%)	(1%)	(0%)	(0%)		(0%)	
Males+Females												
0–34	Sm.	–	–	–	–	–	–	–	–	–	–	–
	Total	11065	205	6	6	193	104	5218	288	70	3649	1531
35–69	Sm.	1924	484	282	102	100	546	16	644	–	234	–
	Total	9991	2007	349	198	1460	1135	76	4089	533	1108	1043
		(19%)	(24%)	(81%)	(52%)	(7%)	(48%)	(21%)	(16%)		(21%)	
70+	Sm.	642	79	53	13	13	435	0	119	–	9	–
	Total	11276	786	87	85	614	2069	61	7660	210	323	167
		(6%)	(10%)	(61%)	(15%)	(2%)	(21%)	(0%)	(2%)		(3%)	
Any age	Sm.	2566	563	335	115	113	981	16	763	–	243	–
	Total	32332	2998	442	289	2267	3308	5355	12037	813	5080	2741
		(8%)	(19%)	(76%)	(40%)	(5%)	(30%)	(0%)	(6%)		(5%)	

(To be conservative, no deaths before age 35, and none from liver cirrhosis or non–medical causes, were attributed to smoking.)

KYRGYZSTAN: 1990

Smoking–attributed deaths (Sm.) and total deaths (Total)

		ALL CAUSES	ALL CANCER	Lung cancer	Upper aero–digestive ca.	Other cancer	COPD	Other respiratory	Vascular disease	Cirrhosis/ other liver	Other medical	Non–medical
Males												
0–34	Sm.	–	–	–	–	–	–	–	–	–	–	–
	Total	5192	152	2	8	142	50	1438	174	41	1644	1693
35–69	Sm.	2020	570	344	112	114	474	16	751	–	209	–
	Total	7092	1365	375	182	808	639	56	2709	352	685	1286
		(28%)	(42%)	(92%)	(62%)	(14%)	(74%)	(29%)	(28%)		(31%)	
70+	Sm.	692	114	76	20	18	389	3	158	–	28	–
	Total	4054	371	90	44	237	674	37	2367	58	443	104
		(17%)	(31%)	(84%)	(45%)	(8%)	(58%)	(8%)	(7%)		(6%)	
Any age	Sm.	2712	684	420	132	132	863	19	909	–	237	–
	Total	16338	1888	467	234	1187	1363	1531	5250	451	2772	3083
		(17%)	(36%)	(90%)	(56%)	(11%)	(63%)	(1%)	(17%)		(9%)	
Females												
0–34	Sm.	–	–	–	–	–	–	–	–	–	–	–
	Total	3362	99	7	4	88	46	1199	123	42	1315	538
35–69	Sm.	168	23	20	2	1	68	1	61	–	15	–
	Total	4235	854	66	42	746	353	30	1963	223	483	329
		(4%)	(3%)	(30%)	(5%)	(0%)	(19%)	(3%)	(3%)		(3%)	
70+	Sm.	335	28	18	8	2	232	0	65	–	10	–
	Total	6645	493	47	50	396	831	51	4348	116	706	100
		(5%)	(6%)	(38%)	(16%)	(1%)	(28%)	(0%)	(1%)		(1%)	
Any age	Sm.	503	51	38	10	3	300	1	126	–	25	–
	Total	14242	1446	120	96	1230	1230	1280	6434	381	2504	967
		(4%)	(4%)	(32%)	(10%)	(0%)	(24%)	(0%)	(2%)		(1%)	
Males+Females												
0–34	Sm.	–	–	–	–	–	–	–	–	–	–	–
	Total	8554	251	9	12	230	96	2637	297	83	2959	2231
35–69	Sm.	2188	593	364	114	115	542	17	812	–	224	–
	Total	11327	2219	441	224	1554	992	86	4672	575	1168	1615
		(19%)	(27%)	(83%)	(51%)	(7%)	(55%)	(20%)	(17%)		(19%)	
70+	Sm.	1027	142	94	28	20	621	3	223	–	38	–
	Total	10699	864	137	94	633	1505	88	6715	174	1149	204
		(10%)	(16%)	(69%)	(30%)	(3%)	(41%)	(3%)	(3%)		(3%)	
Any age	Sm.	3215	735	458	142	135	1163	20	1035	–	262	–
	Total	30580	3334	587	330	2417	2593	2811	11684	832	5276	4050
		(11%)	(22%)	(78%)	(43%)	(6%)	(45%)	(1%)	(9%)		(5%)	

KYRGYZSTAN: 1995

Smoking–attributed deaths (Sm.) and total deaths (Total)

		ALL CAUSES	ALL CANCER	Lung cancer	Upper aero–digestive ca.	Other cancer	COPD	Other respiratory	Vascular disease	Cirrhosis/ other liver	Other medical	Non–medical
Males												
0–34	Sm.	–	–	–	–	–	–	–	–	–	–	–
	Total	4852	181	1	11	169	46	1024	160	42	1225	2174
35–69	Sm.	1999	621	385	115	121	370	18	801	–	189	–
	Total	7662	1433	419	186	828	490	58	2830	348	635	1868
		(26%)	(43%)	(92%)	(62%)	(15%)	(76%)	(31%)	(28%)		(30%)	
70+	Sm.	843	178	118	33	27	375	5	225	–	60	–
	Total	4435	463	133	60	270	564	56	2468	55	677	152
		(19%)	(38%)	(89%)	(55%)	(10%)	(66%)	(9%)	(9%)		(9%)	
Any age	Sm.	2842	799	503	148	148	745	23	1026	–	249	–
	Total	16949	2077	553	257	1267	1100	1138	5458	445	2537	4194
		(17%)	(38%)	(91%)	(58%)	(12%)	(68%)	(2%)	(19%)		(10%)	
Females												
0–34	Sm.	–	–	–	–	–	–	–	–	–	–	–
	Total	2836	95	10	5	80	43	890	107	46	1059	596
35–69	Sm.	269	53	41	7	5	81	1	104	–	30	–
	Total	4334	833	89	43	701	281	35	1937	239	585	424
		(6%)	(6%)	(46%)	(16%)	(1%)	(29%)	(3%)	(5%)		(5%)	
70+	Sm.	551	66	42	18	6	316	3	133	–	33	–
	Total	7078	654	72	65	517	704	78	4305	113	1083	141
		(8%)	(10%)	(58%)	(28%)	(1%)	(45%)	(4%)	(3%)		(3%)	
Any age	Sm.	820	119	83	25	11	397	4	237	–	63	–
	Total	14248	1582	171	113	1298	1028	1003	6349	398	2727	1161
		(6%)	(8%)	(49%)	(22%)	(1%)	(39%)	(0%)	(4%)		(2%)	
Males+Females												
0–34	Sm.	–	–	–	–	–	–	–	–	–	–	–
	Total	7688	276	11	16	249	89	1914	267	88	2284	2770
35–69	Sm.	2268	674	426	122	126	451	19	905	–	219	–
	Total	11996	2266	508	229	1529	771	93	4767	587	1220	2292
		(19%)	(30%)	(84%)	(53%)	(8%)	(58%)	(20%)	(19%)		(18%)	
70+	Sm.	1394	244	160	51	33	691	8	358	–	93	–
	Total	11513	1117	205	125	787	1268	134	6773	168	1760	293
		(12%)	(22%)	(78%)	(41%)	(4%)	(54%)	(6%)	(5%)		(5%)	
Any age	Sm.	3662	918	586	173	159	1142	27	1263	–	312	–
	Total	31197	3659	724	370	2565	2128	2141	11807	843	5264	5355
		(12%)	(25%)	(81%)	(47%)	(6%)	(54%)	(1%)	(11%)		(6%)	

(To be conservative, no deaths before age 35, and none from liver cirrhosis or non–medical causes, were attributed to smoking.)

¶LATVIA: 1990

		No. of deaths			Standardised rates (Defined on p.412)			Annual death rates / 100, 000						
		All ages	0–34	35–69	All ages	0–34	35–69	0–4	5–9	10–14	15–19	20–24	25–29	30–34
ALL CAUSES	M	16951	1702	8526	1633.6	242.8	2042.2	381.5	100.2	79.2	187.1	226.7	322.4	402.2
	F	17861	656	4816	869.2	95.7	817.8	284.1	38.8	31.4	64.5	56.4	94.9	99.8
Tuberculosis	M	142	14	111	13.0	2.0	26.0	1.0	1.0	–	–	–	2.9	8.9
	F	43	1	24	2.4	0.1	4.1	–	–	–	–	–	1.0	–
Other infective	M	61	38	20	4.9	5.3	3.9	26.6	3.0	–	3.2	2.1	1.9	–
and parasitic	F	57	27	24	4.0	3.9	4.0	25.9	–	1.2	–	–	–	–
ALL CANCER	M	2961	86	1955	288.6	12.6	488.8	5.7	21.3	10.2	9.5	15.7	10.6	14.9
	F	2536	76	1407	142.6	11.1	235.9	8.0	7.3	7.0	4.4	6.8	19.6	24.5
Mouth and	M	96	2	76	9.0	0.3	17.5	–	1.0	–	–	1.0	–	–
pharynx cancer	F	22	1	10	1.1	0.1	1.6	–	1.0	–	–	–	–	–
Oesophagus cancer	M	80	–	65	7.6	–	14.7	–	–	–	–	–	–	–
	F	20	–	6	0.9	–	1.0	–	–	–	–	–	–	–
Stomach cancer	M	400	5	272	38.8	0.7	67.4	–	–	–	–	–	2.9	2.0
	F	367	4	182	20.4	0.6	30.9	–	–	–	1.1	–	–	2.9
Colorectal cancer	M	256	3	134	26.1	0.4	34.5	–	–	–	–	1.0	–	2.0
	F	355	3	167	19.0	0.4	28.1	–	–	–	–	–	1.0	2.0
Liver cancer	M	...	...	...	...	...	...	...	...	...	...	...	...	...
	F	...	...	...	...	...	...	...	...	...	...	...	...	...
Pancreas cancer	M	...	...	...	...	...	...	...	...	...	...	...	...	...
	F	...	...	...	...	...	...	...	...	...	...	...	...	...
Larynx cancer	M	97	–	75	9.3	–	17.5	–	–	–	–	–	–	–
	F	9	–	4	0.5	–	0.7	–	–	–	–	–	–	–
Lung cancer	M	928	–	713	89.6	–	179.5	–	–	–	–	–	–	–
	F	179	1	110	9.7	0.1	18.8	–	–	–	–	–	1.0	–
Malignant melanoma	M	...	...	...	...	...	...	...	...	...	...	...	...	...
	F	...	...	...	...	...	...	...	...	...	...	...	...	...
Female breast cancer	F	378	9	265	23.2	1.3	43.4	–	–	–	–	–	2.9	5.9
Cervix cancer	F	107	3	70	6.2	0.4	11.5	–	–	–	–	–	–	2.9
Other uterine cancer	F	135	3	80	7.2	0.4	13.7	–	–	–	–	–	1.0	2.0
Ovarian cancer	F	...	...	...	...	...	...	...	...	...	...	...	...	...
Prostate cancer	M	195	–	63	20.9	–	19.8	–	–	–	–	–	–	–
Bladder cancer	M	...	...	...	...	...	...	...	...	...	...	...	...	...
	F	...	...	...	...	...	...	...	...	...	...	...	...	...
Other and ill-defined	M	712	36	459	68.8	5.2	113.9	1.9	10.1	2.3	4.2	4.2	5.8	7.9
cancer sites	F	779	33	417	43.4	4.8	70.0	4.0	3.1	2.3	2.2	3.4	10.8	7.8
Hodgkin's disease	M	...	...	...	...	...	...	...	...	...	...	...	...	...
	F	...	...	...	...	...	...	...	...	...	...	...	...	...
Myeloma and all	M	84	15	47	7.8	2.3	10.9	–	2.0	4.5	1.1	6.3	1.0	1.0
lymphomas	F	85	8	48	5.0	1.2	8.2	1.0	1.0	1.2	–	3.4	1.0	1.0
Leukaemia	M	113	25	51	10.5	3.7	13.2	3.8	8.1	3.4	4.2	3.1	1.0	2.0
	F	100	11	48	5.8	1.7	7.9	3.0	2.1	3.5	1.1	–	2.0	–
ALL VASCULAR	M	8544	101	3852	861.8	14.3	960.6	1.0	1.0	–	7.4	7.3	29.0	54.6
DISEASE	F	11754	24	2207	529.8	3.5	381.5	2.0	1.0	–	2.2	3.4	5.9	9.8
Rheumatic heart	M	108	4	91	10.0	0.6	20.6	–	–	–	–	1.0	1.9	1.0
disease and fever	F	159	2	129	10.1	0.3	21.2	–	–	–	–	–	1.0	1.0
Hypertensive disease	M	44	2	35	4.1	0.3	6.8	–	–	–	–	–	–	2.0
	F	42	–	27	2.5	–	4.5	–	–	–	–	–	–	–
Ischaemic heart	M	5353	53	2516	538.1	7.5	619.7	–	–	–	1.1	2.1	12.5	36.7
disease	F	6376	7	1099	284.8	1.0	191.4	–	–	–	–	–	1.0	5.9
Pulmonary embolism	M	...	...	...	...	...	...	...	...	...	...	...	...	...
and other venous	F	...	...	...	...	...	...	...	...	...	...	...	...	...
Cerebrovascular	M	2554	19	985	261.5	2.7	259.1	1.0	–	–	5.3	–	1.9	10.9
disease	F	4632	3	832	207.1	0.5	144.4	–	–	–	1.1	1.1	1.0	–
Other vascular	M	485	23	225	48.2	3.3	54.5	–	1.0	–	1.1	4.2	12.5	4.0
disease, incl. venous	F	545	12	120	25.3	1.8	20.1	2.0	1.0	–	1.1	2.3	2.9	2.9
Chronic obstructive	M	594	6	310	59.9	0.9	81.6	1.9	–	1.1	–	–	1.0	2.0
pulmonary disease	F	326	7	109	15.9	1.0	18.7	2.0	–	–	1.1	–	2.9	1.0
Other respiratory	M	162	23	94	14.9	3.2	20.7	11.4	1.0	1.1	1.1	2.1	5.8	–
disease	F	99	18	32	5.6	2.6	5.4	10.0	1.0	–	1.1	1.1	2.9	2.0
Peptic ulcer	M	99	4	63	9.6	0.6	15.1	–	–	–	–	–	1.9	2.0
	F	41	–	15	2.0	–	2.7	–	–	–	–	–	–	–
Liver cirrhosis and	M	115	3	91	11.0	0.4	22.4	–	–	–	–	–	1.0	2.0
other liver disease	F	106	5	70	6.3	0.7	11.8	–	1.0	–	–	–	1.0	2.9
Renal disease	M	142	11	77	13.9	1.6	17.6	–	–	–	3.2	1.0	1.9	5.0
	F	224	10	118	12.3	1.5	20.0	–	–	–	1.1	2.3	4.9	2.0
Pregnancy and birth	F	9	8	1	0.7	1.2	0.2	–	–	–	2.2	2.3	1.0	2.9
Congenital and	M	299	289	9	22.7	39.7	1.6	243.6	13.2	4.5	11.6	–	1.9	3.0
perinatal causes	F	222	201	16	17.3	28.9	2.5	175.5	13.6	5.8	3.3	2.3	–	2.0
Ill-defined causes	M	321	8	–	33.3	1.1	–	7.6	–	–	–	–	–	–
	F	789	11	3	31.0	1.6	0.6	11.0	–	–	–	–	–	–
Other medical causes	M	735	81	423	69.2	11.6	97.5	11.4	7.1	2.3	14.8	5.2	10.6	29.8
	F	703	55	356	40.3	8.1	59.5	7.0	6.3	3.5	3.3	10.2	11.7	14.7
ALL NON-	M	2776	1038	1521	230.8	149.6	306.3	71.4	52.6	60.0	136.4	193.1	253.9	280.0
MEDICAL CAUSES	F	952	213	434	59.1	31.6	71.0	42.9	8.4	14.0	45.6	28.2	44.0	38.2
Motor vehicle	M	813	389	376	65.8	56.6	75.0	6.7	22.3	20.4	70.8	97.6	89.8	88.4
traffic accidents	F	231	80	102	15.3	12.0	16.7	7.0	5.2	5.8	23.4	13.5	21.5	7.8
Fire	M	106	33	58	9.2	4.6	11.6	20.0	3.0	1.1	2.1	2.1	1.9	2.0
	F	56	15	20	3.4	2.1	3.3	11.0	–	–	1.1	–	2.0	1.0
Suicide	M	541	163	317	45.9	23.3	63.3	–	–	5.7	19.0	22.0	52.1	64.5
	F	154	24	85	9.5	3.6	14.0	–	–	2.3	7.8	4.5	7.8	2.9
Homicide	M	181	80	95	14.4	11.4	18.5	1.0	–	–	6.3	14.7	29.0	28.8
	F	64	20	34	4.4	2.9	5.4	–	1.0	1.2	1.1	4.5	4.9	7.8
POPULATION (thousands):	M=males				1243.9	686.5	496.4	105.1	98.8	88.4	94.6	95.3	103.6	100.7
	F=females				1429.7	664.5	617.4	100.3	95.4	85.9	89.9	88.6	102.2	102.2

LATVIA: 1990

Annual death rates / 100, 000 — 9th ICD categories

35–39	40–44	45–49	50–54	55–59	60–64	65–69	70–74	75–79	80+/NK		Cause	ICD
490.5	747.5	1113.4	1624.5	2295.3	3314.2	4710.3	6687.2	9540.7	17463.2	M	ALL CAUSES	001–999
155.8	236.5	425.7	536.2	834.1	1298.0	2238.2	3597.3	6134.8	14479.4	F		
7.8	8.9	25.2	21.7	24.3	35.5	58.5	33.2	19.1	31.6	M	Tuberculosis	010–018, 137
–	1.2	4.5	2.1	4.6	5.5	10.8	11.2	8.0	16.9	F		
1.1	3.8	2.5	4.8	8.6	6.8	–	–	4.8	10.5	M	Other infective	Rest of 001–139
1.1	2.3	3.4	3.1	5.7	4.4	8.1	2.2	6.0	3.7	F	and parasitic	
40.0	85.0	183.9	353.8	596.3	934.1	1228.4	1369.7	1569.4	1594.7	M	ALL CANCER	140–208
39.5	70.3	161.0	167.7	262.0	413.8	537.2	604.0	738.4	779.0	F		
2.2	6.3	6.3	19.3	25.7	32.1	30.6	37.9	23.9	26.3	M	Mouth and	140–149
1.1	1.2	1.1	1.0	1.1	4.4	1.4	–	4.0	16.9	F	pharynx cancer	
2.2	5.1	8.8	16.8	17.1	30.4	22.3	33.2	14.4	26.3	M	Oesophagus cancer	150
–	–	–	1.0	–	2.2	4.1	4.5	8.0	15.0	F		
11.1	12.7	34.0	40.9	88.4	114.9	169.9	161.1	239.2	205.3	M	Stomach cancer	151
5.3	15.2	24.8	14.5	41.2	37.1	78.5	109.6	130.8	125.5	F		
3.3	5.1	10.1	20.5	45.6	59.1	97.5	189.6	196.2	200.0	M	Colorectal cancer	153, 154
2.1	8.2	18.0	21.7	26.3	51.3	69.0	94.0	118.7	157.3	F		
...	...	...	...	...	...	...	...	...	...	M	Liver cancer	Not given separately
...	...	...	...	...	...	...	...	...	...	F		
...	...	...	...	...	...	...	...	...	...	M	Pancreas cancer	Not given separately
...	...	...	...	...	...	...	...	...	...	F		
–	5.1	10.1	15.6	27.1	33.8	30.6	47.4	23.9	36.8	M	Larynx cancer	161
–	–	–	1.0	1.1	1.1	1.4	6.7	–	3.7	F		
2.2	20.3	52.9	131.2	229.7	380.1	440.1	383.9	425.8	236.8	M	Lung cancer	162
2.1	–	4.5	6.2	18.3	42.6	58.2	42.5	60.4	35.6	F		
...	...	...	...	...	...	...	...	...	...	M	Malignant melanoma	Not given
...	...	...	...	...	...	...	...	...	...	F		separately
11.7	21.1	48.4	50.7	50.3	59.0	62.2	64.9	66.4	78.7	F	Female breast cancer	174
2.1	3.5	6.8	11.4	16.0	20.7	20.3	15.7	36.2	16.9	F	Cervix cancer	180
–	–	9.0	6.2	13.7	26.2	40.6	15.7	42.3	44.9	F	Other uterine cancer	179, 182
...	...	...	...	...	...	...	...	...	...	F	Ovarian cancer	Not given separately
–	–	1.3	1.2	11.4	35.5	89.1	156.4	196.2	305.3	M	Prostate cancer	185
...	...	...	...	...	...	...	...	...	...	M	Bladder cancer	Not given separately
...	...	...	...	...	...	...	...	...	...	F		
15.6	20.3	52.9	90.3	131.2	194.3	292.5	289.1	339.7	447.4	M	Other and ill-defined	Rest of 140–208,
7.5	15.2	37.2	47.6	72.1	144.1	166.4	203.6	229.4	232.2	F	cancer sites	incl. 155, 157, 172, 183, 188
...	...	...	...	...	...	...	...	...	...	M	Hodgkin's disease	Not given separately
...	...	...	...	...	...	...	...	...	...	F		
2.2	6.3	3.8	10.8	10.0	23.6	19.5	37.9	33.5	36.8	M	Myeloma and all	200–203,
2.1	1.2	7.9	2.1	12.6	9.8	21.7	20.1	20.1	18.7	F	lymphomas	incl. 201
1.1	3.8	3.8	7.2	10.0	30.4	36.2	33.2	76.6	73.7	M	Leukaemia	204–208
5.3	4.7	3.4	4.1	9.2	15.3	13.5	26.8	22.1	33.7	F		
107.9	242.4	418.1	698.0	1097.0	1670.6	2490.3	4180.1	6311.0	12578.9	M	ALL VASCULAR	390–459
27.7	56.2	114.9	201.9	358.1	622.3	1289.6	2483.2	4533.2	11535.6	F	DISEASE	
6.7	11.4	11.3	21.7	28.5	25.3	39.0	33.2	19.1	10.5	M	Rheumatic heart	390–398
7.5	5.9	15.8	21.7	35.5	29.5	32.5	29.1	18.1	11.2	F	disease and fever	
–	5.1	6.3	13.2	12.8	10.1	–	23.7	4.8	5.3	M	Hypertensive disease	401–405
2.1	3.5	3.4	4.1	6.9	3.3	8.1	8.9	10.1	11.2	F		
82.3	167.5	279.6	472.9	709.0	1094.6	1532.0	2606.6	3818.2	7557.9	M	Ischaemic heart	410–414
8.5	31.6	49.5	80.7	170.5	310.0	688.8	1382.6	2476.9	6406.4	F	disease	
...	...	...	...	...	...	...	...	...	...	M	Pulmonary embolism	Not given
...	...	...	...	...	...	...	...	...	...	F	and other venous	separately
13.3	25.4	81.9	156.4	288.2	462.8	785.5	1298.6	2172.2	4326.3	M	Cerebrovascular	430–438
4.3	9.4	33.8	78.7	129.3	242.4	512.9	973.2	1851.1	4573.0	F	disease	
5.6	33.0	39.0	33.7	58.5	77.7	133.7	218.0	296.7	678.9	M	Other vascular	Rest of 390–459,
5.3	5.9	12.4	16.6	16.0	37.1	47.4	89.5	177.1	533.7	F	disease, incl. venous	incl. 415, 451–3
3.3	14.0	34.0	38.5	99.9	128.4	253.5	289.1	454.5	642.1	M	Chronic obstructive	490–496
2.1	7.0	11.3	11.4	12.6	28.4	58.2	47.0	144.9	219.1	F	pulmonary disease	
6.7	10.2	11.3	20.5	31.4	37.2	27.9	47.4	57.4	121.1	M	Other respiratory	Rest of 460–519
–	4.7	4.5	4.1	5.7	5.5	13.5	17.9	24.1	54.3	F	disease	
–	5.1	7.6	20.5	14.3	22.0	36.2	42.7	47.8	68.4	M	Peptic ulcer	531–533
–	–	–	–	2.3	5.5	10.8	11.2	20.1	20.6	F		
1.1	8.9	16.4	16.8	21.4	33.8	58.5	33.2	28.7	42.1	M	Liver cirrhosis and	570–573, 576,
2.1	7.0	2.3	8.3	17.2	17.5	28.4	22.4	26.2	15.0	F	other liver disease	575.2–579.9
4.4	5.1	15.1	19.3	21.4	22.0	36.2	85.3	71.8	110.5	M	Renal disease	580–590
4.3	4.7	6.8	11.4	22.9	37.1	52.8	49.2	76.5	67.4	F		
1.1	–	–	–	–	–	–	–	–	–	F	Pregnancy and birth	630–676
3.3	1.3	1.3	2.4	1.4	1.7	–	–	4.8	–	M	Congenital and	740–779
3.2	1.2	1.1	6.2	1.1	4.4	–	2.2	6.0	1.9	F	perinatal causes	
–	–	–	–	–	–	–	37.9	258.4	1321.1	M	Ill-defined causes	780–799
–	–	–	–	–	–	4.1	47.0	215.3	1211.6	F		
36.7	55.8	59.2	89.0	94.2	147.0	200.6	251.2	397.1	500.0	M	Other medical causes	Rest of 001–799
19.2	14.1	46.2	47.6	68.6	89.5	131.3	179.0	179.1	230.3	F		
278.1	307.1	338.8	339.4	285.3	275.3	320.3	317.5	315.8	442.1	M	ALL NON-	E800–E999
55.5	67.9	69.8	72.5	73.2	64.4	93.4	120.8	156.9	324.0	F	MEDICAL CAUSES	
83.4	73.6	79.3	81.8	72.8	55.7	78.0	71.1	76.6	89.5	M	Motor vehicle	E810–E819
17.1	21.1	9.0	18.6	17.2	12.0	21.7	29.1	34.2	35.6	F	traffic accidents	
8.9	8.9	12.6	13.2	10.0	22.0	5.6	23.7	19.1	31.6	M	Fire	E890–E899
1.1	2.3	4.5	1.0	4.6	4.4	5.4	6.7	10.1	24.3	F		
62.3	64.7	70.5	66.2	65.6	52.4	61.3	94.8	90.9	115.8	M	Suicide	E950–E959
9.6	9.4	13.5	13.5	13.7	14.2	24.4	20.1	22.1	46.8	F		
18.9	25.4	25.2	16.8	15.7	13.5	13.9	4.7	19.1	5.3	M	Homicide	E960–E969
6.4	4.7	10.1	5.2	4.6	4.4	2.7	6.7	6.0	7.5	F		
89.9	78.8	79.4	83.1	70.1	59.2	35.9	21.1	20.9	19.0	M	POPULATION (thousands)	
93.7	85.4	88.8	96.6	87.4	91.6	73.9	44.7	49.7	53.4	F		

LATVIA: Males

	All ages	0–34	35–69	35–39	40–44	45–49	50–54	55–59	60–64	65–69	70–74	75–79	80+/NK
POPULATION (1000s)													
1985–90	1217.0	673.4	479.1	86.9	76.3	86.2	77.4	71.1	49.8	31.4	25.2	21.4	17.9
1985	1186.9	657.6	460.6	80.0	81.3	87.3	75.8	66.4	42.4	27.4	30.2	21.9	16.6
1990	**1243.9**	**686.5**	**496.4**	**89.9**	**78.8**	**79.4**	**83.1**	**70.1**	**59.2**	**35.9**	**21.1**	**20.9**	**19.0**
1995 projected	*1239.0*	*663.0*	*516.0*	*97.0*	*86.0*	*74.0*	*74.0*	*75.0*	*61.0*	*49.0*	*27.0*	*14.0*	*19.0*
NUMBER OF DEATHS													
All causes													
1985–90	15573	1476	7336	388	522	840	1131	1499	1547	1409	1617	2015	3129
1985	15961	1500	7222	428	630	884	1213	1478	1333	1256	2021	2124	3094
1990	**16951**	**1702**	**8526**	**441**	**589**	**884**	**1350**	**1609**	**1962**	**1691**	**1411**	**1994**	**3318**
1995 projected	*17382*	*1688*	*9455*	*468*	*650*	*848*	*1251*	*1786*	*2097*	*2355*	*1804*	*1280*	*3155*
Lung cancer													
1985–90	898	2	672	6	16	54	103	177	185	131	98	77	49
1985	808	3	584	4	21	58	98	175	130	98	110	58	53
1990	**928**	**–**	**713**	**2**	**16**	**42**	**109**	**161**	**225**	**158**	**81**	**89**	**45**
1995 projected	*1068*	*–*	*826*	*1*	*13*	*36*	*86*	*181*	*259*	*250*	*129*	*62*	*51*
ANNUAL DEATH RATE / 100,000 (*The rates for the age groups 0–34 and 35–69 are the means of seven five-yearly rates, but the all-ages rates are standardised to the conventional "European" age distribution)													
All causes													
1985–90	1550.3*	214.8*	1895.5*	446.5	684.1	974.5	1461.2	2108.3	3106.4	4487.3	6416.7	9415.9	17480.4
1985	1630.2*	225.0*	1982.4*	535.0	774.9	1012.6	1600.3	2225.9	3143.9	4583.9	6692.1	9698.6	18638.6
1990	**1633.6***	**242.8***	**2042.2***	**490.5**	**747.5**	**1113.4**	**1624.5**	**2295.3**	**3314.2**	**4710.3**	**6687.2**	**9540.7**	**17463.2**
1995 projected	*1636.8**	*255.7**	*2100.0**	*482.5*	*755.8*	*1145.9*	*1690.5*	*2381.3*	*3437.7*	*4806.1*	*6681.5*	*9142.9*	*16605.3*
All cancer													
1985–90	286.4*	11.7*	492.7*	40.3	90.4	184.5	352.7	638.5	935.7	1207.0	1357.1	1528.0	1458.1
1985	270.2*	10.9*	465.4*	42.5	93.5	183.3	340.4	629.5	877.4	1091.2	1298.0	1415.5	1301.2
1990	**288.6***	**12.6***	**488.8***	**40.0**	**85.0**	**183.9**	**353.8**	**596.3**	**934.1**	**1228.4**	**1369.7**	**1569.4**	**1594.7**
1995 projected	*306.5**	*13.1**	*510.3**	*37.1*	*82.6*	*182.4*	*348.6*	*608.0*	*996.7*	*1316.3*	*1496.3*	*1671.4*	*1857.9*
Lung cancer													
1985–90	90.3*	0.3*	180.2*	6.9	21.0	62.6	133.1	248.9	371.5	417.2	388.9	359.8	273.7
1985	84.1*	0.5*	164.9*	5.0	25.8	66.4	129.3	263.6	306.6	357.7	364.2	264.8	319.3
1990	**89.6***	**–**	**179.5***	**2.2**	**20.3**	**52.9**	**131.2**	**229.7**	**380.1**	**440.1**	**383.9**	**425.8**	**236.8**
1995 projected	*97.3**	*–*	*193.9**	*1.0*	*15.1*	*48.6*	*116.2*	*241.3*	*424.6*	*510.2*	*477.8*	*442.9*	*268.4*
Upper aerodigestive cancer (mouth, oesophagus, pharynx and larynx)													
1985–90	22.3*	0.4*	44.0*	2.3	11.8	20.9	40.1	63.3	80.3	89.2	87.3	70.1	72.6
1985	16.5*	–	31.5*	3.8	8.6	18.3	23.7	45.2	59.0	62.0	59.6	77.6	60.2
1990	**25.9***	**0.3***	**49.7***	**4.4**	**16.5**	**25.2**	**51.7**	**69.9**	**96.3**	**83.6**	**118.5**	**62.2**	**89.5**
1995 projected	*35.0**	*–*	*69.4**	*6.2*	*22.1*	*35.1*	*73.0*	*98.7*	*134.4*	*116.3*	*155.6*	*78.6*	*94.7*
Other cancer													
1985–90	173.7*	11.0*	268.6*	31.1	57.7	100.9	179.6	326.3	483.9	700.6	881.0	1098.1	1111.7
1985	169.6*	10.4*	269.0*	33.8	59.0	98.5	187.3	320.8	511.8	671.5	874.2	1073.1	921.7
1990	**173.0***	**12.3***	**259.6***	**33.4**	**48.2**	**105.8**	**170.9**	**296.7**	**457.8**	**704.7**	**867.3**	**1081.3**	**1268.4**
1995 projected	*174.2**	*13.1**	*247.0**	*29.9*	*45.3*	*98.6*	*159.5*	*268.0*	*437.7*	*689.8*	*863.0*	*1150.0*	*1494.7*
Chronic obstructive pulmonary disease (COPD)													
1985–90	58.4*	1.6*	72.1*	4.6	9.2	22.0	42.6	80.2	126.5	219.7	309.5	429.9	715.1
1985	69.5*	2.0*	87.3*	7.5	12.3	24.1	60.7	87.3	160.4	259.1	351.0	547.9	801.2
1990	**59.9***	**0.9***	**81.6***	**3.3**	**14.0**	**34.0**	**38.5**	**99.9**	**128.4**	**253.5**	**289.1**	**454.5**	**642.1**
1995 projected	*51.6**	*0.8**	*72.8**	*2.1*	*16.3*	*29.7*	*37.8*	*85.3*	*119.7*	*218.4*	*244.4*	*378.6*	*521.1*
Other respiratory disease													
1985–90	14.2*	5.2*	17.0*	5.8	7.9	13.9	20.7	19.7	22.1	28.7	47.6	60.7	95.0
1985	19.5*	9.1*	20.4*	11.3	12.3	27.5	23.7	22.6	16.5	29.2	66.2	73.1	126.5
1990	**14.9***	**3.2***	**20.7***	**6.7**	**10.2**	**11.3**	**20.5**	**31.4**	**37.2**	**27.9**	**47.4**	**57.4**	**121.1**
1995 projected	*14.4**	*2.5**	*23.1**	*4.1*	*7.0*	*8.1*	*17.6*	*44.0*	*52.5*	*28.6*	*37.0*	*42.9*	*110.5*
Vascular disease													
1985–90	861.0*	13.2*	902.4*	116.2	228.0	378.2	624.0	952.2	1556.2	2461.8	4011.9	6551.4	13770.9
1985	934.4*	13.8*	969.1*	138.8	264.5	395.2	676.8	1052.7	1599.1	2656.9	4225.2	7086.8	15325.3
1990	**861.8***	**14.3***	**960.6***	**107.9**	**242.4**	**418.1**	**698.0**	**1097.0**	**1670.6**	**2490.3**	**4180.1**	**6311.0**	**12578.9**
1995 projected	*790.5**	*12.2**	*949.9**	*90.7*	*226.7*	*418.9*	*718.9*	*1134.7*	*1632.8*	*2426.5*	*3814.8*	*5464.3*	*10605.3*
Liver cirrhosis and other liver disease													
1985–90	11.1*	0.7*	20.1*	4.6	7.9	9.3	16.8	25.3	32.1	44.6	55.6	32.7	39.1
1985	12.8*	1.5*	25.0*	7.5	8.6	11.5	18.5	21.1	49.5	58.4	59.6	13.7	36.1
1990	**11.0***	**0.4***	**22.4***	**1.1**	**8.9**	**16.4**	**16.8**	**21.4**	**33.8**	**58.5**	**33.2**	**28.7**	**42.1**
1995 projected	*10.1**	*0.3**	*19.1**	*1.0*	*8.1*	*17.6*	*17.6*	*17.3*	*29.5*	*42.9*	*29.6*	*21.4*	*63.2*
Other medical causes													
1985–90	130.4*	57.7*	147.0*	52.9	79.9	104.4	134.4	161.7	208.8	286.6	388.9	542.1	966.5
1985	134.5*	69.0*	161.4*	76.3	105.8	119.1	175.5	173.2	217.0	262.8	427.2	365.3	644.6
1990	**166.6***	**61.8***	**161.7***	**53.4**	**79.9**	**110.8**	**157.6**	**164.1**	**234.8**	**331.5**	**450.2**	**803.8**	**2042.1**
1995 projected	*190.7**	*56.4**	*160.8**	*37.1*	*62.8*	*94.6*	*144.6*	*160.0*	*259.0*	*367.3*	*625.9*	*1128.6*	*2889.5*
All non-medical causes													
1985–90	188.9*	124.6*	244.2*	222.1	260.8	262.2	270.0	230.7	224.9	238.9	246.0	271.0	435.8
1985	189.4*	118.7*	253.7*	251.3	278.0	252.0	304.7	239.5	224.1	226.3	264.9	196.3	403.6
1990	**230.8***	**149.6***	**306.3***	**278.1**	**307.1**	**338.8**	**339.4**	**285.3**	**275.3**	**320.3**	**317.5**	**315.8**	**442.1**
1995 projected	*273.1**	*170.5**	*364.0**	*310.3*	*352.3*	*394.6*	*405.4*	*332.0*	*347.5*	*406.1*	*433.3*	*435.7*	*557.9*

LATVIA: Females

	All ages	0–34	35–69	35–39	40–44	45–49	50–54	55–59	60–64	65–69	70–74	75–79	80+/NK
POPULATION (1000s)													
1985–90	1408.4	653.2	603.1	91.4	83.3	96.6	91.3	91.9	88.3	60.3	52.6	48.8	50.7
1985	1383.0	638.3	587.9	85.4	89.5	98.5	89.5	94.9	79.7	50.4	61.4	47.4	48.0
1990	**1429.7**	**664.5**	**617.4**	**93.7**	**85.4**	**88.8**	**96.6**	**87.4**	**91.6**	**73.9**	**44.7**	**49.7**	**53.4**
1995 projected	*1410.0*	*639.0*	*616.0*	*100.0*	*91.0*	*83.0*	*85.0*	*92.0*	*82.0*	*83.0*	*64.0*	*35.0*	*56.0*
NUMBER OF DEATHS													
All causes													
1985–90	17366	629	4418	133	206	340	489	755	1161	1334	1861	3053	7405
1985	18205	661	4417	135	246	374	512	821	1153	1176	2282	3214	7631
1990	**17861**	**656**	**4816**	**146**	**202**	**378**	**518**	**729**	**1189**	**1654**	**1608**	**3049**	**7732**
1995 projected	*16637*	*574*	*4633*	*138*	*217*	*346*	*451*	*712*	*1001*	*1768*	*2147*	*1991*	*7292*
Lung cancer													
1985–90	182	–	100	2	2	3	9	17	35	32	26	32	24
1985	159	2	91	–	1	3	11	23	28	25	29	17	20
1990	**179**	**1**	**110**	**2**	–	**4**	**6**	**16**	**39**	**43**	**19**	**30**	**19**
1995 projected	*195*	*1*	*112*	*2*	–	*3*	*4*	*15*	*37*	*51*	*33*	*24*	*25*
ANNUAL DEATH RATE / 100,000 (*The rates for the age groups 0–34 and 35–69 are the means of seven five-yearly rates, but the all-ages rates are standardised to the conventional "European" age distribution)													
All causes													
1985–90	865.1*	93.5*	804.1*	145.5	247.3	352.0	535.6	821.5	1314.8	2212.3	3538.0	6256.1	14605.5
1985	932.7*	101.7*	861.4*	158.1	274.9	379.7	572.1	865.1	1446.7	2333.3	3716.6	6780.6	15897.9
1990	**869.2***	**95.7***	**817.8***	**155.8**	**236.5**	**425.7**	**536.2**	**834.1**	**1298.0**	**2238.2**	**3597.3**	**6134.8**	**14479.4**
1995 projected	*807.2**	*91.0**	*778.4**	*138.0*	*238.5*	*416.9*	*530.6*	*773.9*	*1220.7*	*2130.1*	*3354.7*	*5688.6*	*13021.4*
All cancer													
1985–90	142.9*	10.6*	239.5*	41.6	84.0	124.2	193.9	281.8	408.8	542.3	610.3	752.0	706.1
1985	145.3*	12.7*	242.5*	35.1	97.2	116.8	212.3	300.3	424.1	511.9	635.2	664.6	729.2
1990	**142.6***	**11.1***	**235.9***	**39.5**	**70.3**	**161.0**	**167.7**	**262.0**	**413.8**	**537.2**	**604.0**	**738.4**	**779.0**
1995 projected	*140.2**	*10.4**	*223.7**	*33.0*	*73.6*	*150.6*	*157.6*	*231.5*	*396.3*	*522.9*	*621.9*	*785.7*	*848.2*
Lung cancer													
1985–90	10.2*	–	18.4*	2.2	2.4	3.1	9.9	18.5	39.6	53.1	49.4	65.6	47.3
1985	9.5*	0.3*	17.9*	–	1.1	3.0	12.3	24.2	35.1	49.6	47.2	35.9	41.7
1990	**9.7***	**0.1***	**18.8***	**2.1**	–	**4.5**	**6.2**	**18.3**	**42.6**	**58.2**	**42.5**	**60.4**	**35.6**
1995 projected	*10.3**	*0.2**	*19.0**	*2.0*	–	*3.6*	*4.7*	*16.3*	*45.1*	*61.4*	*51.6*	*68.6*	*44.6*
Upper aerodigestive cancer (mouth, oesophagus, pharynx and larynx)													
1985–90	2.4*	–	3.8*	–	1.2	1.0	3.3	4.4	6.8	10.0	11.4	12.3	23.7
1985	3.0*	0.2*	4.2*	–	1.1	–	3.4	3.2	10.0	11.9	21.2	19.0	20.8
1990	**2.6***	**0.1***	**3.3***	**1.1**	**1.2**	**1.1**	**3.1**	**2.3**	**7.6**	**6.8**	**11.2**	**12.1**	**35.6**
1995 projected	*2.3**	–	*2.7**	*1.0*	*1.1*	*1.2*	*3.5*	*2.2*	*4.9*	*4.8*	*7.8*	*11.4*	*41.1*
Other cancer													
1985–90	130.3*	10.6*	217.3*	39.4	80.4	120.1	180.7	259.0	362.4	479.3	549.4	674.2	635.1
1985	132.9*	12.2*	220.4*	35.1	95.0	113.7	196.6	272.9	378.9	450.4	566.8	609.7	666.7
1990	**130.2***	**10.8***	**213.8***	**36.3**	**69.1**	**155.4**	**158.4**	**241.4**	**363.5**	**472.3**	**550.3**	**666.0**	**707.9**
1995 projected	*127.5**	*10.3**	*202.0**	*30.0*	*72.5*	*145.8*	*149.4*	*213.0*	*346.3*	*456.6*	*562.5*	*705.7*	*762.5*
Chronic obstructive pulmonary disease (COPD)													
1985–90	16.7*	1.2*	16.8*	2.2	3.6	5.2	11.0	15.2	30.6	49.8	74.1	135.2	262.3
1985	20.8*	1.5*	21.7*	3.5	3.4	6.1	10.1	20.0	45.2	63.5	94.5	151.9	325.0
1990	**15.9***	**1.0***	**18.7***	**2.1**	**7.0**	**11.3**	**11.4**	**12.6**	**28.4**	**58.2**	**47.0**	**144.9**	**219.1**
1995 projected	*12.9**	*0.8**	*15.3**	*2.0*	*9.9*	*15.7*	*10.6*	*8.7*	*20.7*	*39.8*	*37.5*	*111.4*	*167.9*
Other respiratory disease													
1985–90	6.6*	4.2*	6.1*	2.2	3.6	5.2	5.5	6.5	7.9	11.6	17.1	22.5	47.3
1985	9.9*	6.0*	9.3*	5.9	4.5	6.1	7.8	12.6	10.0	17.9	24.4	38.0	70.8
1990	**5.6***	**2.6***	**5.4***	–	**4.7**	**4.5**	**4.1**	**5.7**	**5.5**	**13.5**	**17.9**	**24.1**	**54.3**
1995 projected	*4.2**	*2.3**	*3.8**	–	*3.3*	*3.6*	*2.4*	*4.3*	*3.7*	*9.6*	*12.5*	*17.1*	*39.3*
Vascular disease													
1985–90	559.6*	3.7*	383.1*	24.1	58.8	102.5	187.3	346.0	651.2	1311.8	2490.5	4844.3	12716.0
1985	621.6*	4.3*	425.4*	25.8	62.6	113.7	194.4	376.2	746.5	1458.3	2643.3	5487.3	14222.9
1990	**529.8***	**3.5***	**381.5***	**27.7**	**56.2**	**114.9**	**201.9**	**358.1**	**622.3**	**1289.6**	**2483.2**	**4533.2**	**11535.6**
1995 projected	*448.7**	*2.6**	*340.0**	*25.0*	*53.8*	*115.7*	*196.5*	*315.2*	*534.1*	*1139.8*	*2118.8*	*3857.1*	*9405.4*
Liver cirrhosis and other liver disease													
1985–90	5.4*	0.3*	9.9*	1.1	3.6	4.1	6.6	12.0	17.0	24.9	24.7	24.6	19.7
1985	4.9*	–	9.0*	1.2	2.2	9.1	5.6	7.4	17.6	19.8	21.2	25.3	16.7
1990	**6.3***	**0.7***	**11.8***	**2.1**	**7.0**	**2.3**	**8.3**	**17.2**	**17.5**	**28.4**	**22.4**	**26.2**	**15.0**
1995 projected	*7.4**	*0.6**	*14.8**	*3.0*	*6.6*	*2.4*	*10.6*	*23.9*	*24.4*	*32.5*	*25.0*	*25.7*	*14.3*
Other medical causes													
1985–90	79.1*	42.8*	86.2*	29.5	34.8	53.8	67.9	95.8	129.1	192.4	209.1	311.5	534.5
1985	73.6*	47.1*	83.7*	41.0	41.3	62.9	73.7	79.0	123.0	164.7	177.5	259.5	245.8
1990	**110.0***	**45.3***	**93.4***	**28.8**	**23.4**	**61.9**	**70.4**	**105.3**	**146.3**	**217.9**	**302.0**	**511.1**	**1552.4**
1995 projected	*132.9**	*40.4**	*110.3**	*20.0*	*17.6*	*54.2*	*76.5*	*120.7*	*182.9*	*300.0*	*420.3*	*722.9*	*2194.6*
All non-medical causes													
1985–90	54.8*	30.6*	62.6*	44.9	58.8	56.9	63.5	64.2	70.2	79.6	112.2	166.0	319.5
1985	56.7*	30.1*	69.9*	45.7	63.7	65.0	68.2	69.5	80.3	97.2	120.5	154.0	287.5
1990	**59.1***	**31.6***	**71.0***	**55.5**	**67.9**	**69.8**	**72.5**	**73.2**	**64.4**	**93.4**	**120.8**	**156.9**	**324.0**
1995 projected	*61.1**	*34.0**	*70.5**	*55.0*	*73.6*	*74.7*	*76.5*	*69.6*	*58.5*	*85.5*	*118.8*	*168.6*	*351.8*

LATVIA: 1985–1990

Smoking–attributed deaths (Sm.) and total deaths (Total)

		ALL CAUSES	ALL CANCER	Lung cancer	Upper aero–digestive ca.	Other cancer	COPD	Other respiratory	Vascular disease	Cirrhosis/ other liver	Other medical	Non–medical
Males												
0–34	Sm.	–	–	–	–	–	–	–	–	–	–	–
	Total	1476	79	2	3	74	11	37	90	5	406	848
35–69	Sm.	2922	1012	642	133	237	212	32	1394	–	272	–
	Total	7336	1835	672	173	990	252	73	3309	79	610	1178
		(40%)	(55%)	(96%)	(77%)	(24%)	(84%)	(44%)	(42%)		(45%)	
70+	Sm.	981	291	198	26	67	199	5	449	–	37	–
	Total	6761	930	224	50	656	298	42	4878	28	387	198
		(15%)	(31%)	(88%)	(52%)	(10%)	(67%)	(12%)	(9%)		(10%)	
Any age	Sm.	3903	1303	840	159	304	411	37	1843	–	309	–
	Total	15573	2844	898	226	1720	561	152	8277	112	1403	2224
		(25%)	(46%)	(94%)	(70%)	(18%)	(73%)	(24%)	(22%)		(22%)	
Females												
0–34	Sm.	–	–	–	–	–	–	–	–	–	–	–
	Total	629	71	0	0	71	8	29	25	2	291	203
35–69	Sm.	269	64	51	4	9	33	2	142	–	28	–
	Total	4418	1352	100	21	1231	91	35	2025	55	488	372
		(6%)	(5%)	(51%)	(19%)	(1%)	(36%)	(6%)	(7%)		(6%)	
70+	Sm.	329	49	38	4	7	78	0	191	–	11	–
	Total	12319	1046	82	24	940	238	44	10121	35	533	302
		(3%)	(5%)	(46%)	(17%)	(1%)	(33%)	(0%)	(2%)		(2%)	
Any age	Sm.	598	113	89	8	16	111	2	333	–	39	–
	Total	17366	2469	182	45	2242	337	108	12171	92	1312	877
		(3%)	(5%)	(49%)	(18%)	(1%)	(33%)	(2%)	(3%)		(3%)	
Males+Females												
0–34	Sm.	–	–	–	–	–	–	–	–	–	–	–
	Total	2105	150	2	3	145	19	66	115	7	697	1051
35–69	Sm.	3191	1076	693	137	246	245	34	1536	–	300	–
	Total	11754	3187	772	194	2221	343	108	5334	134	1098	1550
		(27%)	(34%)	(90%)	(71%)	(11%)	(71%)	(31%)	(29%)		(27%)	
70+	Sm.	1310	340	236	30	74	277	5	640	–	48	–
	Total	19080	1976	306	74	1596	536	86	14999	63	920	500
		(7%)	(17%)	(77%)	(41%)	(5%)	(52%)	(6%)	(4%)		(5%)	
Any age	Sm.	4501	1416	929	167	320	522	39	2176	–	348	–
	Total	32939	5313	1080	271	3962	898	260	20448	204	2715	3101
		(14%)	(27%)	(86%)	(62%)	(8%)	(58%)	(15%)	(11%)		(13%)	

LATVIA: 1985

Smoking–attributed deaths (Sm.) and total deaths (Total)

		ALL CAUSES	ALL CANCER	Lung cancer	Upper aero–digestive ca.	Other cancer	COPD	Other respiratory	Vascular disease	Cirrhosis/ other liver	Other medical	Non–medical
Males												
0–34	Sm.	–	–	–	–	–	–	–	–	–	–	–
	Total	1500	72	3	0	69	13	61	91	10	462	791
35–69	Sm.	2805	852	556	85	211	235	43	1371	–	304	–
	Total	7222	1617	584	116	917	280	91	3289	88	663	1194
		(39%)	(53%)	(95%)	(73%)	(23%)	(84%)	(47%)	(42%)		(46%)	
70+	Sm.	936	268	191	21	56	217	5	416	–	30	–
	Total	7239	918	221	45	652	359	57	5372	27	316	190
		(13%)	(29%)	(86%)	(47%)	(9%)	(60%)	(9%)	(8%)		(9%)	
Any age	Sm.	3741	1120	747	106	267	452	48	1787	–	334	–
	Total	15961	2607	808	161	1638	652	209	8752	125	1441	2175
		(23%)	(43%)	(92%)	(66%)	(16%)	(69%)	(23%)	(20%)		(23%)	
Females												
0–34	Sm.	–	–	–	–	–	–	–	–	–	–	–
	Total	661	82	2	1	79	10	39	28	0	306	196
35–69	Sm.	254	53	42	3	8	38	2	134	–	27	–
	Total	4417	1303	91	21	1191	108	51	2051	48	456	400
		(6%)	(4%)	(46%)	(14%)	(1%)	(35%)	(4%)	(7%)		(6%)	
70+	Sm.	86	16	12	2	2	17	0	50	–	3	–
	Total	13127	1055	66	32	957	286	67	11051	33	350	285
		(1%)	(2%)	(18%)	(6%)	(0%)	(6%)	(0%)	(0%)		(1%)	
Any age	Sm.	340	69	54	5	10	55	2	184	–	30	–
	Total	18205	2440	159	54	2227	404	157	13130	81	1112	881
		(2%)	(3%)	(34%)	(9%)	(0%)	(14%)	(1%)	(1%)		(3%)	
Males+Females												
0–34	Sm.	–	–	–	–	–	–	–	–	–	–	–
	Total	2161	154	5	1	148	23	100	119	10	768	987
35–69	Sm.	3059	905	598	88	219	273	45	1505	–	331	–
	Total	11639	2920	675	137	2108	388	142	5340	136	1119	1594
		(26%)	(31%)	(89%)	(64%)	(10%)	(70%)	(32%)	(28%)		(30%)	
70+	Sm.	1022	284	203	23	58	234	5	466	–	33	–
	Total	20366	1973	287	77	1609	645	124	16423	60	666	475
		(5%)	(14%)	(71%)	(30%)	(4%)	(36%)	(4%)	(3%)		(5%)	
Any age	Sm.	4081	1189	801	111	277	507	50	1971	–	364	–
	Total	34166	5047	967	215	3865	1056	366	21882	206	2553	3056
		(12%)	(24%)	(83%)	(52%)	(7%)	(48%)	(14%)	(9%)		(14%)	

(To be conservative, no deaths before age 35, and none from liver cirrhosis or non–medical causes, were attributed to smoking.)

LATVIA: 1990

Smoking-attributed deaths (Sm.) and total deaths (Total)

		ALL CAUSES	ALL CANCER	Lung cancer	Upper aero-digestive ca.	Other cancer	COPD	Other respiratory	Vascular disease	Cirrhosis/ other liver	Other medical	Non-medical
Males												
0–34	Sm.	–	–	–	–	–	–	–	–	–	–	–
	Total	1702	86	0	2	84	6	23	101	3	445	1038
35–69	Sm.	3278	1082	680	162	240	263	42	1589	–	302	–
	Total	8526	1955	713	216	1026	310	94	3852	91	703	1521
		(38%)	(55%)	(95%)	(75%)	(23%)	(85%)	(45%)	(41%)		(43%)	
70+	Sm.	1021	295	192	31	72	193	5	465	–	63	–
	Total	6723	920	215	55	650	278	45	4591	21	651	217
		(15%)	(32%)	(89%)	(56%)	(11%)	(69%)	(11%)	(10%)		(10%)	
Any age	Sm.	4299	1377	872	193	312	456	47	2054	–	365	–
	Total	16951	2961	928	273	1760	594	162	8544	115	1799	2776
		(25%)	(47%)	(94%)	(71%)	(18%)	(77%)	(29%)	(24%)		(20%)	
Females												
0–34	Sm.	–	–	–	–	–	–	–	–	–	–	–
	Total	656	76	1	1	74	7	18	24	5	313	213
35–69	Sm.	300	67	55	3	9	37	2	161	–	33	–
	Total	4816	1407	110	20	1277	109	32	2207	70	557	434
		(6%)	(5%)	(50%)	(15%)	(1%)	(34%)	(6%)	(7%)		(6%)	
70+	Sm.	258	39	28	5	6	60	0	142	–	17	–
	Total	12389	1053	68	30	955	210	49	9523	31	1218	305
		(2%)	(4%)	(41%)	(17%)	(1%)	(29%)	(0%)	(1%)		(1%)	
Any age	Sm.	558	106	83	8	15	97	2	303	–	50	–
	Total	17861	2536	179	51	2306	326	99	11754	106	2088	952
		(3%)	(4%)	(46%)	(16%)	(1%)	(30%)	(2%)	(3%)		(2%)	
Males+Females												
0–34	Sm.	–	–	–	–	–	–	–	–	–	–	–
	Total	2358	162	1	3	158	13	41	125	8	758	1251
35–69	Sm.	3578	1149	735	165	249	300	44	1750	–	335	–
	Total	13342	3362	823	236	2303	419	126	6059	161	1260	1955
		(27%)	(34%)	(89%)	(70%)	(11%)	(72%)	(35%)	(29%)		(27%)	
70+	Sm.	1279	334	220	36	78	253	5	607	–	80	–
	Total	19112	1973	283	85	1605	488	94	14114	52	1869	522
		(7%)	(17%)	(78%)	(42%)	(5%)	(52%)	(5%)	(4%)		(4%)	
Any age	Sm.	4857	1483	955	201	327	553	49	2357	–	415	–
	Total	34812	5497	1107	324	4066	920	261	20298	221	3887	3728
		(14%)	(27%)	(86%)	(62%)	(8%)	(60%)	(19%)	(12%)		(11%)	

LATVIA: 1995

Smoking-attributed deaths (Sm.) and total deaths (Total)

		ALL CAUSES	ALL CANCER	Lung cancer	Upper aero-digestive ca.	Other cancer	COPD	Other respiratory	Vascular disease	Cirrhosis/ other liver	Other medical	Non-medical
Males												
0–34	Sm.	–	–	–	–	–	–	–	–	–	–	–
	Total	1688	88	0	0	88	5	16	82	2	370	1125
35–69	Sm.	3633	1285	789	239	257	265	48	1730	–	305	–
	Total	9455	2209	826	318	1065	310	108	4161	86	725	1856
		(38%)	(58%)	(96%)	(75%)	(24%)	(85%)	(44%)	(42%)		(42%)	
70+	Sm.	1063	347	219	43	85	157	5	457	–	97	–
	Total	6239	991	242	71	678	218	37	3810	23	876	284
		(17%)	(35%)	(90%)	(61%)	(13%)	(72%)	(14%)	(12%)		(11%)	
Any age	Sm.	4696	1632	1008	282	342	422	53	2187	–	402	–
	Total	17382	3288	1068	389	1831	533	161	8053	111	1971	3265
		(27%)	(50%)	(94%)	(72%)	(19%)	(79%)	(33%)	(27%)		(20%)	
Females												
0–34	Sm.	–	–	–	–	–	–	–	–	–	–	–
	Total	574	68	1	0	67	5	14	17	4	253	213
35–69	Sm.	283	68	56	2	10	25	1	146	–	43	–
	Total	4633	1331	112	16	1203	91	23	2011	89	656	432
		(6%)	(5%)	(50%)	(13%)	(1%)	(27%)	(4%)	(7%)		(7%)	
70+	Sm.	318	55	40	7	8	55	0	171	–	37	–
	Total	11430	1148	82	32	1034	157	36	7973	33	1751	332
		(3%)	(5%)	(49%)	(22%)	(1%)	(35%)	(0%)	(2%)		(2%)	
Any age	Sm.	601	123	96	9	18	80	1	317	–	80	–
	Total	16637	2547	195	48	2304	253	73	10001	126	2660	977
		(4%)	(5%)	(49%)	(19%)	(1%)	(32%)	(1%)	(3%)		(3%)	
Males+Females												
0–34	Sm.	–	–	–	–	–	–	–	–	–	–	–
	Total	2262	156	1	0	155	10	30	99	6	623	1338
35–69	Sm.	3916	1353	845	241	267	290	49	1876	–	348	–
	Total	14088	3540	938	334	2268	401	131	6172	175	1381	2288
		(28%)	(38%)	(90%)	(72%)	(12%)	(72%)	(37%)	(30%)		(25%)	
70+	Sm.	1381	402	259	50	93	212	5	628	–	134	–
	Total	17669	2139	324	103	1712	375	73	11783	56	2627	616
		(8%)	(19%)	(80%)	(49%)	(5%)	(57%)	(7%)	(5%)		(5%)	
Any age	Sm.	5297	1755	1104	291	360	502	54	2504	–	482	–
	Total	34019	5835	1263	437	4135	786	234	18054	237	4631	4242
		(16%)	(30%)	(87%)	(67%)	(9%)	(64%)	(23%)	(14%)		(10%)	

(To be conservative, no deaths before age 35, and none from liver cirrhosis or non-medical causes, were attributed to smoking.)

¶LITHUANIA: 1990

		No. of deaths			Standardised rates (Defined on p.418)			Annual death rates / 100, 000						
		All ages	0–34	35–69	All ages	0–34	35–69	0–4	5–9	10–14	15–19	20–24	25–29	30–34
ALL CAUSES	M	20605	1958	10184	1420.8	189.6	1817.0	288.9	55.4	46.3	127.2	205.2	261.8	342.8
	F	19155	773	5391	763.4	77.6	720.6	231.0	34.2	26.8	54.9	42.5	55.5	98.1
Tuberculosis	M	218	15	168	14.6	1.4	26.1	–	–	–	–	–	3.2	6.9
	F	39	3	26	1.8	0.3	3.5	0.7	0.7	–	–	–	–	0.7
Other infective	M	43	22	17	2.7	2.1	2.4	12.7	0.7	0.7	–	0.7	–	–
and parasitic	F	39	14	16	1.9	1.4	2.1	8.4	–	0.8	–	–	–	0.7
ALL CANCER	M	3943	95	2555	284.9	9.3	473.4	4.7	6.3	6.0	7.8	10.5	12.6	17.3
	F	3016	101	1709	138.7	10.1	223.7	5.6	8.7	2.3	7.4	2.2	7.8	36.4
Mouth and	M	136	3	111	9.5	0.3	18.1	–	0.7	–	0.7	–	–	0.7
pharynx cancer	F	29	2	19	1.4	0.2	2.6	0.7	–	–	–	–	–	0.7
Oesophagus cancer	M	104	–	87	7.3	–	15.1	–	–	–	–	–	–	–
	F	15	–	9	0.7	–	1.2	–	–	–	–	–	–	–
Stomach cancer	M	605	5	375	44.2	0.5	69.9	–	–	–	–	–	1.3	2.1
	F	425	9	225	19.0	0.9	30.1	–	–	–	–	–	0.7	5.5
Colorectal cancer	M	352	2	191	25.9	0.2	37.5	–	–	–	–	–	0.6	0.7
	F	357	5	162	15.6	0.5	21.4	–	–	–	–	–	0.7	2.7
Liver cancer	M	...	...	...	...	...	...	...	...	...	...	...	...	...
	F	...	...	...	...	...	...	...	...	...	...	...	...	...
Pancreas cancer	M	...	...	...	...	...	...	...	...	...	...	...	...	...
	F	...	...	...	...	...	...	...	...	...	...	...	...	...
Larynx cancer	M	136	–	109	9.6	–	19.1	–	–	–	–	–	–	–
	F	6	–	2	0.3	–	0.2	–	–	–	–	–	–	–
Lung cancer	M	1213	1	909	88.5	0.1	170.1	–	–	–	–	–	–	0.7
	F	203	3	102	8.9	0.3	13.4	–	–	–	–	0.7	0.7	0.7
Malignant melanoma	M	...	...	...	...	...	...	...	...	...	...	...	...	...
	F	...	...	...	...	...	...	...	...	...	...	...	...	...
Female breast cancer	F	470	11	330	22.8	1.1	42.2	–	–	–	–	–	0.7	6.9
Cervix cancer	F	193	11	131	9.4	1.1	16.9	–	–	–	–	0.7	1.3	5.5
Other uterine cancer	F	136	–	79	6.2	–	10.3	–	–	–	–	–	–	–
Ovarian cancer	F	...	...	...	...	...	...	...	...	...	...	...	...	...
Prostate cancer	M	247	–	59	18.9	–	13.4	–	–	–	–	–	–	–
Bladder cancer	M	...	...	...	...	...	...	...	...	...	...	...	...	...
	F	...	...	...	...	...	...	...	...	...	...	...	...	...
Other and ill-defined	M	905	47	569	64.2	4.6	104.0	2.0	2.8	1.5	4.9	6.3	5.0	9.7
cancer sites	F	966	33	551	44.3	3.3	72.0	2.1	2.9	–	5.9	0.7	2.0	9.6
Hodgkin's disease	M	...	...	...	...	...	...	...	...	...	...	...	...	...
	F	...	...	...	...	...	...	...	...	...	...	...	...	...
Myeloma and all	M	98	15	62	6.5	1.5	11.0	–	0.7	1.5	0.7	2.8	3.2	1.4
lymphomas	F	82	10	43	3.8	1.0	5.8	0.7	1.5	–	0.7	–	1.3	2.7
Leukaemia	M	147	22	83	10.2	2.2	15.3	2.7	2.1	3.0	1.4	1.4	2.5	2.1
	F	134	17	56	6.2	1.7	7.5	2.1	4.4	2.3	0.7	–	0.7	2.1
ALL VASCULAR	M	10157	114	4159	721.3	11.0	782.0	1.3	0.7	0.7	2.1	9.1	23.3	39.4
DISEASE	F	12854	40	2220	472.2	4.0	307.1	0.7	–	0.8	5.2	3.7	6.5	11.0
Rheumatic heart	M	139	10	118	9.5	0.9	19.9	–	–	–	–	1.4	3.2	2.1
disease and fever	F	174	4	135	8.5	0.4	17.5	–	–	–	–	–	0.7	2.1
Hypertensive disease	M	1	–	–	0.1	–	–	–	–	–	–	–	–	–
	F	1	–	–	0.0	–	–	–	–	–	–	–	–	–
Ischaemic heart	M	7699	65	2998	544.8	6.3	561.5	–	–	–	–	2.8	11.4	29.7
disease	F	9244	6	1273	330.6	0.6	178.5	–	–	–	–	–	2.0	2.1
Pulmonary embolism	M	...	...	...	...	...	...	...	...	...	...	...	...	...
and other venous	F	...	...	...	...	...	...	...	...	...	...	...	...	...
Cerebrovascular	M	1887	17	798	136.9	1.6	157.4	–	–	0.7	0.7	2.1	4.4	3.5
disease	F	2967	11	672	114.5	1.1	92.5	–	–	–	1.5	2.2	2.6	1.4
Other vascular	M	431	22	245	30.1	2.1	43.2	1.3	0.7	–	1.4	2.8	4.4	4.1
disease, incl. venous	F	468	19	140	18.5	1.9	18.6	0.7	–	0.8	3.7	1.5	1.3	5.5
Chronic obstructive	M	1077	16	446	77.9	1.6	89.1	–	–	0.7	1.4	2.1	0.6	6.2
pulmonary disease	F	570	8	175	22.6	0.8	24.1	–	–	1.5	2.2	0.7	1.3	–
Other respiratory	M	101	29	59	6.3	2.8	9.4	9.3	2.1	–	3.5	2.1	0.6	2.1
disease	F	70	17	23	3.2	1.7	3.1	6.3	2.2	0.8	1.5	–	1.3	–
Peptic ulcer	M	72	2	47	5.0	0.2	8.6	–	–	–	–	–	0.6	0.7
	F	58	2	20	2.4	0.2	2.8	–	–	–	0.7	0.7	–	–
Liver cirrhosis and	M	210	12	155	14.5	1.2	26.9	–	–	0.7	–	0.7	1.3	5.5
other liver disease	F	129	1	92	6.1	0.1	11.9	–	–	–	–	–	–	0.7
Renal disease	M	178	19	91	12.2	1.8	15.9	–	0.7	–	–	1.4	5.0	5.5
	F	217	13	125	9.9	1.3	16.8	2.1	0.7	–	–	0.7	2.6	2.7
Pregnancy and birth	F	13	7	6	0.7	0.7	0.7	–	–	–	–	0.7	1.3	2.7
Congenital and	M	334	316	15	18.0	30.3	2.5	186.1	6.3	4.5	6.4	3.5	3.2	2.1
perinatal causes	F	273	255	17	15.1	25.5	2.0	159.4	2.9	4.6	4.4	5.2	2.0	–
Ill-defined causes	M	38	7	1	2.4	0.7	0.1	4.7	–	–	–	–	–	–
	F	78	4	–	2.5	0.4	–	2.1	–	–	–	–	0.7	–
Other medical causes	M	795	103	489	53.0	10.0	79.1	15.3	4.2	1.5	3.5	8.4	11.4	25.6
	F	777	66	418	36.3	6.6	54.2	14.6	0.7	5.4	4.4	3.0	7.8	10.3
ALL NON-	M	3439	1208	1982	208.0	117.3	301.4	54.7	34.3	31.3	102.5	166.7	200.0	231.5
MEDICAL CAUSES	F	1022	242	544	50.1	24.5	68.6	31.3	18.2	10.7	28.9	25.4	24.2	32.9
Motor vehicle	M	854	384	399	50.3	37.3	62.2	8.0	12.6	12.7	41.7	64.4	69.4	52.5
traffic accidents	F	293	82	140	14.2	8.4	18.2	4.9	7.3	1.5	16.3	11.2	5.9	11.7
Fire	M	57	20	28	3.6	1.9	4.6	7.3	1.4	–	0.7	1.4	–	2.8
	F	36	14	9	1.7	1.4	1.1	4.9	1.5	1.5	–	0.7	0.7	0.7
Suicide	M	779	203	525	48.4	19.5	80.2	–	–	2.2	14.1	21.7	45.4	53.2
	F	190	34	117	9.3	3.4	14.7	–	–	0.8	4.4	3.7	7.2	7.5
Homicide	M	196	84	104	11.4	8.2	15.1	–	–	–	6.4	15.4	13.2	22.1
	F	85	23	52	4.4	2.3	6.4	0.7	1.5	–	2.2	3.0	2.0	6.9
POPULATION (thousands):	M=males				1755.8	1014.1	656.3	149.9	142.7	134.0	141.5	142.8	158.5	144.7
	F=females				1952.6	979.6	800.0	143.7	137.4	130.6	134.9	134.1	153.1	145.8

LITHUANIA: 1990

Annual death rates / 100, 000

9th ICD categories

35–39	40–44	45–49	50–54	55–59	60–64	65–69	70–74	75–79	80+/NK			
511.9	736.4	1052.0	1418.1	2073.8	2849.9	4076.9	5861.8	7652.7	15287.1	M	**ALL CAUSES**	001–999
160.2	255.6	368.4	456.8	756.4	1179.4	1867.1	3165.4	5234.9	12877.7	F		
22.1	20.6	27.9	20.6	35.8	27.2	28.8	36.4	38.2	47.3	M	**Tuberculosis**	010–018, 137
–	0.9	0.9	1.7	9.4	2.6	8.9	3.9	8.9	4.6	F		
0.8	3.7	5.8	2.9	1.1	2.6	–	14.5	–	–	M	**Other infective**	Rest of 001–139
–	0.9	0.9	1.7	0.9	6.2	4.4	1.9	1.8	10.7	F	**and parasitic**	
41.0	108.4	201.2	335.6	626.5	870.6	1130.8	1516.4	1496.2	1526.8	M	**ALL CANCER**	140–208
50.8	91.2	132.0	181.1	276.0	386.1	448.5	638.1	717.1	726.3	F		
2.5	10.3	20.2	21.6	28.2	20.7	23.1	32.7	30.5	15.8	M	**Mouth and**	140–149
–	1.7	0.9	1.7	2.6	3.5	7.8	3.9	5.3	4.6	F	**pharynx cancer**	
0.8	4.7	7.7	11.8	29.3	28.5	23.1	25.5	11.5	22.1	M	**Oesophagus cancer**	150
–	–	0.9	0.8	1.7	2.6	2.2	1.9	1.8	6.1	F		
9.0	17.8	36.6	52.0	67.3	129.4	176.9	254.5	259.5	274.4	M	**Stomach cancer**	151
9.5	8.6	18.1	21.6	28.1	44.9	79.7	85.6	124.6	117.7	F		
2.5	4.7	9.6	17.7	43.4	75.0	109.6	156.4	187.0	211.4	M	**Colorectal cancer**	153, 154
3.2	6.9	13.8	19.1	23.0	35.2	48.7	83.7	92.5	145.3	F		
...	...	...	...	...	...	...	...	...	...	M	**Liver cancer**	Not given separately
...	...	...	...	...	...	...	...	...	...	F		
...	...	...	...	...	...	...	...	...	...	M	**Pancreas cancer**	Not given separately
...	...	...	...	...	...	...	...	...	...	F		
–	7.5	11.5	19.6	31.5	27.2	36.5	29.1	34.4	31.5	M	**Larynx cancer**	161
–	–	–	–	0.9	0.9	–	7.8	–	–	F		
4.9	24.3	47.2	119.7	244.3	359.6	390.4	483.6	366.4	233.4	M	**Lung cancer**	162
0.8	3.4	6.9	6.6	17.9	30.8	27.7	44.7	69.4	55.0	F		
...	...	...	...	...	...	...	...	...	...	M	**Malignant melanoma**	Not given
...	...	...	...	...	...	...	...	...	...	F		separately
10.3	30.1	32.8	44.0	53.7	66.0	58.7	75.9	71.2	76.5	F	**Female breast cancer**	174
7.9	8.6	11.2	15.0	17.0	31.7	26.6	42.8	21.4	26.0	F	**Cervix cancer**	180
0.8	2.6	2.6	7.5	17.9	21.1	19.9	35.0	28.5	35.2	F	**Other uterine cancer**	179, 182
...	...	...	...	...	...	...	...	...	...	F	**Ovarian cancer**	Not given separately
–	–	1.0	3.9	7.6	18.1	63.5	170.9	190.8	287.1	M	**Prostate cancer**	185
...	...	...	...	...	...	...	...	...	...	M	**Bladder cancer**	Not given separately
...	...	...	...	...	...	...	...	...	...	F		
16.4	29.9	58.7	65.8	145.5	161.7	250.0	294.5	351.1	365.9	M	**Other and ill-defined**	Rest of 140–208,
14.3	26.7	38.8	55.6	96.3	131.9	140.6	198.4	238.4	223.2	F	**cancer sites**	incl. 155, 157, 172, 183, 188
...	...	...	...	...	...	...	...	...	...	M	**Hodgkin's disease**	Not given separately
...	...	...	...	...	...	...	...	...	...	F		
4.1	5.6	1.0	12.8	8.7	22.0	23.1	18.2	26.7	28.4	M	**Myeloma and all**	200–203,
0.8	–	2.6	5.0	6.8	8.8	16.6	17.5	21.4	12.2	F	**lymphomas**	incl. 201
0.8	3.7	7.7	10.8	20.6	28.5	34.6	50.9	38.2	56.8	M	**Leukaemia**	204–208
3.2	2.6	3.5	4.2	10.2	8.8	19.9	40.9	42.7	24.5	F		
102.4	203.7	359.0	548.6	820.8	1341.5	2098.1	3360.0	4904.6	11593.1	M	**ALL VASCULAR**	390–459
15.9	40.4	95.8	140.4	272.6	521.5	1063.1	2087.5	3927.0	11183.5	F	**DISEASE**	
7.4	8.4	20.2	21.6	22.8	20.7	38.5	25.5	7.6	6.3	M	**Rheumatic heart**	390–398
4.0	3.4	12.9	15.8	17.9	38.7	29.9	31.1	16.0	15.3	F	**disease and fever**	
–	–	–	–	–	–	–	3.6	–	–	M	**Hypertensive disease**	401–405
–	–	–	–	–	–	–	–	–	1.5	F		
70.4	143.9	257.0	406.3	621.1	950.8	1480.8	2436.4	3740.5	9419.6	M	**Ischaemic heart**	410–414
5.6	18.1	33.6	64.0	144.0	303.4	681.1	1356.0	2800.7	8706.4	F	**disease**	
...	...	...	...	...	...	...	...	...	...	M	**Pulmonary embolism**	Not given
...	...	...	...	...	...	...	...	...	...	F	**and other venous**	separately
16.4	26.2	56.8	82.4	133.6	296.2	490.4	763.6	1042.0	1858.0	M	**Cerebrovascular**	430–438
5.6	13.8	37.1	45.7	89.4	147.8	307.9	634.2	1021.4	2116.2	F	**disease**	
8.2	25.2	25.0	38.3	43.4	73.7	88.5	130.9	114.5	309.1	M	**Other vascular**	Rest of 390–459,
0.8	5.2	12.1	15.0	21.3	31.7	44.3	66.1	89.0	344.0	F	**disease, incl. venous**	incl. 415, 451–3
5.7	5.6	20.2	41.2	115.1	147.5	288.5	418.2	599.2	1082.0	M	**Chronic obstructive**	490–496
1.6	4.3	9.5	10.0	25.6	36.9	80.8	101.2	190.4	348.6	F	**pulmonary disease**	
3.3	6.5	9.6	10.8	8.7	19.4	7.7	7.3	11.5	25.2	M	**Other respiratory**	Rest of 460–519
1.6	0.9	2.6	0.8	4.3	3.5	7.8	13.6	10.7	26.0	F	**disease**	
2.5	1.9	5.8	6.9	8.7	11.6	23.1	10.9	22.9	44.2	M	**Peptic ulcer**	531–533
0.8	–	0.9	1.7	2.6	3.5	10.0	15.6	12.5	32.1	F		
10.6	15.0	15.4	16.7	29.3	53.0	48.1	47.3	64.9	41.0	M	**Liver cirrhosis and**	570–573, 576,
4.0	6.9	6.9	7.5	12.8	25.5	19.9	21.4	19.6	21.4	F	**other liver disease**	575.2–579.9
8.2	4.7	14.4	12.8	14.1	20.7	36.5	43.6	87.8	104.1	M	**Renal disease**	580–590
3.2	7.7	8.6	10.8	10.2	31.7	45.4	37.0	44.5	53.5	F		
3.2	1.7	–	–	–	–	–	–	–	–	F	**Pregnancy and birth**	630–676
–	2.8	1.9	1.0	4.3	5.2	1.9	7.3	–	3.2	M	**Congenital and**	740–779
4.8	4.3	3.5	0.8	0.9	–	–	–	–	1.5	F	**perinatal causes**	
–	–	1.0	–	–	–	–	3.6	7.6	85.2	M	**Ill-defined causes**	780–799
–	–	–	–	–	–	–	1.9	7.1	105.5	F		
36.0	72.9	70.3	72.6	98.8	93.1	109.6	145.5	206.1	343.8	M	**Other medical causes**	Rest of 001–799
12.7	37.9	36.2	41.5	72.4	82.7	96.3	151.8	167.3	185.0	F		
279.3	290.7	319.5	348.4	310.5	257.4	303.8	250.9	213.7	391.2	M	**ALL NON-**	E800–E999
61.9	58.5	70.8	59.0	69.0	79.2	81.9	91.4	128.1	178.9	F	**MEDICAL CAUSES**	
59.0	47.7	48.1	67.7	77.1	60.8	75.0	72.7	68.7	104.1	M	**Motor vehicle**	E810–E819
11.1	12.9	19.8	17.4	11.9	17.6	36.5	27.2	46.3	47.4	F	**traffic accidents**	
1.6	4.7	7.7	2.9	2.2	5.2	7.7	7.3	7.6	15.8	M	**Fire**	E890–E899
–	–	1.7	0.8	2.6	1.8	1.1	5.8	3.6	12.2	F		
65.5	80.4	92.4	95.2	77.1	66.0	84.6	61.8	45.8	69.4	M	**Suicide**	E950–E959
13.5	11.2	15.5	10.0	13.6	23.7	15.5	17.5	24.9	24.5	F		
18.0	25.2	19.2	14.7	7.6	9.1	11.5	10.9	–	15.8	M	**Homicide**	E960–E969
9.5	9.5	6.9	5.8	3.4	4.4	5.5	5.8	7.1	4.6	F		
122.1	107.0	103.9	101.9	92.1	77.3	52.0	27.5	26.2	31.7	M	**POPULATION (thousands)**	
126.1	116.2	115.9	120.4	117.4	113.7	90.3	51.4	56.2	65.4	F		

LITHUANIA: Males

	All ages	0–34	35–69	35–39	40–44	45–49	50–54	55–59	60–64	65–69	70–74	75–79	80+/NK
POPULATION (1000s)													
1985–90	1708.4	992.3	626.5	115.8	103.1	106.5	100.1	90.9	67.6	42.5	30.6	30.1	28.9
1985	1662.2	970.4	596.7	107.3	105.6	106.4	98.8	85.0	59.7	33.9	34.7	34.2	26.2
1990	**1755.8**	**1014.1**	**656.3**	**122.1**	**107.0**	**103.9**	**101.9**	**92.1**	**77.3**	**52.0**	**27.5**	**26.2**	**31.7**
1995 projected	*1789.0*	*995.0*	*699.0*	*141.0*	*118.0*	*102.0*	*97.0*	*94.0*	*82.0*	*65.0*	*41.0*	*20.0*	*34.0*
NUMBER OF DEATHS													
All causes													
1985–90	19386	1960	8879	550	707	1026	1343	1722	1846	1685	1664	2323	4560
1985	20284	2236	8678	599	794	1104	1425	1678	1695	1383	1982	2944	4444
1990	**20605**	**1958**	**10184**	**625**	**788**	**1093**	**1445**	**1910**	**2203**	**2120**	**1612**	**2005**	**4846**
1995 projected	*21061*	*1595*	*11016*	*671*	*852*	*1065*	*1403*	*1977*	*2365*	*2683*	*2299*	*1440*	*4711*
Lung cancer													
1985–90	1108	3	800	8	26	63	127	207	207	162	119	108	78
1985	995	4	664	15	28	68	129	163	149	112	137	132	58
1990	**1213**	**1**	**909**	**6**	**26**	**49**	**122**	**225**	**278**	**203**	**133**	**96**	**74**
1995 projected	*1527*	*1*	*1154*	*5*	*20*	*40*	*120*	*283*	*371*	*315*	*216*	*78*	*78*
ANNUAL DEATH RATE / 100,000 (*The rates for the age groups 0–34 and 35–69 are the means of seven five-yearly rates, but the all-ages rates are standardised to the conventional "European" age distribution)													
All causes													
1985–90	1384.0*	196.2*	1722.2*	475.0	685.7	963.4	1341.7	1894.4	2730.8	3964.7	5437.9	7717.6	15778.5
1985	1490.0*	232.5*	1811.9*	558.2	751.9	1037.6	1442.3	1974.1	2839.2	4079.6	5711.8	8608.2	16961.8
1990	**1420.8***	**189.6***	**1817.0***	**511.9**	**736.4**	**1052.0**	**1418.1**	**2073.8**	**2849.9**	**4076.9**	**5861.8**	**7652.7**	**15287.1**
1995 projected	*1362.9**	*158.9**	*1829.1**	*475.9*	*722.0*	*1044.1*	*1446.4*	*2103.2*	*2884.1*	*4127.7*	*5607.3*	*7200.0*	*13855.9*
All cancer													
1985–90	268.2*	10.4*	456.5*	44.0	96.0	184.0	346.7	580.9	828.4	1115.3	1277.8	1375.4	1467.1
1985	256.5*	11.0*	435.2*	47.5	90.9	173.9	337.0	544.7	778.9	1073.7	1242.1	1426.9	1263.4
1990	**284.9***	**9.3***	**473.4***	**41.0**	**108.4**	**201.2**	**335.6**	**626.5**	**870.6**	**1130.8**	**1516.4**	**1496.2**	**1526.8**
1995 projected	*314.7**	*8.0**	*524.0**	*48.2*	*124.6*	*216.7*	*359.8*	*693.6*	*956.1*	*1269.2*	*1636.6*	*1720.0*	*1732.4*
Lung cancer													
1985–90	83.9*	0.3*	161.9*	6.9	25.2	59.2	126.9	227.7	306.2	381.2	388.9	358.8	269.9
1985	77.9*	0.4*	143.8*	14.0	26.5	63.9	130.6	191.8	249.6	330.4	394.8	386.0	221.4
1990	**88.5***	**0.1***	**170.1***	**4.9**	**24.3**	**47.2**	**119.7**	**244.3**	**359.6**	**390.4**	**483.6**	**366.4**	**233.4**
1995 projected	*101.1**	*0.1**	*203.1**	*3.5*	*16.9*	*39.2*	*123.7*	*301.1*	*452.4*	*484.6*	*526.8*	*390.0*	*229.4*
Upper aerodigestive cancer (mouth, oesophagus, pharynx and larynx)													
1985–90	22.3*	0.1*	44.8*	5.2	15.5	30.0	50.0	62.7	76.9	72.9	68.6	66.4	65.7
1985	20.7*	0.4*	41.3*	3.7	16.1	23.5	37.4	50.6	72.0	85.5	89.3	67.3	38.2
1990	**26.4***	**0.3***	**52.3***	**3.3**	**22.4**	**39.5**	**53.0**	**89.0**	**76.3**	**82.7**	**87.3**	**76.3**	**69.4**
1995 projected	*32.6**	*0.2**	*64.5**	*4.3*	*31.4*	*53.9*	*73.2*	*118.1*	*89.0*	*81.5*	*85.4*	*95.0*	*94.1*
Other cancer													
1985–90	162.0*	10.0*	249.8*	32.0	55.3	94.8	169.8	290.4	445.3	661.2	820.3	950.2	1131.5
1985	158.0*	10.1*	250.2*	29.8	48.3	86.5	169.0	302.4	457.3	657.8	757.9	973.7	1003.8
1990	**170.0***	**8.9***	**251.1***	**32.8**	**61.7**	**114.5**	**162.9**	**293.2**	**434.7**	**657.7**	**945.5**	**1053.4**	**1224.0**
1995 projected	*181.0**	*7.7**	*256.5**	*40.4*	*76.3*	*123.5*	*162.9*	*274.5*	*414.6*	*703.1*	*1024.4*	*1235.0*	*1408.8*
Chronic obstructive pulmonary disease (COPD)													
1985–90	88.2*	1.0*	98.4*	6.0	11.6	24.4	50.9	106.7	187.9	301.2	490.2	707.6	1224.9
1985	113.3*	1.6*	122.6*	7.5	16.1	38.5	84.0	138.8	227.8	345.1	619.6	967.8	1542.0
1990	**77.9***	**1.6***	**89.1***	**5.7**	**5.6**	**20.2**	**41.2**	**115.1**	**147.5**	**288.5**	**418.2**	**599.2**	**1082.0**
1995 projected	*54.9**	*1.4**	*63.6**	*4.3*	*4.2*	*13.7*	*28.9*	*79.8*	*111.0*	*203.1*	*287.8*	*415.0*	*764.7*
Other respiratory disease													
1985–90	9.0*	5.5*	10.9*	4.3	5.8	7.5	10.0	14.3	17.8	16.5	16.3	23.3	34.6
1985	13.7*	9.9*	15.2*	6.5	8.5	12.2	12.1	16.5	26.8	23.6	25.9	35.1	34.4
1990	**6.3***	**2.8***	**9.4***	**3.3**	**6.5**	**9.6**	**10.8**	**8.7**	**19.4**	**7.7**	**7.3**	**11.5**	**25.2**
1995 projected	*4.7**	*2.5**	*6.5**	*2.1*	*4.2*	*7.8*	*7.2*	*6.4*	*13.4*	*4.6*	*4.9*	*10.0*	*17.6*
Vascular disease													
1985–90	704.6*	11.3*	730.3*	93.3	190.1	322.1	498.5	759.1	1239.6	2009.4	3107.8	4936.9	12093.4
1985	749.2*	13.8*	752.7*	101.6	185.6	332.7	503.0	792.9	1288.1	2064.9	3227.7	5359.6	13259.5
1990	**721.3***	**11.0***	**782.0***	**102.4**	**203.7**	**359.0**	**548.6**	**820.8**	**1341.5**	**2098.1**	**3360.0**	**4904.6**	**11593.1**
1995 projected	*685.2**	*9.2**	*796.3**	*100.0*	*213.6*	*377.5*	*567.0*	*839.4*	*1347.6*	*2129.2*	*3182.9*	*4440.0*	*10270.6*
Liver cirrhosis and other liver disease													
1985–90	12.8*	0.9*	23.8*	8.6	13.6	16.9	23.0	29.7	37.0	37.6	39.2	43.2	41.5
1985	16.0*	1.2*	30.5*	15.8	16.1	21.6	36.4	44.7	55.3	23.6	43.2	43.9	26.7
1990	**14.5***	**1.2***	**26.9***	**10.6**	**15.0**	**15.4**	**16.7**	**29.3**	**53.0**	**48.1**	**47.3**	**64.9**	**41.0**
1995 projected	*14.5**	*0.9**	*24.9**	*9.2*	*11.0*	*10.8*	*11.3*	*20.2*	*54.9*	*56.9*	*65.9*	*85.0*	*58.8*
Other medical causes													
1985–90	111.2*	54.1*	136.3*	65.6	89.2	115.5	119.9	147.4	179.0	237.6	274.5	382.1	581.3
1985	134.4*	72.0*	166.6*	93.2	118.4	143.8	161.9	176.5	201.0	271.4	302.6	494.2	465.6
1990	**107.8***	**46.5***	**134.8***	**69.6**	**106.5**	**127.0**	**116.8**	**162.9**	**160.4**	**200.0**	**261.8**	**362.6**	**627.8**
1995 projected	*86.7**	*31.3**	*107.7**	*53.2*	*89.0*	*102.0*	*95.9*	*129.8*	*126.8*	*156.9*	*197.6*	*340.0*	*647.1*
All non-medical causes													
1985–90	190.1*	112.9*	266.1*	253.0	279.3	293.0	292.7	256.3	241.1	247.1	232.0	249.2	335.6
1985	206.9*	123.0*	289.1*	286.1	316.3	314.8	307.7	260.0	261.3	277.3	250.7	280.7	370.2
1990	**208.0***	**117.3***	**301.4***	**279.3**	**290.7**	**319.5**	**348.4**	**310.5**	**257.4**	**303.8**	**250.9**	**213.7**	**391.2**
1995 projected	*202.2**	*105.7**	*306.1**	*258.9*	*275.4*	*315.7*	*376.3*	*334.0*	*274.4*	*307.7*	*231.7*	*190.0*	*364.7*

LITHUANIA: Females

	All ages	0–34	35–69	35–39	40–44	45–49	50–54	55–59	60–64	65–69	70–74	75–79	80+/NK
POPULATION (1000s)													
1985–90	1909.3	963.6	770.8	122.2	113.0	120.3	119.6	117.6	106.2	71.9	58.4	55.6	60.9
1985	1866.5	947.8	740.8	115.4	115.9	122.3	119.2	115.9	95.2	56.9	67.1	54.4	56.4
1990	**1952.6**	**979.6**	**800.0**	**126.1**	**116.2**	**115.9**	**120.4**	**117.4**	**113.7**	**90.3**	**51.4**	**56.2**	**65.4**
1995 projected	*1980.0*	*959.0*	*829.0*	*144.0*	*124.0*	*114.0*	*113.0*	*116.0*	*112.0*	*106.0*	*80.0*	*42.0*	*70.0*
NUMBER OF DEATHS													
All causes													
1985–90	18542	846	4899	184	272	406	579	876	1220	1362	1788	2989	8020
1985	18885	914	4772	189	310	449	626	933	1148	1117	2078	3182	7939
1990	**19155**	**773**	**5391**	**202**	**297**	**427**	**550**	**888**	**1341**	**1686**	**1627**	**2942**	**8422**
1995 projected	*18764*	*600*	*5462*	*221*	*312*	*393*	*482*	*828*	*1264*	*1962*	*2384*	*2027*	*8291*
Lung cancer													
1985–90	175	1	95	1	3	6	11	16	30	28	25	26	28
1985	173	1	97	1	6	6	22	19	27	16	24	26	25
1990	**203**	**3**	**102**	**1**	**4**	**8**	**8**	**21**	**35**	**25**	**23**	**39**	**36**
1995 projected	*242*	*2*	*104*	*1*	*4*	*6*	*6*	*18*	*36*	*33*	*45*	*39*	*52*

ANNUAL DEATH RATE / 100,000 (*The rates for the age groups 0–34 and 35–69 are the means of seven five-yearly rates, but the all-ages rates are standardised to the conventional "European" age distribution)

	All ages	0–34	35–69	35–39	40–44	45–49	50–54	55–59	60–64	65–69	70–74	75–79	80+/NK
All causes													
1985–90	770.8*	86.8*	714.4*	150.6	240.7	337.5	484.1	744.9	1148.8	1894.3	3061.6	5375.9	13169.1
1985	822.1*	97.0*	756.8*	163.8	267.5	367.1	525.2	805.0	1205.9	1963.1	3096.9	5849.3	14076.2
1990	**763.4***	**77.6***	**720.6***	**160.2**	**255.6**	**368.4**	**456.8**	**756.4**	**1179.4**	**1867.1**	**3165.4**	**5234.9**	**12877.7**
1995 projected	*710.7**	*62.6**	*695.7**	*153.5*	*251.6*	*344.7*	*426.5*	*713.8*	*1128.6*	*1850.9*	*2980.0*	*4826.2*	*11844.3*
All cancer													
1985–90	136.5*	10.2*	229.5*	49.9	85.8	126.4	189.0	272.1	390.8	492.4	585.6	681.7	655.2
1985	138.4*	11.0*	234.0*	43.3	104.4	135.7	199.7	272.6	407.6	474.5	564.8	687.5	631.2
1990	**138.7***	**10.1***	**223.7***	**50.8**	**91.2**	**132.0**	**181.1**	**276.0**	**386.1**	**448.5**	**638.1**	**717.1**	**726.3**
1995 projected	*139.1**	*8.7**	*217.8**	*51.4*	*87.9*	*122.8*	*175.2*	*263.8*	*368.8*	*454.7*	*658.8*	*802.4*	*795.7*
Lung cancer													
1985–90	8.2*	0.1*	14.1*	0.8	2.7	5.0	9.2	13.6	28.2	38.9	42.8	46.8	46.0
1985	8.6*	0.1*	14.6*	0.9	5.2	4.9	18.5	16.4	28.4	28.1	35.8	47.8	44.3
1990	**8.9***	**0.3***	**13.4***	**0.8**	**3.4**	**6.9**	**6.6**	**17.9**	**30.8**	**27.7**	**44.7**	**69.4**	**55.0**
1995 projected	*9.9**	*0.2**	*13.3**	*0.7*	*3.2*	*5.3*	*5.3*	*15.5*	*32.1*	*31.1*	*56.3*	*92.9*	*74.3*
Upper aerodigestive cancer (mouth, oesophagus, pharynx and larynx)													
1985–90	2.0*	–	3.3*	0.8	1.8	0.8	1.7	5.1	5.6	7.0	10.3	9.0	14.8
1985	1.5*	–	2.3*	0.9	0.9	2.5	–	6.0	2.1	3.5	10.4	7.4	8.9
1990	**2.3***	**0.2***	**4.0***	**–**	**1.7**	**1.7**	**2.5**	**5.1**	**7.0**	**10.0**	**13.6**	**7.1**	**10.7**
1995 projected	*2.9**	*0.1**	*5.4**	*–*	*1.6*	*2.6*	*2.7*	*6.9*	*9.8*	*14.2*	*18.8*	*7.1*	*11.4*
Other cancer													
1985–90	126.3*	10.1*	212.2*	48.3	81.4	120.5	178.1	253.4	356.9	446.5	532.5	625.9	594.4
1985	128.3*	10.9*	217.1*	41.6	98.4	128.4	181.2	250.2	377.1	442.9	518.6	632.4	578.0
1990	**127.4***	**9.6***	**206.2***	**50.0**	**86.1**	**123.4**	**171.9**	**253.0**	**348.3**	**410.9**	**579.8**	**640.6**	**660.6**
1995 projected	*126.2**	*8.4**	*199.1**	*50.7*	*83.1*	*114.9*	*167.3*	*241.4*	*326.8*	*409.4*	*583.8*	*702.4*	*710.0*
Chronic obstructive pulmonary disease (COPD)													
1985–90	25.6*	1.0*	23.9*	3.3	3.5	7.5	14.2	25.5	39.5	73.7	125.0	217.6	428.6
1985	34.7*	1.4*	30.3*	6.1	2.6	9.0	14.3	30.2	48.3	101.9	165.4	312.5	611.7
1990	**22.6***	**0.8***	**24.1***	**1.6**	**4.3**	**9.5**	**10.0**	**25.6**	**36.9**	**80.8**	**101.2**	**190.4**	**348.6**
1995 projected	*16.6**	*0.9**	*18.3**	*1.4*	*4.0*	*8.8*	*8.0*	*19.8*	*29.5*	*56.6*	*70.0*	*131.0*	*247.1*
Other respiratory disease													
1985–90	4.3*	3.9*	3.3*	0.8	0.9	2.5	2.5	3.4	4.7	8.3	10.3	10.8	23.0
1985	6.2*	6.5*	4.6*	0.9	2.6	2.5	3.4	3.5	10.5	8.8	10.4	12.9	16.0
1990	**3.2***	**1.7***	**3.1***	**1.6**	**0.9**	**2.6**	**0.8**	**4.3**	**3.5**	**7.8**	**13.6**	**10.7**	**26.0**
1995 projected	*2.9**	*1.3**	*2.4**	*1.4*	*0.8*	*1.8*	*0.9*	*2.6*	*2.7*	*6.6*	*13.8*	*14.3*	*32.9*
Vascular disease													
1985–90	481.8*	4.2*	307.3*	20.5	46.0	82.3	148.0	282.3	515.1	1057.0	2029.1	4084.5	11571.4
1985	511.4*	3.6*	324.7*	24.3	44.9	85.9	156.0	321.0	517.9	1123.0	2049.2	4459.6	12351.1
1990	**472.2***	**4.0***	**307.1***	**15.9**	**40.4**	**95.8**	**140.4**	**272.6**	**521.5**	**1063.1**	**2087.5**	**3927.0**	**11183.5**
1995 projected	*430.6**	*4.1**	*295.8**	*13.9*	*39.5*	*92.1*	*125.7*	*255.2*	*490.2*	*1053.8*	*1903.8*	*3471.4*	*10052.9*
Liver cirrhosis and other liver disease													
1985–90	5.6*	0.2*	11.0*	3.3	5.3	6.7	7.5	13.6	19.8	20.9	18.8	19.8	16.4
1985	6.5*	0.4*	12.3*	1.7	6.0	9.0	12.6	18.1	17.9	21.1	17.9	23.9	21.3
1990	**6.1***	**0.1***	**11.9***	**4.0**	**6.9**	**6.9**	**7.5**	**12.8**	**25.5**	**19.9**	**21.4**	**19.6**	**21.4**
1995 projected	*6.0**	*0.1**	*12.0**	*4.9*	*7.3*	*5.3*	*5.3*	*12.1*	*25.9*	*23.6*	*20.0*	*19.0*	*20.0*
Other medical causes													
1985–90	68.5*	40.6*	77.0*	27.0	43.4	52.4	61.9	85.9	113.0	155.8	198.6	242.8	293.9
1985	73.1*	45.8*	83.7*	35.5	38.0	56.4	76.3	88.0	128.2	163.4	208.6	229.8	244.7
1990	**70.6***	**36.4***	**82.1***	**24.6**	**53.4**	**50.9**	**58.1**	**96.3**	**126.6**	**165.0**	**212.1**	**242.0**	**393.0**
1995 projected	*67.5**	*26.4**	*80.7**	*23.6*	*53.2*	*48.2*	*54.0*	*92.2*	*128.6*	*165.1*	*215.0*	*257.1*	*525.7*
All non-medical causes													
1985–90	48.4*	26.7*	62.4*	45.8	55.8	59.9	61.0	62.1	65.9	86.2	94.2	118.7	180.6
1985	51.9*	28.3*	67.2*	52.0	69.0	68.7	62.9	71.6	75.6	70.3	80.5	123.2	200.4
1990	**50.1***	**24.5***	**68.6***	**61.9**	**58.5**	**70.8**	**59.0**	**69.0**	**79.2**	**81.9**	**91.4**	**128.1**	**178.9**
1995 projected	*48.2**	*21.2**	*68.7**	*56.9*	*58.9*	*65.8*	*57.5*	*68.1*	*83.0*	*90.6*	*98.8*	*131.0*	*170.0*

LITHUANIA: 1985–1990

Smoking–attributed deaths (Sm.) and total deaths (Total)

		ALL CAUSES	ALL CANCER	Lung cancer	Upper aero–digestive ca.	Other cancer	COPD	Other respiratory	Vascular disease	Cirrhosis/ other liver	Other medical	Non–medical
Males												
0–34	Sm.	–	–	–	–	–	–	–	–	–	–	–
	Total	1960	103	3	1	99	10	56	110	9	549	1123
35–69	Sm.	3338	1210	761	181	268	373	26	1396	–	333	–
	Total	8879	2255	800	244	1211	448	61	3528	133	767	1687
		(38%)	(54%)	(95%)	(74%)	(22%)	(83%)	(43%)	(40%)		(43%)	
70+	Sm.	1415	387	270	31	86	475	1	518	–	34	–
	Total	8547	1229	305	60	864	717	22	5932	37	367	243
		(17%)	(31%)	(89%)	(52%)	(10%)	(66%)	(5%)	(9%)		(9%)	
Any age	Sm.	4753	1597	1031	212	354	848	27	1914	–	367	–
	Total	19386	3587	1108	305	2174	1175	139	9570	179	1683	3053
		(25%)	(45%)	(93%)	(70%)	(16%)	(72%)	(19%)	(20%)		(22%)	
Females												
0–34	Sm.	–	–	–	–	–	–	–	–	–	–	–
	Total	846	98	1	0	97	10	38	41	2	398	259
35–69	Sm.	167	39	32	2	5	36	0	76	–	16	–
	Total	4899	1625	95	23	1507	159	23	1992	79	552	469
		(3%)	(2%)	(34%)	(9%)	(0%)	(23%)	(0%)	(4%)		(3%)	
70+	Sm.	196	27	22	1	4	77	0	86	–	6	–
	Total	12797	1120	79	20	1021	455	26	10503	32	430	231
		(2%)	(2%)	(28%)	(5%)	(0%)	(17%)	(0%)	(1%)		(1%)	
Any age	Sm.	363	66	54	3	9	113	0	162	–	22	–
	Total	18542	2843	175	43	2625	624	87	12536	113	1380	959
		(2%)	(2%)	(31%)	(7%)	(0%)	(18%)	(0%)	(1%)		(2%)	
Males+Females												
0–34	Sm.	–	–	–	–	–	–	–	–	–	–	–
	Total	2806	201	4	1	196	20	94	151	11	947	1382
35–69	Sm.	3505	1249	793	183	273	409	26	1472	–	349	–
	Total	13778	3880	895	267	2718	607	84	5520	212	1319	2156
		(25%)	(32%)	(89%)	(69%)	(10%)	(67%)	(31%)	(27%)		(26%)	
70+	Sm.	1611	414	292	32	90	552	1	604	–	40	–
	Total	21344	2349	384	80	1885	1172	48	16435	69	797	474
		(8%)	(18%)	(76%)	(40%)	(5%)	(47%)	(2%)	(4%)		(5%)	
Any age	Sm.	5116	1663	1085	215	363	961	27	2076	–	389	–
	Total	37928	6430	1283	348	4799	1799	226	22106	292	3063	4012
		(13%)	(26%)	(85%)	(62%)	(8%)	(53%)	(12%)	(9%)		(13%)	

LITHUANIA: 1985

Smoking–attributed deaths (Sm.) and total deaths (Total)

		ALL CAUSES	ALL CANCER	Lung cancer	Upper aero–digestive ca.	Other cancer	COPD	Other respiratory	Vascular disease	Cirrhosis/ other liver	Other medical	Non–medical
Males												
0–34	Sm.	–	–	–	–	–	–	–	–	–	–	–
	Total	2236	106	4	4	98	15	97	126	11	700	1181
35–69	Sm.	3092	996	628	144	224	427	33	1254	–	382	–
	Total	8678	1957	664	198	1095	520	79	3299	172	900	1751
		(36%)	(51%)	(95%)	(73%)	(20%)	(82%)	(42%)	(38%)		(42%)	
70+	Sm.	1709	416	291	35	90	645	4	603	–	41	–
	Total	9370	1250	327	64	859	950	30	6427	37	396	280
		(18%)	(33%)	(89%)	(55%)	(10%)	(68%)	(13%)	(9%)		(10%)	
Any age	Sm.	4801	1412	919	179	314	1072	37	1857	–	423	–
	Total	20284	3313	995	266	2052	1485	206	9852	220	1996	3212
		(24%)	(43%)	(92%)	(67%)	(15%)	(72%)	(18%)	(19%)		(21%)	
Females												
0–34	Sm.	–	–	–	–	–	–	–	–	–	–	–
	Total	914	103	1	0	102	13	61	34	4	432	267
35–69	Sm.	210	52	41	2	9	46	1	83	–	28	–
	Total	4772	1549	97	16	1436	177	30	1875	85	562	494
		(4%)	(3%)	(42%)	(13%)	(1%)	(26%)	(3%)	(4%)		(5%)	
70+	Sm.	212	24	20	1	3	103	0	81	–	4	–
	Total	13199	1109	75	16	1018	626	23	10767	37	403	234
		(2%)	(2%)	(27%)	(6%)	(0%)	(16%)	(0%)	(1%)		(1%)	
Any age	Sm.	422	76	61	3	12	149	1	164	–	32	–
	Total	18885	2761	173	32	2556	816	114	12676	126	1397	995
		(2%)	(3%)	(35%)	(9%)	(0%)	(18%)	(1%)	(1%)		(2%)	
Males+Females												
0–34	Sm.	–	–	–	–	–	–	–	–	–	–	–
	Total	3150	209	5	4	200	28	158	160	15	1132	1448
35–69	Sm.	3302	1048	669	146	233	473	34	1337	–	410	–
	Total	13450	3506	761	214	2531	697	109	5174	257	1462	2245
		(25%)	(30%)	(88%)	(68%)	(9%)	(68%)	(31%)	(26%)		(28%)	
70+	Sm.	1921	440	311	36	93	748	4	684	–	45	–
	Total	22569	2359	402	80	1877	1576	53	17194	74	799	514
		(9%)	(19%)	(77%)	(45%)	(5%)	(47%)	(8%)	(4%)		(6%)	
Any age	Sm.	5223	1488	980	182	326	1221	38	2021	–	455	–
	Total	39169	6074	1168	298	4608	2301	320	22528	346	3393	4207
		(13%)	(24%)	(84%)	(61%)	(7%)	(53%)	(12%)	(9%)		(13%)	

(To be conservative, no deaths before age 35, and none from liver cirrhosis or non–medical causes, were attributed to smoking.)

LITHUANIA: 1990

Smoking–attributed deaths (Sm.) and total deaths (Total)

		ALL CAUSES	ALL CANCER	Lung cancer	Upper aero–digestive ca.	Other cancer	COPD	Other respiratory	Vascular disease	Cirrhosis/ other liver	Other medical	Non–medical
Males												
0–34	Sm.	–	–	–	–	–	–	–	–	–	–	–
	Total	1958	95	1	3	91	16	29	114	12	484	1208
35–69	Sm.	3821	1399	865	230	304	374	26	1658	–	364	–
	Total	10184	2555	909	307	1339	446	59	4159	155	828	1982
		(38%)	(55%)	(95%)	(75%)	(23%)	(84%)	(44%)	(40%)		(44%)	
70+	Sm.	1413	409	272	36	101	414	0	554	–	36	–
	Total	8463	1293	303	66	924	615	13	5884	43	366	249
		(17%)	(32%)	(90%)	(55%)	(11%)	(67%)	(0%)	(9%)		(10%)	
Any age	Sm.	5234	1808	1137	266	405	788	26	2212	–	400	–
	Total	20605	3943	1213	376	2354	1077	101	10157	210	1678	3439
		(25%)	(46%)	(94%)	(71%)	(17%)	(73%)	(26%)	(22%)		(24%)	
Females												
0–34	Sm.	–	–	–	–	–	–	–	–	–	–	–
	Total	773	101	3	2	96	8	17	40	1	364	242
35–69	Sm.	181	45	35	4	6	37	0	76	–	23	–
	Total	5391	1709	102	30	1577	175	23	2220	92	628	544
		(3%)	(3%)	(34%)	(13%)	(0%)	(21%)	(0%)	(3%)		(4%)	
70+	Sm.	410	58	46	4	8	135	0	206	–	11	–
	Total	12991	1206	98	18	1090	387	30	10594	36	502	236
		(3%)	(5%)	(47%)	(22%)	(1%)	(35%)	(0%)	(2%)		(2%)	
Any age	Sm.	591	103	81	8	14	172	0	282	–	34	–
	Total	19155	3016	203	50	2763	570	70	12854	129	1494	1022
		(3%)	(3%)	(40%)	(16%)	(1%)	(30%)	(0%)	(2%)		(2%)	
Males+Females												
0–34	Sm.	–	–	–	–	–	–	–	–	–	–	–
	Total	2731	196	4	5	187	24	46	154	13	848	1450
35–69	Sm.	4002	1444	900	234	310	411	26	1734	–	387	–
	Total	15575	4264	1011	337	2916	621	82	6379	247	1456	2526
		(26%)	(34%)	(89%)	(69%)	(11%)	(66%)	(32%)	(27%)		(27%)	
70+	Sm.	1823	467	318	40	109	549	0	760	–	47	–
	Total	21454	2499	401	84	2014	1002	43	16478	79	868	485
		(8%)	(19%)	(79%)	(48%)	(5%)	(55%)	(0%)	(5%)		(5%)	
Any age	Sm.	5825	1911	1218	274	419	960	26	2494	–	434	–
	Total	39760	6959	1416	426	5117	1647	171	23011	339	3172	4461
		(15%)	(27%)	(86%)	(64%)	(8%)	(58%)	(15%)	(11%)		(14%)	

LITHUANIA: 1995

Smoking–attributed deaths (Sm.) and total deaths (Total)

		ALL CAUSES	ALL CANCER	Lung cancer	Upper aero–digestive ca.	Other cancer	COPD	Other respiratory	Vascular disease	Cirrhosis/ other liver	Other medical	Non–medical
Males												
0–34	Sm.	–	–	–	–	–	–	–	–	–	–	–
	Total	1595	81	1	2	78	14	24	95	9	311	1061
35–69	Sm.	4436	1798	1105	316	377	302	22	1984	–	330	–
	Total	11016	3046	1154	406	1486	351	43	4606	149	705	2116
		(40%)	(59%)	(96%)	(78%)	(25%)	(86%)	(51%)	(43%)		(47%)	
70+	Sm.	1520	528	339	50	139	321	0	631	–	40	–
	Total	8450	1604	372	86	1146	461	10	5685	64	369	257
		(18%)	(33%)	(91%)	(58%)	(12%)	(70%)	(0%)	(11%)		(11%)	
Any age	Sm.	5956	2326	1444	366	516	623	22	2615	–	370	–
	Total	21061	4731	1527	494	2710	826	77	10386	222	1385	3434
		(28%)	(49%)	(95%)	(74%)	(19%)	(75%)	(29%)	(25%)		(27%)	
Females												
0–34	Sm.	–	–	–	–	–	–	–	–	–	–	–
	Total	600	88	2	1	85	8	12	40	1	248	203
35–69	Sm.	168	42	33	4	5	29	0	77	–	20	–
	Total	5462	1722	104	42	1576	142	19	2278	96	642	563
		(3%)	(2%)	(32%)	(10%)	(0%)	(20%)	(0%)	(3%)		(3%)	
70+	Sm.	590	101	79	7	15	133	0	333	–	23	–
	Total	12702	1421	136	26	1259	284	40	10018	38	648	253
		(5%)	(7%)	(58%)	(27%)	(1%)	(47%)	(0%)	(3%)		(4%)	
Any age	Sm.	758	143	112	11	20	162	0	410	–	43	–
	Total	18764	3231	242	69	2920	434	71	12336	135	1538	1019
		(4%)	(4%)	(46%)	(16%)	(1%)	(37%)	(0%)	(3%)		(3%)	
Males+Females												
0–34	Sm.	–	–	–	–	–	–	–	–	–	–	–
	Total	2195	169	3	3	163	22	36	135	10	559	1264
35–69	Sm.	4604	1840	1138	320	382	331	22	2061	–	350	–
	Total	16478	4768	1258	448	3062	493	62	6884	245	1347	2679
		(28%)	(39%)	(90%)	(71%)	(12%)	(67%)	(35%)	(30%)		(26%)	
70+	Sm.	2110	629	418	57	154	454	0	964	–	63	–
	Total	21152	3025	508	112	2405	745	50	15703	102	1017	510
		(10%)	(21%)	(82%)	(51%)	(6%)	(61%)	(0%)	(6%)		(6%)	
Any age	Sm.	6714	2469	1556	377	536	785	22	3025	–	413	–
	Total	39825	7962	1769	563	5630	1260	148	22722	357	2923	4453
		(17%)	(31%)	(88%)	(67%)	(10%)	(62%)	(15%)	(13%)		(14%)	

(To be conservative, no deaths before age 35, and none from liver cirrhosis or non-medical causes, were attributed to smoking.)

LUXEMBOURG: 1990

		No. of deaths			Standardised rates (Defined on p.424)			Annual death rates / 100, 000						
		All ages	0–34	35–69	All ages	0–34	35–69	0–4	5–9	10–14	15–19	20–24	25–29	30–34
ALL CAUSES	M	1913	108	727	1061.1	112.7	1106.8	210.1	8.9	18.5	157.9	158.6	119.0	115.9
	F	1920	51	443	630.0	56.4	579.2	157.9	37.4	29.1	9.3	43.2	37.0	80.7
Tuberculosis	M	2	–	1	1.1	–	1.2	–	–	–	–	–	–	–
	F	–	–	–	–	–	–	–	–	–	–	–	–	–
Other infective	M	8	–	4	4.4	–	5.7	–	–	–	–	–	–	–
and parasitic	F	9	1	1	2.6	0.9	1.4	–	–	–	–	–	–	6.2
ALL CANCER	M	527	2	258	295.3	2.6	401.2	–	–	9.3	8.8	–	–	–
	F	442	7	205	168.2	7.2	269.0	–	9.3	9.7	–	–	6.2	24.8
Mouth and	M	31	–	24	17.4	–	34.0	–	–	–	–	–	–	–
pharynx cancer	F	7	–	5	2.9	–	6.5	–	–	–	–	–	–	–
Oesophagus cancer	M	10	–	6	5.6	–	8.7	–	–	–	–	–	–	–
	F	7	–	4	2.9	–	5.0	–	–	–	–	–	–	–
Stomach cancer	M	35	–	17	19.7	–	24.8	–	–	–	–	–	–	–
	F	13	1	5	5.2	0.9	6.8	–	–	–	–	–	–	6.2
Colorectal cancer	M	59	–	29	32.9	–	47.8	–	–	–	–	–	–	–
	F	51	–	18	18.5	–	23.5	–	–	–	–	–	–	–
Liver cancer	M	–	–	–	–	–	–	–	–	–	–	–	–	–
	F	–	–	–	–	–	–	–	–	–	–	–	–	–
Pancreas cancer	M	22	–	15	12.4	–	22.1	–	–	–	–	–	–	–
	F	15	–	3	4.5	–	4.2	–	–	–	–	–	–	–
Larynx cancer	M	15	–	12	8.2	–	17.4	–	–	–	–	–	–	–
	F	1	–	–	0.2	–	–	–	–	–	–	–	–	–
Lung cancer	M	162	–	85	91.3	–	139.3	–	–	–	–	–	–	–
	F	31	–	20	12.2	–	26.2	–	–	–	–	–	–	–
Malignant melanoma	M	1	–	1	0.6	–	1.2	–	–	–	–	–	–	–
	F	7	–	4	2.7	–	5.2	–	–	–	–	–	–	–
Female breast cancer	F	95	1	51	39.5	0.9	65.3	–	–	–	–	–	–	6.2
Cervix cancer	F	12	1	8	5.2	0.9	10.2	–	–	–	–	–	6.2	–
Other uterine cancer	F	26	–	13	9.8	–	17.2	–	–	–	–	–	–	–
Ovarian cancer	F	33	–	18	12.8	–	24.1	–	–	–	–	–	–	–
Prostate cancer	M	48	–	5	27.0	–	8.4	–	–	–	–	–	–	–
Bladder cancer	M	21	–	6	11.7	–	7.8	–	–	–	–	–	–	–
	F	7	–	1	2.1	–	1.3	–	–	–	–	–	–	–
Other and ill–defined	M	84	1	40	46.7	1.3	62.6	–	–	–	8.8	–	–	–
cancer sites	F	104	3	43	38.9	3.6	57.2	–	9.3	9.7	–	–	–	6.2
Hodgkin's disease	M	1	–	1	0.5	–	1.4	–	–	–	–	–	–	–
	F	3	–	3	1.5	–	3.7	–	–	–	–	–	–	–
Myeloma and non–	M	16	–	7	8.9	–	11.2	–	–	–	–	–	–	–
Hodgkin lymphomas	F	19	1	7	6.1	0.9	9.9	–	–	–	–	–	–	6.2
Leukaemia	M	22	1	10	12.5	1.3	14.4	–	–	9.3	–	–	–	–
	F	11	–	2	3.1	–	2.7	–	–	–	–	–	–	–
ALL VASCULAR	M	794	4	240	443.1	3.7	379.4	–	–	–	–	13.8	6.0	6.1
DISEASE	F	985	3	113	286.0	3.2	151.4	–	–	9.7	–	–	6.2	6.2
Rheumatic heart	M	–	–	–	–	–	–	–	–	–	–	–	–	–
disease and fever	F	3	–	2	1.2	–	2.3	–	–	–	–	–	–	–
Hypertensive disease	M	10	–	4	5.9	–	5.9	–	–	–	–	–	–	–
	F	21	–	4	6.4	–	5.1	–	–	–	–	–	–	–
Ischaemic heart	M	284	2	130	160.2	1.9	206.1	–	–	–	–	6.9	–	6.1
disease	F	215	–	34	65.0	–	45.7	–	–	–	–	–	–	–
Pulmonary embolism	M	...	...	...	...	...	...	...	...	...	...	...	...	...
and other venous	F	...	...	...	...	...	...	...	...	...	...	...	...	...
Cerebrovascular	M	241	2	50	133.3	1.8	80.1	–	–	–	–	6.9	6.0	–
disease	F	383	2	35	109.6	2.3	46.4	–	–	9.7	–	–	6.2	–
Other vascular	M	259	–	56	143.8	–	87.2	–	–	–	–	–	–	–
disease, incl. venous	F	363	1	38	103.8	0.9	51.9	–	–	–	–	–	–	6.2
Chronic obstructive	M	94	–	21	52.2	–	32.9	–	–	–	–	–	–	–
pulmonary disease	F	32	1	10	11.7	0.9	12.6	–	–	–	–	–	–	6.2
Other respiratory	M	50	2	11	27.5	2.1	20.3	8.4	–	–	–	–	–	6.1
disease	F	59	1	8	17.3	0.9	10.7	–	–	–	–	–	6.2	–
Peptic ulcer	M	4	–	4	2.3	–	7.9	–	–	–	–	–	–	–
	F	9	–	–	2.6	–	–	–	–	–	–	–	–	–
Liver cirrhosis	M	58	2	47	32.2	1.7	66.3	–	–	–	–	–	–	12.2
	F	35	1	25	16.3	0.9	31.1	–	–	–	–	–	–	6.2
Renal disease	M	7	–	–	3.9	–	–	–	–	–	–	–	–	–
	F	18	–	3	5.2	–	3.8	–	–	–	–	–	–	–
Pregnancy and birth	F	1	1	–	0.4	0.9	–	–	–	–	–	–	–	6.2
Congenital and	M	17	16	1	11.2	19.2	1.0	134.5	–	–	–	–	–	–
perinatal causes	F	8	8	–	5.6	10.0	–	70.2	–	–	–	–	–	–
Ill–defined causes	M	60	6	20	32.6	6.5	28.4	33.6	–	–	–	–	–	12.2
	F	79	8	13	27.6	9.8	16.9	61.4	–	–	–	7.2	–	–
Other medical causes	M	124	6	43	67.3	5.5	65.1	–	–	–	8.8	–	17.9	12.2
	F	173	4	39	56.8	5.0	51.3	8.8	9.3	9.7	–	7.2	–	–
ALL NON–	M	168	70	77	88.0	71.3	97.4	33.6	8.9	9.3	140.4	144.8	95.2	67.1
MEDICAL CAUSES	F	70	16	26	29.8	16.8	31.0	17.5	18.7	–	9.3	28.8	18.5	24.8
Motor vehicle	M	50	30	18	25.9	31.4	22.3	8.4	–	9.3	78.9	69.0	29.8	24.4
traffic accidents	F	18	10	6	8.9	10.6	7.7	–	18.7	–	9.3	21.6	12.3	12.4
Fire	M	4	1	2	2.2	1.2	2.6	8.4	–	–	–	–	–	–
	F	2	–	1	0.9	–	1.3	–	–	–	–	–	–	–
Suicide	M	47	15	24	24.7	14.7	30.1	–	–	–	35.1	13.8	29.8	24.4
	F	21	2	13	9.7	1.8	14.9	–	–	–	–	–	6.2	6.2
Homicide	M	9	1	8	4.9	1.3	9.4	–	–	–	8.8	–	–	–
	F	2	–	2	1.1	–	2.2	–	–	–	–	–	–	–
POPULATION (thousands):	M=males				186.9	93.0	81.5	11.9	11.2	10.8	11.4	14.5	16.8	16.4
	F=females				195.2	89.4	83.4	11.4	10.7	10.3	10.8	13.9	16.2	16.1

LUXEMBOURG: 1990

Annual death rates / 100, 000

9th ICD categories

35–39	40–44	45–49	50–54	55–59	60–64	65–69	70–74	75–79	80+/NK			
206.5	296.6	524.6	663.8	1036.7	1852.9	3166.7	5106.4	7047.6	15485.7	M	ALL CAUSES	001–999
128.4	150.4	215.5	500.0	625.0	839.3	1596.0	2492.8	4138.9	11518.1	F		
–	–	8.2	–	–	–	–	–	–	28.6	M	Tuberculosis	010–018, 137
–	–	–	–	–	–	–	–	–	–	F		
6.5	–	–	8.6	–	9.8	15.2	–	–	114.3	M	Other infective	Rest of 001–139
–	–	–	–	–	–	10.1	–	41.7	48.2	F	and parasitic	
25.8	110.3	180.3	241.4	376.1	647.1	1227.3	1680.9	1714.3	3314.3	M	ALL CANCER	140–208
47.3	37.6	94.8	263.2	312.5	410.7	717.2	594.2	875.0	1518.1	F		
–	20.7	41.0	25.9	55.0	19.6	75.8	42.6	47.6	85.7	M	Mouth and	140–149
–	7.5	–	8.8	–	8.9	20.2	–	13.9	12.0	F	pharynx cancer	
–	–	8.2	8.6	9.2	19.6	15.2	21.3	23.8	57.1	M	Oesophagus cancer	150
–	–	17.2	–	8.9	8.9	–	–	–	36.1	F		
6.5	27.6	8.2	17.2	9.2	29.4	75.8	148.9	71.4	228.6	M	Stomach cancer	151
–	–	8.6	8.8	–	–	30.3	43.5	13.9	36.1	F		
–	20.7	8.2	8.6	36.7	78.4	181.8	148.9	190.5	428.6	M	Colorectal cancer	153, 154
–	–	–	35.1	44.6	44.6	40.4	101.4	97.2	228.9	F		
–	–	–	–	–	–	–	–	–	–	M	Liver cancer	155.0
–	–	–	–	–	–	–	–	–	–	F		
–	–	16.4	17.2	36.7	39.2	45.5	42.6	23.8	114.3	M	Pancreas cancer	157
–	–	–	–	–	8.9	20.2	14.5	41.7	96.4	F		
–	–	24.6	–	27.5	39.2	30.3	21.3	23.8	28.6	M	Larynx cancer	161
–	–	–	–	–	–	–	–	–	12.0	F		
–	13.8	49.2	77.6	128.4	205.9	500.0	617.0	619.0	628.6	M	Lung cancer	162
13.5	–	–	–	35.7	53.6	80.8	29.0	55.6	60.2	F		
–	–	–	8.6	–	–	–	–	–	–	M	Malignant melanoma	172
–	7.5	8.6	–	–	–	20.2	–	–	36.1	F		
20.3	7.5	43.1	87.7	98.2	89.3	111.1	173.9	166.7	228.9	F	Female breast cancer	174
6.8	–	–	17.5	–	26.8	20.2	14.5	13.9	12.0	F	Cervix cancer	180
–	–	8.6	8.8	35.7	26.8	40.4	14.5	55.6	96.4	F	Other uterine cancer	179, 182
–	–	–	26.3	17.9	53.6	70.7	43.5	83.3	72.3	F	Ovarian cancer	183
–	–	–	–	9.2	19.6	30.3	234.0	261.9	600.0	M	Prostate cancer	185
–	–	8.2	8.6	18.3	19.6	–	106.4	119.0	142.9	M	Bladder cancer	188
–	–	–	8.8	–	–	–	–	27.8	48.2	F		
6.5	20.7	8.2	51.7	36.7	117.6	197.0	170.2	261.9	685.7	M	Other and ill-defined	Rest of 140–208
6.8	7.5	–	61.4	71.4	71.4	181.8	159.4	236.1	361.4	F	cancer sites	
–	–	–	–	–	9.8	–	–	–	–	M	Hodgkin's disease	201
–	7.5	8.6	–	–	–	10.1	–	–	–	F		
6.5	–	8.2	8.6	–	9.8	45.5	42.6	71.4	114.3	M	Myeloma and non-	200, 202–203
–	–	–	–	–	8.9	60.6	–	55.6	84.3	F	Hodgkin lymphomas	
6.5	6.9	–	8.6	9.2	39.2	30.3	85.1	–	200.0	M	Leukaemia	204–208
–	–	–	–	–	8.9	10.1	–	13.9	96.4	F		
19.4	27.6	139.3	232.8	330.3	754.9	1151.5	2468.1	3428.6	8285.7	M	ALL VASCULAR	390–459
13.5	22.6	34.5	70.2	151.8	232.1	535.4	1217.4	2555.6	7241.0	F	DISEASE	
–	–	–	–	–	–	–	–	–	–	M	Rheumatic heart	390–398
–	7.5	–	–	–	8.9	–	–	–	12.0	F	disease and fever	
–	–	–	17.2	9.2	–	15.2	21.3	–	142.9	M	Hypertensive disease	401–405
–	7.5	–	–	–	17.9	10.1	29.0	27.8	156.6	F		
–	20.7	90.2	129.3	174.3	392.2	636.4	1085.1	833.3	1885.7	M	Ischaemic heart	410–414
6.8	–	–	–	71.4	80.4	161.6	304.3	791.7	1241.0	F	disease	
...	...	...	...	...	...	...	...	...	...	M	Pulmonary embolism	Not given
...	...	...	...	...	...	...	...	...	...	F	and other venous	separately
6.5	–	32.8	51.7	55.0	156.9	257.6	638.3	1357.1	2914.3	M	Cerebrovascular	430–438
6.8	7.5	–	43.9	53.6	71.4	141.4	478.3	819.4	3060.2	F	disease	
12.9	6.9	16.4	34.5	91.7	205.9	242.4	723.4	1238.1	3342.9	M	Other vascular	Rest of 390–459,
–	–	34.5	26.3	26.8	53.6	222.2	405.8	916.7	2771.1	F	disease, incl. venous	incl. 415, 451–3
–	–	–	25.9	55.0	58.8	90.9	297.9	547.6	1028.6	M	Chronic obstructive	490–496
6.8	–	–	8.8	8.9	53.6	10.1	101.4	41.7	132.5	F	pulmonary disease	
–	–	16.4	–	–	19.6	106.1	21.3	285.7	685.7	M	Other respiratory	Rest of 460–519
–	7.5	–	8.8	8.9	8.9	40.4	72.5	27.8	518.1	F	disease	
–	–	–	–	–	9.8	45.5	–	–	–	M	Peptic ulcer	531–533
–	–	–	–	–	–	–	29.0	13.9	72.3	F		
25.8	6.9	82.0	43.1	91.7	78.4	136.4	106.4	23.8	85.7	M	Liver cirrhosis	571
13.5	30.1	17.2	35.1	35.7	35.7	50.5	72.5	27.8	24.1	F		
–	–	–	–	–	–	–	–	23.8	171.4	M	Renal disease	580–590
–	–	–	8.8	8.9	8.9	–	–	–	180.7	F		
–	–	–	–	–	–	–	–	–	–	F	Pregnancy and birth	630–676
–	6.9	–	–	–	–	–	–	–	–	M	Congenital and	740–779
–	–	–	–	–	–	–	–	–	–	F	perinatal causes	
–	34.5	16.4	–	18.3	68.6	60.6	127.7	333.3	400.0	M	Ill-defined causes	780–799
–	7.5	17.2	26.3	–	26.8	40.4	87.0	180.6	469.9	F		
32.3	27.6	–	17.2	64.2	117.6	197.0	276.6	547.6	1114.3	M	Other medical causes	Rest of 001–799
13.5	15.0	43.1	26.3	53.6	35.7	171.7	246.4	333.3	1072.3	F		
96.8	82.8	82.0	94.8	100.9	88.2	136.4	127.7	142.9	257.1	M	ALL NON-	E800–E999
33.8	30.1	8.6	52.6	44.6	26.8	20.2	72.5	41.7	241.0	F	MEDICAL CAUSES	
25.8	27.6	16.4	17.2	9.2	29.4	30.3	–	–	57.1	M	Motor vehicle	E810–E819
6.8	–	–	8.8	17.9	–	20.2	14.5	13.9	–	F	traffic accidents	
–	–	–	–	18.3	–	–	–	23.8	–	M	Fire	E890–E899
–	–	–	8.8	–	–	–	–	–	12.0	F		
38.7	20.7	24.6	34.5	36.7	9.8	45.5	85.1	47.6	57.1	M	Suicide	E950–E959
20.3	22.6	8.6	26.3	17.9	8.9	–	29.0	13.9	36.1	F		
–	20.7	–	25.9	9.2	9.8	–	–	–	–	M	Homicide	E960–E969
6.8	–	–	8.8	–	–	–	–	–	–	F		
15.5	14.5	12.2	11.6	10.9	10.2	6.6	4.7	4.2	3.5	M	POPULATION (thousands)	
14.8	13.3	11.6	11.4	11.2	11.2	9.9	6.9	7.2	8.3	F		

LUXEMBOURG: Males

	All ages	0–34	35–69	35–39	40–44	45–49	50–54	55–59	60–64	65–69	70–74	75–79	80+/NK
POPULATION (1000s)													
1955	153.0	77.0	67.0	10.0	12.0	12.0	11.0	9.0	7.0	6.0	4.3	2.7	2.0
1965	167.0	86.4	71.2	13.9	10.4	9.1	10.6	10.9	9.4	6.9	4.5	2.7	2.2
1975	178.9	93.8	73.6	13.2	13.0	13.6	9.7	7.7	8.7	7.7	5.6	3.4	2.5
1985	177.9	90.6	74.5	14.2	12.3	11.9	11.8	11.0	7.5	5.8	5.9	4.0	2.9
1990	**186.9**	**93.0**	**81.5**	**15.5**	**14.5**	**12.2**	**11.6**	**10.9**	**10.2**	**6.6**	**4.7**	**4.2**	**3.5**
1995 projected	*183.0*	*84.3*	*86.9*	*15.5*	*15.0*	*14.1*	*11.9*	*11.1*	*10.4*	*8.9*	*5.2*	*3.2*	*3.4*
NUMBER OF DEATHS													
All causes													
1955	1912	223	856	28	56	80	154	116	190	232	243	230	360
1965	2247	168	1049	28	57	65	126	185	301	287	301	285	444
1975	2332	156	1032	21	71	93	101	133	270	343	390	341	413
1985	2100	107	766	31	37	60	96	158	169	215	325	393	509
1990	**1913**	**108**	**727**	**32**	**43**	**64**	**77**	**113**	**189**	**209**	**240**	**296**	**542**
1995 projected	*1641*	*95*	*702*	*32*	*44*	*68*	*64*	*90*	*157*	*247*	*215*	*188*	*441*
Lung cancer													
1955	...	...	...	...	...	...	...	...	...	...	...	...	...
1965	...	...	...	...	...	...	...	...	...	...	...	...	...
1975	161	–	105	3	4	9	11	17	33	28	27	23	6
1985	175	–	85	–	–	2	11	26	22	24	38	29	23
1990	**162**	–	**85**	–	**2**	**6**	**9**	**14**	**21**	**33**	**29**	**26**	**22**
1995 projected	*150*	–	*87*	–	*3*	*8*	*7*	*9*	*18*	*42*	*31*	*15*	*17*
ANNUAL DEATH RATE / 100,000 (*The rates for the age groups 0–34 and 35–69 are the means of seven five-yearly rates, but the all-ages rates are standardised to the conventional "European" age distribution)													
All causes													
1955	1417.1*	287.1*	1526.2*	280.0	466.7	666.7	1400.0	1288.9	2714.3	3866.7	5651.2	8518.5	18000.0
1965	1529.1*	191.8*	1673.0*	201.4	548.1	714.3	1188.7	1697.2	3202.1	4159.4	6688.9	10555.6	20181.8
1975	1433.1*	169.2*	1673.7*	159.1	546.2	683.8	1041.2	1727.3	3103.4	4454.5	6964.3	10029.4	16520.0
1985	1246.8*	114.5*	1319.1*	218.3	300.8	504.2	813.6	1436.4	2253.3	3706.9	5508.5	9825.0	17551.7
1990	**1061.1***	**112.7***	**1106.8***	**206.5**	**296.6**	**524.6**	**663.8**	**1036.7**	**1852.9**	**3166.7**	**5106.4**	**7047.6**	**15485.7**
1995 projected	*899.8**	*112.9**	*945.1**	*206.5*	*293.3*	*482.3*	*537.8*	*810.8*	*1509.6*	*2775.3*	*4134.6*	*5875.0*	*12970.6*
All cancer													
1955	...	...	...	...	...	...	...	...	...	...	...	...	...
1965	...	...	...	...	...	...	...	...	...	...	...	...	...
1975	313.7*	12.2*	461.9*	30.3	115.4	176.5	360.8	519.5	862.1	1168.8	1767.9	2294.1	2000.0
1985	326.7*	9.0*	424.0*	14.1	32.5	126.1	313.6	509.1	800.0	1172.4	1661.0	2525.0	3517.2
1990	**295.3***	**2.6***	**401.2***	**25.8**	**110.3**	**180.3**	**241.4**	**376.1**	**647.1**	**1227.3**	**1680.9**	**1714.3**	**3314.3**
1995 projected	*257.4**	*1.3**	*371.4**	*32.3*	*133.3*	*198.6*	*193.3*	*306.3*	*567.3*	*1168.5*	*1442.3*	*1281.3*	*2764.7*
Lung cancer													
1955	...	...	...	...	...	...	...	...	...	...	...	...	...
1965	...	...	...	...	...	...	...	...	...	...	...	...	...
1975	95.9*	–	171.0*	22.7	30.8	66.2	113.4	220.8	379.3	363.6	482.1	676.5	240.0
1985	102.8*	–	150.5*	–	–	16.8	93.2	236.4	293.3	413.8	644.1	725.0	793.1
1990	**91.3***	–	**139.3***	–	**13.8**	**49.2**	**77.6**	**128.4**	**205.9**	**500.0**	**617.0**	**619.0**	**628.6**
1995 projected	*79.1**	–	*123.1**	–	*20.0*	*56.7*	*58.8*	*81.1*	*173.1*	*471.9*	*596.2*	*468.8*	*500.0*
Upper aerodigestive cancer (mouth, oesophagus, pharynx and larynx)													
1955	...	...	...	...	...	...	...	...	...	...	...	...	...
1965	...	...	...	...	...	...	...	...	...	...	...	...	...
1975	29.3*	1.0*	49.0*	–	–	22.1	61.9	51.9	103.4	103.9	125.0	176.5	160.0
1985	22.9*	–	39.6*	–	8.1	16.8	59.3	36.4	53.3	103.4	118.6	50.0	172.4
1990	**31.2***	–	**60.0***	–	**20.7**	**73.8**	**34.5**	**91.7**	**78.4**	**121.2**	**85.1**	**95.2**	**171.4**
1995 projected	*38.0**	–	*73.7**	–	*26.7*	*92.2*	*50.4*	*117.1*	*105.8*	*123.6*	*96.2*	*93.8*	*205.9*
Other cancer													
1955	...	...	...	...	...	...	...	...	...	...	...	...	...
1965	...	...	...	...	...	...	...	...	...	...	...	...	...
1975	188.6*	11.2*	241.9*	7.6	84.6	88.2	185.6	246.8	379.3	701.3	1160.7	1441.2	1600.0
1985	201.0*	9.0*	233.8*	14.1	24.4	92.4	161.0	236.4	453.3	655.2	898.3	1750.0	2551.7
1990	**172.8***	**2.6***	**201.9***	**25.8**	**75.9**	**57.4**	**129.3**	**156.0**	**362.7**	**606.1**	**978.7**	**1000.0**	**2514.3**
1995 projected	*140.2**	*1.3**	*174.6**	*32.3*	*86.7*	*49.6*	*84.0*	*108.1*	*288.5*	*573.0*	*750.0*	*718.8*	*2058.8*
Chronic obstructive pulmonary disease (COPD)													
1955	...	...	...	...	...	...	...	...	...	...	...	...	...
1965	...	...	...	...	...	...	...	...	...	...	...	...	...
1975	55.3*	1.9*	65.1*	–	–	–	10.3	90.9	172.4	181.8	321.4	411.8	720.0
1985	52.3*	1.0*	48.1*	–	16.3	–	8.5	72.7	66.7	172.4	305.1	350.0	965.5
1990	**52.2***	–	**32.9***	–	–	–	**25.9**	**55.0**	**58.8**	**90.9**	**297.9**	**547.6**	**1028.6**
1995 projected	*54.9**	–	*25.2**	–	–	–	*25.2*	*45.0*	*38.5*	*67.4*	*326.9*	*593.8*	*1205.9*
Other respiratory disease													
1955	...	...	...	...	...	...	...	...	...	...	...	...	...
1965	...	...	...	...	...	...	...	...	...	...	...	...	...
1975	31.0*	–	19.8*	–	–	14.7	–	13.0	46.0	64.9	142.9	441.2	560.0
1985	30.3*	2.3*	16.2*	–	–	–	8.5	9.1	26.7	69.0	152.5	275.0	689.7
1990	**27.5***	**2.1***	**20.3***	–	–	**16.4**	–	–	**19.6**	**106.1**	**21.3**	**285.7**	**685.7**
1995 projected	*24.2**	*2.2**	*15.4**	–	–	*21.3*	–	–	*19.2*	*67.4*	*19.2*	*187.5*	*676.5*
Vascular disease													
1955	...	...	...	...	...	...	...	...	...	...	...	...	...
1965	...	...	...	...	...	...	...	...	...	...	...	...	...
1975	663.6*	8.0*	722.5*	15.2	146.2	257.4	371.1	740.3	1436.8	2090.9	3357.1	5147.1	10040.0
1985	563.0*	3.8*	567.8*	77.5	97.6	193.3	288.1	500.0	973.3	1844.8	2508.5	4925.0	9448.3
1990	**443.1***	**3.7***	**379.4***	**19.4**	**27.6**	**139.3**	**232.8**	**330.3**	**754.9**	**1151.5**	**2468.1**	**3428.6**	**8285.7**
1995 projected	*347.5**	*4.5**	*277.6**	*12.9*	*20.0*	*85.1*	*159.7*	*234.2*	*509.6*	*921.3*	*1846.2*	*3000.0*	*6705.9*
Liver cirrhosis													
1955	...	...	...	...	...	...	...	...	...	...	...	...	...
1965	...	...	...	...	...	...	...	...	...	...	...	...	...
1975	35.2*	–	62.4*	7.6	38.5	51.5	92.8	39.0	103.4	103.9	196.4	176.5	40.0
1985	26.1*	1.0*	42.8*	7.0	24.4	25.2	59.3	72.7	93.3	17.2	67.8	150.0	137.9
1990	**32.2***	**1.7***	**66.3***	**25.8**	**6.9**	**82.0**	**43.1**	**91.7**	**78.4**	**136.4**	**106.4**	**23.8**	**85.7**
1995 projected	*36.3**	*1.9**	*79.2**	*25.8*	*6.7*	*85.1*	*58.8*	*81.1*	*105.8*	*191.0*	*115.4*	*31.3*	*58.8*
Other medical causes													
1955	...	...	...	...	...	...	...	...	...	...	...	...	...
1965	...	...	...	...	...	...	...	...	...	...	...	...	...
1975	218.6*	61.0*	215.7*	22.7	84.6	95.6	123.7	168.8	390.8	623.4	946.4	1323.5	2680.0
1985	154.0*	37.2*	115.2*	21.1	48.8	84.0	59.3	136.4	146.7	310.3	644.1	1375.0	2206.9
1990	**122.9***	**31.3***	**109.3***	**38.7**	**69.0**	**24.6**	**25.9**	**82.6**	**205.9**	**318.2**	**404.3**	**904.8**	**1828.6**
1995 projected	*98.5**	*26.9**	*94.6**	*45.2*	*53.3*	*14.2*	*16.8*	*72.1*	*201.9*	*258.4*	*288.5*	*687.5*	*1382.4*
All non-medical causes													
1955	...	...	...	...	...	...	...	...	...	...	...	...	...
1965	...	...	...	...	...	...	...	...	...	...	...	...	...
1975	115.8*	86.1*	126.3*	83.3	161.5	88.2	82.5	155.8	92.0	220.8	232.1	235.3	480.0
1985	94.5*	60.3*	105.1*	98.6	81.3	75.6	76.3	136.4	146.7	120.7	169.5	225.0	586.2
1990	**88.0***	**71.3***	**97.4***	**96.8**	**82.8**	**82.0**	**94.8**	**100.9**	**88.2**	**136.4**	**127.7**	**142.9**	**257.1**
1995 projected	*81.0**	*76.0**	*81.8**	*90.3*	*80.0*	*78.0*	*84.0*	*72.1*	*67.3*	*101.1*	*96.2*	*93.8*	*176.5*

LUXEMBOURG: Females

	All ages	0–34	35–69	35–39	40–44	45–49	50–54	55–59	60–64	65–69	70–74	75–79	80+/NK
POPULATION (1000s)													
1955	152.0	73.0	68.0	10.0	11.0	12.0	11.0	10.0	8.0	6.0	4.9	3.4	2.7
1965	166.9	78.8	74.9	12.5	11.5	9.5	10.8	11.4	10.8	8.4	6.1	4.0	3.1
1975	181.6	87.0	76.5	11.8	11.8	12.6	11.5	8.8	10.2	9.8	8.1	5.5	4.5
1985	188.1	88.4	77.5	13.0	11.6	11.6	11.7	11.6	10.6	7.4	8.7	7.0	6.5
1990	195.2	89.4	83.4	14.8	13.3	11.6	11.4	11.2	11.2	9.9	6.9	7.2	8.3
1995 projected	193.1	83.0	87.9	15.8	14.7	13.0	11.5	11.3	11.1	10.5	9.0	5.5	7.7

	All ages	0–34	35–69	35–39	40–44	45–49	50–54	55–59	60–64	65–69	70–74	75–79	80+/NK
NUMBER OF DEATHS													
All causes													
1955	1595	146	591	21	38	44	97	79	141	171	204	228	426
1965	1771	94	593	16	29	31	69	83	148	217	258	289	537
1975	2043	62	576	12	20	45	63	66	141	229	327	396	682
1985	1980	61	443	11	35	20	51	85	109	132	279	356	841
1990	1920	51	443	19	20	25	57	70	94	158	172	298	956
1995 projected	1600	40	405	16	21	28	58	64	80	138	183	184	788
Lung cancer													
1955	...	...	...	...	...	...	...	...	...	...	...	...	...
1965	...	...	...	...	...	...	...	...	...	...	...	...	...
1975	18	–	7	1	1	–	–	1	2	2	2	3	6
1985	35	–	17	–	–	2	1	5	5	4	4	8	6
1990	31	–	20	2	–	–	–	4	6	8	2	4	5
1995 projected	27	–	20	–	–	–	–	4	7	9	2	2	3

ANNUAL DEATH RATE / 100,000 (*The rates for the age groups 0–34 and 35–69 are the means of seven five-yearly rates, but the all-ages rates are standardised to the conventional "European" age distribution)

	All ages	0–34	35–69	35–39	40–44	45–49	50–54	55–59	60–64	65–69	70–74	75–79	80+/NK
All causes													
1955	1059.4*	203.7*	1029.5*	210.0	345.5	366.7	881.8	790.0	1762.5	2850.0	4163.3	6705.9	15777.8
1965	988.4*	116.4*	861.0*	128.0	252.2	326.3	638.9	728.1	1370.4	2583.3	4229.5	7225.0	17322.6
1975	899.5*	78.4*	806.5*	101.7	169.5	357.1	547.8	750.0	1382.4	2336.7	4037.0	7200.0	15155.6
1985	729.1*	69.7*	648.5*	84.6	301.7	172.4	435.9	732.8	1028.3	1783.8	3206.9	5085.7	12938.5
1990	630.0*	56.4*	579.2*	128.4	150.4	215.5	500.0	625.0	839.3	1596.0	2492.8	4138.9	11518.1
1995 projected	547.1*	47.3*	509.3*	101.3	142.9	215.4	504.3	566.4	720.7	1314.3	2033.3	3345.5	10233.8
All cancer													
1955	...	...	...	...	...	...	...	...	...	...	...	...	...
1965	...	...	...	...	...	...	...	...	...	...	...	...	...
1975	183.6*	2.3*	266.2*	25.4	50.8	134.9	243.5	363.6	392.2	653.1	851.9	1163.6	1711.1
1985	179.7*	10.1*	250.9*	46.2	77.6	77.6	162.4	396.6	509.4	486.5	965.5	985.7	1584.6
1990	168.2*	7.2*	269.0*	47.3	37.6	94.8	263.2	312.5	410.7	717.2	594.2	875.0	1518.1
1995 projected	154.8*	7.8*	249.0*	25.3	40.8	100.0	269.6	292.0	396.4	619.0	511.1	709.1	1441.6
Lung cancer													
1955	...	...	...	...	...	...	...	...	...	...	...	...	...
1965	...	...	...	...	...	...	...	...	...	...	...	...	...
1975	8.2*	–	9.8*	8.5	8.5	–	–	11.4	19.6	20.4	24.7	54.5	133.3
1985	14.4*	–	24.3*	–	–	17.2	8.5	43.1	47.2	54.1	46.0	114.3	92.3
1990	12.2*	–	26.2*	13.5	–	–	–	35.7	53.6	80.8	29.0	55.6	60.2
1995 projected	10.9*	–	26.3*	–	–	–	–	35.4	63.1	85.7	22.2	36.4	39.0
Upper aerodigestive cancer (mouth, oesophagus, pharynx and larynx)													
1955	...	...	...	...	...	...	...	...	...	...	...	...	...
1965	...	...	...	...	...	...	...	...	...	...	...	...	...
1975	3.9*	–	8.4*	–	–	7.9	–	11.4	29.4	10.2	–	18.2	22.2
1985	4.3*	–	6.3*	–	–	8.6	–	25.9	9.4	–	34.5	–	30.8
1990	6.1*	–	11.5*	–	7.5	17.2	8.8	8.9	17.9	20.2	–	13.9	60.2
1995 projected	7.3*	–	13.0*	–	13.6	23.1	8.7	8.8	18.0	19.0	–	18.2	77.9
Other cancer													
1955	...	...	...	...	...	...	...	...	...	...	...	...	...
1965	...	...	...	...	...	...	...	...	...	...	...	...	...
1975	171.5*	2.3*	248.0*	16.9	42.4	127.0	243.5	340.9	343.1	622.4	827.2	1090.9	1555.6
1985	161.0*	10.1*	220.3*	46.2	77.6	51.7	153.8	327.6	452.8	432.4	885.1	871.4	1461.5
1990	149.9*	7.2*	231.3*	33.8	30.1	77.6	254.4	267.9	339.3	616.2	565.2	805.6	1397.6
1995 projected	136.6*	7.8*	209.7*	25.3	27.2	76.9	260.9	247.8	315.3	514.3	488.9	654.5	1324.7
Chronic obstructive pulmonary disease (COPD)													
1955	...	...	...	...	...	...	...	...	...	...	...	...	...
1965	...	...	...	...	...	...	...	...	...	...	...	...	...
1975	13.4*	1.4*	12.4*	–	16.9	–	–	–	39.2	30.6	98.8	109.1	155.6
1985	15.7*	–	18.2*	15.4	8.6	8.6	8.5	17.2	28.3	40.5	46.0	28.6	338.5
1990	11.7*	0.9*	12.6*	6.8	–	–	8.8	8.9	53.6	10.1	101.4	41.7	132.5
1995 projected	11.5*	0.9*	11.2*	6.3	–	–	8.7	8.8	45.0	9.5	133.3	36.4	103.9
Other respiratory disease													
1955	...	...	...	...	...	...	...	...	...	...	...	...	...
1965	...	...	...	...	...	...	...	...	...	...	...	...	...
1975	16.7*	1.4*	11.1*	–	–	15.9	–	11.4	9.8	40.8	24.7	72.7	488.9
1985	19.7*	2.0*	7.1*	–	–	–	17.1	–	18.9	13.5	80.5	142.9	538.5
1990	17.3*	0.9*	10.7*	–	7.5	–	8.8	8.9	8.9	40.4	72.5	27.8	518.1
1995 projected	13.4*	1.0*	9.2*	–	–	–	8.7	8.8	9.0	38.1	44.4	18.2	402.6
Vascular disease													
1955	...	...	...	...	...	...	...	...	...	...	...	...	...
1965	...	...	...	...	...	...	...	...	...	...	...	...	...
1975	434.8*	–	309.4*	25.4	42.4	134.9	121.7	170.5	568.6	1102.0	2160.5	3890.9	9333.3
1985	347.7*	4.6*	232.2*	15.4	43.1	25.9	136.8	181.0	264.2	959.5	1643.7	3100.0	7800.0
1990	286.0*	3.2*	151.4*	13.5	22.6	34.5	70.2	151.8	232.1	535.4	1217.4	2555.6	7241.0
1995 projected	233.3*	1.9*	104.2*	12.7	20.4	23.1	43.5	115.0	153.2	361.9	888.9	2018.2	6467.5
Liver cirrhosis													
1955	...	...	...	...	...	...	...	...	...	...	...	...	...
1965	...	...	...	...	...	...	...	...	...	...	...	...	...
1975	13.4*	–	28.5*	8.5	8.5	15.9	26.1	11.4	78.4	51.0	24.7	72.7	22.2
1985	13.4*	0.9*	29.0*	–	34.5	34.5	25.6	8.6	18.9	81.1	46.0	14.3	–
1990	16.3*	0.9*	31.1*	13.5	30.1	17.2	35.1	35.7	35.7	50.5	72.5	27.8	24.1
1995 projected	18.9*	0.9*	35.9*	19.0	27.2	15.4	43.5	53.1	36.0	57.1	77.8	36.4	39.0
Other medical causes													
1955	...	...	...	...	...	...	...	...	...	...	...	...	...
1965	...	...	...	...	...	...	...	...	...	...	...	...	...
1975	188.7*	46.4*	140.3*	–	42.4	47.6	104.3	125.0	254.9	408.2	802.5	1690.9	2777.8
1985	110.8*	30.4*	73.3*	7.7	51.7	25.9	25.6	112.1	141.5	148.6	390.8	657.1	2107.7
1990	100.8*	26.6*	73.4*	13.5	22.6	60.3	61.4	62.5	71.4	222.2	362.3	569.4	1843.4
1995 projected	89.6*	21.2*	69.5*	12.7	27.2	69.2	60.9	44.2	63.1	209.5	333.3	490.9	1610.4
All non-medical causes													
1955	...	...	...	...	...	...	...	...	...	...	...	...	...
1965	...	...	...	...	...	...	...	...	...	...	...	...	...
1975	49.0*	26.8*	38.5*	42.4	8.5	7.9	52.2	68.2	39.2	51.0	74.1	200.0	666.7
1985	42.1*	21.6*	37.8*	–	86.2	–	59.8	17.2	47.2	54.1	34.5	157.1	569.2
1990	29.8*	16.8*	31.0*	33.8	30.1	8.6	52.6	44.6	26.8	20.2	72.5	41.7	241.0
1995 projected	25.6*	13.6*	30.2*	25.3	27.2	7.7	69.6	44.2	18.0	19.0	44.4	36.4	168.8

LUXEMBOURG: 1975

Smoking-attributed deaths (Sm.) and total deaths (Total)

		ALL CAUSES	ALL CANCER	Lung cancer	Upper aero-digestive ca.	Other cancer	COPD	Other respiratory	Vascular disease	Liver cirrhosis	Other medical	Non-medical
Males												
0–34	Sm.	–	–	–	–	–	–	–	–	–	–	–
	Total	156	12	0	1	11	2	0	8	0	50	84
35–69	Sm.	403	156	101	22	33	31	4	162	–	50	–
	Total	1032	283	105	30	148	37	12	435	42	134	89
		(39%)	(55%)	(96%)	(73%)	(22%)	(84%)	(33%)	(37%)		(37%)	
70+	Sm.	253	87	52	11	24	39	6	95	–	26	–
	Total	1144	227	56	17	154	50	37	614	18	165	33
		(22%)	(38%)	(93%)	(65%)	(16%)	(78%)	(16%)	(15%)		(16%)	
Any age	Sm.	656	243	153	33	57	70	10	257	–	76	–
	Total	2332	522	161	48	313	89	49	1057	60	349	206
		(28%)	(47%)	(95%)	(69%)	(18%)	(79%)	(20%)	(24%)		(22%)	
Females												
0–34	Sm.	–	–	–	–	–	–	–	–	–	–	–
	Total	62	2	0	0	2	1	1	0	0	35	23
35–69	Sm.	3	0	0	0	0	1	0	1	–	1	–
	Total	576	190	7	6	177	9	8	220	21	100	28
		(1%)	(0%)	(0%)	(0%)	(0%)	(11%)	(0%)	(0%)		(1%)	
70+	Sm.	0	0	0	0	0	0	0	0	–	0	–
	Total	1405	210	11	2	197	21	28	809	7	283	47
		(0%)	(0%)	(0%)	(0%)	(0%)	(0%)	(0%)	(0%)		(0%)	
Any age	Sm.	3	0	0	0	0	1	0	1	–	1	–
	Total	2043	402	18	8	376	31	37	1029	28	418	98
		(0%)	(0%)	(0%)	(0%)	(0%)	(3%)	(0%)	(0%)		(0%)	
Males+Females												
0–34	Sm.	–	–	–	–	–	–	–	–	–	–	–
	Total	218	14	0	1	13	3	1	8	0	85	107
35–69	Sm.	406	156	101	22	33	32	4	163	–	51	–
	Total	1608	473	112	36	325	46	20	655	63	234	117
		(25%)	(33%)	(90%)	(61%)	(10%)	(70%)	(20%)	(25%)		(22%)	
70+	Sm.	253	87	52	11	24	39	6	95	–	26	–
	Total	2549	437	67	19	351	71	65	1423	25	448	80
		(10%)	(20%)	(78%)	(58%)	(7%)	(55%)	(9%)	(7%)		(6%)	
Any age	Sm.	659	243	153	33	57	71	10	258	–	77	–
	Total	4375	924	179	56	689	120	86	2086	88	767	304
		(15%)	(26%)	(85%)	(59%)	(8%)	(59%)	(12%)	(12%)		(10%)	

LUXEMBOURG: 1985

Smoking-attributed deaths (Sm.) and total deaths (Total)

		ALL CAUSES	ALL CANCER	Lung cancer	Upper aero-digestive ca.	Other cancer	COPD	Other respiratory	Vascular disease	Liver cirrhosis	Other medical	Non-medical
Males												
0–34	Sm.	–	–	–	–	–	–	–	–	–	–	–
	Total	107	9	0	0	9	1	2	4	1	31	59
35–69	Sm.	284	123	80	17	26	22	2	111	–	26	–
	Total	766	242	85	24	133	26	8	315	30	70	75
		(37%)	(51%)	(94%)	(71%)	(20%)	(85%)	(25%)	(35%)		(37%)	
70+	Sm.	315	128	85	9	34	48	7	105	–	27	–
	Total	1227	301	90	14	197	60	40	619	14	157	36
		(26%)	(43%)	(94%)	(64%)	(17%)	(80%)	(18%)	(17%)		(17%)	
Any age	Sm.	599	251	165	26	60	70	9	216	–	53	–
	Total	2100	552	175	38	339	87	50	938	45	258	170
		(29%)	(45%)	(94%)	(68%)	(18%)	(80%)	(18%)	(23%)		(21%)	
Females												
0–34	Sm.	–	–	–	–	–	–	–	–	–	–	–
	Total	61	9	0	0	9	0	2	4	1	24	21
35–69	Sm.	41	13	10	1	2	8	0	15	–	5	–
	Total	443	179	17	5	157	13	5	146	20	52	28
		(9%)	(7%)	(59%)	(20%)	(1%)	(62%)	(0%)	(10%)		(10%)	
70+	Sm.	0	0	0	0	0	0	0	0	–	0	–
	Total	1476	256	18	5	233	28	52	867	5	217	51
		(0%)	(0%)	(0%)	(0%)	(0%)	(0%)	(0%)	(0%)		(0%)	
Any age	Sm.	41	13	10	1	2	8	0	15	–	5	–
	Total	1980	444	35	10	399	41	59	1017	26	293	100
		(2%)	(3%)	(29%)	(10%)	(1%)	(20%)	(0%)	(1%)		(2%)	
Males+Females												
0–34	Sm.	–	–	–	–	–	–	–	–	–	–	–
	Total	168	18	0	0	18	1	4	8	2	55	80
35–69	Sm.	325	136	90	18	28	30	2	126	–	31	–
	Total	1209	421	102	29	290	39	13	461	50	122	103
		(27%)	(32%)	(88%)	(62%)	(10%)	(77%)	(15%)	(27%)		(25%)	
70+	Sm.	315	128	85	9	34	48	7	105	–	27	–
	Total	2703	557	108	19	430	88	92	1486	19	374	87
		(12%)	(23%)	(79%)	(47%)	(8%)	(55%)	(8%)	(7%)		(7%)	
Any age	Sm.	640	264	175	27	62	78	9	231	–	58	–
	Total	4080	996	210	48	738	128	109	1955	71	551	270
		(16%)	(27%)	(83%)	(56%)	(8%)	(61%)	(8%)	(12%)		(11%)	

(To be conservative, no deaths before age 35, and none from liver cirrhosis or non-medical causes, were attributed to smoking.)

LUXEMBOURG: 1990

Smoking-attributed deaths (Sm.) and total deaths (Total)

		ALL CAUSES	ALL CANCER	Lung cancer	Upper aero-digestive ca.	Other cancer	COPD	Other respiratory	Vascular disease	Liver cirrhosis	Other medical	Non-medical
Males												
0–34	Sm.	–	–	–	–	–	–	–	–	–	–	–
	Total	108	2	0	0	2	0	2	4	2	28	70
35–69	Sm.	249	131	79	28	24	17	4	74	–	23	–
	Total	727	258	85	42	131	21	11	240	47	73	77
		(34%)	(51%)	(93%)	(67%)	(18%)	(81%)	(36%)	(31%)		(32%)	
70+	Sm.	269	109	71	10	28	56	4	82	–	18	–
	Total	1078	267	77	14	176	73	37	550	9	121	21
		(25%)	(41%)	(92%)	(71%)	(16%)	(77%)	(11%)	(15%)		(15%)	
Any age	Sm.	518	240	150	38	52	73	8	156	–	41	–
	Total	1913	527	162	56	309	94	50	794	58	222	168
		(27%)	(46%)	(93%)	(68%)	(17%)	(78%)	(16%)	(20%)		(18%)	
Females												
0–34	Sm.	–	–	–	–	–	–	–	–	–	–	–
	Total	51	7	0	0	7	1	1	3	1	22	16
35–69	Sm.	40	17	13	2	2	5	1	13	–	4	–
	Total	443	205	20	9	176	10	8	113	25	56	26
		(9%)	(8%)	(65%)	(22%)	(1%)	(50%)	(13%)	(12%)		(7%)	
70+	Sm.	17	3	2	1	0	3	0	9	–	2	–
	Total	1426	230	11	6	213	21	50	869	9	219	28
		(1%)	(1%)	(18%)	(17%)	(0%)	(14%)	(0%)	(1%)		(1%)	
Any age	Sm.	57	20	15	3	2	8	1	22	–	6	–
	Total	1920	442	31	15	396	32	59	985	35	297	70
		(3%)	(5%)	(48%)	(20%)	(1%)	(25%)	(2%)	(2%)		(2%)	
Males+Females												
0–34	Sm.	–	–	–	–	–	–	–	–	–	–	–
	Total	159	9	0	0	9	1	3	7	3	50	86
35–69	Sm.	289	148	92	30	26	22	5	87	–	27	–
	Total	1170	463	105	51	307	31	19	353	72	129	103
		(25%)	(32%)	(88%)	(59%)	(8%)	(71%)	(26%)	(25%)		(21%)	
70+	Sm.	286	112	73	11	28	59	4	91	–	20	–
	Total	2504	497	88	20	389	94	87	1419	18	340	49
		(11%)	(23%)	(83%)	(55%)	(7%)	(63%)	(5%)	(6%)		(6%)	
Any age	Sm.	575	260	165	41	54	81	9	178	–	47	–
	Total	3833	969	193	71	705	126	109	1779	93	519	238
		(15%)	(27%)	(85%)	(58%)	(8%)	(64%)	(8%)	(10%)		(9%)	

LUXEMBOURG: 1995

Smoking-attributed deaths (Sm.) and total deaths (Total)

		ALL CAUSES	ALL CANCER	Lung cancer	Upper aero-digestive ca.	Other cancer	COPD	Other respiratory	Vascular disease	Liver cirrhosis	Other medical	Non-medical
Males												
0–34	Sm.	–	–	–	–	–	–	–	–	–	–	–
	Total	95	1	0	0	1	0	2	4	2	22	64
35–69	Sm.	232	139	80	37	22	14	3	56	–	20	–
	Total	702	273	87	58	128	18	11	197	61	71	71
		(33%)	(51%)	(92%)	(64%)	(17%)	(78%)	(27%)	(28%)		(28%)	
70+	Sm.	207	84	57	9	18	56	3	54	–	10	–
	Total	844	210	63	15	132	77	30	420	9	84	14
		(25%)	(40%)	(90%)	(60%)	(14%)	(73%)	(10%)	(13%)		(12%)	
Any age	Sm.	439	223	137	46	40	70	6	110	–	30	–
	Total	1641	484	150	73	261	95	43	621	72	177	149
		(27%)	(46%)	(91%)	(63%)	(15%)	(74%)	(14%)	(18%)		(17%)	
Females												
0–34	Sm.	–	–	–	–	–	–	–	–	–	–	–
	Total	40	7	0	0	7	1	1	2	1	16	12
35–69	Sm.	34	16	12	2	2	4	1	9	–	4	–
	Total	405	196	20	11	165	9	7	81	30	56	26
		(8%)	(8%)	(60%)	(18%)	(1%)	(44%)	(14%)	(11%)		(7%)	
70+	Sm.	0	0	0	0	0	0	0	0	–	0	–
	Total	1155	196	7	7	182	22	36	689	12	181	19
		(0%)	(0%)	(0%)	(0%)	(0%)	(0%)	(0%)	(0%)		(0%)	
Any age	Sm.	34	16	12	2	2	4	1	9	–	4	–
	Total	1600	399	27	18	354	32	44	772	43	253	57
		(2%)	(4%)	(44%)	(11%)	(1%)	(13%)	(2%)	(1%)		(2%)	
Males+Females												
0–34	Sm.	–	–	–	–	–	–	–	–	–	–	–
	Total	135	8	0	0	8	1	3	6	3	38	76
35–69	Sm.	266	155	92	39	24	18	4	65	–	24	–
	Total	1107	469	107	69	293	27	18	278	91	127	97
		(24%)	(33%)	(86%)	(57%)	(8%)	(67%)	(22%)	(23%)		(19%)	
70+	Sm.	207	84	57	9	18	56	3	54	–	10	–
	Total	1999	406	70	22	314	99	66	1109	21	265	33
		(10%)	(21%)	(81%)	(41%)	(6%)	(57%)	(5%)	(5%)		(4%)	
Any age	Sm.	473	239	149	48	42	74	7	119	–	34	–
	Total	3241	883	177	91	615	127	87	1393	115	430	206
		(15%)	(27%)	(84%)	(53%)	(7%)	(58%)	(8%)	(9%)		(8%)	

(To be conservative, no deaths before age 35, and none from liver cirrhosis or non-medical causes, were attributed to smoking.)

¶Republic of MOLDOVA: 1990

		No. of deaths			Standardised rates (Defined on p.430)			Annual death rates / 100, 000						
		All ages	0–34	35–69	All ages	0–34	35–69	0–4	5–9	10–14	15–19	20–24	25–29	30–34
ALL CAUSES	M	21399	2964	11172	1549.2	227.6	1879.0	505.4	71.1	49.4	112.3	265.6	266.2	323.4
	F	21028	1506	8375	1040.9	110.3	1092.7	387.4	40.6	33.0	61.2	71.6	69.5	109.1
Tuberculosis	M	180	38	131	10.5	3.1	18.3	1.4	–	–	–	2.8	5.9	11.6
	F	34	5	27	1.6	0.4	3.2	–	–	–	–	0.7	1.1	1.0
Other infective and parasitic	M	153	126	24	6.4	8.4	3.8	47.5	3.8	0.5	2.3	1.4	2.4	1.1
	F	103	87	13	4.2	6.1	1.7	32.5	0.5	2.2	–	3.4	2.2	2.1
ALL CANCER	M	3245	152	2415	225.2	12.1	416.5	6.8	11.5	4.7	10.4	13.5	15.9	22.1
	F	2488	149	1676	122.5	11.7	213.4	10.8	5.9	4.9	9.6	14.3	11.0	25.2
Mouth and pharynx cancer	M	180	6	157	12.0	0.5	25.9	–	1.0	–	–	0.7	1.2	0.6
	F	20	1	10	1.0	0.1	1.3	–	–	–	–	0.7	–	–
Oesophagus cancer	M	74	1	56	5.3	0.1	9.1	–	–	–	–	–	–	0.6
	F	21	1	11	1.0	0.1	1.5	–	–	–	–	–	0.6	–
Stomach cancer	M	494	7	374	34.8	0.6	65.7	–	–	–	–	2.1	0.6	1.7
	F	279	7	187	13.8	0.6	23.8	–	–	–	0.6	0.7	0.6	2.1
Colorectal cancer	M	280	2	184	20.9	0.2	33.6	–	–	–	–	–	–	1.1
	F	282	4	189	13.8	0.3	24.5	–	–	–	–	–	0.6	1.6
Liver cancer	M	...	...	...	...	...	...	...	...	...	...	...	...	...
	F	...	...	...	...	...	...	...	...	...	...	...	...	...
Pancreas cancer	M	...	...	...	...	...	...	...	...	...	...	...	...	...
	F	...	...	...	...	...	...	...	...	...	...	...	...	...
Larynx cancer	M	119	2	102	8.0	0.2	16.4	–	–	–	–	–	0.6	0.6
	F	2	–	1	0.1	–	0.1	–	–	–	–	–	–	–
Lung cancer	M	925	10	752	64.1	0.8	129.4	–	–	–	–	–	1.8	3.9
	F	187	4	103	9.2	0.3	13.6	–	–	–	–	–	–	2.1
Malignant melanoma	M	...	...	...	...	...	...	...	...	...	...	...	...	...
	F	...	...	...	...	...	...	...	...	...	...	...	...	...
Female breast cancer	F	404	12	312	20.2	0.9	38.5	–	–	–	–	–	1.1	5.2
Cervix cancer	F	185	7	140	9.2	0.6	17.7	–	–	–	–	0.7	1.7	1.6
Other uterine cancer	F	130	3	87	6.5	0.3	11.3	–	–	–	0.6	0.7	–	0.5
Ovarian cancer	F	...	...	...	...	...	...	...	...	...	...	...	...	...
Prostate cancer	M	102	–	48	8.2	–	8.7	–	–	–	–	–	–	–
Bladder cancer	M	...	...	...	...	...	...	...	...	...	...	...	...	...
	F	...	...	...	...	...	...	...	...	...	...	...	...	...
Other and ill-defined cancer sites	M	852	59	613	58.8	4.8	105.3	2.3	3.4	1.6	1.7	6.4	8.8	9.4
	F	792	54	531	39.0	4.3	68.1	4.7	1.5	1.6	4.8	6.1	3.3	7.9
Hodgkin's disease	M	...	...	...	...	...	...	...	...	...	...	...	...	...
	F	...	...	...	...	...	...	...	...	...	...	...	...	...
Myeloma and all lymphomas	M	109	23	76	6.7	1.7	13.1	2.3	1.9	1.1	2.9	0.7	1.2	2.2
	F	92	20	57	4.4	1.6	7.0	1.4	0.5	1.6	2.4	3.4	2.2	–
Leukaemia	M	110	42	53	6.3	3.3	9.3	2.3	5.3	2.1	5.8	3.5	1.8	2.2
	F	94	36	48	4.3	2.7	6.2	4.7	4.0	1.6	1.2	2.0	1.1	4.2
ALL VASCULAR DISEASE	M	8148	120	4018	660.9	9.9	727.7	3.6	1.0	1.1	4.6	11.3	19.4	28.2
	F	10149	55	3539	508.0	4.4	478.7	0.9	–	1.1	4.2	6.1	6.6	12.1
Rheumatic heart disease and fever	M	138	18	116	8.3	1.5	16.7	–	–	1.1	0.6	2.1	4.7	2.2
	F	160	14	140	8.0	1.1	16.8	–	–	–	0.6	2.0	1.1	4.2
Hypertensive disease	M	85	1	66	6.0	0.1	10.5	–	–	–	–	–	–	0.6
	F	131	1	84	6.6	0.1	10.9	–	–	–	–	–	–	0.5
Ischaemic heart disease	M	4962	42	2287	410.9	3.5	421.2	–	–	–	0.6	3.5	8.8	11.6
	F	6095	9	1790	305.4	0.7	246.8	–	–	–	0.6	1.4	1.1	2.1
Pulmonary embolism and other venous	M	...	...	...	...	...	...	...	...	...	...	...	...	...
	F	...	...	...	...	...	...	...	...	...	...	...	...	...
Cerebrovascular disease	M	2485	25	1301	198.6	2.1	236.5	–	0.5	–	0.6	2.1	4.1	7.2
	F	3324	19	1367	165.7	1.6	184.3	–	–	0.5	1.8	2.7	2.2	3.7
Other vascular disease, incl. venous	M	478	34	248	37.1	2.7	42.8	3.6	0.5	–	2.9	3.5	1.8	6.6
	F	439	12	158	22.4	0.9	19.9	0.9	–	0.5	1.2	–	2.2	1.6
Chronic obstructive pulmonary disease	M	1133	21	658	86.4	1.7	117.5	1.8	0.5	–	0.6	2.1	0.6	6.1
	F	701	12	310	34.6	0.9	41.6	1.4	–	0.5	0.6	–	1.7	2.1
Other respiratory disease	M	604	297	261	31.7	19.8	39.5	119.0	1.9	2.1	3.5	2.8	1.2	7.8
	F	379	231	103	16.2	15.7	12.8	100.4	2.5	–	1.8	–	2.2	3.1
Peptic ulcer	M	158	7	123	10.7	0.6	18.8	–	–	–	–	1.4	1.8	1.1
	F	53	3	27	2.7	0.3	3.4	–	–	–	0.6	0.7	0.6	–
Liver cirrhosis and other liver disease	M	1340	55	1063	91.0	4.4	176.6	1.4	–	1.1	3.5	2.1	5.9	17.2
	F	1804	32	1448	89.0	2.5	185.4	0.5	0.5	0.5	1.8	0.7	3.9	9.4
Renal disease	M	181	29	107	12.4	2.4	17.7	1.4	0.5	–	–	3.5	7.7	3.9
	F	141	17	92	6.9	1.4	11.7	0.9	0.5	0.5	1.8	2.0	1.7	2.1
Pregnancy and birth	F	34	21	13	1.5	1.8	1.3	–	–	–	1.8	4.1	3.3	3.1
Congenital and perinatal causes	M	506	502	4	18.4	32.7	0.5	220.4	1.0	2.1	1.2	1.4	1.2	1.7
	F	366	362	4	13.9	24.7	0.4	159.3	3.5	1.6	2.4	2.7	2.2	1.0
Ill-defined causes	M	1441	3	24	151.4	0.2	5.4	0.9	–	–	0.6	–	–	–
	F	2777	1	47	145.2	0.1	7.0	–	–	–	–	–	–	0.5
Other medical causes	M	1029	202	661	65.9	15.4	103.0	28.1	9.1	7.4	8.7	13.5	14.7	26.6
	F	818	140	472	39.3	10.8	59.3	19.3	5.9	5.4	7.8	12.3	8.8	15.7
ALL NON-MEDICAL CAUSES	M	3281	1412	1683	178.3	116.8	233.8	73.3	41.8	30.5	77.0	209.6	189.6	196.0
	F	1181	391	604	55.4	29.7	72.7	61.3	21.3	16.2	28.8	24.6	24.3	31.5
Motor vehicle traffic accidents	M	971	516	418	50.0	44.0	56.0	14.9	12.5	8.9	31.8	99.9	78.3	61.5
	F	272	119	117	12.4	9.3	13.6	6.6	9.9	4.9	12.6	8.9	9.4	13.1
Fire	M	80	38	31	4.4	2.8	4.2	8.1	1.9	–	0.6	4.2	1.2	3.9
	F	62	15	24	2.9	1.1	3.3	4.2	1.0	0.5	–	1.4	0.6	–
Suicide	M	502	156	323	28.3	13.2	44.8	–	–	3.2	7.5	20.5	25.3	36.0
	F	144	30	90	7.2	2.5	10.8	–	–	1.1	4.8	5.5	2.8	3.7
Homicide	M	272	128	132	14.3	11.0	17.0	2.7	–	0.5	8.7	24.1	20.0	21.0
	F	124	31	81	5.9	2.5	9.3	2.8	–	–	1.2	4.1	5.0	4.2
POPULATION (thousands):	M=males				2076.8	1283.9	719.3	221.0	208.3	190.2	172.8	141.2	169.8	180.6
	F=females				2282.8	1284.5	863.5	212.2	202.2	184.9	166.6	146.6	181.3	190.7

Republic of MOLDOVA: 1990

Annual death rates / 100, 000 — 9th ICD categories

35–39	40–44	45–49	50–54	55–59	60–64	65–69	70–74	75–79	80+/NK		Cause	ICD
445.2	703.4	977.9	1504.6	2071.1	3217.7	4233.0	6320.0	8955.6	17765.1	M	ALL CAUSES	001–999
174.0	309.4	487.8	798.9	1271.4	1811.7	2795.7	4518.0	6530.0	15709.6	F		
16.7	17.2	13.1	24.9	19.7	19.3	17.0	20.0	7.4	18.1	M	Tuberculosis	010–018, 137
2.8	2.5	3.5	0.8	6.2	3.5	3.2	–	4.1	–	F		
0.6	4.5	2.0	3.7	4.4	4.8	6.8	–	7.4	6.0	M	Other infective	Rest of 001–139
–	0.8	2.6	0.8	1.8	2.6	3.2	4.0	–	2.7	F	and parasitic	
38.7	95.8	176.1	346.9	520.8	818.6	918.4	1006.7	900.0	801.2	M	ALL CANCER	140–208
46.0	75.1	113.4	204.2	248.5	371.3	435.7	554.0	424.4	495.9	F		
2.4	9.0	22.1	23.1	36.1	45.9	42.5	26.7	18.5	24.1	M	Mouth and	140–149
1.1	–	–	0.8	1.8	0.9	4.3	4.0	4.1	13.7	F	pharynx cancer	
1.2	3.6	4.0	9.2	10.9	23.0	11.9	30.0	11.1	30.1	M	Oesophagus cancer	150
–	–	0.9	1.5	0.9	1.8	5.4	2.0	6.2	13.7	F		
10.7	13.6	12.1	59.0	64.6	124.5	175.2	176.7	144.4	126.5	M	Stomach cancer	151
5.1	9.1	17.5	18.6	22.0	48.2	46.5	62.0	60.0	68.5	F		
2.4	6.3	14.1	23.1	23.0	64.1	102.0	126.7	125.9	132.5	M	Colorectal cancer	153, 154
2.2	2.5	8.7	27.8	22.9	50.8	56.2	60.0	60.0	82.2	F		
...	...	...	...	...	...	...	...	...	...	M	Liver cancer	Not given separately
...	...	...	...	...	...	...	...	...	...	F		
...	...	...	...	...	...	...	...	...	...	M	Pancreas cancer	Not given separately
...	...	...	...	...	...	...	...	...	...	F		
1.2	2.7	6.0	34.1	15.3	31.4	23.8	26.7	22.2	6.0	M	Larynx cancer	161
–	–	–	–	0.9	–	–	–	–	2.7	F		
7.7	19.9	52.3	91.3	204.6	281.7	248.3	236.7	218.5	198.8	M	Lung cancer	162
2.2	0.8	4.4	9.3	15.9	24.5	37.8	66.0	49.7	63.0	F		
...	...	...	...	...	...	...	...	...	...	M	Malignant melanoma	Not given
...	...	...	...	...	...	...	...	...	...	F		separately
14.0	14.0	28.8	49.5	48.5	56.0	58.4	70.0	49.7	57.5	F	Female breast cancer	174
5.1	6.6	13.1	20.9	14.1	26.3	37.8	36.0	24.8	21.9	F	Cervix cancer	180
1.1	6.6	4.4	6.2	15.9	21.0	23.8	36.0	22.8	30.1	F	Other uterine cancer	179, 182
...	...	...	...	...	...	...	...	...	...	F	Ovarian cancer	Not given separately
–	–	1.0	2.8	14.2	24.2	18.7	86.7	70.4	54.2	M	Prostate cancer	185
...	...	...	...	...	...	...	...	...	...	M	Bladder cancer	Not given separately
...	...	...	...	...	...	...	...	...	...	F		
10.1	32.5	53.3	84.9	131.3	188.6	236.4	263.3	244.4	210.8	M	Other and ill-defined	Rest of 140–208,
11.8	29.7	33.2	52.6	93.4	115.6	140.5	188.0	136.6	128.8	F	cancer sites	incl. 155, 157, 172, 183, 188
...	...	...	...	...	...	...	...	...	...	M	Hodgkin's disease	Not given separately
...	...	...	...	...	...	...	...	...	...	F		
1.8	3.6	8.0	13.8	15.3	13.3	35.7	13.3	14.8	12.0	M	Myeloma and all	200–203,
2.8	2.5	1.7	11.6	5.3	14.0	10.8	14.0	8.3	11.0	F	lymphomas	incl. 201
1.2	4.5	3.0	5.5	5.5	21.8	23.8	20.0	29.6	6.0	M	Leukaemia	204–208
0.6	3.3	0.9	5.4	7.0	12.3	14.1	16.0	2.1	2.7	F		
72.6	146.5	255.5	421.6	723.2	1334.9	2139.5	3556.7	5085.2	9457.8	M	ALL VASCULAR	390–459
27.5	73.4	121.3	242.1	482.8	817.0	1587.0	2794.0	4091.1	8717.8	F	DISEASE	
8.9	15.4	22.1	15.7	25.2	19.3	10.2	6.7	7.4	–	M	Rheumatic heart	390–398
9.0	9.9	16.6	19.3	29.1	18.4	15.1	6.0	4.1	2.7	F	disease and fever	
1.8	4.5	6.0	15.7	10.9	19.3	15.3	26.7	22.2	24.1	M	Hypertensive disease	401–405
–	3.3	3.5	10.8	14.1	21.0	23.8	40.0	26.9	35.6	F		
33.9	79.6	118.7	240.8	382.9	764.2	1328.2	2210.0	3340.7	6433.7	M	Ischaemic heart	410–414
7.9	14.9	44.5	96.7	209.7	422.9	930.8	1756.0	2683.2	5813.7	F	disease	
...	...	...	...	...	...	...	...	...	...	M	Pulmonary embolism	Not given
...	...	...	...	...	...	...	...	...	...	F	and other venous	separately
19.6	37.1	85.5	122.7	254.9	453.4	682.0	1160.0	1492.6	2457.8	M	Cerebrovascular	430–438
3.4	36.3	44.5	96.7	207.0	328.4	574.1	886.0	1248.4	2443.8	F	disease	
8.3	9.9	23.1	26.8	49.2	78.6	103.7	153.3	222.2	542.2	M	Other vascular	Rest of 390–459,
7.3	9.1	12.2	18.6	22.9	26.3	43.2	106.0	128.4	421.9	F	disease, incl. venous	incl. 415, 451–3
10.1	18.1	35.2	79.3	133.5	238.2	307.8	420.0	703.7	831.3	M	Chronic obstructive	490–496
3.4	3.3	12.2	21.7	49.3	72.7	128.6	186.0	256.7	443.8	F	pulmonary disease	
16.7	19.9	39.2	52.6	54.7	42.3	51.0	50.0	63.0	84.3	M	Other respiratory	Rest of 460–519
4.5	7.4	11.3	13.9	11.5	18.4	22.7	26.0	24.8	54.8	F	disease	
7.1	9.0	19.1	27.7	18.6	24.2	25.5	56.7	29.6	18.1	M	Peptic ulcer	531–533
0.6	0.8	2.6	4.6	–	7.9	7.6	24.0	8.3	19.2	F		
33.9	74.1	101.6	145.8	207.9	331.3	341.8	370.0	259.3	247.0	M	Liver cirrhosis and	570–573, 576,
28.1	50.3	104.7	160.9	286.3	307.4	360.0	268.0	260.9	175.3	F	other liver disease	575.2–579.9
5.4	5.4	16.1	14.8	17.5	24.2	40.8	46.7	59.3	90.4	M	Renal disease	580–590
2.2	9.1	8.7	6.2	15.9	20.1	19.5	20.0	31.1	19.2	F		
3.9	4.1	0.9	–	–	–	–	–	–	–	F	Pregnancy and birth	630–676
1.2	–	1.0	–	1.1	–	–	–	–	–	M	Congenital and	740–779
0.6	–	1.7	0.8	–	–	–	–	–	–	F	perinatal causes	
–	–	–	–	–	7.3	30.6	356.7	1474.1	5475.9	M	Ill-defined causes	780–799
–	–	–	–	–	8.8	40.0	400.0	1157.3	5397.3	F		
39.9	46.1	94.6	115.3	123.6	141.5	159.9	186.7	188.9	355.4	M	Other medical causes	Rest of 001–799
15.7	31.4	26.2	59.6	76.7	99.8	105.9	140.0	144.9	180.8	F		
202.4	266.7	224.3	272.1	246.2	231.0	193.9	250.0	177.8	379.5	M	ALL NON-	E800–E999
38.7	51.2	78.5	83.5	92.5	82.3	82.2	102.0	126.3	202.7	F	MEDICAL CAUSES	
65.5	74.1	50.3	59.0	43.8	56.8	42.5	46.7	33.3	84.3	M	Motor vehicle	E810–E819
11.2	10.7	18.3	15.5	13.2	16.6	9.7	30.0	26.9	21.9	F	traffic accidents	
6.0	1.8	3.0	7.4	3.3	1.2	6.8	6.7	11.1	36.1	M	Fire	E890–E899
0.6	1.7	0.9	1.5	3.5	1.8	13.0	8.0	14.5	32.9	F		
39.3	52.4	45.3	50.7	44.9	43.5	37.4	43.3	18.5	30.1	M	Suicide	E950–E959
3.9	8.3	17.5	13.9	15.0	8.8	8.6	18.0	20.7	13.7	F		
22.0	26.2	15.1	14.8	19.7	18.1	3.4	20.0	14.8	12.0	M	Homicide	E960–E969
9.5	8.3	10.5	7.7	9.7	13.1	6.5	10.0	6.2	11.0	F		
168.0	110.6	99.4	108.4	91.4	82.7	58.8	30.0	27.0	16.6	M	**POPULATION (thousands)**	
178.2	121.2	114.6	129.3	113.5	114.2	92.5	50.0	48.3	36.5	F		

Republic of MOLDOVA: Males

	All ages	0–34	35–69	35–39	40–44	45–49	50–54	55–59	60–64	65–69	70–74	75–79	80+/NK
POPULATION (1000s)													
1985–90	2036.8	1279.7	682.8	151.5	94.9	111.1	104.6	95.4	74.9	50.4	34.6	24.2	15.5
1985	1990.7	1271.2	642.7	115.4	104.7	116.4	101.1	93.8	71.4	39.9	40.5	21.5	14.8
1990	**2076.8**	**1283.9**	**719.3**	**168.0**	**110.6**	**99.4**	**108.4**	**91.4**	**82.7**	**58.8**	**30.0**	**27.0**	**16.6**
1995 projected	*2072.3*	*1281.1*	*717.8*	*167.6*	*110.4*	*99.2*	*108.2*	*91.2*	*82.5*	*58.7*	*29.9*	*26.9*	*16.6*
NUMBER OF DEATHS													
All causes													
1985–90	20857	3372	10323	655	614	1078	1508	1954	2315	2199	2125	2266	2771
1985	23036	3939	10956	611	765	1319	1712	2183	2460	1906	2830	2288	3023
1990	**21399**	**2964**	**11172**	**748**	**778**	**972**	**1631**	**1893**	**2661**	**2489**	**1896**	**2418**	**2949**
1995 projected	*19230*	*2596*	*10038*	*675*	*690*	*868*	*1438*	*1719*	*2396*	*2252*	*1645*	*2078*	*2873*
Lung cancer													
1985–90	858	10	701	11	25	63	108	185	188	121	70	53	24
1985	745	6	607	8	31	59	94	165	154	96	67	45	20
1990	**925**	**10**	**752**	**13**	**22**	**52**	**99**	**187**	**233**	**146**	**71**	**59**	**33**
1995 projected	*1021*	*12*	*822*	*10*	*19*	*47*	*104*	*214*	*258*	*170*	*80*	*67*	*40*
ANNUAL DEATH RATE / 100,000 (*The rates for the age groups 0–34 and 35–69 are the means of seven five-yearly rates, but the all-ages rates are standardised to the conventional "European" age distribution)													
All causes													
1985–90	1555.3*	250.4*	1856.2*	432.3	647.0	970.3	1441.7	2048.2	3090.8	4363.1	6141.6	9363.6	17877.4
1985	1773.3*	293.3*	2090.9*	529.5	730.7	1133.2	1693.4	2327.3	3445.4	4776.9	6987.7	10641.9	20425.7
1990	**1549.2***	**227.6***	**1879.0***	**445.2**	**703.4**	**977.9**	**1504.6**	**2071.1**	**3217.7**	**4233.0**	**6320.0**	**8955.6**	**17765.1**
1995 projected	*1407.9**	*205.4**	*1693.9**	*402.7*	*625.0*	*875.0*	*1329.0*	*1884.9*	*2904.2*	*3836.5*	*5501.7*	*7724.9*	*17307.2*
All cancer													
1985–90	208.1*	12.7*	386.2*	44.2	100.1	189.0	337.5	517.8	699.6	815.5	832.4	909.1	651.6
1985	181.5*	11.3*	337.9*	41.6	77.4	177.0	287.8	484.0	588.2	709.3	716.0	851.2	479.7
1990	**225.2***	**12.1***	**416.5***	**38.7**	**95.8**	**176.1**	**346.9**	**520.8**	**818.6**	**918.4**	**1006.7**	**900.0**	**801.2**
1995 projected	*268.7**	*12.0**	*499.6**	*41.2*	*95.1*	*194.6*	*369.7*	*620.6*	*993.9*	*1182.3*	*1234.1*	*1100.4*	*1024.1*
Lung cancer													
1985–90	61.3*	0.8*	125.5*	7.3	26.3	56.7	103.3	193.9	251.0	240.1	202.3	219.0	154.8
1985	55.7*	0.5*	116.1*	6.9	29.6	50.7	93.0	175.9	215.7	240.6	165.4	209.3	135.1
1990	**64.1***	**0.8***	**129.4***	**7.7**	**19.9**	**52.3**	**91.3**	**204.6**	**281.7**	**248.3**	**236.7**	**218.5**	**198.8**
1995 projected	*71.3**	*1.0**	*143.4**	*6.0*	*17.2*	*47.4*	*96.1*	*234.6*	*312.7*	*289.6*	*267.6*	*249.1*	*241.0*
Upper aerodigestive cancer (mouth, oesophagus, pharynx and larynx)													
1985–90	23.6*	0.4*	47.8*	5.3	15.8	36.0	59.3	66.0	82.8	69.4	66.5	74.4	45.2
1985	18.8*	0.2*	38.1*	6.9	6.7	34.4	43.5	54.4	65.8	55.1	69.1	55.8	20.3
1990	**25.3***	**0.7***	**51.4***	**4.8**	**15.4**	**32.2**	**66.4**	**62.4**	**100.4**	**78.2**	**83.3**	**51.9**	**60.2**
1995 projected	*31.9**	*0.7**	*65.6**	*6.0*	*15.4*	*41.3*	*77.6*	*84.4*	*132.1*	*102.2*	*97.0*	*70.6*	*84.3*
Other cancer													
1985–90	123.2*	11.4*	212.9*	31.7	58.0	96.3	175.0	257.9	365.8	506.0	563.6	615.7	451.6
1985	106.9*	10.6*	183.7*	27.7	41.1	91.9	151.3	253.7	306.7	413.5	481.5	586.0	324.3
1990	**135.7***	**10.6***	**235.7***	**26.2**	**60.6**	**91.5**	**189.1**	**253.8**	**436.5**	**591.8**	**686.7**	**629.6**	**542.2**
1995 projected	*165.5**	*10.3**	*290.7**	*29.2*	*62.5*	*105.8*	*195.9*	*301.5*	*549.1*	*790.5*	*869.6*	*780.7*	*698.8*
Chronic obstructive pulmonary disease (COPD)													
1985–90	102.2*	1.7*	130.0*	11.9	21.1	44.1	84.1	147.8	245.7	355.2	505.8	789.3	1187.1
1985	134.0*	1.7*	170.7*	21.7	30.6	65.3	123.6	198.3	329.1	426.1	619.8	958.1	1655.4
1990	**86.4***	**1.7***	**117.5***	**10.1**	**18.1**	**35.2**	**79.3**	**133.5**	**238.2**	**307.8**	**420.0**	**703.7**	**831.3**
1995 projected	*59.1**	*0.9**	*79.4**	*6.6*	*11.8*	*24.2*	*53.6*	*91.0*	*162.4*	*206.1*	*294.3*	*472.1*	*590.4*
Other respiratory disease													
1985–90	39.4*	30.9*	41.4*	14.5	25.3	36.9	54.5	56.6	50.7	51.6	57.8	70.2	103.2
1985	57.6*	47.3*	57.5*	23.4	42.0	47.3	77.2	83.2	64.4	65.2	69.1	107.0	155.4
1990	**31.7***	**19.8***	**39.5***	**16.7**	**19.9**	**39.2**	**52.6**	**54.7**	**42.3**	**51.0**	**50.0**	**63.0**	**84.3**
1995 projected	*21.8**	*14.0**	*26.6**	*10.7*	*12.7*	*26.2*	*36.0*	*37.3*	*29.1*	*34.1*	*33.4*	*40.9*	*60.2*
Vascular disease													
1985–90	776.5*	10.0*	725.2*	67.3	131.7	222.3	405.4	687.6	1308.4	2254.0	3843.9	6400.8	13677.4
1985	926.7*	12.4*	817.7*	68.5	145.2	251.7	460.9	793.2	1508.4	2496.2	4553.1	7790.7	17027.0
1990	**660.9***	**9.9***	**727.7***	**72.6**	**146.5**	**255.5**	**421.6**	**723.2**	**1334.9**	**2139.5**	**3556.7**	**5085.2**	**9457.8**
1995 projected	*498.6**	*7.3**	*602.5**	*64.4*	*138.6*	*235.9*	*378.0*	*623.9*	*1117.6*	*1659.3*	*2541.8*	*3408.9*	*6686.7*
Liver cirrhosis and other liver disease													
1985–90	97.0*	4.5*	190.2*	32.3	62.2	111.6	153.9	220.1	336.4	414.7	343.9	330.6	303.2
1985	123.7*	5.3*	250.5*	50.3	81.2	143.5	234.4	294.2	428.6	521.3	397.5	330.2	351.4
1990	**91.0***	**4.4***	**176.6***	**33.9**	**74.1**	**101.6**	**145.8**	**207.9**	**331.3**	**341.8**	**370.0**	**259.3**	**247.0**
1995 projected	*64.6**	*2.9**	*123.3**	*25.7*	*52.5*	*68.5*	*98.9*	*142.5*	*224.2*	*250.4*	*284.3*	*197.0*	*186.7*
Other medical causes													
1985–90	163.6*	81.4*	159.5*	69.3	94.8	139.5	169.2	182.4	215.0	246.0	332.4	640.5	1612.9
1985	168.5*	109.0*	206.6*	110.1	146.1	214.8	225.5	220.7	263.3	265.7	333.3	381.4	324.3
1990	**275.8***	**62.9***	**167.4***	**70.8**	**82.3**	**145.9**	**186.3**	**184.9**	**221.3**	**280.6**	**666.7**	**1766.7**	**5963.9**
1995 projected	*324.0**	*43.6**	*148.7**	*46.5*	*53.4*	*98.8*	*140.5*	*148.0*	*193.9*	*359.5*	*926.4*	*2368.0*	*8433.7*
All non-medical causes													
1985–90	168.3*	109.2*	223.6*	192.7	211.8	226.8	237.1	235.8	235.0	226.2	225.4	223.1	341.9
1985	181.3*	106.3*	250.0*	214.0	208.2	233.7	283.9	253.7	263.3	293.2	298.8	223.3	432.4
1990	**178.3***	**116.8***	**233.8***	**202.4**	**266.7**	**224.3**	**272.1**	**246.2**	**231.0**	**193.9**	**250.0**	**177.8**	**379.5**
1995 projected	*171.0**	*124.6**	*213.9**	*207.6*	*260.9*	*226.8*	*252.3*	*221.5*	*183.0*	*144.8*	*187.3*	*137.5*	*325.3*

Republic of MOLDOVA: Females

	All ages	0–34	35–69	35–39	40–44	45–49	50–54	55–59	60–64	65–69	70–74	75–79	80+/NK
POPULATION (1000s)													
1985–90	2246.9	1283.6	828.9	160.9	106.6	129.1	124.0	120.4	110.3	77.6	57.1	43.1	34.2
1985	2203.6	1278.2	788.6	123.7	118.4	136.3	120.3	122.4	106.2	61.3	66.1	38.1	32.6
1990	**2282.8**	**1284.5**	**863.5**	**178.2**	**121.2**	**114.6**	**129.3**	**113.5**	**114.2**	**92.5**	**50.0**	**48.3**	**36.5**
1995 projected	*2278.0*	*1281.7*	*861.7*	*177.8*	*120.9*	*114.4*	*129.0*	*113.3*	*114.0*	*92.3*	*49.9*	*48.2*	*36.5*
NUMBER OF DEATHS													
All causes													
1985–90	20868	1858	8259	327	370	688	1050	1526	2045	2253	2514	3015	5222
1985	23039	2221	9047	359	533	895	1158	1753	2307	2042	3204	3009	5558
1990	**21028**	**1506**	**8375**	**310**	**375**	**559**	**1033**	**1443**	**2069**	**2586**	**2259**	**3154**	**5734**
1995 projected	*18623*	*1154*	*7025*	*218*	*264*	*430*	*862*	*1225*	*1751*	*2275*	*1942*	*2888*	*5614*
Lung cancer													
1985–90	192	5	125	5	5	10	18	23	33	31	27	20	15
1985	162	3	117	6	6	10	15	29	28	23	24	11	7
1990	**187**	**4**	**103**	**4**	**1**	**5**	**12**	**18**	**28**	**35**	**33**	**24**	**23**
1995 projected	*213*	*3*	*96*	*2*	*1*	*3*	*8*	*14*	*24*	*44*	*46*	*35*	*33*
ANNUAL DEATH RATE / 100,000 (*The rates for the age groups 0–34 and 35–69 are the means of seven five-yearly rates, but the all-ages rates are standardised to the conventional "European" age distribution)													
All causes													
1985–90	1068.5*	134.1*	1136.4*	203.2	347.1	532.9	846.8	1267.4	1854.0	2903.4	4402.8	6995.4	15269.0
1985	1224.3*	163.1*	1327.9*	290.2	450.2	656.6	962.6	1432.2	2172.3	3331.2	4847.2	7897.6	17049.1
1990	**1040.9***	**110.3***	**1092.7***	**174.0**	**309.4**	**487.8**	**798.9**	**1271.4**	**1811.7**	**2795.7**	**4518.0**	**6530.0**	**15709.6**
1995 projected	*926.3**	*85.9**	*923.9**	*122.6*	*218.4*	*375.9*	*668.2*	*1081.2*	*1536.0*	*2464.8*	*3891.8*	*5991.7*	*15380.8*
All cancer													
1985–90	115.0*	10.9*	206.0*	52.8	78.8	124.7	187.1	239.2	340.9	418.8	444.8	464.0	386.0
1985	105.2*	9.9*	194.1*	62.2	76.0	128.4	153.8	217.3	324.9	396.4	378.2	435.7	282.2
1990	**122.5***	**11.7***	**213.4***	**46.0**	**75.1**	**113.4**	**204.2**	**248.5**	**371.3**	**435.7**	**554.0**	**424.4**	**495.9**
1995 projected	*138.5**	*12.5**	*237.8**	*37.1*	*62.0*	*116.3*	*224.0*	*291.3*	*404.4*	*529.8*	*645.3*	*549.8*	*613.7*
Lung cancer													
1985–90	9.8*	0.4*	17.0*	3.1	4.7	7.7	14.5	19.1	29.9	39.9	47.3	46.4	43.9
1985	8.5*	0.2*	16.8*	4.9	5.1	7.3	12.5	23.7	26.4	37.5	36.3	28.9	21.5
1990	**9.2***	**0.3***	**13.6***	**2.2**	**0.8**	**4.4**	**9.3**	**15.9**	**24.5**	**37.8**	**66.0**	**49.7**	**63.0**
1995 projected	*10.6**	*0.2**	*13.1**	*1.1*	*0.8*	*2.6*	*6.2*	*12.4*	*21.1*	*47.7*	*92.2*	*72.6*	*90.4*
Upper aerodigestive cancer (mouth, oesophagus, pharynx and larynx)													
1985–90	2.3*	0.2*	3.5*	1.2	0.9	1.5	2.4	3.3	7.3	7.7	8.8	13.9	20.5
1985	2.4*	0.2*	4.2*	2.4	2.5	2.9	2.5	3.3	9.4	6.5	1.5	21.0	12.3
1990	**2.1***	**0.2***	**2.9***	**1.1**	**–**	**0.9**	**2.3**	**3.5**	**2.6**	**9.7**	**6.0**	**10.4**	**30.1**
1995 projected	*2.0**	*0.2**	*2.4**	*0.6*	*–*	*0.9*	*1.6*	*2.6*	*1.8*	*9.8*	*6.0*	*10.4*	*35.6*
Other cancer													
1985–90	102.9*	10.4*	185.6*	48.5	73.2	115.4	170.2	216.8	303.7	371.1	388.8	403.7	321.6
1985	94.2*	9.5*	173.2*	55.0	68.4	118.1	138.8	190.4	289.1	352.4	340.4	385.8	248.5
1990	**111.1***	**11.2***	**197.0***	**42.6**	**74.3**	**108.2**	**192.6**	**229.1**	**344.1**	**388.1**	**482.0**	**364.4**	**402.7**
1995 projected	*125.9**	*12.1**	*222.3**	*35.4*	*61.2*	*112.8*	*216.3*	*276.3*	*381.6*	*472.4*	*547.1*	*466.8*	*487.7*
Chronic obstructive pulmonary disease (COPD)													
1985–90	40.7*	0.8*	40.1*	3.7	7.5	11.6	25.0	41.5	66.2	125.0	201.4	343.4	660.8
1985	55.9*	0.9*	57.0*	5.7	11.0	16.1	33.3	57.2	88.5	187.6	295.0	396.3	932.5
1990	**34.6***	**0.9***	**41.6***	**3.4**	**3.3**	**12.2**	**21.7**	**49.3**	**72.7**	**128.6**	**186.0**	**256.7**	**443.8**
1995 projected	*24.7**	*0.5**	*29.9**	*2.2*	*1.7*	*7.9*	*16.3*	*38.8*	*52.6*	*89.9*	*130.3*	*186.7*	*312.3*
Other respiratory disease													
1985–90	22.0*	24.3*	15.1*	5.0	11.3	13.9	14.5	17.4	19.0	24.5	28.0	30.2	49.7
1985	32.4*	35.2*	24.1*	15.4	16.0	23.5	16.6	30.2	24.5	42.4	36.3	42.0	61.3
1990	**16.2***	**15.7***	**12.8***	**4.5**	**7.4**	**11.3**	**13.9**	**11.5**	**18.4**	**22.7**	**26.0**	**24.8**	**54.8**
1995 projected	*11.3**	*10.8**	*8.6**	*2.8*	*5.0*	*7.0*	*9.3*	*7.9*	*12.3*	*16.3*	*18.0*	*20.7*	*43.8*
Vascular disease													
1985–90	626.7*	5.0*	513.4*	28.6	70.4	125.5	256.5	480.1	895.7	1737.1	3120.8	5329.5	12365.5
1985	744.2*	5.5*	600.8*	30.7	75.2	161.4	278.5	565.4	1097.9	1996.7	3502.3	6325.5	15153.4
1990	**508.0***	**4.4***	**478.7***	**27.5**	**73.4**	**121.3**	**242.1**	**482.8**	**817.0**	**1587.0**	**2794.0**	**4091.1**	**8717.8**
1995 projected	*371.8**	*3.5**	*369.4**	*22.5*	*53.8*	*92.7*	*193.0*	*373.3*	*618.4*	*1231.9*	*1984.0*	*2966.8*	*6164.4*
Liver cirrhosis and other liver disease													
1985–90	94.5*	3.1*	192.8*	31.1	69.4	116.2	191.1	281.6	316.4	344.1	269.7	269.1	222.2
1985	125.1*	4.9*	255.4*	64.7	125.0	162.1	273.5	332.5	392.7	437.2	328.3	336.0	263.8
1990	**89.0***	**2.5***	**185.4***	**28.1**	**50.3**	**104.7**	**160.9**	**286.3**	**307.4**	**360.0**	**268.0**	**260.9**	**175.3**
1995 projected	*65.9**	*1.8**	*137.7**	*17.4*	*31.4*	*66.4*	*109.3*	*210.9*	*242.1*	*286.0*	*214.4*	*205.4*	*126.0*
Other medical causes													
1985–90	107.7*	56.1*	87.6*	36.0	48.8	62.7	85.5	102.2	126.9	150.8	225.9	422.3	1362.6
1985	89.3*	67.4*	99.9*	59.8	64.2	77.0	107.2	105.4	135.6	150.1	178.5	194.2	138.0
1990	**215.2***	**45.4***	**88.0***	**25.8**	**48.7**	**46.2**	**72.7**	**100.4**	**142.7**	**179.5**	**588.0**	**1345.8**	**5619.2**
1995 projected	*272.4**	*33.6**	*88.0**	*16.3*	*30.6*	*29.7*	*51.9*	*89.1*	*148.2*	*250.3*	*823.6*	*1952.3*	*7947.9*
All non-medical causes													
1985–90	61.9*	33.9*	81.4*	46.0	61.0	78.2	87.1	105.5	88.8	103.1	112.1	136.9	222.2
1985	72.1*	39.2*	96.5*	51.7	82.8	88.0	99.8	124.2	108.3	120.7	128.6	168.0	217.8
1990	**55.4***	**29.7***	**72.7***	**38.7**	**51.2**	**78.5**	**83.5**	**92.5**	**82.3**	**82.2**	**102.0**	**126.3**	**202.7**
1995 projected	*41.7**	*23.1**	*52.4**	*24.2*	*33.9*	*55.9*	*64.3*	*69.7*	*57.9*	*60.7*	*76.2*	*110.0*	*172.6*

Republic of MOLDOVA: 1985–1990

Smoking–attributed deaths (Sm.) and total deaths (Total)

		ALL CAUSES	ALL CANCER	Lung cancer	Upper aero–digestive ca.	Other cancer	COPD	Other respiratory	Vascular disease	Cirrhosis/ other liver	Other medical	Non–medical
Males												
0–34	Sm.	–	–	–	–	–	–	–	–	–	–	–
	Total	3372	161	10	5	146	21	465	122	55	1180	1368
35–69	Sm.	3281	1073	656	200	217	540	103	1183	–	382	–
	Total	10323	2154	701	285	1168	679	262	3670	1064	986	1508
		(32%)	(50%)	(94%)	(70%)	(19%)	(80%)	(39%)	(32%)		(39%)	
70+	Sm.	749	161	119	17	25	288	3	271	–	26	–
	Total	7162	609	147	48	414	550	53	4999	246	520	185
		(10%)	(26%)	(81%)	(35%)	(6%)	(52%)	(6%)	(5%)		(5%)	
Any age	Sm.	4030	1234	775	217	242	828	106	1454	–	408	–
	Total	20857	2924	858	338	1728	1250	780	8791	1365	2686	3061
		(19%)	(42%)	(90%)	(64%)	(14%)	(66%)	(14%)	(17%)		(15%)	
Females												
0–34	Sm.	–	–	–	–	–	–	–	–	–	–	–
	Total	1858	141	5	2	134	10	355	63	40	798	451
35–69	Sm.	425	76	59	5	12	94	7	206	–	42	–
	Total	8259	1551	125	26	1400	280	117	3515	1466	677	653
		(5%)	(5%)	(47%)	(19%)	(1%)	(34%)	(6%)	(6%)		(6%)	
70+	Sm.	213	21	19	1	1	89	0	95	–	8	–
	Total	10751	586	62	18	506	489	46	8308	346	777	199
		(2%)	(4%)	(31%)	(6%)	(0%)	(18%)	(0%)	(1%)		(1%)	
Any age	Sm.	638	97	78	6	13	183	7	301	–	50	–
	Total	20868	2278	192	46	2040	779	518	11886	1852	2252	1303
		(3%)	(4%)	(41%)	(13%)	(1%)	(23%)	(1%)	(3%)		(2%)	
Males+Females												
0–34	Sm.	–	–	–	–	–	–	–	–	–	–	–
	Total	5230	302	15	7	280	31	820	185	95	1978	1819
35–69	Sm.	3706	1149	715	205	229	634	110	1389	–	424	–
	Total	18582	3705	826	311	2568	959	379	7185	2530	1663	2161
		(20%)	(31%)	(87%)	(66%)	(9%)	(66%)	(29%)	(19%)		(25%)	
70+	Sm.	962	182	138	18	26	377	3	366	–	34	–
	Total	17913	1195	209	66	920	1039	99	13307	592	1297	384
		(5%)	(15%)	(66%)	(27%)	(3%)	(36%)	(3%)	(3%)		(3%)	
Any age	Sm.	4668	1331	853	223	255	1011	113	1755	–	458	–
	Total	41725	5202	1050	384	3768	2029	1298	20677	3217	4938	4364
		(11%)	(26%)	(81%)	(58%)	(7%)	(50%)	(9%)	(8%)		(9%)	

Republic of MOLDOVA: 1985

Smoking–attributed deaths (Sm.) and total deaths (Total)

		ALL CAUSES	ALL CANCER	Lung cancer	Upper aero–digestive ca.	Other cancer	COPD	Other respiratory	Vascular disease	Cirrhosis/ other liver	Other medical	Non–medical
Males												
0–34	Sm.	–	–	–	–	–	–	–	–	–	–	–
	Total	3939	144	6	2	136	21	686	151	64	1520	1353
35–69	Sm.	3361	884	567	149	168	669	135	1195	–	478	–
	Total	10956	1783	607	219	957	849	354	3807	1337	1259	1567
		(31%)	(50%)	(93%)	(68%)	(18%)	(79%)	(38%)	(31%)		(38%)	
70+	Sm.	802	136	103	15	18	348	4	299	–	15	–
	Total	8141	544	132	43	369	702	74	6039	284	265	233
		(10%)	(25%)	(78%)	(35%)	(5%)	(50%)	(5%)	(5%)		(6%)	
Any age	Sm.	4163	1020	670	164	186	1017	139	1494	–	493	–
	Total	23036	2471	745	264	1462	1572	1114	9997	1685	3044	3153
		(18%)	(41%)	(90%)	(62%)	(13%)	(65%)	(12%)	(15%)		(16%)	
Females												
0–34	Sm.	–	–	–	–	–	–	–	–	–	–	–
	Total	2221	127	3	2	122	12	496	70	63	933	520
35–69	Sm.	473	74	55	8	11	120	11	217	–	51	–
	Total	9047	1381	117	31	1233	361	179	3764	1870	749	743
		(5%)	(5%)	(47%)	(26%)	(1%)	(33%)	(6%)	(6%)		(7%)	
70+	Sm.	73	7	6	0	1	31	0	33	–	2	–
	Total	11771	508	42	13	453	650	60	9665	431	237	220
		(1%)	(1%)	(14%)	(0%)	(0%)	(5%)	(0%)	(0%)		(1%)	
Any age	Sm.	546	81	61	8	12	151	11	250	–	53	–
	Total	23039	2016	162	46	1808	1023	735	13499	2364	1919	1483
		(2%)	(4%)	(38%)	(17%)	(1%)	(15%)	(1%)	(2%)		(3%)	
Males+Females												
0–34	Sm.	–	–	–	–	–	–	–	–	–	–	–
	Total	6160	271	9	4	258	33	1182	221	127	2453	1873
35–69	Sm.	3834	958	622	157	179	789	146	1412	–	529	–
	Total	20003	3164	724	250	2190	1210	533	7571	3207	2008	2310
		(19%)	(30%)	(86%)	(63%)	(8%)	(65%)	(27%)	(19%)		(26%)	
70+	Sm.	875	143	109	15	19	379	4	332	–	17	–
	Total	19912	1052	174	56	822	1352	134	15704	715	502	453
		(4%)	(14%)	(63%)	(27%)	(2%)	(28%)	(3%)	(2%)		(3%)	
Any age	Sm.	4709	1101	731	172	198	1168	150	1744	–	546	–
	Total	46075	4487	907	310	3270	2595	1849	23496	4049	4963	4636
		(10%)	(25%)	(81%)	(55%)	(6%)	(45%)	(8%)	(7%)		(11%)	

(To be conservative, no deaths before age 35, and none from liver cirrhosis or non–medical causes, were attributed to smoking.)

Republic of MOLDOVA: 1990

Smoking–attributed deaths (Sm.) and total deaths (Total)

		ALL CAUSES	ALL CANCER	Lung cancer	Upper aero–digestive ca.	Other cancer	COPD	Other respiratory	Vascular disease	Cirrhosis/ other liver	Other medical	Non–medical
Males												
0–34	Sm.	–	–	–	–	–	–	–	–	–	–	–
	Total	2964	152	10	9	133	21	297	120	55	907	1412
35–69	Sm.	3518	1174	705	220	249	525	102	1309	–	408	–
	Total	11172	2415	752	315	1348	658	261	4018	1063	1074	1683
		(31%)	(49%)	(94%)	(70%)	(18%)	(80%)	(39%)	(33%)		(38%)	
70+	Sm.	744	181	132	20	29	242	3	236	–	82	–
	Total	7263	678	163	49	466	454	46	4010	222	1667	186
		(10%)	(27%)	(81%)	(41%)	(6%)	(53%)	(7%)	(6%)		(5%)	
Any age	Sm.	4262	1355	837	240	278	767	105	1545	–	490	–
	Total	21399	3245	925	373	1947	1133	604	8148	1340	3648	3281
		(20%)	(42%)	(90%)	(64%)	(14%)	(68%)	(17%)	(19%)		(13%)	
Females												
0–34	Sm.	–	–	–	–	–	–	–	–	–	–	–
	Total	1506	149	4	2	143	12	231	55	32	636	391
35–69	Sm.	257	39	32	1	6	69	2	126	–	21	–
	Total	8375	1676	103	22	1551	310	103	3539	1448	695	604
		(3%)	(2%)	(31%)	(5%)	(0%)	(22%)	(2%)	(4%)		(3%)	
70+	Sm.	295	39	33	2	4	95	1	122	–	38	–
	Total	11147	663	80	19	564	379	45	6555	324	2995	186
		(3%)	(6%)	(41%)	(11%)	(1%)	(25%)	(2%)	(2%)		(1%)	
Any age	Sm.	552	78	65	3	10	164	3	248	–	59	–
	Total	21028	2488	187	43	2258	701	379	10149	1804	4326	1181
		(3%)	(3%)	(35%)	(7%)	(0%)	(23%)	(1%)	(2%)		(1%)	
Males+Females												
0–34	Sm.	–	–	–	–	–	–	–	–	–	–	–
	Total	4470	301	14	11	276	33	528	175	87	1543	1803
35–69	Sm.	3775	1213	737	221	255	594	104	1435	–	429	–
	Total	19547	4091	855	337	2899	968	364	7557	2511	1769	2287
		(19%)	(30%)	(86%)	(66%)	(9%)	(61%)	(29%)	(19%)		(24%)	
70+	Sm.	1039	220	165	22	33	337	4	358	–	120	–
	Total	18410	1341	243	68	1030	833	91	10565	546	4662	372
		(6%)	(16%)	(68%)	(32%)	(3%)	(40%)	(4%)	(3%)		(3%)	
Any age	Sm.	4814	1433	902	243	288	931	108	1793	–	549	–
	Total	42427	5733	1112	416	4205	1834	983	18297	3144	7974	4462
		(11%)	(25%)	(81%)	(58%)	(7%)	(51%)	(11%)	(10%)		(7%)	

Republic of MOLDOVA: 1995

Smoking–attributed deaths (Sm.) and total deaths (Total)

		ALL CAUSES	ALL CANCER	Lung cancer	Upper aero–digestive ca.	Other cancer	COPD	Other respiratory	Vascular disease	Cirrhosis/ other liver	Other medical	Non–medical
Males												
0–34	Sm.	–	–	–	–	–	–	–	–	–	–	–
	Total	2596	147	12	8	127	11	211	87	36	631	1473
35–69	Sm.	3352	1385	776	287	322	363	72	1194	–	338	–
	Total	10038	2847	822	398	1627	444	175	3369	738	893	1572
		(33%)	(49%)	(94%)	(72%)	(20%)	(82%)	(41%)	(35%)		(38%)	
70+	Sm.	726	225	156	27	42	178	2	190	–	131	–
	Total	6596	835	187	62	586	313	31	2787	169	2314	147
		(11%)	(27%)	(83%)	(44%)	(7%)	(57%)	(6%)	(7%)		(6%)	
Any age	Sm.	4078	1610	932	314	364	541	74	1384	–	469	–
	Total	19230	3829	1021	468	2340	768	417	6243	943	3838	3192
		(21%)	(42%)	(91%)	(67%)	(16%)	(70%)	(18%)	(22%)		(12%)	
Females												
0–34	Sm.	–	–	–	–	–	–	–	–	–	–	–
	Total	1154	158	3	2	153	7	159	43	23	464	300
35–69	Sm.	0	0	0	0	0	0	0	0	–	0	–
	Total	7025	1843	96	18	1729	223	69	2725	1065	668	432
		(0%)	(0%)	(0%)	(0%)	(0%)	(0%)	(0%)	(0%)		(0%)	
70+	Sm.	0	0	0	0	0	0	0	0	–	0	–
	Total	10444	811	114	21	676	269	35	4670	252	4253	154
		(0%)	(0%)	(0%)	(0%)	(0%)	(0%)	(0%)	(0%)		(0%)	
Any age	Sm.	0	0	0	0	0	0	0	0	–	0	–
	Total	18623	2812	213	41	2558	499	263	7438	1340	5385	886
		(0%)	(0%)	(0%)	(0%)	(0%)	(0%)	(0%)	(0%)		(0%)	
Males+Females												
0–34	Sm.	–	–	–	–	–	–	–	–	–	–	–
	Total	3750	305	15	10	280	18	370	130	59	1095	1773
35–69	Sm.	3352	1385	776	287	322	363	72	1194	–	338	–
	Total	17063	4690	918	416	3356	667	244	6094	1803	1561	2004
		(20%)	(30%)	(85%)	(69%)	(10%)	(54%)	(30%)	(20%)		(22%)	
70+	Sm.	726	225	156	27	42	178	2	190	–	131	–
	Total	17040	1646	301	83	1262	582	66	7457	421	6567	301
		(4%)	(14%)	(52%)	(33%)	(3%)	(31%)	(3%)	(3%)		(2%)	
Any age	Sm.	4078	1610	932	314	364	541	74	1384	–	469	–
	Total	37853	6641	1234	509	4898	1267	680	13681	2283	9223	4078
		(11%)	(24%)	(76%)	(62%)	(7%)	(43%)	(11%)	(10%)		(5%)	

(To be conservative, no deaths before age 35, and none from liver cirrhosis or non–medical causes, were attributed to smoking.)

NETHERLANDS: 1990

		No. of deaths			Standardised rates (Defined on p.436)			Annual death rates / 100, 000						
		All ages	0–34	35–69	All ages	0–34	35–69	0–4	5–9	10–14	15–19	20–24	25–29	30–34
ALL CAUSES	M	66628	3006	22495	979.3	77.2	951.7	204.0	22.9	22.3	54.6	67.1	77.6	92.2
	F	62196	1763	12393	559.8	48.7	473.3	160.0	13.6	21.4	24.6	30.7	38.2	52.4
Tuberculosis	M	75	1	19	1.1	0.0	0.9	–	–	–	–	–	–	0.2
	F	61	2	14	0.6	0.0	0.6	–	–	–	–	–	0.2	0.2
Other infective	M	313	45	91	4.6	1.3	3.6	6.3	0.2	0.2	1.1	–	0.5	0.6
and parasitic	F	384	31	60	3.5	0.9	2.3	3.5	0.7	0.9	0.6	0.5	0.2	0.2
ALL CANCER	M	19867	247	8278	293.7	6.0	356.4	2.5	3.5	3.5	6.7	5.7	7.4	12.8
	F	15306	247	6111	161.5	6.3	231.7	3.5	3.0	4.1	3.6	4.2	8.2	17.2
Mouth and	M	264	1	175	4.0	0.0	6.9	–	–	–	–	–	–	0.2
pharynx cancer	F	124	2	62	1.4	0.1	2.3	–	–	0.2	–	–	–	0.2
Oesophagus cancer	M	547	1	297	8.2	0.0	12.5	–	–	–	–	–	0.2	–
	F	286	–	88	2.8	–	3.4	–	–	–	–	–	–	–
Stomach cancer	M	1274	7	495	18.8	0.2	21.2	–	–	–	–	0.3	0.3	0.5
	F	817	7	210	7.6	0.2	8.0	–	–	–	–	0.2	0.2	0.8
Colorectal cancer	M	1772	11	681	26.2	0.3	29.4	–	–	–	0.4	–	0.3	1.1
	F	2135	7	617	20.6	0.2	24.0	–	–	–	0.2	–	0.2	0.8
Liver cancer	M	96	3	58	1.4	0.1	2.5	–	–	–	–	–	0.2	0.3
	F	64	1	27	0.7	0.0	1.0	0.2	–	–	–	–	–	–
Pancreas cancer	M	795	5	363	11.8	0.1	15.5	–	–	–	–	0.2	0.2	0.5
	F	890	2	311	9.0	0.0	12.1	–	–	–	–	–	–	0.3
Larynx cancer	M	179	1	94	2.7	0.0	4.0	–	–	–	–	–	–	0.2
	F	29	–	21	0.4	–	0.8	–	–	–	–	–	–	–
Lung cancer	M	7011	4	3162	104.0	0.1	138.5	–	–	–	–	–	0.3	0.3
	F	1230	8	711	14.7	0.2	27.1	–	–	–	–	–	0.3	1.0
Malignant melanoma	M	171	19	116	2.5	0.4	4.4	–	–	–	0.5	0.2	1.1	1.3
	F	177	8	103	2.1	0.2	3.6	–	–	–	–	–	0.6	0.7
Female breast cancer	F	3293	46	1772	38.2	1.1	65.7	–	–	–	0.2	0.3	1.1	6.0
Cervix cancer	F	288	14	156	3.3	0.3	5.6	–	–	–	–	–	0.6	1.7
Other uterine cancer	F	397	1	121	3.9	0.0	4.8	–	–	–	–	0.2	–	–
Ovarian cancer	F	987	11	501	11.3	0.3	19.2	–	–	–	0.2	0.3	0.5	0.8
Prostate cancer	M	2135	–	392	31.4	–	18.3	–	–	–	–	–	–	–
Bladder cancer	M	827	2	220	12.2	0.1	9.8	–	0.2	–	–	–	–	0.2
	F	302	–	57	2.7	–	2.3	–	–	–	–	–	–	–
Other and ill–defined	M	3391	107	1626	50.2	2.6	68.3	1.7	1.5	1.1	3.3	2.5	3.2	5.1
cancer sites	F	2963	78	930	29.5	2.1	35.7	2.4	1.8	2.3	1.3	1.8	2.4	2.7
Hodgkin's disease	M	73	13	38	1.0	0.3	1.4	–	–	–	0.4	0.5	0.3	1.0
	F	64	12	22	0.7	0.3	0.7	–	–	0.2	0.2	0.5	0.3	0.8
Myeloma and non–	M	777	21	354	11.5	0.5	15.0	0.2	0.9	0.4	0.5	0.6	0.5	0.6
Hodgkin lymphomas	F	805	13	267	8.1	0.3	10.3	–	0.2	0.5	0.4	–	0.9	0.3
Leukaemia	M	555	52	207	8.0	1.3	8.6	0.6	0.9	1.9	1.6	1.5	1.1	1.6
	F	455	37	135	4.6	1.0	5.0	0.9	0.9	0.9	1.1	1.0	1.1	1.0
ALL VASCULAR	M	25887	170	8419	381.9	4.0	364.2	2.1	0.2	1.5	1.5	4.5	5.9	12.2
DISEASE	F	25733	95	3135	211.7	2.3	123.5	2.0	0.5	0.2	1.1	1.3	4.3	7.0
Rheumatic heart	M	12	–	11	0.2	–	0.4	–	–	–	–	–	–	–
disease and fever	F	39	3	24	0.5	0.1	0.9	–	–	–	–	0.2	–	0.3
Hypertensive disease	M	278	–	121	4.1	–	5.2	–	–	–	–	–	–	–
	F	503	1	67	4.2	0.0	2.6	–	–	–	–	–	0.2	–
Ischaemic heart	M	13000	41	5193	192.2	0.9	224.2	–	–	–	–	0.6	1.8	4.0
disease	F	9396	16	1484	81.0	0.4	59.1	0.2	–	–	–	0.2	0.5	1.8
Pulmonary embolism	M	210	2	51	3.1	0.0	2.2	–	–	–	–	–	–	0.3
and other venous	F	330	4	47	2.8	0.1	1.7	–	–	–	–	0.2	0.3	0.2
Cerebrovascular	M	4931	43	1052	72.5	1.0	46.0	0.2	0.2	0.9	0.4	1.4	1.2	2.9
disease	F	7461	38	755	59.9	0.9	29.0	0.2	0.2	–	0.6	0.3	2.2	2.8
Other vascular	M	7456	84	1991	109.8	2.0	86.2	1.9	–	0.6	1.1	2.5	2.9	5.0
disease	F	8004	33	758	63.3	0.9	30.1	1.5	0.2	0.2	0.6	0.5	1.1	1.8
Chronic obstructive	M	4246	10	802	62.1	0.2	37.3	–	0.2	–	0.4	0.5	0.3	0.3
pulmonary disease	F	1814	5	321	15.9	0.1	12.7	–	–	0.2	0.2	0.2	0.3	–
Other respiratory	M	1988	33	227	29.4	0.9	10.1	4.6	0.2	0.4	0.2	–	0.3	0.8
disease	F	2623	15	106	19.4	0.4	4.1	1.7	0.2	–	0.4	0.2	0.5	–
Peptic ulcer	M	202	2	47	3.0	0.0	2.0	–	–	–	–	–	–	0.3
	F	230	–	28	1.9	–	1.1	–	–	–	–	–	–	–
Liver cirrhosis	M	446	13	311	6.6	0.3	12.0	0.2	–	–	–	0.2	0.3	1.4
	F	274	3	180	3.4	0.1	6.5	–	0.2	–	–	–	–	0.3
Renal disease	M	501	2	44	7.4	0.1	2.0	0.2	0.2	–	–	–	–	–
	F	838	3	51	6.3	0.1	2.0	0.2	–	–	–	0.2	0.2	–
Pregnancy and birth	F	15	13	2	0.2	0.3	0.1	–	–	–	–	0.5	0.6	1.0
Congenital and	M	759	693	59	12.3	20.4	2.2	133.4	0.7	1.3	2.9	1.5	1.8	1.3
perinatal causes	F	588	517	52	9.7	15.9	1.8	102.9	1.2	2.0	1.3	1.5	2.1	0.3
Ill–defined causes	M	2838	345	1190	41.5	8.7	47.4	23.2	1.5	2.4	3.8	8.8	12.9	8.3
	F	2600	174	489	23.5	4.8	18.1	17.2	1.2	2.0	1.5	4.2	3.8	3.8
Other medical causes	M	6434	365	1868	94.0	9.3	75.1	17.6	6.4	3.7	7.6	5.1	9.5	15.6
	F	9496	248	1286	79.9	6.8	49.7	19.0	3.2	3.6	4.0	3.9	6.0	8.0
ALL NON–	M	3072	1080	1140	41.6	25.9	38.6	14.0	9.7	9.3	30.4	40.7	38.8	38.2
MEDICAL CAUSES	F	2234	410	558	22.4	10.6	19.2	10.0	3.5	8.2	11.9	14.2	12.0	14.4
Motor vehicle	M	905	474	287	11.8	11.3	10.1	2.3	4.9	4.3	18.2	24.8	15.9	8.8
traffic accidents	F	385	173	127	4.8	4.6	4.5	0.9	2.8	6.1	8.0	6.5	4.7	3.0
Fire	M	37	10	13	0.5	0.3	0.4	1.0	–	–	0.4	0.2	0.2	0.2
	F	34	10	9	0.4	0.3	0.3	1.1	–	–	–	0.5	–	0.3
Suicide	M	909	307	470	12.0	7.0	15.4	–	–	1.1	6.7	9.4	12.6	19.3
	F	541	132	306	6.8	3.1	10.3	–	–	0.5	1.9	5.0	6.0	8.5
Homicide	M	92	53	38	1.2	1.2	1.2	1.0	–	0.4	0.5	1.9	2.4	2.4
	F	43	27	12	0.6	0.7	0.3	1.1	–	0.2	0.9	1.6	0.6	0.3
POPULATION (thousands):	**M=males**				7388.9	3876.5	3030.8	478.4	453.3	461.9	549.8	645.7	664.6	622.8
	F=females				7562.6	3712.9	3038.5	458.8	434.0	440.2	527.7	619.6	633.9	598.7

NETHERLANDS: 1990

Annual death rates / 100, 000 — 9th ICD categories

35–39	40–44	45–49	50–54	55–59	60–64	65–69	70–74	75–79	80+/NK			
122.5	190.9	325.0	536.6	1003.3	1621.7	2862.1	4760.0	7528.1	15399.7	M	ALL CAUSES	001–999
78.9	127.8	208.2	312.7	514.0	803.7	1267.7	2117.6	3845.1	11062.1	F		
–	–	0.2	–	0.3	1.9	3.9	6.4	8.9	21.8	M	Tuberculosis	010–018, 137
–	–	–	0.3	0.3	0.6	2.9	3.3	5.9	7.3	F		
1.0	1.1	2.8	2.5	1.7	6.5	9.9	24.2	28.1	65.4	M	Other infective	Rest of 001–139
0.2	0.7	1.4	1.5	1.4	3.1	7.9	13.1	22.0	68.5	F	and parasitic	
21.5	48.7	108.8	200.7	398.2	636.0	1080.7	1691.9	2293.8	3431.3	M	ALL CANCER	140–208
38.8	66.8	114.8	182.2	283.1	400.6	535.4	691.8	936.5	1612.9	F		
1.4	2.3	3.4	6.2	7.2	16.8	11.3	14.8	14.4	27.8	M	Mouth and	140–149
–	1.2	1.6	2.1	2.5	4.0	5.0	2.5	4.7	14.0	F	pharynx cancer	
0.5	1.6	5.4	7.2	19.4	20.8	32.8	43.0	56.2	60.1	M	Oesophagus cancer	150
0.2	0.5	2.0	2.1	3.8	6.5	8.7	13.1	23.3	35.7	F		
1.7	3.3	7.5	11.7	21.4	38.6	64.2	99.3	145.9	269.0	M	Stomach cancer	151
1.4	2.9	2.9	3.9	9.8	12.8	22.1	31.2	56.7	126.9	F		
1.4	4.6	10.3	17.5	27.7	48.8	95.2	143.7	214.4	357.6	M	Colorectal cancer	153, 154
2.8	4.3	6.6	17.2	28.4	42.8	65.5	104.5	137.1	300.3	F		
0.5	0.2	0.4	1.7	1.7	6.2	6.7	8.4	8.9	3.8	M	Liver cancer	155.0
0.2	0.7	0.5	–	1.1	1.4	3.2	2.5	4.2	6.3	F		
0.7	2.6	5.6	10.2	17.2	22.7	49.7	73.1	82.9	118.7	M	Pancreas cancer	157
1.1	2.2	5.7	5.7	14.7	22.7	32.3	42.5	62.6	104.2	F		
–	0.3	1.7	3.0	5.0	9.0	8.8	14.3	13.0	27.0	M	Larynx cancer	161
–	0.2	0.2	1.3	0.5	1.4	2.0	0.4	0.8	1.7	F		
2.7	11.9	35.2	70.5	157.0	257.3	435.1	676.5	871.9	903.1	M	Lung cancer	162
2.5	7.0	14.3	21.9	35.7	51.3	57.1	62.8	56.3	68.5	F		
1.4	2.4	2.1	4.0	7.5	6.5	6.7	6.4	7.5	9.0	M	Malignant melanoma	172
1.6	2.7	4.5	3.3	3.5	3.4	5.8	6.9	7.2	10.0	F		
14.0	26.5	39.4	66.4	84.5	107.2	122.1	134.7	154.0	247.2	F	Female breast cancer	174
3.0	2.6	3.6	5.9	4.9	7.4	11.9	11.6	14.0	17.7	F	Cervix cancer	180
–	–	1.6	3.1	6.3	7.9	14.9	24.7	27.9	47.1	F	Other uterine cancer	179, 182
1.6	4.8	7.7	14.9	27.0	31.5	47.2	51.2	60.9	63.5	F	Ovarian cancer	183
0.2	–	0.4	3.5	13.9	34.2	75.8	174.8	300.0	714.5	M	Prostate cancer	185
–	0.7	2.6	3.5	11.1	16.2	34.6	65.7	121.9	220.9	M	Bladder cancer	188
0.2	0.2	0.5	0.8	2.5	5.4	6.4	12.0	23.3	52.4	F		
7.0	12.9	24.5	47.5	81.3	118.2	186.5	255.3	316.4	510.1	M	Other and ill-defined	Rest of 140–208
6.2	6.5	17.9	23.4	39.8	63.8	92.0	129.9	202.3	373.7	F	cancer sites	
1.0	0.5	1.3	1.5	1.7	2.5	1.1	4.4	4.1	5.3	M	Hodgkin's disease	201
1.1	0.7	0.2	0.3	1.4	0.9	0.6	2.2	4.2	4.7	F		
1.5	2.6	5.4	8.0	16.4	27.4	44.1	73.1	76.7	106.7	M	Myeloma and non-	200, 202–203
1.4	2.1	3.2	6.4	10.9	20.7	27.7	41.4	64.3	86.5	F	Hodgkin lymphomas	
1.5	2.8	3.0	4.5	9.7	10.6	28.2	39.0	59.6	97.7	M	Leukaemia	204–208
1.6	1.7	2.5	3.6	5.7	9.4	10.8	17.8	32.6	52.4	F		
25.2	51.8	104.9	187.0	379.9	638.8	1161.8	1966.9	3181.5	6513.9	M	ALL VASCULAR	390–459
9.0	18.4	34.2	52.8	112.1	217.9	420.0	887.1	1786.7	5289.6	F	DISEASE	
–	0.2	–	0.7	0.6	0.6	1.1	–	0.7	–	M	Rheumatic heart	390–398
–	0.2	0.5	0.5	3.0	0.9	1.5	1.5	1.3	1.7	F	disease and fever	
0.5	0.8	0.4	3.7	6.7	7.2	17.3	24.7	32.2	45.1	M	Hypertensive disease	401–405
0.2	0.5	0.5	1.3	3.8	2.8	9.3	21.8	36.0	96.9	F		
11.1	30.9	69.1	120.7	244.2	405.1	688.3	1074.1	1603.4	2441.8	M	Ischaemic heart	410–414
2.0	6.0	13.1	24.7	46.6	112.6	208.6	418.1	762.6	1650.6	F	disease	
–	0.7	0.6	1.5	2.2	2.5	7.8	14.3	27.4	66.1	M	Pulmonary embolism	415.1, 451–453
0.7	1.0	1.1	0.8	0.8	2.0	5.5	14.9	19.0	64.5	F	and other venous	
4.1	5.9	9.9	21.5	46.9	75.0	158.7	344.7	661.6	1631.9	M	Cerebrovascular	430–438
5.0	6.7	12.7	14.2	29.7	45.1	90.0	216.0	491.7	1640.3	F	disease	
9.5	13.4	24.9	38.7	79.4	148.4	288.8	509.1	856.2	2329.1	M	Other vascular	Rest of 390–459
1.2	4.0	6.3	11.3	28.1	54.5	105.2	214.9	476.1	1835.7	F	disease	
0.9	1.8	2.1	7.2	23.3	60.7	165.0	337.8	671.2	1329.8	M	Chronic obstructive	490–496
1.4	0.2	3.2	6.4	12.5	27.8	37.6	78.0	129.1	323.3	F	pulmonary disease	
0.9	1.5	2.1	4.0	8.0	12.1	42.0	93.8	207.5	927.9	M	Other respiratory	Rest of 460–519
0.4	1.2	1.6	2.8	3.0	5.1	14.6	38.8	125.7	700.7	F	disease	
0.3	0.3	0.4	0.7	1.9	4.4	6.0	17.3	28.8	57.1	M	Peptic ulcer	531–533
–	0.3	0.7	0.3	1.4	2.0	2.9	6.2	15.7	49.4	F		
3.6	5.6	7.5	10.0	15.3	18.7	23.3	21.2	30.1	26.3	M	Liver cirrhosis	571
1.8	3.8	5.9	7.5	6.8	8.8	10.8	9.1	13.1	11.7	F		
0.2	0.3	0.2	0.5	2.2	2.5	7.8	22.7	59.6	241.9	M	Renal disease	580–590
0.4	–	1.1	0.5	1.6	2.6	7.9	18.9	38.1	214.4	F		
0.4	–	–	–	–	–	–	–	–	–	F	Pregnancy and birth	630–676
1.0	1.0	1.9	2.0	3.3	2.8	3.2	2.0	0.7	1.5	M	Congenital and	740–779
1.1	1.4	1.1	1.3	2.2	3.4	2.3	1.8	2.5	2.7	F	perinatal causes	
11.8	14.7	28.3	39.0	50.8	75.9	111.4	151.6	188.4	541.7	M	Ill-defined causes	780–799
4.4	7.9	12.2	12.9	16.9	26.1	46.6	62.8	114.7	498.7	F		
23.9	26.5	30.9	46.7	80.5	118.2	199.2	356.5	694.5	1852.0	M	Other medical causes	Rest of 001–799
8.2	11.2	17.9	22.9	54.0	81.4	152.1	268.6	584.8	1950.6	F		
32.4	37.7	34.8	36.2	38.0	43.2	48.0	67.7	134.9	389.2	M	ALL NON-	E800–E999
12.9	16.0	14.0	21.4	18.8	24.4	26.8	38.1	70.2	332.3	F	MEDICAL CAUSES	
6.8	8.7	9.4	9.0	8.3	10.9	17.3	15.3	33.6	48.1	M	Motor vehicle	E810–E819
1.8	3.3	3.4	4.4	2.7	6.2	9.9	10.9	10.6	10.0	F	traffic accidents	
0.3	1.1	–	0.5	–	–	0.7	1.0	2.7	6.0	M	Fire	E890–E899
–	0.3	0.2	0.3	0.5	0.3	0.6	0.4	2.5	2.7	F		
13.6	18.6	13.3	16.5	14.7	17.7	13.4	18.3	26.7	42.1	M	Suicide	E950–E959
8.5	8.9	8.2	12.4	10.4	13.9	10.2	8.3	15.2	14.7	F		
2.0	1.1	0.9	1.5	1.4	1.2	–	0.5	–	–	M	Homicide	E960–E969
1.1	0.3	0.2	0.5	0.3	–	–	0.7	0.8	–	F		
586.9	612.3	466.1	400.1	360.4	321.4	283.6	202.5	146.0	133.1	M	**POPULATION (thousands)**	
563.8	582.1	441.5	388.6	366.7	352.5	343.3	275.5	236.3	299.4	F		

NETHERLANDS: Males

	All ages	0–34	35–69	35–39	40–44	45–49	50–54	55–59	60–64	65–69	70–74	75–79	80+/NK
POPULATION (1000s)													
1955	5355.7	3229.9	1861.8	333.1	328.1	309.8	280.9	241.7	203.7	164.5	123.5	82.2	58.3
1965	6134.4	3666.5	2131.4	378.5	374.9	325.5	315.7	289.5	249.1	198.2	150.4	102.2	83.9
1975	6804.3	4050.0	2359.5	424.6	394.1	370.7	359.8	301.5	277.2	231.6	175.6	114.9	104.3
1985	7166.9	3922.2	2787.6	616.5	473.0	411.4	377.0	345.3	318.9	245.5	198.3	135.0	123.8
1990	**7388.9**	**3876.5**	**3030.8**	**586.9**	**612.3**	**466.1**	**400.1**	**360.4**	**321.4**	**283.6**	**202.5**	**146.0**	**133.1**
1995 projected	*7636.8*	*3806.4*	*3302.2*	*632.2*	*591.6*	*609.3*	*457.5*	*385.6*	*338.1*	*287.9*	*235.1*	*149.2*	*143.9*
NUMBER OF DEATHS													
All causes													
1955	43260	5443	15827	491	790	1368	2000	2758	3713	4707	5808	6601	9581
1965	54484	4922	20978	629	978	1411	2480	3789	5234	6457	7504	7933	13147
1975	63526	3903	23867	571	910	1640	2741	3911	5881	8213	9478	9487	16791
1985	65847	3066	22897	744	985	1366	2375	3822	5924	7681	9852	10846	19186
1990	**66628**	**3006**	**22495**	**719**	**1169**	**1515**	**2147**	**3616**	**5212**	**8117**	**9639**	**10991**	**20497**
1995 projected	*68000*	*2869*	*21831*	*754*	*1091*	*1781*	*2213*	*3403*	*4938*	*7651*	*10511*	*10870*	*21919*
Lung cancer													
1955	1767	16	1331	15	51	121	233	299	325	287	209	142	69
1965	3709	15	2536	21	53	119	296	560	706	781	575	366	217
1975	6010	12	3425	17	51	165	332	622	960	1278	1159	802	612
1985	7366	9	3583	29	77	129	356	644	995	1353	1428	1287	1059
1990	**7011**	**4**	**3162**	**16**	**73**	**164**	**282**	**566**	**827**	**1234**	**1370**	**1273**	**1202**
1995 projected	*6667*	*2*	*2739*	*11*	*65*	*169*	*259*	*480*	*689*	*1066*	*1401*	*1249*	*1276*
ANNUAL DEATH RATE / 100,000 (*The rates for the age groups 0–34 and 35–69 are the means of seven five-yearly rates, but the all-ages rates are standardised to the conventional "European" age distribution)													
All causes													
1955	1093.5*	153.8*	1052.4*	147.4	240.8	441.6	712.0	1141.1	1822.8	2861.4	4702.8	8030.4	16434.0
1965	1114.3*	128.0*	1187.7*	166.2	260.9	433.5	785.6	1308.8	2101.2	3257.8	4989.4	7762.2	15669.8
1975	1136.5*	100.3*	1219.2*	134.5	230.9	442.4	761.8	1297.2	2121.6	3546.2	5397.5	8256.7	16098.8
1985	1036.2*	80.7*	1054.9*	120.7	208.2	332.0	630.0	1106.9	1857.6	3128.7	4968.2	8034.1	15497.6
1990	**979.3***	**77.2***	**951.7***	**122.5**	**190.9**	**325.0**	**536.6**	**1003.3**	**1621.7**	**2862.1**	**4760.0**	**7528.1**	**15399.7**
1995 projected	*930.3**	*73.6**	*868.6**	*119.3*	*184.4*	*292.3*	*483.7*	*882.5*	*1460.5*	*2657.5*	*4470.9*	*7285.5*	*15232.1*
All cancer													
1955	222.2*	11.9*	295.7*	30.9	61.3	124.9	216.1	356.6	539.0	741.0	1118.2	1560.8	2161.2
1965	260.2*	11.1*	363.6*	34.9	58.4	115.2	235.0	432.8	660.4	1008.6	1326.5	1781.8	2442.2
1975	298.0*	9.1*	406.6*	29.0	55.3	126.8	237.4	443.1	731.2	1223.7	1621.9	2156.7	2911.8
1985	303.1*	7.6*	387.0*	27.1	59.2	95.5	231.6	409.5	708.1	1178.4	1669.2	2380.7	3277.9
1990	**293.7***	**6.0***	**356.4***	**21.5**	**48.7**	**108.8**	**200.7**	**398.2**	**636.0**	**1080.7**	**1691.9**	**2293.8**	**3431.3**
1995 projected	*282.8**	*4.8**	*331.5**	*17.2*	*46.1*	*98.5*	*188.0*	*358.9*	*583.0*	*1028.5*	*1626.5*	*2284.2*	*3480.9*
Lung cancer													
1955	43.5*	0.6*	85.7*	4.5	15.5	39.1	82.9	123.7	159.5	174.5	169.2	172.7	118.4
1965	76.1*	0.5*	145.8*	5.5	14.1	36.6	93.8	193.4	283.4	394.0	382.3	358.1	258.6
1975	108.2*	0.3*	179.7*	4.0	12.9	44.5	92.3	206.3	346.3	551.8	660.0	698.0	586.8
1985	117.0*	0.2*	170.9*	4.7	16.3	31.4	94.4	186.5	312.0	551.1	720.1	953.3	855.4
1990	**104.0***	**0.1***	**138.5***	**2.7**	**11.9**	**35.2**	**70.5**	**157.0**	**257.3**	**435.1**	**676.5**	**871.9**	**903.1**
1995 projected	*91.6**	*0.0**	*113.7**	*1.7*	*11.0*	*27.7*	*56.6*	*124.5*	*203.8*	*370.3*	*595.9*	*837.1*	*886.7*
Upper aerodigestive cancer (mouth, oesophagus, pharynx and larynx)													
1955	10.5*	0.0*	10.8*	0.6	0.3	5.2	6.8	16.1	19.6	26.7	51.8	101.0	149.2
1965	10.4*	0.1*	12.7*	0.8	2.1	3.4	9.5	14.2	22.9	35.8	48.5	89.0	128.7
1975	10.9*	0.2*	14.2*	0.5	2.0	5.4	12.5	13.6	23.8	41.5	55.2	79.2	123.7
1985	12.1*	0.2*	18.7*	1.3	2.7	5.8	13.3	20.6	38.3	48.9	59.5	73.3	102.6
1990	**14.8***	**0.1***	**23.5***	**1.9**	**4.2**	**10.5**	**16.5**	**31.6**	**46.7**	**52.9**	**72.1**	**83.6**	**115.0**
1995 projected	*17.9**	*0.1**	*28.8**	*2.4*	*5.7*	*14.1*	*22.3*	*40.2*	*55.6*	*61.1*	*81.7*	*101.9*	*130.0*
Other cancer													
1955	168.2*	11.3*	199.3*	25.8	45.4	80.7	126.4	216.8	359.8	539.8	897.2	1287.1	1893.7
1965	173.7*	10.4*	205.1*	28.5	42.1	75.3	131.8	225.2	354.1	578.7	895.6	1334.6	2054.8
1975	179.0*	8.6*	212.7*	24.5	40.3	76.9	132.6	223.2	361.1	630.4	906.6	1379.5	2201.3
1985	174.0*	7.2*	197.4*	21.1	40.2	58.3	123.9	202.4	357.8	578.4	889.6	1354.1	2319.9
1990	**174.9***	**5.9***	**194.3***	**16.9**	**32.5**	**63.1**	**113.7**	**209.5**	**332.0**	**592.7**	**943.2**	**1338.4**	**2413.2**
1995 projected	*173.3**	*4.7**	*189.0**	*13.1*	*29.4*	*56.6*	*109.1*	*194.2*	*323.6*	*597.1*	*949.0*	*1345.2*	*2464.2*
Chronic obstructive pulmonary disease (COPD)													
1955	27.8*	0.8*	32.1*	1.5	4.3	11.9	25.3	38.9	65.8	77.2	119.0	210.5	394.5
1965	44.3*	0.8*	58.6*	1.8	4.5	8.6	30.4	57.3	132.1	175.6	230.7	311.2	523.2
1975	58.9*	0.9*	57.5*	1.6	4.1	6.5	19.7	48.4	105.0	217.2	362.2	544.8	880.2
1985	56.5*	0.4*	39.5*	0.8	1.5	2.4	9.0	28.7	68.0	165.8	325.3	574.8	1113.9
1990	**62.1***	**0.2***	**37.3***	**0.9**	**1.8**	**2.1**	**7.2**	**23.3**	**60.7**	**165.0**	**337.8**	**671.2**	**1329.8**
1995 projected	*69.2**	*0.2**	*35.6**	*0.8*	*1.7*	*1.8*	*5.7*	*19.5*	*56.2*	*163.6*	*367.5*	*764.7*	*1576.1*
Other respiratory disease													
1955	44.9*	7.9*	24.4*	4.2	6.1	10.0	16.4	19.0	45.7	69.3	157.1	322.4	1034.3
1965	24.6*	3.2*	10.7*	0.8	2.9	3.1	9.2	8.3	16.5	34.3	80.5	174.2	657.9
1975	28.2*	1.8*	10.3*	1.4	1.0	2.7	3.9	7.3	16.6	39.3	101.9	214.1	821.7
1985	30.8*	1.7*	11.5*	0.6	1.5	2.2	6.6	10.1	17.2	42.0	103.4	217.8	925.7
1990	**29.4***	**0.9***	**10.1***	**0.9**	**1.5**	**2.1**	**4.0**	**8.0**	**12.1**	**42.0**	**93.8**	**207.5**	**927.9**
1995 projected	*28.3**	*0.7**	*8.6**	*0.9*	*1.5*	*1.5*	*2.8*	*5.4*	*10.6*	*37.5*	*87.6*	*201.1*	*921.5*
Vascular disease													
1955	482.0*	5.6*	410.1*	17.1	47.2	113.6	228.9	396.8	728.0	1339.2	2343.3	4310.2	9025.7
1965	506.6*	4.8*	499.4*	42.3	84.8	162.8	303.5	533.3	880.0	1489.4	2444.8	4031.3	8657.9
1975	502.6*	4.3*	519.1*	31.8	79.9	176.4	333.0	558.5	911.6	1542.3	2498.9	3966.9	8092.0
1985	449.9*	4.3*	447.2*	30.8	63.8	129.3	252.3	481.3	812.2	1360.9	2292.0	3763.0	7323.9
1990	**381.9***	**4.0***	**364.2***	**25.2**	**51.8**	**104.9**	**187.0**	**379.9**	**638.8**	**1161.8**	**1966.9**	**3181.5**	**6513.9**
1995 projected	*321.1**	*3.4**	*291.7**	*19.6*	*40.6*	*77.1*	*138.8*	*287.1*	*513.5*	*965.3*	*1653.3*	*2750.0*	*5697.0*
Liver cirrhosis													
1955	5.2*	0.2*	8.5*	1.2	2.7	6.5	5.7	11.6	14.2	17.6	16.2	35.3	32.6
1965	5.2*	0.2*	6.8*	1.1	4.0	3.7	6.3	6.9	11.6	14.1	27.3	36.2	47.7
1975	7.4*	0.4*	13.5*	1.6	5.8	9.4	12.5	23.5	20.6	21.2	27.3	24.4	29.7
1985	7.6*	0.4*	13.7*	2.4	6.6	9.0	14.6	17.7	22.3	23.2	23.2	27.4	36.3
1990	**6.6***	**0.3***	**12.0***	**3.6**	**5.6**	**7.5**	**10.0**	**15.3**	**18.7**	**23.3**	**21.2**	**30.1**	**26.3**
1995 projected	*5.6**	*0.3**	*10.1**	*3.3*	*4.9*	*5.4*	*7.7*	*11.9*	*16.6*	*21.2*	*21.3*	*25.5*	*23.6*
Other medical causes													
1955	246.6*	89.9*	212.6*	57.3	73.1	117.2	153.1	242.9	341.7	502.7	800.8	1349.1	3346.5
1965	200.3*	65.1*	176.2*	43.3	56.8	88.2	132.1	191.4	295.1	426.3	704.1	1164.4	2743.7
1975	177.9*	45.4*	151.1*	27.1	44.4	66.4	98.4	158.2	264.1	399.0	661.2	1106.2	2817.8
1985	140.3*	37.2*	108.3*	23.4	37.8	46.2	69.0	111.5	173.4	296.9	473.0	910.4	2412.8
1990	**164.0***	**39.9***	**133.2***	**38.2**	**43.9**	**64.8**	**91.5**	**140.7**	**212.2**	**341.3**	**580.7**	**1008.9**	**2781.4**
1995 projected	*188.4**	*42.0**	*160.6**	*48.2*	*58.0*	*80.7*	*114.3*	*171.2*	*247.9*	*404.0*	*659.3*	*1148.8*	*3173.0*
All non-medical causes													
1955	64.8*	37.5*	69.0*	35.1	46.0	57.5	66.6	75.3	88.4	114.3	148.2	242.1	439.1
1965	73.1*	42.7*	72.3*	42.0	49.3	51.9	69.1	78.8	105.6	109.5	175.5	263.2	597.1
1975	63.5*	38.4*	61.1*	41.9	40.3	54.2	57.0	58.0	72.5	103.6	124.1	243.7	545.5
1985	48.1*	29.0*	47.7*	35.5	37.8	47.4	46.9	48.1	56.4	61.5	82.2	160.0	407.1
1990	**41.6***	**25.9***	**38.6***	**32.4**	**37.7**	**34.8**	**36.2**	**38.0**	**43.2**	**48.0**	**67.7**	**134.9**	**389.2**
1995 projected	*34.9**	*22.2**	*30.5**	*29.1*	*31.6*	*27.2*	*26.4*	*28.5*	*32.8*	*37.5*	*55.3*	*111.3*	*360.0*

NETHERLANDS: Females

	All ages	0–34	35–69	35–39	40–44	45–49	50–54	55–59	60–64	65–69	70–74	75–79	80+/NK
POPULATION (1000s)													
1955	5395.2	3132.4	1967.7	342.2	341.8	327.0	298.4	260.7	220.0	177.6	134.7	91.0	69.4
1965	6160.2	3485.4	2266.3	378.8	387.9	337.7	333.9	314.9	280.2	232.9	180.2	122.7	105.6
1975	6862.3	3841.5	2457.6	393.2	380.3	376.4	380.9	326.0	315.5	285.3	235.5	168.6	159.1
1985	7324.7	3760.8	2816.2	582.0	443.3	392.7	374.3	364.0	360.8	299.1	273.4	221.6	252.7
1990	**7562.6**	**3712.9**	**3038.5**	**563.8**	**582.1**	**441.5**	**388.6**	**366.7**	**352.5**	**343.3**	**275.5**	**236.3**	**299.4**
1995 projected	*7772.4*	*3634.3*	*3260.3*	*604.0*	*566.2*	*580.3*	*437.2*	*381.1*	*355.7*	*335.8*	*316.5*	*238.4*	*322.9*
NUMBER OF DEATHS													
All causes													
1955	38104	3729	11985	463	655	991	1370	1934	2677	3895	5439	6358	10593
1965	43542	3059	12543	396	634	930	1342	1946	2945	4350	6002	7519	14419
1975	50211	2257	12605	373	608	959	1474	1848	2933	4410	6631	8589	20129
1985	56857	1768	12016	477	539	828	1365	1942	2925	3940	6276	9035	27762
1990	**62196**	**1763**	**12393**	**445**	**744**	**919**	**1215**	**1885**	**2833**	**4352**	**5834**	**9086**	**33120**
1995 projected	*64925*	*1709*	*12272*	*471*	*723*	*1125*	*1276*	*1868*	*2777*	*4032*	*6300*	*8607*	*36037*
Lung cancer													
1955	180	3	103	5	10	4	9	22	18	35	32	28	14
1965	273	4	161	7	4	26	18	28	34	44	34	38	36
1975	434	4	218	5	12	16	32	54	43	56	78	61	73
1985	928	6	515	9	33	39	88	108	135	103	128	106	173
1990	**1230**	**8**	**711**	**14**	**41**	**63**	**85**	**131**	**181**	**196**	**173**	**133**	**205**
1995 projected	*1603*	*12*	*933*	*16*	*49*	*86*	*107*	*160*	*251*	*264*	*265*	*156*	*237*
ANNUAL DEATH RATE / 100,000 (*The rates for the age groups 0–34 and 35–69 are the means of seven five-yearly rates, but the all-ages rates are standardised to the conventional "European" age distribution)													
All causes													
1955	893.0*	108.3*	748.7*	135.3	191.6	303.1	459.1	741.8	1216.8	2193.1	4037.9	6986.8	15263.7
1965	769.2*	81.6*	640.3*	104.5	163.4	275.4	401.9	618.0	1051.0	1867.8	3330.7	6128.0	13654.4
1975	676.9*	61.9*	562.7*	94.9	159.9	254.8	387.0	566.9	929.6	1545.7	2815.7	5094.3	12651.8
1985	576.4*	50.5*	491.5*	82.0	121.6	210.8	364.7	533.5	810.7	1317.3	2295.5	4077.2	10986.1
1990	**559.8***	**48.7***	**473.3***	**78.9**	**127.8**	**208.2**	**312.7**	**514.0**	**803.7**	**1267.7**	**2117.6**	**3845.1**	**11062.1**
1995 projected	*544.5**	*47.0**	*451.9**	*78.0*	*127.7*	*193.9*	*291.9*	*490.2*	*780.7*	*1200.7*	*1990.5*	*3610.3*	*11160.4*
All cancer													
1955	181.5*	10.1*	252.5*	53.2	84.8	140.1	196.4	290.8	410.9	591.2	856.7	1153.8	1638.3
1965	177.5*	10.7*	245.0*	43.8	83.8	146.0	208.1	275.6	376.2	581.4	813.5	1109.2	1661.9
1975	168.7*	7.6*	232.3*	41.5	71.3	127.0	199.5	280.4	397.8	508.9	751.2	1056.9	1670.6
1985	161.7*	6.4*	227.3*	38.0	65.9	114.6	206.3	267.0	386.9	512.5	711.0	949.0	1631.2
1990	**161.5***	**6.3***	**231.7***	**38.8**	**66.8**	**114.8**	**182.2**	**283.1**	**400.6**	**535.4**	**691.8**	**936.5**	**1612.9**
1995 projected	*159.4**	*6.0**	*231.3**	*38.9*	*66.9*	*106.5*	*176.8*	*280.8*	*414.1*	*535.1*	*682.5*	*891.8*	*1594.0*
Lung cancer													
1955	4.1*	0.1*	6.4*	1.5	2.9	1.2	3.0	8.4	8.2	19.7	23.8	30.8	20.2
1965	4.9*	0.1*	8.0*	1.8	1.0	7.7	5.4	8.9	12.1	18.9	18.9	31.0	34.1
1975	6.3*	0.1*	9.6*	1.3	3.2	4.3	8.4	16.6	13.6	19.6	33.1	36.2	45.9
1985	11.8*	0.2*	20.6*	1.5	7.4	9.9	23.5	29.7	37.4	34.4	46.8	47.8	68.5
1990	**14.7***	**0.2***	**27.1***	**2.5**	**7.0**	**14.3**	**21.9**	**35.7**	**51.3**	**57.1**	**62.8**	**56.3**	**68.5**
1995 projected	*18.2**	*0.3**	*34.5**	*2.6*	*8.7*	*14.8*	*24.5*	*42.0*	*70.6*	*78.6*	*83.7*	*65.4*	*73.4*
Upper aerodigestive cancer (mouth, oesophagus, pharynx and larynx)													
1955	3.9*	0.0*	4.1*	–	0.9	1.5	3.0	3.1	5.9	14.6	17.1	33.0	62.0
1965	3.3*	0.1*	3.8*	–	1.3	2.7	2.4	4.1	8.9	7.3	22.8	21.2	36.9
1975	3.2*	0.1*	3.4*	–	1.3	0.8	1.6	3.7	6.0	10.5	12.7	20.2	55.9
1985	3.8*	0.1*	4.7*	0.9	1.4	2.5	4.8	4.9	8.3	10.0	15.4	27.5	47.1
1990	**4.5***	**0.1***	**6.5***	**0.2**	**1.9**	**3.9**	**5.4**	**6.8**	**11.9**	**15.7**	**16.0**	**28.8**	**51.4**
1995 projected	*5.4**	*0.0**	*8.5**	*0.2*	*2.3*	*4.8*	*6.9*	*8.9*	*16.3*	*20.0*	*18.0*	*28.9*	*55.4*
Other cancer													
1955	173.5*	10.0*	241.9*	51.7	81.0	137.3	190.3	279.2	396.8	556.9	815.9	1090.1	1556.2
1965	169.2*	10.5*	233.2*	42.0	81.5	135.6	200.4	262.6	355.1	555.2	771.9	1057.0	1590.9
1975	159.2*	7.4*	219.4*	40.2	66.8	121.9	189.6	260.1	378.1	478.8	705.3	1000.6	1568.8
1985	146.1*	6.2*	202.1*	35.6	57.1	102.1	177.9	232.4	341.2	468.1	648.9	873.6	1515.6
1990	**142.3***	**6.0***	**198.0***	**36.2**	**57.9**	**96.7**	**154.9**	**240.5**	**337.3**	**462.6**	**613.1**	**851.5**	**1493.0**
1995 projected	*135.8**	*5.7**	*188.3**	*36.1*	*56.0*	*86.9*	*145.5*	*229.9*	*327.2*	*436.6*	*580.7*	*797.4*	*1465.2*
Chronic obstructive pulmonary disease (COPD)													
1955	13.6*	0.6*	9.8*	0.6	1.8	4.6	4.0	8.1	19.5	29.8	64.6	125.3	273.8
1965	12.0*	0.5*	10.6*	1.8	3.6	4.7	5.4	10.2	13.9	34.3	54.4	106.8	211.2
1975	12.6*	0.7*	10.4*	0.8	3.7	3.7	6.3	11.7	16.8	30.1	56.5	113.3	226.3
1985	12.8*	0.4*	11.8*	0.7	0.7	1.8	9.4	14.3	21.1	34.8	55.6	100.6	235.1
1990	**15.9***	**0.1***	**12.7***	**1.4**	**0.2**	**3.2**	**6.4**	**12.5**	**27.8**	**37.6**	**78.0**	**129.1**	**323.3**
1995 projected	*20.0**	*0.1**	*14.2**	*1.0*	*0.2*	*2.6*	*5.5*	*12.9*	*30.1*	*47.1*	*97.9*	*172.4*	*435.7*
Other respiratory disease													
1955	38.5*	7.5*	17.2*	3.5	4.1	4.6	7.7	16.1	20.9	63.6	150.0	318.7	880.4
1965	18.6*	2.4*	6.6*	1.1	2.1	3.6	4.8	6.4	7.5	20.6	51.1	120.6	552.1
1975	19.0*	1.3*	5.7*	1.8	1.3	0.8	1.8	3.4	7.6	23.5	46.7	149.5	600.3
1985	19.8*	1.3*	4.7*	0.5	0.5	1.3	1.1	3.3	8.9	17.7	39.5	127.7	688.2
1990	**19.4***	**0.4***	**4.1***	**0.4**	**1.2**	**1.6**	**2.8**	**3.0**	**5.1**	**14.6**	**38.8**	**125.7**	**700.7**
1995 projected	*19.1**	*0.3**	*3.8**	*0.3*	*1.6*	*2.2*	*3.7*	*2.4*	*3.7*	*12.5*	*36.7*	*114.5*	*709.8*
Vascular disease													
1955	426.0*	4.4*	277.7*	15.8	29.0	56.0	113.3	227.8	467.3	1034.9	2178.2	4085.7	9167.1
1965	364.6*	3.0*	224.3*	18.5	24.5	46.5	83.9	175.0	399.0	822.7	1719.2	3538.7	8262.3
1975	302.0*	3.2*	188.3*	12.7	33.4	56.9	83.2	149.4	305.2	677.5	1426.8	2732.5	6932.7
1985	244.0*	3.2*	151.1*	12.0	20.5	39.7	75.9	149.2	248.6	511.9	1064.0	2104.7	5805.7
1990	**211.7***	**2.3***	**123.5***	**9.0**	**18.4**	**34.2**	**52.8**	**112.1**	**217.9**	**420.0**	**887.1**	**1786.7**	**5289.6**
1995 projected	*180.9**	*1.8**	*98.9**	*7.5*	*15.4*	*25.8*	*38.9*	*88.7*	*174.3*	*341.9*	*729.5*	*1484.1*	*4731.8*
Liver cirrhosis													
1955	3.2*	0.2*	5.2*	0.6	0.9	1.8	3.7	7.7	8.2	13.5	14.1	20.9	18.7
1965	3.2*	0.2*	4.2*	0.5	0.8	0.6	1.8	2.9	9.3	13.3	17.2	22.0	36.9
1975	3.5*	0.4*	4.6*	2.3	1.3	2.1	6.6	6.7	7.3	5.6	17.0	20.8	24.5
1985	3.8*	0.3*	6.5*	1.9	3.6	4.3	7.5	9.1	8.9	10.4	13.2	18.1	16.6
1990	**3.4***	**0.1***	**6.5***	**1.8**	**3.8**	**5.9**	**7.5**	**6.8**	**8.8**	**10.8**	**9.1**	**13.1**	**11.7**
1995 projected	*3.1**	*0.0**	*6.1**	*1.5*	*4.4*	*6.4*	*7.1*	*6.0*	*7.9*	*9.2*	*7.0*	*9.2*	*8.4*
Other medical causes													
1955	200.3*	74.0*	161.9*	52.9	58.8	79.5	113.3	163.4	258.2	407.1	688.9	1133.0	2832.9
1965	154.0*	51.4*	121.5*	26.1	35.8	55.4	73.7	117.8	205.6	335.8	579.4	997.6	2232.0
1975	132.7*	33.7*	91.0*	19.6	27.3	41.2	58.5	86.8	152.5	251.0	445.4	853.5	2543.1
1985	109.4*	28.3*	66.2*	13.9	13.5	29.5	39.8	64.6	110.3	191.6	357.7	685.5	2288.5
1990	**125.5***	**28.9***	**75.6***	**14.5**	**21.5**	**34.4**	**39.6**	**77.7**	**119.1**	**222.5**	**374.6**	**783.7**	**2791.6**
1995 projected	*142.2**	*28.5**	*82.6**	*17.5*	*26.1*	*38.8*	*43.9*	*84.0*	*132.4*	*235.3*	*409.8*	*880.5*	*3356.1*
All non-medical causes													
1955	30.0*	11.5*	24.4*	8.8	12.3	16.5	20.8	28.0	31.8	52.9	85.4	149.5	452.4
1965	39.4*	13.5*	28.3*	12.7	12.9	18.7	24.3	30.2	39.6	59.7	96.0	233.1	697.9
1975	38.4*	15.0*	30.3*	16.3	21.6	23.1	31.0	28.5	42.5	49.1	72.2	167.9	654.3
1985	24.9*	10.6*	23.8*	14.9	16.9	19.6	24.8	26.1	26.1	38.4	54.5	91.6	320.9
1990	**22.4***	**10.6***	**19.2***	**12.9**	**16.0**	**14.0**	**21.4**	**18.8**	**24.4**	**26.8**	**38.1**	**70.2**	**332.3**
1995 projected	*19.8**	*10.3**	*15.0**	*11.3*	*13.1*	*11.5*	*16.0*	*15.5*	*18.3*	*19.7*	*27.2*	*57.9*	*324.6*

NETHERLANDS: 1975

Smoking-attributed deaths (Sm.) and total deaths (Total)

		ALL CAUSES	ALL CANCER	Lung cancer	Upper aero-digestive ca.	Other cancer	COPD	Other respiratory	Vascular disease	Liver cirrhosis	Other medical	Non-medical
Males												
0–34	Sm.	–	–	–	–	–	–	–	–	–	–	–
	Total	3903	360	12	8	340	34	70	167	13	1721	1538
35–69	Sm.	10380	4398	3258	205	935	896	71	3847	–	1168	–
	Total	23867	7862	3425	278	4159	1058	193	10085	287	3023	1359
		(43%)	(56%)	(95%)	(74%)	(22%)	(85%)	(37%)	(38%)		(39%)	
70+	Sm.	9364	3598	2411	216	971	1742	199	2942	–	883	–
	Total	35756	8363	2573	317	5473	2180	1282	17386	107	5371	1067
		(26%)	(43%)	(94%)	(68%)	(18%)	(80%)	(16%)	(17%)		(16%)	
Any age	Sm.	19744	7996	5669	421	1906	2638	270	6789	–	2051	–
	Total	63526	16585	6010	603	9972	3272	1545	27638	407	10115	3964
		(31%)	(48%)	(94%)	(70%)	(19%)	(81%)	(17%)	(25%)		(20%)	
Females												
0–34	Sm.	–	–	–	–	–	–	–	–	–	–	–
	Total	2257	274	4	4	266	27	49	113	14	1216	564
35–69	Sm.	89	34	27	1	6	12	0	25	–	18	–
	Total	12605	5293	218	75	5000	232	124	4091	108	2039	718
		(1%)	(1%)	(12%)	(1%)	(0%)	(5%)	(0%)	(1%)		(1%)	
70+	Sm.	0	0	0	0	0	0	0	0	–	0	–
	Total	35349	6209	212	153	5844	684	1317	18997	114	6534	1494
		(0%)	(0%)	(0%)	(0%)	(0%)	(0%)	(0%)	(0%)		(0%)	
Any age	Sm.	89	34	27	1	6	12	0	25	–	18	–
	Total	50211	11776	434	232	11110	943	1490	23201	236	9789	2776
		(0%)	(0%)	(6%)	(0%)	(0%)	(1%)	(0%)	(0%)		(0%)	
Males+Females												
0–34	Sm.	–	–	–	–	–	–	–	–	–	–	–
	Total	6160	634	16	12	606	61	119	280	27	2937	2102
35–69	Sm.	10469	4432	3285	206	941	908	71	3872	–	1186	–
	Total	36472	13155	3643	353	9159	1290	317	14176	395	5062	2077
		(29%)	(34%)	(90%)	(58%)	(10%)	(70%)	(22%)	(27%)		(23%)	
70+	Sm.	9364	3598	2411	216	971	1742	199	2942	–	883	–
	Total	71105	14572	2785	470	11317	2864	2599	36383	221	11905	2561
		(13%)	(25%)	(87%)	(46%)	(9%)	(61%)	(8%)	(8%)		(7%)	
Any age	Sm.	19833	8030	5696	422	1912	2650	270	6814	–	2069	–
	Total	113737	28361	6444	835	21082	4215	3035	50839	643	19904	6740
		(17%)	(28%)	(88%)	(51%)	(9%)	(63%)	(9%)	(13%)		(10%)	

NETHERLANDS: 1985

Smoking-attributed deaths (Sm.) and total deaths (Total)

		ALL CAUSES	ALL CANCER	Lung cancer	Upper aero-digestive ca.	Other cancer	COPD	Other respiratory	Vascular disease	Liver cirrhosis	Other medical	Non-medical
Males												
0–34	Sm.	–	–	–	–	–	–	–	–	–	–	–
	Total	3066	310	9	7	294	17	57	178	17	1280	1207
35–69	Sm.	9768	4615	3398	298	919	656	86	3502	–	909	–
	Total	22897	8278	3583	408	4287	779	238	9568	327	2440	1267
		(43%)	(56%)	(95%)	(73%)	(21%)	(84%)	(36%)	(37%)		(37%)	
70+	Sm.	12768	5244	3583	253	1408	2346	317	3836	–	1025	–
	Total	39884	10582	3774	344	6464	2800	1645	18692	128	5154	883
		(32%)	(50%)	(95%)	(74%)	(22%)	(84%)	(19%)	(21%)		(20%)	
Any age	Sm.	22536	9859	6981	551	2327	3002	403	7338	–	1934	–
	Total	65847	19170	7366	759	11045	3596	1940	28438	472	8874	3357
		(34%)	(51%)	(95%)	(73%)	(21%)	(83%)	(21%)	(26%)		(22%)	
Females												
0–34	Sm.	–	–	–	–	–	–	–	–	–	–	–
	Total	1768	245	6	3	236	16	43	128	12	913	411
35–69	Sm.	924	388	297	31	60	113	7	279	–	137	–
	Total	12016	5636	515	117	5004	281	111	3572	168	1612	636
		(8%)	(7%)	(58%)	(26%)	(1%)	(40%)	(6%)	(8%)		(8%)	
70+	Sm.	670	177	126	22	29	181	16	218	–	78	–
	Total	43073	8169	407	222	7540	969	2130	22244	118	8280	1163
		(2%)	(2%)	(31%)	(10%)	(0%)	(19%)	(1%)	(1%)		(1%)	
Any age	Sm.	1594	565	423	53	89	294	23	497	–	215	–
	Total	56857	14050	928	342	12780	1266	2284	25944	298	10805	2210
		(3%)	(4%)	(46%)	(15%)	(1%)	(23%)	(1%)	(2%)		(2%)	
Males+Females												
0–34	Sm.	–	–	–	–	–	–	–	–	–	–	–
	Total	4834	555	15	10	530	33	100	306	29	2193	1618
35–69	Sm.	10692	5003	3695	329	979	769	93	3781	–	1046	–
	Total	34913	13914	4098	525	9291	1060	349	13140	495	4052	1903
		(31%)	(36%)	(90%)	(63%)	(11%)	(73%)	(27%)	(29%)		(26%)	
70+	Sm.	13438	5421	3709	275	1437	2527	333	4054	–	1103	–
	Total	82957	18751	4181	566	14004	3769	3775	40936	246	13434	2046
		(16%)	(29%)	(89%)	(49%)	(10%)	(67%)	(9%)	(10%)		(8%)	
Any age	Sm.	24130	10424	7404	604	2416	3296	426	7835	–	2149	–
	Total	122704	33220	8294	1101	23825	4862	4224	54382	770	19679	5567
		(20%)	(31%)	(89%)	(55%)	(10%)	(68%)	(10%)	(14%)		(11%)	

(To be conservative, no deaths before age 35, and none from liver cirrhosis or non-medical causes, were attributed to smoking.)

NETHERLANDS: 1990

Smoking–attributed deaths (Sm.) and total deaths (Total)

	ALL CAUSES	ALL CANCER	Lung cancer	Upper aero–digestive ca.	Other cancer	COPD	Other respiratory	Vascular disease	Liver cirrhosis	Other medical	Non–medical
Males											
0–34 Sm.	–	–	–	–	–	–	–	–	–	–	–
Total	3006	247	4	3	240	10	33	170	13	1453	1080
35–69 Sm.	8623	4168	2962	385	821	651	70	2656	–	1078	–
Total	22495	8278	3162	566	4550	802	227	8419	311	3318	1140
	(38%)	(50%)	(94%)	(68%)	(18%)	(81%)	(31%)	(32%)		(32%)	
70+ Sm.	12994	5376	3633	302	1441	2835	307	3296	–	1180	–
Total	41127	11342	3845	421	7076	3434	1728	17298	122	6351	852
	(32%)	(47%)	(94%)	(72%)	(20%)	(83%)	(18%)	(19%)		(19%)	
Any age Sm.	21617	9544	6595	687	2262	3486	377	5952	–	2258	–
Total	66628	19867	7011	990	11866	4246	1988	25887	446	11122	3072
	(32%)	(48%)	(94%)	(69%)	(19%)	(82%)	(19%)	(23%)		(20%)	
Females											
0–34 Sm.	–	–	–	–	–	–	–	–	–	–	–
Total	1763	247	8	2	237	5	15	95	3	988	410
35–69 Sm.	1420	624	475	58	91	169	13	371	–	243	–
Total	12393	6111	711	171	5229	321	106	3135	180	1982	558
	(11%)	(10%)	(67%)	(34%)	(2%)	(53%)	(12%)	(12%)		(12%)	
70+ Sm.	1299	316	225	40	51	417	33	361	–	172	–
Total	48040	8948	511	266	8171	1488	2502	22503	91	11242	1266
	(3%)	(4%)	(44%)	(15%)	(1%)	(28%)	(1%)	(2%)		(2%)	
Any age Sm.	2719	940	700	98	142	586	46	732	–	415	–
Total	62196	15306	1230	439	13637	1814	2623	25733	274	14212	2234
	(4%)	(6%)	(57%)	(22%)	(1%)	(32%)	(2%)	(3%)		(3%)	
Males+Females											
0–34 Sm.	–	–	–	–	–	–	–	–	–	–	–
Total	4769	494	12	5	477	15	48	265	16	2441	1490
35–69 Sm.	10043	4792	3437	443	912	820	83	3027	–	1321	–
Total	34888	14389	3873	737	9779	1123	333	11554	491	5300	1698
	(29%)	(33%)	(89%)	(60%)	(9%)	(73%)	(25%)	(26%)		(25%)	
70+ Sm.	14293	5692	3858	342	1492	3252	340	3657	–	1352	–
Total	89167	20290	4356	687	15247	4922	4230	39801	213	17593	2118
	(16%)	(28%)	(89%)	(50%)	(10%)	(66%)	(8%)	(9%)		(8%)	
Any age Sm.	24336	10484	7295	785	2404	4072	423	6684	–	2673	–
Total	128824	35173	8241	1429	25503	6060	4611	51620	720	25334	5306
	(19%)	(30%)	(89%)	(55%)	(9%)	(67%)	(9%)	(13%)		(11%)	

NETHERLANDS: 1995

Smoking–attributed deaths (Sm.) and total deaths (Total)

	ALL CAUSES	ALL CANCER	Lung cancer	Upper aero–digestive ca.	Other cancer	COPD	Other respiratory	Vascular disease	Liver cirrhosis	Other medical	Non–medical
Males											
0–34 Sm.	–	–	–	–	–	–	–	–	–	–	–
Total	2869	195	2	3	190	7	26	148	12	1585	896
35–69 Sm.	7483	3699	2525	472	702	613	54	1912	–	1205	–
Total	21831	8158	2739	756	4663	788	202	7091	281	4324	987
	(34%)	(45%)	(92%)	(62%)	(15%)	(78%)	(27%)	(27%)		(28%)	
70+ Sm.	13687	5566	3693	373	1500	3490	311	2931	–	1389	–
Total	43300	12241	3926	531	7784	4273	1832	16188	122	7830	814
	(32%)	(45%)	(94%)	(70%)	(19%)	(82%)	(17%)	(18%)		(18%)	
Any age Sm.	21170	9265	6218	845	2202	4103	365	4843	–	2594	–
Total	68000	20594	6667	1290	12637	5068	2060	23427	415	13739	2697
	(31%)	(45%)	(93%)	(66%)	(17%)	(81%)	(18%)	(21%)		(19%)	
Females											
0–34 Sm.	–	–	–	–	–	–	–	–	–	–	–
Total	1709	241	12	1	228	4	11	73	1	1001	378
35–69 Sm.	1924	905	686	96	123	221	18	412	–	368	–
Total	12272	6345	933	231	5181	360	104	2558	184	2252	469
	(16%)	(14%)	(74%)	(42%)	(2%)	(61%)	(17%)	(16%)		(16%)	
70+ Sm.	2151	507	361	65	81	772	51	501	–	320	–
Total	50944	9433	658	305	8470	2128	2681	21126	71	14233	1272
	(4%)	(5%)	(55%)	(21%)	(1%)	(36%)	(2%)	(2%)		(2%)	
Any age Sm.	4075	1412	1047	161	204	993	69	913	–	688	–
Total	64925	16019	1603	537	13879	2492	2796	23757	256	17486	2119
	(6%)	(9%)	(65%)	(30%)	(1%)	(40%)	(2%)	(4%)		(4%)	
Males+Females											
0–34 Sm.	–	–	–	–	–	–	–	–	–	–	–
Total	4578	436	14	4	418	11	37	221	13	2586	1274
35–69 Sm.	9407	4604	3211	568	825	834	72	2324	–	1573	–
Total	34103	14503	3672	987	9844	1148	306	9649	465	6576	1456
	(28%)	(32%)	(87%)	(58%)	(8%)	(73%)	(24%)	(24%)		(24%)	
70+ Sm.	15838	6073	4054	438	1581	4262	362	3432	–	1709	–
Total	94244	21674	4584	836	16254	6401	4513	37314	193	22063	2086
	(17%)	(28%)	(88%)	(52%)	(10%)	(67%)	(8%)	(9%)		(8%)	
Any age Sm.	25245	10677	7265	1006	2406	5096	434	5756	–	3282	–
Total	132925	36613	8270	1827	26516	7560	4856	47184	671	31225	4816
	(19%)	(29%)	(88%)	(55%)	(9%)	(67%)	(9%)	(12%)		(11%)	

(To be conservative, no deaths before age 35, and none from liver cirrhosis or non–medical causes, were attributed to smoking.)

NEW ZEALAND: 1990

		No. of deaths			Standardised rates (Defined on p.442)			Annual death rates / 100, 000						
		All ages	0–34	35–69	All ages	0–34	35–69	0–4	5–9	10–14	15–19	20–24	25–29	30–34
ALL CAUSES	M	13967	1369	4936	999.0	139.1	1005.0	272.6	28.2	29.9	142.7	208.2	154.6	137.7
	F	12557	636	3242	643.9	66.6	634.2	187.8	16.3	18.3	58.0	57.3	61.1	67.3
Tuberculosis	M	13	–	9	0.9	–	1.7	–	–	–	–	–	–	–
	F	20	1	5	1.0	0.1	0.9	–	–	–	–	–	0.7	–
Other infective	M	71	13	27	5.0	1.3	5.3	5.7	0.8	0.8	0.7	0.7	–	0.7
and parasitic	F	59	5	9	2.8	0.5	1.7	0.8	–	–	1.4	0.7	0.7	–
ALL CANCER	M	3548	97	1598	258.8	10.0	331.7	11.5	3.1	3.8	4.7	7.0	17.9	22.0
	F	3198	81	1517	187.2	8.3	293.5	3.0	4.1	4.0	4.8	4.4	13.9	24.3
Mouth and	M	67	5	40	4.8	0.5	8.2	0.7	–	–	–	0.7	1.4	0.7
pharynx cancer	F	30	–	13	1.7	–	2.5	–	–	–	–	–	–	–
Oesophagus cancer	M	111	1	56	8.1	0.1	12.0	–	–	–	–	–	–	0.7
	F	67	–	22	3.6	–	4.5	–	–	–	–	–	–	–
Stomach cancer	M	186	2	75	13.6	0.2	16.0	–	–	–	–	–	–	1.5
	F	116	4	38	6.1	0.4	7.4	–	–	–	–	–	0.7	2.1
Colorectal cancer	M	517	2	256	38.2	0.2	52.1	–	–	–	–	–	–	1.5
	F	507	2	226	29.3	0.2	44.9	–	–	–	–	0.7	–	0.7
Liver cancer	M	46	2	29	3.3	0.2	5.8	0.7	–	–	–	–	0.7	–
	F	20	2	9	1.2	0.2	1.8	–	–	0.8	0.7	–	–	–
Pancreas cancer	M	153	1	70	11.2	0.1	15.0	–	–	–	–	–	–	0.7
	F	105	–	37	5.7	–	7.4	–	–	–	–	–	–	–
Larynx cancer	M	27	–	16	2.0	–	3.3	–	–	–	–	–	–	–
	F	8	–	5	0.5	–	1.0	–	–	–	–	–	–	–
Lung cancer	M	903	1	455	66.4	0.1	96.2	–	–	–	–	–	–	0.7
	F	433	2	232	26.5	0.2	46.1	–	–	–	–	–	–	1.4
Malignant melanoma	M	115	10	73	8.2	1.0	14.1	–	–	–	–	–	2.1	5.1
	F	73	4	35	4.3	0.4	6.3	–	–	–	–	–	0.7	2.1
Female breast cancer	F	635	13	379	39.5	1.3	70.0	–	–	–	–	–	1.4	7.9
Cervix cancer	F	101	8	73	6.6	0.8	12.8	–	–	–	–	–	2.8	2.9
Other uterine cancer	F	82	–	35	4.6	–	7.2	–	–	–	–	–	–	–
Ovarian cancer	F	181	3	107	11.2	0.3	21.1	–	–	–	–	–	0.7	1.4
Prostate cancer	M	436	–	95	32.1	–	21.3	–	–	–	–	–	–	–
Bladder cancer	M	101	1	26	7.4	0.1	5.7	0.7	–	–	–	–	–	–
	F	48	–	12	2.5	–	2.4	–	–	–	–	–	–	–
Other and ill-defined	M	567	36	267	41.0	3.7	54.4	7.2	1.6	0.8	2.7	2.1	6.4	5.1
cancer sites	F	544	29	198	30.1	3.0	39.0	2.3	4.1	2.4	3.4	0.7	4.9	3.6
Hodgkin's disease	M	4	–	2	0.3	–	0.2	–	–	–	–	–	–	–
	F	9	1	1	0.4	0.1	0.2	–	–	–	–	0.7	–	–
Myeloma and non-	M	195	14	91	14.0	1.4	18.6	–	0.8	–	1.3	0.7	3.6	3.7
Hodgkin lymphomas	F	144	4	61	8.2	0.4	12.5	–	–	–	–	0.7	0.7	1.4
Leukaemia	M	120	22	47	8.3	2.3	8.9	2.2	0.8	3.1	0.7	3.5	3.6	2.2
	F	95	9	34	5.2	0.9	6.4	0.8	–	0.8	0.7	1.5	2.1	0.7
ALL VASCULAR	M	5914	57	2135	434.9	5.8	447.7	4.3	–	1.5	6.7	2.8	11.5	13.9
DISEASE	F	5697	34	984	272.9	3.5	198.9	3.8	0.8	0.8	2.7	1.5	4.9	10.0
Rheumatic heart	M	46	4	27	3.2	0.4	5.2	–	–	–	0.7	–	1.4	0.7
disease and fever	F	80	4	28	4.4	0.4	5.1	–	–	–	–	0.7	–	2.1
Hypertensive disease	M	73	1	26	5.3	0.1	5.2	–	–	–	–	–	–	0.7
	F	112	–	26	5.6	–	5.3	–	–	–	–	–	–	–
Ischaemic heart	M	3884	13	1555	285.3	1.3	326.5	–	–	–	–	0.7	2.9	5.9
disease	F	2923	5	567	142.6	0.5	116.1	–	–	–	0.7	–	0.7	2.1
Pulmonary embolism	M	51	–	21	3.8	–	4.6	–	–	–	–	–	–	–
and other venous	F	73	1	21	3.7	0.1	4.3	–	–	–	–	–	–	0.7
Cerebrovascular	M	1021	8	263	75.3	0.8	56.0	1.4	–	–	2.0	0.7	0.7	0.7
disease	F	1579	7	219	73.9	0.7	43.2	0.8	–	–	–	0.7	1.4	2.1
Other vascular	M	839	31	243	61.9	3.2	50.4	2.9	–	1.5	4.0	1.4	6.4	5.9
disease	F	930	17	123	42.6	1.8	24.8	3.0	0.8	0.8	2.0	–	2.8	2.9
Chronic obstructive	M	842	14	193	61.7	1.4	41.8	1.4	–	0.8	1.3	2.1	0.7	3.7
pulmonary disease	F	527	9	168	28.3	0.9	34.2	1.5	–	–	0.7	1.5	0.7	2.1
Other respiratory	M	487	18	49	36.9	1.8	10.2	10.8	–	0.8	–	0.7	0.7	–
disease	F	724	9	35	30.7	1.0	6.9	3.0	0.8	–	–	0.7	1.4	0.7
Peptic ulcer	M	105	–	28	7.9	–	6.0	–	–	–	–	–	–	–
	F	99	1	12	4.6	0.1	2.5	–	–	–	–	–	0.7	–
Liver cirrhosis	M	71	1	56	5.1	0.1	11.1	–	–	–	–	–	–	0.7
	F	38	2	27	2.5	0.2	5.1	0.8	–	–	–	–	–	0.7
Renal disease	M	137	4	31	10.1	0.4	6.5	–	–	–	–	–	2.1	0.7
	F	143	3	38	7.2	0.3	7.3	0.8	–	–	0.7	–	–	0.7
Pregnancy and birth	F	4	3	1	0.2	0.3	0.1	–	–	–	–	–	0.7	1.4
Congenital and	M	211	196	10	12.3	20.1	1.7	129.8	2.4	3.8	2.0	2.1	–	0.7
perinatal causes	F	148	128	9	8.9	13.8	1.7	88.2	0.8	0.8	3.4	2.9	–	0.7
Ill-defined causes	M	122	95	8	7.5	9.7	1.6	65.3	–	0.8	–	1.4	–	0.7
	F	120	78	6	6.6	8.5	1.2	57.0	–	0.8	0.7	–	–	0.7
Other medical causes	M	1038	87	356	74.5	8.9	68.6	14.3	3.9	2.3	8.7	5.6	12.2	15.4
	F	1207	53	282	60.5	5.5	54.6	9.9	2.4	3.2	5.5	6.5	5.6	5.7
ALL NON-	M	1408	787	436	83.6	79.4	71.1	29.4	18.0	15.3	118.7	185.7	109.5	79.1
MEDICAL CAUSES	F	573	229	149	30.4	23.5	25.4	19.0	7.3	8.7	38.2	39.2	31.9	20.0
Motor vehicle	M	525	388	110	28.8	39.0	17.5	8.6	9.4	10.0	73.3	93.5	50.1	27.8
traffic accidents	F	212	122	64	11.8	12.4	10.8	3.8	4.9	4.8	27.3	23.2	14.6	8.6
Fire	M	20	14	4	1.2	1.4	0.8	4.3	0.8	–	0.7	1.4	2.1	0.7
	F	8	6	1	0.4	0.6	0.2	1.5	0.8	–	0.7	–	0.7	0.7
Suicide	M	363	185	147	21.8	18.6	23.9	–	1.6	–	24.7	52.0	30.8	21.2
	F	92	40	42	5.4	4.0	6.8	–	–	–	4.8	8.7	6.9	7.9
Homicide	M	55	33	19	3.1	3.4	3.0	0.7	2.4	–	2.7	6.3	5.0	6.6
	F	23	15	7	1.3	1.6	1.2	0.8	0.8	1.6	–	2.2	3.5	2.1
POPULATION (thousands):	**M=males**				1671.7	965.8	609.6	139.4	127.5	130.5	150.0	142.2	139.7	136.5
	F=females				1707.6	948.1	610.6	131.5	122.7	125.8	146.5	137.9	144.0	139.7

NEW ZEALAND: 1990

Annual death rates / 100, 000

9th ICD categories

35–39	40–44	45–49	50–54	55–59	60–64	65–69	70–74	75–79	80+/NK			
160.4	225.4	355.3	606.2	1059.7	1731.9	2895.7	4689.7	7738.8	13616.6	M	ALL CAUSES	001–999
91.4	161.1	285.6	464.2	722.1	1054.2	1660.5	2725.2	4086.9	10665.3	F		
–	0.9	2.1	–	–	5.7	3.4	4.8	3.4	4.0	M	Tuberculosis	010–018, 137
–	0.9	1.1	–	–	2.9	1.5	9.3	8.9	9.9	F		
0.8	1.7	3.2	3.9	6.9	8.5	12.0	26.3	34.4	39.5	M	Other infective	Rest of 001–139
0.8	–	1.1	–	7.2	–	3.1	3.7	15.6	71.3	F	and parasitic	
23.8	47.5	93.6	187.8	381.9	646.8	940.2	1389.0	1986.3	2739.1	M	ALL CANCER	140–208
44.1	85.8	154.4	234.0	362.5	496.4	677.4	869.2	957.7	1396.0	F		
–	2.6	2.1	1.3	11.1	19.9	20.5	23.9	24.1	19.8	M	Mouth and	140–149
–	1.8	1.1	2.6	2.9	2.9	6.1	7.5	6.7	19.8	F	pharynx cancer	
0.8	–	2.1	7.8	11.1	22.7	39.3	45.3	51.5	79.1	M	Oesophagus cancer	150
–	–	–	3.8	5.7	10.0	12.3	13.1	40.1	39.6	F		
0.8	1.7	5.3	7.8	15.3	22.7	58.1	90.7	110.0	154.2	M	Stomach cancer	151
1.6	1.8	3.3	5.1	14.3	5.7	20.0	16.8	35.6	97.0	F		
2.5	7.8	18.1	37.6	73.6	112.1	112.8	198.1	299.0	351.8	M	Colorectal cancer	153, 154
2.4	7.9	14.3	46.0	57.3	78.5	107.5	140.2	153.7	267.3	F		
2.5	–	3.2	5.2	6.9	7.1	15.4	16.7	13.7	15.8	M	Liver cancer	155.0
–	0.9	–	2.6	1.4	1.4	6.1	7.5	4.5	5.9	F		
0.8	2.6	3.2	13.0	2.8	22.7	59.8	66.8	79.0	122.5	M	Pancreas cancer	157
–	1.8	2.2	5.1	11.5	11.4	20.0	22.4	40.1	75.2	F		
–	0.9	–	–	6.9	7.1	8.5	11.9	3.4	19.8	M	Larynx cancer	161
–	–	–	1.3	1.4	2.9	1.5	1.9	2.2	2.0	F		
0.8	7.8	16.0	47.9	127.8	201.4	271.8	365.2	525.8	557.3	M	Lung cancer	162
0.8	11.4	23.2	21.7	61.6	84.2	119.8	177.6	95.8	120.8	F		
2.5	5.2	11.7	9.1	18.1	19.9	32.5	35.8	34.4	27.7	M	Malignant melanoma	172
3.3	3.5	4.4	5.1	7.2	7.1	13.8	20.6	20.0	27.7	F		
18.0	32.4	62.8	57.5	94.6	112.7	112.1	132.7	153.7	204.0	F	Female breast cancer	174
5.7	11.4	11.0	12.8	17.2	12.8	18.4	15.0	15.6	9.9	F	Cervix cancer	180
–	1.8	1.1	2.6	5.7	11.4	27.6	33.6	29.0	31.7	F	Other uterine cancer	179, 182
2.4	3.5	6.6	21.7	15.8	51.4	46.1	35.5	55.7	53.5	F	Ovarian cancer	183
–	–	–	1.3	16.7	45.4	85.5	195.7	347.1	624.5	M	Prostate cancer	185
–	–	1.1	–	8.3	8.5	22.2	50.1	79.0	118.6	M	Bladder cancer	188
–	–	1.1	1.3	–	10.0	4.6	18.7	13.4	39.6	F		
7.4	9.5	19.1	40.2	48.6	112.1	143.6	188.5	261.2	430.8	M	Other and ill-defined	Rest of 140–208
5.7	6.1	18.7	30.7	47.3	58.5	106.0	155.1	184.9	299.0	F	cancer sites	
1.6	–	–	–	–	–	–	–	6.9	–	M	Hodgkin's disease	201
–	–	–	–	–	–	1.5	1.9	8.9	4.0	F		
2.5	3.5	6.4	10.4	22.2	34.0	51.3	64.4	103.1	130.4	M	Myeloma and non-	200, 202–203
0.8	0.9	1.1	9.0	12.9	22.8	39.9	43.0	66.8	51.5	F	Hodgkin lymphomas	
1.6	6.0	5.3	6.5	12.5	11.3	18.8	35.8	48.1	87.0	M	Leukaemia	204–208
3.3	0.9	3.3	5.1	5.7	12.8	13.8	26.2	31.2	47.5	F		
24.7	69.1	131.9	259.1	443.1	761.7	1444.4	2272.1	3845.4	6525.7	M	ALL VASCULAR	390–459
12.2	27.1	61.7	116.4	204.9	332.4	637.5	1289.7	2204.9	5938.6	F	DISEASE	
0.8	2.6	4.3	2.6	4.2	8.5	13.7	14.3	10.3	23.7	M	Rheumatic heart	390–398
3.3	0.9	3.3	6.4	4.3	7.1	10.8	28.0	29.0	39.6	F	disease and fever	
–	3.5	–	5.2	4.2	11.3	12.0	35.8	61.9	51.4	M	Hypertensive disease	401–405
–	–	2.2	1.3	10.0	10.0	13.8	22.4	62.4	91.1	F		
17.3	43.2	91.5	187.8	345.8	568.8	1030.8	1570.4	2577.3	3588.9	M	Ischaemic heart	410–414
2.4	13.1	27.6	58.8	111.7	201.1	397.8	760.7	1229.4	2756.4	F	disease	
–	0.9	–	5.2	4.2	2.8	18.8	16.7	13.7	75.1	M	Pulmonary embolism	415.1, 451–453
–	–	2.2	1.3	2.9	7.1	16.9	16.8	29.0	57.4	F	and other venous	
2.5	6.9	18.1	27.2	40.3	95.0	201.7	401.0	738.8	1450.6	M	Cerebrovascular	430–438
5.7	7.9	18.7	34.5	51.6	67.0	116.7	327.1	590.2	1807.9	F	disease	
4.1	12.1	18.1	31.1	44.4	75.2	167.5	233.9	443.3	1336.0	M	Other vascular	Rest of 390–459
0.8	5.3	7.7	14.1	24.4	39.9	81.4	134.6	265.0	1186.1	F	disease	
–	4.3	3.2	13.0	47.2	78.0	147.0	381.9	697.6	1075.1	M	Chronic obstructive	490–496
1.6	2.6	7.7	23.0	38.7	58.5	107.5	173.8	211.6	320.8	F	pulmonary disease	
1.6	2.6	3.2	2.6	4.2	22.7	34.2	81.1	161.5	1339.9	M	Other respiratory	Rest of 460–519
–	0.9	4.4	7.7	7.2	10.0	18.4	52.3	89.1	1211.9	F	disease	
–	–	1.1	3.9	8.3	11.3	17.1	21.5	79.0	177.9	M	Peptic ulcer	531–533
–	–	–	1.3	2.9	5.7	7.7	26.2	49.0	99.0	F		
1.6	4.3	4.3	5.2	15.3	19.9	27.4	21.5	13.7	4.0	M	Liver cirrhosis	571
1.6	1.8	2.2	6.4	2.9	11.4	9.2	3.7	11.1	4.0	F		
–	0.9	3.2	5.2	6.9	7.1	22.2	38.2	123.7	197.6	M	Renal disease	580–590
1.6	2.6	3.3	2.6	7.2	17.1	16.9	24.3	40.1	140.6	F		
0.8	–	–	–	–	–	–	–	–	–	F	Pregnancy and birth	630–676
0.8	1.7	2.1	2.6	1.4	1.4	1.7	7.2	3.4	4.0	M	Congenital and	740–779
–	–	2.2	2.6	2.9	2.9	1.5	9.3	8.9	4.0	F	perinatal causes	
0.8	–	–	1.3	2.8	2.8	3.4	9.5	6.9	51.4	M	Ill-defined causes	780–799
0.8	–	–	–	2.9	1.4	3.1	7.5	2.2	61.4	F		
25.5	25.9	34.0	53.1	72.2	102.1	167.5	334.1	622.0	1083.0	M	Other medical causes	Rest of 001–799
9.0	17.5	23.2	46.0	64.5	88.4	133.6	218.7	387.5	1150.5	F		
80.6	66.5	73.4	68.7	69.4	63.8	75.2	102.6	161.5	375.5	M	ALL NON-	E800–E999
18.8	21.9	24.3	24.3	18.6	27.1	43.0	37.4	100.2	257.4	F	MEDICAL CAUSES	
26.3	13.0	21.3	16.8	15.3	12.8	17.1	21.5	20.6	47.4	M	Motor vehicle	E810–E819
8.2	8.8	14.3	9.0	7.2	14.3	13.8	3.7	22.3	27.7	F	traffic accidents	
–	0.9	–	1.3	1.4	–	1.7	–	3.4	4.0	M	Fire	E890–E899
–	–	1.1	–	–	–	–	–	–	2.0	F		
28.8	19.0	24.5	24.6	27.8	27.0	15.4	23.9	27.5	51.4	M	Suicide	E950–E959
5.7	10.5	4.4	7.7	7.2	4.3	7.7	7.5	11.1	2.0	F		
4.1	5.2	1.1	1.3	1.4	4.3	3.4	2.4	3.4	4.0	M	Homicide	E960–E969
0.8	–	2.2	2.6	–	–	3.1	–	–	2.0	F		
121.6	115.8	94.0	77.2	72.0	70.5	58.5	41.9	29.1	25.3	M	POPULATION (thousands)	
122.5	114.2	90.7	78.2	69.8	70.1	65.1	53.5	44.9	50.5	F		

NEW ZEALAND: Males

	All ages	0–34	35–69	35–39	40–44	45–49	50–54	55–59	60–64	65–69	70–74	75–79	80+/NK
POPULATION (1000s)													
1955	1075.8	645.5	373.8	69.5	70.5	64.4	55.6	44.2	36.5	33.1	27.2	17.5	11.8
1965	1329.7	822.2	448.8	84.1	81.6	70.1	69.6	60.0	48.4	35.0	25.1	18.0	15.6
1975	1544.9	981.2	496.9	85.0	80.2	81.8	78.7	63.9	59.8	47.5	33.2	18.8	14.8
1985	1627.3	973.5	564.6	119.1	95.9	81.8	74.4	74.6	67.7	51.1	42.3	27.0	19.9
1990	**1671.7**	**965.8**	**609.6**	**121.6**	**115.8**	**94.0**	**77.2**	**72.0**	**70.5**	**58.5**	**41.9**	**29.1**	**25.3**
1995 projected	*1752.0*	*976.7*	*667.9*	*132.6*	*120.9*	*117.4*	*92.3*	*77.8*	*64.9*	*62.0*	*49.1*	*31.0*	*27.3*
NUMBER OF DEATHS													
All causes													
1955	10627	1609	3998	172	205	337	508	680	858	1238	1561	1583	1876
1965	12659	1529	5125	186	281	386	654	964	1252	1402	1490	1743	2772
1975	13798	1560	5902	175	251	488	735	941	1520	1792	1972	1640	2724
1985	14534	1303	5416	164	251	357	553	960	1415	1716	2212	2308	3295
1990	**13967**	**1369**	**4936**	**195**	**261**	**334**	**468**	**763**	**1221**	**1694**	**1965**	**2252**	**3445**
1995 projected	*13279*	*1452*	*4450*	*212*	*242*	*341*	*459*	*680*	*947*	*1569*	*2058*	*2116*	*3203*
Lung cancer													
1955	300	2	214	1	5	19	27	45	55	62	42	29	13
1965	489	3	319	6	17	15	32	58	89	102	72	58	37
1975	789	2	473	2	12	20	41	99	148	151	147	104	63
1985	866	1	462	3	8	25	46	89	143	148	146	136	121
1990	**903**	**1**	**455**	**1**	**9**	**15**	**37**	**92**	**142**	**159**	**153**	**153**	**141**
1995 projected	*925*	*1*	*433*	*1*	*6*	*12*	*38*	*92*	*122*	*162*	*177*	*166*	*148*
ANNUAL DEATH RATE / 100,000 (*The rates for the age groups 0–34 and 35–69 are the means of seven five-yearly rates, but the all-ages rates are standardised to the conventional "European" age distribution)													
All causes													
1955	1283.1*	217.9*	1372.1*	247.5	290.8	523.3	913.7	1538.5	2350.7	3740.2	5739.0	9045.7	15898.3
1965	1347.6*	174.2*	1465.0*	221.2	344.4	550.6	939.7	1606.7	2586.8	4005.7	5936.3	9683.3	17769.2
1975	1312.2*	157.8*	1405.2*	205.9	313.0	596.6	933.9	1472.6	2541.8	3772.6	5939.8	8723.4	18405.4
1985	1154.8*	135.2*	1187.7*	137.7	261.7	436.4	743.3	1286.9	2090.1	3358.1	5229.3	8548.1	16557.8
1990	**999.0***	**139.1***	**1005.0***	**160.4**	**225.4**	**355.3**	**606.2**	**1059.7**	**1731.9**	**2895.7**	**4689.7**	**7738.8**	**13616.6**
1995 projected	*878.1**	*146.2**	*858.8**	*159.9*	*200.2*	*290.5*	*497.3*	*874.0*	*1459.2*	*2530.6*	*4191.4*	*6825.8*	*11732.6*
All cancer													
1955	207.4*	11.4*	293.3*	30.2	44.0	119.6	219.4	330.3	515.1	794.6	1025.7	1377.1	1855.9
1965	222.0*	12.3*	302.0*	45.2	74.8	107.0	179.6	330.0	543.4	834.3	1135.5	1616.7	2032.1
1975	261.3*	13.0*	345.6*	41.2	69.8	118.6	217.3	377.2	643.8	951.6	1322.3	1867.0	2682.4
1985	264.0*	9.8*	356.7*	31.1	67.8	123.5	228.5	388.7	663.2	994.1	1338.1	1881.5	2678.4
1990	**258.8***	**10.0***	**331.7***	**23.8**	**47.5**	**93.6**	**187.8**	**381.9**	**646.8**	**940.2**	**1389.0**	**1986.3**	**2739.1**
1995 projected	*251.4**	*9.7**	*306.0**	*16.6*	*33.9*	*69.8*	*163.6*	*350.9*	*599.4*	*908.1*	*1374.7*	*2051.6*	*2849.8*
Lung cancer													
1955	37.5*	0.4*	75.2*	1.4	7.1	29.5	48.6	101.8	150.7	187.3	154.4	165.7	110.2
1965	53.3*	0.5*	95.3*	7.1	20.8	21.4	46.0	96.7	183.9	291.4	286.9	322.2	237.2
1975	74.0*	0.3*	116.3*	2.4	15.0	24.4	52.1	154.9	247.5	317.9	442.8	553.2	425.7
1985	69.2*	0.1*	103.3*	2.5	8.3	30.6	61.8	119.3	211.2	289.6	345.2	503.7	608.0
1990	**66.4***	**0.1***	**96.2***	**0.8**	**7.8**	**16.0**	**47.9**	**127.8**	**201.4**	**271.8**	**365.2**	**525.8**	**557.3**
1995 projected	*63.4**	*0.1**	*89.2**	*0.8*	*5.0*	*10.2*	*41.2*	*118.3*	*188.0*	*261.3*	*360.5*	*535.5*	*542.1*
Upper aerodigestive cancer (mouth, oesophagus, pharynx and larynx)													
1955	13.2*	–	17.7*	–	2.8	4.7	16.2	11.3	46.6	42.3	58.8	91.4	161.0
1965	12.5*	–	17.1*	2.4	2.5	5.7	17.2	25.0	26.9	40.0	79.7	88.9	96.2
1975	15.8*	0.3*	26.9*	–	3.7	12.2	19.1	26.6	56.9	69.5	54.2	95.7	121.6
1985	17.0*	0.1*	27.3*	2.5	4.2	7.3	20.2	44.2	51.7	60.7	75.7	88.9	140.7
1990	**14.9***	**0.6***	**23.5***	**0.8**	**3.5**	**4.3**	**9.1**	**29.2**	**49.6**	**68.4**	**81.1**	**79.0**	**118.6**
1995 projected	*13.3**	*0.6**	*21.4**	*0.8*	*2.5*	*2.6*	*6.5*	*21.9*	*44.7*	*71.0*	*79.4*	*64.5*	*102.6*
Other cancer													
1955	156.7*	11.1*	200.4*	28.8	34.0	85.4	154.7	217.2	317.8	565.0	812.5	1120.0	1584.7
1965	156.2*	11.9*	189.6*	35.7	51.5	79.9	116.4	208.3	332.6	502.9	768.9	1205.6	1698.7
1975	171.5*	12.4*	202.5*	38.8	51.1	81.9	146.1	195.6	339.5	564.2	825.3	1218.1	2135.1
1985	177.8*	9.6*	226.1*	26.0	55.3	85.6	146.5	225.2	400.3	643.8	917.3	1288.9	1929.6
1990	**177.5***	**9.3***	**211.9***	**22.2**	**36.3**	**73.4**	**130.8**	**225.0**	**395.7**	**600.0**	**942.7**	**1381.4**	**2063.2**
1995 projected	*174.8**	*9.0**	*195.4**	*15.1*	*26.5*	*57.1*	*115.9*	*210.8*	*366.7*	*575.8*	*934.8*	*1451.6*	*2205.1*
Chronic obstructive pulmonary disease (COPD)													
1955	54.3*	1.4*	58.6*	4.3	4.3	9.3	32.4	54.3	115.1	190.3	286.8	451.4	788.1
1965	78.9*	2.1*	79.0*	3.6	4.9	8.6	31.6	71.7	161.2	271.4	390.4	783.3	1185.9
1975	88.7*	6.3*	73.7*	1.2	11.2	13.4	44.5	61.0	132.1	252.6	475.9	797.9	1486.5
1985	87.7*	2.4*	73.5*	5.0	5.2	12.2	30.9	71.0	112.3	277.9	484.6	807.4	1552.8
1990	**61.7***	**1.4***	**41.8***	–	**4.3**	**3.2**	**13.0**	**47.2**	**78.0**	**147.0**	**381.9**	**697.6**	**1075.1**
1995 projected	*45.3**	*1.0**	*28.4**	–	*2.5*	*1.7*	*8.7*	*32.1*	*52.4*	*101.6*	*289.2*	*525.8*	*805.9*
Other respiratory disease													
1955	42.5*	18.6*	19.9*	4.3	4.3	6.2	10.8	11.3	30.1	72.5	106.6	285.7	822.0
1965	67.6*	12.6*	31.4*	3.6	7.4	7.1	18.7	30.0	47.5	105.7	235.1	427.8	1705.1
1975	49.5*	7.8*	17.0*	3.5	2.5	11.0	10.2	28.2	21.7	42.1	120.5	297.9	1466.2
1985	64.1*	4.1*	26.5*	0.8	3.1	6.1	10.8	17.4	51.7	95.9	212.8	466.7	1859.3
1990	**36.9***	**1.8***	**10.2***	**1.6**	**2.6**	**3.2**	**2.6**	**4.2**	**22.7**	**34.2**	**81.1**	**161.5**	**1339.9**
1995 projected	*25.8**	*1.2**	*6.9**	*0.8*	*1.7*	*1.7*	*2.2*	*2.6*	*15.4*	*24.2*	*55.0*	*109.7*	*948.7*
Vascular disease													
1955	654.8*	9.6*	704.1*	50.4	122.0	222.0	402.9	816.7	1290.4	2024.2	3371.3	5325.7	9601.7
1965	720.4*	9.7*	818.0*	64.2	123.8	265.3	518.7	923.3	1502.1	2328.6	3402.4	5561.1	10532.1
1975	666.8*	7.2*	739.0*	56.5	123.4	276.3	468.9	790.3	1403.0	2054.7	3337.3	4787.2	10141.9
1985	528.5*	4.7*	557.9*	31.1	79.2	201.7	330.6	623.3	1014.8	1624.3	2628.8	4388.9	8070.4
1990	**434.9***	**5.8***	**447.7***	**24.7**	**69.1**	**131.9**	**259.1**	**443.1**	**761.7**	**1444.4**	**2272.1**	**3845.4**	**6525.7**
1995 projected	*353.6**	*6.8**	*348.6**	*20.4*	*46.3*	*92.0*	*175.5*	*317.5*	*594.8*	*1193.5*	*1922.6*	*3203.2*	*5428.6*
Liver cirrhosis													
1955	4.5*	0.4*	8.1*	–	2.8	1.6	9.0	9.0	16.4	18.1	18.4	11.4	25.4
1965	4.7*	–	9.0*	1.2	3.7	7.1	8.6	11.7	16.5	14.3	23.9	16.7	6.4
1975	11.3*	0.9*	21.1*	5.9	5.0	17.1	22.9	21.9	36.8	37.9	60.2	21.3	20.3
1985	7.1*	0.1*	15.5*	2.5	5.2	7.3	10.8	18.8	32.5	31.3	21.3	11.1	20.1
1990	**5.1***	**0.1***	**11.1***	**1.6**	**4.3**	**4.3**	**5.2**	**15.3**	**19.9**	**27.4**	**21.5**	**13.7**	**4.0**
1995 projected	*3.7**	*0.1**	*7.8**	*1.5*	*2.5*	*2.6*	*3.3*	*10.3*	*13.9*	*21.0*	*20.4*	*9.7*	–
Other medical causes													
1955	227.6*	103.4*	198.1*	66.2	46.8	99.4	131.3	210.4	304.1	528.7	779.4	1377.1	2364.4
1965	159.8*	69.6*	132.3*	33.3	44.1	69.9	69.0	145.0	204.5	360.0	601.6	1044.4	1724.4
1975	140.1*	52.2*	122.0*	22.4	31.2	80.7	88.9	103.3	190.6	336.8	463.9	755.3	1891.9
1985	123.3*	43.3*	87.6*	12.6	28.2	26.9	72.6	89.8	144.8	238.7	444.4	822.2	1899.5
1990	**118.1***	**40.5***	**91.4***	**28.0**	**31.1**	**45.7**	**69.9**	**98.6**	**139.0**	**227.4**	**441.5**	**872.9**	**1557.3**
1995 projected	*112.1**	*37.9**	*91.8**	*36.2*	*40.5*	*48.6*	*74.8*	*95.1*	*131.0*	*216.1*	*437.9*	*790.3*	*1388.3*
All non-medical causes													
1955	92.0*	73.0*	89.9*	92.1	66.7	65.2	107.9	106.3	79.5	111.8	150.7	217.1	440.7
1965	94.2*	67.8*	93.3*	70.2	85.8	85.6	113.5	95.0	111.6	91.4	147.4	233.3	583.3
1975	94.5*	70.5*	86.7*	75.3	69.8	79.5	81.3	90.8	113.7	96.8	159.6	196.8	716.2
1985	80.1*	70.8*	70.0*	54.6	73.0	58.7	59.1	77.7	70.9	95.9	99.3	170.4	477.4
1990	**83.6***	**79.4***	**71.1***	**80.6**	**66.5**	**73.4**	**68.7**	**69.4**	**63.8**	**75.2**	**102.6**	**161.5**	**375.5**
1995 projected	*86.1**	*89.5**	*69.3**	*84.5*	*72.8*	*74.1*	*69.3*	*65.6*	*52.4*	*66.1*	*91.6*	*135.5*	*311.4*

NEW ZEALAND: Females

	All ages	0–34	35–69	35–39	40–44	45–49	50–54	55–59	60–64	65–69	70–74	75–79	80+/NK
POPULATION (1000s)													
1955	1062.6	615.9	380.4	71.1	69.7	61.8	53.2	46.2	41.2	37.2	30.8	20.3	15.2
1965	1317.4	785.2	448.4	78.0	79.2	71.7	69.1	59.3	49.5	41.6	34.5	25.5	23.8
1975	1541.9	941.1	500.2	82.5	76.5	77.5	77.7	68.0	64.6	53.4	42.1	28.8	29.7
1985	1651.3	945.9	570.7	118.9	94.5	80.1	71.1	72.9	72.0	61.2	53.2	39.1	42.4
1990	**1707.6**	**948.1**	**610.6**	**122.5**	**114.2**	**90.7**	**78.2**	**69.8**	**70.1**	**65.1**	**53.5**	**44.9**	**50.5**
1995 projected	*1781.8*	*939.5*	*680.9*	*134.1*	*123.3*	*118.4*	*92.9*	*79.4*	*66.9*	*65.9*	*59.5*	*46.4*	*55.5*
NUMBER OF DEATHS													
All causes													
1955	8598	1022	2831	115	160	256	362	415	593	930	1184	1419	2142
1965	10317	915	3121	98	201	265	398	538	682	939	1205	1593	3483
1975	11317	902	3370	121	161	252	417	532	868	1019	1410	1520	4115
1985	12950	718	3341	138	158	250	332	534	834	1095	1587	1944	5360
1990	**12557**	**636**	**3242**	**112**	**184**	**259**	**363**	**504**	**739**	**1081**	**1458**	**1835**	**5386**
1995 projected	*11881*	*539*	*3243*	*111*	*180*	*325*	*421*	*544*	*659*	*1003*	*1410*	*1674*	*5015*
Lung cancer													
1955	40	–	24	1	2	6	1	3	2	9	5	7	4
1965	70	2	49	1	1	7	9	9	10	12	6	4	9
1975	200	–	134	3	6	6	23	20	43	33	27	22	17
1985	331	–	201	2	6	11	19	45	60	58	54	38	38
1990	**433**	**2**	**232**	**1**	**13**	**21**	**17**	**43**	**59**	**78**	**95**	**43**	**61**
1995 projected	*557*	*3*	*283*	*2*	*19*	*32*	*21*	*46*	*60*	*103*	*134*	*60*	*77*
ANNUAL DEATH RATE / 100,000 (*The rates for the age groups 0–34 and 35–69 are the means of seven five-yearly rates, but the all-ages rates are standardised to the conventional "European" age distribution)													
All causes													
1955	940.9*	139.7*	903.4*	161.7	229.6	414.2	680.5	898.3	1439.3	2500.0	3844.2	6990.1	14092.1
1965	883.4*	103.4*	838.2*	125.6	253.8	369.6	576.0	907.3	1377.8	2257.2	3492.8	6247.1	14634.5
1975	808.7*	95.1*	750.5*	146.7	210.5	325.2	536.7	782.4	1343.7	1908.2	3349.2	5277.8	13855.2
1985	730.5*	78.6*	677.5*	116.1	167.2	312.1	466.9	732.5	1158.3	1789.2	2983.1	4971.9	12641.5
1990	**643.9***	**66.6***	**634.2***	**91.4**	**161.1**	**285.6**	**464.2**	**722.1**	**1054.2**	**1660.5**	**2725.2**	**4086.9**	**10665.3**
1995 projected	*571.5**	*56.9**	*592.7**	*82.8*	*146.0*	*274.5*	*453.2*	*685.1*	*985.1*	*1522.0*	*2369.7*	*3607.8*	*9036.0*
All cancer													
1955	169.7*	9.1*	249.6*	53.4	86.1	163.4	251.9	259.7	373.8	559.1	704.5	1088.7	1335.5
1965	161.8*	12.5*	249.8*	47.4	106.1	142.3	256.2	298.5	385.9	512.0	559.4	843.1	1281.5
1975	173.6*	10.6*	260.6*	55.8	83.7	127.7	244.5	294.1	456.7	561.8	767.2	892.4	1434.3
1985	179.3*	11.0*	272.7*	46.3	81.5	152.3	226.4	348.4	452.8	601.3	802.6	992.3	1344.3
1990	**187.2***	**8.3***	**293.5***	**44.1**	**85.8**	**154.4**	**234.0**	**362.5**	**496.4**	**677.4**	**869.2**	**957.7**	**1396.0**
1995 projected	*191.7**	*6.7**	*305.6**	*41.0*	*84.3*	*155.4*	*239.0*	*375.3*	*524.7*	*719.3*	*885.7*	*989.2*	*1405.4*
Lung cancer													
1955	4.4*	–	7.3*	1.4	2.9	9.7	1.9	6.5	4.9	24.2	16.2	34.5	26.3
1965	6.6*	0.3*	12.8*	1.3	1.3	9.8	13.0	15.2	20.2	28.8	17.4	15.7	37.8
1975	15.6*	–	29.5*	3.6	7.8	7.7	29.6	29.4	66.6	61.8	64.1	76.4	57.2
1985	21.8*	–	41.2*	1.7	6.3	13.7	26.7	61.7	83.3	94.8	101.5	97.2	89.6
1990	**26.5***	**0.2***	**46.1***	**0.8**	**11.4**	**23.2**	**21.7**	**61.6**	**84.2**	**119.8**	**177.6**	**95.8**	**120.8**
1995 projected	*31.1**	*0.3**	*52.9**	*1.5*	*15.4*	*27.0*	*22.6*	*57.9*	*89.7*	*156.3*	*225.2*	*129.3*	*138.7*
Upper aerodigestive cancer (mouth, oesophagus, pharynx and larynx)													
1955	7.3*	–	8.7*	–	–	–	9.4	13.0	14.6	24.2	35.7	54.2	98.7
1965	4.2*	–	6.4*	–	1.3	4.2	4.3	8.4	10.1	16.8	11.6	27.5	46.2
1975	5.7*	0.1*	6.1*	–	1.3	3.9	6.4	10.3	9.3	11.2	21.4	45.1	87.5
1985	5.5*	0.1*	7.1*	–	1.1	1.2	2.8	11.0	12.5	21.2	30.1	46.0	56.6
1990	**5.8***	**–**	**8.0***	**–**	**1.8**	**1.1**	**7.7**	**10.0**	**15.7**	**20.0**	**22.4**	**49.0**	**61.4**
1995 projected	*5.9**	*–*	*8.3**	*–*	*2.4*	*1.7*	*9.7*	*12.6*	*14.9*	*16.7*	*20.2*	*45.3*	*64.9*
Other cancer													
1955	158.0*	9.1*	233.6*	52.0	83.2	153.7	240.6	240.3	354.4	510.8	652.6	1000.0	1210.5
1965	151.0*	12.3*	230.5*	46.2	103.5	128.3	238.8	274.9	355.6	466.3	530.4	800.0	1197.5
1975	152.3*	10.5*	225.0*	52.1	74.5	116.1	208.5	254.4	380.8	488.8	681.7	770.8	1289.6
1985	152.0*	10.9*	224.4*	44.6	74.1	137.3	196.9	275.7	356.9	485.3	671.1	849.1	1198.1
1990	**155.0***	**8.1***	**239.4***	**43.3**	**72.7**	**130.1**	**204.6**	**290.8**	**396.6**	**537.6**	**669.2**	**812.9**	**1213.9**
1995 projected	*154.6**	*6.4**	*244.4**	*39.5*	*66.5*	*126.7*	*206.7*	*304.8*	*420.0*	*546.3*	*640.3*	*814.7*	*1201.8*
Chronic obstructive pulmonary disease (COPD)													
1955	19.2*	0.8*	19.3*	–	1.4	8.1	16.9	17.3	24.3	67.2	87.7	172.4	296.1
1965	23.1*	2.3*	22.0*	6.4	5.1	11.2	21.7	30.4	24.2	55.3	87.0	145.1	403.4
1975	30.0*	4.4*	30.4*	7.3	9.2	14.2	18.0	36.8	52.6	74.9	163.9	128.5	447.8
1985	34.9*	2.0*	45.6*	5.9	2.1	15.0	33.8	54.9	81.9	125.8	212.4	199.5	353.8
1990	**28.3***	**0.9***	**34.2***	**1.6**	**2.6**	**7.7**	**23.0**	**38.7**	**58.5**	**107.5**	**173.8**	**211.6**	**320.8**
1995 projected	*23.9**	*0.6**	*25.4**	*1.5*	*1.6*	*5.1*	*16.1*	*26.4*	*43.3*	*83.5*	*151.3*	*204.7*	*308.1*
Other respiratory disease													
1955	38.7*	15.6*	15.0*	2.8	2.9	1.6	7.5	15.2	26.7	48.4	94.2	221.7	881.6
1965	51.4*	10.0*	19.2*	–	2.5	7.0	8.7	16.9	34.3	64.9	107.2	380.4	1424.4
1975	38.9*	6.9*	12.7*	1.2	2.6	7.7	6.4	10.3	23.2	37.5	83.1	232.6	1171.7
1985	50.0*	2.6*	13.7*	0.8	2.1	2.5	7.0	9.6	26.4	47.4	120.3	299.2	1714.6
1990	**30.7***	**1.0***	**6.9***	**–**	**0.9**	**4.4**	**7.7**	**7.2**	**10.0**	**18.4**	**52.3**	**89.1**	**1211.9**
1995 projected	*21.8**	*0.5**	*5.4**	*–*	*0.8*	*5.1*	*7.5*	*5.0*	*7.5*	*12.1*	*35.3*	*62.5*	*857.7*
Vascular disease													
1955	508.1*	9.2*	436.3*	32.3	66.0	132.7	261.3	430.7	703.9	1427.4	2383.1	4591.1	9381.6
1965	479.3*	8.1*	392.3*	19.2	48.0	117.2	179.5	382.8	725.3	1274.0	2249.3	4145.1	9462.2
1975	408.9*	5.7*	323.2*	37.6	57.5	92.9	172.5	302.9	626.9	971.9	1829.0	3295.1	8585.9
1985	327.6*	4.4*	240.2*	25.2	32.8	84.9	133.6	205.8	426.4	772.9	1454.9	2785.2	7108.5
1990	**272.9***	**3.5***	**198.9***	**12.2**	**27.1**	**61.7**	**116.4**	**204.9**	**332.4**	**637.5**	**1289.7**	**2204.9**	**5938.6**
1995 projected	*222.0**	*2.6**	*162.5**	*8.2*	*18.7*	*49.0*	*103.3*	*170.0*	*267.6*	*520.5*	*1010.1*	*1782.3*	*4888.3*
Liver cirrhosis													
1955	4.0*	0.4*	6.7*	–	1.4	4.9	5.6	6.5	12.1	16.1	26.0	9.9	19.7
1965	3.2*	0.2*	5.9*	1.3	1.3	1.4	2.9	10.1	12.1	12.0	14.5	11.8	12.6
1975	5.1*	0.4*	10.5*	2.4	5.2	7.7	10.3	19.1	15.5	13.1	11.9	–	13.5
1985	2.8*	–	5.9*	1.7	2.1	2.5	4.2	4.1	13.9	13.1	9.4	7.7	7.1
1990	**2.5***	**0.2***	**5.1***	**1.6**	**1.8**	**2.2**	**6.4**	**2.9**	**11.4**	**9.2**	**3.7**	**11.1**	**4.0**
1995 projected	*2.1**	*0.1**	*4.2**	*1.5*	*1.6*	*2.5*	*6.5*	*2.5*	*9.0*	*6.1*	*3.4*	*8.6*	*3.6*
Other medical causes													
1955	166.6*	85.6*	147.3*	64.7	57.4	90.6	109.0	129.9	259.7	319.9	480.5	758.6	1743.4
1965	120.1*	50.7*	111.2*	29.5	69.4	60.0	65.1	138.3	139.4	276.4	371.0	545.1	1424.4
1975	102.1*	43.5*	77.3*	15.8	26.1	42.6	59.2	82.4	133.1	181.6	384.8	541.7	1363.6
1985	99.0*	33.7*	69.8*	15.1	24.3	32.5	39.4	75.4	123.6	178.1	323.3	601.0	1662.7
1990	**91.9***	**29.2***	**70.1***	**13.1**	**21.0**	**30.9**	**52.4**	**87.4**	**118.4**	**167.4**	**299.1**	**512.2**	**1536.6**
1995 projected	*84.0**	*24.6**	*68.3**	*11.2*	*17.8*	*32.9*	*60.3*	*91.9*	*113.6*	*150.2*	*252.1*	*482.8*	*1391.0*
All non-medical causes													
1955	34.6*	19.0*	29.1*	8.4	14.3	12.9	28.2	39.0	38.8	61.8	68.2	147.8	434.2
1965	44.5*	19.6*	37.9*	21.8	21.5	30.7	42.0	30.4	56.6	62.5	104.3	176.5	626.1
1975	50.2*	23.7*	35.8*	26.7	26.1	32.3	25.7	36.8	35.6	67.4	109.3	187.5	838.4
1985	36.9*	24.9*	29.5*	21.0	22.2	22.5	22.5	34.3	33.3	50.7	60.2	87.0	450.5
1990	**30.4***	**23.5***	**25.4***	**18.8**	**21.9**	**24.3**	**24.3**	**18.6**	**27.1**	**43.0**	**37.4**	**100.2**	**257.4**
1995 projected	*26.0**	*21.8**	*21.3**	*19.4*	*21.1*	*24.5*	*20.5*	*13.9*	*19.4*	*30.3*	*31.9*	*77.6*	*182.0*

NEW ZEALAND: 1975

Smoking-attributed deaths (Sm.) and total deaths (Total)

		ALL CAUSES	ALL CANCER	Lung cancer	Upper aero-digestive ca.	Other cancer	COPD	Other respiratory	Vascular disease	Liver cirrhosis	Other medical	Non-medical
Males												
0–34	Sm.	–	–	–	–	–	–	–	–	–	–	–
	Total	1560	120	2	2	116	66	82	61	7	550	674
35–69	Sm.	1917	642	438	72	132	227	22	876	–	150	–
	Total	5902	1437	473	112	852	294	73	3062	95	520	421
		(32%)	(45%)	(93%)	(64%)	(15%)	(77%)	(30%)	(29%)		(29%)	
70+	Sm.	1417	433	287	33	113	395	37	476	–	76	–
	Total	6336	1187	314	54	819	528	313	3509	27	576	196
		(22%)	(36%)	(91%)	(61%)	(14%)	(75%)	(12%)	(14%)		(13%)	
Any age	Sm.	3334	1075	725	105	245	622	59	1352	–	226	–
	Total	13798	2744	789	168	1787	888	468	6632	129	1646	1291
		(24%)	(39%)	(92%)	(63%)	(14%)	(70%)	(13%)	(20%)		(14%)	
Females												
0–34	Sm.	–	–	–	–	–	–	–	–	–	–	–
	Total	902	91	0	1	90	43	70	47	3	427	221
35–69	Sm.	455	125	94	10	21	76	8	196	–	50	–
	Total	3370	1194	134	28	1032	137	56	1411	50	351	171
		(14%)	(10%)	(70%)	(36%)	(2%)	(55%)	(14%)	(14%)		(14%)	
70+	Sm.	309	57	37	11	9	99	11	121	–	21	–
	Total	7045	1006	66	48	892	239	450	4269	9	723	349
		(4%)	(6%)	(56%)	(23%)	(1%)	(41%)	(2%)	(3%)		(3%)	
Any age	Sm.	764	182	131	21	30	175	19	317	–	71	–
	Total	11317	2291	200	77	2014	419	576	5727	62	1501	741
		(7%)	(8%)	(66%)	(27%)	(1%)	(42%)	(3%)	(6%)		(5%)	
Males+Females												
0–34	Sm.	–	–	–	–	–	–	–	–	–	–	–
	Total	2462	211	2	3	206	109	152	108	10	977	895
35–69	Sm.	2372	767	532	82	153	303	30	1072	–	200	–
	Total	9272	2631	607	140	1884	431	129	4473	145	871	592
		(26%)	(29%)	(88%)	(59%)	(8%)	(70%)	(23%)	(24%)		(23%)	
70+	Sm.	1726	490	324	44	122	494	48	597	–	97	–
	Total	13381	2193	380	102	1711	767	763	7778	36	1299	545
		(13%)	(22%)	(85%)	(43%)	(7%)	(64%)	(6%)	(8%)		(7%)	
Any age	Sm.	4098	1257	856	126	275	797	78	1669	–	297	–
	Total	25115	5035	989	245	3801	1307	1044	12359	191	3147	2032
		(16%)	(25%)	(87%)	(51%)	(7%)	(61%)	(7%)	(14%)		(9%)	

NEW ZEALAND: 1985

Smoking-attributed deaths (Sm.) and total deaths (Total)

		ALL CAUSES	ALL CANCER	Lung cancer	Upper aero-digestive ca.	Other cancer	COPD	Other respiratory	Vascular disease	Liver cirrhosis	Other medical	Non-medical
Males												
0–34	Sm.	–	–	–	–	–	–	–	–	–	–	–
	Total	1303	91	1	1	89	24	38	44	1	400	705
35–69	Sm.	1666	647	424	79	144	236	28	648	–	107	–
	Total	5416	1620	462	127	1031	315	114	2506	74	405	382
		(31%)	(40%)	(92%)	(62%)	(14%)	(75%)	(25%)	(26%)		(26%)	
70+	Sm.	1675	546	364	48	134	525	64	451	–	89	–
	Total	7815	1607	403	84	1120	732	586	3903	16	788	183
		(21%)	(34%)	(90%)	(57%)	(12%)	(72%)	(11%)	(12%)		(11%)	
Any age	Sm.	3341	1193	788	127	278	761	92	1099	–	196	–
	Total	14534	3318	866	212	2240	1071	738	6453	91	1593	1270
		(23%)	(36%)	(91%)	(60%)	(12%)	(71%)	(12%)	(17%)		(12%)	
Females												
0–34	Sm.	–	–	–	–	–	–	–	–	–	–	–
	Total	718	101	0	1	100	20	22	41	0	296	238
35–69	Sm.	663	207	158	16	33	147	12	226	–	71	–
	Total	3341	1363	201	34	1128	221	65	1154	30	348	160
		(20%)	(15%)	(79%)	(47%)	(3%)	(67%)	(18%)	(20%)		(20%)	
70+	Sm.	617	129	88	20	21	185	35	218	–	50	–
	Total	8891	1385	130	58	1197	341	908	4877	11	1112	257
		(7%)	(9%)	(68%)	(34%)	(2%)	(54%)	(4%)	(4%)		(4%)	
Any age	Sm.	1280	336	246	36	54	332	47	444	–	121	–
	Total	12950	2849	331	93	2425	582	995	6072	41	1756	655
		(10%)	(12%)	(74%)	(39%)	(2%)	(57%)	(5%)	(7%)		(7%)	
Males+Females												
0–34	Sm.	–	–	–	–	–	–	–	–	–	–	–
	Total	2021	192	1	2	189	44	60	85	1	696	943
35–69	Sm.	2329	854	582	95	177	383	40	874	–	178	–
	Total	8757	2983	663	161	2159	536	179	3660	104	753	542
		(27%)	(29%)	(88%)	(59%)	(8%)	(71%)	(22%)	(24%)		(24%)	
70+	Sm.	2292	675	452	68	155	710	99	669	–	139	–
	Total	16706	2992	533	142	2317	1073	1494	8780	27	1900	440
		(14%)	(23%)	(85%)	(48%)	(7%)	(66%)	(7%)	(8%)		(7%)	
Any age	Sm.	4621	1529	1034	163	332	1093	139	1543	–	317	–
	Total	27484	6167	1197	305	4665	1653	1733	12525	132	3349	1925
		(17%)	(25%)	(86%)	(53%)	(7%)	(66%)	(8%)	(12%)		(9%)	

(To be conservative, no deaths before age 35, and none from liver cirrhosis or non-medical causes, were attributed to smoking.)

NEW ZEALAND: 1990

Smoking–attributed deaths (Sm.) and total deaths (Total)

		ALL CAUSES	ALL CANCER	Lung cancer	Upper aero– digestive ca.	Other cancer	COPD	Other respiratory	Vascular disease	Liver cirrhosis	Other medical	Non– medical
Males												
0–34	Sm.	–	–	–	–	–	–	–	–	–	–	–
	Total	1369	97	1	6	90	14	18	57	1	395	787
35–69	Sm.	1395	616	414	67	135	142	13	508	–	116	–
	Total	4936	1598	455	112	1031	193	49	2135	56	469	436
		(28%)	(39%)	(91%)	(60%)	(13%)	(74%)	(27%)	(24%)		(25%)	
70+	Sm.	1673	622	405	51	166	463	46	444	–	98	–
	Total	7662	1853	447	87	1319	635	420	3722	14	833	185
		(22%)	(34%)	(91%)	(59%)	(13%)	(73%)	(11%)	(12%)		(12%)	
Any age	Sm.	3068	1238	819	118	301	605	59	952	–	214	–
	Total	13967	3548	903	205	2440	842	487	5914	71	1697	1408
		(22%)	(35%)	(91%)	(58%)	(12%)	(72%)	(12%)	(16%)		(13%)	
Females												
0–34	Sm.	–	–	–	–	–	–	–	–	–	–	–
	Total	636	81	2	0	79	9	9	34	2	272	229
35–69	Sm.	667	247	185	20	42	117	7	216	–	80	–
	Total	3242	1517	232	40	1245	168	35	984	27	362	149
		(21%)	(16%)	(80%)	(50%)	(3%)	(70%)	(20%)	(22%)		(22%)	
70+	Sm.	752	198	145	23	30	200	26	264	–	64	–
	Total	8679	1600	199	65	1336	350	680	4679	9	1166	195
		(9%)	(12%)	(73%)	(35%)	(2%)	(57%)	(4%)	(6%)		(5%)	
Any age	Sm.	1419	445	330	43	72	317	33	480	–	144	–
	Total	12557	3198	433	105	2660	527	724	5697	38	1800	573
		(11%)	(14%)	(76%)	(41%)	(3%)	(60%)	(5%)	(8%)		(8%)	
Males+Females												
0–34	Sm.	–	–	–	–	–	–	–	–	–	–	–
	Total	2005	178	3	6	169	23	27	91	3	667	1016
35–69	Sm.	2062	863	599	87	177	259	20	724	–	196	–
	Total	8178	3115	687	152	2276	361	84	3119	83	831	585
		(25%)	(28%)	(87%)	(57%)	(8%)	(72%)	(24%)	(23%)		(24%)	
70+	Sm.	2425	820	550	74	196	663	72	708	–	162	–
	Total	16341	3453	646	152	2655	985	1100	8401	23	1999	380
		(15%)	(24%)	(85%)	(49%)	(7%)	(67%)	(7%)	(8%)		(8%)	
Any age	Sm.	4487	1683	1149	161	373	922	92	1432	–	358	–
	Total	26524	6746	1336	310	5100	1369	1211	11611	109	3497	1981
		(17%)	(25%)	(86%)	(52%)	(7%)	(67%)	(8%)	(12%)		(10%)	

NEW ZEALAND: 1995

Smoking–attributed deaths (Sm.) and total deaths (Total)

		ALL CAUSES	ALL CANCER	Lung cancer	Upper aero– digestive ca.	Other cancer	COPD	Other respiratory	Vascular disease	Liver cirrhosis	Other medical	Non– medical
Males												
0–34	Sm.	–	–	–	–	–	–	–	–	–	–	–
	Total	1452	97	1	6	90	10	12	68	1	370	894
35–69	Sm.	1168	570	391	61	118	97	5	378	–	118	–
	Total	4450	1521	433	103	985	135	34	1726	41	516	477
		(26%)	(37%)	(90%)	(59%)	(12%)	(72%)	(15%)	(22%)		(23%)	
70+	Sm.	1622	687	445	51	191	384	36	415	–	100	–
	Total	7377	2089	491	87	1511	525	320	3419	13	839	172
		(22%)	(33%)	(91%)	(59%)	(13%)	(73%)	(11%)	(12%)		(12%)	
Any age	Sm.	2790	1257	836	112	309	481	41	793	–	218	–
	Total	13279	3707	925	196	2586	670	366	5213	55	1725	1543
		(21%)	(34%)	(90%)	(57%)	(12%)	(72%)	(11%)	(15%)		(13%)	
Females												
0–34	Sm.	–	–	–	–	–	–	–	–	–	–	–
	Total	539	65	3	0	62	6	5	25	1	229	208
35–69	Sm.	714	310	234	25	51	94	7	210	–	93	–
	Total	3243	1688	283	45	1360	130	31	845	25	380	144
		(22%)	(18%)	(83%)	(56%)	(4%)	(72%)	(23%)	(25%)		(24%)	
70+	Sm.	970	297	218	32	47	235	30	322	–	86	–
	Total	8099	1766	271	69	1426	356	526	4141	8	1146	156
		(12%)	(17%)	(80%)	(46%)	(3%)	(66%)	(6%)	(8%)		(8%)	
Any age	Sm.	1684	607	452	57	98	329	37	532	–	179	–
	Total	11881	3519	557	114	2848	492	562	5011	34	1755	508
		(14%)	(17%)	(81%)	(50%)	(3%)	(67%)	(7%)	(11%)		(10%)	
Males+Females												
0–34	Sm.	–	–	–	–	–	–	–	–	–	–	–
	Total	1991	162	4	6	152	16	17	93	2	599	1102
35–69	Sm.	1882	880	625	86	169	191	12	588	–	211	–
	Total	7693	3209	716	148	2345	265	65	2571	66	896	621
		(24%)	(27%)	(87%)	(58%)	(7%)	(72%)	(18%)	(23%)		(24%)	
70+	Sm.	2592	984	663	83	238	619	66	737	–	186	–
	Total	15476	3855	762	156	2937	881	846	7560	21	1985	328
		(17%)	(26%)	(87%)	(53%)	(8%)	(70%)	(8%)	(10%)		(9%)	
Any age	Sm.	4474	1864	1288	169	407	810	78	1325	–	397	–
	Total	25160	7226	1482	310	5434	1162	928	10224	89	3480	2051
		(18%)	(26%)	(87%)	(55%)	(7%)	(70%)	(8%)	(13%)		(11%)	

(To be conservative, no deaths before age 35, and none from liver cirrhosis or non–medical causes, were attributed to smoking.)

NORWAY: 1990

		No. of deaths			Standardised rates (Defined on p.448)			Annual death rates / 100, 000						
		All ages	0–34	35–69	All ages	0–34	35–69	0–4	5–9	10–14	15–19	20–24	25–29	30–34
ALL CAUSES	M	23885	1056	6888	986.7	96.6	964.5	215.9	23.5	28.7	87.0	87.8	106.4	127.2
	F	22156	495	3600	582.1	48.8	471.8	149.3	17.5	19.3	31.8	25.5	49.0	49.1
Tuberculosis	M	47	–	13	1.9	–	1.9	–	–	–	–	–	–	–
	F	29	–	7	0.8	–	0.8	–	–	–	–	–	–	–
Other infective	M	110	14	23	4.7	1.4	3.3	6.3	0.8	0.7	1.2	–	0.6	–
and parasitic	F	122	12	22	3.6	1.2	2.9	2.9	–	0.8	3.2	–	0.6	0.6
ALL CANCER	M	5285	82	1927	221.5	7.5	274.1	2.1	6.1	6.6	6.2	6.9	8.4	16.0
	F	4567	63	1670	150.0	6.0	219.8	4.4	3.2	0.8	5.8	2.4	8.9	16.1
Mouth and	M	109	4	57	4.9	0.3	8.0	–	–	–	0.6	–	1.2	0.6
pharynx cancer	F	41	1	14	1.4	0.1	1.8	–	–	–	–	–	–	0.6
Oesophagus cancer	M	97	–	50	4.5	–	7.4	–	–	–	–	–	–	–
	F	33	–	10	1.0	–	1.2	–	–	–	–	–	–	–
Stomach cancer	M	414	3	137	16.7	0.3	19.7	–	–	–	–	0.6	0.6	0.6
	F	279	1	65	7.8	0.1	8.5	–	–	–	–	–	–	0.6
Colorectal cancer	M	711	4	255	29.8	0.3	36.4	–	–	–	–	0.6	1.2	0.6
	F	755	2	216	22.3	0.2	28.6	–	–	–	0.6	–	0.6	–
Liver cancer	M	30	1	14	1.4	0.1	2.0	–	–	–	–	–	0.6	–
	F	18	–	7	0.6	–	0.9	–	–	–	–	–	–	–
Pancreas cancer	M	260	–	116	11.1	–	16.9	–	–	–	–	–	–	–
	F	288	–	80	8.6	–	10.6	–	–	–	–	–	–	–
Larynx cancer	M	27	–	11	1.1	–	1.6	–	–	–	–	–	–	–
	F	6	–	2	0.2	–	0.3	–	–	–	–	–	–	–
Lung cancer	M	1029	–	491	44.6	–	70.5	–	–	–	–	–	–	–
	F	411	1	212	15.2	0.1	28.4	–	–	–	–	–	–	0.6
Malignant melanoma	M	118	3	65	5.3	0.3	8.6	–	–	–	–	0.6	0.6	0.6
	F	77	6	38	3.0	0.5	4.9	–	–	–	0.6	0.6	0.6	1.9
Female breast cancer	F	760	10	346	27.2	0.9	45.0	–	–	–	–	–	3.2	3.2
Cervix cancer	F	126	4	67	5.1	0.4	8.7	–	–	–	–	0.6	–	1.9
Other uterine cancer	F	126	–	47	4.1	–	6.2	–	–	–	–	–	–	–
Ovarian cancer	F	280	4	138	10.6	0.4	18.5	–	–	–	–	–	1.3	1.3
Prostate cancer	M	951	–	152	36.7	–	22.4	–	–	–	–	–	–	–
Bladder cancer	M	237	–	50	9.5	–	7.4	–	–	–	–	–	–	–
	F	100	–	19	2.7	–	2.5	–	–	–	–	–	–	–
Other and ill-defined	M	835	39	332	35.7	3.6	46.3	0.7	3.8	3.7	1.9	2.3	2.4	10.4
cancer sites	F	824	12	268	26.0	1.2	35.4	2.2	1.6	0.8	1.3	–	1.3	1.3
Hodgkin's disease	M	10	–	8	0.5	–	1.1	–	–	–	–	–	–	–
	F	11	4	4	0.5	0.4	0.5	–	–	–	–	–	1.3	1.3
Myeloma and non-	M	298	8	122	12.8	0.7	16.8	–	0.8	0.7	2.5	–	0.6	0.6
Hodgkin lymphomas	F	291	4	98	9.3	0.4	12.8	0.7	–	–	0.6	–	0.6	0.6
Leukaemia	M	159	20	67	6.9	1.8	9.1	1.4	1.5	2.2	1.2	2.9	1.2	2.5
	F	141	14	39	4.5	1.3	4.9	1.5	1.6	–	2.6	1.2	–	2.6
ALL VASCULAR	M	11169	39	2970	452.7	3.4	425.6	–	–	0.7	3.1	2.9	6.6	10.4
DISEASE	F	10448	18	1009	246.1	1.7	133.6	1.5	–	–	1.3	1.2	5.1	2.6
Rheumatic heart	M	30	–	9	1.2	–	1.3	–	–	–	–	–	–	–
disease and fever	F	60	–	7	1.5	–	1.0	–	–	–	–	–	–	–
Hypertensive disease	M	211	1	60	8.4	0.1	8.8	–	–	–	–	–	–	0.6
	F	226	–	23	5.5	–	3.1	–	–	–	–	–	–	–
Ischaemic heart	M	6613	10	2187	274.1	0.9	313.8	–	–	–	0.6	–	1.2	4.3
disease	F	4633	2	574	113.7	0.2	76.5	–	–	–	–	–	1.3	–
Pulmonary embolism	M	134	1	26	5.4	0.1	3.6	–	–	0.7	–	–	–	–
and other venous	F	143	1	19	3.6	0.1	2.5	–	–	–	–	–	0.6	–
Cerebrovascular	M	2336	11	357	91.2	1.0	51.3	–	–	–	0.6	–	2.4	3.7
disease	F	3286	8	244	74.8	0.7	32.0	–	–	–	0.6	0.6	2.5	1.3
Other vascular	M	1845	16	331	72.6	1.4	46.8	–	–	–	1.9	2.9	3.0	1.8
disease	F	2100	7	142	47.0	0.7	18.6	1.5	–	–	0.6	0.6	0.6	1.3
Chronic obstructive	M	799	8	188	31.7	0.8	27.4	1.4	0.8	0.7	–	–	1.8	0.6
pulmonary disease	F	421	1	114	12.2	0.1	15.2	–	–	–	–	–	0.6	–
Other respiratory	M	1433	13	123	55.1	1.3	17.6	7.7	0.8	–	–	0.6	–	–
disease	F	1962	8	75	41.2	0.8	9.8	4.4	0.8	–	–	–	0.6	–
Peptic ulcer	M	123	1	32	4.9	0.1	4.6	–	–	–	–	–	–	0.6
	F	84	–	13	2.1	–	1.7	–	–	–	–	–	–	–
Liver cirrhosis	M	160	3	121	7.7	0.3	15.8	–	–	–	–	–	–	1.8
	F	80	3	46	3.2	0.3	6.2	–	–	–	–	0.6	0.6	0.6
Renal disease	M	169	–	25	6.6	–	3.6	–	–	–	–	–	–	–
	F	183	1	13	4.3	0.1	1.8	–	–	–	–	–	0.6	–
Pregnancy and birth	F	2	2	–	0.1	0.2	–	–	–	–	–	–	1.3	–
Congenital and	M	225	207	15	12.3	20.5	2.2	130.9	2.3	1.5	3.1	0.6	2.4	2.5
perinatal causes	F	157	135	11	8.7	14.1	1.4	90.0	2.4	4.6	–	1.2	0.6	–
Ill-defined causes	M	883	75	254	37.4	7.2	35.7	38.3	–	–	1.9	1.2	4.8	4.3
	F	823	48	76	20.7	4.9	10.0	28.6	–	0.8	0.6	1.8	1.3	1.3
Other medical causes	M	1803	115	514	74.8	10.4	69.0	13.9	3.0	2.9	3.7	7.5	18.6	22.7
	F	2274	60	299	57.0	5.8	38.7	6.6	3.2	4.6	0.6	4.3	11.5	9.7
ALL NON-	M	1679	499	683	75.3	44.0	83.7	15.3	9.8	15.4	67.7	68.1	63.1	68.2
MEDICAL CAUSES	F	1004	144	245	32.3	13.7	29.9	11.0	8.0	7.7	20.1	14.0	17.2	18.1
Motor vehicle	M	259	138	77	11.6	12.1	9.5	2.8	2.3	2.2	31.1	23.1	10.8	12.3
traffic accidents	F	76	31	31	3.4	2.9	3.7	2.2	0.8	1.5	7.1	3.0	3.2	2.6
Fire	M	48	8	25	2.1	0.7	3.1	0.7	0.8	0.7	–	–	0.6	2.5
	F	21	5	5	0.7	0.5	0.6	0.7	1.6	0.8	–	–	–	0.6
Suicide	M	488	170	259	22.7	14.7	31.5	–	–	2.9	16.8	27.1	29.5	26.4
	F	171	39	107	7.8	3.6	13.0	–	–	–	8.4	4.3	4.5	7.8
Homicide	M	37	16	20	1.8	1.4	2.4	0.7	0.8	–	1.9	2.3	2.4	1.8
	F	12	7	5	0.6	0.6	0.5	0.7	–	–	–	1.2	1.3	1.3
POPULATION (thousands):	M=males				2097.3	1074.9	832.7	143.6	132.0	136.1	161.0	173.2	166.3	162.7
	F=females				2144.2	1022.4	830.9	136.6	125.5	129.6	154.3	164.5	157.1	154.8

NORWAY: 1990

Annual death rates / 100, 000 — 9th ICD categories

35–39	40–44	45–49	50–54	55–59	60–64	65–69	70–74	75–79	80+/NK			
163.2	233.8	362.9	541.0	1030.4	1676.1	2743.9	4609.3	7286.2	15335.2	M	ALL CAUSES	001–999
85.1	127.0	203.1	283.2	491.5	836.5	1276.4	2322.9	4186.4	11602.9	F		
–	–	0.8	–	2.2	2.1	8.1	16.3	19.2	18.9	M	Tuberculosis	010–018, 137
–	0.7	0.8	–	–	–	4.4	4.9	7.2	10.5	F		
–	–	2.4	5.1	3.3	4.2	8.1	17.6	33.2	75.8	M	Other infective	Rest of 001–139
–	1.3	0.8	4.1	3.2	3.0	8.0	12.7	20.3	55.2	F	and parasitic	
24.8	42.5	96.4	144.6	289.9	499.5	821.1	1226.1	1691.1	2520.8	M	ALL CANCER	140–208
41.6	58.9	116.3	161.4	245.7	406.9	507.5	701.6	939.1	1267.6	F		
–	1.2	6.3	7.1	8.7	12.5	20.3	18.8	33.2	26.5	M	Mouth and	140–149
0.7	1.3	0.8	3.0	1.1	2.0	3.5	6.8	9.6	10.5	F	pharynx cancer	
–	–	1.6	8.1	13.0	12.5	16.3	26.4	24.4	22.7	M	Oesophagus cancer	150
0.7	0.7	0.8	1.0	–	2.0	3.5	2.9	13.1	8.6	F		
1.3	1.8	3.1	8.1	11.9	32.4	79.3	82.9	151.8	229.2	M	Stomach cancer	151
–	1.3	7.4	5.1	5.3	11.8	28.3	45.0	52.6	117.1	F		
4.4	5.5	7.8	23.3	41.3	65.8	106.7	134.4	235.6	397.7	M	Colorectal cancer	153, 154
2.7	3.9	11.5	17.3	27.7	53.2	84.1	110.6	170.8	267.6	F		
–	–	1.6	1.0	6.5	2.1	3.0	6.3	8.7	9.5	M	Liver cancer	155.0
–	–	–	1.0	–	3.0	2.7	2.0	2.4	6.7	F		
–	0.6	4.7	7.1	16.3	34.5	54.9	71.6	64.6	94.7	M	Pancreas cancer	157
0.7	1.3	5.7	3.0	12.8	20.7	30.1	59.7	66.9	86.7	F		
–	–	0.8	–	3.3	1.0	6.1	7.5	7.0	11.4	M	Larynx cancer	161
–	–	0.8	–	1.1	–	–	1.0	2.4	1.0	F		
2.5	9.2	21.9	38.4	74.9	135.8	210.4	309.0	279.2	250.0	M	Lung cancer	162
2.7	5.9	7.4	17.3	38.3	60.1	67.3	74.4	69.3	61.0	F		
1.3	5.5	7.8	4.0	10.9	15.7	15.2	23.9	31.4	24.6	M	Malignant melanoma	172
4.7	0.7	4.9	1.0	9.6	7.9	5.3	8.8	10.8	14.3	F		
9.4	19.6	34.4	35.5	50.0	84.7	81.5	107.6	130.2	176.2	F	Female breast cancer	174
3.4	2.6	9.0	13.2	6.4	15.8	10.6	17.6	20.3	19.0	F	Cervix cancer	180
0.7	0.7	4.9	4.1	7.4	10.8	15.1	18.6	29.9	33.3	F	Other uterine cancer	179, 182
1.3	5.2	10.6	18.3	29.8	29.6	34.5	41.1	49.0	52.4	F	Ovarian cancer	183
–	–	0.8	3.0	19.5	41.8	91.5	196.0	410.1	772.7	M	Prostate cancer	185
–	–	0.8	5.1	8.7	13.6	23.4	57.8	90.8	168.6	M	Bladder cancer	188
0.7	0.7	0.8	–	3.2	4.9	7.1	13.7	25.1	43.8	F		
11.4	9.2	19.6	28.3	46.7	82.5	126.0	183.4	244.3	337.1	M	Other and ill-defined	Rest of 140–208
9.4	7.2	11.5	25.4	41.5	68.0	85.0	117.4	178.0	261.9	F	cancer sites	
0.6	–	0.8	1.0	2.2	1.0	2.0	2.5	–	–	M	Hodgkin's disease	201
–	1.3	–	1.0	1.1	–	–	1.0	1.2	1.0	F		
1.9	6.2	11.0	8.1	17.4	32.4	40.7	79.1	82.0	109.8	M	Myeloma and non–	200, 202–203
2.0	4.6	2.5	12.2	8.5	22.7	37.2	52.8	76.5	67.6	F	Hodgkin lymphomas	
1.3	3.1	7.8	2.0	8.7	15.7	25.4	26.4	27.9	66.3	M	Leukaemia	204–208
2.7	2.0	3.3	3.0	2.1	9.9	11.5	20.5	31.1	39.0	F		
28.6	52.3	127.7	210.3	461.5	784.7	1314.0	2386.9	3794.1	7738.6	M	ALL VASCULAR	390–459
8.0	15.7	30.3	50.8	118.1	256.2	456.2	1084.1	2211.5	6154.3	F	DISEASE	
–	–	–	–	–	3.1	6.1	3.8	14.0	18.9	M	Rheumatic heart	390–398
–	–	–	–	1.1	3.0	2.7	14.7	15.5	23.8	F	disease and fever	
–	–	1.6	1.0	5.4	14.6	38.6	40.2	87.3	128.8	M	Hypertensive disease	401–405
–	0.7	–	3.0	5.3	4.9	8.0	21.5	55.0	128.6	F		
16.5	37.5	98.0	166.8	356.1	576.8	945.1	1559.0	2174.5	3653.4	M	Ischaemic heart	410–414
3.4	5.2	13.1	32.5	64.9	158.6	257.8	565.6	1102.7	2434.3	F	disease	
1.3	0.6	1.6	3.0	6.5	4.2	8.1	32.7	54.1	94.7	M	Pulmonary embolism	415.1, 451–453
–	2.0	0.8	1.0	4.3	3.0	6.2	18.6	31.1	74.3	F	and other venous	
4.4	6.2	10.2	22.2	52.1	93.0	170.7	405.8	834.2	2210.2	M	Cerebrovascular	430–438
1.3	5.9	10.6	13.2	24.5	53.2	115.1	297.5	653.5	2079.0	F	disease	
6.3	8.0	16.5	17.2	41.3	93.0	145.3	345.5	630.0	1632.6	M	Other vascular	Rest of 390–459
3.4	2.0	5.7	1.0	18.1	33.5	66.4	166.3	353.6	1414.3	F	disease	
0.6	0.6	3.1	10.1	21.7	53.3	102.6	201.0	338.6	471.6	M	Chronic obstructive	490–496
2.0	1.3	–	9.1	14.9	27.6	51.4	66.5	101.6	145.7	F	pulmonary disease	
0.6	2.5	3.1	11.1	10.9	26.1	69.1	162.1	404.9	1772.7	M	Other respiratory	Rest of 460–519
0.7	1.3	1.6	2.0	8.5	12.8	41.6	78.3	222.2	1536.2	F	disease	
0.6	0.6	–	–	6.5	8.4	16.3	23.9	33.2	98.5	M	Peptic ulcer	531–533
–	–	0.8	2.0	1.1	1.0	7.1	4.9	19.1	47.6	F		
3.8	12.3	12.5	13.1	16.3	24.0	28.5	18.8	17.5	20.8	M	Liver cirrhosis	571
–	1.3	3.3	6.1	8.5	8.9	15.1	13.7	6.0	11.4	F		
–	1.2	0.8	2.0	5.4	5.2	10.2	28.9	47.1	178.0	M	Renal disease	580–590
–	–	0.8	2.0	2.1	3.0	4.4	20.5	33.5	114.3	F		
–	–	–	–	–	–	–	–	–	–	F	Pregnancy and birth	630–676
–	0.6	0.8	2.0	5.4	4.2	2.0	1.3	1.7	1.9	M	Congenital and	740–779
1.3	0.7	0.8	1.0	3.2	2.0	0.9	2.9	6.0	2.9	F	perinatal causes	
5.1	8.6	13.3	22.2	44.5	53.3	102.6	118.1	205.9	647.7	M	Ill-defined causes	780–799
2.0	2.6	1.6	5.1	12.8	18.7	27.5	59.7	109.9	520.0	F		
29.2	31.4	29.0	52.6	66.2	114.9	159.6	257.5	511.3	1280.3	M	Other medical causes	Rest of 001–799
9.4	12.4	13.9	16.2	37.2	64.0	117.8	206.5	412.2	1294.3	F		
69.8	81.2	72.9	67.7	96.6	96.1	101.6	150.8	188.5	509.5	M	ALL NON–	E800–E999
20.1	30.8	31.9	23.4	36.2	32.5	34.5	66.5	98.0	442.9	F	MEDICAL CAUSES	
9.5	5.5	11.8	7.1	11.9	13.6	7.1	16.3	19.2	37.9	M	Motor vehicle	E810–E819
2.7	6.5	1.6	3.0	6.4	3.9	1.8	7.8	1.2	4.8	F	traffic accidents	
3.2	2.5	0.8	2.0	2.2	2.1	9.1	2.5	7.0	17.0	M	Fire	E890–E899
–	1.3	–	–	–	–	2.7	3.9	1.2	5.7	F		
28.6	30.8	29.0	27.3	35.8	32.4	36.6	31.4	34.9	26.5	M	Suicide	E950–E959
8.7	11.8	18.8	8.1	12.8	12.8	17.7	9.8	8.4	7.6	F		
1.9	1.8	4.7	1.0	3.3	1.0	3.0	–	1.7	–	M	Homicide	E960–E969
0.7	1.3	0.8	1.0	–	–	–	–	–	–	F		
157.5	162.5	127.6	98.9	92.1	95.7	98.4	79.6	57.3	52.8	M	POPULATION (thousands)	
149.2	152.7	122.1	98.5	94.0	101.5	112.9	102.2	83.7	105.0	F		

NORWAY: Males

	All ages	0–34	35–69	35–39	40–44	45–49	50–54	55–59	60–64	65–69	70–74	75–79	80+/NK
POPULATION (1000s)													
1955	1706.3	916.7	690.9	128.8	124.4	113.0	102.1	91.7	74.2	56.7	41.6	30.9	26.2
1965	1855.0	971.9	759.7	113.3	130.0	125.0	118.8	105.4	91.2	76.0	56.1	35.9	31.4
1975	1990.5	1095.3	746.2	103.4	100.2	110.6	124.6	116.0	105.1	86.3	65.8	45.1	38.1
1985	2053.3	1075.3	800.0	163.6	129.6	101.5	96.3	102.8	110.5	95.7	77.0	52.8	48.2
1990	**2097.3**	**1074.9**	**832.7**	**157.5**	**162.5**	**127.6**	**98.9**	**92.1**	**95.7**	**98.4**	**79.6**	**57.3**	**52.8**
1995 projected	*2111.2*	*1043.4*	*866.6*	*160.6*	*156.5*	*160.9*	*117.5*	*93.0*	*89.3*	*88.8*	*84.4*	*59.8*	*57.0*
NUMBER OF DEATHS													
All causes													
1955	14841	1704	5448	253	325	435	703	1041	1232	1459	1710	2120	3859
1965	19190	1505	7413	212	406	542	908	1229	1760	2356	2657	2704	4911
1975	21894	1271	7927	176	279	502	908	1385	2040	2637	3309	3508	5879
1985	23783	1096	7535	261	319	402	674	1134	2012	2733	3732	4154	7266
1990	**23885**	**1056**	**6888**	**257**	**380**	**463**	**535**	**949**	**1604**	**2700**	**3669**	**4175**	**8097**
1995 projected	*23732*	*948*	*6246*	*263*	*347*	*497*	*558*	*859*	*1411*	*2311*	*3657*	*4198*	*8683*
Lung cancer													
1955	168	1	134	2	6	6	27	40	30	23	14	9	10
1965	369	2	267	1	12	21	39	38	75	81	53	36	11
1975	683	–	415	2	9	13	56	82	117	136	140	78	50
1985	987	1	520	7	9	14	38	97	157	198	215	148	103
1990	**1029**	–	**491**	**4**	**15**	**28**	**38**	**69**	**130**	**207**	**246**	**160**	**132**
1995 projected	*1073*	–	*473*	*4*	*19*	*40*	*40*	*62*	*114*	*194*	*271*	*176*	*153*
ANNUAL DEATH RATE / 100,000 (*The rates for the age groups 0–34 and 35–69 are the means of seven five-yearly rates, but the all-ages rates are standardised to the conventional "European" age distribution)													
All causes													
1955	1007.9*	174.6*	985.7*	196.4	261.3	385.0	688.5	1135.2	1660.4	2573.2	4110.6	6860.8	14729.0
1965	1093.7*	151.3*	1127.6*	187.1	312.3	433.6	764.3	1166.0	1929.8	3100.0	4736.2	7532.0	15640.1
1975	1080.2*	116.5*	1117.4*	170.2	278.4	453.9	728.7	1194.0	1941.0	3055.6	5028.9	7778.3	15430.4
1985	1034.4*	104.2*	1040.2*	159.5	246.1	396.1	699.9	1103.1	1820.8	2855.8	4846.8	7867.4	15074.7
1990	**986.7***	**96.6***	**964.5***	**163.2**	**233.8**	**362.9**	**541.0**	**1030.4**	**1676.1**	**2743.9**	**4609.3**	**7286.2**	**15335.2**
1995 projected	*941.1**	*89.3**	*896.5**	*163.8*	*221.7*	*308.9*	*474.9*	*923.7*	*1580.1*	*2602.5*	*4332.9*	*7020.1*	*15233.3*
All cancer													
1955	184.6*	12.9*	250.8*	28.0	57.9	78.8	170.4	330.4	451.5	638.4	944.7	1281.6	1637.4
1965	194.8*	13.0*	254.8*	28.2	61.5	100.0	164.1	269.4	461.6	698.7	1021.4	1437.3	1847.1
1975	208.9*	10.0*	265.6*	21.3	52.9	78.7	170.1	300.9	487.2	748.6	1095.7	1598.7	2204.7
1985	228.8*	6.9*	279.1*	27.5	52.5	86.7	171.3	299.6	496.8	819.2	1288.3	1863.6	2506.2
1990	**221.5***	**7.5***	**274.1***	**24.8**	**42.5**	**96.4**	**144.6**	**289.9**	**499.5**	**821.1**	**1226.1**	**1691.1**	**2520.8**
1995 projected	*212.5**	*7.4**	*265.5**	*20.5*	*41.5*	*88.9*	*135.3*	*277.4*	*493.8*	*800.7*	*1161.1*	*1605.4*	*2424.6*
Lung cancer													
1955	11.3*	0.1*	23.2*	1.6	4.8	5.3	26.4	43.6	40.4	40.6	33.7	29.1	38.2
1965	20.4*	0.3*	40.7*	0.9	9.2	16.8	32.8	36.1	82.2	106.6	94.5	100.3	35.0
1975	33.3*	–	58.2*	1.9	9.0	11.8	44.9	70.7	111.3	157.6	212.8	172.9	131.2
1985	43.9*	0.1*	72.5*	4.3	6.9	13.8	39.5	94.4	142.1	206.9	279.2	280.3	213.7
1990	**44.6***	–	**70.5***	**2.5**	**9.2**	**21.9**	**38.4**	**74.9**	**135.8**	**210.4**	**309.0**	**279.2**	**250.0**
1995 projected	*45.2**	–	*69.5**	*2.5*	*12.1*	*24.9*	*34.0*	*66.7*	*127.7*	*218.5*	*321.1*	*294.3*	*268.4*
Upper aerodigestive cancer (mouth, oesophagus, pharynx and larynx)													
1955	11.0*	0.2*	13.8*	1.6	3.2	0.9	5.9	21.8	29.6	33.5	72.1	93.9	95.4
1965	9.8*	–	15.1*	–	3.1	2.4	8.4	24.7	20.8	46.1	53.5	75.2	70.1
1975	9.7*	–	13.3*	–	3.0	7.2	8.0	11.2	25.7	38.2	48.6	71.0	102.4
1985	9.1*	–	14.5*	0.6	–	4.9	15.6	10.7	29.0	40.8	42.9	54.9	76.8
1990	**10.5***	**0.3***	**17.0***	–	**1.2**	**8.6**	**15.2**	**25.0**	**26.1**	**42.7**	**52.8**	**64.6**	**60.6**
1995 projected	*11.8**	*0.1**	*19.8**	–	*1.9*	*10.6*	*20.4*	*29.0*	*30.2*	*46.2*	*60.4*	*68.6*	*56.1*
Other cancer													
1955	162.3*	12.6*	213.7*	24.8	49.8	72.6	138.1	265.0	381.4	564.4	838.9	1158.6	1503.8
1965	164.6*	12.8*	199.1*	27.4	49.2	80.8	122.9	208.7	358.6	546.1	873.4	1261.8	1742.0
1975	165.9*	10.0*	194.1*	19.3	40.9	59.7	117.2	219.0	350.1	552.7	834.3	1354.8	1971.1
1985	175.8*	6.8*	192.0*	22.6	45.5	68.0	116.3	194.6	325.8	571.6	966.2	1528.4	2215.8
1990	**166.4***	**7.1***	**186.7***	**22.2**	**32.0**	**65.8**	**91.0**	**190.0**	**337.5**	**568.1**	**864.3**	**1347.3**	**2210.2**
1995 projected	*155.6**	*7.3**	*176.2**	*18.1*	*27.5*	*53.4*	*80.9*	*181.7*	*335.9*	*536.0*	*779.6*	*1242.5*	*2100.0*
Chronic obstructive pulmonary disease (COPD)													
1955	8.8*	0.4*	12.2*	0.8	2.4	3.5	5.9	10.9	17.5	44.1	31.3	42.1	129.8
1965	12.9*	0.2*	17.4*	–	3.1	3.2	10.1	15.2	29.6	60.5	64.2	103.1	143.3
1975	23.6*	0.1*	26.2*	1.0	5.0	7.2	12.0	23.3	44.7	90.4	148.9	195.1	307.1
1985	35.7*	1.0*	32.9*	1.2	2.3	8.9	10.4	27.2	76.9	103.4	215.6	333.3	541.5
1990	**31.7***	**0.8***	**27.4***	**0.6**	**0.6**	**3.1**	**10.1**	**21.7**	**53.3**	**102.6**	**201.0**	**338.6**	**471.6**
1995 projected	*29.1**	*0.5**	*23.5**	*0.6*	*0.6*	*2.5*	*7.7*	*16.1*	*44.8*	*92.3*	*196.7*	*324.4*	*436.8*
Other respiratory disease													
1955	45.8*	10.8*	18.7*	3.9	3.2	7.1	7.8	16.4	32.3	60.0	117.8	255.7	1232.8
1965	59.5*	4.4*	23.2*	2.6	2.3	7.2	10.9	11.4	25.2	102.6	192.5	454.0	1726.1
1975	71.6*	5.0*	24.6*	1.9	3.0	6.3	9.6	21.6	38.1	91.5	290.3	572.1	2023.6
1985	53.4*	1.9*	11.7*	2.4	0.8	3.9	5.2	7.8	24.4	37.6	151.9	416.7	1771.8
1990	**55.1***	**1.3***	**17.6***	**0.6**	**2.5**	**3.1**	**11.1**	**10.9**	**26.1**	**69.1**	**162.1**	**404.9**	**1772.7**
1995 projected	*56.2**	*1.0**	*22.2**	*0.6*	*1.9*	*4.4*	*15.3*	*14.0*	*37.0*	*82.2*	*169.4*	*386.3*	*1764.9*
Vascular disease													
1955	448.9*	5.8*	434.5*	31.1	46.6	123.0	245.8	460.2	774.9	1359.8	2156.3	3899.7	7568.7
1965	532.2*	5.2*	553.4*	39.7	100.0	156.8	327.4	603.4	997.8	1648.7	2600.7	4270.2	8522.3
1975	530.2*	3.0*	552.4*	30.9	90.8	198.9	310.6	565.5	988.6	1681.3	2712.8	4261.6	8364.8
1985	494.3*	3.7*	498.7*	31.2	71.0	144.8	312.6	530.2	905.9	1495.3	2585.7	4223.5	7713.7
1990	**452.7***	**3.4***	**425.6***	**28.6**	**52.3**	**127.7**	**210.3**	**461.5**	**784.7**	**1314.0**	**2386.9**	**3794.1**	**7738.6**
1995 projected	*413.4**	*3.8**	*364.9**	*22.4*	*42.8*	*92.6*	*165.1*	*378.5*	*679.7*	*1173.4*	*2144.5*	*3571.9*	*7478.9*
Liver cirrhosis													
1955	4.0*	0.1*	6.5*	0.8	–	3.5	7.8	15.3	10.8	7.1	21.6	22.7	11.5
1965	5.5*	0.3*	9.4*	0.9	4.6	2.4	8.4	15.2	20.8	13.2	21.4	22.3	31.8
1975	6.3*	0.1*	13.1*	2.9	2.0	5.4	12.0	14.7	31.4	23.2	21.3	17.7	18.4
1985	10.1*	0.6*	20.1*	6.1	10.0	17.7	23.9	20.4	36.2	26.1	14.3	41.7	20.7
1990	**7.7***	**0.3***	**15.8***	**3.8**	**12.3**	**12.5**	**13.1**	**16.3**	**24.0**	**28.5**	**18.8**	**17.5**	**20.8**
1995 projected	*6.1**	*0.2**	*12.8**	*3.1*	*10.2*	*9.3*	*9.4*	*11.8*	*20.2*	*25.9*	*14.2*	*13.4*	*14.0*
Other medical causes													
1955	239.0*	88.2*	183.8*	73.8	78.0	93.8	165.5	205.0	291.1	379.2	728.4	1181.2	3748.1
1965	209.7*	73.2*	183.7*	60.0	69.2	84.8	154.9	165.1	305.9	446.1	702.3	1069.6	2929.9
1975	157.3*	43.0*	149.0*	35.8	47.9	67.8	122.0	180.2	267.4	322.1	609.4	913.5	2060.4
1985	132.4*	41.4*	111.1*	24.4	40.1	46.3	76.8	124.5	180.1	285.3	479.2	787.9	1946.1
1990	**142.7***	**39.5***	**120.2***	**34.9**	**42.5**	**47.0**	**83.9**	**133.6**	**192.3**	**306.9**	**463.6**	**851.7**	**2301.1**
1995 projected	*153.1**	*36.9**	*126.1**	*44.2*	*46.0*	*49.1*	*86.8*	*140.9*	*204.9*	*310.8*	*482.2*	*941.5*	*2654.4*
All non-medical causes													
1955	76.8*	56.3*	79.4*	58.2	73.2	75.2	85.2	97.1	82.2	84.7	110.6	178.0	400.8
1965	79.1*	54.9*	85.7*	55.6	71.5	79.2	88.4	86.3	88.8	130.3	133.7	175.5	439.5
1975	82.2*	55.4*	86.5*	76.4	76.8	89.5	92.3	87.9	83.7	98.5	150.5	219.5	451.4
1985	79.6*	48.7*	86.6*	66.6	69.4	87.7	99.7	93.4	100.5	88.8	111.7	200.8	574.7
1990	**75.3***	**44.0***	**83.7***	**69.8**	**81.2**	**72.9**	**67.7**	**96.6**	**96.1**	**101.6**	**150.8**	**188.5**	**509.5**
1995 projected	*70.7**	*39.4**	*81.4**	*72.2*	*78.6*	*62.2*	*55.3*	*84.9*	*99.7*	*117.1*	*164.7*	*177.3*	*459.6*

NORWAY: Females

	All ages	0–34	35–69	35–39	40–44	45–49	50–54	55–59	60–64	65–69	70–74	75–79	80+/NK
POPULATION (1000s)													
1955	1722.5	874.8	722.2	127.7	123.2	115.3	108.4	98.9	81.9	66.8	52.2	38.3	35.0
1965	1867.9	926.3	783.8	110.0	128.1	125.6	119.5	110.7	101.4	88.5	67.4	46.6	43.8
1975	2016.7	1037.3	767.3	100.4	97.7	108.7	125.4	121.1	113.0	101.0	86.1	64.6	61.4
1985	2099.3	1024.3	807.1	153.1	123.0	99.8	96.0	105.1	118.8	111.3	97.8	78.2	91.9
1990	**2144.2**	**1022.4**	**830.9**	**149.2**	**152.7**	**122.1**	**98.5**	**94.0**	**101.5**	**112.9**	**102.2**	**83.7**	**105.0**
1995 projected	*2159.7*	*993.7*	*857.8*	*154.5*	*148.5*	*151.9*	*113.8*	*94.8*	*94.2*	*100.1*	*107.1*	*88.9*	*112.2*
NUMBER OF DEATHS													
All causes													
1955	14258	1056	3974	167	226	307	460	636	888	1290	1706	2297	5225
1965	16127	834	4208	114	188	317	404	660	1059	1466	2200	2671	6214
1975	18167	630	4121	76	140	235	468	668	1009	1525	2284	3347	7785
1985	20589	519	3723	116	164	212	317	531	985	1398	2352	3366	10629
1990	**22156**	**495**	**3600**	**127**	**194**	**248**	**279**	**462**	**849**	**1441**	**2374**	**3504**	**12183**
1995 projected	*22973*	*447*	*3404*	*131*	*185*	*278*	*299*	*453*	*794*	*1264*	*2430*	*3611*	*13081*
Lung cancer													
1955	66	3	43	2	1	3	4	6	17	10	7	10	3
1965	65	2	38	1	–	3	6	7	11	10	8	9	8
1975	160	1	93	–	1	8	12	22	25	25	21	17	28
1985	326	–	163	3	3	12	14	42	48	41	63	52	48
1990	**411**	**1**	**212**	**4**	**9**	**9**	**17**	**36**	**61**	**76**	**76**	**58**	**64**
1995 projected	*507*	*1*	*260*	*6*	*8*	*11*	*18*	*44*	*79*	*94*	*99*	*72*	*75*
ANNUAL DEATH RATE / 100,000 (*The rates for the age groups 0–34 and 35–69 are the means of seven five-yearly rates, but the all-ages rates are standardised to the conventional "European" age distribution)													
All causes													
1955	815.5*	109.8*	666.2*	130.8	183.4	266.3	424.4	643.1	1084.2	1931.1	3268.2	5997.4	14928.6
1965	754.3*	84.1*	591.1*	103.6	146.8	252.4	338.1	596.2	1044.4	1656.5	3264.1	5731.8	14187.2
1975	663.4*	60.7*	537.5*	75.7	143.3	216.2	373.2	551.6	892.9	1509.9	2652.7	5181.1	12679.2
1985	592.0*	53.4*	477.5*	75.8	133.3	212.4	330.2	505.2	829.1	1256.1	2404.9	4304.3	11565.8
1990	**582.1***	**48.8***	**471.8***	**85.1**	**127.0**	**203.1**	**283.2**	**491.5**	**836.5**	**1276.4**	**2322.9**	**4186.4**	**11602.9**
1995 projected	*573.2**	*45.4**	*462.7**	*84.8*	*124.6*	*183.0*	*262.7*	*477.8*	*842.9*	*1262.7*	*2268.9*	*4061.9*	*11658.6*
All cancer													
1955	160.1*	14.0*	225.9*	49.3	81.2	124.0	215.9	287.2	356.5	467.1	689.7	968.7	1317.1
1965	142.7*	8.0*	203.9*	43.6	60.1	121.0	149.8	258.4	371.8	422.6	670.6	871.2	1200.9
1975	145.8*	6.7*	219.6*	33.9	73.7	112.2	195.4	278.3	375.2	468.3	602.8	849.8	1210.1
1985	150.6*	7.1*	216.7*	34.0	73.2	111.2	167.7	263.6	405.7	461.8	697.3	923.3	1303.6
1990	**150.0***	**6.0***	**219.8***	**41.6**	**58.9**	**116.3**	**161.4**	**245.7**	**406.9**	**507.5**	**701.6**	**939.1**	**1267.6**
1995 projected	*149.7**	*5.4**	*220.6**	*38.2*	*56.6*	*107.3*	*154.7*	*240.5*	*421.4*	*525.5*	*722.7*	*932.5*	*1255.8*
Lung cancer													
1955	3.9*	0.4*	7.2*	1.6	0.8	2.6	3.7	6.1	20.8	15.0	13.4	26.1	8.6
1965	3.2*	0.2*	5.3*	0.9	–	2.4	5.0	6.3	10.8	11.3	11.9	19.3	18.3
1975	6.7*	0.1*	11.9*	–	1.0	7.4	9.6	18.2	22.1	24.8	24.4	26.3	45.6
1985	12.4*	–	21.2*	2.0	2.4	12.0	14.6	40.0	40.4	36.8	64.4	66.5	52.2
1990	**15.2***	**0.1***	**28.4***	**2.7**	**5.9**	**7.4**	**17.3**	**38.3**	**60.1**	**67.3**	**74.4**	**69.3**	**61.0**
1995 projected	*18.8**	*0.1**	*36.6**	*3.9*	*5.4*	*7.2*	*15.8*	*46.4*	*83.9*	*93.9*	*92.4*	*81.0*	*66.8*
Upper aerodigestive cancer (mouth, oesophagus, pharynx and larynx)													
1955	2.9*	–	2.7*	–	–	–	–	5.1	3.7	10.5	23.0	23.5	42.9
1965	2.7*	–	2.8*	0.9	–	0.8	2.5	4.5	3.9	6.8	16.3	32.2	27.4
1975	2.8*	–	3.6*	1.0	1.0	0.9	4.0	4.1	6.2	7.9	7.0	29.4	30.9
1985	2.7*	–	3.9*	–	1.6	–	3.1	2.9	5.9	13.5	11.2	19.2	30.5
1990	**2.6***	**0.1***	**3.3***	**1.3**	**2.0**	**2.5**	**4.1**	**2.1**	**3.9**	**7.1**	**10.8**	**25.1**	**20.0**
1995 projected	*2.6**	–	*3.4**	*1.9*	*2.7*	*3.3*	*5.3*	*2.1*	*3.2*	*5.0*	*10.3*	*24.7*	*17.8*
Other cancer													
1955	153.3*	13.6*	215.9*	47.8	80.4	121.4	212.2	276.0	332.1	441.6	653.3	919.1	1265.7
1965	136.8*	7.7*	195.9*	41.8	60.1	117.8	142.3	247.5	357.0	404.5	642.4	819.7	1155.3
1975	136.4*	6.6*	204.1*	32.9	71.6	104.0	181.8	256.0	346.9	435.6	571.4	794.1	1133.6
1985	135.5*	7.1*	191.7*	32.0	69.1	99.2	150.0	220.7	359.4	411.5	621.7	837.6	1220.9
1990	**132.2***	**5.8***	**188.1***	**37.5**	**51.1**	**106.5**	**140.1**	**205.3**	**342.9**	**433.1**	**616.4**	**844.7**	**1186.7**
1995 projected	*128.3**	*5.4**	*180.6**	*32.4*	*48.5*	*96.8*	*133.6*	*192.0*	*334.4*	*426.6*	*620.0*	*826.8*	*1171.1*
Chronic obstructive pulmonary disease (COPD)													
1955	6.8*	0.4*	5.7*	–	2.4	0.9	2.8	2.0	12.2	19.5	34.5	44.4	140.0
1965	4.9*	0.6*	4.8*	–	0.8	3.2	1.7	5.4	5.9	16.9	16.3	30.0	89.0
1975	9.5*	0.4*	10.4*	1.0	2.0	2.8	4.8	14.9	19.5	27.7	39.5	88.2	133.6
1985	14.1*	0.7*	15.9*	2.0	0.8	4.0	7.3	20.0	30.3	46.7	77.7	99.7	192.6
1990	**12.2***	**0.1***	**15.2***	**2.0**	**1.3**	–	**9.1**	**14.9**	**27.6**	**51.4**	**66.5**	**101.6**	**145.7**
1995 projected	*11.2**	*0.1**	*14.1**	*2.6*	*0.7*	–	*7.0*	*13.7*	*26.5*	*48.0*	*64.4*	*99.0*	*123.9*
Other respiratory disease													
1955	46.3*	8.8*	15.8*	3.1	5.7	5.2	8.3	7.1	24.4	56.9	97.7	349.9	1305.7
1965	55.3*	5.0*	14.2*	0.9	2.3	2.4	3.3	13.6	23.7	53.1	173.6	409.9	1719.2
1975	58.4*	2.3*	14.9*	3.0	3.1	4.6	9.6	13.2	19.5	51.5	144.0	490.7	1890.9
1985	41.4*	1.4*	7.0*	–	0.8	2.0	–	4.8	12.6	28.8	85.9	236.6	1553.9
1990	**41.2***	**0.8***	**9.8***	**0.7**	**1.3**	**1.6**	**2.0**	**8.5**	**12.8**	**41.6**	**78.3**	**222.2**	**1536.2**
1995 projected	*40.9**	*0.6**	*11.2**	*0.6*	*1.3*	*2.0*	*2.6*	*11.6*	*17.0*	*43.0*	*75.6*	*218.2*	*1508.9*
Vascular disease													
1955	382.3*	3.0*	270.9*	14.9	25.2	56.4	104.2	227.5	486.0	982.0	1858.2	3574.4	8117.1
1965	370.0*	2.2*	237.1*	17.3	28.9	46.2	94.6	202.3	431.0	839.5	1866.5	3478.5	8148.4
1975	313.6*	2.2*	193.5*	7.0	23.5	42.3	78.1	144.5	336.3	722.8	1461.1	3020.1	7167.8
1985	260.3*	2.2*	145.3*	7.8	16.3	38.1	70.8	131.3	239.1	513.9	1187.1	2347.8	6343.9
1990	**246.1***	**1.7***	**133.6***	**8.0**	**15.7**	**30.3**	**50.8**	**118.1**	**256.2**	**456.2**	**1084.1**	**2211.5**	**6154.3**
1995 projected	*231.2**	*1.3**	*121.6**	*7.1*	*13.5*	*23.0*	*41.3*	*112.9*	*237.8*	*415.6*	*997.2*	*2048.4*	*5922.5*
Liver cirrhosis													
1955	4.1*	0.4*	4.9*	–	–	3.5	1.8	6.1	6.1	16.5	24.9	26.1	42.9
1965	2.4*	0.3*	3.0*	0.9	–	1.6	2.5	2.7	8.9	4.5	14.8	8.6	27.4
1975	3.0*	0.3*	3.5*	–	1.0	6.4	4.0	3.3	7.1	3.0	8.1	31.0	24.4
1985	3.9*	0.2*	6.9*	2.6	1.6	3.0	13.5	6.7	10.1	10.8	9.2	15.3	20.7
1990	**3.2***	**0.3***	**6.2***	–	**1.3**	**3.3**	**6.1**	**8.5**	**8.9**	**15.1**	**13.7**	**6.0**	**11.4**
1995 projected	*2.9**	*0.3**	*6.1**	–	*0.7*	*2.0*	*4.4*	*6.3*	*10.6*	*19.0*	*13.1*	*4.5*	*8.0*
Other medical causes													
1955	183.8*	72.6*	122.8*	54.8	56.8	65.0	78.4	102.1	175.8	326.3	488.5	848.6	3354.3
1965	146.2*	55.9*	106.9*	30.9	34.3	62.1	72.8	93.0	180.5	274.6	446.6	770.4	2372.1
1975	98.6*	33.4*	66.5*	14.9	17.4	26.7	51.8	69.4	104.4	181.2	328.7	572.8	1737.8
1985	87.7*	26.0*	57.0*	11.8	17.1	25.1	45.8	45.7	94.3	159.0	287.3	567.8	1640.9
1990	**97.2***	**26.3***	**57.4***	**12.7**	**17.7**	**19.7**	**30.5**	**59.6**	**91.6**	**170.1**	**312.1**	**608.1**	**2044.8**
1995 projected	*106.9**	*25.7**	*58.0**	*13.6*	*16.2*	*14.5*	*28.1*	*58.0*	*97.7*	*177.8*	*333.3*	*679.4*	*2455.4*
All non-medical causes													
1955	32.0*	10.7*	20.3*	8.6	12.2	11.3	12.9	11.1	23.2	62.9	74.7	185.4	651.4
1965	32.8*	12.1*	21.2*	10.0	20.3	15.9	13.4	20.8	22.7	45.2	75.7	163.1	630.1
1975	34.4*	15.4*	29.1*	15.9	22.5	21.2	29.5	28.1	31.0	55.4	68.5	128.5	514.7
1985	34.0*	15.7*	28.7*	17.6	23.6	29.1	25.0	33.3	37.0	35.0	60.3	113.8	510.3
1990	**32.3***	**13.7***	**29.9***	**20.1**	**30.8**	**31.9**	**23.4**	**36.2**	**32.5**	**34.5**	**66.5**	**98.0**	**442.9**
1995 projected	*30.4**	*12.0**	*31.1**	*22.7*	*35.7*	*34.2*	*24.6*	*34.8*	*31.8*	*34.0*	*62.6*	*79.9*	*384.1*

NORWAY: 1975

Smoking–attributed deaths (Sm.) and total deaths (Total)

		ALL CAUSES	ALL CANCER	Lung cancer	Upper aero–digestive ca.	Other cancer	COPD	Other respiratory	Vascular disease	Liver cirrhosis	Other medical	Non–medical
Males												
0–34	Sm.	–	–	–	–	–	–	–	–	–	–	–
	Total	1271	108	0	0	108	1	55	31	1	474	601
35–69	Sm.	1412	507	355	44	108	111	24	594	–	176	–
	Total	7927	1881	415	94	1372	181	168	3876	96	1080	645
		(18%)	(27%)	(86%)	(47%)	(8%)	(61%)	(14%)	(15%)		(16%)	
70+	Sm.	935	334	210	33	91	145	50	330	–	76	–
	Total	12696	2282	268	103	1911	303	1220	6894	29	1598	370
		(7%)	(15%)	(78%)	(32%)	(5%)	(48%)	(4%)	(5%)		(5%)	
Any age	Sm.	2347	841	565	77	199	256	74	924	–	252	–
	Total	21894	4271	683	197	3391	485	1443	10801	126	3152	1616
		(11%)	(20%)	(83%)	(39%)	(6%)	(53%)	(5%)	(9%)		(8%)	
Females												
0–34	Sm.	–	–	–	–	–	–	–	–	–	–	–
	Total	630	66	1	0	65	4	24	21	3	352	160
35–69	Sm.	86	29	23	1	5	13	2	31	–	11	–
	Total	4121	1707	93	28	1586	80	113	1459	28	511	223
		(2%)	(2%)	(25%)	(4%)	(0%)	(16%)	(2%)	(2%)		(2%)	
70+	Sm.	0	0	0	0	0	0	0	0	–	0	–
	Total	13416	1811	66	44	1701	173	1602	7610	42	1720	458
		(0%)	(0%)	(0%)	(0%)	(0%)	(0%)	(0%)	(0%)		(0%)	
Any age	Sm.	86	29	23	1	5	13	2	31	–	11	–
	Total	18167	3584	160	72	3352	257	1739	9090	73	2583	841
		(0%)	(1%)	(14%)	(1%)	(0%)	(5%)	(0%)	(0%)		(0%)	
Males+Females												
0–34	Sm.	–	–	–	–	–	–	–	–	–	–	–
	Total	1901	174	1	0	173	5	79	52	4	826	761
35–69	Sm.	1498	536	378	45	113	124	26	625	–	187	–
	Total	12048	3588	508	122	2958	261	281	5335	124	1591	868
		(12%)	(15%)	(74%)	(37%)	(4%)	(48%)	(9%)	(12%)		(12%)	
70+	Sm.	935	334	210	33	91	145	50	330	–	76	–
	Total	26112	4093	334	147	3612	476	2822	14504	71	3318	828
		(4%)	(8%)	(63%)	(22%)	(3%)	(30%)	(2%)	(2%)		(2%)	
Any age	Sm.	2433	870	588	78	204	269	76	955	–	263	–
	Total	40061	7855	843	269	6743	742	3182	19891	199	5735	2457
		(6%)	(11%)	(70%)	(29%)	(3%)	(36%)	(2%)	(5%)		(5%)	

NORWAY: 1985

Smoking–attributed deaths (Sm.) and total deaths (Total)

		ALL CAUSES	ALL CANCER	Lung cancer	Upper aero–digestive ca.	Other cancer	COPD	Other respiratory	Vascular disease	Liver cirrhosis	Other medical	Non–medical
Males												
0–34	Sm.	–	–	–	–	–	–	–	–	–	–	–
	Total	1096	75	1	0	74	10	18	40	7	401	545
35–69	Sm.	1633	646	458	52	136	159	15	657	–	156	–
	Total	7535	2007	520	103	1384	236	85	3568	150	813	676
		(22%)	(32%)	(88%)	(50%)	(10%)	(67%)	(18%)	(18%)		(19%)	
70+	Sm.	1767	635	396	43	196	361	74	576	–	121	–
	Total	15152	3184	466	99	2619	603	1191	7939	43	1723	469
		(12%)	(20%)	(85%)	(43%)	(7%)	(60%)	(6%)	(7%)		(7%)	
Any age	Sm.	3400	1281	854	95	332	520	89	1233	–	277	–
	Total	23783	5266	987	202	4077	849	1294	11547	200	2937	1690
		(14%)	(24%)	(87%)	(47%)	(8%)	(61%)	(7%)	(11%)		(9%)	
Females												
0–34	Sm.	–	–	–	–	–	–	–	–	–	–	–
	Total	519	74	0	0	74	7	12	23	2	237	164
35–69	Sm.	298	120	94	7	19	51	4	86	–	37	–
	Total	3723	1687	163	30	1494	124	55	1132	53	445	227
		(8%)	(7%)	(58%)	(23%)	(1%)	(41%)	(7%)	(8%)		(8%)	
70+	Sm.	511	115	84	11	20	119	33	195	–	49	–
	Total	16347	2602	163	54	2385	331	1697	8827	40	2233	617
		(3%)	(4%)	(52%)	(20%)	(1%)	(36%)	(2%)	(2%)		(2%)	
Any age	Sm.	809	235	178	18	39	170	37	281	–	86	–
	Total	20589	4363	326	84	3953	462	1764	9982	95	2915	1008
		(4%)	(5%)	(55%)	(21%)	(1%)	(37%)	(2%)	(3%)		(3%)	
Males+Females												
0–34	Sm.	–	–	–	–	–	–	–	–	–	–	–
	Total	1615	149	1	0	148	17	30	63	9	638	709
35–69	Sm.	1931	766	552	59	155	210	19	743	–	193	–
	Total	11258	3694	683	133	2878	360	140	4700	203	1258	903
		(17%)	(21%)	(81%)	(44%)	(5%)	(58%)	(14%)	(16%)		(15%)	
70+	Sm.	2278	750	480	54	216	480	107	771	–	170	–
	Total	31499	5786	629	153	5004	934	2888	16766	83	3956	1086
		(7%)	(13%)	(76%)	(35%)	(4%)	(51%)	(4%)	(5%)		(4%)	
Any age	Sm.	4209	1516	1032	113	371	690	126	1514	–	363	–
	Total	44372	9629	1313	286	8030	1311	3058	21529	295	5852	2698
		(9%)	(16%)	(79%)	(40%)	(5%)	(53%)	(4%)	(7%)		(6%)	

(To be conservative, no deaths before age 35, and none from liver cirrhosis or non–medical causes, were attributed to smoking.)

NORWAY: 1990

Smoking-attributed deaths (Sm.) and total deaths (Total)

		ALL CAUSES	ALL CANCER	Lung cancer	Upper aero-digestive ca.	Other cancer	COPD	Other respiratory	Vascular disease	Liver cirrhosis	Other medical	Non-medical
Males												
0–34	Sm.	–	–	–	–	–	–	–	–	–	–	–
	Total	1056	82	0	4	78	8	13	39	3	412	499
35–69	Sm.	1448	614	430	59	125	127	20	525	–	162	–
	Total	6888	1927	491	118	1318	188	123	2970	121	876	683
		(21%)	(32%)	(88%)	(50%)	(9%)	(68%)	(16%)	(18%)		(18%)	
70+	Sm.	1908	713	460	51	202	364	82	605	–	144	–
	Total	15941	3276	538	111	2627	603	1297	8160	36	2072	497
		(12%)	(22%)	(86%)	(46%)	(8%)	(60%)	(6%)	(7%)		(7%)	
Any age	Sm.	3356	1327	890	110	327	491	102	1130	–	306	–
	Total	23885	5285	1029	233	4023	799	1433	11169	160	3360	1679
		(14%)	(25%)	(86%)	(47%)	(8%)	(61%)	(7%)	(10%)		(9%)	
Females												
0–34	Sm.	–	–	–	–	–	–	–	–	–	–	–
	Total	495	63	1	1	61	1	8	18	3	258	144
35–69	Sm.	434	179	143	10	26	62	8	129	–	56	–
	Total	3600	1670	212	26	1432	114	75	1009	46	441	245
		(12%)	(11%)	(67%)	(38%)	(2%)	(54%)	(11%)	(13%)		(13%)	
70+	Sm.	606	144	108	11	25	120	39	232	–	71	–
	Total	18061	2834	198	53	2583	306	1879	9421	31	2975	615
		(3%)	(5%)	(55%)	(21%)	(1%)	(39%)	(2%)	(2%)		(2%)	
Any age	Sm.	1040	323	251	21	51	182	47	361	–	127	–
	Total	22156	4567	411	80	4076	421	1962	10448	80	3674	1004
		(5%)	(7%)	(61%)	(26%)	(1%)	(43%)	(2%)	(3%)		(3%)	
Males+Females												
0–34	Sm.	–	–	–	–	–	–	–	–	–	–	–
	Total	1551	145	1	5	139	9	21	57	6	670	643
35–69	Sm.	1882	793	573	69	151	189	28	654	–	218	–
	Total	10488	3597	703	144	2750	302	198	3979	167	1317	928
		(18%)	(22%)	(82%)	(48%)	(5%)	(63%)	(14%)	(16%)		(17%)	
70+	Sm.	2514	857	568	62	227	484	121	837	–	215	–
	Total	34002	6110	736	164	5210	909	3176	17581	67	5047	1112
		(7%)	(14%)	(77%)	(38%)	(4%)	(53%)	(4%)	(5%)		(4%)	
Any age	Sm.	4396	1650	1141	131	378	673	149	1491	–	433	–
	Total	46041	9852	1440	313	8099	1220	3395	21617	240	7034	2683
		(10%)	(17%)	(79%)	(42%)	(5%)	(55%)	(4%)	(7%)		(6%)	

NORWAY: 1995

Smoking-attributed deaths (Sm.) and total deaths (Total)

		ALL CAUSES	ALL CANCER	Lung cancer	Upper aero-digestive ca.	Other cancer	COPD	Other respiratory	Vascular disease	Liver cirrhosis	Other medical	Non-medical
Males												
0–34	Sm.	–	–	–	–	–	–	–	–	–	–	–
	Total	948	80	0	1	79	6	10	43	2	376	431
35–69	Sm.	1309	591	412	68	111	102	26	426	–	164	–
	Total	6246	1810	473	139	1198	152	148	2447	99	914	676
		(21%)	(33%)	(87%)	(49%)	(9%)	(67%)	(18%)	(17%)		(18%)	
70+	Sm.	2060	785	517	59	209	376	92	629	–	178	–
	Total	16538	3322	600	124	2598	609	1380	8209	28	2483	507
		(12%)	(24%)	(86%)	(48%)	(8%)	(62%)	(7%)	(8%)		(7%)	
Any age	Sm.	3369	1376	929	127	320	478	118	1055	–	342	–
	Total	23732	5212	1073	264	3875	767	1538	10699	129	3773	1614
		(14%)	(26%)	(87%)	(48%)	(8%)	(62%)	(8%)	(10%)		(9%)	
Females												
0–34	Sm.	–	–	–	–	–	–	–	–	–	–	–
	Total	447	56	1	0	55	1	6	14	3	246	121
35–69	Sm.	538	238	193	11	34	62	13	153	–	72	–
	Total	3404	1633	260	28	1345	99	79	860	44	424	265
		(16%)	(15%)	(74%)	(39%)	(3%)	(63%)	(16%)	(18%)		(17%)	
70+	Sm.	826	205	154	15	36	138	55	311	–	117	–
	Total	19122	3012	246	53	2713	296	1968	9534	27	3716	569
		(4%)	(7%)	(63%)	(28%)	(1%)	(47%)	(3%)	(3%)		(3%)	
Any age	Sm.	1364	443	347	26	70	200	68	464	–	189	–
	Total	22973	4701	507	81	4113	396	2053	10408	74	4386	955
		(6%)	(9%)	(68%)	(32%)	(2%)	(51%)	(3%)	(4%)		(4%)	
Males+Females												
0–34	Sm.	–	–	–	–	–	–	–	–	–	–	–
	Total	1395	136	1	1	134	7	16	57	5	622	552
35–69	Sm.	1847	829	605	79	145	164	39	579	–	236	–
	Total	9650	3443	733	167	2543	251	227	3307	143	1338	941
		(19%)	(24%)	(83%)	(47%)	(6%)	(65%)	(17%)	(18%)		(18%)	
70+	Sm.	2886	990	671	74	245	514	147	940	–	295	–
	Total	35660	6334	846	177	5311	905	3348	17743	55	6199	1076
		(8%)	(16%)	(79%)	(42%)	(5%)	(57%)	(4%)	(5%)		(5%)	
Any age	Sm.	4733	1819	1276	153	390	678	186	1519	–	531	–
	Total	46705	9913	1580	345	7988	1163	3591	21107	203	8159	2569
		(10%)	(18%)	(81%)	(44%)	(5%)	(58%)	(5%)	(7%)		(7%)	

(To be conservative, no deaths before age 35, and none from liver cirrhosis or non-medical causes, were attributed to smoking.)

POLAND: 1990

		No. of deaths			Standardised rates (Defined on p.454)			Annual death rates / 100, 000						
		All ages	0–34	35–69	All ages	0–34	35–69	0–4	5–9	10–14	15–19	20–24	25–29	30–34
ALL CAUSES	M	209333	17601	105138	1482.6	168.7	1814.4	386.6	32.6	34.9	102.2	168.2	187.1	269.3
	F	179107	7846	51545	808.3	77.3	751.3	299.3	21.8	21.9	34.7	37.7	48.5	77.3
Tuberculosis	M	1211	29	833	8.5	0.3	14.0	–	–	–	–	0.2	0.4	1.3
	F	397	17	181	1.9	0.2	2.6	–	–	0.1	0.1	–	0.2	0.7
Other infective	M	811	415	264	5.0	3.9	4.5	23.3	0.6	0.4	0.7	0.9	0.7	0.8
and parasitic	F	656	303	191	3.3	3.0	2.7	17.8	0.5	0.4	0.3	0.9	0.8	0.5
ALL CANCER	M	42076	1018	27699	297.2	9.6	495.7	7.8	5.1	4.7	8.2	10.0	10.5	21.0
	F	30837	836	17086	154.2	8.1	245.9	6.0	4.6	3.4	4.9	6.1	10.8	20.9
Mouth and	M	1275	6	995	8.9	0.1	16.6	–	0.1	–	–	0.1	–	0.2
pharynx cancer	F	340	9	154	1.7	0.1	2.2	–	–	0.1	0.1	–	0.1	0.3
Oesophagus cancer	M	994	1	720	7.0	0.0	12.6	–	–	–	–	–	–	0.1
	F	243	1	114	1.2	0.0	1.7	–	–	–	–	–	0.1	–
Stomach cancer	M	4839	42	2866	34.9	0.4	52.0	–	–	–	0.1	0.1	0.9	1.7
	F	2460	33	1067	11.8	0.3	15.8	–	–	–	0.1	0.2	0.8	1.2
Colorectal cancer	M	3160	42	1827	22.8	0.4	33.3	–	–	–	0.2	0.2	0.6	1.7
	F	3179	17	1498	15.5	0.2	21.9	–	–	–	–	0.2	0.3	0.7
Liver cancer	M	1357	19	853	9.7	0.2	15.8	0.1	0.1	0.1	–	0.4	0.1	0.5
	F	1513	12	676	7.3	0.1	10.0	0.1	0.1	0.1	0.1	0.2	0.2	0.2
Pancreas cancer	M	1691	14	1139	11.9	0.1	20.2	–	–	–	–	0.1	0.1	0.7
	F	1486	7	724	7.2	0.1	10.7	–	0.1	–	–	–	0.2	0.2
Larynx cancer	M	1560	3	1231	10.8	0.0	21.5	–	–	–	–	–	0.1	0.1
	F	124	2	86	0.6	0.0	1.2	–	–	–	–	0.1	–	0.1
Lung cancer	M	14539	46	10784	102.2	0.4	194.2	–	–	–	0.2	0.3	0.3	2.1
	F	2805	36	1703	14.2	0.4	24.9	–	–	0.1	0.4	0.4	0.6	1.0
Malignant melanoma	M	307	24	228	2.1	0.2	3.7	0.1	–	–	0.1	0.2	0.4	0.8
	F	350	24	208	1.8	0.2	2.8	–	–	–	–	0.2	0.7	0.8
Female breast cancer	F	4323	55	2926	22.6	0.5	41.2	–	–	–	–	–	0.8	2.8
Cervix cancer	F	1981	90	1409	10.4	0.8	19.5	–	–	–	–	0.3	1.4	4.1
Other uterine cancer	F	1202	10	697	6.0	0.1	10.2	–	–	–	–	–	0.1	0.6
Ovarian cancer	F	1747	40	1276	9.4	0.4	18.1	–	–	0.1	0.3	0.3	0.6	1.4
Prostate cancer	M	2050	1	711	15.6	0.0	14.4	–	–	–	–	–	–	0.1
Bladder cancer	M	1523	5	822	11.1	0.0	15.5	0.2	0.1	–	–	–	–	0.1
	F	336	–	136	1.6	–	2.0	–	–	–	–	–	–	–
Other and ill–defined	M	6490	486	4147	44.7	4.6	72.3	4.3	2.5	1.9	4.3	4.9	5.4	9.0
cancer sites	F	7065	303	3519	34.6	3.0	50.9	3.5	2.5	1.8	2.3	2.3	3.4	4.7
Hodgkin's disease	M	328	58	219	2.0	0.6	3.4	0.1	0.1	0.1	0.5	1.1	0.7	1.3
	F	176	34	110	0.9	0.3	1.5	0.1	0.1	0.1	0.4	0.4	0.6	0.7
Myeloma and non–	M	784	61	540	5.3	0.6	9.4	0.5	0.3	0.7	0.6	0.6	0.7	0.7
Hodgkin lymphomas	F	578	32	347	3.0	0.3	5.0	0.3	0.5	0.2	–	0.2	0.2	0.7
Leukaemia	M	1179	210	617	7.9	2.0	11.0	2.6	2.0	1.9	2.1	2.0	1.3	1.9
	F	929	131	436	4.6	1.3	6.2	1.9	1.4	0.8	1.3	1.3	0.8	1.4
ALL VASCULAR	M	100443	1355	45415	745.6	12.6	812.1	6.1	0.5	1.3	4.0	9.4	18.8	48.3
DISEASE	F	103171	493	21959	445.9	4.8	327.3	5.8	0.6	0.8	2.5	3.8	5.9	14.1
Rheumatic heart	M	1203	60	951	8.1	0.6	15.6	0.1	–	0.1	0.4	0.5	1.1	1.9
disease and fever	F	1486	35	1087	7.8	0.3	15.7	0.3	–	0.1	0.3	0.2	0.6	0.9
Hypertensive disease	M	3003	36	1915	21.4	0.3	33.6	–	–	–	–	0.2	0.3	1.8
	F	4624	16	1771	21.7	0.2	26.1	–	–	–	0.1	0.3	0.2	0.5
Ischaemic heart	M	27806	527	19414	193.9	4.8	333.5	–	0.1	0.1	0.3	2.1	6.8	24.2
disease	F	13563	59	5873	64.4	0.6	86.7	–	–	–	0.2	0.2	0.9	2.6
Pulmonary embolism	M	920	27	549	6.6	0.3	9.5	0.1	0.1	0.1	0.1	0.2	0.5	0.7
and other venous	F	842	27	428	4.1	0.3	6.2	0.3	–	–	0.1	0.2	0.3	0.9
Cerebrovascular	M	11586	236	5823	84.7	2.2	104.0	0.9	0.1	0.4	1.2	2.6	3.4	7.1
disease	F	13990	151	4232	63.1	1.5	62.5	0.5	0.2	0.4	0.7	1.4	2.0	5.0
Other vascular	M	55925	469	16763	431.0	4.4	315.8	5.0	0.3	0.7	2.0	3.9	6.6	12.6
disease	F	68666	205	8568	284.8	2.0	130.2	4.8	0.4	0.4	1.1	1.4	1.9	4.1
Chronic obstructive	M	6387	33	2670	47.9	0.3	51.2	0.3	0.2	0.3	0.1	0.3	0.4	0.5
pulmonary disease	F	2503	36	790	11.3	0.4	11.8	0.3	–	0.3	0.4	0.3	0.7	0.6
Other respiratory	M	3726	432	1405	26.8	4.1	24.4	19.1	0.5	0.8	1.1	1.8	2.1	3.3
disease	F	3059	328	646	13.7	3.3	9.4	16.9	0.7	0.3	0.9	1.2	1.2	1.5
Peptic ulcer	M	1037	33	593	7.4	0.3	10.3	–	–	0.1	–	0.1	0.4	1.5
	F	637	7	217	2.9	0.1	3.2	–	–	–	–	0.2	–	0.2
Liver cirrhosis	M	2474	92	1780	17.0	0.8	29.9	0.7	0.1	0.1	0.4	0.2	0.8	3.6
	F	1434	36	751	7.1	0.3	10.9	0.1	0.1	0.3	0.1	0.2	0.6	1.0
Renal disease	M	2145	81	1094	15.4	0.8	19.3	0.4	0.2	0.4	0.1	1.2	1.2	2.0
	F	2011	66	908	9.6	0.7	13.3	0.7	0.2	0.1	0.4	0.8	0.8	1.5
Pregnancy and birth	F	70	47	23	0.3	0.5	0.2	–	–	–	0.1	0.8	0.9	1.4
Congenital and	M	4169	4109	46	22.1	38.8	0.6	265.7	0.9	1.0	1.0	1.4	0.7	0.8
perinatal causes	F	3149	3094	42	17.4	30.7	0.5	208.6	1.5	1.1	1.5	0.9	0.8	0.3
Ill–defined causes	M	12522	843	5647	90.4	8.0	87.9	8.5	0.6	0.6	4.1	7.2	13.1	22.2
	F	12865	240	1484	52.7	2.4	20.8	5.8	0.2	0.7	1.3	2.0	2.3	4.3
Other medical causes	M	9862	1213	5430	67.2	11.4	90.9	25.3	4.9	5.8	7.2	7.8	10.1	18.8
	F	10971	816	4657	52.8	8.0	67.9	19.2	3.4	5.7	4.7	5.7	7.2	10.1
ALL NON–	M	22470	7948	12262	132.2	77.7	173.5	29.3	19.2	19.6	75.4	127.7	127.8	145.2
MEDICAL CAUSES	F	7347	1527	2610	34.9	15.1	34.8	18.1	10.1	8.7	17.5	14.5	16.3	20.2
Motor vehicle	M	6587	2867	3204	37.7	28.4	45.2	5.7	8.1	6.6	36.0	55.4	44.0	42.9
traffic accidents	F	1679	536	687	8.4	5.3	9.1	3.5	5.8	4.3	8.3	5.8	4.4	4.8
Fire	M	300	84	171	1.8	0.8	2.4	0.8	0.5	0.2	0.5	1.2	1.1	1.5
	F	122	23	44	0.6	0.2	0.6	0.3	0.1	–	–	0.2	0.3	0.7
Suicide	M	4091	1390	2483	23.7	13.7	35.1	–	0.1	1.9	10.4	22.9	27.7	32.7
	F	879	205	567	4.7	2.1	7.5	–	–	0.4	2.9	2.6	3.3	5.1
Homicide	M	763	251	470	4.4	2.4	6.5	1.3	0.4	0.4	1.0	3.8	4.5	5.7
	F	359	96	196	1.9	0.9	2.6	1.2	0.5	0.4	0.4	0.6	1.6	1.9
POPULATION (thousands):	M=males				18578	10630	7113	1513	1732	1652	1457	1264	1360	1653
	F=females				19541	10209	7796	1441	1659	1579	1392	1204	1318	1616

POLAND: 1990

Annual death rates / 100, 000

9th ICD categories

35–39	40–44	45–49	50–54	55–59	60–64	65–69	70–74	75–79	80+/NK			
387.8	581.3	924.7	1402.6	2078.3	3024.5	4301.7	6139.8	9607.1	17048.7	M	ALL CAUSES	001–999
129.2	215.4	328.5	488.0	784.5	1257.0	2056.6	3393.7	5992.0	13614.7	F		
2.4	5.4	8.9	13.8	19.3	20.9	27.4	41.9	45.9	36.8	M	Tuberculosis	010–018, 137
0.6	1.0	1.8	1.8	2.8	3.4	7.0	8.9	15.3	14.5	F		
1.4	0.8	2.7	4.0	5.3	7.7	9.6	14.8	14.8	18.4	M	Other infective	Rest of 001–139
1.2	1.1	0.9	2.3	3.3	4.0	5.9	5.1	13.1	13.2	F	and parasitic	
39.7	85.9	193.1	371.4	629.1	911.0	1239.9	1461.0	1704.2	1663.5	M	ALL CANCER	140–208
43.6	85.1	136.7	201.3	287.2	411.8	555.7	716.0	872.8	926.3	F		
1.9	5.3	14.0	17.4	25.1	27.7	24.8	27.7	30.4	42.8	M	Mouth and	140–149
0.4	0.9	2.0	1.6	2.7	3.4	4.5	7.5	11.4	15.4	F	pharynx cancer	
0.7	2.8	5.9	13.1	16.1	23.4	26.1	27.1	32.8	40.2	M	Oesophagus cancer	150
0.1	0.3	1.6	0.6	1.4	3.4	4.5	6.3	9.2	9.4	F		
4.1	7.4	21.4	34.5	60.1	97.8	138.8	197.4	255.6	248.0	M	Stomach cancer	151
1.7	2.7	7.1	11.3	15.3	27.1	45.3	66.0	92.3	105.9	F		
2.8	5.6	11.2	24.2	37.4	56.9	94.9	125.3	169.1	177.0	M	Colorectal cancer	153, 154
2.4	4.4	8.9	16.5	25.9	38.9	56.6	88.8	110.8	124.2	F		
0.7	2.0	4.0	9.2	17.9	30.5	45.9	54.2	53.3	69.3	M	Liver cancer	155.0
0.6	1.7	2.9	6.7	10.3	19.1	28.9	44.7	51.2	64.5	F		
2.0	5.9	6.2	15.8	24.8	34.8	51.5	57.3	70.6	66.7	M	Pancreas cancer	157
0.6	2.9	3.2	6.8	11.5	19.0	30.7	39.7	52.9	54.4	F		
1.6	5.3	11.9	18.0	29.9	36.7	47.4	40.6	46.9	27.4	M	Larynx cancer	161
0.2	0.4	0.8	1.3	1.6	2.2	2.2	1.8	2.2	3.0	F		
7.5	22.5	65.8	149.5	268.4	375.2	470.2	498.1	457.1	355.7	M	Lung cancer	162
2.4	5.4	12.9	18.7	29.6	46.4	58.9	68.8	78.8	60.9	F		
1.2	1.8	2.9	4.1	4.3	5.3	6.2	7.6	4.9	7.3	M	Malignant melanoma	172
1.7	1.8	2.7	2.7	3.2	3.8	3.7	6.3	6.3	10.3	F		
9.5	21.8	32.3	42.7	51.6	59.1	71.6	76.3	83.5	101.4	F	Female breast cancer	174
7.8	12.8	15.0	18.4	19.6	28.7	34.1	33.2	34.5	26.7	F	Cervix cancer	180
1.2	2.0	4.8	6.0	12.6	18.9	26.0	31.0	37.1	28.8	F	Other uterine cancer	179, 182
3.4	7.8	15.2	21.2	22.1	26.7	30.6	28.9	32.3	23.1	F	Ovarian cancer	183
0.2	0.2	1.9	4.1	9.7	24.3	60.2	106.7	179.3	209.9	M	Prostate cancer	185
0.6	1.1	3.0	7.9	15.6	32.4	48.0	64.9	91.8	98.3	M	Bladder cancer	188
0.1	0.2	0.4	1.3	1.9	3.9	6.3	7.1	15.5	16.2	F		
11.1	18.6	35.2	57.2	91.5	123.9	168.6	190.5	231.6	254.8	M	Other and ill-defined	Rest of 140–208
8.4	14.8	21.8	37.7	61.2	89.6	122.9	165.1	213.9	251.3	F	cancer sites	
2.3	1.7	2.4	3.1	3.9	5.4	5.0	3.8	10.9	3.4	M	Hodgkin's disease	201
0.9	1.1	1.3	0.6	1.4	2.6	2.4	2.2	2.5	1.5	F		
1.3	2.9	3.4	7.0	13.0	16.3	21.8	23.0	24.7	17.1	M	Myeloma and non-	200, 202–203
0.6	1.2	1.2	3.6	6.9	9.5	12.3	17.6	13.7	7.9	F	Hodgkin lymphomas	
1.8	2.9	3.8	6.3	11.5	20.4	30.6	36.8	45.2	45.7	M	Leukaemia	204–208
1.7	2.9	2.8	3.7	8.4	9.6	14.1	24.9	24.7	21.3	F		
94.1	200.2	339.2	559.2	904.8	1412.9	2174.0	3432.3	5862.7	11185.5	M	ALL VASCULAR	390–459
29.5	59.6	95.1	162.8	308.3	566.6	1069.3	1995.8	3938.1	9549.7	F	DISEASE	
3.3	6.1	10.1	17.1	22.2	26.5	24.1	28.0	21.5	18.0	M	Rheumatic heart	390–398
1.7	4.8	8.4	13.4	23.1	26.6	31.6	28.5	25.3	17.7	F	disease and fever	
3.9	8.3	16.1	26.3	43.3	57.6	80.0	96.0	132.0	159.5	M	Hypertensive disease	401–405
1.9	6.0	10.9	18.0	31.9	42.4	71.6	115.1	174.7	259.0	F		
49.3	113.9	187.3	279.7	416.7	569.4	718.3	810.8	1024.7	1020.5	M	Ischaemic heart	410–414
8.5	16.2	27.7	49.4	94.4	161.5	249.0	365.6	497.4	618.3	F	disease	
1.8	2.4	5.2	6.9	11.9	17.0	21.3	33.1	39.9	53.9	M	Pulmonary embolism	415.1, 451–453
1.1	1.1	3.7	3.9	6.4	12.1	15.3	16.8	25.9	32.4	F	and other venous	
13.1	24.9	41.0	70.6	121.2	177.7	279.6	446.5	660.4	956.8	M	Cerebrovascular	430–438
7.7	15.6	22.4	32.4	59.4	107.5	192.5	320.0	587.9	945.4	F	disease	
22.7	44.6	79.6	158.6	289.4	564.6	1050.9	2017.9	3984.1	8976.9	M	Other vascular	Rest of 390–459
8.7	15.9	22.1	45.8	93.1	216.5	509.2	1149.7	2626.9	7676.8	F	disease	
1.3	2.4	8.1	21.4	52.3	100.9	172.0	286.5	463.1	625.1	M	Chronic obstructive	490–496
1.1	1.8	2.7	5.7	11.7	21.0	38.5	61.5	99.6	162.7	F	pulmonary disease	
5.6	7.3	12.1	20.2	24.9	39.1	61.5	104.8	209.7	411.3	M	Other respiratory	Rest of 460–519
1.9	3.1	4.1	5.5	10.3	15.0	25.8	51.8	100.0	248.1	F	disease	
1.8	3.1	6.4	9.0	9.8	17.8	24.3	34.9	49.8	68.0	M	Peptic ulcer	531–533
0.7	0.8	1.4	2.4	2.8	5.0	9.0	14.6	28.8	36.5	F		
6.3	10.6	18.0	29.8	36.2	51.3	57.3	65.2	78.0	74.4	M	Liver cirrhosis	571
2.1	3.1	4.8	8.5	12.8	17.9	26.7	37.0	45.9	43.3	F		
4.2	5.0	8.8	12.9	21.5	30.7	51.9	73.4	126.0	162.5	M	Renal disease	580–590
2.6	3.0	4.4	8.0	12.6	22.9	39.6	52.4	65.1	83.9	F		
1.1	0.4	–	–	–	–	–	–	–	–	F	Pregnancy and birth	630–676
0.7	0.9	0.3	0.5	0.6	0.2	1.0	0.3	1.1	4.3	M	Congenital and	740–779
0.4	0.4	0.8	0.9	0.8	0.3	0.2	0.8	0.2	1.5	F	perinatal causes	
41.4	54.9	83.8	93.2	98.5	121.1	122.3	171.3	405.6	1855.1	M	Ill-defined causes	780–799
6.9	12.2	15.9	16.2	23.6	28.5	42.7	104.4	279.6	1730.4	F		
29.1	38.0	54.6	72.8	99.9	142.8	199.3	279.9	393.6	519.5	M	Other medical causes	Rest of 001–799
11.8	16.3	28.5	45.2	72.8	117.1	184.0	266.2	377.0	424.9	F		
159.8	166.9	188.6	194.3	175.9	168.3	161.1	173.5	252.7	424.5	M	ALL NON-	E800–E999
25.7	27.5	31.5	27.6	35.5	43.4	52.2	79.3	156.6	379.8	F	MEDICAL CAUSES	
45.1	40.6	45.8	51.3	46.0	45.1	42.2	44.7	64.6	81.7	M	Motor vehicle	E810–E819
6.7	7.2	7.6	9.0	9.1	11.4	12.9	21.0	33.3	34.2	F	traffic accidents	
2.4	2.0	3.2	2.4	3.1	1.6	2.2	2.8	5.3	9.0	M	Fire	E890–E899
0.4	0.4	0.4	0.4	0.4	1.3	0.8	1.2	2.7	6.6	F		
32.5	33.7	40.4	36.5	36.5	35.9	29.9	24.2	25.8	29.1	M	Suicide	E950–E959
5.3	6.8	8.8	6.3	9.3	8.2	7.8	6.1	7.3	7.5	F		
7.5	7.3	6.0	7.3	4.5	5.6	7.0	3.5	5.6	6.4	M	Homicide	E960–E969
2.5	1.9	3.5	2.2	2.8	2.6	2.4	2.6	2.5	7.7	F		
1629	1331	864	942	931	815	602	318	283	234	M	POPULATION (thousands)	
1616	1341	902	1019	1042	1016	860	494	510	532	F		

POLAND: Males

	All ages	0–34	35–69	35–39	40–44	45–49	50–54	55–59	60–64	65–69	70–74	75–79	80+/NK
POPULATION (1000s)													
1955	13094	8764	4008	611	789	822	686	503	343	255	163	92	67
1965	15287	9718	5132	1115	926	603	749	759	591	390	226	131	80
1975	16633	10079	5832	1057	1101	1064	876	552	607	575	385	211	126
1985	18144	10916	6319	1371	900	1000	1012	919	711	406	419	297	192
1990	**18578**	**10630**	**7113**	**1629**	**1331**	**864**	**942**	**931**	**815**	**602**	**318**	**283**	**234**
1995 projected	*19236*	*10484*	*7825*	*1651*	*1621*	*1303*	*830*	*882*	*839*	*700*	*475*	*218*	*234*
NUMBER OF DEATHS													
All causes													
1955	135731	54054	49682	2077	3718	5855	7855	9383	9661	11133	11497	9076	11422
1965	121037	24128	57611	3254	3635	3421	6726	11059	14169	15347	13770	11914	13614
1975	157835	21523	71982	3494	5261	7742	9151	8214	15737	22383	23727	19939	20664
1985	202080	19854	88520	4832	5122	8861	13751	18323	20685	16946	27335	30193	36178
1990	**209333**	**17601**	**105138**	**6317**	**7734**	**7992**	**13218**	**19339**	**24659**	**25879**	**19500**	**27217**	**39877**
1995 projected	*217517*	*16705*	*116378*	*6806*	*9869*	*12444*	*12097*	*19045*	*26297*	*29820*	*28035*	*19510*	*36889*
Lung cancer													
1955	...	...	...	...	...	...	...	...	...	...	...	...	...
1965	3880	39	3082	42	105	150	413	747	832	793	480	211	68
1975	7807	54	5459	80	215	532	763	749	1371	1749	1346	691	257
1985	12619	55	8751	96	224	731	1475	2233	2401	1591	1915	1287	611
1990	**14539**	**46**	**10784**	**122**	**299**	**569**	**1409**	**2497**	**3059**	**2829**	**1582**	**1295**	**832**
1995 projected	*16982*	*39*	*12371*	*116*	*330*	*829*	*1289*	*2560*	*3569*	*3678*	*2596*	*1075*	*901*
ANNUAL DEATH RATE / 100,000 (*The rates for the age groups 0–34 and 35–69 are the means of seven five-yearly rates, but the all-ages rates are standardised to the conventional "European" age distribution)													
All causes													
1955	1627.2*	485.5*	1672.9*	340.2	471.5	712.5	1144.9	1866.9	2815.0	4359.0	7040.4	9919.1	17124.4
1965	1354.5*	254.0*	1419.9*	291.9	392.7	567.2	897.5	1458.0	2399.1	3933.1	6084.8	9129.5	16975.1
1975	1368.5*	213.9*	1507.6*	330.5	477.9	727.8	1044.9	1487.8	2593.4	3890.7	6162.9	9449.8	16374.0
1985	1518.9*	173.1*	1748.9*	352.3	569.0	886.2	1359.3	1993.1	2909.7	4172.9	6517.6	10166.0	18842.7
1990	**1482.6***	**168.7***	**1814.4***	**387.8**	**581.3**	**924.7**	**1402.6**	**2078.3**	**3024.5**	**4301.7**	**6139.8**	**9607.1**	**17048.7**
1995 projected	*1452.8**	*167.0**	*1855.3**	*412.2*	*609.0*	*955.4*	*1457.8*	*2159.1*	*3134.3*	*4259.4*	*5902.1*	*8933.2*	*15751.1*
All cancer													
1955	...	...	...	...	...	...	...	...	...	...	...	...	...
1965	207.3*	10.6*	338.1*	36.3	68.6	114.6	226.6	397.1	612.9	910.8	1129.5	1214.6	1086.0
1975	234.7*	10.2*	377.7*	35.8	80.6	158.6	271.2	409.0	707.0	981.6	1280.5	1433.2	1256.7
1985	284.0*	9.8*	463.2*	38.7	93.1	196.0	363.7	586.6	854.1	1109.8	1418.5	1659.9	1632.3
1990	**297.2***	**9.6***	**495.7***	**39.7**	**85.9**	**193.1**	**371.4**	**629.1**	**911.0**	**1239.9**	**1461.0**	**1704.2**	**1663.5**
1995 projected	*309.6**	*9.5**	*522.4**	*37.8*	*83.4*	*191.9*	*384.6*	*663.2*	*986.2*	*1309.8*	*1520.2*	*1745.0*	*1701.1*
Lung cancer													
1955	...	...	...	...	...	...	...	...	...	...	...	...	...
1965	39.3*	0.5*	76.8*	3.8	11.3	24.9	55.1	98.5	140.9	203.2	212.1	161.7	84.8
1975	64.5*	0.7*	118.5*	7.6	19.5	50.0	87.1	135.7	225.9	304.0	349.6	327.5	203.6
1985	93.7*	0.5*	174.7*	7.0	24.9	73.1	145.8	242.9	337.7	391.8	456.6	433.3	318.2
1990	**102.2***	**0.4***	**194.2***	**7.5**	**22.5**	**65.8**	**149.5**	**268.4**	**375.2**	**470.2**	**498.1**	**457.1**	**355.7**
1995 projected	*111.1**	*0.4**	*212.5**	*7.0*	*20.4*	*63.6*	*155.3*	*290.2*	*425.4*	*525.4*	*546.5*	*492.2*	*384.7*
Upper aerodigestive cancer (mouth, oesophagus, pharynx and larynx)													
1955	...	...	...	...	...	...	...	...	...	...	...	...	...
1965	16.9*	0.2*	27.7*	2.9	5.6	7.1	21.5	35.3	48.8	72.5	92.4	99.6	99.8
1975	19.1*	0.3*	33.5*	2.5	8.5	17.6	29.2	45.5	57.2	74.0	85.7	104.3	87.2
1985	24.7*	0.2*	44.8*	3.4	13.6	26.9	42.3	60.5	72.4	94.6	91.8	108.1	132.3
1990	**26.7***	**0.1***	**50.7***	**4.2**	**13.3**	**31.8**	**48.5**	**71.1**	**87.8**	**98.2**	**95.4**	**110.1**	**110.3**
1995 projected	*28.9**	*0.1**	*56.9**	*4.1*	*14.8*	*35.7*	*56.2*	*83.4*	*98.3*	*105.4*	*97.1*	*102.6*	*101.2*
Other cancer													
1955	...	...	...	...	...	...	...	...	...	...	...	...	...
1965	151.1*	9.9*	233.6*	29.7	51.6	82.6	150.0	263.3	423.3	635.1	825.0	953.3	901.5
1975	151.0*	9.3*	225.6*	25.7	52.5	91.0	154.8	227.9	423.9	603.5	845.2	1001.4	965.9
1985	165.6*	9.1*	243.6*	28.3	54.7	96.0	175.6	283.3	443.9	623.5	870.1	1118.5	1181.8
1990	**168.2***	**9.1***	**250.9***	**28.1**	**50.1**	**95.5**	**173.4**	**289.6**	**447.9**	**671.4**	**867.4**	**1137.0**	**1197.5**
1995 projected	*169.6**	*9.0**	*253.1**	*26.6*	*48.3*	*92.5*	*173.1*	*289.5*	*462.5*	*679.0*	*876.6*	*1150.2*	*1215.2*
Chronic obstructive pulmonary disease (COPD)													
1955	...	...	...	...	...	...	...	...	...	...	...	...	...
1965	39.3*	1.4*	44.1*	1.4	3.6	7.6	19.7	39.7	83.6	153.3	224.5	334.1	507.5
1975	60.4*	1.3*	63.2*	2.2	5.0	13.2	26.4	49.6	123.4	222.7	399.5	610.9	707.6
1985	70.3*	0.6*	74.1*	1.8	4.3	12.2	34.0	77.5	138.8	250.2	436.1	684.2	897.9
1990	**47.9***	**0.3***	**51.2***	**1.3**	**2.4**	**8.1**	**21.4**	**52.3**	**100.9**	**172.0**	**286.5**	**463.1**	**625.1**
1995 projected	*33.6**	*0.2**	*35.8**	*0.9*	*1.7*	*5.7*	*15.1*	*36.6*	*70.7*	*120.0*	*199.8*	*323.7*	*441.9*
Other respiratory disease													
1955	...	...	...	...	...	...	...	...	...	...	...	...	...
1965	54.2*	30.9*	32.1*	5.0	6.7	9.6	14.8	28.7	57.4	102.3	203.3	324.1	659.6
1975	50.2*	17.9*	33.6*	5.6	7.2	12.6	15.9	29.2	59.7	104.8	207.3	394.3	719.5
1985	33.5*	5.9*	28.4*	4.7	7.9	12.1	21.9	30.8	48.8	72.9	142.1	254.5	522.9
1990	**26.8***	**4.1***	**24.4***	**5.6**	**7.3**	**12.1**	**20.2**	**24.9**	**39.1**	**61.5**	**104.8**	**209.7**	**411.3**
1995 projected	*21.6**	*3.2**	*20.3**	*6.1*	*7.3*	*11.4*	*17.6*	*20.5*	*31.9*	*47.3*	*82.7*	*157.1*	*328.8*
Vascular disease													
1955	...	...	...	...	...	...	...	...	...	...	...	...	...
1965	490.3*	14.3*	497.3*	53.8	86.0	156.4	265.9	466.7	883.7	1568.7	2654.4	4017.6	7441.4
1975	603.6*	12.7*	626.0*	80.9	138.3	247.8	385.4	594.1	1112.7	1823.0	3111.2	5039.3	8965.9
1985	749.8*	11.8*	768.0*	88.7	178.3	323.8	541.1	847.9	1335.5	2060.8	3544.6	6052.2	11859.4
1990	**745.6***	**12.6***	**812.1***	**94.1**	**200.2**	**339.2**	**559.2**	**904.8**	**1412.9**	**2174.0**	**3432.3**	**5862.7**	**11185.5**
1995 projected	*735.6**	*13.3**	*835.8**	*104.6*	*213.1*	*354.2*	*583.8*	*946.6*	*1479.9*	*2168.5*	*3331.2*	*5536.6*	*10646.9*
Liver cirrhosis													
1955	...	...	...	...	...	...	...	...	...	...	...	...	...
1965	11.3*	0.4*	17.9*	3.0	5.3	9.9	14.5	22.4	30.0	40.0	60.5	66.7	57.4
1975	17.9*	0.7*	31.9*	5.1	10.6	17.7	25.1	33.5	54.7	76.8	85.7	77.3	73.7
1985	19.4*	0.7*	34.6*	6.1	12.6	20.3	32.0	42.6	60.3	68.2	78.9	89.6	81.8
1990	**17.0***	**0.8***	**29.9***	**6.3**	**10.6**	**18.0**	**29.8**	**36.2**	**51.3**	**57.3**	**65.2**	**78.0**	**74.4**
1995 projected	*14.7**	*0.9**	*25.6**	*6.0*	*9.4*	*16.1*	*26.2*	*31.2*	*42.9*	*47.4*	*54.5*	*67.8*	*66.2*
Other medical causes													
1955	...	...	...	...	...	...	...	...	...	...	...	...	...
1965	464.0*	131.2*	392.0*	98.8	126.5	170.6	257.7	404.7	632.2	1053.3	1674.8	3013.0	6906.5
1975	283.5*	92.4*	230.1*	64.7	93.8	130.1	173.9	236.9	381.7	529.3	913.8	1672.0	4264.7
1985	239.8*	73.5*	224.9*	69.9	110.5	149.0	195.6	254.7	326.1	468.6	713.4	1182.5	3388.0
1990	**215.9***	**63.5***	**227.5***	**81.0**	**108.0**	**165.5**	**206.3**	**255.0**	**341.1**	**435.8**	**616.5**	**1036.7**	**2664.4**
1995 projected	*195.3**	*55.3**	*225.2**	*84.1*	*115.3*	*172.9*	*213.9*	*261.2*	*332.1*	*397.2*	*537.3*	*856.2*	*2157.6*
All non-medical causes													
1955	...	...	...	...	...	...	...	...	...	...	...	...	...
1965	88.2*	65.2*	98.4*	93.5	96.0	98.5	98.2	98.6	99.2	104.8	137.9	159.4	316.7
1975	118.2*	78.6*	145.1*	136.3	142.3	147.9	147.1	135.5	154.3	152.4	164.9	222.7	385.9
1985	122.1*	70.7*	155.7*	142.5	162.3	172.7	170.9	153.1	146.0	142.3	184.1	243.1	460.4
1990	**132.2***	**77.7***	**173.5***	**159.8**	**166.9**	**188.6**	**194.3**	**175.9**	**168.3**	**161.1**	**173.5**	**252.7**	**424.5**
1995 projected	*142.4**	*84.6**	*190.1**	*172.7*	*178.7*	*203.2*	*216.8*	*199.8*	*190.7*	*169.1*	*176.4*	*246.8*	*408.6*

POLAND: Females

	All ages	0–34	35–69	35–39	40–44	45–49	50–54	55–59	60–64	65–69	70–74	75–79	80+/NK
POPULATION (1000s)													
1955	14188	8773	4879	721	939	922	802	645	469	382	258	150	128
1965	16209	9432	6010	1192	1079	706	885	871	725	552	359	237	171
1975	17551	9714	6588	1069	1116	1141	1048	672	785	758	574	384	292
1985	19059	10458	6983	1360	920	1047	1079	1072	936	570	655	513	450
1990	**19541**	**10209**	**7796**	**1616**	**1341**	**902**	**1019**	**1042**	**1016**	**860**	**494**	**510**	**532**
1995 projected	*20129*	*10024*	*8395*	*1605*	*1617*	*1335*	*892*	*998*	*1000*	*947*	*762*	*399*	*549*
NUMBER OF DEATHS													
All causes													
1955	125845	40421	40902	1725	2999	4037	5298	7027	8326	11490	13544	12102	18876
1965	111384	15407	40526	1872	2342	2408	4528	6935	9429	13012	14573	16353	24525
1975	139061	11498	42069	1353	2188	3624	4988	4904	9847	15165	21008	24482	40004
1985	179378	9789	45801	1805	1993	3475	5603	8725	12120	12080	23692	33012	67084
1990	**179107**	**7846**	**51545**	**2089**	**2889**	**2963**	**4970**	**8174**	**12767**	**17693**	**16775**	**30565**	**72376**
1995 projected	*174377*	*6622*	*52224*	*2059*	*3440*	*4236*	*4187*	*7533*	*12184*	*18585*	*24328*	*22208*	*68995*
Lung cancer													
1955	...	...	...	...	...	...	...	...	...	...	...	...	...
1965	813	28	541	21	34	41	66	100	115	164	126	74	44
1975	1367	21	818	17	49	91	103	114	189	255	241	176	111
1985	2205	25	1278	30	46	83	173	294	347	305	329	329	244
1990	**2805**	**36**	**1703**	**38**	**73**	**116**	**190**	**308**	**471**	**507**	**340**	**402**	**324**
1995 projected	*3589*	*44*	*2127*	*40*	*119*	*217*	*196*	*344*	*526*	*685*	*640*	*383*	*395*
ANNUAL DEATH RATE / 100,000 (*The rates for the age groups 0–34 and 35–69 are the means of seven five-yearly rates, but the all-ages rates are standardised to the conventional "European" age distribution)													
All causes													
1955	1203.8*	367.3*	1075.6*	239.3	319.5	438.0	660.7	1090.3	1773.8	3007.9	5247.6	8095.0	14770.0
1965	927.7*	164.6*	811.7*	157.0	217.1	341.0	511.8	796.5	1300.6	2357.7	4055.9	6914.6	14308.6
1975	840.1*	118.8*	729.1*	126.6	196.0	317.7	476.0	730.3	1254.9	2002.0	3659.3	6375.5	13723.5
1985	864.2*	87.4*	775.6*	132.7	216.7	332.0	519.2	814.2	1294.5	2119.7	3617.7	6432.6	14910.9
1990	**808.3***	**77.3***	**751.3***	**129.2**	**215.4**	**328.5**	**488.0**	**784.5**	**1257.0**	**2056.6**	**3393.7**	**5992.0**	**13614.7**
1995 projected	*758.1**	*68.4**	*723.2**	*128.3*	*212.7*	*317.4*	*469.2*	*755.0*	*1218.3*	*1961.9*	*3191.0*	*5571.5*	*12565.1*
All cancer													
1955	...	...	...	...	...	...	...	...	...	...	...	...	...
1965	151.1*	10.2*	239.2*	47.5	75.7	131.4	199.7	280.8	380.4	558.8	735.9	841.0	855.9
1975	144.4*	9.3*	230.2*	41.7	77.0	134.2	201.2	271.5	391.4	494.1	665.4	805.2	813.0
1985	152.3*	8.6*	244.9*	45.3	78.5	131.4	202.2	299.1	412.8	545.2	678.4	836.1	924.0
1990	**154.2***	**8.1***	**245.9***	**43.6**	**85.1**	**136.7**	**201.3**	**287.2**	**411.8**	**555.7**	**716.0**	**872.8**	**926.3**
1995 projected	*156.1**	*7.5**	*247.4**	*44.8*	*87.8*	*139.8*	*197.9*	*281.8*	*409.7*	*570.0*	*741.5*	*907.7*	*946.5*
Lung cancer													
1955	...	...	...	...	...	...	...	...	...	...	...	...	...
1965	6.3*	0.3*	10.7*	1.8	3.2	5.8	7.5	11.5	15.9	29.7	35.1	31.3	25.7
1975	8.3*	0.2*	14.1*	1.6	4.4	8.0	9.8	17.0	24.1	33.7	42.0	45.8	38.1
1985	11.8*	0.2*	21.3*	2.2	5.0	7.9	16.0	27.4	37.1	53.5	50.2	64.1	54.2
1990	**14.2***	**0.4***	**24.9***	**2.4**	**5.4**	**12.9**	**18.7**	**29.6**	**46.4**	**58.9**	**68.8**	**78.8**	**60.9**
1995 projected	*17.1**	*0.5**	*29.6**	*2.5*	*7.4*	*16.3*	*22.0*	*34.5*	*52.6*	*72.3*	*83.9*	*96.1*	*71.9*
Upper aerodigestive cancer (mouth, oesophagus, pharynx and larynx)													
1955	...	...	...	...	...	...	...	...	...	...	...	...	...
1965	3.8*	0.2*	4.5*	0.5	0.8	1.8	3.8	4.6	7.7	12.1	22.0	30.9	40.8
1975	3.4*	0.1*	4.6*	0.1	1.3	1.8	3.6	4.5	8.7	12.1	17.9	22.1	32.9
1985	3.2*	0.1*	4.4*	0.4	1.4	2.7	4.8	5.5	7.3	8.6	15.4	21.0	29.8
1990	**3.5***	**0.1***	**5.1***	**0.6**	**1.6**	**4.3**	**3.4**	**5.8**	**9.1**	**11.3**	**15.6**	**22.7**	**27.8**
1995 projected	*3.8**	*0.1**	*5.8**	*0.7*	*2.2*	*4.5*	*3.6*	*5.9*	*11.0*	*12.9*	*17.1*	*21.8*	*27.7*
Other cancer													
1955	...	...	...	...	...	...	...	...	...	...	...	...	...
1965	141.0*	9.7*	223.9*	45.2	71.7	123.8	188.4	264.7	356.8	516.9	678.8	778.9	789.4
1975	132.7*	9.0*	211.5*	40.0	71.3	124.5	187.8	250.0	358.6	448.3	605.5	737.2	742.0
1985	137.3*	8.3*	219.2*	42.7	72.1	120.8	181.4	266.1	368.5	483.1	612.8	751.0	840.0
1990	**136.5***	**7.6***	**215.9***	**40.6**	**78.1**	**119.5**	**179.2**	**251.9**	**356.4**	**485.5**	**631.6**	**771.2**	**837.5**
1995 projected	*135.3**	*6.9**	*211.9**	*41.6*	*78.3*	*119.0*	*172.3*	*241.4*	*346.1*	*484.9*	*640.5*	*789.8*	*846.8*
Chronic obstructive pulmonary disease (COPD)													
1955	...	...	...	...	...	...	...	...	...	...	...	...	...
1965	12.0*	1.0*	9.7*	1.0	1.5	1.4	3.3	7.4	16.7	37.0	72.4	122.6	181.4
1975	17.1*	0.8*	14.2*	1.1	1.7	3.1	6.0	13.6	24.9	49.4	99.5	166.1	277.9
1985	17.2*	0.5*	18.2*	1.2	3.6	5.9	8.7	20.1	32.6	55.3	88.4	147.1	250.3
1990	**11.3***	**0.4***	**11.8***	**1.1**	**1.8**	**2.7**	**5.7**	**11.7**	**21.0**	**38.5**	**61.5**	**99.6**	**162.7**
1995 projected	*8.0**	*0.3**	*8.3**	*0.8*	*1.2*	*1.9*	*4.0*	*8.2*	*14.7*	*27.0*	*43.2*	*69.7*	*115.1*
Other respiratory disease													
1955	...	...	...	...	...	...	...	...	...	...	...	...	...
1965	37.1*	23.7*	17.6*	1.9	3.5	5.5	7.3	15.4	29.9	59.4	128.9	233.8	462.7
1975	32.7*	14.0*	18.4*	3.5	3.4	4.9	8.6	16.7	31.0	61.0	118.8	235.9	517.3
1985	19.0*	4.4*	12.5*	2.5	3.5	5.2	6.7	12.4	20.8	36.1	66.3	140.1	364.7
1990	**13.7***	**3.3***	**9.4***	**1.9**	**3.1**	**4.1**	**5.5**	**10.3**	**15.0**	**25.8**	**51.8**	**100.0**	**248.1**
1995 projected	*9.9**	*2.4**	*7.1**	*1.5*	*2.5*	*3.4*	*4.5*	*7.8*	*10.9*	*19.2*	*37.6*	*70.0*	*175.4*
Vascular disease													
1955	...	...	...	...	...	...	...	...	...	...	...	...	...
1965	372.3*	10.5*	308.9*	31.0	45.5	83.8	150.7	271.4	515.2	1064.9	1950.7	3436.8	6665.1
1975	398.1*	7.5*	290.2*	28.0	47.3	82.4	140.5	251.1	517.8	964.4	2001.9	3700.5	7991.8
1985	469.3*	5.2*	335.6*	30.3	57.1	99.3	177.4	312.8	573.7	1098.6	2165.7	4210.6	10028.9
1990	**445.9***	**4.8***	**327.3***	**29.5**	**59.6**	**95.1**	**162.8**	**308.3**	**566.6**	**1069.3**	**1995.8**	**3938.1**	**9549.7**
1995 projected	*421.4**	*4.4**	*312.3**	*29.9*	*58.2*	*89.5*	*155.2*	*298.7*	*550.5*	*1004.0*	*1854.1*	*3686.4*	*9045.3*
Liver cirrhosis													
1955	...	...	...	...	...	...	...	...	...	...	...	...	...
1965	6.6*	0.2*	9.0*	1.6	1.9	2.8	5.3	8.6	16.0	26.6	40.4	46.9	55.4
1975	7.6*	0.3*	10.8*	0.7	2.6	4.1	7.4	10.1	20.5	30.0	44.9	47.1	65.2
1985	7.9*	0.3*	11.8*	1.7	3.0	5.0	8.0	13.8	21.0	30.0	41.1	53.6	56.2
1990	**7.1***	**0.3***	**10.9***	**2.1**	**3.1**	**4.8**	**8.5**	**12.8**	**17.9**	**26.7**	**37.0**	**45.9**	**43.3**
1995 projected	*6.4**	*0.4**	*10.0**	*2.5*	*3.2*	*4.9*	*8.3*	*11.6*	*15.7*	*23.5*	*32.3*	*37.9*	*35.1*
Other medical causes													
1955	...	...	...	...	...	...	...	...	...	...	...	...	...
1965	319.9*	103.1*	200.4*	59.2	72.4	94.2	122.1	185.8	306.2	563.0	1062.1	2109.1	5818.6
1975	205.8*	69.8*	132.3*	31.9	41.4	61.8	86.7	132.8	222.9	348.3	643.1	1272.7	3714.2
1985	163.1*	53.0*	119.2*	28.9	42.2	55.3	83.6	125.2	196.7	302.7	490.8	894.8	2870.4
1990	**141.1***	**45.4***	**111.3***	**25.4**	**35.1**	**53.7**	**76.6**	**118.6**	**181.3**	**288.4**	**452.4**	**779.1**	**2304.9**
1995 projected	*121.8**	*38.8**	*102.7**	*22.2*	*31.4*	*48.5*	*71.6*	*109.3*	*169.4*	*266.4*	*403.9*	*647.5*	*1888.0*
All non-medical causes													
1955	...	...	...	...	...	...	...	...	...	...	...	...	...
1965	28.7*	16.0*	26.8*	14.8	16.5	21.8	23.4	27.1	36.1	48.0	65.7	124.3	269.5
1975	34.4*	17.2*	33.0*	19.6	22.7	27.2	25.5	34.5	46.5	54.9	85.7	147.9	344.1
1985	35.5*	15.4*	33.4*	22.9	28.8	30.0	32.7	30.8	36.7	51.8	87.0	150.2	416.3
1990	**34.9***	**15.1***	**34.8***	**25.7**	**27.5**	**31.5**	**27.6**	**35.5**	**43.4**	**52.2**	**79.3**	**156.6**	**379.8**
1995 projected	*34.5**	*14.7**	*35.5**	*26.5*	*28.3*	*29.4*	*27.7*	*37.5*	*47.4*	*51.6*	*78.4*	*152.3*	*359.7*

POLAND: 1975

Smoking-attributed deaths (Sm.) and total deaths (Total)

		ALL CAUSES	ALL CANCER	Lung cancer	Upper aero-digestive ca.	Other cancer	COPD	Other respiratory	Vascular disease	Liver cirrhosis	Other medical	Non-medical
Males												
0–34	Sm.	–	–	–	–	–	–	–	–	–	–	–
	Total	21523	994	54	29	911	127	1857	1152	65	9467	7861
35–69	Sm.	22421	7806	5067	1046	1693	2135	444	8504	–	3532	–
	Total	71982	17522	5459	1587	10476	2753	1537	28909	1538	11293	8430
		(31%)	(45%)	(93%)	(66%)	(16%)	(78%)	(29%)	(29%)		(31%)	
70+	Sm.	10074	2991	2016	338	637	2436	237	3285	–	1125	–
	Total	64330	9540	2294	660	6586	3720	2538	33926	586	12428	1592
		(16%)	(31%)	(88%)	(51%)	(10%)	(65%)	(9%)	(10%)		(9%)	
Any age	Sm.	32495	10797	7083	1384	2330	4571	681	11789	–	4657	–
	Total	157835	28056	7807	2276	17973	6600	5932	63987	2189	33188	17883
		(21%)	(38%)	(91%)	(61%)	(13%)	(69%)	(11%)	(18%)		(14%)	
Females												
0–34	Sm.	–	–	–	–	–	–	–	–	–	–	–
	Total	11498	848	21	11	816	72	1376	681	26	6821	1674
35–69	Sm.	1542	391	296	34	61	193	41	619	–	298	–
	Total	42069	13582	818	263	12501	789	1038	16293	618	7696	2053
		(4%)	(3%)	(36%)	(13%)	(0%)	(24%)	(4%)	(4%)		(4%)	
70+	Sm.	1222	205	150	26	29	342	29	474	–	172	–
	Total	85494	9282	528	284	8470	2019	3096	48999	629	19406	2063
		(1%)	(2%)	(28%)	(9%)	(0%)	(17%)	(1%)	(1%)		(1%)	
Any age	Sm.	2764	596	446	60	90	535	70	1093	–	470	–
	Total	139061	23712	1367	558	21787	2880	5510	65973	1273	33923	5790
		(2%)	(3%)	(33%)	(11%)	(0%)	(19%)	(1%)	(2%)		(1%)	
Males+Females												
0–34	Sm.	–	–	–	–	–	–	–	–	–	–	–
	Total	33021	1842	75	40	1727	199	3233	1833	91	16288	9535
35–69	Sm.	23963	8197	5363	1080	1754	2328	485	9123	–	3830	–
	Total	114051	31104	6277	1850	22977	3542	2575	45202	2156	18989	10483
		(21%)	(26%)	(85%)	(58%)	(8%)	(66%)	(19%)	(20%)		(20%)	
70+	Sm.	11296	3196	2166	364	666	2778	266	3759	–	1297	–
	Total	149824	18822	2822	944	15056	5739	5634	82925	1215	31834	3655
		(8%)	(17%)	(77%)	(39%)	(4%)	(48%)	(5%)	(5%)		(4%)	
Any age	Sm.	35259	11393	7529	1444	2420	5106	751	12882	–	5127	–
	Total	296896	51768	9174	2834	39760	9480	11442	129960	3462	67111	23673
		(12%)	(22%)	(82%)	(51%)	(6%)	(54%)	(7%)	(10%)		(8%)	

POLAND: 1985

Smoking-attributed deaths (Sm.) and total deaths (Total)

		ALL CAUSES	ALL CANCER	Lung cancer	Upper aero-digestive ca.	Other cancer	COPD	Other respiratory	Vascular disease	Liver cirrhosis	Other medical	Non-medical
Males												
0–34	Sm.	–	–	–	–	–	–	–	–	–	–	–
	Total	19854	1094	55	25	1014	64	699	1360	83	8807	7747
35–69	Sm.	37158	12939	8348	1760	2831	2737	595	15566	–	5321	–
	Total	88520	22980	8751	2321	11908	3245	1404	37191	1822	11984	9894
		(42%)	(56%)	(95%)	(76%)	(24%)	(84%)	(42%)	(42%)		(44%)	
70+	Sm.	17302	5139	3451	556	1132	3984	269	6454	–	1456	–
	Total	93706	14013	3813	960	9240	5585	2356	55611	754	13009	2378
		(18%)	(37%)	(91%)	(58%)	(12%)	(71%)	(11%)	(12%)		(11%)	
Any age	Sm.	54460	18078	11799	2316	3963	6721	864	22020	–	6777	–
	Total	202080	38087	12619	3306	22162	8894	4459	94162	2659	33800	20019
		(27%)	(47%)	(94%)	(70%)	(18%)	(76%)	(19%)	(23%)		(20%)	
Females												
0–34	Sm.	–	–	–	–	–	–	–	–	–	–	–
	Total	9789	931	25	6	900	53	506	571	33	6065	1630
35–69	Sm.	3756	957	732	70	155	455	64	1649	–	631	–
	Total	45801	15072	1278	275	13519	1040	726	18875	705	7171	2212
		(8%)	(6%)	(57%)	(25%)	(1%)	(44%)	(9%)	(9%)		(9%)	
70+	Sm.	3340	554	410	61	83	795	51	1552	–	388	–
	Total	123788	12891	902	343	11646	2460	2794	80912	797	20720	3214
		(3%)	(4%)	(45%)	(18%)	(1%)	(32%)	(2%)	(2%)		(2%)	
Any age	Sm.	7096	1511	1142	131	238	1250	115	3201	–	1019	–
	Total	179378	28894	2205	624	26065	3553	4026	100358	1535	33956	7056
		(4%)	(5%)	(52%)	(21%)	(1%)	(35%)	(3%)	(3%)		(3%)	
Males+Females												
0–34	Sm.	–	–	–	–	–	–	–	–	–	–	–
	Total	29643	2025	80	31	1914	117	1205	1931	116	14872	9377
35–69	Sm.	40914	13896	9080	1830	2986	3192	659	17215	–	5952	–
	Total	134321	38052	10029	2596	25427	4285	2130	56066	2527	19155	12106
		(30%)	(37%)	(91%)	(70%)	(12%)	(74%)	(31%)	(31%)		(31%)	
70+	Sm.	20642	5693	3861	617	1215	4779	320	8006	–	1844	–
	Total	217494	26904	4715	1303	20886	8045	5150	136523	1551	33729	5592
		(9%)	(21%)	(82%)	(47%)	(6%)	(59%)	(6%)	(6%)		(5%)	
Any age	Sm.	61556	19589	12941	2447	4201	7971	979	25221	–	7796	–
	Total	381458	66981	14824	3930	48227	12447	8485	194520	4194	67756	27075
		(16%)	(29%)	(87%)	(62%)	(9%)	(64%)	(12%)	(13%)		(12%)	

(To be conservative, no deaths before age 35, and none from liver cirrhosis or non-medical causes, were attributed to smoking.)

POLAND: 1990

Smoking–attributed deaths (Sm.) and total deaths (Total)

		ALL CAUSES	ALL CANCER	Lung cancer	Upper aero–digestive ca.	Other cancer	COPD	Other respiratory	Vascular disease	Liver cirrhosis	Other medical	Non–medical
Males												
0–34	Sm.	–	–	–	–	–	–	–	–	–	–	–
	Total	17601	1018	46	10	962	33	432	1355	92	6723	7948
35–69	Sm.	44608	16075	10318	2272	3485	2282	610	19320	–	6321	–
	Total	105138	27699	10784	2946	13969	2670	1405	45415	1780	13907	12262
		(42%)	(58%)	(96%)	(77%)	(25%)	(85%)	(43%)	(43%)		(45%)	
70+	Sm.	15336	5003	3370	516	1117	2658	212	6212	–	1251	–
	Total	86594	13359	3709	873	8777	3684	1889	53673	602	11127	2260
		(18%)	(37%)	(91%)	(59%)	(13%)	(72%)	(11%)	(12%)		(11%)	
Any age	Sm.	59944	21078	13688	2788	4602	4940	822	25532	–	7572	–
	Total	209333	42076	14539	3829	23708	6387	3726	100443	2474	31757	22470
		(29%)	(50%)	(94%)	(73%)	(19%)	(77%)	(22%)	(25%)		(24%)	
Females												
0–34	Sm.	–	–	–	–	–	–	–	–	–	–	–
	Total	7846	836	36	12	788	36	328	493	36	4590	1527
35–69	Sm.	5116	1420	1083	112	225	392	70	2383	–	851	–
	Total	51545	17086	1703	354	15029	790	646	21959	751	7703	2610
		(10%)	(8%)	(64%)	(32%)	(1%)	(50%)	(11%)	(11%)		(11%)	
70+	Sm.	4421	827	610	86	131	717	60	2293	–	524	–
	Total	119716	12915	1066	341	11508	1677	2085	80719	647	18463	3210
		(4%)	(6%)	(57%)	(25%)	(1%)	(43%)	(3%)	(3%)		(3%)	
Any age	Sm.	9537	2247	1693	198	356	1109	130	4676	–	1375	–
	Total	179107	30837	2805	707	27325	2503	3059	103171	1434	30756	7347
		(5%)	(7%)	(60%)	(28%)	(1%)	(44%)	(4%)	(5%)		(4%)	
Males+Females												
0–34	Sm.	–	–	–	–	–	–	–	–	–	–	–
	Total	25447	1854	82	22	1750	69	760	1848	128	11313	9475
35–69	Sm.	49724	17495	11401	2384	3710	2674	680	21703	–	7172	–
	Total	156683	44785	12487	3300	28998	3460	2051	67374	2531	21610	14872
		(32%)	(39%)	(91%)	(72%)	(13%)	(77%)	(33%)	(32%)		(33%)	
70+	Sm.	19757	5830	3980	602	1248	3375	272	8505	–	1775	–
	Total	206310	26274	4775	1214	20285	5361	3974	134392	1249	29590	5470
		(10%)	(22%)	(83%)	(50%)	(6%)	(63%)	(7%)	(6%)		(6%)	
Any age	Sm.	69481	23325	15381	2986	4958	6049	952	30208	–	8947	–
	Total	388440	72913	17344	4536	51033	8890	6785	203614	3908	62513	29817
		(18%)	(32%)	(89%)	(66%)	(10%)	(68%)	(14%)	(15%)		(14%)	

POLAND: 1995

Smoking–attributed deaths (Sm.) and total deaths (Total)

		ALL CAUSES	ALL CANCER	Lung cancer	Upper aero–digestive ca.	Other cancer	COPD	Other respiratory	Vascular disease	Liver cirrhosis	Other medical	Non–medical
Males												
0–34	Sm.	–	–	–	–	–	–	–	–	–	–	–
	Total	16705	963	39	9	915	23	318	1292	88	5548	8473
35–69	Sm.	50639	18642	11878	2777	3987	1730	593	22471	–	7203	–
	Total	116378	30960	12371	3538	15051	1997	1294	50586	1646	15156	14739
		(44%)	(60%)	(96%)	(78%)	(26%)	(87%)	(46%)	(44%)		(48%)	
70+	Sm.	16873	6145	4205	577	1363	2006	199	7259	–	1264	–
	Total	84434	15016	4572	922	9522	2691	1506	52850	562	9475	2334
		(20%)	(41%)	(92%)	(63%)	(14%)	(75%)	(13%)	(14%)		(13%)	
Any age	Sm.	67512	24787	16083	3354	5350	3736	792	29730	–	8467	–
	Total	217517	46939	16982	4469	25488	4711	3118	104728	2296	30179	25546
		(31%)	(53%)	(95%)	(75%)	(21%)	(79%)	(25%)	(28%)		(28%)	
Females												
0–34	Sm.	–	–	–	–	–	–	–	–	–	–	–
	Total	6622	713	44	13	656	31	230	420	40	3733	1455
35–69	Sm.	6334	1926	1472	157	297	325	71	2983	–	1029	–
	Total	52224	18080	2127	430	15523	579	519	21999	727	7460	2860
		(12%)	(11%)	(69%)	(37%)	(2%)	(56%)	(14%)	(14%)		(14%)	
70+	Sm.	5935	1254	929	121	204	638	65	3295	–	683	–
	Total	115531	14468	1418	369	12681	1239	1529	78498	590	16027	3180
		(5%)	(9%)	(66%)	(33%)	(2%)	(51%)	(4%)	(4%)		(4%)	
Any age	Sm.	12269	3180	2401	278	501	963	136	6278	–	1712	–
	Total	174377	33261	3589	812	28860	1849	2278	100917	1357	27220	7495
		(7%)	(10%)	(67%)	(34%)	(2%)	(52%)	(6%)	(6%)		(6%)	
Males+Females												
0–34	Sm.	–	–	–	–	–	–	–	–	–	–	–
	Total	23327	1676	83	22	1571	54	548	1712	128	9281	9928
35–69	Sm.	56973	20568	13350	2934	4284	2055	664	25454	–	8232	–
	Total	168602	49040	14498	3968	30574	2576	1813	72585	2373	22616	17599
		(34%)	(42%)	(92%)	(74%)	(14%)	(80%)	(37%)	(35%)		(36%)	
70+	Sm.	22808	7399	5134	698	1567	2644	264	10554	–	1947	–
	Total	199965	29484	5990	1291	22203	3930	3035	131348	1152	25502	5514
		(11%)	(25%)	(86%)	(54%)	(7%)	(67%)	(9%)	(8%)		(8%)	
Any age	Sm.	79781	27967	18484	3632	5851	4699	928	36008	–	10179	–
	Total	391894	80200	20571	5281	54348	6560	5396	205645	3653	57399	33041
		(20%)	(35%)	(90%)	(69%)	(11%)	(72%)	(17%)	(18%)		(18%)	

(To be conservative, no deaths before age 35, and none from liver cirrhosis or non–medical causes, were attributed to smoking.)

PORTUGAL: 1990

		No. of deaths			Standardised rates (Defined on p.460)			Annual death rates / 100, 000						
		All ages	0–34	35–69	All ages	0–34	35–69	0–4	5–9	10–14	15–19	20–24	25–29	30–34
ALL CAUSES	M	53439	4185	19351	1181.2	162.3	1204.8	313.4	41.5	49.5	153.6	184.7	179.8	213.3
	F	49676	1821	10444	713.3	76.8	550.8	237.5	32.4	31.3	43.4	54.3	59.1	79.8
Tuberculosis	M	288	17	168	6.5	0.6	10.1	–	–	–	0.2	0.2	1.2	2.8
	F	97	12	43	1.6	0.5	2.2	0.4	–	0.3	0.2	0.7	0.2	1.4
Other infective	M	220	70	91	5.0	3.1	5.5	15.6	1.1	0.2	0.5	1.7	1.0	1.4
and parasitic	F	177	37	66	3.1	1.6	3.4	6.3	1.2	0.5	0.7	1.0	0.7	0.8
ALL CANCER	M	10254	227	5118	226.7	8.5	320.9	5.3	4.5	5.4	8.3	8.9	11.4	15.6
	F	7923	218	3526	128.7	8.6	183.8	9.2	6.0	3.4	6.7	5.5	11.4	17.9
Mouth and	M	366	8	255	8.4	0.3	15.5	0.7	–	0.2	0.2	0.2	–	0.8
pharynx cancer	F	83	1	29	1.3	0.1	1.5	0.4	–	–	–	–	–	–
Oesophagus cancer	M	373	–	234	8.4	–	14.5	–	–	–	–	–	–	–
	F	134	1	40	2.0	0.0	2.1	–	–	–	–	0.2	–	–
Stomach cancer	M	1798	22	902	39.8	0.8	56.7	–	–	–	–	0.5	1.5	4.0
	F	1212	17	434	18.6	0.6	22.9	–	–	–	0.7	0.5	1.2	2.0
Colorectal cancer	M	1204	9	529	26.4	0.3	33.4	–	–	0.2	0.2	0.7	–	1.1
	F	1080	8	382	16.5	0.3	20.1	–	–	–	–	–	0.2	2.0
Liver cancer	M	100	4	67	2.3	0.2	4.3	1.0	–	–	–	–	0.2	–
	F	49	3	25	0.8	0.1	1.3	0.4	–	0.3	–	–	–	0.3
Pancreas cancer	M	395	4	196	8.8	0.2	12.2	–	–	–	–	–	0.2	0.8
	F	328	–	115	5.0	–	6.1	–	–	–	–	–	–	–
Larynx cancer	M	376	1	259	8.6	0.0	15.9	–	–	–	–	–	–	0.3
	F	38	2	15	0.6	0.1	0.8	0.4	–	–	–	–	–	0.3
Lung cancer	M	1825	7	1104	40.3	0.3	69.3	–	–	–	0.5	0.2	0.2	0.8
	F	416	5	185	6.6	0.2	9.7	–	–	–	–	0.2	0.5	0.6
Malignant melanoma	M	43	3	22	1.0	0.1	1.3	–	–	–	–	–	–	0.8
	F	44	6	23	0.8	0.2	1.1	–	0.3	–	–	–	1.2	–
Female breast cancer	F	1410	18	893	25.5	0.7	45.7	–	–	–	–	0.2	1.2	3.4
Cervix cancer	F	181	5	117	3.3	0.2	5.9	–	–	–	–	–	0.5	0.8
Other uterine cancer	F	420	8	214	6.9	0.3	11.2	–	–	–	0.2	–	0.2	1.7
Ovarian cancer	F	271	7	172	4.9	0.3	8.9	–	–	0.3	0.2	0.5	0.2	0.6
Prostate cancer	M	1123	–	256	24.4	–	17.1	–	–	–	–	–	–	–
Bladder cancer	M	372	1	119	8.1	0.0	7.8	–	–	–	–	–	–	0.3
	F	134	2	32	1.9	0.1	1.7	0.4	–	–	–	–	–	0.3
Other and ill-defined	M	1650	80	887	36.6	3.0	55.1	2.0	1.4	2.2	3.1	3.4	4.4	4.2
cancer sites	F	1556	67	616	24.6	2.7	32.5	4.2	2.4	1.8	2.5	1.2	3.2	3.4
Hodgkin's disease	M	28	6	14	0.6	0.2	0.9	–	–	0.2	0.2	0.2	0.7	–
	F	23	4	12	0.4	0.2	0.6	–	–	–	–	–	0.5	0.6
Myeloma and non-	M	301	31	152	6.6	1.1	9.5	0.3	1.1	0.2	1.7	1.7	1.5	1.4
Hodgkin lymphomas	F	268	14	119	4.3	0.5	6.4	0.7	0.3	0.3	1.0	0.2	0.7	0.6
Leukaemia	M	300	51	122	6.4	1.9	7.5	1.3	2.0	2.2	2.4	1.9	2.5	0.8
	F	276	50	103	4.7	2.0	5.3	2.8	3.0	0.8	2.0	2.2	1.5	1.7
ALL VASCULAR	M	20961	159	6049	462.4	6.0	387.5	2.0	2.0	1.5	4.3	7.9	8.2	15.9
DISEASE	F	24565	96	3359	329.0	3.7	180.9	3.9	0.3	2.1	1.7	3.2	5.5	9.5
Rheumatic heart	M	72	5	52	1.6	0.2	3.1	–	–	–	0.2	0.2	0.5	0.3
disease and fever	F	181	7	107	3.1	0.3	5.6	–	–	0.3	–	0.2	0.7	0.6
Hypertensive disease	M	303	1	84	6.8	0.0	5.4	–	–	–	–	–	–	0.3
	F	487	1	53	6.5	0.0	2.9	–	–	–	0.2	–	–	–
Ischaemic heart	M	5288	31	2308	116.6	1.2	145.9	–	0.3	0.5	0.5	1.0	2.0	4.0
disease	F	4202	13	841	58.4	0.5	45.3	0.4	–	0.3	–	0.2	0.5	2.2
Pulmonary embolism	M	437	7	172	9.6	0.2	10.8	–	–	0.2	0.5	0.2	0.5	0.3
and other venous	F	418	4	107	6.0	0.2	5.7	–	–	–	–	0.2	0.2	0.6
Cerebrovascular	M	10750	61	2481	236.3	2.3	161.1	1.0	1.1	0.5	1.9	3.9	2.5	5.1
disease	F	13890	35	1727	184.5	1.4	93.2	1.1	0.3	0.5	0.7	1.0	2.0	3.9
Other vascular	M	4111	54	952	91.6	2.0	61.1	1.0	0.6	0.2	1.2	2.6	2.7	5.9
disease	F	5387	36	524	70.6	1.4	28.2	2.5	–	1.0	0.7	1.5	2.0	2.2
Chronic obstructive	M	1894	27	591	41.5	1.0	38.0	1.7	–	0.2	0.7	1.0	2.2	1.4
pulmonary disease	F	923	17	174	12.9	0.7	9.3	0.7	–	0.3	–	1.0	1.2	1.4
Other respiratory	M	2443	116	618	54.3	4.8	39.2	16.6	1.7	2.0	2.8	2.6	3.0	4.8
disease	F	2208	74	264	30.1	3.3	14.0	13.0	1.8	1.6	1.5	1.0	2.0	2.0
Peptic ulcer	M	257	4	91	5.7	0.2	5.7	–	–	–	–	0.2	0.2	0.6
	F	157	2	27	2.1	0.1	1.5	–	–	–	–	–	0.2	0.3
Liver cirrhosis	M	1741	40	1266	39.9	1.6	76.3	0.3	–	0.2	–	0.5	2.0	7.9
	F	674	28	446	12.3	1.1	22.9	–	–	0.3	–	1.0	1.2	5.0
Renal disease	M	670	17	197	14.7	0.7	12.7	1.3	–	–	0.5	0.7	0.7	1.4
	F	474	8	126	6.9	0.3	6.7	–	0.3	–	0.2	0.2	0.2	1.1
Pregnancy and birth	F	12	8	4	0.2	0.3	0.2	–	–	–	0.2	–	1.0	0.8
Congenital and	M	583	570	11	15.2	26.8	0.6	181.1	1.7	0.5	0.9	1.2	1.5	0.6
perinatal causes	F	437	421	12	11.9	20.9	0.6	139.2	1.8	1.6	0.7	1.0	1.0	0.8
Ill-defined causes	M	5638	642	1618	126.7	24.3	98.2	31.2	4.8	9.9	24.9	32.5	30.6	36.0
	F	6482	217	687	86.6	8.8	36.0	21.5	3.3	2.8	8.6	9.4	7.7	8.4
Other medical causes	M	3572	284	1480	78.3	11.1	91.7	18.6	4.2	6.7	6.2	9.2	12.4	20.4
	F	3729	177	1088	56.0	7.2	57.8	13.7	5.7	6.0	4.2	6.2	6.0	8.4
ALL NON-	M	4918	2012	2053	104.1	73.7	118.4	39.5	21.5	22.8	104.3	118.0	105.5	104.5
MEDICAL CAUSES	F	1818	506	622	31.8	19.9	31.5	29.6	12.0	12.7	18.5	24.1	20.6	21.8
Motor vehicle	M	2178	1063	834	44.6	38.2	48.0	6.3	10.5	11.9	66.5	69.1	55.6	47.3
traffic accidents	F	606	236	219	11.0	9.0	11.0	7.4	6.0	7.3	10.1	13.4	8.4	10.6
Fire	M	58	15	21	1.3	0.6	1.3	2.0	0.8	0.2	0.2	0.2	0.2	0.6
	F	39	7	8	0.6	0.3	0.4	1.8	0.3	–	–	0.2	–	–
Suicide	M	642	173	314	13.9	6.3	18.4	–	–	1.2	3.6	11.3	14.1	13.9
	F	228	52	108	4.1	1.9	5.5	–	–	–	1.2	5.0	2.7	4.5
Homicide	M	118	49	62	2.6	1.8	3.5	1.7	–	–	1.2	3.6	2.2	4.2
	F	47	19	25	1.0	0.8	1.2	1.4	0.9	–	0.2	0.5	1.5	0.8
POPULATION (thousands):	**M=males**				4762.1	2652.9	1778.0	300.9	353.9	403.9	421.1	415.2	404.8	353.1
	F=females				5106.0	2572.1	2013.3	283.8	333.3	386.2	405.9	403.3	402.5	357.1

PORTUGAL: 1990

Annual death rates / 100, 000 — 9th ICD categories

35–39	40–44	45–49	50–54	55–59	60–64	65–69	70–74	75–79	80+/NK			
272.6	372.5	532.9	828.1	1305.7	2007.5	3114.6	4971.2	7962.7	17320.0	M	ALL CAUSES	001–999
117.7	166.4	266.4	374.0	562.2	857.9	1510.9	2761.7	5034.6	14395.9	F		
2.9	3.2	6.5	9.0	14.9	19.8	14.6	24.4	33.7	38.9	M	Tuberculosis	010–018, 137
1.2	0.6	1.4	1.7	2.4	2.5	5.7	6.4	4.8	13.3	F		
3.8	2.5	2.4	3.5	4.8	8.3	13.1	17.3	12.7	25.5	M	Other infective	Rest of 001–139
0.6	2.3	1.1	2.4	3.8	8.4	5.3	9.6	10.1	23.6	F	and parasitic	
38.8	72.1	136.7	222.2	377.3	580.4	818.8	1141.6	1458.6	2090.0	M	ALL CANCER	140–208
42.4	64.5	113.9	148.2	220.0	290.8	407.0	574.1	763.4	1102.3	F		
1.6	4.6	14.5	12.5	24.9	25.0	25.2	33.8	26.4	32.8	M	Mouth and	140–149
0.3	0.6	1.4	1.7	1.4	1.1	4.0	5.9	11.9	13.3	F	pharynx cancer	
1.3	4.6	7.7	10.1	20.5	24.6	32.8	37.4	40.0	52.3	M	Oesophagus cancer	150
0.3	0.6	0.7	0.7	1.4	4.4	6.9	12.3	17.3	24.8	F		
5.4	14.1	23.4	38.6	67.1	99.7	148.4	202.7	261.1	371.0	M	Stomach cancer	151
4.6	5.8	13.3	13.4	24.6	36.4	62.2	101.3	142.4	201.0	F		
4.8	4.9	10.5	24.6	38.6	56.7	93.9	143.8	218.4	274.9	M	Colorectal cancer	153, 154
2.8	6.2	6.5	14.1	25.3	32.4	53.8	86.4	107.9	210.0	F		
0.3	–	1.6	3.5	2.8	10.1	11.6	9.3	1.8	17.0	M	Liver cancer	155.0
–	1.0	0.7		2.1	2.2	3.2	4.3	2.4	5.4	F		
1.0	3.2	6.1	9.0	16.5	20.7	29.3	51.8	45.5	88.8	M	Pancreas cancer	157
1.5	0.6	2.9	3.8	7.6	9.8	16.2	30.4	45.3	48.4	F		
1.0	2.5	11.7	15.6	23.7	28.6	28.3	32.4	36.4	37.7	M	Larynx cancer	161
–	–	0.4	–	1.4	1.1	2.8	0.5	4.2	7.9	F		
8.3	16.2	25.4	44.4	83.2	128.7	179.2	235.1	216.6	181.3	M	Lung cancer	162
1.8	3.6	4.0	6.5	9.0	17.8	25.5	32.5	44.7	54.5	F		
1.3	0.7	0.4	1.2	2.0	1.8	1.5	2.2	7.3	8.5	M	Malignant melanoma	172
0.6	0.6	1.1	1.7	2.1	1.1	0.8	–	3.0	6.1	F		
12.6	21.1	41.5	52.9	63.7	64.3	63.5	84.8	87.6	116.8	F	Female breast cancer	174
3.1	3.2	6.5	4.8	8.3	9.8	5.7	12.3	10.7	10.9	F	Cervix cancer	180
1.8	5.5	6.1	7.2	13.2	18.9	25.5	25.6	39.3	50.8	F	Other uterine cancer	179, 182
2.5	2.6	7.6	8.3	11.4	15.3	14.6	19.7	13.1	20.0	F	Ovarian cancer	183
–	–	1.2	3.9	13.7	30.8	70.2	136.6	256.6	480.5	M	Prostate cancer	185
0.3	–	2.0	2.7	6.4	16.3	26.8	38.1	76.4	139.9	M	Bladder cancer	188
0.9	0.3	–	0.3	2.8	3.3	4.0	9.1	19.1	30.9	F		
9.5	14.8	23.0	44.4	57.5	109.4	127.2	151.0	195.6	313.9	M	Other and ill-defined	Rest of 140–208
5.8	10.4	15.9	22.0	34.6	52.3	86.1	108.2	158.5	244.6	F	cancer sites	
0.3	0.7	0.4	0.4	0.8	0.9	2.5	0.7	1.8	6.1	M	Hodgkin's disease	201
0.3	–	–	0.7	1.0	0.4	2.0	1.1	2.4	0.6	F		
0.6	2.8	5.6	6.2	12.9	16.3	21.7	36.7	35.5	34.1	M	Myeloma and non-	200, 202–203
0.6	1.6	2.5	3.4	4.8	11.6	19.8	24.0	26.8	27.2	F	Hodgkin lymphomas	
3.2	3.2	3.2	5.1	6.8	11.0	20.2	30.2	39.1	51.1	M	Leukaemia	204–208
2.8	0.6	2.9	6.5	5.2	8.7	10.5	16.0	26.8	29.1	F		
40.4	70.3	100.4	210.9	380.1	684.5	1225.6	2233.6	3929.9	8913.6	M	ALL VASCULAR	390–459
14.7	23.0	54.8	89.7	160.0	288.3	635.4	1412.0	2858.2	8271.8	F	DISEASE	
1.3	1.4	0.8	2.7	3.6	7.5	4.5	3.6	8.2	1.2	M	Rheumatic heart	390–398
0.9	1.9	4.0	5.8	5.2	7.6	13.7	8.5	14.3	16.3	F	disease and fever	
0.6	1.1	1.2	3.9	4.8	7.5	18.7	28.0	46.4	155.7	M	Hypertensive disease	401–405
–	0.3	0.7	1.7	1.4	6.5	9.3	32.0	53.6	171.3	F		
18.1	33.8	44.8	93.6	157.9	262.7	410.4	590.9	860.8	1436.7	M	Ischaemic heart	410–414
3.4	4.2	11.5	23.4	43.3	73.4	157.6	304.9	554.8	1116.8	F	disease	
3.2	1.4	2.8	7.0	10.0	22.0	29.3	55.4	65.5	132.6	M	Pulmonary embolism	415.1, 451–453
1.2	1.3	4.3	2.4	4.2	8.0	18.6	27.2	47.1	107.1	F	and other venous	
11.4	18.3	31.5	76.4	147.9	279.0	563.4	1189.1	2224.7	4998.8	M	Cerebrovascular	430–438
7.1	11.0	25.2	43.3	80.0	149.0	336.7	783.6	1643.0	4782.7	F	disease	
5.7	14.4	19.4	27.3	55.8	105.9	199.4	366.6	724.3	2188.6	M	Other vascular	Rest of 390–459
2.2	4.2	9.0	13.1	26.0	43.6	99.4	255.9	545.3	2077.5	F	disease	
1.9	4.9	12.1	17.9	39.8	68.5	121.2	233.6	353.0	684.9	M	Chronic obstructive	490–496
1.5	1.0	5.0	3.8	7.6	16.7	29.5	61.8	111.4	259.7	F	pulmonary disease	
7.0	10.6	14.9	18.3	40.2	62.8	120.6	221.4	420.4	1142.3	M	Other respiratory	Rest of 460–519
2.5	5.2	6.8	7.2	13.9	22.2	40.0	104.5	205.6	804.5	F	disease	
0.3	2.1	2.4	3.9	6.0	9.7	15.6	24.4	43.7	97.3	M	Peptic ulcer	531–533
0.3	0.3	–	0.3	0.7	2.5	6.1	6.4	20.3	49.6	F		
24.5	24.6	51.6	76.0	96.4	133.1	127.7	138.0	128.3	124.1	M	Liver cirrhosis	571
6.1	10.1	15.5	24.8	29.8	37.4	36.8	36.2	40.5	38.7	F		
0.6	2.5	4.8	9.0	9.6	19.8	42.4	62.5	142.9	257.9	M	Renal disease	580–590
1.2	1.9	3.6	4.1	5.5	9.8	20.6	30.9	56.6	113.2	F		
0.9	0.3	–	–	–	–	–	–	–	–	F	Pregnancy and birth	630–676
0.6	0.4	–	0.4	1.2	0.9	1.0	–	1.8	–	M	Congenital and	740–779
0.9	0.6	0.4	–	0.7	0.4	1.2	1.1	–	1.2	F	perinatal causes	
35.3	47.1	62.5	79.1	110.5	138.8	214.0	324.2	631.5	2716.5	M	Ill-defined causes	780–799
12.9	17.2	17.7	25.1	33.3	45.8	100.2	170.6	424.9	2751.2	F		
30.8	33.8	41.1	59.6	88.0	148.5	239.8	362.3	556.9	841.8	M	Other medical causes	Rest of 001–799
13.8	14.6	20.9	34.0	50.9	94.1	175.8	277.7	428.5	740.9	F		
85.8	98.5	97.2	118.1	137.0	132.2	160.0	187.6	249.3	386.9	M	ALL NON-	E800–E999
18.4	24.7	25.2	32.7	33.6	38.9	47.3	70.4	110.3	225.8	F	MEDICAL CAUSES	
37.2	40.1	36.3	44.4	58.7	55.4	64.1	74.0	87.4	99.8	M	Motor vehicle	E810–E819
7.7	11.4	5.8	11.7	12.1	13.4	15.0	24.5	36.4	26.6	F	traffic accidents	
1.0	0.4	1.2	0.8	2.0	–	3.5	6.5	4.5	9.7	M	Fire	E890–E899
–	–	0.4		0.7	0.7	1.2	2.1	4.2	7.9	F		
9.5	14.4	13.7	17.9	23.3	20.7	29.3	31.6	51.0	66.9	M	Suicide	E950–E959
2.5	4.5	5.4	6.2	4.8	6.5	8.5	8.0	17.3	14.5	F		
3.2	4.6	2.4	2.3	4.0	4.4	3.5	1.4	0.9	4.9	M	Homicide	E960–E969
1.2	1.0	1.1	2.4	1.7	0.7	0.4	–	1.2	0.6	F		
314.7	284.3	247.9	256.5	248.9	227.6	198.1	139.1	109.9	82.2	M	POPULATION (thousands)	
325.5	308.3	277.4	290.9	288.7	275.1	247.4	187.6	167.8	165.2	F		

PORTUGAL: Males

	All ages	0–34	35–69	35–39	40–44	45–49	50–54	55–59	60–64	65–69	70–74	75–79	80+/NK
POPULATION (1000s)													
1955	4217.1	2739.9	1334.1	251.1	261.5	232.6	195.4	159.3	129.2	105.0	72.1	42.7	28.3
1965	4346.5	2686.4	1481.8	277.8	261.3	222.5	227.0	206.3	164.3	122.6	85.7	55.7	36.9
1975	4439.8	2614.0	1605.0	250.2	267.9	264.4	249.2	205.5	203.5	164.3	116.8	64.3	39.7
1985	4901.8	2803.9	1778.4	303.7	265.5	273.0	271.9	256.4	231.9	176.0	152.4	99.5	67.6
1990	**4762.1**	**2652.9**	**1778.0**	**314.7**	**284.3**	**247.9**	**256.5**	**248.9**	**227.6**	**198.1**	**139.1**	**109.9**	**82.2**
1995 projected	*5041.5*	*2745.0*	*1928.5*	*365.5*	*322.4*	*290.7*	*250.3*	*250.3*	*238.6*	*210.7*	*170.0*	*105.6*	*92.4*
NUMBER OF DEATHS													
All causes													
1955	50370	18166	16691	986	1462	1832	2212	2665	3383	4151	4708	4958	5847
1965	48928	12608	17912	959	1251	1512	2349	3196	3998	4647	5469	5665	7274
1975	51261	8049	21081	882	1364	1960	2601	3105	4991	6178	6832	6506	8793
1985	50993	4757	18830	733	966	1585	2403	3352	4477	5314	7746	8252	11408
1990	**53439**	**4185**	**19351**	**858**	**1059**	**1321**	**2124**	**3250**	**4569**	**6170**	**6915**	**8751**	**14237**
1995 projected	*57758*	*4435*	*20546*	*1083*	*1194*	*1468*	*1994*	*3284*	*4921*	*6602*	*8274*	*8389*	*16114*
Lung cancer													
1955	283	6	198	3	14	9	39	34	53	46	38	35	6
1965	474	5	336	8	15	22	38	72	108	73	69	39	25
1975	801	6	565	5	26	50	75	94	166	149	112	75	43
1985	1548	10	921	9	21	78	107	218	237	251	288	187	142
1990	**1825**	**7**	**1104**	**26**	**46**	**63**	**114**	**207**	**293**	**355**	**327**	**238**	**149**
1995 projected	*2258*	*8*	*1354*	*42*	*64*	*82*	*110*	*232*	*359*	*465*	*480*	*249*	*167*
ANNUAL DEATH RATE / 100,000 (*The rates for the age groups 0–34 and 35–69 are the means of seven five-yearly rates, but the all-ages rates are standardised to the conventional "European" age distribution)													
All causes													
1955	1753.2*	593.3*	1588.0*	392.7	559.1	787.6	1132.0	1672.9	2618.4	3953.3	6529.8	11611.2	20660.8
1965	1548.6*	400.2*	1473.0*	345.2	478.8	679.6	1034.8	1549.2	2433.4	3790.4	6381.6	10170.6	19712.7
1975	1524.7*	294.5*	1481.5*	352.5	509.1	741.3	1043.7	1510.9	2452.6	3760.2	5849.3	10118.2	22148.6
1985	1187.5*	176.3*	1189.5*	241.4	363.8	580.6	883.8	1307.3	1930.6	3019.3	5082.7	8293.5	16875.7
1990	**1181.2***	**162.3***	**1204.8***	**272.6**	**372.5**	**532.9**	**828.1**	**1305.7**	**2007.5**	**3114.6**	**4971.2**	**7962.7**	**17320.0**
1995 projected	*1177.9**	*157.3**	*1210.9**	*296.3*	*370.3*	*505.0*	*796.6*	*1312.0*	*2062.4*	*3133.4*	*4867.1*	*7944.1*	*17439.4*
All cancer													
1955	134.9*	8.2*	211.5*	24.7	50.5	84.3	164.3	235.4	375.4	545.7	669.9	864.2	802.1
1965	163.2*	10.6*	247.0*	36.4	55.1	106.1	182.8	280.2	469.3	599.5	886.8	992.8	1027.1
1975	185.6*	12.0*	270.1*	35.2	76.5	126.7	199.4	298.3	462.4	692.0	865.6	1199.1	1513.9
1985	206.8*	10.3*	287.9*	35.9	65.2	131.1	227.7	338.9	493.3	723.3	1071.5	1340.7	1831.4
1990	**226.7***	**8.5***	**320.9***	**38.8**	**72.1**	**136.7**	**222.2**	**377.3**	**580.4**	**818.8**	**1141.6**	**1458.6**	**2090.0**
1995 projected	*247.6**	*7.3**	*350.1**	*38.6*	*76.0*	*137.9*	*231.3*	*414.7*	*654.2*	*898.0*	*1238.2*	*1617.4*	*2355.0*
Lung cancer													
1955	11.0*	0.2*	19.5*	1.2	5.4	3.9	20.0	21.3	41.0	43.8	52.7	82.0	21.2
1965	15.5*	0.2*	27.9*	2.9	5.7	9.9	16.7	34.9	65.7	59.5	80.5	70.0	67.8
1975	22.2*	0.3*	39.8*	2.0	9.7	18.9	30.1	45.7	81.6	90.7	95.9	116.6	108.3
1985	35.2*	0.4*	58.4*	3.0	7.9	28.6	39.4	85.0	102.2	142.6	189.0	187.9	210.1
1990	**40.3***	**0.3***	**69.3***	**8.3**	**16.2**	**25.4**	**44.4**	**83.2**	**128.7**	**179.2**	**235.1**	**216.6**	**181.3**
1995 projected	*46.1**	*0.3**	*81.0**	*11.5*	*19.9*	*28.2*	*43.9*	*92.7*	*150.5*	*220.7*	*282.4*	*235.8*	*180.7*
Upper aerodigestive cancer (mouth, oesophagus, pharynx and larynx)													
1955	19.2*	0.4*	33.7*	2.0	6.5	14.2	34.8	43.9	48.8	85.7	70.7	84.3	134.3
1965	22.7*	0.3*	41.3*	3.6	8.4	18.9	33.0	57.2	73.6	94.6	100.4	105.9	100.3
1975	21.8*	0.6*	36.1*	2.0	10.1	17.8	35.3	42.8	58.5	86.4	103.6	115.1	131.0
1985	22.5*	0.2*	38.3*	2.3	9.8	20.1	42.3	51.1	66.4	76.1	112.2	106.5	113.9
1990	**25.4***	**0.4***	**45.9***	**3.8**	**11.6**	**33.9**	**38.2**	**69.1**	**78.2**	**86.3**	**103.5**	**102.8**	**122.9**
1995 projected	*28.1**	*0.3**	*52.4**	*4.7*	*16.1*	*38.2*	*46.7*	*79.1*	*93.0*	*89.2*	*101.8*	*100.4*	*126.6*
Other cancer													
1955	104.7*	7.6*	158.3*	21.5	38.6	66.2	109.5	170.1	285.6	416.2	546.5	697.9	646.6
1965	125.0*	10.1*	177.8*	29.9	40.9	77.3	133.0	188.1	329.9	445.4	706.0	816.9	859.1
1975	141.5*	11.1*	194.1*	31.2	56.7	90.0	134.0	209.7	322.4	514.9	666.1	967.3	1274.6
1985	149.1*	9.7*	191.2*	30.6	47.5	82.4	146.0	202.8	324.7	504.5	770.3	1046.2	1507.4
1990	**161.0***	**7.9***	**205.7***	**26.7**	**44.3**	**77.5**	**139.6**	**225.0**	**373.5**	**553.3**	**803.0**	**1139.2**	**1785.9**
1995 projected	*173.4**	*6.7**	*216.6**	*22.4*	*40.0*	*71.6*	*140.6*	*242.9*	*410.7*	*588.0*	*854.1*	*1281.3*	*2047.6*
Chronic obstructive pulmonary disease (COPD)													
1955	38.7*	1.3*	42.0*	4.8	8.8	12.9	21.5	42.1	87.5	116.2	195.6	381.7	480.6
1965	55.0*	1.7*	67.5*	6.8	12.2	20.7	40.5	76.1	126.6	189.2	312.7	420.1	612.5
1975	64.0*	7.1*	71.4*	4.8	13.8	23.4	37.7	63.7	134.6	221.5	320.2	516.3	763.2
1985	44.3*	1.8*	41.2*	5.6	3.4	12.5	25.0	45.2	71.6	125.0	217.2	387.9	726.3
1990	**41.5***	**1.0***	**38.0***	**1.9**	**4.9**	**12.1**	**17.9**	**39.8**	**68.5**	**121.2**	**233.6**	**353.0**	**684.9**
1995 projected	*38.7**	*0.7**	*35.9**	*1.4*	*4.3*	*10.0*	*14.8*	*34.8*	*64.1*	*122.0*	*224.1*	*327.7*	*638.5*
Other respiratory disease													
1955	118.9*	69.4*	80.3*	16.3	21.4	37.8	53.2	87.3	139.3	206.7	406.4	735.4	1208.5
1965	133.8*	70.9*	94.8*	14.8	26.0	38.2	61.2	95.5	154.6	273.2	459.7	804.3	1528.5
1975	85.8*	33.8*	60.9*	14.0	22.0	24.2	41.7	59.9	96.8	167.4	278.3	496.1	1335.0
1985	54.6*	7.7*	40.9*	5.9	11.7	22.3	27.2	44.9	68.6	105.7	215.9	424.1	1022.2
1990	**54.3***	**4.8***	**39.2***	**7.0**	**10.6**	**14.9**	**18.3**	**40.2**	**62.8**	**120.6**	**221.4**	**420.4**	**1142.3**
1995 projected	*55.4**	*4.1**	*37.2**	*7.4*	*8.4*	*10.3*	*14.0*	*34.0*	*63.3*	*122.9*	*224.1*	*447.0*	*1235.9*
Vascular disease													
1955	533.1*	16.2*	551.7*	50.2	85.7	167.7	295.3	511.6	1011.6	1740.0	2994.5	5208.4	6915.2
1965	512.9*	9.3*	495.7*	34.9	64.7	139.3	226.9	459.5	875.2	1669.7	3101.5	4944.3	7281.8
1975	592.2*	11.5*	566.2*	51.2	91.8	173.2	299.0	536.3	1035.4	1776.6	3102.7	5270.6	9496.2
1985	478.9*	7.5*	406.5*	33.9	58.8	126.4	227.7	394.3	717.1	1287.5	2491.5	4347.7	8554.7
1990	**462.4***	**6.0***	**387.5***	**40.4**	**70.3**	**100.4**	**210.9**	**380.1**	**684.5**	**1225.6**	**2233.6**	**3929.9**	**8913.6**
1995 projected	*441.3**	*5.5**	*357.7**	*45.1*	*66.1*	*90.8*	*191.8*	*356.4*	*643.8*	*1110.1*	*2009.4*	*3757.6*	*8881.0*
Liver cirrhosis													
1955	48.5*	2.6*	89.1*	17.1	34.0	56.7	87.5	120.5	148.6	159.0	183.1	227.2	123.7
1965	57.1*	2.5*	109.0*	25.6	49.0	66.5	115.9	150.3	164.3	191.7	204.2	226.2	116.5
1975	61.5*	2.1*	121.3*	34.0	47.4	98.3	122.4	149.4	201.0	196.6	196.9	196.0	128.5
1985	49.8*	1.9*	95.9*	21.4	38.8	66.3	101.9	131.8	148.3	163.1	175.2	172.9	118.3
1990	**39.9***	**1.6***	**76.3***	**24.5**	**24.6**	**51.6**	**76.0**	**96.4**	**133.1**	**127.7**	**138.0**	**128.3**	**124.1**
1995 projected	*31.3**	*1.6**	*59.5**	*19.4*	*19.2*	*37.2*	*55.9*	*75.9*	*105.6*	*103.0*	*105.3*	*104.2*	*107.1*
Other medical causes													
1955	785.9*	445.5*	493.2*	190.4	270.0	325.5	402.3	531.1	715.2	1018.1	1875.2	3971.9	10735.0
1965	533.3*	252.9*	338.8*	145.8	169.5	218.4	277.5	364.0	486.9	709.6	1241.5	2545.8	8769.6
1975	402.7*	141.3*	223.2*	85.9	122.1	141.5	177.4	234.5	322.4	478.4	875.0	2161.7	8516.4
1985	242.9*	72.4*	185.1*	48.7	79.8	99.3	144.9	210.6	271.2	440.9	706.7	1380.9	4255.9
1990	**252.2***	**66.7***	**224.5***	**74.4**	**91.5**	**119.8**	**164.5**	**235.0**	**345.8**	**540.6**	**815.2**	**1423.1**	**3978.1**
1995 projected	*266.0**	*66.8**	*265.7**	*101.0*	*111.7*	*135.5*	*185.0*	*275.3*	*414.1*	*637.4*	*886.5*	*1429.9*	*3814.9*
All non-medical causes													
1955	93.3*	50.1*	120.3*	89.2	88.7	102.8	108.0	145.0	140.9	167.6	205.3	222.5	395.8
1965	93.4*	52.3*	120.1*	81.0	102.2	90.3	130.0	123.6	156.4	157.4	175.0	237.0	376.7
1975	132.8*	86.7*	168.5*	127.5	135.5	153.9	166.1	168.9	200.0	227.6	210.6	278.4	395.5
1985	110.3*	74.8*	132.0*	89.9	106.2	122.7	129.5	141.6	160.4	173.9	204.7	239.2	366.9
1990	**104.1***	**73.7***	**118.4***	**85.8**	**98.5**	**97.2**	**118.1**	**137.0**	**132.2**	**160.0**	**187.6**	**249.3**	**386.9**
1995 projected	*97.5**	*71.2**	*104.8**	*83.4*	*84.7*	*83.2*	*103.9*	*121.1*	*117.4*	*140.0*	*179.4*	*260.4*	*406.9*

PORTUGAL: Females

	All ages	0–34	35–69	35–39	40–44	45–49	50–54	55–59	60–64	65–69	70–74	75–79	80+/NK
POPULATION (1000s)													
1955	4547.8	2722.5	1585.9	269.8	286.9	266.6	237.5	202.3	172.4	150.4	112.2	68.0	59.2
1965	4769.7	2735.5	1741.5	317.8	294.3	249.7	256.0	244.1	209.4	170.2	128.1	88.0	76.6
1975	5009.0	2727.8	1914.4	300.4	313.3	305.2	288.1	240.1	247.2	220.1	175.6	104.6	86.6
1985	5255.2	2733.9	2017.5	323.5	294.5	304.0	306.9	297.0	273.5	218.1	206.8	156.5	140.5
1990	**5106.0**	**2572.1**	**2013.3**	**325.5**	**308.3**	**277.4**	**290.9**	**288.7**	**275.1**	**247.4**	**187.6**	**167.8**	**165.2**
1995 projected	*5387.8*	*2643.5*	*2167.0*	*373.4*	*336.9*	*317.0*	*286.4*	*292.3*	*290.0*	*271.0*	*232.9*	*162.7*	*181.7*
NUMBER OF DEATHS													
All causes													
1955	49102	15194	12307	623	866	1135	1561	1798	2567	3757	4862	6015	10724
1965	46259	9519	11598	537	720	858	1268	1900	2632	3683	5451	6772	12919
1975	46675	5000	12227	429	668	984	1360	1694	2773	4319	6179	7552	15717
1985	46346	2343	10470	410	511	807	1226	1718	2529	3269	5729	8362	19442
1990	**49676**	**1821**	**10444**	**383**	**513**	**739**	**1088**	**1623**	**2360**	**3738**	**5181**	**8448**	**23782**
1995 projected	*53348*	*1697*	*10839*	*425*	*544*	*811*	*1037*	*1550*	*2428*	*4044*	*6228*	*8030*	*26554*
Lung cancer													
1955	106	4	70	2	7	8	10	10	14	19	10	16	6
1965	119	5	69	2	4	5	7	11	18	22	17	16	12
1975	234	11	135	2	5	8	24	23	31	42	39	27	22
1985	323	12	166	5	7	12	24	37	41	40	41	54	50
1990	**416**	**5**	**185**	**6**	**11**	**11**	**19**	**26**	**49**	**63**	**61**	**75**	**90**
1995 projected	*577*	*4*	*226*	*7*	*14*	*12*	*15*	*25*	*58*	*95*	*105*	*102*	*140*
ANNUAL DEATH RATE / 100,000	(*The rates for the age groups 0–34 and 35–69 are the means of seven five-yearly rates, but the all-ages rates are standardised to the conventional "European" age distribution)												
All causes													
1955	1287.4*	509.3*	927.4*	230.9	301.8	425.7	657.3	888.8	1489.0	2498.0	4333.3	8845.6	18114.9
1965	1068.0*	303.9*	778.8*	169.0	244.6	343.6	495.3	778.4	1256.9	2163.9	4255.3	7695.5	16865.5
1975	964.0*	173.9*	705.7*	142.8	213.2	322.4	472.1	705.5	1121.8	1962.3	3518.8	7219.9	18149.0
1985	723.4*	91.3*	566.7*	126.7	173.5	265.5	399.5	578.5	924.7	1498.9	2770.3	5343.1	13837.7
1990	**713.3***	**76.8***	**550.8***	**117.7**	**166.4**	**266.4**	**374.0**	**562.2**	**857.9**	**1510.9**	**2761.7**	**5034.6**	**14395.9**
1995 projected	*700.6**	*65.0**	*536.1**	*113.8*	*161.5*	*255.8*	*362.1*	*530.3*	*837.2*	*1492.3*	*2674.1*	*4935.5*	*14614.2*
All cancer													
1955	109.9*	8.1*	174.0*	37.4	70.4	111.4	158.7	180.9	295.2	363.7	449.2	613.2	674.0
1965	119.3*	9.1*	185.5*	40.6	68.0	108.9	150.0	212.6	304.2	414.2	564.4	689.8	688.0
1975	119.0*	10.8*	177.3*	37.6	72.5	107.1	156.2	211.2	272.7	383.9	491.5	714.1	839.5
1985	120.1*	8.8*	177.2*	44.5	67.9	97.4	154.4	216.8	309.3	350.3	504.8	682.4	950.2
1990	**128.7***	**8.6***	**183.8***	**42.4**	**64.5**	**113.9**	**148.2**	**220.0**	**290.8**	**407.0**	**574.1**	**763.4**	**1102.3**
1995 projected	*136.1**	*8.2**	*187.6**	*38.3*	*66.5*	*114.2*	*150.5*	*210.4*	*298.3*	*435.1*	*641.5*	*832.8*	*1262.0*
Lung cancer													
1955	3.0*	0.2*	5.2*	0.7	2.4	3.0	4.2	4.9	8.1	12.6	8.9	23.5	10.1
1965	2.9*	0.2*	4.7*	0.6	1.4	2.0	2.7	4.5	8.6	12.9	13.3	18.2	15.7
1975	4.8*	0.4*	7.8*	0.7	1.6	2.6	8.3	9.6	12.5	19.1	22.2	25.8	25.4
1985	5.5*	0.5*	8.8*	1.5	2.4	3.9	7.8	12.5	15.0	18.3	19.8	34.5	35.6
1990	**6.6***	**0.2***	**9.7***	**1.8**	**3.6**	**4.0**	**6.5**	**9.0**	**17.8**	**25.5**	**32.5**	**44.7**	**54.5**
1995 projected	*8.2**	*0.1**	*11.2**	*1.9*	*4.2*	*3.8*	*5.2*	*8.6*	*20.0*	*35.1*	*45.1*	*62.7*	*77.1*
Upper aerodigestive cancer (mouth, oesophagus, pharynx and larynx)													
1955	4.4*	0.3*	6.1*	1.1	1.7	3.4	4.2	7.4	8.1	16.6	16.9	30.9	42.2
1965	4.4*	0.2*	6.2*	1.3	1.4	2.8	6.3	5.3	11.5	15.3	25.0	29.5	31.3
1975	4.6*	0.3*	5.4*	0.3	2.6	2.6	4.2	7.1	10.1	10.9	25.1	34.4	50.8
1985	3.7*	0.1*	4.3*	0.9	0.7	2.3	4.2	5.4	8.0	8.3	19.8	24.3	48.4
1990	**3.8***	**0.2***	**4.5***	**0.6**	**1.3**	**2.5**	**2.4**	**4.2**	**6.5**	**13.7**	**18.7**	**33.4**	**46.0**
1995 projected	*4.0**	*0.1**	*4.4**	*0.8*	*1.5*	*2.2*	*1.7*	*3.1*	*7.2*	*14.4*	*23.2*	*34.4*	*50.1*
Other cancer													
1955	102.6*	7.6*	162.7*	35.6	66.2	105.0	150.3	168.6	279.0	334.4	423.4	558.8	621.6
1965	112.1*	8.7*	174.6*	38.7	65.2	104.1	141.0	202.8	284.1	386.0	526.2	642.0	641.0
1975	109.6*	10.1*	164.1*	36.6	68.3	101.9	143.7	194.5	250.0	353.9	444.2	653.9	763.3
1985	110.8*	8.2*	164.2*	42.0	64.9	91.1	142.4	199.0	286.3	323.7	465.2	623.6	866.2
1990	**118.2***	**8.2***	**169.6***	**39.9**	**59.7**	**107.4**	**139.2**	**206.8**	**266.4**	**367.8**	**522.9**	**685.3**	**1001.8**
1995 projected	*123.9**	*8.0**	*171.9**	*35.6*	*60.8*	*108.2*	*143.5*	*198.8*	*271.0*	*385.6*	*573.2*	*735.7*	*1134.8*
Chronic obstructive pulmonary disease (COPD)													
1955	17.6*	1.5*	17.0*	1.1	3.1	4.5	8.0	13.8	29.6	58.5	107.8	177.9	209.5
1965	23.4*	1.4*	25.8*	4.7	7.5	9.6	12.1	21.3	39.2	86.4	138.2	185.2	285.9
1975	24.8*	4.4*	22.3*	2.3	6.4	6.2	10.4	24.6	42.1	64.1	117.3	212.2	339.5
1985	15.1*	1.0*	12.4*	1.2	1.0	5.9	9.8	15.2	20.8	33.0	66.7	125.2	280.4
1990	**12.9***	**0.7***	**9.3***	**1.5**	**1.0**	**5.0**	**3.8**	**7.6**	**16.7**	**29.5**	**61.8**	**111.4**	**259.7**
1995 projected	*11.2**	*0.5**	*7.5**	*1.6*	*0.9*	*3.5*	*2.8*	*5.5*	*12.8*	*25.8*	*55.0*	*97.1*	*237.8*
Other respiratory disease													
1955	81.4*	64.0*	38.4*	9.6	7.7	14.6	23.2	31.1	67.3	115.0	197.9	445.6	876.7
1965	90.0*	62.7*	38.4*	7.6	11.6	11.6	23.0	34.0	57.3	124.0	275.6	521.6	1152.7
1975	51.7*	27.8*	22.2*	5.7	4.8	9.8	13.5	22.9	34.4	64.5	148.1	319.3	874.1
1985	28.8*	6.6*	14.3*	4.3	4.1	5.9	8.5	12.5	23.4	41.3	96.2	205.8	653.4
1990	**30.1***	**3.3***	**14.0***	**2.5**	**5.2**	**6.8**	**7.2**	**13.9**	**22.2**	**40.0**	**104.5**	**205.6**	**804.5**
1995 projected	*32.7**	*2.1**	*13.8**	*2.1*	*5.0*	*6.9*	*7.3*	*13.3*	*21.4*	*40.2*	*104.8*	*225.6*	*945.5*
Vascular disease													
1955	420.1*	15.6*	371.3*	44.5	62.7	112.2	202.9	334.7	626.5	1215.4	2228.2	4447.1	6348.0
1965	391.9*	8.5*	305.9*	28.6	45.2	82.5	146.9	269.2	505.3	1064.0	2304.4	4083.0	6584.9
1975	419.6*	8.9*	313.9*	27.3	49.2	93.1	153.8	275.7	532.8	1065.4	2083.1	4117.6	8091.2
1985	338.6*	4.6*	207.5*	20.7	29.5	55.9	106.2	173.1	336.0	730.9	1531.4	3236.4	7716.0
1990	**329.0***	**3.7***	**180.9***	**14.7**	**23.0**	**54.8**	**89.7**	**160.0**	**288.3**	**635.4**	**1412.0**	**2858.2**	**8271.8**
1995 projected	*314.9**	*3.0**	*157.0**	*11.2*	*19.6*	*47.0*	*80.0*	*137.9*	*246.6*	*556.5*	*1237.9*	*2711.7*	*8405.1*
Liver cirrhosis													
1955	22.5*	1.2*	41.1*	5.9	18.8	27.8	51.8	50.9	59.7	72.5	81.1	107.4	52.4
1965	23.9*	1.5*	45.3*	6.3	24.1	28.4	43.0	61.5	75.9	78.1	76.5	96.6	60.1
1975	21.2*	0.9*	40.9*	10.3	21.4	31.1	45.5	50.0	57.4	70.9	65.5	59.3	64.7
1985	15.7*	0.9*	29.7*	5.6	17.3	24.7	30.3	35.4	44.2	50.4	49.8	55.6	44.1
1990	**12.3***	**1.1***	**22.9***	**6.1**	**10.1**	**15.5**	**24.8**	**29.8**	**37.4**	**36.8**	**36.2**	**40.5**	**38.7**
1995 projected	*9.6**	*1.2**	*17.5**	*4.8*	*6.8*	*10.7*	*18.9*	*24.6*	*29.3*	*27.3*	*25.8*	*33.2*	*30.3*
Other medical causes													
1955	605.2*	397.7*	258.2*	120.5	127.6	133.5	189.1	248.6	371.8	616.4	1203.2	2929.4	9731.4
1965	390.8*	203.9*	150.2*	65.8	74.1	83.3	91.4	150.3	237.8	349.0	825.1	2000.0	7866.8
1975	293.3*	101.2*	96.8*	40.3	41.5	51.8	60.0	88.7	141.6	254.0	522.8	1644.4	7664.0
1985	170.6*	50.9*	89.9*	26.6	30.9	46.4	57.0	87.5	145.5	235.7	433.8	909.9	3925.3
1990	**168.5***	**39.6***	**108.4***	**32.0**	**38.0**	**45.1**	**67.7**	**97.3**	**163.6**	**314.9**	**502.7**	**945.2**	**3693.1**
1995 projected	*167.5**	*30.4**	*125.1**	*37.0*	*41.0*	*49.5*	*73.3*	*108.8*	*196.6*	*369.4*	*551.3*	*942.2*	*3542.1*
All non-medical causes													
1955	30.7*	21.1*	27.5*	11.9	11.5	21.8	23.6	28.7	38.9	56.5	66.0	125.0	223.0
1965	28.7*	16.8*	27.5*	15.4	14.3	19.2	28.9	29.5	37.2	48.2	71.0	119.3	227.2
1975	34.3*	20.0*	32.2*	19.3	17.6	23.3	32.6	32.5	40.9	59.5	90.5	153.0	276.0
1985	34.4*	18.5*	35.7*	23.8	22.8	29.3	33.2	38.0	45.3	57.3	87.5	127.8	268.3
1990	**31.8***	**19.9***	**31.5***	**18.4**	**24.7**	**25.2**	**32.7**	**33.6**	**38.9**	**47.3**	**70.4**	**110.3**	**225.8**
1995 projected	*28.7**	*19.4**	*27.7**	*18.7*	*21.7*	*24.0*	*29.3*	*29.8*	*32.4*	*38.0*	*58.0*	*92.8*	*191.5*

PORTUGAL: 1975

Smoking–attributed deaths (Sm.) and total deaths (Total)

		ALL CAUSES	ALL CANCER	Lung cancer	Upper aero–digestive ca.	Other cancer	COPD	Other respiratory	Vascular disease	Liver cirrhosis	Other medical	Non–medical
Males												
0–34	Sm.	–	–	–	–	–	–	–	–	–	–	–
	Total	8049	289	6	12	271	197	1022	262	40	4143	2096
35–69	Sm.	2535	765	443	182	140	480	95	802	–	393	–
	Total	21081	3816	565	516	2735	974	857	7705	1816	3282	2631
		(12%)	(20%)	(78%)	(35%)	(5%)	(49%)	(11%)	(10%)		(12%)	
70+	Sm.	976	240	145	49	46	318	28	265	–	125	–
	Total	22131	2383	230	247	1906	1009	1174	10783	407	5793	582
		(4%)	(10%)	(63%)	(20%)	(2%)	(32%)	(2%)	(2%)		(2%)	
Any age	Sm.	3511	1005	588	231	186	798	123	1067	–	518	–
	Total	51261	6488	801	775	4912	2180	3053	18750	2263	13218	5309
		(7%)	(15%)	(73%)	(30%)	(4%)	(37%)	(4%)	(6%)		(4%)	
Females												
0–34	Sm.	–	–	–	–	–	–	–	–	–	–	–
	Total	5000	278	11	6	261	127	828	226	21	2972	548
35–69	Sm.	0	0	0	0	0	0	0	0	–	0	–
	Total	12227	3143	135	95	2913	380	383	5287	742	1704	588
		(0%)	(0%)	(0%)	(0%)	(0%)	(0%)	(0%)	(0%)		(0%)	
70+	Sm.	0	0	0	0	0	0	0	0	–	0	–
	Total	29448	2337	88	124	2125	722	1351	14972	233	9275	558
		(0%)	(0%)	(0%)	(0%)	(0%)	(0%)	(0%)	(0%)		(0%)	
Any age	Sm.	0	0	0	0	0	0	0	0	–	0	–
	Total	46675	5758	234	225	5299	1229	2562	20485	996	13951	1694
		(0%)	(0%)	(0%)	(0%)	(0%)	(0%)	(0%)	(0%)		(0%)	
Males+Females												
0–34	Sm.	–	–	–	–	–	–	–	–	–	–	–
	Total	13049	567	17	18	532	324	1850	488	61	7115	2644
35–69	Sm.	2535	765	443	182	140	480	95	802	–	393	–
	Total	33308	6959	700	611	5648	1354	1240	12992	2558	4986	3219
		(8%)	(11%)	(63%)	(30%)	(2%)	(35%)	(8%)	(6%)		(8%)	
70+	Sm.	976	240	145	49	46	318	28	265	–	125	–
	Total	51579	4720	318	371	4031	1731	2525	25755	640	15068	1140
		(2%)	(5%)	(46%)	(13%)	(1%)	(18%)	(1%)	(1%)		(1%)	
Any age	Sm.	3511	1005	588	231	186	798	123	1067	–	518	–
	Total	97936	12246	1035	1000	10211	3409	5615	39235	3259	27169	7003
		(4%)	(8%)	(57%)	(23%)	(2%)	(23%)	(2%)	(3%)		(2%)	

PORTUGAL: 1985

Smoking–attributed deaths (Sm.) and total deaths (Total)

		ALL CAUSES	ALL CANCER	Lung cancer	Upper aero–digestive ca.	Other cancer	COPD	Other respiratory	Vascular disease	Liver cirrhosis	Other medical	Non–medical
Males												
0–34	Sm.	–	–	–	–	–	–	–	–	–	–	–
	Total	4757	278	10	6	262	48	203	199	46	1903	2080
35–69	Sm.	3331	1326	786	295	245	387	110	978	–	530	–
	Total	18830	4545	921	622	3002	630	644	6163	1595	2970	2283
		(18%)	(29%)	(85%)	(47%)	(8%)	(61%)	(17%)	(16%)		(18%)	
70+	Sm.	2317	763	481	123	159	581	67	669	–	237	–
	Total	27406	4205	617	354	3234	1208	1442	13906	519	5328	798
		(8%)	(18%)	(78%)	(35%)	(5%)	(48%)	(5%)	(5%)		(4%)	
Any age	Sm.	5648	2089	1267	418	404	968	177	1647	–	767	–
	Total	50993	9028	1548	982	6498	1886	2289	20268	2160	10201	5161
		(11%)	(23%)	(82%)	(43%)	(6%)	(51%)	(8%)	(8%)		(8%)	
Females												
0–34	Sm.	–	–	–	–	–	–	–	–	–	–	–
	Total	2343	231	12	4	215	26	169	121	24	1270	502
35–69	Sm.	0	0	0	0	0	0	0	0	–	0	–
	Total	10470	3368	166	81	3121	229	261	3677	573	1665	697
		(0%)	(0%)	(0%)	(0%)	(0%)	(0%)	(0%)	(0%)		(0%)	
70+	Sm.	0	0	0	0	0	0	0	0	–	0	–
	Total	33533	3447	145	147	3155	728	1439	19073	252	7836	758
		(0%)	(0%)	(0%)	(0%)	(0%)	(0%)	(0%)	(0%)		(0%)	
Any age	Sm.	0	0	0	0	0	0	0	0	–	0	–
	Total	46346	7046	323	232	6491	983	1869	22871	849	10771	1957
		(0%)	(0%)	(0%)	(0%)	(0%)	(0%)	(0%)	(0%)		(0%)	
Males+Females												
0–34	Sm.	–	–	–	–	–	–	–	–	–	–	–
	Total	7100	509	22	10	477	74	372	320	70	3173	2582
35–69	Sm.	3331	1326	786	295	245	387	110	978	–	530	–
	Total	29300	7913	1087	703	6123	859	905	9840	2168	4635	2980
		(11%)	(17%)	(72%)	(42%)	(4%)	(45%)	(12%)	(10%)		(11%)	
70+	Sm.	2317	763	481	123	159	581	67	669	–	237	–
	Total	60939	7652	762	501	6389	1936	2881	32979	771	13164	1556
		(4%)	(10%)	(63%)	(25%)	(2%)	(30%)	(2%)	(2%)		(2%)	
Any age	Sm.	5648	2089	1267	418	404	968	177	1647	–	767	–
	Total	97339	16074	1871	1214	12989	2869	4158	43139	3009	20972	7118
		(6%)	(13%)	(68%)	(34%)	(3%)	(34%)	(4%)	(4%)		(4%)	

(To be conservative, no deaths before age 35, and none from liver cirrhosis or non–medical causes, were attributed to smoking.)

PORTUGAL: 1990

Smoking–attributed deaths (Sm.) and total deaths (Total)

		ALL CAUSES	ALL CANCER	Lung cancer	Upper aero–digestive ca.	Other cancer	COPD	Other respiratory	Vascular disease	Liver cirrhosis	Other medical	Non–medical
Males												
0–34	Sm.	–	–	–	–	–	–	–	–	–	–	–
	Total	4185	227	7	9	211	27	116	159	40	1604	2012
35–69	Sm.	3992	1666	969	385	312	388	115	1098	–	725	–
	Total	19351	5118	1104	748	3266	591	618	6049	1266	3656	2053
		(21%)	(33%)	(88%)	(51%)	(10%)	(66%)	(19%)	(18%)		(20%)	
70+	Sm.	2832	947	581	141	225	674	90	804	–	317	–
	Total	29903	4909	714	358	3837	1276	1709	14753	435	5968	853
		(9%)	(19%)	(81%)	(39%)	(6%)	(53%)	(5%)	(5%)		(5%)	
Any age	Sm.	6824	2613	1550	526	537	1062	205	1902	–	1042	–
	Total	53439	10254	1825	1115	7314	1894	2443	20961	1741	11228	4918
		(13%)	(25%)	(85%)	(47%)	(7%)	(56%)	(8%)	(9%)		(9%)	
Females												
0–34	Sm.	–	–	–	–	–	–	–	–	–	–	–
	Total	1821	218	5	4	209	17	74	96	28	882	506
35–69	Sm.	0	0	0	0	0	0	0	0	–	0	–
	Total	10444	3526	185	84	3257	174	264	3359	446	2053	622
		(0%)	(0%)	(0%)	(0%)	(0%)	(0%)	(0%)	(0%)		(0%)	
70+	Sm.	0	0	0	0	0	0	0	0	–	0	–
	Total	37411	4179	226	167	3786	732	1870	21110	200	8630	690
		(0%)	(0%)	(0%)	(0%)	(0%)	(0%)	(0%)	(0%)		(0%)	
Any age	Sm.	0	0	0	0	0	0	0	0	–	0	–
	Total	49676	7923	416	255	7252	923	2208	24565	674	11565	1818
		(0%)	(0%)	(0%)	(0%)	(0%)	(0%)	(0%)	(0%)		(0%)	
Males+Females												
0–34	Sm.	–	–	–	–	–	–	–	–	–	–	–
	Total	6006	445	12	13	420	44	190	255	68	2486	2518
35–69	Sm.	3992	1666	969	385	312	388	115	1098	–	725	–
	Total	29795	8644	1289	832	6523	765	882	9408	1712	5709	2675
		(13%)	(19%)	(75%)	(46%)	(5%)	(51%)	(13%)	(12%)		(13%)	
70+	Sm.	2832	947	581	141	225	674	90	804	–	317	–
	Total	67314	9088	940	525	7623	2008	3579	35863	635	14598	1543
		(4%)	(10%)	(62%)	(27%)	(3%)	(34%)	(3%)	(2%)		(2%)	
Any age	Sm.	6824	2613	1550	526	537	1062	205	1902	–	1042	–
	Total	103115	18177	2241	1370	14566	2817	4651	45526	2415	22793	6736
		(7%)	(14%)	(69%)	(38%)	(4%)	(38%)	(4%)	(4%)		(5%)	

PORTUGAL: 1995

Smoking–attributed deaths (Sm.) and total deaths (Total)

		ALL CAUSES	ALL CANCER	Lung cancer	Upper aero–digestive ca.	Other cancer	COPD	Other respiratory	Vascular disease	Liver cirrhosis	Other medical	Non–medical
Males												
0–34	Sm.	–	–	–	–	–	–	–	–	–	–	–
	Total	4435	208	8	9	191	21	111	161	46	1831	2057
35–69	Sm.	4898	2112	1209	503	400	406	126	1222	–	1032	–
	Total	20546	5857	1354	905	3598	582	614	5889	1040	4606	1958
		(24%)	(36%)	(89%)	(56%)	(11%)	(70%)	(21%)	(21%)		(22%)	
70+	Sm.	3503	1239	752	169	318	742	121	983	–	418	–
	Total	32777	5989	896	396	4697	1317	1995	15590	388	6542	956
		(11%)	(21%)	(84%)	(43%)	(7%)	(56%)	(6%)	(6%)		(6%)	
Any age	Sm.	8401	3351	1961	672	718	1148	247	2205	–	1450	–
	Total	57758	12054	2258	1310	8486	1920	2720	21640	1474	12979	4971
		(15%)	(28%)	(87%)	(51%)	(8%)	(60%)	(9%)	(10%)		(11%)	
Females												
0–34	Sm.	–	–	–	–	–	–	–	–	–	–	–
	Total	1697	221	4	2	215	15	53	84	36	768	520
35–69	Sm.	0	0	0	0	0	0	0	0	–	0	–
	Total	10839	3819	226	89	3504	151	278	3112	360	2532	587
		(0%)	(0%)	(0%)	(0%)	(0%)	(0%)	(0%)	(0%)		(0%)	
70+	Sm.	0	0	0	0	0	0	0	0	–	0	–
	Total	40812	5142	347	201	4594	718	2329	22567	169	9253	634
		(0%)	(0%)	(0%)	(0%)	(0%)	(0%)	(0%)	(0%)		(0%)	
Any age	Sm.	0	0	0	0	0	0	0	0	–	0	–
	Total	53348	9182	577	292	8313	884	2660	25763	565	12553	1741
		(0%)	(0%)	(0%)	(0%)	(0%)	(0%)	(0%)	(0%)		(0%)	
Males+Females												
0–34	Sm.	–	–	–	–	–	–	–	–	–	–	–
	Total	6132	429	12	11	406	36	164	245	82	2599	2577
35–69	Sm.	4898	2112	1209	503	400	406	126	1222	–	1032	–
	Total	31385	9676	1580	994	7102	733	892	9001	1400	7138	2545
		(16%)	(22%)	(77%)	(51%)	(6%)	(55%)	(14%)	(14%)		(14%)	
70+	Sm.	3503	1239	752	169	318	742	121	983	–	418	–
	Total	73589	11131	1243	597	9291	2035	4324	38157	557	15795	1590
		(5%)	(11%)	(60%)	(28%)	(3%)	(36%)	(3%)	(3%)		(3%)	
Any age	Sm.	8401	3351	1961	672	718	1148	247	2205	–	1450	–
	Total	111106	21236	2835	1602	16799	2804	5380	47403	2039	25532	6712
		(8%)	(16%)	(69%)	(42%)	(4%)	(41%)	(5%)	(5%)		(6%)	

(To be conservative, no deaths before age 35, and none from liver cirrhosis or non–medical causes, were attributed to smoking.)

ROMANIA: 1990

		No. of deaths			Standardised rates (Defined on p.466)			Annual death rates / 100, 000						
		All ages	0–34	35–69	All ages	0–34	35–69	0–4	5–9	10–14	15–19	20–24	25–29	30–34
ALL CAUSES	M	131824	13419	62254	1362.8	213.5	1555.3	685.5	71.1	58.1	101.7	139.5	180.8	257.6
	F	115262	8078	35672	929.1	132.9	806.5	556.1	47.5	33.8	46.5	58.0	78.9	109.3
Tuberculosis	M	1373	185	1127	13.2	3.1	24.9	2.1	0.2	0.2	0.1	1.6	6.0	11.8
	F	229	73	129	2.0	1.2	2.7	1.7	–	–	0.5	1.9	1.3	3.1
Other infective and parasitic	M	666	536	102	5.8	8.3	2.4	45.3	2.2	3.5	2.7	1.2	2.0	1.5
	F	493	401	68	4.3	6.5	1.4	38.5	1.1	1.4	1.5	1.1	1.2	0.7
ALL CANCER	M	18753	760	13366	188.2	12.2	332.9	11.1	9.3	8.1	9.5	10.3	14.6	22.7
	F	13809	641	8888	115.6	10.9	195.7	9.4	7.2	4.2	6.1	6.9	14.5	28.1
Mouth and pharynx cancer	M	821	30	661	8.2	0.5	15.8	–	0.1	0.3	0.9	0.5	0.7	0.8
	F	169	8	103	1.4	0.1	2.3	0.1	–	–	0.1	0.1	0.1	0.5
Oesophagus cancer	M	224	–	169	2.3	–	4.0	–	–	–	–	–	–	–
	F	58	1	33	0.5	0.0	0.8	0.1	–	–	–	–	–	–
Stomach cancer	M	2502	26	1690	25.5	0.4	43.3	0.1	–	0.1	0.2	0.3	0.7	1.6
	F	1262	14	715	10.2	0.2	16.2	–	–	–	0.1	0.1	0.3	1.2
Colorectal cancer	M	1384	28	896	14.1	0.5	23.1	0.2	0.1	0.1	–	0.6	1.3	1.0
	F	1258	8	706	10.2	0.1	15.9	–	–	–	–	0.2	–	0.7
Liver cancer	M	466	12	344	4.7	0.2	8.9	0.5	–	–	–	0.2	–	0.6
	F	252	8	160	2.1	0.1	3.5	0.5	0.1	–	–	0.1	0.3	–
Pancreas cancer	M	875	8	619	8.9	0.1	15.7	0.1	–	–	–	–	0.1	0.7
	F	580	6	315	4.7	0.1	7.2	0.1	0.1	–	–	–	0.1	0.4
Larynx cancer	M	793	3	659	7.9	0.0	15.9	–	–	–	0.1	–	–	0.2
	F	61	2	45	0.5	0.0	1.0	–	–	–	–	0.1	–	0.1
Lung cancer	M	5397	46	4560	53.2	0.8	111.7	0.2	–	0.3	0.1	0.4	1.7	2.8
	F	1115	25	778	9.3	0.4	17.3	0.1	0.1	0.3	0.2	0.1	1.0	1.2
Malignant melanoma	M	135	13	93	1.3	0.2	2.2	–	0.1	0.1	–	0.2	0.3	0.8
	F	127	5	75	1.1	0.1	1.6	–	–	–	0.1	–	0.1	0.4
Female breast cancer	F	2399	57	1749	20.6	1.0	37.8	–	–	0.1	–	0.1	1.5	5.4
Cervix cancer	F	1556	98	1123	13.5	1.8	24.0	0.1	–	–	0.1	0.4	4.0	7.7
Other uterine cancer	F	658	13	434	5.5	0.2	9.7	–	0.1	–	–	–	0.3	1.2
Ovarian cancer	F	735	33	587	6.3	0.6	12.8	–	–	–	0.7	0.6	0.9	1.8
Prostate cancer	M	1055	2	348	11.5	0.0	9.9	–	–	–	–	0.1	0.1	–
Bladder cancer	M	694	5	425	7.2	0.1	11.4	0.3	–	–	–	–	–	0.2
	F	247	1	118	2.0	0.0	2.7	–	–	–	–	–	–	0.1
Other and ill-defined cancer sites	M	3290	318	2228	32.7	5.1	54.8	5.3	3.2	2.8	4.7	4.5	5.6	9.6
	F	2569	192	1500	21.4	3.2	33.3	4.1	3.6	2.3	2.4	2.0	3.2	4.9
Hodgkin's disease	M	140	37	95	1.3	0.6	2.2	0.3	0.2	0.3	0.3	0.9	0.4	1.6
	F	84	26	46	0.7	0.4	1.0	–	0.2	–	0.2	1.0	0.7	0.8
Myeloma and non-Hodgkin lymphomas	M	407	70	271	3.9	1.1	6.6	1.2	1.0	1.5	0.6	0.7	1.4	1.4
	F	267	36	175	2.3	0.6	3.8	0.5	0.4	0.7	0.9	0.5	0.3	0.8
Leukaemia	M	570	162	308	5.4	2.6	7.5	2.7	4.5	2.6	2.5	2.0	2.2	1.4
	F	412	108	226	3.5	1.8	4.9	3.8	2.5	0.7	1.3	1.5	1.6	1.0
ALL VASCULAR DISEASE	M	69146	654	27082	747.3	10.9	703.9	6.6	0.5	1.1	3.3	8.2	17.7	39.0
	F	76370	306	17603	603.7	5.3	408.5	4.9	1.0	1.0	2.4	3.4	8.5	15.7
Rheumatic heart disease and fever	M	553	51	444	5.3	0.8	10.1	–	–	0.2	0.5	0.8	1.3	3.1
	F	856	48	656	7.5	0.8	14.1	–	–	–	0.7	0.7	1.5	3.0
Hypertensive disease	M	8185	21	3243	88.3	0.4	86.7	–	–	–	–	0.1	0.8	1.6
	F	11591	15	3079	91.3	0.3	72.0	–	–	–	0.1	0.3	0.7	0.7
Ischaemic heart disease	M	22147	259	10722	234.8	4.4	272.4	–	–	–	0.6	3.3	7.7	19.0
	F	20113	44	5138	158.6	0.8	119.9	–	–	–	0.1	0.7	1.8	2.9
Pulmonary embolism and other venous	M	393	11	277	4.0	0.2	7.0	0.1	–	–	0.1	0.4	0.3	0.3
	F	369	7	216	3.1	0.1	4.8	–	–	0.1	–	0.1	0.1	0.5
Cerebrovascular disease	M	17609	127	7132	189.6	2.1	188.8	0.4	0.1	0.1	0.8	1.7	3.2	8.4
	F	21217	76	5806	168.1	1.3	134.2	0.2	0.1	0.3	0.9	0.6	2.1	5.0
Other vascular disease	M	20259	185	5264	225.4	3.0	138.8	6.1	0.3	0.8	1.2	1.9	4.3	6.5
	F	22224	116	2708	175.0	2.0	63.5	4.6	0.8	0.6	0.7	0.9	2.4	3.7
Chronic obstructive pulmonary disease	M	7563	22	3023	81.3	0.4	80.6	0.2	–	0.1	–	0.5	0.7	1.0
	F	5060	21	1147	39.8	0.4	26.5	0.1	–	0.1	0.1	0.2	0.7	1.3
Other respiratory disease	M	5806	2597	1919	55.8	40.4	46.1	244.0	7.4	4.7	6.2	4.3	4.3	12.1
	F	4159	2085	715	35.4	33.8	15.9	212.5	6.3	4.7	2.2	2.4	4.1	4.6
Peptic ulcer	M	607	27	418	6.1	0.5	10.3	0.1	–	–	0.1	0.2	0.6	2.2
	F	243	8	116	2.0	0.1	2.7	–	–	–	0.1	0.2	–	0.6
Liver cirrhosis	M	4727	163	3635	47.0	2.7	89.4	2.3	0.5	0.9	1.2	0.6	3.6	9.8
	F	2899	92	1893	24.0	1.6	42.1	1.8	0.6	0.4	0.4	1.3	2.2	4.2
Renal disease	M	1181	90	722	12.0	1.4	17.5	0.5	0.5	0.5	1.5	1.8	1.5	3.8
	F	1100	91	653	9.1	1.5	14.6	0.5	0.5	0.7	1.6	1.8	2.5	3.2
Pregnancy and birth	F	263	200	63	2.3	3.5	1.1	–	–	–	1.1	6.0	8.5	8.8
Congenital and perinatal causes	M	1993	1985	8	17.2	30.8	0.2	203.0	4.5	3.0	2.8	0.7	0.6	1.0
	F	1414	1412	2	12.7	22.8	0.0	148.6	5.3	2.1	1.8	1.0	0.6	0.5
Ill-defined causes	M	67	16	35	0.7	0.3	0.8	1.1	0.1	0.2	–	0.1	0.1	0.1
	F	37	13	11	0.3	0.2	0.2	1.4	–	–	–	0.1	–	–
Other medical causes	M	6711	1518	3552	66.0	24.0	85.0	94.3	5.3	7.2	11.1	10.3	14.4	25.1
	F	4657	1087	2274	39.3	17.8	50.1	75.9	4.6	5.8	8.1	7.5	10.3	12.5
ALL NON-MEDICAL CAUSES	M	13231	4866	7265	122.2	78.5	161.3	74.9	40.7	28.8	63.1	99.8	114.6	127.5
	F	4529	1648	2110	38.7	27.2	44.9	61.0	21.0	13.4	20.5	24.1	24.4	26.0
Motor vehicle traffic accidents	M	3311	1182	1842	30.6	19.3	40.9	9.8	15.7	6.6	12.1	25.5	31.4	33.8
	F	1075	399	508	9.0	6.6	10.8	5.8	8.7	4.8	6.0	7.0	7.2	6.9
Fire	M	340	126	157	3.2	2.1	3.5	4.1	1.2	0.5	1.6	1.3	3.5	2.3
	F	263	80	96	2.2	1.3	2.1	4.4	1.2	0.4	0.3	1.0	1.2	0.7
Suicide	M	1523	406	985	14.3	6.6	22.1	–	–	1.9	7.3	10.6	11.1	15.1
	F	556	129	333	4.7	2.2	7.1	–	–	0.3	3.6	3.7	3.5	3.9
Homicide	M	929	331	526	8.6	5.4	11.5	1.8	0.7	0.8	4.1	8.8	9.0	12.4
	F	300	92	170	2.6	1.6	3.5	1.9	0.5	0.3	1.4	1.2	2.6	3.0
POPULATION (thousands):	M=males				11449	6342	4533	921	868	1005	960	1006	714	868
	F=females				11757	6083	4816	884	830	961	919	968	681	841

ROMANIA: 1990

Annual death rates / 100, 000 — 9th ICD categories

35–39	40–44	45–49	50–54	55–59	60–64	65–69	70–74	75–79	80+/NK			
370.6	529.2	851.4	1252.4	1766.0	2506.4	3610.8	5446.9	8641.4	16458.2	M	ALL CAUSES	001–999
159.3	236.4	364.0	533.0	824.4	1306.8	2221.5	3754.6	6762.5	15821.1	F		
19.5	21.3	32.2	32.0	28.3	20.9	20.0	12.2	10.3	9.2	M	Tuberculosis	010–018, 137
3.3	2.5	3.1	2.4	2.4	2.6	2.2	3.8	4.1	1.2	F		
1.8	1.7	2.0	2.4	2.3	1.6	4.9	4.6	4.2	6.1	M	Other infective	Rest of 001–139
1.2	1.7	1.2	1.2	1.1	1.7	2.0	1.4	5.0	1.6	F	and parasitic	
46.2	83.8	168.8	305.2	437.4	577.0	712.2	826.3	856.0	714.1	M	ALL CANCER	140–208
51.8	80.2	121.1	168.2	242.9	315.1	390.7	482.2	520.3	491.3	F		
2.7	5.7	13.2	22.7	20.5	20.7	24.9	18.8	21.0	29.3	M	Mouth and	140–149
0.4	0.6	1.5	1.8	4.0	3.1	4.7	4.5	6.9	9.4	F	pharynx cancer	
0.2	1.3	2.2	4.7	7.2	7.8	4.7	9.6	11.7	6.7	M	Oesophagus cancer	150
–	0.1	0.8	0.7	0.6	0.8	2.4	2.7	3.7	1.6	F		
4.7	9.7	18.3	31.5	48.5	81.2	108.8	132.0	150.1	125.2	M	Stomach cancer	151
2.7	3.5	4.3	8.9	18.9	30.4	44.8	56.6	71.2	56.9	F		
2.8	5.8	8.8	13.4	24.8	45.3	60.9	75.7	89.3	73.3	M	Colorectal cancer	153, 154
3.3	4.9	5.4	10.9	17.0	27.0	42.8	53.5	65.5	72.4	F		
1.2	1.4	4.6	8.3	9.2	12.6	24.9	26.9	19.2	9.8	M	Liver cancer	155.0
0.5	0.8	1.8	3.2	4.1	7.7	6.5	11.7	10.9	6.1	F		
1.4	3.5	7.6	12.2	19.6	28.9	36.7	44.2	48.6	34.8	M	Pancreas cancer	157
0.1	0.4	2.8	4.7	9.0	14.4	18.7	23.7	34.0	32.9	F		
2.1	5.6	11.0	15.0	25.7	27.7	24.2	27.9	25.2	13.4	M	Larynx cancer	161
0.2	0.7	0.5	0.5	1.4	1.1	2.5	0.7	2.2	2.0	F		
10.8	22.0	58.2	122.1	176.4	187.6	205.1	173.2	150.1	78.8	M	Lung cancer	162
2.8	4.0	7.7	15.6	24.7	26.6	39.4	39.5	41.2	26.4	F		
0.9	1.3	2.2	1.9	3.4	2.4	3.3	3.6	5.1	6.7	M	Malignant melanoma	172
0.5	1.5	1.5	1.1	2.0	2.8	2.0	4.1	4.7	8.1	F		
11.8	20.8	32.9	40.3	46.4	58.1	54.4	70.0	68.7	68.7	F	Female breast cancer	174
13.4	17.8	21.4	23.1	28.0	30.0	34.5	42.6	38.4	35.8	F	Cervix cancer	180
1.9	4.9	5.1	8.1	11.6	12.9	23.2	26.4	24.0	23.2	F	Other uterine cancer	179, 182
2.7	4.3	9.0	14.0	17.9	22.0	19.4	15.8	14.4	9.4	F	Ovarian cancer	183
0.1	–	0.8	2.1	6.0	19.5	40.9	86.8	131.4	154.6	M	Prostate cancer	185
0.1	0.7	3.9	5.7	9.9	24.2	35.3	45.7	49.1	42.2	M	Bladder cancer	188
0.2	0.3	0.5	1.2	3.9	3.9	9.1	12.7	17.2	14.6	F		
12.0	19.2	28.8	52.3	67.1	93.1	110.9	142.7	124.8	119.7	M	Other and ill-defined	Rest of 140–208
6.7	11.8	18.1	26.4	40.3	59.9	69.5	95.7	99.3	113.9	F	cancer sites	
1.8	1.4	1.9	2.3	2.1	2.8	2.8	2.0	1.9	–	M	Hodgkin's disease	201
0.9	0.8	0.7	0.5	1.3	1.4	1.1	1.7	1.9	0.4	F		
1.7	2.5	3.9	5.4	8.7	11.2	13.0	16.3	12.2	4.9	M	Myeloma and non-	200, 202–203
1.2	1.0	2.6	3.1	5.1	7.3	6.5	10.0	5.0	4.5	F	Hodgkin lymphomas	
3.7	3.9	3.2	5.4	8.4	11.9	15.8	20.8	16.4	14.7	M	Leukaemia	204–208
2.6	1.8	4.4	3.9	6.7	5.7	9.3	10.3	11.2	4.9	F		
78.6	153.5	268.4	462.0	743.5	1231.1	1989.8	3434.7	6123.4	13163.7	M	ALL VASCULAR	390–459
28.8	58.0	118.8	210.2	370.5	677.2	1395.8	2667.5	5328.0	13671.0	F	DISEASE	
4.7	6.1	9.7	13.7	13.9	12.4	10.2	6.1	13.1	11.0	M	Rheumatic heart	390–398
4.0	8.1	15.1	16.6	20.1	17.8	16.9	16.8	17.5	19.1	F	disease and fever	
4.0	9.9	21.7	44.3	88.7	162.1	276.4	465.2	797.1	1405.0	M	Hypertensive disease	401–405
2.5	5.7	17.8	34.0	63.7	120.0	260.5	484.6	896.7	1712.9	F		
40.2	76.8	128.1	213.1	303.6	462.8	682.4	1038.6	1747.1	3288.9	M	Ischaemic heart	410–414
7.4	13.0	29.8	51.7	106.9	203.2	427.7	720.7	1412.9	3377.0	F	disease	
1.5	2.6	3.9	5.1	7.2	11.7	16.7	17.8	18.7	18.3	M	Pulmonary embolism	415.1, 451–453
1.5	2.2	3.8	4.7	5.6	5.3	10.2	14.8	14.7	22.8	F	and other venous	
15.2	29.9	56.5	103.7	193.5	343.6	579.2	959.4	1612.4	3061.7	M	Cerebrovascular	430–438
8.7	19.9	35.2	75.0	124.3	235.0	441.1	819.5	1478.2	3339.2	F	disease	
12.9	28.2	48.5	82.1	136.6	238.6	424.8	947.7	1935.0	5378.7	M	Other vascular	Rest of 390–459
4.8	9.1	17.1	28.3	49.9	95.9	239.4	611.2	1508.1	5200.1	F	disease	
4.4	8.5	20.0	48.0	80.9	146.9	255.3	399.2	732.6	1322.5	M	Chronic obstructive	490–496
1.9	4.6	7.1	11.9	26.7	48.2	85.1	174.7	383.3	876.4	F	pulmonary disease	
16.6	20.4	35.0	49.0	54.9	61.5	85.3	119.3	196.4	387.9	M	Other respiratory	Rest of 460–519
6.2	7.2	10.0	10.7	14.9	22.3	40.3	62.5	121.7	320.0	F	disease	
2.7	4.9	6.3	7.0	13.5	16.6	21.2	24.9	26.6	34.2	M	Peptic ulcer	531–533
0.2	0.7	1.5	1.5	3.1	3.3	8.3	10.3	14.4	17.5	F		
18.9	30.3	51.7	75.4	119.8	152.3	177.6	186.9	165.5	126.5	M	Liver cirrhosis	571
9.6	15.3	19.7	31.7	48.3	74.2	96.0	105.7	114.2	97.6	F		
5.3	6.8	10.9	17.9	22.0	26.3	33.2	53.8	59.8	82.5	M	Renal disease	580–590
3.3	5.3	7.7	11.3	15.1	24.2	35.2	35.3	40.3	50.4	F		
5.5	2.1	0.2	–	–	–	–	–	–	–	F	Pregnancy and birth	630–676
0.5	0.1	0.2	0.1	0.2	–	–	–	–	–	M	Congenital and	740–779
–	0.1	–	–	–	–	0.2	–	–	–	F	perinatal causes	
0.5	0.6	1.2	0.7	0.5	1.0	1.4	1.0	3.3	4.3	M	Ill-defined causes	780–799
–	0.1	0.2	0.7	0.1	0.5	–	1.0	0.3	3.7	F		
35.4	49.7	66.7	78.1	92.5	118.4	154.4	212.3	283.3	376.9	M	Other medical causes	Rest of 001–799
16.9	25.4	32.4	38.3	52.7	81.0	104.3	141.7	144.2	171.2	F		
140.2	147.7	188.0	174.5	170.2	152.7	155.5	171.7	180.0	230.3	M	ALL NON-	E800–E999
30.5	33.2	41.1	44.9	46.3	56.7	61.5	68.6	86.8	119.2	F	MEDICAL CAUSES	
35.9	36.7	48.5	43.3	43.4	38.7	40.0	44.2	50.5	56.2	M	Motor vehicle	E810–E819
7.3	8.6	8.1	8.5	11.7	16.0	15.8	15.1	20.3	24.0	F	traffic accidents	
2.5	2.4	3.7	3.7	4.6	4.2	3.7	7.6	7.9	15.3	M	Fire	E890–E899
0.8	1.3	1.3	2.7	2.0	2.5	4.0	5.1	8.7	17.9	F		
18.2	17.4	27.3	23.3	22.9	22.0	23.7	17.8	21.5	31.2	M	Suicide	E950–E959
5.0	3.6	7.7	6.9	7.6	8.7	10.3	10.3	11.9	10.6	F		
11.6	12.9	13.7	11.4	12.1	8.9	9.5	10.7	10.3	17.7	M	Homicide	E960–E969
4.1	3.2	3.6	3.6	2.7	3.9	3.4	4.5	5.0	3.7	F		
867	720	589	699	654	574	430	197	214	164	M	**POPULATION (thousands)**	
853	717	608	742	700	646	551	291	320	246	F		

ROMANIA: Males

	All ages	0–34	35–69	35–39	40–44	45–49	50–54	55–59	60–64	65–69	70–74	75–79	80+/NK
POPULATION (1000s)													
1955	8420	5427	2740	386	522	541	453	372	270	196	145	69	39
1965	9316	5584	3391	754	624	349	519	480	396	271	172	108	61
1975	10460	5965	3993	775	765	721	591	316	447	379	269	143	91
1985	11214	6375	4190	738	613	740	707	642	502	248	309	205	136
1990	**11449**	**6342**	**4533**	**867**	**720**	**589**	**699**	**654**	**574**	**430**	**197**	**214**	**164**
1995 projected	*11769*	*6343*	*4777*	*866*	*860*	*705*	*572*	*666*	*604*	*504*	*344*	*137*	*168*
NUMBER OF DEATHS													
All causes													
1955	88309	31624	32605	1106	2132	3376	4539	6162	6983	8307	9756	7185	7139
1965	82111	14315	35959	1874	2123	1646	4393	6360	9307	10256	10022	11697	10118
1975	101725	15692	41788	2134	2875	4090	5104	4417	9758	13410	15198	13305	15742
1985	130178	13579	53255	2495	3299	6195	8230	11121	12640	9275	18204	19728	25412
1990	**131824**	**13419**	**62254**	**3214**	**3809**	**5018**	**8758**	**11546**	**14379**	**15530**	**10725**	**18484**	**26942**
1995 projected	*131729*	*13000*	*65901*	*3351*	*4653*	*6225*	*7419*	*11993*	*14941*	*17319*	*17225*	*10766*	*24837*
Lung cancer													
1955	...	...	...	...	...	...	...	...	...	...	...	...	...
1965	2649	29	2039	44	66	71	268	468	626	496	370	147	64
1975	3446	33	2564	39	129	275	406	349	656	710	529	230	90
1985	4712	60	3739	54	152	488	749	962	862	472	532	285	96
1990	**5397**	**46**	**4560**	**94**	**158**	**343**	**854**	**1153**	**1076**	**882**	**341**	**321**	**129**
1995 projected	*6145*	*45*	*5110*	*92*	*173*	*417*	*767*	*1323*	*1252*	*1086*	*621*	*225*	*144*
ANNUAL DEATH RATE / 100,000 (*The rates for the age groups 0–34 and 35–69 are the means of seven five-yearly rates, but the all-ages rates are standardised to the conventional "European" age distribution)													
All causes													
1955	1614.5*	510.2*	1542.8*	286.9	408.7	623.6	1001.5	1655.1	2590.1	4233.9	6728.3	10382.9	18447.0
1965	1352.2*	271.2*	1339.7*	248.7	340.0	471.6	847.1	1325.8	2353.2	3791.5	5826.7	10830.6	16724.0
1975	1313.7*	246.3*	1314.7*	275.4	376.0	567.3	863.5	1399.1	2184.5	3537.3	5658.2	9310.7	17337.0
1985	1437.9*	219.0*	1552.8*	338.2	538.1	837.4	1163.7	1733.1	2517.4	3741.4	5900.8	9604.7	18657.9
1990	**1362.8***	**213.5***	**1555.3***	**370.6**	**529.2**	**851.4**	**1252.4**	**1766.0**	**2506.4**	**3610.8**	**5446.9**	**8641.4**	**16458.2**
1995 projected	*1298.6**	*209.3**	*1545.3**	*386.9*	*540.8*	*883.0*	*1298.2*	*1801.8*	*2472.0*	*3434.3*	*5008.7*	*7835.5*	*14801.5*
All cancer													
1955	...	...	...	...	...	...	...	...	...	...	...	...	...
1965	185.8*	11.5*	302.8*	28.8	63.6	106.6	212.5	361.5	581.3	765.2	1012.2	971.3	1006.6
1975	179.6*	11.7*	294.7*	33.4	66.2	124.0	217.1	355.7	538.8	728.0	893.9	1022.4	911.9
1985	186.8*	12.6*	326.2*	41.2	83.3	171.5	278.8	420.0	547.5	741.0	829.2	887.5	773.1
1990	**188.2***	**12.2***	**332.9***	**46.2**	**83.8**	**168.8**	**305.2**	**437.4**	**577.0**	**712.2**	**826.3**	**856.0**	**714.1**
1995 projected	*189.6**	*11.9**	*340.7**	*47.0*	*84.7*	*176.5*	*320.9*	*465.1*	*582.7*	*707.9*	*797.3*	*842.8*	*672.2*
Lung cancer													
1955	...	...	...	...	...	...	...	...	...	...	...	...	...
1965	38.8*	0.5*	75.4*	5.8	10.6	20.3	51.7	97.6	158.3	183.4	215.1	136.1	105.8
1975	41.9*	0.7*	81.9*	5.0	16.9	38.1	68.7	110.5	146.9	187.3	196.9	161.0	99.1
1985	49.3*	1.0*	102.3*	7.3	24.8	66.0	105.9	149.9	171.7	190.4	172.4	138.8	70.5
1990	**53.2***	**0.8***	**111.7***	**10.8**	**22.0**	**58.2**	**122.1**	**176.4**	**187.6**	**205.1**	**173.2**	**150.1**	**78.8**
1995 projected	*57.4**	*0.8**	*120.8**	*10.6*	*20.1*	*59.1*	*134.2*	*198.8*	*207.1*	*215.3*	*180.6*	*163.8*	*85.8*
Upper aerodigestive cancer (mouth, oesophagus, pharynx and larynx)													
1955	...	...	...	...	...	...	...	...	...	...	...	...	...
1965	14.2*	0.5*	24.1*	2.0	5.9	12.6	17.2	28.6	45.8	56.9	76.2	50.9	86.0
1975	13.3*	0.4*	24.5*	2.2	6.8	12.9	23.9	32.6	39.0	54.3	60.7	64.4	37.4
1985	16.2*	0.4*	30.9*	4.5	9.8	18.7	33.1	44.9	47.8	57.7	60.3	50.6	58.7
1990	**18.3***	**0.5***	**35.7***	**5.0**	**12.5**	**26.5**	**42.5**	**53.4**	**56.3**	**53.7**	**56.4**	**58.0**	**49.5**
1995 projected	*20.8**	*0.7**	*41.2**	*5.8*	*16.4*	*34.6*	*53.4*	*64.0*	*60.9*	*53.5*	*55.5*	*56.8*	*48.3*
Other cancer													
1955	...	...	...	...	...	...	...	...	...	...	...	...	...
1965	132.8*	10.4*	203.3*	21.0	47.1	73.6	143.7	235.4	377.2	525.0	720.9	784.3	814.9
1975	124.4*	10.7*	188.3*	26.2	42.5	73.0	124.5	212.5	353.0	486.4	636.3	797.1	775.3
1985	121.3*	11.2*	193.0*	29.4	48.8	86.9	139.8	225.2	328.0	492.9	596.4	698.1	643.9
1990	**116.6***	**10.9***	**185.5***	**30.4**	**49.3**	**84.2**	**140.6**	**207.7**	**333.1**	**453.4**	**596.7**	**648.0**	**585.8**
1995 projected	*111.4**	*10.5**	*178.7**	*30.6*	*48.2*	*82.7*	*133.3*	*202.4*	*314.7*	*439.0*	*561.2*	*622.3*	*538.1*
Chronic obstructive pulmonary disease (COPD)													
1955	...	...	...	...	...	...	...	...	...	...	...	...	...
1965	125.5*	1.1*	123.2*	3.5	8.8	30.9	39.9	102.4	203.8	473.2	550.6	1583.3	1785.1
1975	129.8*	1.3*	102.3*	5.5	8.9	21.5	40.4	93.1	179.3	367.2	704.4	1205.7	2467.0
1985	111.0*	0.7*	97.0*	3.9	10.4	26.1	51.5	97.9	171.5	317.9	561.8	1019.5	1991.2
1990	**81.3***	**0.4***	**80.6***	**4.4**	**8.5**	**20.0**	**48.0**	**80.9**	**146.9**	**255.3**	**399.2**	**732.6**	**1322.5**
1995 projected	*60.4**	*0.3**	*64.3**	*3.7*	*6.7*	*17.2*	*40.4*	*69.0*	*120.1*	*193.1*	*288.5*	*512.4*	*935.0*
Other respiratory disease													
1955	...	...	...	...	...	...	...	...	...	...	...	...	...
1965	98.1*	64.9*	47.4*	5.3	11.4	10.6	28.9	42.3	99.4	133.8	331.4	388.9	1375.2
1975	84.4*	67.8*	46.2*	11.1	13.7	21.2	30.1	46.2	75.7	125.3	219.7	387.0	780.8
1985	72.2*	48.1*	58.3*	20.5	31.2	48.0	54.9	63.1	80.5	109.7	173.1	288.7	591.0
1990	**55.8***	**40.4***	**46.1***	**16.6**	**20.4**	**35.0**	**49.0**	**54.9**	**61.5**	**85.3**	**119.3**	**196.4**	**387.9**
1995 projected	*44.0**	*34.4**	*35.8**	*12.6*	*14.5*	*27.0*	*40.8*	*45.4*	*48.6*	*62.1*	*83.5*	*137.6*	*274.1*
Vascular disease													
1955	...	...	...	...	...	...	...	...	...	...	...	...	...
1965	621.1*	12.5*	514.8*	39.9	80.6	127.2	252.6	450.9	926.2	1726.1	3041.3	6603.7	10710.7
1975	667.3*	10.8*	573.8*	59.5	101.6	174.1	306.2	552.1	1000.4	1822.5	3254.3	5956.6	12214.8
1985	784.5*	10.6*	698.9*	77.1	155.1	271.6	428.0	735.5	1227.6	1997.2	3697.9	6599.3	14284.9
1990	**747.3***	**10.9***	**703.9***	**78.6**	**153.5**	**268.4**	**462.0**	**743.5**	**1231.1**	**1989.8**	**3434.7**	**6123.4**	**13163.7**
1995 projected	*707.7**	*11.0**	*692.5**	*78.7*	*150.3*	*274.2*	*470.3*	*751.1*	*1225.0*	*1898.1*	*3193.1*	*5650.7*	*12151.4*
Liver cirrhosis													
1955	...	...	...	...	...	...	...	...	...	...	...	...	...
1965	29.1*	2.0*	49.3*	12.6	17.0	11.5	52.6	64.8	92.8	93.5	127.9	123.1	147.1
1975	35.4*	2.2*	65.7*	10.2	17.0	38.0	57.4	98.5	103.9	135.1	128.4	147.7	121.1
1985	49.5*	2.9*	93.8*	21.6	30.8	54.1	83.3	115.6	161.9	189.6	186.1	180.6	146.8
1990	**47.0***	**2.7***	**89.4***	**18.9**	**30.3**	**51.7**	**75.4**	**119.8**	**152.3**	**177.6**	**186.9**	**165.5**	**126.5**
1995 projected	*44.5**	*2.5**	*85.2**	*17.8*	*28.2*	*47.8*	*73.0*	*114.3*	*145.8*	*169.5*	*176.2*	*152.8*	*112.6*
Other medical causes													
1955	...	...	...	...	...	...	...	...	...	...	...	...	...
1965	209.4*	111.7*	208.5*	69.3	79.3	103.4	156.8	215.1	347.9	488.0	662.8	1062.0	1456.2
1975	121.2*	81.6*	116.1*	46.3	53.4	76.6	93.0	130.8	170.8	241.6	325.0	453.5	645.4
1985	123.9*	73.2*	133.7*	56.5	79.9	102.3	122.2	142.7	180.6	251.3	313.8	446.4	654.2
1990	**121.0***	**68.4***	**141.1***	**65.6**	**85.0**	**119.4**	**138.3**	**159.2**	**184.8**	**235.1**	**308.8**	**387.6**	**513.1**
1995 projected	*119.0**	*64.6**	*148.3**	*71.6*	*94.7*	*132.8*	*155.6*	*170.8*	*185.0*	*227.8*	*281.5*	*343.5*	*419.5*
All non-medical causes													
1955	...	...	...	...	...	...	...	...	...	...	...	...	...
1965	83.3*	67.6*	93.7*	89.3	79.4	81.4	103.7	88.8	101.9	111.6	100.6	98.1	243.0
1975	95.9*	70.9*	115.9*	109.3	115.2	111.9	119.3	122.6	115.5	117.6	132.5	137.9	196.0
1985	110.1*	70.9*	144.9*	117.4	147.3	163.8	145.1	158.2	147.8	134.7	139.1	182.6	216.6
1990	**122.2***	**78.5***	**161.3***	**140.2**	**147.7**	**188.0**	**174.5**	**170.2**	**152.7**	**155.5**	**171.7**	**180.0**	**230.3**
1995 projected	*133.5**	*84.7**	*178.4**	*155.5*	*161.6*	*207.7*	*197.2*	*186.1*	*164.8*	*175.7*	*188.7*	*195.8*	*236.6*

ROMANIA: Females

	All ages	0–34	35–69	35–39	40–44	45–49	50–54	55–59	60–64	65–69	70–74	75–79	80+/NK
POPULATION (1000s)													
1955	8905	5388	3147	463	604	567	464	424	354	271	201	100	69
1965	9712	5426	3771	754	691	429	593	522	432	351	246	160	110
1975	10785	5735	4345	779	764	733	672	399	544	454	338	209	158
1985	11511	6124	4472	729	621	763	729	685	606	340	423	286	206
1990	**11757**	**6083**	**4816**	**853**	**717**	**608**	**742**	**700**	**646**	**551**	**291**	**320**	**246**
1995 projected	*12047*	*6075*	*5007*	*845*	*854*	*713*	*601*	*724*	*672*	*598*	*478*	*222*	*265*
NUMBER OF DEATHS													
All causes													
1955	86393	25938	28958	1216	1936	2725	3409	4498	6514	8660	11287	8983	11227
1965	81282	10086	27689	1192	1785	1462	3539	4370	6494	8847	11939	15313	16255
1975	95813	11279	29476	1166	1674	2416	3524	3222	7294	10180	13915	16179	24964
1985	116492	8541	31754	1159	1511	2671	4070	5886	8413	8044	17793	21742	36662
1990	**115262**	**8078**	**35672**	**1358**	**1696**	**2213**	**3952**	**5769**	**8437**	**12247**	**10941**	**21667**	**38904**
1995 projected	*110049*	*7362*	*35125*	*1311*	*2039*	*2555*	*3118*	*5666*	*8281*	*12155*	*16126*	*13482*	*37954*
Lung cancer													
1955	...	...	...	...	...	...	...	...	...	...	...	...	...
1965	603	15	398	17	24	30	51	99	98	79	99	56	35
1975	778	14	526	13	27	61	76	76	136	137	120	86	32
1985	938	22	610	14	31	56	105	130	156	118	165	85	56
1990	**1115**	**25**	**778**	**24**	**29**	**47**	**116**	**173**	**172**	**217**	**115**	**132**	**65**
1995 projected	*1299*	*28*	*872*	*23*	*35*	*56*	*109*	*201*	*202*	*246*	*215*	*100*	*84*
ANNUAL DEATH RATE / 100,000 (*The rates for the age groups 0–34 and 35–69 are the means of seven five-yearly rates, but the all-ages rates are standardised to the conventional "European" age distribution)													
All causes													
1955	1315.3*	428.7*	1127.4*	262.7	320.7	480.9	734.1	1060.6	1841.7	3190.9	5607.1	8956.1	16318.3
1965	1061.0*	199.7*	888.6*	158.2	258.2	340.6	596.9	837.8	1504.6	2524.1	4861.2	9558.7	14777.3
1975	983.7*	181.8*	802.1*	149.7	219.2	329.5	524.1	807.9	1340.6	2243.8	4119.3	7733.7	15850.2
1985	1018.0*	143.4*	846.1*	159.1	243.2	350.1	558.7	859.6	1389.2	2363.1	4202.4	7607.4	17814.4
1990	**929.1***	**132.9***	**806.5***	**159.3**	**236.4**	**364.0**	**533.0**	**824.4**	**1306.8**	**2221.5**	**3754.6**	**6762.5**	**15821.1**
1995 projected	*853.7**	*124.1**	*760.0**	*155.1*	*238.7*	*358.1*	*518.8*	*782.3*	*1233.2*	*2034.0*	*3374.3*	*6073.0*	*14300.7*
All cancer													
1955	...	...	...	...	...	...	...	...	...	...	...	...	...
1965	131.4*	10.0*	216.4*	50.8	73.9	126.5	209.0	257.9	366.8	430.0	568.0	645.4	660.9
1975	120.6*	10.3*	204.2*	39.5	71.6	116.2	170.6	261.3	350.5	419.9	501.2	590.8	535.2
1985	115.9*	10.8*	197.5*	44.5	72.3	114.8	168.8	241.3	324.1	416.6	486.5	517.8	512.6
1990	**115.6***	**10.9***	**195.7***	**51.8**	**80.2**	**121.1**	**168.2**	**242.9**	**315.1**	**390.7**	**482.2**	**520.3**	**491.3**
1995 projected	*114.3**	*11.1**	*192.7**	*56.3*	*86.4*	*124.2*	*168.6*	*238.6*	*301.3*	*373.3*	*465.4*	*515.3*	*482.3*
Lung cancer													
1955	...	...	...	...	...	...	...	...	...	...	...	...	...
1965	7.3*	0.3*	12.2*	2.3	3.5	7.0	8.6	19.0	22.7	22.5	40.3	35.0	31.8
1975	7.8*	0.3*	14.2*	1.7	3.5	8.3	11.3	19.1	25.0	30.2	35.5	41.1	20.3
1985	8.3*	0.4*	15.4*	1.9	5.0	7.3	14.4	19.0	25.8	34.7	39.0	29.7	27.2
1990	**9.3***	**0.4***	**17.3***	**2.8**	**4.0**	**7.7**	**15.6**	**24.7**	**26.6**	**39.4**	**39.5**	**41.2**	**26.4**
1995 projected	*10.2**	*0.5**	*18.8**	*2.7*	*4.1*	*7.8*	*18.1*	*27.8*	*30.1*	*41.2*	*45.0*	*45.0*	*31.7*
Upper aerodigestive cancer (mouth, oesophagus, pharynx and larynx)													
1955	...	...	...	...	...	...	...	...	...	...	...	...	...
1965	2.9*	0.2*	4.7*	0.5	2.9	2.3	4.0	5.9	8.1	8.8	13.0	6.2	26.4
1975	2.6*	0.2*	3.9*	0.9	0.5	2.5	3.1	4.0	7.5	9.0	11.0	17.7	18.4
1985	2.4*	0.2*	3.9*	1.1	0.8	2.8	3.2	5.5	6.9	6.8	9.9	10.5	17.0
1990	**2.4***	**0.2***	**4.0***	**0.6**	**1.4**	**2.8**	**3.0**	**6.0**	**5.0**	**9.6**	**7.9**	**12.8**	**13.0**
1995 projected	*2.3**	*0.1**	*3.9**	*0.6*	*1.4*	*2.9*	*3.0*	*5.2*	*5.2*	*9.0*	*8.6*	*11.3*	*12.1*
Other cancer													
1955	...	...	...	...	...	...	...	...	...	...	...	...	...
1965	121.1*	9.6*	199.5*	48.0	67.6	117.2	196.3	232.9	336.0	398.6	514.7	604.2	602.7
1975	110.1*	9.8*	186.1*	37.0	67.6	105.4	156.2	238.2	318.0	380.6	454.7	532.0	496.5
1985	105.2*	10.3*	178.2*	41.4	66.5	104.7	151.3	216.7	291.4	375.1	437.6	477.6	468.4
1990	**103.9***	**10.3***	**174.4***	**48.4**	**74.7**	**110.5**	**149.6**	**212.2**	**283.5**	**341.7**	**434.8**	**466.3**	**451.8**
1995 projected	*101.8**	*10.5**	*169.9**	*53.0*	*80.9*	*113.4*	*147.4*	*205.6*	*266.0*	*323.1*	*411.8*	*459.0*	*438.6*
Chronic obstructive pulmonary disease (COPD)													
1955	...	...	...	...	...	...	...	...	...	...	...	...	...
1965	91.1*	0.6*	57.9*	2.4	4.2	7.9	25.0	55.6	81.1	229.4	471.5	998.1	1865.5
1975	82.6*	1.1*	45.5*	1.9	3.0	8.2	18.6	35.6	78.7	172.6	376.6	857.6	1919.4
1985	60.7*	0.5*	35.1*	2.2	3.1	7.6	15.5	29.9	60.4	126.6	269.0	571.4	1455.8
1990	**39.8***	**0.4***	**26.5***	**1.9**	**4.6**	**7.1**	**11.9**	**26.7**	**48.2**	**85.1**	**174.7**	**383.3**	**876.4**
1995 projected	*28.6**	*0.3**	*19.9**	*2.1*	*4.8*	*6.3*	*10.1*	*21.7*	*35.1*	*59.2*	*121.4*	*266.7*	*619.4*
Other respiratory disease													
1955	...	...	...	...	...	...	...	...	...	...	...	...	...
1965	77.9*	59.6*	26.5*	2.8	10.0	7.5	17.0	16.5	60.0	71.9	235.3	497.5	912.7
1975	65.1*	62.5*	23.2*	5.4	8.9	10.4	15.6	20.6	35.8	65.9	132.6	268.2	630.5
1985	47.7*	39.4*	22.7*	7.5	11.6	14.4	17.0	22.6	30.1	55.5	102.7	193.5	520.4
1990	**35.4***	**33.8***	**15.9***	**6.2**	**7.2**	**10.0**	**10.7**	**14.9**	**22.3**	**40.3**	**62.5**	**121.7**	**320.0**
1995 projected	*28.1**	*29.6**	*11.2**	*4.6*	*5.0*	*7.0*	*7.5*	*10.4*	*15.8*	*28.1*	*43.5*	*84.7*	*226.5*
Vascular disease													
1955	...	...	...	...	...	...	...	...	...	...	...	...	...
1965	587.7*	10.1*	432.2*	39.9	65.7	112.3	214.7	356.4	755.8	1480.5	3090.8	6709.1	10360.0
1975	584.7*	8.4*	399.1*	37.5	59.3	105.1	203.5	338.0	692.0	1358.4	2804.3	5645.8	12294.0
1985	658.5*	6.0*	438.0*	34.3	70.0	123.0	224.2	392.7	744.2	1478.0	2979.0	5898.9	14831.9
1990	**603.7***	**5.3***	**408.5***	**28.8**	**58.0**	**118.8**	**210.2**	**370.5**	**677.2**	**1395.8**	**2667.5**	**5328.0**	**13671.0**
1995 projected	*548.8**	*4.5**	*371.2**	*23.3*	*51.6*	*108.8*	*196.0*	*339.1*	*626.4*	*1253.2*	*2378.5*	*4810.4*	*12530.9*
Liver cirrhosis													
1955	...	...	...	...	...	...	...	...	...	...	...	...	...
1965	17.3*	1.3*	26.9*	4.8	9.7	9.6	21.4	36.6	38.7	67.6	84.7	123.6	80.0
1975	17.0*	1.3*	28.1*	4.6	9.8	14.0	23.8	39.4	45.4	59.7	71.6	85.1	93.3
1985	25.1*	1.8*	42.8*	7.7	15.5	19.4	34.6	57.8	75.1	89.6	119.5	119.0	103.0
1990	**24.0***	**1.6***	**42.1***	**9.6**	**15.3**	**19.7**	**31.7**	**48.3**	**74.2**	**96.0**	**105.7**	**114.2**	**97.6**
1995 projected	*22.7**	*1.5**	*40.1**	*10.1*	*15.8*	*18.8*	*28.0*	*44.0*	*72.1*	*91.7*	*100.0*	*105.4*	*93.1*
Other medical causes													
1955	...	...	...	...	...	...	...	...	...	...	...	...	...
1965	125.5*	92.5*	100.8*	39.7	68.0	55.2	84.0	85.3	162.9	210.8	355.9	527.5	762.7
1975	79.6*	72.6*	65.9*	35.2	38.0	42.8	57.4	72.2	98.1	117.7	168.7	198.9	263.5
1985	75.8*	60.2*	71.4*	36.6	34.1	37.2	62.7	76.1	108.7	144.2	189.4	225.0	281.3
1990	**72.0***	**53.7***	**72.9***	**30.4**	**37.9**	**46.2**	**55.4**	**74.7**	**113.2**	**152.2**	**193.5**	**208.2**	**245.6**
1995 projected	*68.4**	*48.4**	*73.4**	*27.6*	*39.6*	*47.5*	*54.7*	*72.8*	*115.9*	*155.6*	*188.7*	*191.0*	*220.4*
All non-medical causes													
1955	...	...	...	...	...	...	...	...	...	...	...	...	...
1965	30.2*	25.5*	27.8*	17.8	26.8	21.7	25.8	29.5	39.4	34.0	55.0	57.4	135.5
1975	34.1*	25.7*	36.0*	25.5	28.5	32.7	34.7	40.9	40.1	49.6	64.2	87.5	114.3
1985	34.3*	24.6*	38.7*	26.2	36.7	33.7	35.8	39.1	46.6	52.6	56.2	81.9	109.3
1990	**38.7***	**27.2***	**44.9***	**30.5**	**33.2**	**41.1**	**44.9**	**46.3**	**56.7**	**61.5**	**68.6**	**86.8**	**119.2**
1995 projected	*42.7**	*28.7**	*51.6**	*31.1*	*35.5*	*45.6*	*53.9*	*55.8*	*66.7*	*72.8*	*76.8*	*99.5*	*128.1*

ROMANIA: 1975

Smoking-attributed deaths (Sm.) and total deaths (Total)

Age		ALL CAUSES	ALL CANCER	Lung cancer	Upper aero-digestive ca.	Other cancer	COPD	Other respiratory	Vascular disease	Liver cirrhosis	Other medical	Non-medical
Males												
0–34	Sm.	–	–	–	–	–	–	–	–	–	–	–
	Total	15692	667	33	21	613	74	4632	581	124	5447	4167
35–69	Sm.	10582	3432	2300	448	684	2060	344	3741	–	1005	–
	Total	41788	9232	2564	786	5882	2992	1481	17424	2109	3961	4589
		(25%)	(37%)	(90%)	(57%)	(12%)	(69%)	(23%)	(21%)		(25%)	
70+	Sm.	5130	934	662	99	173	2670	88	1327	–	111	–
	Total	44245	4690	849	289	3552	5855	1852	28344	666	2107	731
		(12%)	(20%)	(78%)	(34%)	(5%)	(46%)	(5%)	(5%)		(5%)	
Any age	Sm.	15712	4366	2962	547	857	4730	432	5068	–	1116	–
	Total	101725	14589	3446	1096	10047	8921	7965	46349	2899	11515	9487
		(15%)	(30%)	(86%)	(50%)	(9%)	(53%)	(5%)	(11%)		(10%)	
Females												
0–34	Sm.	–	–	–	–	–	–	–	–	–	–	–
	Total	11279	560	14	13	533	61	4081	445	69	4534	1529
35–69	Sm.	1309	256	198	20	38	366	35	537	–	115	–
	Total	29476	7708	526	148	7034	1576	867	14160	1049	2620	1496
		(4%)	(3%)	(38%)	(14%)	(1%)	(23%)	(4%)	(4%)		(4%)	
70+	Sm.	866	54	43	5	6	577	11	215	–	9	–
	Total	55058	3772	238	103	3431	6089	2002	40647	567	1401	580
		(2%)	(1%)	(18%)	(5%)	(0%)	(9%)	(1%)	(1%)		(1%)	
Any age	Sm.	2175	310	241	25	44	943	46	752	–	124	–
	Total	95813	12040	778	264	10998	7726	6950	55252	1685	8555	3605
		(2%)	(3%)	(31%)	(9%)	(0%)	(12%)	(1%)	(1%)		(1%)	
Males+Females												
0–34	Sm.	–	–	–	–	–	–	–	–	–	–	–
	Total	26971	1227	47	34	1146	135	8713	1026	193	9981	5696
35–69	Sm.	11891	3688	2498	468	722	2426	379	4278	–	1120	–
	Total	71264	16940	3090	934	12916	4568	2348	31584	3158	6581	6085
		(17%)	(22%)	(81%)	(50%)	(6%)	(53%)	(16%)	(14%)		(17%)	
70+	Sm.	5996	988	705	104	179	3247	99	1542	–	120	–
	Total	99303	8462	1087	392	6983	11944	3854	68991	1233	3508	1311
		(6%)	(12%)	(65%)	(27%)	(3%)	(27%)	(3%)	(2%)		(3%)	
Any age	Sm.	17887	4676	3203	572	901	5673	478	5820	–	1240	–
	Total	197538	26629	4224	1360	21045	16647	14915	101601	4584	20070	13092
		(9%)	(18%)	(76%)	(42%)	(4%)	(34%)	(3%)	(6%)		(6%)	

ROMANIA: 1985

Smoking-attributed deaths (Sm.) and total deaths (Total)

Age		ALL CAUSES	ALL CANCER	Lung cancer	Upper aero-digestive ca.	Other cancer	COPD	Other respiratory	Vascular disease	Liver cirrhosis	Other medical	Non-medical
Males												
0–34	Sm.	–	–	–	–	–	–	–	–	–	–	–
	Total	13579	789	60	24	705	46	2982	651	183	4553	4375
35–69	Sm.	16759	5252	3462	751	1039	2197	756	6812	–	1742	–
	Total	53255	11337	3739	1136	6462	2927	2166	22391	3362	4974	6098
		(31%)	(46%)	(93%)	(66%)	(16%)	(75%)	(35%)	(30%)		(35%)	
70+	Sm.	5419	957	679	110	168	2631	74	1641	–	116	–
	Total	63344	5434	913	370	4151	6539	1932	44419	1145	2776	1099
		(9%)	(18%)	(74%)	(30%)	(4%)	(40%)	(4%)	(4%)		(4%)	
Any age	Sm.	22178	6209	4141	861	1207	4828	830	8453	–	1858	–
	Total	130178	17560	4712	1530	11318	9512	7080	67461	4690	12303	11572
		(17%)	(35%)	(88%)	(56%)	(11%)	(51%)	(12%)	(13%)		(15%)	
Females												
0–34	Sm.	–	–	–	–	–	–	–	–	–	–	–
	Total	8541	655	22	12	621	27	2343	354	108	3571	1483
35–69	Sm.	1644	336	263	26	47	348	46	760	–	154	–
	Total	31754	7912	610	160	7142	1208	887	15483	1708	2890	1666
		(5%)	(4%)	(43%)	(16%)	(1%)	(29%)	(5%)	(5%)		(5%)	
70+	Sm.	544	61	50	4	7	227	8	233	–	15	–
	Total	76197	4595	306	107	4182	5768	2059	59996	1058	2024	697
		(1%)	(1%)	(16%)	(4%)	(0%)	(4%)	(0%)	(0%)		(1%)	
Any age	Sm.	2188	397	313	30	54	575	54	993	–	169	–
	Total	116492	13162	938	279	11945	7003	5289	75833	2874	8485	3846
		(2%)	(3%)	(33%)	(11%)	(0%)	(8%)	(1%)	(1%)		(2%)	
Males+Females												
0–34	Sm.	–	–	–	–	–	–	–	–	–	–	–
	Total	22120	1444	82	36	1326	73	5325	1005	291	8124	5858
35–69	Sm.	18403	5588	3725	777	1086	2545	802	7572	–	1896	–
	Total	85009	19249	4349	1296	13604	4135	3053	37874	5070	7864	7764
		(22%)	(29%)	(86%)	(60%)	(8%)	(62%)	(26%)	(20%)		(24%)	
70+	Sm.	5963	1018	729	114	175	2858	82	1874	–	131	–
	Total	139541	10029	1219	477	8333	12307	3991	104415	2203	4800	1796
		(4%)	(10%)	(60%)	(24%)	(2%)	(23%)	(2%)	(2%)		(3%)	
Any age	Sm.	24366	6606	4454	891	1261	5403	884	9446	–	2027	–
	Total	246670	30722	5650	1809	23263	16515	12369	143294	7564	20788	15418
		(10%)	(22%)	(79%)	(49%)	(5%)	(33%)	(7%)	(7%)		(10%)	

(To be conservative, no deaths before age 35, and none from liver cirrhosis or non-medical causes, were attributed to smoking.)

ROMANIA: 1990

Smoking–attributed deaths (Sm.) and total deaths (Total)

		ALL CAUSES	ALL CANCER	Lung cancer	Upper aero–digestive ca.	Other cancer	COPD	Other respiratory	Vascular disease	Liver cirrhosis	Other medical	Non–medical
Males												
0–34	Sm.	–	–	–	–	–	–	–	–	–	–	–
	Total	13419	760	46	33	681	22	2597	654	163	4357	4866
35–69	Sm.	19629	6444	4232	1004	1208	2277	676	8084	–	2148	–
	Total	62254	13366	4560	1489	7317	3023	1919	27082	3635	5964	7265
		(32%)	(48%)	(93%)	(67%)	(17%)	(75%)	(35%)	(30%)		(36%)	
70+	Sm.	4217	815	583	91	141	1850	45	1416	–	91	–
	Total	56151	4627	791	316	3520	4518	1290	41410	929	2277	1100
		(8%)	(18%)	(74%)	(29%)	(4%)	(41%)	(3%)	(3%)		(4%)	
Any age	Sm.	23846	7259	4815	1095	1349	4127	721	9500	–	2239	–
	Total	131824	18753	5397	1838	11518	7563	5806	69146	4727	12598	13231
		(18%)	(39%)	(89%)	(60%)	(12%)	(55%)	(12%)	(14%)		(18%)	
Females												
0–34	Sm.	–	–	–	–	–	–	–	–	–	–	–
	Total	8078	641	25	11	605	21	2085	306	92	3285	1648
35–69	Sm.	2159	479	377	36	66	383	46	1034	–	217	–
	Total	35672	8888	778	181	7929	1147	715	17603	1893	3316	2110
		(6%)	(5%)	(48%)	(20%)	(1%)	(33%)	(6%)	(6%)		(7%)	
70+	Sm.	776	75	62	5	8	380	6	300	–	15	–
	Total	71512	4280	312	96	3872	3892	1359	58461	914	1835	771
		(1%)	(2%)	(20%)	(5%)	(0%)	(10%)	(0%)	(1%)		(1%)	
Any age	Sm.	2935	554	439	41	74	763	52	1334	–	232	–
	Total	115262	13809	1115	288	12406	5060	4159	76370	2899	8436	4529
		(3%)	(4%)	(39%)	(14%)	(1%)	(15%)	(1%)	(2%)		(3%)	
Males+Females												
0–34	Sm.	–	–	–	–	–	–	–	–	–	–	–
	Total	21497	1401	71	44	1286	43	4682	960	255	7642	6514
35–69	Sm.	21788	6923	4609	1040	1274	2660	722	9118	–	2365	–
	Total	97926	22254	5338	1670	15246	4170	2634	44685	5528	9280	9375
		(22%)	(31%)	(86%)	(62%)	(8%)	(64%)	(27%)	(20%)		(25%)	
70+	Sm.	4993	890	645	96	149	2230	51	1716	–	106	–
	Total	127663	8907	1103	412	7392	8410	2649	99871	1843	4112	1871
		(4%)	(10%)	(58%)	(23%)	(2%)	(27%)	(2%)	(2%)		(3%)	
Any age	Sm.	26781	7813	5254	1136	1423	4890	773	10834	–	2471	–
	Total	247086	32562	6512	2126	23924	12623	9965	145516	7626	21034	17760
		(11%)	(24%)	(81%)	(53%)	(6%)	(39%)	(8%)	(7%)		(12%)	

ROMANIA: 1995

Smoking–attributed deaths (Sm.) and total deaths (Total)

		ALL CAUSES	ALL CANCER	Lung cancer	Upper aero–digestive ca.	Other cancer	COPD	Other respiratory	Vascular disease	Liver cirrhosis	Other medical	Non–medical
Males												
0–34	Sm.	–	–	–	–	–	–	–	–	–	–	–
	Total	13000	733	45	42	646	16	2140	646	147	4002	5316
35–69	Sm.	21269	7321	4761	1256	1304	1991	575	8847	–	2535	–
	Total	65901	14402	5110	1804	7488	2601	1566	28571	3648	6664	8449
		(32%)	(51%)	(93%)	(70%)	(17%)	(77%)	(37%)	(31%)		(38%)	
70+	Sm.	4369	1051	763	114	174	1466	41	1699	–	112	–
	Total	52828	5028	990	350	3688	3265	936	39135	1005	2144	1315
		(8%)	(21%)	(77%)	(33%)	(5%)	(45%)	(4%)	(4%)		(5%)	
Any age	Sm.	25638	8372	5524	1370	1478	3457	616	10546	–	2647	–
	Total	131729	20163	6145	2196	11822	5882	4642	68352	4800	12810	15080
		(19%)	(42%)	(90%)	(62%)	(13%)	(59%)	(13%)	(15%)		(21%)	
Females												
0–34	Sm.	–	–	–	–	–	–	–	–	–	–	–
	Total	7362	638	28	7	603	17	1754	258	87	2875	1733
35–69	Sm.	2369	581	458	42	81	342	40	1140	–	266	–
	Total	35125	9095	872	183	8040	912	526	16743	1873	3474	2502
		(7%)	(6%)	(53%)	(23%)	(1%)	(38%)	(8%)	(7%)		(8%)	
70+	Sm.	1186	149	123	10	16	456	10	541	–	30	–
	Total	67562	4648	399	98	4151	2816	997	55303	959	1911	928
		(2%)	(3%)	(31%)	(10%)	(0%)	(16%)	(1%)	(1%)		(2%)	
Any age	Sm.	3555	730	581	52	97	798	50	1681	–	296	–
	Total	110049	14381	1299	288	12794	3745	3277	72304	2919	8260	5163
		(3%)	(5%)	(45%)	(18%)	(1%)	(21%)	(2%)	(2%)		(4%)	
Males+Females												
0–34	Sm.	–	–	–	–	–	–	–	–	–	–	–
	Total	20362	1371	73	49	1249	33	3894	904	234	6877	7049
35–69	Sm.	23638	7902	5219	1298	1385	2333	615	9987	–	2801	–
	Total	101026	23497	5982	1987	15528	3513	2092	45314	5521	10138	10951
		(23%)	(34%)	(87%)	(65%)	(9%)	(66%)	(29%)	(22%)		(28%)	
70+	Sm.	5555	1200	886	124	190	1922	51	2240	–	142	–
	Total	120390	9676	1389	448	7839	6081	1933	94438	1964	4055	2243
		(5%)	(12%)	(64%)	(28%)	(2%)	(32%)	(3%)	(2%)		(4%)	
Any age	Sm.	29193	9102	6105	1422	1575	4255	666	12227	–	2943	–
	Total	241778	34544	7444	2484	24616	9627	7919	140656	7719	21070	20243
		(12%)	(26%)	(82%)	(57%)	(6%)	(44%)	(8%)	(9%)		(14%)	

(To be conservative, no deaths before age 35, and none from liver cirrhosis or non–medical causes, were attributed to smoking.)

¶RUSSIAN FEDERATION: 1990

		No. of deaths			Standardised rates (Defined on p.472)			Annual death rates / 100, 000						
		All ages	0–34	35–69	All ages	0–34	35–69	0–4	5–9	10–14	15–19	20–24	25–29	30–34
ALL CAUSES	M	802400	102081	459812	1676.0	248.2	2123.2	435.4	69.7	59.3	162.3	259.5	321.2	430.2
	F	853593	39696	250806	869.5	100.1	830.8	319.6	37.2	29.2	63.3	71.1	74.9	105.5
Tuberculosis	M	10294	1391	8179	17.2	3.2	31.8	0.3	0.0	0.1	0.4	2.5	6.5	12.6
	F	1615	255	908	1.9	0.6	2.8	0.4	0.0	0.0	0.2	0.9	1.3	1.5
Other infective and parasitic	M	3219	2260	824	4.8	5.4	3.4	31.3	1.2	0.6	1.4	1.0	1.1	1.4
	F	2814	1806	692	3.7	4.5	2.2	26.5	0.8	0.5	0.7	1.2	1.0	1.0
ALL CANCER	M	157427	4408	116146	320.4	10.7	560.0	8.8	7.6	5.7	9.4	9.6	12.9	21.2
	F	126979	3953	71604	141.5	9.8	233.5	7.6	5.9	4.9	6.5	8.1	12.5	23.1
Mouth and pharynx cancer	M	6216	64	5265	11.9	0.2	23.7	0.1	0.1	0.1	0.2	0.2	0.1	0.4
	F	1356	44	674	1.5	0.1	2.2	0.1	0.0	0.0	0.1	0.1	0.1	0.3
Oesophagus cancer	M	6213	12	4864	12.6	0.0	23.3	–	0.0	–	0.0	0.1	–	0.1
	F	2608	6	1045	2.7	0.0	3.5	–	–	–	0.0	–	0.0	0.0
Stomach cancer	M	29860	343	21845	61.7	0.8	104.8	0.0	0.0	–	0.1	0.6	1.3	3.5
	F	24485	343	12267	26.4	0.8	40.4	0.0	–	0.1	0.1	0.7	1.6	3.2
Colorectal cancer	M	11831	191	7472	26.2	0.5	38.1	0.1	0.0	0.1	0.3	0.4	0.9	1.5
	F	16870	157	8552	18.1	0.4	28.2	–	–	0.0	0.1	0.1	0.7	1.6
Liver cancer	M	...	...	...	...	...	...	...	...	...	...	...	...	...
	F	...	...	...	...	...	...	...	...	...	...	...	...	...
Pancreas cancer	M	...	...	...	...	...	...	...	...	...	...	...	...	...
	F	...	...	...	...	...	...	...	...	...	...	...	...	...
Larynx cancer	M	5782	23	4887	11.1	0.1	22.2	–	–	0.0	–	0.1	0.1	0.2
	F	332	6	197	0.4	0.0	0.7	0.0	–	–	0.0	0.0	0.0	0.0
Lung cancer	M	52954	249	42401	105.6	0.6	206.0	0.1	–	0.1	0.2	0.4	0.7	2.6
	F	9893	91	5520	10.8	0.2	18.3	0.1	0.0	0.0	0.2	0.1	0.2	0.8
Malignant melanoma	M	...	...	...	...	...	...	...	...	...	...	...	...	...
	F	...	...	...	...	...	...	...	...	...	...	...	...	...
Female breast cancer	F	16067	352	11498	19.2	0.8	36.6	0.0	–	–	0.0	0.3	1.2	4.1
Cervix cancer	F	6152	184	3695	7.0	0.4	12.0	–	–	–	0.0	0.1	0.7	2.1
Other uterine cancer	F	5982	89	3632	6.7	0.2	11.9	0.0	0.0	–	0.1	0.1	0.4	0.8
Ovarian cancer	F	...	...	...	...	...	...	...	...	...	...	...	...	...
Prostate cancer	M	4310	19	1988	10.8	0.0	11.5	–	–	–	–	0.0	0.1	0.2
Bladder cancer	M	...	...	...	...	...	...	...	...	...	...	...	...	...
	F	...	...	...	...	...	...	...	...	...	...	...	...	...
Other and ill-defined cancer sites	M	32769	1850	22901	66.7	4.5	109.3	4.5	3.0	2.2	3.8	4.2	5.5	8.4
	F	36535	1492	20834	40.9	3.7	67.8	4.0	2.5	2.3	2.9	2.9	4.8	6.9
Hodgkin's disease	M	...	...	...	...	...	...	...	...	...	...	...	...	...
	F	...	...	...	...	...	...	...	...	...	...	...	...	...
Myeloma and all lymphomas	M	3745	720	2421	6.9	1.8	11.1	1.2	1.4	1.2	2.1	2.1	2.4	2.2
	F	2963	397	1705	3.4	1.0	5.6	0.8	0.7	0.5	1.0	1.9	1.1	1.3
Leukaemia	M	3747	937	2102	7.0	2.3	9.9	2.9	3.1	2.1	2.7	1.6	1.8	2.1
	F	3736	792	1985	4.4	2.0	6.4	2.5	2.7	1.9	1.9	1.6	1.7	2.0
ALL VASCULAR DISEASE	M	353002	5666	186778	846.5	13.2	925.3	2.5	0.7	1.0	6.0	10.0	20.9	51.5
	F	562494	1824	118447	542.6	4.5	402.8	2.1	0.8	0.9	3.3	5.2	6.9	12.3
Rheumatic heart disease and fever	M	4203	416	3529	7.2	1.0	14.3	0.1	0.1	0.1	0.7	0.9	2.0	2.9
	F	6905	271	5624	8.4	0.7	17.9	0.1	0.1	0.2	0.7	0.7	1.0	2.0
Hypertensive disease	M	4500	93	3287	9.2	0.2	15.3	0.0	0.0	0.1	0.1	0.1	0.4	0.8
	F	7403	36	3346	7.8	0.1	11.0	–	0.0	0.0	0.0	0.1	0.1	0.3
Ischaemic heart disease	M	193451	2512	111442	450.1	5.7	539.8	–	–	0.0	0.8	2.2	7.9	28.9
	F	252392	313	50817	242.2	0.7	174.3	–	–	–	0.4	0.4	1.0	3.3
Pulmonary embolism and other venous	M	...	...	...	...	...	...	...	...	...	...	...	...	...
	F	...	...	...	...	...	...	...	...	...	...	...	...	...
Cerebrovascular disease	M	111312	970	50874	281.7	2.3	270.2	0.4	0.1	0.3	1.3	2.4	3.8	7.9
	F	226241	514	48294	218.1	1.3	164.8	0.4	0.2	0.2	0.8	1.7	2.4	3.2
Other vascular disease, incl. venous	M	39536	1675	17646	98.2	4.0	85.8	1.9	0.5	0.5	3.2	4.4	6.8	11.0
	F	69553	690	10366	66.0	1.7	34.8	1.7	0.5	0.5	1.3	2.3	2.5	3.4
Chronic obstructive pulmonary disease	M	42442	681	23457	99.9	1.7	122.3	1.9	0.4	0.5	1.7	1.6	2.0	3.5
	F	29203	408	8125	29.0	1.0	27.4	1.3	0.2	0.3	0.9	1.4	1.4	1.8
Other respiratory disease	M	9891	4292	4309	17.1	10.3	18.6	59.9	2.1	0.8	1.9	2.3	1.7	3.5
	F	6434	3001	1413	7.8	7.5	4.6	46.4	1.5	0.9	1.1	0.8	0.8	1.0
Peptic ulcer	M	4247	178	3161	8.5	0.4	14.6	–	–	–	0.2	0.5	0.7	1.6
	F	1847	33	873	2.0	0.1	2.9	–	0.0	–	0.1	0.1	0.1	0.2
Liver cirrhosis and other liver disease	M	8609	372	6617	16.8	0.9	30.3	0.6	0.1	0.3	0.4	0.9	1.1	2.7
	F	7117	234	4030	7.9	0.6	13.1	0.5	0.2	0.3	0.5	1.0	0.6	1.1
Renal disease	M	5502	738	3462	10.8	1.8	15.3	0.5	0.4	0.5	1.5	3.2	3.2	3.6
	F	6453	462	4056	7.5	1.2	13.1	0.3	0.2	0.4	1.3	1.3	1.9	2.7
Pregnancy and birth	F	943	666	277	1.2	1.7	0.7	–	–	–	1.7	3.8	2.8	3.7
Congenital and perinatal causes	M	15783	15467	301	21.1	37.0	1.1	247.8	4.0	2.0	1.7	1.4	1.2	1.0
	F	10981	10630	328	15.2	26.5	1.0	175.4	3.5	1.8	1.5	1.4	0.9	0.9
Ill-defined causes	M	12249	1953	5454	28.1	4.7	21.2	9.2	0.5	0.6	2.5	4.7	6.3	9.2
	F	20084	789	1847	19.0	2.0	5.9	7.3	0.3	0.4	1.1	1.5	1.5	1.8
Other medical causes	M	27110	4954	15472	53.4	12.1	69.4	21.7	8.3	6.3	9.1	9.7	11.0	18.5
	F	30945	3487	15023	34.7	8.9	48.8	16.2	6.3	5.5	7.2	8.2	7.9	10.9
ALL NON-MEDICAL CAUSES	M	152625	59721	85652	231.6	146.7	309.9	50.9	44.4	40.8	126.1	212.2	252.6	299.8
	F	45684	12148	23183	55.8	31.2	72.0	35.5	17.4	13.4	37.1	36.0	35.3	43.5
Motor vehicle traffic accidents	M	28283	14521	12653	41.2	36.3	45.2	6.3	13.3	10.4	38.6	62.8	61.2	61.3
	F	8093	3046	3509	10.0	8.0	10.9	4.6	6.7	4.9	12.3	10.5	8.0	8.9
Fire	M	3098	1116	1711	5.0	2.7	6.6	5.1	1.4	1.1	1.7	2.3	3.1	4.4
	F	1675	451	615	1.9	1.1	2.0	3.8	1.3	0.4	0.4	0.5	0.8	0.7
Suicide	M	30392	10002	18165	48.0	24.4	67.5	–	0.2	4.6	23.5	34.0	48.3	60.2
	F	8758	1603	4937	10.5	4.1	15.5	–	0.1	0.9	6.5	6.9	6.6	8.1
Homicide	M	16038	7727	7911	22.7	18.9	26.7	1.3	0.7	1.5	13.5	33.4	38.6	43.6
	F	5107	1667	2795	6.4	4.2	8.4	1.2	0.9	1.1	3.8	5.8	7.8	8.8
POPULATION (thousands):	**M=males**				69112	39980	26809	5982	5894	5426	5165	4887	6124	6502
	F=females				78550	38707	32591	5748	5710	5270	4967	4670	5938	6405

RUSSIAN FEDERATION: 1990

Annual death rates / 100, 000 — 9th ICD categories

35–39	40–44	45–49	50–54	55–59	60–64	65–69	70–74	75–79	80+/NK			
562.3	813.4	1089.8	1623.1	2314.2	3496.0	4963.7	6667.3	9823.1	17758.7	M	ALL CAUSES	001–999
156.4	251.8	350.2	543.9	845.9	1355.2	2312.5	3643.0	6132.9	14157.5	F		
20.5	25.6	30.3	36.5	35.9	38.0	36.1	32.3	27.9	34.4	M	Tuberculosis	010–018, 137
2.4	2.2	2.0	2.8	2.8	3.3	4.3	5.4	6.3	7.1	F		
1.8	2.5	2.5	3.1	3.7	4.8	5.7	4.6	6.5	7.0	M	Other infective	Rest of 001–139
1.0	1.6	1.6	1.5	2.8	3.4	3.6	3.6	4.2	5.4	F	and parasitic	
43.8	106.2	217.1	412.4	695.9	1055.9	1388.3	1543.7	1670.8	1533.7	M	ALL CANCER	140–208
44.1	84.6	120.5	186.5	265.0	383.0	550.8	652.1	753.8	719.0	F		
2.2	7.5	14.6	24.1	31.0	39.9	46.8	39.0	36.6	39.3	M	Mouth and	140–149
0.4	1.0	1.1	1.4	2.4	3.8	5.5	5.3	8.8	12.5	F	pharynx cancer	
0.5	3.5	10.4	18.6	31.0	44.5	54.6	52.3	59.7	63.6	M	Oesophagus cancer	150
0.1	0.3	1.0	1.8	3.9	7.1	10.2	14.6	22.1	28.2	F		
9.0	21.6	40.6	78.5	131.8	195.1	256.9	305.1	360.6	327.1	M	Stomach cancer	151
6.8	12.5	16.8	26.9	41.6	70.0	108.2	147.5	182.3	159.8	F		
3.1	6.1	11.6	22.2	40.3	70.5	113.3	151.1	197.4	201.5	M	Colorectal cancer	153, 154
3.2	6.7	10.6	20.0	31.8	48.7	76.5	95.2	120.9	121.7	F		
...	...	...	...	...	...	...	...	...	...	M	Liver cancer	Not given separately
...	...	...	...	...	...	...	...	...	...	F		
...	...	...	...	...	...	...	...	...	...	M	Pancreas cancer	Not given separately
...	...	...	...	...	...	...	...	...	...	F		
1.4	5.9	11.9	20.2	31.4	41.5	43.2	42.5	37.5	29.0	M	Larynx cancer	161
0.1	0.3	0.3	0.4	0.7	1.0	1.8	2.0	1.5	1.8	F		
7.7	25.7	70.6	149.6	268.6	409.3	510.2	505.9	456.7	312.3	M	Lung cancer	162
1.7	3.6	6.3	11.7	21.4	32.4	51.0	60.5	63.4	52.5	F		
...	...	...	...	...	...	...	...	...	...	M	Malignant melanoma	Not given
...	...	...	...	...	...	...	...	...	...	F		separately
10.1	21.8	31.1	41.2	43.9	50.8	57.1	54.7	56.8	63.5	F	Female breast cancer	174
3.8	6.6	7.5	9.4	12.5	17.6	26.6	31.1	34.1	28.4	F	Cervix cancer	180
1.7	3.5	5.5	9.4	14.5	20.2	28.2	30.8	33.8	28.5	F	Other uterine cancer	179, 182
...	...	...	...	...	...	...	...	...	...	F	Ovarian cancer	Not given separately
0.1	0.4	1.3	3.6	9.3	21.4	44.7	68.6	111.7	133.6	M	Prostate cancer	185
...	...	...	...	...	...	...	...	...	...	M	Bladder cancer	Not given separately
...	...	...	...	...	...	...	...	...	...	F		
14.6	27.9	46.6	79.6	128.2	199.1	269.3	320.5	351.2	379.8	M	Other and ill-defined	Rest of 140–208,
12.0	22.9	33.7	55.2	79.9	113.0	158.0	182.9	201.8	203.3	F	cancer sites	incl. 155, 157, 172, 183, 188
...	...	...	...	...	...	...	...	...	...	M	Hodgkin's disease	Not given separately
...	...	...	...	...	...	...	...	...	...	F		
2.7	4.2	5.3	9.0	12.6	18.9	24.8	28.7	26.4	20.7	M	Myeloma and all	200–203,
1.9	2.3	2.5	4.2	6.1	8.1	13.8	13.5	12.5	9.3	F	lymphomas	incl. 201
2.4	3.4	4.2	7.0	11.9	15.7	24.6	30.2	33.1	26.9	M	Leukaemia	204–208
2.3	3.0	4.2	5.0	6.4	10.2	13.8	14.1	15.6	9.4	F		
112.6	231.4	362.4	608.1	946.7	1629.8	2586.1	3919.8	6432.4	12998.7	M	ALL VASCULAR	390–459
24.0	54.0	97.8	190.2	370.1	701.7	1381.7	2499.3	4635.6	11723.5	F	DISEASE	
5.7	8.5	11.5	16.6	21.2	18.2	18.7	15.9	8.7	6.4	M	Rheumatic heart	390–398
3.7	6.1	12.8	20.6	26.2	27.0	28.6	17.9	14.5	8.9	F	disease and fever	
2.0	4.8	7.0	11.7	20.4	27.4	33.5	34.2	50.5	69.6	M	Hypertensive disease	401–405
0.8	2.1	4.0	8.7	13.6	19.0	28.7	38.8	50.1	79.8	F		
69.5	152.4	240.2	392.1	576.3	933.3	1414.7	2028.3	3220.4	6224.0	M	Ischaemic heart	410–414
7.0	18.3	33.0	68.4	149.8	307.4	636.4	1160.6	2129.2	5287.6	F	disease	
...	...	...	...	...	...	...	...	...	...	M	Pulmonary embolism	Not given
...	...	...	...	...	...	...	...	...	...	F	and other venous	separately
16.6	36.9	64.7	130.8	249.8	509.6	882.7	1428.1	2404.9	4820.9	M	Cerebrovascular	430–438
6.7	17.3	35.0	72.4	149.2	293.0	579.8	1044.1	1920.1	4588.6	F	disease	
18.9	28.9	38.9	56.9	79.0	141.4	236.5	413.3	747.9	1877.7	M	Other vascular	Rest of 390–459,
5.8	10.1	13.0	20.0	31.3	55.3	108.2	238.0	521.7	1758.4	F	disease, incl. venous	incl. 415, 451–3
6.1	12.9	28.5	62.9	134.2	235.0	376.4	527.8	797.4	1235.9	M	Chronic obstructive	490–496
2.8	5.1	8.5	14.9	27.6	45.9	86.8	139.6	240.0	495.9	F	pulmonary disease	
5.4	9.7	15.9	18.6	20.9	26.8	33.3	39.2	52.6	89.4	M	Other respiratory	Rest of 460–519
1.4	1.7	2.8	3.4	5.0	7.1	10.7	17.0	23.3	45.0	F	disease	
3.1	5.3	8.2	11.8	16.3	24.3	33.3	33.6	41.1	45.7	M	Peptic ulcer	531–533
0.3	0.9	1.3	2.2	2.8	4.4	8.3	9.2	14.0	16.0	F		
5.6	11.8	17.4	26.1	32.7	52.1	66.3	67.0	70.9	72.8	M	Liver cirrhosis and	570–573, 576,
2.6	4.1	6.0	10.1	16.0	22.2	30.8	33.1	39.5	46.0	F	other liver disease	575.2–579.9
5.4	7.3	9.4	13.3	16.5	23.6	31.9	40.4	59.8	77.9	M	Renal disease	580–590
4.0	5.6	7.8	10.7	15.3	20.7	27.3	26.2	28.0	25.7	F		
3.4	1.5	0.1	–	–	0.1	0.1	–	–	–	F	Pregnancy and birth	630–676
0.9	1.5	0.9	1.3	1.4	0.8	0.9	0.4	0.7	0.9	M	Congenital and	740–779
1.0	1.1	1.0	1.1	1.1	0.8	0.9	0.3	0.3	0.3	F	perinatal causes	
12.8	17.7	20.9	24.4	24.9	24.7	23.2	37.7	105.5	675.9	M	Ill-defined causes	780–799
2.7	4.0	4.7	5.3	6.2	8.0	10.5	23.1	84.8	659.3	F		
24.5	35.2	42.7	55.3	71.3	105.1	151.7	188.8	296.0	450.7	M	Other medical causes	Rest of 001–799
14.6	20.5	26.3	37.5	52.5	76.7	113.6	135.2	174.9	206.9	F		
319.9	346.4	333.7	349.3	313.9	275.3	230.6	232.1	261.4	535.7	M	ALL NON–	E800–E999
52.2	65.0	69.9	77.7	78.6	77.9	83.0	98.9	128.2	207.6	F	MEDICAL CAUSES	
55.5	53.0	43.7	47.3	42.6	38.2	36.0	36.5	43.3	74.9	M	Motor vehicle	E810–E819
8.9	10.0	9.2	11.0	11.4	11.8	13.9	19.4	22.2	22.0	F	traffic accidents	
4.7	6.3	6.5	7.0	6.8	7.2	7.9	7.5	10.9	20.3	M	Fire	E890–E899
1.2	1.6	1.6	1.6	2.3	2.3	3.2	4.5	8.0	13.1	F		
63.6	69.5	71.3	71.2	67.6	67.4	62.0	79.7	90.5	132.8	M	Suicide	E950–E959
9.3	11.6	13.8	16.3	15.8	19.5	22.1	24.5	29.2	38.8	F		
42.0	39.3	28.9	26.3	20.5	17.0	12.8	13.3	11.3	33.5	M	Homicide	E960–E969
10.5	11.6	8.5	8.6	7.2	6.8	5.7	6.9	7.9	12.2	F		
5928	4468	3133	4786	3475	3492	1527	945	846	532	M	POPULATION (thousands)	
5962	4607	3456	5538	4359	5192	3478	2423	2602	2227	F		

RUSSIAN FEDERATION: Males

	All ages	0–34	35–69	35–39	40–44	45–49	50–54	55–59	60–64	65–69	70–74	75–79	80+/NK
POPULATION (1000s)													
1985–90	67663	40021	25278	5439	3368	4473	4093	3931	2657	1317	1108	780	476
1985	66079	39776	23872	4601	3264	5098	3810	3998	1847	1254	1288	711	432
1990	**69112**	**39980**	**26809**	**5928**	**4468**	**3133**	**4786**	**3475**	**3492**	**1527**	**945**	**846**	**532**
1995 projected	*70084*	*40543*	*27187*	*6011*	*4531*	*3177*	*4853*	*3524*	*3541*	*1549*	*958*	*858*	*539*
NUMBER OF DEATHS													
All causes													
1985–90	746840	102782	405443	27801	25283	45735	64076	88161	91522	62865	74466	79218	84931
1985	777425	115959	411464	28315	27065	60778	66212	100423	67767	60904	92051	77550	80401
1990	**802400**	**102081**	**459812**	**33334**	**36342**	**34144**	**77680**	**80427**	**122089**	**75796**	**62979**	**83123**	**94405**
1995 projected	*764572*	*91993*	*443479*	*32158*	*34460*	*32480*	*72770*	*76558*	*120852*	*74201*	*59818*	*78999*	*90283*
Lung cancer													
1985–90	48417	242	38118	428	890	3079	6168	10648	10733	6172	5220	3444	1393
1985	43118	247	33345	338	905	3403	5698	10878	6776	5347	5587	2894	1045
1990	**52954**	**249**	**42401**	**458**	**1149**	**2212**	**7161**	**9335**	**14295**	**7791**	**4779**	**3865**	**1660**
1995 projected	*58139*	*238*	*45818*	*425*	*1157*	*2207*	*7146*	*9800*	*16005*	*9078*	*5565*	*4524*	*1994*
ANNUAL DEATH RATE / 100,000													
All causes													
1985–90	1655.1*	246.9*	2044.3*	511.2	750.6	1022.5	1565.5	2242.7	3444.4	4773.3	6722.6	10157.5	17835.2
1985	1782.8*	279.5*	2201.7*	615.4	829.2	1192.2	1737.7	2512.0	3669.2	4856.0	7144.6	10905.6	18628.6
1990	**1676.0***	**248.2***	**2123.2***	**562.3**	**813.4**	**1089.8**	**1623.1**	**2314.2**	**3496.0**	**4963.7**	**6667.3**	**9823.1**	**17758.7**
1995 projected	*1577.9**	*221.5**	*2027.7**	*535.0*	*760.6*	*1022.3*	*1499.4*	*2172.3*	*3412.6*	*4791.8*	*6244.7*	*9206.3*	*16747.0*
All cancer													
1985–90	313.0*	11.0*	546.4*	46.1	105.3	213.3	412.5	686.6	1051.9	1309.3	1492.0	1656.1	1450.7
1985	299.6*	11.2*	524.8*	47.6	102.7	210.2	403.7	698.3	1001.0	1210.3	1427.1	1578.3	1288.5
1990	**320.4***	**10.7***	**560.0***	**43.8**	**106.2**	**217.1**	**412.4**	**695.9**	**1055.9**	**1388.3**	**1543.7**	**1670.8**	**1533.7**
1995 projected	*339.6**	*9.3**	*590.6**	*41.3*	*106.0*	*220.6*	*412.7*	*709.4*	*1132.4*	*1511.6*	*1669.5*	*1816.8*	*1711.6*
Lung cancer													
1985–90	102.1*	0.6*	199.6*	7.9	26.4	68.8	150.7	270.9	403.9	468.6	471.2	441.6	292.5
1985	95.6*	0.6*	188.1*	7.3	27.7	66.8	149.5	272.1	366.9	426.3	433.6	407.0	242.1
1990	**105.6***	**0.6***	**206.0***	**7.7**	**25.7**	**70.6**	**149.6**	**268.6**	**409.3**	**510.2**	**505.9**	**456.7**	**312.3**
1995 projected	*115.8**	*0.5**	*223.7**	*7.1*	*25.5*	*69.5*	*147.2*	*278.1*	*452.0*	*586.2*	*581.0*	*527.2*	*369.9*
Upper aerodigestive cancer (mouth, oesophagus, pharynx and larynx)													
1985–90	33.3*	0.3*	63.7*	4.7	15.2	31.0	58.0	85.0	121.1	130.6	127.7	135.0	130.8
1985	30.4*	0.3*	57.1*	4.7	13.6	27.1	49.1	82.4	110.5	112.3	119.9	129.5	124.2
1990	**35.6***	**0.2***	**69.2***	**4.1**	**16.9**	**36.9**	**62.9**	**93.4**	**125.9**	**144.5**	**133.7**	**133.8**	**131.9**
1995 projected	*41.2**	*0.2**	*81.7**	*4.4*	*21.0*	*46.9*	*75.4*	*107.4*	*148.6*	*168.5*	*150.4*	*142.4*	*138.0*
Other cancer													
1985–90	177.6*	10.2*	283.2*	33.6	63.7	113.4	203.8	330.7	526.9	710.1	893.1	1079.5	1027.3
1985	173.6*	10.3*	279.6*	35.6	61.4	116.4	205.0	343.8	523.6	671.7	873.6	1041.8	922.2
1990	**179.2***	**9.9***	**284.8***	**32.0**	**63.6**	**109.6**	**199.9**	**334.0**	**520.7**	**733.6**	**904.1**	**1080.2**	**1089.5**
1995 projected	*182.6**	*8.6**	*285.2**	*29.8*	*59.5*	*104.2*	*190.1*	*324.0*	*531.9*	*756.9*	*938.1*	*1147.2*	*1203.7*
Chronic obstructive pulmonary disease (COPD)													
1985–90	104.1*	1.9*	123.7*	7.1	15.6	32.5	72.4	138.3	238.3	361.9	544.7	842.5	1312.9
1985	126.4*	2.4*	153.6*	11.0	24.3	45.8	102.2	180.1	298.8	412.6	640.7	1010.5	1530.4
1990	**99.9***	**1.7***	**122.3***	**6.1**	**12.9**	**28.5**	**62.9**	**134.2**	**235.0**	**376.4**	**527.8**	**797.4**	**1235.9**
1995 projected	*79.5**	*1.1**	*97.6**	*4.1*	*8.9*	*19.6*	*43.7*	*98.4*	*194.5*	*313.6*	*429.8*	*636.3*	*989.1*
Other respiratory disease													
1985–90	20.9*	16.1*	19.7*	6.0	10.2	15.0	20.0	24.8	29.3	32.7	41.5	55.6	90.3
1985	30.4*	23.8*	30.4*	12.2	18.6	25.0	32.1	38.0	43.5	43.6	51.8	64.5	105.0
1990	**17.1***	**10.3***	**18.6***	**5.4**	**9.7**	**15.9**	**18.6**	**20.9**	**26.8**	**33.3**	**39.2**	**52.6**	**89.4**
1995 projected	*12.0**	*6.6**	*13.0**	*3.6*	*6.7*	*11.0*	*12.9*	*14.6*	*18.8*	*23.6*	*30.3*	*41.5*	*74.8*
Vascular disease													
1985–90	859.8*	13.1*	901.3*	107.6	214.0	340.7	583.5	913.8	1617.2	2532.5	4037.6	6792.9	13609.6
1985	923.1*	14.8*	954.8*	123.5	217.7	370.4	614.3	1001.4	1745.1	2611.5	4364.9	7431.3	14581.6
1990	**846.5***	**13.2***	**925.3***	**112.6**	**231.4**	**362.4**	**608.1**	**946.7**	**1629.8**	**2586.1**	**3919.8**	**6432.4**	**12998.7**
1995 projected	*766.5**	*10.9**	*869.4**	*106.6*	*223.2*	*353.6*	*577.1*	*884.9*	*1554.6*	*2385.6*	*3476.6*	*5641.8*	*11474.1*
Liver cirrhosis and other liver disease													
1985–90	17.2*	0.9*	31.1*	5.5	10.8	17.0	26.0	36.5	55.3	66.4	68.9	75.0	69.7
1985	21.8*	1.4*	41.3*	10.1	15.6	24.7	35.2	50.1	74.1	79.3	75.8	81.4	63.9
1990	**16.8***	**0.9***	**30.3***	**5.6**	**11.8**	**17.4**	**26.1**	**32.7**	**52.1**	**66.3**	**67.0**	**70.9**	**72.8**
1995 projected	*13.2**	*0.6**	*22.4**	*3.8*	*8.1*	*12.4*	*18.2*	*22.8*	*38.3*	*53.1*	*57.2*	*65.8*	*72.0*
Other medical causes													
1985–90	139.0*	75.1*	153.0*	69.5	94.1	114.6	142.7	169.2	213.8	266.8	329.0	479.9	901.3
1985	157.7*	94.1*	184.6*	109.0	129.0	156.3	182.3	209.6	239.7	266.2	346.9	462.7	621.6
1990	**143.8***	**64.7***	**156.9***	**68.9**	**94.9**	**114.9**	**145.8**	**169.9**	**221.2**	**282.8**	**337.7**	**537.6**	**1292.5**
1995 projected	*137.9**	*44.7**	*133.5**	*46.5*	*65.2*	*85.4*	*112.6*	*142.5*	*206.2*	*276.0*	*359.1*	*746.3*	*1827.9*
All non-medical causes													
1985–90	201.2*	128.7*	269.0*	269.3	300.4	289.3	308.4	273.5	238.6	203.7	208.8	255.3	400.7
1985	223.9*	131.8*	312.1*	302.0	321.3	359.9	367.7	334.6	267.0	232.5	237.4	276.9	437.7
1990	**231.6***	**146.7***	**309.9***	**319.9**	**346.4**	**333.7**	**349.3**	**313.9**	**275.3**	**230.6**	**232.1**	**261.4**	**535.7**
1995 projected	*229.2**	*148.2**	*301.3**	*329.1*	*342.5*	*319.7*	*322.2*	*299.7*	*267.8*	*228.4*	*222.3*	*257.8*	*597.7*

(*The rates for the age groups 0–34 and 35–69 are the means of seven five-yearly rates, but the all-ages rates are standardised to the conventional "European" age distribution)

RUSSIAN FEDERATION: Females

	All ages	0–34	35–69	35–39	40–44	45–49	50–54	55–59	60–64	65–69	70–74	75–79	80+/NK
POPULATION (1000s)													
1985–90	77587	38809	31419	5486	3520	4983	4762	5063	4624	2981	2892	2422	2046
1985	76460	38621	30385	4657	3500	5683	4490	5445	3804	2807	3335	2247	1873
1990	**78550**	**38707**	**32591**	**5962**	**4607**	**3456**	**5538**	**4359**	**5192**	**3478**	**2423**	**2602**	**2227**
1995 projected	*79655*	*39252*	*33050*	*6046*	*4672*	*3504*	*5615*	*4420*	*5265*	*3527*	*2458*	*2638*	*2258*
NUMBER OF DEATHS													
All causes													
1985–90	830472	43987	235260	8507	8469	17025	26193	42631	64263	68172	106579	155053	289593
1985	847841	48596	240242	8788	8873	22467	27492	50923	57823	63876	128975	152142	277886
1990	**853593**	**39696**	**250806**	**9326**	**11601**	**12101**	**30121**	**36868**	**70365**	**80424**	**88284**	**159547**	**315260**
1995 projected	*804772*	*33133*	*237102*	*8625*	*10652*	*11149*	*27357*	*33455*	*68070*	*77794*	*83798*	*151940*	*298799*
Lung cancer													
1985–90	9374	97	5221	92	123	319	561	1088	1580	1458	1603	1490	963
1985	8658	98	4835	89	104	396	515	1210	1306	1215	1706	1244	775
1990	**9893**	**91**	**5520**	**103**	**167**	**219**	**646**	**931**	**1682**	**1772**	**1465**	**1649**	**1168**
1995 projected	*10951*	*77*	*5773*	*111*	*164*	*221*	*628*	*901*	*1771*	*1977*	*1699*	*1984*	*1418*
ANNUAL DEATH RATE / 100,000 (*The rates for the age groups 0–34 and 35–69 are the means of seven five-yearly rates, but the all-ages rates are standardised to the conventional "European" age distribution)													
All causes													
1985–90	880.9*	109.6*	829.4*	155.1	240.6	341.7	550.0	842.0	1389.8	2286.9	3684.8	6402.7	14156.2
1985	937.4*	122.3*	883.0*	188.7	253.6	395.3	612.3	935.2	1520.3	2276.0	3867.7	6771.2	14840.4
1990	**869.5***	**100.1***	**830.8***	**156.4**	**251.8**	**350.2**	**543.9**	**845.9**	**1355.2**	**2312.5**	**3643.0**	**6132.9**	**14157.5**
1995 projected	*805.7**	*83.0**	*775.9**	*142.6*	*228.0*	*318.2*	*487.2*	*756.9*	*1292.8*	*2205.9*	*3409.9*	*5759.4*	*13232.3*
All cancer													
1985–90	139.0*	9.9*	231.1*	44.8	78.8	118.1	185.0	268.7	392.8	529.4	631.3	740.3	676.5
1985	135.1*	10.3*	225.3*	47.2	70.7	118.2	181.4	276.4	399.6	483.5	613.8	694.0	629.3
1990	**141.5***	**9.8***	**233.5***	**44.1**	**84.6**	**120.5**	**186.5**	**265.0**	**383.0**	**550.8**	**652.1**	**753.8**	**719.0**
1995 projected	*146.9**	*8.9**	*238.1**	*46.3*	*87.9*	*125.6*	*183.3*	*255.8*	*392.0*	*575.5*	*699.4*	*828.0*	*800.4*
Lung cancer													
1985–90	10.5*	0.2*	18.3*	1.7	3.5	6.4	11.8	21.5	34.2	48.9	55.4	61.5	47.1
1985	10.0*	0.2*	17.6*	1.9	3.0	7.0	11.5	22.2	34.3	43.3	51.2	55.4	41.4
1990	**10.8***	**0.2***	**18.3***	**1.7**	**3.6**	**6.3**	**11.7**	**21.4**	**32.4**	**51.0**	**60.5**	**63.4**	**52.5**
1995 projected	*11.7**	*0.2**	*19.0**	*1.8*	*3.5*	*6.3*	*11.2*	*20.4*	*33.6*	*56.1*	*69.1*	*75.2*	*62.8*
Upper aerodigestive cancer (mouth, oesophagus, pharynx and larynx)													
1985–90	4.7*	0.1*	6.3*	0.6	1.2	2.1	3.9	7.3	11.6	17.5	24.4	34.9	44.2
1985	4.7*	0.1*	6.3*	0.6	0.8	2.0	4.3	7.3	11.8	17.0	25.2	34.7	45.3
1990	**4.5***	**0.1***	**6.4***	**0.6**	**1.5**	**2.3**	**3.5**	**7.0**	**11.9**	**17.6**	**21.9**	**32.5**	**42.6**
1995 projected	*4.3**	*0.1**	*6.2**	*0.8*	*2.0*	*2.4*	*3.3*	*6.6*	*11.9*	*16.5*	*20.1*	*30.1*	*39.9*
Other cancer													
1985–90	123.9*	9.6*	206.5*	42.5	74.1	109.6	169.3	239.9	347.1	463.0	551.4	643.9	585.2
1985	120.5*	9.9*	201.4*	44.7	66.9	109.2	165.6	246.9	353.4	423.2	537.4	603.9	542.6
1990	**126.1***	**9.4***	**208.8***	**41.8**	**79.4**	**111.8**	**171.3**	**236.7**	**338.7**	**482.3**	**569.7**	**657.9**	**624.0**
1995 projected	*131.0**	*8.5**	*212.9**	*43.7*	*82.4*	*116.9*	*168.8*	*228.8*	*346.4*	*503.0*	*610.2*	*722.8*	*697.6*
Chronic obstructive pulmonary disease (COPD)													
1985–90	31.9*	1.3*	28.6*	3.2	5.5	8.5	16.6	28.7	49.7	87.8	151.5	265.5	566.8
1985	39.5*	1.6*	35.3*	4.3	6.9	10.9	21.3	35.8	61.2	106.4	181.2	329.3	709.2
1990	**29.0***	**1.0***	**27.4***	**2.8**	**5.1**	**8.5**	**14.9**	**27.6**	**45.9**	**86.8**	**139.6**	**240.0**	**495.9**
1995 projected	*21.2**	*0.8**	*20.8**	*2.0*	*3.7*	*6.1*	*11.0*	*20.4*	*35.8*	*66.8*	*103.5*	*171.1*	*351.4*
Other respiratory disease													
1985–90	10.5*	12.0*	5.1*	1.8	2.1	2.8	3.8	5.8	7.8	11.6	16.7	25.7	43.1
1985	14.5*	17.4*	7.1*	3.0	2.7	4.6	5.6	8.4	11.3	14.2	19.2	30.6	49.8
1990	**7.8***	**7.5***	**4.6***	**1.4**	**1.7**	**2.8**	**3.4**	**5.0**	**7.1**	**10.7**	**17.0**	**23.3**	**45.0**
1995 projected	*5.5**	*4.8**	*3.3**	*1.0*	*1.2*	*1.9*	*2.4*	*3.5*	*5.0*	*8.2*	*13.3*	*20.0*	*38.2*
Vascular disease													
1985–90	564.8*	4.9*	410.9*	25.2	52.8	97.4	199.2	370.4	732.2	1399.4	2592.2	4968.8	12212.9
1985	605.4*	5.4*	442.2*	31.6	56.4	117.1	227.8	417.1	820.8	1424.5	2770.4	5352.4	12960.1
1990	**542.6***	**4.5***	**402.8***	**24.0**	**54.0**	**97.8**	**190.2**	**370.1**	**701.7**	**1381.7**	**2499.3**	**4635.6**	**11723.5**
1995 projected	*481.8**	*3.7**	*358.8**	*20.7*	*45.5*	*82.2*	*162.6*	*316.1*	*640.1*	*1244.2*	*2185.1*	*4124.5*	*10472.9*
Liver cirrhosis and other liver disease													
1985–90	7.7*	0.6*	12.9*	2.2	4.1	6.1	10.1	16.2	22.5	29.1	32.2	38.8	40.9
1985	8.9*	0.7*	15.6*	3.3	6.1	8.6	13.4	22.3	26.2	29.4	31.2	38.1	41.1
1990	**7.9***	**0.6***	**13.1***	**2.6**	**4.1**	**6.0**	**10.1**	**16.0**	**22.2**	**30.8**	**33.1**	**39.5**	**46.0**
1995 projected	*7.2**	*0.5**	*11.2**	*1.8*	*2.8*	*4.2*	*7.3*	*12.4*	*19.5*	*30.1*	*33.9*	*42.6*	*49.6*
Other medical causes													
1985–90	74.9*	52.4*	73.0*	29.9	36.9	43.0	61.1	79.3	111.2	149.9	171.7	237.8	419.4
1985	74.6*	57.3*	74.9*	38.7	39.5	51.5	67.3	84.1	111.8	131.2	160.0	203.3	254.6
1990	**85.0***	**45.5***	**77.5***	**29.4**	**37.4**	**44.7**	**61.1**	**83.5**	**117.4**	**168.7**	**202.9**	**312.6**	**920.6**
1995 projected	*91.1**	*33.0**	*81.1**	*24.3*	*31.6*	*39.9*	*56.4*	*82.5*	*131.3*	*201.7*	*275.2*	*438.8*	*1301.9*
All non-medical causes													
1985–90	52.1*	28.5*	67.8*	47.9	60.3	65.8	74.2	72.9	73.6	79.7	89.2	125.7	196.6
1985	59.4*	29.7*	82.7*	60.6	71.2	84.5	95.5	91.1	89.4	86.8	91.9	123.4	196.4
1990	**55.8***	**31.2***	**72.0***	**52.2**	**65.0**	**69.9**	**77.7**	**78.6**	**77.9**	**83.0**	**98.9**	**128.2**	**207.6**
1995 projected	*52.0**	*31.4**	*62.7**	*46.5*	*55.3*	*58.3*	*64.1*	*66.2*	*69.2*	*79.3*	*99.5*	*134.5*	*217.9*

RUSSIAN FEDERATION: 1985–1990

Smoking–attributed deaths (Sm.) and total deaths (Total)

		ALL CAUSES	ALL CANCER	Lung cancer	Upper aero–digestive ca.	Other cancer	COPD	Other respiratory	Vascular disease	Cirrhosis/ other liver	Other medical	Non–medical
Males												
0–34	Sm.	–	–	–	–	–	–	–	–	–	–	–
	Total	102782	4520	242	123	4155	807	6761	5600	400	31471	53223
35–69	Sm.	172275	60682	36577	9999	14106	18922	2106	74203	–	16362	–
	Total	405443	104666	38118	12809	53739	21865	4347	164431	6266	33765	70103
		(42%)	(58%)	(96%)	(78%)	(26%)	(87%)	(48%)	(45%)		(48%)	
70+	Sm.	48478	13888	9128	1822	2938	13538	169	19438	–	1445	–
	Total	238615	36351	10057	3090	23204	18857	1324	162512	1680	11679	6212
		(20%)	(38%)	(91%)	(59%)	(13%)	(72%)	(13%)	(12%)		(12%)	
Any age	Sm.	220753	74570	45705	11821	17044	32460	2275	93641	–	17807	–
	Total	746840	145537	48417	16022	81098	41529	12432	332543	8346	76915	129538
		(30%)	(51%)	(94%)	(74%)	(21%)	(78%)	(18%)	(28%)		(23%)	
Females												
0–34	Sm.	–	–	–	–	–	–	–	–	–	–	–
	Total	43987	4032	97	55	3880	514	4867	1984	248	21121	11221
35–69	Sm.	15449	3456	2586	369	501	2905	94	7626	–	1368	–
	Total	235260	67485	5221	1796	60468	7952	1499	111904	3776	21611	21033
		(7%)	(5%)	(50%)	(21%)	(1%)	(37%)	(6%)	(7%)		(6%)	
70+	Sm.	18666	2620	1867	434	319	7063	42	8522	–	419	–
	Total	551225	50027	4056	2456	43515	22408	1986	445146	2707	19304	9647
		(3%)	(5%)	(46%)	(18%)	(1%)	(32%)	(2%)	(2%)		(2%)	
Any age	Sm.	34115	6076	4453	803	820	9968	136	16148	–	1787	–
	Total	830472	121544	9374	4307	107863	30874	8352	559034	6731	62036	41901
		(4%)	(5%)	(48%)	(19%)	(1%)	(32%)	(2%)	(3%)		(3%)	
Males+Females												
0–34	Sm.	–	–	–	–	–	–	–	–	–	–	–
	Total	146769	8552	339	178	8035	1321	11628	7584	648	52592	64444
35–69	Sm.	187724	64138	39163	10368	14607	21827	2200	81829	–	17730	–
	Total	640703	172151	43339	14605	114207	29817	5846	276335	10042	55376	91136
		(29%)	(37%)	(90%)	(71%)	(13%)	(73%)	(38%)	(30%)		(32%)	
70+	Sm.	67144	16508	10995	2256	3257	20601	211	27960	–	1864	–
	Total	789840	86378	14113	5546	66719	41265	3310	607658	4387	30983	15859
		(9%)	(19%)	(78%)	(41%)	(5%)	(50%)	(6%)	(5%)		(6%)	
Any age	Sm.	254868	80646	50158	12624	17864	42428	2411	109789	–	19594	–
	Total	1577312	267081	57791	20329	188961	72403	20784	891577	15077	138951	171439
		(16%)	(30%)	(87%)	(62%)	(9%)	(59%)	(12%)	(12%)		(14%)	

RUSSIAN FEDERATION: 1985

Smoking–attributed deaths (Sm.) and total deaths (Total)

		ALL CAUSES	ALL CANCER	Lung cancer	Upper aero–digestive ca.	Other cancer	COPD	Other respiratory	Vascular disease	Cirrhosis/ other liver	Other medical	Non–medical
Males												
0–34	Sm.	–	–	–	–	–	–	–	–	–	–	–
	Total	115959	4536	247	132	4157	1000	9736	6282	597	38738	55070
35–69	Sm.	169421	52790	31942	8253	12595	21879	3196	71768	–	19788	–
	Total	411464	93226	33345	10654	49227	25426	6533	160095	7939	40280	77965
		(41%)	(57%)	(96%)	(77%)	(26%)	(86%)	(49%)	(45%)		(49%)	
70+	Sm.	50063	13023	8592	1720	2711	15509	199	20004	–	1328	–
	Total	250002	35171	9526	3002	22643	22046	1579	172016	1831	10442	6917
		(20%)	(37%)	(90%)	(57%)	(12%)	(70%)	(13%)	(12%)		(13%)	
Any age	Sm.	219484	65813	40534	9973	15306	37388	3395	91772	–	21116	–
	Total	777425	132933	43118	13788	76027	48472	17848	338393	10367	89460	139952
		(28%)	(50%)	(94%)	(72%)	(20%)	(77%)	(19%)	(27%)		(24%)	
Females												
0–34	Sm.	–	–	–	–	–	–	–	–	–	–	–
	Total	48596	4141	98	51	3992	632	6855	2212	289	22698	11769
35–69	Sm.	14982	3097	2320	329	448	3228	125	7222	–	1310	–
	Total	240242	63352	4835	1686	56831	9279	2031	114241	4492	21650	25197
		(6%)	(5%)	(48%)	(20%)	(1%)	(35%)	(6%)	(6%)		(6%)	
70+	Sm.	16972	2147	1531	365	251	7127	42	7358	–	298	–
	Total	559003	47846	3725	2470	41651	26719	2261	455326	2666	14670	9515
		(3%)	(4%)	(41%)	(15%)	(1%)	(27%)	(2%)	(2%)		(2%)	
Any age	Sm.	31954	5244	3851	694	699	10355	167	14580	–	1608	–
	Total	847841	115339	8658	4207	102474	36630	11147	571779	7447	59018	46481
		(4%)	(5%)	(44%)	(16%)	(1%)	(28%)	(1%)	(3%)		(3%)	
Males+Females												
0–34	Sm.	–	–	–	–	–	–	–	–	–	–	–
	Total	164555	8677	345	183	8149	1632	16591	8494	886	61436	66839
35–69	Sm.	184403	55887	34262	8582	13043	25107	3321	78990	–	21098	–
	Total	651706	156578	38180	12340	106058	34705	8564	274336	12431	61930	103162
		(28%)	(36%)	(90%)	(70%)	(12%)	(72%)	(39%)	(29%)		(34%)	
70+	Sm.	67035	15170	10123	2085	2962	22636	241	27362	–	1626	–
	Total	809005	83017	13251	5472	64294	48765	3840	627342	4497	25112	16432
		(8%)	(18%)	(76%)	(38%)	(5%)	(46%)	(6%)	(4%)		(6%)	
Any age	Sm.	251438	71057	44385	10667	16005	47743	3562	106352	–	22724	–
	Total	1625266	248272	51776	17995	178501	85102	28995	910172	17814	148478	186433
		(15%)	(29%)	(86%)	(59%)	(9%)	(56%)	(12%)	(12%)		(15%)	

(To be conservative, no deaths before age 35, and none from liver cirrhosis or non–medical causes, were attributed to smoking.)

RUSSIAN FEDERATION: 1990

Smoking–attributed deaths (Sm.) and total deaths (Total)

		ALL CAUSES	ALL CANCER	Lung cancer	Upper aero–digestive ca.	Other cancer	COPD	Other respiratory	Vascular disease	Cirrhosis/ other liver	Other medical	Non–medical
Males												
0–34	Sm.	–	–	–	–	–	–	–	–	–	–	–
	Total	102081	4408	249	99	4060	681	4292	5666	372	26941	59721
35–69	Sm.	191878	67999	40710	11751	15538	20346	2060	83822	–	17651	–
	Total	459812	116146	42401	15016	58729	23457	4309	186778	6617	36853	85652
		(42%)	(59%)	(96%)	(78%)	(26%)	(87%)	(48%)	(45%)		(48%)	
70+	Sm.	48641	14285	9380	1851	3054	13250	163	19216	–	1727	–
	Total	240507	36873	10304	3096	23473	18304	1290	160558	1620	14610	7252
		(20%)	(39%)	(91%)	(60%)	(13%)	(72%)	(13%)	(12%)		(12%)	
Any age	Sm.	240519	82284	50090	13602	18592	33596	2223	103038	–	19378	–
	Total	802400	157427	52954	18211	86262	42442	9891	353002	8609	78404	152625
		(30%)	(52%)	(95%)	(75%)	(22%)	(79%)	(22%)	(29%)		(25%)	
Females												
0–34	Sm.	–	–	–	–	–	–	–	–	–	–	–
	Total	39696	3953	91	56	3806	408	3001	1824	234	18128	12148
35–69	Sm.	16402	3677	2746	396	535	2997	90	8112	–	1526	–
	Total	250806	71604	5520	1916	64168	8125	1413	118447	4030	24004	23183
		(7%)	(5%)	(50%)	(21%)	(1%)	(37%)	(6%)	(7%)		(6%)	
70+	Sm.	19347	2859	2063	437	359	6858	45	8898	–	687	–
	Total	563091	51422	4282	2324	44816	20670	2020	442223	2853	33550	10353
		(3%)	(6%)	(48%)	(19%)	(1%)	(33%)	(2%)	(2%)		(2%)	
Any age	Sm.	35749	6536	4809	833	894	9855	135	17010	–	2213	–
	Total	853593	126979	9893	4296	112790	29203	6434	562494	7117	75682	45684
		(4%)	(5%)	(49%)	(19%)	(1%)	(34%)	(2%)	(3%)		(3%)	
Males+Females												
0–34	Sm.	–	–	–	–	–	–	–	–	–	–	–
	Total	141777	8361	340	155	7866	1089	7293	7490	606	45069	71869
35–69	Sm.	208280	71676	43456	12147	16073	23343	2150	91934	–	19177	–
	Total	710618	187750	47921	16932	122897	31582	5722	305225	10647	60857	108835
		(29%)	(38%)	(91%)	(72%)	(13%)	(74%)	(38%)	(30%)		(32%)	
70+	Sm.	67988	17144	11443	2288	3413	20108	208	28114	–	2414	–
	Total	803598	88295	14586	5420	68289	38974	3310	602781	4473	48160	17605
		(8%)	(19%)	(78%)	(42%)	(5%)	(52%)	(6%)	(5%)		(5%)	
Any age	Sm.	276268	88820	54899	14435	19486	43451	2358	120048	–	21591	–
	Total	1655993	284406	62847	22507	199052	71645	16325	915496	15726	154086	198309
		(17%)	(31%)	(87%)	(64%)	(10%)	(61%)	(14%)	(13%)		(14%)	

RUSSIAN FEDERATION: 1995

Smoking–attributed deaths (Sm.) and total deaths (Total)

		ALL CAUSES	ALL CANCER	Lung cancer	Upper aero–digestive ca.	Other cancer	COPD	Other respiratory	Vascular disease	Cirrhosis/ other liver	Other medical	Non–medical
Males												
0–34	Sm.	–	–	–	–	–	–	–	–	–	–	–
	Total	91993	3883	238	76	3569	473	2778	4758	260	18874	60967
35–69	Sm.	190498	74733	44104	14277	16352	16302	1483	83234	–	14746	–
	Total	443479	122835	45818	18019	58998	18609	3038	178946	4849	30526	84676
		(43%)	(61%)	(96%)	(79%)	(28%)	(88%)	(49%)	(47%)		(48%)	
70+	Sm.	50537	17041	11138	2163	3740	11236	149	19579	–	2532	–
	Total	229100	40809	12083	3407	25319	14909	1049	143571	1501	19698	7563
		(22%)	(42%)	(92%)	(63%)	(15%)	(75%)	(14%)	(14%)		(13%)	
Any age	Sm.	241035	91774	55242	16440	20092	27538	1632	102813	–	17278	–
	Total	764572	167527	58139	21502	87886	33991	6865	327275	6610	69098	153206
		(32%)	(55%)	(95%)	(76%)	(23%)	(81%)	(24%)	(31%)		(25%)	
Females												
0–34	Sm.	–	–	–	–	–	–	–	–	–	–	–
	Total	33133	3626	77	59	3490	301	1953	1484	201	13331	12237
35–69	Sm.	16014	3944	2951	412	581	2401	68	7898	–	1703	–
	Total	237102	73843	5773	1912	66158	6271	1028	106938	3433	25184	20405
		(7%)	(5%)	(51%)	(22%)	(1%)	(38%)	(7%)	(7%)		(7%)	
70+	Sm.	22317	3920	2851	529	540	6149	51	10881	–	1316	–
	Total	534537	57105	5101	2188	49816	14993	1716	398995	3078	47738	10912
		(4%)	(7%)	(56%)	(24%)	(1%)	(41%)	(3%)	(3%)		(3%)	
Any age	Sm.	38331	7864	5802	941	1121	8550	119	18779	–	3019	–
	Total	804772	134574	10951	4159	119464	21565	4697	507417	6712	86253	43554
		(5%)	(6%)	(53%)	(23%)	(1%)	(40%)	(3%)	(4%)		(4%)	
Males+Females												
0–34	Sm.	–	–	–	–	–	–	–	–	–	–	–
	Total	125126	7509	315	135	7059	774	4731	6242	461	32205	73204
35–69	Sm.	206512	78677	47055	14689	16933	18703	1551	91132	–	16449	–
	Total	680581	196678	51591	19931	125156	24880	4066	285884	8282	55710	105081
		(30%)	(40%)	(91%)	(74%)	(14%)	(75%)	(38%)	(32%)		(30%)	
70+	Sm.	72854	20961	13989	2692	4280	17385	200	30460	–	3848	–
	Total	763637	97914	17184	5595	75135	29902	2765	542566	4579	67436	18475
		(10%)	(21%)	(81%)	(48%)	(6%)	(58%)	(7%)	(6%)		(6%)	
Any age	Sm.	279366	99638	61044	17381	21213	36088	1751	121592	–	20297	–
	Total	1569344	302101	69090	25661	207350	55556	11562	834692	13322	155351	196760
		(18%)	(33%)	(88%)	(68%)	(10%)	(65%)	(15%)	(15%)		(13%)	

(To be conservative, no deaths before age 35, and none from liver cirrhosis or non–medical causes, were attributed to smoking.)

¶SLOVAKIA: 1990

		No. of deaths			Standardised rates (Defined on p.478)			Annual death rates / 100, 000						
		All ages	0–34	35–69	All ages	0–34	35–69	0–4	5–9	10–14	15–19	20–24	25–29	30–34
ALL CAUSES	M	30263	2003	15240	1504.0	136.3	1942.7	310.7	30.6	27.1	84.4	130.9	148.4	222.2
	F	24356	960	7227	815.6	67.0	773.6	230.6	21.0	22.1	36.8	40.9	49.3	68.4
Tuberculosis	M	47	1	33	2.4	0.1	4.2	–	–	–	–	–	–	0.5
	F	29	–	9	1.0	–	1.0	–	–	–	–	–	–	–
Other infective	M	29	6	14	1.4	0.4	1.6	1.9	0.4	–	0.5	–	–	–
and parasitic	F	26	4	11	1.0	0.3	1.1	1.5	–	0.4	–	–	–	–
ALL CANCER	M	6276	153	4024	315.0	10.3	522.2	8.1	8.7	3.3	8.2	8.9	12.9	21.8
	F	4030	120	2206	148.3	8.4	233.2	3.9	1.8	4.8	4.7	8.7	14.4	20.7
Mouth and	M	436	2	383	22.1	0.1	45.8	–	–	–	–	–	0.5	0.5
pharynx cancer	F	37	3	18	1.2	0.2	1.9	–	–	–	–	–	1.0	0.5
Oesophagus cancer	M	182	1	146	9.1	0.1	18.2	–	–	–	–	–	–	0.5
	F	22	1	11	0.8	0.1	1.2	–	–	–	–	0.5	–	–
Stomach cancer	M	592	5	344	29.9	0.3	45.8	–	–	–	–	–	1.5	0.9
	F	417	3	182	14.8	0.2	19.2	–	–	–	–	–	1.0	0.5
Colorectal cancer	M	694	5	385	35.0	0.3	50.9	–	–	–	–	–	0.5	1.9
	F	584	6	273	20.9	0.4	29.4	–	–	–	0.5	–	0.5	1.9
Liver cancer	M	453	7	278	22.8	0.5	36.5	1.0	–	–	–	0.5	–	1.9
	F	284	5	159	10.4	0.3	17.2	1.0	–	–	–	–	–	1.4
Pancreas cancer	M	268	5	175	13.4	0.3	22.5	–	–	–	–	0.5	1.0	0.9
	F	216	1	119	7.6	0.1	12.9	–	–	–	–	–	0.5	–
Larynx cancer	M	195	1	157	9.7	0.1	19.7	–	–	–	–	–	–	0.5
	F	12	–	8	0.5	–	0.8	–	–	–	–	–	–	–
Lung cancer	M	1930	8	1389	97.9	0.5	183.4	–	–	–	–	–	0.5	3.2
	F	274	1	143	9.9	0.1	15.3	–	–	–	–	–	–	0.5
Malignant melanoma	M	53	5	32	2.6	0.3	3.9	–	–	–	–	0.5	1.0	0.9
	F	38	4	19	1.3	0.3	2.0	–	–	–	–	0.5	–	1.4
Female breast cancer	F	614	12	396	23.5	0.8	41.1	–	–	–	–	0.5	0.5	4.8
Cervix cancer	F	187	13	134	7.3	0.9	13.3	–	–	–	–	–	1.0	5.3
Other uterine cancer	F	212	2	133	7.9	0.1	14.1	–	–	–	–	–	0.5	0.5
Ovarian cancer	F	220	7	165	8.7	0.5	17.4	–	–	0.4	0.5	1.1	1.0	0.5
Prostate cancer	M	343	–	115	17.6	–	16.4	–	–	–	–	–	–	–
Bladder cancer	M	195	–	104	9.8	–	14.3	–		–	–	–	–	–
	F	47	1	20	1.7	0.1	2.1	–	–	–	–	–	–	0.5
Other and ill-defined	M	653	72	382	31.4	4.9	47.9	6.2	3.1	1.6	5.0	5.8	6.9	5.6
cancer sites	F	659	40	325	24.0	2.8	34.7	2.0	1.4	2.6	0.9	4.9	5.7	2.4
Hodgkin's disease	M	20	3	12	0.9	0.2	1.3	–	–	–	–	–	–	1.4
	F	15	1	6	0.6	0.1	0.6	–	–	–	–	–	0.5	–
Myeloma and non-	M	96	13	51	4.7	0.8	6.5	–	1.7	–	1.8	–	1.0	1.4
Hodgkin lymphomas	F	83	3	40	3.0	0.2	4.3	–	–	0.4	0.9	–	–	–
Leukaemia	M	166	26	71	8.0	1.7	8.9	1.0	3.9	1.6	1.4	1.6	–	2.3
	F	109	17	55	4.1	1.2	5.7	1.0	0.5	1.3	1.9	1.1	2.1	0.5
ALL VASCULAR	M	14735	143	6510	753.0	9.7	862.8	1.0	0.9	1.6	5.0	8.9	15.8	34.8
DISEASE	F	14393	58	3237	463.6	4.1	354.1	3.4	0.9	0.4	3.3	4.9	6.2	9.6
Rheumatic heart	M	62	4	49	3.0	0.3	6.0	–	–	0.4	0.5	0.5	–	0.5
disease and fever	F	75	1	55	3.0	0.1	5.9	–	–	–	–	–	–	0.5
Hypertensive disease	M	332	–	184	16.8	–	24.3	–	–	–	–	–	–	–
	F	409	1	133	13.7	0.1	14.7	–	–	–	–	–	–	0.5
Ischaemic heart	M	8212	63	3768	420.1	4.3	499.5	–	–	–	0.5	2.6	6.4	20.4
disease	F	7234	8	1512	231.2	0.6	166.4	–	–	–	–	0.5	1.0	2.4
Pulmonary embolism	M	40	–	27	1.9	–	3.6	–	–	–	–	–	–	–
and other venous	F	43	–	16	1.5	–	1.7	–	–	–	–	–	–	–
Cerebrovascular	M	3112	22	1265	159.5	1.5	168.9	–	–	–	1.8	2.6	2.5	3.7
disease	F	3623	9	863	118.0	0.6	94.3	1.0	–	–	0.9	–	1.0	1.4
Other vascular	M	2977	54	1217	151.7	3.7	160.5	1.0	0.9	1.2	2.3	3.2	6.9	10.2
disease	F	3009	39	658	96.3	2.8	71.1	2.4	0.9	0.4	2.4	4.4	4.1	4.8
Chronic obstructive	M	420	6	171	21.5	0.4	23.1	–	–	0.4	0.5	–	1.0	0.9
pulmonary disease	F	198	2	47	6.5	0.1	5.1	0.5	–	0.4	–	–	–	–
Other respiratory	M	1775	142	587	88.8	9.4	74.7	37.1	4.4	5.3	7.7	2.1	2.5	7.0
disease	F	1586	109	274	50.6	7.6	29.8	35.7	2.3	3.5	0.5	2.2	5.7	3.4
Peptic ulcer	M	119	3	70	5.9	0.2	8.5	0.5	–	–	–	–	–	0.9
	F	66	1	23	2.2	0.1	2.5	0.5	–	–	–	–	–	–
Liver cirrhosis	M	1271	46	1067	61.9	3.1	127.1	0.5	–	–	–	0.5	5.9	14.8
	F	412	14	302	16.5	1.0	31.0	0.5	0.5	–	0.5	–	1.5	3.9
Renal disease	M	436	16	239	21.5	1.1	30.4	1.9	–	–	0.9	–	1.0	3.7
	F	443	16	225	16.2	1.1	24.1	2.0	0.9	0.4	0.9	1.1	1.0	1.4
Pregnancy and birth	F	5	2	3	0.2	0.1	0.2	–	–	–	–	–	0.5	0.5
Congenital and	M	465	465	–	17.7	31.6	–	219.3	1.3	–	–	0.5	–	–
perinatal causes	F	318	318	–	12.3	22.1	–	150.0	2.3	1.7	0.9	–	–	–
Ill-defined causes	M	465	34	125	23.4	2.3	14.7	5.7	–	–	0.9	1.1	3.5	5.1
	F	614	19	55	18.5	1.4	5.5	3.9	–	–	0.9	1.6	2.1	1.0
Other medical causes	M	1321	125	750	63.9	8.3	90.6	10.5	5.7	3.3	5.0	3.7	9.4	20.9
	F	1199	79	483	42.3	5.5	51.1	9.3	3.2	3.9	3.8	4.9	3.6	9.6
ALL NON-	M	2904	863	1650	127.7	59.4	182.8	24.3	9.2	13.1	55.8	105.2	96.4	111.8
MEDICAL CAUSES	F	1037	218	352	36.4	15.2	34.8	19.5	9.1	6.5	21.2	17.4	14.4	18.3
Motor vehicle	M	631	304	278	26.1	21.1	30.2	6.7	4.8	4.9	22.2	51.5	26.7	30.6
traffic accidents	F	203	83	68	7.3	5.8	6.7	2.9	5.5	2.2	12.7	6.0	6.7	4.3
Fire	M	44	6	24	2.0	0.4	2.8	–	–	–	–	2.1	1.0	–
	F	26	4	6	0.9	0.3	0.7	0.5	0.5	–	0.5	0.5	–	–
Suicide	M	648	161	415	28.8	11.1	44.9	–	–	1.2	8.6	14.7	23.7	29.2
	F	153	33	94	5.9	2.3	9.1	–	–	0.9	2.8	4.9	2.1	5.8
Homicide	M	74	27	39	3.1	1.9	4.1	1.9	–	–	0.5	2.6	4.5	3.7
	F	35	11	15	1.3	0.8	1.4	1.0	0.5	–	0.5	–	1.5	1.9
POPULATION (thousands):	M=males				2590.6	1511.4	954.2	210.2	229.0	243.9	220.3	190.2	202.2	215.6
	F=females				2707.4	1452.5	1051.9	204.7	219.4	230.8	212.0	183.4	194.6	207.6

SLOVAKIA: 1990

Annual death rates / 100, 000

9th ICD categories

35–39	40–44	45–49	50–54	55–59	60–64	65–69	70–74	75–79	80+/NK			
344.1	589.8	990.3	1570.2	2183.2	3282.5	4639.1	6289.7	9403.5	16601.6	M	ALL CAUSES	001–999
127.7	198.4	316.2	516.0	828.7	1256.9	2171.6	3497.6	6191.7	13561.6	F		
–	1.7	4.5	6.0	2.6	3.8	10.7	9.2	6.7	16.5	M	Tuberculosis	010–018, 137
–	–	–	0.8	2.2	3.8	–	3.2	7.2	18.2	F		
0.5	0.6	3.0	0.9	1.7	3.8	1.1	6.9	2.2	13.7	M	Other infective	Rest of 001–139
0.5	0.6	2.1	–	1.5	0.8	2.4	4.9	4.3	7.0	F	and parasitic	
49.8	117.6	228.5	458.9	659.7	909.6	1230.9	1441.4	1753.9	1870.9	M	ALL CANCER	140–208
49.0	78.0	118.1	191.3	279.7	388.0	528.3	641.8	879.8	970.6	F		
6.5	24.3	50.9	69.3	61.6	49.0	59.1	48.3	26.6	49.5	M	Mouth and	140–149
0.9	0.6	–	–	2.2	3.0	6.4	1.6	5.7	15.4	F	pharynx cancer	
1.4	7.0	13.5	22.3	24.3	29.2	30.1	23.0	44.3	13.7	M	Oesophagus cancer	150
–	–	–	0.8	1.5	3.8	2.4	–	5.7	8.4	F		
2.3	7.0	13.5	37.7	55.6	80.0	124.6	142.5	215.1	230.8	M	Stomach cancer	151
4.7	6.9	7.6	13.0	22.4	31.3	48.7	84.3	128.8	126.1	F		
5.5	6.4	18.0	41.1	53.0	95.1	137.5	172.4	279.4	283.0	M	Colorectal cancer	153, 154
3.8	5.7	8.3	22.1	40.4	48.8	76.6	110.2	166.0	169.5	F		
4.2	9.3	9.7	29.1	39.9	63.1	99.9	126.4	128.6	151.1	M	Liver cancer	155.0
2.4	1.7	3.5	7.6	20.9	38.9	45.5	58.3	65.8	53.2	F		
2.3	6.4	10.5	23.1	26.9	35.8	52.6	52.9	90.9	65.9	M	Pancreas cancer	157
0.9	2.9	4.2	3.8	12.0	29.7	36.7	24.3	61.5	53.2	F		
1.8	6.4	16.5	20.5	24.3	33.9	34.4	20.7	44.3	22.0	M	Larynx cancer	161
0.5	–	–	3.0	1.5	–	0.8	1.6	–	4.2	F		
5.5	29.0	62.9	152.4	256.9	345.6	431.8	464.4	394.7	420.3	M	Lung cancer	162
2.8	4.0	2.8	10.7	20.9	23.6	42.3	50.2	67.2	72.8	F		
0.9	2.3	0.7	5.1	3.5	9.4	5.4	11.5	11.1	16.5	M	Malignant melanoma	172
0.5	0.6	2.1	1.5	2.2	2.3	4.8	1.6	4.3	15.4	F		
8.0	21.2	41.0	40.4	51.6	60.2	65.4	64.8	118.7	116.2	F	Female breast cancer	174
9.0	10.3	9.7	13.0	14.2	18.3	18.4	21.1	18.6	19.6	F	Cervix cancer	180
3.3	2.9	6.3	9.9	14.2	29.7	32.7	37.3	48.6	28.0	F	Other uterine cancer	179, 182
2.4	7.5	10.4	19.8	21.7	25.2	35.1	25.9	17.2	28.0	F	Ovarian cancer	183
–	–	1.5	3.4	13.9	27.3	68.7	117.2	188.5	252.7	M	Prostate cancer	185
0.5	1.7	3.0	4.3	14.8	25.4	50.5	52.9	66.5	104.4	M	Bladder cancer	188
0.9	1.1	0.7	1.5	3.0	0.8	6.4	13.0	8.6	16.8	F		
13.8	13.9	21.0	33.4	65.1	82.9	105.3	121.8	155.2	208.8	M	Other and ill-defined	Rest of 140–208
4.2	9.2	18.1	35.8	40.4	54.9	80.6	97.2	125.9	204.5	F	cancer sites	
0.9	0.6	2.2	–	1.7	2.8	1.1	–	6.7	5.5	M	Hodgkin's disease	201
0.9	–	0.7		1.5	0.8	–	6.5	4.3	1.4	F		
1.4	0.6	2.2	10.3	6.1	15.1	9.7	27.6	37.7	8.2	M	Myeloma and non-	200, 202–203
0.5	1.7	2.1	2.3	4.5	7.6	11.2	19.4	20.0	19.6	F	Hodgkin lymphomas	
2.8	2.9	2.2	6.8	12.2	15.1	20.4	59.8	64.3	38.5	M	Leukaemia	204–208
3.3	1.7	0.7	6.1	4.5	9.1	14.4	24.3	12.9	18.2	F		
68.3	161.1	330.3	566.8	922.7	1547.1	2443.6	3579.3	5638.6	10939.6	M	ALL VASCULAR	390–459
21.7	45.9	86.9	181.4	333.6	589.2	1220.3	2137.8	4164.5	9619.0	F	DISEASE	
0.5	4.6	1.5	5.1	13.9	5.6	10.7	2.3	6.7	13.7	M	Rheumatic heart	390–398
–	2.3	4.2	6.1	7.5	8.4	12.8	9.7	11.4	7.0	F	disease and fever	
1.4	4.6	12.7	19.7	24.3	38.6	68.7	78.2	130.8	151.1	M	Hypertensive disease	401–405
–	0.6	2.1	9.1	21.7	22.9	46.3	63.2	107.3	225.5	F		
33.2	91.0	188.8	330.5	557.3	927.5	1368.4	2000.0	3022.2	5901.1	M	Ischaemic heart	410–414
5.2	16.1	27.1	62.5	157.1	301.8	595.4	1097.2	2025.8	5071.4	F	disease	
0.5	–	3.0	1.7	4.3	4.7	10.7	2.3	15.5	13.7	M	Pulmonary embolism	415.1, 451–453
–	1.1	–	1.5	0.7	2.3	6.4	11.3	11.4	16.8	F	and other venous	
13.4	30.1	62.9	99.3	161.5	297.6	517.7	857.5	1348.1	2318.7	M	Cerebrovascular	430–438
8.0	10.9	25.0	47.3	87.5	155.5	325.6	604.5	1148.8	2205.9	F	disease	
19.4	30.7	61.4	110.4	161.5	273.1	467.2	639.1	1115.3	2541.2	M	Other vascular	Rest of 390–459
8.5	14.9	28.5	54.9	59.1	98.3	233.8	351.7	859.8	2092.4	F	disease	
0.5	4.1	6.7	10.3	23.4	49.0	67.7	105.7	164.1	337.9	M	Chronic obstructive	490–496
0.5	1.1	2.8	1.5	5.2	8.4	16.0	35.7	44.3	134.5	F	pulmonary disease	
13.4	31.9	30.0	53.9	66.0	145.0	182.6	381.6	747.2	1491.8	M	Other respiratory	Rest of 460–519
2.4	6.3	10.4	16.0	19.4	48.8	105.3	189.6	406.3	1123.2	F	disease	
2.3	4.6	7.5	5.1	7.8	14.1	18.3	25.3	37.7	49.5	M	Peptic ulcer	531–533
0.5	–	–	–	3.7	4.6	8.8	9.7	21.5	29.4	F		
42.9	57.9	107.9	136.1	162.3	212.8	169.7	147.1	115.3	115.4	M	Liver cirrhosis	571
9.9	14.9	27.8	33.5	55.3	33.5	42.3	47.0	32.9	61.6	F		
7.8	8.7	12.7	24.0	39.9	37.7	81.6	75.9	159.6	208.8	M	Renal disease	580–590
2.8	6.3	9.0	15.2	30.7	45.7	59.1	90.8	91.6	114.8	F		
0.9	–	0.7	–	–	–	–	–	–	–	F	Pregnancy and birth	630–676
–	–	–	–	–	–	–	–	–	–	M	Congenital and	740–779
–	–	–	–	–	–	–	–	–	–	F	perinatal causes	
7.4	7.5	12.7	13.7	8.7	27.3	25.8	27.6	117.5	662.1	M	Ill-defined causes	780–799
2.8	4.0	6.3	3.0	2.2	11.4	8.8	37.3	87.3	638.7	F		
31.4	49.2	61.4	82.2	85.1	139.4	185.8	273.6	350.3	464.3	M	Other medical causes	Rest of 001–799
14.6	12.6	20.2	39.6	57.6	82.3	130.9	207.5	280.4	438.4	F		
119.9	144.8	185.0	212.3	203.1	193.0	221.3	216.1	310.4	431.3	M	ALL NON-	E800–E999
22.1	28.7	32.0	33.5	37.4	40.4	49.5	92.4	171.7	406.2	F	MEDICAL CAUSES	
20.3	31.9	22.5	40.2	33.9	35.8	26.9	46.0	39.9	30.2	M	Motor vehicle	E810–E819
5.2	5.7	3.5	6.9	6.7	10.7	8.0	19.4	27.2	29.4	F	traffic accidents	
2.3	1.7	–	2.6	1.7	4.7	6.4	4.6	13.3	16.5	M	Fire	E890–E899
–	–	0.7	0.8	–	0.8	2.4	3.2	8.6	11.2	F		
32.7	35.9	53.9	62.5	56.4	33.0	39.7	29.9	82.0	60.4	M	Suicide	E950–E959
6.6	8.6	10.4	9.1	10.5	8.4	10.4	9.7	11.4	16.8	F		
4.6	4.1	3.7	1.7	3.5	4.7	6.4	4.6	2.2	13.7	M	Homicide	E960–E969
1.9	1.7	–	1.5	1.5	3.0	–	1.6	2.9	8.4	F		
216.8	172.6	133.5	116.8	115.2	106.2	93.1	43.5	45.1	36.4	M	**POPULATION (thousands)**	
212.2	174.4	143.9	131.2	133.7	131.2	125.3	61.7	69.9	71.4	F		

SLOVAKIA: Males

	All ages	0–34	35–69	35–39	40–44	45–49	50–54	55–59	60–64	65–69	70–74	75–79	80+/NK
POPULATION (1000s)													
1955	1815.6	1166.6	585.2	82.1	114.1	114.3	100.0	79.8	54.1	40.8	30.1	19.9	13.8
1965	2163.5	1313.3	769.3	146.5	148.8	83.1	118.0	112.7	92.5	67.7	39.9	23.3	17.7
1975	2334.8	1412.4	805.9	131.1	138.1	138.1	137.3	73.8	100.9	86.6	60.5	35.3	20.7
1985	2531.6	1534.9	854.9	176.3	138.7	123.9	125.8	121.0	112.6	56.6	66.1	44.9	30.8
1990	2590.6	1511.4	954.2	216.8	172.6	133.5	116.8	115.2	106.2	93.1	43.5	45.1	36.4
1995 projected	2620.0	1499.4	985.4	202.7	180.5	160.9	138.8	107.1	104.5	90.9	71.5	27.3	36.4
NUMBER OF DEATHS													
All causes													
1955	16917	4369	6530	194	458	691	1035	1248	1405	1499	1708	1777	2533
1965	18975	2947	8497	391	539	449	981	1488	2123	2526	2280	2113	3138
1975	25023	3008	10920	436	719	1045	1609	1216	2466	3429	3760	3575	3760
1985	28613	2366	12346	554	736	1115	1807	2349	3426	2359	4178	4380	5343
1990	30263	2003	15240	746	1018	1322	1834	2515	3486	4319	2736	4241	6043
1995 projected	31848	1854	16883	764	1175	1750	2417	2561	3787	4429	4517	2494	6100
Lung cancer													
1955	248	8	208	3	13	18	47	50	49	28	21	7	4
1965	759	8	589	11	15	18	65	121	171	188	103	42	17
1975	1174	7	781	14	32	70	120	95	173	277	232	120	34
1985	1749	6	1173	15	48	94	213	240	350	213	275	196	99
1990	1930	8	1389	12	50	84	178	296	367	402	202	178	153
1995 projected	2117	7	1501	9	42	86	222	300	414	428	335	109	165
ANNUAL DEATH RATE / 100,000 (*The rates for the age groups 0–34 and 35–69 are the means of seven five-yearly rates, but the all-ages rates are standardised to the conventional "European" age distribution)													
All causes													
1955	1412.8*	314.3*	1444.6*	236.3	401.4	604.5	1035.0	1563.9	2597.0	3674.0	5674.4	8929.6	18355.1
1965	1307.0*	221.6*	1335.3*	266.9	362.2	540.3	831.4	1320.3	2295.1	3731.2	5714.3	9068.7	17728.8
1975	1435.7*	209.0*	1547.6*	332.6	520.6	756.7	1171.9	1647.7	2444.0	3959.6	6214.9	10127.5	18164.3
1985	1468.8*	152.8*	1761.9*	314.2	530.6	899.9	1436.4	1941.3	3042.6	4167.8	6320.7	9755.0	17347.4
1990	1504.0*	136.3*	1942.7*	344.1	589.8	990.3	1570.2	2183.2	3282.5	4639.1	6289.7	9403.5	16601.6
1995 projected	1560.7*	125.5*	2106.3*	376.9	651.0	1087.6	1741.4	2391.2	3623.9	4872.4	6317.5	9135.5	16758.2
All cancer													
1955	170.9*	9.6*	291.5*	29.2	64.0	123.4	246.0	340.9	573.0	664.2	840.5	799.0	840.6
1965	224.3*	12.2*	349.9*	36.2	67.9	111.9	228.0	374.4	672.4	958.6	1243.1	1412.0	1355.9
1975	259.1*	12.8*	398.8*	51.9	98.5	168.7	292.1	460.7	675.9	1043.9	1330.6	1739.4	1603.9
1985	284.4*	10.9*	464.8*	45.4	114.6	219.5	416.5	527.3	838.4	1091.9	1399.4	1625.8	1577.9
1990	315.0*	10.3*	522.2*	49.8	117.6	228.5	458.9	659.7	909.6	1230.9	1441.4	1753.9	1870.9
1995 projected	341.8*	9.5*	572.5*	50.8	123.5	249.8	526.7	743.2	1021.1	1292.6	1488.1	1798.5	2126.4
Lung cancer													
1955	20.2*	0.8*	42.8*	3.7	11.4	15.7	47.0	62.7	90.6	68.6	69.8	35.2	29.0
1965	47.0*	0.7*	94.9*	7.5	10.1	21.7	55.1	107.4	184.9	277.7	258.1	180.3	96.0
1975	63.0*	0.6*	113.1*	10.7	23.2	50.7	87.4	128.7	171.5	319.9	383.5	339.9	164.3
1985	90.5*	0.4*	167.7*	8.5	34.6	75.9	169.3	198.3	310.8	376.3	416.0	436.5	321.4
1990	97.9*	0.5*	183.4*	5.5	29.0	62.9	152.4	256.9	345.6	431.8	464.4	394.7	420.3
1995 projected	103.7*	0.5*	198.3*	4.4	23.3	53.4	159.9	280.1	396.2	470.8	468.5	399.3	453.3
Upper aerodigestive cancer (mouth, oesophagus, pharynx and larynx)													
1955	14.1*	–	19.3*	2.4	4.4	8.7	14.0	22.6	31.4	51.5	76.4	90.5	144.9
1965	12.7*	0.2*	19.2*	0.7	6.7	9.6	16.1	17.7	29.2	54.7	55.1	107.3	90.4
1975	19.9*	0.4*	30.8*	3.8	12.3	22.4	28.4	52.8	43.6	52.0	82.6	119.0	135.3
1985	29.5*	0.2*	55.6*	7.9	25.2	46.0	78.7	75.2	81.7	74.2	102.9	102.4	84.4
1990	40.9*	0.3*	83.7*	9.7	37.7	80.9	112.2	110.2	112.1	123.5	92.0	115.3	85.2
1995 projected	53.6*	0.3*	113.4*	13.3	52.6	111.2	156.3	153.1	155.0	151.8	104.9	106.2	93.4
Other cancer													
1955	136.6*	8.9*	229.4*	23.1	48.2	98.9	185.0	255.6	451.0	544.1	694.4	673.4	666.7
1965	164.6*	11.3*	235.8*	28.0	51.1	80.6	156.8	249.3	458.4	626.3	929.8	1124.5	1169.5
1975	176.2*	11.7*	254.9*	37.4	63.0	95.6	176.3	279.1	460.9	672.1	864.5	1280.5	1304.3
1985	164.3*	10.3*	241.5*	28.9	54.8	97.7	168.5	253.7	445.8	641.3	880.5	1086.9	1172.1
1990	176.2*	9.5*	255.0*	34.6	51.0	84.6	194.3	292.5	452.0	675.6	885.1	1243.9	1365.4
1995 projected	184.5*	8.7*	260.9*	33.1	47.6	85.1	210.4	310.0	469.9	670.0	914.7	1293.0	1579.7
Chronic obstructive pulmonary disease (COPD)													
1955	38.2*	1.4*	50.1*	4.9	8.8	11.4	39.0	57.6	94.3	134.8	215.9	271.4	376.8
1965	101.5*	0.8*	99.1*	4.8	3.4	8.4	38.1	97.6	203.2	338.3	533.8	1021.5	1565.0
1975	126.3*	0.5*	113.5*	5.3	15.9	29.7	59.7	97.6	177.4	408.8	738.8	1238.0	2014.5
1985	60.8*	0.5*	36.3*	0.6	5.8	8.9	16.7	35.5	70.2	116.6	316.2	643.7	1282.5
1990	21.5*	0.4*	23.1*	0.5	4.1	6.7	10.3	23.4	49.0	67.7	105.7	164.1	337.9
1995 projected	14.8*	0.3*	15.8*	0.5	2.8	4.4	7.2	15.9	33.5	46.2	71.3	109.9	239.0
Other respiratory disease													
1955	90.9*	47.2*	57.8*	7.3	15.8	14.0	23.0	60.2	105.4	178.9	392.0	527.6	1108.7
1965	65.1*	20.4*	36.4*	4.1	6.0	9.6	13.6	23.1	67.0	131.5	238.1	416.3	1299.4
1975	91.5*	26.5*	55.4*	9.2	11.6	22.4	21.8	55.6	90.2	176.7	358.7	787.5	1550.7
1985	114.1*	15.9*	101.8*	15.9	18.0	42.0	75.5	96.7	176.7	288.0	467.5	922.0	1818.2
1990	88.8*	9.4*	74.7*	13.4	31.9	30.0	53.9	66.0	145.0	182.6	381.6	747.2	1491.8
1995 projected	69.9*	6.9*	56.3*	16.3	31.6	24.9	37.5	49.5	100.5	134.2	286.7	608.1	1219.8
Vascular disease													
1955	493.3*	23.3*	552.2*	42.6	93.8	171.5	318.0	561.4	1018.5	1659.3	2697.7	3738.7	6550.7
1965	540.1*	14.0*	491.0*	61.4	100.1	186.5	267.8	447.2	854.1	1519.9	2571.4	4527.9	9598.9
1975	644.8*	10.9*	621.6*	80.9	137.6	244.0	429.0	643.6	1073.3	1742.5	3054.5	5209.6	10961.4
1985	704.8*	8.7*	764.0*	80.5	157.9	297.8	532.6	823.1	1403.2	2053.0	3354.0	5521.2	10652.6
1990	753.0*	9.7*	862.8*	68.3	161.1	330.3	566.8	922.7	1547.1	2443.6	3579.3	5638.6	10939.6
1995 projected	785.5*	9.7*	937.3*	64.6	166.8	344.9	614.6	996.3	1741.6	2632.6	3669.9	5542.1	11214.3
Liver cirrhosis													
1955	8.3*	0.4*	12.4*	2.4	5.3	7.0	15.0	12.5	22.2	22.1	29.9	60.3	58.0
1965	12.1*	0.7*	20.3*	3.4	4.7	26.5	23.7	22.2	21.6	39.9	60.2	51.5	39.5
1975	36.4*	2.4*	66.9*	17.5	47.1	57.2	68.5	78.6	78.3	121.2	99.2	127.5	144.9
1985	44.0*	2.0*	86.1*	26.7	44.0	74.3	88.2	106.6	139.4	123.7	127.1	133.6	97.4
1990	61.9*	3.1*	127.1*	42.9	57.9	107.9	136.1	162.3	212.8	169.7	147.1	115.3	115.4
1995 projected	82.2*	4.2*	174.5*	59.2	81.4	148.5	189.5	225.0	294.7	223.3	159.4	124.5	112.6
Other medical causes													
1955	525.3*	164.0*	383.7*	76.7	119.2	182.0	291.0	426.1	661.7	928.9	1388.7	3402.0	9195.7
1965	257.6*	98.5*	216.3*	39.6	69.9	86.6	150.8	230.7	342.7	593.8	909.8	1420.6	3446.3
1975	153.5*	79.7*	135.8*	46.5	60.1	81.8	122.4	162.6	185.3	292.1	429.8	750.7	1468.6
1985	145.8*	57.2*	152.8*	45.4	63.4	94.4	127.2	175.2	244.2	319.8	444.8	643.7	1490.3
1990	136.1*	44.0*	150.1*	49.4	72.4	101.9	131.8	145.8	226.0	323.3	418.4	674.1	1414.8
1995 projected	126.8*	33.6*	143.6*	54.3	79.2	106.9	123.9	131.7	208.6	300.3	404.2	644.7	1384.6
All non-medical causes													
1955	85.9*	68.2*	97.0*	73.1	94.7	95.4	103.0	105.3	122.0	85.8	109.6	130.7	224.6
1965	106.3*	74.9*	122.3*	117.4	110.2	110.7	109.3	125.1	134.1	149.2	157.9	218.9	423.7
1975	124.0*	76.3*	155.6*	121.3	149.9	152.8	178.4	149.1	163.5	174.4	203.3	274.8	420.3
1985	114.8*	57.6*	156.0*	99.8	126.9	163.0	179.7	176.9	170.5	174.9	211.8	265.0	428.6
1990	127.7*	59.4*	182.8*	119.9	144.8	185.0	212.3	203.1	193.0	221.3	216.1	310.4	431.3
1995 projected	139.8*	61.4*	206.3*	131.2	165.7	208.2	242.1	229.7	223.9	243.1	237.8	307.7	461.5

SLOVAKIA: Females

	All ages	0–34	35–69	35–39	40–44	45–49	50–54	55–59	60–64	65–69	70–74	75–79	80+/NK
POPULATION (1000s)													
1955	1911.0	1160.0	661.5	87.1	124.6	122.3	109.3	94.2	68.1	55.9	40.6	25.5	23.4
1965	2210.0	1277.5	814.4	149.9	154.0	86.1	122.1	117.7	102.1	82.5	55.1	35.0	28.0
1975	2404.6	1365.6	868.6	136.7	143.1	145.5	148.5	80.3	112.3	102.2	79.9	53.2	37.3
1985	2630.3	1473.0	939.4	176.0	145.8	133.9	138.1	138.2	136.5	70.9	89.1	68.9	59.9
1990	**2707.4**	**1452.5**	**1051.9**	**212.2**	**174.4**	**143.9**	**131.2**	**133.7**	**131.2**	**125.3**	**61.7**	**69.9**	**71.4**
1995 projected	*2732.3*	*1441.2*	*1071.9*	*198.2*	*182.4*	*170.2*	*152.7*	*123.5*	*125.7*	*119.2*	*103.3*	*43.6*	*72.3*
NUMBER OF DEATHS													
All causes													
1955	16005	3075	5304	163	357	487	718	875	1162	1542	2045	2190	3391
1965	16935	1850	5610	194	327	278	602	885	1351	1973	2343	2690	4442
1975	20225	1632	6021	178	259	464	760	653	1491	2216	3067	3724	5781
1985	23851	1194	6122	226	281	462	718	1187	1759	1489	3412	4508	8615
1990	**24356**	**960**	**7227**	**271**	**346**	**455**	**677**	**1108**	**1649**	**2721**	**2158**	**4328**	**9683**
1995 projected	*23269*	*829*	*6958*	*262*	*348*	*524*	*760*	*998*	*1582*	*2484*	*3435*	*2529*	*9518*
Lung cancer													
1955	80	3	60	–	5	10	13	10	11	11	10	4	3
1965	144	6	80	1	2	5	11	18	17	26	23	19	16
1975	168	2	95	–	7	5	16	14	27	26	36	18	17
1985	235	5	123	7	9	8	12	26	32	29	40	32	35
1990	**274**	**1**	**143**	**6**	**7**	**4**	**14**	**28**	**31**	**53**	**31**	**47**	**52**
1995 projected	*310*	*1*	*141*	*4*	*5*	*4*	*17*	*27*	*31*	*53*	*61*	*37*	*70*
ANNUAL DEATH RATE / 100,000 (*The rates for the age groups 0–34 and 35–69 are the means of seven five-yearly rates, but the all-ages rates are standardised to the conventional "European" age distribution)													
All causes													
1955	1090.0*	221.7*	988.9*	187.1	286.5	398.2	656.9	928.9	1706.3	2758.5	5036.9	8588.2	14491.5
1965	960.9*	138.8*	803.5*	129.4	212.3	322.9	493.0	751.9	1323.2	2391.5	4252.3	7685.7	15864.3
1975	908.0*	113.8*	778.7*	130.2	181.0	318.9	511.8	813.2	1327.7	2168.3	3838.5	7000.0	15498.7
1985	858.4*	79.2*	776.3*	128.4	192.7	345.0	519.9	858.9	1288.6	2100.1	3829.4	6542.8	14382.3
1990	**815.6***	**67.0***	**773.6***	**127.7**	**198.4**	**316.2**	**516.0**	**828.7**	**1256.9**	**2171.6**	**3497.6**	**6191.7**	**13561.6**
1995 projected	*782.8**	*57.8**	*754.2**	*132.2*	*190.8*	*307.9*	*497.7*	*808.1*	*1258.6*	*2083.9*	*3325.3*	*5800.5*	*13164.6*
All cancer													
1955	130.4*	9.5*	224.3*	41.3	90.7	126.7	199.5	259.0	402.3	450.8	625.6	580.4	474.4
1965	144.4*	10.9*	220.3*	35.4	76.0	126.6	175.3	241.3	346.7	540.6	682.4	885.7	921.4
1975	146.8*	8.9*	222.7*	35.1	59.4	120.3	189.9	286.4	374.0	494.1	688.4	887.2	1002.7
1985	145.5*	9.7*	225.0*	46.6	71.3	135.9	171.6	313.3	372.2	464.0	656.6	807.0	953.3
1990	**148.3***	**8.4***	**233.2***	**49.0**	**78.0**	**118.1**	**191.3**	**279.7**	**388.0**	**528.3**	**641.8**	**879.8**	**970.6**
1995 projected	*149.7**	*7.8**	*234.0**	*51.0*	*74.6*	*118.1*	*180.1*	*272.9*	*400.2*	*541.1*	*667.0*	*883.0*	*1024.9*
Lung cancer													
1955	5.4*	0.3*	10.1*	–	4.0	8.2	11.9	10.6	16.2	19.7	24.6	15.7	12.8
1965	7.9*	0.5*	11.5*	0.7	1.3	5.8	9.0	15.3	16.7	31.5	41.7	54.3	57.1
1975	7.6*	0.1*	12.3*	–	4.9	3.4	10.8	17.4	24.0	25.4	45.1	33.8	45.6
1985	9.3*	0.3*	15.4*	4.0	6.2	6.0	8.7	18.8	23.4	40.9	44.9	46.4	58.4
1990	**9.9***	**0.1***	**15.3***	**2.8**	**4.0**	**2.8**	**10.7**	**20.9**	**23.6**	**42.3**	**50.2**	**67.2**	**72.8**
1995 projected	*11.0**	*0.1**	*15.6**	*2.0*	*2.7*	*2.4*	*11.1*	*21.9*	*24.7*	*44.5*	*59.1*	*84.9*	*96.8*
Upper aerodigestive cancer (mouth, oesophagus, pharynx and larynx)													
1955	2.8*	0.3*	4.1*	1.1	0.8	2.5	3.7	5.3	4.4	10.7	17.2	15.7	17.1
1965	2.6*	0.2*	4.0*	–	3.2	–	2.5	1.7	5.9	14.5	5.4	11.4	39.3
1975	2.3*	–	3.1*	0.7	–	2.1	0.7	7.5	2.7	7.8	8.8	22.6	24.1
1985	2.9*	0.3*	3.0*	–	2.7	1.5	2.9	5.8	5.1	2.8	16.8	20.3	30.1
1990	**2.5***	**0.3***	**3.9***	**1.4**	**0.6**	–	**3.8**	**5.2**	**6.9**	**9.6**	**3.2**	**11.4**	**28.0**
1995 projected	*2.1**	–	*3.9**	*1.0*	*0.5*	–	*3.3*	*5.7*	*9.5*	*7.6*	*1.9*	*6.9*	*22.1*
Other cancer													
1955	122.2*	9.0*	210.2*	40.2	85.9	116.1	183.9	243.1	381.8	420.4	583.7	549.0	444.4
1965	133.8*	10.2*	204.8*	34.7	71.4	120.8	163.8	224.3	324.2	494.5	635.2	820.0	825.0
1975	136.9*	8.8*	207.4*	34.4	54.5	114.8	178.5	261.5	347.3	460.9	634.5	830.8	933.0
1985	133.4*	9.1*	206.6*	42.6	62.4	128.5	160.0	288.7	343.6	420.3	594.8	740.2	864.8
1990	**135.9***	**8.1***	**214.0***	**44.8**	**73.4**	**115.4**	**176.8**	**253.6**	**357.5**	**476.5**	**588.3**	**801.1**	**869.7**
1995 projected	*136.6**	*7.8**	*214.4**	*47.9*	*71.3*	*115.7*	*165.7*	*245.3*	*366.0*	*489.1*	*606.0*	*791.3*	*905.9*
Chronic obstructive pulmonary disease (COPD)													
1955	18.6*	1.6*	18.7*	1.1	3.2	5.7	10.1	15.9	33.8	60.8	133.0	149.0	213.7
1965	49.5*	0.7*	35.3*	1.3	1.9	10.5	9.8	24.6	51.9	146.7	274.0	542.9	921.4
1975	50.0*	0.7*	27.9*	1.5	6.3	9.6	11.4	28.6	52.5	85.1	212.8	428.6	1246.6
1985	21.8*	0.6*	11.7*	1.1	0.7	7.5	10.1	6.5	20.5	35.3	84.2	207.5	532.6
1990	**6.5***	**0.1***	**5.1***	**0.5**	**1.1**	**2.8**	**1.5**	**5.2**	**8.4**	**16.0**	**35.7**	**44.3**	**134.5**
1995 projected	*4.4**	*0.1**	*3.4**	*0.5*	*0.5*	*1.8*	*1.3*	*3.2*	*5.6*	*10.9*	*24.2*	*29.8*	*94.1*
Other respiratory disease													
1955	78.7*	41.7*	48.2*	8.0	12.0	13.9	18.3	39.3	79.3	166.4	369.5	545.1	846.2
1965	54.9*	18.3*	19.8*	4.0	3.2	5.8	13.9	13.6	36.2	61.8	228.7	454.3	1096.4
1975	67.4*	20.3*	30.5*	2.9	6.3	6.9	12.1	21.2	52.5	111.5	249.1	509.4	1410.2
1985	66.4*	9.9*	35.9*	8.5	6.2	6.0	21.0	33.3	52.0	124.1	292.9	593.6	1399.0
1990	**50.6***	**7.6***	**29.8***	**2.4**	**6.3**	**10.4**	**16.0**	**19.4**	**48.8**	**105.3**	**189.6**	**406.3**	**1123.2**
1995 projected	*38.2**	*6.0**	*22.8**	*1.5*	*5.5*	*10.0*	*11.8*	*15.4*	*39.8*	*75.5*	*129.7*	*295.9*	*863.1*
Vascular disease													
1955	440.8*	18.3*	438.9*	45.9	76.2	118.6	230.6	380.0	791.5	1429.3	2820.2	4039.2	5683.8
1965	473.3*	8.1*	336.5*	30.7	59.7	89.4	154.0	295.7	598.4	1127.3	2364.8	4454.3	9657.1
1975	476.0*	3.8*	339.7*	29.3	46.1	97.6	172.4	295.1	610.0	1127.2	2200.3	4434.2	10099.2
1985	476.3*	3.7*	352.5*	25.0	47.3	111.3	184.6	331.4	608.8	1159.4	2313.1	4238.0	9894.8
1990	**463.6***	**4.1***	**354.1***	**21.7**	**45.9**	**86.9**	**181.4**	**333.6**	**589.2**	**1220.3**	**2137.8**	**4164.5**	**9619.0**
1995 projected	*443.6**	*3.5**	*339.8**	*19.7*	*37.3*	*77.0*	*172.2*	*319.0*	*595.9*	*1157.7*	*2021.3*	*3850.9*	*9380.4*
Liver cirrhosis													
1955	3.4*	0.5*	5.9*	–	2.4	3.3	7.3	4.2	5.9	17.9	14.8	11.8	12.8
1965	6.7*	0.4*	11.2*	2.7	2.6	3.5	10.6	11.0	16.7	31.5	29.0	34.3	42.9
1975	11.0*	0.4*	18.2*	5.9	4.2	11.7	23.6	22.4	28.5	31.3	32.5	54.5	75.1
1985	11.2*	0.4*	21.1*	8.0	13.7	12.7	30.4	26.0	30.0	26.8	32.5	29.0	38.4
1990	**16.5***	**1.0***	**31.0***	**9.9**	**14.9**	**27.8**	**33.5**	**55.3**	**33.5**	**42.3**	**47.0**	**32.9**	**61.6**
1995 projected	*22.3**	*1.1**	*42.2**	*12.1*	*20.3*	*35.8*	*47.2*	*76.1*	*46.9*	*57.0*	*62.9*	*45.9*	*85.8*
Other medical causes													
1955	391.0*	133.5*	229.6*	80.4	85.1	108.7	162.9	207.0	364.2	599.3	1007.4	3160.8	7012.8
1965	197.4*	83.7*	149.6*	37.4	47.4	62.7	97.5	141.0	237.0	424.2	606.2	1165.7	2789.3
1975	117.4*	61.2*	101.1*	25.6	34.2	50.2	72.7	114.6	167.4	242.7	361.7	511.3	1254.7
1985	103.8*	42.1*	97.0*	18.2	27.4	46.3	68.1	110.0	169.2	239.8	372.6	502.2	1185.3
1990	**93.7***	**30.6***	**85.6***	**22.1**	**23.5**	**38.2**	**58.7**	**98.0**	**148.6**	**209.9**	**353.3**	**492.1**	**1246.5**
1995 projected	*85.7**	*22.6**	*75.2**	*22.2*	*20.8*	*31.1*	*50.4*	*84.2*	*129.7*	*187.9*	*324.3*	*511.5*	*1284.9*
All non-medical causes													
1955	27.1*	16.5*	23.4*	10.3	16.9	21.3	28.4	23.4	29.4	34.0	66.5	102.0	247.9
1965	34.6*	16.8*	30.9*	18.0	21.4	24.4	31.9	24.6	36.2	59.4	67.2	148.6	435.7
1975	39.2*	18.5*	38.7*	30.0	24.5	22.7	29.6	44.8	42.7	76.3	93.9	174.8	410.2
1985	33.3*	12.9*	33.1*	21.0	26.1	25.4	34.0	38.4	35.9	50.8	77.4	165.5	379.0
1990	**36.4***	**15.2***	**34.8***	**22.1**	**28.7**	**32.0**	**33.5**	**37.4**	**40.4**	**49.5**	**92.4**	**171.7**	**406.2**
1995 projected	*38.8**	*16.8**	*36.8**	*25.2*	*31.8*	*34.1*	*34.7*	*37.2*	*40.6*	*53.7*	*95.8*	*183.5*	*431.5*

SLOVAKIA: 1975

Smoking–attributed deaths (Sm.) and total deaths (Total)

		ALL CAUSES	ALL CANCER	Lung cancer	Upper aero–digestive ca.	Other cancer	COPD	Other respiratory	Vascular disease	Liver cirrhosis	Other medical	Non–medical
Males												
0–34	Sm.	–	–	–	–	–	–	–	–	–	–	–
	Total	3008	173	7	5	161	6	405	131	28	1221	1044
35–69	Sm.	3341	1135	722	142	271	582	104	1215	–	305	–
	Total	10920	2764	781	220	1763	757	374	4289	503	985	1248
		(31%)	(41%)	(92%)	(65%)	(15%)	(77%)	(28%)	(28%)		(31%)	
70+	Sm.	2140	529	342	62	125	862	77	590	–	82	–
	Total	11095	1751	386	120	1245	1301	816	5956	135	829	307
		(19%)	(30%)	(89%)	(52%)	(10%)	(66%)	(9%)	(10%)		(10%)	
Any age	Sm.	5481	1664	1064	204	396	1444	181	1805	–	387	–
	Total	25023	4688	1174	345	3169	2064	1595	10376	666	3035	2599
		(22%)	(35%)	(91%)	(59%)	(12%)	(70%)	(11%)	(17%)		(13%)	
Females												
0–34	Sm.	–	–	–	–	–	–	–	–	–	–	–
	Total	1632	113	2	0	111	10	301	47	5	901	255
35–69	Sm.	160	33	26	1	6	36	5	65	–	21	–
	Total	6021	1745	95	22	1628	211	231	2578	148	793	315
		(3%)	(2%)	(27%)	(5%)	(0%)	(17%)	(2%)	(3%)		(3%)	
70+	Sm.	128	18	14	1	3	47	6	49	–	8	–
	Total	12572	1396	71	28	1297	863	996	7884	83	1029	321
		(1%)	(1%)	(20%)	(4%)	(0%)	(5%)	(1%)	(1%)		(1%)	
Any age	Sm.	288	51	40	2	9	83	11	114	–	29	–
	Total	20225	3254	168	50	3036	1084	1528	10509	236	2723	891
		(1%)	(2%)	(24%)	(4%)	(0%)	(8%)	(1%)	(1%)		(1%)	
Males+Females												
0–34	Sm.	–	–	–	–	–	–	–	–	–	–	–
	Total	4640	286	9	5	272	16	706	178	33	2122	1299
35–69	Sm.	3501	1168	748	143	277	618	109	1280	–	326	–
	Total	16941	4509	876	242	3391	968	605	6867	651	1778	1563
		(21%)	(26%)	(85%)	(59%)	(8%)	(64%)	(18%)	(19%)		(18%)	
70+	Sm.	2268	547	356	63	128	909	83	639	–	90	–
	Total	23667	3147	457	148	2542	2164	1812	13840	218	1858	628
		(10%)	(17%)	(78%)	(43%)	(5%)	(42%)	(5%)	(5%)		(5%)	
Any age	Sm.	5769	1715	1104	206	405	1527	192	1919	–	416	–
	Total	45248	7942	1342	395	6205	3148	3123	20885	902	5758	3490
		(13%)	(22%)	(82%)	(52%)	(7%)	(49%)	(6%)	(9%)		(7%)	

SLOVAKIA: 1985

Smoking–attributed deaths (Sm.) and total deaths (Total)

		ALL CAUSES	ALL CANCER	Lung cancer	Upper aero–digestive ca.	Other cancer	COPD	Other respiratory	Vascular disease	Liver cirrhosis	Other medical	Non–medical
Males												
0–34	Sm.	–	–	–	–	–	–	–	–	–	–	–
	Total	2366	166	6	3	157	8	252	131	30	911	868
35–69	Sm.	4813	1815	1116	326	373	192	271	2060	–	475	–
	Total	12346	3235	1173	430	1632	229	679	5138	667	1113	1285
		(39%)	(56%)	(95%)	(76%)	(23%)	(84%)	(40%)	(40%)		(43%)	
70+	Sm.	2558	764	514	80	170	629	141	905	–	119	–
	Total	13901	2141	570	140	1431	893	1283	7977	174	1042	391
		(18%)	(36%)	(90%)	(57%)	(12%)	(70%)	(11%)	(11%)		(11%)	
Any age	Sm.	7371	2579	1630	406	543	821	412	2965	–	594	–
	Total	28613	5542	1749	573	3220	1130	2214	13246	871	3066	2544
		(26%)	(47%)	(93%)	(71%)	(17%)	(73%)	(19%)	(22%)		(19%)	
Females												
0–34	Sm.	–	–	–	–	–	–	–	–	–	–	–
	Total	1194	143	5	4	134	9	150	53	6	644	189
35–69	Sm.	259	63	50	4	9	26	12	121	–	37	–
	Total	6122	1875	123	27	1725	89	266	2628	189	781	294
		(4%)	(3%)	(41%)	(15%)	(1%)	(29%)	(5%)	(5%)		(5%)	
70+	Sm.	269	41	32	4	5	90	14	109	–	15	–
	Total	16535	1712	107	47	1558	537	1508	10908	72	1388	410
		(2%)	(2%)	(30%)	(9%)	(0%)	(17%)	(1%)	(1%)		(1%)	
Any age	Sm.	528	104	82	8	14	116	26	230	–	52	–
	Total	23851	3730	235	78	3417	635	1924	13589	267	2813	893
		(2%)	(3%)	(35%)	(10%)	(0%)	(18%)	(1%)	(2%)		(2%)	
Males+Females												
0–34	Sm.	–	–	–	–	–	–	–	–	–	–	–
	Total	3560	309	11	7	291	17	402	184	36	1555	1057
35–69	Sm.	5072	1878	1166	330	382	218	283	2181	–	512	–
	Total	18468	5110	1296	457	3357	318	945	7766	856	1894	1579
		(27%)	(37%)	(90%)	(72%)	(11%)	(69%)	(30%)	(28%)		(27%)	
70+	Sm.	2827	805	546	84	175	719	155	1014	–	134	–
	Total	30436	3853	677	187	2989	1430	2791	18885	246	2430	801
		(9%)	(21%)	(81%)	(45%)	(6%)	(50%)	(6%)	(5%)		(6%)	
Any age	Sm.	7899	2683	1712	414	557	937	438	3195	–	646	–
	Total	52464	9272	1984	651	6637	1765	4138	26835	1138	5879	3437
		(15%)	(29%)	(86%)	(64%)	(8%)	(53%)	(11%)	(12%)		(11%)	

(To be conservative, no deaths before age 35, and none from liver cirrhosis or non-medical causes, were attributed to smoking.)

SLOVAKIA: 1990

Smoking-attributed deaths (Sm.) and total deaths (Total)

		ALL CAUSES	ALL CANCER	Lung cancer	Upper aero-digestive ca.	Other cancer	COPD	Other respiratory	Vascular disease	Liver cirrhosis	Other medical	Non-medical
Males												
0–34	Sm.	–	–	–	–	–	–	–	–	–	–	–
	Total	2003	153	8	4	141	6	142	143	46	650	863
35–69	Sm.	5833	2316	1326	526	464	145	243	2597	–	532	–
	Total	15240	4024	1389	686	1949	171	587	6510	1067	1231	1650
		(38%)	(58%)	(95%)	(77%)	(24%)	(85%)	(41%)	(40%)		(43%)	
70+	Sm.	1900	706	477	68	161	167	102	825	–	100	–
	Total	13020	2099	533	123	1443	243	1046	8082	158	1001	391
		(15%)	(34%)	(89%)	(55%)	(11%)	(69%)	(10%)	(10%)		(10%)	
Any age	Sm.	7733	3022	1803	594	625	312	345	3422	–	632	–
	Total	30263	6276	1930	813	3533	420	1775	14735	1271	2882	2904
		(26%)	(48%)	(93%)	(73%)	(18%)	(74%)	(19%)	(23%)		(22%)	
Females												
0–34	Sm.	–	–	–	–	–	–	–	–	–	–	–
	Total	960	120	1	4	115	2	109	58	14	439	218
35–69	Sm.	291	73	57	5	11	15	13	153	–	37	–
	Total	7227	2206	143	37	2026	47	274	3237	302	809	352
		(4%)	(3%)	(40%)	(14%)	(1%)	(32%)	(5%)	(5%)		(5%)	
70+	Sm.	399	79	61	6	12	51	23	217	–	29	–
	Total	16169	1704	130	30	1544	149	1203	11098	96	1452	467
		(2%)	(5%)	(47%)	(20%)	(1%)	(34%)	(2%)	(2%)		(2%)	
Any age	Sm.	690	152	118	11	23	66	36	370	–	66	–
	Total	24356	4030	274	71	3685	198	1586	14393	412	2700	1037
		(3%)	(4%)	(43%)	(15%)	(1%)	(33%)	(2%)	(3%)		(2%)	
Males+Females												
0–34	Sm.	–	–	–	–	–	–	–	–	–	–	–
	Total	2963	273	9	8	256	8	251	201	60	1089	1081
35–69	Sm.	6124	2389	1383	531	475	160	256	2750	–	569	–
	Total	22467	6230	1532	723	3975	218	861	9747	1369	2040	2002
		(27%)	(38%)	(90%)	(73%)	(12%)	(73%)	(30%)	(28%)		(28%)	
70+	Sm.	2299	785	538	74	173	218	125	1042	–	129	–
	Total	29189	3803	663	153	2987	392	2249	19180	254	2453	858
		(8%)	(21%)	(81%)	(48%)	(6%)	(56%)	(6%)	(5%)		(5%)	
Any age	Sm.	8423	3174	1921	605	648	378	381	3792	–	698	–
	Total	54619	10306	2204	884	7218	618	3361	29128	1683	5582	3941
		(15%)	(31%)	(87%)	(68%)	(9%)	(61%)	(11%)	(13%)		(13%)	

SLOVAKIA: 1995

Smoking-attributed deaths (Sm.) and total deaths (Total)

		ALL CAUSES	ALL CANCER	Lung cancer	Upper aero-digestive ca.	Other cancer	COPD	Other respiratory	Vascular disease	Liver cirrhosis	Other medical	Non-medical
Males												
0–34	Sm.	–	–	–	–	–	–	–	–	–	–	–
	Total	1854	140	7	4	129	4	104	141	59	498	908
35–69	Sm.	6559	2712	1439	764	509	101	202	2987	–	557	–
	Total	16883	4497	1501	982	2014	117	462	7120	1521	1229	1937
		(39%)	(60%)	(96%)	(78%)	(25%)	(86%)	(44%)	(42%)		(45%)	
70+	Sm.	2114	821	551	81	189	118	89	974	–	112	–
	Total	13111	2329	609	138	1582	168	815	8219	189	969	422
		(16%)	(35%)	(90%)	(59%)	(12%)	(70%)	(11%)	(12%)		(12%)	
Any age	Sm.	8673	3533	1990	845	698	219	291	3961	–	669	–
	Total	31848	6966	2117	1124	3725	289	1381	15480	1769	2696	3267
		(27%)	(51%)	(94%)	(75%)	(19%)	(76%)	(21%)	(26%)		(25%)	
Females												
0–34	Sm.	–	–	–	–	–	–	–	–	–	–	–
	Total	829	110	1	0	109	1	85	49	15	325	244
35–69	Sm.	277	76	58	6	12	9	10	150	–	32	–
	Total	6958	2198	141	36	2021	31	207	3024	415	703	380
		(4%)	(3%)	(41%)	(17%)	(1%)	(29%)	(5%)	(5%)		(5%)	
70+	Sm.	568	120	96	6	18	46	27	328	–	47	–
	Total	15482	1815	168	21	1626	106	887	10549	147	1487	491
		(4%)	(7%)	(57%)	(29%)	(1%)	(43%)	(3%)	(3%)		(3%)	
Any age	Sm.	845	196	154	12	30	55	37	478	–	79	–
	Total	23269	4123	310	57	3756	138	1179	13622	577	2515	1115
		(4%)	(5%)	(50%)	(21%)	(1%)	(40%)	(3%)	(4%)		(3%)	
Males+Females												
0–34	Sm.	–	–	–	–	–	–	–	–	–	–	–
	Total	2683	250	8	4	238	5	189	190	74	823	1152
35–69	Sm.	6836	2788	1497	770	521	110	212	3137	–	589	–
	Total	23841	6695	1642	1018	4035	148	669	10144	1936	1932	2317
		(29%)	(42%)	(91%)	(76%)	(13%)	(74%)	(32%)	(31%)		(30%)	
70+	Sm.	2682	941	647	87	207	164	116	1302	–	159	–
	Total	28593	4144	777	159	3208	274	1702	18768	336	2456	913
		(9%)	(23%)	(83%)	(55%)	(6%)	(60%)	(7%)	(7%)		(6%)	
Any age	Sm.	9518	3729	2144	857	728	274	328	4439	–	748	–
	Total	55117	11089	2427	1181	7481	427	2560	29102	2346	5211	4382
		(17%)	(34%)	(88%)	(73%)	(10%)	(64%)	(13%)	(15%)		(14%)	

(To be conservative, no deaths before age 35, and none from liver cirrhosis or non-medical causes, were attributed to smoking.)

¶SLOVENIA: 1990

		No. of deaths			Standardised rates (Defined on p.484)			Annual death rates / 100, 000						
		All ages	**0–34**	**35–69**	**All ages**	**0–34**	**35–69**	**0–4**	**5–9**	**10–14**	**15–19**	**20–24**	**25–29**	**30–34**
ALL CAUSES	**M**	9517	588	4542	1232.5	115.2	1422.4	226.0	31.2	29.4	77.5	138.6	135.2	168.7
	F	9038	248	2287	682.1	51.7	573.7	147.0	22.4	14.9	32.2	48.8	38.1	58.6
Tuberculosis	**M**	36	2	25	4.2	0.4	6.5	–	–	–	–	–	–	2.5
	F	14	–	3	1.0	–	0.8	–	–	–	–	–	–	–
Other infective	**M**	31	8	8	4.2	1.7	2.1	8.0	1.4	–	–	–	–	2.5
and parasitic	**F**	30	4	9	2.5	0.9	2.2	5.1	–	1.4	–	–	–	–
ALL CANCER	**M**	2271	43	1436	291.1	7.9	460.1	–	7.1	5.1	4.0	6.8	6.4	26.1
	F	1817	36	889	151.3	6.8	221.9	3.4	1.5	2.7	1.4	5.4	7.6	25.5
Mouth and	**M**	128	1	106	15.3	0.2	29.7	–	–	–	–	–	–	1.2
pharynx cancer	**F**	15	–	6	1.2	–	1.5	–	–	–	–	–	–	–
Oesophagus cancer	**M**	63	–	46	7.6	–	13.4	–	–	–	–	–	–	–
	F	15	–	8	1.4	–	2.0	–	–	–	–	–	–	–
Stomach cancer	**M**	279	2	175	36.9	0.4	58.5	–	–	–	–	1.4	1.3	–
	F	167	–	58	12.8	–	14.6	–	–	–	–	–	–	–
Colorectal cancer	**M**	241	1	123	31.7	0.2	40.6	–	–	–	–	–	–	1.2
	F	247	1	94	19.5	0.2	23.9	–	–	–	–	–	–	1.3
Liver cancer	**M**	33	1	21	4.2	0.2	6.5	–	1.4	–	–	–	–	–
	F	27	1	13	2.4	0.2	3.3	–	–	–	–	–	–	1.3
Pancreas cancer	**M**	91	–	46	12.3	–	15.0	–	–	–	–	–	–	–
	F	96	–	47	8.1	–	11.7	–	–	–	–	–	–	–
Larynx cancer	**M**	67	–	51	8.3	–	16.3	–	–	–	–	–	–	–
	F	3	–	2	0.2	–	0.5	–	–	–	–	–	–	–
Lung cancer	**M**	714	6	542	89.8	1.1	173.8	–	–	–	1.3	–	–	6.2
	F	139	–	86	12.1	–	21.7	–	–	–	–	–	–	–
Malignant melanoma	**M**	34	5	19	4.1	0.9	5.6	–	–	–	–	1.4	1.3	3.7
	F	32	3	15	2.6	0.5	3.6	–	–	–	–	–	–	3.8
Female breast cancer	**F**	326	3	206	28.7	0.5	50.8	–	–	–	–	–	2.5	1.3
Cervix cancer	**F**	51	5	32	4.8	0.9	7.7	–	–	–	–	–	1.3	5.1
Other uterine cancer	**F**	98	1	42	8.0	0.2	10.5	–	–	–	–	–	–	1.3
Ovarian cancer	**F**	119	2	77	10.7	0.4	19.0	–	–	–	–	–	1.3	1.3
Prostate cancer	**M**	158	–	45	22.0	–	17.4	–	–	–	–	–	–	–
Bladder cancer	**M**	68	–	32	9.5	–	11.9	–	–	–	–	–	–	–
	F	31	–	11	2.5	–	2.8	–	–	–	–	–	–	–
Other and ill–defined	**M**	280	17	163	34.7	3.1	49.1	–	2.8	1.3	2.7	4.1	–	11.2
cancer sites	**F**	341	9	147	27.4	1.7	37.1	–	1.5	1.4	–	4.1	–	5.1
Hodgkin's disease	**M**	3	1	–	0.4	0.2	–	–	–	–	–	–	1.3	–
	F	10	–	4	0.7	–	1.1	–	–	–	–	–	–	–
Myeloma and non–	**M**	54	2	35	7.1	0.4	11.4	–	1.4	1.3	–	–	–	–
Hodgkin lymphomas	**F**	50	3	22	3.8	0.6	5.9	–	–	–	1.4	–	1.3	1.3
Leukaemia	**M**	58	7	32	7.1	1.3	10.9	–	1.4	2.6	–	–	2.6	2.5
	F	50	8	19	4.4	1.6	4.4	3.4	–	1.4	–	1.4	1.3	3.8
ALL VASCULAR	**M**	3875	28	1434	526.1	5.3	480.7	8.0	–	2.6	1.3	4.1	5.1	16.1
DISEASE	**F**	4921	13	717	347.5	2.5	183.9	3.4	–	1.4	–	2.7	3.8	6.4
Rheumatic heart	**M**	22	1	14	2.7	0.2	4.0	–	–	–	–	–	–	1.2
disease and fever	**F**	38	–	14	3.0	–	3.6	–	–	–	–	–	–	–
Hypertensive disease	**M**	132	–	52	18.1	–	19.2	–	–	–	–	–	–	–
	F	247	–	51	17.8	–	13.2	–	–	–	–	–	–	–
Ischaemic heart	**M**	1179	6	563	156.2	1.1	180.5	–	–	–	–	–	2.6	5.0
disease	**F**	1253	–	208	88.8	–	53.2	–	–	–	–	–	–	–
Pulmonary embolism	**M**	46	–	19	6.1	–	6.1	–	–	–	–	–	–	–
and other venous	**F**	72	–	15	5.3	–	3.9	–	–	–	–	–	–	–
Cerebrovascular	**M**	1129	8	395	154.9	1.5	139.3	1.6	–	1.3	1.3	2.7	–	3.7
disease	**F**	1418	6	236	102.5	1.1	60.3	–	–	–	–	2.7	–	5.1
Other vascular	**M**	1367	13	391	188.0	2.5	131.6	6.4	–	1.3	–	1.4	2.6	6.2
disease	**F**	1893	7	193	130.1	1.4	49.7	3.4	–	1.4	–	–	3.8	1.3
Chronic obstructive	**M**	478	2	145	65.5	0.4	51.5	1.6	–	1.3	–	–	–	–
pulmonary disease	**F**	197	3	41	14.3	0.6	10.3	–	–	–	1.4	–	–	2.5
Other respiratory	**M**	239	10	67	32.4	2.0	20.9	8.0	–	–	–	1.4	–	5.0
disease	**F**	251	2	30	17.5	0.4	8.0	1.7	–	–	1.4	–	–	–
Peptic ulcer	**M**	58	–	28	7.8	–	8.8	–	–	–	–	–	–	–
	F	47	–	10	3.4	–	2.5	–	–	–	–	–	–	–
Liver cirrhosis	**M**	434	4	371	51.8	0.7	106.7	–	–	–	–	–	3.8	1.2
	F	212	3	165	19.8	0.5	40.8	–	–	–	–	–	–	3.8
Renal disease	**M**	93	3	27	12.8	0.6	9.5	1.6	–	–	–	–	1.3	1.2
	F	103	1	30	7.9	0.2	7.4	–	–	–	–	1.4	–	–
Pregnancy and birth	**F**	2	2	–	0.2	0.4	–	–	–	–	1.4	1.4	–	–
Congenital and	**M**	99	93	6	12.4	21.1	1.6	141.0	2.8	–	1.3	–	1.3	1.2
perinatal causes	**F**	73	69	3	9.3	16.3	0.7	101.4	4.5	4.1	–	1.4	1.3	1.3
Ill–defined causes	**M**	178	31	80	21.7	6.4	20.5	25.6	1.4	1.3	2.7	2.7	5.1	6.2
	F	249	10	36	17.4	2.2	8.7	8.4	–	–	–	4.1	2.5	–
Other medical causes	**M**	513	32	243	66.3	6.1	74.0	4.8	4.3	2.6	10.7	6.8	2.6	11.2
	F	604	16	159	45.8	3.2	40.2	5.1	–	–	2.8	5.4	5.1	3.8
ALL NON–	**M**	1212	332	672	136.2	62.5	179.5	27.2	14.2	16.6	57.5	116.8	109.7	95.5
MEDICAL CAUSES	**F**	518	89	195	44.4	17.8	46.2	18.6	16.4	5.4	23.8	27.1	17.8	15.3
Motor vehicle	**M**	327	153	148	34.1	28.9	38.7	8.0	9.9	10.2	34.8	62.5	38.3	38.5
traffic accidents	**F**	115	46	44	10.7	9.1	10.3	3.4	11.9	1.4	16.8	12.2	11.4	6.4
Fire	**M**	7	1	4	0.8	0.2	1.4	–	–	–	–	1.4	–	–
	F	5	1	1	0.4	0.2	0.2	1.7	–	–	–	–	–	–
Suicide	**M**	423	96	276	46.5	17.7	70.9	–	–	1.3	9.4	28.5	49.7	34.7
	F	130	17	81	12.1	3.2	18.9	–	–	1.4	4.2	6.8	5.1	5.1
Homicide	**M**	30	15	15	3.1	2.9	4.1	6.4	–	–	–	2.7	3.8	7.4
	F	11	5	5	1.0	1.0	1.2	–	–	–	1.4	2.7	1.3	1.3
POPULATION (thousands):	**M=males**				970.3	518.5	406.7	62.4	70.5	78.2	74.8	73.6	78.4	80.6
	F=females				1029.7	502.5	437.3	59.2	67.1	73.7	71.5	73.8	78.7	78.5

SLOVENIA: 1990

Annual death rates / 100, 000

9th ICD categories

35–39	40–44	45–49	50–54	55–59	60–64	65–69	70–74	75–79	80+/NK			
222.2	346.3	676.2	1006.8	1855.3	2342.9	3506.7	5105.3	9263.8	15448.5	M	ALL CAUSES	001–999
96.9	153.2	256.5	405.5	610.0	929.7	1564.0	2833.3	5659.0	12382.7	F		
1.2	5.4	10.1	5.1	14.8	2.2	6.7	6.6	24.5	29.4	M	Tuberculosis	010–018, 137
–	–	–	–	1.7	–	3.9	–	26.2	9.3	F		
–	2.7	1.7	–	5.6	4.4	–	32.9	6.1	66.2	M	Other infective and parasitic	Rest of 001–139
1.2	–	–	3.4	5.0	1.7	3.9	3.7	16.4	34.0	F		
35.1	69.8	161.9	336.8	634.5	831.9	1151.0	1348.7	1901.8	2036.8	M	ALL CANCER	140–208
31.1	70.9	123.1	170.4	248.3	368.8	540.7	681.5	983.6	1259.3	F		
2.3	8.1	11.8	47.9	53.8	57.5	26.8	46.1	67.5	22.1	M	Mouth and pharynx cancer	140–149
–	–	3.5	–	1.7	5.1	–	3.7	13.1	12.3	F		
2.3	5.4	8.4	10.3	20.4	26.5	20.1	19.7	55.2	36.8	M	Oesophagus cancer	150
–	1.4	–	3.4	3.3	1.7	3.9	11.1	6.6	6.2	F		
–	4.0	16.9	37.6	81.6	101.8	167.8	230.3	202.5	250.0	M	Stomach cancer	151
5.0	4.3	6.9	6.8	8.3	22.3	48.4	59.3	118.0	175.9	F		
2.3	14.8	11.8	30.8	35.3	61.9	127.5	151.3	312.9	316.2	M	Colorectal cancer	153, 154
1.2	4.3	8.7	17.0	20.0	48.0	67.8	100.0	157.4	237.7	F		
–	–	6.7	6.8	7.4	11.1	13.4	13.2	24.5	36.8	M	Liver cancer	155.0
–	–	–	3.4	5.0	8.6	5.8	18.5	13.1	12.3	F		
1.2	1.3	3.4	12.0	22.3	24.3	40.3	98.7	116.6	80.9	M	Pancreas cancer	157
2.5	–	1.7	6.8	21.7	22.3	27.1	59.3	39.3	64.8	F		
2.3	1.3	5.1	12.0	29.7	19.9	43.6	19.7	36.8	51.5	M	Larynx cancer	161
–	–	–	–	–	3.4	–	–	3.3	–	F		
4.7	16.1	55.6	109.4	269.0	369.5	392.6	414.5	404.9	272.1	M	Lung cancer	162
1.2	2.8	12.1	25.6	21.7	34.3	54.3	48.1	68.9	58.6	F		
5.8	1.3	3.4	3.4	3.7	4.4	16.8	19.7	24.5	22.1	M	Malignant melanoma	172
1.2	2.8	1.7	3.4	–	8.6	7.8	7.4	13.1	24.7	F		
3.7	28.4	45.1	40.9	71.7	66.9	98.8	92.6	114.8	175.9	F	Female breast cancer	174
1.2	8.5	6.9	5.1	6.7	15.4	9.7	25.9	9.8	12.3	F	Cervix cancer	180
1.2	2.8	5.2	6.8	13.3	18.9	25.2	40.7	88.5	52.5	F	Other uterine cancer	179, 182
5.0	5.7	12.1	17.0	26.7	27.4	38.8	55.6	36.1	43.2	F	Ovarian cancer	183
1.2	1.3	–	5.1	7.4	26.5	80.5	111.8	263.8	389.7	M	Prostate cancer	185
1.2	–	3.4	6.8	7.4	11.1	53.7	65.8	61.3	117.6	M	Bladder cancer	188
1.2	–	–	–	5.0	3.4	9.7	18.5	29.5	18.5	F		
9.4	14.8	21.9	46.2	74.2	73.0	104.0	85.5	239.3	352.9	M	Other and ill-defined cancer sites	Rest of 140–208
3.7	5.7	12.1	27.3	41.7	68.6	100.8	111.1	219.7	271.6	F		
–	–	–	–	–	–	–	6.6	6.1	–	M	Hodgkin's disease	201
–	–	–	–	–	1.7	5.8	3.7	6.6	9.3	F		
1.2	1.3	3.4	6.8	14.8	22.1	30.2	52.6	30.7	29.4	M	Myeloma and non-Hodgkin lymphomas	200, 202–203
1.2	–	–	1.7		3.4	34.9	11.1	29.5	40.1	F		
1.2	–	10.1	1.7	7.4	22.1	33.6	13.2	55.2	58.8	M	Leukaemia	204–208
2.5	4.3	6.9	5.1	1.7	8.6	1.9	14.8	16.4	43.2	F		
36.3	72.5	156.8	254.7	534.3	847.3	1463.1	2381.6	4797.5	9330.9	M	ALL VASCULAR DISEASE	390–459
17.4	27.0	39.9	86.9	150.0	317.3	649.2	1551.9	3426.2	8416.7	F		
–	1.3	5.1	3.4	3.7	11.1	3.4	13.2	18.4	14.7	M	Rheumatic heart disease and fever	390–398
–	–	1.7	1.7	–	12.0	9.7	22.2	32.8	24.7	F		
–	4.0	–	13.7	13.0	19.9	83.9	98.7	190.2	250.0	M	Hypertensive disease	401–405
–	2.8	–	3.4	10.0	25.7	50.4	85.2	186.9	358.0	F		
15.2	34.9	64.1	114.5	246.8	331.9	456.4	671.1	1220.9	2272.1	M	Ischaemic heart disease	410–414
5.0	4.3	3.5	22.1	50.0	113.2	174.4	388.9	914.8	2040.1	F		
1.2	–	3.4	1.7	11.1	8.8	16.8	26.3	67.5	88.2	M	Pulmonary embolism and other venous	415.1, 451–453
–	–		3.4	6.7	–	17.4	25.9	45.9	111.1	F		
7.0	9.4	40.5	68.4	120.6	232.3	496.6	835.5	1644.2	2433.8	M	Cerebrovascular disease	430–438
6.2	11.3	15.6	37.5	43.3	102.9	205.4	537.0	1065.6	2179.0	F		
12.9	22.8	43.8	53.0	139.1	243.4	406.0	736.8	1656.4	4272.1	M	Other vascular disease	Rest of 390–459
6.2	8.5	19.1	18.7	40.0	63.5	191.9	492.6	1180.3	3703.7	F		
2.3	2.7	5.1	34.2	46.4	81.9	187.9	309.2	816.0	1110.3	M	Chronic obstructive pulmonary disease	490–496
5.0	–	3.5	1.7	11.7	17.2	32.9	63.0	144.3	284.0	F		
3.5	1.3	8.4	22.2	29.7	31.0	50.3	131.6	349.7	625.0	M	Other respiratory disease	Rest of 460–519
–	–	–	5.1	3.3	6.9	40.7	74.1	173.8	450.6	F		
2.3	2.7	1.7	5.1	13.0	13.3	23.5	46.1	55.2	102.9	M	Peptic ulcer	531–533
–	2.8	1.7		3.3	1.7	7.8	7.4	52.5	58.6	F		
23.4	28.2	67.5	104.3	204.1	154.9	164.4	157.9	153.4	73.5	M	Liver cirrhosis	571
5.0	7.1	29.5	40.9	61.7	72.0	69.8	70.4	26.2	52.5	F		
–	4.0	6.7	–	13.0	2.2	40.3	72.4	141.1	213.2	M	Renal disease	580–590
1.2	1.4	5.2	3.4	13.3	13.7	13.6	29.6	88.5	114.2	F		
–	–	–	–	–	–	–	–	–	–	F	Pregnancy and birth	630–676
1.2	2.7	–	–	1.9	2.2	3.4	–	–	–	M	Congenital and perinatal causes	740–779
–	–	–	–	3.3	1.7	–	–	3.3	–	F		
9.4	17.4	21.9	22.2	31.5	24.3	16.8	13.2	98.2	360.3	M	Ill-defined causes	780–799
2.5	7.1	–	13.6	11.7	10.3	15.5	14.8	65.6	552.5	F		
21.1	24.2	42.2	44.4	102.0	106.2	177.9	322.4	496.9	794.1	M	Other medical causes	Rest of 001–799
2.5	9.9	13.9	23.9	55.0	58.3	118.2	203.7	439.3	740.7	F		
86.5	112.8	192.2	177.8	224.5	241.2	221.5	282.9	423.3	705.9	M	ALL NON-MEDICAL CAUSES	E800–E999
31.1	27.0	39.9	56.2	41.7	60.0	67.8	133.3	213.1	410.5	F		
29.2	21.5	37.1	32.5	46.4	64.2	40.3	39.5	67.5	66.2	M	Motor vehicle traffic accidents	E810–E819
9.9	5.7	12.1	6.8	5.0	18.9	13.6	33.3	29.5	21.6	F		
–	–	–	–	1.9	4.4	3.4	–	6.1	7.4	M	Fire	E890–E899
1.2								9.8		F		
35.1	61.7	97.8	66.7	81.6	86.3	67.1	85.5	116.6	139.7	M	Suicide	E950–E959
14.9	12.8	15.6	25.6	21.7	22.3	19.4	33.3	49.2	24.7	F		
4.7	2.7	–	1.7	9.3	–	10.1	–	–	–	M	Homicide	E960–E969
1.2	1.4	–	–	–	1.7	3.9	–	3.3	–	F		
85.5	74.5	59.3	58.5	53.9	45.2	29.8	15.2	16.3	13.6	M	POPULATION (thousands)	
80.5	70.5	57.7	58.7	60.0	58.3	51.6	27.0	30.5	32.4	F		

SLOVENIA: Males

	All ages	0–34	35–69	35–39	40–44	45–49	50–54	55–59	60–64	65–69	70–74	75–79	80+/NK
POPULATION (1000s)													
1955	...	...	...	...	...	...	...	...	...	...	...	...	...
1965	789.4	482.6	276.3	58.7	44.4	26.8	42.9	42.3	36.3	24.9	14.8	9.1	6.6
1975	861.5	502.1	317.5	63.9	63.9	55.7	41.3	24.2	36.3	32.2	22.8	12.2	6.9
1985	958.4	539.8	366.2	77.1	62.1	62.5	59.0	51.0	35.2	19.3	23.7	17.2	11.5
1990	**970.3**	**518.5**	**406.7**	**85.5**	**74.5**	**59.3**	**58.5**	**53.9**	**45.2**	**29.8**	**15.2**	**16.3**	**13.6**
1995 projected	*943.7*	*482.8*	*412.6*	*78.9*	*80.1*	*60.9*	*56.3*	*52.2*	*48.2*	*36.0*	*22.9*	*10.1*	*15.3*
NUMBER OF DEATHS													
All causes													
1955	...	...	...	...	...	...	...	...	...	...	...	...	...
1965	8488	1460	3751	233	260	174	445	668	934	1037	968	1034	1275
1975	9651	971	4297	233	353	446	478	443	976	1368	1561	1328	1494
1985	10228	839	4345	204	282	477	735	960	955	732	1407	1658	1979
1990	**9517**	**588**	**4542**	**190**	**258**	**401**	**589**	**1000**	**1059**	**1045**	**776**	**1510**	**2101**
1995 projected	*8728*	*415*	*4240*	*139*	*233*	*339*	*516*	*864*	*1037*	*1112*	*1079*	*835*	*2159*
Lung cancer													
1955	...	...	...	...	...	...	...	...	...	...	...	...	...
1965	...	...	...	...	...	...	...	...	...	...	...	...	...
1975	495	1	315	2	16	33	37	38	74	115	103	59	17
1985	619	2	405	4	17	27	84	108	91	74	84	90	38
1990	**714**	**6**	**542**	**4**	**12**	**33**	**64**	**145**	**167**	**117**	**63**	**66**	**37**
1995 projected	*812*	*6*	*647*	*3*	*13*	*28*	*67*	*167*	*208*	*161*	*91*	*35*	*33*
ANNUAL DEATH RATE / 100,000 (*The rates for the age groups 0–34 and 35–69 are the means of seven five-yearly rates, but the all-ages rates are standardised to the conventional "European" age distribution)													
All causes													
1955	...	...	...	...	...	...	...	...	...	...	...	...	...
1965	1544.7*	305.4*	1569.4*	396.9	585.6	649.3	1037.3	1579.2	2573.0	4164.7	6540.5	11362.6	19318.2
1975	1571.5*	193.3*	1663.3*	364.6	552.4	800.7	1157.4	1830.6	2688.7	4248.4	6846.5	10885.2	21652.2
1985	1386.3*	156.1*	1588.0*	264.6	454.1	763.2	1245.8	1882.4	2713.1	3792.7	5936.7	9639.5	17208.7
1990	**1232.5***	**115.2***	**1422.4***	**222.2**	**346.3**	**676.2**	**1006.8**	**1855.3**	**2342.9**	**3506.7**	**5105.3**	**9263.8**	**15448.5**
1995 projected	*1099.6**	*87.5**	*1262.2**	*176.2*	*290.9*	*556.7*	*916.5*	*1655.2*	*2151.5*	*3088.9*	*4711.8*	*8267.3*	*14111.1*
All cancer													
1955	...	...	...	...	...	...	...	...	...	...	...	...	...
1965	...	...	...	...	...	...	...	...	...	...	...	...	...
1975	273.6*	10.2*	400.4*	39.1	89.2	150.8	283.3	421.5	691.5	1127.3	1530.7	2041.0	1869.6
1985	298.9*	9.7*	455.2*	38.9	93.4	172.8	357.6	588.2	795.5	1139.9	1375.5	2064.0	2226.1
1990	**291.1***	**7.9***	**460.1***	**35.1**	**69.8**	**161.9**	**336.8**	**634.5**	**831.9**	**1151.0**	**1348.7**	**1901.8**	**2036.8**
1995 projected	*283.4**	*6.3**	*459.4**	*29.2*	*59.9*	*147.8*	*337.5*	*653.3*	*854.8*	*1133.3*	*1296.9*	*1782.2*	*1915.0*
Lung cancer													
1955	...	...	...	...	...	...	...	...	...	...	...	...	...
1965	...	...	...	...	...	...	...	...	...	...	...	...	...
1975	74.6*	0.2*	127.9*	3.1	25.0	59.2	89.6	157.0	203.9	357.1	451.8	483.6	246.4
1985	84.1*	0.3*	153.1*	5.2	27.4	43.2	142.4	211.8	258.5	383.4	354.4	523.3	330.4
1990	**89.8***	**1.1***	**173.8***	**4.7**	**16.1**	**55.6**	**109.4**	**269.0**	**369.5**	**392.6**	**414.5**	**404.9**	**272.1**
1995 projected	*95.3**	*1.1**	*197.7**	*3.8*	*16.2*	*46.0*	*119.0*	*319.9*	*431.5*	*447.2*	*397.4*	*346.5*	*215.7*
Upper aerodigestive cancer (mouth, oesophagus, pharynx and larynx)													
1955	...	...	...	...	...	...	...	...	...	...	...	...	...
1965	...	...	...	...	...	...	...	...	...	...	...	...	...
1975	25.4*	0.2*	46.2*	1.6	12.5	23.3	36.3	45.5	101.9	102.5	100.9	114.8	144.9
1985	38.4*	0.3*	69.3*	6.5	20.9	41.6	79.7	125.5	96.6	114.0	109.7	180.2	200.0
1990	**31.3***	**0.2***	**59.4***	**7.0**	**14.8**	**25.3**	**70.1**	**103.9**	**104.0**	**90.6**	**85.5**	**159.5**	**110.3**
1995 projected	*25.6**	*0.2**	*50.1**	*5.1*	*10.0*	*19.7*	*55.1*	*93.9*	*89.2*	*77.8*	*69.9*	*118.8*	*78.4*
Other cancer													
1955	...	...	...	...	...	...	...	...	...	...	...	...	...
1965	...	...	...	...	...	...	...	...	...	...	...	...	...
1975	173.6*	9.8*	226.3*	34.4	51.6	68.2	157.4	219.0	385.7	667.7	978.1	1442.6	1478.3
1985	176.4*	9.1*	232.8*	27.2	45.1	88.0	135.6	251.0	440.3	642.5	911.4	1360.5	1695.7
1990	**169.9***	**6.7***	**226.9***	**23.4**	**38.9**	**80.9**	**157.3**	**261.6**	**358.4**	**667.8**	**848.7**	**1337.4**	**1654.4**
1995 projected	*162.4**	*4.9**	*211.6**	*20.3*	*33.7*	*82.1*	*163.4*	*239.5*	*334.0*	*608.3*	*829.7*	*1316.8*	*1620.9*
Chronic obstructive pulmonary disease (COPD)													
1955	...	...	...	...	...	...	...	...	...	...	...	...	...
1965	...	...	...	...	...	...	...	...	...	...	...	...	...
1975	70.7*	0.6*	63.5*	6.3	4.7	10.8	36.3	33.1	126.7	226.7	486.8	672.1	1043.5
1985	33.2*	0.5*	45.8*	1.3	1.6	11.2	27.1	43.1	122.2	114.0	253.2	226.7	234.8
1990	**65.5***	**0.4***	**51.5***	**2.3**	**2.7**	**5.1**	**34.2**	**46.4**	**81.9**	**187.9**	**309.2**	**816.0**	**1110.3**
1995 projected	*85.8**	–	*55.1**	*2.5*	*1.2*	*4.9*	*35.5*	*38.3*	*89.2*	*213.9*	*436.7*	*1138.6*	*1575.2*
Other respiratory disease													
1955	...	...	...	...	...	...	...	...	...	...	...	...	...
1965	...	...	...	...	...	...	...	...	...	...	...	...	...
1975	55.5*	6.7*	32.1*	6.3	6.3	7.2	36.3	20.7	55.1	93.2	241.2	459.0	1188.4
1985	46.9*	6.0*	41.7*	3.9	14.5	19.2	28.8	39.2	82.4	103.6	223.6	407.0	678.3
1990	**32.4***	**2.0***	**20.9***	**3.5**	**1.3**	**8.4**	**22.2**	**29.7**	**31.0**	**50.3**	**131.6**	**349.7**	**625.0**
1995 projected	*26.1**	*1.8**	*14.5**	*2.5*	*1.2*	*6.6*	*16.0*	*21.1*	*20.7*	*33.3*	*96.1*	*277.2*	*562.1*
Vascular disease													
1955	...	...	...	...	...	...	...	...	...	...	...	...	...
1965	...	...	...	...	...	...	...	...	...	...	...	...	...
1975	712.6*	8.9*	601.3*	43.8	97.0	193.9	283.3	686.0	1013.8	1891.3	3482.5	6155.7	13492.8
1985	642.4*	4.3*	579.5*	40.2	99.8	176.0	362.7	609.8	1011.4	1756.5	3122.4	5412.8	11669.6
1990	**526.1***	**5.3***	**480.7***	**36.3**	**72.5**	**156.8**	**254.7**	**534.3**	**847.3**	**1463.1**	**2381.6**	**4797.5**	**9330.9**
1995 projected	*426.8**	*5.7**	*380.3**	*27.9*	*59.9*	*116.6*	*207.8*	*431.0*	*690.9*	*1127.8*	*1995.6*	*3772.3*	*7712.4*
Liver cirrhosis													
1955	...	...	...	...	...	...	...	...	...	...	...	...	...
1965	...	...	...	...	...	...	...	...	...	...	...	...	...
1975	45.0*	1.2*	85.2*	20.3	54.8	48.5	77.5	144.6	126.7	124.2	201.8	98.4	115.9
1985	65.0*	2.9*	125.8*	27.2	35.4	70.4	145.8	215.7	235.8	150.3	173.0	267.4	139.1
1990	**51.8***	**0.7***	**106.7***	**23.4**	**28.2**	**67.5**	**104.3**	**204.1**	**154.9**	**164.4**	**157.9**	**153.4**	**73.5**
1995 projected	*41.5**	*0.6**	*86.7**	*16.5*	*25.0*	*52.5*	*90.6*	*155.2*	*130.7*	*136.1*	*126.6*	*108.9*	*52.3*
Other medical causes													
1955	...	...	...	...	...	...	...	...	...	...	...	...	...
1965	...	...	...	...	...	...	...	...	...	...	...	...	...
1975	230.2*	75.2*	232.3*	87.6	117.4	172.4	196.1	227.3	349.9	475.2	570.2	967.2	3130.4
1985	137.8*	53.1*	138.2*	44.1	46.7	86.4	94.9	166.7	233.0	295.3	405.1	796.5	1417.4
1990	**129.4***	**36.3***	**122.9***	**35.1**	**59.1**	**84.3**	**76.9**	**181.8**	**154.9**	**268.5**	**493.4**	**822.1**	**1566.2**
1995 projected	*123.0**	*25.5**	*111.8**	*34.2*	*57.4*	*80.5*	*74.6*	*149.4*	*130.7*	*255.6*	*519.7*	*851.5*	*1686.3*
All non-medical causes													
1955	...	...	...	...	...	...	...	...	...	...	...	...	...
1965	...	...	...	...	...	...	...	...	...	...	...	...	...
1975	183.8*	90.4*	248.5*	161.2	183.1	217.2	244.6	297.5	325.1	310.6	333.3	491.8	811.6
1985	162.1*	79.6*	201.9*	108.9	162.6	227.2	228.8	219.6	233.0	233.2	384.0	465.1	843.5
1990	**136.2***	**62.5***	**179.5***	**86.5**	**112.8**	**192.2**	**177.8**	**224.5**	**241.2**	**221.5**	**282.9**	**423.3**	**705.9**
1995 projected	*113.0**	*47.7**	*154.6**	*63.4*	*86.1*	*147.8*	*154.5*	*206.9*	*234.4*	*188.9*	*240.2*	*336.6*	*607.8*

SLOVENIA: Females

	All ages	0–34	35–69	35–39	40–44	45–49	50–54	55–59	60–64	65–69	70–74	75–79	80+/NK
POPULATION (1000s)													
1955	...	...	...	...	...	...	...	...	...	...	...	...	...
1965	858.2	467.5	340.7	64.8	60.0	34.3	51.2	49.9	45.1	35.4	23.2	15.5	11.3
1975	916.7	473.9	369.9	60.2	64.3	63.3	58.2	32.7	47.5	43.7	35.0	22.8	15.1
1985	1016.9	520.2	400.4	72.0	59.1	60.4	62.1	61.1	55.4	30.3	37.8	30.9	27.6
1990	**1029.7**	**502.5**	**437.3**	**80.5**	**70.5**	**57.7**	**58.7**	**60.0**	**58.3**	**51.6**	**27.0**	**30.5**	**32.4**
1995 projected	*1007.2*	*468.8*	*437.3*	*76.7*	*75.3*	*59.9*	*57.7*	*55.8*	*58.4*	*53.5*	*44.2*	*20.1*	*36.8*
NUMBER OF DEATHS													
All causes													
1955	...	...	...	...	...	...	...	...	...	...	...	...	...
1965	7499	666	2613	110	133	122	287	411	613	937	1036	1377	1807
1975	8648	451	2589	76	160	211	306	284	581	971	1398	1682	2528
1985	9626	327	2304	82	94	172	305	438	624	589	1326	1869	3800
1990	**9038**	**248**	**2287**	**78**	**108**	**148**	**238**	**366**	**542**	**807**	**765**	**1726**	**4012**
1995 projected	*8336*	*189*	*1914*	*69*	*106*	*136*	*198*	*284*	*444*	*677*	*1095*	*972*	*4166*
Lung cancer													
1955	...	...	...	...	...	...	...	...	...	...	...	...	...
1965	...	...	...	...	...	...	...	...	...	...	...	...	...
1975	76	–	43	–	3	5	5	3	15	12	15	13	5
1985	114	–	61	4	–	3	9	9	17	19	18	25	10
1990	**139**	–	**86**	**1**	**2**	**7**	**15**	**13**	**20**	**28**	**13**	**21**	**19**
1995 projected	*153*	–	*98*	*1*	*3*	*10*	*20*	*16*	*20*	*28*	*19*	*13*	*23*
ANNUAL DEATH RATE / 100,000 (*The rates for the age groups 0–34 and 35–69 are the means of seven five-yearly rates, but the all-ages rates are standardised to the conventional "European" age distribution)													
All causes													
1955	...	...	...	...	...	...	...	...	...	...	...	...	...
1965	1021.2*	140.4*	876.8*	169.8	221.7	355.7	560.5	823.6	1359.2	2646.9	4465.5	8883.9	15991.2
1975	941.4*	96.1*	792.5*	126.2	248.8	333.3	525.8	868.5	1223.2	2222.0	3994.3	7377.2	16741.7
1985	786.1*	64.9*	690.9*	113.9	159.1	284.8	491.1	716.9	1126.4	1943.9	3507.9	6048.5	13768.1
1990	**682.1***	**51.7***	**573.7***	**96.9**	**153.2**	**256.5**	**405.5**	**610.0**	**929.7**	**1564.0**	**2833.3**	**5659.0**	**12382.7**
1995 projected	*594.3**	*42.1**	*476.5**	*90.0*	*140.8*	*227.0*	*343.2*	*509.0*	*760.3*	*1265.4*	*2477.4*	*4835.8*	*11320.7*
All cancer													
1955	...	...	...	...	...	...	...	...	...	...	...	...	...
1965	...	...	...	...	...	...	...	...	...	...	...	...	...
1975	156.5*	9.3*	240.3*	28.2	71.5	128.0	195.9	296.6	414.7	546.9	760.0	894.7	1053.0
1985	155.3*	6.2*	236.0*	36.1	64.3	101.0	167.5	276.6	422.4	584.2	772.5	967.6	1137.7
1990	**151.3***	**6.8***	**221.9***	**31.1**	**70.9**	**123.1**	**170.4**	**248.3**	**368.8**	**540.7**	**681.5**	**983.6**	**1259.3**
1995 projected	*144.3**	*6.3**	*202.4**	*31.3*	*73.0*	*123.5*	*164.6*	*220.4*	*327.1*	*476.6*	*642.5*	*950.2*	*1339.7*
Lung cancer													
1955	...	...	...	...	...	...	...	...	...	...	...	...	...
1965	...	...	...	...	...	...	...	...	...	...	...	...	...
1975	7.8*	–	12.8*	–	4.7	7.9	8.6	9.2	31.6	27.5	42.9	57.0	33.1
1985	10.4*	–	19.0*	5.6	–	5.0	14.5	14.7	30.7	62.7	47.6	80.9	36.2
1990	**12.1***	–	**21.7***	**1.2**	**2.8**	**12.1**	**25.6**	**21.7**	**34.3**	**54.3**	**48.1**	**68.9**	**58.6**
1995 projected	*13.3**	–	*24.6**	*1.3*	*4.0*	*16.7*	*34.7*	*28.7*	*34.2*	*52.3*	*43.0*	*64.7*	*62.5*
Upper aerodigestive cancer (mouth, oesophagus, pharynx and larynx)													
1955	...	...	...	...	...	...	...	...	...	...	...	...	...
1965	...	...	...	...	...	...	...	...	...	...	...	...	...
1975	2.9*	–	3.7*	–	–	1.6	1.7	9.2	6.3	6.9	11.4	30.7	26.5
1985	2.7*	–	4.6*	–	–	–	3.2	6.5	12.6	9.9	10.6	16.2	21.7
1990	**2.8***	–	**3.9***	–	**1.4**	**3.5**	**3.4**	**5.0**	**10.3**	**3.9**	**14.8**	**23.0**	**18.5**
1995 projected	*2.7**	–	*3.2**	–	–	*5.0*	*3.5*	*3.6*	*6.8*	*3.7*	*15.8*	*24.9*	*21.7*
Other cancer													
1955	...	...	...	...	...	...	...	...	...	...	...	...	...
1965	...	...	...	...	...	...	...	...	...	...	...	...	...
1975	145.8*	9.3*	223.8*	28.2	66.9	118.5	185.6	278.3	376.8	512.6	705.7	807.0	993.4
1985	142.1*	6.2*	212.4*	30.6	64.3	96.0	149.8	255.3	379.1	511.6	714.3	870.6	1079.7
1990	**136.4***	**6.8***	**196.2***	**29.8**	**66.7**	**107.5**	**141.4**	**221.7**	**324.2**	**482.6**	**618.5**	**891.8**	**1182.1**
1995 projected	*128.3**	*6.3**	*174.6**	*30.0*	*69.1*	*101.8*	*126.5*	*188.2*	*286.0*	*420.6*	*583.7*	*860.7*	*1255.4*
Chronic obstructive pulmonary disease (COPD)													
1955	...	...	...	...	...	...	...	...	...	...	...	...	...
1965	...	...	...	...	...	...	...	...	...	...	...	...	...
1975	15.4*	–	13.1*	–	1.6	3.2	6.9	24.5	14.7	41.2	108.6	157.9	218.5
1985	6.8*	–	9.0*	1.4	–	1.7	4.8	4.9	10.8	39.6	55.6	51.8	54.3
1990	**14.3***	**0.6***	**10.3***	**5.0**	–	**3.5**	**1.7**	**11.7**	**17.2**	**32.9**	**63.0**	**144.3**	**284.0**
1995 projected	*18.9**	*0.4**	*11.5**	*6.5*	–	*3.3*	*1.7*	*16.1*	*18.8*	*33.6*	*88.2*	*199.0*	*399.5*
Other respiratory disease													
1955	...	...	...	...	...	...	...	...	...	...	...	...	...
1965	...	...	...	...	...	...	...	...	...	...	...	...	...
1975	35.2*	3.8*	12.3*	–	1.6	3.2	8.6	15.3	21.1	36.6	137.1	271.9	960.3
1985	22.3*	3.1*	12.4*	1.4	1.7	6.6	9.7	6.5	14.4	46.2	124.3	187.7	438.4
1990	**17.5***	**0.4***	**8.0***	–	–	–	**5.1**	**3.3**	**6.9**	**40.7**	**74.1**	**173.8**	**450.6**
1995 projected	*15.4**	*0.2**	*5.5**	–	–	–	*3.5*	*1.8*	*5.1*	*28.0*	*58.8*	*139.3*	*451.1*
Vascular disease													
1955	...	...	...	...	...	...	...	...	...	...	...	...	...
1965	...	...	...	...	...	...	...	...	...	...	...	...	...
1975	521.4*	4.4*	322.3*	23.3	60.7	69.5	139.2	287.5	515.8	1160.2	2422.9	5236.8	11589.4
1985	426.1*	3.7*	249.7*	11.1	30.5	67.9	111.1	216.0	413.4	897.7	1957.7	3880.3	10148.6
1990	**347.5***	**2.5***	**183.9***	**17.4**	**27.0**	**39.9**	**86.9**	**150.0**	**317.3**	**649.2**	**1551.9**	**3426.2**	**8416.7**
1995 projected	*282.0**	*2.1**	*135.4**	*15.6*	*19.9*	*26.7*	*58.9*	*109.3*	*227.7*	*489.7*	*1285.1*	*2711.4*	*7106.0*
Liver cirrhosis													
1955	...	...	...	...	...	...	...	...	...	...	...	...	...
1965	...	...	...	...	...	...	...	...	...	...	...	...	...
1975	17.3*	1.4*	31.4*	6.6	6.2	20.5	27.5	52.0	61.1	45.8	62.9	70.2	53.0
1985	26.6*	0.7*	54.6*	15.3	13.5	39.7	83.7	70.4	86.6	72.6	60.8	77.7	39.9
1990	**19.8***	**0.5***	**40.8***	**5.0**	**7.1**	**29.5**	**40.9**	**61.7**	**72.0**	**69.8**	**70.4**	**26.2**	**52.5**
1995 projected	*15.3**	*0.4**	*32.7**	*3.9*	*5.3*	*20.0*	*27.7*	*43.0*	*63.4*	*65.4*	*54.3*	*19.9*	*38.0*
Other medical causes													
1955	...	...	...	...	...	...	...	...	...	...	...	...	...
1965	...	...	...	...	...	...	...	...	...	...	...	...	...
1975	143.2*	52.0*	113.1*	28.2	56.0	71.1	92.8	134.6	138.9	270.0	391.4	596.5	2397.4
1985	96.4*	31.2*	74.3*	23.6	15.2	34.8	54.8	85.1	95.7	211.2	425.9	657.0	1308.0
1990	**87.4***	**23.1***	**62.5***	**7.5**	**21.3**	**20.8**	**44.3**	**93.3**	**87.5**	**162.8**	**259.3**	**691.8**	**1509.3**
1995 projected	*81.5**	*17.7**	*49.7**	*5.2*	*14.6*	*16.7*	*38.1*	*86.0*	*75.3*	*112.1*	*221.7*	*646.8*	*1690.2*
All non-medical causes													
1955	...	...	...	...	...	...	...	...	...	...	...	...	...
1965	...	...	...	...	...	...	...	...	...	...	...	...	...
1975	52.5*	25.2*	60.0*	39.9	51.3	37.9	55.0	58.1	56.8	121.3	111.4	149.1	470.2
1985	52.6*	20.0*	54.9*	25.0	33.8	33.1	59.6	57.3	83.0	92.4	111.1	226.5	641.3
1990	**44.4***	**17.8***	**46.2***	**31.1**	**27.0**	**39.9**	**56.2**	**41.7**	**60.0**	**67.8**	**133.3**	**213.1**	**410.5**
1995 projected	*36.9**	*15.0**	*39.3**	*27.4*	*27.9*	*36.7*	*48.5*	*32.3*	*42.8*	*59.8*	*126.7*	*169.2*	*296.2*

SLOVENIA: 1975

Smoking-attributed deaths (Sm.) and total deaths (Total)

			ALL CAUSES	ALL CANCER	Lung cancer	Upper aero-digestive ca.	Other cancer	COPD	Other respiratory	Vascular disease	Liver cirrhosis	Other medical	Non-medical
Males													
	0-34	Sm.	–	–	–	–	–	–	–	–	–	–	–
		Total	971	51	1	1	49	3	34	42	6	380	455
	35-69	Sm.	1271	470	294	80	96	121	26	437	–	217	–
		Total	4297	999	315	118	566	155	82	1458	228	643	732
			(30%)	(47%)	(93%)	(68%)	(17%)	(78%)	(32%)	(30%)		(34%)	
	70+	Sm.	851	258	164	28	66	195	24	317	–	57	–
		Total	4383	727	179	47	501	265	193	2476	66	464	192
			(19%)	(35%)	(92%)	(60%)	(13%)	(74%)	(12%)	(13%)		(12%)	
	Any age	Sm.	2122	728	458	108	162	316	50	754	–	274	–
		Total	9651	1777	495	166	1116	423	309	3976	300	1487	1379
			(22%)	(41%)	(93%)	(65%)	(15%)	(75%)	(16%)	(19%)		(18%)	
Females													
	0-34	Sm.	–	–	–	–	–	–	–	–	–	–	–
		Total	451	42	0	0	42	0	18	20	6	246	119
	35-69	Sm.	62	17	13	1	3	7	1	29	–	8	–
		Total	2589	791	43	11	737	40	39	1024	103	380	212
			(2%)	(2%)	(30%)	(9%)	(0%)	(18%)	(3%)	(3%)		(2%)	
	70+	Sm.	114	17	12	2	3	27	4	56	–	10	–
		Total	5608	629	33	15	581	107	255	3792	46	635	144
			(2%)	(3%)	(36%)	(13%)	(1%)	(25%)	(2%)	(1%)		(2%)	
	Any age	Sm.	176	34	25	3	6	34	5	85	–	18	–
		Total	8648	1462	76	26	1360	147	312	4836	155	1261	475
			(2%)	(2%)	(33%)	(12%)	(0%)	(23%)	(2%)	(2%)		(1%)	
Males+Females													
	0-34	Sm.	–	–	–	–	–	–	–	–	–	–	–
		Total	1422	93	1	1	91	3	52	62	12	626	574
	35-69	Sm.	1333	487	307	81	99	128	27	466	–	225	–
		Total	6886	1790	358	129	1303	195	121	2482	331	1023	944
			(19%)	(27%)	(86%)	(63%)	(8%)	(66%)	(22%)	(19%)		(22%)	
	70+	Sm.	965	275	176	30	69	222	28	373	–	67	–
		Total	9991	1356	212	62	1082	372	448	6268	112	1099	336
			(10%)	(20%)	(83%)	(48%)	(6%)	(60%)	(6%)	(6%)		(6%)	
	Any age	Sm.	2298	762	483	111	168	350	55	839	–	292	–
		Total	18299	3239	571	192	2476	570	621	8812	455	2748	1854
			(13%)	(24%)	(85%)	(58%)	(7%)	(61%)	(9%)	(10%)		(11%)	

SLOVENIA: 1985

Smoking-attributed deaths (Sm.) and total deaths (Total)

			ALL CAUSES	ALL CANCER	Lung cancer	Upper aero-digestive ca.	Other cancer	COPD	Other respiratory	Vascular disease	Liver cirrhosis	Other medical	Non-medical
Males													
	0-34	Sm.	–	–	–	–	–	–	–	–	–	–	–
		Total	839	55	2	2	51	3	30	25	17	268	441
	35-69	Sm.	1505	665	384	156	125	94	42	541	–	163	–
		Total	4345	1207	405	211	591	112	110	1423	395	397	701
			(35%)	(55%)	(95%)	(74%)	(21%)	(84%)	(38%)	(38%)		(41%)	
	70+	Sm.	833	318	191	47	80	91	24	354	–	46	–
		Total	5044	937	212	80	645	126	201	3013	103	396	268
			(17%)	(34%)	(90%)	(59%)	(12%)	(72%)	(12%)	(12%)		(12%)	
	Any age	Sm.	2338	983	575	203	205	185	66	895	–	209	–
		Total	10228	2199	619	293	1287	241	341	4461	515	1061	1410
			(23%)	(45%)	(93%)	(69%)	(16%)	(77%)	(19%)	(20%)		(20%)	
Females													
	0-34	Sm.	–	–	–	–	–	–	–	–	–	–	–
		Total	327	34	0	0	34	0	15	20	4	150	104
	35-69	Sm.	117	36	29	2	5	10	2	54	–	15	–
		Total	2304	809	61	16	732	26	38	769	208	250	204
			(5%)	(4%)	(48%)	(13%)	(1%)	(38%)	(5%)	(7%)		(6%)	
	70+	Sm.	205	40	28	4	8	19	5	122	–	19	–
		Total	6995	905	53	15	837	52	226	4740	58	725	289
			(3%)	(4%)	(53%)	(27%)	(1%)	(37%)	(2%)	(3%)		(3%)	
	Any age	Sm.	322	76	57	6	13	29	7	176	–	34	–
		Total	9626	1748	114	31	1603	78	279	5529	270	1125	597
			(3%)	(4%)	(50%)	(19%)	(1%)	(37%)	(3%)	(3%)		(3%)	
Males+Females													
	0-34	Sm.	–	–	–	–	–	–	–	–	–	–	–
		Total	1166	89	2	2	85	3	45	45	21	418	545
	35-69	Sm.	1622	701	413	158	130	104	44	595	–	178	–
		Total	6649	2016	466	227	1323	138	148	2192	603	647	905
			(24%)	(35%)	(89%)	(70%)	(10%)	(75%)	(30%)	(27%)		(28%)	
	70+	Sm.	1038	358	219	51	88	110	29	476	–	65	–
		Total	12039	1842	265	95	1482	178	427	7753	161	1121	557
			(9%)	(19%)	(83%)	(54%)	(6%)	(62%)	(7%)	(6%)		(6%)	
	Any age	Sm.	2660	1059	632	209	218	214	73	1071	–	243	–
		Total	19854	3947	733	324	2890	319	620	9990	785	2186	2007
			(13%)	(27%)	(86%)	(65%)	(8%)	(67%)	(12%)	(11%)		(11%)	

(To be conservative, no deaths before age 35, and none from liver cirrhosis or non-medical causes, were attributed to smoking.)

SLOVENIA: 1990

Smoking–attributed deaths (Sm.) and total deaths (Total)

		ALL CAUSES	ALL CANCER	Lung cancer	Upper aero–digestive ca.	Other cancer	COPD	Other respiratory	Vascular disease	Liver cirrhosis	Other medical	Non–medical
Males												
0–34	Sm.	–	–	–	–	–	–	–	–	–	–	–
	Total	588	43	6	1	36	2	10	28	4	169	332
35–69	Sm.	1720	829	517	153	159	122	26	564	–	179	–
	Total	4542	1436	542	203	691	145	67	1434	371	417	672
		(38%)	(58%)	(95%)	(75%)	(23%)	(84%)	(39%)	(39%)		(43%)	
70+	Sm.	758	240	148	30	62	227	16	232	–	43	–
	Total	4387	792	166	54	572	331	162	2413	59	422	208
		(17%)	(30%)	(89%)	(56%)	(11%)	(69%)	(10%)	(10%)		(10%)	
Any age	Sm.	2478	1069	665	183	221	349	42	796	–	222	–
	Total	9517	2271	714	258	1299	478	239	3875	434	1008	1212
		(26%)	(47%)	(93%)	(71%)	(17%)	(73%)	(18%)	(21%)		(22%)	
Females												
0–34	Sm.	–	–	–	–	–	–	–	–	–	–	–
	Total	248	36	0	0	36	3	2	13	3	102	89
35–69	Sm.	169	65	50	5	10	17	2	61	–	24	–
	Total	2287	889	86	16	787	41	30	717	165	250	195
		(7%)	(7%)	(58%)	(31%)	(1%)	(41%)	(7%)	(9%)		(10%)	
70+	Sm.	190	34	25	3	6	54	4	83	–	15	–
	Total	6503	892	53	17	822	153	219	4191	44	770	234
		(3%)	(4%)	(47%)	(18%)	(1%)	(35%)	(2%)	(2%)		(2%)	
Any age	Sm.	359	99	75	8	16	71	6	144	–	39	–
	Total	9038	1817	139	33	1645	197	251	4921	212	1122	518
		(4%)	(5%)	(54%)	(24%)	(1%)	(36%)	(2%)	(3%)		(3%)	
Males+Females												
0–34	Sm.	–	–	–	–	–	–	–	–	–	–	–
	Total	836	79	6	1	72	5	12	41	7	271	421
35–69	Sm.	1889	894	567	158	169	139	28	625	–	203	–
	Total	6829	2325	628	219	1478	186	97	2151	536	667	867
		(28%)	(38%)	(90%)	(72%)	(11%)	(75%)	(29%)	(29%)		(30%)	
70+	Sm.	948	274	173	33	68	281	20	315	–	58	–
	Total	10890	1684	219	71	1394	484	381	6604	103	1192	442
		(9%)	(16%)	(79%)	(46%)	(5%)	(58%)	(5%)	(5%)		(5%)	
Any age	Sm.	2837	1168	740	191	237	420	48	940	–	261	–
	Total	18555	4088	853	291	2944	675	490	8796	646	2130	1730
		(15%)	(29%)	(87%)	(66%)	(8%)	(62%)	(10%)	(11%)		(12%)	

SLOVENIA: 1995

Smoking–attributed deaths (Sm.) and total deaths (Total)

		ALL CAUSES	ALL CANCER	Lung cancer	Upper aero–digestive ca.	Other cancer	COPD	Other respiratory	Vascular disease	Liver cirrhosis	Other medical	Non–medical
Males												
0–34	Sm.	–	–	–	–	–	–	–	–	–	–	–
	Total	415	32	6	1	25	0	8	27	3	106	239
35–69	Sm.	1776	924	619	134	171	142	22	510	–	178	–
	Total	4240	1512	647	175	690	166	49	1222	309	397	585
		(42%)	(61%)	(96%)	(77%)	(25%)	(86%)	(45%)	(42%)		(45%)	
70+	Sm.	761	219	142	21	56	299	12	187	–	44	–
	Total	4073	770	159	40	571	456	136	2018	48	463	182
		(19%)	(28%)	(89%)	(53%)	(10%)	(66%)	(9%)	(9%)		(10%)	
Any age	Sm.	2537	1143	761	155	227	441	34	697	–	222	–
	Total	8728	2314	812	216	1286	622	193	3267	360	966	1006
		(29%)	(49%)	(94%)	(72%)	(18%)	(71%)	(18%)	(21%)		(23%)	
Females												
0–34	Sm.	–	–	–	–	–	–	–	–	–	–	–
	Total	189	32	0	0	32	2	1	10	2	71	71
35–69	Sm.	174	75	62	4	9	23	1	51	–	24	–
	Total	1914	817	98	13	706	46	21	533	131	199	167
		(9%)	(9%)	(63%)	(31%)	(1%)	(50%)	(5%)	(10%)		(12%)	
70+	Sm.	187	33	24	4	5	71	4	65	–	14	–
	Total	6233	968	55	20	893	226	220	3728	42	850	199
		(3%)	(3%)	(44%)	(20%)	(1%)	(31%)	(2%)	(2%)		(2%)	
Any age	Sm.	361	108	86	8	14	94	5	116	–	38	–
	Total	8336	1817	153	33	1631	274	242	4271	175	1120	437
		(4%)	(6%)	(56%)	(24%)	(1%)	(34%)	(2%)	(3%)		(3%)	
Males+Females												
0–34	Sm.	–	–	–	–	–	–	–	–	–	–	–
	Total	604	64	6	1	57	2	9	37	5	177	310
35–69	Sm.	1950	999	681	138	180	165	23	561	–	202	–
	Total	6154	2329	745	188	1396	212	70	1755	440	596	752
		(32%)	(43%)	(91%)	(73%)	(13%)	(78%)	(33%)	(32%)		(34%)	
70+	Sm.	948	252	166	25	61	370	16	252	–	58	–
	Total	10306	1738	214	60	1464	682	356	5746	90	1313	381
		(9%)	(14%)	(78%)	(42%)	(4%)	(54%)	(4%)	(4%)		(4%)	
Any age	Sm.	2898	1251	847	163	241	535	39	813	–	260	–
	Total	17064	4131	965	249	2917	896	435	7538	535	2086	1443
		(17%)	(30%)	(88%)	(65%)	(8%)	(60%)	(9%)	(11%)		(12%)	

(To be conservative, no deaths before age 35, and none from liver cirrhosis or non–medical causes, were attributed to smoking.)

SPAIN: 1990

		No. of deaths			Standardised rates (Defined on p.490)			Annual death rates / 100, 000						
		All ages	**0–34**	**35–69**	**All ages**	**0–34**	**35–69**	**0–4**	**5–9**	**10–14**	**15–19**	**20–24**	**25–29**	**30–34**
ALL CAUSES	**M**	176779	12825	62931	935.3	124.9	942.3	197.3	27.8	29.8	94.7	156.7	179.5	188.8
	F	156363	5210	29108	537.3	57.1	395.2	164.0	19.4	20.5	36.0	44.0	53.4	62.2
Tuberculosis	**M**	705	62	342	3.8	0.6	5.0	0.2	–	0.1	0.2	0.7	0.9	2.0
	F	275	16	88	1.0	0.1	1.2	–	–	–	–	0.2	0.5	0.4
Other infective	**M**	1498	208	485	8.0	2.1	7.1	5.3	0.8	0.6	0.9	2.0	2.3	3.1
and parasitic	**F**	1412	141	318	5.3	1.6	4.3	5.6	0.6	0.6	0.8	0.9	1.1	1.8
ALL CANCER	**M**	47242	848	23343	252.1	8.1	352.1	5.4	5.5	5.0	6.6	6.5	11.0	16.8
	F	29581	654	12292	117.7	6.5	165.4	4.2	3.8	3.5	4.8	5.3	7.9	15.9
Mouth and	**M**	1612	11	1165	9.0	0.1	16.8	–	–	–	0.1	0.1	0.2	0.4
pharynx cancer	**F**	288	9	127	1.2	0.1	1.7	–	–	–	0.1	0.1	0.3	0.1
Oesophagus cancer	**M**	1494	4	992	8.2	0.0	14.6	–	–	–	–	–	0.1	0.1
	F	267	–	84	1.0	–	1.1	–	–	–	–	–	–	–
Stomach cancer	**M**	4102	24	1908	21.8	0.2	29.0	–	–	–	–	0.1	0.4	1.0
	F	2786	27	859	10.2	0.3	11.7	–	–	–	0.1	0.2	0.4	1.1
Colorectal cancer	**M**	4204	27	1771	22.3	0.3	26.9	0.1	–	–	–	0.2	0.3	1.3
	F	3760	19	1321	14.1	0.2	17.9	–	–	–	–	0.2	0.2	0.9
Liver cancer	**M**	1066	11	602	5.7	0.1	9.2	0.2	0.1	0.1	0.1	0.1	0.1	0.2
	F	503	6	210	2.0	0.1	2.9	–	0.1	–	0.1	0.1	–	0.1
Pancreas cancer	**M**	1622	9	870	8.7	0.1	13.1	–	–	–	0.1	0.1	0.2	0.2
	F	1326	8	422	4.9	0.1	5.8	–	–	–	0.1	0.1	0.1	0.2
Larynx cancer	**M**	1919	2	1282	10.5	0.0	19.0	–	0.1	–	–	–	0.1	–
	F	57	–	14	0.2	–	0.2	–	–	–	–	–	–	–
Lung cancer	**M**	12662	62	7337	67.9	0.6	110.9	–	–	–	0.2	0.2	1.2	2.5
	F	1320	20	545	5.2	0.2	7.3	–	–	–	0.1	0.1	0.2	1.0
Malignant melanoma	**M**	265	20	159	1.4	0.2	2.3	–	–	–	0.1	0.3	0.4	0.6
	F	203	9	91	0.8	0.1	1.2	–	–	–	0.1	–	0.3	0.3
Female breast cancer	**F**	5398	79	3204	24.1	0.8	42.4	–	–	–	0.1	0.2	1.4	3.7
Cervix cancer	**F**	521	16	335	2.4	0.2	4.4	–	–	–	–	0.1	0.1	0.9
Other uterine cancer	**F**	1290	6	598	5.2	0.1	8.1	0.1	–	–	–	–	0.1	0.3
Ovarian cancer	**F**	1148	27	705	5.1	0.3	9.4	0.1	–	–	0.3	0.2	0.4	0.8
Prostate cancer	**M**	4314	6	860	22.4	0.1	14.0	–	–	0.1	0.1	0.1	–	0.2
Bladder cancer	**M**	2492	3	886	13.0	0.0	13.9	–	–	–	0.1	–	–	0.1
	F	611	1	142	2.1	0.0	2.0	–	–	–	0.1	–	–	–
Other and ill–defined	**M**	8592	336	4165	45.8	3.2	62.6	3.3	2.3	1.8	3.2	2.9	4.1	5.0
cancer sites	**F**	7734	190	2734	29.4	1.9	37.2	1.6	1.3	1.4	1.4	1.7	2.0	3.8
Hodgkin's disease	**M**	198	53	105	1.0	0.5	1.5	–	–	0.3	0.4	0.5	1.1	1.2
	F	117	21	50	0.5	0.2	0.7	–	–	0.1	0.3	0.4	0.4	0.2
Myeloma and non–	**M**	1409	85	725	7.5	0.8	10.8	0.5	0.8	0.5	0.7	0.7	1.3	1.3
Hodgkin lymphomas	**F**	1146	42	481	4.6	0.4	6.5	0.3	0.2	0.4	0.2	0.4	0.6	0.8
Leukaemia	**M**	1291	195	516	6.8	1.9	7.6	1.4	2.3	2.3	1.8	1.4	1.4	2.5
	F	1106	174	370	4.6	1.8	4.9	2.2	2.2	1.7	1.9	1.4	1.5	1.7
ALL VASCULAR	**M**	61174	1024	17517	322.2	9.8	266.6	9.1	1.9	2.3	4.6	11.8	16.0	23.0
DISEASE	**F**	74413	450	7642	233.7	4.6	105.4	7.4	1.5	2.5	2.8	4.4	5.8	7.9
Rheumatic heart	**M**	462	15	272	2.5	0.1	4.0	0.1	–	0.1	–	0.3	0.3	0.2
disease and fever	**F**	1139	11	520	4.6	0.1	7.1	–	–	0.1	–	0.2	0.1	0.4
Hypertensive disease	**M**	1047	9	309	5.5	0.1	4.8	0.2	–	0.1	0.1	–	0.1	0.1
	F	1753	4	201	5.6	0.0	2.8	–	–	–	0.1	0.1	0.1	–
Ischaemic heart	**M**	19674	130	8240	104.4	1.2	125.1	–	0.1	0.1	0.2	0.8	2.0	5.6
disease	**F**	14209	34	2176	46.5	0.3	30.2	0.2	–	–	0.2	0.4	0.6	0.9
Pulmonary embolism	**M**	1280	41	417	6.7	0.4	6.3	0.4	–	0.1	0.3	0.5	0.7	0.8
and other venous	**F**	1643	20	312	5.6	0.2	4.2	–	–	–	0.2	0.3	0.3	0.6
Cerebrovascular	**M**	17728	192	3776	92.9	1.8	58.1	1.3	0.5	0.6	1.1	2.5	2.2	4.7
disease	**F**	25535	140	2242	79.5	1.4	31.0	0.9	0.8	1.3	0.9	1.6	1.5	2.8
Other vascular	**M**	20983	637	4503	110.2	6.1	68.2	7.2	1.3	1.4	3.0	7.7	10.7	11.6
disease	**F**	30134	241	2191	91.9	2.6	30.2	6.3	0.8	1.1	1.5	1.9	3.2	3.2
Chronic obstructive	**M**	10522	38	2472	54.9	0.4	39.1	0.4	0.2	0.2	0.4	0.4	0.3	0.8
pulmonary disease	**F**	4239	28	599	13.8	0.3	8.3	0.4	0.3	0.2	0.3	0.1	0.4	0.4
Other respiratory	**M**	9103	472	2122	47.8	4.6	32.5	7.7	0.7	0.8	2.3	4.9	8.1	7.9
disease	**F**	8473	205	821	26.9	2.3	11.3	6.5	0.8	0.7	1.4	1.5	1.9	3.0
Peptic ulcer	**M**	672	6	195	3.5	0.1	3.0	–	–	–	–	0.2	0.1	0.1
	F	460	1	68	1.5	0.0	0.9	–	–	–	–	–	–	0.1
Liver cirrhosis	**M**	5525	157	3814	30.3	1.5	55.6	–	–	–	0.1	0.6	2.2	7.7
	F	2367	54	1218	10.0	0.5	16.4	0.2	0.1	0.1	0.1	0.3	0.8	2.2
Renal disease	**M**	2900	61	691	15.2	0.6	10.6	1.1	0.1	0.1	0.3	0.7	0.7	1.3
	F	2961	47	463	9.8	0.5	6.4	1.2	0.5	0.2	0.1	0.3	0.3	1.1
Pregnancy and birth	**F**	22	16	6	0.1	0.2	0.1	–	–	–	–	0.2	0.3	0.5
Congenital and	**M**	1535	1469	53	10.9	18.9	0.7	124.3	2.9	1.1	1.4	1.0	0.8	0.9
perinatal causes	**F**	1210	1127	52	9.0	15.6	0.7	103.4	1.3	1.6	0.9	0.7	0.5	0.4
Ill–defined causes	**M**	3142	306	660	16.7	3.3	10.0	10.9	0.8	0.6	1.4	2.9	3.1	3.1
	F	3838	130	255	12.0	1.6	3.5	8.0	0.2	0.3	0.3	0.7	0.7	1.1
Other medical causes	**M**	18752	1947	5703	98.5	18.6	84.4	13.4	4.4	6.8	6.7	12.9	39.5	46.5
	F	22254	829	3574	74.9	8.5	48.9	13.7	4.3	3.1	3.9	7.6	14.4	12.6
ALL NON–	**M**	14009	6227	5534	71.4	56.4	75.7	19.5	10.7	12.2	69.8	112.4	94.2	75.7
MEDICAL CAUSES	**F**	4858	1512	1712	21.6	14.7	22.5	13.2	6.1	7.6	20.6	21.7	18.9	15.1
Motor vehicle	**M**	6164	3284	2195	30.7	29.3	29.7	5.7	5.5	5.6	45.4	64.4	44.5	34.1
traffic accidents	**F**	1825	808	655	8.5	7.7	8.6	3.9	3.5	4.2	14.3	12.9	8.4	6.8
Fire	**M**	155	53	68	0.8	0.5	0.9	0.9	–	0.1	0.2	1.0	0.7	0.7
	F	121	24	35	0.5	0.3	0.5	0.6	0.3	–	0.1	0.2	0.3	0.4
Suicide	**M**	2135	584	999	11.1	5.2	14.0	–	–	1.2	4.9	9.4	11.4	9.8
	F	804	150	407	3.6	1.4	5.3	–	–	0.4	1.3	2.1	3.5	2.5
Homicide	**M**	275	116	140	1.5	1.1	1.9	0.4	0.2	0.1	0.8	1.7	2.0	2.4
	F	106	44	46	0.5	0.4	0.6	0.2	0.3	0.3	0.3	0.6	0.6	0.7
POPULATION (thousands):				**M=males**	19122	10390	7398	1086	1286	1593	1688	1684	1621	1433
				F=females	19837	9923	7793	1012	1197	1505	1597	1610	1580	1422

SPAIN: 1990

Annual death rates / 100, 000 9th ICD categories

35–39	40–44	45–49	50–54	55–59	60–64	65–69	70–74	75–79	80+/NK			
198.7	276.3	405.1	648.8	999.4	1551.2	2516.8	3950.1	6487.6	13933.9	M	ALL CAUSES	001–999
81.3	112.3	167.3	269.9	404.3	642.0	1089.4	1957.1	3797.3	11445.6	F		
1.5	3.0	3.4	4.8	4.4	7.7	10.0	16.2	24.3	29.9	M	Tuberculosis	010–018, 137
0.3	0.7	0.2	0.8	1.3	1.4	3.8	4.3	7.6	12.4	F		
2.5	3.4	3.1	4.8	6.9	12.6	16.6	35.5	54.0	102.8	M	Other infective	Rest of 001–139
1.3	1.2	1.8	3.1	4.5	6.4	11.9	17.3	33.5	83.9	F	and parasitic	
36.3	78.4	135.4	252.7	395.6	615.1	951.3	1309.9	1757.3	2297.0	M	ALL CANCER	140–208
36.2	54.0	86.9	135.6	190.1	273.6	381.1	510.9	725.2	1122.3	F		
2.5	6.9	10.5	21.8	23.4	24.5	28.3	31.5	32.2	34.9	M	Mouth and	140–149
0.4	1.0	1.0	1.8	2.0	2.6	3.0	5.0	4.9	11.4	F	pharynx cancer	
0.8	4.3	7.0	15.8	19.9	25.6	28.8	32.9	38.9	42.0	M	Oesophagus cancer	150
0.1	0.4	0.6	0.8	2.1	1.7	2.2	3.3	7.7	15.0	F		
2.7	6.5	11.2	19.2	28.3	50.9	84.2	115.5	164.2	228.8	M	Stomach cancer	151
1.8	3.2	4.7	6.9	12.6	20.5	32.1	50.7	78.6	139.8	F		
2.8	6.2	9.9	15.1	28.6	47.1	78.7	120.6	178.6	268.1	M	Colorectal cancer	153, 154
2.8	3.9	6.4	12.7	19.1	35.3	45.0	64.8	106.4	172.5	F		
0.7	0.8	3.2	5.2	11.9	16.0	26.4	37.7	34.7	27.8	M	Liver cancer	155.0
0.1	0.6	0.8	1.5	2.8	5.9	8.5	10.8	12.9	16.9	F		
1.7	3.6	5.6	8.5	14.2	23.1	34.8	46.2	56.5	68.5	M	Pancreas cancer	157
0.7	1.0	1.8	3.4	5.7	10.8	16.9	27.3	41.2	58.8	F		
1.0	3.9	11.5	18.1	25.5	31.8	41.2	45.3	46.8	51.7	M	Larynx cancer	161
–	–	–	0.4	0.3	0.2	0.5	1.0	1.4	3.6	F		
8.2	19.8	39.1	80.7	128.4	201.7	298.7	373.5	425.0	391.9	M	Lung cancer	162
2.1	2.7	3.4	4.2	8.2	11.9	19.0	23.1	36.8	47.7	F		
0.7	1.6	1.7	1.7	2.5	3.3	4.6	4.7	6.9	8.4	M	Malignant melanoma	172
0.9	0.6	0.7	0.7	1.3	2.1	2.1	2.9	6.3	5.6	F		
13.5	22.0	35.4	45.2	53.9	59.4	67.2	77.4	91.1	130.6	F	Female breast cancer	174
2.8	2.0	3.3	5.1	4.6	5.9	7.3	8.7	7.7	7.6	F	Cervix cancer	180
1.2	1.6	2.6	5.0	11.3	14.2	20.7	24.8	31.6	40.9	F	Other uterine cancer	179, 182
1.3	3.1	5.3	10.2	11.8	16.0	18.4	18.9	19.9	20.1	F	Ovarian cancer	183
–	0.2	0.9	3.0	8.1	23.2	62.4	125.2	238.7	471.1	M	Prostate cancer	185
0.3	0.7	1.9	6.2	13.3	26.5	48.1	73.5	126.8	180.2	M	Bladder cancer	188
0.1	0.1	0.3	0.9	1.7	4.8	5.8	10.5	19.4	36.5	F		
9.5	16.6	22.2	43.2	71.8	106.1	169.0	234.4	306.3	410.8	M	Other and ill-defined	Rest of 140–208
4.7	8.0	14.5	27.4	40.9	62.8	102.2	136.9	202.7	342.0	F	cancer sites	
1.4	0.8	1.5	1.1	1.2	2.5	1.7	3.1	3.0	2.9	M	Hodgkin's disease	201
0.4	0.5	0.5	0.2	0.5	0.6	2.0	2.0	3.3	1.4	F		
1.8	3.3	5.6	8.2	10.8	19.9	25.9	36.8	53.7	47.2	M	Myeloma and non–	200, 202–203
1.4	1.7	2.9	4.6	5.8	11.6	17.8	25.6	29.1	33.6	F	Hodgkin lymphomas	
2.3	3.2	3.7	5.0	7.7	12.9	18.5	28.9	45.1	62.7	M	Leukaemia	204–208
2.0	1.6	2.7	4.6	5.8	7.4	10.4	17.4	24.0	38.2	F		
32.9	59.4	95.6	163.3	267.7	453.6	793.6	1370.3	2530.7	6527.5	M	ALL VASCULAR	390–459
12.3	17.8	29.3	50.7	91.4	175.2	361.5	829.1	1864.7	6639.4	F	DISEASE	
0.7	0.8	2.1	3.7	4.7	7.0	9.2	9.5	13.4	18.1	M	Rheumatic heart	390–398
1.3	1.3	2.7	5.4	7.7	11.8	19.4	25.6	26.8	33.5	F	disease and fever	
0.2	0.5	1.0	1.9	5.8	8.4	15.6	24.7	47.3	105.5	M	Hypertensive disease	401–405
0.2	0.2	0.9	1.3	2.3	5.6	8.9	24.1	44.1	149.5	F		
13.9	26.7	46.9	81.6	128.8	216.1	361.8	522.9	795.9	1368.3	M	Ischaemic heart	410–414
1.5	3.7	5.6	12.4	26.0	53.6	108.4	224.6	429.5	1042.4	F	disease	
0.6	2.2	2.4	4.0	6.1	10.4	18.5	30.4	55.5	113.1	M	Pulmonary embolism	415.1, 451–453
1.0	0.5	2.3	2.0	4.0	8.5	11.4	25.0	46.6	113.7	F	and other venous	
5.3	11.1	19.5	31.6	53.8	98.4	186.9	385.4	824.2	2181.0	M	Cerebrovascular	430–438
4.1	5.3	8.9	15.8	26.0	48.3	108.4	285.6	689.7	2288.1	F	disease	
12.2	18.1	23.6	40.4	68.6	113.2	201.6	397.4	794.5	2741.6	M	Other vascular	Rest of 390–459
4.2	6.7	8.8	13.8	25.5	47.3	105.0	244.2	628.0	3012.3	F	disease	
1.3	2.3	5.2	14.2	31.9	69.6	149.4	309.3	541.9	1081.8	M	Chronic obstructive	490–496
0.7	1.5	1.1	4.6	8.4	13.5	27.9	59.5	114.8	334.9	F	pulmonary disease	
6.4	8.1	11.1	17.9	27.6	50.5	105.8	176.3	350.7	1081.8	M	Other respiratory	Rest of 460–519
2.6	2.4	4.6	6.5	8.9	17.6	36.3	79.3	183.3	782.7	F	disease	
0.6	0.7	1.3	1.6	2.9	4.5	9.2	15.6	27.5	71.9	M	Peptic ulcer	531–533
–	0.1	0.6	0.4	0.5	1.9	3.1	6.0	11.5	37.5	F		
12.6	19.5	33.1	52.1	72.3	90.9	108.4	116.3	125.3	107.3	M	Liver cirrhosis	571
3.1	5.2	7.7	13.3	19.3	27.9	38.1	45.2	56.8	53.7	F		
0.7	2.4	3.2	5.7	10.5	17.4	34.6	61.5	121.1	346.5	M	Renal disease	580–590
0.6	1.2	2.0	3.3	4.7	10.9	21.9	41.8	78.2	225.5	F		
0.3	0.2	–	–	–	–	–	–	–	–	F	Pregnancy and birth	630–676
0.4	0.3	0.5	1.4	0.6	1.4	0.6	0.2	1.0	2.1	M	Congenital and	740–779
0.6	0.6	0.5	1.0	0.7	0.7	0.7	1.6	0.9	1.8	F	perinatal causes	
2.3	3.0	4.4	6.3	9.3	15.5	28.9	48.4	102.3	392.7	M	Ill-defined causes	780–799
1.3	1.0	1.2	2.3	2.1	6.0	10.4	20.1	56.4	405.5	F		
33.0	33.8	42.9	51.7	83.3	124.0	221.8	379.4	691.4	1633.0	M	Other medical causes	Rest of 001–799
9.1	11.1	15.6	25.9	45.7	79.7	155.6	294.0	597.5	1629.2	F		
68.1	61.9	66.1	72.4	86.5	88.5	86.7	111.4	160.2	259.4	M	ALL NON–	E800–E999
13.0	15.5	15.8	22.5	26.5	27.1	37.0	47.9	66.8	116.6	F	MEDICAL CAUSES	
31.4	25.2	27.8	28.2	33.2	33.2	29.0	38.9	48.5	72.1	M	Motor vehicle	E810–E819
5.4	6.4	6.8	8.8	9.9	10.3	12.2	14.6	18.9	18.0	F	traffic accidents	
0.8	0.7	0.7	1.0	1.0	1.1	1.2	1.6	2.0	4.5	M	Fire	E890–E899
0.2	0.2	0.4	0.2	0.7	0.5	1.0	1.4	1.7	5.5	F		
9.6	9.4	10.9	13.2	16.0	17.8	21.1	26.9	43.8	59.5	M	Suicide	E950–E959
3.1	3.3	3.8	4.9	7.9	5.5	8.8	9.4	11.2	14.3	F		
2.0	2.3	1.7	2.6	1.6	1.3	1.6	0.9	1.2	2.4	M	Homicide	E960–E969
0.6	0.6	0.3	0.5	0.7	0.8	0.7	0.7	0.8	0.8	F		
1256	1208	1073	989	1088	978	807	550	404	381	M	**POPULATION (thousands)**	
1248	1216	1086	1034	1163	1088	958	763	633	726	F		

SPAIN: Males

	All ages	0–34	35–69	35–39	40–44	45–49	50–54	55–59	60–64	65–69	70–74	75–79	80+/NK
POPULATION (1000s)													
1955	14084	8746	4800	885	856	817	738	631	480	393	273	159	106
1965	15407	9095	5622	1104	1030	826	789	740	635	498	328	208	154
1975	17190	10089	6222	984	1153	1092	991	741	681	579	422	246	210
1985	18911	10633	7060	1224	1093	1018	1137	1046	896	647	528	378	314
1990	**19122**	**10390**	**7398**	**1256**	**1208**	**1073**	**989**	**1088**	**978**	**807**	**550**	**404**	**381**
1995 projected	*19695*	*10362*	*7847*	*1467*	*1260*	*1201*	*1077*	*928*	*1019*	*896*	*693*	*410*	*384*
NUMBER OF DEATHS													
All causes													
1955	135251	31962	51734	2571	3396	4893	6929	8676	11213	14056	15851	15611	20093
1965	137503	20691	55225	2539	3535	4134	6224	9543	13458	15792	17921	18436	25230
1975	155471	15535	61758	2123	3642	5363	7846	9461	13998	19325	23370	22176	32632
1985	164834	10476	60274	2164	2885	4394	7801	11136	15263	16631	22734	26737	44613
1990	**176779**	**12825**	**62931**	**2496**	**3338**	**4345**	**6413**	**10876**	**15165**	**20298**	**21710**	**26197**	**53116**
1995 projected	*181343*	*16877*	*62825*	*3425*	*3511*	*4683*	*6572*	*8586*	*14999*	*21049*	*25407*	*24668*	*51566*
Lung cancer													
1955	1664	21	1217	15	38	85	174	284	341	280	237	117	72
1965	3232	53	2152	25	81	101	228	458	656	603	520	336	171
1975	5894	47	3678	47	115	231	458	608	987	1232	1123	641	405
1985	10085	42	5812	73	146	353	741	1166	1690	1643	1756	1440	1035
1990	**12662**	**62**	**7337**	**103**	**239**	**419**	**798**	**1397**	**1972**	**2409**	**2053**	**1716**	**1494**
1995 projected	*15248*	*100*	*8594*	*173*	*303*	*569*	*999*	*1312*	*2289*	*2949*	*2860*	*1966*	*1728*
ANNUAL DEATH RATE / 100,000 (*The rates for the age groups 0–34 and 35–69 are the means of seven five-yearly rates, but the all-ages rates are standardised to the conventional "European" age distribution)													
All causes													
1955	1429.1*	340.0*	1358.9*	290.5	396.7	598.9	938.9	1375.0	2336.0	3576.6	5806.2	9818.2	18955.7
1965	1219.3*	207.0*	1206.1*	230.0	343.2	500.5	788.8	1289.6	2119.4	3171.1	5463.7	8846.4	16425.8
1975	1174.5*	149.2*	1211.6*	215.7	315.8	491.2	791.8	1276.8	2054.9	3335.3	5539.2	9007.3	15516.9
1985	969.3*	103.8*	985.6*	176.8	264.1	431.8	686.0	1064.5	1704.4	2571.7	4308.9	7082.6	14208.0
1990	**935.3***	**124.9***	**942.3***	**198.7**	**276.3**	**405.1**	**648.8**	**999.4**	**1551.2**	**2516.8**	**3950.1**	**6487.6**	**13933.9**
1995 projected	*904.8**	*153.1**	*894.3**	*233.5*	*278.7*	*389.9*	*610.4*	*925.4*	*1471.9*	*2350.5*	*3664.6*	*6022.5*	*13435.6*
All cancer													
1955	155.3*	6.7*	229.2*	24.7	45.7	95.2	158.4	265.1	433.1	582.2	823.4	1040.3	1146.2
1965	194.4*	11.3*	269.3*	29.3	56.7	99.8	180.4	327.2	513.7	677.9	1053.4	1417.5	1537.8
1975	222.4*	10.9*	316.8*	31.2	62.1	112.3	212.4	354.0	582.6	863.1	1211.7	1557.3	1764.1
1985	235.0*	8.2*	327.7*	31.3	62.3	136.1	234.2	369.7	598.5	861.9	1240.5	1651.1	2083.8
1990	**252.1***	**8.1***	**352.1***	**36.3**	**78.4**	**135.4**	**252.7**	**395.6**	**615.1**	**951.3**	**1309.9**	**1757.3**	**2297.0**
1995 projected	*266.8**	*8.5**	*370.5**	*44.7*	*83.9*	*145.1*	*266.0*	*409.8*	*650.0*	*994.0*	*1369.8*	*1851.1*	*2492.7*
Lung cancer													
1955	17.5*	0.3*	32.5*	1.7	4.4	10.4	23.6	45.0	71.0	71.2	86.8	73.6	67.9
1965	27.8*	0.7*	48.2*	2.3	7.9	12.2	28.9	61.9	103.3	121.1	158.5	161.2	111.3
1975	43.7*	0.5*	74.5*	4.8	10.0	21.2	46.2	82.1	144.9	212.6	266.2	260.4	192.6
1985	59.0*	0.4*	96.2*	6.0	13.4	34.7	65.2	111.5	188.7	254.1	332.8	381.5	329.6
1990	**67.9***	**0.6***	**110.9***	**8.2**	**19.8**	**39.1**	**80.7**	**128.4**	**201.7**	**298.7**	**373.5**	**425.0**	**391.9**
1995 projected	*76.6**	*0.9**	*124.5**	*11.8*	*24.0*	*47.4*	*92.8*	*141.4*	*224.6*	*329.3*	*412.5*	*480.0*	*450.2*
Upper aerodigestive cancer (mouth, oesophagus, pharynx and larynx)													
1955	16.4*	0.2*	26.7*	1.8	5.5	14.7	23.7	34.1	46.3	61.1	71.8	86.2	119.8
1965	19.3*	0.3*	31.8*	3.2	6.6	12.7	29.7	43.1	57.0	70.1	91.2	107.5	121.1
1975	25.1*	0.3*	42.6*	2.6	8.9	20.9	37.4	55.7	77.4	95.4	118.3	151.1	121.3
1985	25.2*	0.3*	43.7*	4.4	11.5	28.0	44.4	58.9	77.3	81.2	105.8	117.4	133.8
1990	**27.7***	**0.2***	**50.4***	**4.3**	**15.1**	**29.0**	**55.6**	**68.8**	**81.9**	**98.2**	**109.7**	**117.9**	**128.5**
1995 projected	*30.1**	*0.2**	*56.2**	*5.2*	*16.3*	*33.9*	*63.7*	*77.1*	*92.1*	*105.4*	*114.5*	*113.5*	*126.1*
Other cancer													
1955	121.5*	6.3*	170.0*	21.2	35.7	70.1	111.1	186.1	315.8	449.9	664.8	880.5	958.5
1965	147.2*	10.4*	189.3*	23.8	42.2	74.8	121.8	222.2	353.4	486.7	803.7	1148.8	1305.3
1975	153.6*	10.0*	199.7*	23.8	43.2	70.2	128.8	216.2	360.4	555.1	827.2	1145.8	1450.3
1985	150.9*	7.5*	187.8*	20.9	37.4	73.4	124.6	199.3	332.6	526.7	801.9	1152.3	1620.4
1990	**156.5***	**7.4***	**190.7***	**23.8**	**43.5**	**67.3**	**116.3**	**198.4**	**331.4**	**554.4**	**826.6**	**1214.5**	**1776.5**
1995 projected	*160.1**	*7.5**	*189.8**	*27.7*	*43.6*	*63.9*	*109.5*	*191.3*	*333.2*	*559.2*	*842.8*	*1257.6*	*1916.4*
Chronic obstructive pulmonary disease (COPD)													
1955	65.9*	7.4*	66.7*	6.3	9.5	23.3	40.2	70.7	121.5	195.7	340.3	523.3	877.4
1965	62.9*	3.3*	62.6*	6.9	14.3	18.8	28.8	66.2	114.0	189.2	334.1	527.4	926.4
1975	79.5*	2.1*	75.1*	6.7	10.1	19.6	32.9	72.5	133.3	250.3	463.1	750.2	1180.7
1985	48.4*	0.5*	37.1*	1.3	3.2	6.6	14.4	31.5	66.9	135.9	248.9	494.6	917.5
1990	**54.9***	**0.4***	**39.1***	**1.3**	**2.3**	**5.2**	**14.2**	**31.9**	**69.6**	**149.4**	**309.3**	**541.9**	**1081.8**
1995 projected	*61.1**	*0.4**	*42.4**	*1.1*	*1.8*	*4.6*	*13.6*	*32.0*	*73.1*	*171.0*	*343.0*	*592.0*	*1243.9*
Other respiratory disease													
1955	103.9*	49.7*	64.7*	10.4	15.7	23.1	41.1	62.0	108.3	192.1	333.3	690.6	1480.2
1965	63.3*	26.1*	35.6*	6.2	10.4	13.1	19.8	32.6	63.9	103.0	214.6	440.0	1048.8
1975	67.3*	10.6*	43.4*	6.7	11.0	15.5	21.9	39.9	77.4	131.3	281.8	574.3	1310.5
1985	53.6*	4.1*	38.0*	5.2	7.6	14.6	22.6	36.9	64.9	114.4	236.7	436.0	1105.1
1990	**47.8***	**4.6***	**32.5***	**6.4**	**8.1**	**11.1**	**17.9**	**27.6**	**50.5**	**105.8**	**176.3**	**350.7**	**1081.8**
1995 projected	*42.3**	*5.8**	*26.4**	*9.3*	*7.4*	*9.0*	*13.4*	*20.8*	*42.2*	*82.7*	*138.2*	*289.8*	*1005.5*
Vascular disease													
1955	459.9*	26.0*	426.0*	46.1	74.3	123.3	247.3	391.9	763.8	1335.1	2298.2	4138.4	7275.5
1965	442.5*	17.0*	400.3*	44.7	84.3	125.8	205.8	370.9	720.8	1249.8	2289.3	3981.3	7257.8
1975	495.1*	12.5*	447.2*	50.0	84.5	143.7	257.6	442.9	761.2	1390.7	2543.5	4558.1	8177.8
1985	384.1*	11.3*	324.4*	37.8	68.2	115.9	198.4	332.8	578.3	939.5	1738.4	3184.1	7334.1
1990	**322.2***	**9.8***	**266.6***	**32.9**	**59.4**	**95.6**	**163.3**	**267.7**	**453.6**	**793.6**	**1370.3**	**2530.7**	**6527.5**
1995 projected	*265.2**	*9.5**	*212.2**	*30.3*	*49.3*	*78.2*	*130.1*	*209.1*	*364.4*	*624.1*	*1069.5*	*2007.8*	*5621.4*
Liver cirrhosis													
1955	23.3*	1.2*	40.3*	7.2	14.8	23.5	40.0	49.9	70.8	75.8	102.6	95.6	107.5
1965	32.4*	0.9*	58.4*	6.4	14.4	36.0	56.0	74.5	97.5	124.1	135.4	150.7	132.2
1975	39.7*	1.4*	73.8*	11.1	22.2	45.2	67.8	96.8	123.2	150.2	158.8	172.2	126.5
1985	34.7*	1.5*	64.7*	12.2	24.1	38.2	62.1	84.6	110.7	120.9	137.2	132.2	111.8
1990	**30.3***	**1.5***	**55.6***	**12.6**	**19.5**	**33.1**	**52.1**	**72.3**	**90.9**	**108.4**	**116.3**	**125.3**	**107.3**
1995 projected	*26.2**	*1.8**	*46.6**	*12.1*	*16.7*	*27.4*	*43.5*	*59.3*	*76.6*	*90.8*	*101.5*	*113.8*	*102.1*
Other medical causes													
1955	556.4*	210.3*	457.2*	129.2	172.1	237.0	339.2	463.1	755.6	1104.6	1794.5	3184.3	7703.8
1965	364.6*	109.0*	308.2*	83.5	111.4	143.0	226.5	335.0	519.1	738.8	1319.2	2208.7	5337.9
1975	201.9*	69.4*	174.2*	41.8	57.0	84.8	126.7	186.1	281.4	442.0	737.6	1205.9	2654.3
1985	150.0*	34.6*	121.4*	28.8	34.1	53.2	83.1	124.6	205.0	321.3	592.1	1032.3	2422.3
1990	**156.6***	**44.1***	**120.8***	**41.1**	**46.6**	**58.6**	**76.2**	**117.9**	**183.1**	**321.8**	**556.8**	**1021.5**	**2579.0**
1995 projected	*160.7**	*51.1**	*118.1**	*59.0*	*57.5*	*61.4*	*72.3*	*105.6*	*171.9*	*298.8*	*529.9*	*1009.5*	*2687.6*
All non-medical causes													
1955	64.4*	38.8*	74.8*	66.6	64.7	73.6	72.8	72.3	82.9	91.1	113.9	145.9	365.1
1965	59.1*	39.5*	71.8*	53.0	51.8	64.2	71.6	83.2	90.4	88.4	117.7	120.9	184.9
1975	68.9*	42.2*	81.1*	68.3	68.9	70.2	72.5	84.6	95.9	107.7	142.7	189.3	302.9
1985	63.3*	43.6*	72.2*	60.1	64.6	67.1	71.2	84.6	80.1	77.6	115.0	152.3	233.4
1990	**71.4***	**56.4***	**75.7***	**68.1**	**61.9**	**66.1**	**72.4**	**86.5**	**88.5**	**86.7**	**111.4**	**160.2**	**259.4**
1995 projected	*82.5**	*76.1**	*78.1**	*77.0*	*62.0*	*64.2*	*71.6*	*88.8*	*93.7*	*89.1*	*112.6*	*158.4*	*282.4*

SPAIN: Females

	All ages	0–34	35–69	35–39	40–44	45–49	50–54	55–59	60–64	65–69	70–74	75–79	80+/NK
POPULATION (1000s)													
1955	14972	8659	5460	980	949	902	799	741	594	495	392	253	208
1965	16541	9122	6376	1166	1141	949	908	852	733	627	459	307	277
1975	18029	9823	6852	1027	1190	1139	1051	875	837	733	588	380	386
1985	19593	10191	7491	1222	1094	1046	1183	1118	1002	826	738	581	594
1990	**19837**	**9923**	**7793**	**1248**	**1216**	**1086**	**1034**	**1163**	**1088**	**958**	**763**	**633**	**726**
1995 projected	*20220*	*9815*	*8171*	*1455*	*1250*	*1208*	*1104*	*986*	*1120*	*1048*	*875*	*624*	*735*
NUMBER OF DEATHS													
All causes													
1955	134047	25380	40272	2206	2798	3497	4677	5949	8803	12342	16028	18859	33508
1965	129904	14104	38172	1738	2278	2898	4172	5890	8857	12339	16520	20475	40633
1975	142721	9767	36845	1186	1977	2975	4122	5511	8355	12719	19210	24111	52788
1985	147698	5114	29924	935	1304	1911	3348	4954	7277	10195	16669	25021	70970
1990	**156363**	**5210**	**29108**	**1015**	**1365**	**1816**	**2792**	**4702**	**6985**	**10433**	**14925**	**24048**	**83072**
1995 projected	*148366*	*5976*	*27186*	*1208*	*1336*	*1900*	*2758*	*3614*	*6390*	*9980*	*15029*	*21053*	*79122*
Lung cancer													
1955	487	19	313	18	24	43	44	56	62	66	64	54	37
1965	783	21	461	13	21	52	71	88	92	124	118	91	92
1975	1066	16	586	18	34	54	82	81	130	187	183	141	140
1985	1264	19	518	12	19	38	67	96	129	157	205	226	296
1990	**1320**	**20**	**545**	**26**	**33**	**37**	**43**	**95**	**129**	**182**	**176**	**233**	**346**
1995 projected	*1274*	*27*	*532*	*42*	*43*	*38*	*39*	*70*	*124*	*176*	*183*	*199*	*333*
ANNUAL DEATH RATE / 100,000 (*The rates for the age groups 0–34 and 35–69 are the means of seven five-yearly rates, but the all-ages rates are standardised to the conventional "European" age distribution)													
All causes													
1955	1070.4*	279.7*	895.9*	225.1	294.8	387.7	585.4	802.8	1482.0	2493.3	4088.8	7454.2	16109.6
1965	867.8*	139.5*	711.6*	149.1	199.6	305.4	459.5	691.3	1208.3	1967.9	3599.1	6667.2	14669.0
1975	771.4*	94.1*	614.0*	115.5	166.1	261.2	392.1	629.9	998.4	1734.5	3269.8	6348.3	13686.3
1985	579.9*	54.3*	437.8*	76.5	119.3	182.6	283.0	443.2	726.5	1233.7	2260.2	4306.5	11951.8
1990	**537.3***	**57.1***	**395.2***	**81.3**	**112.3**	**167.3**	**269.9**	**404.3**	**642.0**	**1089.4**	**1957.1**	**3797.3**	**11445.6**
1995 projected	*495.9**	*60.7**	*355.2**	*83.0*	*106.9*	*157.3*	*249.9*	*366.5*	*570.4*	*952.2*	*1717.2*	*3373.9*	*10764.9*
All cancer													
1955	115.1*	6.5*	173.7*	33.7	62.7	97.8	147.8	183.1	291.4	399.6	514.8	691.3	854.3
1965	130.0*	7.8*	184.5*	36.6	61.7	104.8	161.8	215.3	301.9	409.3	535.3	809.2	1194.6
1975	129.6*	9.1*	185.1*	39.8	62.6	105.9	151.0	220.9	289.6	425.6	590.3	837.3	1034.5
1985	115.1*	6.9*	158.9*	33.6	53.5	87.1	129.5	188.2	260.0	360.7	528.3	736.5	1055.1
1990	**117.7***	**6.5***	**165.4***	**36.2**	**54.0**	**86.9**	**135.6**	**190.1**	**273.6**	**381.1**	**510.9**	**725.2**	**1122.3**
1995 projected	*117.9**	*6.3**	*165.6**	*36.1*	*54.3*	*87.2*	*135.1*	*191.7*	*277.3*	*377.4*	*500.2*	*713.5*	*1158.0*
Lung cancer													
1955	3.9*	0.2*	6.6*	1.8	2.5	4.8	5.5	7.6	10.4	13.3	16.3	21.3	17.8
1965	5.3*	0.2*	8.4*	1.1	1.8	5.5	7.8	10.3	12.6	19.8	25.7	29.6	33.2
1975	6.0*	0.2*	9.6*	1.8	2.9	4.7	7.8	9.3	15.5	25.5	31.1	37.1	36.3
1985	5.5*	0.2*	7.5*	1.0	1.7	3.6	5.7	8.6	12.9	19.0	27.8	38.9	49.8
1990	**5.2***	**0.2***	**7.3***	**2.1**	**2.7**	**3.4**	**4.2**	**8.2**	**11.9**	**19.0**	**23.1**	**36.8**	**47.7**
1995 projected	*4.9**	*0.2**	*6.9**	*2.9*	*3.4*	*3.1*	*3.5*	*7.1*	*11.1*	*16.8*	*20.9*	*31.9*	*45.3*
Upper aerodigestive cancer (mouth, oesophagus, pharynx and larynx)													
1955	2.4*	0.1*	2.9*	0.5	0.7	1.4	2.0	3.5	4.5	7.3	12.5	19.0	25.0
1965	3.5*	0.1*	3.9*	0.3	1.1	2.3	2.4	5.3	4.8	10.8	12.6	28.0	53.1
1975	2.8*	0.1*	3.4*	0.6	0.9	1.1	2.7	3.2	7.3	8.3	15.3	20.0	29.8
1985	2.3*	0.1*	2.6*	0.7	0.6	0.4	1.9	3.5	5.4	5.6	12.1	18.9	25.6
1990	**2.4***	**0.1***	**3.0***	**0.5**	**1.4**	**1.6**	**3.0**	**4.3**	**4.5**	**5.7**	**9.3**	**14.1**	**30.0**
1995 projected	*2.4**	*0.1**	*3.2**	*0.6*	*1.9*	*2.2*	*4.2*	*4.6*	*4.4*	*4.8*	*7.3*	*13.3*	*29.8*
Other cancer													
1955	108.8*	6.2*	164.3*	31.3	59.4	91.6	140.3	172.1	276.4	379.0	486.0	651.0	811.5
1965	121.2*	7.5*	172.2*	35.2	58.7	97.0	151.5	199.6	284.6	378.6	496.9	751.5	1108.3
1975	120.8*	8.8*	172.0*	37.5	58.8	100.1	140.5	208.5	266.7	391.8	543.8	780.1	968.4
1985	107.4*	6.6*	148.9*	32.0	51.1	83.0	122.0	176.1	241.7	336.2	488.4	678.7	979.6
1990	**110.2***	**6.2***	**155.0***	**33.6**	**49.9**	**81.9**	**128.4**	**177.6**	**257.3**	**356.4**	**478.5**	**674.4**	**1044.6**
1995 projected	*110.6**	*6.0**	*155.5**	*32.6*	*48.9*	*81.9*	*127.4*	*180.1*	*261.8*	*355.9*	*472.0*	*668.3*	*1082.9*
Chronic obstructive pulmonary disease (COPD)													
1955	34.0*	6.3*	25.3*	4.9	4.7	6.0	11.3	19.6	43.3	87.5	151.8	291.7	576.9
1965	30.0*	2.9*	20.4*	2.1	3.2	4.3	7.7	13.8	39.0	72.4	137.3	272.9	600.4
1975	33.1*	1.5*	21.6*	3.1	4.0	6.1	10.0	16.3	34.1	77.5	154.2	331.8	683.7
1985	13.7*	0.3*	7.8*	0.9	1.6	2.2	3.6	7.6	11.6	27.0	55.3	120.0	339.2
1990	**13.8***	**0.3***	**8.3***	**0.7**	**1.5**	**1.1**	**4.6**	**8.4**	**13.5**	**27.9**	**59.5**	**114.8**	**334.9**
1995 projected	*13.6**	*0.2**	*8.6**	*0.7*	*1.0*	*1.1*	*4.8*	*9.5*	*14.1*	*29.2*	*58.5*	*110.9*	*328.0*
Other respiratory disease													
1955	82.0*	44.9*	35.6*	7.8	8.7	12.4	19.1	25.1	60.4	115.6	236.2	515.8	1363.5
1965	49.2*	21.7*	16.8*	4.1	3.7	6.2	9.5	14.7	23.2	56.5	143.8	334.1	1012.6
1975	48.0*	8.3*	20.4*	3.8	4.5	7.2	9.4	20.9	32.4	64.6	168.7	392.0	1167.2
1985	29.4*	2.5*	13.5*	1.7	3.1	4.1	7.0	10.6	25.5	42.8	95.2	221.5	805.8
1990	**26.9***	**2.3***	**11.3***	**2.6**	**2.4**	**4.6**	**6.5**	**8.9**	**17.6**	**36.3**	**79.3**	**183.3**	**782.7**
1995 projected	*24.2**	*2.2**	*9.3**	*3.2*	*2.5*	*4.3*	*5.8*	*6.7*	*13.6*	*28.9*	*64.8*	*155.8*	*736.1*
Vascular disease													
1955	381.1*	24.5*	318.9*	52.0	68.4	93.0	165.1	270.3	548.0	1035.2	1811.7	3435.2	6708.7
1965	359.5*	10.7*	265.7*	29.6	49.8	80.6	131.5	227.8	470.8	869.5	1707.6	3378.7	7145.1
1975	368.4*	8.9*	235.7*	25.6	43.0	70.8	113.4	211.1	396.6	789.0	1690.0	3596.9	7976.1
1985	277.8*	6.3*	141.8*	13.5	23.6	39.2	67.7	119.0	240.0	489.8	1051.5	2323.4	7388.3
1990	**233.7***	**4.6***	**105.4***	**12.3**	**17.8**	**29.3**	**50.7**	**91.4**	**175.2**	**361.5**	**829.1**	**1864.7**	**6639.4**
1995 projected	*194.1**	*3.6**	*77.7**	*9.7*	*13.6*	*21.6*	*37.4*	*66.0*	*125.7*	*270.2*	*644.1*	*1492.8*	*5813.6*
Liver cirrhosis													
1955	12.7*	0.8*	20.5*	4.9	7.6	11.8	15.6	24.7	34.3	44.2	46.4	65.6	93.8
1965	13.8*	0.6*	22.8*	4.0	7.4	13.8	19.8	25.6	41.1	47.7	61.4	80.1	69.3
1975	14.6*	0.7*	23.2*	4.8	8.1	13.3	20.4	30.3	37.4	48.0	59.7	84.3	92.6
1985	11.4*	0.7*	19.8*	3.9	5.7	10.3	16.2	23.7	35.6	43.2	48.9	52.5	54.7
1990	**10.0***	**0.5***	**16.4***	**3.1**	**5.2**	**7.7**	**13.3**	**19.3**	**27.9**	**38.1**	**45.2**	**56.8**	**53.7**
1995 projected	*8.7**	*0.4**	*13.3**	*2.7*	*4.1*	*6.2*	*10.4*	*15.1*	*22.6*	*32.3*	*43.1*	*54.5*	*55.5*
Other medical causes													
1955	424.3*	186.1*	298.2*	106.6	125.6	148.7	204.0	260.2	473.1	768.9	1267.3	2366.0	6383.7
1965	267.3*	84.8*	181.5*	56.6	58.2	80.4	112.4	171.9	306.5	484.1	974.7	1733.6	4549.5
1975	152.7*	54.3*	105.3*	27.5	31.8	42.1	65.8	104.9	175.1	289.6	531.7	988.2	2450.1
1985	113.1*	25.8*	74.5*	11.2	17.1	25.1	40.4	71.3	123.3	233.1	431.7	792.3	2197.7
1990	**113.7***	**28.1***	**66.0***	**13.5**	**16.0**	**21.8**	**36.7**	**59.6**	**107.1**	**207.5**	**385.1**	**785.6**	**2395.8**
1995 projected	*113.6**	*29.8**	*57.4**	*16.3*	*15.0*	*19.4*	*30.9*	*50.1*	*90.9*	*179.6*	*358.0*	*780.4*	*2549.1*
All non-medical causes													
1955	21.1*	10.7*	23.8*	15.2	17.1	18.1	22.4	19.8	31.5	42.4	60.5	88.5	128.8
1965	18.1*	11.0*	20.0*	16.0	15.7	15.2	16.7	22.2	25.8	28.5	39.0	58.6	97.5
1975	25.0*	11.3*	22.8*	10.9	12.2	15.9	22.2	25.4	33.3	40.1	75.1	118.0	282.1
1985	19.4*	11.8*	21.4*	11.6	14.7	14.6	18.5	22.8	30.6	37.0	49.2	60.4	111.0
1990	**21.6***	**14.7***	**22.5***	**13.0**	**15.5**	**15.8**	**22.5**	**26.5**	**27.1**	**37.0**	**47.9**	**66.8**	**116.6**
1995 projected	*23.8**	*18.2**	*23.1**	*14.4*	*16.4*	*17.6*	*25.5*	*27.3*	*26.3*	*34.5*	*48.6*	*66.0*	*124.6*

SPAIN: 1975

Smoking-attributed deaths (Sm.) and total deaths (Total)

		ALL CAUSES	ALL CANCER	Lung cancer	Upper aero-digestive ca.	Other cancer	COPD	Other respiratory	Vascular disease	Liver cirrhosis	Other medical	Non-medical
Males												
0–34	Sm.	–	–	–	–	–	–	–	–	–	–	–
	Total	15535	1051	47	29	975	211	1183	1168	120	7803	3999
35–69	Sm.	14412	5417	3245	1162	1010	2444	420	4293	–	1838	–
	Total	61758	15947	3678	2221	10048	3618	2163	22113	3956	9106	4855
		(23%)	(34%)	(88%)	(52%)	(10%)	(68%)	(19%)	(19%)		(20%)	
70+	Sm.	10527	2993	1828	493	672	3655	353	2721	–	805	–
	Total	78178	12656	2169	1126	9361	6284	5359	39151	1360	11663	1705
		(13%)	(24%)	(84%)	(44%)	(7%)	(58%)	(7%)	(7%)		(7%)	
Any age	Sm.	24939	8410	5073	1655	1682	6099	773	7014	–	2643	–
	Total	155471	29654	5894	3376	20384	10113	8705	62432	5436	28572	10559
		(16%)	(28%)	(86%)	(49%)	(8%)	(60%)	(9%)	(11%)		(9%)	
Females												
0–34	Sm.	–	–	–	–	–	–	–	–	–	–	–
	Total	9767	837	16	8	813	152	904	831	65	5854	1124
35–69	Sm.	0	0	0	0	0	0	0	0	–	0	–
	Total	36845	11424	586	207	10631	1250	1201	13726	1441	6339	1464
		(0%)	(0%)	(0%)	(0%)	(0%)	(0%)	(0%)	(0%)		(0%)	
70+	Sm.	0	0	0	0	0	0	0	0	–	0	–
	Total	96109	10638	464	281	9893	4803	6982	54354	1028	16327	1977
		(0%)	(0%)	(0%)	(0%)	(0%)	(0%)	(0%)	(0%)		(0%)	
Any age	Sm.	0	0	0	0	0	0	0	0	–	0	–
	Total	142721	22899	1066	496	21337	6205	9087	68911	2534	28520	4565
		(0%)	(0%)	(0%)	(0%)	(0%)	(0%)	(0%)	(0%)		(0%)	
Males+Females												
0–34	Sm.	–	–	–	–	–	–	–	–	–	–	–
	Total	25302	1888	63	37	1788	363	2087	1999	185	13657	5123
35–69	Sm.	14412	5417	3245	1162	1010	2444	420	4293	–	1838	–
	Total	98603	27371	4264	2428	20679	4868	3364	35839	5397	15445	6319
		(15%)	(20%)	(76%)	(48%)	(5%)	(50%)	(12%)	(12%)		(12%)	
70+	Sm.	10527	2993	1828	493	672	3655	353	2721	–	805	–
	Total	174287	23294	2633	1407	19254	11087	12341	93505	2388	27990	3682
		(6%)	(13%)	(69%)	(35%)	(3%)	(33%)	(3%)	(3%)		(3%)	
Any age	Sm.	24939	8410	5073	1655	1682	6099	773	7014	–	2643	–
	Total	298192	52553	6960	3872	41721	16318	17792	131343	7970	57092	15124
		(8%)	(16%)	(73%)	(43%)	(4%)	(37%)	(4%)	(5%)		(5%)	

SPAIN: 1985

Smoking-attributed deaths (Sm.) and total deaths (Total)

		ALL CAUSES	ALL CANCER	Lung cancer	Upper aero-digestive ca.	Other cancer	COPD	Other respiratory	Vascular disease	Liver cirrhosis	Other medical	Non-medical
Males												
0–34	Sm.	–	–	–	–	–	–	–	–	–	–	–
	Total	10476	850	42	26	782	48	402	1129	140	3303	4604
35–69	Sm.	17374	8485	5296	1694	1495	1538	566	4874	–	1911	–
	Total	60274	19913	5812	2803	11298	2089	2260	19380	4165	7428	5039
		(29%)	(43%)	(91%)	(60%)	(13%)	(74%)	(25%)	(25%)		(26%)	
70+	Sm.	15804	5826	3731	744	1351	4043	574	4023	–	1338	–
	Total	94084	19321	4231	1421	13669	6061	6365	44221	1574	14627	1915
		(17%)	(30%)	(88%)	(52%)	(10%)	(67%)	(9%)	(9%)		(9%)	
Any age	Sm.	33178	14311	9027	2438	2846	5581	1140	8897	–	3249	–
	Total	164834	40084	10085	4250	25749	8198	9027	64730	5879	25358	11558
		(20%)	(36%)	(90%)	(57%)	(11%)	(68%)	(13%)	(14%)		(13%)	
Females												
0–34	Sm.	–	–	–	–	–	–	–	–	–	–	–
	Total	5114	677	19	11	647	33	232	600	69	2309	1194
35–69	Sm.	0	0	0	0	0	0	0	0	–	0	–
	Total	29924	11128	518	180	10430	518	908	9416	1389	5023	1542
		(0%)	(0%)	(0%)	(0%)	(0%)	(0%)	(0%)	(0%)		(0%)	
70+	Sm.	0	0	0	0	0	0	0	0	–	0	–
	Total	112660	14440	727	351	13362	3119	6774	65126	991	20837	1373
		(0%)	(0%)	(0%)	(0%)	(0%)	(0%)	(0%)	(0%)		(0%)	
Any age	Sm.	0	0	0	0	0	0	0	0	–	0	–
	Total	147698	26245	1264	542	24439	3670	7914	75142	2449	28169	4109
		(0%)	(0%)	(0%)	(0%)	(0%)	(0%)	(0%)	(0%)		(0%)	
Males+Females												
0–34	Sm.	–	–	–	–	–	–	–	–	–	–	–
	Total	15590	1527	61	37	1429	81	634	1729	209	5612	5798
35–69	Sm.	17374	8485	5296	1694	1495	1538	566	4874	–	1911	–
	Total	90198	31041	6330	2983	21728	2607	3168	28796	5554	12451	6581
		(19%)	(27%)	(84%)	(57%)	(7%)	(59%)	(18%)	(17%)		(15%)	
70+	Sm.	15804	5826	3731	744	1351	4043	574	4023	–	1338	–
	Total	206744	33761	4958	1772	27031	9180	13139	109347	2565	35464	3288
		(8%)	(17%)	(75%)	(42%)	(5%)	(44%)	(4%)	(4%)		(4%)	
Any age	Sm.	33178	14311	9027	2438	2846	5581	1140	8897	–	3249	–
	Total	312532	66329	11349	4792	50188	11868	16941	139872	8328	53527	15667
		(11%)	(22%)	(80%)	(51%)	(6%)	(47%)	(7%)	(6%)		(6%)	

(To be conservative, no deaths before age 35, and none from liver cirrhosis or non-medical causes, were attributed to smoking.)

SPAIN: 1990

Smoking-attributed deaths (Sm.) and total deaths (Total)

		ALL CAUSES	ALL CANCER	Lung cancer	Upper aero-digestive ca.	Other cancer	COPD	Other respiratory	Vascular disease	Liver cirrhosis	Other medical	Non-medical
Males												
0–34	Sm.	–	–	–	–	–	–	–	–	–	–	–
	Total	12825	848	62	17	769	38	472	1024	157	4059	6227
35–69	Sm.	20516	10875	6770	2209	1896	1889	579	4842	–	2331	–
	Total	62931	23343	7337	3439	12567	2472	2122	17517	3814	8129	5534
		(33%)	(47%)	(92%)	(64%)	(15%)	(76%)	(27%)	(28%)		(29%)	
70+	Sm.	19440	7352	4702	869	1781	5554	629	4218	–	1687	–
	Total	101023	23051	5263	1569	16219	8012	6509	42633	1554	17016	2248
		(19%)	(32%)	(89%)	(55%)	(11%)	(69%)	(10%)	(10%)		(10%)	
Any age	Sm.	39956	18227	11472	3078	3677	7443	1208	9060	–	4018	–
	Total	176779	47242	12662	5025	29555	10522	9103	61174	5525	29204	14009
		(23%)	(39%)	(91%)	(61%)	(12%)	(71%)	(13%)	(15%)		(14%)	
Females												
0–34	Sm.	–	–	–	–	–	–	–	–	–	–	–
	Total	5210	654	20	9	625	28	205	450	54	2307	1512
35–69	Sm.	0	0	0	0	0	0	0	0	–	0	–
	Total	29108	12292	545	225	11522	599	821	7642	1218	4824	1712
		(0%)	(0%)	(0%)	(0%)	(0%)	(0%)	(0%)	(0%)		(0%)	
70+	Sm.	0	0	0	0	0	0	0	0	–	0	–
	Total	122045	16635	755	378	15502	3612	7447	66321	1095	25301	1634
		(0%)	(0%)	(0%)	(0%)	(0%)	(0%)	(0%)	(0%)		(0%)	
Any age	Sm.	0	0	0	0	0	0	0	0	–	0	–
	Total	156363	29581	1320	612	27649	4239	8473	74413	2367	32432	4858
		(0%)	(0%)	(0%)	(0%)	(0%)	(0%)	(0%)	(0%)		(0%)	
Males+Females												
0–34	Sm.	–	–	–	–	–	–	–	–	–	–	–
	Total	18035	1502	82	26	1394	66	677	1474	211	6366	7739
35–69	Sm.	20516	10875	6770	2209	1896	1889	579	4842	–	2331	–
	Total	92039	35635	7882	3664	24089	3071	2943	25159	5032	12953	7246
		(22%)	(31%)	(86%)	(60%)	(8%)	(62%)	(20%)	(19%)		(18%)	
70+	Sm.	19440	7352	4702	869	1781	5554	629	4218	–	1687	–
	Total	223068	39686	6018	1947	31721	11624	13956	108954	2649	42317	3882
		(9%)	(19%)	(78%)	(45%)	(6%)	(48%)	(5%)	(4%)		(4%)	
Any age	Sm.	39956	18227	11472	3078	3677	7443	1208	9060	–	4018	–
	Total	333142	76823	13982	5637	57204	14761	17576	135587	7892	61636	18867
		(12%)	(24%)	(82%)	(55%)	(6%)	(50%)	(7%)	(7%)		(7%)	

SPAIN: 1995

Smoking-attributed deaths (Sm.) and total deaths (Total)

		ALL CAUSES	ALL CANCER	Lung cancer	Upper aero-digestive ca.	Other cancer	COPD	Other respiratory	Vascular disease	Liver cirrhosis	Other medical	Non-medical
Males												
0–34	Sm.	–	–	–	–	–	–	–	–	–	–	–
	Total	16877	926	100	17	809	38	645	1065	207	5357	8639
35–69	Sm.	22697	12859	8003	2668	2188	2201	552	4388	–	2697	–
	Total	62825	25646	8594	3972	13080	2813	1845	14647	3329	8515	6030
		(36%)	(50%)	(93%)	(67%)	(17%)	(78%)	(30%)	(30%)		(32%)	
70+	Sm.	23003	9214	5933	1021	2260	6901	655	4188	–	2045	–
	Total	101641	26646	6554	1743	18349	9577	6004	37214	1562	18124	2514
		(23%)	(35%)	(91%)	(59%)	(12%)	(72%)	(11%)	(11%)		(11%)	
Any age	Sm.	45700	22073	13936	3689	4448	9102	1207	8576	–	4742	–
	Total	181343	53218	15248	5732	32238	12428	8494	52926	5098	31996	17183
		(25%)	(41%)	(91%)	(64%)	(14%)	(73%)	(14%)	(16%)		(15%)	
Females												
0–34	Sm.	–	–	–	–	–	–	–	–	–	–	–
	Total	5976	652	27	8	617	24	220	369	43	2791	1877
35–69	Sm.	0	0	0	0	0	0	0	0	–	0	–
	Total	27186	12700	532	249	11919	647	714	5876	1021	4394	1834
		(0%)	(0%)	(0%)	(0%)	(0%)	(0%)	(0%)	(0%)		(0%)	
70+	Sm.	0	0	0	0	0	0	0	0	–	0	–
	Total	115204	17341	715	366	16260	3615	6949	57682	1125	26739	1753
		(0%)	(0%)	(0%)	(0%)	(0%)	(0%)	(0%)	(0%)		(0%)	
Any age	Sm.	0	0	0	0	0	0	0	0	–	0	–
	Total	148366	30693	1274	623	28796	4286	7883	63927	2189	33924	5464
		(0%)	(0%)	(0%)	(0%)	(0%)	(0%)	(0%)	(0%)		(0%)	
Males+Females												
0–34	Sm.	–	–	–	–	–	–	–	–	–	–	–
	Total	22853	1578	127	25	1426	62	865	1434	250	8148	10516
35–69	Sm.	22697	12859	8003	2668	2188	2201	552	4388	–	2697	–
	Total	90011	38346	9126	4221	24999	3460	2559	20523	4350	12909	7864
		(25%)	(34%)	(88%)	(63%)	(9%)	(64%)	(22%)	(21%)		(21%)	
70+	Sm.	23003	9214	5933	1021	2260	6901	655	4188	–	2045	–
	Total	216845	43987	7269	2109	34609	13192	12953	94896	2687	44863	4267
		(11%)	(21%)	(82%)	(48%)	(7%)	(52%)	(5%)	(4%)		(5%)	
Any age	Sm.	45700	22073	13936	3689	4448	9102	1207	8576	–	4742	–
	Total	329709	83911	16522	6355	61034	16714	16377	116853	7287	65920	22647
		(14%)	(26%)	(84%)	(58%)	(7%)	(54%)	(7%)	(7%)		(7%)	

(To be conservative, no deaths before age 35, and none from liver cirrhosis or non-medical causes, were attributed to smoking.)

SWEDEN: 1990

		No. of deaths			Standardised rates (Defined on p.496)			Annual death rates / 100, 000						
		All ages	0–34	35–69	All ages	0–34	35–69	0–4	5–9	10–14	15–19	20–24	25–29	30–34
ALL CAUSES	M	49050	1645	13006	885.9	80.1	832.9	174.1	18.5	16.5	62.6	85.2	95.9	107.8
	F	46092	882	7453	547.9	45.8	448.4	135.3	13.1	16.5	26.8	32.1	43.3	53.7
Tuberculosis	M	58	–	8	1.0	–	0.5	–	–	–	–	–	–	–
	F	58	–	10	0.7	–	0.6	–	–	–	–	–	–	–
Other infective	M	258	19	75	4.8	0.9	4.7	3.2	0.4	–	1.0	0.3	0.6	1.0
and parasitic	F	252	12	34	3.0	0.6	2.1	3.3	–	0.4	–	0.3	–	0.4
ALL CANCER	M	10682	115	3706	197.4	5.7	241.4	3.9	7.2	1.2	3.8	6.1	8.0	9.5
	F	9649	111	3489	143.8	5.8	210.2	3.3	5.1	3.3	4.0	2.4	9.9	12.4
Mouth and	M	187	3	102	3.8	0.1	6.6	–	–	–	0.3	0.3	0.3	–
pharynx cancer	F	115	1	28	1.5	0.1	1.7	–	–	–	–	–	–	0.4
Oesophagus cancer	M	222	1	90	4.3	0.0	6.0	–	–	–	–	–	–	0.3
	F	108	–	25	1.4	–	1.5	–	–	–	–	–	–	–
Stomach cancer	M	722	4	240	13.2	0.2	15.8	–	–	–	–	–	0.3	1.0
	F	505	3	141	6.8	0.2	8.5	–	–	–	–	–	0.3	0.7
Colorectal cancer	M	1233	9	399	22.5	0.4	26.1	–	–	–	0.3	0.6	1.0	1.0
	F	1299	5	357	17.5	0.3	21.9	0.4	–	–	–	–	0.7	0.7
Liver cancer	M	198	2	88	3.8	0.1	5.8	0.4	–	–	–	–	0.3	–
	F	152	1	58	2.3	0.0	3.5	–	–	–	–	–	0.3	–
Pancreas cancer	M	646	–	255	12.1	–	16.7	–	–	–	–	–	–	–
	F	736	–	211	10.0	–	12.9	–	–	–	–	–	–	–
Larynx cancer	M	57	–	24	1.1	–	1.6	–	–	–	–	–	–	–
	F	6	–	3	0.1	–	0.2	–	–	–	–	–	–	–
Lung cancer	M	1851	3	812	35.7	0.1	53.5	–	–	–	–	–	–	1.0
	F	836	6	407	14.0	0.3	24.6	–	–	–	–	–	0.7	1.4
Malignant melanoma	M	178	3	95	3.6	0.1	5.7	–	–	–	–	0.6	0.3	–
	F	132	4	71	2.3	0.2	4.1	–	–	–	–	–	1.0	0.4
Female breast cancer	F	1477	13	740	25.2	0.7	43.9	–	–	–	–	–	1.4	3.2
Cervix cancer	F	191	7	92	3.3	0.3	5.2	–	–	–	–	–	1.0	1.4
Other uterine cancer	F	291	1	99	4.2	0.1	6.2	–	–	–	–	–	–	0.4
Ovarian cancer	F	620	1	315	10.6	0.0	19.1	–	–	–	–	–	0.3	–
Prostate cancer	M	2093	–	363	35.2	–	24.5	–	–	–	–	–	–	–
Bladder cancer	M	390	–	83	6.7	–	5.6	–	–	–	–	–	–	–
	F	183	–	40	2.3	–	2.5	–	–	–	–	–	–	–
Other and ill-defined	M	1877	49	763	35.8	2.4	48.7	1.1	3.6	–	2.8	1.9	3.5	4.1
cancer sites	F	2147	46	683	30.7	2.4	41.4	2.2	2.1	2.1	2.9	1.7	2.7	3.2
Hodgkin's disease	M	22	2	7	0.4	0.1	0.4	–	–	–	–	–	0.3	0.3
	F	11	–	6	0.2	–	0.4	–	–	–	–	–	–	–
Myeloma and non-	M	646	11	262	12.3	0.6	16.7	0.4	0.8	0.4	0.3	0.3	1.0	0.7
Hodgkin lymphomas	F	542	4	143	7.2	0.2	8.6	–	0.4	–	0.4	–	0.7	–
Leukaemia	M	360	28	123	6.9	1.4	7.7	2.1	2.8	0.8	–	2.2	1.0	1.0
	F	298	19	70	4.1	1.0	4.2	0.7	2.5	1.2	0.7	0.7	0.7	0.7
ALL VASCULAR	M	24725	72	5554	430.1	3.5	365.2	2.8	1.2	1.2	2.4	2.6	5.5	8.8
DISEASE	F	23837	43	2034	247.5	2.2	124.0	2.2	0.4	1.2	1.1	2.7	3.4	4.3
Rheumatic heart	M	85	1	23	1.5	0.0	1.5	–	–	–	–	–	0.3	–
disease and fever	F	184	2	22	2.1	0.1	1.3	–	–	–	–	0.3	–	0.4
Hypertensive disease	M	219	–	34	3.7	–	2.2	–	–	–	–	–	–	–
	F	295	–	16	2.9	–	1.0	–	–	–	–	–	–	–
Ischaemic heart	M	14882	13	3911	263.0	0.6	258.2	–	–	–	0.3	0.3	0.6	3.0
disease	F	10937	3	1151	117.0	0.2	70.4	–	–	–	–	–	0.3	0.7
Pulmonary embolism	M	544	7	131	9.6	0.3	8.4	0.4	0.4	–	–	0.3	0.3	1.0
and other venous	F	735	2	107	8.4	0.1	6.5	–	–	–	–	0.3	–	0.4
Cerebrovascular	M	4284	16	708	72.5	0.8	46.1	0.7	–	–	0.7	0.6	1.3	2.0
disease	F	6010	15	441	61.7	0.8	26.8	0.4	–	0.4	0.7	0.3	2.0	1.4
Other vascular	M	4711	35	747	79.8	1.7	48.8	1.8	0.8	1.2	1.4	1.3	2.9	2.7
disease	F	5676	21	297	55.3	1.1	18.0	1.9	0.4	0.8	0.4	1.7	1.0	1.4
Chronic obstructive	M	1280	14	259	22.1	0.7	17.2	–	–	0.4	0.7	1.6	1.3	0.7
pulmonary disease	F	784	9	205	10.3	0.5	12.6	–	–	–	0.7	0.3	1.0	1.1
Other respiratory	M	2508	12	235	41.3	0.6	15.1	2.1	–	–	0.3	0.3	–	1.4
disease	F	2572	17	108	24.6	0.9	6.5	2.2	–	0.4	0.4	0.3	0.7	2.1
Peptic ulcer	M	291	1	72	5.2	0.0	4.7	–	–	–	–	0.3	–	–
	F	252	–	31	2.8	–	1.9	–	–	–	–	–	–	–
Liver cirrhosis	M	424	5	293	9.2	0.2	18.1	–	–	–	–	0.3	–	1.4
	F	225	4	122	4.1	0.2	7.4	–	–	–	–	–	0.3	1.1
Renal disease	M	325	2	43	5.5	0.1	2.8	0.4	–	–	–	0.3	–	–
	F	316	5	41	3.6	0.3	2.5	0.7	–	0.4	–	–	0.3	0.4
Pregnancy and birth	F	4	4	–	0.1	0.2	–	–	–	–	–	0.3	0.7	0.4
Congenital and	M	379	337	24	10.3	17.0	1.5	108.2	3.6	2.4	1.7	1.3	1.3	0.7
perinatal causes	F	294	251	28	8.2	13.3	1.7	86.6	0.8	0.4	1.5	–	2.7	1.1
Ill-defined causes	M	605	119	121	12.0	5.9	7.4	34.9	–	–	0.3	0.6	1.3	4.4
	F	846	66	35	9.2	3.5	2.0	22.3	–	–	–	0.7	1.4	–
Other medical causes	M	4330	167	1175	78.8	8.1	71.9	10.2	1.6	2.8	4.2	7.4	13.5	16.9
	F	5193	83	744	60.0	4.3	44.5	7.8	1.7	4.5	1.5	3.7	4.8	6.4
ALL NON-	M	3185	782	1441	68.2	37.3	82.5	8.5	4.4	8.6	48.1	63.9	64.4	63.2
MEDICAL CAUSES	F	1810	277	572	29.9	14.1	32.5	6.7	5.1	5.8	17.8	21.3	18.1	24.2
Motor vehicle	M	504	243	173	11.2	11.6	9.9	2.1	2.4	2.0	24.9	21.2	17.4	11.5
traffic accidents	F	243	102	79	5.2	5.2	4.6	1.1	2.5	3.7	11.2	8.1	7.2	2.8
Fire	M	77	15	36	1.6	0.7	2.1	0.4	–	1.2	0.7	0.6	1.0	1.4
	F	25	4	11	0.4	0.2	0.6	0.7	–	–	0.4	0.3	–	–
Suicide	M	1020	249	552	22.5	11.7	31.3	–	–	1.6	8.0	20.9	24.8	27.0
	F	451	94	264	9.7	4.7	14.9	–	–	0.4	4.4	6.1	8.2	13.9
Homicide	M	70	30	33	1.6	1.4	1.8	0.4	0.8	0.4	1.0	2.6	2.6	2.4
	F	38	18	12	0.9	1.0	0.6	1.9	1.7	0.4	–	1.4	–	1.4
POPULATION (thousands):	M=males				4227.9	1994.3	1797.8	283.7	249.2	254.5	289.1	311.2	310.6	296.0
	F=females				4330.6	1893.5	1802.8	269.1	236.3	242.1	275.8	295.6	293.2	281.4

SWEDEN: 1990

Annual death rates / 100, 000

9th ICD categories

35–39	40–44	45–49	50–54	55–59	60–64	65–69	70–74	75–79	80+/NK			
137.0	209.7	320.5	501.3	903.3	1439.5	2319.2	4008.0	6811.4	14383.3	M	ALL CAUSES	001–999
77.5	124.1	203.4	288.0	508.7	730.7	1206.5	2078.9	3832.2	11060.2	F		
–	–	–	–	–	1.9	1.9	8.6	9.7	17.4	M	Tuberculosis	010–018, 137
–	–	–	–	0.9	0.9	2.5	5.2	8.1	9.3	F		
1.7	0.9	3.6	2.1	4.4	6.8	13.2	20.1	28.2	71.8	M	Other infective	Rest of 001–139
0.7	0.3	0.7	1.3	1.4	4.5	5.4	9.5	21.6	61.5	F	and parasitic	
23.3	39.5	73.2	135.6	268.4	439.5	710.0	1106.7	1521.9	2272.9	M	ALL CANCER	140–208
27.8	60.7	107.4	148.8	264.1	342.1	520.5	675.8	885.1	1254.8	F		
0.3	0.6	3.9	4.3	6.3	17.0	13.7	16.6	21.5	18.9	M	Mouth and	140–149
0.7	0.3	0.3	1.8	3.3	2.3	3.3	4.7	11.3	23.2	F	pharynx cancer	
–	0.3	0.3	6.0	6.3	13.6	15.5	27.5	28.2	35.5	M	Oesophagus cancer	150
0.3	–	1.0	1.3	1.4	1.8	4.6	8.0	15.7	15.6	F		
1.0	3.0	3.0	6.9	19.0	30.6	47.1	73.4	101.0	168.8	M	Stomach cancer	151
–	2.5	4.8	5.3	8.5	15.8	22.6	35.0	45.3	85.5	F		
2.3	3.6	7.6	12.9	30.1	50.6	75.8	126.2	199.7	265.0	M	Colorectal cancer	153, 154
2.1	2.5	6.9	11.4	30.2	39.3	61.0	87.0	126.3	218.6	F		
0.7	0.6	1.3	3.0	7.3	7.8	19.8	17.8	20.8	38.6	M	Liver cancer	155.0
0.7	0.6	2.1	1.8	4.7	4.5	10.0	13.7	15.7	14.7	F		
0.3	1.8	5.9	11.2	15.6	30.1	51.8	78.6	86.9	108.0	M	Pancreas cancer	157
0.7	1.8	3.5	10.1	13.2	20.8	40.1	57.2	83.6	104.9	F		
–	–	0.3	0.9	2.4	3.9	3.8	6.9	6.7	9.5	M	Larynx cancer	161
–	–	–	–	–	–	1.3	0.5	1.1	–	F		
3.0	4.2	15.1	33.0	71.0	97.2	150.7	219.2	231.6	269.7	M	Lung cancer	162
1.0	6.2	15.5	17.5	33.5	38.4	59.8	67.6	71.8	61.9	F		
2.0	2.1	5.3	7.3	4.9	4.9	13.7	18.9	15.6	20.5	M	Malignant melanoma	172
1.0	3.4	3.5	2.2	3.3	6.3	8.8	6.6	10.8	9.7	F		
10.4	19.4	34.5	37.2	65.2	67.8	72.7	88.4	99.3	148.7	F	Female breast cancer	174
2.8	4.3	4.1	4.4	5.2	5.4	10.5	13.7	17.8	12.6	F	Cervix cancer	180
0.7	0.3	0.7	2.6	10.9	11.3	16.7	22.7	23.7	41.7	F	Other uterine cancer	179, 182
1.4	5.2	10.4	19.3	25.0	31.6	40.6	49.1	50.7	44.7	F	Ovarian cancer	183
–	–	1.6	4.7	16.5	43.3	105.5	207.7	357.8	698.7	M	Prostate cancer	185
–	0.6	0.3	1.7	6.8	12.6	16.9	33.8	75.7	115.1	M	Bladder cancer	188
–	–	0.7	1.8	1.9	4.5	8.4	11.3	22.7	32.4	F		
8.0	14.6	19.4	26.2	57.4	85.6	129.9	177.3	256.9	323.3	M	Other and ill-defined	Rest of 140–208
3.8	10.8	13.5	25.4	45.3	72.3	118.7	149.8	206.7	302.4	F	cancer sites	
0.3	0.9	–	–	–	1.5	–	4.6	2.2	1.6	M	Hodgkin's disease	201
–	0.3	–	–	0.5	0.9	0.8	0.9	0.5	0.8	F		
3.3	5.1	5.6	11.6	19.9	27.2	44.3	63.1	70.5	132.5	M	Myeloma and non-	200, 202–203
1.7	1.5	3.5	3.5	8.0	13.6	28.4	42.5	57.7	83.4	F	Hodgkin lymphomas	
2.0	2.4	3.6	6.0	4.9	13.6	21.7	35.0	46.8	67.0	M	Leukaemia	204–208
0.3	1.5	2.4	3.5	3.8	5.4	12.1	17.0	24.3	53.9	F		
16.3	46.6	93.3	174.7	374.8	671.9	1178.9	2156.6	3797.3	8063.9	M	ALL VASCULAR	390–459
10.1	15.7	28.7	48.6	117.6	211.5	436.0	950.9	2092.3	6685.3	F	DISEASE	
–	–	–	0.9	0.5	1.0	8.5	9.2	14.8	19.7	M	Rheumatic heart	390–398
–	–	0.7	0.4	0.5	2.7	5.0	15.1	27.5	32.4	F	disease and fever	
–	0.9	1.0	0.9	2.4	6.3	3.8	18.9	40.8	76.5	M	Hypertensive disease	401–405
–	–	–	–	1.4	0.9	4.6	9.5	27.0	88.0	F		
6.3	25.5	63.4	126.2	265.9	477.9	842.3	1459.6	2297.7	4194.8	M	Ischaemic heart	410–414
2.4	6.5	13.5	21.9	60.0	126.1	262.5	526.0	1054.5	2829.0	F	disease	
–	2.4	4.3	5.2	7.8	13.6	25.4	47.6	91.3	157.7	M	Pulmonary embolism	415.1, 451–453
1.4	0.9	1.4	2.2	9.0	7.2	23.4	39.2	79.9	166.4	F	and other venous	
4.0	9.2	12.5	20.6	47.6	81.2	147.8	319.6	728.3	1594.6	M	Cerebrovascular	430–438
3.5	4.9	6.9	16.2	28.3	44.7	83.2	225.4	529.4	1725.4	F	disease	
6.0	8.6	12.2	21.0	50.6	91.9	151.1	301.8	624.4	2020.5	M	Other vascular	Rest of 390–459
2.8	3.4	6.2	7.9	18.4	29.8	57.3	135.6	374.0	1844.1	F	disease	
1.0	1.8	3.3	5.2	19.9	32.6	56.5	118.2	204.9	414.0	M	Chronic obstructive	490–496
1.4	0.6	2.4	6.6	12.8	19.9	44.3	53.4	83.6	127.2	F	pulmonary disease	
1.7	4.8	4.6	9.4	20.4	25.8	39.1	104.4	369.0	1247.6	M	Other respiratory	Rest of 460–519
1.4	1.8	1.7	5.3	4.7	7.2	23.0	45.4	167.8	859.3	F	disease	
0.7	0.3	1.0	4.7	5.3	6.8	14.1	20.7	36.4	104.9	M	Peptic ulcer	531–533
0.7	0.6	–	1.3	1.4	3.2	5.9	14.7	21.6	63.2	F		
2.3	7.4	14.8	16.3	22.4	35.5	27.8	27.0	33.4	26.8	M	Liver cirrhosis	571
2.1	2.5	3.1	7.4	11.3	15.4	10.0	14.7	17.3	15.2	F		
0.3	0.3	–	3.4	2.4	4.9	8.5	18.9	46.8	145.1	M	Renal disease	580–590
0.7	–	0.7	0.4	3.3	2.7	9.6	14.7	32.4	75.4	F		
–	–	–	–	–	–	–	–	–	–	F	Pregnancy and birth	630–676
0.7	–	1.0	0.9	2.9	1.0	4.2	2.3	1.5	9.5	M	Congenital and	740–779
0.3	0.3	1.4	1.3	2.4	3.2	2.9	1.9	2.2	2.9	F	perinatal causes	
2.7	4.5	3.3	8.6	13.1	10.7	8.9	11.5	28.2	242.1	M	Ill-defined causes	780–799
1.0	0.9	1.4	1.8	1.4	3.6	4.2	5.7	22.1	291.5	F		
26.7	36.8	41.1	57.1	79.7	101.6	160.1	297.2	544.2	1369.9	M	Other medical causes	Rest of 001–799
12.5	12.6	22.8	33.3	45.3	75.9	109.1	227.3	392.9	1329.8	F		
59.7	66.8	81.4	83.3	89.5	100.6	96.0	115.9	190.1	397.5	M	ALL NON-	E800–E999
18.8	28.0	33.1	31.9	42.0	40.7	33.0	60.0	85.3	284.8	F	MEDICAL CAUSES	
7.0	7.4	11.2	7.3	9.7	13.6	13.2	14.3	22.3	26.0	M	Motor vehicle	E810–E819
1.0	3.4	5.5	4.8	7.6	6.8	2.9	8.5	8.1	12.2	F	traffic accidents	
1.0	2.4	1.3	1.3	1.9	2.4	4.2	2.3	5.2	11.8	M	Fire	E890–E899
–	0.9	0.3	0.4	0.5	0.5	1.7	–	0.5	3.8	F		
27.7	26.7	29.2	33.5	29.2	36.5	36.3	43.0	50.5	59.9	M	Suicide	E950–E959
12.5	13.2	13.8	16.2	17.9	16.3	14.2	14.2	18.9	11.8	F		
1.7	2.4	2.3	2.1	1.9	0.5	1.4	–	1.5	3.9	M	Homicide	E960–E969
–	1.5	1.4	0.4	0.5	–	0.4	0.9	1.6	1.3	F		
299.9	336.6	304.5	233.0	205.7	205.7	212.4	174.3	134.7	126.8	M	POPULATION (thousands)	
287.8	324.7	289.6	228.5	211.7	221.3	239.2	211.6	185.3	237.4	F		

SWEDEN: Males

	All ages	0–34	35–69	35–39	40–44	45–49	50–54	55–59	60–64	65–69	70–74	75–79	80+/NK
POPULATION (1000s)													
1955	3619.6	1840.6	1550.9	267.8	274.5	265.2	234.1	202.2	168.2	138.9	104.4	71.4	52.3
1965	3861.6	1923.8	1662.6	238.9	273.0	262.1	264.0	248.1	208.9	167.6	123.5	83.4	68.3
1975	4074.7	2085.5	1650.5	244.3	222.4	233.8	262.1	245.1	236.6	206.2	153.6	100.9	84.2
1985	4123.8	1957.5	1753.6	337.7	307.5	237.5	213.0	218.4	234.5	205.0	176.7	127.8	108.2
1990	4227.9	1994.3	1797.8	299.9	336.6	304.5	233.0	205.7	205.7	212.4	174.3	134.7	126.8
1995 projected	4205.0	1928.0	1823.8	288.7	293.2	327.7	307.2	227.9	193.6	185.5	178.2	136.9	138.1
NUMBER OF DEATHS													
All causes													
1955	35542	2811	13387	507	703	1080	1575	2363	3123	4036	5054	5709	8581
1965	42031	2559	15293	473	681	984	1784	2581	3820	4970	6166	6744	11269
1975	48322	2236	17041	477	654	1059	1798	2646	4231	6176	7420	8075	13550
1985	50034	1596	14903	511	681	864	1274	2201	3825	5547	7716	9240	16579
1990	49050	1645	13006	411	706	976	1168	1858	2961	4926	6986	9175	18238
1995 projected	47027	1551	11270	367	558	916	1349	1808	2433	3839	6561	8673	18972
Lung cancer													
1955	537	4	375	7	5	26	52	92	121	72	86	53	19
1965	990	6	605	6	18	31	62	93	173	222	192	112	75
1975	1678	6	843	8	14	39	86	135	213	348	351	274	204
1985	1879	3	907	7	22	41	76	137	252	372	368	317	284
1990	1851	3	812	9	14	46	77	146	200	320	382	312	342
1995 projected	1786	4	739	7	10	42	102	155	167	256	362	316	365
ANNUAL DEATH RATE / 100,000 (*The rates for the age groups 0–34 and 35–69 are the means of seven five-yearly rates, but the all-ages rates are standardised to the conventional "European" age distribution)													
All causes													
1955	1098.8*	152.5*	1065.2*	189.3	256.1	407.2	672.8	1168.6	1856.7	2905.7	4841.0	7995.8	16407.3
1965	1087.8*	132.8*	1047.6*	198.0	249.5	375.4	675.8	1040.3	1828.6	2965.4	4992.7	8086.3	16499.3
1975	1069.6*	107.3*	1070.2*	195.3	294.1	453.0	686.0	1079.6	1788.3	2995.2	4830.7	8003.0	16092.6
1985	967.8*	82.2*	954.2*	151.3	221.5	363.8	598.1	1007.8	1631.1	2705.9	4366.7	7230.0	15322.6
1990	885.9*	80.1*	832.9*	137.0	209.7	320.5	501.3	903.3	1439.5	2319.2	4008.0	6811.4	14383.3
1995 projected	817.7*	78.2*	736.5*	127.1	190.3	279.5	439.1	793.3	1256.7	2069.5	3681.8	6335.3	13737.9
All cancer													
1955	177.4*	10.8*	228.2*	25.0	42.6	70.1	139.7	262.1	431.0	627.1	967.4	1348.7	1711.3
1965	192.5*	10.7*	235.7*	33.1	41.8	77.1	146.6	233.0	446.1	672.4	1064.8	1539.6	2014.6
1975	226.8*	8.8*	261.7*	24.2	51.3	102.7	157.6	267.2	468.3	760.4	1244.8	1792.9	2794.5
1985	200.8*	6.9*	250.9*	20.4	39.3	73.7	145.5	262.4	460.6	754.1	1041.3	1614.2	2268.9
1990	197.4*	5.7*	241.4*	23.3	39.5	73.2	135.6	268.4	439.5	710.0	1106.7	1521.9	2272.9
1995 projected	190.6*	4.7*	232.0*	23.2	40.2	69.3	131.2	254.9	412.7	692.2	1065.1	1485.0	2223.0
Lung cancer													
1955	15.7*	0.2*	29.4*	2.6	1.8	9.8	22.2	45.5	71.9	51.8	82.4	74.2	36.3
1965	24.5*	0.3*	42.5*	2.5	6.6	11.8	23.5	37.5	82.8	132.5	155.5	134.3	109.8
1975	36.0*	0.3*	53.3*	3.3	6.3	16.7	32.8	55.1	90.0	168.8	228.5	271.6	242.3
1985	37.3*	0.1*	59.1*	2.1	7.2	17.3	35.7	62.7	107.5	181.5	208.3	248.0	262.5
1990	35.7*	0.1*	53.5*	3.0	4.2	15.1	33.0	71.0	97.2	150.7	219.2	231.6	269.7
1995 projected	33.6*	0.2*	49.2*	2.4	3.4	12.8	33.2	68.0	86.3	138.0	203.1	230.8	264.3
Upper aerodigestive cancer (mouth, oesophagus, pharynx and larynx)													
1955	7.9*	0.3*	10.5*	0.4	0.4	4.1	6.4	12.9	20.8	28.8	40.2	47.6	89.9
1965	8.7*	0.1*	13.1*	0.4	2.6	4.2	4.9	16.1	26.8	37.0	47.8	60.0	67.3
1975	9.4*	0.1*	13.2*	–	1.8	5.1	8.8	16.3	23.7	36.4	46.2	72.3	87.9
1985	9.6*	0.0*	15.1*	0.6	1.3	2.9	6.1	21.5	25.2	47.8	46.4	66.5	81.3
1990	9.2*	0.2*	14.2*	0.3	0.9	4.6	11.2	15.1	34.5	33.0	51.1	56.4	63.9
1995 projected	8.5*	0.2*	13.9*	0.3	1.0	6.4	11.1	17.1	29.4	31.8	43.8	48.9	51.4
Other cancer													
1955	153.7*	10.2*	188.3*	22.0	40.4	56.2	111.1	203.8	338.3	546.4	844.8	1226.9	1585.1
1965	159.3*	10.3*	180.1*	30.1	32.6	61.0	118.2	179.4	336.5	503.0	861.5	1345.3	1837.5
1975	181.5*	8.5*	195.2*	20.9	43.2	80.8	116.0	195.8	354.6	555.3	970.1	1449.0	2464.4
1985	153.9*	6.7*	176.7*	17.8	30.9	53.5	103.8	178.1	327.9	524.9	786.6	1299.7	1925.1
1990	152.5*	5.3*	173.7*	20.0	34.5	53.5	91.4	182.3	307.7	526.4	836.5	1233.9	1939.3
1995 projected	148.4*	4.4*	168.9*	20.4	35.8	50.0	86.9	169.8	297.0	522.4	818.2	1205.3	1907.3
Chronic obstructive pulmonary disease (COPD)													
1955	6.9*	1.1*	7.2*	2.6	1.8	0.8	3.0	7.4	13.1	21.6	35.4	42.0	91.8
1965	13.5*	0.5*	13.0*	0.8	1.1	4.2	5.3	12.5	22.5	44.7	71.3	113.9	221.1
1975	23.9*	0.9*	23.2*	1.6	3.6	6.8	12.6	18.0	41.8	77.6	126.3	239.8	344.4
1985	25.7*	0.7*	22.4*	1.5	4.2	3.4	9.9	20.6	40.5	77.1	131.9	219.1	466.7
1990	22.1*	0.7*	17.2*	1.0	1.8	3.3	5.2	19.9	32.6	56.5	118.2	204.9	414.0
1995 projected	19.1*	0.7*	13.6*	0.7	1.4	2.1	4.2	15.8	25.3	45.8	103.3	177.5	373.6
Other respiratory disease													
1955	52.4*	9.2*	26.2*	4.5	4.4	9.8	12.8	24.7	49.3	77.8	197.3	438.4	1174.0
1965	59.9*	3.5*	26.3*	2.1	4.8	6.9	8.0	18.9	53.1	90.7	212.1	562.4	1573.9
1975	30.4*	2.0*	15.3*	3.3	6.7	8.1	8.4	18.0	21.1	41.2	110.0	246.8	774.3
1985	52.4*	1.4*	24.4*	3.6	4.2	8.0	16.4	25.6	42.2	70.7	167.5	430.4	1466.7
1990	41.3*	0.6*	15.1*	1.7	4.8	4.6	9.4	20.4	25.8	39.1	104.4	369.0	1247.6
1995 projected	33.5*	0.5*	10.5*	1.4	3.4	3.1	6.5	14.0	18.1	27.0	78.6	291.5	1062.3
Vascular disease													
1955	554.0*	6.2*	508.0*	27.3	59.7	128.2	261.9	538.6	918.0	1622.8	2787.4	4805.3	9732.3
1965	561.5*	5.1*	502.6*	33.5	60.8	116.0	271.2	481.7	922.9	1631.9	2859.1	4645.1	10313.3
1975	552.3*	4.4*	514.5*	22.1	59.8	130.9	282.3	503.9	923.1	1679.4	2701.2	4702.7	9839.7
1985	509.2*	4.8*	465.3*	26.7	46.2	114.9	253.5	477.1	840.5	1498.0	2580.6	4219.9	9175.6
1990	430.1*	3.5*	365.2*	16.3	46.6	93.3	174.7	374.8	671.9	1178.9	2156.6	3797.3	8063.9
1995 projected	362.5*	2.8*	284.2*	13.2	38.2	69.3	129.2	284.8	519.6	935.3	1822.7	3284.1	7136.1
Liver cirrhosis													
1955	5.1*	0.3*	9.1*	2.6	2.9	5.7	8.5	14.8	10.1	18.7	21.1	21.0	17.2
1965	7.3*	0.4*	12.5*	3.3	4.8	3.4	14.8	20.2	21.1	19.7	24.3	30.0	42.5
1975	16.5*	0.5*	32.2*	11.9	20.7	27.4	30.5	42.8	48.2	44.1	41.7	45.6	51.1
1985	8.8*	0.4*	17.5*	5.0	7.8	12.6	15.5	27.9	27.3	26.3	23.8	24.3	23.1
1990	9.2*	0.2*	18.1*	2.3	7.4	14.8	16.3	22.4	35.5	27.8	27.0	33.4	26.8
1995 projected	9.7*	0.2*	18.7*	1.7	7.2	15.6	15.3	22.8	36.7	31.8	31.4	37.3	34.0
Other medical causes													
1955	214.1*	71.5*	179.2*	60.9	60.5	98.0	131.6	196.3	293.1	414.0	648.5	1145.7	3265.8
1965	163.9*	59.7*	144.4*	42.3	49.1	66.4	106.4	149.5	227.9	369.3	598.4	973.6	2014.6
1975	124.3*	37.1*	107.0*	38.1	50.4	59.9	82.0	107.7	157.2	253.6	446.6	753.2	1760.1
1985	99.3*	29.5*	84.1*	24.0	41.6	52.6	72.3	92.9	120.3	184.9	303.3	545.4	1550.8
1990	117.5*	32.1*	93.5*	32.7	42.8	49.9	76.8	107.9	133.7	210.9	379.2	694.9	1960.6
1995 projected	138.2*	34.5*	103.2*	36.7	44.7	49.7	80.4	117.6	148.8	244.2	463.5	858.3	2482.3
All non-medical causes													
1955	89.1*	53.4*	107.3*	66.5	84.2	94.6	115.3	124.6	142.1	123.8	183.9	194.7	414.9
1965	89.2*	52.9*	113.0*	82.9	87.2	101.5	123.5	124.5	135.0	136.6	162.8	221.8	319.2
1975	95.3*	53.6*	116.4*	94.1	101.6	117.2	112.6	122.0	128.5	138.7	160.2	222.0	528.5
1985	71.5*	38.5*	89.6*	70.2	78.0	98.5	85.0	101.2	99.8	94.6	118.3	176.8	370.6
1990	68.2*	37.3*	82.5*	59.7	66.8	81.4	83.3	89.5	100.6	96.0	115.9	190.1	397.5
1995 projected	64.1*	34.8*	74.3*	50.2	55.3	70.5	72.3	83.4	95.6	93.3	117.3	201.6	426.5

SWEDEN: Females

	All ages	0–34	35–69	35–39	40–44	45–49	50–54	55–59	60–64	65–69	70–74	75–79	80+/NK
POPULATION (1000s)													
1955	3642.7	1783.1	1591.0	262.5	268.8	264.2	240.3	212.9	185.0	157.3	119.9	82.9	65.8
1965	3872.3	1831.8	1691.9	236.1	269.5	258.6	261.8	253.0	224.0	188.9	150.0	106.4	92.2
1975	4118.2	1978.8	1675.7	232.4	218.7	234.4	264.1	249.4	247.3	229.4	189.0	137.8	136.9
1985	4226.6	1867.2	1766.9	324.1	290.6	230.3	214.9	227.1	250.7	229.2	214.3	177.7	200.5
1990	**4330.6**	**1893.5**	**1802.8**	**287.8**	**324.7**	**289.6**	**228.5**	**211.7**	**221.3**	**239.2**	**211.6**	**185.3**	**237.4**
1995 projected	*4304.3*	*1832.4*	*1812.9*	*276.6*	*283.3*	*318.2*	*295.0*	*226.7*	*203.8*	*209.3*	*217.4*	*187.6*	*254.0*
NUMBER OF DEATHS													
All causes													
1955	33092	1806	10606	365	562	854	1243	1691	2353	3538	4814	5786	10080
1965	36163	1520	10008	272	491	699	1095	1606	2342	3503	5002	6549	13084
1975	39880	1189	9387	228	366	614	1025	1416	2209	3529	5154	7160	16990
1985	43979	910	7910	298	358	435	711	1165	1957	2986	4787	7519	22853
1990	**46092**	**882**	**7453**	**223**	**403**	**589**	**658**	**1077**	**1617**	**2886**	**4399**	**7101**	**26257**
1995 projected	*45968*	*772*	*6821*	*193*	*352*	*619*	*823*	*1084*	*1402*	*2348*	*4141*	*6694*	*27540*
Lung cancer													
1955	182	6	108	1	5	8	13	24	29	28	29	25	14
1965	271	3	136	3	4	15	22	23	29	40	46	43	43
1975	495	2	223	1	10	17	30	34	59	72	88	84	98
1985	706	4	335	9	12	24	41	50	102	97	103	94	170
1990	**836**	**6**	**407**	**3**	**20**	**45**	**40**	**71**	**85**	**143**	**143**	**133**	**147**
1995 projected	*968*	*6*	*478*	*3*	*23*	*56*	*66*	*82*	*96*	*152*	*197*	*135*	*152*
ANNUAL DEATH RATE / 100,000 (*The rates for the age groups 0–34 and 35–69 are the means of seven five-yearly rates, but the all-ages rates are standardised to the conventional "European" age distribution)													
All causes													
1955	903.9*	100.7*	786.3*	139.0	209.1	323.2	517.3	794.3	1271.9	2249.2	4015.0	6979.5	15319.1
1965	784.1*	82.6*	645.8*	115.2	182.2	270.3	418.3	634.8	1045.5	1854.4	3334.7	6155.1	14190.9
1975	669.7*	60.6*	559.3*	98.1	167.4	261.9	388.1	567.8	893.2	1538.4	2727.0	5195.9	12410.5
1985	579.2*	50.5*	475.9*	91.9	123.2	188.9	330.9	513.0	780.6	1302.8	2233.8	4231.3	11398.0
1990	**547.9***	**45.8***	**448.4***	**77.5**	**124.1**	**203.4**	**288.0**	**508.7**	**730.7**	**1206.5**	**2078.9**	**3832.2**	**11060.2**
1995 projected	*521.6**	*41.5**	*422.2**	*69.8*	*124.2*	*194.5*	*279.0*	*478.2*	*687.9*	*1121.8*	*1904.8*	*3568.2*	*10842.5*
All cancer													
1955	161.9*	11.1*	238.8*	47.6	81.5	131.3	192.3	285.6	397.3	535.9	744.8	932.4	1258.4
1965	153.5*	8.8*	221.6*	34.3	75.3	133.4	191.0	256.1	356.7	504.5	722.7	923.9	1259.2
1975	165.1*	8.0*	230.0*	35.3	74.1	115.2	190.8	273.9	379.7	541.0	725.9	1065.3	1593.1
1985	146.7*	6.6*	211.7*	32.7	53.7	100.3	185.2	254.5	362.2	493.0	658.0	883.5	1342.1
1990	**143.8***	**5.8***	**210.2***	**27.8**	**60.7**	**107.4**	**148.8**	**264.1**	**342.1**	**520.5**	**675.8**	**885.1**	**1254.8**
1995 projected	*139.4**	*5.1**	*204.4**	*26.4*	*62.8*	*99.0*	*143.1*	*246.6*	*340.0*	*512.7*	*673.9*	*851.3*	*1207.5*
Lung cancer													
1955	4.8*	0.3*	7.9*	0.4	1.9	3.0	5.4	11.3	15.7	17.8	24.2	30.2	21.3
1965	6.0*	0.2*	8.6*	1.3	1.5	5.8	8.4	9.1	12.9	21.2	30.7	40.4	46.6
1975	9.0*	0.1*	13.2*	0.4	4.6	7.3	11.4	13.6	23.9	31.4	46.6	61.0	71.6
1985	11.9*	0.2*	20.2*	2.8	4.1	10.4	19.1	22.0	40.7	42.3	48.1	52.9	84.8
1990	**14.0***	**0.3***	**24.6***	**1.0**	**6.2**	**15.5**	**17.5**	**33.5**	**38.4**	**59.8**	**67.6**	**71.8**	**61.9**
1995 projected	*16.4**	*0.3**	*29.3**	*1.1*	*8.1*	*17.6*	*22.4*	*36.2*	*47.1*	*72.6*	*90.6*	*72.0*	*59.8*
Upper aerodigestive cancer (mouth, oesophagus, pharynx and larynx)													
1955	4.8*	0.0*	6.1*	0.4	1.1	1.5	4.6	8.9	10.3	15.9	29.2	43.4	39.5
1965	3.8*	0.1*	4.3*	–	–	1.2	3.1	5.5	8.5	11.6	22.0	29.1	52.1
1975	3.5*	–	4.0*	0.4	–	0.9	2.7	4.8	8.1	10.9	15.3	29.8	51.1
1985	2.6*	0.1*	3.0*	0.6	0.7	1.3	1.4	4.8	5.6	6.5	10.7	20.8	36.9
1990	**3.0***	**0.1***	**3.4***	**1.0**	**0.3**	**1.4**	**3.1**	**4.7**	**4.1**	**9.2**	**13.2**	**28.1**	**38.8**
1995 projected	*3.5**	*0.0**	*3.8**	*1.1*	*0.4*	*1.9*	*3.7*	*4.9*	*4.4*	*10.0*	*17.0*	*33.6*	*44.9*
Other cancer													
1955	152.3*	10.7*	224.8*	46.9	78.5	126.8	182.3	265.4	371.4	502.2	691.4	858.9	1197.6
1965	143.7*	8.6*	208.8*	33.0	73.8	126.5	179.5	241.5	335.3	471.7	670.0	854.3	1160.5
1975	152.6*	7.9*	212.8*	34.4	69.5	107.1	176.8	255.4	347.8	498.7	664.0	974.6	1470.4
1985	132.2*	6.3*	188.5*	29.3	48.9	88.6	164.7	227.7	315.9	444.2	599.2	809.8	1220.4
1990	**126.8***	**5.4***	**182.2***	**25.7**	**54.2**	**90.5**	**128.2**	**225.8**	**299.6**	**451.5**	**595.0**	**785.2**	**1154.2**
1995 projected	*119.5**	*4.7**	*171.3**	*24.2*	*54.4*	*79.5*	*116.9*	*205.6*	*288.5*	*430.0*	*566.2*	*745.7*	*1102.8*
Chronic obstructive pulmonary disease (COPD)													
1955	4.1*	0.6*	3.2*	0.4	1.5	1.1	2.1	2.8	7.0	7.6	15.0	26.5	83.6
1965	5.7*	0.4*	4.2*	0.4	1.9	0.8	0.4	3.6	8.5	13.8	31.3	62.0	93.3
1975	9.6*	0.7*	10.8*	2.2	2.7	2.1	6.8	10.8	18.2	32.7	43.4	59.5	146.8
1985	11.1*	0.5*	14.1*	0.6	1.0	4.3	10.7	16.3	26.7	39.3	53.7	74.3	136.2
1990	**10.3***	**0.5***	**12.6***	**1.4**	**0.6**	**2.4**	**6.6**	**12.8**	**19.9**	**44.3**	**53.4**	**83.6**	**127.2**
1995 projected	*10.0**	*0.5**	*11.1**	*1.4*	*0.4*	*1.6*	*4.7*	*9.3*	*18.2*	*42.0*	*55.7*	*90.1*	*127.6*
Other respiratory disease													
1955	46.1*	7.4*	21.6*	3.0	4.1	7.2	13.3	17.8	30.3	75.7	189.3	430.6	1013.7
1965	47.3*	2.8*	17.9*	2.5	3.3	3.9	5.7	14.6	28.1	67.2	158.0	416.4	1335.1
1975	17.5*	0.8*	5.4*	1.7	1.8	3.4	3.0	5.6	6.1	16.1	43.9	147.3	539.8
1985	31.0*	1.0*	10.8*	1.9	3.1	6.1	4.2	7.0	18.3	35.3	79.3	217.2	994.0
1990	**24.6***	**0.9***	**6.5***	**1.4**	**1.8**	**1.7**	**5.3**	**4.7**	**7.2**	**23.0**	**45.4**	**167.8**	**859.3**
1995 projected	*20.4**	*1.0**	*4.5**	*1.4*	*1.4*	*1.3*	*3.7*	*3.1*	*4.9*	*15.8*	*31.3*	*137.0*	*728.7*
Vascular disease													
1955	479.7*	4.6*	354.4*	19.0	40.2	92.4	161.9	300.6	599.5	1267.0	2470.4	4513.9	9618.5
1965	409.8*	3.4*	253.1*	19.1	33.0	52.6	118.0	204.3	417.0	927.5	1868.7	3834.6	9477.2
1975	338.9*	2.7*	194.4*	12.0	26.5	52.9	87.5	152.0	327.9	701.8	1482.0	3125.5	8225.7
1985	283.3*	2.0*	148.2*	13.9	15.8	27.4	55.8	122.4	246.9	555.4	1161.5	2513.8	7369.1
1990	**247.5***	**2.2***	**124.0***	**10.1**	**15.7**	**28.7**	**48.6**	**117.6**	**211.5**	**436.0**	**950.9**	**2092.3**	**6685.3**
1995 projected	*212.6**	*2.3**	*101.3**	*8.3*	*14.8*	*26.1*	*45.4*	*103.2*	*170.3*	*341.1*	*753.0*	*1758.0*	*5937.0*
Liver cirrhosis													
1955	4.0*	0.8*	6.2*	0.8	0.4	1.5	6.2	8.9	8.1	17.2	17.5	26.5	13.7
1965	4.4*	0.1*	6.7*	2.5	3.7	2.3	5.7	6.7	12.9	13.2	22.0	27.3	28.2
1975	6.2*	0.3*	10.4*	4.3	8.2	6.0	11.4	11.2	16.6	14.8	13.8	36.3	33.6
1985	4.3*	0.3*	7.8*	2.8	3.1	3.9	7.0	11.4	14.4	11.8	9.8	19.7	20.0
1990	**4.1***	**0.2***	**7.4***	**2.1**	**2.5**	**3.1**	**7.4**	**11.3**	**15.4**	**10.0**	**14.7**	**17.3**	**15.2**
1995 projected	*3.9**	*0.2**	*7.2**	*1.8*	*1.8*	*2.8*	*7.1*	*11.5*	*14.7*	*11.0*	*14.3*	*15.5*	*12.2*
Other medical causes													
1955	175.4*	62.7*	133.4*	49.9	58.4	69.6	113.2	145.6	192.4	304.5	497.9	918.0	2873.9
1965	128.5*	49.9*	105.4*	28.8	36.0	46.0	62.3	104.7	183.9	276.3	474.0	770.7	1657.3
1975	88.9*	28.6*	67.7*	13.8	21.0	35.0	49.6	68.6	102.3	184.0	327.5	579.8	1349.2
1985	71.3*	25.1*	48.3*	14.8	14.1	20.4	31.6	62.1	74.6	120.4	207.2	426.0	1248.4
1990	**87.6***	**22.2***	**55.3***	**16.0**	**14.8**	**26.9**	**39.4**	**56.2**	**94.0**	**139.6**	**278.8**	**500.8**	**1833.6**
1995 projected	*107.2**	*19.2**	*63.2**	*14.8*	*16.9*	*32.1*	*41.7*	*62.6*	*103.0*	*171.0*	*327.5*	*631.7*	*2555.9*
All non-medical causes													
1955	32.8*	13.5*	28.7*	18.3	23.1	20.1	28.3	32.9	37.3	41.3	80.1	131.5	457.4
1965	34.8*	17.2*	36.8*	27.5	28.9	31.3	35.1	44.7	38.4	51.9	58.0	120.3	340.6
1975	43.6*	19.5*	40.6*	28.8	32.9	47.4	39.0	45.7	42.5	48.0	90.5	182.1	522.3
1985	31.5*	14.9*	35.0*	25.3	32.3	26.5	36.3	39.2	37.5	47.6	64.4	96.8	288.3
1990	**29.9***	**14.1***	**32.5***	**18.8**	**28.0**	**33.1**	**31.9**	**42.0**	**40.7**	**33.0**	**60.0**	**85.3**	**284.8**
1995 projected	*28.1**	*13.2**	*30.5**	*15.5*	*26.1*	*31.7*	*33.2*	*41.9*	*36.8*	*28.2*	*49.2*	*84.8*	*273.6*

SWEDEN: 1975

Smoking-attributed deaths (Sm.) and total deaths (Total)

Age		ALL CAUSES	ALL CANCER	Lung cancer	Upper aero-digestive ca.	Other cancer	COPD	Other respiratory	Vascular disease	Liver cirrhosis	Other medical	Non-medical
Males												
0–34	Sm.	–	–	–	–	–	–	–	–	–	–	–
	Total	2236	187	6	2	179	18	42	96	12	749	1132
35–69	Sm.	2579	1012	704	90	218	212	33	1080	–	242	–
	Total	17041	4157	843	210	3104	364	243	8115	529	1719	1914
		(15%)	(24%)	(84%)	(43%)	(7%)	(58%)	(14%)	(13%)		(14%)	
70+	Sm.	2915	1127	691	92	344	418	65	1115	–	190	–
	Total	29045	6074	829	218	5027	726	1070	17179	153	2928	915
		(10%)	(19%)	(83%)	(42%)	(7%)	(58%)	(6%)	(6%)		(6%)	
Any age	Sm.	5494	2139	1395	182	562	630	98	2195	–	432	–
	Total	48322	10418	1678	430	8310	1108	1355	25390	694	5396	3961
		(11%)	(21%)	(83%)	(42%)	(7%)	(57%)	(7%)	(9%)		(8%)	
Females												
0–34	Sm.	–	–	–	–	–	–	–	–	–	–	–
	Total	1189	162	2	0	160	14	15	55	7	547	389
35–69	Sm.	274	93	71	8	14	38	2	105	–	36	–
	Total	9387	3881	223	67	3591	181	90	3241	175	1137	682
		(3%)	(2%)	(32%)	(12%)	(0%)	(21%)	(2%)	(3%)		(3%)	
70+	Sm.	647	166	114	23	29	108	16	301	–	56	–
	Total	29304	5021	270	140	4611	365	1025	18369	122	3265	1137
		(2%)	(3%)	(42%)	(16%)	(1%)	(30%)	(2%)	(2%)		(2%)	
Any age	Sm.	921	259	185	31	43	146	18	406	–	92	–
	Total	39880	9064	495	207	8362	560	1130	21665	304	4949	2208
		(2%)	(3%)	(37%)	(15%)	(1%)	(26%)	(2%)	(2%)		(2%)	
Males+Females												
0–34	Sm.	–	–	–	–	–	–	–	–	–	–	–
	Total	3425	349	8	2	339	32	57	151	19	1296	1521
35–69	Sm.	2853	1105	775	98	232	250	35	1185	–	278	–
	Total	26428	8038	1066	277	6695	545	333	11356	704	2856	2596
		(11%)	(14%)	(73%)	(35%)	(3%)	(46%)	(11%)	(10%)		(10%)	
70+	Sm.	3562	1293	805	115	373	526	81	1416	–	246	–
	Total	58349	11095	1099	358	9638	1091	2095	35548	275	6193	2052
		(6%)	(12%)	(73%)	(32%)	(4%)	(48%)	(4%)	(4%)		(4%)	
Any age	Sm.	6415	2398	1580	213	605	776	116	2601	–	524	–
	Total	88202	19482	2173	637	16672	1668	2485	47055	998	10345	6169
		(7%)	(12%)	(73%)	(33%)	(4%)	(47%)	(5%)	(6%)		(5%)	

SWEDEN: 1985

Smoking-attributed deaths (Sm.) and total deaths (Total)

Age		ALL CAUSES	ALL CANCER	Lung cancer	Upper aero-digestive ca.	Other cancer	COPD	Other respiratory	Vascular disease	Liver cirrhosis	Other medical	Non-medical
Males												
0–34	Sm.	–	–	–	–	–	–	–	–	–	–	–
	Total	1596	136	3	1	132	15	26	99	8	526	786
35–69	Sm.	2633	1096	773	107	216	213	56	1056	–	212	–
	Total	14903	3874	907	230	2737	345	379	7129	283	1352	1541
		(18%)	(28%)	(85%)	(47%)	(8%)	(62%)	(15%)	(15%)		(16%)	
70+	Sm.	3219	1210	792	101	317	560	129	1157	–	163	–
	Total	33535	6358	969	255	5134	1018	2433	19881	98	2911	836
		(10%)	(19%)	(82%)	(40%)	(6%)	(55%)	(5%)	(6%)		(6%)	
Any age	Sm.	5852	2306	1565	208	533	773	185	2213	–	375	–
	Total	50034	10368	1879	486	8003	1378	2838	27109	389	4789	3163
		(12%)	(22%)	(83%)	(43%)	(7%)	(56%)	(7%)	(8%)		(8%)	
Females												
0–34	Sm.	–	–	–	–	–	–	–	–	–	–	–
	Total	910	126	4	2	120	10	18	39	5	423	289
35–69	Sm.	594	234	186	14	34	95	14	186	–	65	–
	Total	7910	3507	335	50	3122	232	181	2444	131	808	607
		(8%)	(7%)	(56%)	(28%)	(1%)	(41%)	(8%)	(8%)		(8%)	
70+	Sm.	635	174	133	16	25	125	28	263	–	45	–
	Total	35159	5671	367	134	5170	520	2549	21731	96	3704	888
		(2%)	(3%)	(36%)	(12%)	(0%)	(24%)	(1%)	(1%)		(1%)	
Any age	Sm.	1229	408	319	30	59	220	42	449	–	110	–
	Total	43979	9304	706	186	8412	762	2748	24214	232	4935	1784
		(3%)	(4%)	(45%)	(16%)	(1%)	(29%)	(2%)	(2%)		(2%)	
Males+Females												
0–34	Sm.	–	–	–	–	–	–	–	–	–	–	–
	Total	2506	262	7	3	252	25	44	138	13	949	1075
35–69	Sm.	3227	1330	959	121	250	308	70	1242	–	277	–
	Total	22813	7381	1242	280	5859	577	560	9573	414	2160	2148
		(14%)	(18%)	(77%)	(43%)	(4%)	(53%)	(13%)	(13%)		(13%)	
70+	Sm.	3854	1384	925	117	342	685	157	1420	–	208	–
	Total	68694	12029	1336	389	10304	1538	4982	41612	194	6615	1724
		(6%)	(12%)	(69%)	(30%)	(3%)	(45%)	(3%)	(3%)		(3%)	
Any age	Sm.	7081	2714	1884	238	592	993	227	2662	–	485	–
	Total	94013	19672	2585	672	16415	2140	5586	51323	621	9724	4947
		(8%)	(14%)	(73%)	(35%)	(4%)	(46%)	(4%)	(5%)		(5%)	

(To be conservative, no deaths before age 35, and none from liver cirrhosis or non-medical causes, were attributed to smoking.)

SWEDEN: 1990

Smoking-attributed deaths (Sm.) and total deaths (Total)

		ALL CAUSES	ALL CANCER	Lung cancer	Upper aero-digestive ca.	Other cancer	COPD	Other respiratory	Vascular disease	Liver cirrhosis	Other medical	Non-medical
Males												
0–34	Sm.	–	–	–	–	–	–	–	–	–	–	–
	Total	1645	115	3	4	108	14	12	72	5	645	782
35–69	Sm.	2127	961	679	92	190	153	35	750	–	228	–
	Total	13006	3706	812	216	2678	259	235	5554	293	1518	1441
		(16%)	(26%)	(84%)	(43%)	(7%)	(59%)	(15%)	(14%)		(15%)	
70+	Sm.	3180	1268	841	95	332	538	110	1048	–	216	–
	Total	34399	6861	1036	246	5579	1007	2261	19099	126	4083	962
		(9%)	(18%)	(81%)	(39%)	(6%)	(53%)	(5%)	(5%)		(5%)	
Any age	Sm.	5307	2229	1520	187	522	691	145	1798	–	444	–
	Total	49050	10682	1851	466	8365	1280	2508	24725	424	6246	3185
		(11%)	(21%)	(82%)	(40%)	(6%)	(54%)	(6%)	(7%)		(7%)	
Females												
0–34	Sm.	–	–	–	–	–	–	–	–	–	–	–
	Total	882	111	6	1	104	9	17	43	4	421	277
35–69	Sm.	738	316	256	16	44	99	13	210	–	100	–
	Total	7453	3489	407	56	3026	205	108	2034	122	923	572
		(10%)	(9%)	(63%)	(29%)	(1%)	(48%)	(12%)	(10%)		(11%)	
70+	Sm.	1252	322	229	39	54	224	52	514	–	140	–
	Total	37757	6049	423	172	5454	570	2447	21760	99	5871	961
		(3%)	(5%)	(54%)	(23%)	(1%)	(39%)	(2%)	(2%)		(2%)	
Any age	Sm.	1990	638	485	55	98	323	65	724	–	240	–
	Total	46092	9649	836	229	8584	784	2572	23837	225	7215	1810
		(4%)	(7%)	(58%)	(24%)	(1%)	(41%)	(3%)	(3%)		(3%)	
Males+Females												
0–34	Sm.	–	–	–	–	–	–	–	–	–	–	–
	Total	2527	226	9	5	212	23	29	115	9	1066	1059
35–69	Sm.	2865	1277	935	108	234	252	48	960	–	328	–
	Total	20459	7195	1219	272	5704	464	343	7588	415	2441	2013
		(14%)	(18%)	(77%)	(40%)	(4%)	(54%)	(14%)	(13%)		(13%)	
70+	Sm.	4432	1590	1070	134	386	762	162	1562	–	356	–
	Total	72156	12910	1459	418	11033	1577	4708	40859	225	9954	1923
		(6%)	(12%)	(73%)	(32%)	(3%)	(48%)	(3%)	(4%)		(4%)	
Any age	Sm.	7297	2867	2005	242	620	1014	210	2522	–	684	–
	Total	95142	20331	2687	695	16949	2064	5080	48562	649	13461	4995
		(8%)	(14%)	(75%)	(35%)	(4%)	(49%)	(4%)	(5%)		(5%)	

SWEDEN: 1995

Smoking-attributed deaths (Sm.) and total deaths (Total)

		ALL CAUSES	ALL CANCER	Lung cancer	Upper aero-digestive ca.	Other cancer	COPD	Other respiratory	Vascular disease	Liver cirrhosis	Other medical	Non-medical
Males												
0–34	Sm.	–	–	–	–	–	–	–	–	–	–	–
	Total	1551	96	4	3	89	14	9	56	4	673	699
35–69	Sm.	1752	859	609	87	163	109	22	528	–	234	–
	Total	11270	3479	739	214	2526	196	161	4164	306	1656	1308
		(16%)	(25%)	(82%)	(41%)	(6%)	(56%)	(14%)	(13%)		(14%)	
70+	Sm.	3056	1257	841	83	333	499	96	926	–	278	–
	Total	34206	7001	1043	216	5742	943	2006	17599	154	5429	1074
		(9%)	(18%)	(81%)	(38%)	(6%)	(53%)	(5%)	(5%)		(5%)	
Any age	Sm.	4808	2116	1450	170	496	608	118	1454	–	512	–
	Total	47027	10576	1786	433	8357	1153	2176	21819	464	7758	3081
		(10%)	(20%)	(81%)	(39%)	(6%)	(53%)	(5%)	(7%)		(7%)	
Females												
0–34	Sm.	–	–	–	–	–	–	–	–	–	–	–
	Total	772	96	6	1	89	10	19	44	4	351	248
35–69	Sm.	858	404	331	21	52	94	11	209	–	140	–
	Total	6821	3313	478	62	2773	170	73	1577	119	1024	545
		(13%)	(12%)	(69%)	(34%)	(2%)	(55%)	(15%)	(13%)		(14%)	
70+	Sm.	1440	400	285	53	62	255	48	518	–	219	–
	Total	38375	6129	484	214	5431	614	2176	20015	91	8389	961
		(4%)	(7%)	(59%)	(25%)	(1%)	(42%)	(2%)	(3%)		(3%)	
Any age	Sm.	2298	804	616	74	114	349	59	727	–	359	–
	Total	45968	9538	968	277	8293	794	2268	21636	214	9764	1754
		(5%)	(8%)	(64%)	(27%)	(1%)	(44%)	(3%)	(3%)		(4%)	
Males+Females												
0–34	Sm.	–	–	–	–	–	–	–	–	–	–	–
	Total	2323	192	10	4	178	24	28	100	8	1024	947
35–69	Sm.	2610	1263	940	108	215	203	33	737	–	374	–
	Total	18091	6792	1217	276	5299	366	234	5741	425	2680	1853
		(14%)	(19%)	(77%)	(39%)	(4%)	(55%)	(14%)	(13%)		(14%)	
70+	Sm.	4496	1657	1126	136	395	754	144	1444	–	497	–
	Total	72581	13130	1527	430	11173	1557	4182	37614	245	13818	2035
		(6%)	(13%)	(74%)	(32%)	(4%)	(48%)	(3%)	(4%)		(4%)	
Any age	Sm.	7106	2920	2066	244	610	957	177	2181	–	871	–
	Total	92995	20114	2754	710	16650	1947	4444	43455	678	17522	4835
		(8%)	(15%)	(75%)	(34%)	(4%)	(49%)	(4%)	(5%)		(5%)	

(To be conservative, no deaths before age 35, and none from liver cirrhosis or non-medical causes, were attributed to smoking.)

SWITZERLAND: 1990

		No. of deaths			Standardised rates (Defined on p.502)			Annual death rates / 100, 000						
		All ages	0–34	35–69	All ages	0–34	35–69	0–4	5–9	10–14	15–19	20–24	25–29	30–34
ALL CAUSES	M	32492	1987	10009	914.4	117.1	878.4	196.9	19.5	20.3	101.2	154.9	165.2	162.0
	F	31247	850	5232	522.2	54.8	405.3	159.2	16.1	15.8	34.6	43.5	53.2	61.2
Tuberculosis	M	63	–	22	1.8	–	1.9	–	–	–	–	–	–	–
	F	23	–	5	0.4	–	0.4	–	–	–	–	–	–	–
Other infective	M	471	179	188	13.2	9.8	13.0	10.0	–	–	0.5	2.7	25.8	29.4
and parasitic	F	247	75	37	5.2	4.4	2.7	7.9	0.5	0.5	1.0	4.0	10.9	6.2
ALL CANCER	M	9072	113	3571	260.1	6.6	320.9	2.5	3.6	5.7	7.3	6.6	10.4	10.4
	F	7302	86	2541	146.0	5.2	196.2	4.7	2.1	2.7	2.9	4.7	6.9	11.9
Mouth and	M	307	3	207	9.3	0.2	17.2	–	–	–	0.5	–	0.4	0.4
pharynx cancer	F	78	1	27	1.6	0.1	2.0	–	–	–	0.5	–	–	–
Oesophagus cancer	M	278	–	137	8.1	–	11.8	–	–	–	–	–	–	–
	F	74	–	18	1.4	–	1.4	–	–	–	–	–	–	–
Stomach cancer	M	534	4	194	15.2	0.2	17.7	–	–	–	–	0.4	–	1.1
	F	371	4	82	6.4	0.2	6.5	–	–	–	–	–	0.7	0.8
Colorectal cancer	M	1024	3	324	28.8	0.2	29.4	–	–	–	0.5	–	0.4	0.4
	F	926	2	246	16.9	0.1	19.4	–	–	–	–	–	–	0.8
Liver cancer	M	242	2	121	7.1	0.1	11.4	–	–	–	–	–	–	0.7
	F	102	4	40	2.2	0.2	3.1	–	–	–	–	–	0.7	0.8
Pancreas cancer	M	411	–	189	11.9	–	17.0	–	–	–	–	–	–	–
	F	439	–	134	8.3	–	10.8	–	–	–	–	–	–	–
Larynx cancer	M	116	–	66	3.5	–	5.7	–	–	–	–	–	–	–
	F	17	–	5	0.4	–	0.4	–	–	–	–	–	–	–
Lung cancer	M	2242	5	1174	66.6	0.3	106.9	–	–	–	–	–	1.1	0.7
	F	491	2	235	11.1	0.1	18.0	–	–	–	–	–	0.4	0.4
Malignant melanoma	M	124	5	60	3.6	0.3	4.8	–	–	–	–	1.2	0.4	0.4
	F	110	8	49	2.4	0.5	3.6	–	–	–	0.5	0.8	–	1.9
Female breast cancer	F	1675	10	736	35.6	0.5	55.8	–	–	–	–	–	1.5	2.3
Cervix cancer	F	148	–	73	3.3	–	5.3	–	–	–	–	–	–	–
Other uterine cancer	F	289	1	87	5.5	0.1	6.9	–	–	–	–	–	–	0.4
Ovarian cancer	F	485	1	217	10.7	0.1	16.8	–	–	–	–	0.4	–	–
Prostate cancer	M	1478	–	205	39.5	–	20.6	–	–	–	–	–	–	–
Bladder cancer	M	328	–	93	9.2	–	8.6	–	–	–	–	–	–	–
	F	165	–	34	2.9	–	2.7	–	–	–	–	–	–	–
Other and ill-defined	M	1184	51	527	34.4	3.1	45.9	2.5	1.0	3.6	4.1	1.6	5.7	3.0
cancer sites	F	1203	26	361	23.3	1.7	27.9	3.7	1.6	1.1	0.5	1.6	2.6	0.8
Hodgkin's disease	M	43	6	18	1.2	0.3	1.3	–	–	–	–	0.8	0.4	1.1
	F	39	5	14	0.9	0.3	1.0	–	–	–	–	0.8	0.4	0.8
Myeloma and non-	M	506	8	166	14.2	0.5	15.0	–	0.5	–	0.5	0.8	0.7	0.7
Hodgkin lymphomas	F	440	5	119	8.3	0.3	9.5	–	–	–	–	0.8	0.4	0.8
Leukaemia	M	255	26	90	7.2	1.6	7.7	–	2.0	2.1	1.8	1.9	1.4	1.9
	F	250	17	64	4.9	1.1	4.9	1.0	0.5	1.6	1.4	0.4	0.4	2.3
ALL VASCULAR	M	13068	82	3226	360.1	4.6	295.8	4.0	–	0.5	3.2	6.2	9.7	8.6
DISEASE	F	14951	46	1140	216.0	2.8	91.4	2.1	1.1	1.6	1.9	3.6	2.2	6.9
Rheumatic heart	M	32	1	10	0.9	0.1	1.0	–	–	–	–	–	0.4	–
disease and fever	F	34	–	11	0.7	–	0.9	–	–	–	–	–	–	–
Hypertensive disease	M	466	1	142	13.0	0.1	13.0	–	–	–	–	0.4	–	–
	F	811	–	58	11.9	–	4.7	–	–	–	–	–	–	–
Ischaemic heart	M	5657	20	1814	159.0	1.1	166.6	–	–	–	–	0.4	2.1	4.8
disease	F	4569	3	459	69.0	0.2	37.3	–	–	–	0.5	–	0.4	0.4
Pulmonary embolism	M	233	3	64	6.5	0.2	6.0	–	–	–	–	0.8	–	0.4
and other venous	F	442	5	55	6.9	0.3	4.4	–	–	–	0.5	–	0.4	1.2
Cerebrovascular	M	2353	12	361	63.2	0.6	33.3	–	–	–	0.5	0.8	2.5	0.7
disease	F	3431	8	226	48.8	0.5	17.6	–	0.5	–	–	0.8	0.7	1.2
Other vascular	M	4327	45	835	117.5	2.6	75.9	4.0	–	0.5	2.7	3.9	4.6	2.6
disease	F	5664	30	331	78.7	1.9	26.5	2.1	0.5	1.6	1.0	2.8	0.7	4.2
Chronic obstructive	M	1555	9	397	43.2	0.6	38.5	1.0	0.5	–	0.9	0.4	0.4	0.7
pulmonary disease	F	693	11	143	12.0	0.7	11.5	–	0.5	1.1	0.5	0.4	0.4	1.9
Other respiratory	M	1203	26	141	32.1	1.7	12.9	6.5	–	–	1.4	2.3	0.7	0.7
disease	F	1729	13	81	23.7	0.9	6.5	4.7	–	0.5	–	0.4	–	0.8
Peptic ulcer	M	108	2	27	3.0	0.1	2.3	–	–	–	–	–	0.4	0.4
	F	172	–	20	2.6	–	1.6	–	–	–	–	–	–	–
Liver cirrhosis	M	466	5	321	14.1	0.3	26.5	–	–	–	–	0.4	0.7	0.7
	F	215	3	154	5.5	0.2	11.3	–	–	–	–	0.4	–	0.8
Renal disease	M	40	–	12	1.1	–	1.1	–	–	–	–	–	–	–
	F	47	1	11	0.8	0.1	0.9	0.5	–	–	–	–	–	–
Pregnancy and birth	F	5	4	1	0.1	0.2	0.1	–	–	–	–	–	0.7	0.8
Congenital and	M	230	228	2	9.1	16.2	0.1	110.2	0.5	0.5	0.9	0.4	–	1.1
perinatal causes	F	201	199	2	8.3	14.8	0.1	97.4	2.1	1.6	1.4	–	1.1	–
Ill-defined causes	M	600	134	245	18.1	8.5	20.0	32.6	1.0	1.0	1.8	7.8	7.2	7.8
	F	398	63	111	8.7	4.5	8.4	25.1	0.5	–	1.4	0.8	1.8	1.5
Other medical causes	M	2344	89	644	65.3	5.5	55.8	9.0	4.6	2.1	5.5	3.9	4.3	8.9
	F	3242	70	498	53.4	4.4	39.5	8.9	3.2	1.1	3.4	3.2	3.6	7.7
ALL NON-	M	3272	1120	1213	93.3	63.4	89.4	21.0	9.2	10.4	79.8	124.1	105.9	93.1
MEDICAL CAUSES	F	2022	279	488	39.5	16.7	34.8	7.9	5.9	6.6	22.1	26.1	25.5	22.7
Motor vehicle	M	699	385	197	20.1	22.3	13.9	5.5	6.1	6.8	37.8	48.2	30.4	21.2
traffic accidents	F	231	77	80	5.9	4.8	5.6	1.6	3.2	3.3	9.6	9.5	3.6	3.1
Fire	M	15	6	4	0.4	0.4	0.3	0.5	–	–	0.5	0.8	–	0.7
	F	8	–	1	0.2	–	0.1	–	–	–	–	–	–	–
Suicide	M	1032	300	542	29.8	16.4	39.8	–	–	–	16.9	31.5	32.9	33.5
	F	435	91	248	11.5	5.2	17.5	–	–	2.2	4.8	7.5	9.8	11.9
Homicide	M	53	27	20	1.6	1.6	1.3	2.5	0.5	0.5	0.5	2.3	0.4	4.5
	F	46	18	25	1.4	1.1	1.6	2.1	1.6	–	0.5	1.6	1.1	1.2
POPULATION (thousands):				M=males	3277.9	1611.4	1409.6	199.6	195.3	191.9	219.4	257.0	279.6	268.6
				F=females	3434.3	1555.5	1455.3	191.0	186.4	183.2	208.0	252.8	274.4	259.7

SWITZERLAND: 1990

Annual death rates / 100, 000

9th ICD categories

35–39	40–44	45–49	50–54	55–59	60–64	65–69	70–74	75–79	80+/NK			
166.1	221.0	319.6	524.5	887.6	1522.3	2507.5	3930.5	6545.2	14516.0	M	ALL CAUSES	001–999
80.9	118.5	201.1	286.8	405.3	680.8	1063.7	1925.1	3529.5	10822.1	F		
0.4	0.8	0.8	1.5	1.1	3.9	4.5	10.2	17.3	21.7	M	Tuberculosis	010–018, 137
–	–	–	–	1.6	–	1.2	1.5	3.2	7.1	F		
22.5	12.7	9.3	11.2	10.7	11.1	13.6	17.4	35.9	74.1	M	Other infective	Rest of 001–139
2.4	0.4	2.2	1.5	5.4	2.9	4.2	12.4	19.9	55.8	F	and parasitic	
22.9	48.1	99.9	189.6	351.3	595.7	938.9	1344.2	1977.7	3162.2	M	ALL CANCER	140–208
34.4	57.4	94.1	162.4	216.9	354.1	453.9	671.0	949.8	1551.0	F		
0.8	6.5	9.7	17.8	23.0	32.8	29.4	29.6	39.7	46.0	M	Mouth and	140–149
0.4	1.6	–	2.5	2.7	4.0	3.0	6.9	12.8	14.8	F	pharynx cancer	
0.4	3.1	7.2	8.2	14.1	20.3	29.4	39.8	55.8	72.8	M	Oesophagus cancer	150
0.4	–	0.4	0.5	3.2	2.3	3.0	8.5	8.0	20.8	F		
0.8	1.5	4.2	10.7	19.1	34.1	53.5	85.8	116.5	201.8	M	Stomach cancer	151
1.2	1.6	1.7	2.5	5.4	13.1	20.0	25.5	58.2	106.2	F		
2.4	4.2	5.1	17.8	34.9	53.1	88.2	146.1	255.3	444.4	M	Colorectal cancer	153, 154
2.0	4.8	7.3	11.1	18.3	32.6	60.1	88.8	113.2	249.7	F		
–	0.8	1.7	4.1	9.6	27.5	36.2	34.7	57.0	49.8	M	Liver cancer	155.0
1.2	0.4	0.9	0.5	4.8	7.4	6.7	11.6	12.8	16.0	F		
0.8	3.1	5.1	11.7	17.4	29.5	51.3	57.2	75.6	134.1	M	Pancreas cancer	157
0.8	0.4	1.7	10.6	7.5	21.7	32.8	43.2	59.0	103.8	F		
–	1.5	2.5	6.1	7.9	7.2	14.3	16.3	13.6	29.4	M	Larynx cancer	161
–	–	–	1.0	0.5	1.1	–	3.1	2.4	3.0	F		
1.6	10.4	31.6	56.6	115.2	227.4	305.4	415.7	432.5	392.1	M	Lung cancer	162
2.8	5.9	10.8	13.7	21.5	33.7	37.6	56.4	75.0	51.6	F		
2.8	1.9	1.7	4.1	8.4	5.2	9.8	17.4	24.8	28.1	M	Malignant melanoma	172
1.6	1.2	3.9	3.5	2.7	5.1	7.3	6.2	13.6	16.6	F		
12.1	17.4	35.8	57.2	72.5	88.5	106.8	117.4	187.4	321.5	F	Female breast cancer	174
2.4	4.4	3.5	6.6	3.2	6.3	10.9	13.1	14.4	23.7	F	Cervix cancer	180
–	1.6	2.2	2.5	7.0	17.1	18.2	28.6	47.0	62.3	F	Other uterine cancer	179, 182
1.6	5.9	5.2	15.7	22.5	29.7	37.0	57.9	59.8	69.4	F	Ovarian cancer	183
–	0.4	1.3	3.1	10.1	28.8	100.3	181.8	449.8	934.9	M	Prostate cancer	185
–	0.8	1.7	2.0	10.7	20.3	24.9	55.2	70.6	158.4	M	Bladder cancer	188
0.4	0.4	0.4	1.5	3.2	6.3	6.7	17.0	27.1	44.5	F		
6.7	8.1	19.4	33.1	60.7	70.1	122.9	157.3	205.7	365.3	M	Other and ill-defined	Rest of 140–208
3.6	8.3	15.1	20.2	30.6	52.5	64.9	110.4	157.9	281.7	F	cancer sites	
2.4	0.4	–	2.5	0.6	2.6	0.8	5.1	7.4	10.2	M	Hodgkin's disease	201
0.8	0.8	1.7	1.0	0.5	0.6	1.2	3.9	3.2	6.5	F		
2.8	3.1	3.4	7.6	12.9	24.2	51.3	76.6	128.9	195.4	M	Myeloma and non–	200, 202–203
1.6	1.6	1.3	5.6	8.1	22.8	25.5	45.6	72.6	98.5	F	Hodgkin lymphomas	
1.6	2.3	5.5	4.1	6.7	12.5	21.1	25.5	44.6	99.6	M	Leukaemia	204–208
1.2	1.2	2.2	6.1	2.7	9.1	12.1	27.0	25.5	60.5	F		
24.1	41.2	78.8	138.1	267.0	538.0	983.4	1658.8	2940.5	7360.2	M	ALL VASCULAR	390–459
6.9	15.1	32.8	38.4	73.5	155.3	318.0	771.4	1677.0	6324.4	F	DISEASE	
–	–	–	1.0	0.6	–	5.3	9.2	7.4	7.7	M	Rheumatic heart	390–398
–	0.4	–	0.5	1.6	1.1	2.4	2.3	7.2	6.5	F	disease and fever	
0.8	2.3	3.8	5.1	12.4	22.3	44.5	61.3	102.9	229.9	M	Hypertensive disease	401–405
–	0.4	0.9	4.0	4.3	8.6	14.6	56.4	103.7	326.2	F		
13.4	24.3	41.7	76.5	148.4	306.0	555.8	865.2	1297.4	2463.6	M	Ischaemic heart	410–414
0.4	4.8	10.4	10.6	32.2	65.1	137.7	304.2	619.6	1741.4	F	disease	
0.8	–	1.3	2.0	7.3	8.5	21.9	32.7	59.5	109.8	M	Pulmonary embolism	415.1, 451–453
0.4	1.6	0.9	2.5	3.2	5.1	17.0	33.2	47.0	166.1	F	and other venous	
1.2	6.2	8.9	15.8	24.2	60.3	116.9	253.3	572.5	1622.0	M	Cerebrovascular	430–438
3.6	4.8	10.8	10.1	9.1	26.8	58.3	156.8	410.7	1470.3	F	disease	
7.9	8.5	23.2	37.7	74.2	140.9	239.1	437.2	900.9	2927.2	M	Other vascular	Rest of 390–459
2.4	3.2	9.9	10.6	23.1	48.5	88.0	218.5	488.8	2613.9	F	disease	
0.8	0.8	3.0	11.7	27.5	71.4	154.6	254.3	408.9	728.0	M	Chronic obstructive	490–496
1.2	2.0	2.6	4.6	10.7	21.7	37.6	57.9	88.5	209.4	F	pulmonary disease	
2.0	1.2	3.8	3.6	14.6	22.3	43.0	93.0	235.4	964.2	M	Other respiratory	Rest of 460–519
0.4	1.6	1.7	2.5	6.4	11.4	21.2	53.3	156.3	812.6	F	disease	
0.4	0.4	0.8	1.5	3.9	3.3	6.0	8.2	28.5	61.3	M	Peptic ulcer	531–533
0.4	–	0.4	–	2.1	2.9	5.5	6.9	19.9	70.0	F		
4.7	11.6	15.6	18.3	40.5	40.6	54.3	47.0	49.6	69.0	M	Liver cirrhosis	571
2.4	7.5	11.2	10.6	11.3	20.0	15.8	10.0	13.6	16.6	F		
–	0.4	–	0.5	1.7	2.0	3.0	8.2	13.6	11.5	M	Renal disease	580–590
–	–	0.4	0.5	0.5	1.1	3.6	2.3	10.4	11.3	F		
0.4	–	–	–	–	–	–	–	–	–	F	Pregnancy and birth	630–676
0.4	–	–	0.5	–	–	–	–	–	–	M	Congenital and	740–779
0.4	–	–	0.5	–	–	–	–	–	–	F	perinatal causes	
8.3	8.5	11.8	14.3	21.4	36.7	39.2	59.2	69.4	136.7	M	Ill–defined causes	780–799
2.0	4.8	3.9	7.6	9.7	10.9	20.0	18.5	32.7	94.3	F		
10.3	17.3	20.2	41.8	55.1	96.3	149.3	261.5	469.6	1246.5	M	Other medical causes	Rest of 001–799
4.4	7.1	17.3	22.8	31.7	63.4	129.9	240.2	388.4	1112.7	F		
69.5	78.2	75.5	91.7	92.7	100.9	117.6	168.5	298.6	680.7	M	ALL NON–	E800–E999
25.5	22.6	34.5	35.4	35.4	37.1	52.8	79.5	169.9	556.9	F	MEDICAL CAUSES	
11.0	17.7	13.5	17.3	10.7	12.5	14.3	30.6	48.3	61.3	M	Motor vehicle	E810–E819
5.3	2.4	7.8	4.6	4.8	8.6	6.1	13.9	19.9	18.4	F	traffic accidents	
–	0.8	–	–	0.6	–	0.8	–	2.5	3.8	M	Fire	E890–E899
–	–	–	0.5	–	–	–	2.3	1.6	1.2	F		
32.4	32.0	37.1	41.3	42.7	42.6	50.5	53.1	66.9	107.3	M	Suicide	E950–E959
12.5	13.1	17.7	21.8	18.8	13.7	24.9	20.8	27.1	20.8	F		
2.8	0.8	1.3	2.5	1.1	0.7	–	5.1	1.2	–	M	Homicide	E960–E969
2.8	1.2	2.6	1.5	1.6	1.7	–	0.8	0.8	0.6	F		
253.4	259.7	237.2	196.2	177.9	152.6	132.6	97.9	80.7	78.3	M	**POPULATION (thousands)**	
247.3	252.4	231.7	197.7	186.3	175.1	164.8	129.5	125.4	168.6	F		

SWITZERLAND: Males

	All ages	0–34	35–69	35–39	40–44	45–49	50–54	55–59	60–64	65–69	70–74	75–79	80+/NK
POPULATION (1000s)													
1955	2417.4	1326.5	964.8	159.6	168.6	170.0	153.7	129.1	102.9	80.9	61.9	39.4	24.8
1965	2853.1	1626.1	1076.4	186.8	181.6	153.9	164.7	156.2	132.1	101.1	70.9	44.8	34.9
1975	3096.1	1705.0	1194.6	216.5	202.9	185.2	175.9	144.2	144.5	125.4	93.7	58.4	44.4
1985	3152.8	1585.0	1319.9	257.5	239.3	201.6	187.8	167.0	150.7	116.0	105.3	77.3	65.3
1990	3277.9	1611.4	1409.6	253.4	259.7	237.2	196.2	177.9	152.6	132.6	97.9	80.7	78.3
1995 projected	3264.4	1493.2	1487.7	257.7	242.9	252.5	236.1	190.3	168.3	139.9	114.8	77.9	90.8
NUMBER OF DEATHS													
All causes													
1955	25726	2981	10707	342	571	949	1453	1907	2440	3045	3544	3919	4575
1965	29051	2728	11910	353	567	774	1278	2171	2964	3803	4038	4170	6205
1975	29689	2104	11452	340	543	839	1263	1730	2692	4045	4622	4589	6922
1985	30934	1704	10155	397	497	701	1104	1743	2505	3208	4422	5295	9358
1990	32492	1987	10009	421	574	758	1029	1579	2323	3325	3848	5282	11366
1995 projected	34367	2097	9909	498	533	750	1083	1504	2303	3238	4242	4900	13219
Lung cancer													
1955	810	1	610	4	17	55	109	139	154	132	108	55	36
1965	1245	4	895	8	22	37	101	211	269	247	165	122	59
1975	2000	3	1254	7	35	74	135	215	340	448	374	226	143
1985	2321	3	1228	8	22	53	129	223	352	441	426	381	283
1990	2242	5	1174	4	27	75	111	205	347	405	407	349	307
1995 projected	2204	6	1148	4	28	74	117	199	330	396	429	304	317
ANNUAL DEATH RATE / 100,000 (*The rates for the age groups 0–34 and 35–69 are the means of seven five-yearly rates, but the all-ages rates are standardised to the conventional "European" age distribution)													
All causes													
1955	1354.8*	216.6*	1381.3*	214.3	338.7	558.2	945.3	1477.1	2371.2	3763.9	5725.4	9946.7	18447.6
1965	1267.2*	160.7*	1310.8*	189.0	312.2	502.9	776.0	1389.9	2243.8	3761.6	5695.3	9308.0	17779.4
1975	1088.2*	127.5*	1126.3*	157.0	267.6	453.0	718.0	1199.7	1863.0	3225.7	4932.8	7857.9	15590.1
1985	950.6*	105.8*	967.0*	154.2	207.7	347.7	587.9	1043.7	1662.2	2765.5	4199.4	6849.9	14330.8
1990	914.4*	117.1*	878.4*	166.1	221.0	319.6	524.5	887.6	1522.3	2507.5	3930.5	6545.2	14516.0
1995 projected	884.4*	131.3*	805.9*	193.2	219.4	297.0	458.7	790.3	1368.4	2314.5	3695.1	6290.1	14558.4
All cancer													
1955	255.3*	11.2*	359.9*	21.9	56.9	106.5	236.2	427.6	680.3	990.1	1294.0	1835.0	2270.2
1965	256.2*	11.0*	354.5*	27.8	61.1	109.8	213.1	412.9	649.5	1006.9	1365.3	1825.9	2343.8
1975	268.7*	11.5*	360.9*	28.6	59.1	136.1	216.6	397.4	638.1	1050.2	1458.9	1893.8	2637.4
1985	277.1*	7.6*	351.4*	24.1	43.9	112.1	203.9	403.6	635.7	1036.2	1444.4	2117.7	3165.4
1990	260.1*	6.6*	320.9*	22.9	48.1	99.9	189.6	351.3	595.7	938.9	1344.2	1977.7	3162.2
1995 projected	243.3*	6.5*	292.5*	23.3	44.9	92.3	165.6	318.4	539.5	863.5	1239.5	1875.5	3099.1
Lung cancer													
1955	39.5*	0.1*	76.6*	2.5	10.1	32.4	70.9	107.7	149.7	163.2	174.5	139.6	145.2
1965	51.1*	0.3*	97.8*	4.3	12.1	24.0	61.3	135.1	203.6	244.3	232.7	272.3	169.1
1975	70.8*	0.2*	125.5*	3.2	17.2	40.0	76.7	149.1	235.3	357.3	399.1	387.0	322.1
1985	73.2*	0.2*	122.1*	3.1	9.2	26.3	68.7	133.5	233.6	380.2	404.6	492.9	433.4
1990	66.6*	0.3*	106.9*	1.6	10.4	31.6	56.6	115.2	227.4	305.4	415.7	432.5	392.1
1995 projected	60.0*	0.3*	96.5*	1.6	11.5	29.3	49.6	104.6	196.1	283.1	373.7	390.2	349.1
Upper aerodigestive cancer (mouth, oesophagus, pharynx and larynx)													
1955	34.8*	0.2*	54.1*	–	3.0	8.2	31.9	68.2	111.8	155.7	177.7	233.5	290.3
1965	31.0*	0.1*	45.4*	0.5	6.1	9.7	35.2	49.3	90.1	126.6	177.7	214.3	257.9
1975	25.0*	0.2*	38.1*	2.3	4.9	13.5	28.4	48.5	67.1	102.1	139.8	149.0	198.2
1985	21.7*	0.3*	33.9*	0.8	5.9	22.8	34.1	49.7	54.4	69.8	83.6	130.7	173.0
1990	20.9*	0.2*	34.6*	1.2	11.2	19.4	32.1	45.0	60.3	73.2	85.8	109.0	148.1
1995 projected	20.0*	0.2*	34.8*	1.9	11.5	19.0	28.4	44.1	61.8	76.5	81.0	93.7	125.6
Other cancer													
1955	180.9*	10.9*	229.2*	19.4	43.9	65.9	133.4	251.7	418.9	671.2	941.8	1461.9	1834.7
1965	174.1*	10.6*	211.3*	23.0	43.0	76.0	116.6	228.6	355.8	636.0	954.9	1339.3	1916.9
1975	172.9*	11.2*	197.2*	23.1	37.0	82.6	111.4	199.7	335.6	590.9	920.0	1357.9	2117.1
1985	182.3*	7.1*	195.4*	20.2	28.8	63.0	101.2	220.4	347.7	586.2	956.3	1494.2	2559.0
1990	172.6*	6.2*	179.4*	20.1	26.6	48.9	100.9	191.1	308.0	560.3	842.7	1436.2	2622.0
1995 projected	163.4*	6.0*	161.2*	19.8	21.8	44.0	87.7	169.7	281.6	503.9	784.8	1391.5	2624.4
Chronic obstructive pulmonary disease (COPD)													
1955	23.7*	1.1*	23.0*	2.5	4.2	7.1	22.1	21.7	36.9	66.7	87.2	203.0	407.3
1965	31.1*	1.2*	36.2*	–	4.4	13.0	15.8	39.1	64.3	116.7	160.8	274.6	378.2
1975	38.6*	0.9*	40.2*	1.4	4.9	7.6	16.5	34.7	87.9	128.4	233.7	337.3	533.8
1985	39.0*	0.9*	37.4*	2.3	3.3	8.9	9.6	30.5	70.3	137.1	218.4	345.4	624.8
1990	43.2*	0.6*	38.5*	0.8	0.8	3.0	11.7	27.5	71.4	154.6	254.3	408.9	728.0
1995 projected	48.9*	0.4*	41.4*	0.8	0.4	2.0	9.7	27.3	76.1	173.7	295.3	475.0	853.5
Other respiratory disease													
1955	55.3*	13.4*	35.6*	3.1	7.1	16.5	28.0	30.2	50.5	113.7	174.5	378.2	1129.0
1965	38.3*	4.8*	20.5*	2.1	3.3	7.1	13.4	16.6	31.8	69.2	126.9	328.1	908.3
1975	36.0*	3.5*	20.3*	2.3	2.5	4.9	13.6	27.7	33.9	57.4	137.7	270.5	862.6
1985	19.6*	1.5*	8.8*	1.9	2.1	1.0	8.0	5.4	22.6	20.7	71.2	130.7	545.2
1990	32.1*	1.7*	12.9*	2.0	1.2	3.8	3.6	14.6	22.3	43.0	93.0	235.4	964.2
1995 projected	44.7*	2.3*	16.9*	1.6	1.6	2.8	5.1	16.3	31.5	59.3	130.7	331.2	1363.4
Vascular disease													
1955	602.6*	7.8*	523.4*	37.6	79.5	148.8	281.7	499.6	945.6	1671.2	2919.2	5510.2	10927.4
1965	580.7*	6.7*	504.5*	40.1	79.3	138.4	265.9	490.4	858.4	1658.8	2833.6	5031.3	10819.5
1975	490.6*	5.5*	436.3*	28.6	68.5	141.5	257.0	430.0	732.9	1395.5	2308.4	4126.7	9157.7
1985	399.7*	3.9*	349.8*	25.6	49.3	90.8	182.1	352.1	631.7	1117.2	1846.2	3274.3	7758.0
1990	360.1*	4.6*	295.8*	24.1	41.2	78.8	138.1	267.0	538.0	983.4	1658.8	2940.5	7360.2
1995 projected	323.0*	5.5*	251.0*	21.0	34.6	61.8	105.0	213.9	455.7	864.9	1478.2	2634.1	6871.1
Liver cirrhosis													
1955	25.6*	0.1*	49.1*	3.1	7.1	17.6	40.3	63.5	99.1	112.5	108.2	132.0	80.6
1965	28.5*	0.2*	48.9*	5.4	7.7	18.2	29.1	64.7	93.9	123.6	163.6	183.0	106.0
1975	21.8*	0.2*	40.2*	4.2	8.4	16.2	40.9	47.9	60.2	103.7	101.4	99.3	87.8
1985	17.9*	0.3*	33.4*	4.7	12.5	20.3	31.4	50.9	52.4	61.2	60.8	81.5	65.8
1990	14.1*	0.3*	26.5*	4.7	11.6	15.6	18.3	40.5	40.6	54.3	47.0	49.6	69.0
1995 projected	10.9*	0.2*	20.6*	4.7	9.5	10.7	13.1	29.4	33.3	43.6	34.8	42.4	55.1
Other medical causes													
1955	265.7*	110.6*	240.8*	53.9	81.3	136.5	191.9	280.4	364.4	577.3	851.4	1522.8	2951.6
1965	210.4*	73.5*	197.8*	29.4	54.0	83.2	105.0	215.7	346.0	550.9	764.5	1310.3	2487.1
1975	130.4*	42.0*	112.9*	16.6	32.0	41.6	68.2	125.5	178.5	327.8	504.8	851.0	1738.7
1985	106.8*	32.6*	91.2*	15.1	26.3	36.2	66.6	100.0	141.3	252.6	372.3	652.0	1589.6
1990	111.6*	40.0*	94.2*	42.2	40.0	43.0	71.4	93.9	153.3	215.7	364.7	634.4	1551.7
1995 projected	115.1*	46.7*	97.7*	62.5	54.8	50.3	72.0	96.2	143.2	205.1	345.8	605.9	1513.2
All non-medical causes													
1955	126.6*	72.4*	149.4*	92.1	102.6	125.3	145.1	154.1	194.4	232.4	290.8	365.5	681.5
1965	122.0*	63.3*	148.4*	84.0	102.4	133.2	133.6	150.4	199.8	235.4	280.7	354.9	736.4
1975	102.1*	63.9*	115.5*	75.3	92.2	105.3	105.2	136.6	131.5	162.7	187.8	279.1	572.1
1985	90.5*	59.0*	95.0*	80.4	70.2	78.4	86.3	101.2	108.2	140.5	186.1	248.4	581.9
1990	93.3*	63.4*	89.4*	69.5	78.2	75.5	91.7	92.7	100.9	117.6	168.5	298.6	680.7
1995 projected	98.3*	69.6*	85.8*	79.5	73.7	77.2	88.1	88.8	89.1	104.4	170.7	326.1	802.9

SWITZERLAND: Females

	All ages	0–34	35–69	35–39	40–44	45–49	50–54	55–59	60–64	65–69	70–74	75–79	80+/NK
POPULATION (1000s)													
1955	2585.3	1328.1	1078.0	164.8	178.0	182.4	171.1	151.8	126.6	103.3	81.6	56.7	40.9
1965	3004.2	1581.4	1192.3	195.4	191.6	160.3	175.9	175.9	159.4	133.8	101.2	69.2	60.1
1975	3252.9	1662.4	1274.2	209.8	202.2	194.7	188.2	154.7	165.7	158.9	133.5	96.2	86.6
1985	3317.5	1537.2	1373.9	250.4	232.5	200.8	192.6	183.4	174.2	140.0	143.5	123.6	139.3
1990	3434.3	1555.5	1455.3	247.3	252.4	231.7	197.7	186.3	175.1	164.8	129.5	125.4	168.6
1995 projected	3417.6	1444.7	1522.5	257.6	243.0	248.3	231.4	194.2	180.6	167.4	152.9	114.3	183.2
NUMBER OF DEATHS													
All causes													
1955	24640	1935	8106	259	415	714	985	1337	1819	2577	3554	4409	6636
1965	26496	1614	7700	211	352	439	776	1213	1993	2716	3655	4604	8923
1975	26235	1069	6300	201	299	437	680	872	1398	2413	3495	4811	10560
1985	28649	830	5279	211	301	394	578	856	1233	1706	2894	4721	14925
1990	31247	850	5232	200	299	466	567	755	1192	1753	2493	4426	18246
1995 projected	31962	802	5071	193	282	485	616	732	1104	1659	2719	3743	19627
Lung cancer													
1955	112	1	69	1	3	3	8	20	15	19	19	15	8
1965	147	1	88	1	2	8	9	20	21	27	26	19	13
1975	234	3	133	3	6	13	13	17	40	41	34	40	24
1985	391	4	193	8	12	22	25	28	44	54	78	56	60
1990	491	2	235	7	15	25	27	40	59	62	73	94	87
1995 projected	621	2	275	7	14	28	37	53	69	67	104	106	134
ANNUAL DEATH RATE / 100,000													
All causes													
1955	1005.2*	140.7*	881.4*	157.2	233.1	391.4	575.7	880.8	1436.8	2494.7	4355.4	7776.0	16224.9
1965	845.3*	96.6*	710.9*	108.0	183.7	273.9	441.2	689.6	1250.3	2029.9	3611.7	6653.2	14846.9
1975	652.4*	67.5*	536.5*	95.8	147.9	224.4	361.3	563.7	843.7	1518.6	2618.0	5001.0	12194.0
1985	541.9*	55.7*	443.3*	84.3	129.5	196.2	300.1	466.7	707.8	1218.6	2016.7	3819.6	10714.3
1990	522.2*	54.8*	405.3*	80.9	118.5	201.1	286.8	405.3	680.8	1063.7	1925.1	3529.5	10822.1
1995 projected	500.0*	54.5*	376.0*	74.9	116.0	195.3	266.2	376.9	611.3	991.0	1778.3	3274.7	10713.4
All cancer													
1955	178.0*	9.7*	250.2*	46.1	74.2	139.3	198.7	315.5	421.0	556.6	806.4	1153.4	1577.0
1965	167.1*	7.1*	240.5*	31.7	71.5	118.5	184.8	261.5	432.2	583.0	770.8	1070.8	1497.5
1975	154.1*	7.7*	215.0*	36.7	58.9	109.4	167.9	261.2	347.0	524.2	704.9	1014.6	1436.5
1985	152.2*	6.7*	210.1*	33.5	57.2	94.6	172.4	243.2	355.3	514.3	675.3	958.7	1573.6
1990	146.0*	5.2*	196.2*	34.4	57.4	94.1	162.4	216.9	354.1	453.9	671.0	949.8	1551.0
1995 projected	139.5*	4.5*	183.7*	33.0	56.0	90.6	150.4	204.9	321.2	429.5	646.2	929.1	1530.0
Lung cancer													
1955	4.4*	0.1*	7.4*	0.6	1.7	1.6	4.7	13.2	11.8	18.4	23.3	26.5	19.6
1965	4.8*	0.1*	8.1*	0.5	1.0	5.0	5.1	11.4	13.2	20.2	25.7	27.5	21.6
1975	6.4*	0.2*	11.3*	1.4	3.0	6.7	6.9	11.0	24.1	25.8	25.5	41.6	27.7
1985	9.5*	0.2*	15.9*	3.2	5.2	11.0	13.0	15.3	25.3	38.6	54.4	45.3	43.1
1990	11.1*	0.1*	18.0*	2.8	5.9	10.8	13.7	21.5	33.7	37.6	56.4	75.0	51.6
1995 projected	13.1*	0.1*	20.2*	2.7	5.8	11.3	16.0	27.3	38.2	40.0	68.0	92.7	73.1
Upper aerodigestive cancer (mouth, oesophagus, pharynx and larynx)													
1955	4.6*	0.1*	3.9*	1.2	1.1	2.2	2.9	5.9	5.5	8.7	31.9	37.0	68.5
1965	3.6*	0.1*	4.7*	–	0.5	1.2	3.4	4.0	6.3	17.2	26.7	26.0	31.6
1975	3.3*	0.1*	5.0*	–	0.5	1.0	2.7	7.8	8.4	14.5	9.7	15.6	45.0
1985	3.7*	0.1*	6.0*	–	0.4	2.5	4.7	8.2	8.6	17.9	9.1	13.8	45.2
1990	3.3*	0.1*	3.8*	0.8	1.6	0.4	4.0	6.4	7.4	6.1	18.5	23.1	38.6
1995 projected	3.3*	0.1*	3.1*	1.2	1.6	0.4	3.0	5.1	5.0	5.4	21.6	31.5	40.4
Other cancer													
1955	169.0*	9.5*	238.8*	44.3	71.3	135.4	191.1	296.4	403.6	529.5	751.2	1089.9	1489.0
1965	158.8*	7.0*	227.7*	31.2	69.9	112.3	176.2	246.2	412.8	545.6	718.4	1017.3	1444.3
1975	144.4*	7.5*	198.8*	35.3	55.4	101.7	158.3	242.4	314.4	484.0	669.7	957.4	1363.7
1985	139.0*	6.3*	188.1*	30.4	51.6	81.2	154.7	219.7	321.5	457.9	611.8	899.7	1485.3
1990	131.6*	5.0*	174.3*	30.7	49.9	82.9	144.7	188.9	313.0	410.2	596.1	851.7	1460.9
1995 projected	123.1*	4.3*	160.4*	29.1	48.6	78.9	131.4	172.5	278.0	384.1	556.6	804.9	1416.5
Chronic obstructive pulmonary disease (COPD)													
1955	11.4*	0.6*	4.4*	1.8	2.2	–	2.9	2.6	6.3	14.5	45.3	111.1	295.8
1965	9.2*	0.8*	6.6*	–	1.0	1.9	3.4	6.8	10.0	23.2	42.5	57.8	201.3
1975	9.4*	0.5*	9.0*	1.4	3.0	2.6	8.0	8.4	14.5	25.2	39.7	74.8	158.2
1985	9.3*	0.8*	8.1*	0.4	0.4	2.0	3.6	7.1	16.1	27.1	46.7	74.4	163.0
1990	12.0*	0.7*	11.5*	1.2	2.0	2.6	4.6	10.7	21.7	37.6	57.9	88.5	209.4
1995 projected	15.2*	0.8*	15.2*	1.6	2.9	3.6	6.5	14.4	29.3	48.4	71.3	104.1	263.1
Other respiratory disease													
1955	47.2*	13.1*	23.9*	3.0	6.7	5.5	14.0	17.8	38.7	81.3	152.0	317.5	1046.5
1965	28.6*	4.2*	9.6*	1.0	2.1	2.5	7.4	7.4	16.3	30.6	98.8	225.4	770.4
1975	23.1*	2.9*	9.5*	4.3	2.5	4.1	4.8	5.8	18.7	26.4	60.7	193.3	621.2
1985	14.1*	1.3*	5.1*	–	0.9	2.0	5.2	4.4	7.5	15.7	32.1	84.1	444.4
1990	23.7*	0.9*	6.5*	0.4	1.6	1.7	2.5	6.4	11.4	21.2	53.3	156.3	812.6
1995 projected	32.7*	0.6*	8.4*	0.4	2.1	1.2	2.2	7.7	15.5	29.9	74.6	218.7	1149.0
Vascular disease													
1955	510.5*	4.9*	363.4*	25.5	38.2	95.9	166.6	299.7	629.5	1288.5	2582.1	4943.6	10396.1
1965	428.9*	3.9*	262.9*	16.9	33.4	57.4	104.6	214.3	473.7	940.2	1963.4	4161.8	9790.3
1975	315.6*	3.2*	173.3*	13.8	27.7	41.1	78.6	139.0	289.1	623.7	1284.6	2795.2	8027.7
1985	235.9*	2.1*	112.1*	9.2	14.2	25.9	43.1	97.6	176.8	417.9	855.7	1966.8	6598.0
1990	216.0*	2.8*	91.4*	6.9	15.1	32.8	38.4	73.5	155.3	318.0	771.4	1677.0	6324.4
1995 projected	194.0*	3.0*	77.2*	7.4	16.5	33.8	33.3	60.8	119.0	269.4	651.4	1405.1	5907.8
Liver cirrhosis													
1955	5.2*	0.2*	10.1*	1.2	3.4	2.2	11.1	8.6	19.7	24.2	12.3	21.2	26.9
1965	6.3*	0.2*	11.5*	1.0	5.2	6.2	9.7	15.9	17.6	24.7	18.8	34.7	28.3
1975	5.9*	0.3*	10.4*	2.4	4.5	7.7	10.1	16.8	14.5	17.0	17.2	28.1	26.6
1985	5.2*	0.6*	9.3*	1.2	6.0	8.0	9.3	12.5	11.5	16.4	15.3	21.0	17.9
1990	5.5*	0.2*	11.3*	2.4	7.5	11.2	10.6	11.3	20.0	15.8	10.0	13.6	16.6
1995 projected	6.1*	0.1*	13.2*	2.7	10.3	14.1	11.7	13.9	22.7	16.7	7.2	10.5	12.6
Other medical causes													
1955	204.9*	92.8*	183.7*	59.5	80.9	105.8	127.4	189.1	269.4	454.0	653.2	1005.3	2286.1
1965	158.1*	60.6*	140.4*	33.3	46.5	59.3	98.9	146.1	237.1	361.7	604.7	910.4	1846.9
1975	99.0*	29.8*	80.4*	15.3	20.8	31.8	55.3	87.3	111.0	241.0	412.0	694.4	1376.4
1985	81.3*	24.3*	58.4*	13.2	15.5	27.9	31.7	56.7	99.3	164.3	305.9	560.7	1333.8
1990	79.5*	28.4*	53.7*	10.1	12.3	24.2	32.9	51.0	81.1	164.4	281.9	474.5	1351.1
1995 projected	76.6*	31.4*	48.6*	9.7	9.9	22.2	30.3	44.3	73.1	150.5	249.2	442.7	1301.9
All non-medical causes													
1955	48.1*	19.4*	45.8*	20.0	27.5	42.8	54.9	47.4	52.1	75.5	104.2	224.0	596.6
1965	47.2*	19.8*	39.4*	24.1	24.0	28.1	32.4	37.5	63.4	66.5	112.6	192.2	712.1
1975	45.3*	23.1*	38.9*	21.9	30.7	27.7	36.7	45.2	48.9	61.0	98.9	200.6	547.3
1985	43.8*	20.0*	40.3*	26.8	35.3	35.9	34.8	45.3	41.3	62.9	85.7	153.7	583.6
1990	39.5*	16.7*	34.8*	25.5	22.6	34.5	35.4	35.4	37.1	52.8	79.5	169.9	556.9
1995 projected	35.9*	14.1*	29.8*	20.2	18.5	29.8	32.0	30.9	30.5	46.6	78.5	164.5	549.1

(*The rates for the age groups 0–34 and 35–69 are the means of seven five-yearly rates, but the all-ages rates are standardised to the conventional "European" age distribution)

SWITZERLAND: 1975

Smoking-attributed deaths (Sm.) and total deaths (Total)

		ALL CAUSES	ALL CANCER	Lung cancer	Upper aero-digestive ca.	Other cancer	COPD	Other respiratory	Vascular disease	Liver cirrhosis	Other medical	Non-medical
Males												
0–34	Sm.	–	–	–	–	–	–	–	–	–	–	–
	Total	2104	198	3	3	192	14	56	94	3	662	1077
35–69	Sm.	3767	1759	1169	257	333	311	62	1287	–	348	–
	Total	11452	3627	1254	385	1988	394	204	4344	414	1148	1321
		(33%)	(48%)	(93%)	(67%)	(17%)	(79%)	(30%)	(30%)		(30%)	
70+	Sm.	2679	1107	663	168	276	448	64	879	–	181	–
	Total	16133	3644	743	306	2595	653	670	8639	192	1742	593
		(17%)	(30%)	(89%)	(55%)	(11%)	(69%)	(10%)	(10%)		(10%)	
Any age	Sm.	6446	2866	1832	425	609	759	126	2166	–	529	–
	Total	29689	7469	2000	694	4775	1061	930	13077	609	3552	2991
		(22%)	(38%)	(92%)	(61%)	(13%)	(72%)	(14%)	(17%)		(15%)	
Females												
0–34	Sm.	–	–	–	–	–	–	–	–	–	–	–
	Total	1069	131	3	1	127	8	44	54	5	448	379
35–69	Sm.	99	33	26	3	4	12	2	37	–	15	–
	Total	6300	2537	133	57	2347	106	113	1998	125	942	479
		(2%)	(1%)	(20%)	(5%)	(0%)	(11%)	(2%)	(2%)		(2%)	
70+	Sm.	0	0	0	0	0	0	0	0	–	0	–
	Total	18866	3161	98	67	2996	262	805	11356	73	2410	799
		(0%)	(0%)	(0%)	(0%)	(0%)	(0%)	(0%)	(0%)		(0%)	
Any age	Sm.	99	33	26	3	4	12	2	37	–	15	–
	Total	26235	5829	234	125	5470	376	962	13408	203	3800	1657
		(0%)	(1%)	(11%)	(2%)	(0%)	(3%)	(0%)	(0%)		(0%)	
Males+Females												
0–34	Sm.	–	–	–	–	–	–	–	–	–	–	–
	Total	3173	329	6	4	319	22	100	148	8	1110	1456
35–69	Sm.	3866	1792	1195	260	337	323	64	1324	–	363	–
	Total	17752	6164	1387	442	4335	500	317	6342	539	2090	1800
		(22%)	(29%)	(86%)	(59%)	(8%)	(65%)	(20%)	(21%)		(17%)	
70+	Sm.	2679	1107	663	168	276	448	64	879	–	181	–
	Total	34999	6805	841	373	5591	915	1475	19995	265	4152	1392
		(8%)	(16%)	(79%)	(45%)	(5%)	(49%)	(4%)	(4%)		(4%)	
Any age	Sm.	6545	2899	1858	428	613	771	128	2203	–	544	–
	Total	55924	13298	2234	819	10245	1437	1892	26485	812	7352	4648
		(12%)	(22%)	(83%)	(52%)	(6%)	(54%)	(7%)	(8%)		(7%)	

SWITZERLAND: 1985

Smoking-attributed deaths (Sm.) and total deaths (Total)

		ALL CAUSES	ALL CANCER	Lung cancer	Upper aero-digestive ca.	Other cancer	COPD	Other respiratory	Vascular disease	Liver cirrhosis	Other medical	Non-medical
Males												
0–34	Sm.	–	–	–	–	–	–	–	–	–	–	–
	Total	1704	124	3	6	115	15	22	67	5	464	1007
35–69	Sm.	3316	1700	1139	238	323	285	29	1017	–	285	–
	Total	10155	3610	1228	372	2010	366	94	3545	377	973	1190
		(33%)	(47%)	(93%)	(64%)	(16%)	(78%)	(31%)	(29%)		(29%)	
70+	Sm.	3664	1641	987	178	476	655	58	1090	–	220	–
	Total	19075	5225	1090	302	3833	905	532	9541	170	1934	768
		(19%)	(31%)	(91%)	(59%)	(12%)	(72%)	(11%)	(11%)		(11%)	
Any age	Sm.	6980	3341	2126	416	799	940	87	2107	–	505	–
	Total	30934	8959	2321	680	5958	1286	648	13153	552	3371	2965
		(23%)	(37%)	(92%)	(61%)	(13%)	(73%)	(13%)	(16%)		(15%)	
Females												
0–34	Sm.	–	–	–	–	–	–	–	–	–	–	–
	Total	830	106	4	2	100	12	18	33	9	327	325
35–69	Sm.	241	113	86	12	15	26	3	63	–	36	–
	Total	5279	2524	193	70	2261	92	59	1263	117	693	531
		(5%)	(4%)	(45%)	(17%)	(1%)	(28%)	(5%)	(5%)		(5%)	
70+	Sm.	307	88	64	8	16	68	6	113	–	32	–
	Total	22540	4346	194	93	4059	386	769	12850	73	2990	1126
		(1%)	(2%)	(33%)	(9%)	(0%)	(18%)	(1%)	(1%)		(1%)	
Any age	Sm.	548	201	150	20	31	94	9	176	–	68	–
	Total	28649	6976	391	165	6420	490	846	14146	199	4010	1982
		(2%)	(3%)	(38%)	(12%)	(0%)	(19%)	(1%)	(1%)		(2%)	
Males+Females												
0–34	Sm.	–	–	–	–	–	–	–	–	–	–	–
	Total	2534	230	7	8	215	27	40	100	14	791	1332
35–69	Sm.	3557	1813	1225	250	338	311	32	1080	–	321	–
	Total	15434	6134	1421	442	4271	458	153	4808	494	1666	1721
		(23%)	(30%)	(86%)	(57%)	(8%)	(68%)	(21%)	(22%)		(19%)	
70+	Sm.	3971	1729	1051	186	492	723	64	1203	–	252	–
	Total	41615	9571	1284	395	7892	1291	1301	22391	243	4924	1894
		(10%)	(18%)	(82%)	(47%)	(6%)	(56%)	(5%)	(5%)		(5%)	
Any age	Sm.	7528	3542	2276	436	830	1034	96	2283	–	573	–
	Total	59583	15935	2712	845	12378	1776	1494	27299	751	7381	4947
		(13%)	(22%)	(84%)	(52%)	(7%)	(58%)	(6%)	(8%)		(8%)	

(To be conservative, no deaths before age 35, and none from liver cirrhosis or non-medical causes, were attributed to smoking.)

SWITZERLAND: 1990

Smoking–attributed deaths (Sm.) and total deaths (Total)

Age		ALL CAUSES	ALL CANCER	Lung cancer	Upper aero–digestive ca.	Other cancer	COPD	Other respiratory	Vascular disease	Liver cirrhosis	Other medical	Non–medical
Males												
0–34	Sm.	–	–	–	–	–	–	–	–	–	–	–
	Total	1987	113	5	3	105	9	26	82	5	632	1120
35–69	Sm.	3090	1614	1077	253	284	302	36	830	–	308	–
	Total	10009	3571	1174	410	1987	397	141	3226	321	1140	1213
		(31%)	(45%)	(92%)	(62%)	(14%)	(76%)	(26%)	(26%)		(27%)	
70+	Sm.	3687	1572	955	162	455	805	99	997	–	214	–
	Total	20496	5388	1063	288	4037	1149	1036	9760	140	2084	939
		(18%)	(29%)	(90%)	(56%)	(11%)	(70%)	(10%)	(10%)		(10%)	
Any age	Sm.	6777	3186	2032	415	739	1107	135	1827	–	522	–
	Total	32492	9072	2242	701	6129	1555	1203	13068	466	3856	3272
		(21%)	(35%)	(91%)	(59%)	(12%)	(71%)	(11%)	(14%)		(14%)	
Females												
0–34	Sm.	–	–	–	–	–	–	–	–	–	–	–
	Total	850	86	2	1	83	11	13	46	3	412	279
35–69	Sm.	320	148	117	11	20	51	5	72	–	44	–
	Total	5232	2541	235	50	2256	143	81	1140	154	685	488
		(6%)	(6%)	(50%)	(22%)	(1%)	(36%)	(6%)	(6%)		(6%)	
70+	Sm.	850	203	135	27	41	213	36	320	–	78	–
	Total	25165	4675	254	118	4303	539	1635	13765	58	3238	1255
		(3%)	(4%)	(53%)	(23%)	(1%)	(40%)	(2%)	(2%)		(2%)	
Any age	Sm.	1170	351	252	38	61	264	41	392	–	122	–
	Total	31247	7302	491	169	6642	693	1729	14951	215	4335	2022
		(4%)	(5%)	(51%)	(22%)	(1%)	(38%)	(2%)	(3%)		(3%)	
Males+Females												
0–34	Sm.	–	–	–	–	–	–	–	–	–	–	–
	Total	2837	199	7	4	188	20	39	128	8	1044	1399
35–69	Sm.	3410	1762	1194	264	304	353	41	902	–	352	–
	Total	15241	6112	1409	460	4243	540	222	4366	475	1825	1701
		(22%)	(29%)	(85%)	(57%)	(7%)	(65%)	(18%)	(21%)		(19%)	
70+	Sm.	4537	1775	1090	189	496	1018	135	1317	–	292	–
	Total	45661	10063	1317	406	8340	1688	2671	23525	198	5322	2194
		(10%)	(18%)	(83%)	(47%)	(6%)	(60%)	(5%)	(6%)		(5%)	
Any age	Sm.	7947	3537	2284	453	800	1371	176	2219	–	644	–
	Total	63739	16374	2733	870	12771	2248	2932	28019	681	8191	5294
		(12%)	(22%)	(84%)	(52%)	(6%)	(61%)	(6%)	(8%)		(8%)	

SWITZERLAND: 1995

Smoking–attributed deaths (Sm.) and total deaths (Total)

Age		ALL CAUSES	ALL CANCER	Lung cancer	Upper aero–digestive ca.	Other cancer	COPD	Other respiratory	Vascular disease	Liver cirrhosis	Other medical	Non–medical
Males												
0–34	Sm.	–	–	–	–	–	–	–	–	–	–	–
	Total	2097	104	6	3	95	7	33	90	4	734	1125
35–69	Sm.	2958	1555	1044	261	250	338	45	691	–	329	–
	Total	9909	3515	1148	443	1924	454	194	2926	266	1302	1252
		(30%)	(44%)	(91%)	(59%)	(13%)	(74%)	(23%)	(24%)		(25%)	
70+	Sm.	3809	1528	932	151	445	1006	141	924	–	210	–
	Total	22361	5698	1050	280	4368	1484	1646	9988	123	2243	1179
		(17%)	(27%)	(89%)	(54%)	(10%)	(68%)	(9%)	(9%)		(9%)	
Any age	Sm.	6767	3083	1976	412	695	1344	186	1615	–	539	–
	Total	34367	9317	2204	726	6387	1945	1873	13004	393	4279	3556
		(20%)	(33%)	(90%)	(57%)	(11%)	(69%)	(10%)	(12%)		(13%)	
Females												
0–34	Sm.	–	–	–	–	–	–	–	–	–	–	–
	Total	802	71	2	1	68	13	8	47	2	445	216
35–69	Sm.	401	189	153	12	24	79	6	77	–	50	–
	Total	5071	2491	275	43	2173	197	107	1004	190	644	438
		(8%)	(8%)	(56%)	(28%)	(1%)	(40%)	(6%)	(8%)		(8%)	
70+	Sm.	1300	315	211	43	61	345	80	447	–	113	–
	Total	26089	4853	344	143	4366	710	2469	13425	46	3272	1314
		(5%)	(6%)	(61%)	(30%)	(1%)	(49%)	(3%)	(3%)		(3%)	
Any age	Sm.	1701	504	364	55	85	424	86	524	–	163	–
	Total	31962	7415	621	187	6607	920	2584	14476	238	4361	1968
		(5%)	(7%)	(59%)	(29%)	(1%)	(46%)	(3%)	(4%)		(4%)	
Males+Females												
0–34	Sm.	–	–	–	–	–	–	–	–	–	–	–
	Total	2899	175	8	4	163	20	41	137	6	1179	1341
35–69	Sm.	3359	1744	1197	273	274	417	51	768	–	379	–
	Total	14980	6006	1423	486	4097	651	301	3930	456	1946	1690
		(22%)	(29%)	(84%)	(56%)	(7%)	(64%)	(17%)	(20%)		(19%)	
70+	Sm.	5109	1843	1143	194	506	1351	221	1371	–	323	–
	Total	48450	10551	1394	423	8734	2194	4115	23413	169	5515	2493
		(11%)	(17%)	(82%)	(46%)	(6%)	(62%)	(5%)	(6%)		(6%)	
Any age	Sm.	8468	3587	2340	467	780	1768	272	2139	–	702	–
	Total	66329	16732	2825	913	12994	2865	4457	27480	631	8640	5524
		(13%)	(21%)	(83%)	(51%)	(6%)	(62%)	(6%)	(8%)		(8%)	

(To be conservative, no deaths before age 35, and none from liver cirrhosis or non–medical causes, were attributed to smoking.)

¶TAJIKISTAN: 1990

		No. of deaths			Standardised rates (Defined on p.508)			Annual death rates / 100, 000						
		All ages	0–34	35–69	All ages	0–34	35–69	0–4	5–9	10–14	15–19	20–24	25–29	30–34
ALL CAUSES	M	17664	8576	5234	1197.0	310.8	1312.7	1468.1	90.8	60.6	76.0	94.8	174.9	210.0
	F	15356	6879	3691	855.6	250.5	814.4	1241.7	57.0	36.3	56.7	99.0	115.3	147.5
Tuberculosis	M	99	27	57	8.3	1.7	13.1	0.9	–	0.7	0.7	1.3	3.2	5.2
	F	103	37	55	6.6	2.4	10.3	0.4	–	0.3	1.1	3.8	4.0	7.4
Other infective and parasitic	M	2035	1976	48	39.8	61.6	9.9	405.0	8.4	6.3	4.1	2.2	3.2	2.3
	F	1785	1735	40	36.0	57.4	8.3	357.5	4.7	1.0	4.8	11.8	12.4	9.1
ALL CANCER	M	1505	194	987	145.2	10.6	245.3	9.2	7.9	4.6	5.5	8.3	14.5	24.2
	F	1145	137	645	90.6	7.5	139.6	8.1	3.9	2.7	3.4	5.1	11.5	17.7
Mouth and pharynx cancer	M	58	5	41	5.7	0.3	9.8	0.2	–	–	–	–	0.9	1.2
	F	27	3	18	2.2	0.2	4.2	–	–	0.3	–	–	0.4	0.6
Oesophagus cancer	M	124	2	81	13.8	0.2	21.6	–	–	–	–	–	–	1.2
	F	113	5	60	9.4	0.3	13.4	0.4	–	–	–	0.4	0.4	0.6
Stomach cancer	M	430	10	319	45.4	0.7	82.1	0.2	–	–	–	1.3	1.4	1.7
	F	227	11	142	18.8	0.8	32.0	0.2	–	–	–	0.4	1.8	2.9
Colorectal cancer	M	107	34	61	8.2	1.7	13.6	3.6	–	0.3	0.7	0.9	2.3	4.0
	F	64	25	22	3.9	1.0	4.7	4.6	–	–	–	–	–	2.3
Liver cancer	M	...	...	...	...	...	...	...	...	...	...	...	...	...
	F	...	...	...	...	...	...	...	...	...	...	...	...	...
Pancreas cancer	M	...	...	...	...	...	...	...	...	...	...	...	...	...
	F	...	...	...	...	...	...	...	...	...	...	...	...	...
Larynx cancer	M	8	–	6	0.9	–	1.8	–	–	–	–	–	–	–
	F	5	–	4	0.4	–	0.7	–	–	–	–	–	–	–
Lung cancer	M	208	11	153	21.1	0.7	37.1	–	–	0.3	0.4	0.9	1.8	1.7
	F	76	7	40	6.2	0.5	9.2	–	–	–	0.4	0.8	0.9	1.1
Malignant melanoma	M	...	...	...	...	...	...	...	...	...	...	...	...	...
	F	...	...	...	...	...	...	...	...	...	...	...	...	...
Female breast cancer	F	102	8	67	8.5	0.6	13.2	–	–	–	–	–	0.9	3.4
Cervix cancer	F	80	4	51	6.8	0.3	11.4	–	–	–	–	0.4	0.4	1.1
Other uterine cancer	F	23	1	18	1.9	0.1	3.4	–	–	–	–	0.4	–	–
Ovarian cancer	F	...	...	...	...	...	...	...	...	...	...	...	...	...
Prostate cancer	M	35	1	17	4.2	0.1	4.5	–	–	–	–	–	–	0.6
Bladder cancer	M	...	...	...	...	...	...	...	...	...	...	...	...	...
	F	...	...	...	...	...	...	...	...	...	...	...	...	...
Other and ill-defined cancer sites	M	327	56	207	30.1	3.2	51.4	1.7	2.7	1.3	2.6	2.6	3.2	8.1
	F	290	28	165	23.2	1.6	34.3	0.4	2.0	0.7	1.1	1.3	2.7	2.9
Hodgkin's disease	M	...	...	...	...	...	...	...	...	...	...	...	...	...
	F	...	...	...	...	...	...	...	...	...	...	...	...	...
Myeloma and all lymphomas	M	124	21	76	11.5	1.1	17.9	0.6	1.4	0.7	0.4	0.9	2.3	1.7
	F	90	19	42	6.7	1.0	9.7	0.7	0.6	1.0	1.1	0.8	1.8	1.1
Leukaemia	M	84	54	26	4.2	2.6	5.5	2.8	3.8	2.0	1.5	1.7	2.7	4.0
	F	48	26	16	2.6	1.3	3.3	1.8	1.4	0.7	0.7	0.4	2.2	1.7
ALL VASCULAR DISEASE	M	4845	134	2179	569.6	8.5	592.4	4.3	1.6	2.0	3.0	6.5	12.2	30.0
	F	5128	137	1661	430.0	8.5	383.1	3.7	1.4	1.7	4.1	11.4	14.1	22.9
Rheumatic heart disease and fever	M	104	34	64	7.3	2.2	12.7	0.2	0.3	1.0	1.8	2.6	3.2	6.3
	F	165	52	102	10.9	3.4	19.1	0.2	0.3	0.7	0.7	5.5	7.5	9.1
Hypertensive disease	M	411	8	238	46.7	0.5	62.8	0.4	–	0.3	–	–	–	2.9
	F	451	7	223	38.3	0.4	49.4	0.2	–	–	0.4	1.3	–	1.1
Ischaemic heart disease	M	2826	30	1226	339.3	2.3	337.9	–	–	–	–	0.9	3.2	12.1
	F	2753	17	761	233.9	1.3	183.2	–	–	–	0.7	0.8	0.9	6.3
Pulmonary embolism and other venous	M	...	...	...	...	...	...	...	...	...	...	...	...	...
	F	...	...	...	...	...	...	...	...	...	...	...	...	...
Cerebrovascular disease	M	1225	22	543	146.9	1.4	152.4	0.4	0.3	0.3	–	1.3	3.2	4.6
	F	1462	12	490	124.3	0.8	112.5	0.2	–	–	0.7	0.4	1.3	2.9
Other vascular disease, incl. venous	M	279	40	108	29.3	2.0	26.6	3.2	1.1	0.3	1.1	1.7	2.7	4.0
	F	297	49	85	22.5	2.6	18.9	3.1	1.1	1.0	1.5	3.4	4.4	3.4
Chronic obstructive pulmonary disease	M	764	48	289	88.8	2.4	81.2	4.7	0.3	0.7	0.7	2.2	2.3	6.3
	F	737	52	268	60.1	2.9	61.6	4.2	0.3	–	0.7	2.1	3.5	9.7
Other respiratory disease	M	3162	2927	135	77.4	91.6	32.5	596.1	16.9	6.3	7.0	5.2	5.9	4.0
	F	2793	2562	120	65.2	82.8	24.1	532.4	18.1	6.7	3.4	6.3	6.6	6.3
Peptic ulcer	M	63	10	43	5.7	0.7	10.6	–	–	–	0.7	0.4	1.4	2.3
	F	29	3	12	2.3	0.2	3.1	–	–	0.3	–	–	0.4	0.6
Liver cirrhosis and other liver disease	M	356	41	248	34.3	2.4	62.0	1.1	0.8	1.3	2.6	2.2	4.5	4.0
	F	285	40	164	22.0	2.5	36.3	0.7	0.6	1.0	1.9	2.9	4.0	6.3
Renal disease	M	199	79	80	15.0	4.1	18.1	4.9	2.4	1.0	3.0	6.1	5.9	5.2
	F	214	77	97	13.3	4.3	18.9	3.7	0.8	2.7	4.1	5.1	3.1	10.9
Pregnancy and birth	F	86	54	32	3.9	3.6	4.3	–	–	–	0.7	8.0	8.4	8.0
Congenital and perinatal causes	M	1144	1144	–	19.6	35.0	–	242.1	0.5	1.0	0.7	–	0.9	–
	F	799	799	–	14.1	25.2	–	173.3	1.1	1.0	–	0.4	0.4	–
Ill-defined causes	M	1019	558	279	60.9	21.5	64.0	87.9	7.6	4.3	5.5	9.1	15.0	20.8
	F	883	468	168	44.1	18.0	35.6	76.1	5.9	3.7	6.7	8.0	14.1	11.4
Other medical causes	M	708	334	289	45.6	13.9	69.4	40.1	8.4	8.6	11.4	7.4	9.1	12.1
	F	633	276	249	36.8	12.8	53.4	28.3	5.6	3.4	9.3	16.4	12.4	14.3
ALL NON-MEDICAL CAUSES	M	1765	1104	600	86.8	56.8	114.4	72.1	35.9	24.0	31.0	43.9	97.0	93.5
	F	736	502	180	30.8	22.4	35.9	53.3	14.5	11.8	16.4	17.7	20.3	22.9
Motor vehicle traffic accidents	M	544	336	186	28.3	19.7	36.3	6.2	14.7	7.2	11.1	17.4	41.7	39.8
	F	148	75	51	8.0	3.7	10.9	3.9	4.5	3.7	1.9	2.5	4.4	5.1
Fire	M	66	52	12	2.3	1.9	2.3	7.9	1.1	1.3	1.1	–	0.9	1.2
	F	81	65	13	2.9	3.3	2.3	4.2	1.1	2.4	3.4	3.8	4.9	3.4
Suicide	M	141	57	79	9.1	3.9	13.9	–	–	1.0	2.2	3.5	9.1	11.5
	F	91	41	46	5.2	2.5	8.8	–	–	1.0	5.6	4.2	2.7	4.0
Homicide	M	93	55	36	5.1	3.8	6.9	0.2	–	0.3	–	4.8	11.8	9.2
	F	30	15	13	1.7	0.9	2.5	0.7	–	–	0.7	–	3.5	1.1
POPULATION (thousands):	M=males				2599.9	2035.1	518.0	468.9	367.7	303.6	271.0	229.9	220.7	173.3
	F=females				2632.0	2018.1	537.1	455.9	358.2	297.3	268.1	237.4	226.3	174.9

TAJIKISTAN: 1990

Annual death rates / 100, 000

9th ICD categories

35–39	40–44	45–49	50–54	55–59	60–64	65–69	70–74	75–79	80+/NK			
288.6	445.1	555.7	1002.4	1442.1	2258.3	3196.6	4890.2	7027.8	12750.0	M	**ALL CAUSES**	001–999
220.2	306.6	378.6	599.3	810.6	1450.6	1934.6	3456.7	5125.0	10518.2	F		
0.8	10.0	7.0	13.0	23.7	16.7	20.3	24.4	48.6	25.0	M	**Tuberculosis**	010–018, 137
10.3	10.2	6.4	11.8	12.2	6.2	15.3	17.3	8.6	16.2	F		
4.8	6.2	4.2	14.2	16.3	13.3	10.2	–	20.8	50.0	M	**Other infective**	Rest of 001–139
4.7	8.9	11.2	5.9	4.1	7.7	15.3	10.4	21.6	8.1	F	**and parasitic**	
31.4	58.6	94.7	196.0	301.2	520.0	515.3	689.0	756.9	637.5	M	**ALL CANCER**	140–208
28.4	56.0	92.7	140.7	147.5	233.0	278.9	453.3	456.9	510.1	F		
0.8	6.2	4.2	8.3	10.4	21.7	16.9	24.4	41.7	12.5	M	**Mouth and**	140–149
–	2.5	3.2	5.9	2.7	–	15.3	3.5	4.3	16.2	F	**pharynx cancer**	
2.4	1.2	5.6	17.7	25.2	38.3	61.0	61.0	138.9	68.8	M	**Oesophagus cancer**	150
0.8	2.5	6.4	10.6	20.3	24.7	28.3	51.9	47.4	89.1	F		
4.0	10.0	26.5	64.9	97.9	185.0	186.4	213.4	215.3	218.8	M	**Stomach cancer**	151
3.2	6.4	9.6	27.2	33.8	67.9	76.3	86.5	94.8	109.3	F		
2.4	7.5	5.6	10.6	20.8	35.0	13.6	42.7	20.8	12.5	M	**Colorectal cancer**	153, 154
1.6	2.5	3.2	5.9	1.4	9.3	8.7	24.2	8.6	32.4	F		
...	...	...	...	...	...	...	...	...	...	M	**Liver cancer**	Not given separately
...	...	...	...	...	...	...	...	...	...	F		
...	...	...	...	...	...	...	...	...	...	M	**Pancreas cancer**	Not given separately
...	...	...	...	...	...	...	...	...	...	F		
–	–	1.4	1.2	1.5	1.7	6.8	6.1	–	6.3	M	**Larynx cancer**	161
–	1.3	–	1.2	2.7	–	–	–	4.3	–	F		
1.6	2.5	23.7	29.5	56.4	85.0	61.0	97.6	118.1	68.8	M	**Lung cancer**	162
0.8	2.5	6.4	7.1	5.4	20.1	21.8	38.1	25.9	48.6	F		
...	...	...	...	...	...	...	...	...	...	M	**Malignant melanoma**	Not given
...	...	...	...	...	...	...	...	...	...	F		separately
5.5	12.7	17.6	21.3	8.1	13.9	13.1	41.5	43.1	20.2	F	**Female breast cancer**	174
0.8	6.4	8.0	8.3	17.6	10.8	28.3	31.1	34.5	32.4	F	**Cervix cancer**	180
3.9	1.3	6.4	2.4	2.7	3.1	4.4	6.9	4.3	4.0	F	**Other uterine cancer**	179, 182
...	...	...	...	...	...	...	...	...	...	F	**Ovarian cancer**	Not given separately
0.8	–	–	1.2	5.9	13.3	10.2	42.7	41.7	25.0	M	**Prostate cancer**	185
...	...	...	...	...	...	...	...	...	...	M	**Bladder cancer**	Not given separately
...	...	...	...	...	...	...	...	...	...	F		
10.5	20.0	20.9	41.3	50.4	98.3	118.6	122.0	118.1	168.8	M	**Other and ill-defined**	Rest of 140–208,
11.0	15.3	22.4	39.0	37.9	60.2	54.5	117.6	150.9	113.4	F	**cancer sites**	incl. 155, 157, 172, 183, 188
...	...	...	...	...	...	...	...	...	...	M	**Hodgkin's disease**	Not given separately
...	...	...	...	...	...	...	...	...	...	F		
5.6	5.0	4.2	16.5	28.2	31.7	33.9	61.0	62.5	50.0	M	**Myeloma and all**	200–203,
0.8	–	8.0	8.3	10.8	13.9	26.1	38.1	34.5	40.5	F	**lymphomas**	incl. 201
3.2	6.2	2.8	4.7	4.5	10.0	6.8	18.3	–	6.3	M	**Leukaemia**	204–208
–	2.5	1.6	3.5	4.1	9.3	2.2	13.8	4.3	4.0	F		
52.3	116.0	186.6	392.0	642.4	1011.7	1745.8	3018.3	4472.2	8706.3	M	**ALL VASCULAR**	390–459
46.6	95.4	127.8	242.3	370.8	753.1	1045.8	2152.2	3581.9	7599.2	F	**DISEASE**	
11.3	8.7	11.1	13.0	16.3	15.0	13.6	12.2	6.9	18.8	M	**Rheumatic heart**	390–398
14.2	19.1	12.8	23.6	21.7	29.3	13.1	17.3	21.6	4.0	F	**disease and fever**	
4.8	13.7	20.9	53.1	77.2	96.7	172.9	262.2	250.0	537.5	M	**Hypertensive disease**	401–405
5.5	14.0	30.4	41.4	55.5	98.8	100.2	197.2	215.5	461.5	F		
22.5	67.3	104.5	219.6	357.6	563.3	1030.5	1774.4	2638.9	5618.8	M	**Ischaemic heart**	410–414
11.8	24.2	36.7	87.5	167.8	359.6	594.8	1166.1	2159.5	4603.2	F	**disease**	
...	...	...	...	...	...	...	...	...	...	M	**Pulmonary embolism**	Not given
...	...	...	...	...	...	...	...	...	...	F	**and other venous**	separately
8.0	17.5	33.4	88.5	163.2	285.0	471.2	823.2	1319.4	2093.8	M	**Cerebrovascular**	430–438
9.5	29.3	41.5	75.7	113.7	228.4	289.8	636.7	1034.5	2170.0	F	**disease**	
5.6	8.7	16.7	17.7	28.2	51.7	57.6	146.3	256.9	437.5	M	**Other vascular**	Rest of 390–459,
5.5	8.9	6.4	14.2	12.2	37.0	47.9	134.9	150.9	360.3	F	**disease, incl. venous**	incl. 415, 451–3
8.0	10.0	22.3	44.9	92.0	130.0	261.0	451.2	729.2	1550.0	M	**Chronic obstructive**	490–496
7.1	20.4	20.8	43.7	52.8	118.8	167.8	318.3	418.1	923.1	F	**pulmonary disease**	
8.8	12.5	13.9	24.8	46.0	53.3	67.8	128.0	236.1	281.3	M	**Other respiratory**	Rest of 460–519
17.4	10.2	12.8	21.3	28.4	37.0	41.4	103.8	107.8	226.7	F	**disease**	
1.6	3.7	2.8	8.3	7.4	30.0	20.3	24.4	–	37.5	M	**Peptic ulcer**	531–533
–	–	–	–	5.4	3.1	13.1	6.9	21.6	28.3	F		
8.0	24.9	29.2	57.9	71.2	93.3	149.2	122.0	145.8	162.5	M	**Liver cirrhosis and**	570–573, 576,
7.9	11.5	25.6	21.3	36.5	77.2	74.1	69.2	94.8	157.9	F	**other liver disease**	575.2–579.9
7.2	10.0	13.9	20.1	14.8	26.7	33.9	73.2	62.5	118.8	M	**Renal disease**	580–590
14.2	16.5	8.0	14.2	24.4	30.9	24.0	24.2	43.1	93.1	F		
17.4	11.5	1.6	–	–	–	–	–	–	–	F	**Pregnancy and birth**	630–676
–	–	–	–	–	–	–	–	–	–	M	**Congenital and**	740–779
–	–	–	–	–	–	–	–	–	–	F	**perinatal causes**	
19.3	38.7	37.6	62.6	57.9	120.0	111.9	128.0	256.9	775.0	M	**Ill-defined causes**	780–799
15.8	19.1	12.8	30.7	37.9	52.5	80.6	110.7	150.9	728.7	F		
23.3	36.2	29.2	51.9	60.8	135.0	149.2	128.0	187.5	231.3	M	**Other medical causes**	Rest of 001–799
22.9	22.9	31.9	37.8	55.5	84.9	117.6	141.9	120.7	157.9	F		
123.0	118.5	114.2	116.9	108.3	108.3	111.9	103.7	111.1	175.0	M	**ALL NON–**	E800–E999
27.6	24.2	27.2	29.6	35.2	46.3	61.0	48.4	99.1	68.8	F	**MEDICAL CAUSES**	
40.2	31.2	34.8	39.0	31.2	30.0	47.5	36.6	34.7	68.8	M	**Motor vehicle**	E810–E819
4.7	6.4	6.4	7.1	13.5	12.3	26.1	20.8	43.1	24.3	F	**traffic accidents**	
4.0	1.2	2.8	–	1.5	3.3	3.4	6.1	–	6.3	M	**Fire**	E890–E899
3.2	2.5	–	2.4	4.1	1.5	2.2	3.5	8.6	–	F		
15.3	24.9	12.5	16.5	14.8	10.0	3.4	12.2	13.9	6.3	M	**Suicide**	E950–E959
7.1	5.1	4.8	10.6	12.2	10.8	10.9	–	8.6	8.1	F		
8.8	5.0	8.4	3.5	5.9	10.0	6.8	–	13.9	–	M	**Homicide**	E960–E969
3.2	2.5	4.8	–	1.4	1.5	4.4	3.5	4.3	–	F		
124.4	80.2	71.8	84.7	67.4	60.0	29.5	16.4	14.4	16.0	M	**POPULATION (thousands)**	
126.7	78.6	62.6	84.6	73.9	64.8	45.9	28.9	23.2	24.7	F		

TAJIKISTAN: Males

	All ages	0–34	35–69	35–39	40–44	45–49	50–54	55–59	60–64	65–69	70–74	75–79	80+/NK
POPULATION (1000s)													
1985–90	2414.7	1888.1	477.6	105.1	70.2	85.5	77.7	68.9	46.0	24.2	18.0	14.2	16.8
1985	2226.9	1735.6	439.9	83.0	74.6	89.5	72.3	66.0	34.3	20.2	20.4	13.9	17.1
1990	**2599.9**	**2035.1**	**518.0**	**124.4**	**80.2**	**71.8**	**84.7**	**67.4**	**60.0**	**29.5**	**16.4**	**14.4**	**16.0**
1995 projected	*2984.0*	*2335.8*	*594.6*	*142.8*	*92.0*	*82.4*	*97.2*	*77.4*	*68.9*	*33.9*	*18.8*	*16.5*	*18.3*
NUMBER OF DEATHS													
All causes													
1985–90	17584	9122	4587	300	285	508	736	963	1015	780	900	1038	1937
1985	16820	8894	4098	232	304	554	700	935	714	659	1087	963	1778
1990	**17664**	**8576**	**5234**	**359**	**357**	**399**	**849**	**972**	**1355**	**943**	**802**	**1012**	**2040**
1995 projected	*18615*	*7702*	*6069*	*417*	*404*	*460*	*973*	*1177*	*1588*	*1050*	*897*	*1215*	*2732*
Lung cancer													
1985–90	249	8	185	4	6	18	33	52	45	27	26	17	13
1985	214	3	146	3	3	15	38	51	13	23	40	12	13
1990	**208**	**11**	**153**	**2**	**2**	**17**	**25**	**38**	**51**	**18**	**16**	**17**	**11**
1995 projected	*211*	*17*	*148*	*2*	*3*	*14*	*21*	*43*	*51*	*14*	*13*	*18*	*15*
ANNUAL DEATH RATE / 100,000 (*The rates for the age groups 0–34 and 35–69 are the means of seven five-yearly rates, but the all-ages rates are standardised to the conventional "European" age distribution)													
All causes													
1985–90	1197.5*	354.4*	1294.3*	285.4	406.0	594.2	947.2	1397.7	2206.5	3223.1	5000.0	7309.9	11529.8
1985	1194.8*	388.4*	1290.7*	279.5	407.5	619.0	968.2	1416.7	2081.6	3262.4	5328.4	6928.1	10397.7
1990	**1197.0***	**310.8***	**1312.7***	**288.6**	**445.1**	**555.7**	**1002.4**	**1442.1**	**2258.3**	**3196.6**	**4890.2**	**7027.8**	**12750.0**
1995 projected	*1213.0**	*249.4**	*1316.2**	*292.0*	*439.1*	*558.3*	*1001.0*	*1520.7*	*2304.8*	*3097.3*	*4771.3*	*7363.6*	*14929.0*
All cancer													
1985–90	153.6*	9.3*	262.1*	30.4	55.6	115.8	203.3	326.6	491.3	611.6	766.7	831.0	619.0
1985	158.9*	8.8*	271.8*	20.5	56.3	120.7	215.8	328.8	472.3	688.1	843.1	870.5	602.3
1990	**145.2***	**10.6***	**245.3***	**31.4**	**58.6**	**94.7**	**196.0**	**301.2**	**520.0**	**515.3**	**689.0**	**756.9**	**637.5**
1995 projected	*135.6**	*12.4**	*229.0**	*38.5*	*56.5*	*85.0*	*185.2*	*320.4*	*471.7*	*445.4*	*553.2*	*703.0*	*628.4*
Lung cancer													
1985–90	27.8*	0.6*	51.5*	3.8	8.5	21.1	42.5	75.5	97.8	111.6	144.4	119.7	77.4
1985	25.7*	0.2*	43.7*	3.6	4.0	16.8	52.6	77.3	37.9	113.9	196.1	86.3	76.0
1990	**21.1***	**0.7***	**37.1***	**1.6**	**2.5**	**23.7**	**29.5**	**56.4**	**85.0**	**61.0**	**97.6**	**118.1**	**68.8**
1995 projected	*18.1**	*1.0**	*30.6**	*1.4*	*3.3*	*17.0*	*21.6*	*55.6*	*74.0*	*41.3*	*69.1*	*109.1*	*82.0*
Upper aerodigestive cancer (mouth, oesophagus, pharynx and larynx)													
1985–90	27.1*	0.5*	46.9*	3.8	8.5	17.5	36.0	55.2	91.3	115.7	127.8	162.0	131.0
1985	31.9*	0.2*	53.6*	3.6	12.1	22.3	49.8	68.2	125.4	94.1	137.3	194.2	175.4
1990	**20.5***	**0.5***	**33.2***	**3.2**	**7.5**	**11.1**	**27.2**	**37.1**	**61.7**	**84.7**	**91.5**	**180.6**	**87.5**
1995 projected	*14.7**	*0.6**	*22.9**	*2.1*	*5.4*	*7.3*	*18.5*	*25.8*	*42.1*	*59.0*	*74.5*	*127.3*	*65.6*
Other cancer													
1985–90	98.8*	8.2*	163.7*	22.8	38.5	77.2	124.8	195.9	302.2	384.3	494.4	549.3	410.7
1985	101.3*	8.3*	174.4*	13.3	40.2	81.6	113.4	183.3	309.0	480.2	509.8	589.9	350.9
1990	**103.6***	**9.4***	**175.0***	**26.5**	**48.6**	**59.9**	**139.3**	**207.7**	**373.3**	**369.5**	**500.0**	**458.3**	**481.3**
1995 projected	*102.8**	*10.8**	*175.5**	*35.0*	*47.8*	*60.7*	*145.1*	*239.0*	*355.6*	*345.1*	*409.6*	*466.7*	*480.9*
Chronic obstructive pulmonary disease (COPD)													
1985–90	100.1*	2.3*	97.0*	8.6	12.8	24.6	55.3	94.3	160.9	322.3	550.0	908.5	1529.8
1985	116.9*	1.7*	117.1*	12.0	20.1	25.7	69.2	116.7	209.9	366.3	676.5	1057.6	1678.4
1990	**88.8***	**2.4***	**81.2***	**8.0**	**10.0**	**22.3**	**44.9**	**92.0**	**130.0**	**261.0**	**451.2**	**729.2**	**1550.0**
1995 projected	*67.5**	*2.7**	*56.3**	*5.6*	*6.5*	*15.8*	*32.9*	*63.3*	*90.0*	*179.9*	*313.8*	*557.6*	*1289.6*
Other respiratory disease													
1985–90	82.4*	107.5*	27.3*	6.7	12.8	16.4	23.2	30.5	43.5	57.9	111.1	183.1	267.9
1985	90.1*	123.9*	28.6*	4.8	13.4	16.8	26.3	31.8	37.9	69.3	122.5	151.1	187.1
1990	**77.4***	**91.6***	**32.5***	**8.8**	**12.5**	**13.9**	**24.8**	**46.0**	**53.3**	**67.8**	**128.0**	**236.1**	**281.3**
1995 projected	*70.3**	*67.5**	*35.5**	*7.7*	*12.0*	*12.1*	*26.7*	*56.8*	*62.4*	*70.8*	*159.6*	*327.3*	*398.9*
Vascular disease													
1985–90	547.0*	8.1*	575.4*	58.0	105.4	195.3	355.2	589.3	1030.4	1694.2	2972.2	4542.3	7916.7
1985	506.1*	7.6*	538.2*	53.0	104.6	188.8	358.2	574.2	909.6	1579.2	3044.1	4122.3	6807.0
1990	**569.6***	**8.5***	**592.4***	**52.3**	**116.0**	**186.6**	**392.0**	**642.4**	**1011.7**	**1745.8**	**3018.3**	**4472.2**	**8706.3**
1995 projected	*624.6**	*7.6**	*619.5**	*53.9*	*116.3*	*193.0*	*414.6*	*689.9*	*1095.8*	*1772.9*	*3117.0*	*4793.9*	*10497.3*
Liver cirrhosis and other liver disease													
1985–90	31.8*	2.2*	53.6*	8.6	19.9	30.4	51.5	62.4	87.0	115.7	116.7	154.9	184.5
1985	35.6*	2.6*	57.3*	19.3	16.1	36.9	58.1	65.2	81.6	123.8	112.7	187.1	257.3
1990	**34.3***	**2.4***	**62.0***	**8.0**	**24.9**	**29.2**	**57.9**	**71.2**	**93.3**	**149.2**	**122.0**	**145.8**	**162.5**
1995 projected	*33.7**	*2.3**	*65.4**	*6.3*	*20.7*	*29.1*	*55.6*	*74.9*	*106.0*	*165.2*	*117.0*	*127.3*	*114.8*
Other medical causes													
1985–90	201.8*	168.6*	174.1*	62.8	92.6	106.4	157.0	193.0	284.8	322.3	383.3	584.5	910.7
1985	207.4*	187.4*	174.6*	66.3	99.2	131.8	148.0	195.5	259.5	321.8	397.1	460.4	760.2
1990	**194.9***	**138.4***	**185.0***	**57.1**	**104.7**	**94.7**	**170.0**	**181.0**	**341.7**	**345.8**	**378.0**	**576.4**	**1237.5**
1995 projected	*189.7**	*101.8**	*189.0**	*48.3*	*89.1*	*89.8*	*155.3*	*201.6*	*373.0*	*365.8*	*409.6*	*727.3*	*1748.6*
All non-medical causes													
1985–90	80.6*	56.3*	104.8*	110.4	106.8	105.3	101.7	101.6	108.7	99.2	100.0	105.6	101.2
1985	79.9*	56.4*	103.1*	103.6	97.9	98.3	92.7	104.5	110.8	113.9	132.4	79.1	105.3
1990	**86.8***	**56.8***	**114.4***	**123.0**	**118.5**	**114.2**	**116.9**	**108.3**	**108.3**	**111.9**	**103.7**	**111.1**	**175.0**
1995 projected	*91.7**	*55.1**	*121.5**	*131.7*	*138.0*	*133.5*	*130.7*	*113.7*	*106.0*	*97.3*	*101.1*	*127.3*	*251.4*

TAJIKISTAN: Females

	All ages	0–34	35–69	35–39	40–44	45–49	50–54	55–59	60–64	65–69	70–74	75–79	80+/NK
POPULATION (1000s)													
1985–90	2445.4	1868.9	501.0	106.4	63.3	80.6	80.0	72.9	58.0	39.8	29.2	21.9	24.4
1985	2258.3	1716.4	466.9	81.4	64.9	88.3	77.2	68.5	52.0	34.6	30.4	20.8	23.8
1990	**2632.0**	**2018.1**	**537.1**	**126.7**	**78.6**	**62.6**	**84.6**	**73.9**	**64.8**	**45.9**	**28.9**	**23.2**	**24.7**
1995 projected	*3020.7*	*2316.2*	*616.4*	*145.4*	*90.2*	*71.8*	*97.1*	*84.8*	*74.4*	*52.7*	*33.2*	*26.6*	*28.3*
NUMBER OF DEATHS													
All causes													
1985–90	15660	7529	3516	257	210	318	469	645	781	836	996	1124	2495
1985	15194	7497	3305	237	207	380	475	645	681	680	1061	1035	2296
1990	**15356**	**6879**	**3691**	**279**	**241**	**237**	**507**	**599**	**940**	**888**	**999**	**1189**	**2598**
1995 projected	*15820*	*5879*	*4092*	*279*	*242*	*256*	*524*	*686*	*1074*	*1031*	*1155*	*1429*	*3265*
Lung cancer													
1985–90	102	5	58	3	2	6	5	12	16	14	17	10	12
1985	96	3	58	5	1	9	5	12	20	6	21	5	9
1990	**76**	**7**	**40**	**1**	**2**	**4**	**6**	**4**	**13**	**10**	**11**	**6**	**12**
1995 projected	*72*	*8*	*33*	*1*	*2*	*4*	*5*	*3*	*10*	*8*	*9*	*5*	*17*

ANNUAL DEATH RATE / 100,000 (*The rates for the age groups 0–34 and 35–69 are the means of seven five-yearly rates, but the all-ages rates are standardised to the conventional "European" age distribution)

	All ages	0–34	35–69	35–39	40–44	45–49	50–54	55–59	60–64	65–69	70–74	75–79	80+/NK
All causes													
1985–90	883.5*	297.4*	840.8*	241.5	331.8	394.5	586.3	884.8	1346.6	2100.5	3411.0	5132.4	10225.4
1985	892.5*	330.3*	838.9*	291.2	319.0	430.4	615.3	941.6	1309.6	1965.3	3490.1	4976.0	9647.1
1990	**855.6***	**250.5***	**814.4***	**220.2**	**306.6**	**378.6**	**599.3**	**810.6**	**1450.6**	**1934.6**	**3456.7**	**5125.0**	**10518.2**
1995 projected	*838.2**	*189.1**	*795.0**	*191.9*	*268.3*	*356.5*	*539.6*	*809.0*	*1443.5*	*1956.4*	*3478.9*	*5372.2*	*11537.1*
All cancer													
1985–90	93.2*	7.5*	151.4*	37.6	66.4	89.3	131.3	174.2	251.7	309.0	434.9	461.2	450.8
1985	89.8*	7.3*	146.0*	51.6	52.4	73.6	120.5	192.7	276.9	254.3	444.1	451.9	369.7
1990	**90.6***	**7.5***	**139.6***	**28.4**	**56.0**	**92.7**	**140.7**	**147.5**	**233.0**	**278.9**	**453.3**	**456.9**	**510.1**
1995 projected	*92.0**	*6.8**	*133.8**	*26.1*	*58.8*	*107.2*	*137.0*	*128.5*	*205.6*	*273.2*	*451.8*	*552.6*	*600.7*
Lung cancer													
1985–90	9.0*	0.4*	14.1*	2.8	3.2	7.4	6.3	16.5	27.6	35.2	58.2	45.7	49.2
1985	8.8*	0.3*	14.0*	6.1	1.5	10.2	6.5	17.5	38.5	17.3	69.1	24.0	37.8
1990	**6.2***	**0.5***	**9.2***	**0.8**	**2.5**	**6.4**	**7.1**	**5.4**	**20.1**	**21.8**	**38.1**	**25.9**	**48.6**
1995 projected	*5.1**	*0.5**	*6.5**	*0.7*	*2.2*	*5.6*	*5.1*	*3.5*	*13.4*	*15.2*	*27.1*	*18.8*	*60.1*
Upper aerodigestive cancer (mouth, oesophagus, pharynx and larynx)													
1985–90	11.6*	0.6*	19.7*	3.8	7.9	11.2	17.5	23.3	29.3	45.2	51.4	50.2	65.6
1985	12.8*	0.6*	18.8*	2.5	10.8	12.5	20.7	27.7	28.8	28.9	59.2	62.5	96.6
1990	**12.0***	**0.5***	**18.3***	**0.8**	**6.4**	**9.6**	**17.7**	**25.7**	**24.7**	**43.6**	**55.4**	**56.0**	**105.3**
1995 projected	*11.6**	*0.3**	*16.7**	*0.7*	*4.4*	*7.0*	*14.4*	*21.2*	*25.5*	*43.6*	*54.2*	*75.2*	*106.0*
Other cancer													
1985–90	72.5*	6.6*	117.5*	31.0	55.3	70.7	107.5	134.4	194.8	228.6	325.3	365.3	336.1
1985	68.2*	6.4*	113.2*	43.0	40.1	51.0	93.3	147.4	209.6	208.1	315.8	365.4	235.3
1990	**72.3***	**6.6***	**112.1***	**26.8**	**47.1**	**76.7**	**115.8**	**116.4**	**188.3**	**213.5**	**359.9**	**375.0**	**356.3**
1995 projected	*75.4**	*6.1**	*110.5**	*24.8*	*52.1*	*94.7*	*117.4*	*103.8*	*166.7*	*214.4*	*370.5*	*458.6*	*434.6*
Chronic obstructive pulmonary disease (COPD)													
1985–90	73.2*	2.5*	78.1*	9.4	19.0	31.0	50.0	85.0	125.9	226.1	352.7	529.7	1135.2
1985	91.4*	1.8*	98.8*	9.8	26.2	38.5	68.7	112.4	161.5	274.6	457.2	668.3	1378.2
1990	**60.1***	**2.9***	**61.6***	**7.1**	**20.4**	**20.8**	**43.7**	**52.8**	**118.8**	**167.8**	**318.3**	**418.1**	**923.1**
1995 projected	*42.3**	*3.5**	*42.0**	*6.2*	*14.4*	*13.9*	*29.9*	*35.4*	*80.6*	*113.9*	*216.9*	*289.5*	*653.7*
Other respiratory disease													
1985–90	73.8*	101.2*	23.5*	14.1	11.1	14.9	18.8	26.1	29.3	50.3	75.3	109.6	209.0
1985	83.5*	119.7*	26.1*	12.3	7.7	27.2	24.6	39.4	25.0	46.2	59.2	57.7	189.1
1990	**65.2***	**82.8***	**24.1***	**17.4**	**10.2**	**12.8**	**21.3**	**28.4**	**37.0**	**41.4**	**103.8**	**107.8**	**226.7**
1995 projected	*54.7**	*58.0**	*24.4**	*20.6*	*8.9*	*9.7*	*14.4*	*27.1*	*34.9*	*55.0*	*141.6*	*142.9*	*307.4*
Vascular disease													
1985–90	429.3*	9.2*	389.2*	52.6	97.9	129.0	223.8	381.3	674.1	1165.8	2130.1	3534.2	7586.1
1985	405.4*	9.9*	370.0*	65.1	106.3	131.4	218.9	388.3	625.0	1054.9	2102.0	3298.1	6911.8
1990	**430.0***	**8.5***	**383.1***	**46.6**	**95.4**	**127.8**	**242.3**	**370.8**	**753.1**	**1045.8**	**2152.2**	**3581.9**	**7599.2**
1995 projected	*446.8**	*6.7**	*383.7**	*37.8*	*83.1*	*124.0*	*231.7*	*395.0*	*760.8*	*1053.1*	*2186.7*	*3710.5*	*8321.6*
Liver cirrhosis and other liver disease													
1985–90	21.4*	2.2*	34.3*	10.3	14.2	19.9	28.8	39.8	56.9	70.4	75.3	95.9	147.5
1985	22.8*	1.6*	33.0*	16.0	9.2	26.0	31.1	32.1	55.8	60.7	92.1	120.2	197.5
1990	**22.0***	**2.5***	**36.3***	**7.9**	**11.5**	**25.6**	**21.3**	**36.5**	**77.2**	**74.1**	**69.2**	**94.8**	**157.9**
1995 projected	*21.1**	*2.6**	*38.1**	*6.9*	*10.0*	*20.9*	*18.5*	*40.1*	*94.1*	*75.9*	*57.2*	*75.2*	*127.2*
Other medical causes													
1985–90	161.0*	151.0*	129.9*	91.2	94.8	80.6	102.5	142.7	169.0	228.6	277.4	319.6	618.9
1985	165.7*	166.8*	125.4*	99.5	90.9	104.2	114.0	144.5	125.0	199.4	250.0	288.5	525.2
1990	**156.9***	**123.9***	**133.9***	**85.2**	**89.1**	**71.9**	**100.5**	**139.4**	**185.2**	**265.8**	**311.4**	**366.4**	**1032.4**
1995 projected	*153.7**	*91.0**	*142.5**	*70.8*	*73.2*	*58.5*	*82.4*	*148.6*	*224.5*	*339.7*	*385.5*	*503.8*	*1459.4*
All non-medical causes													
1985–90	31.7*	23.8*	34.5*	26.3	28.4	29.8	31.3	35.7	39.7	50.3	65.1	82.2	77.9
1985	33.9*	23.2*	39.7*	36.9	26.2	29.4	37.6	32.1	40.4	75.1	85.5	91.3	75.6
1990	**30.8***	**22.4***	**35.9***	**27.6**	**24.2**	**27.2**	**29.6**	**35.2**	**46.3**	**61.0**	**48.4**	**99.1**	**68.8**
1995 projected	*27.4**	*20.5**	*30.6**	*23.4*	*20.0*	*22.3*	*25.7*	*34.2*	*43.0*	*45.5*	*39.2*	*97.7*	*67.1*

TAJIKISTAN: 1985–1990

Smoking-attributed deaths (Sm.) and total deaths (Total)

		ALL CAUSES	ALL CANCER	Lung cancer	Upper aero-digestive ca.	Other cancer	COPD	Other respiratory	Vascular disease	Cirrhosis/other liver	Other medical	Non-medical
Males												
0–34	Sm.	–	–	–	–	–	–	–	–	–	–	–
	Total	9122	154	8	7	139	40	3134	113	35	4651	995
35–69	Sm.	901	272	156	71	45	176	20	307	–	126	–
	Total	4587	927	185	161	581	299	103	1868	200	686	504
		(20%)	(29%)	(84%)	(44%)	(8%)	(59%)	(19%)	(16%)		(18%)	
70+	Sm.	310	63	39	16	8	167	1	70	–	9	–
	Total	3875	360	56	68	236	485	91	2510	74	305	50
		(8%)	(18%)	(70%)	(24%)	(3%)	(34%)	(1%)	(3%)		(3%)	
Any age	Sm.	1211	335	195	87	53	343	21	377	–	135	–
	Total	17584	1441	249	236	956	824	3328	4491	309	5642	1549
		(7%)	(23%)	(78%)	(37%)	(6%)	(42%)	(1%)	(8%)		(2%)	
Females												
0–34	Sm.	–	–	–	–	–	–	–	–	–	–	–
	Total	7529	119	5	8	106	41	2844	131	33	3867	494
35–69	Sm.	186	30	20	9	1	73	3	59	–	21	–
	Total	3516	655	58	84	513	312	105	1534	149	597	164
		(5%)	(5%)	(34%)	(11%)	(0%)	(23%)	(3%)	(4%)		(4%)	
70+	Sm.	165	21	14	6	1	96	1	43	–	4	–
	Total	4615	338	39	42	257	496	97	3247	79	302	56
		(4%)	(6%)	(36%)	(14%)	(0%)	(19%)	(1%)	(1%)		(1%)	
Any age	Sm.	351	51	34	15	2	169	4	102	–	25	–
	Total	15660	1112	102	134	876	849	3046	4912	261	4766	714
		(2%)	(5%)	(33%)	(11%)	(0%)	(20%)	(0%)	(2%)		(1%)	
Males+Females												
0–34	Sm.	–	–	–	–	–	–	–	–	–	–	–
	Total	16651	273	13	15	245	81	5978	244	68	8518	1489
35–69	Sm.	1087	302	176	80	46	249	23	366	–	147	–
	Total	8103	1582	243	245	1094	611	208	3402	349	1283	668
		(13%)	(19%)	(72%)	(33%)	(4%)	(41%)	(11%)	(11%)		(11%)	
70+	Sm.	475	84	53	22	9	263	2	113	–	13	–
	Total	8490	698	95	110	493	981	188	5757	153	607	106
		(6%)	(12%)	(56%)	(20%)	(2%)	(27%)	(1%)	(2%)		(2%)	
Any age	Sm.	1562	386	229	102	55	512	25	479	–	160	–
	Total	33244	2553	351	370	1832	1673	6374	9403	570	10408	2263
		(5%)	(15%)	(65%)	(28%)	(3%)	(31%)	(0%)	(5%)		(2%)	

TAJIKISTAN: 1985

Smoking-attributed deaths (Sm.) and total deaths (Total)

		ALL CAUSES	ALL CANCER	Lung cancer	Upper aero-digestive ca.	Other cancer	COPD	Other respiratory	Vascular disease	Cirrhosis/other liver	Other medical	Non-medical
Males												
0–34	Sm.	–	–	–	–	–	–	–	–	–	–	–
	Total	8894	132	3	3	126	20	3204	89	31	4514	904
35–69	Sm.	768	226	122	69	35	169	17	242	–	114	–
	Total	4098	841	146	175	520	321	96	1560	199	637	444
		(19%)	(27%)	(84%)	(39%)	(7%)	(53%)	(18%)	(16%)		(18%)	
70+	Sm.	325	70	45	18	7	169	2	74	–	10	–
	Total	3828	396	65	85	246	572	78	2358	93	275	56
		(8%)	(18%)	(69%)	(21%)	(3%)	(30%)	(3%)	(3%)		(4%)	
Any age	Sm.	1093	296	167	87	42	338	19	316	–	124	–
	Total	16820	1369	214	263	892	913	3378	4007	323	5426	1404
		(6%)	(22%)	(78%)	(33%)	(5%)	(37%)	(1%)	(8%)		(2%)	
Females												
0–34	Sm.	–	–	–	–	–	–	–	–	–	–	–
	Total	7497	103	3	7	93	26	2989	121	22	3797	439
35–69	Sm.	216	38	24	12	2	88	4	61	–	25	–
	Total	3305	598	58	80	460	368	114	1363	138	553	171
		(7%)	(6%)	(41%)	(15%)	(0%)	(24%)	(4%)	(4%)		(5%)	
70+	Sm.	0	0	0	0	0	0	0	0	–	0	–
	Total	4392	317	35	54	228	606	75	2970	100	261	63
		(0%)	(0%)	(0%)	(0%)	(0%)	(0%)	(0%)	(0%)		(0%)	
Any age	Sm.	216	38	24	12	2	88	4	61	–	25	–
	Total	15194	1018	96	141	781	1000	3178	4454	260	4611	673
		(1%)	(4%)	(25%)	(9%)	(0%)	(9%)	(0%)	(1%)		(1%)	
Males+Females												
0–34	Sm.	–	–	–	–	–	–	–	–	–	–	–
	Total	16391	235	6	10	219	46	6193	210	53	8311	1343
35–69	Sm.	984	264	146	81	37	257	21	303	–	139	–
	Total	7403	1439	204	255	980	689	210	2923	337	1190	615
		(13%)	(18%)	(72%)	(32%)	(4%)	(37%)	(10%)	(10%)		(12%)	
70+	Sm.	325	70	45	18	7	169	2	74	–	10	–
	Total	8220	713	100	139	474	1178	153	5328	193	536	119
		(4%)	(10%)	(45%)	(13%)	(1%)	(14%)	(1%)	(1%)		(2%)	
Any age	Sm.	1309	334	191	99	44	426	23	377	–	149	–
	Total	32014	2387	310	404	1673	1913	6556	8461	583	10037	2077
		(4%)	(14%)	(62%)	(25%)	(3%)	(22%)	(0%)	(4%)		(1%)	

(To be conservative, no deaths before age 35, and none from liver cirrhosis or non-medical causes, were attributed to smoking.)

TAJIKISTAN: 1990

Smoking-attributed deaths (Sm.) and total deaths (Total)

		ALL CAUSES	ALL CANCER	Lung cancer	Upper aero-digestive ca.	Other cancer	COPD	Other respiratory	Vascular disease	Cirrhosis/ other liver	Other medical	Non-medical
Males												
0–34	Sm.	–	–	–	–	–	–	–	–	–	–	–
	Total	8576	194	11	7	176	48	2927	134	41	4128	1104
35–69	Sm.	724	206	122	46	38	139	19	255	–	105	–
	Total	5234	987	153	128	706	289	135	2179	248	796	600
		(14%)	(21%)	(80%)	(36%)	(5%)	(48%)	(14%)	(12%)		(13%)	
70+	Sm.	247	45	28	11	6	135	2	57	–	8	–
	Total	3854	324	44	55	225	427	100	2532	67	343	61
		(6%)	(14%)	(64%)	(20%)	(3%)	(32%)	(2%)	(2%)		(2%)	
Any age	Sm.	971	251	150	57	44	274	21	312	–	113	–
	Total	17664	1505	208	190	1107	764	3162	4845	356	5267	1765
		(5%)	(17%)	(72%)	(30%)	(4%)	(36%)	(1%)	(6%)		(2%)	
Females												
0–34	Sm.	–	–	–	–	–	–	–	–	–	–	–
	Total	6879	137	7	8	122	52	2562	137	40	3449	502
35–69	Sm.	0	0	0	0	0	0	0	0	–	0	–
	Total	3691	645	40	82	523	268	120	1661	164	653	180
		(0%)	(0%)	(0%)	(0%)	(0%)	(0%)	(0%)	(0%)		(0%)	
70+	Sm.	0	0	0	0	0	0	0	0	–	0	–
	Total	4786	363	29	55	279	417	111	3330	81	430	54
		(0%)	(0%)	(0%)	(0%)	(0%)	(0%)	(0%)	(0%)		(0%)	
Any age	Sm.	0	0	0	0	0	0	0	0	–	0	–
	Total	15356	1145	76	145	924	737	2793	5128	285	4532	736
		(0%)	(0%)	(0%)	(0%)	(0%)	(0%)	(0%)	(0%)		(0%)	
Males+Females												
0–34	Sm.	–	–	–	–	–	–	–	–	–	–	–
	Total	15455	331	18	15	298	100	5489	271	81	7577	1606
35–69	Sm.	724	206	122	46	38	139	19	255	–	105	–
	Total	8925	1632	193	210	1229	557	255	3840	412	1449	780
		(8%)	(13%)	(63%)	(22%)	(3%)	(25%)	(7%)	(7%)		(7%)	
70+	Sm.	247	45	28	11	6	135	2	57	–	8	–
	Total	8640	687	73	110	504	844	211	5862	148	773	115
		(3%)	(7%)	(38%)	(10%)	(1%)	(16%)	(1%)	(1%)		(1%)	
Any age	Sm.	971	251	150	57	44	274	21	312	–	113	–
	Total	33020	2650	284	335	2031	1501	5955	9973	641	9799	2501
		(3%)	(9%)	(53%)	(17%)	(2%)	(18%)	(0%)	(3%)		(1%)	

TAJIKISTAN: 1995

Smoking-attributed deaths (Sm.) and total deaths (Total)

		ALL CAUSES	ALL CANCER	Lung cancer	Upper aero-digestive ca.	Other cancer	COPD	Other respiratory	Vascular disease	Cirrhosis/ other liver	Other medical	Non-medical
Males												
0–34	Sm.	–	–	–	–	–	–	–	–	–	–	–
	Total	7702	261	17	9	235	66	2477	126	49	3502	1221
35–69	Sm.	649	179	111	30	38	96	17	258	–	99	–
	Total	6069	1081	148	101	832	231	169	2636	293	913	746
		(11%)	(17%)	(75%)	(30%)	(5%)	(42%)	(10%)	(10%)		(11%)	
70+	Sm.	218	40	27	8	5	106	4	58	–	10	–
	Total	4844	335	46	47	242	387	157	3298	64	517	86
		(5%)	(12%)	(59%)	(17%)	(2%)	(27%)	(3%)	(2%)		(2%)	
Any age	Sm.	867	219	138	38	43	202	21	316	–	109	–
	Total	18615	1677	211	157	1309	684	2803	6060	406	4932	2053
		(5%)	(13%)	(65%)	(24%)	(3%)	(30%)	(1%)	(5%)		(2%)	
Females												
0–34	Sm.	–	–	–	–	–	–	–	–	–	–	–
	Total	5879	155	8	5	142	72	2058	133	49	2891	521
35–69	Sm.	0	0	0	0	0	0	0	0	–	0	–
	Total	4092	707	33	84	590	211	137	1900	196	763	178
		(0%)	(0%)	(0%)	(0%)	(0%)	(0%)	(0%)	(0%)		(0%)	
70+	Sm.	0	0	0	0	0	0	0	0	–	0	–
	Total	5849	467	31	68	368	334	172	4068	75	675	58
		(0%)	(0%)	(0%)	(0%)	(0%)	(0%)	(0%)	(0%)		(0%)	
Any age	Sm.	0	0	0	0	0	0	0	0	–	0	–
	Total	15820	1329	72	157	1100	617	2367	6101	320	4329	757
		(0%)	(0%)	(0%)	(0%)	(0%)	(0%)	(0%)	(0%)		(0%)	
Males+Females												
0–34	Sm.	–	–	–	–	–	–	–	–	–	–	–
	Total	13581	416	25	14	377	138	4535	259	98	6393	1742
35–69	Sm.	649	179	111	30	38	96	17	258	–	99	–
	Total	10161	1788	181	185	1422	442	306	4536	489	1676	924
		(6%)	(10%)	(61%)	(16%)	(3%)	(22%)	(6%)	(6%)		(6%)	
70+	Sm.	218	40	27	8	5	106	4	58	–	10	–
	Total	10693	802	77	115	610	721	329	7366	139	1192	144
		(2%)	(5%)	(35%)	(7%)	(1%)	(15%)	(1%)	(1%)		(1%)	
Any age	Sm.	867	219	138	38	43	202	21	316	–	109	–
	Total	34435	3006	283	314	2409	1301	5170	12161	726	9261	2810
		(3%)	(7%)	(49%)	(12%)	(2%)	(16%)	(0%)	(3%)		(1%)	

(To be conservative, no deaths before age 35, and none from liver cirrhosis or non-medical causes, were attributed to smoking.)

¶TURKMENISTAN: 1990

		No. of deaths			Standardised rates (Defined on p.514)			Annual death rates / 100, 000						
		All ages	0–34	35–69	All ages	0–34	35–69	0–4	5–9	10–14	15–19	20–24	25–29	30–34
ALL CAUSES	M	13890	6139	5094	1561.1	358.9	1882.1	1567.3	93.3	64.9	117.0	182.4	221.4	266.2
	F	11865	4448	3368	1029.7	257.4	1039.9	1233.5	66.2	41.0	74.2	106.3	113.9	166.5
Tuberculosis	M	256	69	166	27.8	6.1	44.8	2.1	0.8	0.5	1.6	6.0	17.6	14.5
	F	133	51	69	11.6	4.5	18.4	0.7	1.7	0.5	2.2	6.1	9.0	11.1
Other infective	M	1146	1093	44	38.4	55.4	13.7	355.9	6.7	3.8	6.4	6.6	5.0	3.1
and parasitic	F	957	912	30	32.0	48.5	8.0	295.5	8.1	5.8	3.3	8.5	7.8	10.3
ALL CANCER	M	1259	119	868	194.2	8.9	331.7	8.3	6.7	8.6	4.8	8.3	14.5	11.4
	F	1041	93	632	116.2	7.8	190.4	5.0	2.6	4.3	4.9	8.5	5.4	23.6
Mouth and	M	69	3	54	10.6	0.3	19.5	–	–	–	0.5	–	0.6	0.8
pharynx cancer	F	20	1	10	2.4	0.1	2.7	–	–	–	–	0.6	–	–
Oesophagus cancer	M	306	1	205	54.4	0.1	82.5	–	–	–	–	–	–	0.8
	F	289	3	177	34.3	0.3	55.7	–	–	–	–	–	–	2.2
Stomach cancer	M	194	5	140	32.3	0.5	54.3	–	–	–	–	1.2	0.6	1.5
	F	144	6	86	16.9	0.6	27.4	–	–	–	0.5	1.2	–	2.2
Colorectal cancer	M	54	11	31	8.0	1.0	12.4	–	–	–	0.5	1.8	3.1	1.5
	F	33	–	25	3.8	–	7.7	–	–	–	–	–	–	–
Liver cancer	M	...	...	...	...	...	...	...	...	...	...	...	...	...
	F	...	...	...	...	...	...	...	...	...	...	...	...	...
Pancreas cancer	M	...	...	...	...	...	...	...	...	...	...	...	...	...
	F	...	...	...	...	...	...	...	...	...	...	...	...	...
Larynx cancer	M	38	2	28	6.4	0.2	12.3	–	–	–	–	–	0.6	0.8
	F	3	–	2	0.4	–	0.7	–	–	–	–	–	–	–
Lung cancer	M	203	5	168	31.1	0.4	63.1	0.7	–	–	–	0.6	1.3	–
	F	42	2	27	5.0	0.2	8.6	–	–	–	–	–	–	1.5
Malignant melanoma	M	...	...	...	...	...	...	...	...	...	...	...	...	...
	F	...	...	...	...	...	...	...	...	...	...	...	...	...
Female breast cancer	F	110	9	80	12.2	0.9	21.8	–	–	–	–	–	1.8	4.4
Cervix cancer	F	56	1	43	6.4	0.1	12.2	–	–	–	–	–	–	0.7
Other uterine cancer	F	36	4	19	4.0	0.3	6.0	0.7	–	–	–	–	–	1.5
Ovarian cancer	F	...	...	...	...	...	...	...	...	...	...	...	...	...
Prostate cancer	M	13	1	8	2.3	0.1	4.2	–	–	–	–	0.6	–	–
Bladder cancer	M	...	...	...	...	...	...	...	...	...	...	...	...	...
	F	...	...	...	...	...	...	...	...	...	...	...	...	...
Other and ill-defined	M	289	44	195	40.9	3.1	72.0	4.5	2.9	3.8	2.1	1.2	3.8	3.1
cancer sites	F	250	36	140	26.7	2.9	41.7	2.1	1.3	1.0	2.2	4.3	2.4	7.4
Hodgkin's disease	M	...	...	...	...	...	...	...	...	...	...	...	...	...
	F	...	...	...	...	...	...	...	...	...	...	...	...	...
Myeloma and all	M	50	17	27	5.6	1.3	8.3	0.7	0.8	1.9	1.1	0.6	1.9	2.3
lymphomas	F	24	10	11	2.0	0.8	2.9	0.4	–	1.4	0.5	1.2	–	2.2
Leukaemia	M	43	30	12	2.7	2.1	3.2	2.4	2.9	2.9	0.5	2.4	2.5	0.8
	F	34	21	12	2.2	1.5	3.0	1.8	1.3	1.9	1.6	1.2	1.2	1.5
ALL VASCULAR	M	4626	261	2520	835.5	20.0	999.6	30.6	4.2	4.3	12.8	16.7	25.2	46.5
DISEASE	F	4984	211	1807	587.6	16.0	584.4	25.2	4.3	2.4	12.0	12.8	21.0	34.6
Rheumatic heart	M	63	23	35	7.0	2.0	11.5	–	–	1.0	1.6	4.2	4.4	3.1
disease and fever	F	86	44	38	6.6	3.9	9.4	0.4	0.9	–	4.4	4.9	5.4	11.8
Hypertensive disease	M	509	11	312	92.6	1.0	126.2	–	0.4	–	1.1	1.2	0.6	3.8
	F	591	11	314	69.9	1.0	97.4	0.7	–	–	0.5	0.6	0.6	4.4
Ischaemic heart	M	2971	68	1542	565.9	6.5	609.3	1.0	0.4	0.5	2.1	5.4	8.8	27.5
disease	F	3083	22	914	375.5	1.9	305.9	0.7	–	0.5	0.5	0.6	5.4	5.9
Pulmonary embolism	M	...	...	...	...	...	...	...	...	...	...	...	...	...
and other venous	F	...	...	...	...	...	...	...	...	...	...	...	...	...
Cerebrovascular	M	788	39	515	135.0	2.9	208.2	6.2	0.4	–	0.5	2.4	3.8	6.9
disease	F	972	35	462	114.2	2.6	149.0	4.3	0.9	–	2.7	3.6	3.0	3.7
Other vascular	M	295	120	116	35.0	7.6	44.5	23.4	2.9	2.9	7.4	3.6	7.5	5.3
disease, incl. venous	F	252	99	79	21.5	6.6	22.7	19.1	2.6	1.9	3.8	3.0	6.6	8.8
Chronic obstructive	M	580	159	221	86.5	9.0	89.5	44.4	1.3	1.0	1.6	4.8	3.8	6.1
pulmonary disease	F	571	128	169	57.6	7.6	53.9	34.7	0.9	1.4	1.6	2.4	4.2	8.1
Other respiratory	M	1889	1802	61	65.1	90.1	23.3	596.2	15.1	5.2	4.3	3.0	2.5	4.6
disease	F	1498	1407	46	51.3	72.5	13.7	477.3	10.7	6.3	4.4	3.0	3.0	2.9
Peptic ulcer	M	43	1	34	6.7	0.1	12.5	–	–	–	–	–	–	0.8
	F	16	3	8	1.7	0.3	2.6	–	0.4	–	–	–	0.6	0.7
Liver cirrhosis and	M	467	75	314	65.7	5.6	112.2	9.0	1.7	2.9	3.2	1.8	9.4	11.4
other liver disease	F	345	45	206	36.8	3.5	61.3	4.3	0.9	–	2.2	4.9	6.0	6.6
Renal disease	M	96	33	51	10.6	2.4	16.4	3.8	1.7	0.5	2.7	2.4	2.5	3.1
	F	94	36	41	7.8	2.8	10.7	2.8	0.4	1.4	3.3	3.6	3.6	4.4
Pregnancy and birth	F	53	38	15	3.0	3.4	2.7	–	–	–	1.1	7.3	8.4	7.4
Congenital and	M	844	842	2	23.6	41.8	0.7	285.0	1.3	1.0	2.7	1.8	0.6	–
perinatal causes	F	604	600	4	17.5	30.9	0.8	205.5	3.4	1.4	–	1.2	3.0	1.5
Ill-defined causes	M	380	193	93	42.8	11.5	32.2	49.9	1.3	1.4	1.6	6.0	8.8	11.4
	F	333	149	30	27.1	8.6	8.2	42.2	2.6	0.5	2.7	2.4	3.6	5.9
Other medical causes	M	591	352	193	49.3	21.4	69.2	80.9	5.9	9.5	9.0	12.5	10.7	21.4
	F	500	253	159	37.0	15.8	46.6	57.8	5.6	4.3	6.5	11.5	12.0	12.5
ALL NON-	M	1713	1140	527	114.9	86.6	136.1	101.2	46.8	26.2	66.5	112.6	120.8	132.0
MEDICAL CAUSES	F	736	522	152	42.5	35.3	38.1	82.6	24.8	12.6	30.0	34.0	26.4	36.8
Motor vehicle	M	429	271	147	29.9	22.0	37.8	10.0	13.8	7.6	14.4	41.7	31.4	35.1
traffic accidents	F	123	71	39	8.6	5.1	10.0	6.4	6.8	1.4	4.4	4.9	5.4	6.6
Fire	M	63	40	19	4.5	2.8	4.5	5.9	1.7	–	1.6	1.8	5.0	3.8
	F	110	96	7	5.1	6.9	1.5	11.3	4.3	1.9	9.3	10.3	3.6	7.4
Suicide	M	216	123	87	16.8	11.0	22.6	–	–	2.9	13.3	18.5	19.5	22.9
	F	82	43	23	6.5	3.7	6.0	–	–	–	8.2	7.3	4.8	5.9
Homicide	M	193	108	80	15.1	10.0	19.6	–	0.4	0.5	9.0	8.9	25.2	25.9
	F	52	24	26	3.9	2.1	6.0	0.7	0.4	–	1.6	1.2	4.2	6.6
POPULATION (thousands):	M=males				1779.9	1385.2	366.9	290.5	239.1	209.6	188.1	167.8	159.0	131.1
	F=females				1831.2	1374.1	401.6	282.2	234.2	207.1	183.4	164.7	166.8	135.7

TURKMENISTAN: 1990

Annual death rates / 100, 000

9th ICD categories

35–39	40–44	45–49	50–54	55–59	60–64	65–69	70–74	75–79	80+/NK			
456.1	568.4	848.2	1453.0	1995.6	3149.1	4704.1	6118.2	8591.4	15800.0	M	ALL CAUSES	001–999
219.0	259.2	413.4	773.4	1146.0	1829.5	2638.8	4255.7	5966.7	13096.2	F		
41.8	19.8	33.3	70.1	61.5	61.7	25.5	100.0	53.8	66.7	M	Tuberculosis	010–018, 137
11.0	6.4	16.7	24.6	28.4	21.1	20.9	22.8	5.6	44.9	F		
8.4	11.5	4.2	15.4	15.4	15.4	25.5	18.2	32.3	53.3	M	Other infective	Rest of 001–139
3.0	6.4	8.4	13.1	10.1	6.3	9.0	22.8	33.3	25.6	F	and parasitic	
38.7	49.4	101.9	285.5	411.0	604.1	831.6	1009.1	1010.8	893.3	M	ALL CANCER	140–208
31.0	70.4	100.2	175.7	198.8	360.0	397.0	648.4	516.7	519.2	F		
–	1.6	8.3	27.4	33.0	25.7	40.8	45.5	64.5	13.3	M	Mouth and	140–149
1.0	–	4.2	1.6	8.1	4.2	–	27.4	16.7	–	F	pharynx cancer	
3.1	9.9	24.9	58.1	92.3	164.5	224.5	354.5	430.1	280.0	M	Oesophagus cancer	150
3.0	17.6	14.6	47.6	58.8	105.3	143.3	228.3	188.9	160.3	F		
7.3	6.6	10.4	30.8	63.7	133.7	127.6	236.4	139.8	133.3	M	Stomach cancer	151
1.0	3.2	10.4	16.4	40.6	54.7	65.7	105.0	77.8	96.2	F		
1.0	4.9	4.2	5.1	17.6	18.0	35.7	54.5	43.0	26.7	M	Colorectal cancer	153, 154
2.0	1.6	2.1	4.9	6.1	18.9	17.9	9.1	5.6	32.1	F		
...	...	...	...	...	...	...	...	...	...	M	Liver cancer	Not given separately
...	...	...	...	...	...	...	...	...	...	F		
...	...	...	...	...	...	...	...	...	...	M	Pancreas cancer	Not given separately
...	...	...	...	...	...	...	...	...	...	F		
–	–	2.1	13.7	8.8	15.4	45.9	36.4	10.8	40.0	M	Larynx cancer	161
–	–	–	–	–	2.1	3.0	4.6	–	–	F		
5.2	4.9	18.7	61.5	90.1	118.3	142.9	136.4	107.5	66.7	M	Lung cancer	162
–	–	4.2	13.1	6.1	12.6	23.9	41.1	16.7	6.4	F		
...	...	...	...	...	...	...	...	...	...	M	Malignant melanoma	Not given
...	...	...	...	...	...	...	...	...	...	F		separately
7.0	16.0	16.7	39.4	18.3	25.3	29.9	22.8	22.2	76.9	F	Female breast cancer	174
6.0	12.8	12.5	6.6	8.1	12.6	26.9	27.4	22.2	12.8	F	Cervix cancer	180
–	3.2	6.3	1.6	2.0	16.8	11.9	27.4	22.2	19.2	F	Other uterine cancer	179, 182
...	...	...	...	...	...	...	...	...	...	F	Ovarian cancer	Not given separately
–	–	–	1.7	4.4	2.6	20.4	9.1	21.5	13.3	M	Prostate cancer	185
...	...	...	...	...	...	...	...	...	...	M	Bladder cancer	Not given separately
...	...	...	...	...	...	...	...	...	...	F		
18.8	13.2	27.0	71.8	81.3	102.8	188.8	109.1	172.0	293.3	M	Other and ill-defined	Rest of 140–208,
6.0	14.4	23.0	39.4	40.6	96.8	71.6	150.7	138.9	102.6	F	cancer sites	incl. 155, 157, 172, 183, 188
...	...	...	...	...	...	...	...	...	...	M	Hodgkin's disease	Not given separately
...	...	...	...	...	...	...	...	...	...	F		
1.0	8.2	4.2	6.8	17.6	15.4	5.1	18.2	21.5	26.7	M	Myeloma and all	200–203,
2.0	–	2.1	1.6	6.1	8.4	–	–	5.6	12.8	F	lymphomas	incl. 201
2.1	–	2.1	8.5	2.2	7.7	–	9.1	–	–	M	Leukaemia	204–208
3.0	1.6	4.2	3.3	4.1	2.1	3.0	4.6	–	–	F		
110.9	222.4	399.2	676.9	980.2	1771.2	2836.7	3945.5	5989.2	11386.7	M	ALL VASCULAR	390–459
53.0	97.6	171.2	339.9	630.8	1111.6	1686.6	2780.8	4316.7	10128.2	F	DISEASE	
4.2	4.9	12.5	10.3	15.4	12.9	20.4	27.3	–	26.7	M	Rheumatic heart	390–398
9.0	12.8	10.4	8.2	8.1	8.4	9.0	4.6	–	19.2	F	disease and fever	
7.3	13.2	62.4	71.8	145.1	231.4	352.0	436.4	612.9	1080.0	M	Hypertensive disease	401–405
11.0	22.4	29.2	88.7	113.6	181.1	235.8	319.6	388.9	807.7	F		
68.0	136.7	232.8	430.8	556.0	1141.4	1699.0	2790.9	4430.1	8560.0	M	Ischaemic heart	410–414
15.0	33.6	77.2	141.2	288.0	583.2	1003.0	1812.8	3083.3	7660.3	F	disease	
...	...	...	...	...	...	...	...	...	...	M	Pulmonary embolism	Not given
...	...	...	...	...	...	...	...	...	...	F	and other venous	separately
18.8	49.4	72.8	133.3	224.2	331.6	627.6	581.8	741.9	1346.7	M	Cerebrovascular	430–438
11.0	17.6	39.7	83.7	198.8	286.3	406.0	593.6	744.4	1352.6	F	disease	
12.6	18.1	18.7	30.8	39.6	54.0	137.8	109.1	204.3	373.3	M	Other vascular	Rest of 390–459,
7.0	11.2	14.6	18.1	22.3	52.6	32.8	50.2	100.0	288.5	F	disease, incl. venous	incl. 415, 451–3
13.6	9.9	37.4	51.3	94.5	149.1	270.4	354.5	763.4	1200.0	M	Chronic obstructive	490–496
12.0	12.8	10.4	32.8	60.9	77.9	170.1	328.8	450.0	775.6	F	pulmonary disease	
5.2	4.9	6.2	18.8	15.4	51.4	61.2	81.8	86.0	120.0	M	Other respiratory	Rest of 460–519
5.0	–	10.4	9.9	26.4	14.7	29.9	54.8	66.7	134.6	F	disease	
1.0	–	8.3	8.5	13.2	36.0	20.4	18.2	32.3	40.0	M	Peptic ulcer	531–533
–	–	–	–	8.1	4.2	6.0	13.7	5.6	6.4	F		
14.6	57.7	60.3	92.3	138.5	187.7	234.7	263.6	204.3	400.0	M	Liver cirrhosis and	570–573, 576,
16.0	11.2	18.8	69.0	85.2	94.7	134.3	109.6	172.2	250.0	F	other liver disease	575.2–579.9
12.6	9.9	10.4	13.7	4.4	28.3	35.7	27.3	32.3	80.0	M	Renal disease	580–590
11.0	12.8	–	6.6	8.1	12.6	23.9	22.8	22.2	51.3	F		
10.0	4.8	4.2	–	–	–	–	–	–	–	F	Pregnancy and birth	630–676
–	–	–	–	–	5.1	–	–	–	–	M	Congenital and	740–779
2.0	1.6	–	–	–	2.1	–	–	–	–	F	perinatal causes	
19.9	4.9	20.8	25.6	26.4	46.3	81.6	90.9	129.0	960.0	M	Ill-defined causes	780–799
8.0	4.8	4.2	6.6	–	12.6	20.9	41.1	133.3	775.6	F		
14.6	24.7	31.2	65.0	87.9	102.8	158.2	127.3	129.0	266.7	M	Other medical causes	Rest of 001–799
22.0	9.6	31.3	36.1	46.7	75.8	104.5	123.3	166.7	198.7	F		
174.7	153.2	135.1	129.9	147.3	90.0	122.4	81.8	129.0	333.3	M	ALL NON-	E800–E999
35.0	20.8	37.6	59.1	42.6	35.8	35.8	86.8	77.8	185.9	F	MEDICAL CAUSES	
57.5	29.7	29.1	29.1	52.7	30.8	35.7	36.4	43.0	40.0	M	Motor vehicle	E810–E819
6.0	8.0	10.4	14.8	16.2	8.4	6.0	13.7	27.8	32.1	F	traffic accidents	
9.4	3.3	2.1	5.1	6.6	–	5.1	–	10.8	40.0	M	Fire	E890–E899
3.0	1.6	–	–	2.0	4.2	–	22.8	–	12.8	F		
25.1	28.0	20.8	23.9	22.0	23.1	15.3	9.1	32.3	26.7	M	Suicide	E950–E959
5.0	3.2	12.5	8.2	2.0	2.1	9.0	18.3	11.1	64.1	F		
30.3	29.7	24.9	13.7	15.4	7.7	15.3	9.1	–	53.3	M	Homicide	E960–E969
8.0	4.8	–	13.1	4.1	6.3	6.0	–	–	12.8	F		
95.6	60.7	48.1	58.5	45.5	38.9	19.6	11.0	9.3	7.5	M	**POPULATION (thousands)**	
100.0	62.5	47.9	60.9	49.3	47.5	33.5	21.9	18.0	15.6	F		

TURKMENISTAN: Males

	All ages	0–34	35–69	35–39	40–44	45–49	50–54	55–59	60–64	65–69	70–74	75–79	80+/NK
POPULATION (1000s)													
1985–90	1670.6	1304.0	337.8	81.1	50.2	59.1	53.2	46.8	31.0	16.4	12.3	8.9	7.6
1985	1565.1	1224.3	310.9	63.8	50.4	63.1	50.2	44.9	23.9	14.6	13.9	8.3	7.7
1990	**1779.9**	**1385.2**	**366.9**	**95.6**	**60.7**	**48.1**	**58.5**	**45.5**	**38.9**	**19.6**	**11.0**	**9.3**	**7.5**
1995 projected	*2048.8*	*1594.3*	*422.4*	*110.0*	*69.9*	*55.4*	*67.3*	*52.4*	*44.8*	*22.6*	*12.7*	*10.7*	*8.7*
NUMBER OF DEATHS													
All causes													
1985–90	14323	6971	4594	349	286	516	737	979	967	760	779	823	1156
1985	13874	6752	4303	300	290	601	679	1031	694	708	894	803	1122
1990	**13890**	**6139**	**5094**	**436**	**345**	**408**	**850**	**908**	**1225**	**922**	**673**	**799**	**1185**
1995 projected	*14258*	*5513*	*5699*	*464*	*371*	*470*	*913*	*1052*	*1382*	*1047*	*718*	*926*	*1402*
Lung cancer													
1985–90	192	5	156	4	6	16	29	43	35	23	19	9	3
1985	194	4	151	5	8	20	24	49	24	21	27	7	5
1990	**203**	**5**	**168**	**5**	**3**	**9**	**36**	**41**	**46**	**28**	**15**	**10**	**5**
1995 projected	*216*	*4*	*181*	*4*	*2*	*9*	*37*	*49*	*51*	*29*	*15*	*9*	*7*
ANNUAL DEATH RATE / 100,000 (*The rates for the age groups 0–34 and 35–69 are the means of seven five-yearly rates, but the all-ages rates are standardised to the conventional "European" age distribution)													
All causes													
1985–90	1603.5*	426.5*	1872.0*	430.3	569.7	873.1	1385.3	2091.9	3119.4	4634.1	6333.3	9247.2	15210.5
1985	1632.5*	451.8*	1914.3*	470.2	575.4	952.5	1352.6	2296.2	2903.8	4849.3	6431.7	9674.7	14571.4
1990	**1561.1***	**358.9***	**1882.1***	**456.1**	**568.4**	**848.2**	**1453.0**	**1995.6**	**3149.1**	**4704.1**	**6118.2**	**8591.4**	**15800.0**
1995 projected	*1499.5**	*290.1**	*1840.4**	*421.8*	*530.8*	*848.4*	*1356.6*	*2007.6*	*3084.8*	*4632.7*	*5653.5*	*8654.2*	*16114.9*
All cancer													
1985–90	206.8*	10.4*	362.1*	34.5	63.7	142.1	274.4	474.4	661.3	884.1	1065.0	1033.7	802.6
1985	215.9*	13.8*	382.4*	34.5	67.5	163.2	280.9	530.1	648.5	952.1	1136.7	915.7	805.2
1990	**194.2***	**8.9***	**331.7***	**38.7**	**49.4**	**101.9**	**285.5**	**411.0**	**604.1**	**831.6**	**1009.1**	**1010.8**	**893.3**
1995 projected	*177.7**	*6.4**	*284.9**	*31.8*	*34.3*	*84.8*	*231.8*	*368.3*	*513.4*	*730.1*	*944.9*	*1130.8*	*988.5*
Lung cancer													
1985–90	31.4*	0.5*	63.4*	4.9	12.0	27.1	54.5	91.9	112.9	140.2	154.5	101.1	39.5
1985	33.6*	0.5*	65.2*	7.8	15.9	31.7	47.8	109.1	100.4	143.8	194.2	84.3	64.9
1990	**31.1***	**0.4***	**63.1***	**5.2**	**4.9**	**18.7**	**61.5**	**90.1**	**118.3**	**142.9**	**136.4**	**107.5**	**66.7**
1995 projected	*28.9**	*0.3**	*59.1**	*3.6*	*2.9*	*16.2*	*55.0*	*93.5*	*113.8*	*128.3*	*118.1*	*84.1*	*80.5*
Upper aerodigestive cancer (mouth, oesophagus, pharynx and larynx)													
1985–90	77.9*	0.5*	136.3*	4.9	17.9	38.9	101.5	166.7	264.5	359.8	439.0	415.7	355.3
1985	81.4*	1.0*	145.8*	9.4	19.8	39.6	117.5	171.5	292.9	369.9	410.1	361.4	428.6
1990	**71.4***	**0.6***	**114.3***	**3.1**	**11.5**	**35.3**	**99.1**	**134.1**	**205.7**	**311.2**	**436.4**	**505.4**	**333.3**
1995 projected	*66.0**	*0.4**	*91.9**	*1.8*	*7.2*	*28.9*	*80.2*	*99.2*	*156.3*	*269.9*	*464.6*	*607.5*	*344.8*
Other cancer													
1985–90	97.6*	9.4*	162.4*	24.7	33.9	76.1	118.4	215.8	283.9	384.1	471.5	516.9	407.9
1985	101.0*	12.3*	171.4*	17.2	31.7	91.9	115.5	249.4	255.2	438.4	532.4	469.9	311.7
1990	**91.7***	**8.0***	**154.4***	**30.3**	**32.9**	**47.8**	**124.8**	**186.8**	**280.2**	**377.6**	**436.4**	**397.8**	**493.3**
1995 projected	*82.8**	*5.7**	*134.0**	*26.4*	*24.3*	*39.7*	*96.6*	*175.6*	*243.3*	*331.9*	*362.2*	*439.3*	*563.2*
Chronic obstructive pulmonary disease (COPD)													
1985–90	96.3*	6.0*	99.1*	13.6	12.0	30.5	63.9	111.1	158.1	304.9	471.5	797.8	1394.7
1985	118.7*	3.7*	131.6*	9.4	15.9	44.4	83.7	144.8	205.0	417.8	568.3	1108.4	1558.4
1990	**86.5***	**9.0***	**89.5***	**13.6**	**9.9**	**37.4**	**51.3**	**94.5**	**149.1**	**270.4**	**354.5**	**763.4**	**1200.0**
1995 projected	*63.8**	*9.9**	*62.1**	*11.8*	*8.6*	*25.3*	*35.7*	*64.9*	*102.7*	*185.8*	*244.1*	*560.7*	*885.1*
Other respiratory disease													
1985–90	104.8*	148.1*	30.6*	9.9	10.0	15.2	22.6	32.1	51.6	73.2	97.6	146.1	250.0
1985	118.6*	187.2*	19.8*	11.0	15.9	12.7	10.0	20.0	20.9	47.9	64.7	96.4	129.9
1990	**65.1***	**90.1***	**23.3***	**5.2**	**4.9**	**6.2**	**18.8**	**15.4**	**51.4**	**61.2**	**81.8**	**86.0**	**120.0**
1995 projected	*45.3**	*50.9**	*29.5**	*3.6*	*2.9*	*5.4*	*17.8*	*21.0*	*71.4*	*84.1*	*86.6*	*93.5*	*114.9*
Vascular disease													
1985–90	839.2*	20.6*	975.3*	118.4	217.1	367.2	641.0	1032.1	1725.8	2725.6	4056.9	6449.4	11342.1
1985	823.5*	15.3*	944.2*	123.8	222.2	345.5	609.6	1106.9	1543.9	2657.5	4036.0	6747.0	10948.1
1990	**835.5***	**20.0***	**999.6***	**110.9**	**222.4**	**399.2**	**676.9**	**980.2**	**1771.2**	**2836.7**	**3945.5**	**5989.2**	**11386.7**
1995 projected	*826.7**	*21.1**	*1016.6**	*99.1*	*216.0*	*426.0*	*664.2*	*1013.4*	*1812.5*	*2885.0*	*3661.4*	*5878.5*	*11172.4*
Liver cirrhosis and other liver disease													
1985–90	52.7*	4.2*	92.5*	19.7	35.9	55.8	77.1	111.1	171.0	176.8	187.0	236.0	236.8
1985	49.7*	4.3*	84.7*	26.6	37.7	57.1	63.7	113.6	150.6	143.8	151.1	277.1	220.8
1990	**65.7***	**5.6***	**112.2***	**14.6**	**57.7**	**60.3**	**92.3**	**138.5**	**187.7**	**234.7**	**263.6**	**204.3**	**400.0**
1995 projected	*81.8**	*5.4**	*144.1**	*14.5*	*57.2*	*77.6*	*112.9*	*173.7*	*250.0*	*323.0*	*315.0*	*289.7*	*482.8*
Other medical causes													
1985–90	197.8*	155.7*	184.0*	83.8	95.6	125.2	178.6	203.0	248.4	353.7	374.0	449.4	1000.0
1985	202.9*	150.4*	224.9*	122.3	113.1	183.8	179.3	236.1	246.9	493.2	417.3	397.6	649.4
1990	**199.1***	**138.6***	**189.6***	**98.3**	**70.8**	**108.1**	**198.3**	**208.8**	**295.6**	**346.9**	**381.8**	**408.6**	**1466.7**
1995 projected	*184.0**	*107.9**	*161.5**	*65.5*	*45.8*	*83.0*	*167.9*	*217.6*	*250.0*	*300.9*	*322.8*	*532.7*	*2080.5*
All non-medical causes													
1985–90	105.8*	81.4*	128.3*	150.4	135.5	137.1	127.8	128.2	103.2	115.9	81.3	134.8	184.2
1985	103.2*	77.1*	126.7*	142.6	103.2	145.8	125.5	144.8	87.9	137.0	57.6	132.5	259.7
1990	**114.9***	**86.6***	**136.1***	**174.7**	**153.2**	**135.1**	**129.9**	**147.3**	**90.0**	**122.4**	**81.8**	**129.0**	**333.3**
1995 projected	*120.2**	*88.5**	*141.6**	*195.5*	*166.0*	*146.2*	*126.3*	*148.9*	*84.8*	*123.9*	*78.7*	*168.2*	*390.8*

TURKMENISTAN: Females

	All ages	0–34	35–69	35–39	40–44	45–49	50–54	55–59	60–64	65–69	70–74	75–79	80+/NK
POPULATION (1000s)													
1985–90	1724.2	1296.1	374.0	84.2	50.3	60.0	54.8	52.3	42.9	29.5	22.9	16.4	14.8
1985	1619.8	1217.7	349.0	65.4	49.8	63.9	52.5	52.0	38.4	27.0	24.1	14.8	14.2
1990	**1831.2**	**1374.1**	**401.6**	**100.0**	**62.5**	**47.9**	**60.9**	**49.3**	**47.5**	**33.5**	**21.9**	**18.0**	**15.6**
1995 projected	*2107.8*	*1581.7*	*462.2*	*115.1*	*71.9*	*55.1*	*70.1*	*56.7*	*54.7*	*38.6*	*25.2*	*20.7*	*18.0*
NUMBER OF DEATHS													
All causes													
1985–90	12610	5372	3255	189	157	268	415	619	790	817	983	1058	1942
1985	12206	5367	3021	142	142	298	398	624	664	753	1005	998	1815
1990	**11865**	**4448**	**3368**	**219**	**162**	**198**	**471**	**565**	**869**	**884**	**932**	**1074**	**2043**
1995 projected	*12248*	*3844*	*3823*	*246*	*171*	*218*	*522*	*662*	*983*	*1021*	*1006*	*1226*	*2349*
Lung cancer													
1985–90	55	3	36	–	2	4	5	8	10	7	8	4	4
1985	61	1	41	–	1	4	5	8	15	8	11	2	6
1990	**42**	**2**	**27**	–	–	**2**	**8**	**3**	**6**	**8**	**9**	**3**	**1**
1995 projected	*36*	*3*	*22*	–	–	*2*	*7*	*2*	*5*	*6*	*9*	*2*	–
ANNUAL DEATH RATE / 100,000 (*The rates for the age groups 0–34 and 35–69 are the means of seven five-yearly rates, but the all-ages rates are standardised to the conventional "European" age distribution)													
All causes													
1985–90	1092.3*	325.8*	1076.4*	224.5	312.1	446.7	757.3	1183.6	1841.5	2769.5	4292.6	6451.2	13121.6
1985	1097.4*	351.5*	1063.5*	217.1	285.1	466.4	758.1	1200.0	1729.2	2788.9	4170.1	6743.2	12781.7
1990	**1029.7***	**257.4***	**1039.9***	**219.0**	**259.2**	**413.4**	**773.4**	**1146.0**	**1829.5**	**2638.8**	**4255.7**	**5966.7**	**13096.2**
1995 projected	*982.6**	*199.0**	*1028.8**	*213.7*	*237.8*	*395.6*	*744.7*	*1167.5*	*1797.1*	*2645.1*	*3992.1*	*5922.7*	*13050.0*
All cancer													
1985–90	127.7*	8.8*	217.7*	35.6	69.6	106.7	180.7	256.2	393.9	481.4	602.6	603.7	567.6
1985	129.2*	7.9*	226.0*	27.5	58.2	95.5	177.1	311.5	419.3	492.6	580.9	655.4	514.1
1990	**116.2***	**7.8***	**190.4***	**31.0**	**70.4**	**100.2**	**175.7**	**198.8**	**360.0**	**397.0**	**648.4**	**516.7**	**519.2**
1995 projected	*105.4**	*7.4**	*169.4**	*38.2*	*76.5*	*107.1*	*145.5*	*160.5*	*285.2*	*373.1*	*587.3*	*507.2*	*472.2*
Lung cancer													
1985–90	6.6*	0.3*	11.7*	–	4.0	6.7	9.1	15.3	23.3	23.7	34.9	24.4	27.0
1985	7.9*	0.1*	14.6*	–	2.0	6.3	9.5	15.4	39.1	29.6	45.6	13.5	42.3
1990	**5.0***	**0.2***	**8.6***	–	–	**4.2**	**13.1**	**6.1**	**12.6**	**23.9**	**41.1**	**16.7**	**6.4**
1995 projected	*3.6**	*0.3**	*6.0**	–	–	*3.6*	*10.0*	*3.5*	*9.1*	*15.5*	*35.7*	*9.7*	–
Upper aerodigestive cancer (mouth, oesophagus, pharynx and larynx)													
1985–90	41.8*	0.7*	71.8*	4.8	13.9	25.0	54.7	84.1	130.5	189.8	222.7	213.4	223.0
1985	41.9*	0.7*	77.6*	1.5	14.1	21.9	70.5	109.6	114.6	211.1	157.7	236.5	190.1
1990	**37.0***	**0.4***	**59.2***	**4.0**	**17.6**	**18.8**	**49.3**	**66.9**	**111.6**	**146.3**	**260.3**	**205.6**	**160.3**
1995 projected	*33.2**	*0.3**	*51.4**	*4.3*	*18.1*	*14.5*	*34.2*	*51.1*	*82.3*	*155.4*	*261.9*	*202.9*	*138.9*
Other cancer													
1985–90	79.2*	7.8*	134.1*	30.9	51.7	75.0	116.8	156.8	240.1	267.8	345.0	365.9	317.6
1985	79.4*	7.0*	133.8*	26.0	42.2	67.3	97.1	186.5	265.6	251.9	377.6	405.4	281.7
1990	**74.2***	**7.1***	**122.7***	**27.0**	**52.8**	**77.2**	**113.3**	**125.8**	**235.8**	**226.9**	**347.0**	**294.4**	**352.6**
1995 projected	*68.5**	*6.8**	*112.0**	*33.9*	*58.4*	*88.9*	*101.3*	*105.8*	*193.8*	*202.1*	*289.7*	*294.7*	*333.3*
Chronic obstructive pulmonary disease (COPD)													
1985–90	61.9*	5.8*	57.9*	11.9	9.9	20.0	32.8	57.4	107.2	166.1	288.2	469.5	1006.8
1985	75.5*	4.2*	65.1*	12.2	10.0	28.2	32.4	69.2	114.6	188.9	336.1	547.3	1450.7
1990	**57.6***	**7.6***	**53.9***	**12.0**	**12.8**	**10.4**	**32.8**	**60.9**	**77.9**	**170.1**	**328.8**	**450.0**	**775.6**
1995 projected	*46.3**	*8.2**	*45.2**	*13.0*	*8.3*	*7.3*	*25.7*	*47.6*	*64.0*	*150.3*	*289.7*	*318.8*	*550.0*
Other respiratory disease													
1985–90	83.7*	126.4*	17.1*	7.1	6.0	11.7	10.9	15.3	21.0	47.5	52.4	91.5	182.4
1985	97.7*	162.3*	9.1*	3.1	10.0	9.4	5.7	5.8	7.8	22.2	8.3	67.6	98.6
1990	**51.3***	**72.5***	**13.7***	**5.0**	–	**10.4**	**9.9**	**26.4**	**14.7**	**29.9**	**54.8**	**66.7**	**134.6**
1995 projected	*37.7**	*42.6**	*17.9**	*3.5*	–	*9.1*	*14.3*	*37.0*	*20.1*	*41.5*	*75.4*	*91.8*	*161.1*
Vascular disease													
1985–90	605.4*	17.5*	584.7*	61.8	107.4	178.3	344.9	625.2	1046.6	1728.8	2903.9	4707.3	10391.9
1985	595.7*	15.6*	575.1*	67.3	96.4	187.8	369.5	592.3	953.1	1759.3	2892.1	4804.1	10056.3
1990	**587.6***	**16.0***	**584.4***	**53.0**	**97.6**	**171.2**	**339.9**	**630.8**	**1111.6**	**1686.6**	**2780.8**	**4316.7**	**10128.2**
1995 projected	*572.0**	*14.3**	*583.1**	*46.9*	*86.2*	*154.3*	*332.4*	*666.7*	*1137.1*	*1658.0*	*2575.4*	*4193.2*	*9850.0*
Liver cirrhosis and other liver disease													
1985–90	37.3*	3.8*	57.6*	11.9	19.9	28.3	52.9	80.3	90.9	118.6	144.1	195.1	256.8
1985	31.3*	2.7*	51.7*	9.2	16.1	40.7	49.5	82.7	59.9	103.7	74.7	202.7	176.1
1990	**36.8***	**3.5***	**61.3***	**16.0**	**11.2**	**18.8**	**69.0**	**85.2**	**94.7**	**134.3**	**109.6**	**172.2**	**250.0**
1995 projected	*43.1**	*4.4**	*74.6**	*17.4*	*7.0*	*16.3*	*68.5*	*107.6*	*118.8*	*186.5*	*119.0*	*207.7*	*283.3*
Other medical causes													
1985–90	137.2*	132.6*	101.7*	64.1	71.6	63.3	89.4	110.9	139.9	172.9	222.7	298.8	587.8
1985	129.1*	127.1*	98.8*	73.4	72.3	70.4	89.5	98.1	125.0	163.0	224.1	331.1	345.1
1990	**137.8***	**114.6***	**98.1***	**67.0**	**46.4**	**64.7**	**87.0**	**101.4**	**134.7**	**185.1**	**246.6**	**366.7**	**1102.6**
1995 projected	*134.3**	*87.0**	*96.8**	*53.9*	*36.2*	*54.4*	*84.2*	*102.3*	*144.4*	*202.1*	*273.8*	*516.9*	*1555.6*
All non-medical causes													
1985–90	39.2*	30.9*	39.8*	32.1	27.8	38.3	45.6	38.2	42.0	54.2	78.6	85.4	128.4
1985	38.9*	31.7*	37.8*	24.5	22.1	34.4	34.3	40.4	49.5	59.3	53.9	135.1	140.8
1990	**42.5***	**35.3***	**38.1***	**35.0**	**20.8**	**37.6**	**59.1**	**42.6**	**35.8**	**35.8**	**86.8**	**77.8**	**185.9**
1995 projected	*43.8**	*35.2**	*41.8**	*40.8*	*23.6*	*47.2*	*74.2*	*45.9*	*27.4*	*33.7*	*71.4*	*87.0*	*177.8*

TURKMENISTAN: 1985–1990

Smoking–attributed deaths (Sm.) and total deaths (Total)

		ALL CAUSES	ALL CANCER	Lung cancer	Upper aero–digestive ca.	Other cancer	COPD	Other respiratory	Vascular disease	Cirrhosis/ other liver	Other medical	Non–medical
Males												
0–34	Sm.	–	–	–	–	–	–	–	–	–	–	–
	Total	6971	126	5	6	115	94	2757	241	52	2697	1004
35–69	Sm.	1067	331	136	156	39	144	15	458	–	119	–
	Total	4594	862	156	309	397	220	77	2228	242	515	450
		(23%)	(38%)	(87%)	(50%)	(10%)	(65%)	(19%)	(21%)		(23%)	
70+	Sm.	191	55	22	29	4	75	1	55	–	5	–
	Total	2758	284	31	118	135	235	44	1935	62	162	36
		(7%)	(19%)	(71%)	(25%)	(3%)	(32%)	(2%)	(3%)		(3%)	
Any age	Sm.	1258	386	158	185	43	219	16	513	–	124	–
	Total	14323	1272	192	433	647	549	2878	4404	356	3374	1490
		(9%)	(30%)	(82%)	(43%)	(7%)	(40%)	(1%)	(12%)		(4%)	
Females												
0–34	Sm.	–	–	–	–	–	–	–	–	–	–	–
	Total	5372	102	3	7	92	85	2290	211	46	2204	434
35–69	Sm.	102	27	10	17	0	28	0	40	–	7	–
	Total	3255	673	36	212	425	170	53	1688	182	346	143
		(3%)	(4%)	(28%)	(8%)	(0%)	(16%)	(0%)	(2%)		(2%)	
70+	Sm.	23	5	2	3	0	9	0	8	–	1	–
	Total	3983	321	16	119	186	292	54	2975	103	187	51
		(1%)	(2%)	(13%)	(3%)	(0%)	(3%)	(0%)	(0%)		(1%)	
Any age	Sm.	125	32	12	20	0	37	0	48	–	8	–
	Total	12610	1096	55	338	703	547	2397	4874	331	2737	628
		(1%)	(3%)	(22%)	(6%)	(0%)	(7%)	(0%)	(1%)		(0%)	
Males+Females												
0–34	Sm.	–	–	–	–	–	–	–	–	–	–	–
	Total	12343	228	8	13	207	179	5047	452	98	4901	1438
35–69	Sm.	1169	358	146	173	39	172	15	498	–	126	–
	Total	7849	1535	192	521	822	390	130	3916	424	861	593
		(15%)	(23%)	(76%)	(33%)	(5%)	(44%)	(12%)	(13%)		(15%)	
70+	Sm.	214	60	24	32	4	84	1	63	–	6	–
	Total	6741	605	47	237	321	527	98	4910	165	349	87
		(3%)	(10%)	(51%)	(14%)	(1%)	(16%)	(1%)	(1%)		(2%)	
Any age	Sm.	1383	418	170	205	43	256	16	561	–	132	–
	Total	26933	2368	247	771	1350	1096	5275	9278	687	6111	2118
		(5%)	(18%)	(69%)	(27%)	(3%)	(23%)	(0%)	(6%)		(2%)	

TURKMENISTAN: 1985

Smoking–attributed deaths (Sm.) and total deaths (Total)

		ALL CAUSES	ALL CANCER	Lung cancer	Upper aero–digestive ca.	Other cancer	COPD	Other respiratory	Vascular disease	Cirrhosis/ other liver	Other medical	Non–medical
Males												
0–34	Sm.	–	–	–	–	–	–	–	–	–	–	–
	Total	6752	150	4	9	137	46	3200	145	41	2292	878
35–69	Sm.	1103	330	133	157	40	171	12	444	–	146	–
	Total	4303	832	151	301	380	259	49	1969	212	578	404
		(26%)	(40%)	(88%)	(52%)	(11%)	(66%)	(24%)	(23%)		(25%)	
70+	Sm.	219	63	27	30	6	86	1	64	–	5	–
	Total	2819	296	39	120	137	291	27	1964	61	141	39
		(8%)	(21%)	(69%)	(25%)	(4%)	(30%)	(4%)	(3%)		(4%)	
Any age	Sm.	1322	393	160	187	46	257	13	508	–	151	–
	Total	13874	1278	194	430	654	596	3276	4078	314	3011	1321
		(10%)	(31%)	(82%)	(43%)	(7%)	(43%)	(0%)	(12%)		(5%)	
Females												
0–34	Sm.	–	–	–	–	–	–	–	–	–	–	–
	Total	5367	90	1	6	83	51	2705	157	29	1918	417
35–69	Sm.	155	41	15	25	1	41	0	62	–	11	–
	Total	3021	657	41	217	399	179	28	1555	160	319	123
		(5%)	(6%)	(37%)	(12%)	(0%)	(23%)	(0%)	(4%)		(3%)	
70+	Sm.	56	11	4	6	1	23	0	20	–	2	–
	Total	3818	310	19	100	191	368	26	2836	73	152	53
		(1%)	(4%)	(21%)	(6%)	(1%)	(6%)	(0%)	(1%)		(1%)	
Any age	Sm.	211	52	19	31	2	64	0	82	–	13	–
	Total	12206	1057	61	323	673	598	2759	4548	262	2389	593
		(2%)	(5%)	(31%)	(10%)	(0%)	(11%)	(0%)	(2%)		(1%)	
Males+Females												
0–34	Sm.	–	–	–	–	–	–	–	–	–	–	–
	Total	12119	240	5	15	220	97	5905	302	70	4210	1295
35–69	Sm.	1258	371	148	182	41	212	12	506	–	157	–
	Total	7324	1489	192	518	779	438	77	3524	372	897	527
		(17%)	(25%)	(77%)	(35%)	(5%)	(48%)	(16%)	(14%)		(18%)	
70+	Sm.	275	74	31	36	7	109	1	84	–	7	–
	Total	6637	606	58	220	328	659	53	4800	134	293	92
		(4%)	(12%)	(53%)	(16%)	(2%)	(17%)	(2%)	(2%)		(2%)	
Any age	Sm.	1533	445	179	218	48	321	13	590	–	164	–
	Total	26080	2335	255	753	1327	1194	6035	8626	576	5400	1914
		(6%)	(19%)	(70%)	(29%)	(4%)	(27%)	(0%)	(7%)		(3%)	

(To be conservative, no deaths before age 35, and none from liver cirrhosis or non–medical causes, were attributed to smoking.)

TURKMENISTAN: 1990

Smoking–attributed deaths (Sm.) and total deaths (Total)

		ALL CAUSES	ALL CANCER	Lung cancer	Upper aero–digestive ca.	Other cancer	COPD	Other respiratory	Vascular disease	Cirrhosis/ other liver	Other medical	Non–medical
Males												
0–34	Sm.	–	–	–	–	–	–	–	–	–	–	–
	Total	6139	119	5	6	108	159	1802	261	75	2583	1140
35–69	Sm.	1100	330	146	145	39	141	12	490	–	127	–
	Total	5094	868	168	287	413	221	61	2520	314	583	527
		(22%)	(38%)	(87%)	(51%)	(9%)	(64%)	(20%)	(19%)		(22%)	
70+	Sm.	166	50	20	26	4	62	1	48	–	5	–
	Total	2657	272	30	120	122	200	26	1845	78	190	46
		(6%)	(18%)	(67%)	(22%)	(3%)	(31%)	(4%)	(3%)		(3%)	
Any age	Sm.	1266	380	166	171	43	203	13	538	–	132	–
	Total	13890	1259	203	413	643	580	1889	4626	467	3356	1713
		(9%)	(30%)	(82%)	(41%)	(7%)	(35%)	(1%)	(12%)		(4%)	
Females												
0–34	Sm.	–	–	–	–	–	–	–	–	–	–	–
	Total	4448	93	2	4	87	128	1407	211	45	2042	522
35–69	Sm.	0	0	0	0	0	0	0	0	–	0	–
	Total	3368	632	27	189	416	169	46	1807	206	356	152
		(0%)	(0%)	(0%)	(0%)	(0%)	(0%)	(0%)	(0%)		(0%)	
70+	Sm.	0	0	0	0	0	0	0	0	–	0	–
	Total	4049	316	13	119	184	274	45	2966	94	292	62
		(0%)	(0%)	(0%)	(0%)	(0%)	(0%)	(0%)	(0%)		(0%)	
Any age	Sm.	0	0	0	0	0	0	0	0	–	0	–
	Total	11865	1041	42	312	687	571	1498	4984	345	2690	736
		(0%)	(0%)	(0%)	(0%)	(0%)	(0%)	(0%)	(0%)		(0%)	
Males+Females												
0–34	Sm.	–	–	–	–	–	–	–	–	–	–	–
	Total	10587	212	7	10	195	287	3209	472	120	4625	1662
35–69	Sm.	1100	330	146	145	39	141	12	490	–	127	–
	Total	8462	1500	195	476	829	390	107	4327	520	939	679
		(13%)	(22%)	(75%)	(30%)	(5%)	(36%)	(11%)	(11%)		(14%)	
70+	Sm.	166	50	20	26	4	62	1	48	–	5	–
	Total	6706	588	43	239	306	474	71	4811	172	482	108
		(2%)	(9%)	(47%)	(11%)	(1%)	(13%)	(1%)	(1%)		(1%)	
Any age	Sm.	1266	380	166	171	43	203	13	538	–	132	–
	Total	25755	2300	245	725	1330	1151	3387	9610	812	6046	2449
		(5%)	(17%)	(68%)	(24%)	(3%)	(18%)	(0%)	(6%)		(2%)	

TURKMENISTAN: 1995

Smoking–attributed deaths (Sm.) and total deaths (Total)

		ALL CAUSES	ALL CANCER	Lung cancer	Upper aero–digestive ca.	Other cancer	COPD	Other respiratory	Vascular disease	Cirrhosis/ other liver	Other medical	Non–medical
Males												
0–34	Sm.	–	–	–	–	–	–	–	–	–	–	–
	Total	5513	95	4	5	86	203	1164	323	87	2344	1297
35–69	Sm.	1101	318	158	125	35	113	15	541	–	114	–
	Total	5699	850	181	260	409	179	83	2938	451	557	641
		(19%)	(37%)	(87%)	(48%)	(9%)	(63%)	(18%)	(18%)		(20%)	
70+	Sm.	132	47	18	26	3	39	1	40	–	5	–
	Total	3046	327	31	154	142	168	31	2066	113	279	62
		(4%)	(14%)	(58%)	(17%)	(2%)	(23%)	(3%)	(2%)		(2%)	
Any age	Sm.	1233	365	176	151	38	152	16	581	–	119	–
	Total	14258	1272	216	419	637	550	1278	5327	651	3180	2000
		(9%)	(29%)	(81%)	(36%)	(6%)	(28%)	(1%)	(11%)		(4%)	
Females												
0–34	Sm.	–	–	–	–	–	–	–	–	–	–	–
	Total	3844	98	3	4	91	162	943	227	63	1779	572
35–69	Sm.	0	0	0	0	0	0	0	0	–	0	–
	Total	3823	651	22	184	445	163	67	2074	280	392	196
		(0%)	(0%)	(0%)	(0%)	(0%)	(0%)	(0%)	(0%)		(0%)	
70+	Sm.	0	0	0	0	0	0	0	0	–	0	–
	Total	4581	338	11	133	194	238	67	3290	124	456	68
		(0%)	(0%)	(0%)	(0%)	(0%)	(0%)	(0%)	(0%)		(0%)	
Any age	Sm.	0	0	0	0	0	0	0	0	–	0	–
	Total	12248	1087	36	321	730	563	1077	5591	467	2627	836
		(0%)	(0%)	(0%)	(0%)	(0%)	(0%)	(0%)	(0%)		(0%)	
Males+Females												
0–34	Sm.	–	–	–	–	–	–	–	–	–	–	–
	Total	9357	193	7	9	177	365	2107	550	150	4123	1869
35–69	Sm.	1101	318	158	125	35	113	15	541	–	114	–
	Total	9522	1501	203	444	854	342	150	5012	731	949	837
		(12%)	(21%)	(78%)	(28%)	(4%)	(33%)	(10%)	(11%)		(12%)	
70+	Sm.	132	47	18	26	3	39	1	40	–	5	–
	Total	7627	665	42	287	336	406	98	5356	237	735	130
		(2%)	(7%)	(43%)	(9%)	(1%)	(10%)	(1%)	(1%)		(1%)	
Any age	Sm.	1233	365	176	151	38	152	16	581	–	119	–
	Total	26506	2359	252	740	1367	1113	2355	10918	1118	5807	2836
		(5%)	(15%)	(70%)	(20%)	(3%)	(14%)	(1%)	(5%)		(2%)	

(To be conservative, no deaths before age 35, and none from liver cirrhosis or non–medical causes, were attributed to smoking.)

¶UKRAINE: 1990

		No. of deaths			Standardised rates (Defined on p.520)			Annual death rates / 100, 000						
		All ages	0–34	35–69	All ages	0–34	35–69	0–4	5–9	10–14	15–19	20–24	25–29	30–34
ALL CAUSES	M	297584	26370	159171	1533.7	201.6	1907.7	349.8	57.7	53.7	118.7	228.7	255.0	347.8
	F	332018	11074	92606	851.6	86.0	792.1	260.5	33.2	26.6	54.7	61.1	69.5	96.7
Tuberculosis	M	3818	360	3108	17.5	2.7	32.8	0.4	0.1	–	0.2	1.1	5.1	11.9
	F	703	66	425	2.2	0.5	3.5	0.4	0.2	0.2	0.1	0.7	0.8	1.2
Other infective and parasitic	M	791	482	273	3.4	3.7	2.9	19.8	0.7	0.7	0.9	1.2	1.3	1.1
	F	654	347	224	2.4	2.7	1.9	15.4	0.7	0.3	0.6	0.8	0.6	0.7
ALL CANCER	M	56801	1676	41502	279.1	12.8	501.8	11.8	9.4	7.4	9.5	13.4	14.9	23.3
	F	44569	1474	26688	130.9	11.2	224.9	9.3	6.9	5.2	6.2	7.6	15.1	27.9
Mouth and pharynx cancer	M	2624	37	2269	12.2	0.3	25.3	0.1	0.2	0.1	0.2	0.2	0.4	0.7
	F	426	16	202	1.2	0.1	1.7	0.1	0.1	0.1	–	0.1	0.4	0.2
Oesophagus cancer	M	1717	1	1402	8.3	0.0	16.5	–	–	–	–	–	–	0.1
	F	351	1	130	0.9	0.0	1.1	–	–	–	–	–	0.1	–
Stomach cancer	M	9009	105	6479	44.8	0.8	78.7	–	0.1	0.1	0.4	0.7	1.5	2.8
	F	6432	112	3480	18.2	0.8	29.5	–	–	0.1	0.2	0.4	1.4	3.7
Colorectal cancer	M	4817	65	2974	25.0	0.5	38.1	0.2	–	0.2	0.2	0.4	0.8	1.7
	F	5985	48	3110	16.6	0.4	26.4	0.1	–	–	–	0.2	0.6	1.6
Liver cancer	M	...	...	...	...	...	...	...	...	...	...	...	...	...
	F	...	...	...	...	...	...	...	...	...	...	...	...	...
Pancreas cancer	M	...	...	...	...	...	...	...	...	...	...	...	...	...
	F	...	...	...	...	...	...	...	...	...	...	...	...	...
Larynx cancer	M	2193	5	1883	10.4	0.0	21.6	–	–	–	–	–	–	0.3
	F	91	2	52	0.3	0.0	0.5	–	–	–	–	–	0.1	–
Lung cancer	M	18673	97	14747	90.9	0.7	179.4	0.2	0.1	0.1	0.3	0.7	0.9	2.9
	F	3792	48	2063	10.6	0.4	17.5	0.2	–	0.1	0.1	0.2	1.0	0.9
Malignant melanoma	M	...	...	...	...	...	...	...	...	...	...	...	...	...
	F	...	...	...	...	...	...	...	...	...	...	...	...	...
Female breast cancer	F	6671	143	4917	21.1	1.0	40.9	–	–	–	0.1	0.2	1.4	5.5
Cervix cancer	F	2670	77	1675	8.0	0.6	14.2	–	–	–	–	0.3	0.6	3.0
Other uterine cancer	F	2261	24	1443	6.6	0.2	12.2	0.1	–	–	0.1	0.1	0.4	0.7
Ovarian cancer	F	...	...	...	...	...	...	...	...	...	...	...	...	...
Prostate cancer	M	1969	9	927	10.8	0.1	12.8	–	–	–	0.1	0.2	0.2	0.1
Bladder cancer	M	...	...	...	...	...	...	...	...	...	...	...	...	...
	F	...	...	...	...	...	...	...	...	...	...	...	...	...
Other and ill-defined cancer sites	M	12765	693	8924	62.6	5.3	107.5	6.0	3.5	2.6	3.4	6.0	5.9	9.8
	F	13451	582	8175	39.7	4.5	68.8	4.9	2.8	3.0	3.1	3.6	5.6	8.3
Hodgkin's disease	M	...	...	...	...	...	...	...	...	...	...	...	...	...
	F	...	...	...	...	...	...	...	...	...	...	...	...	...
Myeloma and all lymphomas	M	1377	275	910	6.4	2.1	10.3	1.4	2.1	1.1	1.9	2.9	2.8	2.6
	F	1011	169	604	3.2	1.3	5.0	1.1	0.8	0.5	1.2	1.3	2.2	2.0
Leukaemia	M	1657	389	987	7.7	3.0	11.7	4.0	3.4	3.2	3.1	2.3	2.3	2.5
	F	1428	252	837	4.5	2.0	7.1	3.0	3.3	1.6	1.5	1.0	1.3	2.0
ALL VASCULAR DISEASE	M	133592	1671	64130	729.0	12.6	813.5	5.0	0.8	1.4	4.8	12.2	20.2	44.1
	F	199301	576	45106	484.8	4.4	391.4	3.7	0.5	1.2	2.9	4.7	6.8	10.9
Rheumatic heart disease and fever	M	1886	144	1653	8.5	1.1	17.6	–	0.1	0.2	0.6	1.1	1.8	3.8
	F	2471	95	2149	8.2	0.7	17.9	–	–	0.3	0.6	0.9	1.5	1.8
Hypertensive disease	M	891	26	703	4.3	0.2	7.9	–	–	0.1	–	0.2	0.3	0.9
	F	997	4	610	2.9	0.0	5.2	–	0.1	–	–	–	0.1	0.1
Ischaemic heart disease	M	77474	684	38536	421.0	5.1	488.6	–	–	–	0.9	3.5	8.1	23.4
	F	102127	125	22190	246.5	0.9	193.8	–	–	–	0.3	0.9	2.0	3.4
Pulmonary embolism and other venous	M	...	...	...	...	...	...	...	...	...	...	...	...	...
	F	...	...	...	...	...	...	...	...	...	...	...	...	...
Cerebrovascular disease	M	38979	328	17557	215.4	2.5	229.6	0.1	0.2	0.4	1.1	3.4	4.3	8.0
	F	69632	128	16639	170.1	1.0	144.1	0.2	0.2	0.4	0.8	1.3	1.1	2.9
Other vascular disease, incl. venous	M	14362	489	5681	79.8	3.7	69.8	4.9	0.6	0.8	2.2	4.0	5.7	7.9
	F	24074	224	3518	57.0	1.7	30.4	3.6	0.3	0.6	1.2	1.7	2.2	2.7
Chronic obstructive pulmonary disease	M	20145	198	10081	109.4	1.5	133.1	1.3	0.3	0.1	0.8	1.4	2.0	4.5
	F	13221	117	3575	32.9	0.9	31.1	0.9	0.2	0.4	0.8	1.2	1.3	1.6
Other respiratory disease	M	2437	876	1243	11.2	6.6	13.6	37.8	0.9	0.7	1.1	1.0	1.7	3.0
	F	1455	635	422	5.1	5.0	3.6	30.1	0.7	0.5	0.8	0.7	1.4	0.6
Peptic ulcer	M	1422	46	1005	7.0	0.3	11.9	–	–	–	0.2	0.2	0.5	1.5
	F	578	6	243	1.6	0.0	2.1	0.1	–	–	0.1	0.1	0.1	0.1
Liver cirrhosis and other liver disease	M	4752	184	3784	22.7	1.4	43.6	0.5	0.2	0.3	0.9	1.1	1.8	4.9
	F	2947	93	1950	8.9	0.7	16.4	0.3	0.1	0.4	0.6	0.8	0.9	1.8
Renal disease	M	1880	231	1264	9.0	1.8	14.2	0.6	0.3	0.5	1.2	2.3	2.8	4.6
	F	2061	171	1378	6.5	1.3	11.6	0.4	0.2	0.4	0.9	2.3	1.8	3.3
Pregnancy and birth	F	213	160	53	0.8	1.3	0.4	–	–	–	1.1	3.7	2.3	1.9
Congenital and perinatal causes	M	3934	3806	116	16.6	28.7	1.2	190.2	2.4	2.5	1.6	1.7	1.3	1.3
	F	2829	2706	113	12.2	21.3	0.9	138.5	2.7	2.1	1.5	1.7	0.9	1.4
Ill-defined causes	M	15284	322	1319	95.9	2.5	15.2	7.7	0.1	0.1	1.0	2.2	2.8	3.4
	F	40933	157	615	90.4	1.2	5.4	5.3	0.3	0.3	0.6	0.8	0.4	0.9
Other medical causes	M	9907	1724	5947	47.5	13.1	67.5	27.7	8.5	7.1	9.5	10.2	12.0	17.1
	F	9739	1274	5159	29.9	9.9	43.6	21.1	6.1	4.5	7.4	8.0	9.9	12.1
ALL NON-MEDICAL CAUSES	M	42821	14794	25399	185.4	113.9	256.3	47.0	34.1	32.9	87.3	180.4	188.7	227.0
	F	12815	3292	6655	43.1	25.6	55.3	34.9	14.6	11.1	31.3	28.1	27.0	32.5
Motor vehicle traffic accidents	M	9291	4628	4197	39.2	36.0	42.7	6.8	10.5	9.4	35.5	74.2	61.0	54.8
	F	2647	1043	1118	9.1	8.2	9.2	5.4	6.2	5.0	13.9	10.3	8.3	8.2
Fire	M	664	239	349	3.0	1.8	3.6	4.6	0.8	0.8	0.5	1.6	1.6	2.9
	F	401	109	132	1.3	0.9	1.1	3.0	0.8	0.4	0.5	0.5	0.3	0.5
Suicide	M	8270	2162	5355	36.7	16.5	54.8	–	0.4	2.8	12.2	23.2	33.0	44.2
	F	2423	374	1406	7.8	2.9	11.7	–	–	0.3	4.5	5.2	4.5	5.8
Homicide	M	2881	1222	1518	12.2	9.4	14.9	0.9	0.3	0.8	7.6	15.6	18.5	22.2
	F	1260	370	689	4.4	2.8	5.7	1.6	0.7	0.6	3.0	3.2	4.7	6.1
POPULATION (thousands):	M=males				23845	13026	9727	1896	1913	1838	1860	1662	1920	1938
	F=females				27739	12802	12054	1818	1846	1781	1789	1643	1935	1990

UKRAINE: 1990

Annual death rates / 100, 000

9th ICD categories

35–39	40–44	45–49	50–54	55–59	60–64	65–69	70–74	75–79	80+/NK			
468.3	702.8	991.1	1487.0	2100.8	3099.1	4504.7	6217.0	9119.5	17292.3	M	ALL CAUSES	001–999
144.1	231.2	340.6	539.4	806.4	1280.5	2202.2	3644.1	6115.1	14343.4	F		
19.3	28.2	35.8	35.8	38.9	35.4	36.4	35.2	31.3	28.9	M	Tuberculosis	010–018, 137
2.9	2.0	2.4	3.5	4.2	4.6	5.0	8.2	7.0	6.9	F		
2.3	2.0	2.2	3.2	2.9	3.5	4.4	2.0	3.3	5.1	M	Other infective	Rest of 001–139
0.7	1.0	1.4	1.7	2.1	2.7	3.6	2.8	2.7	3.1	F	and parasitic	
47.8	107.4	215.5	413.3	634.9	919.2	1174.3	1287.4	1342.6	1067.0	M	ALL CANCER	140–208
48.5	85.3	123.7	197.4	253.6	369.4	496.7	587.8	607.7	505.6	F		
3.7	10.6	20.0	29.4	32.7	41.9	38.5	29.7	29.8	27.5	M	Mouth and	140–149
0.3	0.3	0.9	1.1	2.1	3.1	4.2	5.1	6.7	9.9	F	pharynx cancer	
0.4	3.7	9.8	16.4	21.7	29.4	34.3	32.2	28.3	24.8	M	Oesophagus cancer	150
0.1	–	0.5	0.5	1.1	2.1	3.7	5.9	8.1	8.9	F		
7.7	18.2	34.0	63.2	98.3	140.9	188.5	224.8	252.6	177.4	M	Stomach cancer	151
5.6	10.0	13.6	22.1	29.5	50.3	75.6	99.3	112.2	81.8	F		
2.7	5.7	11.9	25.0	39.3	69.0	112.8	146.5	180.3	161.5	M	Colorectal cancer	153, 154
3.6	5.7	10.4	20.4	30.0	45.1	69.7	91.7	106.7	94.6	F		
...	...	...	...	...	...	...	...	...	...	M	Liver cancer	Not given separately
...	...	...	...	...	...	...	...	...	...	F		
...	...	...	...	...	...	...	...	...	...	M	Pancreas cancer	Not given separately
...	...	...	...	...	...	...	...	...	...	F		
2.2	6.4	12.2	24.4	31.7	34.9	39.2	39.8	22.8	19.0	M	Larynx cancer	161
0.1	–	0.1	0.1	1.0	0.8	1.1	1.3	0.8	1.9	F		
7.8	24.6	64.4	143.8	245.5	351.6	418.0	419.1	367.8	235.6	M	Lung cancer	162
1.7	4.5	7.4	12.3	17.9	32.5	46.1	60.4	65.9	47.3	F		
...	...	...	...	...	...	...	...	...	...	M	Malignant melanoma	Not given
...	...	...	...	...	...	...	...	...	...	F		separately
12.8	27.3	33.1	48.5	47.7	56.1	60.9	62.5	53.2	52.3	F	Female breast cancer	174
5.0	7.3	9.0	12.0	14.3	20.5	31.2	35.2	34.1	25.9	F	Cervix cancer	180
1.4	2.3	4.8	10.1	16.2	22.4	28.0	32.1	27.8	22.6	F	Other uterine cancer	179, 182
...	...	...	...	...	...	...	...	...	...	F	Ovarian cancer	Not given separately
0.4	0.3	1.5	4.0	10.8	26.7	45.8	70.2	102.5	116.9	M	Prostate cancer	185
...	...	...	...	...	...	...	...	...	...	M	Bladder cancer	Not given separately
...	...	...	...	...	...	...	...	...	...	F		
16.5	29.1	50.1	86.9	129.4	188.7	251.4	274.4	318.3	266.8	M	Other and ill-defined	Rest of 140–208,
13.3	22.8	36.0	59.9	82.1	117.7	149.9	169.8	170.7	146.6	F	cancer sites	incl. 155, 157, 172, 183, 188
...	...	...	...	...	...	...	...	...	...	M	Hodgkin's disease	Not given separately
...	...	...	...	...	...	...	...	...	...	F		
2.8	5.5	5.5	10.3	11.8	17.6	18.9	23.7	13.8	14.6	M	Myeloma and all	200–203,
2.0	1.7	3.2	5.1	5.1	7.8	10.4	9.5	9.1	6.1	F	lymphomas	incl. 201
3.5	3.3	6.1	10.1	13.6	18.5	26.9	27.2	26.5	22.8	M	Leukaemia	204–208
2.6	3.4	4.7	5.3	6.5	11.1	16.0	15.0	12.3	7.8	F		
96.3	187.5	306.4	518.8	818.5	1413.4	2353.6	3613.4	5634.9	10503.4	M	ALL VASCULAR	390–459
20.6	52.8	96.1	186.1	359.1	674.5	1350.4	2483.9	4337.6	9357.4	F	DISEASE	
6.5	10.8	16.4	22.2	26.4	21.8	18.8	11.6	6.5	5.8	M	Rheumatic heart	390–398
3.2	8.0	14.2	23.6	29.4	23.9	22.8	11.4	7.5	4.7	F	disease and fever	
1.8	3.7	6.0	8.0	11.6	11.6	12.8	15.6	14.5	14.3	M	Hypertensive disease	401–405
0.5	1.5	2.9	4.7	7.4	7.6	11.7	14.0	13.7	12.0	F		
55.7	114.0	182.0	316.7	480.5	856.1	1415.1	2131.4	3201.6	5772.6	M	Ischaemic heart	410–414
6.1	18.5	32.8	68.4	159.7	345.0	725.8	1334.8	2285.2	4780.1	F	disease	
...	...	...	...	...	...	...	...	...	...	M	Pulmonary embolism	Not given
...	...	...	...	...	...	...	...	...	...	F	and other venous	separately
16.0	33.3	63.5	120.8	231.0	422.3	720.3	1121.8	1764.9	3255.9	M	Cerebrovascular	430–438
6.2	16.5	33.9	71.6	138.9	251.4	490.4	885.5	1512.2	3166.5	F	disease	
16.3	25.6	38.4	51.2	69.0	101.6	186.7	333.0	647.4	1454.8	M	Other vascular	Rest of 390–459,
4.6	8.2	12.4	17.8	23.7	46.6	99.7	238.2	519.0	1394.1	F	disease, incl. venous	incl. 415, 451–3
6.2	13.0	30.1	66.3	147.0	244.5	424.8	610.6	884.5	1326.6	M	Chronic obstructive	490–496
3.6	4.4	8.0	15.1	30.7	49.1	106.8	173.2	295.9	529.9	F	pulmonary disease	
4.9	8.9	13.2	14.7	16.8	17.0	19.9	20.9	28.8	40.8	M	Other respiratory	Rest of 460–519
1.1	1.7	2.6	2.9	4.1	5.1	7.5	9.9	13.0	18.7	F	disease	
2.5	4.2	6.7	10.3	13.1	19.7	27.0	28.9	40.8	31.6	M	Peptic ulcer	531–533
0.2	0.6	1.0	1.9	2.3	3.3	5.1	9.6	10.8	14.0	F		
8.8	20.0	30.1	39.3	54.0	71.6	81.3	81.6	70.3	60.8	M	Liver cirrhosis and	570–573, 576,
3.0	6.1	10.1	15.4	21.1	26.6	32.4	35.2	35.1	23.1	F	other liver disease	575.2–579.9
5.3	8.2	9.4	12.4	19.7	21.2	23.5	32.7	35.8	38.1	M	Renal disease	580–590
3.4	5.0	8.0	11.0	14.4	17.7	21.5	24.6	18.7	9.8	F		
2.3	0.6	–	–	–	–	–	–	–	–	F	Pregnancy and birth	630–676
1.0	1.4	0.8	1.7	1.5	0.7	1.1	1.3	0.8	1.4	M	Congenital and	740–779
1.2	0.8	1.3	0.9	1.0	0.6	0.8	0.2	0.5	0.3	F	perinatal causes	
4.8	9.6	11.3	13.4	16.4	20.2	31.0	156.6	635.4	3562.2	M	Ill-defined causes	780–799
0.7	1.8	1.9	3.5	5.2	6.5	17.9	132.3	576.7	3616.7	F		
28.0	39.6	48.9	59.8	73.6	97.6	124.7	166.4	215.8	242.0	M	Other medical causes	Rest of 001–799
15.5	21.0	27.2	37.5	52.0	63.0	89.0	104.4	116.4	123.1	F		
241.1	273.0	280.4	298.0	263.7	235.0	202.6	180.0	195.5	384.4	M	ALL NON-	E800–E999
40.3	48.1	56.8	62.5	56.9	57.2	65.6	72.0	93.0	134.8	F	MEDICAL CAUSES	
48.7	44.7	42.0	41.8	44.1	38.3	39.1	30.0	41.8	61.2	M	Motor vehicle	E810–E819
8.3	7.7	8.2	10.1	9.0	10.0	11.4	12.3	17.9	20.3	F	traffic accidents	
3.2	3.1	3.8	4.0	3.8	3.5	3.7	3.3	6.3	12.9	M	Fire	E890–E899
0.8	0.6	1.2	0.8	1.1	1.2	2.2	3.2	4.2	9.6	F		
47.0	54.9	58.9	61.8	58.0	53.4	49.5	54.9	59.0	101.6	M	Suicide	E950–E959
6.3	9.4	10.7	12.8	12.1	14.4	16.3	20.0	20.8	26.3	F		
21.1	21.3	17.3	12.9	11.6	11.6	8.4	8.6	8.3	25.2	M	Homicide	E960–E969
7.8	7.9	6.7	4.6	4.2	4.2	4.8	6.0	5.6	9.6	F		
1821	1443	1334	1840	1228	1333	729	397	400	294	M	POPULATION (thousands)	
1907	1566	1518	2139	1505	1944	1476	919	1056	909	F		

UKRAINE: Males

	All ages	0–34	35–69	35–39	40–44	45–49	50–54	55–59	60–64	65–69	70–74	75–79	80+/NK
POPULATION (1000s)													
1985–90	23600	13092	9374	1727	1265	1732	1518	1429	1106	597	480	383	270
1985	23359	13165	8997	1486	1370	1940	1335	1493	862	512	585	362	249
1990	**23845**	**13026**	**9727**	**1821**	**1443**	**1334**	**1840**	**1228**	**1333**	**729**	**397**	**400**	**294**
1995 projected	*24219*	*13231*	*9880*	*1850*	*1466*	*1355*	*1869*	*1247*	*1353*	*740*	*404*	*406*	*299*
NUMBER OF DEATHS													
All causes													
1985–90	278372	26072	139634	7266	8016	15816	21180	28018	33340	25998	29448	36020	47198
1985	287346	27688	138183	7058	9633	19795	19738	31539	27680	22740	37732	36685	47058
1990	**297584**	**26370**	**159171**	**8527**	**10141**	**13225**	**27354**	**25790**	**41295**	**32839**	**24700**	**36469**	**50874**
1995 projected	*291612*	*26346*	*159928*	*8730*	*10127*	*13338*	*27586*	*25752*	*41700*	*32695*	*23676*	*34382*	*47280*
Lung cancer													
1985–90	16885	94	13005	139	319	1130	2091	3355	3690	2281	1858	1349	579
1985	14681	94	10969	94	367	1215	1631	3370	2590	1702	2066	1122	430
1990	**18673**	**97**	**14747**	**142**	**355**	**859**	**2645**	**3014**	**4685**	**3047**	**1665**	**1471**	**693**
1995 projected	*21858*	*101*	*16965*	*134*	*353*	*935*	*2905*	*3431*	*5542*	*3665*	*2023*	*1889*	*880*
ANNUAL DEATH RATE / 100,000 (*The rates for the age groups 0–34 and 35–69 are the means of seven five-yearly rates, but the all-ages rates are standardised to the conventional "European" age distribution)													
All causes													
1985–90	1500.1*	196.4*	1813.3*	420.9	633.5	913.0	1395.7	1960.9	3013.4	4355.5	6133.7	9397.3	17487.2
1985	1602.2*	207.5*	1919.9*	474.9	703.4	1020.6	1479.1	2111.9	3211.1	4437.9	6449.9	10134.0	18868.5
1990	**1533.7***	**201.6***	**1907.7***	**468.3**	**702.8**	**991.1**	**1487.0**	**2100.8**	**3099.1**	**4504.7**	**6217.0**	**9119.5**	**17292.3**
1995 projected	*1470.1**	*198.9**	*1883.7**	*472.0*	*691.0*	*984.1*	*1476.4*	*2065.3*	*3081.1*	*4415.9*	*5867.7*	*8464.3*	*15823.3*
All cancer													
1985–90	266.8*	12.4*	480.4*	47.4	104.6	211.5	392.9	611.9	886.3	1108.1	1221.4	1282.8	1000.4
1985	246.4*	12.3*	445.3*	46.0	99.0	206.2	358.3	598.4	815.9	993.4	1122.4	1167.4	856.5
1990	**279.1***	**12.8***	**501.8***	**47.8**	**107.4**	**215.5**	**413.3**	**634.9**	**919.2**	**1174.3**	**1287.4**	**1342.6**	**1067.0**
1995 projected	*314.1**	*12.1**	*558.6**	*48.6*	*111.7*	*235.5*	*446.2*	*697.8*	*1033.8*	*1336.6*	*1478.1*	*1617.2*	*1268.7*
Lung cancer													
1985–90	85.9*	0.7*	169.5*	8.1	25.2	65.2	137.8	234.8	333.5	382.1	387.0	351.9	214.5
1985	77.7*	0.7*	153.8*	6.3	26.8	62.6	122.2	225.7	300.5	332.2	353.2	309.9	172.4
1990	**90.9***	**0.7***	**179.4***	**7.8**	**24.6**	**64.4**	**143.8**	**245.5**	**351.6**	**418.0**	**419.1**	**367.8**	**235.6**
1995 projected	*105.3**	*0.8**	*205.1**	*7.2*	*24.1*	*69.0*	*155.5*	*275.2*	*409.5*	*495.0*	*501.4*	*465.0*	*294.5*
Upper aerodigestive cancer (mouth, oesophagus, pharynx and larynx)													
1985–90	27.6*	0.3*	56.0*	5.5	17.6	36.4	60.8	76.0	94.8	100.7	88.9	79.6	69.3
1985	23.1*	0.3*	45.9*	5.0	13.5	29.0	46.7	68.0	78.8	80.6	79.8	73.2	64.2
1990	**31.0***	**0.3***	**63.4***	**6.3**	**20.7**	**42.0**	**70.1**	**86.2**	**106.2**	**112.1**	**101.7**	**80.8**	**71.4**
1995 projected	*40.4**	*0.3**	*84.5**	*8.5*	*28.3*	*57.9*	*94.7*	*114.7*	*140.0*	*147.2*	*126.6*	*93.3*	*79.0*
Other cancer													
1985–90	153.3*	11.3*	254.9*	33.8	61.7	109.9	194.3	301.1	458.0	625.2	745.5	851.3	716.6
1985	145.6*	11.3*	245.6*	34.7	58.7	114.5	189.4	304.7	436.7	580.6	689.4	784.3	619.9
1990	**157.3***	**11.8***	**259.0***	**33.7**	**62.1**	**109.1**	**199.4**	**303.2**	**461.5**	**644.3**	**766.7**	**894.0**	**760.0**
1995 projected	*168.3**	*11.0**	*269.1**	*32.8*	*59.3*	*108.6*	*196.0*	*308.0*	*484.3*	*694.4*	*850.1*	*1058.8*	*895.2*
Chronic obstructive pulmonary disease (COPD)													
1985–90	117.7*	1.7*	131.7*	6.9	15.6	33.9	72.2	139.3	246.4	407.6	605.1	998.7	1634.7
1985	132.1*	2.2*	148.0*	9.4	23.5	46.0	96.9	161.0	292.9	406.5	648.4	1097.5	1833.6
1990	**109.4***	**1.5***	**133.1***	**6.2**	**13.0**	**30.1**	**66.3**	**147.0**	**244.5**	**424.8**	**610.6**	**884.5**	**1326.6**
1995 projected	*92.0**	*1.0**	*118.6**	*4.1*	*8.9*	*20.7*	*51.9*	*119.8*	*228.5*	*396.3*	*538.3*	*743.5*	*1001.0*
Other respiratory disease													
1985–90	12.3*	9.8*	12.2*	4.8	8.2	10.8	13.8	15.0	15.8	17.3	22.1	27.7	36.3
1985	18.3*	14.5*	18.0*	7.4	14.2	16.2	22.2	20.6	22.0	23.6	29.6	41.7	57.7
1990	**11.2***	**6.6***	**13.6***	**4.9**	**8.9**	**13.2**	**14.7**	**16.8**	**17.0**	**19.9**	**20.9**	**28.8**	**40.8**
1995 projected	*7.9**	*4.3**	*10.1**	*3.3*	*6.1*	*9.1*	*10.9*	*12.4*	*13.6*	*15.0*	*15.1*	*20.7*	*28.8*
Vascular disease													
1985–90	790.4*	12.0*	790.9*	89.0	170.2	285.7	496.3	769.0	1403.2	2323.2	3744.6	6326.9	13173.0
1985	893.3*	13.5*	866.4*	100.7	180.0	322.9	543.9	841.3	1576.5	2499.2	4129.9	7227.3	15427.0
1990	**729.0***	**12.6***	**813.5***	**96.3**	**187.5**	**306.4**	**518.8**	**818.5**	**1413.4**	**2353.6**	**3613.4**	**5634.9**	**10503.4**
1995 projected	*599.3**	*11.0**	*738.3**	*90.8*	*177.6*	*288.8*	*488.4*	*745.4*	*1298.1*	*2079.3*	*2989.8*	*4427.4*	*7482.3*
Liver cirrhosis and other liver disease													
1985–90	22.1*	1.2*	43.4*	8.7	17.1	25.7	39.5	53.3	73.9	85.4	78.7	72.0	51.9
1985	27.9*	1.9*	56.2*	16.5	25.1	34.9	54.8	71.2	97.0	93.7	85.3	72.9	43.7
1990	**22.7***	**1.4***	**43.6***	**8.8**	**20.0**	**30.1**	**39.3**	**54.0**	**71.6**	**81.3**	**81.6**	**70.3**	**60.8**
1995 projected	*18.6**	*1.0**	*33.7**	*5.9*	*14.9*	*22.9*	*29.5*	*39.1*	*55.7*	*67.9*	*74.6*	*74.1*	*68.3*
Other medical causes													
1985–90	133.6*	60.7*	140.7*	63.8	89.4	109.3	135.7	156.2	192.5	237.6	294.9	489.7	1299.0
1985	127.7*	74.4*	162.3*	96.3	120.8	140.6	158.8	180.3	206.6	233.0	262.9	317.1	359.3
1990	**196.8***	**52.8***	**145.8***	**63.2**	**93.1**	**115.3**	**136.6**	**165.9**	**198.3**	**248.0**	**423.1**	**963.0**	**3909.2**
1995 projected	*228.8**	*36.7**	*137.6**	*42.3*	*68.5*	*92.2*	*116.4*	*149.3*	*192.8*	*301.5*	*591.3*	*1388.0*	*5528.8*
All non-medical causes													
1985–90	157.1*	98.6*	214.0*	200.2	228.3	236.0	245.3	216.2	195.2	176.4	166.8	199.6	292.0
1985	156.6*	88.7*	223.6*	198.6	240.7	253.8	244.2	239.1	200.2	188.5	171.5	209.9	290.7
1990	**185.4***	**113.9***	**256.3***	**241.1**	**273.0**	**280.4**	**298.0**	**263.7**	**235.0**	**202.6**	**180.0**	**195.5**	**384.4**
1995 projected	*209.4**	*132.8**	*286.8**	*277.0*	*303.2*	*314.9*	*333.1*	*301.4*	*258.6*	*219.3*	*180.4*	*193.5*	*445.4*

UKRAINE: Females

	All ages	0–34	35–69	35–39	40–44	45–49	50–54	55–59	60–64	65–69	70–74	75–79	80+/NK
POPULATION (1000s)													
1985–90	27623	12866	11818	1817	1397	1973	1744	1828	1831	1228	1130	982	827
1985	27483	12921	11553	1582	1531	2189	1551	2030	1610	1061	1356	903	751
1990	**27739**	**12802**	**12054**	**1907**	**1566**	**1518**	**2139**	**1505**	**1944**	**1476**	**919**	**1056**	**909**
1995 projected	*28175*	*13003*	*12243*	*1937*	*1591*	*1542*	*2172*	*1529*	*1974*	*1499*	*933*	*1072*	*923*
NUMBER OF DEATHS													
All causes													
1985–90	321661	12063	86917	2579	3066	6495	9386	14438	23885	27068	41010	62399	119272
1985	330202	13224	86483	2519	3525	7907	8886	17248	22362	24036	51606	61579	117310
1990	**332018**	**11074**	**92606**	**2747**	**3621**	**5169**	**11535**	**12137**	**24890**	**32507**	**33471**	**64557**	**130310**
1995 projected	*311855*	*9694*	*89406*	*2691*	*3508*	*5010*	*11074*	*11513*	*24070*	*31540*	*31537*	*60320*	*120898*
Lung cancer													
1985–90	3523	42	1943	37	56	135	222	353	590	550	600	605	333
1985	3132	34	1756	26	61	161	192	384	489	443	631	452	259
1990	**3792**	**48**	**2063**	**33**	**70**	**113**	**264**	**270**	**632**	**681**	**555**	**696**	**430**
1995 projected	*4570*	*63*	*2228*	*36*	*74*	*115*	*258*	*276*	*670*	*799*	*704*	*990*	*585*
ANNUAL DEATH RATE / 100,000 (*The rates for the age groups 0–34 and 35–69 are the means of seven five-yearly rates, but the all-ages rates are standardised to the conventional "European" age distribution)													
All causes													
1985–90	859.7*	92.6*	789.7*	141.9	219.5	329.2	538.1	789.8	1304.2	2205.1	3627.9	6354.9	14422.2
1985	920.2*	101.7*	832.7*	159.2	230.2	361.2	573.0	849.9	1389.2	2265.8	3805.8	6823.2	15620.5
1990	**851.6***	**86.0***	**792.1***	**144.1**	**231.2**	**340.6**	**539.4**	**806.4**	**1280.5**	**2202.2**	**3644.1**	**6115.1**	**14343.4**
1995 projected	*788.0**	*74.1**	*752.9**	*138.9*	*220.5*	*325.0*	*509.8*	*753.2*	*1219.2*	*2103.6*	*3380.5*	*5625.3*	*13101.2*
All cancer													
1985–90	126.9*	11.4*	220.8*	47.9	80.0	122.6	192.4	256.9	366.6	478.9	537.5	590.5	468.7
1985	120.5*	11.1*	212.9*	50.5	76.5	122.0	178.7	258.3	355.7	448.3	502.8	518.8	420.2
1990	**130.9***	**11.2***	**224.9***	**48.5**	**85.3**	**123.7**	**197.4**	**253.6**	**369.4**	**496.7**	**587.8**	**607.7**	**505.6**
1995 projected	*142.0**	*10.6**	*236.5**	*50.1*	*87.2*	*131.1*	*200.3*	*259.0*	*382.8*	*544.8*	*678.9*	*754.0*	*599.7*
Lung cancer													
1985–90	10.1*	0.3*	17.4*	2.0	4.0	6.8	12.7	19.3	32.2	44.8	53.1	61.6	40.3
1985	9.3*	0.3*	16.6*	1.6	4.0	7.4	12.4	18.9	30.4	41.8	46.5	50.1	34.5
1990	**10.6***	**0.4***	**17.5***	**1.7**	**4.5**	**7.4**	**12.3**	**17.9**	**32.5**	**46.1**	**60.4**	**65.9**	**47.3**
1995 projected	*12.3**	*0.5**	*18.7**	*1.9*	*4.7*	*7.5*	*11.9*	*18.1*	*33.9*	*53.3*	*75.5*	*92.3*	*63.4*
Upper aerodigestive cancer (mouth, oesophagus, pharynx and larynx)													
1985–90	2.4*	0.2*	3.4*	0.6	0.9	1.6	2.2	4.0	6.3	8.5	11.9	16.0	19.6
1985	2.2*	0.2*	3.2*	0.3	0.6	1.6	2.1	4.0	5.7	8.1	11.9	15.0	16.0
1990	**2.4***	**0.1***	**3.3***	**0.5**	**0.3**	**1.5**	**1.7**	**4.2**	**5.9**	**8.9**	**12.3**	**15.5**	**20.7**
1995 projected	*2.5**	*0.2**	*3.3**	*0.4*	*0.3*	*1.2*	*1.7*	*4.2*	*6.2*	*9.3*	*13.0*	*18.0*	*24.3*
Other cancer													
1985–90	114.3*	10.9*	199.9*	45.3	75.1	114.2	177.5	233.6	328.0	425.6	472.6	512.9	408.8
1985	109.0*	10.7*	193.0*	48.6	71.9	113.0	164.2	235.4	319.7	398.5	444.3	453.7	369.8
1990	**117.9***	**10.7***	**204.1***	**46.3**	**80.5**	**114.8**	**183.3**	**231.4**	**330.9**	**441.6**	**515.1**	**526.2**	**437.5**
1995 projected	*127.1**	*9.9**	*214.4**	*47.9*	*82.2*	*122.4*	*186.7*	*236.8*	*342.7*	*482.2*	*590.4*	*643.7*	*512.0*
Chronic obstructive pulmonary disease (COPD)													
1985–90	41.1*	1.1*	32.6*	3.2	5.3	9.0	16.7	30.3	53.9	109.8	198.4	376.3	789.7
1985	49.4*	1.6*	37.2*	3.9	6.1	11.2	21.2	33.8	65.3	119.1	232.1	447.6	981.6
1990	**32.9***	**0.9***	**31.1***	**3.6**	**4.4**	**8.0**	**15.1**	**30.7**	**49.1**	**106.8**	**173.2**	**295.9**	**529.9**
1995 projected	*24.4**	*0.6**	*24.6**	*2.7*	*3.3*	*5.6*	*12.1*	*23.9*	*41.3*	*83.2*	*125.2*	*217.8*	*374.7*
Other respiratory disease													
1985–90	6.2*	7.4*	3.2*	1.5	1.7	2.1	2.6	3.5	4.4	6.4	9.0	12.4	18.5
1985	9.0*	10.7*	4.5*	2.0	2.5	2.7	3.9	5.2	6.2	8.6	12.5	16.2	31.7
1990	**5.1***	**5.0***	**3.6***	**1.1**	**1.7**	**2.6**	**2.9**	**4.1**	**5.1**	**7.5**	**9.9**	**13.0**	**18.7**
1995 projected	*3.6**	*3.3**	*2.8**	*0.8*	*1.3*	*2.0*	*2.3*	*3.2*	*4.2*	*6.1*	*8.1*	*9.5*	*13.2*
Vascular disease													
1985–90	556.6*	5.0*	401.4*	23.3	48.1	93.2	194.5	352.2	706.5	1391.8	2627.7	4957.8	11941.1
1985	629.6*	5.7*	442.2*	27.3	51.7	108.9	230.3	393.8	789.7	1493.4	2844.5	5588.3	13875.6
1990	**484.8***	**4.4***	**391.4***	**20.6**	**52.8**	**96.1**	**186.1**	**359.1**	**674.5**	**1350.4**	**2483.9**	**4337.6**	**9357.4**
1995 projected	*380.1**	*3.3**	*339.0**	*18.0*	*47.0*	*81.0*	*160.6*	*305.7*	*590.7*	*1170.3*	*2049.3*	*3423.4*	*6616.6*
Liver cirrhosis and other liver disease													
1985–90	8.5*	0.7*	16.0*	3.0	6.2	9.0	14.7	20.7	26.3	32.3	30.2	31.3	25.3
1985	9.7*	0.9*	19.0*	4.7	9.7	13.0	17.4	27.2	29.9	30.7	28.0	24.5	24.1
1990	**8.9***	**0.7***	**16.4***	**3.0**	**6.1**	**10.1**	**15.4**	**21.1**	**26.6**	**32.4**	**35.2**	**35.1**	**23.1**
1995 projected	*8.5**	*0.6**	*14.6**	*2.1*	*4.3*	*7.8*	*12.3*	*17.6*	*23.9*	*33.9*	*43.5*	*46.5*	*27.7*
Other medical causes													
1985–90	80.6*	43.7*	65.2*	27.6	34.0	43.1	61.1	72.8	92.9	124.6	154.6	294.5	1045.0
1985	61.2*	49.5*	63.3*	33.6	35.7	49.0	64.2	71.3	82.9	106.5	114.5	138.6	143.9
1990	**146.1***	**38.2***	**69.3***	**27.0**	**32.8**	**43.3**	**59.9**	**81.1**	**98.5**	**142.8**	**282.1**	**732.8**	**3773.9**
1995 projected	*184.6**	*27.4**	*79.4**	*22.9*	*28.2*	*38.9*	*59.1*	*87.7*	*119.7*	*199.0*	*399.8*	*1078.9*	*5337.0*
All non-medical causes													
1985–90	39.8*	23.4*	50.6*	35.3	44.3	50.2	56.1	53.3	53.6	61.3	70.5	92.1	134.0
1985	40.8*	22.2*	53.7*	37.2	47.9	54.4	57.3	60.2	59.5	59.2	71.3	89.2	143.3
1990	**43.1***	**25.6***	**55.3***	**40.3**	**48.1**	**56.8**	**62.5**	**56.9**	**57.2**	**65.6**	**72.0**	**93.0**	**134.8**
1995 projected	*44.8**	*28.4**	*56.0**	*42.3*	*49.4*	*58.6*	*63.2*	*56.0*	*56.5*	*66.2*	*75.7*	*95.1*	*132.2*

UKRAINE: 1985–1990

Smoking–attributed deaths (Sm.) and total deaths (Total)

		ALL CAUSES	ALL CANCER	Lung cancer	Upper aero–digestive ca.	Other cancer	COPD	Other respiratory	Vascular disease	Cirrhosis/ other liver	Other medical	Non– medical
Males												
0–34	Sm.	–	–	–	–	–	–	–	–	–	–	–
	Total	26072	1632	94	46	1492	224	1324	1598	165	8149	12980
35–69	Sm.	56667	20361	12388	3476	4497	7704	488	22771	–	5343	–
	Total	139634	36930	13005	4607	19318	9149	1076	56551	3502	11967	20459
		(41%)	(55%)	(95%)	(75%)	(23%)	(84%)	(45%)	(40%)		(45%)	
70+	Sm.	20012	4740	3351	490	899	7380	31	7243	–	618	–
	Total	112666	13481	3786	919	8776	11145	310	77783	794	6799	2354
		(18%)	(35%)	(89%)	(53%)	(10%)	(66%)	(10%)	(9%)		(9%)	
Any age	Sm.	76679	25101	15739	3966	5396	15084	519	30014	–	5961	–
	Total	278372	52043	16885	5572	29586	20518	2710	135932	4461	26915	35793
		(28%)	(48%)	(93%)	(71%)	(18%)	(74%)	(19%)	(22%)		(22%)	
Females												
0–34	Sm.	–	–	–	–	–	–	–	–	–	–	–
	Total	12063	1495	42	22	1431	147	968	655	91	5685	3022
35–69	Sm.	5535	1178	928	74	176	1218	20	2677	–	442	–
	Total	86917	25051	1943	385	22723	3491	363	42788	1833	7455	5936
		(6%)	(5%)	(48%)	(19%)	(1%)	(35%)	(6%)	(6%)		(6%)	
70+	Sm.	8287	874	696	79	99	3878	8	3292	–	235	–
	Total	222681	15750	1538	453	13759	12469	377	177137	857	13282	2809
		(4%)	(6%)	(45%)	(17%)	(1%)	(31%)	(2%)	(2%)		(2%)	
Any age	Sm.	13822	2052	1624	153	275	5096	28	5969	–	677	–
	Total	321661	42296	3523	860	37913	16107	1708	220580	2781	26422	11767
		(4%)	(5%)	(46%)	(18%)	(1%)	(32%)	(2%)	(3%)		(3%)	
Males+Females												
0–34	Sm.	–	–	–	–	–	–	–	–	–	–	–
	Total	38135	3127	136	68	2923	371	2292	2253	256	13834	16002
35–69	Sm.	62202	21539	13316	3550	4673	8922	508	25448	–	5785	–
	Total	226551	61981	14948	4992	42041	12640	1439	99339	5335	19422	26395
		(27%)	(35%)	(89%)	(71%)	(11%)	(71%)	(35%)	(26%)		(30%)	
70+	Sm.	28299	5614	4047	569	998	11258	39	10535	–	853	–
	Total	335347	29231	5324	1372	22535	23614	687	254920	1651	20081	5163
		(8%)	(19%)	(76%)	(41%)	(4%)	(48%)	(6%)	(4%)		(4%)	
Any age	Sm.	90501	27153	17363	4119	5671	20180	547	35983	–	6638	–
	Total	600033	94339	20408	6432	67499	36625	4418	356512	7242	53337	47560
		(15%)	(29%)	(85%)	(64%)	(8%)	(55%)	(12%)	(10%)		(12%)	

UKRAINE: 1985

Smoking–attributed deaths (Sm.) and total deaths (Total)

		ALL CAUSES	ALL CANCER	Lung cancer	Upper aero–digestive ca.	Other cancer	COPD	Other respiratory	Vascular disease	Cirrhosis/ other liver	Other medical	Non– medical
Males												
0–34	Sm.	–	–	–	–	–	–	–	–	–	–	–
	Total	27688	1626	94	42	1490	293	1945	1790	246	9963	11825
35–69	Sm.	53658	16862	10409	2630	3823	8039	683	22062	–	6012	–
	Total	138183	31881	10969	3553	17359	9659	1535	56442	4376	13599	20691
		(39%)	(53%)	(95%)	(74%)	(22%)	(83%)	(44%)	(39%)		(44%)	
70+	Sm.	20425	4419	3168	454	797	7855	45	7740	–	366	–
	Total	121475	12928	3618	892	8418	12339	468	88798	872	3582	2488
		(17%)	(34%)	(88%)	(51%)	(9%)	(64%)	(10%)	(9%)		(10%)	
Any age	Sm.	74083	21281	13577	3084	4620	15894	728	29802	–	6378	–
	Total	287346	46435	14681	4487	27267	22291	3948	147030	5494	27144	35004
		(26%)	(46%)	(92%)	(69%)	(17%)	(71%)	(18%)	(20%)		(23%)	
Females												
0–34	Sm.	–	–	–	–	–	–	–	–	–	–	–
	Total	13224	1456	34	21	1401	205	1383	756	113	6428	2883
35–69	Sm.	5111	1006	797	61	148	1216	27	2478	–	384	–
	Total	86483	23135	1756	339	21040	3730	488	43726	2137	7060	6207
		(6%)	(4%)	(45%)	(18%)	(1%)	(33%)	(6%)	(6%)		(5%)	
70+	Sm.	6150	583	471	50	62	3108	8	2386	–	65	–
	Total	230495	14656	1342	417	12897	14559	553	193212	782	3885	2848
		(3%)	(4%)	(35%)	(12%)	(0%)	(21%)	(1%)	(1%)		(2%)	
Any age	Sm.	11261	1589	1268	111	210	4324	35	4864	–	449	–
	Total	330202	39247	3132	777	35338	18494	2424	237694	3032	17373	11938
		(3%)	(4%)	(40%)	(14%)	(1%)	(23%)	(1%)	(2%)		(3%)	
Males+Females												
0–34	Sm.	–	–	–	–	–	–	–	–	–	–	–
	Total	40912	3082	128	63	2891	498	3328	2546	359	16391	14708
35–69	Sm.	58769	17868	11206	2691	3971	9255	710	24540	–	6396	–
	Total	224666	55016	12725	3892	38399	13389	2023	100168	6513	20659	26898
		(26%)	(32%)	(88%)	(69%)	(10%)	(69%)	(35%)	(24%)		(31%)	
70+	Sm.	26575	5002	3639	504	859	10963	53	10126	–	431	–
	Total	351970	27584	4960	1309	21315	26898	1021	282010	1654	7467	5336
		(8%)	(18%)	(73%)	(39%)	(4%)	(41%)	(5%)	(4%)		(6%)	
Any age	Sm.	85344	22870	14845	3195	4830	20218	763	34666	–	6827	–
	Total	617548	85682	17813	5264	62605	40785	6372	384724	8526	44517	46942
		(14%)	(27%)	(83%)	(61%)	(8%)	(50%)	(12%)	(9%)		(15%)	

(To be conservative, no deaths before age 35, and none from liver cirrhosis or non–medical causes, were attributed to smoking.)

UKRAINE: 1990

Smoking-attributed deaths (Sm.) and total deaths (Total)

		ALL CAUSES	ALL CANCER	Lung cancer	Upper aero-digestive ca.	Other cancer	COPD	Other respiratory	Vascular disease	Cirrhosis/ other liver	Other medical	Non-medical
Males												
0–34	Sm.	–	–	–	–	–	–	–	–	–	–	–
	Total	26370	1676	97	43	1536	198	876	1671	184	6971	14794
35–69	Sm.	64443	23377	14072	4230	5075	8541	569	26104	–	5852	–
	Total	159171	41502	14747	5554	21201	10081	1243	64130	3784	13032	25399
		(40%)	(56%)	(95%)	(76%)	(24%)	(85%)	(46%)	(41%)		(45%)	
70+	Sm.	19497	4856	3404	512	940	6646	31	6535	–	1429	–
	Total	112043	13623	3829	937	8857	9866	318	67791	784	17033	2628
		(17%)	(36%)	(89%)	(55%)	(11%)	(67%)	(10%)	(10%)		(8%)	
Any age	Sm.	83940	28233	17476	4742	6015	15187	600	32639	–	7281	–
	Total	297584	56801	18673	6534	31594	20145	2437	133592	4752	37036	42821
		(28%)	(50%)	(94%)	(73%)	(19%)	(75%)	(25%)	(24%)		(20%)	
Females												
0–34	Sm.	–	–	–	–	–	–	–	–	–	–	–
	Total	11074	1474	48	19	1407	117	635	576	93	4887	3292
35–69	Sm.	5909	1258	993	76	189	1265	25	2870	–	491	–
	Total	92606	26688	2063	384	24241	3575	422	45106	1950	8210	6655
		(6%)	(5%)	(48%)	(20%)	(1%)	(35%)	(6%)	(6%)		(6%)	
70+	Sm.	8541	1045	832	92	121	3320	10	3334	–	832	–
	Total	228338	16407	1681	465	14261	9529	398	153619	904	44613	2868
		(4%)	(6%)	(49%)	(20%)	(1%)	(35%)	(3%)	(2%)		(2%)	
Any age	Sm.	14450	2303	1825	168	310	4585	35	6204	–	1323	–
	Total	332018	44569	3792	868	39909	13221	1455	199301	2947	57710	12815
		(4%)	(5%)	(48%)	(19%)	(1%)	(35%)	(2%)	(3%)		(2%)	
Males+Females												
0–34	Sm.	–	–	–	–	–	–	–	–	–	–	–
	Total	37444	3150	145	62	2943	315	1511	2247	277	11858	18086
35–69	Sm.	70352	24635	15065	4306	5264	9806	594	28974	–	6343	–
	Total	251777	68190	16810	5938	45442	13656	1665	109236	5734	21242	32054
		(28%)	(36%)	(90%)	(73%)	(12%)	(72%)	(36%)	(27%)		(30%)	
70+	Sm.	28038	5901	4236	604	1061	9966	41	9869	–	2261	–
	Total	340381	30030	5510	1402	23118	19395	716	221410	1688	61646	5496
		(8%)	(20%)	(77%)	(43%)	(5%)	(51%)	(6%)	(4%)		(4%)	
Any age	Sm.	98390	30536	19301	4910	6325	19772	635	38843	–	8604	–
	Total	629602	101370	22465	7402	71503	33366	3892	332893	7699	94746	55636
		(16%)	(30%)	(86%)	(66%)	(9%)	(59%)	(16%)	(12%)		(9%)	

UKRAINE: 1995

Smoking-attributed deaths (Sm.) and total deaths (Total)

		ALL CAUSES	ALL CANCER	Lung cancer	Upper aero-digestive ca.	Other cancer	COPD	Other respiratory	Vascular disease	Cirrhosis/ other liver	Other medical	Non-medical
Males												
0–34	Sm.	–	–	–	–	–	–	–	–	–	–	–
	Total	26346	1610	101	44	1465	132	581	1477	135	4922	17489
35–69	Sm.	67980	28014	16282	5907	5825	7759	446	26226	–	5535	–
	Total	159928	46653	16965	7541	22147	8978	927	59580	2934	11915	28941
		(43%)	(60%)	(96%)	(78%)	(26%)	(86%)	(48%)	(44%)		(46%)	
70+	Sm.	21233	6386	4360	680	1346	5941	29	6315	–	2562	–
	Total	105338	16324	4792	1126	10406	8183	231	52405	806	24544	2845
		(20%)	(39%)	(91%)	(60%)	(13%)	(73%)	(13%)	(12%)		(10%)	
Any age	Sm.	89213	34400	20642	6587	7171	13700	475	32541	–	8097	–
	Total	291612	64587	21858	8711	34018	17293	1739	113462	3875	41381	49275
		(31%)	(53%)	(94%)	(76%)	(21%)	(79%)	(27%)	(29%)		(20%)	
Females												
0–34	Sm.	–	–	–	–	–	–	–	–	–	–	–
	Total	9694	1418	63	25	1330	82	427	441	75	3557	3694
35–69	Sm.	6097	1449	1138	86	225	1111	23	2877	–	637	–
	Total	89406	28414	2228	394	25792	2884	341	39715	1745	9462	6845
		(7%)	(5%)	(51%)	(22%)	(1%)	(39%)	(7%)	(7%)		(7%)	
70+	Sm.	11801	1841	1432	163	246	3410	11	4393	–	2146	–
	Total	212755	19952	2279	538	17135	6962	300	116885	1161	64549	2946
		(6%)	(9%)	(63%)	(30%)	(1%)	(49%)	(4%)	(4%)		(3%)	
Any age	Sm.	17898	3290	2570	249	471	4521	34	7270	–	2783	–
	Total	311855	49784	4570	957	44257	9928	1068	157041	2981	77568	13485
		(6%)	(7%)	(56%)	(26%)	(1%)	(46%)	(3%)	(5%)		(4%)	
Males+Females												
0–34	Sm.	–	–	–	–	–	–	–	–	–	–	–
	Total	36040	3028	164	69	2795	214	1008	1918	210	8479	21183
35–69	Sm.	74077	29463	17420	5993	6050	8870	469	29103	–	6172	–
	Total	249334	75067	19193	7935	47939	11862	1268	99295	4679	21377	35786
		(30%)	(39%)	(91%)	(76%)	(13%)	(75%)	(37%)	(29%)		(29%)	
70+	Sm.	33034	8227	5792	843	1592	9351	40	10708	–	4708	–
	Total	318093	36276	7071	1664	27541	15145	531	169290	1967	89093	5791
		(10%)	(23%)	(82%)	(51%)	(6%)	(62%)	(8%)	(6%)		(5%)	
Any age	Sm.	107111	37690	23212	6836	7642	18221	509	39811	–	10880	–
	Total	603467	114371	26428	9668	78275	27221	2807	270503	6856	118949	62760
		(18%)	(33%)	(88%)	(71%)	(10%)	(67%)	(18%)	(15%)		(9%)	

(To be conservative, no deaths before age 35, and none from liver cirrhosis or non-medical causes, were attributed to smoking.)

UNITED KINGDOM: 1990

		No. of deaths			Standardised rates (Defined on p.526)			Annual death rates / 100, 000						
		All ages	0–34	35–69	All ages	0–34	35–69	0–4	5–9	10–14	15–19	20–24	25–29	30–34
ALL CAUSES	M	314601	13108	106638	1021.5	89.5	1071.9	217.9	20.1	23.0	73.9	94.6	94.7	101.8
	F	327198	6870	67970	649.7	49.8	625.7	168.0	14.0	16.4	28.0	31.3	38.7	52.5
Tuberculosis	M	420	8	178	1.4	0.1	1.8	0.1	0.1	–	–	–	0.1	0.1
	F	231	8	91	0.5	0.1	0.8	–	–	–	–	0.1	0.1	0.1
Other infective	M	1012	237	361	3.5	1.7	3.4	6.3	0.7	0.5	1.1	0.9	0.8	1.4
and parasitic	F	1122	160	277	2.7	1.2	2.5	4.4	0.8	0.3	0.8	0.7	0.6	0.7
ALL CANCER	M	84144	1020	35286	274.8	6.9	357.8	3.9	4.2	4.2	5.5	6.9	9.9	13.8
	F	77086	969	30687	185.0	6.8	281.5	3.2	4.0	3.5	3.4	4.3	9.2	19.9
Mouth and	M	1201	20	724	4.1	0.1	7.2	–	0.1	–	0.2	0.1	0.2	0.4
pharynx cancer	F	731	3	278	1.7	0.0	2.6	–	0.1	–	–	0.0	–	–
Oesophagus cancer	M	3564	10	1789	11.9	0.1	18.1	–	–	–	–	–	0.2	0.3
	F	2429	6	700	5.2	0.0	6.5	–	–	–	–	–	0.0	0.2
Stomach cancer	M	5858	16	2363	19.0	0.1	24.1	–	–	0.1	0.0	0.0	0.1	0.5
	F	3950	11	958	8.0	0.1	8.9	–	–	–	–	–	0.1	0.4
Colorectal cancer	M	9573	42	3918	31.2	0.3	39.8	–	–	0.1	0.1	0.2	0.6	0.9
	F	9836	28	2930	21.2	0.2	27.1	–	–	–	0.1	0.1	0.6	0.5
Liver cancer	M	536	14	284	1.8	0.1	2.9	0.2	0.1	–	0.1	–	0.1	0.1
	F	234	8	110	0.6	0.1	1.0	–	0.1	0.1	–	0.1	0.1	0.0
Pancreas cancer	M	3375	11	1531	11.2	0.1	15.4	0.1	–	–	–	0.0	0.1	0.3
	F	3579	6	1198	8.0	0.0	11.1	–	–	–	0.1	0.1	–	0.1
Larynx cancer	M	739	–	387	2.5	–	3.9	–	–	–	–	–	–	–
	F	191	–	95	0.5	–	0.9	–	–	–	–	–	–	–
Lung cancer	M	26924	15	12120	87.8	0.1	124.4	–	–	–	–	0.1	0.0	0.6
	F	12345	19	5685	30.8	0.1	52.9	0.1	–	–	–	0.0	0.2	0.6
Malignant melanoma	M	622	34	390	2.2	0.2	3.6	–	–	–	–	0.1	0.6	0.8
	F	665	38	347	1.8	0.2	3.1	–	–	–	–	0.4	0.6	0.7
Female breast cancer	F	15179	162	7639	40.1	1.1	69.2	–	–	–	–	0.1	1.6	6.1
Cervix cancer	F	1981	108	1143	5.7	0.7	10.0	–	–	–	–	0.2	1.3	3.5
Other uterine cancer	F	1618	4	567	3.7	0.0	5.3	–	–	–	–	–	0.0	0.1
Ovarian cancer	F	4513	38	2485	12.4	0.3	22.8	–	0.1	–	0.3	0.2	0.5	0.8
Prostate cancer	M	8938	1	1844	27.8	0.0	19.4	–	–	–	–	–	–	0.0
Bladder cancer	M	3668	2	1124	11.7	0.0	11.6	–	–	–	–	0.0	–	0.0
	F	1816	3	421	3.6	0.0	3.9	–	–	0.1	–	–	–	0.1
Other and ill–defined	M	13521	481	6342	45.0	3.3	63.1	2.2	2.1	1.7	2.4	3.2	4.5	6.6
cancer sites	F	12984	302	4383	29.7	2.2	40.3	1.8	2.3	2.1	1.8	1.6	2.1	3.7
Hodgkin's disease	M	236	58	131	0.8	0.4	1.2	–	0.1	–	0.2	0.6	1.0	0.7
	F	189	44	81	0.5	0.3	0.7	–	–	–	0.3	0.4	0.7	0.6
Myeloma and non–	M	3307	95	1555	11.0	0.6	15.4	0.2	0.1	0.6	0.3	0.9	1.0	1.3
Hodgkin lymphomas	F	3047	31	1096	7.1	0.2	10.1	0.2	0.1	–	0.1	0.2	0.3	0.6
Leukaemia	M	2082	221	784	6.9	1.6	7.7	1.2	1.8	1.8	2.0	1.5	1.4	1.1
	F	1799	158	571	4.3	1.2	5.2	1.2	1.3	1.3	0.8	0.9	1.0	1.5
ALL VASCULAR	M	142773	613	48681	460.3	4.1	494.3	3.9	0.5	0.7	2.7	3.6	5.5	12.0
DISEASE	F	153054	381	22146	276.2	2.6	206.1	3.0	0.7	0.9	1.7	2.7	3.8	5.7
Rheumatic heart	M	632	7	262	2.1	0.0	2.6	0.1	–	–	0.0	0.0	–	0.2
disease and fever	F	1823	9	597	4.1	0.1	5.6	0.1	–	–	0.1	–	0.2	0.1
Hypertensive disease	M	1522	6	597	4.9	0.0	6.0	–	0.1	–	–	0.0	0.0	0.1
	F	2088	2	400	4.1	0.0	3.7	–	–	–	–	–	–	0.1
Ischaemic heart	M	93104	179	36613	302.9	1.2	371.2	0.7	0.1	–	0.2	0.4	1.5	5.6
disease	F	76416	49	13530	143.7	0.3	126.4	0.4	–	–	–	0.2	0.4	1.4
Pulmonary embolism	M	1527	18	489	4.9	0.1	4.9	0.1	0.1	–	0.0	0.1	0.2	0.3
and other venous	F	2822	32	503	5.4	0.2	4.6	–	–	–	0.3	0.3	0.6	0.3
Cerebrovascular	M	28507	154	6267	89.9	1.0	64.1	0.7	0.1	0.2	0.7	1.2	1.3	3.0
disease	F	47913	144	5043	82.1	1.0	46.6	0.7	0.2	0.1	0.5	1.0	1.8	2.6
Other vascular	M	17481	249	4453	55.6	1.7	45.3	2.4	0.2	0.5	1.7	1.8	2.5	2.7
disease	F	21992	145	2073	36.8	1.0	19.2	1.9	0.5	0.8	0.9	1.2	0.9	1.1
Chronic obstructive	M	19831	134	4746	62.3	0.9	49.5	1.1	0.3	0.7	1.0	0.8	1.1	1.5
pulmonary disease	F	11388	103	3269	24.3	0.7	30.5	0.9	0.1	0.4	1.3	0.9	0.7	0.9
Other respiratory	M	15568	398	2331	49.3	2.8	23.4	10.8	0.6	0.6	0.9	0.9	2.3	3.3
disease	F	24291	252	1490	38.6	1.8	13.8	8.6	0.2	0.4	0.7	0.9	1.3	0.9
Peptic ulcer	M	2235	15	677	7.2	0.1	6.9	0.1	–	0.1	–	0.1	0.2	0.3
	F	2580	8	386	4.7	0.1	3.6	0.1	–	–	0.1	0.1	0.1	0.1
Liver cirrhosis	M	1995	53	1483	7.2	0.4	13.9	0.1	–	–	0.0	0.1	0.6	1.7
	F	1628	47	1062	4.9	0.3	9.5	0.1	–	–	0.1	0.1	0.7	1.2
Renal disease	M	2445	58	441	7.8	0.4	4.5	1.5	0.2	0.1	0.1	0.2	0.1	0.6
	F	3014	30	347	5.2	0.2	3.2	0.9	–	–	0.1	0.3	0.1	0.2
Pregnancy and birth	F	61	54	7	0.2	0.4	0.1	–	–	–	0.3	0.6	0.8	0.8
Congenital and	M	2980	2621	235	11.8	18.9	2.2	121.6	1.5	1.5	1.9	2.7	1.6	1.7
perinatal causes	F	2389	2008	232	9.5	15.2	2.1	98.4	2.0	1.3	1.3	1.3	1.4	1.2
Ill–defined causes	M	1815	862	213	6.6	6.2	2.0	40.9	0.1	–	0.2	0.8	0.6	1.0
	F	3584	546	87	6.7	4.1	0.8	28.3	–	–	–	0.2	0.3	0.2
Other medical causes	M	25572	1510	6361	82.2	10.3	62.5	15.1	3.5	5.0	11.1	9.8	12.6	15.0
	F	39286	856	5591	72.0	6.2	51.3	12.5	2.5	4.0	6.3	5.0	6.1	6.7
ALL NON–	M	13811	5579	5645	47.4	36.7	49.8	12.7	8.6	9.7	49.3	67.9	59.3	49.4
MEDICAL CAUSES	F	7484	1448	2298	19.2	10.1	20.0	7.7	3.7	5.7	12.1	14.2	13.5	13.8
Motor vehicle	M	4009	2246	1190	13.6	14.9	10.5	3.4	5.0	5.4	29.3	28.7	19.1	13.6
traffic accidents	F	1619	553	498	4.7	3.9	4.4	1.7	2.4	3.6	7.1	5.8	3.9	3.0
Fire	M	384	130	152	1.3	0.9	1.4	1.7	0.6	0.3	0.3	1.1	1.2	0.9
	F	332	75	104	0.9	0.5	0.9	1.8	0.4	0.3	0.1	0.6	0.3	0.3
Suicide	M	3524	1293	1836	12.2	8.3	16.0	–	–	0.1	5.9	17.6	18.2	16.0
	F	1119	265	624	3.5	1.8	5.4	–	–	–	1.4	2.6	3.7	4.6
Homicide	M	293	154	127	1.0	1.0	1.1	0.8	0.3	0.5	1.2	1.7	1.4	1.3
	F	120	57	50	0.4	0.4	0.4	0.6	–	0.2	0.3	0.5	0.6	0.7
POPULATION (thousands):	M=males	28013	14376	11349				1968	1870	1762	2011	2321	2389	2055
	F=females	29398	13823	11717				1873	1779	1668	1907	2234	2330	2032

UNITED KINGDOM: 1990
9th ICD categories

Annual death rates / 100, 000

35–39	40–44	45–49	50–54	55–59	60–64	65–69	70–74	75–79	80+/NK			
142.8	208.5	355.8	610.8	1074.0	1893.7	3217.8	4975.9	7934.5	14371.2	M	ALL CAUSES	001–999
88.4	135.9	228.7	374.6	645.2	1115.5	1792.0	2797.3	4588.7	11193.2	F		
0.1	0.3	0.9	0.8	2.1	2.6	5.6	7.2	10.2	14.7	M	Tuberculosis	010–018, 137
0.2	0.0	0.3	0.3	0.9	1.4	2.9	2.3	3.3	4.4	F		
2.1	1.8	2.4	2.4	3.2	5.2	6.6	11.2	15.7	30.9	M	Other infective	Rest of 001–139
0.6	0.9	1.1	2.3	3.6	4.0	5.2	6.1	12.9	31.3	F	and parasitic	
24.7	48.9	102.5	199.4	366.1	677.4	1085.9	1533.5	2128.0	2863.9	M	ALL CANCER	140–208
42.9	73.7	126.5	207.8	330.3	495.3	693.8	859.6	1077.6	1521.6	F		
0.9	1.1	3.4	5.7	10.1	12.6	16.6	17.2	18.8	25.4	M	Mouth and	140–149
0.4	0.6	1.0	1.3	3.4	5.4	5.8	7.0	10.4	16.5	F	pharynx cancer	
1.0	1.8	6.5	11.8	20.5	34.1	51.0	64.1	81.9	90.8	M	Oesophagus cancer	150
0.2	0.6	1.6	4.6	6.4	13.3	19.0	27.9	39.8	62.5	F		
1.2	2.6	6.3	11.8	24.3	45.2	77.3	113.0	157.7	202.7	M	Stomach cancer	151
1.0	1.4	2.0	4.7	9.5	16.0	27.6	43.1	63.4	116.7	F		
2.1	5.3	10.3	21.2	40.8	77.0	122.0	171.0	240.2	360.0	M	Colorectal cancer	153, 154
2.4	5.3	9.6	15.2	32.7	47.5	76.6	105.4	146.4	264.0	F		
0.2	0.3	0.5	1.5	3.2	6.1	8.5	11.5	9.9	9.3	M	Liver cancer	155.0
0.1	0.4	0.5	0.5	1.6	1.6	2.3	2.4	3.3	3.3	F		
0.4	2.3	6.1	10.6	17.7	28.5	42.3	62.7	85.5	99.5	M	Pancreas cancer	157
0.7	1.1	3.1	7.2	13.8	19.9	32.2	44.5	55.7	80.4	F		
0.1	0.4	1.5	2.9	4.4	7.2	10.9	13.0	13.4	21.2	M	Larynx cancer	161
–	0.1	0.2	0.4	1.1	2.3	2.2	2.8	2.3	2.4	F		
3.1	9.8	26.5	57.6	122.1	250.5	401.0	546.3	680.1	753.8	M	Lung cancer	162
2.1	6.6	14.3	27.9	51.8	109.6	157.8	181.8	189.2	150.8	F		
1.8	2.3	2.8	3.2	4.0	5.7	5.6	5.4	9.1	12.9	M	Malignant melanoma	172
1.2	2.5	2.5	2.7	3.5	4.3	4.7	5.4	6.3	9.6	F		
14.0	27.7	47.0	69.3	89.5	110.6	126.3	139.7	162.6	256.7	F	Female breast cancer	174
7.6	7.2	8.6	8.6	8.7	11.5	17.6	18.8	18.9	19.0	F	Cervix cancer	180
0.4	0.4	1.3	3.3	6.5	10.7	14.4	18.8	24.8	36.0	F	Other uterine cancer	179, 182
2.3	5.4	11.5	23.0	30.0	39.5	48.1	51.9	51.0	51.8	F	Ovarian cancer	183
0.1	0.3	1.2	3.6	12.5	34.4	83.8	165.7	297.4	535.9	M	Prostate cancer	185
0.2	0.6	2.0	5.4	10.5	23.6	38.9	65.4	105.2	184.7	M	Bladder cancer	188
0.2	0.4	0.7	1.5	3.8	6.9	14.0	18.9	31.1	54.3	F		
8.4	14.4	25.2	44.3	70.0	111.7	167.9	209.8	307.9	396.8	M	Other and ill-defined	Rest of 140–208
6.9	9.5	16.2	26.2	49.5	69.8	103.9	135.6	198.3	294.8	F	cancer sites	
1.1	0.8	0.9	0.9	1.7	1.4	1.5	1.9	2.3	1.9	M	Hodgkin's disease	201
0.5	0.2	0.4	0.4	0.7	1.0	1.8	1.6	1.9	1.5	F		
2.6	4.1	6.1	13.1	16.7	27.2	37.6	55.7	73.9	95.2	M	Myeloma and non-	200, 202–203
1.2	2.7	4.1	6.3	11.8	17.6	26.8	37.0	49.2	60.9	F	Hodgkin lymphomas	
1.6	2.8	3.1	5.7	7.5	12.3	20.9	31.0	44.5	73.6	M	Leukaemia	204–208
1.8	1.6	1.9	4.5	5.8	7.9	12.9	16.9	23.0	40.4	F		
32.2	68.0	141.2	270.3	505.7	892.7	1549.7	2441.5	3885.0	6724.6	M	ALL VASCULAR	390–459
11.1	20.2	42.6	86.2	177.8	383.5	721.7	1315.3	2378.7	5895.5	F	DISEASE	
0.4	0.2	0.6	2.0	2.4	5.2	7.6	11.9	18.5	18.6	M	Rheumatic heart	390–398
0.2	0.3	1.4	3.8	5.7	9.5	18.0	24.0	30.2	38.9	F	disease and fever	
0.6	0.8	2.1	3.1	5.6	11.5	18.6	27.6	40.8	57.8	M	Hypertensive disease	401–405
0.3	0.4	0.9	2.0	4.2	6.6	11.6	23.9	34.1	67.7	F		
21.4	50.7	108.3	214.0	396.4	680.5	1127.5	1668.8	2429.0	3658.5	M	Ischaemic heart	410–414
3.3	8.2	19.8	48.0	107.7	249.5	448.2	774.6	1282.2	2613.4	F	disease	
0.5	1.1	1.3	2.3	4.7	9.4	15.3	23.8	47.2	72.2	M	Pulmonary embolism	415.1, 451–453
0.3	0.8	1.6	2.4	3.9	8.1	15.3	24.4	47.8	97.4	F	and other venous	
4.6	8.0	16.8	28.3	55.4	108.0	227.7	438.8	872.6	1843.5	M	Cerebrovascular	430–438
5.2	7.7	13.4	21.5	41.0	76.0	161.4	338.9	712.2	2058.1	F	disease	
4.6	7.3	12.0	20.6	41.3	78.2	153.0	270.6	477.0	1074.1	M	Other vascular	Rest of 390–459
1.7	2.6	5.5	8.4	15.3	33.8	67.1	129.4	272.2	1020.1	F	disease	
1.3	2.7	5.2	14.0	33.3	91.1	198.9	357.8	613.6	1132.5	M	Chronic obstructive	490–496
1.5	2.2	5.9	11.6	28.6	60.6	103.1	140.3	190.3	277.9	F	pulmonary disease	
4.8	5.1	7.1	13.6	19.7	36.5	77.0	156.9	377.6	1364.4	M	Other respiratory	Rest of 460–519
1.7	2.5	3.3	6.8	10.6	24.6	46.8	95.4	224.6	1273.5	F	disease	
0.5	0.8	1.5	4.3	7.2	12.5	21.4	35.4	59.8	123.2	M	Peptic ulcer	531–533
0.2	0.9	1.0	1.3	2.9	6.9	11.8	22.3	35.2	102.1	F		
4.0	8.0	12.3	14.6	18.3	18.4	21.8	23.0	18.8	17.2	M	Liver cirrhosis	571
2.9	4.6	9.2	7.7	10.8	16.4	15.0	16.9	13.9	10.2	F		
0.5	0.7	1.5	1.9	5.3	6.8	14.6	27.3	65.4	192.3	M	Renal disease	580–590
0.3	0.7	0.8	2.0	3.2	5.3	10.3	19.3	40.4	131.1	F		
0.3	0.1	–	–	–	–	–	–	–	–	F	Pregnancy and birth	630–676
1.7	1.3	1.4	2.9	2.4	2.4	3.0	4.0	4.6	8.5	M	Congenital and	740–779
1.4	1.3	1.1	1.5	3.4	2.7	3.0	3.5	3.8	4.3	F	perinatal causes	
1.1	1.1	2.1	1.7	1.8	2.5	3.5	3.3	8.1	102.6	M	Ill-defined causes	780–799
0.2	0.1	0.5	0.7	1.1	1.4	1.4	2.6	9.6	190.3	F		
19.3	20.9	27.9	36.0	58.8	99.0	175.9	311.7	645.9	1597.5	M	Other medical causes	Rest of 001–799
10.6	12.7	18.8	28.4	52.6	89.7	146.3	271.6	529.8	1586.2	F		
50.6	48.9	49.6	48.9	50.0	46.7	54.0	63.3	101.9	198.8	M	ALL NON-	E800–E999
14.5	16.2	17.5	17.9	19.4	23.7	30.8	42.1	68.6	164.8	F	MEDICAL CAUSES	
11.2	11.0	9.0	10.6	9.9	9.9	11.8	16.1	29.4	33.2	M	Motor vehicle	E810–E819
3.6	3.0	3.3	3.6	4.9	4.7	7.4	10.6	15.8	17.3	F	traffic accidents	
0.7	1.0	1.5	1.0	1.2	1.5	3.1	2.1	3.9	8.5	M	Fire	E890–E899
0.2	0.4	1.1	1.1	0.8	1.1	1.8	2.7	2.8	6.0	F		
17.8	17.2	17.9	16.2	16.3	12.1	14.1	14.1	15.9	23.5	M	Suicide	E950–E959
4.6	4.6	6.6	4.3	4.8	6.2	6.5	6.1	6.2	5.6	F		
1.8	0.9	1.0	1.2	1.6	0.7	0.5	0.4	0.8	0.3	M	Homicide	E960–E969
0.4	0.6	0.4	0.5	0.3	0.3	0.4	0.4	0.3	0.3	F		
1885	2062	1696	1551	1450	1395	1310	931	725	633	M	POPULATION (thousands)	
1882	2061	1691	1562	1488	1502	1531	1236	1146	1476	F		

UNITED KINGDOM: Males

	All ages	0–34	35–69	35–39	40–44	45–49	50–54	55–59	60–64	65–69	70–74	75–79	80+/NK
POPULATION (1000s)													
1955	24510	12748	10342	1657	1853	1839	1674	1340	1094	887	676	440	304
1965	26444	13909	11049	1727	1879	1628	1750	1651	1414	999	698	443	346
1975	27221	14643	10804	1645	1588	1635	1733	1453	1488	1262	900	497	377
1985	27574	14305	11051	2075	1722	1589	1514	1507	1494	1150	1016	691	510
1990	28013	14376	11349	1885	2062	1696	1551	1450	1395	1310	931	725	633
1995 projected	28321	14306	11652	2056	1869	2024	1656	1484	1340	1225	1063	662	637
NUMBER OF DEATHS													
All causes													
1955	306166	23321	130096	3299	5899	10244	17277	23338	30878	39161	45906	47884	58959
1965	323083	22676	145841	3255	5930	8757	16683	27076	39854	44286	46696	44793	63077
1975	335006	16936	141668	2576	4430	8627	16003	21634	36947	51451	58675	49459	68268
1985	331562	12802	116684	2826	3902	6343	10973	19312	33190	40138	57320	61400	83356
1990	314601	13108	106638	2692	4299	6034	9473	15575	26408	42157	46301	57541	91013
1995 projected	280597	13132	92297	2908	3616	6266	8578	13491	22435	35003	47352	46582	81234
Lung cancer													
1955	16568	101	12826	144	475	1068	2065	2972	3178	2924	2115	1084	442
1965	25072	81	17891	166	420	930	2095	3767	5302	5211	3741	2214	1145
1975	29507	55	17197	95	243	778	1848	2831	5001	6401	6059	3831	2365
1985	29543	28	13844	93	188	488	1075	2500	4458	5042	6085	5397	4189
1990	26924	15	12120	58	202	450	893	1770	3493	5254	5083	4932	4774
1995 projected	23488	12	9983	50	151	431	712	1428	2844	4367	5161	4034	4298
ANNUAL DEATH RATE / 100,000													
All causes													
1955	1473.1*	177.6*	1584.3*	199.1	318.4	557.1	1032.3	1742.3	2823.8	4417.0	6794.8	10875.3	19400.8
1965	1403.0*	149.6*	1555.1*	188.4	315.7	537.9	953.2	1639.6	2818.9	4431.7	6688.1	10120.4	18251.4
1975	1327.9*	119.3*	1419.5*	156.6	278.9	527.7	923.4	1488.8	2483.8	4077.3	6521.6	9959.5	18113.0
1985	1152.4*	90.8*	1211.6*	136.2	226.5	399.2	724.6	1281.9	2221.1	3491.5	5644.0	8883.1	16334.7
1990	1021.5*	89.5*	1071.9*	142.8	208.5	355.8	610.8	1074.0	1893.7	3217.8	4975.9	7934.5	14371.2
1995 projected	909.3*	89.7*	943.5*	141.4	193.5	309.6	518.1	909.2	1674.6	2858.3	4453.7	7037.6	12756.6
All cancer													
1955	252.7*	11.5*	384.8*	37.2	73.5	144.8	278.4	479.7	710.1	969.8	1258.7	1623.0	1813.1
1965	272.7*	11.7*	410.7*	39.0	70.2	137.8	262.1	473.5	767.7	1124.4	1442.1	1757.1	2052.4
1975	282.6*	10.4*	393.2*	31.4	55.6	128.5	245.1	430.3	724.6	1137.2	1594.0	2071.1	2420.0
1985	284.1*	7.5*	372.6*	29.3	53.1	102.5	212.8	414.3	716.0	1079.9	1574.8	2164.1	2906.1
1990	274.8*	6.9*	357.8*	24.7	48.9	102.5	199.4	366.1	677.4	1085.9	1533.5	2128.0	2863.9
1995 projected	265.8*	6.3*	341.1*	21.3	45.0	94.9	180.5	337.2	650.4	1058.1	1505.4	2084.2	2839.7
Lung cancer													
1955	73.8*	0.8*	151.2*	8.7	25.6	58.1	123.4	221.9	290.6	329.8	313.1	246.2	145.4
1965	100.9*	0.7*	190.5*	9.6	22.4	57.1	119.7	228.1	375.0	521.5	535.8	500.2	331.3
1975	109.4*	0.4*	173.4*	5.8	15.3	47.6	106.6	194.8	336.2	507.3	673.4	771.4	627.5
1985	100.7*	0.2*	145.7*	4.5	10.9	30.7	71.0	165.9	298.3	438.6	599.2	780.8	820.9
1990	87.8*	0.1*	124.4*	3.1	9.8	26.5	57.6	122.1	250.5	401.0	546.3	680.1	753.8
1995 projected	76.2*	0.1*	105.7*	2.4	8.1	21.3	43.0	96.2	212.3	356.6	485.4	609.5	674.9
Upper aerodigestive cancer (mouth, oesophagus, pharynx and larynx)													
1955	19.1*	0.2*	22.5*	2.0	3.0	6.1	10.6	24.3	43.2	68.1	110.9	173.5	215.9
1965	15.0*	0.1*	19.7*	2.0	3.1	6.9	11.3	21.0	36.1	57.7	82.9	108.5	162.0
1975	15.0*	0.2*	20.9*	1.5	2.9	8.4	14.5	25.7	37.2	56.1	78.7	110.1	141.4
1985	17.4*	0.2*	26.7*	1.2	4.6	9.3	19.3	35.3	51.7	65.6	88.3	107.3	138.7
1990	18.5*	0.2*	29.2*	1.9	3.3	11.4	20.4	35.0	53.9	78.5	94.3	114.0	137.4
1995 projected	19.4*	0.2*	31.0*	1.7	3.5	11.6	20.7	35.3	58.4	85.8	102.7	116.5	140.4
Other cancer													
1955	159.8*	10.5*	211.1*	26.5	44.9	80.5	144.4	233.5	376.3	571.8	834.8	1203.3	1451.8
1965	156.8*	10.9*	200.5*	27.4	44.7	73.8	131.1	224.4	356.6	545.2	823.4	1148.4	1559.0
1975	158.1*	9.8*	199.0*	24.2	37.4	72.6	124.0	209.7	351.1	573.8	841.8	1189.5	1651.1
1985	165.9*	7.1*	200.2*	23.6	37.6	62.6	122.5	213.1	366.0	575.8	887.4	1275.9	1946.5
1990	168.6*	6.6*	204.3*	19.7	35.8	64.6	121.4	209.0	373.0	606.4	893.0	1333.8	1972.7
1995 projected	170.2*	6.0*	204.4*	17.2	33.4	62.0	116.9	205.6	379.7	615.7	917.2	1358.2	2024.3
Chronic obstructive pulmonary disease (COPD)													
1955	109.0*	2.1*	153.8*	7.2	14.7	34.5	87.3	176.1	299.7	457.1	582.0	758.1	1070.7
1965	116.6*	2.1*	145.5*	3.9	9.8	22.4	62.2	135.6	291.2	493.5	711.3	967.0	1276.6
1975	94.8*	2.0*	89.7*	3.9	6.4	15.8	37.2	78.8	169.2	316.5	589.8	928.1	1361.9
1985	78.2*	1.0*	66.0*	1.9	3.6	9.4	21.1	55.6	130.7	239.8	440.7	765.6	1360.2
1990	62.3*	0.9*	49.5*	1.3	2.7	5.2	14.0	33.3	91.1	198.9	357.8	613.6	1132.5
1995 projected	49.8*	0.8*	37.9*	0.9	1.9	3.6	9.6	23.1	68.4	157.6	287.5	495.2	930.1
Other respiratory disease													
1955	76.8*	14.8*	61.4*	7.2	9.9	18.4	36.0	63.6	109.9	184.8	317.1	593.9	1282.3
1965	81.3*	12.5*	46.1*	6.0	8.2	13.2	20.1	39.8	78.5	156.9	332.3	674.6	1752.9
1975	104.9*	8.5*	50.9*	4.4	6.8	16.1	23.4	45.1	81.1	179.3	424.7	893.1	2611.6
1985	57.1*	3.7*	24.5*	3.2	3.5	5.8	11.4	21.9	42.8	83.2	178.0	420.6	1647.3
1990	49.3*	2.8*	23.4*	4.8	5.1	7.1	13.6	19.7	36.5	77.0	156.9	377.6	1364.4
1995 projected	42.7*	2.6*	21.9*	6.6	6.6	8.5	13.6	17.7	32.5	67.9	139.8	315.5	1149.5
Vascular disease													
1955	734.3*	8.8*	704.1*	50.7	100.2	203.7	404.4	714.4	1274.0	2181.5	3720.7	6425.8	12144.8
1965	710.5*	7.5*	756.7*	64.0	134.1	248.0	460.3	785.0	1385.6	2220.0	3562.4	5653.2	10908.6
1975	668.3*	6.3*	728.8*	49.5	127.7	266.0	490.0	771.7	1278.1	2118.3	3400.1	5236.6	9909.3
1985	551.1*	4.7*	600.1*	35.1	88.5	187.1	366.2	639.6	1117.8	1766.4	2893.0	4487.4	7996.7
1990	460.3*	4.1*	494.3*	32.2	68.0	141.2	270.3	505.7	892.7	1549.7	2441.5	3885.0	6724.6
1995 projected	383.7*	3.7*	401.1*	25.2	50.9	101.6	201.6	389.9	738.8	1299.5	2087.8	3303.8	5715.1
Liver cirrhosis													
1955	3.2*	0.1*	5.9*	1.2	2.5	2.8	5.9	6.2	9.5	13.3	12.3	15.0	10.5
1965	3.5*	0.2*	6.2*	1.2	2.3	4.5	5.3	7.8	10.3	11.8	13.2	13.1	15.3
1975	4.3*	0.2*	8.5*	2.3	3.5	6.3	8.8	11.8	12.7	14.1	11.2	11.5	14.3
1985	6.1*	0.3*	11.8*	2.9	4.6	8.6	12.5	13.6	19.3	20.7	22.4	17.8	16.1
1990	7.2*	0.4*	13.9*	4.0	8.0	12.3	14.6	18.3	18.4	21.8	23.0	18.8	17.2
1995 projected	8.3*	0.5*	16.1*	5.4	10.9	16.1	18.4	20.3	19.8	21.9	23.8	19.9	18.2
Other medical causes													
1955	230.5*	99.2*	204.0*	52.9	69.0	99.9	154.9	225.4	327.5	498.6	763.8	1231.4	2639.0
1965	153.8*	71.8*	124.0*	30.1	38.6	55.0	83.2	126.4	200.9	333.5	505.7	862.0	1837.1
1975	118.5*	51.6*	94.2*	22.1	30.5	44.7	65.7	97.1	152.5	246.6	414.1	678.4	1482.4
1985	128.0*	39.7*	86.1*	17.9	24.8	37.6	50.8	87.2	139.9	244.3	459.2	909.9	2165.2
1990	120.3*	37.7*	83.2*	25.3	26.9	37.8	50.0	80.8	130.9	230.5	400.0	809.7	2069.8
1995 projected	112.1*	35.8*	78.0*	30.7	29.0	36.9	46.6	74.7	121.5	206.4	354.6	734.9	1938.3
All non-medical causes													
1955	66.5*	41.0*	70.2*	42.6	48.5	53.1	65.4	77.0	93.1	111.9	140.3	228.0	440.3
1965	64.7*	43.8*	65.9*	44.2	52.4	57.0	60.0	71.5	84.7	91.6	121.0	193.4	408.6
1975	54.4*	40.1*	54.2*	43.0	48.3	50.3	53.1	54.1	65.6	65.2	87.7	140.8	313.6
1985	47.7*	33.9*	50.5*	45.9	48.3	48.3	49.8	49.7	54.5	57.2	75.7	117.8	243.2
1990	47.4*	36.7*	49.8*	50.6	48.9	49.6	48.9	50.0	46.7	54.0	63.3	101.9	198.8
1995 projected	46.9*	40.0*	47.5*	51.4	49.2	48.2	47.7	46.4	43.1	46.8	54.9	84.2	165.7

(*The rates for the age groups 0–34 and 35–69 are the means of seven five-yearly rates, but the all-ages rates are standardised to the conventional "European" age distribution)

UNITED KINGDOM: Females

	All ages	0–34	35–69	35–39	40–44	45–49	50–54	55–59	60–64	65–69	70–74	75–79	80+/NK
POPULATION (1000s)													
1955	26437	12630	11568	1715	1922	1896	1790	1607	1418	1220	990	694	555
1965	27997	13387	11924	1697	1882	1676	1859	1791	1631	1387	1115	811	760
1975	28722	14043	11455	1600	1566	1655	1800	1575	1690	1569	1313	950	962
1985	29044	13751	11493	2069	1701	1582	1526	1573	1651	1391	1385	1135	1281
1990	29398	13823	11717	1882	2061	1691	1562	1488	1502	1531	1236	1146	1476
1995 projected	29543	13706	11964	2029	1864	2047	1670	1524	1424	1406	1381	1030	1463
NUMBER OF DEATHS													
All causes													
1955	289750	16635	90589	2630	4585	7181	10519	14394	20766	30514	42632	51138	88756
1965	304715	14785	88945	2315	4234	5878	9894	14683	21485	30456	41996	51654	107335
1975	327471	10378	85208	1809	3088	5509	9545	12702	21202	31353	44106	54758	133021
1985	339094	7477	73028	1878	2519	4013	6568	11697	20313	26040	42465	57156	158968
1990	327198	6870	67970	1663	2800	3866	5852	9598	16752	27439	34580	52577	165201
1995 projected	293267	6169	60334	1676	2328	4159	5471	8734	14665	23301	35527	42604	148633
Lung cancer													
1955	2775	49	1812	46	96	178	266	355	413	458	408	291	215
1965	4719	33	3118	59	143	253	487	609	740	827	649	473	446
1975	7652	29	4545	38	108	289	669	849	1247	1345	1259	934	885
1985	11317	20	5460	57	101	227	403	970	1755	1947	2238	1812	1787
1990	12345	19	5685	39	136	241	436	771	1646	2416	2248	2168	2225
1995 projected	13219	15	5657	40	121	299	422	762	1601	2412	2838	2203	2506
ANNUAL DEATH RATE / 100,000 (*The rates for the age groups 0–34 and 35–69 are the means of seven five-yearly rates, but the all-ages rates are standardised to the conventional "European" age distribution)													
All causes													
1955	986.9*	128.7*	888.4*	153.4	238.6	378.8	587.6	895.9	1464.0	2500.3	4308.4	7367.5	15989.2
1965	866.1*	100.3*	796.7*	136.4	224.9	350.7	532.1	819.8	1317.4	2195.3	3766.8	6370.7	14119.3
1975	806.4*	76.6*	747.5*	113.1	197.2	332.8	530.2	806.6	1254.8	1998.0	3360.2	5763.4	13833.3
1985	716.4*	56.8*	681.3*	90.8	148.1	253.6	430.3	743.8	1230.1	1872.7	3067.0	5037.1	12407.7
1990	649.7*	49.8*	625.7*	88.4	135.9	228.7	374.6	645.2	1115.5	1792.0	2797.3	4588.7	11193.2
1995 projected	590.1*	44.3*	571.2*	82.6	124.9	203.2	327.6	573.0	1030.2	1657.0	2573.3	4135.5	10160.9
All cancer													
1955	169.6*	10.5*	256.7*	45.4	90.3	149.6	228.7	307.0	417.6	557.9	744.2	943.8	1275.6
1965	167.9*	10.0*	257.5*	48.3	94.9	154.7	233.4	316.2	411.2	543.4	717.4	913.8	1233.9
1975	176.2*	8.6*	273.2*	45.0	90.7	154.2	249.3	337.0	452.7	583.2	744.0	955.3	1330.4
1985	187.2*	7.5*	287.5*	45.2	77.1	137.8	220.7	352.6	518.3	660.5	847.9	1043.5	1500.2
1990	185.0*	6.8*	281.5*	42.9	73.7	126.5	207.8	330.3	495.3	693.8	859.6	1077.6	1521.6
1995 projected	182.1*	6.1*	272.4*	40.0	68.3	116.3	191.8	309.3	487.0	694.3	877.7	1097.9	1551.5
Lung cancer													
1955	9.6*	0.4*	17.2*	2.7	5.0	9.4	14.9	22.1	29.1	37.5	41.2	41.9	38.7
1965	14.6*	0.3*	27.3*	3.5	7.6	15.1	26.2	34.0	45.4	59.6	58.2	58.3	58.7
1975	21.6*	0.2*	39.6*	2.4	6.9	17.5	37.2	53.9	73.8	85.7	95.9	98.3	92.0
1985	29.0*	0.2*	51.1*	2.8	5.9	14.3	26.4	61.7	106.3	140.0	161.6	159.7	139.5
1990	30.8*	0.1*	52.9*	2.1	6.6	14.3	27.9	51.8	109.6	157.8	181.8	189.2	150.8
1995 projected	32.8*	0.1*	54.6*	2.0	6.5	14.6	25.3	50.0	112.5	171.5	205.6	213.8	171.3
Upper aerodigestive cancer (mouth, oesophagus, pharynx and larynx)													
1955	7.3*	0.2*	9.9*	2.0	2.4	5.6	8.1	11.2	17.0	22.7	35.8	52.2	68.1
1965	6.5*	0.2*	9.0*	1.3	1.9	4.0	6.2	10.7	15.8	22.8	30.9	45.1	65.2
1975	6.6*	0.1*	9.0*	0.9	2.0	3.4	6.9	10.0	15.9	24.0	32.8	42.7	73.8
1985	7.3*	0.1*	10.4*	0.8	1.8	2.8	5.6	13.4	20.8	27.6	35.7	47.9	75.6
1990	7.4*	0.1*	10.0*	0.6	1.3	2.8	6.3	10.9	20.9	27.0	37.7	52.5	81.4
1995 projected	7.5*	0.1*	9.6*	0.4	1.1	2.8	5.7	10.3	19.7	27.1	39.2	59.0	88.3
Other cancer													
1955	152.7*	10.0*	229.5*	40.7	82.9	134.6	205.8	273.7	371.5	497.7	667.2	849.7	1168.8
1965	146.9*	9.6*	221.2*	43.6	85.4	135.7	201.0	271.5	350.0	461.0	628.3	810.3	1110.0
1975	148.0*	8.3*	224.5*	41.7	81.7	133.3	205.1	273.1	363.0	473.5	615.3	814.2	1164.5
1985	150.9*	7.3*	226.0*	41.7	69.4	120.6	188.7	277.5	391.3	492.8	650.6	836.0	1285.1
1990	146.9*	6.6*	218.6*	40.2	65.7	109.5	173.6	267.6	364.8	509.1	640.0	835.9	1289.4
1995 projected	141.8*	5.9*	208.2*	37.6	60.6	98.9	160.8	249.0	354.9	495.7	632.9	825.1	1291.9
Chronic obstructive pulmonary disease (COPD)													
1955	33.3*	1.6*	30.3*	3.1	5.7	9.6	14.9	27.0	53.9	97.9	156.8	277.2	582.8
1965	26.7*	1.5*	27.2*	4.0	6.1	9.8	16.5	26.6	48.6	78.6	125.7	208.3	410.0
1975	23.7*	1.3*	26.4*	2.8	6.1	12.5	18.4	32.5	45.9	66.5	102.8	165.9	347.0
1985	25.3*	0.9*	32.2*	1.9	3.3	6.3	17.9	37.5	63.1	95.1	135.9	167.3	306.1
1990	24.3*	0.7*	30.5*	1.5	2.2	5.9	11.6	28.6	60.6	103.1	140.3	190.3	277.9
1995 projected	23.9*	0.6*	29.1*	1.1	1.8	4.2	8.6	24.0	58.9	105.2	150.7	195.8	274.9
Other respiratory disease													
1955	53.9*	12.1*	32.4*	5.8	6.5	11.8	17.9	29.3	54.5	101.0	203.5	406.3	1079.1
1965	55.0*	10.1*	27.2*	5.0	6.3	9.0	13.5	21.3	43.5	91.8	194.3	402.4	1308.3
1975	71.0*	6.0*	31.0*	4.3	5.7	8.6	15.8	28.4	50.4	103.9	236.7	545.0	1949.5
1985	42.7*	2.5*	14.6*	1.8	2.2	4.5	6.6	12.7	26.6	47.7	108.0	261.0	1388.9
1990	38.6*	1.8*	13.8*	1.7	2.5	3.3	6.8	10.6	24.6	46.8	95.4	224.6	1273.5
1995 projected	34.5*	1.6*	12.5*	1.6	2.1	3.1	5.9	9.6	23.0	42.2	82.8	189.2	1156.5
Vascular disease													
1955	533.0*	7.9*	406.1*	32.5	60.7	111.7	202.9	367.2	694.9	1372.5	2625.1	4809.8	10699.3
1965	460.4*	5.3*	351.3*	30.6	55.5	96.9	167.9	313.2	619.1	1175.7	2257.7	4049.6	9386.3
1975	405.0*	3.9*	304.4*	23.8	44.4	88.0	157.6	286.5	532.8	997.5	1891.2	3440.6	8588.4
1985	326.2*	2.9*	245.0*	13.0	27.3	54.3	111.6	230.7	456.1	822.2	1549.5	2775.9	6937.9
1990	276.2*	2.6*	206.1*	11.1	20.2	42.6	86.2	177.8	383.5	721.7	1315.3	2378.7	5895.5
1995 projected	232.6*	2.4*	171.1*	8.6	15.6	32.2	65.8	142.8	322.9	609.8	1112.6	1996.4	5021.8
Liver cirrhosis													
1955	2.2*	0.2*	4.1*	0.6	1.3	2.0	4.1	4.9	6.3	9.8	8.3	9.4	6.7
1965	2.5*	0.2*	4.3*	0.9	1.4	2.4	3.8	5.6	6.7	9.4	10.2	12.0	8.7
1975	3.3*	0.3*	6.1*	1.6	2.6	5.4	5.3	8.1	10.3	9.4	10.9	10.8	9.4
1985	4.2*	0.3*	8.1*	1.6	3.4	4.6	8.0	11.4	13.3	14.5	13.5	12.6	11.7
1990	4.9*	0.3*	9.5*	2.9	4.6	9.2	7.7	10.8	16.4	15.0	16.9	13.9	10.2
1995 projected	5.7*	0.4*	11.1*	4.1	6.4	12.2	8.9	11.5	17.6	17.3	18.8	15.6	10.1
Other medical causes													
1955	160.2*	83.9*	128.6*	52.9	58.5	72.6	92.2	128.7	194.4	301.0	472.5	731.6	1861.6
1965	117.8*	58.5*	94.9*	30.6	38.6	52.4	65.7	96.8	145.0	234.8	368.3	617.0	1349.8
1975	96.1*	42.6*	76.5*	18.1	26.9	38.7	54.9	81.3	123.8	191.7	305.2	517.7	1246.4
1985	107.1*	32.0*	68.6*	12.4	18.4	24.6	43.0	70.1	119.7	191.9	357.5	684.6	2028.1
1990	101.6*	27.4*	64.3*	13.8	16.6	23.6	36.5	67.7	111.3	180.8	327.8	634.9	2049.7
1995 projected	95.5*	23.5*	59.2*	13.0	16.1	20.6	33.4	62.0	103.9	165.3	299.5	591.3	2028.5
All non-medical causes													
1955	34.7*	12.5*	30.2*	13.0	15.5	21.5	26.8	31.9	42.5	60.2	98.0	189.5	484.1
1965	35.8*	14.7*	34.4*	17.0	22.1	25.4	31.4	40.1	43.3	61.6	93.3	167.6	422.3
1975	31.1*	13.9*	30.0*	17.5	20.7	25.3	29.0	32.6	38.8	45.8	69.3	128.1	362.3
1985	23.8*	10.7*	25.4*	14.8	16.5	21.6	22.5	28.7	33.0	40.8	54.7	92.3	234.9
1990	19.2*	10.1*	20.0*	14.5	16.2	17.5	17.9	19.4	23.7	30.8	42.1	68.6	164.8
1995 projected	15.6*	9.7*	15.8*	14.2	14.6	14.6	13.3	13.8	16.9	22.9	31.2	49.2	117.6

UNITED KINGDOM: 1975

Smoking–attributed deaths (Sm.) and total deaths (Total)

		ALL CAUSES	ALL CANCER	Lung cancer	Upper aero–digestive ca.	Other cancer	COPD	Other respiratory	Vascular disease	Liver cirrhosis	Other medical	Non–medical
Males												
0–34	Sm.	–	–	–	–	–	–	–	–	–	–	–
	Total	16936	1473	55	22	1396	292	1208	852	32	7366	5713
35–69	Sm.	62142	22266	16342	1544	4380	7344	1811	27111	–	3610	–
	Total	141668	39129	17197	2094	19838	8724	4975	72640	888	9509	5803
		(44%)	(57%)	(95%)	(74%)	(22%)	(84%)	(36%)	(37%)		(38%)	
70+	Sm.	52039	16557	11537	1254	3766	12237	3165	17735	–	2345	–
	Total	176402	33747	12255	1788	19704	15048	18099	93944	212	12682	2670
		(30%)	(49%)	(94%)	(70%)	(19%)	(81%)	(17%)	(19%)		(18%)	
Any age	Sm.	114181	38823	27879	2798	8146	19581	4976	44846	–	5955	–
	Total	335006	74349	29507	3904	40938	24064	24282	167436	1132	29557	14186
		(34%)	(52%)	(94%)	(72%)	(20%)	(81%)	(20%)	(27%)		(20%)	
Females												
0–34	Sm.	–	–	–	–	–	–	–	–	–	–	–
	Total	10378	1156	29	10	1117	174	815	519	40	5768	1906
35–69	Sm.	15393	4715	3500	475	740	1970	648	6381	–	1679	–
	Total	85208	31289	4545	1032	25712	3010	3515	34538	700	8722	3434
		(18%)	(15%)	(77%)	(46%)	(3%)	(65%)	(18%)	(18%)		(19%)	
70+	Sm.	14874	3073	2079	528	466	3316	1122	6390	–	973	–
	Total	231885	31635	3078	1546	27011	6263	27031	140099	336	20910	5611
		(6%)	(10%)	(68%)	(34%)	(2%)	(53%)	(4%)	(5%)		(5%)	
Any age	Sm.	30267	7788	5579	1003	1206	5286	1770	12771	–	2652	–
	Total	327471	64080	7652	2588	53840	9447	31361	175156	1076	35400	10951
		(9%)	(12%)	(73%)	(39%)	(2%)	(56%)	(6%)	(7%)		(7%)	
Males+Females												
0–34	Sm.	–	–	–	–	–	–	–	–	–	–	–
	Total	27314	2629	84	32	2513	466	2023	1371	72	13134	7619
35–69	Sm.	77535	26981	19842	2019	5120	9314	2459	33492	–	5289	–
	Total	226876	70418	21742	3126	45550	11734	8490	107178	1588	18231	9237
		(34%)	(38%)	(91%)	(65%)	(11%)	(79%)	(29%)	(31%)		(29%)	
70+	Sm.	66913	19630	13616	1782	4232	15553	4287	24125	–	3318	–
	Total	408287	65382	15333	3334	46715	21311	45130	234043	548	33592	8281
		(16%)	(30%)	(89%)	(53%)	(9%)	(73%)	(9%)	(10%)		(10%)	
Any age	Sm.	144448	46611	33458	3801	9352	24867	6746	57617	–	8607	–
	Total	662477	138429	37159	6492	94778	33511	55643	342592	2208	64957	25137
		(22%)	(34%)	(90%)	(59%)	(10%)	(74%)	(12%)	(17%)		(13%)	

UNITED KINGDOM: 1985

Smoking–attributed deaths (Sm.) and total deaths (Total)

		ALL CAUSES	ALL CANCER	Lung cancer	Upper aero–digestive ca.	Other cancer	COPD	Other respiratory	Vascular disease	Liver cirrhosis	Other medical	Non–medical
Males												
0–34	Sm.	–	–	–	–	–	–	–	–	–	–	–
	Total	12802	1080	28	30	1022	145	495	662	36	5313	5071
35–69	Sm.	45848	18484	13018	1809	3657	4997	750	18846	–	2771	–
	Total	116684	35730	13844	2602	19284	6117	2317	57414	1200	8379	5527
		(39%)	(52%)	(94%)	(70%)	(19%)	(82%)	(32%)	(33%)		(33%)	
70+	Sm.	58989	21467	14707	1626	5134	13501	2155	18098	–	3768	–
	Total	202076	45782	15671	2347	27764	16709	13121	101205	433	22002	2824
		(29%)	(47%)	(94%)	(69%)	(18%)	(81%)	(16%)	(18%)		(17%)	
Any age	Sm.	104837	39951	27725	3435	8791	18498	2905	36944	–	6539	–
	Total	331562	82592	29543	4979	48070	22971	15933	159281	1669	35694	13422
		(32%)	(48%)	(94%)	(69%)	(18%)	(81%)	(18%)	(23%)		(18%)	
Females												
0–34	Sm.	–	–	–	–	–	–	–	–	–	–	–
	Total	7477	1030	20	10	1000	131	316	396	40	4062	1502
35–69	Sm.	17026	5985	4473	603	909	2476	382	6399	–	1784	–
	Total	73028	31084	5460	1116	24508	3422	1549	25887	885	7364	2837
		(23%)	(19%)	(82%)	(54%)	(4%)	(72%)	(25%)	(25%)		(24%)	
70+	Sm.	28555	6850	4682	1010	1158	5324	1622	11675	–	3084	–
	Total	258589	42802	5837	2006	34959	7702	22250	141840	480	38702	4813
		(11%)	(16%)	(80%)	(50%)	(3%)	(69%)	(7%)	(8%)		(8%)	
Any age	Sm.	45581	12835	9155	1613	2067	7800	2004	18074	–	4868	–
	Total	339094	74916	11317	3132	60467	11255	24115	168123	1405	50128	9152
		(13%)	(17%)	(81%)	(52%)	(3%)	(69%)	(8%)	(11%)		(10%)	
Males+Females												
0–34	Sm.	–	–	–	–	–	–	–	–	–	–	–
	Total	20279	2110	48	40	2022	276	811	1058	76	9375	6573
35–69	Sm.	62874	24469	17491	2412	4566	7473	1132	25245	–	4555	–
	Total	189712	66814	19304	3718	43792	9539	3866	83301	2085	15743	8364
		(33%)	(37%)	(91%)	(65%)	(10%)	(78%)	(29%)	(30%)		(29%)	
70+	Sm.	87544	28317	19389	2636	6292	18825	3777	29773	–	6852	–
	Total	460665	88584	21508	4353	62723	24411	35371	243045	913	60704	7637
		(19%)	(32%)	(90%)	(61%)	(10%)	(77%)	(11%)	(12%)		(11%)	
Any age	Sm.	150418	52786	36880	5048	10858	26298	4909	55018	–	11407	–
	Total	670656	157508	40860	8111	108537	34226	40048	327404	3074	85822	22574
		(22%)	(34%)	(90%)	(62%)	(10%)	(77%)	(12%)	(17%)		(13%)	

(To be conservative, no deaths before age 35, and none from liver cirrhosis or non–medical causes, were attributed to smoking.)

UNITED KINGDOM: 1990

Smoking-attributed deaths (Sm.) and total deaths (Total)

		ALL CAUSES	ALL CANCER	Lung cancer	Upper aero-digestive ca.	Other cancer	COPD	Other respiratory	Vascular disease	Liver cirrhosis	Other medical	Non-medical
Males												
0–34	Sm.	–	–	–	–	–	–	–	–	–	–	–
	Total	13108	1020	15	30	975	134	398	613	53	5311	5579
35–69	Sm.	37212	16488	11267	1893	3328	3765	662	13867	–	2430	–
	Total	106638	35286	12120	2900	20266	4746	2331	48681	1483	8466	5645
		(35%)	(47%)	(93%)	(65%)	(16%)	(79%)	(28%)	(28%)		(29%)	
70+	Sm.	52147	20526	13761	1712	5053	11754	1851	14634	–	3382	–
	Total	194855	47838	14789	2574	30475	14951	12839	93479	459	22702	2587
		(27%)	(43%)	(93%)	(67%)	(17%)	(79%)	(14%)	(16%)		(15%)	
Any age	Sm.	89359	37014	25028	3605	8381	15519	2513	28501	–	5812	–
	Total	314601	84144	26924	5504	51716	19831	15568	142773	1995	36479	13811
		(28%)	(44%)	(93%)	(65%)	(16%)	(78%)	(16%)	(20%)		(16%)	
Females												
0–34	Sm.	–	–	–	–	–	–	–	–	–	–	–
	Total	6870	969	19	9	941	103	252	381	47	3670	1448
35–69	Sm.	16393	6182	4687	589	906	2406	380	5695	–	1730	–
	Total	67970	30687	5685	1073	23929	3269	1490	22146	1062	7018	2298
		(24%)	(20%)	(82%)	(55%)	(4%)	(74%)	(26%)	(26%)		(25%)	
70+	Sm.	32119	8190	5505	1247	1438	5854	1937	12340	–	3798	–
	Total	252358	45430	6641	2269	36520	8016	22549	130527	519	41579	3738
		(13%)	(18%)	(83%)	(55%)	(4%)	(73%)	(9%)	(9%)		(9%)	
Any age	Sm.	48512	14372	10192	1836	2344	8260	2317	18035	–	5528	–
	Total	327198	77086	12345	3351	61390	11388	24291	153054	1628	52267	7484
		(15%)	(19%)	(83%)	(55%)	(4%)	(73%)	(10%)	(12%)		(11%)	
Males+Females												
0–34	Sm.	–	–	–	–	–	–	–	–	–	–	–
	Total	19978	1989	34	39	1916	237	650	994	100	8981	7027
35–69	Sm.	53605	22670	15954	2482	4234	6171	1042	19562	–	4160	–
	Total	174608	65973	17805	3973	44195	8015	3821	70827	2545	15484	7943
		(31%)	(34%)	(90%)	(62%)	(10%)	(77%)	(27%)	(28%)		(27%)	
70+	Sm.	84266	28716	19266	2959	6491	17608	3788	26974	–	7180	–
	Total	447213	93268	21430	4843	66995	22967	35388	224006	978	64281	6325
		(19%)	(31%)	(90%)	(61%)	(10%)	(77%)	(11%)	(12%)		(11%)	
Any age	Sm.	137871	51386	35220	5441	10725	23779	4830	46536	–	11340	–
	Total	641799	161230	39269	8855	113106	31219	39859	295827	3623	88746	21295
		(21%)	(32%)	(90%)	(61%)	(9%)	(76%)	(12%)	(16%)		(13%)	

UNITED KINGDOM: 1995

Smoking-attributed deaths (Sm.) and total deaths (Total)

		ALL CAUSES	ALL CANCER	Lung cancer	Upper aero-digestive ca.	Other cancer	COPD	Other respiratory	Vascular disease	Liver cirrhosis	Other medical	Non-medical
Males												
0–34	Sm.	–	–	–	–	–	–	–	–	–	–	–
	Total	13132	945	12	34	899	119	383	562	79	5130	5914
35–69	Sm.	28401	13744	9138	1833	2773	2654	539	9506	–	1958	–
	Total	92297	32862	9983	3033	19846	3475	2188	38460	1778	7955	5579
		(31%)	(42%)	(92%)	(60%)	(14%)	(76%)	(25%)	(25%)		(25%)	
70+	Sm.	44256	18953	12446	1758	4749	9387	1440	11623	–	2853	–
	Total	175168	47883	13493	2757	31633	12258	10894	80459	501	20977	2196
		(25%)	(40%)	(92%)	(64%)	(15%)	(77%)	(13%)	(14%)		(14%)	
Any age	Sm.	72657	32697	21584	3591	7522	12041	1979	21129	–	4811	–
	Total	280597	81690	23488	5824	52378	15852	13465	119481	2358	34062	13689
		(26%)	(40%)	(92%)	(62%)	(14%)	(76%)	(15%)	(18%)		(14%)	
Females												
0–34	Sm.	–	–	–	–	–	–	–	–	–	–	–
	Total	6169	907	15	8	884	85	217	349	64	3183	1364
35–69	Sm.	14871	6091	4677	552	862	2212	339	4660	–	1569	–
	Total	60334	29077	5657	1000	22420	2968	1304	17571	1267	6292	1855
		(25%)	(21%)	(83%)	(55%)	(4%)	(75%)	(26%)	(27%)		(25%)	
70+	Sm.	33835	9495	6414	1431	1650	6170	1977	12007	–	4186	–
	Total	226764	46123	7547	2440	36136	8118	20009	109387	569	39900	2658
		(15%)	(21%)	(85%)	(59%)	(5%)	(76%)	(10%)	(11%)		(10%)	
Any age	Sm.	48706	15586	11091	1983	2512	8382	2316	16667	–	5755	–
	Total	293267	76107	13219	3448	59440	11171	21530	127307	1900	49375	5877
		(17%)	(20%)	(84%)	(58%)	(4%)	(75%)	(11%)	(13%)		(12%)	
Males+Females												
0–34	Sm.	–	–	–	–	–	–	–	–	–	–	–
	Total	19301	1852	27	42	1783	204	600	911	143	8313	7278
35–69	Sm.	43272	19835	13815	2385	3635	4866	878	14166	–	3527	–
	Total	152631	61939	15640	4033	42266	6443	3492	56031	3045	14247	7434
		(28%)	(32%)	(88%)	(59%)	(9%)	(76%)	(25%)	(25%)		(25%)	
70+	Sm.	78091	28448	18860	3189	6399	15557	3417	23630	–	7039	–
	Total	401932	94006	21040	5197	67769	20376	30903	189846	1070	60877	4854
		(19%)	(30%)	(90%)	(61%)	(9%)	(76%)	(11%)	(12%)		(12%)	
Any age	Sm.	121363	48283	32675	5574	10034	20423	4295	37796	–	10566	–
	Total	573864	157797	36707	9272	111818	27023	34995	246788	4258	83437	19566
		(21%)	(31%)	(89%)	(60%)	(9%)	(76%)	(12%)	(15%)		(13%)	

(To be conservative, no deaths before age 35, and none from liver cirrhosis or non-medical causes, were attributed to smoking.)

UNITED STATES: 1990

		No. of deaths			Standardised rates (Defined on p.532)			Annual death rates / 100, 000						
		All ages	0–34	35–69	All ages	0–34	35–69	0–4	5–9	10–14	15–19	20–24	25–29	30–34
ALL CAUSES	M	1113417	102882	415118	1013.7	146.9	1118.8	269.0	25.6	31.6	127.2	166.3	184.9	223.4
	F	1035046	47660	257081	615.3	71.0	618.7	212.4	18.5	20.2	46.4	51.3	63.9	84.3
Tuberculosis	M	1254	102	603	1.1	0.1	1.5	0.0	0.0	–	0.0	0.1	0.3	0.6
	F	770	80	274	0.5	0.1	0.6	0.0	0.0	0.0	0.0	0.1	0.2	0.3
Other infective	M	13682	1586	5127	12.3	2.3	13.1	5.9	0.6	0.4	0.9	1.2	2.6	4.1
and parasitic	F	14718	1052	3557	8.8	1.6	8.4	5.0	0.6	0.5	0.7	1.0	1.5	1.7
ALL CANCER	M	268283	4737	123325	251.5	6.7	348.9	3.4	3.5	3.4	4.8	6.5	9.6	15.5
	F	237039	4206	104239	163.1	6.0	252.0	3.0	2.8	2.7	3.7	4.5	8.2	16.8
Mouth and	M	5636	68	3494	5.5	0.1	9.7	–	0.0	0.0	0.0	0.1	0.2	0.3
pharynx cancer	F	2769	26	1188	1.9	0.0	2.9	0.0	–	0.0	0.1	0.0	0.1	0.1
Oesophagus cancer	M	7213	18	4236	7.0	0.0	12.0	–	–	–	–	0.0	0.1	0.1
	F	2506	3	1103	1.7	0.0	2.8	–	–	–	–	–	–	0.0
Stomach cancer	M	8336	62	3789	7.8	0.1	10.5	–	–	–	0.0	0.1	0.1	0.3
	F	5737	72	1870	3.6	0.1	4.5	–	–	–	0.0	0.0	0.2	0.4
Colorectal cancer	M	28173	186	11671	26.3	0.2	33.3	–	–	–	0.1	0.2	0.5	1.0
	F	28352	163	8967	17.6	0.2	22.0	–	–	–	0.1	0.1	0.5	0.9
Liver cancer	M	2814	71	1509	2.7	0.1	4.2	0.2	0.0	0.0	0.1	0.1	0.1	0.2
	F	1314	46	587	0.9	0.1	1.4	0.1	0.0	0.0	0.0	0.1	0.0	0.1
Pancreas cancer	M	12199	47	5871	11.5	0.1	16.7	–	–	–	–	0.0	0.1	0.3
	F	12883	28	4413	8.2	0.0	11.0	–	0.0	0.0	0.0	0.0	0.1	0.1
Larynx cancer	M	2977	4	1714	2.9	0.0	4.9	–	–	–	–	–	–	0.0
	F	733	3	425	0.6	0.0	1.1	–	–	0.0	–	–	0.0	0.0
Lung cancer	M	91091	212	48371	86.7	0.3	138.9	0.0	–	0.0	0.0	0.1	0.4	1.4
	F	50194	122	26173	36.7	0.2	64.9	0.0	0.0	0.0	0.0	0.0	0.3	0.8
Malignant melanoma	M	3844	221	2290	3.6	0.3	5.8	0.0	–	–	0.1	0.3	0.5	1.2
	F	2576	149	1327	1.9	0.2	3.0	–	0.0	0.0	0.1	0.1	0.5	0.7
Female breast cancer	F	43391	643	23807	32.1	0.8	55.8	–	–	–	0.0	0.1	1.1	4.6
Cervix cancer	F	4627	324	2902	3.6	0.4	6.4	–	–	–	0.0	0.2	0.7	2.1
Other uterine cancer	F	6028	24	2366	4.0	0.0	5.9	–	–	–	0.0	–	0.0	0.2
Ovarian cancer	F	12762	149	6280	9.1	0.2	15.3	–	–	0.1	0.1	0.2	0.4	0.7
Prostate cancer	M	32378	7	6979	29.2	0.0	21.1	0.0	–	–	0.0	–	0.0	0.0
Bladder cancer	M	6910	14	2055	6.3	0.0	6.0	–	–	–	–	–	0.0	0.1
	F	3431	10	778	2.0	0.0	1.9	–	–	–	–	–	0.0	0.1
Other and ill–defined	M	41208	1917	20426	38.7	2.7	56.2	2.0	2.0	1.4	1.9	2.8	3.6	5.4
cancer sites	F	37499	1340	14433	24.9	2.0	34.9	1.8	1.8	1.6	1.6	1.5	2.0	3.5
Hodgkin's disease	M	956	284	461	0.8	0.4	1.1	–	0.0	0.0	0.3	0.5	0.9	1.0
	F	676	159	267	0.5	0.2	0.6	0.0	0.0	0.0	0.1	0.4	0.6	0.4
Myeloma and non–	M	14356	563	6536	13.3	0.8	17.9	0.1	0.3	0.4	0.4	0.8	1.4	2.2
Hodgkin lymphomas	F	13179	229	4609	8.5	0.3	11.3	0.1	0.0	0.2	0.2	0.4	0.5	0.8
Leukaemia	M	10192	1063	3923	9.3	1.6	10.7	1.1	1.2	1.5	1.9	1.5	1.8	1.9
	F	8382	716	2744	5.4	1.1	6.4	1.0	0.9	0.8	1.2	1.2	1.1	1.4
ALL VASCULAR	M	444763	4617	152846	411.7	6.4	429.2	7.7	1.0	1.5	3.2	5.0	8.8	17.9
DISEASE	F	475482	2993	77913	255.6	4.3	192.2	6.8	0.9	1.4	1.8	3.4	5.7	9.9
Rheumatic heart	M	1830	71	862	1.7	0.1	2.3	0.0	0.0	0.0	0.1	0.1	0.1	0.3
disease and fever	F	4188	83	1388	2.7	0.1	3.4	0.1	0.0	0.0	0.1	0.1	0.2	0.3
Hypertensive disease	M	13614	168	5776	12.8	0.2	15.8	0.0	0.0	–	0.0	0.2	0.4	1.0
	F	19004	92	4170	10.8	0.1	10.2	0.1	0.0	0.0	0.0	0.1	0.2	0.4
Ischaemic heart	M	252597	919	90154	234.7	1.2	254.8	0.2	0.0	0.1	0.2	0.6	1.9	5.6
disease	F	236574	311	37637	126.6	0.4	94.0	0.2	0.0	0.1	0.1	0.3	0.6	1.6
Pulmonary embolism	M	5166	175	2258	4.8	0.2	6.2	0.1	0.0	0.0	0.2	0.3	0.4	0.7
and other venous	F	6099	189	1927	3.8	0.3	4.6	0.0	0.0	0.1	0.2	0.4	0.4	0.7
Cerebrovascular	M	56697	729	14669	51.8	1.0	40.9	1.1	0.2	0.2	0.5	0.9	1.4	2.8
disease	F	87391	708	13042	46.3	1.0	31.6	0.9	0.2	0.3	0.3	0.8	1.7	2.8
Other vascular	M	114859	2555	39127	106.0	3.6	109.2	6.2	0.7	1.1	2.3	2.9	4.6	7.5
disease	F	122226	1610	19749	65.5	2.4	48.5	5.5	0.6	0.9	1.1	1.7	2.6	4.1
Chronic obstructive	M	49416	389	14206	44.9	0.6	42.0	0.8	0.3	0.5	0.5	0.5	0.7	0.8
pulmonary disease	F	37263	314	10837	22.9	0.5	27.2	0.4	0.1	0.4	0.4	0.5	0.6	0.7
Other respiratory	M	50659	1843	10900	45.9	2.6	30.0	8.6	0.8	0.7	0.7	1.4	2.3	4.1
disease	F	54867	1389	6540	28.3	2.1	15.7	6.9	0.7	0.7	0.8	1.2	1.8	2.4
Peptic ulcer	M	2973	57	958	2.7	0.1	2.7	0.1	0.0	0.0	0.0	0.1	0.2	0.2
	F	3213	27	553	1.7	0.0	1.4	0.1	–	0.0	0.0	0.0	0.1	0.1
Liver cirrhosis	M	16627	592	12324	16.0	0.8	30.9	0.1	0.0	0.0	0.1	0.2	1.2	4.0
	F	9188	371	5600	7.1	0.5	13.0	0.1	0.0	0.0	0.0	0.2	0.7	2.4
Renal disease	M	10409	293	2650	9.4	0.4	7.2	1.1	0.1	0.0	0.1	0.3	0.5	0.9
	F	11651	198	2356	6.5	0.3	5.7	0.9	0.0	0.1	0.1	0.2	0.3	0.4
Pregnancy and birth	F	343	267	76	0.2	0.4	0.1	–	–	–	0.5	0.7	0.7	0.8
Congenital and	M	17106	15853	788	14.3	23.6	1.9	156.5	1.8	1.1	1.6	1.6	1.3	1.2
perinatal causes	F	13653	12370	714	11.7	19.3	1.6	128.1	1.6	1.1	0.9	1.2	1.0	1.0
Ill–defined causes	M	13533	5796	4205	11.7	8.4	9.9	42.2	0.3	0.6	1.8	3.3	4.8	6.1
	F	10604	3410	2059	7.0	5.2	4.5	28.7	0.2	0.3	0.9	1.6	2.1	2.7
Other medical causes	M	116713	14032	47291	104.0	19.3	114.2	16.5	4.1	3.5	5.9	10.6	33.9	60.5
	F	124043	5635	28458	71.9	8.2	67.2	13.2	3.2	3.4	4.1	6.2	11.0	16.0
ALL NON–	M	107999	52985	39895	88.1	75.6	87.3	26.2	13.2	19.9	107.8	135.7	119.0	107.6
MEDICAL CAUSES	F	42212	15348	13905	29.9	22.7	29.2	19.3	8.3	9.5	32.4	30.4	30.0	29.0
Motor vehicle	M	31647	18495	10184	25.3	26.6	22.1	5.5	6.2	7.2	44.9	52.4	38.9	31.2
traffic accidents	F	14180	6903	4851	10.7	10.4	10.2	4.9	4.1	5.0	19.9	15.8	12.7	10.2
Fire	M	2571	1105	950	2.2	1.6	2.3	4.1	1.3	0.6	0.7	1.4	1.4	1.7
	F	1604	631	452	1.2	1.0	1.0	2.8	1.2	0.5	0.6	0.5	0.5	0.7
Suicide	M	24724	9694	11125	20.7	13.6	24.9	–	0.0	2.2	18.1	25.7	24.9	24.6
	F	6182	1989	3359	4.8	2.8	7.0	–	0.0	0.8	3.7	4.1	4.9	6.3
Homicide	M	19298	12808	5966	14.8	18.2	11.8	4.0	0.8	2.6	27.8	36.9	31.2	24.4
	F	5316	3207	1675	4.0	4.7	3.2	3.5	1.0	1.5	5.4	7.0	7.4	6.9
POPULATION (thousands):	M=males				121239	68050	45205	9599	9232	8739	9173	9743	10703	10862
	F=females				127471	65977	48465	9159	8803	8322	8709	9389	10625	10971

UNITED STATES: 1990

Annual death rates / 100, 000 — 9th ICD categories

35–39	40–44	45–49	50–54	55–59	60–64	65–69	70–74	75–79	80+/NK			
280.7	344.2	491.1	756.5	1208.5	1902.7	2847.6	4345.3	6608.6	13192.2	M	ALL CAUSES	001–999
114.8	163.9	267.8	432.9	681.5	1069.1	1600.8	2465.0	3856.8	10017.3	F		
0.7	0.8	1.1	1.2	1.7	2.2	2.9	4.2	6.4	11.5	M	Tuberculosis	010–018, 137
0.2	0.2	0.3	0.5	0.7	1.1	1.5	2.2	2.6	4.6	F		
5.8	6.8	7.5	9.2	12.2	19.8	30.3	47.6	74.8	162.2	M	Other infective	Rest of 001–139
2.3	3.1	4.2	6.0	9.2	13.9	20.0	31.8	52.5	141.6	F	and parasitic	
26.7	51.9	111.5	225.2	405.1	662.3	959.9	1337.5	1752.1	2407.8	M	ALL CANCER	140–208
33.8	64.1	118.3	200.3	304.3	443.7	599.7	771.7	940.2	1232.2	F		
0.8	1.9	4.4	7.8	13.2	19.2	20.3	23.0	24.4	32.3	M	Mouth and	140–149
0.2	0.5	1.0	2.3	4.0	5.4	7.1	9.8	11.1	14.7	F	pharynx cancer	
0.5	1.7	4.4	9.4	15.0	22.7	30.0	34.9	37.1	40.3	M	Oesophagus cancer	150
0.1	0.2	0.6	1.8	3.5	5.9	7.2	8.6	10.3	13.2	F		
1.0	2.3	4.1	8.0	12.5	18.1	27.8	41.2	55.6	79.9	M	Stomach cancer	151
0.6	1.1	2.1	3.4	4.8	8.4	11.2	17.3	25.9	43.1	F		
2.4	4.3	9.6	20.5	36.4	62.1	97.6	138.4	200.4	310.6	M	Colorectal cancer	153, 154
1.8	3.8	8.0	15.3	24.7	40.0	60.5	88.4	125.3	222.3	F		
0.5	0.9	1.4	3.0	5.2	8.0	10.5	14.2	16.3	16.5	M	Liver cancer	155.0
0.2	0.4	0.6	0.8	1.6	2.6	3.7	4.2	6.0	5.6	F		
1.0	2.2	5.9	10.4	19.7	31.1	46.5	63.3	80.7	100.1	M	Pancreas cancer	157
0.5	1.2	3.6	6.8	12.4	20.4	31.9	45.1	59.7	87.8	F		
0.1	0.5	1.4	4.1	6.0	9.7	12.2	14.7	15.4	17.8	M	Larynx cancer	161
0.0	0.1	0.2	0.8	1.3	2.3	2.7	2.8	2.8	1.6	F		
4.3	13.3	38.2	86.2	168.9	277.7	383.7	492.3	567.7	555.8	M	Lung cancer	162
3.0	7.8	22.9	48.5	82.4	126.9	162.5	195.9	200.8	157.8	F		
2.1	3.1	4.0	4.9	7.0	9.4	10.4	13.9	16.8	20.9	M	Malignant melanoma	172
1.2	1.8	2.4	2.9	3.6	4.1	5.1	6.8	7.1	11.0	F		
12.0	24.4	37.3	55.1	70.3	86.6	105.1	119.7	139.4	175.0	F	Female breast cancer	174
3.5	4.8	5.9	7.2	7.2	7.9	8.1	9.2	9.1	13.5	F	Cervix cancer	180
0.3	0.9	1.7	3.7	6.4	10.5	17.4	23.3	27.8	32.6	F	Other uterine cancer	179, 182
1.5	3.4	7.8	12.4	18.7	26.6	36.3	44.2	50.0	51.8	F	Ovarian cancer	183
0.1	0.2	0.7	4.7	15.4	39.5	87.2	169.7	288.6	579.4	M	Prostate cancer	185
0.2	0.6	0.9	2.9	5.4	12.8	19.2	33.7	58.0	105.1	M	Bladder cancer	188
0.1	0.2	0.4	0.8	1.9	4.0	6.3	9.1	16.3	34.2	F		
7.7	13.0	24.1	41.7	67.9	100.7	138.5	183.3	234.1	320.4	M	Other and ill-defined	Rest of 140–208
5.1	8.6	15.6	25.9	41.4	61.5	86.3	116.8	152.3	226.5	F	cancer sites	
0.9	0.7	0.8	0.8	1.4	1.5	1.5	2.4	2.3	3.4	M	Hodgkin's disease	201
0.4	0.5	0.3	0.4	0.6	0.7	1.2	1.3	2.2	2.3	F		
2.9	4.6	7.5	13.3	19.9	31.7	45.5	67.4	91.2	126.9	M	Myeloma and non-	200, 202–203
1.3	2.0	4.3	7.3	12.4	19.7	32.0	45.9	60.7	84.1	F	Hodgkin lymphomas	
2.3	2.7	4.2	7.4	11.3	18.2	29.1	45.2	63.4	98.2	M	Leukaemia	204–208
2.0	2.4	3.5	4.8	7.2	10.3	15.0	23.4	33.4	55.1	F		
38.1	80.0	158.4	277.9	476.3	770.6	1203.5	1922.4	3058.7	6776.6	M	ALL VASCULAR	390–459
16.1	30.0	60.6	109.4	196.4	346.2	586.4	1037.6	1856.0	5875.6	F	DISEASE	
0.6	0.7	1.0	1.2	2.6	4.1	6.2	8.2	10.3	16.9	M	Rheumatic heart	390–398
0.5	0.9	1.2	2.8	3.8	5.5	8.7	12.6	19.3	30.1	F	disease and fever	
2.1	4.3	7.3	12.3	19.6	26.3	38.8	54.2	81.4	176.8	M	Hypertensive disease	401–405
0.9	2.0	4.3	7.1	11.3	17.8	28.0	45.6	76.8	207.1	F		
16.3	42.3	90.7	164.4	288.0	464.0	718.1	1137.8	1759.9	3678.0	M	Ischaemic heart	410–414
3.9	9.1	22.7	46.8	93.8	175.5	306.0	547.6	969.7	2905.5	F	disease	
1.3	1.7	2.6	3.8	7.2	10.3	16.4	21.8	33.2	54.6	M	Pulmonary embolism	415.1, 451–453
1.0	1.7	2.4	3.3	5.0	7.4	11.2	16.0	25.3	48.8	F	and other venous	
5.1	8.7	16.1	25.8	42.3	66.6	121.9	226.5	426.8	1065.4	M	Cerebrovascular	430–438
4.5	7.9	14.0	20.7	32.1	52.1	89.8	171.9	330.8	1129.9	F	disease	
12.8	22.4	40.7	70.3	116.7	199.3	302.2	474.0	747.2	1784.9	M	Other vascular	Rest of 390–459
5.2	8.5	16.0	28.7	50.4	87.9	142.7	243.9	434.1	1554.3	F	disease	
1.2	2.3	6.0	13.7	37.1	80.3	153.1	271.6	438.2	688.2	M	Chronic obstructive	490–496
1.0	2.1	5.0	13.3	27.2	52.9	88.7	140.9	198.3	259.7	F	pulmonary disease	
6.1	8.4	10.8	16.7	27.0	52.4	88.3	172.2	339.1	1090.7	M	Other respiratory	Rest of 460–519
3.4	4.2	6.5	9.4	15.6	26.6	44.3	85.9	175.4	770.9	F	disease	
0.4	0.6	1.0	1.7	2.9	4.4	7.5	13.9	19.8	46.1	M	Peptic ulcer	531–533
0.1	0.3	0.6	0.8	1.2	2.6	3.9	7.2	13.2	38.3	F		
11.5	17.4	24.2	29.5	39.2	46.5	48.0	48.1	46.7	43.7	M	Liver cirrhosis	571
4.4	5.9	8.4	11.3	16.6	19.9	24.1	25.2	26.9	22.5	F		
1.7	2.1	2.8	4.3	6.5	12.2	20.9	41.0	73.6	196.4	M	Renal disease	580–590
1.0	1.3	2.1	3.4	5.8	10.2	16.2	27.8	45.4	129.7	F		
0.5	0.2	0.0	–	–	–	–	–	–	–	F	Pregnancy and birth	630–676
1.5	1.4	1.5	1.6	1.9	2.2	2.9	3.5	5.1	10.1	M	Congenital and	740–779
0.9	1.1	1.3	1.5	1.8	2.0	2.4	3.5	3.2	6.1	F	perinatal causes	
7.9	7.7	6.9	7.9	9.8	12.8	16.6	22.6	34.2	88.6	M	Ill-defined causes	780–799
3.1	2.9	3.3	3.9	4.3	6.1	8.1	13.4	20.2	79.6	F		
78.7	78.2	78.7	87.8	107.6	148.4	220.0	343.9	590.6	1346.8	M	Other medical causes	Rest of 001–799
20.2	23.0	30.9	46.1	68.8	112.7	168.6	269.7	448.1	1287.7	F		
100.4	86.6	80.9	79.9	81.0	88.6	93.8	116.8	169.2	323.5	M	ALL NON-	E800–E999
27.6	25.5	26.3	27.0	29.6	31.4	36.9	48.0	74.8	168.7	F	MEDICAL CAUSES	
26.5	21.5	21.6	21.3	20.9	21.5	21.7	26.0	35.8	55.9	M	Motor vehicle	E810–E819
9.4	8.8	9.2	9.8	10.2	11.1	12.9	15.3	20.9	20.1	F	traffic accidents	
1.7	1.5	1.6	2.1	2.3	3.2	3.3	4.1	5.9	10.8	M	Fire	E890–E899
0.6	0.7	0.9	1.0	0.9	1.0	1.9	2.5	3.2	6.1	F		
24.5	23.2	23.5	22.8	25.0	26.5	28.9	36.6	51.8	64.8	M	Suicide	E950–E959
6.8	6.8	6.8	7.0	8.0	6.7	6.5	7.0	6.0	6.1	F		
20.9	16.0	12.9	10.7	8.2	7.7	6.0	5.5	5.7	9.2	M	Homicide	E960–E969
5.4	4.0	3.5	2.7	2.5	2.0	2.1	2.4	3.1	4.4	F		
9833	8677	6739	5493	5008	4947	4508	3399	2389	2197	M	POPULATION (thousands)	
10013	8913	7004	5820	5479	5679	5558	4580	3714	4733	F		

UNITED STATES: Males

	All ages	0–34	35–69	35–39	40–44	45–49	50–54	55–59	60–64	65–69	70–74	75–79	80+/NK
POPULATION (1000s)													
1955	81068	46731	30333	5746	5410	4998	4314	3829	3322	2714	1928	1171	905
1965	95115	56477	33577	5828	6033	5570	5146	4420	3710	2870	2283	1545	1233
1975	104876	63625	35582	5654	5475	5705	5736	5048	4368	3596	2441	1653	1575
1985	116161	67537	41343	8741	6888	5678	5282	5382	5117	4255	3217	2137	1927
1990	**121239**	**68050**	**45205**	**9833**	**8677**	**6739**	**5493**	**5008**	**4947**	**4508**	**3399**	**2389**	**2197**
1995 projected	*126002*	*66076*	*50933*	*11076*	*10128*	*8646*	*6660*	*5303*	*4689*	*4430*	*3773*	*2667*	*2554*
NUMBER OF DEATHS													
All causes													
1955	872638	119117	403118	16685	25371	37788	52905	70519	90872	108978	110803	100061	139539
1965	1035200	117506	460089	17639	28045	41408	62553	83438	104026	122980	137059	130494	190052
1975	1050819	108653	457216	15567	22869	38166	60151	81142	108960	130361	135835	129830	219285
1985	1097758	98200	424790	20561	22933	29181	44139	72223	105488	130265	152752	152649	269367
1990	**1113417**	**102882**	**415118**	**27601**	**29861**	**33097**	**41557**	**60527**	**94119**	**128356**	**147711**	**157873**	**289833**
1995 projected	*1147355*	*102796*	*413859*	*34802*	*35949*	*40173*	*45980*	*58472*	*82236*	*116247*	*151306*	*162236*	*317158*
Lung cancer													
1955	22704	182	17271	293	660	1553	2545	3647	4434	4139	2775	1565	911
1965	40879	172	28381	446	1135	2252	4004	5910	7097	7537	6391	3724	2211
1975	63413	190	40836	389	1168	2958	5555	7952	10936	11878	10158	6813	5416
1985	83854	169	47675	412	1148	2433	4933	9424	13789	15536	15007	11464	9539
1990	**91091**	**212**	**48371**	**425**	**1151**	**2573**	**4733**	**8458**	**13736**	**17295**	**16736**	**13561**	**12211**
1995 projected	*100337*	*216*	*49336*	*405*	*1135*	*2848*	*5312*	*8788*	*13225*	*17623*	*19393*	*15930*	*15462*
ANNUAL DEATH RATE / 100,000 (*The rates for the age groups 0–34 and 35–69 are the means of seven five-yearly rates, but the all-ages rates are standardised to the conventional "European" age distribution)													
All causes													
1955	1370.1*	226.7*	1619.2*	290.4	469.0	756.1	1226.4	1841.7	2735.5	4015.4	5747.0	8544.9	15418.7
1965	1377.9*	202.0*	1671.9*	302.7	464.9	743.4	1215.6	1887.7	2803.9	4285.0	6003.5	8446.2	15413.8
1975	1228.9*	178.3*	1448.3*	275.3	417.7	669.0	1048.7	1607.4	2494.5	3625.2	5564.7	7854.2	13922.9
1985	1077.7*	142.1*	1197.5*	235.2	332.9	513.9	835.6	1341.9	2061.5	3061.5	4748.3	7143.1	13978.6
1990	**1013.7***	**146.9***	**1118.8***	**280.7**	**344.2**	**491.1**	**756.5**	**1208.5**	**1902.7**	**2847.6**	**4345.3**	**6608.6**	**13192.2**
1995 projected	*954.5**	*153.6**	*1043.5**	*314.2*	*355.0*	*464.6*	*690.4*	*1102.6*	*1753.7*	*2623.8*	*4010.8*	*6084.2*	*12417.1*
All cancer													
1955	201.6*	12.1*	296.9*	33.6	59.0	118.7	216.1	349.8	537.9	763.4	974.3	1268.2	1629.1
1965	218.8*	11.2*	330.4*	37.0	67.4	124.9	230.7	393.2	591.2	868.5	1113.4	1324.6	1660.7
1975	236.8*	8.9*	343.5*	31.1	64.1	133.9	241.9	398.3	635.5	899.6	1273.0	1545.6	1931.7
1985	246.6*	7.3*	347.8*	28.7	59.5	119.8	233.3	416.4	651.7	925.5	1297.3	1685.6	2242.9
1990	**251.5***	**6.7***	**348.9***	**26.7**	**51.9**	**111.5**	**225.2**	**405.1**	**662.3**	**959.9**	**1337.5**	**1752.1**	**2407.8**
1995 projected	*254.4**	*6.2**	*347.0**	*24.2*	*46.3*	*100.8*	*213.5*	*398.7*	*667.2*	*978.4*	*1371.9*	*1795.7*	*2546.4*
Lung cancer													
1955	35.2*	0.4*	69.8*	5.1	12.2	31.1	59.0	95.2	133.5	152.5	143.9	133.6	100.7
1965	55.2*	0.4*	104.6*	7.7	18.8	40.4	77.8	133.7	191.3	262.6	279.9	241.0	179.3
1975	75.3*	0.4*	130.7*	6.9	21.3	51.8	96.8	157.5	250.4	330.3	416.1	412.2	343.9
1985	84.4*	0.2*	138.2*	4.7	16.7	42.8	93.4	175.1	269.5	365.1	466.5	536.5	495.0
1990	**86.7***	**0.3***	**138.9***	**4.3**	**13.3**	**38.2**	**86.2**	**168.9**	**277.7**	**383.7**	**492.3**	**567.7**	**555.8**
1995 projected	*88.5**	*0.3**	*139.0**	*3.7*	*11.2*	*32.9*	*79.8*	*165.7*	*282.0*	*397.8*	*514.1*	*597.4*	*605.4*
Upper aerodigestive cancer (mouth, oesophagus, pharynx and larynx)													
1955	15.6*	0.2*	25.6*	1.4	4.2	9.7	20.9	32.8	46.5	63.8	69.7	89.7	114.4
1965	15.6*	0.1*	27.2*	1.5	4.4	11.7	22.6	38.1	50.0	62.5	71.1	76.8	90.3
1975	16.2*	0.1*	28.3*	1.2	4.5	13.1	23.3	38.1	53.3	64.8	77.9	75.5	90.0
1985	15.1*	0.1*	26.5*	1.3	4.4	11.2	20.8	37.1	49.8	60.7	70.9	75.9	83.0
1990	**15.3***	**0.1***	**26.5***	**1.5**	**4.1**	**10.2**	**21.3**	**34.2**	**51.6**	**62.5**	**72.5**	**76.9**	**90.5**
1995 projected	*15.3**	*0.1**	*26.2**	*1.4*	*3.7*	*9.6*	*20.0*	*33.7*	*51.4*	*63.7*	*73.3*	*78.1*	*95.3*
Other cancer													
1955	150.7*	11.5*	201.5*	27.1	42.7	77.9	136.2	221.7	357.9	547.1	760.7	1044.9	1414.0
1965	147.9*	10.7*	198.5*	27.9	44.2	72.8	130.3	221.4	349.9	543.3	762.3	1006.8	1391.0
1975	145.2*	8.4*	184.4*	23.0	38.2	69.0	121.7	202.7	331.8	504.4	779.0	1057.9	1497.8
1985	147.1*	6.9*	183.2*	22.7	38.4	65.8	119.2	204.2	332.4	499.7	759.8	1073.2	1664.8
1990	**149.5***	**6.3***	**183.6***	**20.9**	**34.5**	**63.0**	**117.7**	**202.1**	**333.0**	**513.7**	**772.7**	**1107.5**	**1761.5**
1995 projected	*150.6**	*5.7**	*181.8**	*19.1*	*31.4*	*58.2*	*113.8*	*199.3*	*333.8*	*517.0*	*784.5*	*1120.2*	*1845.7*
Chronic obstructive pulmonary disease (COPD)													
1955	16.6*	2.9*	23.7*	2.0	3.7	6.9	14.3	27.3	46.4	65.6	76.9	92.3	119.1
1965	37.0*	2.2*	52.0*	2.6	5.1	11.6	25.6	52.7	97.6	169.1	220.3	269.1	292.1
1975	47.0*	1.6*	55.4*	2.9	5.1	10.8	23.7	51.8	106.1	187.0	307.0	414.8	488.3
1985	45.9*	0.5*	43.9*	1.2	2.2	6.1	16.8	39.0	82.3	160.0	287.7	444.5	670.2
1990	**44.9***	**0.6***	**42.0***	**1.2**	**2.3**	**6.0**	**13.7**	**37.1**	**80.3**	**153.1**	**271.6**	**438.2**	**688.2**
1995 projected	*43.7**	*0.7**	*39.5**	*1.3*	*2.3*	*5.0*	*12.4*	*34.9*	*76.5*	*144.3*	*259.9*	*423.3*	*695.4*
Other respiratory disease													
1955	40.0*	13.0*	33.2*	7.3	11.3	17.8	24.4	35.8	52.6	83.4	134.1	234.7	590.8
1965	47.6*	11.1*	39.1*	8.0	11.8	17.0	27.1	40.5	60.5	109.0	181.9	311.7	780.5
1975	38.2*	4.8*	29.7*	5.4	9.2	13.3	20.3	31.0	50.4	78.1	150.4	286.8	724.1
1985	46.2*	3.0*	30.9*	5.4	7.4	11.6	17.9	30.4	53.0	90.6	176.8	345.2	1069.5
1990	**45.9***	**2.6***	**30.0***	**6.1**	**8.4**	**10.8**	**16.7**	**27.0**	**52.4**	**88.3**	**172.2**	**339.1**	**1090.7**
1995 projected	*45.2**	*2.4**	*28.7**	*6.8*	*8.4*	*10.0*	*14.9*	*25.4*	*50.1*	*85.3*	*166.7*	*334.1*	*1102.3*
Vascular disease													
1955	773.1*	12.4*	898.5*	87.7	190.0	356.7	638.2	1021.2	1580.5	2415.3	3656.8	5698.8	10868.3
1965	763.4*	10.3*	897.9*	85.2	182.2	343.0	616.1	1004.4	1565.5	2489.1	3660.8	5436.9	10789.1
1975	630.5*	8.2*	710.3*	62.0	141.7	275.4	485.2	793.3	1277.7	1936.8	3124.9	4658.6	9148.9
1985	488.5*	7.2*	518.6*	45.2	98.8	192.8	351.9	581.3	926.6	1433.6	2316.1	3624.0	7808.4
1990	**411.7***	**6.4***	**429.2***	**38.1**	**80.0**	**158.4**	**277.9**	**476.3**	**770.6**	**1203.5**	**1922.4**	**3058.7**	**6776.6**
1995 projected	*343.6**	*5.7**	*350.5**	*31.7*	*63.9*	*121.8*	*221.4*	*387.0*	*635.9*	*992.1*	*1595.3*	*2545.2*	*5829.9*
Liver cirrhosis													
1955	16.7*	0.7*	32.2*	8.5	17.5	27.2	35.3	39.1	44.0	54.0	50.4	51.8	46.4
1965	21.1*	1.3*	42.5*	13.4	23.1	34.3	49.0	56.4	59.7	61.7	51.8	47.6	37.9
1975	24.7*	1.7*	50.2*	16.6	29.0	43.7	54.7	63.6	73.9	69.9	61.0	49.3	33.0
1985	17.7*	1.2*	34.6*	11.0	18.1	26.5	36.0	44.6	52.5	53.6	51.1	46.3	38.4
1990	**16.0***	**0.8***	**30.9***	**11.5**	**17.4**	**24.2**	**29.5**	**39.2**	**46.5**	**48.0**	**48.1**	**46.7**	**43.7**
1995 projected	*14.4**	*0.7**	*27.2**	*10.7*	*16.2*	*20.5*	*25.2*	*33.6*	*40.8*	*43.1*	*45.0*	*46.4*	*46.6*
Other medical causes													
1955	205.7*	106.4*	204.7*	54.2	79.7	114.8	167.9	233.4	319.9	462.8	647.6	911.8	1613.1
1965	174.2*	82.5*	179.8*	45.6	63.9	96.3	136.3	200.4	285.1	430.8	589.5	811.7	1387.9
1975	140.5*	63.1*	139.9*	40.3	54.4	76.0	107.0	153.2	227.3	320.9	489.3	693.8	1244.6
1985	143.3*	48.8*	131.0*	50.3	57.1	70.5	95.2	137.8	203.6	302.3	493.1	816.1	1810.5
1990	**155.6***	**54.2***	**150.4***	**96.6**	**97.5**	**99.4**	**113.7**	**142.7**	**201.9**	**301.1**	**476.7**	**804.6**	**1861.8**
1995 projected	*166.9**	*60.0**	*168.0**	*136.7*	*134.2*	*133.0*	*131.1*	*148.5*	*200.6*	*292.1*	*463.2*	*783.8*	*1890.0*
All non-medical causes													
1955	116.3*	79.1*	129.9*	97.2	107.7	114.0	130.2	135.1	154.1	170.9	206.9	287.4	551.8
1965	115.9*	83.5*	130.1*	110.9	111.4	116.2	130.8	140.2	144.4	156.9	185.8	244.7	465.5
1975	111.3*	90.0*	119.4*	117.0	114.2	115.9	115.9	116.2	123.7	132.8	159.1	205.3	352.3
1985	89.5*	74.1*	90.6*	93.5	89.8	86.6	84.5	92.5	91.8	95.9	126.2	181.5	338.7
1990	**88.1***	**75.6***	**87.3***	**100.4**	**86.6**	**80.9**	**79.9**	**81.0**	**88.6**	**93.8**	**116.8**	**169.2**	**323.5**
1995 projected	*86.3**	*78.0**	*82.5**	*102.8*	*83.7*	*73.5*	*72.0*	*74.5*	*82.5*	*88.4*	*108.7*	*155.6*	*306.4*

UNITED STATES: Females

	All ages	0–34	35–69	35–39	40–44	45–49	50–54	55–59	60–64	65–69	70–74	75–79	80+/NK
POPULATION (1000s)													
1955	83240	46961	31460	5997	5578	5118	4379	3938	3497	2953	2193	1394	1232
1965	98703	55871	36035	6092	6378	5879	5424	4736	4099	3427	2906	2054	1837
1975	110590	62592	39103	5931	5700	6072	6235	5598	5031	4536	3344	2593	2958
1985	122579	65981	44775	8967	7167	5968	5661	5959	5877	5176	4354	3359	4110
1990	**127471**	**65977**	**48465**	**10013**	**8913**	**7004**	**5820**	**5479**	**5679**	**5558**	**4580**	**3714**	**4733**
1995 projected	*132160*	*63762*	*53977*	*11076*	*10260*	*8958*	*7080*	*5806*	*5369*	*5429*	*5041*	*4038*	*5343*
NUMBER OF DEATHS													
All causes													
1955	656079	79365	240725	11332	16354	22148	29425	38725	52176	70565	82683	88907	164399
1965	792936	74105	264511	11335	17802	24851	34036	43432	56569	76486	98867	114653	240800
1975	842060	55996	262043	8698	13558	22195	33830	45262	60360	78140	98160	118500	307361
1985	988682	47889	260888	9878	12443	17073	26241	42969	65800	86484	113145	137500	429260
1990	**1035046**	**47660**	**257081**	**11492**	**14608**	**18759**	**25195**	**37338**	**60712**	**88977**	**112905**	**143241**	**474159**
1995 projected	*1076640*	*44528*	*255217*	*12741*	*16127*	*22467*	*28804*	*37490*	*54788*	*82800*	*117703*	*144837*	*514355*
Lung cancer													
1955	4123	92	2577	102	171	267	357	459	568	653	577	471	406
1965	7604	83	5073	165	387	671	880	976	977	1017	980	725	743
1975	18627	89	12737	215	599	1276	2012	2732	3061	2842	2216	1614	1971
1985	38702	137	22720	257	643	1402	2658	4456	6369	6935	6562	4635	4648
1990	**50194**	**122**	**26173**	**296**	**692**	**1606**	**2823**	**4514**	**7207**	**9035**	**8973**	**7459**	**7467**
1995 projected	*66185*	*109*	*30567*	*289*	*749*	*2033*	*3613*	*5316*	*7881*	*10686*	*12723*	*10867*	*11919*
ANNUAL DEATH RATE / 100,000 (*The rates for the age groups 0–34 and 35–69 are the means of seven five-yearly rates, but the all-ages rates are standardised to the conventional "European" age distribution)													
All causes													
1955	924.6*	144.8*	921.7*	189.0	293.2	432.7	672.0	983.4	1492.0	2389.6	3770.3	6377.8	13344.1
1965	860.6*	123.9*	863.5*	186.1	279.1	422.7	627.5	917.1	1380.1	2231.9	3402.2	5581.9	13108.3
1975	705.3*	95.6*	717.7*	146.7	237.9	365.5	542.6	808.5	1199.8	1722.7	2935.4	4570.0	10390.8
1985	645.0*	72.7*	649.3*	110.2	173.6	286.1	463.5	721.1	1119.6	1670.9	2598.6	4093.5	10444.3
1990	**615.3***	**71.0***	**618.7***	**114.8**	**163.9**	**267.8**	**432.9**	**681.5**	**1069.1**	**1600.8**	**2465.0**	**3856.8**	**10017.3**
1995 projected	*586.3**	*69.6**	*588.8**	*115.0*	*157.2*	*250.8*	*406.8*	*645.8*	*1020.4*	*1525.3*	*2335.1*	*3586.9*	*9627.1*
All cancer													
1955	163.1*	11.0*	250.8*	55.0	98.7	152.4	223.3	305.6	398.2	522.7	670.6	898.1	1164.3
1965	154.3*	10.4*	241.3*	47.8	88.6	144.7	219.3	296.3	381.4	511.1	638.4	793.8	1090.9
1975	151.3*	7.7*	237.1*	39.7	77.9	139.3	212.1	304.6	402.7	483.5	665.4	794.2	1053.4
1985	159.9*	6.4*	251.8*	35.0	66.8	124.2	206.0	311.7	447.5	571.1	731.9	868.1	1162.7
1990	**163.1***	**6.0***	**252.0***	**33.8**	**64.1**	**118.3**	**200.3**	**304.3**	**443.7**	**599.7**	**771.7**	**940.2**	**1232.2**
1995 projected	*166.2**	*5.6**	*251.7**	*31.7*	*60.7*	*113.4*	*193.4*	*298.3*	*447.7*	*616.8*	*814.6*	*986.8*	*1318.3*
Lung cancer													
1955	5.9*	0.2*	9.7*	1.7	3.1	5.2	8.2	11.7	16.2	22.1	26.3	33.8	33.0
1965	8.8*	0.2*	15.8*	2.7	6.1	11.4	16.2	20.6	23.8	29.7	33.7	35.3	40.4
1975	17.8*	0.2*	34.2*	3.6	10.5	21.0	32.3	48.8	60.8	62.7	66.3	62.2	66.6
1985	30.7*	0.2*	57.1*	2.9	9.0	23.5	47.0	74.8	108.4	134.0	150.7	138.0	113.1
1990	**36.7***	**0.2***	**64.9***	**3.0**	**7.8**	**22.9**	**48.5**	**82.4**	**126.9**	**162.5**	**195.9**	**200.8**	**157.8**
1995 projected	*44.1**	*0.2**	*74.1**	*2.6*	*7.3*	*22.7*	*51.0*	*91.6*	*146.8*	*196.8*	*252.4*	*269.1*	*223.1*
Upper aerodigestive cancer (mouth, oesophagus, pharynx and larynx)													
1955	3.3*	0.1*	4.6*	0.6	1.4	2.8	4.0	5.4	7.7	10.6	14.9	20.0	33.8
1965	3.6*	0.1*	5.9*	0.8	1.6	3.4	6.7	8.1	9.5	11.4	14.2	17.3	27.5
1975	4.4*	0.1*	7.8*	0.5	1.4	4.1	7.4	11.5	14.7	14.7	17.0	18.1	26.8
1985	4.2*	0.1*	7.2*	0.4	1.2	3.0	5.4	9.2	13.9	17.5	18.8	20.1	27.2
1990	**4.2***	**0.0***	**6.7***	**0.4**	**0.8**	**1.8**	**4.9**	**8.7**	**13.6**	**16.9**	**21.1**	**24.2**	**29.5**
1995 projected	*4.2**	*0.0**	*6.4**	*0.3*	*0.6*	*1.4*	*4.3*	*8.3*	*13.0*	*17.1*	*22.6*	*26.6*	*33.4*
Other cancer													
1955	153.8*	10.7*	236.5*	52.7	94.2	144.4	211.1	288.6	374.3	490.0	629.4	844.3	1097.5
1965	141.9*	10.1*	219.6*	44.3	81.0	129.8	196.4	267.6	348.1	470.0	590.5	741.2	1022.9
1975	129.1*	7.5*	195.1*	35.5	66.0	114.2	172.5	244.3	327.1	406.1	582.1	713.8	959.9
1985	125.0*	6.1*	187.5*	31.8	56.6	97.7	153.7	227.7	325.2	419.6	562.4	709.9	1022.4
1990	**122.3***	**5.7***	**180.4***	**30.5**	**55.5**	**93.6**	**146.9**	**213.2**	**303.2**	**420.2**	**554.7**	**715.2**	**1045.0**
1995 projected	*118.0**	*5.4**	*171.2**	*28.8*	*52.8*	*89.2*	*138.1*	*198.4*	*288.0*	*402.9*	*539.5*	*691.1*	*1061.8*
Chronic obstructive pulmonary disease (COPD)													
1955	5.4*	2.0*	4.5*	1.4	1.7	2.0	3.4	5.0	6.4	11.5	19.4	29.0	75.0
1965	8.1*	1.7*	9.5*	1.7	3.1	5.2	7.3	10.5	16.1	22.6	29.8	46.7	89.8
1975	12.9*	1.2*	18.1*	2.4	4.3	7.4	12.4	21.6	34.4	44.4	64.7	75.0	106.9
1985	19.2*	0.4*	24.6*	1.0	2.0	5.6	12.9	25.9	46.8	78.0	116.0	154.9	191.9
1990	**22.9***	**0.5***	**27.2***	**1.0**	**2.1**	**5.0**	**13.3**	**27.2**	**52.9**	**88.7**	**140.9**	**198.3**	**259.7**
1995 projected	*27.4**	*0.5**	*30.2**	*1.0*	*1.9*	*5.0*	*13.5*	*29.5*	*58.4*	*102.1*	*168.3*	*246.8*	*343.0*
Other respiratory disease													
1955	27.3*	10.8*	16.4*	4.9	6.1	8.1	11.9	15.7	24.4	43.7	77.7	156.0	493.6
1965	29.1*	8.9*	18.1*	5.8	7.7	9.4	12.7	17.4	28.1	45.8	84.7	165.9	581.1
1975	20.8*	3.9*	13.5*	4.0	5.2	6.9	8.8	14.7	22.4	32.2	67.7	128.2	451.0
1985	26.3*	2.2*	15.1*	2.8	4.6	6.3	10.2	15.3	25.3	41.5	81.9	164.1	692.3
1990	**28.3***	**2.1***	**15.7***	**3.4**	**4.2**	**6.5**	**9.4**	**15.6**	**26.6**	**44.3**	**85.9**	**175.4**	**770.9**
1995 projected	*30.1**	*2.0**	*16.0**	*3.4*	*4.3*	*6.1*	*9.3*	*15.7*	*27.6*	*45.7*	*88.8*	*180.6*	*851.8*
Vascular disease													
1955	528.2*	9.6*	460.0*	45.2	85.7	148.5	276.5	457.0	789.2	1418.2	2448.9	4460.4	9911.2
1965	485.0*	8.2*	404.2*	42.9	73.5	130.5	224.3	386.3	690.3	1281.6	2148.6	3848.6	9880.7
1975	368.5*	5.8*	291.4*	29.1	56.0	95.7	171.0	294.4	515.9	877.9	1704.2	2963.2	7600.9
1985	296.8*	4.6*	225.0*	18.1	37.8	69.1	129.1	226.1	399.1	695.7	1240.0	2220.5	6687.8
1990	**255.6***	**4.3***	**192.2***	**16.1**	**30.0**	**60.6**	**109.4**	**196.4**	**346.2**	**586.4**	**1037.6**	**1856.0**	**5875.6**
1995 projected	*216.3**	*3.9**	*161.3**	*13.4*	*25.3*	*50.9*	*93.8*	*168.4*	*291.9*	*485.3*	*846.0*	*1500.8*	*5099.4*
Liver cirrhosis													
1955	8.0*	0.8*	14.3*	6.3	10.2	13.4	16.5	15.9	17.4	20.1	23.0	23.2	28.7
1965	10.3*	1.1*	20.0*	9.4	14.1	21.3	24.5	25.4	21.7	23.2	21.1	19.4	16.8
1975	11.1*	0.9*	22.4*	7.6	14.6	21.6	25.8	30.0	31.3	25.7	23.1	18.1	15.2
1985	8.0*	0.6*	15.1*	4.6	6.9	11.2	15.7	19.6	21.8	26.2	25.2	25.2	20.8
1990	**7.1***	**0.5***	**13.0***	**4.4**	**5.9**	**8.4**	**11.3**	**16.6**	**19.9**	**24.1**	**25.2**	**26.9**	**22.5**
1995 projected	*6.2**	*0.4**	*11.1**	*3.7*	*4.9*	*6.3*	*8.8*	*13.8*	*17.6*	*22.3*	*24.3*	*27.2*	*24.2*
Other medical causes													
1955	146.9*	87.5*	136.3*	50.8	61.2	76.3	103.0	142.3	209.1	311.3	432.8	621.1	1109.8
1965	128.3*	67.4*	124.8*	42.9	53.9	69.5	95.6	134.8	191.9	285.0	394.6	567.9	1056.3
1975	101.1*	48.5*	93.7*	28.8	38.7	54.1	72.1	102.8	149.8	209.9	343.4	495.0	946.0
1985	103.9*	35.5*	86.8*	21.9	27.2	40.8	60.6	92.7	145.4	218.8	347.6	584.3	1519.5
1990	**108.4***	**35.0***	**89.5***	**28.4**	**32.1**	**42.8**	**62.3**	**91.8**	**148.4**	**220.8**	**355.7**	**585.3**	**1687.6**
1995 projected	*111.5**	*34.9**	*91.3**	*34.7*	*36.4*	*45.3*	*62.8*	*92.2*	*147.6*	*220.4*	*349.6*	*577.0*	*1823.1*
All non-medical causes													
1955	45.7*	23.1*	39.4*	25.3	29.4	32.1	37.4	41.9	47.4	62.1	97.9	190.0	561.4
1965	45.4*	26.2*	45.6*	35.6	38.3	42.2	43.7	46.3	50.6	62.6	84.9	139.6	392.7
1975	39.7*	27.6*	41.4*	34.9	41.1	40.6	40.4	40.6	43.2	49.1	66.9	96.2	217.3
1985	31.0*	23.0*	30.9*	26.8	28.2	28.9	29.1	29.8	33.8	39.5	56.0	76.4	169.3
1990	**29.9***	**22.7***	**29.2***	**27.6**	**25.5**	**26.3**	**27.0**	**29.6**	**31.4**	**36.9**	**48.0**	**74.8**	**168.7**
1995 projected	*28.5**	*22.3**	*27.1**	*27.1*	*23.8*	*23.8*	*25.3*	*27.9*	*29.5*	*32.6*	*43.4*	*67.6*	*167.1*

UNITED STATES: 1975

Smoking-attributed deaths (Sm.) and total deaths (Total)

		ALL CAUSES	ALL CANCER	Lung cancer	Upper aero-digestive ca.	Other cancer	COPD	Other respiratory	Vascular disease	Liver cirrhosis	Other medical	Non-medical
Males												
0-34	Sm.	–	–	–	–	–	–	–	–	–	–	–
	Total	108653	5399	190	74	5135	936	2832	4716	902	37000	56868
35-69	Sm.	156800	54456	38191	6138	10127	13035	3043	71117	–	15149	–
	Total	457216	106997	40836	8984	57177	16396	9303	220305	17105	44938	42172
		(34%)	(51%)	(94%)	(68%)	(18%)	(80%)	(33%)	(32%)		(34%)	
70+	Sm.	83592	29392	20081	2566	6745	15432	1994	32047	–	4727	–
	Total	484950	87047	22387	4566	60094	22041	19818	297381	2823	43015	12825
		(17%)	(34%)	(90%)	(56%)	(11%)	(70%)	(10%)	(11%)		(11%)	
Any age	Sm.	240392	83848	58272	8704	16872	28467	5037	103164	–	19876	–
	Total	1050819	199443	63413	13624	122406	39373	31953	522402	20830	124953	111865
		(23%)	(42%)	(92%)	(64%)	(14%)	(72%)	(16%)	(20%)		(16%)	
Females												
0-34	Sm.	–	–	–	–	–	–	–	–	–	–	–
	Total	55996	4532	89	43	4400	702	2260	3363	482	27485	17172
35-69	Sm.	40067	12516	9449	1240	1827	3997	845	16687	–	6022	–
	Total	262043	87715	12737	2871	72107	6568	4920	103648	8618	34506	16068
		(15%)	(14%)	(74%)	(43%)	(3%)	(61%)	(17%)	(16%)		(17%)	
70+	Sm.	15761	3781	2869	364	548	2548	377	7780	–	1275	–
	Total	524021	74003	5801	1831	66371	7274	18932	358660	1693	52301	11158
		(3%)	(5%)	(49%)	(20%)	(1%)	(35%)	(2%)	(2%)		(2%)	
Any age	Sm.	55828	16297	12318	1604	2375	6545	1222	24467	–	7297	–
	Total	842060	166250	18627	4745	142878	14544	26112	465671	10793	114292	44398
		(7%)	(10%)	(66%)	(34%)	(2%)	(45%)	(5%)	(5%)		(6%)	
Males+Females												
0-34	Sm.	–	–	–	–	–	–	–	–	–	–	–
	Total	164649	9931	279	117	9535	1638	5092	8079	1384	64485	74040
35-69	Sm.	196867	66972	47640	7378	11954	17032	3888	87804	–	21171	–
	Total	719259	194712	53573	11855	129284	22964	14223	323953	25723	79444	58240
		(27%)	(34%)	(89%)	(62%)	(9%)	(74%)	(27%)	(27%)		(27%)	
70+	Sm.	99353	33173	22950	2930	7293	17980	2371	39827	–	6002	–
	Total	1008971	161050	28188	6397	126465	29315	38750	656041	4516	95316	23983
		(10%)	(21%)	(81%)	(46%)	(6%)	(61%)	(6%)	(6%)		(6%)	
Any age	Sm.	296220	100145	70590	10308	19247	35012	6259	127631	–	27173	–
	Total	1892879	365693	82040	18369	265284	53917	58065	988073	31623	239245	156263
		(16%)	(27%)	(86%)	(56%)	(7%)	(65%)	(11%)	(13%)		(11%)	

UNITED STATES: 1985

Smoking-attributed deaths (Sm.) and total deaths (Total)

		ALL CAUSES	ALL CANCER	Lung cancer	Upper aero-digestive ca.	Other cancer	COPD	Other respiratory	Vascular disease	Liver cirrhosis	Other medical	Non-medical
Males												
0-34	Sm.	–	–	–	–	–	–	–	–	–	–	–
	Total	98200	5071	169	95	4807	322	2019	5040	885	32407	52456
35-69	Sm.	153739	62926	44725	6423	11778	11750	3519	59028	–	16516	–
	Total	424790	120869	47675	9270	63924	14604	10793	179991	12985	48060	37488
		(36%)	(52%)	(94%)	(69%)	(18%)	(80%)	(33%)	(33%)		(34%)	
70+	Sm.	122996	47230	32956	3385	10889	23618	4125	39260	–	8763	–
	Total	574768	120974	36010	5504	79460	31670	33674	302422	3374	68190	14464
		(21%)	(39%)	(92%)	(62%)	(14%)	(75%)	(12%)	(13%)		(13%)	
Any age	Sm.	276735	110156	77681	9808	22667	35368	7644	98288	–	25279	–
	Total	1097758	246914	83854	14869	148191	46596	46486	487453	17244	148657	104408
		(25%)	(45%)	(93%)	(66%)	(15%)	(76%)	(16%)	(20%)		(17%)	
Females												
0-34	Sm.	–	–	–	–	–	–	–	–	–	–	–
	Total	47889	4406	137	52	4217	294	1429	3137	454	22496	15673
35-69	Sm.	66122	24043	19076	1655	3312	7196	1638	23702	–	9543	–
	Total	260888	101432	22720	2873	75839	9635	6077	88702	6272	35166	13604
		(25%)	(24%)	(84%)	(58%)	(4%)	(75%)	(27%)	(27%)		(27%)	
70+	Sm.	65473	16145	12336	1224	2585	11923	2443	27983	–	6979	–
	Total	679905	108811	15845	2611	90355	18137	37535	403447	2797	97215	11963
		(10%)	(15%)	(78%)	(47%)	(3%)	(66%)	(7%)	(7%)		(7%)	
Any age	Sm.	131595	40188	31412	2879	5897	19119	4081	51685	–	16522	–
	Total	988682	214649	38702	5536	170411	28066	45041	495286	9523	154877	41240
		(13%)	(19%)	(81%)	(52%)	(3%)	(68%)	(9%)	(10%)		(11%)	
Males+Females												
0-34	Sm.	–	–	–	–	–	–	–	–	–	–	–
	Total	146089	9477	306	147	9024	616	3448	8177	1339	54903	68129
35-69	Sm.	219861	86969	63801	8078	15090	18946	5157	82730	–	26059	–
	Total	685678	222301	70395	12143	139763	24239	16870	268693	19257	83226	51092
		(32%)	(39%)	(91%)	(67%)	(11%)	(78%)	(31%)	(31%)		(31%)	
70+	Sm.	188469	63375	45292	4609	13474	35541	6568	67243	–	15742	–
	Total	1254673	229785	51855	8115	169815	49807	71209	705869	6171	165405	26427
		(15%)	(28%)	(87%)	(57%)	(8%)	(71%)	(9%)	(10%)		(10%)	
Any age	Sm.	408330	150344	109093	12687	28564	54487	11725	149973	–	41801	–
	Total	2086440	461563	122556	20405	318602	74662	91527	982739	26767	303534	145648
		(20%)	(33%)	(89%)	(62%)	(9%)	(73%)	(13%)	(15%)		(14%)	

(To be conservative, no deaths before age 35, and none from liver cirrhosis or non-medical causes, were attributed to smoking.)

UNITED STATES: 1990

Smoking–attributed deaths (Sm.) and total deaths (Total)

		ALL CAUSES	ALL CANCER	Lung cancer	Upper aero–digestive ca.	Other cancer	COPD	Other respiratory	Vascular disease	Liver cirrhosis	Other medical	Non–medical
Males												
0–34	Sm.	–	–	–	–	–	–	–	–	–	–	–
	Total	102882	4737	212	90	4435	389	1843	4617	592	37719	52985
35–69	Sm.	150009	63899	45367	6522	12010	11461	3533	49642	–	21474	–
	Total	415118	123325	48371	9444	65510	14206	10900	152846	12324	61622	39895
		(36%)	(52%)	(94%)	(69%)	(18%)	(81%)	(32%)	(32%)		(35%)	
70+	Sm.	136252	56195	39085	3954	13156	26336	4838	38712	–	10171	–
	Total	595417	140221	42508	6292	91421	34821	37916	287300	3711	76329	15119
		(23%)	(40%)	(92%)	(63%)	(14%)	(76%)	(13%)	(13%)		(13%)	
Any age	Sm.	286261	120094	84452	10476	25166	37797	8371	88354	–	31645	–
	Total	1113417	268283	91091	15826	161366	49416	50659	444763	16627	175670	107999
		(26%)	(45%)	(93%)	(66%)	(16%)	(76%)	(17%)	(20%)		(18%)	
Females												
0–34	Sm.	–	–	–	–	–	–	–	–	–	–	–
	Total	47660	4206	122	32	4052	314	1389	2993	371	23039	15348
35–69	Sm.	72730	27830	22451	1657	3722	8409	1947	23188	–	11356	–
	Total	257081	104239	26173	2716	75350	10837	6540	77913	5600	38047	13905
		(28%)	(27%)	(86%)	(61%)	(5%)	(78%)	(30%)	(30%)		(30%)	
70+	Sm.	102136	26305	20096	1870	4339	19490	4504	39705	–	12132	–
	Total	730305	128594	23899	3260	101435	26112	46938	394576	3217	117909	12959
		(14%)	(20%)	(84%)	(57%)	(4%)	(75%)	(10%)	(10%)		(10%)	
Any age	Sm.	174866	54135	42547	3527	8061	27899	6451	62893	–	23488	–
	Total	1035046	237039	50194	6008	180837	37263	54867	475482	9188	178995	42212
		(17%)	(23%)	(85%)	(59%)	(4%)	(75%)	(12%)	(13%)		(13%)	
Males+Females												
0–34	Sm.	–	–	–	–	–	–	–	–	–	–	–
	Total	150542	8943	334	122	8487	703	3232	7610	963	60758	68333
35–69	Sm.	222739	91729	67818	8179	15732	19870	5480	72830	–	32830	–
	Total	672199	227564	74544	12160	140860	25043	17440	230759	17924	99669	53800
		(33%)	(40%)	(91%)	(67%)	(11%)	(79%)	(31%)	(32%)		(33%)	
70+	Sm.	238388	82500	59181	5824	17495	45826	9342	78417	–	22303	–
	Total	1325722	268815	66407	9552	192856	60933	84854	681876	6928	194238	28078
		(18%)	(31%)	(89%)	(61%)	(9%)	(75%)	(11%)	(12%)		(11%)	
Any age	Sm.	461127	174229	126999	14003	33227	65696	14822	151247	–	55133	–
	Total	2148463	505322	141285	21834	342203	86679	105526	920245	25815	354665	150211
		(21%)	(34%)	(90%)	(64%)	(10%)	(76%)	(14%)	(16%)		(16%)	

UNITED STATES: 1995

Smoking–attributed deaths (Sm.) and total deaths (Total)

		ALL CAUSES	ALL CANCER	Lung cancer	Upper aero–digestive ca.	Other cancer	COPD	Other respiratory	Vascular disease	Liver cirrhosis	Other medical	Non–medical
Males												
0–34	Sm.	–	–	–	–	–	–	–	–	–	–	–
	Total	102796	4230	216	92	3922	449	1615	3924	490	40297	51791
35–69	Sm.	149288	65082	46244	6669	12169	10868	3558	42094	–	27686	–
	Total	413859	126084	49336	9715	67033	13462	10949	129549	11877	79180	42758
		(36%)	(52%)	(94%)	(69%)	(18%)	(81%)	(32%)	(32%)		(35%)	
70+	Sm.	153749	67564	46880	4662	16022	29746	5746	38717	–	11976	–
	Total	630700	164677	50785	7285	106607	38854	43355	276961	4127	86648	16078
		(24%)	(41%)	(92%)	(64%)	(15%)	(77%)	(13%)	(14%)		(14%)	
Any age	Sm.	303037	132646	93124	11331	28191	40614	9304	80811	–	39662	–
	Total	1147355	294991	100337	17092	177562	52765	55919	410434	16494	206125	110627
		(26%)	(45%)	(93%)	(66%)	(16%)	(77%)	(17%)	(20%)		(19%)	
Females												
0–34	Sm.	–	–	–	–	–	–	–	–	–	–	–
	Total	44528	3772	109	24	3639	319	1290	2606	299	21936	14306
35–69	Sm.	80173	32617	26719	1690	4208	9705	2263	22111	–	13477	–
	Total	255217	108430	30567	2626	75237	12100	6895	67082	5063	41317	14330
		(31%)	(30%)	(87%)	(64%)	(6%)	(80%)	(33%)	(33%)		(33%)	
70+	Sm.	146088	40373	31232	2608	6533	29557	7336	50092	–	18730	–
	Total	776895	151345	35509	4004	111832	36776	57282	375699	3618	138330	13845
		(19%)	(27%)	(88%)	(65%)	(6%)	(80%)	(13%)	(13%)		(14%)	
Any age	Sm.	226261	72990	57951	4298	10741	39262	9599	72203	–	32207	–
	Total	1076640	263547	66185	6654	190708	49195	65467	445387	8980	201583	42481
		(21%)	(28%)	(88%)	(65%)	(6%)	(80%)	(15%)	(16%)		(16%)	
Males+Females												
0–34	Sm.	–	–	–	–	–	–	–	–	–	–	–
	Total	147324	8002	325	116	7561	768	2905	6530	789	62233	66097
35–69	Sm.	229461	97699	72963	8359	16377	20573	5821	64205	–	41163	–
	Total	669076	234514	79903	12341	142270	25562	17844	196631	16940	120497	57088
		(34%)	(42%)	(91%)	(68%)	(12%)	(80%)	(33%)	(33%)		(34%)	
70+	Sm.	299837	107937	78112	7270	22555	59303	13082	88809	–	30706	–
	Total	1407595	316022	86294	11289	218439	75630	100637	652660	7745	224978	29923
		(21%)	(34%)	(91%)	(64%)	(10%)	(78%)	(13%)	(14%)		(14%)	
Any age	Sm.	529298	205636	151075	15629	38932	79876	18903	153014	–	71869	–
	Total	2223995	558538	166522	23746	368270	101960	121386	855821	25474	407708	153108
		(24%)	(37%)	(91%)	(66%)	(11%)	(78%)	(16%)	(18%)		(18%)	

(To be conservative, no deaths before age 35, and none from liver cirrhosis or non–medical causes, were attributed to smoking.)

¶Former USSR: 1990

		No. of deaths			Standardised rates (Defined on p.538)			Annual death rates / 100, 000						
		All ages	0–34	35–69	All ages	0–34	35–69	0–4	5–9	10–14	15–19	20–24	25–29	30–34
ALL CAUSES	M	1462389	214760	787317	1592.7	252.6	1984.1	617.7	69.0	58.8	134.3	225.8	282.2	380.7
	F	1522769	105756	444516	873.1	124.2	822.6	479.1	40.1	30.9	59.8	72.8	78.5	107.9
Tuberculosis	M	18569	2542	14546	17.0	3.1	31.3	0.5	0.1	0.1	0.4	2.3	6.1	12.1
	F	3979	754	2284	2.6	0.9	4.0	0.5	0.1	0.1	0.4	1.4	1.9	2.2
Other infective	M	13716	11822	1622	9.0	12.8	3.6	79.7	2.4	1.6	1.7	1.5	1.4	1.5
and parasitic	F	11725	9821	1342	7.4	11.1	2.4	67.7	1.7	1.1	1.2	2.3	1.9	1.6
ALL CANCER	M	267064	8983	195257	288.5	10.9	508.0	8.7	7.6	5.8	8.7	10.5	13.4	21.5
	F	213257	7888	123418	134.4	9.7	224.4	7.1	5.4	4.7	6.2	7.8	12.6	24.0
Mouth and	M	10712	181	9047	10.9	0.2	21.9	0.1	0.1	0.1	0.2	0.3	0.3	0.5
pharynx cancer	F	2325	99	1160	1.4	0.1	2.1	0.1	0.0	0.0	0.1	0.2	0.2	0.3
Oesophagus cancer	M	11496	47	8798	12.5	0.1	22.8	0.0	0.0	–	0.0	0.1	0.0	0.2
	F	5502	43	2554	3.3	0.1	4.7	0.0	0.0	–	0.0	0.0	0.1	0.2
Stomach cancer	M	48133	639	34999	52.9	0.8	91.0	0.0	0.0	0.0	0.2	0.7	1.2	3.3
	F	37548	629	19484	23.0	0.8	35.8	0.0	–	0.1	0.2	0.6	1.4	3.1
Colorectal cancer	M	20126	440	12608	23.4	0.5	34.7	0.3	0.0	0.1	0.2	0.4	1.0	1.7
	F	26932	322	13864	16.4	0.4	25.6	0.2	0.0	0.0	0.1	0.2	0.6	1.6
Liver cancer	M	...	...	...	...	...	...	...	...	...	...	...	...	...
	F	...	...	...	...	...	...	...	...	...	...	...	...	...
Pancreas cancer	M	...	...	...	...	...	...	...	...	...	...	...	...	...
	F	...	...	...	...	...	...	...	...	...	...	...	...	...
Larynx cancer	M	9694	40	8202	10.0	0.0	20.3	0.0	–	0.0	0.0	0.0	0.1	0.2
	F	584	10	354	0.4	0.0	0.7	0.0	–	–	0.0	0.0	0.0	0.0
Lung cancer	M	86345	474	68955	92.2	0.6	180.3	0.1	0.0	0.1	0.2	0.5	0.8	2.4
	F	16690	230	9402	10.3	0.3	17.4	0.1	0.0	0.0	0.2	0.3	0.5	0.9
Malignant melanoma	M	...	...	...	...	...	...	...	...	...	...	...	...	...
	F	...	...	...	...	...	...	...	...	...	...	...	...	...
Female breast cancer	F	28270	705	20517	19.0	0.9	36.3	0.0	0.0	0.0	0.0	0.2	1.2	4.5
Cervix cancer	F	11158	364	6936	7.2	0.4	12.5	–	–	–	0.0	0.2	0.6	2.3
Other uterine cancer	F	10156	166	6299	6.4	0.2	11.5	0.0	0.0	0.0	0.1	0.2	0.4	0.7
Ovarian cancer	F	...	...	...	...	...	...	...	...	...	...	...	...	...
Prostate cancer	M	8037	39	3628	10.4	0.0	11.2	0.0	–	–	0.0	0.1	0.1	0.2
Bladder cancer	M	...	...	...	...	...	...	...	...	...	...	...	...	...
	F	...	...	...	...	...	...	...	...	...	...	...	...	...
Other and ill-defined	M	58591	3678	40820	62.9	4.5	105.3	4.0	2.8	2.2	3.4	4.5	5.7	8.6
cancer sites	F	62276	2941	36379	39.3	3.6	66.0	3.4	2.2	2.1	2.8	3.0	4.7	7.2
Hodgkin's disease	M	...	...	...	...	...	...	...	...	...	...	...	...	...
	F	...	...	...	...	...	...	...	...	...	...	...	...	...
Myeloma and all	M	6861	1445	4375	6.6	1.8	10.7	1.2	1.5	1.2	1.8	2.1	2.3	2.4
lymphomas	F	5240	870	2985	3.4	1.1	5.4	0.9	0.7	0.6	1.0	1.6	1.3	1.5
Leukaemia	M	7069	2000	3825	6.7	2.4	9.7	2.9	3.2	2.2	2.5	1.9	2.0	2.2
	F	6576	1509	3484	4.2	1.8	6.3	2.4	2.4	1.8	1.7	1.4	1.5	1.9
ALL VASCULAR	M	634580	10805	323956	788.2	13.2	871.6	4.2	1.1	1.4	6.0	10.5	20.8	48.4
DISEASE	F	944105	4615	211120	519.3	5.7	401.3	3.6	1.0	1.2	4.1	6.8	9.1	14.3
Rheumatic heart	M	8390	1017	6875	7.7	1.3	15.2	0.2	0.1	0.3	0.9	1.3	2.5	3.4
disease and fever	F	12430	894	9936	8.5	1.1	17.5	0.1	0.2	0.3	1.0	1.3	2.0	2.9
Hypertensive disease	M	9284	225	6460	10.3	0.3	16.3	0.1	0.0	0.1	0.1	0.2	0.4	1.0
	F	13215	112	6292	8.0	0.1	11.5	0.1	0.0	0.0	0.1	0.2	0.2	0.4
Ischaemic heart	M	364444	4491	195192	448.4	5.5	518.8	0.0	0.0	0.1	1.0	2.7	7.8	26.7
disease	F	460417	925	96285	251.6	1.1	185.0	0.1	0.0	0.1	0.5	1.2	1.9	4.2
Pulmonary embolism	M	...	...	...	...	...	...	...	...	...	...	...	...	...
and other venous	F	...	...	...	...	...	...	...	...	...	...	...	...	...
Cerebrovascular	M	189312	2026	87470	242.7	2.5	248.1	0.8	0.2	0.3	1.4	2.5	4.2	8.0
disease	F	354039	1153	81992	195.1	1.4	156.1	0.7	0.3	0.3	1.0	2.0	2.4	3.5
Other vascular	M	63150	3046	27959	79.0	3.7	73.2	3.1	0.6	0.6	2.6	3.8	6.0	9.3
disease, incl. venous	F	104004	1531	16615	56.1	1.9	31.2	2.7	0.4	0.5	1.5	2.1	2.6	3.4
Chronic obstructive	M	81278	1636	42530	100.3	1.9	120.4	3.6	0.5	0.5	1.3	1.7	2.1	3.9
pulmonary disease	F	57406	1242	16316	32.4	1.5	30.7	2.8	0.4	0.4	0.9	1.6	2.0	2.4
Other respiratory	M	35275	25579	7309	25.8	27.6	17.1	176.6	4.4	2.1	2.3	2.3	2.1	3.3
disease	F	26628	20476	2776	16.4	22.9	5.0	147.9	4.0	2.1	1.8	1.6	1.6	1.3
Peptic ulcer	M	7365	332	5370	7.8	0.4	13.4	0.0	0.0	0.0	0.2	0.4	0.7	1.5
	F	3157	79	1463	1.9	0.1	2.7	0.0	0.0	0.0	0.1	0.1	0.2	0.3
Liver cirrhosis and	M	21819	1239	16693	22.5	1.5	41.2	1.4	0.5	0.7	1.0	1.2	1.8	3.9
other liver disease	F	17446	813	10668	11.1	1.0	19.3	1.0	0.4	0.5	0.8	1.3	1.2	2.0
Renal disease	M	11079	1763	6784	11.3	2.2	16.3	1.4	0.7	0.7	1.5	3.2	3.5	4.2
	F	12272	1402	7485	7.9	1.8	13.4	1.2	0.5	0.7	1.5	2.4	2.5	3.5
Pregnancy and birth	F	1973	1399	574	1.3	1.8	0.8	–	–	–	1.3	4.0	3.2	4.1
Congenital and	M	33662	33122	506	20.3	35.5	1.0	238.3	3.1	1.9	1.8	1.4	1.2	1.0
perinatal causes	F	23472	22883	539	14.6	25.5	0.9	169.6	2.8	1.7	1.5	1.4	0.8	0.9
Ill-defined causes	M	37083	4017	8640	49.9	4.7	19.2	13.3	0.7	0.7	2.0	3.7	5.1	7.2
	F	76641	2236	3340	39.5	2.6	6.1	11.0	0.6	0.4	1.2	1.6	1.6	1.9
Other medical causes	M	51259	11162	28493	51.3	13.2	69.1	28.9	8.0	6.7	9.3	10.1	11.5	17.7
	F	54375	8376	26401	34.0	10.2	47.8	21.9	6.4	5.3	7.4	9.2	9.3	11.6
ALL NON-	M	249640	101758	135611	200.8	125.7	271.9	61.2	40.2	36.5	98.1	177.1	212.4	254.4
MEDICAL CAUSES	F	76333	23772	36790	50.2	29.3	63.7	44.8	16.8	12.5	31.6	31.3	30.5	37.7
Motor vehicle	M	51564	26899	22510	39.6	33.7	45.0	7.0	12.5	9.8	31.5	58.3	58.0	58.6
traffic accidents	F	14528	5799	6146	9.5	7.3	10.6	5.1	6.3	4.3	10.7	9.1	7.3	8.4
Fire	M	5110	2117	2540	4.3	2.5	5.4	5.7	1.2	0.9	1.2	2.1	2.5	3.7
	F	3169	1203	1001	2.0	1.4	1.8	4.4	1.3	0.6	0.8	0.9	1.0	0.9
Suicide	M	46902	15282	28179	39.7	19.1	57.7	–	0.2	3.8	17.0	26.1	38.0	48.7
	F	13886	2846	7722	9.2	3.7	13.5	–	0.0	0.9	6.0	6.4	5.6	6.8
Homicide	M	24165	11757	11702	18.4	14.7	22.0	0.9	0.5	1.1	10.2	25.0	30.5	35.0
	F	7901	2623	4283	5.4	3.3	7.2	1.1	0.7	0.8	2.9	4.3	6.1	7.2
POPULATION (thousands):	**M=males**				135682	82526	48629	13392	12645	11552	11008	10155	11884	11890
	F=females				151759	80570	58581	12879	12253	11233	10602	9893	11799	11912

Former USSR: 1990

Annual death rates / 100, 000

9th ICD categories

35–39	40–44	45–49	50–54	55–59	60–64	65–69	70–74	75–79	80+/NK			
506.1	750.3	1011.4	1531.1	2174.7	3275.8	4639.3	6403.6	9291.0	16950.8	M	ALL CAUSES	001–999
155.8	248.7	351.2	550.4	842.4	1347.6	2261.8	3629.8	6034.8	13904.7	F		
19.3	25.0	30.3	35.1	36.0	37.1	36.1	34.9	29.6	33.7	M	Tuberculosis	010–018, 137
3.2	2.7	3.0	3.9	4.4	4.7	5.8	7.3	7.0	8.1	F		
2.0	2.6	2.7	3.5	4.1	5.0	5.6	4.5	6.1	8.2	M	Other infective	Rest of 001–139
1.1	1.7	2.0	1.9	2.6	3.4	4.0	3.7	4.3	5.5	F	and parasitic	
42.8	101.1	201.7	389.6	633.3	959.6	1227.6	1400.2	1470.4	1255.8	M	ALL CANCER	140–208
44.5	82.4	119.2	184.5	252.6	371.9	515.6	618.3	690.1	638.0	F		
2.3	7.5	14.6	23.2	28.7	36.8	40.0	34.4	32.9	30.3	M	Mouth and	140–149
0.4	0.8	1.1	1.4	2.4	3.5	5.3	5.7	8.3	11.6	F	pharynx cancer	
0.6	3.5	10.2	19.0	30.2	43.2	52.8	55.4	58.7	63.0	M	Oesophagus cancer	150
0.2	0.6	1.7	3.0	5.4	9.1	13.1	17.8	22.9	28.8	F		
8.3	19.7	35.6	69.0	114.0	170.2	220.2	268.0	303.4	250.2	M	Stomach cancer	151
6.3	11.3	15.5	24.9	37.0	62.2	93.7	127.1	154.6	131.7	F		
2.7	5.8	10.4	21.3	36.1	64.8	102.0	138.9	172.8	159.5	M	Colorectal cancer	153, 154
3.1	6.2	10.0	18.5	28.0	44.5	68.7	87.9	109.0	106.1	F		
...	...	...	...	...	...	...	...	...	...	M	Liver cancer	Not given separately
...	...	...	...	...	...	...	...	...	...	F		
...	...	...	...	...	...	...	...	...	...	M	Pancreas cancer	Not given separately
...	...	...	...	...	...	...	...	...	...	F		
1.4	5.2	10.5	19.7	28.4	37.3	39.5	38.2	30.6	25.1	M	Larynx cancer	161
0.1	0.2	0.3	0.5	0.9	1.0	1.6	1.9	1.4	1.9	F		
7.3	24.0	62.8	136.8	238.8	361.9	430.8	442.6	391.8	246.7	M	Lung cancer	162
1.8	3.7	6.6	11.5	19.5	31.6	47.1	57.7	61.0	48.5	F		
...	...	...	...	...	...	...	...	...	...	M	Malignant melanoma	Not given
...	...	...	...	...	...	...	...	...	...	F		separately
10.7	22.1	30.7	41.3	42.6	50.5	56.2	55.6	54.6	57.6	F	Female breast cancer	174
4.0	6.6	7.9	10.4	13.1	18.6	27.1	32.1	32.9	26.4	F	Cervix cancer	180
1.6	3.3	5.4	9.0	14.1	20.1	27.0	30.0	31.2	26.3	F	Other uterine cancer	179, 182
...	...	...	...	...	...	...	...	...	...	F	Ovarian cancer	Not given separately
0.2	0.3	1.2	3.3	9.2	21.8	42.5	70.2	105.4	123.4	M	Prostate cancer	185
...	...	...	...	...	...	...	...	...	...	M	Bladder cancer	Not given separately
...	...	...	...	...	...	...	...	...	...	F		
14.7	27.3	47.0	80.3	124.3	189.7	253.7	296.9	324.2	315.0	M	Other and ill-defined	Rest of 140–208,
12.2	22.5	33.4	54.7	77.3	112.5	149.7	175.7	188.8	181.2	F	cancer sites	incl. 155, 157, 172, 183, 188
...	...	...	...	...	...	...	...	...	...	M	Hodgkin's disease	Not given separately
...	...	...	...	...	...	...	...	...	...	F		
2.8	4.5	5.1	9.5	12.4	18.3	22.5	27.2	21.7	18.6	M	Myeloma and all	200–203,
1.9	2.2	2.7	4.4	6.0	8.2	12.4	12.5	11.4	9.0	F	lymphomas	incl. 201
2.5	3.3	4.3	7.4	11.3	15.7	23.7	28.4	28.9	24.1	M	Leukaemia	204–208
2.3	2.9	4.0	4.8	6.2	10.1	13.7	14.4	14.0	9.0	F		
104.5	215.5	339.4	575.3	896.8	1535.3	2434.1	3762.0	5981.0	11743.3	M	ALL VASCULAR	390–459
25.8	56.8	101.9	196.1	372.7	699.8	1356.2	2471.9	4455.6	10746.3	F	DISEASE	
6.2	9.3	13.2	18.0	22.0	18.9	18.6	14.6	8.9	8.6	M	Rheumatic heart	390–398
4.8	7.4	13.3	20.8	25.6	25.3	25.3	16.1	12.6	9.2	F	disease and fever	
2.2	4.9	7.8	13.3	21.1	29.1	35.7	41.2	53.0	87.4	M	Hypertensive disease	401–405
1.0	2.6	4.8	9.5	14.9	19.7	28.3	39.2	46.4	78.2	F		
63.8	138.6	217.5	365.7	544.8	900.7	1400.9	2090.2	3261.7	6454.1	M	Ischaemic heart	410–414
7.7	19.4	35.2	72.4	158.7	328.5	673.3	1241.7	2218.6	5352.8	F	disease	
...	...	...	...	...	...	...	...	...	...	M	Pulmonary embolism	Not given
...	...	...	...	...	...	...	...	...	...	F	and other venous	separately
16.2	36.6	65.6	127.7	239.1	467.8	783.5	1274.4	2042.9	3806.0	M	Cerebrovascular	430–438
7.2	18.3	36.5	74.6	146.1	276.9	533.0	961.9	1716.7	3884.7	F	disease	
16.1	26.0	35.3	50.6	69.8	118.8	195.4	341.6	614.5	1387.2	M	Other vascular	Rest of 390–459,
5.2	9.0	12.1	18.8	27.4	49.4	96.4	212.9	461.3	1421.5	F	disease, incl. venous	incl. 415, 451–3
6.2	13.1	28.9	62.1	131.4	227.2	373.9	538.1	804.6	1257.8	M	Chronic obstructive	490–496
3.4	5.6	9.1	17.0	31.4	51.5	97.2	159.1	267.4	536.2	F	pulmonary disease	
5.3	9.2	14.2	17.0	20.0	24.9	29.4	36.1	49.0	82.6	M	Other respiratory	Rest of 460–519
1.8	2.2	3.1	3.9	5.9	7.6	10.6	16.9	21.7	42.9	F	disease	
3.0	5.0	7.5	11.2	15.2	22.2	29.6	31.9	39.7	39.8	M	Peptic ulcer	531–533
0.3	0.8	1.2	2.0	2.8	4.2	7.7	9.7	13.1	15.7	F		
7.6	16.7	25.3	36.3	47.5	69.0	86.3	86.0	83.1	89.5	M	Liver cirrhosis and	570–573, 576,
3.8	6.3	10.3	16.6	25.3	31.3	41.5	42.3	46.9	53.0	F	other liver disease	575.2–579.9
5.7	8.0	10.1	14.7	18.4	24.7	32.6	42.2	56.8	75.1	M	Renal disease	580–590
4.4	6.2	8.3	11.5	15.6	21.0	27.0	26.7	27.6	26.1	F		
3.8	1.8	0.1	0.0	0.1	0.0	0.0	–	–	–	F	Pregnancy and birth	630–676
0.9	1.3	0.8	1.3	1.3	0.8	1.0	0.6	0.6	1.1	M	Congenital and	740–779
1.0	1.0	1.0	1.0	1.0	0.7	0.7	0.3	0.5	0.4	F	perinatal causes	
10.0	14.2	16.8	20.8	21.5	23.7	27.5	78.3	280.9	1578.7	M	Ill-defined causes	780–799
2.3	3.4	3.7	5.0	6.0	8.0	14.1	56.9	228.8	1474.8	F		
24.7	35.9	44.4	57.0	73.9	103.2	144.5	181.9	262.3	358.3	M	Other medical causes	Rest of 001–799
14.7	20.6	26.7	37.8	53.9	74.3	106.7	128.0	157.4	182.0	F		
274.1	302.9	289.5	307.1	275.4	243.2	211.0	206.8	226.9	427.1	M	ALL NON-	E800–E999
45.7	57.2	61.7	69.0	68.3	69.2	74.7	88.5	114.4	175.7	F	MEDICAL CAUSES	
52.9	51.3	43.3	46.0	43.7	38.1	39.5	36.4	43.5	69.9	M	Motor vehicle	E810–E819
8.6	9.3	9.2	11.1	11.0	11.5	13.6	17.8	21.4	22.2	F	traffic accidents	
4.1	5.0	5.4	5.7	5.4	5.9	5.9	6.5	9.1	16.4	M	Fire	E890–E899
1.2	1.4	1.5	1.3	2.1	2.0	3.0	4.2	7.1	11.9	F		
53.2	59.7	61.4	62.3	58.5	56.7	51.8	64.6	70.6	100.4	M	Suicide	E950–E959
8.0	10.3	12.2	14.5	13.6	17.0	18.6	21.8	25.2	32.3	F		
33.7	32.7	23.7	21.2	17.0	14.8	11.1	11.3	10.2	29.3	M	Homicide	E960–E969
8.8	10.0	7.6	7.1	5.9	5.8	5.3	6.6	6.8	10.5	F		
10490	7823	6067	8694	6299	6260	2996	1738	1616	1174	M	POPULATION (thousands)	
10700	8181	6673	9967	7730	9042	6289	4169	4476	3963	F		

Former USSR: Males

	All ages	0–34	35–69	35–39	40–44	45–49	50–54	55–59	60–64	65–69	70–74	75–79	80+/NK
POPULATION (1000s)													
1955	87291	62061	22962	4002	4645	4427	3369	2684	2159	1676	1173	672	423
1965	105602	71089	31294	8895	5442	3797	4308	3960	2820	2072	1554	958	707
1975	118145	72886	40876	10076	7896	8125	4796	3056	3720	3207	2082	1208	1093
1985	128965	80555	43534	8081	6306	9254	6897	7117	3597	2282	2410	1446	1021
1990	**135682**	**82526**	**48629**	**10490**	**7823**	**6067**	**8694**	**6299**	**6260**	**2996**	**1738**	**1616**	**1174**
1995 projected	*140105*	*85514*	*49946*	*10804*	*8045*	*6220*	*8890*	*6468*	*6417*	*3101*	*1800*	*1637*	*1208*
NUMBER OF DEATHS													
All causes													
1955	787640	230890	349580	24490	33650	44620	51450	58230	65980	71160	71130	57137	78903
1965	826415	200134	374061	42286	31599	28719	53339	66140	75712	76266	80932	72196	99092
1975	1174935	227765	582790	59603	61245	90007	68052	64368	112927	126588	120358	98758	145264
1985	1424395	241379	692667	44556	47007	100819	109645	164223	121328	105089	162343	147405	180601
1990	**1462389**	**214760**	**787317**	**53092**	**58694**	**61366**	**133112**	**136996**	**205055**	**139002**	**111262**	**150115**	**198935**
1995 projected	*1422216*	*196227*	*780671*	*52723*	*57277*	*60399*	*128953*	*134822*	*206425*	*140072*	*108579*	*143426*	*193313*
Lung cancer													
1955	...	...	...	...	...	...	...	...	...	...	...	...	...
1965	30894	389	24622	650	945	1433	4010	5779	6415	5390	3504	1699	680
1975	45750	353	35980	731	1703	4758	4803	5607	9465	8913	5701	2597	1119
1985	69723	469	53437	566	1630	5680	8972	16947	11301	8341	9085	4818	1914
1990	**86345**	**474**	**68955**	**767**	**1878**	**3810**	**11897**	**15040**	**22655**	**12908**	**7691**	**6330**	**2895**
1995 projected	*97165*	*469*	*76292*	*720*	*1872*	*3900*	*12242*	*16314*	*25848*	*15396*	*9226*	*7608*	*3570*
ANNUAL DEATH RATE / 100,000 (*The rates for the age groups 0–34 and 35–69 are the means of seven five-yearly rates, but the all-ages rates are standardised to the conventional "European" age distribution)													
All causes													
1955	1629.0*	347.3*	1906.1*	611.9	724.4	1007.9	1527.2	2169.5	3056.0	4245.8	6063.9	8502.5	18653.2
1965	1325.4*	276.2*	1583.8*	475.4	580.7	756.4	1238.1	1670.2	2684.8	3680.8	5208.0	7536.1	14013.9
1975	1481.3*	327.5*	1854.7*	591.5	775.6	1107.8	1418.9	2106.3	3035.7	3947.2	5780.9	8175.3	13290.4
1985	1679.7*	288.8*	2037.5*	551.4	745.4	1089.4	1589.7	2307.4	3373.5	4605.9	6736.8	10194.0	17695.6
1990	**1592.7***	**252.6***	**1984.1***	**506.1**	**750.3**	**1011.4**	**1531.1**	**2174.7**	**3275.8**	**4639.3**	**6403.6**	**9291.0**	**16950.8**
1995 projected	*1511.5**	*225.5**	*1919.9**	*488.0*	*712.0*	*971.0*	*1450.5*	*2084.4*	*3216.7*	*4516.7*	*6032.5*	*8763.7*	*16002.7*
All cancer													
1955	...	...	...	...	...	...	...	...	...	...	...	...	...
1965	238.9*	11.4*	430.4*	49.6	89.5	169.7	353.5	516.5	814.9	1019.4	1096.7	1118.2	954.3
1975	232.7*	11.8*	427.0*	47.8	98.1	207.8	326.4	559.1	808.6	941.1	1074.4	1021.4	746.6
1985	266.8*	11.1*	473.6*	46.0	96.9	198.9	367.9	633.0	880.9	1091.7	1268.4	1347.7	1045.4
1990	**288.5***	**10.9***	**508.0***	**42.8**	**101.1**	**201.7**	**389.6**	**633.3**	**959.6**	**1227.6**	**1400.2**	**1470.4**	**1255.8**
1995 projected	*308.5**	*9.8**	*539.6**	*41.0*	*100.3*	*206.9*	*394.7*	*656.1*	*1032.4*	*1345.8*	*1529.6*	*1640.4*	*1407.5*
Lung cancer													
1955	...	...	...	...	...	...	...	...	...	...	...	...	...
1965	54.0*	0.6*	112.7*	7.3	17.4	37.7	93.1	145.9	227.5	260.1	225.5	177.3	96.2
1975	62.8*	0.6*	129.1*	7.3	21.6	58.6	100.1	183.5	254.4	277.9	273.8	215.0	102.4
1985	82.3*	0.6*	163.2*	7.0	25.8	61.4	130.1	238.1	314.2	365.6	377.0	333.2	187.5
1990	**92.2***	**0.6***	**180.3***	**7.3**	**24.0**	**62.8**	**136.8**	**238.8**	**361.9**	**430.8**	**442.6**	**391.8**	**246.7**
1995 projected	*102.1**	*0.6**	*197.4**	*6.7*	*23.3*	*62.7*	*137.7*	*252.2*	*402.8*	*496.5*	*512.6*	*464.9*	*295.5*
Upper aerodigestive cancer (mouth, oesophagus, pharynx and larynx)													
1955	...	...	...	...	...	...	...	...	...	...	...	...	...
1965	25.1*	0.4*	42.0*	3.9	7.7	18.1	32.7	46.6	78.7	106.6	128.1	143.3	143.8
1975	23.4*	0.3*	41.0*	3.5	10.3	22.3	36.5	53.8	73.3	87.0	106.0	118.7	109.0
1985	28.8*	0.4*	53.9*	4.9	12.6	27.3	47.6	77.8	100.8	106.2	113.6	121.9	116.0
1990	**33.4***	**0.3***	**64.9***	**4.4**	**16.3**	**35.2**	**61.9**	**87.3**	**117.2**	**132.2**	**127.9**	**122.2**	**118.4**
1995 projected	*38.8**	*0.3**	*76.9**	*4.8*	*20.0*	*44.4*	*74.3*	*101.6*	*138.7*	*154.8*	*143.4*	*130.8*	*121.4*
Other cancer													
1955	...	...	...	...	...	...	...	...	...	...	...	...	...
1965	159.8*	10.4*	275.7*	38.4	64.5	113.8	227.7	324.0	508.7	652.7	743.1	797.5	714.3
1975	146.5*	10.8*	257.0*	37.0	66.3	126.9	189.7	321.8	480.8	576.2	694.6	687.7	535.2
1985	155.7*	10.2*	256.6*	34.2	58.5	110.2	190.2	317.0	465.9	620.0	777.8	892.7	741.8
1990	**162.9***	**10.0***	**262.7***	**31.2**	**60.8**	**103.7**	**190.9**	**307.3**	**480.5**	**664.6**	**829.6**	**956.4**	**890.8**
1995 projected	*167.7**	*8.9**	*265.2**	*29.5*	*57.0*	*99.8*	*182.6*	*302.3*	*490.8*	*694.5*	*873.6*	*1044.7*	*990.6*
Chronic obstructive pulmonary disease (COPD)													
1955	...	...	...	...	...	...	...	...	...	...	...	...	...
1965	102.5*	2.3*	131.3*	10.9	20.9	38.9	81.1	139.0	254.4	373.8	534.2	756.7	1176.5
1975	131.7*	2.7*	158.4*	13.1	30.1	56.2	98.5	172.4	295.8	442.9	719.0	1039.2	1564.4
1985	127.3*	2.5*	147.7*	10.7	23.5	44.6	97.8	167.5	285.9	403.7	645.8	1032.2	1657.2
1990	**100.3***	**1.9***	**120.4***	**6.2**	**13.1**	**28.9**	**62.1**	**131.4**	**227.2**	**373.9**	**538.1**	**804.6**	**1257.8**
1995 projected	*80.2**	*1.6**	*97.8**	*4.3*	*9.3*	*20.2*	*44.9*	*98.9*	*192.1*	*315.1*	*438.2*	*648.8*	*981.2*
Other respiratory disease													
1955	...	...	...	...	...	...	...	...	...	...	...	...	...
1965	37.1*	44.1*	16.7*	4.4	6.2	9.1	13.0	18.4	28.0	37.8	54.2	80.3	157.4
1975	55.4*	69.8*	26.5*	10.1	15.1	19.6	22.6	31.0	41.3	45.7	62.2	80.6	136.6
1985	41.8*	48.6*	25.5*	10.4	15.7	20.6	27.0	31.5	35.3	37.7	45.9	58.9	99.1
1990	**25.8***	**27.6***	**17.1***	**5.3**	**9.2**	**14.2**	**17.0**	**20.0**	**24.9**	**29.4**	**36.1**	**49.0**	**82.6**
1995 projected	*19.2**	*19.5**	*13.1**	*3.8*	*6.6*	*10.3*	*12.7*	*15.6*	*19.6*	*23.1*	*30.1*	*42.2*	*75.2*
Vascular disease													
1955	...	...	...	...	...	...	...	...	...	...	...	...	...
1965	572.1*	12.1*	550.1*	63.8	108.8	176.3	343.0	534.2	1012.8	1611.5	2770.3	4578.4	9796.4
1975	685.9*	15.0*	741.6*	103.9	174.9	303.8	477.6	796.6	1344.3	1990.1	3345.8	5394.1	10074.9
1985	874.6*	14.3*	900.4*	114.9	201.5	348.0	577.5	932.6	1624.3	2504.3	4153.2	7011.2	13926.6
1990	**788.2***	**13.2***	**871.6***	**104.5**	**215.5**	**339.4**	**575.3**	**896.8**	**1535.3**	**2434.1**	**3762.0**	**5981.0**	**11743.3**
1995 projected	*707.3**	*11.3**	*820.8**	*98.6*	*207.1*	*331.6*	*551.2*	*848.3*	*1462.5*	*2246.3*	*3315.7*	*5190.3*	*10070.2*
Liver cirrhosis and other liver disease													
1955	...	...	...	...	...	...	...	...	...	...	...	...	...
1965	14.6*	1.4*	22.5*	5.9	8.9	12.7	20.3	24.4	36.7	48.7	57.8	75.2	105.5
1975	19.7*	1.7*	34.9*	10.4	15.8	25.4	37.2	47.8	54.0	53.5	62.2	73.2	78.4
1985	27.4*	1.8*	51.9*	13.1	20.4	31.8	46.8	62.9	91.6	96.9	90.5	94.5	91.3
1990	**22.5***	**1.5***	**41.2***	**7.6**	**16.7**	**25.3**	**36.3**	**47.5**	**69.0**	**86.3**	**86.0**	**83.1**	**89.5**
1995 projected	*19.4**	*1.3**	*34.2**	*5.8*	*13.1*	*20.4*	*28.7*	*38.6*	*57.4*	*75.8*	*77.8*	*81.4*	*88.8*
Other medical causes													
1955	...	...	...	...	...	...	...	...	...	...	...	...	...
1965	209.5*	92.3*	244.5*	104.5	135.8	156.8	222.7	264.5	381.1	446.1	561.4	771.0	1595.4
1975	139.7*	84.0*	170.1*	80.1	100.9	134.3	159.2	205.6	243.9	267.0	324.2	374.7	443.1
1985	154.8*	100.3*	176.9*	102.0	121.0	149.1	173.0	200.5	229.7	263.3	325.9	415.0	543.3
1990	**166.5***	**71.8***	**153.9***	**65.5**	**91.8**	**112.5**	**143.7**	**170.3**	**216.6**	**277.0**	**374.4**	**676.0**	**2094.8**
1995 projected	*170.4**	*51.3**	*137.3**	*44.8*	*65.6*	*87.0*	*115.6*	*148.0*	*206.4*	*293.7*	*438.1*	*932.3*	*2896.3*
All non-medical causes													
1955	...	...	...	...	...	...	...	...	...	...	...	...	...
1965	150.6*	112.7*	188.3*	236.3	210.6	192.9	204.6	173.2	157.0	143.3	133.5	156.5	228.4
1975	216.1*	142.5*	296.2*	326.2	340.7	360.7	297.5	293.8	247.8	206.9	193.1	192.1	246.4
1985	186.9*	110.3*	261.5*	254.2	266.5	296.4	299.6	279.4	225.9	208.4	207.0	234.4	332.7
1990	**200.8***	**125.7***	**271.9***	**274.1**	**302.9**	**289.5**	**307.1**	**275.4**	**243.2**	**211.0**	**206.8**	**226.9**	**427.1**
1995 projected	*206.5**	*130.8**	*277.1**	*289.8*	*310.2*	*294.6*	*302.8*	*278.9*	*246.5*	*217.0*	*203.0*	*228.3*	*483.4*

Former USSR: Females

	All ages	0–34	35–69	35–39	40–44	45–49	50–54	55–59	60–64	65–69	70–74	75–79	80+/NK
POPULATION (1000s)													
1955	108868	64848	38301	6280	7395	6904	6033	4863	3784	3042	2787	1741	1191
1965	125338	69752	48173	10171	8017	6191	7212	6626	5625	4331	3404	2117	1892
1975	136324	70918	54795	10483	8422	9989	7645	5402	6806	6048	4842	2945	2824
1985	146396	78759	54597	8303	6783	10260	7989	9503	6914	4847	5757	3899	3385
1990	**151759**	**80570**	**58581**	**10700**	**8181**	**6673**	**9967**	**7730**	**9042**	**6289**	**4169**	**4476**	**3963**
1995 projected	*156448*	*83502*	*60042*	*11019*	*8404*	*6833*	*10179*	*7920*	*9230*	*6457*	*4317*	*4529*	*4058*
NUMBER OF DEATHS													
All causes													
1955	870060	164840	305860	17010	23860	32620	41240	50350	61130	79650	101850	107104	190406
1965	863419	122994	306217	18882	20586	21503	39422	50259	69797	85768	102308	120065	211835
1975	1188460	125253	394866	20226	22255	39173	45042	47873	94065	126232	165292	173413	329636
1985	1522673	130308	419746	15417	17044	40145	48128	86985	101951	110076	218822	258999	494798
1990	**1522769**	**105756**	**444516**	**16672**	**20342**	**23437**	**54855**	**65117**	**121850**	**142243**	**151325**	**270101**	**551071**
1995 projected	*1449949*	*89193*	*429075*	*15824*	*19064*	*22195*	*51283*	*61331*	*119123*	*140255*	*147004*	*257434*	*527243*
Lung cancer													
1955	...	...	...	...	...	...	...	...	...	...	...	...	...
1965	8457	208	5871	209	307	417	889	1221	1404	1424	1132	761	485
1975	11382	182	7340	210	313	754	890	1047	1952	2174	1909	1209	742
1985	14414	193	8147	161	220	718	898	1956	2180	2014	2795	1999	1280
1990	**16690**	**230**	**9402**	**188**	**301**	**439**	**1143**	**1511**	**2856**	**2964**	**2406**	**2728**	**1924**
1995 projected	*19006*	*249*	*10049*	*205*	*309*	*453*	*1132*	*1528*	*3042*	*3380*	*2881*	*3422*	*2405*
ANNUAL DEATH RATE / 100,000 (*The rates for the age groups 0–34 and 35–69 are the means of seven five-yearly rates, but the all-ages rates are standardised to the conventional "European" age distribution)													
All causes													
1955	1045.2*	232.6*	1002.7*	270.9	322.7	472.5	683.6	1035.4	1615.5	2618.3	3654.5	6151.9	15987.1
1965	795.7*	166.3*	759.4*	185.6	256.8	347.3	546.6	758.5	1240.8	1980.3	3005.5	5671.5	11196.4
1975	854.4*	176.7*	827.7*	192.9	264.2	392.2	589.2	886.2	1382.1	2087.2	3413.7	5888.4	11672.7
1985	942.6*	156.8*	870.3*	185.7	251.3	391.3	602.4	915.4	1474.6	2271.1	3801.2	6643.0	14619.1
1990	**873.1***	**124.2***	**822.6***	**155.8**	**248.7**	**351.2**	**550.4**	**842.4**	**1347.6**	**2261.8**	**3629.8**	**6034.8**	**13904.7**
1995 projected	*811.0**	*102.0**	*776.6**	*143.6*	*226.8*	*324.8*	*503.8*	*774.4*	*1290.6*	*2172.1*	*3404.9*	*5683.7*	*12994.3*
All cancer													
1955	...	...	...	...	...	...	...	...	...	...	...	...	...
1965	135.4*	10.0*	238.9*	46.8	85.3	134.6	224.0	284.9	397.7	499.2	517.7	627.2	555.6
1975	126.7*	10.3*	225.0*	45.1	73.8	128.0	198.4	281.6	392.5	455.8	513.6	566.9	445.9
1985	128.0*	10.1*	217.5*	47.3	71.6	118.5	177.1	266.4	378.4	462.9	566.9	626.8	552.3
1990	**134.4***	**9.7***	**224.4***	**44.5**	**82.4**	**119.2**	**184.5**	**252.6**	**371.9**	**515.6**	**618.3**	**690.1**	**638.0**
1995 projected	*140.5**	*9.0**	*229.1**	*46.2*	*84.2*	*123.2*	*181.1*	*246.0*	*378.6*	*544.4*	*672.6*	*781.5*	*717.2*
Lung cancer													
1955	...	...	...	...	...	...	...	...	...	...	...	...	...
1965	7.8*	0.3*	14.5*	2.1	3.8	6.7	12.3	18.4	25.0	32.9	33.3	35.9	25.6
1975	8.5*	0.3*	15.6*	2.0	3.7	7.5	11.6	19.4	28.7	35.9	39.4	41.1	26.3
1985	9.5*	0.2*	16.7*	1.9	3.2	7.0	11.2	20.6	31.5	41.6	48.6	51.3	37.8
1990	**10.3***	**0.3***	**17.4***	**1.8**	**3.7**	**6.6**	**11.5**	**19.5**	**31.6**	**47.1**	**57.7**	**61.0**	**48.5**
1995 projected	*11.4**	*0.3**	*18.3**	*1.9*	*3.7*	*6.6*	*11.1*	*19.3*	*33.0*	*52.3*	*66.7*	*75.6*	*59.3*
Upper aerodigestive cancer (mouth, oesophagus, pharynx and larynx)													
1955	...	...	...	...	...	...	...	...	...	...	...	...	...
1965	8.4*	0.2*	12.8*	1.4	2.4	4.7	8.4	14.3	24.0	34.7	39.9	59.3	64.9
1975	6.2*	0.2*	9.6*	1.1	3.1	4.4	6.8	11.6	18.4	21.9	30.7	40.2	41.9
1985	5.2*	0.2*	7.8*	0.7	1.5	3.2	6.3	9.5	13.9	19.3	25.9	33.2	43.0
1990	**5.1***	**0.2***	**7.5***	**0.7**	**1.6**	**3.1**	**4.9**	**8.8**	**13.6**	**19.9**	**25.4**	**32.5**	**42.3**
1995 projected	*5.0**	*0.2**	*7.3**	*0.8*	*1.7*	*2.8*	*4.3*	*8.1*	*13.7*	*19.9*	*25.4*	*32.9*	*42.6*
Other cancer													
1955	...	...	...	...	...	...	...	...	...	...	...	...	...
1965	119.2*	9.5*	211.6*	43.3	79.1	123.2	203.3	252.2	348.7	431.7	444.5	531.9	465.1
1975	112.0*	9.8*	199.8*	41.9	67.0	116.0	179.9	250.6	345.4	397.9	443.5	485.6	377.7
1985	113.3*	9.7*	193.0*	44.6	66.9	108.2	159.5	236.3	333.0	402.1	492.4	542.3	471.4
1990	**119.0***	**9.2***	**199.5***	**42.0**	**77.1**	**109.5**	**168.1**	**224.2**	**326.7**	**448.5**	**535.2**	**596.6**	**547.2**
1995 projected	*124.1**	*8.5**	*203.5**	*43.5*	*78.7*	*113.8*	*165.7*	*218.6*	*331.9*	*472.1*	*580.4*	*673.1*	*615.3*
Chronic obstructive pulmonary disease (COPD)													
1955	...	...	...	...	...	...	...	...	...	...	...	...	...
1965	42.6*	1.4*	39.5*	2.8	4.9	10.4	19.7	36.1	73.4	129.0	205.4	402.0	702.8
1975	58.0*	1.8*	49.8*	5.0	8.1	13.6	24.6	47.3	90.8	159.1	287.1	517.4	1039.6
1985	45.2*	1.8*	39.0*	5.0	7.3	12.5	23.5	38.5	67.6	118.7	208.0	376.2	833.1
1990	**32.4***	**1.5***	**30.7***	**3.4**	**5.6**	**9.1**	**17.0**	**31.4**	**51.5**	**97.2**	**159.1**	**267.4**	**536.2**
1995 projected	*24.3**	*1.3**	*23.9**	*2.6*	*4.2*	*6.7*	*13.2*	*24.4*	*41.1*	*75.2*	*117.8*	*196.0*	*387.0*
Other respiratory disease													
1955	...	...	...	...	...	...	...	...	...	...	...	...	...
1965	27.3*	37.3*	7.3*	2.0	2.6	3.1	4.9	7.0	12.1	19.3	28.2	50.7	100.1
1975	40.9*	59.4*	11.0*	4.7	5.3	6.0	8.5	12.9	17.3	22.5	32.9	48.9	86.7
1985	27.4*	40.6*	6.8*	2.9	3.2	4.6	5.5	7.9	10.5	13.2	18.5	28.2	51.0
1990	**16.4***	**22.9***	**5.0***	**1.8**	**2.2**	**3.1**	**3.9**	**5.9**	**7.6**	**10.6**	**16.9**	**21.7**	**42.9**
1995 projected	*12.3**	*16.4**	*4.2**	*1.6*	*1.7*	*2.5*	*3.3*	*5.2*	*6.3*	*9.2*	*14.8*	*19.5*	*38.6*
Vascular disease													
1955	...	...	...	...	...	...	...	...	...	...	...	...	...
1965	427.4*	9.7*	320.6*	33.0	56.0	86.8	163.3	277.8	558.4	1068.9	1926.7	4029.5	8658.9
1975	494.1*	7.9*	390.6*	37.4	66.2	112.0	205.3	370.3	696.0	1246.9	2345.5	4454.9	9718.2
1985	597.9*	6.5*	440.4*	33.3	58.7	119.0	230.2	411.4	800.0	1430.3	2734.1	5266.9	12727.9
1990	**519.3***	**5.7***	**401.3***	**25.8**	**56.8**	**101.9**	**196.1**	**372.7**	**699.8**	**1356.2**	**2471.9**	**4455.6**	**10746.3**
1995 projected	*452.4**	*4.9**	*359.7**	*22.3*	*48.5*	*87.3*	*171.5*	*327.4*	*638.9*	*1221.8*	*2149.7*	*3887.4*	*9208.3*
Liver cirrhosis and other liver disease													
1955	...	...	...	...	...	...	...	...	...	...	...	...	...
1965	9.4*	1.0*	13.3*	2.8	4.6	6.1	10.2	13.7	22.8	32.8	39.8	61.5	79.1
1975	9.7*	0.9*	15.6*	4.2	6.6	9.4	15.2	22.0	23.8	27.9	35.4	44.7	57.0
1985	12.3*	1.1*	22.1*	5.3	9.7	13.4	20.1	30.3	35.9	40.2	39.1	45.2	53.7
1990	**11.1***	**1.0***	**19.3***	**3.8**	**6.3**	**10.3**	**16.6**	**25.3**	**31.3**	**41.5**	**42.3**	**46.9**	**53.0**
1995 projected	*10.6**	*1.0**	*17.6**	*3.1*	*4.9*	*8.4*	*13.9*	*22.3*	*29.2*	*41.5*	*44.2*	*52.0*	*56.3*
Other medical causes													
1955	...	...	...	...	...	...	...	...	...	...	...	...	...
1965	116.4*	78.9*	99.1*	63.8	64.6	65.1	78.7	97.4	135.8	188.0	238.4	421.0	980.8
1975	74.5*	65.9*	69.7*	45.7	45.4	51.1	63.9	78.3	92.2	111.6	128.9	158.3	191.3
1985	79.7*	68.3*	74.9*	41.0	41.4	53.2	68.7	83.4	106.2	130.1	151.1	189.6	229.8
1990	**109.3***	**54.0***	**78.1***	**30.8**	**38.2**	**46.0**	**63.2**	**86.4**	**116.4**	**166.0**	**232.8**	**438.8**	**1712.6**
1995 projected	*123.1**	*40.1**	*83.7**	*25.3*	*31.9*	*41.0*	*59.6*	*88.5*	*133.0*	*207.0*	*315.4*	*628.5*	*2406.0*
All non-medical causes													
1955	...	...	...	...	...	...	...	...	...	...	...	...	...
1965	37.1*	28.0*	40.8*	34.5	38.9	41.3	45.8	41.6	40.7	43.2	49.3	79.6	119.0
1975	50.6*	30.5*	66.0*	50.9	58.9	72.1	73.3	73.8	69.6	63.4	70.4	97.2	134.1
1985	52.1*	28.4*	69.5*	50.8	59.3	70.0	77.4	77.5	75.9	75.6	83.5	110.0	171.3
1990	**50.2***	**29.3***	**63.7***	**45.7**	**57.2**	**61.7**	**69.0**	**68.3**	**69.2**	**74.7**	**88.5**	**114.4**	**175.7**
1995 projected	*47.9**	*29.3**	*58.3**	*42.5*	*51.5*	*55.8*	*61.2*	*60.6*	*63.5*	*73.1*	*90.4*	*118.9*	*180.9*

Former USSR: 1975

Smoking-attributed deaths (Sm.) and total deaths (Total)

		ALL CAUSES	ALL CANCER	Lung cancer	Upper aero-digestive ca.	Other cancer	COPD	Other respiratory	Vascular disease	Cirrhosis/ other liver	Other medical	Non-medical
Males												
0–34	Sm.	–	–	–	–	–	–	–	–	–	–	–
	Total	227765	7815	353	195	7267	1725	53554	8686	1027	61894	93064
35–69	Sm.	185053	55532	33663	8180	13689	34544	3288	69479	–	22210	–
	Total	582790	122444	35980	11892	74572	43462	8829	210037	11337	58505	128176
		(32%)	(45%)	(94%)	(69%)	(18%)	(79%)	(37%)	(33%)		(38%)	
70+	Sm.	53484	11859	7856	1999	2004	24458	260	15695	–	1212	–
	Total	364380	42868	9417	4832	28619	44622	3763	244939	3036	16119	9033
		(15%)	(28%)	(83%)	(41%)	(7%)	(55%)	(7%)	(6%)		(8%)	
Any age	Sm.	238537	67391	41519	10179	15693	59002	3548	85174	–	23422	–
	Total	1174935	173127	45750	16919	110458	89809	66146	463662	15400	136518	230273
		(20%)	(39%)	(91%)	(60%)	(14%)	(66%)	(5%)	(18%)		(17%)	
Females												
0–34	Sm.	–	–	–	–	–	–	–	–	–	–	–
	Total	125253	6612	182	118	6312	1224	43637	4956	598	47197	21029
35–69	Sm.	21952	4452	3108	731	613	6688	271	8732	–	1809	–
	Total	394866	108377	7340	4545	96492	22804	5425	179158	7586	35858	35658
		(6%)	(4%)	(42%)	(16%)	(1%)	(29%)	(5%)	(5%)		(5%)	
70+	Sm.	11139	1206	847	243	116	6394	41	3349	–	149	–
	Total	668341	54152	3860	3853	46439	58497	5479	519210	4639	16305	10059
		(2%)	(2%)	(22%)	(6%)	(0%)	(11%)	(1%)	(1%)		(1%)	
Any age	Sm.	33091	5658	3955	974	729	13082	312	12081	–	1958	–
	Total	1188460	169141	11382	8516	149243	82525	54541	703324	12823	99360	66746
		(3%)	(3%)	(35%)	(11%)	(0%)	(16%)	(1%)	(2%)		(2%)	
Males+Females												
0–34	Sm.	–	–	–	–	–	–	–	–	–	–	–
	Total	353018	14427	535	313	13579	2949	97191	13642	1625	109091	114093
35–69	Sm.	207005	59984	36771	8911	14302	41232	3559	78211	–	24019	–
	Total	977656	230821	43320	16437	171064	66266	14254	389195	18923	94363	163834
		(21%)	(26%)	(85%)	(54%)	(8%)	(62%)	(25%)	(20%)		(25%)	
70+	Sm.	64623	13065	8703	2242	2120	30852	301	19044	–	1361	–
	Total	1032721	97020	13277	8685	75058	103119	9242	764149	7675	32424	19092
		(6%)	(13%)	(66%)	(26%)	(3%)	(30%)	(3%)	(2%)		(4%)	
Any age	Sm.	271628	73049	45474	11153	16422	72084	3860	97255	–	25380	–
	Total	2363395	342268	57132	25435	259701	172334	120687	1166986	28223	235878	297019
		(11%)	(21%)	(80%)	(44%)	(6%)	(42%)	(3%)	(8%)		(11%)	

Former USSR: 1985

Smoking-attributed deaths (Sm.) and total deaths (Total)

		ALL CAUSES	ALL CANCER	Lung cancer	Upper aero-digestive ca.	Other cancer	COPD	Other respiratory	Vascular disease	Cirrhosis/ other liver	Other medical	Non-medical
Males												
0–34	Sm.	–	–	–	–	–	–	–	–	–	–	–
	Total	241379	8901	469	274	8158	1991	42991	11196	1425	86020	88855
35–69	Sm.	271865	83909	50859	13918	19132	37568	4534	113861	–	31993	–
	Total	692667	155249	53437	18582	83230	44637	9973	275963	18501	70137	118207
		(39%)	(54%)	(95%)	(75%)	(23%)	(84%)	(45%)	(41%)		(46%)	
70+	Sm.	87155	20923	13979	2977	3967	31115	308	32738	–	2071	–
	Total	490349	60722	15817	5683	39222	47401	2970	343601	4481	19400	11774
		(18%)	(34%)	(88%)	(52%)	(10%)	(66%)	(10%)	(10%)		(11%)	
Any age	Sm.	359020	104832	64838	16895	23099	68683	4842	146599	–	34064	–
	Total	1424395	224872	69723	24539	130610	94029	55934	630760	24407	175557	218836
		(25%)	(47%)	(93%)	(69%)	(18%)	(73%)	(9%)	(23%)		(19%)	
Females												
0–34	Sm.	–	–	–	–	–	–	–	–	–	–	–
	Total	130308	7929	193	136	7600	1480	34794	5089	842	57406	22768
35–69	Sm.	24788	5059	3698	673	688	5914	193	11502	–	2120	–
	Total	419746	109003	8147	3793	97063	18165	3489	201079	11394	38732	37884
		(6%)	(5%)	(45%)	(18%)	(1%)	(33%)	(6%)	(6%)		(5%)	
70+	Sm.	26790	3121	2247	539	335	12519	59	10673	–	418	–
	Total	972619	75764	6074	4243	65447	54837	3892	793529	5834	23869	14894
		(3%)	(4%)	(37%)	(13%)	(1%)	(23%)	(2%)	(1%)		(2%)	
Any age	Sm.	51578	8180	5945	1212	1023	18433	252	22175	–	2538	–
	Total	1522673	192696	14414	8172	170110	74482	42175	999697	18070	120007	75546
		(3%)	(4%)	(41%)	(15%)	(1%)	(25%)	(1%)	(2%)		(2%)	
Males+Females												
0–34	Sm.	–	–	–	–	–	–	–	–	–	–	–
	Total	371687	16830	662	410	15758	3471	77785	16285	2267	143426	111623
35–69	Sm.	296653	88968	54557	14591	19820	43482	4727	125363	–	34113	–
	Total	1112413	264252	61584	22375	180293	62802	13462	477042	29895	108869	156091
		(27%)	(34%)	(89%)	(65%)	(11%)	(69%)	(35%)	(26%)		(31%)	
70+	Sm.	113945	24044	16226	3516	4302	43634	367	43411	–	2489	–
	Total	1462968	136486	21891	9926	104669	102238	6862	1137130	10315	43269	26668
		(8%)	(18%)	(74%)	(35%)	(4%)	(43%)	(5%)	(4%)		(6%)	
Any age	Sm.	410598	113012	70783	18107	24122	87116	5094	168774	–	36602	–
	Total	2947068	417568	84137	32711	300720	168511	98109	1630457	42477	295564	294382
		(14%)	(27%)	(84%)	(55%)	(8%)	(52%)	(5%)	(10%)		(12%)	

(To be conservative, no deaths before age 35, and none from liver cirrhosis or non-medical causes, were attributed to smoking.)

Former USSR: 1990

Smoking-attributed deaths (Sm.) and total deaths (Total)

		ALL CAUSES	ALL CANCER	Lung cancer	Upper aero-digestive ca.	Other cancer	COPD	Other respiratory	Vascular disease	Cirrhosis/ other liver	Other medical	Non-medical
Males												
0–34	Sm.	–	–	–	–	–	–	–	–	–	–	–
	Total	214760	8983	474	268	8241	1636	25579	10805	1239	64760	101758
35–69	Sm.	313359	109676	65827	19791	24058	36161	3276	134710	–	29536	–
	Total	787317	195257	68955	26047	100255	42530	7309	323956	16693	65961	135611
		(40%)	(56%)	(95%)	(76%)	(24%)	(85%)	(45%)	(42%)		(45%)	
70+	Sm.	83524	22840	15160	3121	4559	25561	258	30846	–	4019	–
	Total	460312	62824	16916	5587	40321	37112	2387	299819	3887	42012	12271
		(18%)	(36%)	(90%)	(56%)	(11%)	(69%)	(11%)	(10%)		(10%)	
Any age	Sm.	396883	132516	80987	22912	28617	61722	3534	165556	–	33555	–
	Total	1462389	267064	86345	31902	148817	81278	35275	634580	21819	172733	249640
		(27%)	(50%)	(94%)	(72%)	(19%)	(76%)	(10%)	(26%)		(19%)	
Females												
0–34	Sm.	–	–	–	–	–	–	–	–	–	–	–
	Total	105756	7888	230	152	7506	1242	20476	4615	813	46950	23772
35–69	Sm.	27568	6061	4454	775	832	5650	161	13179	–	2517	–
	Total	444516	123418	9402	4068	109948	16316	2776	211120	10668	43428	36790
		(6%)	(5%)	(47%)	(19%)	(1%)	(35%)	(6%)	(6%)		(6%)	
70+	Sm.	32206	4497	3241	738	518	12441	71	13525	–	1672	–
	Total	972497	81951	7058	4191	70702	39848	3376	728370	5965	97216	15771
		(3%)	(5%)	(46%)	(18%)	(1%)	(31%)	(2%)	(2%)		(2%)	
Any age	Sm.	59774	10558	7695	1513	1350	18091	232	26704	–	4189	–
	Total	1522769	213257	16690	8411	188156	57406	26628	944105	17446	187594	76333
		(4%)	(5%)	(46%)	(18%)	(1%)	(32%)	(1%)	(3%)		(2%)	
Males+Females												
0–34	Sm.	–	–	–	–	–	–	–	–	–	–	–
	Total	320516	16871	704	420	15747	2878	46055	15420	2052	111710	125530
35–69	Sm.	340927	115737	70281	20566	24890	41811	3437	147889	–	32053	–
	Total	1231833	318675	78357	30115	210203	58846	10085	535076	27361	109389	172401
		(28%)	(36%)	(90%)	(68%)	(12%)	(71%)	(34%)	(28%)		(29%)	
70+	Sm.	115730	27337	18401	3859	5077	38002	329	44371	–	5691	–
	Total	1432809	144775	23974	9778	111023	76960	5763	1028189	9852	139228	28042
		(8%)	(19%)	(77%)	(39%)	(5%)	(49%)	(6%)	(4%)		(4%)	
Any age	Sm.	456657	143074	88682	24425	29967	79813	3766	192260	–	37744	–
	Total	2985158	480321	103035	40313	336973	138684	61903	1578685	39265	360327	325973
		(15%)	(30%)	(86%)	(61%)	(9%)	(58%)	(6%)	(12%)		(10%)	

Former USSR: 1995

Smoking-attributed deaths (Sm.) and total deaths (Total)

		ALL CAUSES	ALL CANCER	Lung cancer	Upper aero-digestive ca.	Other cancer	COPD	Other respiratory	Vascular disease	Cirrhosis/ other liver	Other medical	Non-medical
Males												
0–34	Sm.	–	–	–	–	–	–	–	–	–	–	–
	Total	196227	8330	469	245	7616	1398	18783	9514	1121	48205	108876
35–69	Sm.	319749	123719	73085	24548	26086	30092	2618	137136	–	26184	–
	Total	780671	210871	76292	31773	102806	34944	5684	315326	14023	57731	142092
		(41%)	(59%)	(96%)	(77%)	(25%)	(86%)	(46%)	(43%)		(45%)	
70+	Sm.	89030	28211	18595	3731	5885	22057	266	32126	–	6370	–
	Total	445318	71380	20404	6188	44788	30359	2140	266273	3806	58130	13230
		(20%)	(40%)	(91%)	(60%)	(13%)	(73%)	(12%)	(12%)		(11%)	
Any age	Sm.	408779	151930	91680	28279	31971	52149	2884	169262	–	32554	–
	Total	1422216	290581	97165	38206	155210	66701	26607	591113	18950	164066	264198
		(29%)	(52%)	(94%)	(74%)	(21%)	(78%)	(11%)	(29%)		(20%)	
Females												
0–34	Sm.	–	–	–	–	–	–	–	–	–	–	–
	Total	89193	7527	249	163	7115	1154	15193	4085	812	36161	24261
35–69	Sm.	27936	6732	4965	831	936	4766	148	13311	–	2979	–
	Total	429075	128601	10049	4064	114488	13017	2399	193753	9892	46983	34430
		(7%)	(5%)	(49%)	(20%)	(1%)	(37%)	(6%)	(7%)		(6%)	
70+	Sm.	40124	6742	4838	1044	860	12148	91	17570	–	3573	–
	Total	931681	93531	8708	4315	80508	29670	3091	642507	6548	139706	16628
		(4%)	(7%)	(56%)	(24%)	(1%)	(41%)	(3%)	(3%)		(3%)	
Any age	Sm.	68060	13474	9803	1875	1796	16914	239	30881	–	6552	–
	Total	1449949	229659	19006	8542	202111	43841	20683	840345	17252	222850	75319
		(5%)	(6%)	(52%)	(22%)	(1%)	(39%)	(1%)	(4%)		(3%)	
Males+Females												
0–34	Sm.	–	–	–	–	–	–	–	–	–	–	–
	Total	285420	15857	718	408	14731	2552	33976	13599	1933	84366	133137
35–69	Sm.	347685	130451	78050	25379	27022	34858	2766	150447	–	29163	–
	Total	1209746	339472	86341	35837	217294	47961	8083	509079	23915	104714	176522
		(29%)	(38%)	(90%)	(71%)	(12%)	(73%)	(34%)	(30%)		(28%)	
70+	Sm.	129154	34953	23433	4775	6745	34205	357	49696	–	9943	–
	Total	1376999	164911	29112	10503	125296	60029	5231	908780	10354	197836	29858
		(9%)	(21%)	(80%)	(45%)	(5%)	(57%)	(7%)	(5%)		(5%)	
Any age	Sm.	476839	165404	101483	30154	33767	69063	3123	200143	–	39106	–
	Total	2872165	520240	116171	46748	357321	110542	47290	1431458	36202	386916	339517
		(17%)	(32%)	(87%)	(65%)	(9%)	(62%)	(7%)	(14%)		(10%)	

(To be conservative, no deaths before age 35, and none from liver cirrhosis or non-medical causes, were attributed to smoking.)

¶UZBEKISTAN: 1990

		No. of deaths			Standardised rates (Defined on p.544)			Annual death rates / 100, 000						
		All ages	**0–34**	**35–69**	**All ages**	**0–34**	**35–69**	**0–4**	**5–9**	**10–14**	**15–19**	**20–24**	**25–29**	**30–34**
ALL CAUSES	M	66659	26329	23867	1311.9	280.2	1527.5	1129.4	79.8	66.0	87.1	147.5	191.0	260.4
	F	57894	18838	15930	871.8	197.4	875.8	890.8	51.7	45.4	58.1	92.7	101.4	141.6
Tuberculosis	M	828	131	616	18.3	2.2	34.5	0.5	0.1	0.3	0.5	2.2	3.6	8.2
	F	509	140	309	8.6	2.3	15.4	0.3	0.1	0.2	0.7	2.9	4.7	7.5
Other infective	M	3342	3188	132	19.7	28.9	7.4	174.9	8.6	6.5	3.9	3.1	2.0	3.4
and parasitic	F	2823	2683	109	16.9	26.1	5.2	145.3	4.9	4.8	4.5	8.4	7.7	6.8
ALL CANCER	M	5924	651	4012	153.4	9.4	264.6	7.1	4.3	5.4	6.4	9.5	11.8	21.0
	F	5093	519	3093	96.9	7.7	165.5	4.9	3.1	4.3	4.5	7.9	10.3	18.8
Mouth and	M	224	18	164	5.8	0.3	10.3	0.1	0.1	–	0.4	0.2	0.4	0.7
pharynx cancer	F	113	18	58	2.1	0.3	3.1	0.2	0.1	–	0.1	0.3	0.4	0.8
Oesophagus cancer	M	914	14	612	26.7	0.2	43.3	0.2	–	–	0.1	0.3	0.2	0.7
	F	638	13	406	12.8	0.2	23.5	–	–	–	–	0.2	0.6	0.8
Stomach cancer	M	1066	34	755	30.1	0.6	50.0	–	–	0.2	0.3	0.6	0.6	2.6
	F	723	26	443	14.3	0.4	24.2	0.1	–	0.1	0.2	0.7	0.3	1.8
Colorectal cancer	M	270	54	150	6.8	0.8	10.0	1.2	0.1	0.1	0.1	0.4	1.2	2.3
	F	301	23	173	5.8	0.3	9.3	0.4	0.1	–	–	0.4	0.7	0.8
Liver cancer	M	...	...	...	...	...	...	...	...	...	...	...	...	...
	F	...	...	...	...	...	...	...	...	...	...	...	...	...
Pancreas cancer	M	...	...	...	...	...	...	...	...	...	...	...	...	...
	F	...	...	...	...	...	...	...	...	...	...	...	...	...
Larynx cancer	M	135	4	110	3.6	0.0	7.6	0.2	–	–	0.1	–	–	–
	F	23	–	16	0.5	–	0.8	–	–	–	–	–	–	–
Lung cancer	M	1078	25	874	29.0	0.4	58.0	0.2	–	0.1	0.4	0.3	0.6	1.2
	F	394	14	248	7.8	0.2	13.4	–	0.1	0.1	0.1	0.1	0.7	0.4
Malignant melanoma	M	...	...	...	...	...	...	...	...	...	...	...	...	...
	F	...	...	...	...	...	...	...	...	...	...	...	...	...
Female breast cancer	F	543	34	393	10.6	0.6	19.8	–	–	0.1	–	0.2	0.9	3.1
Cervix cancer	F	235	12	167	4.7	0.2	8.7	–	–	–	–	0.2	0.1	1.2
Other uterine cancer	F	204	15	124	4.0	0.3	6.6	–	–	–	–	0.4	0.7	0.7
Ovarian cancer	F	...	...	...	...	...	...	...	...	...	...	...	...	...
Prostate cancer	M	122	–	60	4.0	–	5.0	–	–	–	–	–	–	–
Bladder cancer	M	...	...	...	...	...	...	...	...	...	...	...	...	...
	F	...	...	...	...	...	...	...	...	...	...	...	...	...
Other and ill–defined	M	1631	255	1081	39.9	3.8	68.5	2.4	1.6	1.7	2.0	4.5	4.9	9.3
cancer sites	F	1547	196	899	29.0	2.9	47.9	1.9	1.3	1.8	1.6	2.8	3.9	6.9
Hodgkin's disease	M	...	...	...	...	...	...	...	...	...	...	...	...	...
	F	...	...	...	...	...	...	...	...	...	...	...	...	...
Myeloma and all	M	199	66	112	3.9	0.9	6.8	0.5	0.8	0.9	1.0	0.9	0.9	1.4
lymphomas	F	109	28	62	1.8	0.4	3.2	0.3	0.2	0.3	0.4	0.7	0.1	0.9
Leukaemia	M	285	181	94	3.7	2.4	5.1	2.4	1.8	2.4	2.1	2.2	2.9	2.9
	F	263	140	104	3.3	1.8	4.9	2.1	1.3	1.9	2.1	1.7	2.0	1.4
ALL VASCULAR	M	24291	840	11021	718.6	13.1	759.0	8.0	1.5	2.3	6.6	10.6	21.3	41.6
DISEASE	F	26891	706	7767	512.9	10.9	448.7	5.8	1.5	2.3	7.3	13.4	17.6	28.6
Rheumatic heart	M	529	191	297	9.4	3.0	14.8	0.8	0.4	1.1	2.6	3.0	5.8	7.3
disease and fever	F	707	237	395	11.1	3.8	17.8	0.4	0.6	1.0	3.7	4.5	7.1	9.2
Hypertensive disease	M	1009	35	647	28.2	0.5	42.9	0.6	0.1	0.2	0.3	0.3	0.6	1.5
	F	1028	18	549	20.6	0.3	30.2	0.2	0.1	–	0.2	0.4	0.3	0.7
Ischaemic heart	M	15432	247	6390	468.9	4.4	446.3	–	0.1	–	1.1	2.9	6.6	20.4
disease	F	16402	141	3806	313.7	2.4	229.2	0.3	–	0.2	1.0	2.6	4.3	8.4
Pulmonary embolism	M	...	...	...	...	...	...	...	...	...	...	...	...	...
and other venous	F	...	...	...	...	...	...	...	...	...	...	...	...	...
Cerebrovascular	M	6250	188	3215	184.9	2.8	225.0	2.5	0.3	0.5	1.6	2.1	4.7	8.0
disease	F	7718	151	2714	149.5	2.4	154.8	1.1	0.6	0.2	1.2	3.6	3.1	6.8
Other vascular	M	1071	179	472	27.2	2.4	30.1	4.1	0.7	0.5	1.1	2.3	3.6	4.4
disease, incl. venous	F	1036	159	303	18.1	2.1	16.7	3.8	0.2	0.9	1.3	2.3	2.8	3.5
Chronic obstructive	M	2848	228	1298	82.3	2.9	93.3	6.6	0.5	0.8	1.3	2.6	3.6	4.8
pulmonary disease	F	2758	236	1010	51.5	3.1	57.3	5.6	1.2	0.9	1.5	2.6	4.3	5.7
Other respiratory	M	8947	8509	302	53.6	75.3	17.5	494.5	11.6	5.9	3.9	3.5	2.9	4.5
disease	F	7294	6937	198	42.3	63.6	10.1	412.4	10.5	6.4	3.7	4.7	4.3	3.1
Peptic ulcer	M	278	27	202	7.0	0.5	12.4	–	–	0.1	0.5	0.3	0.8	1.5
	F	128	16	66	2.4	0.3	3.8	0.1	0.1	0.1	–	0.2	0.4	0.8
Liver cirrhosis and	M	1898	257	1368	44.9	3.4	83.1	4.3	1.8	2.7	3.5	2.4	2.7	6.7
other liver disease	F	1600	191	1004	30.1	2.7	53.5	2.9	1.0	1.5	2.0	2.0	3.4	6.1
Renal disease	M	887	282	480	17.6	4.0	27.8	3.5	1.8	2.3	1.9	5.2	6.4	6.5
	F	831	296	404	12.8	4.3	19.6	3.3	1.5	1.7	3.0	4.9	6.1	9.9
Pregnancy and birth	F	236	163	73	2.5	2.8	2.4	–	–	–	0.5	4.9	5.2	8.9
Congenital and	M	4667	4660	7	22.9	40.7	0.4	278.8	1.7	0.9	1.3	1.0	0.7	0.4
perinatal causes	F	3163	3157	3	16.0	28.5	0.1	194.4	1.0	1.4	1.3	1.0	0.1	0.4
Ill–defined causes	M	773	312	325	14.0	3.6	18.1	11.0	1.0	0.9	1.8	2.4	3.6	4.6
	F	512	242	131	6.8	2.7	6.6	9.5	1.0	0.4	1.6	1.5	2.4	2.8
Other medical causes	M	2879	1419	1139	47.6	16.5	70.4	43.2	9.8	8.8	9.9	13.5	13.5	16.9
	F	2630	1212	960	36.1	14.8	49.7	33.7	8.7	7.5	8.4	14.9	14.8	15.4
ALL NON–	M	9097	5825	2965	112.1	79.8	139.0	96.8	37.2	29.2	45.6	90.9	118.3	140.3
MEDICAL CAUSES	F	3426	2340	803	35.8	27.6	38.0	72.6	17.1	14.0	19.4	23.4	20.0	26.7
Motor vehicle	M	2610	1656	862	33.5	24.8	41.3	10.7	13.0	8.3	14.3	34.2	41.2	51.7
traffic accidents	F	644	381	199	7.7	4.8	9.6	6.3	6.4	3.1	4.2	4.7	4.1	5.0
Fire	M	213	153	53	2.3	1.8	2.5	4.8	1.0	0.9	0.9	1.2	2.0	1.6
	F	224	171	44	2.1	2.1	2.0	4.1	1.2	1.2	1.9	2.1	2.4	1.9
Suicide	M	1013	516	460	14.9	8.4	21.1	–	0.1	3.5	8.3	11.6	15.0	20.3
	F	454	242	165	6.1	3.8	7.8	–	–	1.7	6.9	7.0	4.4	6.4
Homicide	M	976	493	442	14.1	8.2	19.1	0.4	0.2	0.5	4.7	12.3	17.2	22.3
	F	269	115	123	3.9	1.8	5.5	0.7	0.4	0.6	1.0	2.1	3.0	4.9
POPULATION (thousands):	**M=males**				9997	7750	2068	1648	1367	1167	1039	902	893	735
	F=females				10231	7669	2220	1596	1338	1144	1032	916	906	738

UZBEKISTAN: 1990

9th ICD categories

Annual death rates / 100, 000

35–39	40–44	45–49	50–54	55–59	60–64	65–69	70–74	75–79	80+/NK			
331.5	562.9	714.3	1221.2	1698.1	2591.5	3573.1	5528.5	7511.0	13736.5	M	**ALL CAUSES**	001–999
180.4	293.8	378.7	616.5	931.5	1570.8	2159.1	3580.7	5235.3	11521.3	F		
14.8	26.1	27.0	32.9	38.2	47.0	55.8	58.7	42.3	35.9	M	**Tuberculosis**	010–018, 137
7.4	9.4	12.8	13.3	17.9	23.7	23.6	24.7	12.3	14.8	F		
3.9	5.2	4.0	5.6	9.6	11.5	11.9	8.6	9.2	18.0	M	**Other infective**	Rest of 001–139
3.9	4.5	4.1	5.2	3.2	7.9	7.5	4.1	9.5	13.9	F	**and parasitic**	
29.3	64.9	96.8	206.1	331.9	507.3	616.1	846.3	689.3	592.8	M	**ALL CANCER**	140–208
35.7	65.7	90.8	139.2	178.4	307.8	340.7	398.7	500.9	407.5	F		
1.5	3.7	5.8	7.7	15.8	16.8	21.0	29.4	29.4	13.5	M	**Mouth and**	140–149
1.1	0.9	2.3	2.6	2.8	5.3	6.4	9.1	14.2	9.6	F	**pharynx cancer**	
0.8	4.6	12.6	29.9	50.5	87.7	117.0	164.1	117.6	193.1	M	**Oesophagus cancer**	150
0.9	3.3	9.0	14.4	26.7	44.8	65.0	47.0	75.9	71.2	F		
3.9	12.9	18.4	34.9	67.5	99.7	112.4	191.7	172.8	107.8	M	**Stomach cancer**	151
4.1	6.1	10.2	21.3	23.5	49.4	54.8	66.7	77.8	79.1	F		
0.9	3.1	3.6	7.4	9.6	21.7	23.8	46.6	46.0	21.0	M	**Colorectal cancer**	153, 154
2.0	4.8	4.9	5.8	9.5	18.8	19.3	28.0	38.0	26.9	F		
...	...	...	...	...	...	...	...	...	...	M	**Liver cancer**	Not given separately
...	...	...	...	...	...	...	...	...	...	F		
...	...	...	...	...	...	...	...	...	...	M	**Pancreas cancer**	Not given separately
...	...	...	...	...	...	...	...	...	...	F		
0.6	1.2	1.8	5.0	10.0	15.1	19.2	10.4	18.4	7.5	M	**Larynx cancer**	161
–	0.6	0.8	0.6	1.4	1.9	0.5	2.5	2.8	0.9	F		
4.5	10.5	17.6	51.8	70.5	115.6	135.3	134.7	99.3	70.4	M	**Lung cancer**	162
2.0	4.5	4.5	9.2	16.5	30.9	26.3	32.9	52.2	32.1	F		
...	...	...	...	...	...	...	...	...	...	M	**Malignant melanoma**	Not given separately
...	...	...	...	...	...	...	...	...	...	F		
7.2	13.0	17.3	19.6	19.7	32.0	30.1	27.2	45.5	30.4	F	**Female breast cancer**	174
2.2	3.9	4.9	9.5	9.1	14.3	17.2	19.8	18.0	11.3	F	**Cervix cancer**	180
1.8	2.7	4.9	4.9	8.4	9.4	14.0	22.2	20.9	13.9	F	**Other uterine cancer**	179, 182
...	...	...	...	...	...	...	...	...	...	F	**Ovarian cancer**	Not given separately
0.2	0.3	0.4	0.9	5.0	8.9	19.2	31.1	38.6	34.4	M	**Prostate cancer**	185
...	...	...	...	...	...	...	...	...	...	M	**Bladder cancer**	Not given separately
...	...	...	...	...	...	...	...	...	...	F		
11.7	24.0	28.8	57.4	86.7	124.9	146.3	219.3	150.7	128.7	M	**Other and ill-defined**	Rest of 140–208,
10.2	21.8	26.4	43.2	48.5	87.8	97.3	131.8	145.2	120.8	F	**cancer sites**	incl. 155, 157, 172, 183, 188
...	...	...	...	...	...	...	...	...	...	M	**Hodgkin's disease**	Not given separately
...	...	...	...	...	...	...	...	...	...	F		
1.9	2.2	4.7	6.2	8.5	10.6	13.7	10.4	12.9	12.0	M	**Myeloma and all**	200–203,
0.6	0.6	1.9	2.6	6.7	6.0	4.3	4.1	4.7	7.8	F	**lymphomas**	incl. 201
3.4	2.5	3.2	4.7	7.7	6.2	8.2	8.6	3.7	4.5	M	**Leukaemia**	204–208
3.5	3.3	3.8	5.5	5.6	7.2	5.4	7.4	5.7	3.5	F		
80.1	182.3	279.6	533.9	783.7	1385.0	2068.6	3568.2	5507.4	11029.9	M	**ALL VASCULAR**	390–459
44.5	84.2	132.3	255.5	453.8	856.4	1313.8	2485.2	3918.4	9792.4	F	**DISEASE**	
8.8	15.1	16.6	18.7	18.9	12.8	12.8	17.3	23.9	26.9	M	**Rheumatic heart**	390–398
15.2	15.4	20.0	23.6	20.0	17.0	13.4	15.7	17.1	33.0	F	**disease and fever**	
4.7	7.4	14.0	36.1	50.9	86.4	100.5	139.9	176.5	224.6	M	**Hypertensive disease**	401–405
1.8	8.8	11.3	25.9	38.6	59.5	65.6	109.6	103.4	190.3	F		
43.2	103.6	167.3	308.9	424.4	809.9	1266.9	2309.2	3735.3	8122.8	M	**Ischaemic heart**	410–414
12.4	25.4	37.3	90.8	199.5	463.8	774.9	1581.5	2502.8	6861.0	F	**disease**	
...	...	...	...	...	...	...	...	...	...	M	**Pulmonary embolism**	Not given
...	...	...	...	...	...	...	...	...	...	F	**and other venous**	separately
16.7	45.8	66.9	144.5	257.9	424.0	618.8	984.5	1391.5	2275.4	M	**Cerebrovascular**	430–438
10.5	29.1	55.4	104.3	178.4	290.9	414.8	702.6	1172.7	2401.4	F	**disease**	
6.6	10.5	14.8	25.8	31.6	51.8	69.5	117.4	180.1	380.2	M	**Other vascular**	Rest of 390–459,
4.6	5.5	8.3	10.9	17.2	25.2	45.1	75.8	122.4	306.7	F	**disease, incl. venous**	incl. 415, 451–3
7.9	15.1	27.0	55.7	104.9	161.3	281.5	462.9	634.2	1061.4	M	**Chronic obstructive**	490–496
6.7	10.6	17.0	37.7	65.3	108.1	155.8	281.7	346.3	699.4	F	**pulmonary disease**	
5.1	9.5	10.8	18.1	22.0	28.8	28.3	41.5	60.7	118.3	M	**Other respiratory**	Rest of 460–519
4.3	7.3	6.8	6.9	12.6	15.4	17.2	30.5	29.4	79.1	F	**disease**	
2.3	5.5	7.2	13.3	14.6	18.2	25.6	29.4	31.3	22.5	M	**Peptic ulcer**	531–533
0.4	0.9	1.5	3.5	3.5	4.9	11.8	10.7	15.2	14.8	F		
12.8	27.7	52.2	86.2	111.0	143.1	149.0	176.2	139.7	142.2	M	**Liver cirrhosis and**	570–573, 576,
9.6	21.5	29.0	54.5	67.1	82.5	110.2	112.9	107.2	134.7	F	**other liver disease**	575.2–579.9
8.6	18.1	14.0	30.8	33.9	40.3	48.4	48.4	66.2	91.3	M	**Renal disease**	580–590
11.5	14.5	15.1	18.7	22.8	27.5	27.4	32.1	37.0	46.0	F		
8.5	7.6	0.4	–	0.4	–	–	–	–	–	F	**Pregnancy and birth**	630–676
0.2	–	–	0.9	0.4	0.4	0.9	–	–	–	M	**Congenital and**	740–779
–	0.9	–	–	–	–	–	0.8	0.9	0.9	F	**perinatal causes**	
6.0	12.9	15.1	22.2	20.4	22.6	27.4	36.3	42.3	137.7	M	**Ill-defined causes**	780–799
2.2	4.5	4.1	7.8	6.0	11.3	10.2	23.9	30.4	67.8	F		
19.5	29.8	38.9	60.1	85.2	105.4	153.6	153.7	150.7	224.6	M	**Other medical causes**	Rest of 001–799
18.9	23.3	29.8	37.7	65.7	79.9	92.4	110.4	145.2	148.6	F		
141.0	165.7	141.8	155.5	142.3	120.5	106.0	98.4	137.9	262.0	M	**ALL NON–**	E800–E999
27.0	38.8	35.0	36.6	34.8	45.2	48.4	65.1	82.5	101.7	F	**MEDICAL CAUSES**	
41.3	47.0	42.1	40.9	42.8	35.4	39.3	29.4	49.6	71.9	M	**Motor vehicle**	E810–E819
5.7	8.5	9.0	9.5	10.2	11.3	12.9	16.5	23.7	16.5	F	**traffic accidents**	
2.6	2.2	3.2	3.0	3.1	1.3	1.8	3.5	3.7	4.5	M	**Fire**	E890–E899
1.8	3.3	1.1	0.9	2.8	2.3	1.6	1.6	1.9	4.3	F		
22.9	24.9	21.6	23.7	25.4	16.4	12.8	20.7	22.1	19.5	M	**Suicide**	E950–E959
5.4	7.3	8.3	8.6	5.3	10.6	9.1	14.0	11.4	15.6	F		
25.9	27.1	18.4	24.3	16.6	14.2	7.3	5.2	7.4	50.9	M	**Homicide**	E960–E969
5.9	7.6	4.9	5.8	2.8	4.9	6.4	7.4	9.5	10.4	F		
532	325	278	338	259	226	109	58	54	67	M	**POPULATION (thousands)**	
541	330	265	347	285	265	186	121	105	115	F		

UZBEKISTAN: Males

	All ages	0–34	35–69	35–39	40–44	45–49	50–54	55–59	60–64	65–69	70–74	75–79	80+/NK
POPULATION (1000s)													
1985–90	9418	7314	1909	447	277	345	306	267	178	89	66	59	69
1985	8815	6851	1753	344	292	366	286	257	133	76	78	62	71
1990	**9997**	**7750**	**2068**	**532**	**325**	**278**	**338**	**259**	**226**	**109**	**58**	**54**	**67**
1995 projected	*11283*	*8747*	*2333*	*601*	*367*	*314*	*381*	*293*	*255*	*124*	*65*	*61*	*75*
NUMBER OF DEATHS													
All causes													
1985–90	68689	30300	21028	1567	1372	2474	3513	4425	4536	3141	3579	4493	9289
1985	69599	31471	19565	1463	1375	2896	3355	4442	3274	2760	4211	4648	9704
1990	**66659**	**26329**	**23867**	**1764**	**1831**	**1985**	**4124**	**4405**	**5849**	**3909**	**3201**	**4086**	**9176**
1995 projected	*68782*	*22689*	*27010*	*1943*	*1967*	*2298*	*4577*	*5101*	*6630*	*4494*	*3644*	*4872*	*10567*
Lung cancer													
1985–90	1085	30	835	19	27	82	152	218	215	122	105	71	44
1985	934	24	710	13	25	101	136	209	139	87	104	60	36
1990	**1078**	**25**	**874**	**24**	**34**	**49**	**175**	**183**	**261**	**148**	**78**	**54**	**47**
1995 projected	*1233*	*23*	*985*	*29*	*30*	*51*	*174*	*208*	*312*	*181*	*94*	*69*	*62*
ANNUAL DEATH RATE / 100,000 (*The rates for the age groups 0–34 and 35–69 are the means of seven five-yearly rates, but the all-ages rates are standardised to the conventional "European" age distribution)													
All causes													
1985–90	1316.2*	329.9*	1493.9*	350.6	495.5	716.9	1147.3	1654.8	2551.2	3541.1	5398.2	7589.5	13384.7
1985	1357.7*	372.8*	1527.0*	425.3	471.4	792.3	1171.4	1731.1	2470.9	3626.8	5384.9	7448.7	13725.6
1990	**1311.9***	**280.2***	**1527.5***	**331.5**	**562.9**	**714.3**	**1221.2**	**1698.1**	**2591.5**	**3573.1**	**5528.5**	**7511.0**	**13736.5**
1995 projected	*1298.8**	*221.8**	*1539.6**	*323.6*	*535.8*	*732.8*	*1201.0*	*1742.1*	*2603.1*	*3638.9*	*5580.4*	*7934.9*	*14014.6*
All cancer													
1985–90	163.4*	10.0*	283.1*	34.7	60.3	115.0	219.1	356.8	534.3	661.8	841.6	802.4	623.9
1985	160.9*	10.4*	279.1*	39.2	60.7	119.0	222.4	375.7	482.3	654.4	798.0	775.6	628.0
1990	**153.4***	**9.4***	**264.6***	**29.3**	**64.9**	**96.8**	**206.1**	**331.9**	**507.3**	**616.1**	**846.3**	**689.3**	**592.8**
1995 projected	*145.4**	*7.5**	*253.6**	*27.0*	*55.0*	*85.8*	*180.0*	*317.6*	*486.5*	*623.5*	*813.2*	*688.9*	*542.4*
Lung cancer													
1985–90	31.2*	0.5*	61.1*	4.3	9.8	23.8	49.6	81.5	120.9	137.5	158.4	119.9	63.4
1985	28.0*	0.5*	55.4*	3.8	8.6	27.6	47.5	81.4	104.9	114.3	133.0	96.2	50.9
1990	**29.0***	**0.4***	**58.0***	**4.5**	**10.5**	**17.6**	**51.8**	**70.5**	**115.6**	**135.3**	**134.7**	**99.3**	**70.4**
1995 projected	*29.9**	*0.3**	*59.3**	*4.8*	*8.2*	*16.3*	*45.7*	*71.0*	*122.5*	*146.6*	*144.0*	*112.4*	*82.2*
Upper aerodigestive cancer (mouth, oesophagus, pharynx and larynx)													
1985–90	38.8*	0.5*	64.7*	4.5	9.4	23.5	48.0	84.5	125.4	157.8	205.1	226.4	208.9
1985	38.2*	0.7*	62.3*	6.1	8.6	24.4	53.4	89.6	107.2	147.2	199.5	243.6	196.6
1990	**36.1***	**0.5***	**61.2***	**2.8**	**9.5**	**20.2**	**42.6**	**76.3**	**119.6**	**157.2**	**203.8**	**165.4**	**214.1**
1995 projected	*33.7**	*0.4**	*59.9**	*2.2*	*7.6*	*16.3*	*34.9*	*72.1*	*121.7*	*164.4*	*180.7*	*156.4*	*184.4*
Other cancer													
1985–90	93.4*	8.9*	157.4*	26.0	41.2	67.8	121.5	190.7	288.0	366.4	478.1	456.1	351.6
1985	94.7*	9.2*	161.3*	29.4	43.5	67.0	121.5	204.6	270.2	392.9	465.5	435.9	380.5
1990	**88.4***	**8.4***	**145.5***	**22.0**	**44.9**	**59.0**	**111.6**	**185.0**	**272.0**	**323.6**	**507.8**	**424.6**	**308.4**
1995 projected	*81.9**	*6.8**	*134.5**	*20.0*	*39.2*	*53.3*	*99.4*	*174.5*	*242.2*	*312.6*	*488.5*	*420.2*	*275.9*
Chronic obstructive pulmonary disease (COPD)													
1985–90	93.5*	2.7*	100.6*	9.6	17.3	29.8	63.7	110.7	180.0	293.1	517.3	782.1	1259.4
1985	110.6*	2.9*	121.2*	9.3	19.9	38.6	90.8	126.3	219.6	344.3	638.1	876.6	1452.6
1990	**82.3***	**2.9***	**93.3***	**7.9**	**15.1**	**27.0**	**55.7**	**104.9**	**161.3**	**281.5**	**462.9**	**634.2**	**1061.4**
1995 projected	*61.0**	*2.7**	*69.8**	*6.0*	*10.9*	*18.5*	*40.1*	*76.5*	*126.8*	*209.7*	*340.0*	*465.8*	*771.9*
Other respiratory disease													
1985–90	67.3*	102.9*	14.7*	5.1	7.2	9.3	14.4	17.6	23.1	25.9	37.7	52.4	100.9
1985	80.5*	127.5*	13.8*	7.3	5.8	10.9	12.6	16.0	20.4	23.7	29.4	36.9	114.6
1990	**53.6***	**75.3***	**17.5***	**5.1**	**9.5**	**10.8**	**18.1**	**22.0**	**28.8**	**28.3**	**41.5**	**60.7**	**118.3**
1995 projected	*43.9**	*51.9**	*22.5**	*5.5*	*9.8*	*13.7*	*22.8*	*30.4*	*37.7*	*37.2*	*58.2*	*84.7*	*140.6*
Vascular disease													
1985–90	687.6*	11.8*	730.3*	86.8	162.9	268.9	485.3	758.0	1321.7	2028.2	3429.9	5288.9	10507.2
1985	688.7*	13.3*	739.6*	106.4	151.2	275.2	469.3	784.9	1289.1	2101.2	3381.1	5145.8	10601.1
1990	**718.6***	**13.1***	**759.0***	**80.1**	**182.3**	**279.6**	**533.9**	**783.7**	**1385.0**	**2068.6**	**3568.2**	**5507.4**	**11029.9**
1995 projected	*750.0**	*11.2**	*777.3**	*74.9*	*180.6*	*302.3*	*548.4*	*823.1*	*1391.8*	*2119.8*	*3707.5*	*6014.7*	*11583.6*
Liver cirrhosis and other liver disease													
1985–90	42.8*	3.1*	79.0*	14.1	27.8	47.2	79.7	98.7	138.9	146.6	146.3	155.4	161.4
1985	42.2*	2.9*	77.5*	21.8	35.3	61.8	77.2	94.3	112.5	139.3	129.2	141.0	174.0
1990	**44.9***	**3.4***	**83.1***	**12.8**	**27.7**	**52.2**	**86.2**	**111.0**	**143.1**	**149.0**	**176.2**	**139.7**	**142.2**
1995 projected	*48.6**	*3.5**	*92.3**	*8.7*	*21.0*	*48.5*	*90.5*	*131.5*	*164.9*	*181.4*	*197.5*	*154.7*	*127.3*
Other medical causes													
1985–90	160.9*	124.7*	162.3*	65.1	90.3	117.6	152.2	191.1	240.2	279.6	312.2	385.1	573.5
1985	176.5*	143.1*	174.0*	93.3	91.9	149.7	170.0	214.3	247.5	251.0	303.1	367.0	596.9
1990	**146.9***	**96.4***	**170.9***	**55.4**	**97.8**	**106.2**	**165.8**	**202.4**	**245.5**	**323.6**	**335.1**	**341.9**	**529.9**
1995 projected	*126.6**	*65.0**	*166.9**	*39.5*	*73.8*	*92.8*	*144.8*	*194.3*	*263.1*	*360.3*	*361.4*	*350.2*	*478.8*
All non-medical causes													
1985–90	100.7*	74.6*	123.9*	135.1	129.6	128.9	132.9	121.9	113.0	106.0	113.1	123.3	158.5
1985	98.3*	72.5*	121.9*	148.0	106.6	137.1	129.2	119.6	99.6	113.0	106.1	105.8	158.4
1990	**112.1***	**79.8***	**139.0***	**141.0**	**165.7**	**141.8**	**155.5**	**142.3**	**120.5**	**106.0**	**98.4**	**137.9**	**262.0**
1995 projected	*123.4**	*79.9**	*157.2**	*162.0*	*184.7*	*171.2*	*174.2*	*168.7*	*132.3*	*106.9*	*102.6*	*175.9*	*370.0*

UZBEKISTAN: Females

	All ages	0–34	35–69	35–39	40–44	45–49	50–54	55–59	60–64	65–69	70–74	75–79	80+/NK
POPULATION (1000s)													
1985–90	9656	7218	2084	452	269	341	315	298	244	164	132	106	116
1985	9053	6740	1951	344	278	366	304	291	219	150	146	103	114
1990	**10231**	**7669**	**2220**	**541**	**330**	**265**	**347**	**285**	**265**	**186**	**121**	**105**	**115**
1995 projected	*11546*	*8655*	*2505*	*611*	*373*	*300*	*392*	*321*	*300*	*210*	*137*	*119*	*130*
NUMBER OF DEATHS													
All causes													
1985–90	61976	23131	15239	934	786	1322	1998	2851	3636	3712	4600	5727	13279
1985	62087	24348	14471	862	783	1559	1889	2843	3181	3354	4893	5492	12883
1990	**57894**	**18838**	**15930**	**976**	**970**	**1005**	**2140**	**2652**	**4169**	**4018**	**4347**	**5518**	**13261**
1995 projected	*60232*	*15558*	*17814*	*970*	*972*	*1099*	*2298*	*3060*	*4702*	*4713*	*4926*	*6726*	*15208*
Lung cancer													
1985–90	372	16	229	8	10	17	27	47	67	53	52	44	31
1985	337	15	188	6	10	8	24	50	46	44	66	40	28
1990	**394**	**14**	**248**	**11**	**15**	**12**	**32**	**47**	**82**	**49**	**40**	**55**	**37**
1995 projected	*499*	*15*	*312*	*13*	*23*	*18*	*40*	*65*	*101*	*52*	*44*	*73*	*55*
ANNUAL DEATH RATE / 100,000													
All causes													
1985–90	906.2*	251.8*	890.0*	206.8	291.8	387.2	634.1	955.7	1489.6	2264.8	3487.5	5423.3	11437.6
1985	920.3*	287.5*	892.3*	250.9	282.2	426.4	622.4	975.6	1452.5	2236.0	3344.5	5352.8	11320.7
1990	**871.8***	**197.4***	**875.8***	**180.4**	**293.8**	**378.7**	**616.5**	**931.5**	**1570.8**	**2159.1**	**3580.7**	**5235.3**	**11521.3**
1995 projected	*854.7**	*146.5**	*877.1**	*158.9*	*260.8*	*366.9*	*586.7*	*952.4*	*1569.9*	*2244.3*	*3595.6*	*5652.1*	*11707.5*
All cancer													
1985–90	101.2*	8.7*	174.1*	38.5	66.8	94.0	149.8	205.5	301.9	362.4	436.7	468.8	405.7
1985	95.1*	8.4*	166.0*	45.4	62.0	96.6	136.4	206.6	279.9	335.3	388.9	394.7	388.4
1990	**96.9***	**7.7***	**165.5***	**35.7**	**65.7**	**90.8**	**139.2**	**178.4**	**307.8**	**340.7**	**398.7**	**500.9**	**407.5**
1995 projected	*99.8**	*6.7**	*165.1**	*32.6*	*61.4*	*91.2*	*129.7*	*179.3*	*308.5*	*352.9*	*439.4*	*574.8*	*472.7*
Lung cancer													
1985–90	7.6*	0.3*	13.5*	1.8	3.7	5.0	8.6	15.8	27.4	32.3	39.4	41.7	26.7
1985	7.1*	0.3*	11.8*	1.7	3.6	2.2	7.9	17.2	21.0	29.3	45.1	39.0	24.6
1990	**7.8***	**0.2***	**13.4***	**2.0**	**4.5**	**4.5**	**9.2**	**16.5**	**30.9**	**26.3**	**32.9**	**52.2**	**32.1**
1995 projected	*8.7**	*0.2**	*14.7**	*2.1*	*6.2*	*6.0*	*10.2*	*20.2*	*33.7*	*24.8*	*32.1*	*61.3*	*42.3*
Upper aerodigestive cancer (mouth, oesophagus, pharynx and larynx)													
1985–90	17.1*	0.4*	29.5*	3.3	5.9	14.6	24.4	37.5	52.4	68.3	79.6	84.3	92.2
1985	16.9*	0.4*	30.0*	3.5	6.8	17.8	28.3	34.7	54.8	64.0	73.1	60.4	98.4
1990	**15.4***	**0.5***	**27.3***	**2.0**	**4.8**	**12.1**	**17.6**	**30.9**	**52.0**	**72.0**	**58.5**	**93.0**	**81.7**
1995 projected	*14.7**	*0.6**	*24.6**	*1.5*	*3.2*	*8.3*	*13.0*	*26.1*	*52.1*	*68.1*	*65.7*	*98.3*	*90.1*
Other cancer													
1985–90	76.5*	7.9*	131.1*	33.4	57.2	74.4	116.8	152.2	222.0	261.7	317.7	342.8	286.8
1985	71.1*	7.7*	124.2*	40.2	51.5	76.6	100.2	154.8	204.1	242.0	270.7	295.3	265.4
1990	**73.7***	**7.0***	**124.7***	**31.6**	**56.3**	**74.2**	**112.4**	**131.0**	**224.9**	**242.3**	**307.2**	**355.8**	**293.7**
1995 projected	*76.3**	*6.0**	*125.7**	*29.0*	*52.1*	*76.8*	*106.5*	*132.9*	*222.7*	*260.0*	*341.6*	*415.1*	*340.3*
Chronic obstructive pulmonary disease (COPD)													
1985–90	57.8*	2.8*	62.2*	8.4	13.7	20.2	38.7	62.7	109.4	182.4	283.5	417.6	868.2
1985	68.0*	3.2*	73.5*	15.4	17.3	29.3	42.8	71.4	124.7	213.3	308.3	492.2	1048.3
1990	**51.5***	**3.1***	**57.3***	**6.7**	**10.6**	**17.0**	**37.7**	**65.3**	**108.1**	**155.8**	**281.7**	**346.3**	**699.4**
1995 projected	*39.8**	*2.9**	*47.0**	*4.6*	*7.2*	*12.0*	*31.1*	*57.3*	*86.5*	*130.5*	*216.1*	*252.9*	*494.2*
Other respiratory disease													
1985–90	56.0*	89.4*	8.9*	4.2	5.6	5.9	6.7	9.4	13.1	17.7	22.7	36.0	67.2
1985	65.9*	109.0*	7.2*	3.2	5.0	7.7	5.3	4.5	14.6	10.0	15.0	23.4	66.8
1990	**42.3***	**63.6***	**10.1***	**4.3**	**7.3**	**6.8**	**6.9**	**12.6**	**15.4**	**17.2**	**30.5**	**29.4**	**79.1**
1995 projected	*34.3**	*45.2**	*13.5**	*5.1*	*8.0*	*7.7*	*9.7*	*17.7*	*21.7*	*24.3*	*43.1*	*41.2*	*95.5*
Vascular disease													
1985–90	512.2*	11.1*	455.3*	49.6	83.9	140.9	267.2	462.6	798.4	1384.4	2408.6	4092.8	9584.8
1985	507.6*	13.0*	459.5*	59.1	91.9	156.5	286.7	471.2	768.5	1382.7	2328.8	4058.5	9329.5
1990	**512.9***	**10.9***	**448.7***	**44.5**	**84.2**	**132.3**	**255.5**	**453.8**	**856.4**	**1313.8**	**2485.2**	**3918.4**	**9792.4**
1995 projected	*519.3**	*8.9**	*445.7**	*35.9*	*68.7*	*113.2*	*232.6*	*462.8*	*852.1*	*1354.8*	*2447.4*	*4238.7*	*10028.5*
Liver cirrhosis and other liver disease													
1985–90	28.6*	2.9*	49.9*	11.1	17.4	27.8	48.9	65.0	79.9	98.8	99.3	112.7	137.8
1985	26.8*	2.8*	46.0*	12.2	15.9	26.8	40.9	66.6	76.7	82.7	91.6	123.8	118.6
1990	**30.1***	**2.7***	**53.5***	**9.6**	**21.5**	**29.0**	**54.5**	**67.1**	**82.5**	**110.2**	**112.9**	**107.2**	**134.7**
1995 projected	*33.4**	*2.5**	*61.3**	*10.2*	*22.5*	*35.4*	*60.5*	*73.8*	*94.2*	*132.9*	*124.1*	*114.3*	*134.7*
Other medical causes													
1985–90	115.1*	108.0*	103.7*	66.6	71.3	68.2	87.3	116.7	142.6	173.3	181.2	215.0	280.8
1985	120.5*	120.0*	103.7*	81.5	62.3	76.0	82.7	118.4	137.0	168.0	160.6	192.0	268.9
1990	**102.2***	**81.8***	**102.9***	**52.7**	**65.7**	**67.8**	**86.1**	**119.4**	**155.2**	**173.0**	**206.8**	**250.5**	**306.7**
1995 projected	*92.7**	*56.7**	*104.5**	*41.8*	*53.4*	*65.4*	*84.0*	*126.7*	*163.3*	*197.1*	*248.2*	*331.1*	*371.1*
All non-medical causes													
1985–90	35.2*	29.0*	35.9*	28.3	33.0	30.2	35.5	33.9	44.2	45.8	55.3	80.5	93.0
1985	36.3*	31.1*	36.5*	34.1	27.7	33.6	27.7	37.1	51.1	44.0	51.3	68.2	100.2
1990	**35.8***	**27.6***	**38.0***	**27.0**	**38.8**	**35.0**	**36.6**	**34.8**	**45.2**	**48.4**	**65.1**	**82.5**	**101.7**
1995 projected	*35.4**	*23.6**	*40.0**	*28.8*	*39.4*	*42.1*	*39.1*	*34.9*	*43.7*	*51.9*	*77.4*	*99.2*	*110.9*

(*The rates for the age groups 0–34 and 35–69 are the means of seven five-yearly rates, but the all-ages rates are standardised to the conventional "European" age distribution)

UZBEKISTAN: 1985–1990

Smoking–attributed deaths (Sm.) and total deaths (Total)

		ALL CAUSES	ALL CANCER	Lung cancer	Upper aero–digestive ca.	Other cancer	COPD	Other respiratory	Vascular disease	Cirrhosis/other liver	Other medical	Non–medical
Males												
0–34	Sm.	–	–	–	–	–	–	–	–	–	–	–
	Total	30300	659	30	31	598	199	11002	659	207	12303	5271
35–69	Sm.	4586	1348	724	426	198	811	50	1822	–	555	–
	Total	21028	3881	835	863	2183	1265	230	9429	1188	2599	2436
		(22%)	(35%)	(87%)	(49%)	(9%)	(64%)	(22%)	(19%)		(21%)	
70+	Sm.	1258	282	152	102	28	589	5	356	–	26	–
	Total	17361	1466	220	415	831	1680	126	12697	301	833	258
		(7%)	(19%)	(69%)	(25%)	(3%)	(35%)	(4%)	(3%)		(3%)	
Any age	Sm.	5844	1630	876	528	226	1400	55	2178	–	581	–
	Total	68689	6006	1085	1309	3612	3144	11358	22785	1696	15735	7965
		(9%)	(27%)	(81%)	(40%)	(6%)	(45%)	(0%)	(10%)		(4%)	
Females												
0–34	Sm.	–	–	–	–	–	–	–	–	–	–	–
	Total	23131	546	16	25	505	189	9267	639	180	9929	2381
35–69	Sm.	680	138	74	55	9	222	5	253	–	62	–
	Total	15239	3091	229	510	2352	1019	164	7371	897	1981	716
		(4%)	(4%)	(32%)	(11%)	(0%)	(22%)	(3%)	(3%)		(3%)	
70+	Sm.	373	49	27	19	3	205	1	111	–	7	–
	Total	23606	1542	127	301	1114	1823	146	18627	410	792	266
		(2%)	(3%)	(21%)	(6%)	(0%)	(11%)	(1%)	(1%)		(1%)	
Any age	Sm.	1053	187	101	74	12	427	6	364	–	69	–
	Total	61976	5179	372	836	3971	3031	9577	26637	1487	12702	3363
		(2%)	(4%)	(27%)	(9%)	(0%)	(14%)	(0%)	(1%)		(1%)	
Males+Females												
0–34	Sm.	–	–	–	–	–	–	–	–	–	–	–
	Total	53431	1205	46	56	1103	388	20269	1298	387	22232	7652
35–69	Sm.	5266	1486	798	481	207	1033	55	2075	–	617	–
	Total	36267	6972	1064	1373	4535	2284	394	16800	2085	4580	3152
		(15%)	(21%)	(75%)	(35%)	(5%)	(45%)	(14%)	(12%)		(13%)	
70+	Sm.	1631	331	179	121	31	794	6	467	–	33	–
	Total	40967	3008	347	716	1945	3503	272	31324	711	1625	524
		(4%)	(11%)	(52%)	(17%)	(2%)	(23%)	(2%)	(1%)		(2%)	
Any age	Sm.	6897	1817	977	602	238	1827	61	2542	–	650	–
	Total	130665	11185	1457	2145	7583	6175	20935	49422	3183	28437	11328
		(5%)	(16%)	(67%)	(28%)	(3%)	(30%)	(0%)	(5%)		(2%)	

UZBEKISTAN: 1985

Smoking–attributed deaths (Sm.) and total deaths (Total)

		ALL CAUSES	ALL CANCER	Lung cancer	Upper aero–digestive ca.	Other cancer	COPD	Other respiratory	Vascular disease	Cirrhosis/other liver	Other medical	Non–medical
Males												
0–34	Sm.	–	–	–	–	–	–	–	–	–	–	–
	Total	31471	628	24	35	569	185	12432	646	157	12587	4836
35–69	Sm.	4245	1158	611	372	175	854	44	1607	–	582	–
	Total	19565	3485	710	772	2003	1368	204	8478	1122	2692	2216
		(22%)	(33%)	(86%)	(48%)	(9%)	(62%)	(22%)	(19%)		(22%)	
70+	Sm.	1159	239	127	89	23	603	2	294	–	21	–
	Total	18563	1552	200	447	905	2073	127	13350	312	888	261
		(6%)	(15%)	(64%)	(20%)	(3%)	(29%)	(2%)	(2%)		(2%)	
Any age	Sm.	5404	1397	738	461	198	1457	46	1901	–	603	–
	Total	69599	5665	934	1254	3477	3626	12763	22474	1591	16167	7313
		(8%)	(25%)	(79%)	(37%)	(6%)	(40%)	(0%)	(8%)		(4%)	
Females												
0–34	Sm.	–	–	–	–	–	–	–	–	–	–	–
	Total	24348	487	15	21	451	189	10340	662	155	10103	2412
35–69	Sm.	451	87	45	36	6	172	1	153	–	38	–
	Total	14471	2813	188	499	2126	1139	129	7030	794	1879	687
		(3%)	(3%)	(24%)	(7%)	(0%)	(15%)	(1%)	(2%)		(2%)	
70+	Sm.	389	52	31	19	2	208	1	121	–	7	–
	Total	23268	1416	134	281	1001	2149	122	18188	396	738	259
		(2%)	(4%)	(23%)	(7%)	(0%)	(10%)	(1%)	(1%)		(1%)	
Any age	Sm.	840	139	76	55	8	380	2	274	–	45	–
	Total	62087	4716	337	801	3578	3477	10591	25880	1345	12720	3358
		(1%)	(3%)	(23%)	(7%)	(0%)	(11%)	(0%)	(1%)		(0%)	
Males+Females												
0–34	Sm.	–	–	–	–	–	–	–	–	–	–	–
	Total	55819	1115	39	56	1020	374	22772	1308	312	22690	7248
35–69	Sm.	4696	1245	656	408	181	1026	45	1760	–	620	–
	Total	34036	6298	898	1271	4129	2507	333	15508	1916	4571	2903
		(14%)	(20%)	(73%)	(32%)	(4%)	(41%)	(14%)	(11%)		(14%)	
70+	Sm.	1548	291	158	108	25	811	3	415	–	28	–
	Total	41831	2968	334	728	1906	4222	249	31538	708	1626	520
		(4%)	(10%)	(47%)	(15%)	(1%)	(19%)	(1%)	(1%)		(2%)	
Any age	Sm.	6244	1536	814	516	206	1837	48	2175	–	648	–
	Total	131686	10381	1271	2055	7055	7103	23354	48354	2936	28887	10671
		(5%)	(15%)	(64%)	(25%)	(3%)	(26%)	(0%)	(4%)		(2%)	

(To be conservative, no deaths before age 35, and none from liver cirrhosis or non–medical causes, were attributed to smoking.)

UZBEKISTAN: 1990

Smoking-attributed deaths (Sm.) and total deaths (Total)

		ALL CAUSES	ALL CANCER	Lung cancer	Upper aero-digestive ca.	Other cancer	COPD	Other respiratory	Vascular disease	Cirrhosis/ other liver	Other medical	Non-medical
Males												
0–34	Sm.	–	–	–	–	–	–	–	–	–	–	–
	Total	26329	651	25	36	590	228	8509	840	257	10019	5825
35–69	Sm.	4724	1355	749	417	189	805	59	1946	–	559	–
	Total	23867	4012	874	886	2252	1298	302	11021	1368	2901	2965
		(20%)	(34%)	(86%)	(47%)	(8%)	(62%)	(20%)	(18%)		(19%)	
70+	Sm.	880	205	114	71	20	387	3	266	–	19	–
	Total	16463	1261	179	351	731	1322	136	12430	273	734	307
		(5%)	(16%)	(64%)	(20%)	(3%)	(29%)	(2%)	(2%)		(3%)	
Any age	Sm.	5604	1560	863	488	209	1192	62	2212	–	578	–
	Total	66659	5924	1078	1273	3573	2848	8947	24291	1898	13654	9097
		(8%)	(26%)	(80%)	(38%)	(6%)	(42%)	(1%)	(9%)		(4%)	
Females												
0–34	Sm.	–	–	–	–	–	–	–	–	–	–	–
	Total	18838	519	14	31	474	236	6937	706	191	7909	2340
35–69	Sm.	748	155	86	58	11	226	9	286	–	72	–
	Total	15930	3093	248	480	2365	1010	198	7767	1004	2055	803
		(5%)	(5%)	(35%)	(12%)	(0%)	(22%)	(5%)	(4%)		(4%)	
70+	Sm.	530	67	37	25	5	287	1	167	–	8	–
	Total	23126	1481	132	263	1086	1512	159	18418	405	868	283
		(2%)	(5%)	(28%)	(10%)	(0%)	(19%)	(1%)	(1%)		(1%)	
Any age	Sm.	1278	222	123	83	16	513	10	453	–	80	–
	Total	57894	5093	394	774	3925	2758	7294	26891	1600	10832	3426
		(2%)	(4%)	(31%)	(11%)	(0%)	(19%)	(0%)	(2%)		(1%)	
Males+Females												
0–34	Sm.	–	–	–	–	–	–	–	–	–	–	–
	Total	45167	1170	39	67	1064	464	15446	1546	448	17928	8165
35–69	Sm.	5472	1510	835	475	200	1031	68	2232	–	631	–
	Total	39797	7105	1122	1366	4617	2308	500	18788	2372	4956	3768
		(14%)	(21%)	(74%)	(35%)	(4%)	(45%)	(14%)	(12%)		(13%)	
70+	Sm.	1410	272	151	96	25	674	4	433	–	27	–
	Total	39589	2742	311	614	1817	2834	295	30848	678	1602	590
		(4%)	(10%)	(49%)	(16%)	(1%)	(24%)	(1%)	(1%)		(2%)	
Any age	Sm.	6882	1782	986	571	225	1705	72	2665	–	658	–
	Total	124553	11017	1472	2047	7498	5606	16241	51182	3498	24486	12523
		(6%)	(16%)	(67%)	(28%)	(3%)	(30%)	(0%)	(5%)		(3%)	

UZBEKISTAN: 1995

Smoking-attributed deaths (Sm.) and total deaths (Total)

		ALL CAUSES	ALL CANCER	Lung cancer	Upper aero-digestive ca.	Other cancer	COPD	Other respiratory	Vascular disease	Cirrhosis/ other liver	Other medical	Non-medical
Males												
0–34	Sm.	–	–	–	–	–	–	–	–	–	–	–
	Total	22689	599	23	34	542	271	6602	860	323	7672	6362
35–69	Sm.	5026	1485	845	447	193	680	82	2222	–	557	–
	Total	27010	4258	985	949	2324	1093	430	12724	1655	3035	3815
		(19%)	(35%)	(86%)	(47%)	(8%)	(62%)	(19%)	(17%)		(18%)	
70+	Sm.	1009	256	150	81	25	358	5	365	–	25	–
	Total	19083	1363	225	353	785	1090	196	14848	320	812	454
		(5%)	(19%)	(67%)	(23%)	(3%)	(33%)	(3%)	(2%)		(3%)	
Any age	Sm.	6035	1741	995	528	218	1038	87	2587	–	582	–
	Total	68782	6220	1233	1336	3651	2454	7228	28432	2298	11519	10631
		(9%)	(28%)	(81%)	(40%)	(6%)	(42%)	(1%)	(9%)		(5%)	
Females												
0–34	Sm.	–	–	–	–	–	–	–	–	–	–	–
	Total	15558	512	15	40	457	277	5519	684	216	6188	2162
35–69	Sm.	1010	221	132	72	17	250	16	407	–	116	–
	Total	17814	3450	312	480	2658	930	295	8609	1287	2289	954
		(6%)	(6%)	(42%)	(15%)	(1%)	(27%)	(5%)	(5%)		(5%)	
70+	Sm.	721	111	62	42	7	310	3	281	–	16	–
	Total	26860	1900	172	324	1404	1239	232	21424	481	1216	368
		(3%)	(6%)	(36%)	(13%)	(0%)	(25%)	(1%)	(1%)		(1%)	
Any age	Sm.	1731	332	194	114	24	560	19	688	–	132	–
	Total	60232	5862	499	844	4519	2446	6046	30717	1984	9693	3484
		(3%)	(6%)	(39%)	(14%)	(1%)	(23%)	(0%)	(2%)		(1%)	
Males+Females												
0–34	Sm.	–	–	–	–	–	–	–	–	–	–	–
	Total	38247	1111	38	74	999	548	12121	1544	539	13860	8524
35–69	Sm.	6036	1706	977	519	210	930	98	2629	–	673	–
	Total	44824	7708	1297	1429	4982	2023	725	21333	2942	5324	4769
		(13%)	(22%)	(75%)	(36%)	(4%)	(46%)	(14%)	(12%)		(13%)	
70+	Sm.	1730	367	212	123	32	668	8	646	–	41	–
	Total	45943	3263	397	677	2189	2329	428	36272	801	2028	822
		(4%)	(11%)	(53%)	(18%)	(1%)	(29%)	(2%)	(2%)		(2%)	
Any age	Sm.	7766	2073	1189	642	242	1598	106	3275	–	714	–
	Total	129014	12082	1732	2180	8170	4900	13274	59149	4282	21212	14115
		(6%)	(17%)	(69%)	(29%)	(3%)	(33%)	(1%)	(6%)		(3%)	

(To be conservative, no deaths before age 35, and none from liver cirrhosis or non-medical causes, were attributed to smoking.)

¶Former YUGOSLAVIA: 1990

		No. of deaths			Standardised rates (Defined on p.550)			Annual death rates / 100, 000						
		All ages	**0–34**	**35–69**	**All ages**	**0–34**	**35–69**	**0–4**	**5–9**	**10–14**	**15–19**	**20–24**	**25–29**	**30–34**
ALL CAUSES	**M**	112832	9091	54092	1217.4	141.9	1389.6	457.9	37.2	31.4	71.0	109.7	128.0	158.5
	F	99316	5376	31267	790.9	90.0	692.9	399.1	26.3	21.0	32.1	38.3	47.3	65.7
Tuberculosis	**M**	848	45	547	8.8	0.7	13.2	0.3	0.2	–	0.4	0.7	0.8	2.3
	F	376	29	176	3.0	0.5	3.8	0.5	0.2	0.1	0.1	0.5	1.1	0.8
Other infective	**M**	539	360	108	5.1	5.8	2.6	37.9	0.9	0.1	0.4	0.2	0.6	0.3
and parasitic	**F**	506	353	92	4.6	6.1	2.0	40.2	0.5	0.6	0.3	0.5	0.1	0.2
ALL CANCER	**M**	21840	533	14860	229.6	8.2	384.2	6.3	5.4	4.0	6.4	7.2	9.1	18.7
	F	15728	453	9303	129.0	7.3	201.5	4.5	4.0	3.1	5.2	4.3	10.2	19.6
Mouth and	**M**	985	8	804	10.0	0.1	19.3	–	0.1	–	–	0.2	0.1	0.4
pharynx cancer	**F**	169	7	80	1.4	0.1	1.8	0.1	–	–	0.1	0.1	0.2	0.2
Oesophagus cancer	**M**	503	5	386	5.1	0.1	9.5	–	–	–	–	0.1	–	0.4
	F	116	1	51	0.9	0.0	1.1	0.1	–	–	–	–	–	–
Stomach cancer	**M**	2373	24	1525	25.6	0.4	40.5	–	0.2	–	–	0.3	0.4	1.6
	F	1431	20	745	11.7	0.3	16.4	0.1	–	0.2	0.2	0.2	1.0	0.4
Colorectal cancer	**M**	1871	25	1116	20.3	0.4	29.8	–	–	–	–	0.5	0.2	1.9
	F	1748	15	898	14.2	0.2	19.9	0.1	–	–	0.1	–	0.6	0.9
Liver cancer	**M**	...	...	...	...	...	...	...	...	...	...	...	...	...
	F	...	...	...	...	...	...	...	...	...	...	...	...	...
Pancreas cancer	**M**	903	5	601	9.7	0.1	15.5	–	–	0.1	0.1	–	0.1	0.2
	F	713	5	390	5.8	0.1	8.6	–	–	–	–	–	0.3	0.2
Larynx cancer	**M**	896	3	683	9.3	0.0	17.4	–	–	0.1	–	0.1	0.1	–
	F	84	1	49	0.7	0.0	1.1	–	–	–	–	–	0.1	–
Lung cancer	**M**	6898	29	5376	71.0	0.4	138.2	–	0.1	–	0.4	0.2	0.2	2.1
	F	1304	15	843	10.8	0.2	18.3	–	–	0.1	0.1	–	0.4	1.0
Malignant melanoma	**M**	199	16	133	2.0	0.2	3.1	–	–	–	–	0.1	0.6	1.0
	F	188	16	105	1.5	0.3	2.2	–	0.1	–	–	0.1	0.6	1.0
Female breast cancer	**F**	2642	43	1875	22.1	0.7	39.7	–	–	–	–	0.1	1.7	3.0
Cervix cancer	**F**	688	31	516	5.8	0.5	10.9	–	–	–	–	–	0.8	2.7
Other uterine cancer	**F**	798	15	503	6.5	0.2	10.9	–	–	–	–	0.1	0.4	1.1
Ovarian cancer	**F**	796	16	581	6.7	0.3	12.4	–	–	–	0.2	0.1	0.4	1.0
Prostate cancer	**M**	1266	–	418	14.8	–	12.4	–	–	–	–	–	–	–
Bladder cancer	**M**	648	2	332	7.3	0.0	9.3	–	–	–	–	–	–	0.2
	F	220	–	87	1.8	–	2.0	–	–	–	–	–	–	–
Other and ill-defined	**M**	4156	265	2766	43.0	4.1	70.8	3.7	2.7	2.0	3.5	4.1	4.6	7.8
cancer sites	**F**	3937	149	2101	32.0	2.4	46.0	1.8	2.0	1.5	2.6	1.8	2.3	4.6
Hodgkin's disease	**M**	110	12	82	1.1	0.2	1.9	–	–	–	0.1	0.2	0.5	0.4
	F	84	17	43	0.7	0.3	0.9	–	–	0.1	0.5	0.3	0.3	0.7
Myeloma and non–	**M**	415	37	285	4.2	0.6	7.3	0.2	1.1	0.4	0.3	0.1	0.8	1.0
Hodgkin lymphomas	**F**	363	27	214	2.9	0.4	4.7	0.4	0.1	0.2	0.6	0.1	0.6	1.1
Leukaemia	**M**	617	102	353	6.2	1.6	9.0	2.4	1.3	1.4	1.9	1.1	1.4	1.6
	F	447	75	222	3.7	1.2	4.8	1.8	1.7	0.9	0.8	1.3	0.4	1.7
ALL VASCULAR	**M**	52774	627	21117	597.7	9.7	567.0	16.3	2.0	2.2	6.3	8.0	11.2	21.5
DISEASE	**F**	57907	368	13696	452.3	6.0	311.3	12.9	2.0	3.3	2.7	3.8	6.1	11.2
Rheumatic heart	**M**	191	9	151	1.9	0.1	3.6	–	–	0.1	–	0.3	0.4	0.1
disease and fever	**F**	250	5	161	2.1	0.1	3.5	–	–	0.1	–	0.1	0.2	0.1
Hypertensive disease	**M**	1943	9	651	22.5	0.1	18.1	–	–	–	–	0.3	0.1	0.5
	F	3231	4	713	25.3	0.1	16.4	–	–	–	–	–	0.2	0.2
Ischaemic heart	**M**	11963	138	7927	127.0	2.1	202.7	–	–	–	0.6	1.2	3.7	9.1
disease	**F**	7249	43	3103	58.0	0.7	69.2	–	–	–	0.1	0.8	0.9	3.0
Pulmonary embolism	**M**	...	...	...	...	...	...	...	...	...	...	...	...	...
and other venous	**F**	...	...	...	...	...	...	...	...	...	...	...	...	...
Cerebrovascular	**M**	13969	160	5614	159.2	2.5	154.4	3.9	0.4	0.6	1.6	2.5	2.3	5.8
disease	**F**	16768	108	4740	132.4	1.8	108.1	3.0	0.5	1.0	1.1	1.5	1.1	4.1
Other vascular	**M**	24708	311	6774	287.0	4.8	188.2	12.4	1.6	1.5	4.1	3.7	4.7	5.9
disease, incl. venous	**F**	30409	208	4979	234.6	3.4	114.2	9.9	1.6	2.2	1.5	1.4	3.6	3.8
Chronic obstructive	**M**	3783	16	1435	43.5	0.2	40.6	0.2	0.3	0.2	–	0.2	0.4	0.3
pulmonary disease	**F**	2249	18	656	17.7	0.3	15.0	0.6	0.1	0.1	0.2	0.3	0.2	0.4
Other respiratory	**M**	1860	443	590	19.7	7.1	14.8	40.0	2.0	1.6	1.9	1.1	1.1	1.7
disease	**F**	1717	444	320	14.1	7.6	7.2	45.2	1.6	1.0	1.6	0.9	1.5	1.1
Peptic ulcer	**M**	498	9	278	5.5	0.1	7.3	–	–	–	0.2	0.2	0.1	0.4
	F	289	1	101	2.3	0.0	2.2	–	–	–	–	–	0.1	–
Liver cirrhosis	**M**	2878	42	2404	28.8	0.6	57.3	–	–	–	0.3	0.2	1.4	2.5
	F	1093	18	839	9.0	0.3	18.0	0.2	0.1	0.2	0.1	0.1	0.3	0.9
Renal disease	**M**	1292	44	667	14.0	0.7	17.6	1.0	0.2	–	0.2	1.0	1.1	1.3
	F	1177	37	550	9.5	0.6	12.1	0.6	0.1	0.3	0.3	0.9	0.7	1.2
Pregnancy and birth	**F**	36	29	7	0.3	0.5	0.1	–	–	–	0.3	1.0	0.8	1.1
Congenital and	**M**	2303	2278	22	20.7	36.6	0.5	250.1	1.8	0.8	0.7	0.3	1.4	1.1
perinatal causes	**F**	1738	1709	19	16.6	29.4	0.4	200.6	1.3	1.3	0.9	0.5	0.6	0.4
Ill-defined causes	**M**	7890	1007	3126	84.9	15.8	75.4	63.3	4.5	3.7	6.6	8.6	11.8	12.3
	F	7103	725	1472	56.3	12.2	31.9	62.8	3.2	1.5	2.1	5.2	4.3	6.4
Other medical causes	**M**	6343	613	3517	66.8	9.5	88.9	26.0	3.3	3.7	6.5	4.9	7.6	14.6
	F	5476	420	2331	44.2	6.9	52.0	21.2	3.6	2.9	2.9	4.9	6.6	6.3
ALL NON–	**M**	9984	3074	5421	92.4	47.0	120.2	16.3	16.5	15.2	40.9	77.2	81.3	81.4
MEDICAL CAUSES	**F**	3921	772	1705	32.0	12.5	35.2	9.8	9.6	6.5	15.1	15.4	14.7	16.1
Motor vehicle	**M**	3095	1312	1536	27.1	20.0	33.0	3.8	8.7	7.2	19.6	37.6	32.0	31.4
traffic accidents	**F**	875	334	394	7.2	5.4	8.0	2.4	5.8	2.8	7.2	7.2	6.8	5.4
Fire	**M**	137	51	50	1.3	0.8	1.2	1.1	0.3	–	0.3	1.3	1.5	1.0
	F	85	10	25	0.7	0.2	0.5	0.5	0.3	–	0.1	0.1	–	0.1
Suicide	**M**	2549	523	1578	24.3	8.0	35.7	–	–	2.1	6.4	12.8	15.9	18.6
	F	1104	164	680	9.2	2.6	14.0	–	–	1.0	3.3	3.9	4.6	5.5
Homicide	**M**	344	139	188	3.0	2.1	3.9	0.9	–	0.4	1.7	2.7	4.2	4.9
	F	128	37	78	1.1	0.6	1.5	0.5	0.3	–	0.5	0.8	0.8	1.3
POPULATION (thousands):	**M=males**				11781	6526	4734	888	936	958	935	922	944	943
	F=females				12037	6187	5030	830	879	905	885	877	906	905

Former YUGOSLAVIA: 1990

Annual death rates / 100, 000

9th ICD categories

35–39	40–44	45–49	50–54	55–59	60–64	65–69	70–74	75–79	80+/NK			
243.2	353.7	603.3	976.6	1610.6	2408.6	3531.0	5249.0	8575.6	15180.9	M	**ALL CAUSES**	001–999
110.1	169.1	281.6	438.0	689.8	1171.2	1990.7	3428.6	6136.7	13389.2	F		
3.9	5.9	8.7	10.6	16.4	21.4	25.9	36.6	52.4	58.9	M	**Tuberculosis**	010–018, 137
1.0	1.9	1.9	1.9	4.3	5.9	9.9	14.0	24.9	23.1	F		
0.9	1.3	1.1	2.1	3.5	4.2	5.0	10.3	12.0	19.0	M	**Other infective**	Rest of 001–139
0.2	0.8	0.6	1.2	2.2	4.2	4.9	4.5	5.9	11.9	F	**and parasitic**	
36.3	69.4	144.3	270.7	494.1	721.1	953.3	1099.6	1312.1	1300.4	M	**ALL CANCER**	140–208
38.3	69.1	114.6	162.2	229.1	332.4	464.8	591.4	712.5	877.2	F		
1.6	6.2	11.6	23.0	29.1	32.1	31.4	33.8	32.2	33.7	M	**Mouth and**	140–149
0.2	0.4	1.1	1.0	1.9	3.0	4.9	6.1	9.0	14.9	F	**pharynx cancer**	
0.5	2.0	4.6	8.9	13.4	21.2	15.8	17.2	28.9	17.8	M	**Oesophagus cancer**	150
0.2	0.1	0.8	0.8	1.6	1.5	2.7	5.3	8.3	9.7	F		
2.9	6.8	13.8	25.1	49.0	70.4	115.5	146.0	168.6	159.4	M	**Stomach cancer**	151
2.8	4.0	6.9	11.8	15.5	30.9	42.7	68.9	81.3	92.9	F		
2.6	5.0	9.9	19.6	32.6	51.4	87.6	113.3	159.8	146.5	M	**Colorectal cancer**	153, 154
2.1	4.4	10.4	13.1	22.4	32.5	54.1	72.3	95.5	137.3	F		
...	...	...	...	...	...	...	...	...	...	M	**Liver cancer**	Not given separately
...	...	...	...	...	...	...	...	...	...	F		
2.1	2.9	6.1	12.8	16.3	30.0	38.2	58.4	56.2	56.4	M	**Pancreas cancer**	157
0.8	1.4	2.0	5.3	11.6	16.5	22.5	38.6	34.9	42.9	F		
1.7	3.2	7.6	12.7	23.1	34.6	39.0	42.9	38.2	39.9	M	**Larynx cancer**	161
0.2	0.1	0.8	0.4	0.5	3.3	2.2	4.9	3.8	3.7	F		
8.5	20.1	47.2	94.7	200.8	272.6	323.9	313.1	318.6	221.9	M	**Lung cancer**	162
2.9	4.0	8.3	19.2	21.4	30.0	42.0	51.5	58.8	52.2	F		
1.6	1.4	2.7	3.2	2.7	4.6	5.8	7.4	7.6	14.1	M	**Malignant melanoma**	172
0.8	2.9	1.6	2.0	2.0	1.9	4.2	3.4	6.6	14.6	F		
8.8	22.2	34.6	41.8	44.1	58.0	68.5	66.6	90.3	107.1	F	**Female breast cancer**	174
4.0	6.1	9.2	9.0	12.1	16.8	19.0	18.9	15.9	16.8	F	**Cervix cancer**	180
2.3	3.2	5.6	8.6	14.1	16.6	25.8	27.6	37.7	36.6	F	**Other uterine cancer**	179, 182
2.3	5.1	8.6	12.4	15.2	20.2	23.0	26.9	24.2	21.6	F	**Ovarian cancer**	183
0.3	0.4	0.6	3.4	8.6	23.7	50.1	90.4	164.2	238.5	M	**Prostate cancer**	185
0.4	0.8	1.3	4.1	10.2	16.4	31.9	44.6	62.2	74.8	M	**Bladder cancer**	188
0.1	0.4	0.3	0.8	1.9	2.8	7.7	11.7	14.9	22.0	F		
9.9	15.3	31.5	51.8	86.8	129.0	171.5	184.9	220.4	244.0	M	**Other and ill-defined**	Rest of 140–208,
8.1	11.8	19.8	30.1	52.9	81.1	118.2	160.5	193.4	262.7	F	**cancer sites**	incl. 155
0.5	1.8	1.1	1.7	2.3	2.8	3.2	3.4	4.9	0.6	M	**Hodgkin's disease**	201
0.8	0.6	0.3	0.3	1.1	1.8	1.3	2.7	1.7	4.5	F		
1.3	1.1	2.7	4.9	8.9	14.8	17.4	17.7	21.8	13.5	M	**Myeloma and non-**	200, 202–203
1.1	0.5	1.2	2.9	5.4	7.7	14.4	11.7	15.6	17.2	F	**Hodgkin lymphomas**	
2.5	2.5	3.6	4.7	10.2	17.5	21.9	26.3	28.4	39.2	M	**Leukaemia**	204–208
0.8	1.8	3.3	2.9	5.5	8.0	11.7	13.6	20.4	20.5	F		
49.2	88.7	185.2	334.7	611.1	1023.8	1676.3	2820.3	5203.5	10156.3	M	**ALL VASCULAR**	390–459
22.3	40.3	77.2	152.4	277.5	542.6	1067.0	2104.1	4174.7	9784.0	F	**DISEASE**	
0.5	1.1	3.5	3.7	4.9	5.5	6.3	6.3	6.5	4.9	M	**Rheumatic heart**	390–398
0.9	0.9	2.3	2.6	4.2	5.6	7.9	9.8	11.4	9.3	F	**disease and fever**	
0.5	2.4	4.2	10.6	17.0	31.8	59.9	118.5	217.1	415.7	M	**Hypertensive disease**	401–405
0.8	1.8	3.0	8.0	14.5	25.7	60.8	129.9	260.2	529.5	F		
22.9	43.9	91.9	151.6	256.8	368.4	483.5	597.6	752.9	903.7	M	**Ischaemic heart**	410–414
5.5	9.6	17.9	40.3	75.3	133.8	202.0	326.0	457.8	716.0	F	**disease**	
...	...	...	...	...	...	...	...	...	...	M	**Pulmonary embolism**	Not given
...	...	...	...	...	...	...	...	...	...	F	**and other venous**	separately
11.4	19.9	40.1	82.0	154.9	271.1	501.2	896.4	1560.8	2310.2	M	**Cerebrovascular**	430–438
6.9	14.7	29.0	51.6	92.5	183.6	378.6	734.2	1294.1	2328.7	F	**disease**	
13.9	21.3	45.5	86.8	177.4	347.0	625.4	1201.5	2666.1	6521.8	M	**Other vascular**	Rest of 390–459,
8.3	13.4	25.1	50.0	91.1	193.9	417.7	904.2	2151.2	6200.4	F	**disease, incl. venous**	incl. 415, 451–3
1.5	2.1	3.8	15.9	40.4	80.7	139.8	252.4	423.9	683.0	M	**Chronic obstructive**	490–496
0.8	1.0	3.3	6.3	12.4	30.3	50.8	96.2	178.5	300.4	F	**pulmonary disease**	
3.1	4.8	7.2	11.6	17.4	25.2	34.3	63.5	152.8	267.3	M	**Other respiratory**	Rest of 460–519
1.4	1.2	3.4	3.0	6.0	11.0	24.7	40.5	83.0	226.1	F	**disease**	
1.0	2.4	2.5	4.5	8.5	11.5	20.3	32.6	35.5	54.6	M	**Peptic ulcer**	531–533
0.2	0.8	0.8	1.4	2.8	2.8	6.9	12.5	22.1	33.6	F		
12.7	21.1	40.6	58.2	83.0	88.8	96.5	100.7	93.3	52.1	M	**Liver cirrhosis**	571
2.1	4.7	9.0	17.1	23.7	33.7	36.0	29.9	30.1	26.1	F		
1.4	6.1	5.2	10.7	19.9	30.0	49.9	64.7	118.9	153.3	M	**Renal disease**	580–590
2.2	2.5	4.2	6.3	12.1	24.9	32.9	54.5	77.5	82.8	F		
0.4	0.1	–	0.1	0.1	–	–	–	–	–	F	**Pregnancy and birth**	630–676
0.4	0.9	–	0.6	0.3	0.4	0.8	–	–	1.8	M	**Congenital and**	740–779
0.7	0.3	0.2	0.4	0.4	0.4	0.2	0.8	1.0	1.9	F	**perinatal causes**	
23.0	33.1	47.3	71.1	87.3	119.9	146.1	272.5	476.8	1475.8	M	**Ill-defined causes**	780–799
8.3	13.9	14.8	25.0	35.9	43.6	82.0	156.8	349.1	1299.6	F		
23.1	29.9	47.7	62.8	97.1	141.2	220.8	299.9	416.3	567.7	M	**Other medical causes**	Rest of 001–799
8.6	11.8	21.5	26.5	47.3	92.9	155.3	227.9	334.9	431.0	F		
86.8	88.1	109.8	123.1	131.4	140.5	162.0	195.8	278.2	390.6	M	**ALL NON-**	E800–E999
23.6	20.7	30.2	34.0	36.0	46.6	55.3	95.4	142.2	291.4	F	**MEDICAL CAUSES**	
28.3	28.3	32.2	37.7	34.7	34.1	35.6	34.9	49.6	58.2	M	**Motor vehicle**	E810–E819
7.6	5.4	8.3	7.5	6.3	9.5	11.5	17.8	18.7	17.2	F	**traffic accidents**	
0.6	0.8	0.3	1.0	1.6	1.2	2.9	2.3	6.5	12.3	M	**Fire**	E890–E899
0.1	0.1	0.2	0.1	0.8	1.3	1.1	4.2	4.2	10.1	F		
22.3	24.2	31.9	36.0	37.8	43.4	54.3	61.2	91.7	106.1	M	**Suicide**	E950–E959
8.7	8.4	11.8	14.6	15.6	18.2	20.6	29.9	35.3	29.5	F		
4.4	5.2	2.5	4.0	4.0	3.0	4.2	2.3	2.7	4.9	M	**Homicide**	E960–E969
2.5	1.3	1.1	1.1	1.6	1.2	1.8	1.5	1.4	1.9	F		
958	792	636	709	694	567	379	175	183	163	M	**POPULATION (thousands)**	
916	771	642	735	744	674	548	264	289	268	F		

Former YUGOSLAVIA: Males

	All ages	0–34	35–69	35–39	40–44	45–49	50–54	55–59	60–64	65–69	70–74	75–79	80+/NK
POPULATION (1000s)													
1955	8514	5794	2455	325	475	501	432	324	218	181	132	76	56
1965	9535	6160	3074	724	541	300	442	451	374	241	139	91	72
1975	10503	6288	3760	764	793	690	509	273	380	352	250	125	80
1985	11433	6630	4219	804	652	738	742	626	440	218	262	191	132
1990	**11781**	**6526**	**4734**	**958**	**792**	**636**	**709**	**694**	**567**	**379**	**175**	**183**	**163**
1995 projected	*12081*	*6389*	*5096*	*936*	*947*	*777*	*614*	*672*	*647*	*503*	*304*	*122*	*170*
NUMBER OF DEATHS													
All causes													
1955	99796	44672	30187	1009	2161	3349	4639	5574	5853	7602	8195	7183	9559
1965	86108	24340	33502	1830	2024	1613	3790	6397	8649	9199	8325	8436	11505
1975	96124	15273	39647	1960	3117	4219	4716	3916	8797	12922	14736	12269	14199
1985	112440	12143	45688	1965	2556	4823	8005	10106	10476	7757	15037	17972	21600
1990	**112832**	**9091**	**54092**	**2330**	**2803**	**3835**	**6919**	**11174**	**13645**	**13386**	**9170**	**15719**	**24760**
1995 projected	*114589*	*7347*	*58436*	*2130*	*3117*	*4261*	*5719*	*10657*	*15556*	*16996*	*14792*	*9697*	*24317*
Lung cancer													
1955	...	...	...	...	...	...	...	...	...	...	...	...	...
1965	1927	24	1461	23	47	49	168	319	437	418	254	120	68
1975	3501	26	2328	35	109	237	314	279	606	748	662	350	135
1985	5566	37	3886	53	114	338	817	1018	1004	542	754	596	293
1990	**6898**	**29**	**5376**	**81**	**159**	**300**	**671**	**1393**	**1544**	**1228**	**547**	**584**	**362**
1995 projected	*8636*	*30*	*6786*	*91*	*204*	*340*	*620*	*1506*	*2142*	*1883*	*1044*	*394*	*382*
ANNUAL DEATH RATE / 100,000													
All causes													
1955	1643.7*	639.4*	1588.4*	310.3	455.0	668.9	1075.1	1718.8	2686.1	4204.6	6227.2	9426.5	16978.7
1965	1381.2*	373.7*	1366.5*	252.7	374.2	537.1	857.3	1419.0	2314.4	3810.7	5989.2	9260.2	15979.2
1975	1360.5*	241.5*	1373.1*	256.5	393.3	611.4	926.9	1433.4	2315.0	3675.2	5887.3	9846.7	17815.6
1985	1310.1*	183.5*	1418.2*	244.3	392.3	653.5	1079.4	1613.9	2382.5	3561.5	5748.1	9434.1	16388.5
1990	**1217.4***	**141.9***	**1389.6***	**243.2**	**353.7**	**603.3**	**976.6**	**1610.6**	**2408.6**	**3531.0**	**5249.0**	**8575.6**	**15180.9**
1995 projected	*1143.9**	*117.4**	*1343.8**	*227.6*	*329.1*	*548.7*	*930.8*	*1585.2*	*2406.2*	*3378.9*	*4859.4*	*7935.4*	*14278.9*
All cancer													
1955	...	...	...	...	...	...	...	...	...	...	...	...	...
1965	142.2*	9.2*	229.0*	25.7	47.7	74.9	144.3	265.3	419.1	625.9	818.7	829.9	702.8
1975	185.2*	8.7*	286.0*	31.1	58.4	119.9	212.1	326.1	509.2	745.4	962.4	1207.9	1175.7
1985	216.7*	9.4*	347.4*	33.9	67.4	145.0	291.1	438.0	629.3	827.4	1055.0	1306.6	1289.8
1990	**229.6***	**8.2***	**384.2***	**36.3**	**69.4**	**144.3**	**270.7**	**494.1**	**721.1**	**953.3**	**1099.6**	**1312.1**	**1300.4**
1995 projected	*240.5**	*7.2**	*413.9**	*37.5*	*70.2*	*138.2*	*279.3*	*534.1*	*810.2*	*1027.8*	*1132.4*	*1317.5*	*1309.5*
Lung cancer													
1955	...	...	...	...	...	...	...	...	...	...	...	...	...
1965	31.9*	0.4*	61.0*	3.2	8.7	16.3	38.0	70.8	116.9	173.2	182.7	131.7	94.4
1975	47.8*	0.5*	84.1*	4.6	13.8	34.3	61.7	102.1	159.5	212.7	264.5	280.9	169.4
1985	63.3*	0.6*	117.1*	6.6	17.5	45.8	110.2	162.6	228.3	248.9	288.2	312.9	222.3
1990	**71.0***	**0.4***	**138.2***	**8.5**	**20.1**	**47.2**	**94.7**	**200.8**	**272.6**	**323.9**	**313.1**	**318.6**	**221.9**
1995 projected	*78.7**	*0.5**	*157.9**	*9.7*	*21.5*	*43.8*	*100.9*	*224.0*	*331.3*	*374.4*	*343.0*	*322.4*	*224.3*
Upper aerodigestive cancer (mouth, oesophagus, pharynx and larynx)													
1955	...	...	...	...	...	...	...	...	...	...	...	...	...
1965	11.2*	0.3*	20.3*	1.7	5.9	6.3	12.7	24.6	35.3	55.9	56.8	58.2	44.4
1975	16.5*	0.2*	29.3*	2.1	7.6	15.1	24.6	35.5	49.7	70.5	73.1	73.8	94.1
1985	22.4*	0.2*	40.5*	2.0	10.0	22.4	41.3	58.1	67.1	82.6	91.4	108.1	97.9
1990	**24.4***	**0.2***	**46.2***	**3.8**	**11.4**	**23.8**	**44.6**	**65.6**	**87.9**	**86.3**	**93.9**	**99.3**	**91.4**
1995 projected	*26.1**	*0.3**	*51.5**	*4.7*	*12.8*	*25.5*	*48.7*	*76.8*	*98.8*	*93.2*	*90.7*	*94.1*	*84.6*
Other cancer													
1955	...	...	...	...	...	...	...	...	...	...	...	...	...
1965	99.1*	8.5*	147.6*	20.8	33.1	52.3	93.6	169.9	266.8	396.9	579.1	640.0	563.9
1975	120.9*	8.1*	172.6*	24.5	37.1	70.4	125.8	188.5	300.0	462.2	624.9	853.1	912.2
1985	130.9*	8.6*	189.8*	25.4	39.9	76.8	139.7	217.3	333.9	495.9	675.5	885.6	969.7
1990	**134.2***	**7.5***	**199.8***	**24.1**	**38.0**	**73.3**	**131.4**	**227.7**	**360.6**	**543.1**	**692.6**	**894.2**	**987.1**
1995 projected	*135.7**	*6.4**	*204.5**	*23.1*	*35.9*	*68.9*	*129.7*	*233.4*	*380.0*	*560.2*	*698.8*	*901.0*	*1000.6*
Chronic obstructive pulmonary disease (COPD)													
1955	...	...	...	...	...	...	...	...	...	...	...	...	...
1965	25.6*	1.1*	31.6*	1.7	3.3	6.0	15.8	35.5	60.7	98.2	155.4	195.4	272.2
1975	45.2*	0.8*	47.4*	2.7	5.4	9.7	22.4	45.8	96.1	149.9	267.7	451.8	564.6
1985	37.1*	0.4*	37.2*	1.5	2.6	7.6	18.2	39.4	73.9	117.1	230.1	361.7	496.2
1990	**43.5***	**0.2***	**40.6***	**1.5**	**2.1**	**3.8**	**15.9**	**40.4**	**80.7**	**139.8**	**252.4**	**423.9**	**683.0**
1995 projected	*50.9**	*0.2**	*43.3**	*1.2*	*1.5*	*2.8*	*14.5*	*41.4*	*89.1*	*152.7*	*283.2*	*512.3*	*881.4*
Other respiratory disease													
1955	...	...	...	...	...	...	...	...	...	...	...	...	...
1965	52.7*	43.0*	26.6*	4.0	6.1	7.0	11.5	29.1	44.2	84.1	131.7	232.7	540.3
1975	56.6*	31.1*	31.1*	3.5	5.7	13.2	15.9	24.2	52.4	102.7	181.4	365.2	786.7
1985	44.9*	18.0*	33.9*	5.6	6.3	12.6	22.8	32.4	58.7	99.2	168.6	298.2	592.6
1990	**19.7***	**7.1***	**14.8***	**3.1**	**4.8**	**7.2**	**11.6**	**17.4**	**25.2**	**34.3**	**63.5**	**152.8**	**267.3**
1995 projected	*13.7**	*4.8**	*10.3**	*2.2*	*3.4*	*5.0*	*8.1*	*12.2*	*17.5*	*23.7*	*43.7*	*105.6*	*189.1*
Vascular disease													
1955	...	...	...	...	...	...	...	...	...	...	...	...	...
1965	445.1*	9.9*	437.3*	30.4	63.8	110.6	229.6	419.0	789.7	1418.4	2428.1	4054.9	6722.2
1975	564.3*	11.1*	536.3*	48.9	94.0	179.0	306.0	530.7	937.6	1657.6	2794.6	5038.5	9256.0
1985	631.2*	8.9*	586.8*	53.8	109.1	197.6	373.2	642.6	1026.2	1705.2	3105.1	5534.4	10673.7
1990	**597.7***	**9.7***	**567.0***	**49.2**	**88.7**	**185.2**	**334.7**	**611.1**	**1023.8**	**1676.3**	**2820.3**	**5203.5**	**10156.3**
1995 projected	*558.2**	*10.4**	*528.0**	*41.2*	*79.0*	*164.5*	*309.1*	*579.9*	*980.0*	*1542.3*	*2576.9*	*4799.5*	*9624.8*
Liver cirrhosis													
1955	...	...	...	...	...	...	...	...	...	...	...	...	...
1965	16.9*	0.6*	32.4*	5.5	12.2	17.3	28.3	44.4	53.5	65.9	72.7	69.2	31.9
1975	26.0*	1.1*	48.6*	8.5	19.7	27.2	46.6	68.8	84.7	84.8	108.7	85.9	80.3
1985	30.7*	1.1*	58.3*	12.1	24.9	38.5	60.9	83.5	98.0	90.4	108.6	113.4	79.7
1990	**28.8***	**0.6***	**57.3***	**12.7**	**21.1**	**40.6**	**58.2**	**83.0**	**88.8**	**96.5**	**100.7**	**93.3**	**52.1**
1995 projected	*26.8**	*0.5**	*54.4**	*11.0*	*20.7*	*38.8*	*57.3*	*77.5*	*85.4*	*90.5*	*91.3*	*74.5*	*39.3*
Other medical causes													
1955	...	...	...	...	...	...	...	...	...	...	...	...	...
1965	607.3*	256.8*	487.9*	98.7	144.0	203.8	300.2	499.8	800.9	1367.9	2218.0	3694.8	7430.6
1975	378.3*	130.5*	286.2*	60.7	97.8	144.8	190.3	283.7	466.3	760.0	1369.2	2431.8	5584.7
1985	257.5*	97.3*	235.1*	55.1	81.8	129.7	187.0	254.1	364.6	573.5	873.5	1570.6	2923.4
1990	**205.8***	**69.2***	**205.5***	**53.7**	**79.5**	**112.5**	**162.5**	**233.1**	**328.5**	**468.7**	**716.7**	**1111.8**	**2331.1**
1995 projected	*162.5**	*49.8**	*175.8**	*50.9*	*72.7*	*99.3*	*143.2*	*206.2*	*276.9*	*381.1*	*531.5*	*836.3*	*1786.3*
All non-medical causes													
1955	...	...	...	...	...	...	...	...	...	...	...	...	...
1965	91.5*	53.1*	121.7*	86.7	97.1	117.5	127.6	126.0	146.4	150.4	164.7	183.3	279.2
1975	104.8*	58.3*	137.5*	100.9	112.3	117.7	133.6	154.1	168.7	174.9	203.4	265.7	367.6
1985	92.0*	48.5*	119.4*	82.3	100.2	122.6	126.1	123.8	131.9	148.8	207.2	249.3	333.1
1990	**92.4***	**47.0***	**120.2***	**86.8**	**88.1**	**109.8**	**123.1**	**131.4**	**140.5**	**162.0**	**195.8**	**278.2**	**390.6**
1995 projected	*91.4**	*44.5**	*118.1**	*83.6*	*81.6*	*100.2*	*119.3*	*133.9*	*147.1*	*160.8*	*200.4*	*289.7*	*448.6*

(*The rates for the age groups 0–34 and 35–69 are the means of seven five-yearly rates, but the all-ages rates are standardised to the conventional "European" age distribution)

Former YUGOSLAVIA: Females

	All ages	0–34	35–69	35–39	40–44	45–49	50–54	55–59	60–64	65–69	70–74	75–79	80+/NK
POPULATION (1000s)													
1955	9006	5783	2846	396	547	519	460	382	288	255	184	109	85
1965	9950	5967	3525	770	661	365	516	484	425	304	199	142	116
1975	10849	6020	4183	768	796	745	639	346	475	415	322	183	141
1985	11691	6289	4546	777	650	749	767	708	594	303	370	267	219
1990	**12037**	**6187**	**5030**	**916**	**771**	**642**	**735**	**744**	**674**	**548**	**264**	**289**	**268**
1995 projected	*12308*	*6052*	*5269*	*902*	*911*	*764*	*633*	*714*	*714*	*631*	*480*	*209*	*298*
NUMBER OF DEATHS													
All causes													
1955	100186	41328	27834	1190	1980	2566	3381	4646	5628	8443	9544	8974	12506
1965	84441	20473	26370	1430	1606	1339	2974	4320	6262	8439	9353	11310	16935
1975	88783	11080	27608	1056	1717	2458	3218	2842	6454	9863	13256	14368	22471
1985	100443	7816	27424	902	1252	2268	3645	5433	7449	6475	14286	18759	32158
1990	**99316**	**5376**	**31267**	**1008**	**1304**	**1809**	**3218**	**5133**	**7896**	**10899**	**9055**	**17735**	**35883**
1995 projected	*97249*	*3944*	*30491*	*894*	*1412*	*1970*	*2528*	*4530*	*7738*	*11419*	*14627*	*11704*	*36483*
Lung cancer													
1955	...	...	...	...	...	...	...	...	...	...	...	...	...
1965	428	17	300	13	23	22	42	63	65	72	52	38	21
1975	738	21	446	9	33	51	65	50	114	124	122	101	48
1985	1122	17	686	24	28	61	98	148	200	127	158	146	115
1990	**1304**	**15**	**843**	**27**	**31**	**53**	**141**	**159**	**202**	**230**	**136**	**170**	**140**
1995 projected	*1475*	*14*	*906*	*24*	*35*	*77*	*139*	*157*	*203*	*271*	*264*	*130*	*161*
ANNUAL DEATH RATE / 100,000 (*The rates for the age groups 0–34 and 35–69 are the means of seven five-yearly rates, but the all-ages rates are standardised to the conventional "European" age distribution)													
All causes													
1955	1384.8*	613.2*	1196.9*	300.7	362.1	494.7	735.0	1217.2	1957.6	3311.0	5192.6	8271.0	14730.3
1965	1103.6*	326.4*	931.3*	185.6	243.0	366.6	576.1	893.3	1474.5	2779.6	4692.9	7948.0	14586.6
1975	993.7*	183.3*	821.0*	137.5	215.7	330.1	503.7	821.4	1359.9	2378.9	4111.7	7855.7	15925.6
1985	887.9*	125.6*	749.6*	116.1	192.6	303.0	475.5	767.8	1254.9	2137.0	3861.1	7015.3	14690.7
1990	**790.9***	**90.0***	**692.9***	**110.1**	**169.1**	**281.6**	**438.0**	**689.8**	**1171.2**	**1990.7**	**3428.6**	**6136.7**	**13389.2**
1995 projected	*713.2**	*68.1**	*634.2**	*99.1*	*155.0*	*257.8*	*399.4*	*634.6*	*1084.2*	*1809.1*	*3044.8*	*5610.7*	*12250.8*
All cancer													
1955	...	...	...	...	...	...	...	...	...	...	...	...	...
1965	102.8*	8.2*	167.9*	36.5	66.9	105.7	144.5	194.4	256.4	371.2	474.2	527.1	493.5
1975	117.6*	7.9*	184.7*	34.0	66.3	104.5	159.0	217.6	310.8	400.6	523.9	688.4	703.8
1985	124.8*	8.1*	195.5*	39.0	68.1	109.1	150.8	240.2	331.4	429.7	564.9	715.0	782.1
1990	**129.0***	**7.3***	**201.5***	**38.3**	**69.1**	**114.6**	**162.2**	**229.1**	**332.4**	**464.8**	**591.4**	**712.5**	**877.2**
1995 projected	*131.2**	*6.3**	*203.4**	*36.7*	*69.7*	*117.9*	*161.8*	*226.3*	*335.2*	*476.4*	*596.4*	*756.5*	*931.5*
Lung cancer													
1955	...	...	...	...	...	...	...	...	...	...	...	...	...
1965	5.7*	0.3*	10.2*	1.7	3.5	6.0	8.1	13.0	15.3	23.7	26.1	26.7	18.1
1975	7.9*	0.4*	13.0*	1.2	4.1	6.8	10.2	14.5	24.0	29.9	37.8	55.2	34.0
1985	10.2*	0.3*	17.8*	3.1	4.3	8.1	12.8	20.9	33.7	41.9	42.7	54.6	52.5
1990	**10.8***	**0.2***	**18.3***	**2.9**	**4.0**	**8.3**	**19.2**	**21.4**	**30.0**	**42.0**	**51.5**	**58.8**	**52.2**
1995 projected	*11.2**	*0.2**	*18.8**	*2.7*	*3.8*	*10.1*	*22.0*	*22.0*	*28.4*	*42.9*	*55.0*	*62.3*	*54.1*
Upper aerodigestive cancer (mouth, oesophagus, pharynx and larynx)													
1955	...	...	...	...	...	...	...	...	...	...	...	...	...
1965	2.4*	0.2*	3.2*	0.4	1.2	3.3	1.9	4.1	4.9	6.3	15.6	15.5	14.6
1975	2.5*	0.1*	3.5*	0.8	0.6	1.7	3.0	4.6	6.5	7.5	9.9	16.9	26.2
1985	3.2*	0.1*	5.2*	1.3	1.8	2.3	3.1	5.1	9.9	12.5	11.9	20.9	25.1
1990	**3.0***	**0.1***	**4.0***	**0.7**	**0.6**	**2.6**	**2.2**	**4.0**	**7.7**	**9.9**	**16.3**	**21.1**	**28.4**
1995 projected	*2.9**	*0.1**	*3.3**	*0.4*	*0.4*	*2.0*	*1.7*	*3.1*	*5.9*	*9.5*	*16.4*	*24.9*	*30.6*
Other cancer													
1955	...	...	...	...	...	...	...	...	...	...	...	...	...
1965	94.8*	7.7*	154.6*	34.4	62.2	96.4	134.4	177.2	236.2	341.2	432.5	484.9	460.8
1975	107.1*	7.4*	168.2*	32.0	61.6	95.9	145.9	198.6	280.2	363.2	476.1	616.2	643.5
1985	111.4*	7.7*	172.5*	34.6	62.0	98.7	134.9	214.2	287.7	375.2	510.3	639.5	704.4
1990	**115.2***	**6.9***	**179.3***	**34.7**	**64.5**	**103.7**	**140.9**	**203.7**	**294.7**	**413.0**	**523.7**	**632.5**	**796.6**
1995 projected	*117.1**	*5.9**	*181.3**	*33.6*	*65.4*	*105.9*	*138.1*	*201.2*	*300.8*	*424.0*	*525.0*	*669.2*	*846.9*
Chronic obstructive pulmonary disease (COPD)													
1955	...	...	...	...	...	...	...	...	...	...	...	...	...
1965	12.7*	1.2*	13.9*	1.3	2.0	4.7	7.7	10.5	21.7	49.4	74.8	90.7	161.1
1975	20.0*	0.8*	20.3*	1.8	3.3	5.9	10.8	14.2	35.0	71.2	111.7	191.9	271.4
1985	15.2*	0.4*	14.2*	1.0	1.2	3.6	7.6	11.9	19.7	54.5	79.2	154.5	234.4
1990	**17.7***	**0.3***	**15.0***	**0.8**	**1.0**	**3.3**	**6.3**	**12.4**	**30.3**	**50.8**	**96.2**	**178.5**	**300.4**
1995 projected	*20.5**	*0.3**	*16.4**	*0.6*	*0.9*	*2.7*	*5.8*	*15.1*	*32.2*	*57.4*	*106.0*	*211.4*	*369.7*
Other respiratory disease													
1955	...	...	...	...	...	...	...	...	...	...	...	...	...
1965	45.9*	41.4*	16.1*	1.8	2.0	3.8	8.9	17.2	25.7	53.7	102.4	215.0	491.0
1975	48.0*	30.8*	18.9*	2.5	5.0	6.8	11.4	14.5	25.9	65.8	130.9	293.6	725.0
1985	31.8*	17.3*	15.9*	2.6	3.2	5.6	8.9	16.0	25.3	49.8	100.0	207.6	476.0
1990	**14.1***	**7.6***	**7.2***	**1.4**	**1.2**	**3.4**	**3.0**	**6.0**	**11.0**	**24.7**	**40.5**	**83.0**	**226.1**
1995 projected	*9.8**	*5.1**	*5.0**	*1.0*	*0.8*	*2.4*	*2.1*	*4.2*	*7.6*	*17.1*	*27.9*	*57.5*	*159.8*
Vascular disease													
1955	...	...	...	...	...	...	...	...	...	...	...	...	...
1965	393.6*	8.8*	348.6*	30.9	45.7	79.7	175.3	307.3	591.9	1209.2	2162.6	3778.6	6456.5
1975	469.0*	9.0*	354.8*	29.2	54.1	92.9	173.0	314.5	620.1	1200.2	2291.6	4628.2	9041.1
1985	494.9*	6.8*	339.7*	25.4	48.9	90.7	166.7	309.6	589.1	1147.5	2337.8	4672.8	10536.8
1990	**452.3***	**6.0***	**311.3***	**22.3**	**40.3**	**77.2**	**152.4**	**277.5**	**542.6**	**1067.0**	**2104.1**	**4174.7**	**9784.0**
1995 projected	*408.9**	*5.7**	*277.7**	*18.0*	*33.4*	*66.5*	*133.5*	*249.2*	*491.7*	*951.4*	*1846.4*	*3790.5*	*8977.8*
Liver cirrhosis													
1955	...	...	...	...	...	...	...	...	...	...	...	...	...
1965	6.8*	0.3*	11.7*	1.9	3.3	6.3	10.8	18.0	19.3	22.4	32.6	33.7	21.5
1975	9.1*	0.6*	15.7*	3.6	5.2	10.6	13.3	23.1	28.0	25.8	35.4	43.7	39.0
1985	11.1*	0.4*	20.2*	4.1	7.5	12.3	22.2	25.3	36.4	33.7	45.4	52.4	27.9
1990	**9.0***	**0.3***	**18.0***	**2.1**	**4.7**	**9.0**	**17.1**	**23.7**	**33.7**	**36.0**	**29.9**	**30.1**	**26.1**
1995 projected	*7.4**	*0.2**	*15.5**	*1.4*	*3.2*	*6.4*	*14.1*	*20.6*	*32.4*	*30.4*	*21.2*	*20.6*	*18.5*
Other medical causes													
1955	...	...	...	...	...	...	...	...	...	...	...	...	...
1965	512.1*	249.0*	340.8*	90.1	101.5	141.0	202.1	310.2	517.1	1023.4	1772.2	3198.2	6779.5
1975	296.2*	116.8*	187.3*	40.6	57.4	77.5	104.6	190.2	293.3	547.5	947.0	1892.3	4906.4
1985	178.8*	79.2*	128.5*	26.5	39.5	51.4	83.8	127.8	205.0	365.7	651.1	1085.3	2367.3
1990	**136.8***	**56.1***	**104.6***	**21.6**	**32.0**	**43.9**	**62.9**	**105.1**	**174.7**	**292.1**	**471.0**	**815.6**	**1884.0**
1995 projected	*103.5**	*39.3**	*81.6**	*17.0*	*26.0*	*34.0*	*49.6*	*85.0*	*140.5*	*219.3*	*344.7*	*623.7*	*1472.8*
All non-medical causes													
1955	...	...	...	...	...	...	...	...	...	...	...	...	...
1965	29.9*	17.4*	32.2*	23.1	21.6	25.5	26.7	35.8	42.4	50.4	74.3	104.7	183.5
1975	33.9*	17.4*	39.4*	25.8	24.4	31.8	31.6	47.4	46.8	67.8	71.3	117.6	238.8
1985	31.5*	13.4*	35.5*	17.5	24.0	30.2	35.6	37.0	48.0	56.1	82.7	127.9	266.3
1990	**32.0***	**12.5***	**35.2***	**23.6**	**20.7**	**30.2**	**34.0**	**36.0**	**46.6**	**55.3**	**95.4**	**142.2**	**291.4**
1995 projected	*32.0**	*11.2**	*34.6**	*24.5*	*21.1*	*27.9*	*32.5*	*34.2*	*44.7*	*57.2*	*102.2*	*150.5*	*320.7*

Former YUGOSLAVIA: 1975

Smoking–attributed deaths (Sm.) and total deaths (Total)

		ALL CAUSES	ALL CANCER	Lung cancer	Upper aero–digestive ca.	Other cancer	COPD	Other respiratory	Vascular disease	Liver cirrhosis	Other medical	Non–medical
Males												
0–34	Sm.	–	–	–	–	–	–	–	–	–	–	–
	Total	15273	527	26	10	491	48	2026	643	59	8425	3545
35–69	Sm.	9398	3138	2092	476	570	890	188	3223	–	1959	–
	Total	39647	8054	2328	839	4887	1262	870	14752	1454	8425	4830
		(24%)	(39%)	(90%)	(57%)	(12%)	(71%)	(22%)	(22%)		(23%)	
70+	Sm.	4916	1390	974	159	257	1012	113	1582	–	819	–
	Total	41204	4851	1147	350	3354	1683	1536	20650	443	10908	1133
		(12%)	(29%)	(85%)	(45%)	(8%)	(60%)	(7%)	(8%)		(8%)	
Any age	Sm.	14314	4528	3066	635	827	1902	301	4805	–	2778	–
	Total	96124	13432	3501	1199	8732	2993	4432	36045	1956	27758	9508
		(15%)	(34%)	(88%)	(53%)	(9%)	(64%)	(7%)	(13%)		(10%)	
Females												
0–34	Sm.	–	–	–	–	–	–	–	–	–	–	–
	Total	11080	445	21	5	419	48	1884	508	31	7119	1045
35–69	Sm.	872	175	139	13	23	133	19	351	–	194	–
	Total	27608	6472	446	121	5905	663	629	11459	553	6334	1498
		(3%)	(3%)	(31%)	(11%)	(0%)	(20%)	(3%)	(3%)		(3%)	
70+	Sm.	897	114	87	12	15	245	24	351	–	163	–
	Total	50095	3941	271	100	3570	1094	1982	28610	249	13437	782
		(2%)	(3%)	(32%)	(12%)	(0%)	(22%)	(1%)	(1%)		(1%)	
Any age	Sm.	1769	289	226	25	38	378	43	702	–	357	–
	Total	88783	10858	738	226	9894	1805	4495	40577	833	26890	3325
		(2%)	(3%)	(31%)	(11%)	(0%)	(21%)	(1%)	(2%)		(1%)	
Males+Females												
0–34	Sm.	–	–	–	–	–	–	–	–	–	–	–
	Total	26353	972	47	15	910	96	3910	1151	90	15544	4590
35–69	Sm.	10270	3313	2231	489	593	1023	207	3574	–	2153	–
	Total	67255	14526	2774	960	10792	1925	1499	26211	2007	14759	6328
		(15%)	(23%)	(80%)	(51%)	(5%)	(53%)	(14%)	(14%)		(15%)	
70+	Sm.	5813	1504	1061	171	272	1257	137	1933	–	982	–
	Total	91299	8792	1418	450	6924	2777	3518	49260	692	24345	1915
		(6%)	(17%)	(75%)	(38%)	(4%)	(45%)	(4%)	(4%)		(4%)	
Any age	Sm.	16083	4817	3292	660	865	2280	344	5507	–	3135	–
	Total	184907	24290	4239	1425	18626	4798	8927	76622	2789	54648	12833
		(9%)	(20%)	(78%)	(46%)	(5%)	(48%)	(4%)	(7%)		(6%)	

Former YUGOSLAVIA: 1985

Smoking–attributed deaths (Sm.) and total deaths (Total)

		ALL CAUSES	ALL CANCER	Lung cancer	Upper aero–digestive ca.	Other cancer	COPD	Other respiratory	Vascular disease	Liver cirrhosis	Other medical	Non–medical
Males												
0–34	Sm.	–	–	–	–	–	–	–	–	–	–	–
	Total	12143	624	37	14	573	24	1188	592	73	6414	3228
35–69	Sm.	15278	5610	3627	945	1038	822	339	5806	–	2701	–
	Total	45688	11253	3886	1391	5976	1047	1025	17620	2146	7763	4834
		(33%)	(50%)	(93%)	(68%)	(17%)	(79%)	(33%)	(33%)		(35%)	
70+	Sm.	6721	2081	1413	273	395	1212	140	2571	–	717	–
	Total	54609	6949	1643	574	4732	1945	1790	32734	605	9130	1456
		(12%)	(30%)	(86%)	(48%)	(8%)	(62%)	(8%)	(8%)		(8%)	
Any age	Sm.	21999	7691	5040	1218	1433	2034	479	8377	–	3418	–
	Total	112440	18826	5566	1979	11281	3016	4003	50946	2824	23307	9518
		(20%)	(41%)	(91%)	(62%)	(13%)	(67%)	(12%)	(16%)		(15%)	
Females												
0–34	Sm.	–	–	–	–	–	–	–	–	–	–	–
	Total	7816	512	17	7	488	24	1070	429	27	4908	846
35–69	Sm.	1723	439	342	40	57	166	36	771	–	311	–
	Total	27424	7688	686	196	6806	467	565	11637	840	4719	1508
		(6%)	(6%)	(50%)	(20%)	(1%)	(36%)	(6%)	(7%)		(7%)	
70+	Sm.	1237	195	150	20	25	294	26	580	–	142	–
	Total	65203	5714	419	155	5140	1219	1967	44210	369	10493	1231
		(2%)	(3%)	(36%)	(13%)	(0%)	(24%)	(1%)	(1%)		(1%)	
Any age	Sm.	2960	634	492	60	82	460	62	1351	–	453	–
	Total	100443	13914	1122	358	12434	1710	3602	56276	1236	20120	3585
		(3%)	(5%)	(44%)	(17%)	(1%)	(27%)	(2%)	(2%)		(2%)	
Males+Females												
0–34	Sm.	–	–	–	–	–	–	–	–	–	–	–
	Total	19959	1136	54	21	1061	48	2258	1021	100	11322	4074
35–69	Sm.	17001	6049	3969	985	1095	988	375	6577	–	3012	–
	Total	73112	18941	4572	1587	12782	1514	1590	29257	2986	12482	6342
		(23%)	(32%)	(87%)	(62%)	(9%)	(65%)	(24%)	(22%)		(24%)	
70+	Sm.	7958	2276	1563	293	420	1506	166	3151	–	859	–
	Total	119812	12663	2062	729	9872	3164	3757	76944	974	19623	2687
		(7%)	(18%)	(76%)	(40%)	(4%)	(48%)	(4%)	(4%)		(4%)	
Any age	Sm.	24959	8325	5532	1278	1515	2494	541	9728	–	3871	–
	Total	212883	32740	6688	2337	23715	4726	7605	107222	4060	43427	13103
		(12%)	(25%)	(83%)	(55%)	(6%)	(53%)	(7%)	(9%)		(9%)	

(To be conservative, no deaths before age 35, and none from liver cirrhosis or non–medical causes, were attributed to smoking.)

Former YUGOSLAVIA: 1990

Smoking-attributed deaths (Sm.) and total deaths (Total)

		ALL CAUSES	ALL CANCER	Lung cancer	Upper aero-digestive ca.	Other cancer	COPD	Other respiratory	Vascular disease	Liver cirrhosis	Other medical	Non-medical
Males												
0–34	Sm.	–	–	–	–	–	–	–	–	–	–	–
	Total	9091	533	29	16	488	16	443	627	42	4356	3074
35–69	Sm.	19354	7820	5055	1320	1445	1155	214	7163	–	3002	–
	Total	54092	14860	5376	1873	7611	1435	590	21117	2404	8265	5421
		(36%)	(53%)	(94%)	(70%)	(19%)	(80%)	(36%)	(34%)		(36%)	
70+	Sm.	6301	1908	1290	239	379	1459	61	2331	–	542	–
	Total	49649	6447	1493	495	4459	2332	827	31030	432	7092	1489
		(13%)	(30%)	(86%)	(48%)	(8%)	(63%)	(7%)	(8%)		(8%)	
Any age	Sm.	25655	9728	6345	1559	1824	2614	275	9494	–	3544	–
	Total	112832	21840	6898	2384	12558	3783	1860	52774	2878	19713	9984
		(23%)	(45%)	(92%)	(65%)	(15%)	(69%)	(15%)	(18%)		(18%)	
Females												
0–34	Sm.	–	–	–	–	–	–	–	–	–	–	–
	Total	5376	453	15	9	429	18	444	368	18	3303	772
35–69	Sm.	2027	544	431	37	76	237	22	899	–	325	–
	Total	31267	9303	843	180	8280	656	320	13696	839	4748	1705
		(6%)	(6%)	(51%)	(21%)	(1%)	(36%)	(7%)	(7%)		(7%)	
70+	Sm.	1559	252	189	29	34	453	15	697	–	142	–
	Total	62673	5972	446	180	5346	1575	953	43843	236	8650	1444
		(2%)	(4%)	(42%)	(16%)	(1%)	(29%)	(2%)	(2%)		(2%)	
Any age	Sm.	3586	796	620	66	110	690	37	1596	–	467	–
	Total	99316	15728	1304	369	14055	2249	1717	57907	1093	16701	3921
		(4%)	(5%)	(48%)	(18%)	(1%)	(31%)	(2%)	(3%)		(3%)	
Males+Females												
0–34	Sm.	–	–	–	–	–	–	–	–	–	–	–
	Total	14467	986	44	25	917	34	887	995	60	7659	3846
35–69	Sm.	21381	8364	5486	1357	1521	1392	236	8062	–	3327	–
	Total	85359	24163	6219	2053	15891	2091	910	34813	3243	13013	7126
		(25%)	(35%)	(88%)	(66%)	(10%)	(67%)	(26%)	(23%)		(26%)	
70+	Sm.	7860	2160	1479	268	413	1912	76	3028	–	684	–
	Total	112322	12419	1939	675	9805	3907	1780	74873	668	15742	2933
		(7%)	(17%)	(76%)	(40%)	(4%)	(49%)	(4%)	(4%)		(4%)	
Any age	Sm.	29241	10524	6965	1625	1934	3304	312	11090	–	4011	–
	Total	212148	37568	8202	2753	26613	6032	3577	110681	3971	36414	13905
		(14%)	(28%)	(85%)	(59%)	(7%)	(55%)	(9%)	(10%)		(11%)	

Former YUGOSLAVIA: 1995

Smoking-attributed deaths (Sm.) and total deaths (Total)

		ALL CAUSES	ALL CANCER	Lung cancer	Upper aero-digestive ca.	Other cancer	COPD	Other respiratory	Vascular disease	Liver cirrhosis	Other medical	Non-medical
Males												
0–34	Sm.	–	–	–	–	–	–	–	–	–	–	–
	Total	7347	460	30	19	411	13	286	658	35	3009	2886
35–69	Sm.	22573	9913	6424	1665	1824	1448	174	7992	–	3046	–
	Total	58436	17804	6786	2286	8732	1758	456	22303	2480	7909	5726
		(39%)	(56%)	(95%)	(73%)	(21%)	(82%)	(38%)	(36%)		(39%)	
70+	Sm.	7412	2327	1595	272	460	1914	49	2616	–	506	–
	Total	48806	7287	1820	535	4932	2989	584	30100	436	5682	1728
		(15%)	(32%)	(88%)	(51%)	(9%)	(64%)	(8%)	(9%)		(9%)	
Any age	Sm.	29985	12240	8019	1937	2284	3362	223	10608	–	3552	–
	Total	114589	25551	8636	2840	14075	4760	1326	53061	2951	16600	10340
		(26%)	(48%)	(93%)	(68%)	(16%)	(71%)	(17%)	(20%)		(21%)	
Females												
0–34	Sm.	–	–	–	–	–	–	–	–	–	–	–
	Total	3944	388	14	8	366	17	288	336	14	2216	685
35–69	Sm.	2057	594	475	34	85	279	17	883	–	284	–
	Total	30491	9905	906	158	8841	771	239	13112	750	3958	1756
		(7%)	(6%)	(52%)	(22%)	(1%)	(36%)	(7%)	(7%)		(7%)	
70+	Sm.	2067	350	260	42	48	662	15	887	–	153	–
	Total	62814	7217	555	222	6440	2051	730	43513	200	7343	1760
		(3%)	(5%)	(47%)	(19%)	(1%)	(32%)	(2%)	(2%)		(2%)	
Any age	Sm.	4124	944	735	76	133	941	32	1770	–	437	–
	Total	97249	17510	1475	388	15647	2839	1257	56961	964	13517	4201
		(4%)	(5%)	(50%)	(20%)	(1%)	(33%)	(3%)	(3%)		(3%)	
Males+Females												
0–34	Sm.	–	–	–	–	–	–	–	–	–	–	–
	Total	11291	848	44	27	777	30	574	994	49	5225	3571
35–69	Sm.	24630	10507	6899	1699	1909	1727	191	8875	–	3330	–
	Total	88927	27709	7692	2444	17573	2529	695	35415	3230	11867	7482
		(28%)	(38%)	(90%)	(70%)	(11%)	(68%)	(27%)	(25%)		(28%)	
70+	Sm.	9479	2677	1855	314	508	2576	64	3503	–	659	–
	Total	111620	14504	2375	757	11372	5040	1314	73613	636	13025	3488
		(8%)	(18%)	(78%)	(41%)	(4%)	(51%)	(5%)	(5%)		(5%)	
Any age	Sm.	34109	13184	8754	2013	2417	4303	255	12378	–	3989	–
	Total	211838	43061	10111	3228	29722	7599	2583	110022	3915	30117	14541
		(16%)	(31%)	(87%)	(62%)	(8%)	(57%)	(10%)	(11%)		(13%)	

(To be conservative, no deaths before age 35, and none from liver cirrhosis or non-medical causes, were attributed to smoking.)